ELSEVIER

You now have access to...

Access your content when, where and how you want.

on evolve

GET STARTED

To activate your Elsevier eBook on VitalSource:

1. Visit **evolve.elsevier.com**
2. Enter your eBook ACCESS CODE, click **Submit** and **follow the prompts**

eBook ACCESS CODE
(scratch here to reveal your code)

evolve.elsevier.com

HAVARD'S NURSING GUIDE TO DRUGS

HAVARD'S

NURSING GUIDE TO DRUGS

ADRIANA TIZIANI

RN, BSC (MON), DIPED (MELB), MEDST (MON)

11e

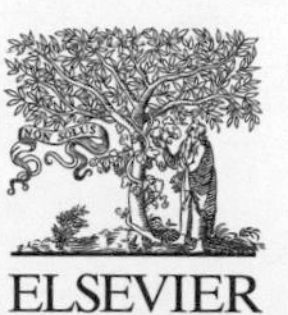

ADRIANA TIZIANI

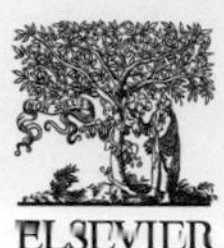

Elsevier Australia. ACN 001 002 357
(a division of Reed International Books Australia Pty Ltd)
Tower 1, 475 Victoria Avenue, Chatswood, NSW 2067

Copyright 2022 Elsevier Australia.

All rights reserved. No part of this publication may be reproduced or transmitted in any form or by any means, electronic or mechanical, including photocopying, recording, or any information storage and retrieval system, without permission in writing from the publisher. Details on how to seek permission, further information about the Publisher's permissions policies and our arrangements with organisations such as the Copyright Clearance Center and the Copyright Licensing Agency, can be found at our website: www.elsevier.com/permissions.

This book and the individual contributions contained in it are protected under copyright by the Publisher (other than as may be noted herein).

ISBN 978-0-7295-4359-0

Notice

Practitioners and researchers must always rely on their own experience and knowledge in evaluating and using any information, methods, compounds or experiments described herein. Because of rapid advances in the medical sciences, in particular, independent verification of diagnoses and drug dosages should be made. To the fullest extent of the law, no responsibility is assumed by Elsevier, authors, editors or contributors for any injury and/or damage to persons or property as a matter of product liability, negligence or otherwise, or from any use or operation of any methods, products, instructions or ideas contained in the material herein.

National Library of Australia Cataloguing-in-Publication Data

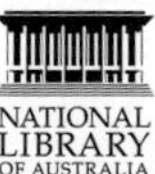

A catalogue record for this book is available from the National Library of Australia

Senior Content Strategist: Natalie Hunt
Content Project Manager: Fariha Nadeem
Edited by Margaret Trudgeon
Proofread by Annabel Adair
Cover and internal design by Georgette Hall
Typeset by GW Tech
Printed in Singapore by KHL Printing Co Pte Ltd

To all my 'boys'.
You are the 'wind beneath my wings'.
Thank you for your love and support through this difficult journey.
Love you

AT

CONTENTS BY THERAPEUTIC CLASS

CONTENTS BY BODY SYSTEM

Cardiac and Vascular Systems

Central Nervous System

Peripheral Nervous System

Respiratory System

Alimentary System

Musculoskeletal System

Endocrine System

Urinary System

Reproductive System

Integumentary System

Immune System

Special Senses

Infection and Infestations

Miscellaneous

INTRODUCTION

As with the original aim of the book, *Havard's Nursing Guide to Drugs* continues to be a guide only. This book is meant to be a companion guide to pharmacology texts, something smaller and easier to transport around and reference in the clinical setting, given its availability as an eBook as well.

The Nurse's Role in Drug Therapy

The aims of administering medication are to do it in a safe and efficient manner while observing the patient for both desirable and undesirable effects. Therefore, the nurse needs to:

- assess the patient, including medication history
- have an understanding of the legal requirements associated with the administration of drugs
- have pharmacological knowledge of the medication(s)
- be able to safely administer medications.

Assessing the Patient

Patient assessment should be holistic, looking at the patient's condition and personal circumstances as an entirety, rather than simply as a disease to be treated. It should include:

- all current medical problems
- co-morbidities
- relevant past history
- physical assessment
- medication history (including current medications, over-the-counter (OTC) preparations, herbal preparations, vitamin and mineral supplements)
- alcohol or tobacco use (and in some cases, illicit drug use).

Medical history, co-morbidities and medication history are intertwined, as a person with co-morbidities is often prescribed multiple medications concurrently (polypharmacy), which increases the risk of adverse effects and interactions. Sometimes a person sees more than one medical practitioner (e.g. general practitioner (GP) plus specialist/s), which increases the risk of medications not being regularly reviewed.

People may become confused because medications can have more than one brand/trade name for the same generic drug and they can potentially end up taking the same drug twice (e.g. a patient taking Urex and Lasix (both trade names for furosemide (frusemide)) may become quickly dehydrated).

Unfortunately, people do not always complete courses of medications, especially antibiotics, and 'keep the rest for next time' with no understanding of the ramifications of doing this (e.g. bacteria becoming resistant to that antibiotic and the agent becoming ineffective in treating that same infection if it recurs). Other reasons for not completing courses of medications (or getting prescriptions refilled) include adverse effects, costs or failing to see any obvious benefits from the medication.

Some people believe they are allergic to medications. It is important for the nurse to explore what form the allergy takes (e.g. someone may mistakenly believe that they are allergic to morphine because they were nauseous and vomited after taking it (a common side-effect), whereas another patient may correctly describe an anaphylactic reaction with breathing difficulties after administration of an antibiotic).

Many people take OTC preparations or alternative medicines, including herbal preparations, either concurrently or instead of traditional medication. OTC preparations are those that are non-prescription and are generally intended for short-term use only in self-limiting illnesses, such as headache, heartburn and constipation. OTCs also include vitamins, minerals, herbal drugs and remedies (e.g. St John's wort, ginseng), and unfortunately many people consider them to be 'safe' because they are natural. However, many herbal drugs and remedies interact with prescription medications (e.g. St John's wort interacts with warfarin, increasing its metabolism and decreasing its effectiveness); antacids can interfere with some oral medications if not taken 2 hours apart; and non-prescription medications such as aspirin and ibuprofen can cause gastrointestinal bleeding and must only be taken at recommended doses. OTCs are readily available in pharmacies and supermarkets, with the buyer not needing to seek advice before purchasing these products.

It is essential for the nurse to establish if the patient is compliant/adherent/concordant with his or her medication regimen, and if not, why not. While these terms are sometimes used interchangeably, there are some important differences between them. *Compliance* suggests that the patient has little input into their management strategy and follows doctor's orders (power lies with the doctor), while *concordance* is at the other end of the spectrum, and is based on equality and respect between the patient and the healthcare practitioner. *Adherence* falls somewhere in between as there is negotiation between the patient and the healthcare professional that is based around the therapy. Intentional non-adherence describes a patient deciding to reject their treatment, which may seem rational from their perspective, although the clinician may not agree (Anderson 2013).

Adherence is a very complex issue. Some of the factors that may lead to a patient being non-adherent with a medication regimen may include:

- multiple medications required
- complex dosing schedules (a person is more likely to remember a once-daily dosing schedule, compared to a 3–4 times daily regimen)
- the medication is difficult to take or administer (e.g. medications that have an unpleasant taste or are large in size; eye and ear drops that are difficult to instil)
- impairments, including:
  - sight (e.g. unable to read directions)
  - dexterity (e.g. arthritis) may make it difficult to open containers with childproof lids or blister packs
  - memory (e.g. unable to remember instructions of how or when to take medication)
- adverse effects (i.e. the person may decide that the side-effects of the medications are worse than the disease itself)
- feeling 'better' and therefore not needing to take the medication any longer
- not 'seeing' any effects from the medication (e.g. effects of lipid-lowering agents are not visible and these are commonly discontinued by patients)
- the cost and ease of filling prescriptions (e.g. decreased mobility or lack

of transport to be able to get to the pharmacy)
- lack of knowledge/understanding of the disease process and the role of medication in disease management
- language, cultural and/or religious issues
- attitude towards medication, disease and/or health (e.g. a 'devil may care' attitude or thoughts such as 'I have to die of something')
- inconsistency in the messages that healthcare providers are giving (e.g. one nurse advises the patient to take certain medications 30–60 minutes before food, while another nurse says that it doesn't matter when the medication is taken). Not only are these inconsistent messages confusing for the patient, but they damage the trust the patient may have in the nurse(s), as well as potentially affecting the absorption and effectiveness of the medication.

Armed with all this information, the nurse is in an ideal position to support and educate the patient (see section on General Patient teaching and advice, p. xxvii).

Children and the Elderly

Children and the elderly require highly specialised nursing care and knowledge regarding the administration of medications. Special care should be taken with dosages because an overdose can occur easily due to smaller weights (and surface ratios), and differences in kidney and liver capacity. There are many specialised texts available that cover both these groups in detail and take into account the differences in drug administration. Specific paediatric and geriatric dosages are not generally included in this book. Doses are for the 'average' adult patient. The only exceptions are when a particular drug is mainly or specifically used in paediatrics (e.g. drugs used for attention deficit disorder, growth hormone).

Many older people require assistance with the administration of medications and the nurse may consider splitting or crushing tablets in order to make them easier to take. Before doing this, investigate whether the medication is available in a different oral form (e.g. liquid rather than solid) or a non-oral form (e.g. dermal, rectal, intranasal). Tablets with an enteric coating should not be crushed as these are formulated to ensure the medication passes through the stomach intact (e.g. enteric aspirin is formulated to prevent gastric irritation). Extended-release medications (often marked as CD, CR, SA, SR) are designed to release the active components over an extended period and therefore should not be crushed. Further discussion on crushing or dispersing medication for easier administration can be found on p. xxi.

Drugs in Sport

The World Anti-Doping Agency (WADA) was established in 1999 to foster a doping-free culture in sport by:
- conducting scientific research to develop new detection methods
- educating athletes and support personnel
- raising awareness and providing information about doping and its consequences
- conducting an unannounced out-of-competition testing program that complements the programs of the International Sports Federations
- developing an independent observer program (which randomly monitors

and reports on all phases of doping control in an unbiased manner)

- monitoring acceptance and compliance with the World Anti-Doping Code, which ensures all athletes in all sports are governed by the same anti-doping rules and regulations.

WADA classifies drugs or methods into those that are prohibited at all times and those that may be prohibited in-competition and out-of-competition in some sports. Prohibited at all times include:

- anabolic steroids (e.g. stanozolol, testosterone)
- peptide hormones (e.g. erythropoietin), growth factors and related substances (e.g. growth hormone)
- beta-2 agonists (e.g. formoterol, NOT inhaled salbutamol or salmeterol)
- hormone antagonists and modulators (e.g. clomiphene, aminoglutethimide, tamoxifen)
- diuretics (e.g. furosemide (frusemide), acetazolamide) and other masking agents (e.g. probenecid)
- manipulation of blood and blood components, including substances that enhance oxygen transfer (e.g. haemoglobin products), blood doping (e.g. red blood cell product of any origin) and sample manipulation methods (e.g. tampering with samples or urine substitution)
- gene or cell doping (e.g. use of genetically modified cells)
- narcotics (opioids) (e.g. heroin, morphine, fentanyl) and cannabinoids (e.g. marijuana)
- glucocorticosteroids (oral, IV, IM or rectal) (e.g. dexamethasone, prednisolone) (WADA 2020).

Prohibited in-competition are stimulants (e.g. amphetamines, epinephrine (adrenaline), pseudoephedrine), while prohibited in-competition and out-of-competition in some sports only (e.g. archery, shooting) includes the beta2 adrenoceptor blocking agents (e.g. propranolol) (WADA 2020).

It is imperative that athletes (and the athlete's team) are aware of substances and methods that are prohibited at all times, substances that are prohibited in-competition and substances that are prohibited in particular sports. Important also is the need to know when and how to apply for a therapeutic use exemption (TUE), as well as understanding that sport supplements are largely unregulated and hence may contain substances prohibited by WADA (WADA 2020).

Pregnancy

Any medication (including OTCs, herbal preparations, alternative therapies or chemicals such as alcohol) has the potential to reach the developing fetus via the maternal circulation if taken during pregnancy. The risk to the fetus is dependent on a number of factors, including fetal gestational age on exposure (i.e. the fetus is most at risk during the first trimester when cells are rapidly proliferating and organs, muscles, CNS, arms, legs, toes and fingers are developing), duration of therapy (including dose, frequency and length of therapy), as well as any other medication taken concurrently (Bryant et al 2019). Animal studies have shown considerable differences in species' response with regard to the teratogenic effects of drugs and it may not be possible to extrapolate this data to humans. Fetal abnormalities include missing digits, excessive development or duplication of parts, splitting of parts abnormally, non-splitting of parts, fusion failure or over-fusion of some parts, openings failing to close or open adequately or abnormal placement of parts.

If possible, medications should be avoided during pregnancy. However, this is not always possible or practicable. The woman who is pregnant (or considering pregnancy) should work in partnership with her medical practitioner to develop a medication regimen that balances the benefits to the mother against the potential risks to the fetus. For example, a woman with epilepsy may need to consider the potentially life-threatening risks associated with uncontrolled epilepsy versus the benefits of controlling epilepsy with an agent that has an increased risk of causing fetal abnormalities.

Breastfeeding

Most drugs taken by a mother who is breastfeeding will be excreted to some extent in the breastmilk; however, the amount ingested by the infant will generally be extremely small, dependent on the age of the infant and the amount of breastmilk consumed (Hotham & Hotham 2015). Some drugs are concentrated in breastmilk relative to the maternal plasma concentration because of their chemical properties, including fat solubility, and may be toxic to the infant because of immaturity of the liver and kidney detoxification systems. Drugs contraindicated during breastfeeding include amiodarone, antineoplastic agents, gold salts, iodine, lithium, oral retinoids and radiopharmaceuticals. Further contraindications during breastfeeding include those very toxic agents where even very small amounts will affect the infant, if the drug has highly allergenic potential, if the maternal renal function is compromised (as this may lead to higher levels being excreted into breastmilk or the mother having a medical condition requiring prolonged administration of a drug (e.g. cancer) (Bryant et al 2019; Hotham & Hotham 2015).

Administering the drug when or immediately after the infant feeds will result in the lowest amount of drug being in the milk at subsequent feedings. If a drug is essential for the mother but of uncertain effect on the infant, it may be necessary to temporarily discontinue breastfeeding and remove contaminated breastmilk (via breast pump), which should be discarded (Bryant et al 2019).

If medication is taken during breastfeeding, the infant should always be closely observed for any side-effects, including poor feeding, listlessness, withdrawal symptoms and other abnormal behaviours, which should be reported if they occur.

Renal and Liver Impairment

Dose reduction is often required in those with any type of kidney and/or liver impairment because these organs are the main sites of drug metabolism and excretion. Monitoring of kidney and liver function throughout any drug therapy may be recommended to ensure that there is no further deterioration caused by the therapy. Furthermore, some medications may damage the liver or kidneys (e.g. large doses of paracetamol are hepatotoxic, NSAIDs may be nephrotoxic). If potentially nephrotoxic or hepatotoxic agents are given to those with renal or liver impairment, the risk of further damage is greatly increased.

Legal Requirements

Before a drug can be administered safely, the nurse needs to be aware of the legal aspects of drug administration. This includes knowledge of the laws governing the possession, use and dispensation of drugs and of the directives of the nurse's registering body on the administration of medications to clients. It also means observing the employing healthcare facility's occupational health and safety (OHS) regulations which are designed to promote safe storage, handling and use of drugs.

The Nursing and Midwifery Board of Australia (NMBA) is one of the national boards of the Australian Health Practitioner Regulation Agency (AHPRA). With the changes to registration of nurses by AHPRA from 2010, it was decided that enrolled nurses no longer required endorsement for medication administration. The NMBA's goal is for all enrolled nurses to undertake relevant units of study that will enable them to administer medicines safely as part of their education program. However, for enrolled nurses who have not completed the required units, a notation reading 'Does not hold Board-approved qualifications in administration of medicines' will appear on the national nursing register against that nurse's name (NMBA AHPRA 2020b). Jurisdictional legislation and policy specifies the routes and schedules of medicines that the enrolled nurse is able to administer and it is therefore of paramount importance that the nurse and employer understand and comply with the drugs and poisons legislation and policy. Furthermore, to administer intravenous medication, the enrolled nurse (Division 2) is required to have completed a separate NMBA-approved unit on the administration and monitoring of intravenous medications (NMBA AHPRA 2020b).

Legal Acts concerning poisons and the poisons regulatory bodies in New Zealand and each state and territory in Australia deal with the control of all drugs, from prescription medication through to agricultural poisons and research drugs. The Standard for the Uniform Scheduling of Medicines and Poisons (SUSMP) applies to sale, supply, containers, disposal, record keeping, storage, labelling, possession, use and advertising. The drugs and poisons contained in the schedules are divided into groups according to their mode of action, therapeutic use, potency, potential for abuse and addiction and safety. In Australia, there are currently 10 schedules with most medications being listed in Schedules 2, 3, 4 or 8 (Therapeutic Goods Administration 2020). Unscheduled substances (i.e. those not contained in these 10 schedules) are not considered a poison by definition and can be supplied to the public; these include laxatives, sunscreens, baby formula, herbal remedies and vitamins (Bryant et al 2019).

While medical practitioners are the main health professionals that advise and prescribe medications, there are members of other health disciplines who have limited prescribing rights. Nurse practitioners, as defined by the *Nurses Act 1993*, are those whose registration has been endorsed as being qualified to obtain and have in their possession and to use, sell or supply Schedule 2, 3, 4 or 8 poisons, as described under the *Drugs, Poisons and Controlled Substances Act 1981* (Version No. 065, 1/12/2003). The approved list of medications (scheduled poisons) is dependent on nurse practitioners' scope of practice (e.g. an acute care nurse practitioner list will be different to that of a paediatric care nurse practitioner). Dentists are able to prescribe drugs related to their practice (e.g. antibiotics, analgesics); podiatrists with endorsement may prescribe a limited range of Schedule 4 drugs related to podiatry practice (e.g. antibiotics, analgesics); optometrists (in some states, with extra training) are also able to prescribe a limited range of optometry-related Schedule 4 drugs (e.g. eye drops, drugs to treat glaucoma); midwives (with endorsement for scheduled medicines) are qualified to prescribe medications related to midwifery practice (Bryant et al 2019; NMBA AHPRA 2020a).

Storage

All medications in a ward or department should be kept in a locked cupboard, medication trolley or some other type of locked container, the key of which is kept by a nurse at all times. Victoria's Drugs, Poisons and Controlled Substances Regulations 2017 are very specific about the storage requirements for Schedule 8 or Schedule 9 poisons (e.g. constructed of steel 10 millimetres thick; fitted with a 6 lever lock; able to resist attack by hand tools for 30 minutes or power tools for 5 minutes) (Victorian Government 2017), with other states having similar requirements.

Drugs or preparations for external use should be stored apart from those intended for internal use, so that errors in administration do not occur. Suppositories, pessaries, insulins, antisera, vaccines, some blood products, some intravenous solutions and some antibiotics (particularly if reconstituted) should be stored in the refrigerator. Nothing else should be stored in the refrigerator (e.g. food) and it should also be kept locked.

The trend towards single-dose units being dispensed contributes to accuracy in dosage, better economy and less risk of product contamination. Many institutions have policies that discourage the use of multi-dose vials because of the risk of cross-contamination between patients.

Drug Orders

In 2004 Australian health ministers advised that 'to reduce the harm to patients from medication errors, by June 2006, all public hospitals will be using a common medication chart. This means that the same chart will be used wherever a doctor or nurse works and wherever the patient is within a hospital' (ACSQHC 2019a). The result was the National Inpatient Medication Chart (NIMC). Since then, additional national charts have been developed, including the National Residential Medication Chart (NRMC), National Subcutaneous Insulin Chart, Paediatric National Inpatient Medication Chart, Clozapine Titration Chart, NIMC (acute), NIMC (long stay), NIMC (day surgery) and NIMC (day surgery, private hospital) (ACSQHC 2019b).

A drug or preparation may be given only on written or verbal order from a medical officer, and must be clearly written and/or understood verbally. The law in all states requires that a legal drug order must be legibly written in ink, dated and signed by the prescriber and must include the patient's name and identification number (if applicable), the name and strength of the drug, the dose, route of administration, frequency of administration and duration of administration (if applicable). Any alteration to a drug order should be initialled. An unusual dose, drug strength or quantity should be underlined and initialled by the prescriber. If there is any doubt about the meaning of the order, the medical officer should be contacted immediately for clarification before administration.

The policy of the institution should be consulted before taking telephone orders for drugs. A telephone order should only be taken 'if in the opinion of the registered medical practitioner, dentist or nurse practitioner, an emergency exists' (Drugs, Poisons and Controlled Substances Regulations 2006, Reg. 47, 2 (C)). Errors may be eliminated if the nurse ensures that the drug has been ordered for the correct patient, writes it on the correct patient's medication chart, then asks a second nurse to read the drug order back over the telephone to the medical officer. The order should be confirmed in writing by the prescriber as soon 'as practicable'. However, institutions may have their own policies that require their medical officers to sign the order within 24 hours. If any doubt at all exists (e.g. the patient is unwell and requires reviewing, the nurse is unsure about the drug, dose etc.), the nurse should not take the telephone order and should ask the medical officer to review the patient or medication order as soon as practicable.

Legal Responsibility

Following a medical officer's order was once thought by many to absolve the nurse from all responsibility. However, legal judgements have shown that this is not always the case. The question that is often asked in situations of a drug error occurring is, 'What would the *reasonable* nurse do in this situation?'

Given that administering drugs is an everyday part of the role of most nurses, it is therefore not an unfair expectation that they will have some knowledge of the drugs they are administering. This includes the class of drug, why it is prescribed (purpose), how it works (action), recommended or usual dose range, how it is administered, contraindications, side-effects, potential for causing allergic reactions, any interactions with foods or other drugs and compatibility (especially when multiple intravenous drugs are to be administered).

It is not necessary for the nurse to memorise all this information; however, what is important is that the nurse has ready access to information and knows where or how to readily do so *before* administration. Information on any drug or preparation may be obtained from a pharmacist, textbooks or *reliable* internet sources. Once in possession of this knowledge, the nurse can question an unclear order, assess what skills are required to carry out the order and will understand what to observe in the patient in terms of beneficial and adverse effects.

Drug Incidents (Errors)

Drug incidents (or errors) are any preventable events involving medications that may result in harm and are related to the prescribing, dispensing or administering stages of the process (Jokanovic et al 2019). An audit of inpatient medication charts found that about 56% of errors were prescribing errors, 6% transcribing errors, 4% dispensing errors and 34% were administration errors (Atik 2012). Drug errors can cause adverse effects in patients, including death, as well as adding costs to the healthcare budget. A 2002 study by the Australian Commission on Safety and Quality in Health Care (ACSQHC), before the introduction of the National Inpatient Medication Chart, found that drug therapy errors occurred in 5–20% of drug administrations within

Australia, with a later 2006 study by ACSQHC finding that more than 700,000 hospital admissions each year were related to medication adverse effects, resulting in about $350 million in costs, and more importantly, 8000 deaths (ACSQHC 2019).

Administration incidents (errors) occur when:

- the wrong drug is administered, including the administration of the wrong intravenous fluid (e.g. drugs with similar names; use of abbreviations for names)
- the wrong dose is given (e.g. misreading dosage or units; misinterpreting abbreviations used for units, such as micrograms)
- the drug is given via the wrong route (e.g. an oral drug given intravenously)
- the drug is given to the wrong patient
- the drug is given at the wrong time or frequency, including omission, and/or
- an intravenous infusion is administered at the wrong rate.

Since 2008, standard prescribing terminology, abbreviations and symbols have been introduced in an attempt to reduce the number of associated errors. Abbreviations are used when referring to strength of medications, such as grams (g) and milligrams (mg). For example, the abbreviation for micrograms using the Greek letter μ (mu), that is, μg, is not recommended, nor is mcg, as these may lead to errors; microg is the preferred and recommended abbreviation, or the whole word (microgram) should be used. Other error-prone abbreviations and symbols that should be avoided include IU (international units – can be mistaken for IV), IVI (intravenous injection – mistaken for IV 1) and qd (every day – mistaken as qid (4 times daily)) (ACSQHC 2016a).

The use of 'dose administration aids' (DAAs), commonly found in the community and some residential aged care facilities, may not necessarily reduce the number of administration errors. A 2006 study found that DAAs contained a significant number of errors (incident rate 4.3% of packs and 12% of residents), which included missing medications, the wrong medication or wrong strength of medication dispensed, incorrect dosage instructions supplied or medications being supplied that had been ceased by a doctor (Carruthers et al 2008). A 2016 study by Gilmartin and colleagues also found similar results with a proportion of inspected DAAs having additional medications added to them, medications missing, incorrect or inappropriate division of tablets amongst identified errors. Furthermore, while the majority of errors were classified as minor or insignificant, there were also a number of potential major or catastrophic errors (Gilmartin et al 2016). Although on the surface this would appear to be a dispensing and pharmacy-related problem, it is also the responsibility of the nurse administering the medications to have some idea of what medication a patient has been prescribed (or no longer prescribed), and what the medication(s) actually looks like. DAAs are not suitable for all patients and require careful patient selection (e.g. the community-based patients should be motivated and willing to take the medication, have adequate vision, dexterity and cognition) and awareness of the limitations of the aid selected (e.g. increase in cost, including set-up costs; doses missed if medication spilled during administration and no back-up available;

if home delivered, no opportunity for pharmacist review and counselling; many medicines cannot be packed into a dosing aid; do not address intentional non-adherence, poor motivation or forgetfulness) (Elliott 2014).

An administration error may or may not have an adverse effect. The seriousness of the outcome (e.g. the adverse effect or lack of effect) does not absolve the nurse from the mistake that was made. It is important to clearly document the error and outcome. Some institutions may also have policies regarding further documentation requirements when an error has occurred (e.g. a 'drug incident' form).

It is important for nurses to practise within their own limitations and within the policies and protocols of the institution. If this is not done and an error occurs (especially a serious one), the nurse may find that the institution (and its insurers) may abrogate any responsibility because the nurse did not follow its policies. The nurse may also be liable under common law.

A Little Pharmacology

For extensive pharmacokinetics and pharmacology, refer to pharmacology texts. Here are some basic concepts that nurses need to understand.

Drug dosage

Dosage depends on the age, weight, sex, renal and liver function and general condition of the patient, and can be based on age, body weight or body surface area. As children usually require smaller doses than adults, various rules are used to estimate the fraction of the adult dose (see inside front cover).

Dose interval is important (e.g. anti-infective agents are given at regular intervals, 4-, 6- or 8-hourly, to maintain adequate blood levels, while hormones are given at the same time each day for uniform effect). The time of day must be suitable to the individual's lifestyle. For example, diuretics may be ordered twice daily and normal convention would see them administered at regular intervals (e.g. 8–10-hourly during the day); however, for an older person it may be more practicable to administer the diuretic in the morning and at lunchtime, so that sleep is not disturbed by frequent micturition, increasing the risk of falls.

Drug half-life

The half-life of a drug is a function of both distribution and elimination. In general terms, it is the time required for one-half of the amount of drug in the body to be eliminated. It is of practical use in calculating the frequency with which multiple doses of a drug can be administered to keep the blood level between the minimum effective concentration and the threshold for toxicity (e.g. a drug with a very short half-life may need to be administered intravenously to maintain levels, while another drug with a long half-life may be suitable for once-daily administration). Furthermore, a drug with a very long half-life may require patient monitoring for some time after the drug has been discontinued, or may require a 'washout' period to allow the drug to be removed from the system before the introduction of another agent.

Therapeutic drug monitoring

Some drugs have a narrow therapeutic range (i.e. the difference between overdosing and underdosing). Therapeutic drug monitoring involves measuring drug concentration in the blood. Information accompanying a request form should include the time the blood sample was taken, the time the last dose of the drug was given and its route of administration. The main aim of therapeutic drug monitoring is to optimise drug therapy by achieving adequate drug levels while minimising toxicity. It is especially important in those at the extremes of age (i.e. babies and the elderly).

Why measure drug levels?

Drug levels are measured for a number of reasons, which include:

- to individualise the dose (e.g. lithium, phenytoin, warfarin, levothyroxine)
- to assess the adequacy of loading dose (e.g. phenytoin) or to check levels after dose adjustment
- to avoid or diagnose toxicity (e.g. digoxin, vancomycin)
- to ensure effective blood levels (e.g. prophylactic antiepileptics, gentamicin)
- to check adherence to regimen (e.g. antipsychotic agents)
- to check that co-morbidities that may alter drug metabolism and elimination (e.g. renal impairment, hepatic failure, shock, sepsis) are not affecting blood levels
- to ensure that concurrent drug administration is not affecting blood levels
- to diagnose sub-therapeutic or failed therapy (to distinguish between ineffective drug treatment, non-adherence and adverse effects that mimic underlying disease)
- to change the route of administration or dosage (e.g. from IV or IM to oral administration) if necessary while maintaining adequate serum levels
- to guide withdrawal of therapy (Bryant et al 2019).

Drug route

The effectiveness of a drug often depends on the route of administration. A drug may have a systemic or local effect depending on whether it is taken orally, injected or applied topically (see Glossary, pp. 1657–58 for forms of preparations). Drugs are formulated to meet the requirements for rapid or slow absorption, metabolism or excretion in order to obtain the required therapeutic blood levels. The two most common routes of drug administration are oral and parenteral.

Oral administration

Many oral preparations are given on an empty stomach because food may decrease the absorption; however, if gastric irritation is a problem they may be given with or immediately after food.

It is recommended that a capsule is preceded by a small amount of water and then taken with half a glass of water to prevent it becoming lodged in the oesophagus. A number of medications known to cause oesophageal ulceration include aspirin, bisphosphonates (e.g. alendronate), doxycycline, iron tablets, potassium chloride and zidovudine (Gowan & Roller 2010). Enteric-coated, slow-release, extended-release, modified-release, sustained-release and controlled-dosage tablets should be swallowed whole, not crushed or chewed, for a number of reasons, which may include:

- absorption will be altered (e.g. MS Contin, Keflor CD, Efexor XR, Dilantin)
- the medication may become unstable (e.g. Augmentin Duo, Nimotop)
- they may cause local irritation (e.g. Cartia, Roaccutane)

- they will not reach the site of the intended action (e.g. Creon, Dipentum)
- unacceptable taste (e.g. Neoral, Coloxyl)
- being hazardous (e.g. Imuran, Myleran, Leukeran).

Care must be taken to select the correct formulation of tablets when several different formulations and/or dosages exist (e.g. Isoptin (verapamil) is available in 40 mg, 80 mg, 120 mg or 160 mg tablets; Isoptin SR is available as 180 mg or 240 mg), because the consequences may be very serious if the wrong formulation is administered (e.g. substituting Isoptin 80 mg (3 tablets), which will act quickly compared with Isoptin SR 240 mg, which is a sustained-release preparation and will act over 24 hours). It is important to check whether different formulations are interchangeable or not (e.g. olapatib is available as a tablet or capsule. However, the strengths are different as are the recommended dosages and are therefore not interchangeable).

Crushing or dispersing medications

It is important to check if the medication can be dispersed or crushed. As previously stated, sustained- or modified-release medications should not be crushed or dispersed. Important considerations include:

- assessing whether the patient has any swallowing difficulties or is 'at risk' of aspiration. If there are any concerns, referral to a speech pathologist is recommended to determine appropriate fluids or soft foods (e.g. apple puree, yoghurt) that can be used to administer crushed or dispersed medication
- checking if the medication is available in a different formulation which is easier to administer (e.g. syrup or solution rather than tablet form)
- only preparing one medication at a time (i.e. only one tablet should be crushed and prepared at a time, not the patient's entire medications)
- any fluid restriction when dispersing medication (e.g. how much fluid should be used to disperse the medication, which should be considered in the patient's overall fluid intake)
- using a closed tablet crusher for medications which are hazardous, cytotoxic or teratogenic
- use of safety glasses, mask and gloves for handling of medications which are hazardous, cytotoxic or teratogenic
- reducing pregnant staff contact with medications that are hazardous, cytotoxic or teratogenic
- ensuring mortar and pestle/tablet crusher are cleaned between medications and between patients (Society of Hospital Pharmacists of Australia 2018).

Parenteral administration

Parenteral medications are given either as injections or by infusion. The most common routes are intramuscular (IM), subcutaneous (SC) and intravenous (IV).

Intramuscular

The three main muscles used for intramuscular injections are:

- the lateral aspect of the thigh (middle third when the thigh is divided into three)
- the upper outer quadrant of the dorsogluteal
- the deltoid.

No more than 5 mL should be administered by intramuscular injection, and less into the deltoid muscle. If a volume > 5 mL is required, the dose should be divided and given into different sites.

Furthermore, the deltoid muscle is not recommended for intramuscular injection in children.

Subcutaneous

Subcutaneous injection sites include:

- upper outer aspect (middle third) of the upper arm
- upper anterior thigh
- abdomen below the costal margins to the iliac crests (avoiding the area around the navel by about 5 cm).

When frequent administration is required (e.g. insulin administration in a patient with diabetes mellitus, daily heparin injections), administration sites should be rotated and documented on the medication chart to prevent atrophy of the subcutaneous tissue, increased risk of infection and pain.

Intravenous

A drug may be given by direct IV injection as a bolus in a volume of 20 mL or less in under 1 minute, or by slow IV injection over 5–15 minutes. It is important to check and adhere to the manufacturer's information regarding the required administration time, because administering some drugs too quickly can cause pain, damage the blood vessel, as well as other adverse effects, such as flushing, hyper- or hypotension, syncope, arrhythmias, feelings of warmth or anxiety, depending on the drug administered. IV injection (bolus or slow injection) is used when an immediate effect is required or the drug becomes unstable on reconstitution or dilution. The intermittent infusion method is used when a drug is diluted, when interval dosing is desired and when slow administration is required. The drug is diluted in 50–250 mL and infused over 15 minutes to 2 hours. This minimises stability and incompatibility problems and gives the 'peak' and 'trough' effect in antibiotic therapy. One of the advantages of intermittent IV administration is that the patient can have an intermittent venous access port, which increases client mobility, comfort and safety, as well as providing a cost benefit from not having continuous IV therapy; also the nurse does not have to continuously monitor flow rates.

When a drug must be highly diluted and a steady-state blood level is to be maintained, the continuous infusion method is used, in which the drug is diluted in 500–1000 mL and infused over 4–24 hours (e.g. potassium chloride requires high dilution and constant blood levels to prevent depression of cardiac function).

The IV flow rate may be controlled by using an infusion pump, a microdrip set or a burette. When a drug is added to the burette during intermittent infusion, details of the additive are indicated on a label that is attached to the burette. Any IV drug admixture must be prepared aseptically, mixed thoroughly and labelled with the name and amount of the additive, the name of the person adding the agent, the name of the person checking the addition and the time of starting the infusion. National recommendations for user-applied labelling of injectable medicines, fluids and lines now exist and it is imperative that nurses understand and comply with these as consequences of non-labelling can result in a potentially life-threatening situation for the patient. These recommendations include colour coding the route of administration (e.g. red for intra-arterial, blue for intravenous, yellow for epidural or intrathecal and beige for subcutaneous), the process for medicine and label preparation (including label placement), when to discard containers of injectable medicines and special circumstances (ACSQHC 2016a). While these labelling recommendations do not apply to enteral, topical or inhalation routes, the general principles still apply as a way of improving practice and decreasing the risk of errors occurring.

An IV admixture should not be administered if there are signs of physical incompatibility such as a colour change, loss of clarity or precipitate formation. Chemical and physical compatibility and stability of admixtures should be checked *before* administration. If in any doubt, consult a pharmacist, textbooks, manufacturer's information or a drug information centre.

Other administration routes

Drugs generally should not be mixed with blood or blood products.

Other methods of administering medications include the following:

- Transdermal patches, which deliver drugs through the skin at a steady concentration, avoiding first-pass metabolism in the liver and any gastric side-effects. Several types of drugs, including glyceryl trinitrate, hormones and nicotine, are available as transdermal patches. Advantages include ease of application and frequency of application (once daily or longer), but the disadvantages include some skin reactions and the low number of drugs available via this route.
- Intradermal implants, which are surgically implanted subcutaneously. Advantages include the frequency of administration (some may be implanted for 6–8 weeks or longer); however, they require surgical implanting and removal (e.g. etonogestrel (long-term contraception) is left in situ for 3 years before replacement).

Guide for Safe Administration

Some drugs, such as Schedule 8, require double-checking; however, it is important that the double-checking procedure is an independent cognitive task (i.e. the nurse independently calculates the amount required as opposed to checking or glancing at someone else's calculations), rather than it being a superficial routine task. While double-checking is time consuming, it is central to patient safety and reducing drug errors (Ramasamy et al 2013).

Check the order

- Check that the information on the drug name (preferably generic rather than trade name), dose, route, frequency, time due and when the drug was last given are all legible (if any doubt exists, withhold the drug and check with the medical officer) and that the order is signed by the medical officer.
- Check that patient details are correct, including any known allergies (it is important to discuss any allergy/sensitivity history with the patient as cross-sensitivity between products does occur).

Check the drug

- Check the container label against the medication order when selecting the preparation, before measuring out and when replacing the preparation.
- Check the expiry date of the drug.
- Complete the drug calculation and then check the answer with another registered nurse, a pharmacist or medical officer (ask the second person to do the calculation independently, then compare answers, remembering

that it is rare to give less than half a tablet or more than 2 tablets or 1 ampoule at a time).
- Mix liquid contents thoroughly, but rotate or swirl protein preparations gently to prevent denaturation and frothing. If the reconstituted solution containing protein is further diluted, it should be gently inverted (not shaken) to ensure even mixing.
- Note any discolouration, precipitate or foreign bodies (and do not administer if they are present).

Check the patient

- Check the patient's identity carefully (check wrist identity band or verbally), taking extra care if there are patients with the same or similar names, or if the patient is unknown to the nurse. An observational study of nurses administering medications found that 79% did not check the patient's identity before administration (Westbrook et al 2015).
- Check if the patient has any known allergies.
- Check that the patient knows the reason for the medication and discuss any query with the medical officer before giving it.
- Only give medications that you, the nurse, have prepared or seen a pharmacist prepare (i.e. do not administer an IV drug that was drawn up by someone else without you present).
- Give the correct drug and dose.
- Give to the correct patient.
- Give at the correct time.
- Give medication by the prescribed route.
- Do not handle tablets.
- Wait until oral medications are swallowed (never leave medications on bedside tables, lockers or dinner trays).

Documentation

- Ensure that the drug administration sheet is signed after administration.
- Document any discrepancies (e.g. patient unable or refuses to take medication, patient absent, medication not available).
- If Schedule 8 drugs are involved, ensure that the drug register is correctly filled in (date, time, patient, drug (form, strength, amount to be administered), persons administering drug, balance of drug remaining, any drug discarded).
- Observe the patient and document in the patient's history.
- Note beneficial effects and/or report and chart any adverse effects (see brief discussion below).

Disposal

- Correctly and safely dispose of equipment used (e.g. do not recap syringes, dispose of them safely in a sharps container; return unused medications to pharmacy).

Drug effects

A drug may produce more than one effect, which may be beneficial or not.

- The *desired action* is the physiological response the drug is expected to cause (e.g. antihypertensive medications are expected to lower blood pressure).
- *Adverse effects* refer to an unwanted effect which may or may not be dose related and is usually via a different mechanism to its pharmacological action.

- *Toxic effects* develop after prolonged administration of high doses of medication, or when a drug accumulates in the blood because of impaired metabolism or excretion. Some drugs, such as digoxin and lithium, have a very narrow safety margin and toxicity can occur at recommended or therapeutic doses.
- *Allergic reactions* are unpredictable responses to a drug that acts as an antigen, triggering the release of antibodies. Allergic reactions may be mild (such as urticaria (hives) and pruritus (itching)), or they may be severe (e.g. severe wheezing and respiratory distress), or life threatening (e.g. anaphylactic reaction). Some reactions occur within minutes of the drug being given (e.g. penicillin, streptomycin, radiological contrast media), while other allergic reactions may be delayed for hours or days (e.g. contact sensitivity to local anaesthetic cream).
- *Idiosyncratic reactions* are those where the patient's body either overreacts or underreacts to a drug, or when the reaction is unusual and there is no known cause (e.g. the antihistamine promethazine (Phenergan) is sometimes used for sedation; however, in some people (especially children) it can cause insomnia and agitation).
- *Pharmacogenetic reactions* occur because a person may have a genetic trait which leads to abnormal reactions to drugs (e.g. those with glucose-6-phosphate dehydrogenase (G6PD) deficiency may experience haemolysis if given dapsone, nitrofurantoin, primaquine or sulfamethoxazole) (Bryant et al 2019).
- *Drug tolerance* may also occur where a person has a decreased response to a drug over time, necessitating an increase in dosage to achieve the required response (Bryant et al 2019).
- *Drug interactions* occur when one drug modifies the action of another drug (e.g. a drug may either increase or decrease the action of other drugs). A drug interaction may be synergistic (enhances the effects of another drug) (e.g. probenecid may be given orally before IM procaine penicillin to increase and prolong the serum level of penicillin), antagonistic (opposes the effects of another drug) (e.g. protamine sulphate can be given to neutralise the anticoagulant effects of heparin) or additive (where the two drug actions are added together (e.g. when alcohol is consumed by a person on heparin, the risk of bleeding is significantly increased)).

Summary

Administering medication is one of the nurse's most important responsibilities and should be treated with the due care it demands. It is not a task merely to be completed, but rather an opportunity for nurses to increase their own knowledge, to ensure that patients have been educated regarding their medications and to observe patients for both expected and unexpected responses – part of holistic nursing care. The right patient has a right to receive the right dose of the right medication in the right form at the right time by the right route for the right duration of therapy. If any doubt exists, the medication should be withheld; remember, WHEN IN DOUBT, DON'T!!

AT A GLANCE

Available Forms

This section outlines the various formulations for the medication.

Action

Because this is not a pharmacology text, only a brief description of the action of each agent is included. For more detailed information, a pharmacology text should be consulted.

Use

The most common uses of drugs (including both hospital and community uses).

Dose

Dosages listed in this book are those for the *average adult* (unless otherwise stated). Occasionally a paediatric dose may be included if that particular agent is used predominantly in children (e.g. growth hormone, agents used to treat attention deficit hyperactivity disorder (ADHD)).

Adverse effects

Adverse effects are generally unwanted effects, some of which are predictable and often dose related. Other adverse effects may be unpredictable and occur less frequently (e.g. anaphylaxis, anaphylactoid reaction). Very common adverse effects are considered to be those that occur in 10% or more of study participants. Common adverse effects are found in 1–10%, uncommon in 1–0.1%, and rare adverse effects occur in less than 0.1%. The adverse effects listed in this book are generally those that are common or very common, and rare or less common adverse effects are listed when they require some action to be taken. For example, thrombocytopenia may be a rare adverse effect, but there is a requirement for regular monitoring of blood counts.

Interactions

Interactions occur when one drug alters the action of the second drug, or both agents affect each other. As with the adverse effects, the interactions listed are those that occur commonly or are the most dangerous. It should be noted, however, that interactions between any agents are always possible and caution should be taken when multiple agents are given. For detailed explanations of how and why interactions occur, a pharmacological text should be consulted.

Nursing points/Cautions

The points in this section are those most directly applicable to nurses and include:

- IV administration rate
- monitoring advice
- reconstitution and dilution requirements
- incompatibilities
- any specific storage requirements (e.g. refrigeration)
- cautions (e.g. particular patient groups that may need extra monitoring) and contraindications.

Patient teaching and advice

Included in this section is important information that the patient should receive about their medication and includes:

- taking with food or fluids
- dividing of tablets
- grapefruit juice incompatibility

- driving warning
- when to seek medical advice (see following section for detailed patient teaching and advice information)
- advice regarding contraception if medication causes problems during pregnancy (e.g. teratogenic causing fetal malformations; use of effective contraception during and for some time after last dose).

It is assumed that the nurse will:

- use an aseptic technique when reconstituting medication
- inspect the solution for any particulate matter or cloudiness
- not use the medication if either particulates or cloudiness are present
- administer the medication using a safe, aseptic and correct technique
- dispose of sharps in a safe and responsible manner.

These points *are not* made for every parenteral agent in the text.

- 'Cautions' are the equivalent of amber traffic lights – go slow and take care. For example, a person with renal impairment may not excrete the medication at the same rate as someone with normal renal function, thus increasing the risk of adverse effects and toxicity. Therefore, a reduced dose may be required and/or close monitoring of renal function and drug excretion, as well as monitoring for adverse effects.
- 'Contraindications' are the equivalent of red traffic lights – no go!
  - hypersensitivity to the agent itself is not listed for every agent as it is assumed that this will be checked routinely before administration (i.e. the patient will be asked 'Have you had this medication before? Did you have any problems with it?'). Although cautions and contraindications are often more relevant to the person prescribing the medication, it is important that the nurse is also aware of these factors.

GENERAL PATIENT TEACHING AND ADVICE

Patient teaching and advice regarding medications is an essential part of care, which often involves the nurse, in addition to the pharmacist, doctor and/or other members of a multidisciplinary team. If possible, take the time to build a rapport with the patient (and their significant other/carer/family member, if appropriate). It is easier to learn from and ask questions of someone you are comfortable with. Also, given the extent of this educational task, it should start on admission rather than a few days before (or on the day of) discharge.

There are a number of factors which may impact on a person's ability to learn (Roach 2005), including the following:

- *Environment and available time:* It may be difficult to teach and/or learn in an area where there are constant distractions or interruptions. Consider using a small room where the door can be closed and at a time when the nurse knows there will not be any interruptions (e.g. not during meal breaks or at other times of reduced staffing or during visiting hours). Although accessing a small room may not be possible, pulling the curtain around the person's bed may alert others that something is taking place, even if it doesn't really afford privacy (curtains are not soundproof). The nurse should also consider how much time they have available to conduct the session. A short session crammed with too much information may cause confusion for the patient, as well as potentially leading to important information being overlooked.

- *Pain and/or discomfort:* Are you able to concentrate if you are tired, in pain, need to go to the toilet, are hungry or thirsty? All of these impact on a person's capacity to concentrate and should be eliminated or minimised before starting a teaching session.
- *Sensory deficits:* Does the patient have a hearing impairment? Do they have a hearing aid? Do they have it in (and is it turned on)? Can the person read the label on the medication bottle or graduations on a syringe? Is the person dexterous enough to open medication bottles or operate an injector pen or glucometer? Does the person have sufficient coordination to use an inhaler or is a spacer device required?
- *Anxiety/stress/fear:* These are similar to pain and discomfort and should be minimised or alleviated before starting a teaching session.
- *Learning styles:* Not everyone learns in the same manner. Some people learn by reading, others require demonstration, while others may require both (e.g. to demonstrate an injection or puffer technique get the patient to practise, as well as leaving literature for them to read). Consider your own learning style(s) – how do you prefer to learn about a new piece of equipment: play with it until you work out how it works, have it demonstrated to you, read the instruction manual from cover to cover or a combination of two or more methods? We often teach others in the manner we like to learn, therefore we should also consider teaching using the other, less comfortable ways. Allowing the patient to practise the skills (e.g. injection technique, blood glucose monitoring, puffer technique) gives the nurse an opportunity to observe and anticipate any problems (e.g. the patient may require follow-up by a district nurse on discharge to ensure the technique is correct).
- *Literacy:* Information should be presented at a level that takes into account the patient's education and reading level.
- *Language and culture:* Is an interpreter required? Does consideration need to be given to the nature of the material (e.g. contraception) and the genders of the teacher and patient? It is very difficult to give important information to someone who does not speak the same language as yourself, or who may be able to understand but not able to ask questions. Furthermore, it is important to use a professional interpreter if possible, as using family members (especially children or adults of the opposite sex) can put them into situations where they are not comfortable (e.g. a teenage son interpreting for his mother who is taking medication for gynaecological problems).

There are also issues of privacy and patient confidentiality to consider, as well as possible misinterpretation, giving incorrect drug and dosing information, or family members withholding information. It is also necessary to remember these issues of language and culture if giving the patient written information.

Before starting any teaching session, it is important to lay down the 'ground rules' (e.g. how long the session will last, what is going to be discussed, follow-up). Factors which can be alleviated or minimised should be attended to before starting the session. Other general considerations may include the following:

- *Use of appropriate language:* Nurses (and medical professionals in general) often use jargon (e.g. doing 'obs' or the 'meds'), which can be confusing (and daunting or overwhelming) for non-medical people.
- *Speed of conversation:* It is important to consider how quickly the information is delivered (i.e. how quickly does the nurse/doctor/pharmacist/allied health professional talk?) as this can lead to misunderstandings, especially if the patient is elderly, has a hearing impairment or is from a non-English speaking background (e.g. a patient may be too embarrassed to say they have not understood information because the person is speaking too quickly). Furthermore, when the health professional is feeling rushed, they may also speak faster.
- *Previous knowledge and skills of the person:* Even if the patient has been prescribed the medication before, assessing knowledge and any misunderstandings can be important as this may improve the patient's motivation to take the medication, thereby improving adherence with the regimen. If the medication is new, it is important to determine if the information and/or skill (such as using an inhaler or administration of insulin) requires more than one session, making discharge planning essential. This extra time gives the patient time not only to practise skills (supervised and/or unsupervised), but also to ask questions and seek clarification on anything that they have not understood (Roach 2005).
- It is important to return at an agreed time to review information and follow up on any other questions the person may have.

Consideration should be given to including the following as part of patient teaching and advice:

- Why is the person taking the medication (including the benefits)? If the person has any concerns about taking the medication, they should be encouraged to discuss these with their doctor before starting.
- Provide a simplified explanation of how the medication works (however, it is important not to be condescending).
- The importance of telling other health professionals (e.g. dentist, specialist, surgeon, anaesthetist) that they are taking medications (e.g. it may be necessary to discontinue some medications before a procedure). This should also include the patient reminding the health professional of any allergies (including to food(s) or latex) or other medical conditions (past or present) (such as kidney impairment, asthma, tuberculosis, hepatitis B, heart failure, cancer, blood disorders, gastric ulcer

or bleeding, diabetes, high blood pressure), whether they smoke or regularly drink alcohol.

- The importance of telling the doctor if the patient is pregnant, planning to become pregnant, breastfeeding or planning to breastfeed as many medications cross the placental barrier and/or are excreted in breastmilk.
- Ensuring prescriptions are filled in a timely manner so that the medication does not run out.
- A recommendation that the patient carries a list of current medications (with exact names) in their wallet/purse so that they can ensure that any other health professional knows what is being taken rather than a general description (e.g. 'small blue pill for my heart'). This may also be important in the event of an emergency.

Dosage

- Name and strength of the medication (including information about differing strengths and trade names).
- What the medication looks like (e.g. capsules, tablets, liquid, injection).
- Dose – this may be straightforward (e.g. patient is ordered 10 mg and tablets are supplied as 10 mg) or not (e.g. patient is ordered 15 mg and tablets are supplied as 10 mg which means splitting one tablet. Depending on the dexterity of the person or the size of the tablet, this may not be a simple task. Is a pill splitter required?)
- When to take (e.g. morning, evening, same time every day, in relation to food or other tablets, once per week, once per month). It can be useful to specify a day. This can make adherence to the regimen simpler.
- Not increasing, decreasing or stopping medication without seeking advice from the doctor.

How to Take

- Swallow whole with glass of water (or other fluids as recommended). Some fluids may interfere with the medication and it is important to know which ones to avoid.
- Importance of taking with or without food. Some medications need to be taken on an empty stomach, so instructions will include an hour before or 2 hours after food.
- Tablets/capsules should generally not be chewed (unless the tablets are chewable), broken, opened or crushed (however, this is dependent on specific medication).
- Techniques (such as inhalation using a puffer or injection) will need to be demonstrated and taught. If the patient is unable to manage, consideration should be given to teaching a carer/family member/significant other, involving a community-based service (e.g. district nursing service) or discussing with a doctor the appropriateness of the medication and the risk of non-adherence with the regimen.
- What to do if a dose is forgotten, omitted or vomiting occurs soon after an oral medication (e.g. seeking advice from a pharmacist or doctor; not taking a double dose to 'catch up').
- What to do if too much medication is taken (e.g. contacting doctor, pharmacist or Poisons Information Centre (131 126 in Australia or 0800 764 766 in New Zealand), going to the nearest Accident and Emergency Department).

- Length of time that the medication will be required (including emphasis on completing the course and not stopping the medication abruptly or without seeking medical advice).
- Whether there is anything that should be avoided while taking the medication (e.g. certain foods or fluids, alcohol, standing up quickly, not lying down after taking medication).

Adverse Effects

- All medications cause some side/adverse effects. Some of these may be common, mild and transient in nature, while others are more serious (and life threatening). It is important for the patient to be made aware of any potential side/adverse effects that may require immediate medical attention. Caution should be taken with explaining side-effects (e.g. some patients may become anxious or frightened by potential side-effects and not take medications at all). It may be safer and simpler to suggest seeing a doctor immediately if anything unusual occurs. However, sometimes it is important to give specific directions, such as 'report to your doctor immediately if you develop any yellowing of the skin or whites of the eyes, your urine looks darker than usual, you develop nausea, vomiting or abdominal pain'.
- Life-threatening side-effects (such as allergic reaction, including development of wheezing, shortness of breath, rash, skin blistering, difficulty swallowing) should be emphasised as requiring urgent and immediate medical attention (e.g. call an ambulance rather than going to a medical centre).

Storage

- All medications should be kept out of reach of children.
- Medications should be correctly stored. If there are special storage requirements (such as refrigeration) these should be emphasised (e.g. not using if left out of the fridge for 12 hours or more).
- Medications should not be stored in a bathroom, near a sink, on a windowsill or in the car as heat and dampness may destroy them.
- Most medications should not be frozen.
- Medications should be kept in the original containers/packets with labels intact. Medication should not be taken if the packaging/container is torn or has signs of being tampered with.
- If the medication changes colour, becomes cloudy, has foreign particles present or develops an odour, it should not be used and a pharmacist should be consulted immediately.
- Medications have a 'use by' (or expiry) date and should not be used after this date. It is important to show the patient where this information is located (it can be difficult to see on some containers). Some medications, such as eye drops, ointments and oral suspensions/mixtures, may have a very short life and deteriorate chemically with time, so it is important to write the date opened so that the person knows when to dispose of them.
- Expired medications or medications that are no longer needed should not be disposed of in general waste or sewerage as they end up in landfill and may be damaging to the

environment by ending up in waterways or may be found by children or animals. The Australian Government has established a National Return and Disposal of Unwanted Medicines program, which collects medicines returned to pharmacies and incinerates them according to Environmental Protection Authority (EPA) requirements (The National Return and Disposal of Unwanted Medicines Ltd 2020).

Other Issues

- Follow all instructions on package/container (e.g. 'shake well before use', 'keep refrigerated', 'take 1 hour before meals').
- Seek advice from doctor if symptoms do not improve or worsen.
- Attend doctor's appointments as requested, including the need for regular blood or other tests to monitor drug levels (e.g. some medications, such as warfarin, require regular monitoring of the therapeutic blood level and the dosage may need to be adjusted accordingly).
- The importance of having a current prescription and getting it filled/refilled before the medication runs out (especially if planning to take a holiday).
- Medications should not be given to others with similar conditions, nor kept for next time the condition recurs (e.g. antibiotics used to treat respiratory infection).
- OTC medications (such as simple analgesics, antacids, laxatives, cold and flu preparations) and herbal preparations or vitamins/minerals may interact with prescribed medications. It is important to consult with the doctor or pharmacist before taking any of these preparations (including those bought from the supermarket or health food stores).
- Consideration should be given to wearing a MedicAlert pendant or bracelet or some other form of identification for some conditions/medications (e.g. diabetes, anticoagulants, corticosteroids, insulin) in case of an emergency.
- Is the patient able to manage the medications alone (e.g. it may be appropriate to suggest using a dose administration aid (DAA) (e.g. Dosette box)? (See discussion on p. xviii regarding the suitability of patients for administration aids.) Involve a carer in any discussions or refer the patient to a community-based agency (such as the district nursing service) for monitoring). This may also include the ability to open containers or split tablets if needed. Most pharmacies will provide a unit-dose packing service on request at a cost.
- Warn patient against driving or operating machinery until they know how the medication will affect them. This is particularly important if the medication has known side-effects that affect vision, balance, coordination or reaction time or increases the effects of alcohol. If this is a known occurrence, extra labels will be attached to containers/packages (e.g. 'this medication may cause drowsiness and may increase the effects of alcohol. If affected, do not drive a motor vehicle or operate machinery').
- Other medication-specific considerations are discussed under patient teaching and advice in each section.

REVIEWERS

Swapnali Gazula
RN, GradCertEd(TertEd), MSc(Nurs), PhD
International Nursing Coordinator, Lecturer, School of Health, Federation University, Ballarat, VIC, Australia

Tanya Langtree
RN, GradCertNursSc(IntCare), GradDipAdvClinNurs(NeuroSc), MNursSt, PhD, CHIA, JP(Qual)
Lecturer/Academic Lead: Practice Integration
Nursing and Midwifery, College of Healthcare Sciences, James Cook University, Townsville, QLD, Australia

Giselle M. Mitchell
RN, BNurs(Hons), GradDipEd(Nurs), CertTAE
Operational Manager – Diploma of Nursing, Faculty of Health, Community & Life Sciences, Box Hill Institute, VIC, Australia

Nicole M. Norman
RN, MNurs
Academic Lead Undergraduate Nursing, College of Nursing and Midwifery, Charles Darwin University, NT, Australia

Daniel Wadsworth
BSc(Hons), MPhil, PhD
Lecturer in Applied Science, School of Nursing, Midwifery & Paramedicine, University of the Sunshine Coast, QLD, Australia

Technical reviewers

Jerry Perkins
BPharm, BSc

Lynne Margaret Perkins
BPharm, BVA

Sompal Gumi
RN, GradCertDiabEd&Mgt, MSc(Nurs), PhD

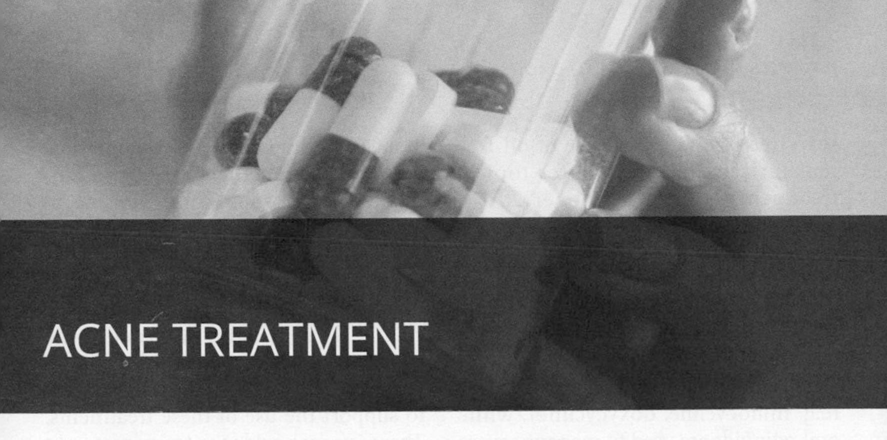

ACNE TREATMENT

Although a small number of adults (often women) continue to experience acne vulgaris, it is commonly a disorder of teenagers and young adults. After puberty there is an increased sebum production, and blocked follicles result in small cysts (comedones) containing sebum and keratinous material. *P. acnes* acts on the sebum leading to release of free fatty acids, which results in inflammation and cyst rupture (Lawley et al 2018; Harris & Cooper 2017).

There are a number of types of lesions that appear in acne vulgaris, including comedones (closed – whiteheads, open – blackheads), papules, pustules, nodules, cysts and scars. Distribution follows the areas of the body with the greatest number of pilosebaceous glands, namely face, neck, chest and back (Harris & Cooper 2017). Comedones are most common on the forehead and cheeks. Papules may evolve quickly over a few hours, are often itchy or painful and become pustules which resolve over a few days (Lawley et al 2018). Nodules and cysts, however, are a sign of deeper inflammation, are more uncomfortable and take longer to resolve. Scarring is a common result, especially if the lesions are scratched, picked or squeezed. For the person experiencing acne, the number or severity of the lesions may not be in proportion to the emotional impact it has on them. It has been found that the severity of the acne tends to be underestimated by the doctor and overestimated by the patient, and a few 'zits/spots' are likely to cause as much angst as many lesions in a teenager. Regardless of the severity of the acne, patients are at greater risk of anxiety and depression compared to those with no acne (Lawley et al 2018; Harris & Cooper 2017; Zaenglein et al 2016).

A number of medications can cause eruptions or worsen pre-existing acne. These include glucocorticoids (topical and systemic), phenytoin, lithium, isoniazid, oral contraceptive pills and androgenic steroids. Genetic factors and polycystic disease may also play a role in the development of secondary acne. Other factors known to aggravate acne include friction and trauma to the area (e.g. chin straps, headbands), some topical preparations (e.g. cosmetics, hair preparations) or exposure to certain industrial compounds (Lawley et al 2018).

Management of acne should always commence with face hygiene using a soap-free face wash and use of oil-free moisturisers, especially after topical treatments (Harris & Cooper 2017). Treatment of mild-to-moderate acne is usually topical (e.g. topical retinoids, benzoyl peroxide, azelaic acid or salicylic acid), while topical antibacterial agents (e.g. erythromycin, clindamycin) are used as adjuncts. Moderate-to-severe acne is managed with systemic therapy (e.g. minocycline, doxycycline), while oral retinoids are used to manage severe nodulocystic acne that is unresponsive to other therapies. Therapy can be one agent alone (monotherapy) or a combination, with combination therapy being recommended for most patients with acne, as a number of aspects of the disease process are treated simultaneously (Lawley et al 2018; Zaenglein et al 2016). Other therapies for acne management include chemical peels, light, laser and radio frequency; however, there is little long-term research or evidence in these areas to support the use of these treatments. There is some evidence to suggest light therapy is both safe and effective in acne treatment (Harris & Cooper 2017).

RETINOIDS

General Actions of retinoids

- analogues of vitamin A
- cause epidermal hyperplasia, decreased hyperkeratosis, inhibit sebum production and decrease size of sebaceous glands
- (acne) assist in the extrusion of fatty substance from comedones and prevent reblocking and formation of new lesions
- some anti-inflammatory action

General Adverse effects of oral retinoids

- pruritus, rash, skin thinning and scaling (especially palms, soles), dermatitis, sticky skin, dry skin, erythema, skin fragility, bullous eruptions
- eye irritation, decreased night vision, conjunctivitis, dry eyes, blurred vision, contact lens intolerance, xerophthalmia
- headache, depression, fatigue, somnolence, anxiety, mood swings
- cheilitis, dry mouth and/or lips, taste disturbance, cracked corners of mouth and lips
- nausea, vomiting, abdominal pain, inflammatory bowel disease, diarrhoea, stomatitis, gingivitis
- flushing
- paronychia, nail fragility
- tinnitus, hearing impairment
- arthralgia, arthritis, myalgia (with or without elevated creatinine phosphokinase (CPK)), joint and bone pain
- drying of mucous membranes, leading to epistaxis or rhinitis
- reversible alopecia, abnormal hair texture
- increased serum cholesterol and triglycerides, raised liver enzymes
- alteration to blood glucose levels
- (uncommon) photosensitivity
- (rare, high dose) corneal opacities, erosions or ulceration
- (rare) benign intracranial hypertension (pseudotumour celebri), skeletal hyperostosis, allergy, suicide, suicidal ideation, pancreatitis, gynaecomastia
- (overdose, hypervitaminosis A) transient headache, vomiting, facial

flushing, dizziness, cheilosis, abdominal pain, ataxia

General Interactions of oral retinoids

- contraindicated with tetracyclines because of risk of benign intracranial hypertension
- contraindicated with other retinoids or vitamin A due to increased risk of hypervitaminosis A
- not recommended with alcohol (especially in women of childbearing potential)
- may reduce efficacy of progestogen-only oral contraceptives

General Nursing points/Cautions for retinoids

- before starting therapy, patient should be assessed for any family history of lipid disorders or obesity, alcohol abuse, diabetes or smoking
- liver function should be monitored before starting therapy, weekly during the first 2 months and then at 3-monthly intervals during therapy
- blood lipids (triglycerides and cholesterol) should be monitored before starting and then 1–2 weekly until lipid response is determined (usually 4–8 weeks), then regularly throughout therapy (especially if there is a predisposition to lipid disorders, including family history, diabetes mellitus, obesity or increased alcohol intake)
- exacerbation of cystic acne or psoriasis may occur during initial stages of treatment
- (long-term therapy) patient should have regular X-rays during therapy to monitor for signs of new, or changes in, bony abnormalities of the spine
- if used in those under 18 years, bone growth and development should be regularly monitored by X-ray and measurement
- caution if used in those with diabetes as glucose tolerance may be affected. Blood glucose levels should be closely monitored, especially at the start of therapy, as they may be elevated
- caution if used in those who have been previously exposed to topical retinoids as this increases the risk of allergic reactions (purpura, allergic vasculitis)
- caution if used in those who have not reached puberty as retinoids may cause premature closure of epiphyseal plates
- caution if used in those with pre-existing or history of depression, psychosis or intestinal disorders
- contraindicated in those with hypersensitivity to any retinoid products, severe liver or kidney impairment, chronically elevated blood lipids or pre-existing hypervitaminosis A

General Patient teaching and advice for retinoids

Topical therapy

- warn patient that condition may initially appear worse
- advise patient to avoid excess sunlight or sunlamps and wear protective clothing and sunscreen with high protective factor (SPF 30+) when going outdoors
- patient should be advised to avoid extremes of weather/temperature (e.g. wind, extreme cold) during therapy
- if patient becomes sunburnt, therapy should be discontinued until the skin has completely recovered

- patient should be warned to wash hands before and after applying gel/cream
- instruct patient to use moisturising cream/lotion on skin and use lip balm, lubricating eye ointment or tear replacement therapy to overcome some drying of skin, lips and eyes caused by the retinoid therapy
- advise patient to first wash skin with mild soap and dry before applying gel or cream as per directions, but avoid excessive application
- moisturisers and emollients may be used with retinoid cream, but should be allowed to dry before applying second cream
- avoid application of gel or cream to mucous membranes, eyes, mouth, corners of nose or broken skin. If contact occurs, area should be thoroughly rinsed with water
- to avoid risk of dermatitis, scarring or epidermal stripping, wax epilation should be avoided during and for 5–6 months after stopping therapy
- dermabrasion and laser therapy should be avoided during and for 5–6 months after stopping therapy, because there is an increased risk of hypertrophic scarring and/or skin pigmentation changes
- warn patient not to apply gel/cream more frequently or in greater quantity than prescribed as this may cause redness, stinging and discomfort and does not increase effect
- if other topical acne products (e.g. benzoyl peroxide) are also used, they should be applied at different times (e.g. retinoid gel/cream in the evening, other therapy in the morning)
- if severe redness, peeling or discomfort occurs, patient should be advised to decrease frequency of application or use cream/gel of lower strength (if available)

Oral therapy

- warn patient that condition may initially appear worse
- patient should be instructed to swallow capsule whole. If capsule is opened, absorption will be altered
- instruct patient to immediately report any:
  - abdominal pain, rectal bleeding or severe diarrhoea (especially containing blood)
  - visual disturbances, such as blurred vision, decreased night vision or eye irritation
  - hearing loss or ringing in ears
  - skin reactions
  - headache, nausea, vomiting or visual disturbances (if they occur, patient should be screened for papilloedema)
  - sadness, crying, sleeping too much or not being able to fall asleep, change in appetite, trouble with concentration, withdrawal from family, friends and/or previously pleasurable activities, lack of energy and/or thoughts of self-harm
- patient should be advised to avoid driving or operating machinery if vision (especially night vision) is affected
- instruct patient not to take vitamin A supplements (or other vitamin supplements containing vitamin A) during therapy
- patients wearing contact lenses should be warned of decreased tolerance during initial therapy
- patient should be instructed not to donate blood during and for 1 month

(isotretinoin) or 3 years (acitretin) after stopping therapy
- patients with diabetes mellitus may find their glucose tolerance is affected and therefore regular monitoring of blood glucose is suggested
- patient should be advised to avoid alcohol (as a drink or in food or medicine) during and for 2 months after stopping therapy, because alcohol slows the elimination of retinoids
- male patients should be reminded to not share medications, especially with women of childbearing potential or if pregnant
- all women (including those who are not sexually active or have amenorrhoea) should be counselled regarding the importance of using effective contraception
- women of childbearing potential should be given both oral and written information regarding the teratogenic and embryotoxic potential of retinoids. The woman needs to agree to use effective contraception (preferably two different complementary methods, such as oral contraceptive plus condom/diaphragm), starting 1 month before commencement, during and for 3 years following therapy. A negative serum or urine pregnancy test should be completed within 1 week of starting therapy. Monthly pregnancy testing is recommended throughout therapy and for 1–3 months after stopping. Therapy should be started on day 2 or 3 of the menstrual period. Women should also be advised that taking acitretin with alcohol produces etretinate, which is teratogenic, and therefore alcohol should be avoided during therapy and for 2 weeks after stopping. If pregnancy occurs, patient should be counselled regarding continuation or termination given the possible teratogenic effects on the fetus
- pregnant patient should be warned to avoid opening capsules and making contact with powder
- see also General Patient teaching and advice (p. xxvii)

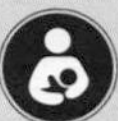

contraindicated during pregnancy and breastfeeding

ACITRETIN (Neotigason, Zetin)

Available forms

Capsules: 10 mg, 25 mg

Action

- see General Actions of retinoids (p. 2)
- metabolite is teratogenic
- half-life 50 hours

Use

- psoriasis
- severe keratinisation disorders

Dose

- (psoriasis) initially 25–30 mg orally once daily with food for 2–4 weeks, followed by 25–50 mg daily for 6–8 weeks **OR**
- (keratinisation disorders) 20 mg orally daily, adjusting dose according to clinical response (daily maximum 50 mg)

Adverse effects

- peripheral oedema
- see also General Adverse effects of oral retinoids (p. 2)

Interactions

- contraindicated with methotrexate due to increased risk of hepatitis

- not recommended with minocycline or doxycycline due to risk of additive toxicity
- see also General Interactions of oral retinoids (p. 3)

Nursing points/Cautions

- see General Nursing points/Cautions for retinoids (p. 3)
- (psoriasis) therapy should be stopped when lesions have resolved and any relapses treated as previously

Patient teaching and advice

- patients should be advised to take capsules with milk or food
- (psoriasis) patient should be warned that psoriasis may appear worse during early treatment
- see General Patient teaching and advice for retinoids (oral therapy) (p. 3)

ISOTRETINOIN (Dermatane, Oratane, Roaccutane, Rocta)

Available forms

Capsules: 5 mg, 10 mg, 20 mg, 40 mg

Action

- see General Actions of retinoids (p. 2)
- half-life 10–20 hours (half-life of major metabolite 11–50 hours)

Use

- severe cystic acne (unresponsive to conventional therapy including systemic antibiotics)

Dose

- (severe cystic acne) initially up to 0.5 mg/kg orally daily as a single or 2 divided doses with food for 2–4 weeks, then dose adjusted according to clinical response (for total of 16 weeks)

Adverse effects

- see General Adverse effects of oral retinoids (p. 2)
- (rare) inflammatory bowel disease

Interactions

- see General Interactions of oral retinoids (p. 3)

Nursing points/Cautions

- see General Nursing points/Cautions for retinoids (p. 3)
- (cystic acne) second course of treatment should not be within 8 weeks of first course

Patient teaching and advice

- capsules contain soy, so caution should be used in those with soy or peanut allergy
- see General Patient teaching and advice for retinoids (p. 3)

TAZAROTENE (Zorac Cream)

Available forms

Cream: 0.5 mg/g, 1.0 mg/g

Action

- retinoid prodrug which is converted to active tazarotenic acid
- see General Actions of retinoids (p. 2)

Use

- plaque psoriasis
- mild-to-moderate acne

Dose

- (plaque psoriasis) apply thin film over lesions nightly, starting with 0.5 mg/g strength cream and, if tolerated, increasing to 1.0 mg/g strength OR
- (acne) apply thin film over acne lesions nightly (1 mg/g only)

Adverse effects

- dry skin, erythema, peeling, burning, pruritus, irritation, stinging, skin discolouration, rash, contact dermatitis
- face pain
- temporary worsening of acne or psoriasis

Interactions

- caution if used with other agents known to cause photosensitivity (e.g.

thiazides, phenothiazines, sulfonamides)
- (gel) not recommended with other topical medication, especially peeling agents such as resorcinol, benzoyl peroxide, sulfur or salicylic acid

Nursing points/Cautions

- see General Nursing points/Cautions for retinoids (p. 3)
- contraindicated on eczematous skin

Patient teaching and advice

- patient should be warned that skin may sting or have a burning sensation at the start of treatment
- see General Patient teaching and advice for retinoids (topical therapy) (p. 3)

TRETINOIN (ReTrieve Cream, Stieva-A, Vesanoid)

Available forms

Cream: 0.25 mg/g, 0.5 mg/g, 1 mg/g; Capsules: 10 mg

Action

- see General Actions of retinoids (p. 2)

Use

- acne vulgaris where comedones, papules and/or pustules predominate
- dry skin due to photoageing
- acute promyelocytic leukaemia (Vesanoid only)

Dose

- (acne vulgaris) applied to acne lesion(s) nightly for at least 6–8 weeks; frequency may be decreased when acne responds satisfactorily to treatment (Stieva-A) **OR**
- (dry skin due to photoageing) wash and dry skin, then:
  - night 1: apply cream to skin and leave for 5 minutes, then wash off
  - night 2: apply to skin and leave for 10 minutes, then wash off
  - nights 3–6: increasing time by 30 minutes per night until left on for 120 minutes. If no redness or irritation occurs next day, cream can be left on overnight and washed off in the morning. If skin reaction occurs, apply every second night until skin tolerance increases (ReTrieve Cream)

Adverse effects

- transient stinging, feeling of warmth, peeling, erythema, temporary changes to skin pigmentation
- photosensitivity
- reversible elevation of liver enzymes and bilirubin
- (rare) allergy, contact dermatitis

Interactions

- not recommended with other topical medication, especially peeling agents such as resorcinol, benzoyl peroxide, sulfur or salicylic acid
- caution if used with other agents known to cause photosensitivity (e.g. thiazides, phenothiazines, sulfonamides) or those containing high concentrations of alcohol, menthol, lime or spices

Nursing points/Cautions

- not recommended as monotherapy for deep cystic nodular acne or severe pustular acne
- caution if applied to neck or other sensitive areas
- not recommended for eczematous skin
- not recommended in those with personal or family history of skin cancer
- see General Nursing points/Cautions for retinoids (p. 3)

Patient teaching and advice

- advise patient that it may take more than 6 weeks for effects to be seen and treatment should be continued for at least 12 weeks

- see General Patient teaching and advice for retinoids (topical therapy) (p. 3)

Note

- Vesanoid is used as an antineoplastic agent (p. 707), not as a general dermatological agent
- contained in Acnatac with clindamycin

TOPICAL AGENTS USED IN ACNE MANAGEMENT

ADAPALENE (Differin Topical Cream, Differin Topical Gel)

Available forms

Cream: 0.1%; Gel: 0.1%

Action

- retinoid-like properties
- modulates cellular differentiation, keratinisation and inflammatory processes
- normalises differentiation of follicular epithelial cells resulting in decreased microcomedone formation

Use

- acne vulgaris (with comedones, papules and pustules) of face, chest and back

Dose

- apply thin film to affected areas at night

Adverse effects

- redness, dry skin, burning sensation, scaling, skin irritation, pruritus, sunburn
- (uncommon) contact dermatitis, flu-like syndrome, headache

Interactions

- not recommended with abrasive cleansers, astringents, strong drying agents or irritants or other topical retinoids as there may be increased skin irritation

Nursing points/Cautions

- not recommended for those with eczema or seborrheic dermatitis

Patient teaching and advice

- advise patient to wash and dry affected area(s) thoroughly before applying cream/gel
- patient should be warned to avoid contact with eyes, lips and mucous membranes and if contact occurs, area should be washed immediately with copious amounts of water
- warn patients that preparation should not be applied to broken skin, reddened areas or sunburnt sites, or on skin with eczema or seborrhoeic dermatitis or if acne covers a large body area
- instruct patient to stop therapy if severe skin reaction occurs
- patient should be warned to use only oil-free moisturisers to manage dry facial skin
- advise patient to avoid excess sunlight or sunlamps and wear protective clothing and sunscreen with high protective factor (SPF 30+) when going outdoors

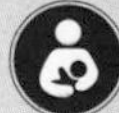

not recommended during pregnancy or in women who plan to become pregnant

caution if used during breastfeeding and should not be used in chest area

Note

- contained in Epiduo and Epiduo Forte with benzoyl peroxide (both are contraindicated during pregnancy or in women planning to become pregnant)

AZELAIC ACID (Azclear Medicated Lotion, Finacea)

Available forms
Gel: 15%; Lotion: 20%

Action
- antibacterial action that acts on *P. acnes*, reducing number of bacteria, as well as reducing free fatty acids in the skin surface lipids
- penetrates damaged skin more rapidly than intact skin
- unknown action in rosacea, although thought to be anti-inflammatory

Use
- mild-to-moderate acne vulgaris
- papulopustular rosacea

Dose
- apply sparingly to affected area twice daily (morning and night) and massage into skin until it vanishes

Adverse effects
- skin burning, pruritus, stinging, tingling, erythema, irritation, dry skin, scaling, rash
- skin discolouration/depigmentation (especially in darker skin)
- (uncommon) contact dermatitis, folliculitis, skin disorder, acne
- (rare) allergic reaction

Nursing points/Cautions
- duration of therapy depends on the severity of disorder, but improvement is commonly seen in 4–8 weeks
- contraindicated in those with hypersensitivity to propylene glycol

Patient teaching and advice
- instruct patient to wash skin thoroughly with water before applying gel or cream
- warn patients that adverse effects usually occur at the start of therapy. If adverse effects are severe, therapy should be stopped and the number of applications per day reduced
- advise patient to avoid contact with eyes and if this occurs eyes should be immediately rinsed with copious amounts of water
- patient should be warned that any skin discolouration or depigmentation is temporary
- see General Patient teaching and advice (p. xxvii)

BENZOYL PEROXIDE (Benzac, Benzac AC Wash, Clean & Clear Continuous Control Acne Cleanser, Oxy Cream, Oxy Vanishing Cream)

Available forms
Gel: 2.5%, 5%, 10%; Cream: 40 mg/g, 50 mg/g, 100 mg/g

Action
- action not totally understood
- antibacterial action against *P. acnes*
- reduces lipids and fatty acids with mild drying and peeling action

Use
- acne vulgaris

Dose
- (days 1–3) wash and dry affected areas, apply gel once daily and leave on skin for 2 hours, then wash gel off
- (days 4–6) if no discomfort occurs, apply gel and leave overnight
- if no discomfort occurs and acne is resisting treatment, apply twice daily, once in the morning (and leave on all day), then wash the affected area and reapply at night (and leave overnight) OR
- (Benzac AC Wash, Clean & Clear Continuous Control Acne Cleanser) apply twice daily to affected area using the following instructions. Wet area to be treated and preparation applied to hands; wash affected area with solution, allowing skin contact for 30 seconds, followed by thoroughly rinsing area with water and drying

Adverse effects
- skin dryness, erythema, peeling, pruritus
- allergic contact dermatitis

Interactions
- not recommended with tretinoin, isotretinoin and tazarotene, as these may cause increased irritation and decrease retinoid efficacy
- caution if used with topical sulfonamide as skin or facial hair may turn orange/yellow temporarily

Patient teaching and advice
- patient should be warned to wash hands before and after applying gel/cream
- advise patient that mild burning sensation occurs on application of gel/cream and moderate skin reddening and peeling will occur within a few days. Increased peeling and reddening will occur in the first week and then subside within 1–2 days
- warn fair-haired patients that they may be more prone to skin irritation
- if severe irritation occurs, advise patient to stop therapy until it clears and then restart at a decreased frequency
- warn patient to avoid contact with coloured material (e.g. material, hair) as bleaching or discolouration may occur
- cool compresses should be recommended to help reduce irritation
- if used with retinoid gel/cream, advise patient to apply at different times (e.g. benzoyl peroxide in the morning, retinoid in the evening)
- advise patient to avoid contact with eyes, mouth, sensitive neck areas, mucous membranes and angles of nose; if contact occurs, area should be washed thoroughly with water
- warn patient that preparation should only be applied to intact skin
- advise patient to avoid excess sunlight or sunlamps and wear protective clothing and sunscreen with high protective factor (SPF 30+) when going outdoors
- if patient becomes sunburnt, therapy should be discontinued until the skin has completely recovered
- warm patient that use with other topical acne preparations is not recommended due to added skin irritation
- see General Patient teaching and advice (p. xxvii)

Note
- contained in Clearasil Ultra Acne Treatment Cream, Duac Once Daily Gel, Epiduo Gel and Epiduo Forte Gel

ANALGESICS AND NON-STEROIDAL ANTI-INFLAMMATORY DRUGS (NSAIDs)

The NSAIDs are a diverse group of compounds, often chemically unrelated, that share some therapeutic actions and side-effects because of their non-selective inhibition of cyclo-oxygenase (COX). Not all drugs in this class possess the anti-inflammatory, antipyretic and analgesic characteristics to the same degree. For example, paracetamol has antipyretic and analgesic properties, but is not useful as an anti-inflammatory. When used as analgesics, these drugs are usually effective against low-to-moderate intensity pain only. As anti-inflammatory agents, they are used in treating musculoskeletal disorders, providing symptomatic relief from pain and inflammation, but leaving the progression of the disease course unchanged. As antipyretics, they are thought to inhibit hypothalamic prostaglandins that act on the thermoregulatory centre in the hypothalamus. The COX-2 inhibitors are a newer class of agents with similar properties to those of other NSAIDs without having the same side-effects (especially gastrointestinal (GI)) because of their selective inhibition (Grosser et al 2018).

Most NSAIDs are taken orally, while some are applied topically to relieve muscular and/or rheumatic pain. Some are used in ophthalmic preparations to reduce ocular inflammation. A systematic review of the literature found that topical NSAIDs provide a good level of pain relief in acute conditions such as sprains, strains and overuse injuries, with gel preparations providing the best effects with minimal adverse effects (Derry et al 2019).

Simple analgesics are those that contain only one compound (e.g. 500 mg paracetamol), while compound analgesics combine two or more preparations. While this might be an advantage to the patient because only one tablet is taken, it can have its disadvantages as it is difficult for the clinician to titrate the dose or interval, may be more expensive and/or produce more adverse effects than the individual compounds (Bryant et al 2019).

In 2018, the Department of Therapeutic Goods Administration (TGA) amended previously Schedule 2 (Pharmacy Only) and Schedule 3 (Pharmacist Only) preparations containing codeine (e.g. Panadeine = paracetamol plus codeine) to become prescription-only (Schedule 4) (Therapeutic Goods Administration [TGA] 2018). This has resulted in a number of these codeine-containing products no longer being produced by some manufacturers.

General Actions of NSAIDs (not paracetamol)

During the inflammatory response, arachidonic acid is converted by the enzyme cyclo-oxygenase (COX) to prostaglandins and thromboxane A2, and by the enzyme lipoxygenase to leukotrienes, which produce the pain, swelling, redness and heat associated with inflammation (Brenner & Stevens 2013). Cyclo-oxygenase is present in two forms that have distinct properties. Cyclo-oxygenase 1 (COX-1) is found in the stomach, intestines, kidneys and platelets, and appears to be responsible for functions involving prostaglandins, such as renal function, platelet aggregation and cytoprotection of the stomach. NSAIDs inhibit COX-1 non-selectively, resulting in the common side-effects of gastric ulceration and, to a lesser extent, renal toxicity and increased risk of bleeding. Cyclo-oxygenase 2 (COX-2) is found in fewer tissues (including the brain, renal glomeruli and vasculature) at low levels; however, during inflammation, pro-inflammatory substances lead to an increase in COX-2 levels. Selectively inhibiting COX-2 decreases the signs and symptoms of inflammation and pain, with less likelihood of causing gastric or renal problems (Grosser et al 2018).

General Adverse effects of NSAIDs (not paracetamol)

- epigastric pain, anorexia, nausea, vomiting, diarrhoea, abdominal pain/cramps, heartburn, dyspepsia, flatulence, constipation, gastritis
- rash, pruritus, erythema, urticaria, dermatitis, sweating, photosensitivity
- tinnitus, temporary deafness
- headache, dizziness, vertigo, fatigue, drowsiness, insomnia
- prolonged bleeding time, increased risk of bruising and bleeding
- fluid retention, peripheral oedema
- hypertension (new, or worsening of existing), palpitations, premature closure of ductus arteriosis
- increased risk of cardiovascular thrombotic events (COX-2 inhibitors)
- elevated liver enzymes (ALT, AST), decreased serum urea, hyperkalaemia
- blood dyscrasias, iron-deficiency anaemia
- may mask signs and symptoms of infection
- (females) may impair fertility by delaying or preventing rupture of ovarian follicles
- inhibition of labour, prolongation of gestation
- increased risk of myocardial infarction and stroke
- (prolonged therapy, high dose) visual disturbances (including blurred vision), acute interstitial nephritis with haematuria, proteinuria, nephrotic syndrome
- (rare) anaphylactoid reactions, angioedema, serious skin reactions, hypersensitivity reactions (especially in those with asthma or family history), aseptic meningitis
- (rare) GI bleeding and/or ulceration
- (rare) renal papillary necrosis, jaundice, hepatitis, liver toxicity

General Interactions of NSAIDs (not paracetamol)

- may increase blood lithium or digoxin levels (except ketoprofen), thereby increasing the risk of toxicity; lithium or digoxin levels should be closely monitored, especially when starting or stopping therapy with NSAIDs

- use with aspirin or other NSAIDs is not recommended because of increased risk of GI side-effects
- use caution and close monitoring if warfarin is given with NSAIDs because of increased risk of haemorrhage
- increased risk of nephrotoxicity if tenofovir, ciclosporin or tacrolimus are given with NSAIDs
- methotrexate toxicity may occur if NSAIDs are given within 24 hours of methotrexate therapy
- use of quinolone antibiotics and NSAIDs may lead to convulsions (not celecoxib)
- risk of gastric ulceration is increased if aspirin or NSAIDs are taken with alcohol and/or corticosteroids
- not recommended with alendronate or nicorandil due to increased risk of gastric ulceration
- increased risk of bleeding if given with SSRIs, zidovudine, fibrinolytic or antiplatelet agents
- use of antacids may reduce absorption of aspirin or NSAIDs (except ketoprofen, ketorolac trometamol, sulindac and piroxicam)
- may decrease excretion of aminoglycoside antibiotics, increasing risk of toxicity
- avoid use with other nephrotoxic agents
- plasma levels may be increased if given with probenecid
- may increase serum potassium levels if given with potassium-sparing diuretics, increasing risk of nephrotoxicity. Renal function, potassium serum levels and blood pressure should be closely monitored if used together
- may decrease diuretic, natriuretic and antihypertensive effects of loop, potassium-sparing and thiazide diuretics by inhibiting the synthesis of renal prostaglandin
- may potentiate effects of sulfonylureas, therefore blood glucose levels should be closely monitored during therapy to prevent hypoglycaemia
- may reduce antihypertensive effects of beta-adrenergic blocking agents, ACE inhibitors and angiotensin II antagonists
- risk of renal impairment is increased if NSAIDs, thiazide diuretics and ACE inhibitors/angiotensin II antagonists are given together, especially in the elderly or those with pre-existing renal impairment
- may decrease efficacy of intrauterine device (IUD)
- not recommended within 8–10 days of mifepristone
- increased elimination if given with colestyramine
- increased risk of bleeding if given with *Ginkgo biloba*

General Nursing points/Cautions for NSAIDs (not paracetamol)

- before starting therapy, the patient should be assessed for:
  - any allergic reactions after prior aspirin or other NSAID therapy, as cross-sensitivity occurs
  - any history of asthma (may induce asthma attack in susceptible individuals) or gastric ulceration/bleeding (due to increased risk of both) should be assessed before starting therapy
  - cardiovascular risk factors (such as hypertension, hyperlipidaemia, smoking, diabetes)

- if administered preoperatively, patient should be carefully monitored for any signs of bleeding intra- or postoperatively
- signs of infection such as fever can be masked by NSAID therapy
- regular ophthalmological examination, haematological and liver enzyme monitoring should all be performed during prolonged therapy
- in patients with concurrent hypertension managed with antihypertensive agents (beta-adrenergic blocking agents, ACE inhibitors and angiotensin II antagonists) regular measurement of BP is recommended before starting therapy and then at regular intervals
- caution if used in those with pre-existing oedema because of increased potential for fluid retention, peripheral oedema and increased blood pressure
- caution if given to those with pre-existing renal disease, uraemia or bleeding disorders
- caution if used in those with inflammatory bowel disease (IBD) as NSAIDs have been associated with exacerbation of IBD-associated spondyloarthropathies
- not recommended in those with uncontrolled hypertension, congestive cardiac failure, ischaemic heart disease or peripheral arterial disease
- contraindicated in those with a history of peptic or GI ulceration or bleeding
- contraindicated in those with bleeding disorders (e.g. haemophilia, von Willebrand disease)
- contraindicated in those with severe liver or kidney insufficiency or severe cardiac failure
- contraindicated in those with salicylate hypersensitivity (as cross-sensitivity between aspirin and other NSAIDs exists)
- contraindicated in those with 'aspirin triad' (person with asthma who experiences rhinitis with/without nasal polyps, or experiences severe bronchospasm after taking aspirin or NSAIDs)
- contraindicated post coronary artery bypass graft (CABG) surgery

General Patient teaching and advice for NSAIDs (not paracetamol)

- instruct patient to take NSAIDs with food or milk (e.g. after meals) to reduce gastric irritation
- warn patient to avoid alcohol during therapy with NSAIDs to reduce risk of GI adverse effects
- patient should be warned to immediately report to their doctor any:
  - changes in hearing or visual disturbances
  - nausea, tiredness, lack of appetite, lethargy, itching, yellowing of skin, eyes, pale bowel motions and dark urine, flu-like symptoms or abdominal tenderness (in upper outer right quadrant) (as these are signs of impending liver toxicity)
  - breathlessness, difficulty breathing when lying down, any swelling in feet or legs (signs of cardiac failure)
  - sudden and oppressive chest pain (may be sign of heart attack)
  - severe stomach or throat pain, vomiting blood or black vomit, bleeding from rectum, sticky bowel motions
  - skin rash, hives, blistering or peeling skin, mouth ulcers or swelling

  of face, lips, mouth, tongue or throat, or wheezing/difficulty breathing occurs
  - changes to the amount or colour of urine passed, any blood in urine
- caution patients not to drive or operate machinery if dizziness, drowsiness or visual disturbances occur
- warn patients with diabetes using oral hypoglycaemic agents to monitor blood glucose levels carefully during therapy to prevent hypoglycaemia
- advise female patient if she is having a problem becoming pregnant, NSAID therapy should be stopped
- counsel female patients not to take NSAIDs during pregnancy, especially during third trimester. If the patient becomes pregnant, she should be advised to tell her doctor immediately

Topical gel/solution

- advise patient to avoid excess sunlight or sunlamps and wear protective clothing and sunscreen with high protective factor (SPF 30+) when going outdoors as some topical gels can increase skin sensitivity and therefore risk of burning
- instruct patient to wash hands before and after applying gel and avoid contact with eyes or mouth
- warn patient to avoid contact with eyes, mouth, mucous membrane, angles of the nose or skin which is broken, abraded or infected, or has eczema. If contact occurs, area should be washed with copious amounts of water
- advise patient to not use gel under occlusive dressing or on a large area

Eye drops

- should not be instilled if soft or gas-permeable contact lenses are in situ as many eye drops contain benzalkonium chloride as a preservative, which may cause discolouration of soft contact lenses. Lenses should be removed before instillation and reinserted after at least a 15-minute interval
- advise patient not to use drops if they are cloudy or change colour
- instruct patient in correct technique for instilling eye drops, including:
  - not allowing tip of dispensing container to touch the eye as it may cause injury and/or contaminate the eye drops
  - if the container is new, remove protective seal, otherwise check expiry date
  - wash hands thoroughly with soap and water
  - remove lid/cap and hold container upside down in one hand between thumb and forefinger or index finger
  - using other hand, gently pull down on lower eyelid to form a pouch/pocket and tilt head back, looking up
  - place tip of container close to lower eyelid (taking care not to make contact between tip and eye). Squeezing bottle gently, release one drop into pouch/pocket formed between eye and eyelid
  - gently close eye, but do not blink or rub eye
  - while eye is closed, place index finger against inside corner of eye and press against nose for about 2 minutes (this stops medicine from draining through tear duct into nose and throat)
  - replace lid/cap tightly
  - wash hands again to remove any residue

- warn patient that vision may be blurred for a few minutes after eye drops have been instilled and it is therefore advisable not to drive or use machinery during this time
- patient should be advised to write expiry date on eye drops when opened and not use beyond this date (usually 28 days)

Suppositories

- instruct adult patient in correct technique for suppository insertion, including:
  - the need to empty bowel if possible before suppository insertion
  - wash hands with soap and water
  - if suppository feels soft, place it (unwrapped) in the fridge or hold it under cold water to firm it up
  - put on disposable glove if wanted
  - remove wrapper from suppository and moisten slightly by dipping in cool water
  - lie on side with knees raised to chest
  - push suppository (blunt end first) gently into rectum, taking care not to break suppository
  - remain lying down for a few minutes to allow suppository to dissolve
  - wash hands thoroughly after insertion
- advise patient not to use bowels for at least 1 hour (if possible) after suppository insertion
- see General Patient teaching and advice (p. xxvii)

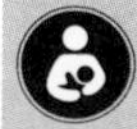

use of these agents during the latter stages of pregnancy may cause closure of the fetal ductus arteriosus, fetal renal impairment, inhibition of platelet aggregation and may delay labour and birth. Therefore, continuous treatment with these agents during the third trimester of pregnancy is generally contraindicated

not recommended during labour or delivery

not recommended during breastfeeding as some NSAIDs and/or their metabolites are excreted in breastmilk and their actions on the newborn may be unknown

ASPIRIN (Aspro Clear, Aspro Clear Extra Strength, Astrix 100, Astrix Tablets, Cardasa, Cardiprin 100, Cartia, Disprin preparations, Solprin, Spren)

Available forms

Capsules: 100 mg; Tablets: 100 mg, 300 mg, 320 mg, 500 mg; Tablets (enteric-coated): 100 mg; Tablets (effervescent): 300 mg, 500 mg

Action

- see General Actions of NSAIDs (p. 12)
- aspirin is converted to salicylic acid mainly in the GI tract
- absorption is dependent on formulation (e.g. soluble formulation increases rate of absorption)
- irreversibly inhibits COX platelet activity (needed for thromboxane synthesis) resulting in prolonged action. It may take 8–12 days (platelet turnover time) after therapy is stopped to fully recover
- half-life of aspirin is about 20–60 minutes, half-life of salicylate acid is about 6 hours

Use

- relief of mild-to-moderate non-visceral pain
- headache, migraine

- acute febrile illnesses (not for children or teenagers)
- dysmenorrhoea
- rheumatic pain, including juvenile rheumatoid arthritis
- inflammation associated with back or muscular pain/strain
- cold and flu symptoms
- toothache
- antiplatelet therapy (only on medical advice) for prophylaxis against myocardial infarction, unstable angina, transient ischaemic attacks (TIAs) and stroke

Dose

- (analgesic, antipyretic) 300–1000 mg orally with food 4–6-hourly as required (up to 4 g/day) **OR**
- (effervescent tablets) 300–1000 mg orally dissolved in 1/2 glass of water 4-hourly as required (up to 4 g/day) **OR**
- (antiplatelet) 100 mg daily

Adverse effects

- increase in respiratory rate
- (very high salicylate level) depresses respiration
- (prolonged therapy, high dose) hypoprothrombinaemia
- see General Adverse effects of NSAIDs (p. 12)

Interactions

- may increase blood levels of sodium valproate and methotrexate, increasing risk of toxicity and/or adverse effects
- caution if used with anticoagulants due to increased risk of bleeding
- action of probenecid may be reduced if given with aspirin
- hypoglycaemic action of sulfonylureas may be increased if given with high-dose aspirin; therefore blood glucose levels should be closely monitored
- excretion is increased if given with urinary alkalinisers
- rate and extent of absorption is increased by caffeine
- hydrocortisone may increase metabolism and/or clearance of aspirin. Further, when hydrocortisone is ceased, blood levels of aspirin may rise significantly, increasing risk of adverse effects and/or toxicity
- increased risk of gastrointestinal bleeding if aspirin is given with high dose corticosteroids
- may interfere with a number of laboratory tests, including measurement of heparin activity and urinary glucose oxidase test in the presence of glycosuria

Nursing points/Cautions

- see General Nursing points/Cautions for NSAIDs (p. 13)
- soluble, effervescent, buffered and enteric-coated salicylate preparations reduce gastric irritation
- enteric-coated and sustained-action preparations have delayed absorption, which is useful for regular long-term therapy
- elderly patients are at greater risk of adverse effects, including tinnitus, nausea, anorexia and gastric irritation
- tinnitus (with normal hearing) is a reliable index of therapeutic plasma level, but may not be detected in patients with hearing loss
- therapy should be stopped 1 week before scheduled surgery
- symptoms of salicylism (chronic salicylate intoxication) are hyperventilation, tremor, papilloedema, agitation, paranoia, bizarre behaviour, memory deficits, confusion and stupor, and, rarely, pulmonary oedema, seizures and renal failure
- symptoms of acute salicylate poisoning include nausea, vomiting, tinnitus, hearing loss, sweating and hyperventilation, followed by mixed acid–base disturbance of respiratory alkalosis

and metabolic acidosis. Uncommonly, fever, neurological dysfunction, renal failure, acute lung injury (non-cardiogenic pulmonary oedema), cardiac dysrhythmias and hypoglycaemia may occur. Rarely, other complications include rhabdomyolysis, gastric perforation and GI haemorrhage
- there is no specific antidote for salicylate toxicity. Treatment of acute salicylate poisoning involves stabilisation of airway, breathing and circulation, correction of volume depletion and metabolic disturbance, GI decontamination and reduction in levels of salicylate. This involves:
  - gastric lavage, followed by single dose of activated charcoal/sorbitol (whole bowel irrigation may be necessary if overdose involves large amounts of enteric-coated or modified-release tablets)
  - assessment of patient's volume and electrolytes. Volume replacement is usually with normal saline with potassium supplementation, as hypokalaemia is common
  - urine alkalisation with IV sodium bicarbonate is more effective than forced diuresis or forced alkaline diuresis
  - urine output should be 1–2 mL/kg/hour
  - serum salicylate and electrolytes should be monitored 1–2-hourly
  - if condition worsens, haemodialysis, peritoneal dialysis or exchange transfusion may be necessary
- not recommended in infants, children and adolescents, including for the treatment of fever and/or muscle pain associated with febrile, viral illness because of the association with Reye's syndrome (see Glossary)

Patient teaching and advice

- see General Patient teaching and advice for NSAIDs (p. 14)
- stopping aspirin for any reason (e.g. donation of blood) should be discussed with doctor before discontinuing therapy
- effervescent and soluble preparations should be dissolved in ½–1 glass of water for more rapid absorption
- warn patients that sustained-release and enteric-coated preparations should be swallowed whole and not crushed or broken
- advise patient to avoid aspirin within 30 minutes of alcohol
- instruct patient to discuss the need to stop before any surgical procedure with the surgeon
- blood donors should be advised not to take aspirin in the week preceding the donation
- if patient is on a low-sodium diet, he/she should be cautioned that effervescent preparations contain sodium

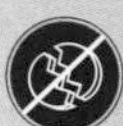

enteric-coated tablets/capsules should not be crushed. Tablets are available in dispersible form

Note

- contained in Alka-Seltzer, Aspalgin, Clopidogrel/Aspirin 75/100 Tablets, Clopidogrel Winthrop Plus Aspirin, CoPlavix, Diasp SR, DuoCover, DuoPlidogrel, Dipyridamole/Aspirin, Piax-Plus Aspirin

BENZYDAMINE (Difflam Anti-inflammatory Gel, Difflam Sore Throat Gargle and Mouth Solution, Difflam Sore Throat Spray, Difflam Sore Throat Spray Forte)

Available forms

Throat spray: 1.5 mg/mL, 3 mg/mL; Gel: 3%, 5%; Solution: 22.5 mg/15 mL

Action

- analgesic, anti-inflammatory
- chemically unrelated to other NSAIDs

Use

- relief of inflammatory conditions of the mouth and throat (e.g. tonsillitis, radiation mucositis)
- (topically) inflammatory disorders (e.g. sprains, strains, acute phases of myalgia and bursitis)

Dose

- (inflammatory disorders) 3% or 5% gel massaged into affected area 3–6 times daily (maximum 6 times daily in severe conditions) for up to 14 days **OR**
- (throat spray) 4–8 sprays or 2–4 sprays (forte solution) on inflamed area and swallowed gently 1.5–3-hourly for up to 7 days **OR**
- 15 mL (undiluted solution) gargled or swirled in mouth for 30 seconds 1.5–3-hourly for up to 7 days

Adverse effects

- (gel) erythema, rash, photosensitivity
- (throat spray, solution) numbness, stinging, tingling, burning, thirst, dryness, altered taste sensation, warm feeling in mouth

Nursing points/Cautions

- if sore throat is due to bacterial infection, antibacterial therapy should also be considered
- (throat spray) not recommended for children under 6 years

Patient teaching and advice

- see p. 15 for topical gel application advice
- advise patient that oral solution should be used as a rinse or gargled and not swallowed
- if stinging occurs while rinsing or gargling, oral solution can be diluted with water for gargling
- (throat spray) instruct patient to prime spray before first use or after a period of non-use. Spray nozzle should be cleaned after each use to prevent clogging

Note

- contained in Difflam C Sore Throat Gargle and Mouthwash Solution, Difflam Sore Throat Lozenges, Difflam C Anti-Inflammatory Antiseptic Solution, Difflam Mouth Gel, Difflam Plus Sore Throat and Cough Lozenges, Difflam Sugar Free Lozenges

CELECOXIB (Celaxib, Celebrex, Celexi)

Available forms

Capsules: 100 mg, 200 mg

Action

- COX-2 inhibitor preventing prostaglandin synthesis with actions similar to other NSAIDs with analgesic, antipyretic and anti-inflammatory activity
- half-life 4–15 hours

Use

- osteoarthritis, rheumatoid arthritis, ankylosing spondylitis
- primary dysmenorrhoea
- (short-term) pain management post-surgery or musculoskeletal/soft tissue injury

Dose

- (osteoarthritis, ankylosing spondylitis) 200 mg orally daily as single dose or 2 divided doses **OR**
- (rheumatoid arthritis) 200 mg orally daily in 2 divided doses, increasing to 400 mg daily for short-term management of disease flares/exacerbations **OR**
- (primary dysmenorrhoea) 400 mg orally daily as single dose or 2 divided doses (first day), then 200 mg daily on following days for up to 5 days maximum **OR**
- (acute postsurgical pain, musculoskeletal and/or soft tissue injury) initially 400 mg orally daily, then 200 mg 1–2 times daily on following days for up to 5 days maximum

Adverse effects
- see General Adverse effects of NSAIDs (p. 12); however, GI adverse effects occur less frequently
- pharyngitis, rhinitis, sinusitis
- back pain
- (rare) increased risk of cardiac and thrombotic events, serious skin reactions

Interactions
- increased plasma levels may occur if given with fluconazole
- increased risk of renal impairment if given with ACE inhibitor/angiotensin receptor antagonist and thiazide diuretic at same time (especially in the elderly)
- may decrease antihypertensive effects of ACE inhibitor, angiotensin receptor antagonist, thiazide diuretics and beta-adrenoceptor blocking agents
- may decrease natriuretic effect of furosemide (frusemide) and thiazide diuretics because of renal prostaglandin synthesis inhibition
- increased risk of GI adverse effects if given with oral glucocorticoids, especially in the elderly
- increased risk of GI adverse effects if given with aspirin
- increased risk of nephrotoxicity if given with ciclosporin
- may increase plasma levels of digoxin, lithium and warfarin, thereby increasing risk of toxicity; digoxin, lithium and warfarin levels should be closely monitored, especially when starting, stopping or altering doses of celecoxib
- may increase plasma levels of metoprolol and dextromethorphan
- decreased plasma levels may occur if given with aluminium or magnesium-containing antacids, rifampicin, carbamazepine and barbiturates
- contraindicated with other NSAIDs

Nursing points/Cautions

- any dehydration should be corrected before starting therapy
- blood pressure should be regularly monitored during therapy
- any skin reactions usually occur within 4 weeks of starting therapy
- to lessen the risk of cardiovascular events, the lowest effective dose should be used for the shortest possible duration
- (long-term treatment) haemoglobin or haematocrit levels should be regularly monitored for signs of anaemia
- caution if used in those with high risk of cardiovascular disease or multiple risk factors such as diabetes, hypertension, smoking, cardiac failure or hypercholesterolaemia
- contraindicated in those with sensitivity to sulfonamides
- contraindicated in the treatment of pain in those undergoing coronary artery bypass graft (CABG) surgery
- contraindicated in those with unstable or significant ischaemic heart disease, peripheral arterial disease and/or cerebrovascular disease; congestive heart failure; severe liver or kidney impairment or creatinine clearance < 30 mL/min
- see General Nursing points/Cautions for NSAIDs (p. 13)

Patient teaching and advice

- advise patient to take antacids 2 hours before or after celecoxib
- warn patient to seek medical advice immediately if the following occurs:
  - fainting, collapse, shortness of breath, tiredness, chest pain or irregular heart beat
  - skin reactions
- see General Patient teaching and advice for NSAIDs (p. 14)

capsules can be opened and dispersed in water or mixed with spoonful of yoghurt or apple puree

CHOLINE SALICYLATE (Bonjela Mouth Ulcer Gel, Bonjela Teething Gel)

Available form
Oral gel: 87 mg/g

Action
- local analgesic

Use
- painful oral irritation (e.g. teething)
- lesions of the mouth

Dose
- (adult) massage 1 cm gel into painful area 3-hourly **OR**
- (infant > 4 months) massage 0.5 cm gel into painful area 3-hourly if required (up to 6 applications/24 hours)

Adverse effects
- transient stinging on application

Nursing points/Cautions
- not recommended in those with salicylate hypersensitivity
- contraindicated in babies less than 4 months old or children under 12 in combination with aspirin-containing products (to avoid excessive salicylate levels)

Patient teaching and advice
- advise patient to wash hands before and after applying gel
- warn patient that gel should not be applied directly to dentures
- (mouth ulcers) advise patient to wipe mucus from ulcer surface before applying gel

Note
- contained in Seda-Gel

DICLOFENAC DIETHYLAMINE (DICLOFENAC DIETHYLAMMONIUM) (Voltaren Emulgel, Voltaren Osteo Gel 12-hourly)

DICLOFENAC POTASSIUM (Voltaren Rapid)

DICLOFENAC SODIUM (Clonac, Dencorub Anti-Inflammatory Gel, Fenac, Solaraze 3% Gel, Viclofen, Voltaren, Voltaren Ophtha)

Available forms
Gel: 1%, 3%; Tablets (enteric-coated): 25 mg, 50 mg; Tablets (rapid-release): 12.5 mg, 25 mg, 50 mg; Capsules (liquid, rapid-release): 12.5 mg; Suppositories: 12.5 mg, 25 mg, 50 mg, 100 mg; Eye drops: 1 mg/mL

Action
- see General Actions of NSAIDs (p. 12)
- selectively inhibits COX-2 at therapeutic doses
- more potent analgesic, antipyretic and anti-inflammatory than aspirin

Use
- rheumatoid arthritis, osteoarthritis
- acute or chronic pain with inflammatory conditions
- primary dysmenorrhoea
- acute migraine, headache
- cold and flu symptoms
- dental pain, back ache, muscle pain
- postoperative pain management in children (suppositories)
- management of actinic keratosis (where other treatment is inappropriate)
- postoperative inflammation following eye surgery

Dose
- (primary dysmenorrhoea) initially 50–100 mg orally daily, starting with

onset of symptoms, followed by 50 mg orally 3 times daily for 3 days **OR**
- (arthritis, inflammatory conditions) initially 75–150 mg orally daily in 2–3 divided doses, reducing to 75–100 mg orally in divided doses for long-term therapy (enteric-coated tablets, rapid-release tablets) **OR**
- (arthritis, inflammatory conditions, dental pain, backache) initially 25 mg orally, followed by 12.5–25 mg orally 4–6-hourly if needed (daily maximum 75 mg) (12.5 mg rapid-release tablets) **OR**
- (acute migraine) 50 mg orally at first sign of migraine, followed by 50 mg 2 hours later if pain is not relieved. If needed, further 50 mg can be taken at 4–6-hourly intervals (daily maximum 200 mg) **OR**
- (postoperative pain management in children aged 12 months and above) initially 1–2 mg/kg, followed by 1 mg/kg 3 times daily for up to 3 days if needed (daily maximum 3 mg/kg) (suppositories) **OR**
- (local pain, soft tissue injury, soft tissue rheumatism) apply gel to affected area and rub gently 3–4 times daily for up to 14 days **OR**
- (pain, inflammation) apply cherry-size amount of gel to affected area and rub gently twice daily for up to 21 days (12-hourly gel) **OR**
- (actinic keratosis) apply to skin twice daily for 30–90 days (daily maximum 8 g) (Solaraze 3% Gel) **OR**
- (cataract surgery) up to 5 drops to affected eye(s) 3 hours preoperatively, then 1 drop 3 times on day of surgery, then 1 drop 3–5 times daily for 2–4 weeks

Adverse effects
- see General Adverse effects of NSAIDs (p. 12)
- (suppositories) discomfort, worsening of haemorrhoids
- (gel, rare) itching, reddened or scaly skin, photosensitivity
- (gel) contact dermatitis, redness, peeling, skin dryness, numbness, itching, rash, eczema, paraesthesia, hyperaesthesia
- (eye drops) eye irritation, keratitis, increase in intraocular pressure, blurred vision, delayed corneal healing

Interactions
- (eye drops) not recommended with topical corticosteroids in patients with corneal inflammation due to increased risk of delayed healing
- increased plasma levels may occur if given with voriconazole
- decreased plasma levels may occur if given with rifampicin
- see General Interactions of NSAIDs (p. 12)

Nursing points/Cautions
- care should be taken when selecting tablets as rapid-release and slow-release forms are available
- effects may not be seen for up to 30 days after therapy has been stopped
- (gel) 0.5 g gel (size of pea) is sufficient to cover area 5 cm × 5 cm
- (gel) duration of treatment varies with condition (14 days for soft tissue injuries, 21 days for osteoarthritis)
- (gel) not recommended for treatment of bruises
- tablets contain lactose and are therefore not recommended in galactose intolerance, severe Lapp lactase deficiency or glucose–galactose malabsorption
- (100 mg suppositories) should not be used for children or teenagers
- (suppositories) not recommended in infants under 12 months
- (suppositories) contraindicated in those with proctitis
- (gel) contraindicated in those with hypersensitivity to diclofenac, propylene glycol or isopropyl alcohol
- see General Nursing points/Cautions for NSAIDs (p. 13)

Patient teaching and advice

- instruct patient that enteric-coated tablets should be swallowed whole (not divided or chewed) with fluids, preferably before food for better absorption and efficacy, but can be taken with food if stomach is upset
- advise patient that diclofenac should not be used to prevent migraine (prophylaxis), only for management, and should be taken at first sign of headache
- patients who experience night pain and/or morning stiffness should be advised to take oral treatment during the day and suppositories at bedtime for better control of symptoms (daily maximum 150 mg)
- see suppository insertion advice (p. 16)
- see eye drop instillation advice (p. 15)
- see General Patient teaching and advice for NSAIDs (p. 14)

rapid-release tablets can be crushed and mixed with water or spoonful of yoghurt or apple puree

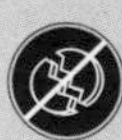

enteric-coated tablets should not be crushed

Note

- contained in Anthrotec 50 with misoprostol

ETORICOXIB (Arcoxia)

Available forms

Tablets: 30 mg, 60 mg, 120 mg

Action

- COX-2 inhibitor preventing prostaglandin synthesis with actions similar to other NSAIDs
- no effect on platelet function
- half-life 22 hours

Use

- osteoarthritis
- acute gouty arthritis
- primary dysmenorrhoea
- minor dental pain

Dose

- (osteoarthritis) initially 30 mg orally daily, increasing to 60 mg orally daily if needed (daily maximum 60 mg) **OR**
- (acute gouty arthritis, primary dysmenorrhoea, dental pain) 120 mg orally daily (maximum 8 days) **OR**
- (dental pain) 90 mg orally daily (up to 8 days maximum)

Adverse effects

- dizziness, headache
- dyspepsia, upper abdominal pain, diarrhoea, nausea, altered taste
- nasopharyngitis, upper respiratory tract infection
- dyspnoea
- urinary tract infection
- peripheral oedema, fluid retention
- hypertension
- increased risk of myocardial infarction and stroke, new or worsened congestive cardiac failure
- (rare) jaundice, renal injury, serious skin reactions, breast malignant neoplasm

Interactions

- may increase levels of ethinylestradiol, resulting in an increased risk of adverse effects, such as venous thromboembolic events in at-risk women
- may decrease antihypertensive effects of ACE inhibitor or angiotensin receptor antagonist
- increased risk of renal injury if given with ACE inhibitor or angiotensin receptor antagonist, especially in the elderly and if treated with diuretics
- caution if given with warfarin, especially when starting or stopping therapy. INR should be closely monitored
- may decrease natriuretic effect of furosemide (frusemide) and thiazide diuretics because of renal prostaglandin synthesis inhibition
- contraindicated with aspirin or other NSAIDs

- increased risk of GI adverse effects if given with aspirin
- may reduce clearance of lithium, increasing plasma levels and risk of toxicity, therefore monitoring during therapy is recommended
- decreased levels (and therefore decreased analgesic effect) may occur if given with rifampicin
- caution if given with methotrexate at doses ≥ 90 mg, therefore monitoring of methotrexate levels is recommended

Nursing points/Cautions

- any dehydration should be corrected before starting therapy
- hypertension should be controlled before starting therapy. BP should be monitored every 2 weeks throughout therapy and stopped if there is a significant increase
- to lessen the risk of cardiovascular events, the lowest effective dose should be used for the shortest possible duration
- caution if used in those with increased risk factors for cerebrovascular events (diabetes, hypertension, hypercholesterolaemia, family history of ischaemic heart disease, cardiac failure, left ventricular dysfunction and/or smokers) or pre-existing oedema
- contraindicated in those who have recently undergone CABG surgery or angioplasty
- contraindicated in those with unstable or significant ischaemic heart disease, peripheral arterial disease and/or cerebrovascular disease; hypertension which is not adequately controlled (above 140/90 mmHg); congestive heart failure; severe liver or kidney impairment or creatinine clearance < 30 mL/min; active peptic ulceration or GI bleeding; history of asthma, urticaria or other allergic reaction after taking aspirin or NSAIDs
- see General Nursing points/Cautions for NSAIDs (p. 13)

Patient teaching and advice

- advise patient against driving or operating machinery if dizziness occurs
- see General Patient teaching and advice for NSAIDs (p. 14)

tablets can be dispersed in water or crushed and mixed with spoonful of yoghurt or apple puree

FLURBIPROFEN (Strepfen Intensive Lozenges, Strepfen Throat Spray)

Available form

Lozenges: 8.75 mg; Throat spray: 8.75 mg/ 3 sprays

Action

- anti-inflammatory

Use

- pain, swelling, inflammation associated with severe sore throat

Dose

- 3 sprays to back of throat every 3–6 hours for 3 days maximum (daily maximum 15 sprays) **OR**
- 1 lozenge allowed to dissolve slowly, 3–6-hourly (maximum 8 lozenges/day)

Adverse effects

- (lozenge) warm sensation/tingling in mouth, taste alteration and rarely, nausea, vomiting, diarrhoea, dyspepsia, abdominal pain
- (rare) allergic reaction, hypersensitivity

Interactions

- not recommended with other NSAIDs

Nursing points/ Cautions

- not recommended in those with heart failure

- not recommended in children < 12 years
- (throat spray) not recommended in those < 18 years

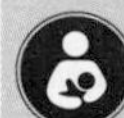

should only be used in first and second trimester of pregnancy on medical advice. Not recommended during third trimester

Patient teaching and advice

- advise patient to seek medical advice if symptoms persist
- (throat spray) instruct patient to:
  - prime pump with four or more sprays before first use, and one spray if unused recently, until fine mist is produced
  - depress pump fully with each spray
  - hold breath during administration
  - do not eat or drink immediately after using spray
  - discard pump 6 months after opening (write opening date on pump)

IBUPROFEN (Advil preparations, Brufen, Bugesic Oral Suspension, Caldolor, FenPaed Oral Liquid, FenPaed Double Strength Oral Liquid, Nurofen, Nurofen for Children, Nurofen Gel, Nurofen Liquid Capsules, Pedea Solution for Infusion, Nurofen Zavance, Rafen)

IBUPROFEN LYSINE (Nurofen QuikZorb)

Available forms

Capsules (liquid): 200 mg; Caplets: 200 mg, 342 mg; Tablets: 200 mg, 400 mg; Tablets (chewable): 100 mg; Syrup/Suspension: 40 mg/mL, 100 mg/5 mL; Gel: 5%; Vial: 800 mg/8 mL

Action

- see General Actions of NSAIDs (p. 12)
- analgesic, antipyretic and anti-inflammatory properties similar to those of other NSAIDs
- half-life about 2 hours

Use

- rheumatoid arthritis, including juvenile rheumatoid arthritis, osteoarthritis
- primary dysmenorrhea
- headache
- migraine
- acute/chronic pain with inflammatory component, including muscle, dental and sinus pain
- fever reduction
- (IV) acute mild-to-moderate post-operative pain, or moderate-to-severe postoperative pain as an adjunct to morphine
- (topical gel) sprains, strains, sports injuries

Dose

- (rheumatoid arthritis, osteoarthritis (acute exacerbation)) initially 1200–2400 mg orally daily in 3–4 divided doses with food, reducing to 1600 mg when symptoms stabilise **OR**
- (primary dysmenorrhoea) 400–800 mg orally with food at the first sign of pain or menstrual bleeding, then 400 mg 4–6-hourly (maximum daily dose 1.6 g) **OR**
- (minor aches and pains, dental pain, headache) 684 mg (2 caplets) with food initially, then 342–684 mg 4–6-hourly as needed (daily maximum 6 caplets) (342 mg caplets) **OR**
- (minor aches and pains, dental pain, headache) 200–400 mg orally 4–6-hourly as needed (daily maximum 1.2 g) **OR**
- (analgesia) 400–600 mg by IV infusion over 30 minutes 6-hourly, as needed (daily maximum 3.2 g for ≤ 2 days) **OR**

- (fever) initially 400 mg by IV infusion over 30 minutes, then 400 mg IV 4–6-hourly as needed (daily maximum 3.2 g) **OR**
- (topical gel) apply 4–10 cm of gel 4-hourly (as needed) to affected area and rub gently (maximum 4 applications daily)

Adverse effects

- (rare) aseptic meningitis with fever and coma
- see General Adverse effects of NSAIDs (p. 12)

Interactions

- colestyramine may decrease absorption of ibuprofen
- see General Interactions of NSAIDs (p. 12)

Nursing points/Cautions

- (IV) patient must be well hydrated before IV ibuprofen is used to decrease risk of kidney damage
- (IV) must be diluted with sodium chloride 0.9% or glucose 5% to a concentration of 4 mg/mL before administration
- (Nurofen QuikZorb) each caplet contains 342 mg ibuprofen lysine, which is the equivalent of 200 mg ibuprofen
- chewable tablets contain aspartame and are therefore not recommended in those with phenylketouria
- caution if used in patient undergoing spinal or epidural analgesia
- caution if used in patients with SLE due to risk of aseptic meningitis
- see General Nursing points/Cautions for NSAIDs (p. 13)

Patient teaching and advice

- (oral solution) advise patient to shake well before use and syringe/measuring spoon should be used to measure dose
- (chewable tablet) instruct patient to chew tablet, not swallow whole
- see p. 15 for topical gel administration advice
- see General Patient teaching and advice for NSAIDs (p. 14)

liquid preparation and chewable tablets are available. Tablet can be crushed and mixed with water or spoonful of yoghurt or apple puree

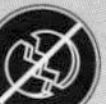

liquid-filled capsules should not be opened or crushed

Note

- contained in Combigesic, Ibudeine, Ibupane, Maxigesic, Mersynofen, Nurofen Cold and Flu PE, Nurofen Plus, Nurofen Sinus Pain PE, Nuromol, Sudafed Sinus+ Anti-Inflammatory Pain Relief Caplets

INDOMETACIN (INDOMETHACIN) (Arthrexin, Indocid)

Available forms

Capsules: 25 mg; Suppositories: 100 mg

Action

- see General Actions of NSAIDs (p. 12)
- more potent analgesic, antipyretic and anti-inflammatory properties than aspirin
- (oral) half-life about 4.5 hours

Use

- rheumatoid arthritis, osteoarthritis, ankylosing spondylitis
- degenerative hip disease
- gout
- bursitis, capsulitis, tenosynovitis, tendonitis
- sprains and strains
- low back pain (lumbago)
- inflammation, pain and oedema following orthopaedic surgery or reduction and immobilisation of fractures and dislocations
- primary dysmenorrhoea

Dose

- 50–200 mg orally daily with food in divided doses (daily maximum 200 mg) **OR**

- 100 mg rectal suppository once or twice daily if oral therapy not tolerated **OR**
- in combination (e.g. 25 mg orally 2–4 times daily and 100 mg rectal suppository at night (to a total of 200 mg)) **OR**
- (acute gouty arthritis) 150–200 mg orally daily with food in divided doses until symptoms subside **OR**
- (primary dysmenorrhoea) 25 mg orally 3 times daily with food at the first sign of pain or menstrual bleeding and continuing for as long as the symptoms usually last

Adverse effects
- see General Adverse effects of NSAIDs (p. 12)
- (oral) headache, may aggravate pre-existing psychiatric disturbances, epilepsy or Parkinsonism
- (prolonged therapy) corneal deposits, retinal disturbances
- (suppository) burning, pain, discomfort, rectal bleeding, proctitis, tenesmus

Interactions
- may cause false negative in dexamethasone suppression test
- see General Interactions of NSAIDs (p. 12)

Nursing points/Cautions
- see General Nursing points/Cautions for NSAIDs (p. 13)
- (rheumatic conditions) loading dose not required
- capsules contain lactose, therefore are not recommended in those with hereditary galactose intolerance, Lapp lactase deficiency or glucose–galactose malabsorption
- caution if used in those with psychiatric disturbances, epilepsy or Parkinsonism as condition may be aggravated
- (suppository) contraindicated in those with proctitis or recent rectal bleeding

Patient teaching and advice
- see General Patient teaching and advice for NSAIDs (p. 14)
- patients who experience night pain and/or morning stiffness should be advised to take oral treatment during the day and suppositories at bedtime for better control of symptoms
- warn patient that headache may occur early in treatment. If severe, dose can be decreased or therapy stopped if headache persists
- instruct patient to seek medical advice if vision becomes blurred or disturbed

capsules can be opened and contents dispersed in water or mixed with spoonful of yoghurt or apple puree

KETOPROFEN (Orudis SR Capsules and Suppositories, Oruvail SR)

Available forms
Capsules (sustained-release): 200 mg; Suppositories: 100 mg

Action
- see General Actions of NSAIDs (p. 12)
- half-life less than 2 hours

Use
- rheumatoid arthritis, osteoarthritis

Dose
- 100 mg rectal suppository at night supplemented as required with 100 mg orally 1–2 times daily **OR**
- 100–200 mg orally in 2–4 divided doses daily with food (sustained-release capsules)

Adverse effects
- see General Adverse effects of NSAIDs (p. 12)
- non-bacterial cystitis (bladder pain, dysuria, haematuria, increased micturition and frequency)

- (suppositories) pain, burning, itching, tenesmus and rarely, rectal bleeding

Interactions
- see General Interactions of NSAIDs (p. 12)
- may reduce efficacy of gemeprost and intrauterine contraceptive devices, increasing risk of pregnancy
- increased risk of bleeding if given with pentoxifylline (oxpentifylline)

Nursing points/Cautions
- suppositories provide more consistent control of overnight symptoms than oral medication
- (suppositories) contraindicated in those with haemorrhoids, recent proctitis or rectal bleeding
- see General Nursing points/Cautions for NSAIDs (p. 13)

Patient teaching and advice
- patients who experience night pain and/or morning stiffness should be advised to take oral treatment during the day and suppositories at bedtime for better control of symptoms
- recommend that slow-release capsules should not be broken, crushed or chewed but swallowed whole
- warn patient about symptoms of non-bacterial urinary tract infection symptoms, including change in colour, amount or frequency of urine, blood in urine or burning feeling when passing urine
- (suppositories) see p. 16 for suppository insertion advice
- see General Patient teaching and advice for NSAIDs (p. 14)

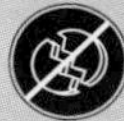

capsules or contents (sustained-release pellets) should not be crushed or chewed. Pellets can be mixed with spoonful of yoghurt or apple puree but must not be chewed

KETOROLAC TROMETAMOL (Acular Eye Drops, Ketorolac Solution for Injection, Toradol)

Available forms

Tablets: 10 mg; Ampoule: 10 mg/mL, 30 mg/mL; Eye drops: 5 mg/mL

Action
- inhibits prostaglandin synthesis by inhibiting COX
- potent peripherally-acting analgesic with poor anti-inflammatory properties
- half-life 5–6 hours
- platelet inhibition reverses 24–48 hours after stopping

Use
- moderate-to-severe postoperative pain (short term not exceeding 5 days)
- seasonal allergic conjunctivitis (short term); prophylaxis and reduction of inflammation after cataract surgery

Dose
- (under 65 years) initially 10–30 mg IM, followed by 10–30 mg 4–6-hourly (maximum 90 mg daily) **OR**
- (65 years and over, less than 50 kg or less severe pain) initially 10–15 mg IM, followed by 10–15 mg 4–6-hourly (maximum 60 mg daily) **OR**
- (under 65 years) 10 mg orally 4–6-hourly (maximum 40 mg daily) **OR**
- (65 years and over) 10 mg orally 6–8-hourly (maximum 30–40 mg daily) **OR**
- (seasonal allergic conjunctivitis) 1 drop 4 times daily for up to 4 weeks **OR**
- (prophylaxis and postoperative inflammation) 1–2 drops 4 times daily, starting 24 hours before surgery and for up to 2–4 weeks

Adverse effects
- (injection site) pain, ecchymosis, bruising, tingling and, rarely, haematoma, tingling

- (rare, but fatal) haemorrhage
- (eye drops) transient stinging, burning, itching, erythema, keratitis, scratching, foreign body sensation
- see General Adverse effects of NSAIDs (p. 12)

Interactions

- increased risk of seizure activity if given with anti-epileptic agents (e.g. phenytoin, carbamazepine)
- may be used with opioid analgesics to achieve optimal analgesia or when the sedative or anxiolytic effect of the opioid is wanted
- increased risk of hallucinations if given with fluoxetine or alprazolam
- contraindicated with aspirin, NSAIDs, pentoxifylline (oxpentifylline), lithium or probenecid
- (eye drops) increased risk of delayed corneal healing if given with topical corticosteroids
- see General Interactions of NSAIDs (p. 12)

Nursing points/Cautions

- any hypovolaemia should be corrected before administration of ketorolac trometamol
- IM injection should be given deeply and slowly into large muscle
- pressure should be applied to injection site for 15–30 seconds to decrease local effects
- total duration of use should not exceed 5 days because the risk of adverse effects increases with prolonged use
- conversion from parenteral to oral route should occur as soon as practicable and total combined dose (IM, oral) should not exceed 90 mg (or 60 mg in those aged 65 years and over)
- (eye drops) contain benzalkonium chloride (preservative) which may discolour soft contact lenses
- contraindicated via epidural or intrathecal route
- contraindicated in those with dehydration, hypovolaemia, moderate/severe kidney impairment, coagulation disorders or on anticoagulant therapy, surgical procedures with high risk of bleeding, history of bleeding (GI or intracranial)
- see General Nursing points/Cautions for NSAIDs (p. 13)

Patient teaching and advice

- (eye drops) see p. 15 for eye drop instillation advice
- see General Patient teaching and advice for NSAIDs (p. 14)

tablet can be crushed and mixed with water or spoonful of yoghurt or apple puree

MEFENAMIC ACID (Ponstan)

Available form

Capsules: 250 mg

Action

- see General Actions of NSAIDs (p. 12)
- half-life 2 hours

Use

- primary dysmenorrhoea
- primary menorrhagia
- mild-to-moderate pain (e.g. dental and soft tissue pain)

Dose

- (primary dysmenorrhoea) 500 mg orally 3 times daily with food from onset of pain for usual duration of pain **OR**
- (primary menorrhagia) 500 mg orally 3 times daily with food from onset of menses and continued according to doctor's advice, not exceeding 7 days (except on doctor's advice) **OR**
- (other indications) 500 mg orally 3 times daily with food

Adverse effects

- see General Adverse effects of NSAIDs (p. 12), particularly severe diarrhoea

Interactions

- see General Interactions of NSAIDs (p. 12)
- may cause false positive reaction for urinary bile. Other diagnostic procedures for bilirubinuria are recommended

Nursing points/Cautions

- see General Nursing points/Cautions for NSAIDs (p. 13)
- contraindicated in those who have previously experienced mefenamic acid-induced diarrhoea

Patient teaching and advice

- advise patient that diarrhoea is dose dependent and disappears when medication is stopped
- see General Patient teaching and advice for NSAIDs (p. 14)

MELOXICAM (Melobic, Melox Capsules, Meloxibell, Mobic, Moxicam)

Available forms

Tablets: 7.5 mg, 15 mg; Capsules: 7.5 mg, 15 mg

Action

- selective COX-2 inhibitor
- half-life 20 hours
- see General Actions of NSAIDs (p. 12)

Use

- osteoarthritis, rheumatoid arthritis

Dose

- (osteoarthritis) 7.5 mg orally daily with food, increasing to 15 mg daily if needed (daily maximum 15 mg) **OR**
- (rheumatoid arthritis) 15 mg orally daily with food, decreasing to 7.5 mg daily if condition allows

Adverse effects

- see General Adverse effects of NSAIDs (p. 12)

Interactions

- caution if given with itraconazole, erythromycin, ciclosporin and amiodarone
- not recommended with pemetrexed. If creatinine clearance is between 45–79 mL/min, meloxicam should be stopped for 5 days before, day of and 2 days after pemetrexed administration
- see also General Interactions of NSAIDs (p. 12)

Nursing points/Cautions

- contains lactose, therefore is contraindicated in those with hereditary galactose intolerance, Lapp lactase deficiency or glucose–galactose malabsorption
- see General Nursing points/Cautions for NSAIDs (p. 13)

Patient teaching and advice

- see General Patient teaching and advice for NSAIDs (p. 14)

tablets can be crushed or capsules can be opened and contents dispersed in water or mixed with spoonful of yoghurt or apple puree

METHYL SALICYLATE (Methyl Salicylate Liniment, Cream and Ointment)

Available forms

Cream, Liniment and Ointment

Action

- salicylate
- topical analgesic properties

Use

- relief of pain and inflammation associated with rheumatic conditions, lumbago, musculoskeletal disorders, sprains and strains

Dose
- massage small amount into affected area 2–3 times daily

Adverse effects
- acute poisoning can occur if taken orally
- mild skin irritation, erythema

Interactions
- excessive use may increase risk of bleeding in those taking warfarin or other anticoagulants

Nursing points/Cautions
- wash hands after use and avoid contact with eyes or mucous membranes

Patient teaching and advice
- see p. 15 for topical gel/solution application advice
- ensure patient understands preparation is only for external use
- warn patient to avoid vigorous rubbing
- instruct patient not to bandage area tightly or apply heating pads while preparation is on skin
- caution patient to keep medication away from open flame

Note
- contained in Bosisto's Eucalyptus Rub, Deep Heat, Dencorub Extra Strength Heat Gel, Dencorub Pain Relieving Cream, Goanna Heat Cream, Metsal Heat Rub Cream

NAPROXEN (Inza, Naprosyn, Naprosyn SR, Naproxen Suspension, Proxen SR)

NAPROXEN SODIUM (Aleve, Anaprox, Crysanal, Naprogesic)

Available forms

Tablets: 250 mg, 275 mg, 500 mg, 550 mg; Tablets (sustained-release): 750 mg, 1000 mg; Suspension: 125 mg/5 mL

Action
- see General Actions of NSAIDs (p. 12)
- half-life 14 hours

Use
- rheumatoid arthritis, osteoarthritis, ankylosing spondylitis, gout
- acute/chronic inflammatory pain
- acute migraine
- primary dysmenorrhoea

Dose
- (arthritis, spondylitis) initially 500–1100 mg orally daily in 2 divided doses with food, then 375–1000 mg daily (maintenance) **OR**
- (arthritis, spondylitis) 750–1000 mg orally once daily (SR) (daily maximum 1000 mg) **OR**
- (primary dysmenorrhoea) 500–550 mg orally with food at the first sign of pain or bleeding, then 250–275 mg 6–8-hourly as required (daily maximum 1250–1375 mg) **OR**
- (migraine) initially 750–825 mg orally at first sign of impending headache, then 250–550 mg throughout day, but not before 1 hour of initial dose (daily maximum 1250–1375 mg) **OR**
- (acute inflammatory pain) initially 500–550 mg orally with food, then 250–275 mg 6–8-hourly (daily maximum 1375 mg)
- (migraine, 550 mg tablets) 825 mg orally at first sign of impending headache, then 275–550 mg at least 1 hour after initial dose (daily maximum 1375 mg)

Adverse effects
- see General Adverse effects of NSAIDs (p. 12)

Interactions
- see General Interactions of NSAIDs (p. 12)
- may increase serum levels of zidovudine
- may interfere with some tests for 7-ketogenic steroids and some urinary assays for 5-hydroxy-indoleacetic acid

Nursing points/Cautions

- sustained-release preparations should not be used for acute conditions
- suspension contains 8 mg sodium per mL and tablets (Anaprox, Crysanal) contain 50 mg of sodium per 550 mg tablet, which should be considered if patient requires sodium restriction
- see General Nursing points/Cautions for NSAIDs (p. 13)

Patient teaching and advice

- instruct patient to discontinue medication 72 hours before adrenal function tests
- advise patients that sustained-release tablets should be taken whole, not crushed or chewed
- warn patient that slow-release (SR) tablets are not recommended for acute conditions such as migraine
- patient should be instructed to shake suspension well before use
- see General Patient teaching and advice for NSAIDs (p. 14)

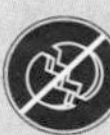

sustained-release tablets should not be crushed; however, it is available as an oral suspension. Some formulations are very difficult to crush and/or do not disperse easily in water

PARACETAMOL (Dymadon, Dymadon Suspension, Febridol, Lemsip Cold & Flu, Lemsip Max, Mendeleev, Osteomol, Panadol preparations, Panamax, Paracetamol preparations, Paracetamol Solution for Infusion, Paralgin)

Available forms

Tablets: 500 mg; Tablets/caplets (modified-release): 665 mg; Tablets (soluble): 250 mg, 500 mg; Tablets (chewable): 120 mg; Caplets: 500 mg; Suppositories: 125 mg, 250 mg, 500 mg; Sachets (powder): 500 mg, 1 g; Syrup/Suspension/Elixir: 120 mg/5 mL, 240 mg/5 mL, 50 mg/mL, 250 mg/5 mL; Drops: 50 mg/mL, 100 mg/mL; IV solution: 10 mg/mL

Action

- known as acetaminophen in the USA
- analgesic, antipyretic but has no useful anti-inflammatory properties
- analgesic and antipyretic actions are thought to be related to prostaglandin synthesis inhibition in the CNS
- half-life 1–3 hours

Use

- mild-to-moderate pain
- headache, migraine, tension headache, sinus pain
- muscle ache
- osteoarthritis
- toothache, dental pain post-procedure
- cold and flu symptoms
- fever
- (IV) mild-to-moderate pain when IV route is clinically indicated
- suitable alternative for those with aspirin allergy (including those with asthma), dyspepsia or peptic ulceration or children with fever caused by viral illness

Dose

- 0.5–1 g orally 4–6-hourly as required (up to 4 g/day) **OR**
- 1330 mg (2 tablets) orally 3 times daily as required (up to 4 g/day (6 tablets)) (modified-release tablets) **OR**
- 0.5–1 g rectal suppository 4–6-hourly as required (up to 4 g/day) **OR**
- (patient weight $>$ 50 kg) 1 g IV 4-hourly, up to 4 g/day **OR**
- (patient weight $>$ 33 kg but $\leq$ 50 kg) 15 mg/kg IV 4-hourly, up to 3 g/day **OR**
- (patient weight $>$ 10 kg but $\leq$ 33 kg) 15 mg/kg IV 6-hourly, up to 2 g/day

Adverse effects

- (rarely) nausea, dyspepsia, allergic or haematological reaction, hypersensitivity, serious skin reactions

- (10–15 g or more) hepatic necrosis, renal dysfunction
- (IV) nausea, vomiting, diarrhoea, dyspepsia, headache, dizziness, increase in liver enzymes, injection site pain and pruritus

Interactions

- (immediate-release preparations) absorption rate may be increased by metoclopramide but decreased for sustained-release preparations
- prolonged use may require reduction in anticoagulant dose, therefore INR should be closely monitored during therapy and 7 days after stopping therapy
- large or chronic doses of paracetamol increase the likelihood of hepatotoxicity if given with concurrent use of alcohol, other hepatotoxic agents or anti-epileptic drugs
- may decrease clearance of busulfan
- increase risk of hepatotoxicity and decrease effectiveness if given with phenytoin
- products containing paracetamol should not be given together (e.g. oral and IV) to avoid risk of overdose and hepatic damage. All routes should be considered when calculating total daily dose
- probenecid reduces clearance
- increased serum levels may result if given with diflusinal
- (IV) metabolism may be increased (therefore increasing level of hepatoxic metabolites) by barbiturates, anticoagulants, isoniazid, zidovudine, amoxicillin with clavulanic acid and carbamazepine
- absorption may be decreased by agents that decrease gastric emptying (e.g. opioids, propantheline, antidepressants with anticholinergic properties)

Nursing points/Cautions

- when estimating total daily dose, <u>all</u> routes (e.g. oral, IV, PR) and prescribed and over-the-counter paracetamol-containing products should be considered. Total daily dose should not exceed 4 g (patient weight $\geq$ 50 kg), 60 mg/kg up to 3 g for patient weight $<$ 50 kg to $\geq$ 33 kg, and 60 mg/kg for patient weight $<$ 33 kg to $\geq$ 10 kg
- administer alone IV
- IV infusion given over 15 minutes
- IV solution has slight yellow colour
- IV administration should be changed to oral administration as soon as practicable
- early overdose symptoms: sweating, pallor, anorexia, nausea, vomiting, abdominal pain or cramping and/or diarrhoea occurring 6–14 hours after ingestion, and lasting about 24 hours
- late overdose symptoms include tenderness or pain in abdominal area, indicating liver necrosis/failure (jaundice, hypoglycaemia, metabolic acidosis) and confusion
- symptoms of overdose in first 48 hours may not reflect potential seriousness, as symptoms of liver failure may not manifest for at least 72 hours. Absorption of SR formulations will be prolonged in overdose
- overdose management: after taking blood for paracetamol assay, overdose should be treated promptly (within 10 hours) with activated charcoal and sorbitol or gastric lavage to reduce gastric absorption and with IV acetylcysteine to protect against liver damage (see Antidotes, antagonists and chelating agents, p. 332) if 10–15 g or more of paracetamol has been ingested. Liver tests are recommended at the start of overdose management, then daily
- (Febridol tablets) contain sodium metabisulfite, which may cause a hypersensitivity reaction in sensitive individuals
- (Panadol Soluble) may contain sorbitol, which is not recommended in those with fructose intolerance
- (soluble/effervescent preparations) contain sodium, which should be considered in sodium-restricted diets

- (soluble/effervescent preparations) contain aspartame and should not be used in those with glucose-6-phosphate dehydrogenase (G6PD) deficiency as haemolytic anaemia may result
- (IV) if patient has liver disease, daily dose should not exceed 3 g
- (IV) caution if used in those with dehydration, hypovolaemia, chronic malnutrition (including anorexia, bulimia or cachexia) or chronic alcoholism (> 3 drinks/day)
- not recommended for infants under 1 month of age
- caution if used in those with liver or kidney dysfunction
- contraindicated in those with severe liver disease/failure

Patient teaching and advice

- instruct patient to dissolve effervescent and soluble preparations in ½–1 glass of water for more rapid absorption
- warn patient to avoid alcohol during therapy
- advise patient to swallow modified-release tablets whole, not chewed or crushed
- patient should be cautioned regarding risk of overdose if taking multiple paracetamol-containing preparations
- (powder) instruct patient to pour sachet into mug, fill with hot (not boiling) water and stir until dissolved. May be sweetened with sugar or honey if required
- (drops/suspension) can be administered to infant mixed with water or fruit juice
- advise patient to seek medical advice if skin reaction occurs
- see p. 16 for suppository insertion advice

Note

- contained in Anagraine, Codalgin Forte, Codapane Forte 500/30, Codral Original Cold & Flu + Cough Day and Night Capsules, Codral Original Day & Night Cold & Flu Tablets, Combigesic, Comfarol Forte, Demazin Cold and Flu Tablets, Dimetapp Cough Cold and Flu Daytime Nighttime Liquid Capsules, Dimetapp PE Sinus Day + Night Tablets, Dimetapp PE Sinus Pain Tablets, Dolased Forte, Ibupane, Lemsip Max Cold & Flu with Decongestant, Lemsip Multi-Relief Cold & Flu, Maxi Clear Cold & Flu Relief, Maxi Clear, Maxi Clear Sinus & Pain Relief, Maxigesic, Mersyndol, Mersyndol Day Strength, Mersyndol Forte, Mersynofen, Metomax, Mydol 15, Norgesic, Nuromol, Painstop for Children Day-Time Pain Relief, Painstop Day-Time Pain Reliever, Painstop Night-Time Pain Reliever, Panadeine Forte, Panadol Cold & Flu + Decongestant, Panadol Cold & Flu Max + Decongestant Hot Lemon, Panadol Cold & Flu Relief PE, Panadol Cold & Flu Relief + Cough, Panadol Extra, Panadol Extra Optizorb, Panadol Night, Paracetamol/Codeine GH 500/30, Panamax Co, Prodeine, Prodeine Forte, Prodeinextra, Sudafed PE Sinus + Allergy & Pain Relief, Sudafed PE Sinus & Pain Relief, Sudafed Sinus + Allergy & Pain Relief Tablets, Sudafed Sinus Day + Night, Zaldiar

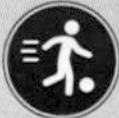

any combination products containing dextromethorphan or pseudoephedrine are banned in sport

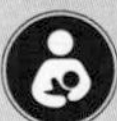

safe to use during pregnancy and breastfeeding at analgesic doses

available as an oral suspension or soluble or chewable tablets. Plain tablet can be dispersed in water or crushed and mixed with spoonful of yoghurt or apple puree

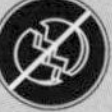

modified-release tablet should not be crushed

PARECOXIB SODIUM (Dynastat)

Available form
Vial: 40 mg

Action
- selective COX-2 inhibitor
- rapidly converted to valdecoxib, which is the active component
- onset of analgesia 7–14 minutes, peak reached within 2 hours, duration of action 6–24 hours, half-life about 8 hours
- see also General Actions of NSAIDs (p. 12)

Use
- postoperative pain (single dose)

Dose
- 40 mg IV or IM as once-only dose

Adverse effects
- severe hypotension
- hypoaesthesia, dizziness, insomnia
- hypokalaemia
- nausea, vomiting, abdominal pain, constipation, dyspepsia
- postoperative anaemia
- peripheral oedema
- respiratory insufficiency
- increased sweating, pruritus
- oliguria
- (injection site) pain, redness
- (rare) serious skin reactions
- (very rare) myocardial infarction
- see also General Adverse effects of NSAIDs (p. 12)

Interactions
- increased serum levels may occur if given with ketoconazole or fluconazole
- caution if given with warfarin, therefore international normalised ratio (INR) should be closely monitored
- may decrease clearance of lithium, therefore blood levels should be closely monitored
- caution if given with ACE inhibitors, angiotensin II receptor antagonists, diuretics and beta-adrenoceptor blocking agents
- caution if given with ciclosporin

Nursing points/Cautions
- patient should be adequately hydrated before starting therapy
- monitor for any signs of hypotension
- reconstituted using sodium chloride 0.9% (not sterile water for injections) 2 mL (40 mg) or 1 mL (20 mg)
- administer alone
- may be given as IV bolus
- IM injection should be given slowly into large muscle
- incompatible with lactated Ringer's or glucose 5% in lactated Ringer's as precipitate will form and therefore should not be reconstituted with these fluids or added into IV lines with these fluids already running
- contraindicated in those with known allergy to sulfonamides
- see General Nursing points/Cautions for NSAIDs (p. 13)

Patient teaching and advice
- advise patient to seek medical advice if any skin reaction occurs. This could occur 1–2 weeks after administration

PIROXICAM (Feldene, Feldene D, Feldene Gel, Mobilis, Mobilis D)

Available forms
Capsules: 10 mg, 20 mg; Tablets (dispersible): 10 mg, 20 mg; Gel: 5 mg/g

Action
- see General Actions of NSAIDs (p. 12)
- half-life 36–45 hours

Use
- rheumatoid arthritis, osteoarthritis, ankylosing spondylitis
- acute soft tissue injuries (e.g. sprains, strains, tendonitis)

Dose
- initially 10 mg orally daily, increasing to 20 mg if needed **OR**
- 1 g (3 cm of gel) to affected area 3–4 times daily for up to 2 weeks

Adverse effects
- (gel) mild skin irritation (erythema, rash, pruritus), transient skin discolouration, photosensitivity, contact dermatitis, eczema
- see General Adverse effects of NSAIDs (p. 12)

Interactions
- see General Interactions of NSAIDs (p. 12)

Nursing points/Cautions
- (oral) once daily dose required because of long plasma half-life
- see General Nursing points/Cautions for NSAIDs (p. 13)

Patient teaching and advice
- see p. 15 for topical gel administration advice
- advise patient that gel should be completely rubbed in to prevent skin discolouration or staining of clothes
- see General Patient teaching and advice for NSAIDs (p. 14)

available as dispersible tablets or capsule can be opened and contents mixed with spoonful of yoghurt or apple puree

ANORECTICS AND WEIGHT-LOSS AGENTS

National survey figures in 2017–18 showed that more than 67% of Australian adults aged 18 years and over were either overweight (35.6%) or obese (31.3%), 31.7% are normal weight and about 1.3% were underweight (ABS 2019).

A thorough patient assessment should include an obesity-focused history (e.g. factors contributing to obesity, impact on health, patient goals, expectations and barriers to weight management, motivation), physical examination to determine degree and type of obesity, assessment of co-morbid conditions and the patient's willingness to engage in lifestyle changes (Kushner 2018).

To evaluate the degree of obesity, height, weight and waist circumference should be measured (Kushner 2018). Body mass index (BMI) is calculated by dividing the person's weight (kg) by the person's height (in metres squared (m^2)) and is an estimate of body fat, which is related to risk of disease. It should be noted, however, that BMI is a less useful measure in the elderly and those who are fit and muscular (Kushner 2018). A person is classified as obese if their BMI is equal to or greater than 30, while 25–29.9 is considered to be overweight. Waist circumference is a good indicator of visceral fat and is associated with an increased risk of cardiovascular disease and diabetes (Kushner 2018).

The overall goal of therapy is to reduce weight in order to reduce the risk of related co-morbidities including cardiovascular disease, type 2 diabetes mellitus, cancer, bone and joint disease, reproductive disorder and increased mortality (Kushner 2018). Management should always start with lifestyle management (diet, physical activity, behaviour modification).

Anorectic and weight-loss agents are considered adjunctive in the management of obesity where other regimens (lifestyle management) have not been successful in achieving an adequate response (e.g. greater than 5% weight loss within 3 months) (Kushner 2018). Sometimes a person who is classified as overweight with a BMI of 27 may be prescribed anorectic and weight-loss agents if they have other obesity-related risk factors such as hypertension, diabetes or dyslipidaemia. Bariatric surgery, such as laparoscopic sleeve gastrectomy or laparoscopic adjustable gastric banding, may be recommended for those with co-morbidities and a BMI of 35 kg/m^2 or greater or those with severe obesity (≥ 40 kg/m^2) (Kushner 2018).

The use of anorectic and weight-loss agents should be limited because tolerance and habituation are known to develop. They should be used in conjunction with a well-balanced, calorie-modified diet, appropriate exercise regimen and behaviour modification (Kushner 2018). Secondary causes of obesity should be eliminated before commencing on any weight-loss agent.

BUPROPION HYDROCHLORIDE and NALTREXONE HYDROCHLORIDE (Contrave 8/90)

Available form

Tablets (naltrexone hydrochloride 8 mg and bupropion hydrochloride 90 mg) (modified-release)

Action

- naltrexone hydrochloride is a mu-opioid antagonist used as part of alcohol dependence programs and as an adjunct in maintaining abstinence from opioids (see Drug Dependence, p. 1039)
- buproion hydrochloride selectively inhibits neuronal reuptake of dopamine and norepinephrine and is used as an adjunct to counselling in management of nicotine dependence (see Drug Dependence, p. 1035)
- the exact mode of action of this combination medication on appetite suppression is not totally understood, although it is thought to increase the firing rate of hypothalamic pro-opiomelancortin neurons involved in appetite regulation. Furthermore, in animal studies, a reduced food intake was observed when injected directly into the ventral tegmental area of the mesolimbic circuit, which is associated with reward pathway regulation
- action of the combinated two agents is thought to be greater than either single agent alone in reducing food intake
- elimination half-life was about 5 hours for naltrexone hydrochloride and 21 hours for bupropion hydrochloride

Use

- as an adjunct in weight management in adults (≥ 18 years) with an initial BMI ≥ 30 kg/m^2 (obese) or ≥ 27 kg/m^2 to < 30 kg/m^2 (overweight with one or more related co-morbidities including type 2 diabetes, dyslipidaemia or controlled hypertension) with reduced calorie diet and increased exercise program

Dose

- (week 1) 1 tablet orally daily mane
- (week 2) 1 tablet orally mane and nocte
- (week 3) 2 tablets orally mane, 1 table orally nocte
- (week 4 and onwards) 2 tablets orally mane and nocte

Adverse effects

- nausea, vomiting, constipation, upper abdominal pain, altered taste
- dry mouth, toothache
- dizziness, headache, insomnia, feeling jittery, tremor, lethargy, attention disturbance
- palpitations
- tinnitus, vertigo
- hot flush, pruritus, excessive sweating
- alopecia
- (rare) seizures, angioedema

Interactions

- contraindicated with or within 14 days of stopping MAOIs
- contraindicated with other treatments using naltrexone hydrochloride or bupropion hydrochloride

- caution if used with agents that may lower seizure threshold, including antipsychotics, antidepressants, antimalarials, tramadol, theophylline, systemic corticosteroids, quinolones and sedating antihistamine
- may increase levels of antiarrhythmics, antidepressants, TCAs, SSRIs, antipsychotics and beta-adrenergic blocking agents increasing risk of adverse effects
- concentration may be increased if given with ticlopidine or clopidogrel
- if patient is undergoing intermittent opioid treatment, therapy should be stopped temporarily or dose of opioid reduced
- efficacy may be reduced if given with ritonavir, lopinavir or efavirenz
- caution if given with metformin
- CNS toxicity may result if given with levodopa or amantadine
- may produce a false positive in urinary screening test for amphetamines. Further testing is required to differentiate between bupropion and amphetamines
- not recommended with alcohol

Nursing points/Cautions

- blood pressure and pulse should be measured before starting and regularly throughout therapy
- therapy should be reviewed after 16 weeks and then annually. If patient has not lost at least 5% of the initial body weight after 16 weeks, therapy should be discontinued
- blood glucose levels should be closely monitored in those with type 2 diabetes at the start of therapy
- if patient experiences seizure, therapy should be stopped and not restarted
- caution if used in those with diabetes as blood glucose levels may be affected, increasing risk of hypoglycaemia and seizure
- caution if used in those with controlled hypertension
- caution if used in those with risk of seizure, including head trauma history, excessive alcohol use, addiction of cocaine or stimulants
- caution if used in those with a history of depression, suicide attempt or suicide ideation
- caution if used in those over 65 years and not recommended in those over 75 years
- not recommended in those with history of myocardial infarction, unstable heart disease or congestive heart failure
- contraindicated in those with severe liver impairment or end-stage kidney failure
- contraindicated in those with uncontrolled hypertension, seizure disorder or history of seizures, known presence of central nervous system tumour, history of bipolar disorder, current or past history of an eating disorder or mania
- contraindicated in those with current dependency on opioids or opioid antagonists (e.g. methadone) or currently withdrawing from opioids
- contraindicated in those with rare hereditary problems of galactose intolerance, Lapp lactase deficiency or glucose–galactose malabsorption
- contraindicated in those with hypersensitivity to naltrexone hydrochloride or bupropion hydrochloride

Patient teaching and advice

- counsel patient to avoid or minimise intake of alcohol during therapy
- patient should be advised that adverse effects generally resolve within 4 weeks of starting therapy
- advise patient to take tablets whole (should not be cut, chewed or crushed)
- patients with type 2 diabetes mellitus should be warned that they may be more likely to experience gastrointestinal adverse effects, including

nausea, vomiting and diarrhoea. They should also be advised to closely monitor blood glucose levels at the start of therapy to prevent hypoglycaemia
- instruct patient to immediately report any:
  - sadness, crying, sleeping too much or not being able to fall asleep, change in appetite, trouble with concentration, withdrawal from family, friends and/or previously pleasurable activities, lack of energy and/or thoughts of self-harm
  - rash, hives, itching, shortness of breath, chest pain, swelling (oedema) (signs of anaphylactic/anaphylactoid reaction)
  - fever, rash, muscle pain, bone pain (signs of delayed hypersensitive reaction)
  - unusual tiredness, persistent loss of appetite, upper abdominal pain, yellowing of eyes or skin, dark urine (signs of hepatitis)
- carers and/or family members should be alerted to the need to monitor the patient's mood or any unusual behaviours in relation to depression or suicidal ideation
- warn patient that may be more sensitive to opioids (even low doses) when therapy is stopped increasing the risk of overdose
- encourage patient to participate in regular exercise, such as swimming or walking (approved by doctor) in addition to medication for sustained weight loss
- see General Patient teaching and advice (p. xxvii)

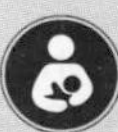

contraindicated during pregnancy, not recommended during breastfeeding

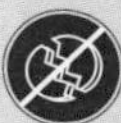

tablets should not be crushed

LIRAGUTIDE (Saxenda, Victoza)

Available form

Prefilled pen: 6 mg/mL

Action

- glucagon-like peptide-1 (GLP-1) analogue
- protracted release is due to self-association (resulting in slow absorption), binding to albumin and enzymatic stability, resulting in long plasma half-life
- physiological regulator of appetite and calorie intake as GLP-1 receptors are present in the brain in areas involved in appetite regulation, as well as being present in the intestine
- increases satiety and decreases hunger signals
- peak effect 8–12 hours, duration of action 24 hours, half-life about 13 hours

Use

- type 2 diabetes, chronic weight management in those with BMI $\geq$ 30 kg/m^2 (obese) or $\geq$ 27 kg/m^2 and $<$ 30 kg/m^2 (overweight) with $\geq$ 1 weight-related co-morbidity (e.g. dyslipidaemia, hypertension, obstructive sleep apnoea) (adjunct to reduced calorie diet and increased physical activity) (see Antidiabetic agents, p. 322)

ORLISTAT (Prolistat, Xenical)

Available form

Capsules: 120 mg

Action

- peripherally acting agent that specifically and reversibly inhibits lipase in the gut by approximately 30% resulting in weight loss

Use

- management of obesity (BMI $\geq$ 30) or overweight (BMI $\geq$ 27 with other risk factors, such as hypertension or high cholesterol) in conjunction with a mild hypocaloric diet

Dose

- 120 mg orally 3 times daily with meals

Adverse effects

- fatty/oily stools, loose stools, faecal urgency, flatulence, oily spotting from rectum, increased frequency of defecation, faecal incontinence
- abdominal pain, nausea, dyspepsia
- headache, asthenia
- (rare) hepatitis, liver failure, pancreatitis, hypersensitivity skin reaction

Interactions

- because vitamin K absorption may be altered, warfarin plasma levels may also be altered and therefore INR should be closely monitored
- may decrease ciclosporin plasma levels necessitating monitoring of ciclosporin levels
- may decrease effect of amiodarone
- a decreased oral hypoglycaemic dose may be required with weight loss
- decreases absorption of fat-soluble vitamins A, D, E and beta carotene
- caution if used with anti-epileptic agents
- not recommended with acarbose
- not recommended with other anorectic or weight-loss agents

Nursing points/Cautions

- effects become obvious within 1–2 days of starting therapy because fatty stools start to appear. Stools return to normal within 48–72 hours of stopping therapy
- those with epilepsy should be monitored for any changes in frequency and/or severity of seizures
- caution if used in those with active peptic ulcer disease, symptomatic cholelithiasis, postsurgical adhesions, eating disorders, psychiatric or neurological disorders, nephrolithiasis, deficiency of fat-soluble vitamins (A, D, E, K), or in those with significant cardiac, liver, kidney, gastrointestinal or endocrine disorders
- contraindicated in those with cholestasis, chronic malabsorption syndrome, chronic pancreatic enzyme deficiency, chronic pancreatitis or after major gastrointestinal surgery

Patient teaching and advice

- advise patient that weight loss is usually seen within 2 weeks of starting and continues for 6–12 months during therapy
- instruct patient that capsules should be swallowed whole and taken with meals or up to 1 hour after meals. If a meal is missed or contains no fat, capsules may be omitted. Daily intake of fat should be spread over 3 main meals rather than concentrated in 1 meal
- advise patients that the risk of gastrointestinal adverse effects is greater if the meal contains a high fat content
- explain to patients that some symptoms (e.g. increased wind, abdominal pain, urgent need to open bowels or fatty, oily or liquid stools) will decrease as therapy continues; however, if a meal containing high fat is eaten, symptoms will return
- counsel patient regarding the benefits of undertaking a nutritionally balanced, calorie-reduced diet and exercise program for continued weight loss. The diet should be nutritionally balanced and rich in fruit and vegetables, with fat making up 30% of the calorie value (≤ 67 g fat/day) and adequate intake of fat-soluble vitamins. Patient should also be counselled to avoid fat-containing foods such as biscuits and chocolate as between-meal snacks
- encourage patient to read food labels to determine fat content of food
- multivitamin supplement may be needed and should be taken 2 hours before or after medication

- encourage patient to participate in regular exercise such as swimming or walking (approved by doctor) in addition to medication for sustained weight loss
- advise patient with type 2 diabetes mellitus that weight loss may require adjustment to oral hypoglycaemic agent in order to maintain stable blood glucose levels and prevent hypoglycaemia
- see General Patient teaching and advice (p. xxvii)

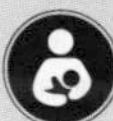

not recommended during pregnancy and breastfeeding

capsule can be opened and contents dispersed in water or fruit juice, or given with spoonful of yoghurt

PHENTERMINE (Duromine, Metermine)

Available forms

Capsules, Extended/modified-release capsules: 15 mg, 30 mg, 40 mg

Action

- sympathomimetic agent thought to suppress appetite through action on the hypothalamus
- has effects on the dopaminergic and noradrenergic nervous systems
- long half-life (about 25 hours)

Use

- short-term management of obesity (BMI $\geq$ 30) or overweight (BMI $\geq$ 27) with other risk factors (such as hypertension or high cholesterol) in conjunction with a mild hypocaloric diet and exercise program

Dose

- initially 30–40 mg orally daily, then 15–40 mg as maintenance

Adverse effects

- insomnia, restlessness, tremor, headache, nervousness, dizziness
- dry mouth, diarrhoea/constipation, nausea, vomiting, unpleasant taste, abdominal cramps
- palpitations, hypertension, tachycardia, precordial pain
- impotence, disturbed micturition, changes in libido
- rash
- facial oedema
- (rare) valvular heart disease, primary pulmonary hypertension

Interactions

- contraindicated with MAOIs or within 14 days of stopping MAOI therapy
- may antagonise clonidine and methyldopa sesquihydrate, reducing their antihypertensive actions
- may cause effects of insulin and oral hypoglycaemic agents to vary; therefore blood glucose levels should be closely monitored in those with diabetes
- use cautiously with other sympathomimetics or psychotropic agents, including sedatives
- should not be used with any other anorectic or weight-loss agents
- concurrent use with thyroid agents may cause CNS stimulation
- alcohol may increase CNS effects (e.g. dizziness, confusion)
- not recommended with SSRIs, ergot-related agents or clomipramine

Nursing points/Cautions

- cause of obesity should be determined before start of therapy to exclude any organic cause
- blood pressure should be monitored regularly throughout therapy (especially at the start) in those with mild hypertension
- course of treatment should be continued for 12 weeks and then reviewed by doctor
- caution if used in those with mild hypertension, diabetes, epilepsy (may increase frequency/severity of seizure) or if receiving antihypertensive therapy

- not recommended in the elderly
- contraindicated in those with glaucoma, moderate-to-severe or uncontrolled hypertension, pulmonary artery hypertension, hyperthyroidism, advanced arteriosclerosis, heart valve abnormalities or heart murmurs, cerebrovascular disease, severe cardiac disease, history of drug/alcohol abuse/dependence or psychiatric illness (including depression or eating disorders)
- contraindicated in those with hypersensitivity to sympathomimetic agents

Patient teaching and advice

- instruct patients to swallow capsule whole with a glass of water. Capsules should not be chewed or opened
- warn patients to avoid alcohol during therapy
- advise patients not to drive or use machinery if they experience dizziness, tremor or confusion
- to avoid any sleep disturbances at night, suggest taking medication in morning rather than later in the day
- caution patients with diabetes that blood glucose levels should be monitored more frequently as weight loss may necessitate a reduction in dose of insulin and/or oral hypoglycaemic agents increasing risk of hypoglycaemia
- see General Patient teaching and advice (p. xxvii)

banned in sport

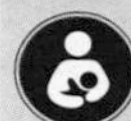

not recommended during pregnancy and breastfeeding

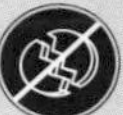

capsules should not be opened or crushed

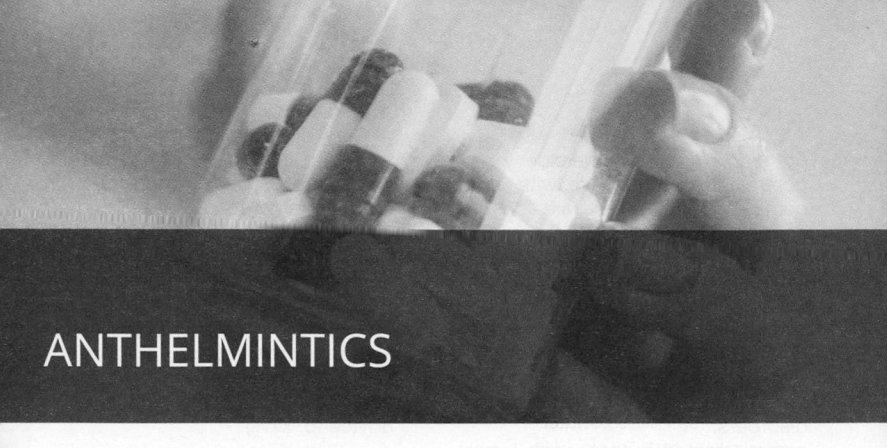

ANTHELMINTICS

It is from the Greek word *helmins* that the term 'helminth' (meaning worm) is derived. Helminths can be subdivided into nematodes (roundworms, hookworms, threadworms, whipworms and filariae), trematodes (flukes) and cestodes (tapeworms) (Keiser, McCarthy & Hotez 2018).

Helminth infestations are thought to be present in more than 1.5 billion people worldwide (24% of the world's population), with the greatest prevalence appearing to be in tropical and subtropical areas (World Health Organization [WHO] 2019d) where there is poor faecal sanitation and poor resources. Adult worms live in human intestines and produce thousands of eggs daily, which are then passed in faeces contaminating the soil. Transmission can then occur via vegetables grown in contaminated soil that are not adequately washed, from water sources or playing in contaminated soil and not washing hands. Transmission is not person-to-person or via fresh faeces as the eggs require about 3 weeks to mature and become infective in the soil. Furthermore, hookworm eggs can hatch in soil and mature larvae can penetrate the skin when a person walks barefoot on contaminated soil (WHO 2019d).

These helminths not only cause ill health, but also have major economic and social consequences in areas where these infestations are endemic. Children in developing countries are particularly at risk of helminth infestation (often mixed), which may lead to impaired growth and physical development, malnutrition, vitamin deficiency, diarrhoea, anaemia and pneumonia (WHO 2019d). In 2017, WHO set a global target of reaching 75% of children in need of treatment by 2020 (WHO 2019d).

Anthelmintics are drugs used to treat worm infestation. Their actions are selective, by taking advantage of the differences between the worm and host (e.g. different transmitter substances at the neuromuscular junction). These drugs must first be able to penetrate the cuticle of the worm, or its alimentary tract, to be effective. This heterogeneous group works in a variety of ways, including damaging or killing the worm directly, causing the worm to become paralysed and thus expelled in the faeces, damaging the worm in such a way that the host defences then take over, or interfering with the worm's metabolism (Keiser et al 2018).

General Patient teaching and advice for helminth infestation

- as parasites generally enter the body by the mouth, hygiene is a very important issue for control. Other affected members of a household may require concurrent treatment to prevent reinfection, even if they appear asymptomatic
- eggs are very small and stick to whatever they come into contact with
- everyone in the household should be advised to wear shoes to prevent infestation or reinfestation by eggs
- fingernails should be cut short to avoid scratching anal area and causing reinfestation (see point below about not shaking linen)
- shower or bathe daily
- underwear should be changed daily
- hands and fingernails should be washed thoroughly with soap and water after using the toilet and especially before preparing food or eating
- toilet seats should be thoroughly cleaned after use
- after treatment, bed linen, bed clothes and towels should be washed thoroughly. It is important not to shake bed clothes, bed linen or towels as eggs floating in the air may be swallowed, causing infestation or reinfestation
- bedroom floor should be vacuumed or damp-mopped (not swept) for 3 days post-treatment

ALBENDAZOLE (Eskazole, Zentel)

Available forms

Tablets (chewable): 200 mg, 400 mg

Action

- benzimidazole
- disrupts metabolism, immobilising and killing the worm
- larvicidal, ovicidal and vermicidal
- poorly absorbed and remains in the gastrointestinal (GI) tract
- active metabolite (albendazole sulfoxide) has half-life of 8.5 hours

Use

- hydatid disease caused by the tapeworm *Echinococcus granulosus* (where surgery is not possible, multiple cysts are present or as an adjunct pre- or post-surgery)
- cysticercosis (especially with neurological involvement (neurocysticercosis))
- capillariasis (*Capillaria philippinensis*)
- pinworm/threadworm (*Enterobius vermicularis*), roundworm (*Ascaris lumbricoides*), hookworm (*Ancylostoma duodenale*, *Necator americanus*), whipworm (*Trichuris trichiura*), strongyloides, liver flukes (*Opisthorchis viverrini*, *Clonorchis sinensis*)
- cutaneous larva migrans
- tapeworm (*Hymenolepis nana* or *Taenia* sp. with other species also present)

Dose

Hydatid disease

- 400 mg orally twice daily with food (for 28 days), which may be repeated for 3 cycles with a 14-day drug-free break between cycles **OR**
- (under 60 kg) 15 mg/kg/day in divided doses with food (for 28 days), which may be repeated for 3 cycles with a 14-day drug-free break between cycles **OR**
- (preoperatively) 2 × 28-day cycles as above **OR**
- (postoperatively) 2 × 28-day cycles as above (if preoperative dose was given less than 14 days, operation was in emergency theatre or if cysts were viable after preoperative treatment) **OR**
- (inoperable or multiple cysts) 400 mg orally twice daily with food (for 28 days) repeated for 3 cycles with

a 14-day drug-free break between cycles

Neurocysticercosis

- 400 mg orally twice daily with food for 3–7 days, which may be repeated for 1 cycle with a 14-day drug-free break between cycles **OR**
- (under 60 kg) 15 mg/kg/day in divided doses with food, as above

Capillariasis

- 400 mg orally daily with food for 10 days

Pinworm, threadworm, roundworm, hookworm, whipworm

- 400 mg orally on an empty stomach as a single dose

Strongyloides

- 400 mg orally daily on an empty stomach for 3 consecutive days

Cutaneous larva migrans

- 400 mg orally daily with food for 1–3 days

Mixed worm infestation (including liver flukes)

- 400 mg orally twice daily with food for 3 days

Tape worm

- 400 mg orally daily on an empty stomach for 3 days. If ineffective after 21 days, course can be repeated

Adverse effects

- abdominal pain, nausea, vomiting
- dizziness, headache
- leucopenia
- rash, pruritus, urticaria
- reversible alopecia (hair thinning and moderate hair loss)
- fever
- transient elevation of liver enzymes
- (rare) bone pain, proteinuria, hepatitis, pancytopenia, thrombocytopenia
- (neurocysticercosis) headache, nausea, visual changes, neurological events (including increased intracranial pressure and convulsions) (due to death of parasite)

Interactions

- plasma levels of active metabolite may be increased by cimetidine, praziquantel and dexamethasone
- plasma levels of active metabolite may be decreased by ritonavir, phenytoin, carbamazepine and phenobarbital (phenobarbitone), resulting in decreased efficacy

Nursing points/Cautions

- (neurocysticercosis) oral/IV corticosteroids will prevent increased intracranial pressure if given during the week of treatment. Also recommended are appropriate antihistamines and/or antiepileptics to prevent hypersensitivity reaction
- (neurocysticercosis) second course is recommended after 14-day drug-free interval if no response to the first course
- (hydatid cyst) if there are no signs of cyst shrinkage (X-ray, ultrasound or CT) within 3 cycles, further improvement of cysts in the liver, lung or peritoneum are unlikely with repeated treatment; bone or brain cysts may require more prolonged treatment
- (hydatid cyst) blood counts and liver function should be monitored before start of treatment and then 2-weekly during the 28-day cycle
- (tapeworm) if tapeworm is due to *Hymenolepis nana* infestation, retreatment in 10–21 days is recommended
- therapy should be stopped if liver enzymes reach twice normal level. Therapy can be restarted when levels return to normal, but liver function must be regularly monitored during repeat therapy
- patients should be followed up after 14 days to ensure infestation has been eradicated

- patients with hydatid disease should be monitored for 2 years to detect recurrent cysts
- symptoms of neurocysticercosis may be exacerbated, or neurological symptoms, such as headaches, nausea, convulsions and visual disturbances, may be precipitated
- not recommended in children under 6 years of age
- caution if given to those with liver disease as there will be an increased risk of bone marrow depression
- caution if used in those with abnormal liver function
- contraindicated in those with hypersensitivity to albendazole or other benzimadizoles

Patient teaching and advice

- advise patients that chewable tablets can be crushed, chewed or swallowed whole and that tablets are better absorbed if taken with a fatty meal
- patient should be advised that fever may occur in the first few days of therapy
- patients should be warned against driving or operating machinery if dizziness occurs
- (neurocysticercosis) patients should be warned that neurological disturbances, such as headache, nausea, visual disturbances and seizures, may occur or initially become worse
- women of childbearing years should be counselled to use adequate contraception while taking albendazole and for 4 weeks after finishing therapy to prevent pregnancy occurring. If pregnancy is suspected, patient should be advised to consult doctor immediately. Breastfeeding should also be avoided
- see General Patient teaching and advice for helminth infestation (p. 45)

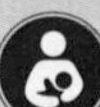

contraindicated during pregnancy

breastfeeding is not advised during or within 1 month of stopping treatment

tablets are chewable and can be crushed

IVERMECTIN (Soolantra, Stromectol)

Available forms

Tablets: 3 mg; Cream: 10 mg/g (1%)

Action

- avermectin
- inhibits signal transmission in nematodes by stimulating release of the inhibitory neurotransmitter GABA, without having any effect on mammalian neurotransmission
- half-life 12 hours; active metabolite has long half-life (3 days)
- (topical) thought to have anti-inflammatory action

Use

- onchocerciasis (*Onchocerca volvulus*) (also known as river blindness)
- intestinal strongyloidiasis (*Strongyloides stercoralis*)
- crusted scabies (with topical therapy)
- human sarcoptic scabies (where topical treatment is contraindicated or has been ineffective)
- rosacea (papulopustular) in adults > 18 years

Dose

- (strongyloidiasis) 200 microgram/kg orally as a single dose **OR**
- (onchocerciasis) 150 microgram/kg orally as a single dose (with repeated dose after 6–12 months) **OR**

- (sarcoptic scabies, mild crusted scabies) 200 microgram/kg orally given once on day 1 and repeated (second dose) between day 8 and 15 **OR**
- (moderate to severe crusted scabies) as above with third dose **OR**
- (rosacea) apply thin layer as 5 pea-sized amounts on forehead, chin, nose and each cheek (less than 1 g total) daily for up to 16 weeks

Adverse effects

Strongyloidiasis

- asthenia, fatigue
- anorexia, constipation, diarrhoea, nausea, vomiting, abdominal pain
- dizziness, somnolence, vertigo, tremor
- pruritus, rash, urticaria
- elevated liver enzymes, decreased leucocyte count

Onchocerciasis

- tachycardia, orthostatic hypotension
- headache, myalgia, peripheral and facial oedema
- abnormal eye sensation, eyelid oedema, conjunctivitis, keratitis, ocular limbitis, anterior uveitis
- eosinophilia, increased haemoglobin level
- Mazzotti reaction (pruritus, rash, urticaria, fever, oedema, lymph node enlargement and tenderness, arthralgia, synovitis)

Scabies

- exacerbation of pruritis
- headache, lethargy, listlessness, dizziness
- arthralgia
- anorexia, abdominal discomfort

Rosacea

- skin-burning sensation, skin irritation, pruritus, dry skin

Interaction

- (oral) caution if given with warfarin as INR may be increased

Nursing points/Cautions

- Mazzotti reaction is thought to be an allergic and immune response to the dead organisms. The degree of reaction may be partially determined by the type of organism, as well as the degree of infestation
- dose interval 6–12 months depending on prevalence and/or density of skin microfilariae
- (scabies) pregnant female mite burrows under stratum corneum laying eggs that mature in 14 days and emerge as adults, which can then reinvade the same host or the other host. Transmission is via intimate contact with infected person or via contaminated objects. Signs of infestation include blisters, lumps and intense pruritus. Common sites include between fingers, wrists, under arms, female breasts (particularly nipples), stomach, penis, scrotum and buttocks. In children, common sites are face, scalp, palms and soles of the feet
- (scabies) therapy should only be started when a definitive diagnosis has been made and not based solely on presence of pruritus
- (crusted scabies) scaling (harbouring mites) can be reduced by using keratolytics (e.g. 6% salicylic acid) when not treated with topical scarbicide (e.g. permethrin) (Lyclear)
- (rosacea) if no improvement is seen in 12 weeks, therapy should be discontinued
- (rosacea) course can be repeated if needed
- (cream) contains cetyl alcohol, stearyl alcohol, methyl hydroxybenzoate and propyl hydroxybenzoate, which can all cause local skin or allergic reactions
- (cream) caution if used in those with liver or kidney impairment

- caution if used in those with liver impairment
- not recommended in children under 5 years or under 15 kg
- (rosacea) only recommended for papulopustular rosacea and not other forms of rosacea or facial dermatoses
- (onchocerciasis) contraindicated in African regions where *O. volvulus* is co-endemic with *Loa loa* due to the risk of severe post-therapy encephalopathy

Patient teaching and advice

- patients should be warned against driving or operating machinery if dizziness, sleepiness, fatigue, tremor or vertigo occur
- women of childbearing years should be counselled to use adequate contraception while taking ivermectin to prevent pregnancy occurring as animal studies have shown fetal damage. If pregnancy is suspected, patient should be advised to consult doctor immediately. Breastfeeding should also be avoided
- see General Patient teaching and advice for helminth infestation (p. 45)

Scabies

- personal garments, towels and bedclothes should be washed in hot water and dried in a tumble dryer for 30 minutes on hot setting
- blankets should be drycleaned or placed in tumble dryer for 30 minutes on hot setting
- shoes and non-washable items should be placed in a tightly sealed plastic bag for 3 days
- patient should be warned that itch (pruritus) may continue for 1–2 weeks (sometimes months) after treatment has been completed and mites eliminated

Rosacea

- instruct patient to:
  - avoid eyes, eyelids, mouth and lips when applying cream to face
  - apply small amount (pea size) of cream evenly to forehead, chin, nose and each cheek
  - apply sunscreen with high protection factor (SPF 50+) to treated areas after cream has dried
  - cosmetics can also be applied once cream has dried
  - wash hands thoroughly after applying cream

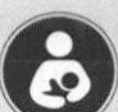

safety during pregnancy has not been established; animal studies have shown some fetal damage

only recommended during breastfeeding if benefits outweigh risks. If mother intends to breastfeed, treatment should be delayed until at least 1 week after delivery

tablets can be dispersed in water or crushed and given with a water or spoonful of yoghurt or apple puree

MEBENDAZOLE (Combantrin-1 with Mebendazole, Combantrin-1 with Mebendazole Chocolate Squares, DeWorm Chewable Tablets, Vermox)

Available forms

Tablets (chewable): 100 mg; Chocolate squares: 100 mg/square; Suspension: 100 mg/5 mL

Action

- thought to interfere with glucose uptake by worm cells during metabolism, resulting in death of worm

Use

- whipworm, roundworm and/or threadworm infestation, including mixed infestations

- hookworm (under medical supervision)

Dose (adults and children over 2 years)

Threadworm

- 100 mg orally (tablet or suspension) as single dose, repeated in 2–4 weeks to prevent reinfestation

Hookworm, roundworm, whipworm or mixed infestations

- 100 mg orally twice daily for 3 consecutive days. A second course may be necessary after 3 weeks, **OR**
- single 500 mg oral dose

Adverse effects

- nausea, abdominal pain, diarrhoea, vomiting (in those with large numbers of parasites)
- dizziness

Interaction

- plasma levels may be increased by cimetidine

Nursing points/Cautions

- course can be repeated after 2–4 weeks if infestation recurs
- caution if used in those with Crohn's disease or ulcerative colitis, as absorption may be increased. Caution also in those with liver impairment as half-life may be prolonged
- contraindicated in children under 2 years

Patient teaching and advice

- tablets may be chewed or swallowed whole
- shake suspension before use
- advise patient that it can take up to 3 days for dead worms to pass through body
- patients should be warned against driving or operating machinery if dizziness or drowsiness occurs
- women of childbearing years should be counselled to use adequate contraception while taking mebendazole. If pregnancy is suspected, patient should be advised to consult doctor immediately. Breastfeeding should also be avoided
- see General Patient teaching and advice for helminth infestation (p. 45)

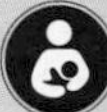

safety during pregnancy has not been established and mebendazole is therefore best avoided, especially during the first trimester. Animal studies have found it to be embryotoxic and teratogenic

not recommended during breastfeeding

tablets can be chewed

PRAZIQUANTEL (Biltricide)

Available form

Tablets: 600 mg

Action

- increases permeability of worm cell membrane to calcium, resulting in paralysis and detachment
- effect is greater in adult rather than immature worms
- treatment during acute phase of infection may not prevent progression to chronic phase

Use

- schistosoma infection (flukes)

Dose

- 20 mg/kg orally after food every 4 hours for 3 doses

Adverse effects

- headache, dizziness, drowsiness, somnolence, vertigo
- nausea, vomiting, abdominal pain, anorexia, diarrhoea
- malaise, asthenia, fever, fatigue
- myalgia

- urticaria, rash
- (rare) cardiac arrhythmias, seizures, bloody diarrhoea, mild increases in liver enzymes

Interactions

- plasma levels may be increased by cimetidine, erythromycin and itraconazole
- plasma levels may be decreased by dexamethasone, anti-epileptic agents and hydroxychloroquine
- not recommended with rifampicin
- not recommended with grapefruit juice

Nursing points/Cautions

- patient may show clinical deterioration if treatment is given during acute phase of schistosomiasis when adult worms begin to produce eggs. This deterioration can include paradoxical reactions, serum sickness and Jarisch-Herxheimer-like reaction and may be life threatening
- adverse effects may occur earlier and more frequently if infestation is severe. Adverse effects are also dependent on the species present, extent and duration of infestation and location of parasites
- if patient has cardiac irregularities, cardiac monitoring is recommended during therapy as cardiac arrhythmias may occur (although rarely)
- extra care and monitoring should occur if there is a potential for the patient to have undiagnosed neurocysticosis
- patients with known neurocysticosis should be treated in hospital setting
- tablets are triple scored to allow precise amounts to be given (¼ tablet = 150 mg)
- caution if used in those with impaired kidney or liver function
- not recommended in those with epilepsy
- contraindicated in those with ocular cysticosis as destruction of parasite may result in permanent damage

Patient teaching and advice

- warn patient against driving or operating machinery on day of treatment and the following 24 hours
- patient should be advised that tablets have a bitter taste that may result in gagging or vomiting
- tablets should be swallowed whole
- tablets are triple scored to allow precise amounts to be given (¼ tablet = 150 mg) and aid in swallowing
- warn patient to avoid grapefruit juice during therapy
- women of childbearing years should be counselled to use adequate contraception while taking praziquantel. If pregnancy is suspected, patient should be advised to consult doctor immediately. Breastfeeding should also be avoided during therapy and within 72 hours of stopping
- see General Patient teaching and advice for helminth infestation (p. 45)

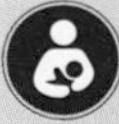

safety during pregnancy has not been established and breastfeeding should be avoided during treatment and within 72 hours of stopping treatment

PYRANTEL EMBONATE (Anthel, Combantrin Chocolate Squares, Early Bird)

Available forms

Tablets: 125 mg, 250 mg; Chocolate squares: 100 mg/square

Action

- acts at the neuromuscular junction, resulting in paralysis and immobilisation of the worm, which is then excreted in the faeces

Use

- threadworm, roundworm or hookworm infestation (ineffective against whipworm)

Dose

- 10 mg pyrantel base/kg for adults and children given in a single oral dose as tablets or chocolate squares (e.g. 70 kg adult = 7 squares)

Adverse effects

- nausea, vomiting, abdominal cramps, diarrhoea, anorexia
- dizziness, drowsiness, insomnia, headache, fatigue
- rash
- (occasionally) elevated liver enzyme levels

Nursing points/Cautions

- all family or group members should be treated, even if asymptomatic
- retreatment may be required in 7–10 days if infestation recurs after initial treatment
- (chocolate squares) dose for children and adults is based on age and weight with 1 square = 10 kg
- contraindicated in those with acute liver disease or in children under 12 months

Patient teaching and advice

- all family or group members should be treated even if asymptomatic
- may be given at any time of day, with or without food and without the need for purging
- tablets may be crushed and mixed with honey or jam for administration to young children if necessary
- see General Patient teaching and advice for helminth infestation (p. 45)

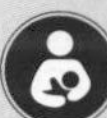

best avoided during pregnancy if possible, although animal studies have not shown teratogenic effects

safety during breastfeeding has not been established

tablets may be crushed and mixed with honey or jam for administration to young children if necessary

ANTI-ALZHEIMER'S AGENTS

In 1906, Alois Alzheimer first described the brain changes that would become known as Alzheimer's disease (AD). Dementia is an umbrella term that describes a number of conditions that result in a decline in brain functioning (AIHW 2019c). AD is the most common type of dementia, accounting for more than half of those experiencing memory loss (Seeley & Miller 2018). It appears that the cholinergic system in the cortex and limbic systems (especially the hippocampus, amygdala and basal forebrain) are damaged and destroyed by structural changes, such as atrophy, neurofibrillary tangles and beta-amyloid protein plaques (Seeley & Miller 2018). Risk factors for the development of AD include age (prevalence increases with each decade of adult life), female gender and a positive family history. A history of head trauma with concussion also appears to increase the risk of AD; however, the exact cause still remains unknown (Seeley & Miller 2018).

AD generally progresses in three stages. During the first stage there is an accumulation of protein plaques and tangles and it is usually asymptomatic. During the second stage cognitive changes start to be noticeable, although not sufficient to impair daily functioning. These changes can include repeated questions, misplacing items and memory loss. In these early stages it is often put down to 'old age'. However, once these changes become noticeable and are evident on a standardised memory test, this is considered mild cognitive impairment or early symptomatic AD. With time the disease progresses to interfere with daily activities, driving, shopping and environmental changes (such as travel, hospitalisation), making these activities problematic. Language becomes impaired over time, the person may become easily lost and confused; performing tasks that require a sequential order, solving simple puzzles or copying diagrams becomes increasing difficult. In the late stages, some people wander aimlessly, lose their ability to reason and for some, delusions, disinhibition and belligerent behaviour become increasingly common. End-stage results in the person becoming bedridden, rigid, mute, incontinent and requiring full care (Roberson 2018; Seeley & Miller 2018).

Typical duration of symptomatic AD is 8–10 years, but can range from

1–25 years. Death is usually related to complications related to immobility, such as pneumonia (Roberson 2018; Seeley & Miller 2018).

A number of drugs prevent the symptoms from worsening for a period of time, but to date there is no treatment that will prevent the progress of AD (Roberson 2018).

General Actions of anti-Alzheimer's agents (anticholinesterases)

- loss of cholinergic neurons in the central nervous system (CNS) (especially those that input from basal forebrain to hippocampus and cerebral cortex) appear to be related to impaired memory and learning, associated with AD. Centrally acting reversible anticholinesterases (cholinesterase inhibitors) increase and prolong acetylcholine levels in the brain, thereby improving cognitive function and slowing decline in function in some patients (but not all).

General Adverse effects of anti-Alzheimer's agents (anticholinesterases)

- headache, fatigue, malaise
- bradycardia, hypertension, SA/AV heart block
- nausea, diarrhoea, vomiting, abdominal disturbance, decreased appetite, constipation
- weight loss
- urinary incontinence/frequency, nocturia
- muscle cramps, muscle weakness
- increased sweating
- syncope, insomnia, dizziness, depression, somnolence, abnormal dreams, tremor
- confusion, anxiety, agitation, aggression
- (rare) extrapyramidal symptoms (especially in those with existing Parkinson's disease)

General Interactions of anti-Alzheimer's agents (anticholinesterases)

- may increase or prolong muscle relaxation if given with suxamethonium
- may antagonise action of anticholinergic agents
- not recommended with other cholinesterase inhibitors or cholinomimetic agents
- may increase risk of gastric bleeding or ulceration if given with NSAIDs
- caution if given with digoxin or beta-adrenoreceptor blocking agents as heart rate may be further decreased

General Nursing points/Cautions for anti-Alzheimer's agents (anticholinesterases)

- therapy should be supervised by a doctor who is experienced in diagnosing and caring for patients with AD
- patient requires a caregiver to supervise medication administration
- patient should be reassessed after 4 weeks of therapy to determine its effectiveness
- if patient is taking digoxin and/or beta-adrenoreceptor blocking agents concurrently, his/her pulse should be monitored to detect any decrease in heart rate
- not recommended in those recovering from GI surgery or with GI obstruction because cholinesterase inhibitors increase gastric acid secretion

- not recommended in those recovering from bladder surgery or with urinary outflow obstruction due to urinary tract adverse effects, including urinary frequency, nocturia and increased risk of urinary tract infection and incontinence
- caution if used in the immediate post-myocardial infarction period or in those with newly diagnosed atrial fibrillation, heart block (second degree or greater), unstable angina, hypokalaemia, hyperkalaemia, congestive cardiac failure, sick sinus syndrome or supraventricular cardiac conduction disorders
- caution if used in those with gastric ulcers, severe asthma, seizures, active pneumonia or chronic obstructive lung disease
- AD rarely occurs during child-bearing years, therefore pregnancy and breastfeeding advice has been omitted from this section

General Patient/Carer teaching and advice for anti-Alzheimer's agents (anticholinesterases)

- carer should be included in the patient teaching and advice as the person with AD may not remember the information
- patient should be advised not to drive or operate machinery if fatigue, dizziness or somnolence occur. AD may already compromise a person's ability to drive or operate machinery safely
- carer should be advised of the high incidence of anorexia, nausea and vomiting at the start of therapy (usually resolves in 1–2 days). Carer should be advised of the importance of close monitoring of weight during therapy, and reporting any symptoms that persist
- patient should be monitored for any fainting (syncope) or bradycardia as cardiac arrhythmias may occur
- advise patient (and carer) to report any:
  - severe and persist vomiting or diarrhoea
  - weight loss
  - difficulty passing urine or more frequent urination
  - heartburn, indigestion or stomach pain
  - new or worsening agitation or aggressive behaviour

DONEPEZIL HYDROCHLORIDE (Arazil, Aricept, Aridon APN, Donepezil AN, Donepezil-DRLA, Donepezil-GH)

Available forms
Tablets: 5 mg, 10 mg

Action
- reversible specific cholinesterase inhibitor
- see General Actions of anti-Alzheimer's agents (anticholinesterases) (p. 54)
- active metabolites
- very long half-life (about 70 hours)

Use
- mild-to-severe AD

Dose
- initially 5 mg orally nightly before retiring for 4 weeks, then increased to 10 mg orally at night if needed (daily maximum 10 mg)

Adverse effects
- (very rare) neuroleptic malignant syndrome (NMS)
- see General Adverse effects of anti-Alzheimer's agents (anticholinesterases) (p. 54)

Interactions
- see also General Interactions of anti-Alzheimer's agents (anticholinesterases) (p. 54)
- elimination may be increased by phenytoin, phenobarbital (phenobarbitone), rifampicin, dexamethasone, carbamazepine
- may increase the effects of neuromuscular blocking agents or beta-adrenoceptor blocking agents that affect cardiac conduction

Nursing points and Cautions
- see also General Nursing points/Cautions for anti-Alzheimer's agents (anticholinesterases) (p. 54)
- caution if used in those with risk of aggression as it may worsen during therapy, especially in those with severe AD
- contraindicated in those with a hypersensitivity to piperidine products

Patient/Carer teaching and advice
- carer should be advised to immediately report any unexpected high fever, muscle rigidity and altered consciousness (which may be signs of NMS)
- see also General Patient/Carer teaching and advice for anti-Alzheimer's agents (p. 55)

tablet can be dispersed in water or crushed and mixed with water or spoonful of yoghurt or apple puree

GALANTAMINE HYDROBROMIDE (Galantamine MR, Galantyl, Gamine XR, Reminyl)

Available forms
Capsules (prolonged/modified-release): 8 mg, 16 mg, 24 mg

Action
- reversible cholinesterase inhibitor
- see General Actions of anti-Alzheimer's agents (anticholinesterases) (p. 54)
- active metabolites
- half-life 7–8 hours

Use
- mild-to-moderately severe AD

Dose
- initially 8 mg orally daily with meals for 4 weeks, increasing to 16 mg daily for at least 4 weeks, increasing further to 24 mg daily if needed

Adverse effects
- see General Adverse effects of anti-Alzheimer's agents (anticholinesterases) (p. 54)
- (rare) serious skin reaction

Interactions
- bioavailability may increase if given with erythromycin, paroxetine, fluoxetine or fluvoxamine, increasing risk of cholinergic side-effects, including nausea and vomiting
- see also General Interactions of anti-Alzheimer's agents (anticholinesterases) (p. 54)

Nursing points/Cautions
- any electrolyte imbalance should be corrected before therapy is started
- if therapy is stopped for more than 2 days it should be restarted at lowest dose and gradually increased
- increasing dose slowly should decrease side-effects
- contraindicated in those with severe liver or kidney impairment
- see also General Nursing points/Cautions for anti-Alzheimer's agents (anticholinesterases) (p. 54)

Patient/Carer teaching and advice
- prolonged-release capsules should be swallowed whole, not crushed or

chewed. Capsules should not be opened
- advise patient/carer to immediately report any skin rash
- see also General Patient/Carer teaching and advice for anti-Alzheimer's agents (p. 55)

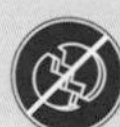

prolonged-release capsules should be swallowed whole, not crushed or chewed. Capsules should not be opened

MEMANTINE HYDROCHLORIDE (Ebixa, Memanxa)

Available forms

Tablets: 10 mg, 20 mg

Action

- N-methyl-D-aspartate (NMDA) receptor antagonist (it is thought that malfunctioning glutamatergic neurotransmission and especially NMDA receptors may be responsible for neuronal degeneration in dementia)
- protects against chronically raised levels of glutamate in the brain
- metabolites are not active
- half-life 60–100 hours

Use

- moderately severe to severe AD

Dose

- initially 5 mg orally daily for 1 week, then 10 mg daily for 1 week, then 15 mg daily (given as a 10 mg and 5 mg dose) for 1 week, then 20 mg daily as maintenance

Adverse effects

- fatigue
- peripheral oedema
- dizziness, headache, confusion
- diarrhoea, vomiting, anorexia, nausea, constipation, faecal incontinence
- agitation, insomnia, hallucinations, somnolence, sleep disorders, delusions, anxiety, depression
- abnormal gait, increased falls risk
- conjunctivitis
- coughing, bronchitis, pneumonia
- urinary incontinence, urinary tract infection
- (rare) cataract formation

Interactions

- not recommended with other NMDA receptor antagonists (e.g. ketamine, amantadine, dextromethorphan)
- may potentiate effects of levodopa, bromocriptine, amantadine or anticholinergics
- caution if given with barbiturates, antipsychotics, anti-epileptics, dantrolene or baclofen
- increased levels may occur if given with cimetidine, ranitidine, quinine and nicotine
- caution if given with warfarin as INR may be increased

Nursing points/Cautions

- therapy should be supervised by a doctor who is experienced in diagnosing and caring for patients with AD
- patient requires a caregiver to supervise medication administration
- patient should be reassessed after 4 weeks of therapy to determine its effectiveness
- dose reduction required in those with renal impairment (where creatinine clearance is less than or equal to 50 mL/minute)
- caution if used in those with recent myocardial infarction, congestive heart failure or uncontrolled hypertension
- caution if used in those with predisposing factors for seizures or epilepsy
- not recommended in those with severe liver impairment
- contraindicated in those with epilepsy (or other seizure disorders)

Patient/Carer teaching and advice

- see General Patient/Carer teaching and advice for anti-Alzheimer's agents (p. 55)

- patients/caregiver should be advised about factors that may increase urinary pH and therefore affect the elimination of memantine (e.g. change to vegetarian diet, severe urinary tract infection)

tablet can be dispersed in water or crushed and mixed with water or spoonful of yoghurt or apple puree

RIVASTIGMINE (Exelon, Exelon Patch)

Available forms

Capsules: 1.5 mg, 3 mg, 4.5 mg, 6 mg; Oral solution: 2 mg/mL; Transdermal patch: 5 (releases 4.6 mg/24 hours), 10 (releases 9.5 mg/24 hours); 15 (releases 13.3 mg/24 hours)

Action

- 'pseudo irreversible' selective cholinesterase inhibitor
- see General Actions of anti-Alzheimer's agents (anticholinesterases) (p. 54)
- half-life about 1 hour, duration of action 9 hours

Use

- mild-to-moderately severe AD

Dose

- initially 1.5 mg orally twice daily with food, increasing dose gradually every 2–4 weeks to a maximum of 6 mg twice daily if necessary, then 1.5–6 mg orally twice daily as maintenance **OR**
- initially 4.6 mg/24-hour patch applied daily for minimum of 4 weeks. If tolerated, dose is increased to 9.5 mg/24-hour patch. In moderate-to-severe AD, if well tolerated after a minimum of 4 weeks, dose can be increased to 13.3 mg/24-hour patch (transdermal patch)

Adverse effects

- (transdermal patch) erythema, pruritus
- see also General Adverse effects of anti-Alzheimer's agents (anticholinesterases) (p. 54)

Interactions

- clearance may be increased by smoking
- not recommended with metoclopramide due to increased risk of extrapyramidal symptoms
- see also General Interactions of anti-Alzheimer's agents (anticholinesterases) (p. 54)

Nursing points/Cautions

- capsules and oral solution are interchangeable (bioequivalent)
- if therapy is stopped for more than 3 days, it should be restarted at the lowest dose
- if adverse effects, such as nausea, vomiting and abdominal pain persist, dose should be reduced to previously tolerated level
- (switching from oral solution or capsules to transdermal patch) total oral daily dose 3–6 mg, switch to 4.6 mg/24-hour patch. If well tolerated after 4 weeks, dose can be increased to 9.5 mg/24-hour patch daily. If daily oral dose is 9–12 mg, switch to 9.5 mg/24-hour patch daily. If daily oral dose is 9 mg but not well tolerated, switch to 4.6 mg/24-hour patch daily and increase to 9.5 mg/24-hour patch if well tolerated after 4 weeks. First patch should be applied the day following the last oral dose
- caution if used in those with very low body weight, as adverse effects may be more pronounced
- contraindicated in those with severe liver disease or with hypersensitivity to carbamates
- (transdermal patch) contraindicated if allergic contact dermatitis has previously occurred
- see General Nursing points/Cautions for anti-Alzheimer's agents (anticholinesterases) (p. 54)

Patient/Carer teaching and advice

- see General Patient/Carer teaching and advice for anti-Alzheimer's agents (p. 55)

- if therapy is interrupted for 3 days or more, advice should be sought from doctor before giving next dose
- capsules should be swallowed whole
- oral solution can be taken directly from the dosing syringe provided or diluted with water, cola or cold orange/apple juice
- ensure patient (and carer) understands application instructions regarding transdermal patches, including:
    - ensuring previous day's patch has been removed before applying new one (to avoid overdose)
    - only one patch should be worn at a time; it is advisable to date patch
    - if patch falls off, new patch should be applied to same site for the remainder of 24-hour period
    - should be applied once daily to dry, clean, intact, hairless skin
    - any reddened, irritated or broken skin areas should be avoided
    - application sites include upper and lower back, upper arm and chest and should be rotated
    - areas that may be rubbed by tight clothing should be avoided
    - press transdermal patch firmly onto skin for at least 30 seconds until sides stick well
    - patch should not be cut into pieces
    - it is important to safely dispose of used patches (fold adhesive sides together)
- patient (and carer) should be advised to immediately report any increasing redness at patch application site, especially if it extends beyond patch size; if there is any swelling, papules or vesicles present; or if there is no improvement in skin condition 48 hours after patch removal
- if switching from oral solution or drops to patch, the first patch should be applied on the day after the last oral dose
- oral solution contains sodium benzoate, which is mildly irritating to skin, eyes and mucous membranes, and therefore care should be taken not to splash the solution and to wash area well if contact occurs

capsule can be opened and contents dispersed in water or sprinkled on spoonful of yoghurt or apple puree. Oral solution is also available

ANTIANGINAL AGENTS

Coronary artery disease is caused by an imbalance in the heart between myocardial oxygen demand and supply. Atherosclerosis causes a narrowing of the arteries due to an accumulation of plaques in the arteries, resulting in blood-flow obstruction, which is particularly evident when there is an increased demand during activity, resulting in myocardial ischaemia. Angina pectoris is a condition where myocardial blood flow is temporarily reduced, resulting in transient myocardial ischaemia. It is characterised by chest pain or discomfort described as heaviness, pressure, choking or squeezing, and rarely flank pain. It can radiate to either shoulders, both arms, jaw, neck, teeth and epigastrium. However, symptoms may be atypical in women or those with diabetes (Antman & Loscalzo 2019; Bryant et al 2019).

Angina may be subdivided into stable angina, unstable angina and variant (Prinzmetal's) angina. *Chronic stable angina* is precipitated by a known cause (e.g. exercise, heavy meal, exposure to the cold, emotional stress), and eased by rest and nitrate treatment. *Unstable angina* has symptoms that are intermediate, between those of stable angina and myocardial infarction; that is, previously stable angina occurs more frequently, lasts longer, is of greater intensity, and/or nitrate treatment is no longer as effective. The coronary artery/arteries have become so occluded that they can no longer meet the heart's oxygen demand, increasing the person's risk of myocardial infarction, especially if angina occurs at rest. *Variant* (*Prinzmetal's* or *vasospastic*) angina is caused by coronary artery spasm, which may or may not be related to atherosclerosis. This type of angina often occurs at rest and usually during the night or in the early hours of the day with chest discomfort that is more severe than with stable angina. In some people, it is related to the atherosclerotic lesion being near the site of the spasm. Prolonged vasospasm may lead to heart block, ventricular arrhythmias or death (Jameson et al 2020; Katzung 2018).

The main aims of antianginal treatment are to manage the acute pain and prevent further attacks by improving perfusion (by relaxing the smooth muscle of the coronary artery) or by reducing the metabolic demand on the heart, or both (Bryant et al 2019). However, the antianginal agents treat the symptoms, not the cause of the problem. The main pharmacological agents used to treat angina include the organic nitrates (glyceryl trinitrate, isosorbide dinitrate and isosorbide mononitrate) and calcium-channel blockers (verapamil, diltiazem and amlodipine) (see Antihypertensive agents, p. 520).

General Patient teaching and advice for antianginal agents

- ensure that patient understands the importance of lifestyle (diet, exercise, weight reduction, smoking cessation) and risk factors (blood pressure, cholesterol/lipid and diabetes control, sleep apnoea treatment) modification as an important part of overall management of chronic stable angina
- emphasise the importance of the patient telling his/her doctor or healthcare professional if angina attacks continue or become more frequent despite taking medication as prescribed
- warn patient against driving or operating machinery if dizziness or lightheadedness occurs
- instruct patient to take care when first taking medication, not to overdo physical activities and to be especially careful when standing up or getting out of bed, as dizziness, lightheadedness or fainting can occur
- ensure that patient understands the difference between medications that are used to treat sudden (acute) angina attack and those that are meant to reduce the frequency of attacks
- alcohol should generally be avoided as this increases the feeling of being dizzy or faint
- ensure that patient understands the importance of having a sufficient supply of medication, especially over a weekend or during holidays
- see also General Patient teaching and advice (p. xxvii)

GLYCERYL TRINITRATE (often abbreviated to GTN) (known as nitroglycerin in USA) (DBL Glyceryl Trinitrate Concentrate Injection, Minitran, Nitrolingual Pump Spray, Nitrostat, Transiderm-Nitro)

Available forms

Sublingual tablets: 300 microgram, 600 microgram; Metered dose pump spray: 400 microgram/dose; Transdermal patch: 5 mg/24 hrs, 10 mg/24 hrs, 15 mg/24 hrs; Ampoules: 50 mg/10 mL

Action

- organic nitrate relaxes smooth muscle, including vascular muscle, causing vasodilation of peripheral arteries and veins. At low doses, the effect is venodilation, whereas at higher doses, arterial dilation occurs
- decreases cardiac output and arterial pressure, which results in decreased oxygen demand on myocardium
- also dilates normal coronary and coronary collateral vessels, increasing perfusion and oxygen delivery to ensure efficient distribution to ischaemic areas of heart
- does not change contractility or heart rate
- may relieve variant angina by relaxing coronary arteries that are in spasm
- (sublingual tablets) onset of action 1–3 minutes, duration 30–60 minutes
- (sublingual spray) onset of action 2–4 minutes, duration less than 60 minutes
- sublingual spray absorbed rapidly from the oral mucosa, bypassing the liver to reach the vascular system

- (transdermal) onset of action greater than 4 hours, duration 8–24 hours
- transdermally, drug is continuously absorbed through the skin and reaches target organs before being inactivated by the liver
- (IV) onset of action 1–2 minutes, duration 3–5 minutes (although this is dependent on duration of infusion)

Use

- prophylaxis and treatment of angina pectoris (symptom preventer (transdermal patch) and reliever (sublingual tablets and spray, IV))
- (IV) angina pectoris refractory to other treatments, left ventricular failure or congestive heart failure associated with acute myocardial infarction, or control of perioperative hypertension associated with surgical procedures, to produce controlled hypotension during neurosurgery and orthopaedic surgery

Dose

Treatment of acute attack

- (sublingual tablets) 600–900 microgram under the tongue (300 microgram in elderly) or in the cheek (buccal) pouch and allowed to dissolve, at the first sign of an attack or if about to undertake an activity known to cause an attack. Dose may be repeated at 5-minute intervals during acute attack (maximum 1200–1800 microgram) **OR**
- (sublingual spray) (therapeutic) 1 spray (400 microgram) under the tongue from a metered dose aerosol at the first sign of an attack, followed by a second spray if pain is not relieved within 5 minutes **OR**
- initially 5 microgram/min (if using a non-adsorbing set), increasing by 5 microgram/min every 3–5 minutes until response is noted; maintain adequate systemic blood pressure and coronary perfusion pressure. If no response at 20 microgram/min, increases of 10 microgram/min can be made. Once a partial BP response is seen, dose should be decreased and interval between doses lengthened

Prophylaxis

- (sublingual spray) (prophylactic) 1–2 sprays (400–800 microgram) under the tongue from a metered dose aerosol before engaging in activities known to cause an attack **OR**
- (transdermal patch) initially patch releasing 5 mg/24 hours is applied once daily and left in situ for 12 hours (dose can then be titrated according to clinical response)

Adverse effects

- throbbing headache (requires dose reduction)
- flushing of the face and neck
- tachycardia, dizziness, restlessness
- orthostatic hypotension, syncope
- nausea, vomiting
- (rare) bradycardia, rash, blurred vision, dry mouth, severe/prolonged headache, methaemoglobinaemia
- tolerance, cross-tolerance to other nitrates/nitrites
- (abrupt withdrawal) angina, exacerbation of Raynaud's phenomenon (in susceptible people) (see Glossary)
- (transdermal patch/pad) skin irritation, erythema, pruritus, burning sensation, sensitisation phenomena
- (IV) bradycardia, hypotension retrosternal discomfort, abdominal pain, apprehension, restlessness, muscle twitching, alcohol intoxication, hyperosmolarity, nausea, vomiting, dizziness

Interactions

- contraindicated with phosphodiesterase-5 (PDE-5) inhibitors (sildenafil, vardenafil or tadalafil)
- increased risk of orthostatic hypotension and syncope if used with alcohol, calcium-channel blockers, antihypertensive agents, hydralazine, levodopa, opioid analgesics, phenothiazines, prazosin, minoxidil, antipsychotics or TCAs

- effect may be decreased if given with aspirin and other NSAIDs, levodopa, opioid analgesics and hydralazine
- ergot alkaloids may antagonise effects leading to coronary vasoconstriction
- antianginal effects may be reduced by sympathomimetic agents
- hypotension may occur if given with sympathomimetic agents
- may potentiate anticholinergic effects of TCAs
- may decrease effects of heparin
- (IV) may slow morphine metabolism, increasing the risk of overdose and respiratory depression
- may decrease the effect of noradrenaline (norepinephrine)
- (IV) increases neuromuscular blockade induced by pancuronium
- may cause false result on serum cholesterol test (ZlatkisZak colour reaction)
- may give falsely elevated serum triglyceride results

Nursing points/Cautions

- any hypovolemia should be corrected before starting therapy to decrease risk of hypotension
- tolerance may occur, although less likely with intermittent therapy
- ensure the patient receives written instructions and understands the 'Patient teaching and advice' information
- withdrawal should be gradual, reducing dose over 4–6 weeks to prevent withdrawal reaction
- sublingual medication ineffective if swallowed because the bioavailability is reduced by extensive first-pass metabolism
- patient may sit or lie down for 10–20 minutes after taking tablets to avoid dizziness
- sublingual spray is more stable than sublingual tablets and patient may therefore receive a higher dose, increasing the risk of possible side-effects such as headache when transferring from tablet to spray medication
- (transdermal patch) if there are any signs of hypotension or collapse, remove transdermal patch and place patient in a recumbent position with legs raised
- (transdermal patch) should be removed before cardioversion, DC defibrillation or diathermy to prevent burning
- (IV) continuously monitor heart rate, blood pressure, pulmonary capillary wedge pressure and chest pain, especially at the start of infusion and after a dose increase
- (IV) significant amounts of glyceryl trinitrate are adsorbed by PVC plastics, so dilute and store in glass parenteral solution bottles only and avoid using filters
- (IV) greatest adsorption by PVC occurs when the concentration of glyceryl trinitrate is high, the rate is low and the tubing is long
- (IV) if using a peristaltic action pump, follow the manufacturer's instructions closely, especially if non-adsorbing (non-PVC) tubing is used, as it is less pliable
- (IV) check the administration set for compatibility with the IV infusion solution and that it is recommended for use
- (IV) line should be flushed or replaced if concentration of solution is altered
- (IV) dosage must be carefully titrated to prevent profound fall in BP
- (IV) must be further diluted before infusing by adding 50 mg (10 mL) ampoule to 490 mL of either glucose 5% or sodium chloride 0.9% to make a concentration of 100 microgram/mL; invert prepared solution several times for uniform dilution

- (IV) administer alone
- (IV) solution diluted with sodium chloride 0.9% or dextrose 5% is stable
- (IV) not given by direct IV injection
- caution if used in industrial workers who may have had long-term high-dose exposure to organic nitrates as tolerance may occur
- cross-tolerance between organic nitrates or nitrites may occur
- increased risk of methaemoglobinaemia if used in those with impaired liver function or if given in high doses
- abrupt withdrawal may precipitate angina and also Raynaud's phenomenon in those who are susceptible
- caution if used in those with increased intraocular pressure (glaucoma), impaired liver function, recent head trauma, lung disease, cor pulmonale, anaemia, hyperthyroidism, hypothyroidism, hypothermia, hypoxaemia, ventilation perfusion imbalance, malnutrition, cerebral vascular disease or severe coronary atherosclerosis
- not recommended within 24 hours of myocardial infarction as severe arterial hypotension with bradycardia may occur
- contraindicated in severe hypotension (systolic BP < 90mm Hg), marked anaemia, uncorrected hypovolaemia, hypertrophic obstructive cardiomyopathy, cardiogenic shock, arterial hypoxaemia, cerebral haemorrhage or raised intracranial pressure caused by head trauma, constrictive pericarditis and pericardial tamponade, cardiogenic shock, primary pulmonary hypertension, obstructive myocardial failure (including aortic or mitral valve stenosis), acute circulatory failure or hypersensitivity to nitrates
- (transdermal patch) contraindicated in those with allergy to adhesive

Patient teaching and advice

- see also General Patient teaching and advice for antifungal agents (p. 58)

Sublingual tablets

- take tablet as early in the attack as possible, preferably while sitting down
- if preventing an attack, take tablet just before exercise or other situation which is a known trigger
- do not swallow tablet, but allow to dissolve under the tongue or in pouch of cheek (ineffective if swallowed)
- do not eat, drink or smoke while tablet is dissolving
- 1/2 tablet (300 microgram) may be adequate early in onset or for an elderly person; tablets are scored and easily broken in half
- once pain is relieved or if headache becomes severe, the tablet may be removed or swallowed
- if angina is not relieved in 5 minutes, take a second tablet
- if 2 fresh tablets and resting do not relieve the chest pain within 10 minutes, an ambulance should be called
- it is important that the tablets/spray are carried with the person at all times
- ensure that the patient understands that the tablets can lose their strength if not stored correctly and therefore will not work during an angina attack. It is important to keep tablets airtight in the manufacturer's bottle (do not place tablets in other pill containers) and do not put other drugs or any materials apart from the manufacturer's packing into the bottle
- lid should be kept tightly closed
- store in a cool place; do not keep close to the body (e.g. in a pocket) or in direct sunlight

- unopened bottle has shelf-life of 2 years if stored below 25°C
- if tablets are unused 3 months after first opening, the bottle should be discarded and a fresh supply obtained; it is important to write the date of opening on the bottle as a reminder
- tell anyone else who lives in the house or visits regularly where the main supply is kept in case they need to find the medication in an emergency

Sublingual spray

- advise patient that spray pump should be primed by pressing nozzle 5 times before first use
- if pump has not been used for 7 days, priming with 1 spray may be necessary; if pump has been unused for more than 4 months, it should be primed with up to 5 sprays until spray is even
- spray under the tongue at the onset of the attack, preferably while sitting down
- keep canister vertical with nozzle uppermost and the nozzle opening as close to the mouth as possible
- spray under the tongue or onto the oral mucosa, then close the mouth immediately after each dose
- the spray should not be inhaled
- avoid swallowing immediately after spraying dose
- replace plastic cap after use
- if pain persists after 2 metered doses, an ambulance should be called immediately
- store canister in cool, dry place at < 20°C

Transdermal patch

- ensure patient understands that transdermal patches are not suitable for acute angina attacks
- it is important to allow a 12-hour nitrate-free period (usually at night) per 24 hours to decrease the risk of nitrate tolerance developing (leading to decreased effectiveness of nitrate); however, nocturnal angina may occur in some patients
- ensure that the old patch is removed before applying a new one. Skin may feel warm or dry or look red when old patch is removed, but this will quickly disappear
- instruct patient to wash skin with soap and water and dry thoroughly before applying patch. Skin should be cool (wait a few minutes after bath or shower) and free from any creams, lotions or oils
- separate the protective foil cover and apply to a hairless skin site not subject to excessive movement/ sweating, preferably the chest or inner aspect of arm (shave if necessary). Skin folds, scars, burned or irritated areas should not be used
- patch is designed to be used as a complete unit and should not be cut or trimmed
- patch is applied once each day only; if it loosens or falls off for any reason, apply a new one
- wash hands thoroughly before and after applying patch
- patient can bathe or shower with patch in place
- rotate application site each day to avoid undue skin irritation
- if the patch is forgotten, apply as soon as it is remembered (elderly patients may be advised to write the date on the patch before applying). Two patches should not be used if a dose is forgotten
- used patch should be disposed of appropriately as they still contain glyceryl trinitrate
- used and unused patches should be kept out of the reach of children at all times
- store patches in cool place to avoid extremes of temperature and humidity but do not refrigerate

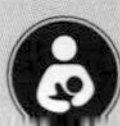
only recommended during pregnancy if benefits are thought to outweigh risks

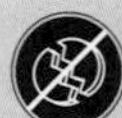
sublingual tablets should not be crushed

Note
- glyceryl trinitrate is also available as a topical rectal agent (Rectogesic) used for treatment of anal fissure and post-haemorrhoidectomy

ISOSORBIDE DINITRATE (Isordil)

ISOSORBIDE MONONITRATE (Duride, Imdur Durules, Isobide MR, Isomonit, Monodur Durules)

Available forms
Tablets: 10 mg; Tablets (sustained-release): 60 mg, 120 mg; Sublingual tablets: 5 mg

Action
- organic nitrate
- isosorbide mononitrate is an active metabolite of isosorbide dinitrate
- relaxes vascular smooth muscle producing arterial and venodilation
- may redistribute coronary blood flow, selectively dilating coronary or coronary collateral vessels, increasing perfusion and oxygen delivery, ensuring efficient distribution to ischaemic areas of the heart
- reduces myocardial oxygen demand
- slower onset of action but longer duration than glyceryl trinitrate
- (sublingual) onset of action within 2–5 minutes, duration of 1–2 hours
- (oral) onset of action 15–40 minutes, duration of 4–6 hours
- (controlled-release tablets) onset of action within 1–2 hours, duration up to 24 hours
- half-life is biphasic (first phase 1.1 hours, second phase 7.7 hours)

Use
- prophylaxis and treatment of angina pectoris
- myocardial ischaemia due to ischaemic heart disease
- acute and chronic congestive heart failure
- (adjunctive therapy) left ventricular failure

Dose
Acute angina
- 5–10 mg sublingually 2–3-hourly

Prophylactic treatment of angina pectoris, myocardial ischaemia
- initially 60 mg orally daily increasing to 120 mg if needed (sustained-release tablets) **OR**
- 5–30 mg orally 4 times daily

Acute left ventricular failure
- 5–10 mg sublingually every 2 hours or as needed

Chronic left ventricular failure
- initially 5–10 mg sublingually every 2 hours or as needed, then 20–40 mg orally 4 times daily (maintenance)

Adverse effects
- headache, flushing of face
- vertigo, fainting
- dizziness
- postural hypotension, tachycardia, peripheral oedema
- nausea, vomiting, diarrhoea, dyspepsia, poor appetite, gastrointestinal disturbances
- sleep disturbances, tiredness
- rash, pruritus
- (abrupt withdrawal) increased frequency of angina tolerance
- (uncommon) haemolytic anaemia (in those with glucose-6-phosphate dehydrogenase (G6PD))

Interactions
- contraindicated with phosphodiesterase type 5 (PDE-5) inhibitors (sildenafil, vardenafil or tadalafil)
- increased risk of hypotension if given with TCAs, anticholinergics,

phenothiazines or antihypertensive agents, including calcium-channel blocker
- alcohol may increase vasodilation, leading to hypotension
- effect may be decreased if given with aspirin and other NSAIDs, levodopa, opioid analgesics and hydralazine
- (sustained-release) action may be enhanced if given with methionine, captopril or acetylcysteine, including risk of hypotension
- caution if used with propranolol in those with cirrhosis and portal hypertension
- improved left ventricular function may occur if the SR preparation is given with verapamil-like calcium-channel blockers

Nursing points/Cautions

- any hypovolemia should be corrected before starting therapy
- ensure that correct tablet is administered via the correct route (i.e. some brands have formulations that are sublingual, immediate-release or sustained-release)
- sustained-release (SR) preparations are only recommended for stable chronic angina (not variant angina or management of acute angina)
- (sustained-release) if headache occurs, dose may be reduced
- caution if used in industrial workers who may have had long-term high-dose exposure to organic nitrates as tolerance may occur
- cross-tolerance between organic nitrates or nitrites may occur
- tolerance may be prevented by having a 10–12-hour nitrate-free period in every 24 hours
- withdrawal should be gradual over 2 weeks to prevent increase in frequency of angina
- (cardiac failure) pulmonary capillary pressure should not be allowed to fall below 15 mmHg or systolic BP below physiological range for normal or hypertensive patient. If patient has pre-existing hypotension, range should be 90–100 mmHg
- caution if used in those with G6PD as haemolytic anaemia may occur
- caution if used in patients with hypoxia
- caution if used in those with kidney impairment as accumulation of active metabolite may occur
- caution if given to those with severe coronary or cerebral arteriosclerosis, or pronounced mitral stenosis
- not recommended in those with acute myocardial infarction or congestive cardiac failure
- contraindicated in those with hypersensitivity to nitrates, cardiogenic shock, hypotension, obstructive hypertrophic cardiomyopathy, constrictive pericardial tamponade or pericarditis, isolated right ventricular failure, uncorrected hypovolaemia, severe anaemia, intracranial hypertension or arterial hypoxaemia

Patient teaching and advice

- see General Patient teaching and advice for antianginal agents (p. 58)
- if angina attack is not relieved after taking 1–2 sublingual tablets and resting, an ambulance should be called immediately
- instruct patient that only sublingual tablets should be used for acute attack, whereas oral tablets are used to reduce the number of angina attacks
- SR preparations should only be taken once daily and are used to reduce the number of angina attacks
- sustained-release tablets should not be crushed, broken or chewed; however, 60 mg SR preparations (but NOT 120 mg SR preparations) are scored and may be halved without

altering properties if not crushed during the splitting process
- advise patient that reducing the dose, plus simple analgesics (such as paracetamol) may be required if headache is severe

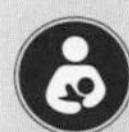

safety during pregnancy and breastfeeding has not been established, therefore not recommended unless the expected benefit outweighs any potential risk

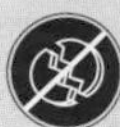

sublingual and sustained-release tablets should not be crushed

IVABRADINE (Coralan)

Available forms
Tablets: 5 mg, 7.5 mg

Action
- selective I_f channel inhibitor that slows heart rate (by about 10 beats/min) by selectively inhibiting cardiac pacemaker in the sinus node, reducing cardiac workload and therefore myocardial oxygen consumption
- may also interact with retinal current I_h which resembles cardiac I_f resulting in visual adverse effects
- no effect on intra-atrial, AV or intraventricular conduction times, myocardial contractility or ventricular repolarisation
- half-life about 11 hours

Use
- chronic stable angina (in those with normal sinus rhythm who cannot take beta-adrenergic blocking agents or with atenolol when heart rate is ≥ 70 bpm but angina is not controlled)
- chronic heart failure (with left ventricular injection fraction ≤ 35%, sinus rhythm and HR ≥ 77 bpm)

Dose
- (angina) initially 5 mg orally twice daily with meals, increasing after 3–4 weeks depending on HR and response (alone or with atenolol 50 mg) **OR**
- (chronic heart failure) initially 5 mg orally twice daily with meals, increasing/decreasing dose after 2 weeks (depending on HR)

Adverse effects
- blurred vision, transient luminous phenomena (transient enhanced brightness in a limited area of the visual field triggered by sudden variations in light intensity, halo, stroboscopic effects, coloured bright lights, multiple images)
- bradycardia, ventricular extrasystole, tachycardia, AV first-degree block, unstable or aggravated angina, cardiac failure, atrial fibrillation, inadequate BP control
- headache, dizziness
- (uncommon) prolonged QT interval

Interactions
- contraindicated with itraconazole, clarithromycin, macrolide antibiotics, ciclosporin, gestodene and antiretroviral agents
- contraindicated with calcium-channel blockers such as diltiazem or verapamil, as further heart rate lowering may occur
- not recommended with agents that prolong QT interval (e.g. disopyramide, sotalol, amiodarone, TCAs, antipsychotic agents, IV erythromycin, pentamidine, mefloquine) or agents that cause hypokalaemia (e.g. diuretics, stimulant laxatives, corticosteroids, amphotericin B (amphotericin))
- should not be taken with grapefruit or grapefruit juice as increased serum levels may occur
- metabolism may be increased if given with rifampicin, barbiturates, phenytoin or St John's wort requiring a dose adjustment
- bioavailability may be reduced if given with carbamazepine

Nursing points/Cautions

- any heart failure should be stabilised before starting therapy
- serial HR, ECG or ambulatory BP monitoring is recommended before starting or titrating therapy
- therapy should not be started if resting HR < 70 bpm
- dose titration is according to resting HR:
    - if persistently ≥ 60 bpm (still symptomatic, initial dose well tolerated), dose should be increased to 7.5 mg
    - if 50–60 bpm, dose should be maintained
    - if < 50 bpm rest or patient has symptoms of bradycardia (e.g. dizziness, fatigue, hypotension), dose should be reduced (minimum daily dose 2.5 mg). If bradycardia or heart rate continues below 50 bpm, therapy should be stopped
- transient luminous phenomena usually occur in the first 8 weeks of therapy and last about 12 weeks
- (angina) if no response and angina continues after 12 weeks, therapy should be stopped
- caution in those with aortic stenosis, second-degree heart block, hypertrophic cardiomyopathy, mild-to-moderate hypotension, heart failure, asymptomatic left ventricular dysfunction, end-stage renal failure, moderate liver impairment or retinitis pigmentosa
- not recommended in those with atrial fibrillation or other cardiac arrhythmias that interfere with sinus node function, immediately after stroke or surgery (cardiac or non-cardiac), or QT prolongation (if used, cardiac monitoring is strongly recommended)
- contraindicated in those with galactose intolerance, Lapp lactase deficiency or glucose–galactose malabsorption as tablets contain lactose
- contraindicated in those with artificial pacemaker or sick sinus syndrome, third-degree AV block, unstable or acute heart failure, resting heart rate less than 70 bpm, severe hypotension (less than 90/50), unstable angina, cardiogenic shock, acute myocardial infarction, sinoatrial block, severe liver impairment, hypertrophic cardiomyopathy (unless co-existing coronary artery disease is proven)

Patient teaching and advice

- see General Patient teaching and advice for antianginal agents (p. 58)
- patient should be advised to report immediately any:
    - fatigue or dizziness (signs of bradycardia)
    - sudden changes in vision including blurred vision, halo, coloured flashes, multiple/distorted images or bright spots of light (especially when moving quickly between dim and bright light)
    - palpitations or abnormal heartbeat
- warn patients not to drive or operate machinery in situations where light intensity may vary suddenly, including at night, if visual changes (transient luminous phenomena) occur
- advise patient to avoid grapefruit and grapefruit juice during therapy
- ensure that patient understands that this medication is not to be used in the event of an acute angina attack
- female patient of childbearing potential should be counselled to use adequate contraception during therapy to avoid pregnancy

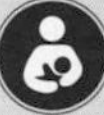

contraindicated during pregnancy and breastfeeding

tablet does not disperse easily, but can be crushed to fine powder and mixed with spoonful of yoghurt or apple puree

NICORANDIL (Ikorel, Ikotab)

Available forms

Tablets: 10 mg, 20 mg

Action

- nitrate properties
- opens ATP-dependent potassium channels in blood vessels, leading to arterial dilation and reduced myocardial afterload
- relaxes vascular smooth muscle, improves blood flow and oxygenation
- reduces coronary artery spasm
- rapidly absorbed with biphasic half-life (first phase about 1 hour, second phase 8–24 hours)

Use

- chronic stable angina pectoris

Dose

- initially 5–10 mg orally twice daily increasing to 10–20 mg twice daily if needed

Adverse effects

- headache, dizziness, vertigo, weakness, lethargy
- infection
- vasodilation/flush, palpitations, hypertension, chest pain, angina
- dyspepsia, nausea, vomiting, abdominal pain, weight loss
- myalgia, back pain
- dyspnoea, bronchitis, respiratory disorder
- hyperkalaemia
- (uncommon) ulceration (skin, gastrointestinal, mucosal, corneal, conjunctival)
- (rare) gastrointestinal bleeding, tinnitus, hepatitis, jaundice
- (high dose) hypotension

Interactions

- contraindicated with PDE-5 inhibitors (sildenafil, vardenafil or tadalafil)
- increased risk of gastric ulceration or gastrointestinal perforation if given with corticosteroids, NSAIDs or aspirin
- caution if given with nitrates due to risk of additive hypotension occurring
- caution if given with other agents causing hyperkalaemia
- caution if given with antihypertensive agents

Nursing points/Cautions

- risk of headache may be decreased by starting at a low dose, or if headache is severe the dosage is reduced
- caution in patients with low blood volume, low systolic BP (below 100 mmHg) or liver impairment
- caution if used in those with diverticular disease due to increased risk of fistula formation or bowel perforation
- contraindicated in those with cardiogenic shock, hypotension, acute myocardial infarction with left ventricular failure (with low filling pressure and hypovolaemia) or hypersensitivity to nicotinamide or nicotinic acid

Patient teaching and advice

- see General Patient teaching and advice for antianginal agents (p. 58)
- warn patient that headache commonly occurs at the start, but usually goes with continued therapy. If headache continues or worsens, patient should be advised to seek medical advice
- patients should be advised to immediately report any:
  - skin ulceration, mouth, genital or anal ulcers
  - ringing in ears
  - dark bowel motions, bloody diarrhoea
- ensure that patient understands that this medication is not to be used in the event of an acute angina attack

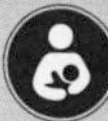

safety during pregnancy and breastfeeding has not been established, therefore not recommended unless the expected benefit outweighs any potential risk

tablet can be dispersed in water (6 minutes) or crushed and mixed with spoonful of yoghurt or apple puree

PERHEXILINE MALEATE (Pexsig)

Available form

Tablets: 100 mg

Action

- non-selective calcium-channel blocker
- appears to increase glucose utilisation, thereby decreasing oxygen demand and increasing myocardial efficiency
- reduces exercise-induced tachycardia, but does not affect resting heart rate
- mild diuretic properties
- half-life 2–6 days, but is variable (up to 30 days)
- narrow therapeutic index

Use

- reduce frequency of moderate-to-severe angina attacks resistant to conventional treatment and not suitable for coronary bypass surgery

Dose

- initially 100 mg orally daily, then adjust dose up or down at 2–4-week intervals depending on response and plasma levels (daily maximum 300–400 mg)

Adverse effects

Short term (within 24 hours)

- anorexia, nausea, vomiting, weight loss
- transient dizziness, headache, gait disorders, unsteadiness, drunken sensation
- hypoglycaemia (patients with diabetes)

Long term (≥ 12 weeks of continuous therapy)

- cirrhosis, hepatotoxicity (severe and occasionally fatal), elevated liver enzymes, bilirubin, total lipids and triglycerides
- peripheral neuropathy, muscle weakness, ataxia
- extrapyramidal dysfunction
- alterations to ECG

Interactions

- hypoglycaemia may occur if given with hypoglycaemic agents such as insulin or sulfonylureas or beta-adrenoceptor blocking agents
- concurrent use with doxorubicin may lead to doxorubicin toxicity
- increased risk of perhexiline toxicity if given with SSRIs
- increased serum transaminases may occur if given with warfarin
- caution if given with TCAs, tetracyclic antidepressants, antiviral agents, antimalarial agents, antiemetics, antiarrhythmic agents, opioid analgesics, cytotoxic agents or neuroleptic agents
- may interfere with ECG, with a slight depression of the T wave and prolonged QT interval

Nursing points/Cautions

- serum liver enzymes should be measured before therapy and monitored monthly thereafter
- plasma perhexiline levels should be monitored at the end of the first week and then monthly and maintained between 0.15 and 0.6 microgram/mL
- monitor at least monthly and stop therapy if any of the following occur:
  - peripheral neuropathy (e.g. numbness or tingling of feet/hands, muscle weakness, paraesthesia)
  - papilloedema
  - hepatic toxicity (e.g. weakness, loss of appetite, weight loss, persistent

- elevation of serum enzymes or abnormal liver function tests)
  - excessive weight loss
  - persistent or marked hypoglycaemia
- dose increases should only occur if plasma level is subtherapeutic and therapy has been in place for 2–4 weeks
- doses > 100 mg daily are administered as divided dose
- caution if used in ventricular conduction disturbances after myocardial infarction as they may be aggravated
- caution if used in those with diabetes mellitus
- contraindicated in those with porphyria, kidney or liver impairment or if plasma level monitoring is not available

Patient teaching and advice

- see General Patient teaching and advice for antianginal agents (p. 58)
- ensure patient understands the importance of regular blood tests
- advise patient to seek medical advice immediately if any of the following occur:
  - muscle weakness, numbness or tingling of hands or feet, difficulty walking
  - loss of appetite, nausea, yellowing of eyes/skin, dark urine, upper abdominal pain
  - excessive weight loss
- patients with diabetes (especially if taking insulin and/or sulfonylureas) should be instructed to closely monitor blood glucose levels for hypoglycaemia throughout therapy, especially in first 3 days
- ensure patient understands this medication is not to be used for an acute angina attack

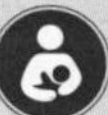

not recommended during pregnancy or breastfeeding unless expected benefit outweighs any potential risk

tablet can be crushed and mixed with water or spoonful of yoghurt or apple puree

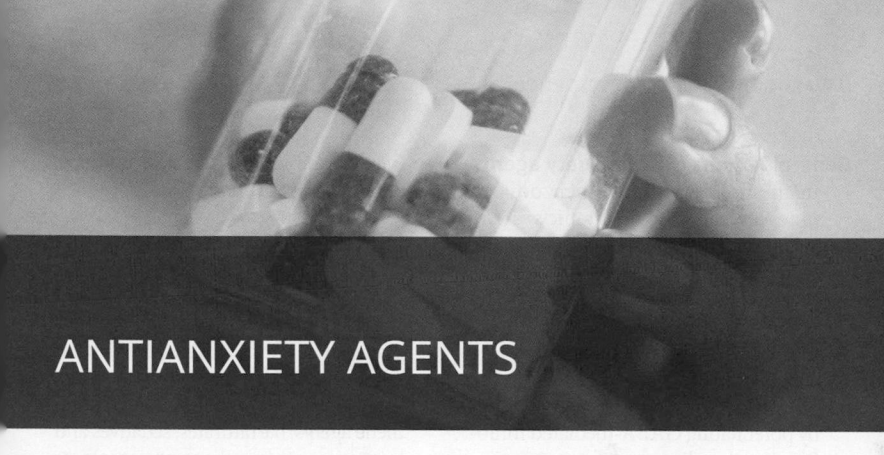

ANTIANXIETY AGENTS

In 2017–18 there were 4.8 million Australians (20.1%) who reported a mental or behavioural condition, with anxiety being the most frequently reported (3.2 million, 13.1% of the population), up from 2.6 million in 2014–15. About 1 in 20 (5.1% Australians) had both an anxiety-related condition and mood (affective) disorder (such as depression). Women reported anxiety-related conditions more commonly than males (15.7% compared with 10.6%), with younger women (15–24 years) reporting anxiety at a rate of almost 19% (ABS 2019).

Anxiety is a normal human response to a personally threatening situation, such as a threat to one's health, loved ones, job or lifestyle (e.g. performance in exams, moving house, changing job, illness), and can in some instances improve a person's performance because of the increased alertness (e.g. exams, sport, job interview). However, in some instances high levels of anxiety can decrease a person's ability to think clearly, plan or carry out complex tasks, leading to distress and disability (Andrews et al 2018).

Anxiety disorders include generalised anxiety disorder, obsessive-compulsive disorder (OCD), panic disorder, social anxiety disorder, specific phobias, separation anxiety, post-traumatic stress disorder (PTSD) and acute stress. Anxiety can also be experienced as part of other psychiatric or mental disorders such as depression (Shelton 2019).

Management can be either pharmacological with antianxiety (or anxiolytic) agents and/or non-pharmacological, including counselling, stress management, relaxation techniques, graded exposure (e.g. to the cause of the specific phobia) and cognitive behaviour therapy (Shelton 2019).

The main pharmacological agents used to manage anxiety are the selective serotonin reuptake inhibitors (SSRIs) and serotonin and norepinephrine reuptake inhibitors (SNRI) venlafaxine (see Antidepressants p. 287) and benzodiazepines. The choice of agent is dependent on the specific anxiety disorder. For example, benzodiazepines are prescribed for acute situations (rather than chronic) in the treatment of generalised anxiety disorder, to control symptoms and allow the person to return to normal functioning, and should then be discontinued gradually (Shelton 2019).

It should be noted that antianxiety agents are not recommended for the management of everyday stress or tension.

General Actions of antianxiety agents

- main sites of action of benzodiazepines appear to be the limbic system, thalamus and spinal cord
- suppression of the limbic system is thought to prevent stimulation of the reticular activating centre, resulting in drowsiness
- agents bind to specific receptors in the central nervous system (CNS), either by potentiating GABA-mediated inhibition or by directly affecting action potential
- agents produce muscle relaxation, sedative-hypnotic effect, antegrade amnesia, anti-convulsant properties and decreased anxiety

General Adverse effects of antianxiety agents

- (most common) drowsiness, fatigue, dizziness, light-headedness, muscle weakness/spasm, ataxia, nervousness, irritability
- headache, tremor, confusion, transient amnesia, insomnia, slurred speech, blurred vision, diplopia, reduced alertness, decreased coordination, slowed reaction time
- depression, irritability, disturbed dreams, anxiety, altered mood
- nausea, vomiting, anorexia, diarrhoea, dry mouth
- urinary retention/incontinence
- altered libido, sexual dysfunction
- menstrual irregularities
- rash, dermatitis, pruritus
- risk of dependence (physical and psychological) and tolerance (with chronic use)
- (rare) hypotension, respiratory depression, paradoxical reaction (e.g. excitation, stimulation, acute rage, agitation, increased anxiety), increased intraocular pressure
- (very rare) blood dyscrasias, jaundice, abnormal liver function

General Interactions of antianxiety agents

- may increase CNS depression if given with alcohol (acute intake), opioid analgesics, some antihistamines, antidepressants (tricyclic, non-selective MAOIs), muscle relaxants, antipsychotics, anaesthetic agents, barbiturates, sedatives and hypnotics, other antianxiety agents or phenothiazines
- increased plasma level may result if given with amiodarone, azole antifungals, calcium-blocking agents (e.g. verapamil, nifedipine), ciclosporin, cimetidine, diltiazem, disulfiram, ergotamine, fluvoxamine, HIV protease inhibitors (e.g. ritonavir), isoniazid, macrolide antibiotics (e.g. erythromycin), grapefruit juice, oestrogens, oral contraceptives
- benzodiazepines may increase the anticholinergic effects of atropine or atropine-like agents, antihistamines or antidepressants
- serum levels of both benzodiazepine and anti-epileptic agents may be altered if given together, therefore serum levels of anti-epileptic agents should be closely monitored
- may increase euphoria if given with opioid analgesics, increasing the risk of psychological dependence

General Nursing points/Cautions for antianxiety agents

- regular reassessment of anxiety level is recommended
- ambulant patients should be started on the lowest possible dose to decrease the risk of falls
- benzodiazepines should only be prescribed for 2–4 weeks (unless used

for management of panic disorders, where therapy is usually prolonged); physical and psychological dependence on benzodiazepines may occur after 4–6 weeks and generally results in withdrawal symptoms if they are stopped abruptly

- tolerance of the sedating effect may develop
- withdrawal from benzodiazepines should be gradual (over 4–16 weeks depending on the indication for use) to prevent withdrawal symptoms
- withdrawal symptoms may occur if the patient has developed a physical dependence from taking excessive doses of the benzodiazepine agent over a prolonged period; symptoms may include insomnia, rebound anxiety, palpitations, panic attacks, vertigo, dysphoria, akinesia, myoclonus, metallic taste, hypersensitivity to light, sound and/or touch, delusions, confusion, delirium, abdominal and muscle cramps, tremor, vomiting, sweating, hallucinations, hyperthermia, psychosis and convulsions
- sudden withdrawal of benzodiazepines may result in a temporary increase in the frequency and severity of seizures in patients with epilepsy, or increase in sleep disturbance in other patients
- 'rebound phenomena' refers to a return to the original presenting symptoms (e.g. anxiety, panic attacks, insomnia) combined with withdrawal symptoms when the benzodiazepine is stopped
- blood counts and liver function tests are advisable during prolonged administration, especially in those with pre-existing kidney or liver impairment
- note and report paradoxical reactions, such as excitement, muscle spasticity, sleep disturbance or acute rage; the benzodiazepine should be stopped if any of these occur
- overdosage is treated with activated charcoal (oral or nasogastric) and flumazenil (see Antidotes, antagonists and chelating agents, p. 346), as well as general supportive measures as appropriate
- risk of accumulation of active metabolites exists in the elderly because of age-related changes to the renal and hepatic systems that alter drug metabolism and excretion
- extreme caution should be taken when using benzodiazepines in the elderly because of an associated increased risk of hypotension, falls, confusion, drowsiness and oversedation
- short-acting benzodiazepines with no active metabolites are the safest option for the elderly
- not recommended as primary treatment in those with depression or psychosis as benzodiazepines may increase depression, unmask suicidal tendencies or contribute to deterioration of severe schizophrenia
- caution if used in those with epilepsy as an increase in frequency and/or severity of seizures may occur, requiring an increase in dosage of anti-epileptic agent. Risk of seizure is increased if withdrawal is abrupt and should therefore be avoided
- caution if used in those where decreased blood pressure may lead to cardiac or cerebral complications
- caution should be taken if giving benzodiazepines to patients with

narrow angle glaucoma, pre-existing muscle weakness or spinal/cerebellar ataxia, respiratory depression, impaired liver or kidney function

- contraindicated in those with myasthenia gravis, sleep apnoea, chronic obstructive airways disease with incipient respiratory failure, severe liver impairment, a personal or family history of alcohol or drug dependence or hypersensitivity to other benzodiazepines

General Patient teaching and advice for antianxiety agents

- warn patient against driving a vehicle or operating machinery if drowsy, dizzy or fatigued
- warn patient about the reduced tolerance to alcohol or other CNS depressants and advise against large intakes of alcohol
- advise patient to avoid grapefruit juice during therapy
- patient should be informed that adverse effects are often seen at the beginning of therapy but usually disappear with continued use or a decrease in dosage
- patient should be warned not to stop benzodiazepines abruptly or alter the prescribed dose
- instruct patient to immediately seek medical advice if any of the following occurs:
  - aggressive behaviour, hostility, anger, violence, hallucinations or sudden anxiety
  - involuntary movements, tremor, shakiness, muscle weakness
  - unexplained nausea, vomiting, abdominal pain, yellowing of skin or eyes, dark urine
- women should be counselled to use adequate contraception to avoid pregnancy
- see General Patient teaching and advice (p. xxvii)

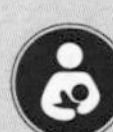

benzodiazepines cross the placenta. If taken during the first trimester they may result in congenital abnormalities. If taken late in third trimester or during labour they may cause hypotonia (floppy baby), respiratory depression, difficult drinking or sucking and hypothermia in the newborn. Withdrawal symptoms have been reported in the newborn

benzodiazepines are secreted in breastmilk and may cause hypotonia (floppy baby) and problems with sucking and drinking; therefore they are not recommended while breastfeeding

ALPRAZOLAM (Alprax, Kalma)

Available forms

Tablets: 0.25 mg, 0.5 mg, 1 mg, 2 mg

Action

- see General Actions of antianxiety agents (p. 74)
- short-acting benzodiazepine with active metabolite
- half-life 11–16 hours; half-life of active metabolite 10–15 hours

Use

- anxiety disorder
- panic disorders

Dose

- (anxiety) 0.5–4 mg/day orally daily in 2–3 divided doses **OR**
- (anxiety with depressive symptoms) 1.5–4.5 mg orally daily in divided doses **OR**
- (panic disorder) initially 0.5–1 mg orally at bedtime, increasing by 0.25–1 mg every 3 days until adequate response is achieved (daily maximum 10 mg)

Adverse effects
- see General Adverse effects of anti-anxiety agents (p. 74)

Interactions
- may cause a small increase in serum lithium, therefore blood levels should be monitored to prevent toxicity
- may increase plasma levels of imipramine
- concentration reduced by smoking
- see also General Interactions of anti-anxiety agents (p. 74)

Nursing points and Cautions/ Patient teaching and advice
- half-life is prolonged in Asians and decreased in smokers
- see General Nursing points/Cautions for antianxiety agents (p. 74) and General Patient teaching and advice for antianxiety agents (p. 76)

tablets can be dispersed in water, placed under the tongue and allowed to dissolve or crushed and mixed with spoonful of yoghurt or apple puree

BROMAZEPAM (Lexotan)

Available forms
Tablets: 3 mg, 6 mg

Action
- see General Actions of antianxiety agents (p. 74)
- medium-acting benzodiazepine with active metabolite
- half-life 12–24 hours; half-life of active metabolite 20 hours

Use
- tension, anxiety and agitation

Dose
- (ambulant patients) 3 mg orally 2–3 times daily before food (daily maximum 60 mg) **OR**
- (severe hospitalised patients) 6–12 mg orally 2–3 times daily before food

Adverse effects/Interactions
- see General Adverse effects and General Interactions of antianxiety agents (p. 74)

Nursing points/Cautions
- see General Nursing points/Cautions for antianxiety agents (p. 74)
- tablets contain lactose and therefore not recommended in those with galactose intolerance, Lapp lactase deficiency or glucose–galactose malabsorption
- it may be an advantage to divide the dosage in such a way as to give a larger dose in the evening or, if the dosage is small (3–6 mg), give as a single dose in the evening

Patient teaching and advice
- advise patient to take tablets before meals
- see General Patient teaching and advice for antianxiety agents (p. 76)

tablets can be dispersed in water or crushed and mixed with spoonful of yoghurt or apple puree

CLOBAZAM (Frisium)

Available form
Tablets: 10 mg

Action
- anxiolytic agent, chemically distinguishable from other benzodiazepines with some characteristics similar to diazepam
- long-acting benzodiazepine with active metabolite
- does not produce muscle relaxation at normal dosage
- long half-life (18–48 hours); active metabolite long half-life (2–5 days)

Use
- short-term (1 month) treatment of anxiety or sleep disturbances associated with anxiety

- epilepsy (adjunct therapy for partial refractory epilepsy or Lennox-Gastaut epilepsy not stabilised on current antiepileptic therapy in children over 4 years)

Dose
- (anxiety) 10–30 mg orally daily in 1–2 divided doses **OR**
- (epilepsy) initially 5 mg orally daily, then 0.3–1.0 mg/kg (maintenance)

Adverse effects
- serious skin reactions (Stevens-Johnson syndrome, toxic epidermal necrolysis)
- see General Adverse effects of anti-anxiety agents (p. 74)

Interactions
- see General Interactions of anti-anxiety agents (p. 74)
- increased conversion to metabolite may occur if given with carbamazepine or phenytoin

Nursing points/Cautions
- patient should be carefully monitored for skin signs and symptoms, especially in the first 8 weeks of therapy
- (epilepsy) patient should be reassessed after 4 weeks of therapy for improvement in seizure control
- if dose is divided, higher proportion should be given at night. Doses of up to 30 mg can be given as a single nightly dose
- see General Nursing points/Cautions for antianxiety agents (p. 74)

Patient teaching and advice
- advise patient/carer to seek medical advice immediately if severe blisters and/or bleeding of lips, eyes, mouth, nose and/or genitals occurs
- see General Patient teaching and advice for antianxiety agents (p. 76)

tablet can be dispersed in water or crushed and mixed with spoonful of yoghurt or apple puree

DIAZEPAM (Antenex, Diazepam Elixir, Diazepam Solution for Injection, Noumed Diazepam, Ranzepam, Valium, Valpam)

Available forms

Tablets: 2 mg, 5 mg; Ampoule: 10 mg/2 mL; Elixir: 10 mg/10 mL; Suppository: 10 mg

Action
- see General Actions of antianxiety agents (p. 74)
- long-acting benzodiazepine
- long duration of action because of active metabolites (desmethyldiazepam (half-life 20–70 hours and temazepam (half-life 30–100 hours)) which are then finally metabolised to oxazepam) (half-life 5–15 hours)
- crosses the blood–brain and placental barriers
- half-life increases with age and liver or kidney disease
- (IM) onset of action is variable depending on muscle mass

Use
- anxiety disorders (short-term management)
- allay anxiety before surgery (premedication), cardioversion, endoscopy, orthopaedic or dental procedures
- relieve acute withdrawal symptoms of alcohol
- status epilepticus (IV)
- tetanus spasm (IV)
- muscle spasm, spasticity

Dose
- (ambulant patient) 2 mg orally 3 times daily **OR**
- (ambulant patient) 2 mg orally 1–2 times daily plus 5 mg in the evening **OR**

- (muscle spasm) 10–30 mg orally daily **OR**
- (hospitalised patient, acute tension, excitation or motor unrest) 10–15 mg orally 3 times daily until acute symptoms subside **OR**
- (premedication) 10–20 mg orally at least 30 minutes before procedure **OR**
- (endoscopic procedures) 10–20 mg by slow IV (immediately before) or 5–10 mg IM (30 minutes before procedure) (if IV route is not available) **OR**
- (status epilepticus, convulsive seizure) initially 5–10 mg by slow IV, repeated in 10–15 minutes if necessary (to a maximum of 30 mg) **OR**
- (cardioversion) 5–15 mg by slow IV 5–10 minutes before procedure

Adverse effects

- see General Adverse effects of antianxiety agents (p. 74)
- (IV) cardiovascular and respiratory depression (due to propylene glycol)
- (rapid IV) phlebitis, local irritation, swelling, venous thrombosis, pain, syncope, hypotension, bradycardia, cardiac/respiratory arrest
- (IM) tenderness, local pain, erythema

Interactions

- see General Interactions of antianxiety agents (p. 74)
- plasma levels may be increased if given with isoniazid
- plasma levels may be decreased if given with rifampicin
- may reduce the effects of levodopa, decreasing control of Parkinsonian symptoms
- can inhibit binding of thyroxine and liothyronine resulting in false thyroid function test results

- (oral) to offset some of the adverse effects, doctor may order most of the daily dose (2/3) at night and the other 1/3 in the morning
- (acute alcohol withdrawal) dose may be readministered over next 2–7 days if withdrawal symptoms return
- injectable diazepam forms an incompatible precipitate when mixed with other drugs and therefore should be administered alone
- (IV) monitor vital signs, noting hypotension, bradycardia, respiratory depression/apnoea, syncope or muscle weakness
- resuscitation equipment should be available during IV administration
- (IV/IM) maximum dose in 8 hours should not be greater than 30 mg
- if possible, IM administration should be avoided because absorption is erratic
- IV injection administered slowly (5 mg/min) should be into a blood vessel with a large lumen, taking care to avoid extravasation and accidental IA administration. Small vessels should not be used
- hangover effect may occur (mainly in the elderly) as a result of the accumulation of diazepam and its metabolites
- (tablets) contain lactose and are therefore not recommended for those with rare hereditary problems of galactose intolerance, including Lapp lactase deficiency or glucose–galactose malabsorption
- (elixir) not recommended for control status epilepticus or other acute conditions
- (IV) contraindicated in those in shock or coma, acute alcohol intoxication with depressed vital signs or those with respiratory or cardiac insufficiency

Nursing points/Cautions

- see General Nursing points/Cautions for antianxiety agents (p. 74)

Patient teaching and advice

- see General Patient teaching and advice for antianxiety agents (p. 76)

elixir is available. Tablets can be dispersed in water or crushed and mixed with spoonful of yoghurt or apple puree

LORAZEPAM (Ativan)

Available form

Tablets: 1 mg, 2.5 mg

Action

- medium-acting benzodiazepine with no active metabolites
- half-life 10–20 hours
- see General Actions of antianxiety agents (p. 74)

Use

- anxiety disorders
- premedication (1–2 hours before procedure)

Dose

- (anxiety) 2–3 mg orally daily in divided doses (range 1–10 mg) **OR**
- (insomnia because of anxiety or stress) 1–2 mg orally at bedtime **OR**
- (premedication) 2–4 mg orally the night before surgery and/or 1–2 hours before surgery

Adverse effects/Interactions/ Nursing points/Cautions/Patient teaching and advice

- see General Actions of antianxiety agents (p. 74)

tablets can be dispersed in water or placed under the tongue and allowed to dissolve or crushed and mixed with spoonful of yoghurt or apple puree

OXAZEPAM (Alepam, Murelax, Serepax)

Available forms

Tablets: 15 mg, 30 mg

Action

- see General Actions of antianxiety agents (p. 74)
- short-acting benzodiazepine with no active metabolites
- half-life 5–15 hours

Use

- anxiety disorders
- alcohol withdrawal

Dose

- (mild-to-moderate anxiety) 7.5–15 mg orally 3–4 times daily **OR**
- (severe anxiety) 15–30 mg orally 3–4 times daily **OR**
- (alcohol withdrawal) 15–30 mg orally 3–4 times daily

Adverse effects/Interactions/ Nursing points/Cautions/Patient teaching and advice

- see General Actions of antianxiety agents (p. 74)
- should not be given if person undergoing alcohol withdrawal is acutely inebriated

tablets can be dispersed in water (although Serepax formulation does not disperse easily)

tablets can be crushed and mixed with spoonful of yoghurt or apple puree

ANTIARRHYTHMIC AGENTS

If the conducting system of the heart becomes disrupted, the effect on the electrical activity results in a rhythm disorder, which can be classified as a bradyarrhythmia (HR < 60 bpm) or tachyarrhythmias (HR > 100 bpm). Bradyarrhythmias include sinus bradycardia and atrioventricular (AV) blocks, while tachyarrhythmias include both atrial (e.g. supraventricular tachycardia, atrial fibrillation, atrial flutter) and ventricular tachycardia (e.g. ventricular tachycardia, premature ventricular ectopics, torsades de pointes). Tachyarrhythmias can be classified according to rhythm regularity, site of the rhythm's origin (atrium or ventricle), duration of QRS complex (narrow or wide), and the mechanism involved in the arrhythmia. Bradyarrhythmias are generally managed by reversing the cause of the bradycardia or pacemaker implantation, while tachyarrhythmias are treated by reversing the cause if possible, medications (e.g. antiarrhythmic agents) or ablation (Banga & Chalfoun 2018).

Antiarrhythmic agents are divided into four classes according to their mode of action and effect on the cardiac action potential. They may be broadly divided into agents that act mainly on supraventricular arrhythmias, those that act mainly on ventricular arrhythmias and those that act on both. Class I agents are further subdivided by their effect on the duration of the action potential (Bryant et al 2019). Some drugs have multiple actions and so belong in more than one class. Adenosine is unique as it is not classified under this system.

CLASS I

- inhibit the fast inward sodium channels responsible for phase 0 of the action potential (sodium channel blockade) and slow membrane repolarisation
- bind to the sodium channel when open or in the refractory phase, therefore the greater the frequency of sodium channels being open, the greater the degree of block by Class I agents
- in slowing conduction speed, may promote tachycardias via re-entry mechanisms
- minor differences are discussed under specific subclasses (Ia, Ib, Ic)

CLASS IA

DISOPYRAMIDE (Rythmodan)

Available forms
Capsules: 100 mg, 150 mg

Action
- depresses myocardial excitability, prolongs cardiac muscle refractory period of atria and ventricles, prolongs the action potential and refractory period, decreases conduction velocity
- decreases cardiac output, increases peripheral resistance
- slight, transient myocardial depression
- AV node conduction unchanged
- anticholinergic effects
- onset of action 3 minutes to 3 hours
- half-life 4–10 hours

Use
- management of life-threatening ventricular arrhythmias

Dose
- initially 800–600 mg orally daily in 3 divided doses, reducing to 300–400 mg orally in 3 divided doses

Adverse effects
- difficulty in micturition (hesitancy, frequency), urinary retention; dry mouth, eyes, nose and throat; blurred vision; constipation (anticholinergic effects)
- anorexia, nausea, indigestion, vomiting, diarrhoea, flatulence, bad taste in mouth
- dizziness, fatigue, vertigo, drowsiness
- hypotension, prolongation of QT interval, widening of QRS interval, bradycardia, AV block, severe cardiac failure, disturbance of cardiac conduction, chest pain, oedema, cyanosis, dyspnoea, cardiac arrest, worsening or provoking ventricular arrhythmias
- rash, pruritus, urticaria, photosensitivity
- profuse sweating
- elevated AST levels
- hypoglycaemia
- aggravation of pre-existing congestive cardiac failure

Interactions
- contraindicated with other antiarrhythmic agents, erythromycin IV, TCAs, tetracyclic antidepressants or pentamidine because of risk of prolongation of QT interval and 'torsades de pointes' (see Glossary)
- not recommended with stimulant laxatives, amphotericin B (amphotericin), tetracosactide (tetracosactrin), glucocorticoids, mineralocorticoids or diuretics because of risk of potassium imbalance
- not recommended with phosphodiesterase-5 (PDE-5) inhibitors (sildenafil, vardenafil or tadalafil) used for erectile dysfunction due to risk of QT interval prolongation
- use with extreme caution with atropine, phenothiazines and other anticholinergic (antimuscarinic) agents due to increased anticholinergic effects
- serum levels may be decreased by rifampicin, phenytoin, primidone or carbamazepine and should not be given together
- not recommended with macrolide or azole antifungal agents and roxithromycin because it may increase disopyramide serum levels, therefore increasing the risk of adverse effects
- may increase serum levels of theophylline, HIV protease inhibitors, warfarin and ciclosporin, therefore increasing the risk of adverse effects and/or toxicity

Nursing points/Cautions

- serum potassium should be measured before starting and regularly during therapy
- any potassium imbalance should be corrected before starting treatment
- frequent monitoring of ECG (especially for prolongation of PR or QT intervals or QRS widening) and blood pressure is recommended
- if patient is to undergo cardioversion, disopyramide should be started 1–2 days beforehand
- blood glucose levels should be monitored regularly throughout therapy (especially in the elderly or in those with pre-existing diabetes or kidney insufficiency)
- if a family history of glaucoma exists, intraocular pressure measurement is recommended before starting therapy
- monitor closely for hypotension and congestive cardiac failure
- not recommended in those who have had a recent myocardial infarction (within 2 years), structural heart disease and associated heart failure (unless treated and able to be closely monitored during therapy), uncompensated heart failure or hypotension
- not recommended in those with chronic closed angle glaucoma, urinary retention, benign prostatic hypertrophy or prostatic adenoma due to anticholinergic effects
- caution if used in those with kidney or liver impairment, family history of glaucoma or myasthenia gravis (may precipitate myasthenic crisis)
- caution if used in the elderly, malnourished or those with diabetes mellitus or kidney insufficiency due to increased risk of hypoglycaemia
- contraindicated in those with cardiogenic shock, second/third degree A-V block (without pacemaker), bundle branch block, double block, pre-existing QT interval prolongation, sinus node dysfunction, cardiac insufficiency or those taking medication that might provoke ventricular arrhythmias or prolong QT interval

Patient teaching and advice

- patients should be warned not to drive or operate heavy machinery if dizziness or light-headedness occurs
- if patient has diabetes, he/she should be instructed to monitor blood glucose levels more frequently because of the risk of hypoglycaemia occurring
- warn patient that dry mouth and throat commonly occur at the start of therapy and may be alleviated by melting chips of ice in the mouth
- advise patient to immediately report any of the following:
  - difficulty urinating
  - fast or irregular heartbeat
  - ongoing dizziness or light-headedness
  - chills, cold sweat, confusion, cool/pale skin, drowsiness, headache, excessive hunger, nausea, shakiness, unusual weakness/tiredness (signs of low blood sugar)
- if patient is opening capsules for ease of swallowing, advise them to rinse their mouth carefully as powder can cause mouth ulcers
- see also General Patient teaching and advice (p. xxvii)

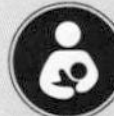

not used in pregnancy unless the expected benefit outweighs any potential risk as disopyramide may stimulate the pregnant uterus as well as passing into fetal circulation

not recommended during breastfeeding

capsules can be opened and contents dispersed in water or given with spoonful of apple puree or yoghurt

CLASS IB

- shorten action potential duration (usually shorten repolarisation)
- increases effective refractory period

LIDOCAINE (LIGNOCAINE) HYDROCHLORIDE (Lignocaine HCl Injection, Min-I-Jet Lignocaine Hydrochloride, Xylocard)

Available forms

Ampoule: 50 mg/5 mL (1%), 100 mg/5 mL (2%), 200 mg/20 mL (1%), 400 mg/20 mL (2%), 500 mg/5 mL (10%); Prefilled syringe: 20 mg/mL (2%)

Action

- amide
- depresses electrical activity reversibly in nerve, muscle and secretory cell membranes
- decreases slow spontaneous depolarisation
- decreases action potential duration and effective refractory period of Purkinje and ventricular cells
- little effect on conduction speed, membrane responsiveness or cardiac output
- less active metabolites
- onset of action 1 minute (IV) or 3–15 minutes (IM)
- half-life 1.6 hours
- therapeutic range 5–20 micromol/L (1.5–6 microgram/mL)

Use

- treatment or prophylaxis of ventricular arrhythmias and tachycardias associated with acute myocardial infarction, digoxin toxicity, cardiac surgery and after cardiac arrest
- local anaesthetic (see Local anaesthetics, p. 1269)

Dose

- 1 mg/kg slowly IV over 1–2 minutes initially, followed by IV infusion within 10 minutes **OR**
- 50–100 mg IV at a rate of 25–50 mg/min (2.5–5 mL of 1% solution or 1.25–2.5 mL 2% solution) initially, repeated after 5 minutes if needed, not exceeding 200–300 mg in 1 hour (with ECG monitoring) **OR**
- 20–50 microgram/kg/minute (4 mg/min) by IV infusion (with ECG monitoring) after initial injection

Adverse effects

- light-headedness, apprehension, euphoria, nervousness, dizziness, tremors, twitching, drowsiness, agitation, confusion, disorientation, paraesthesia, numbness
- blurred vision, double vision
- dyspnoea
- slurred speech
- tinnitus
- sensations of heat or cold
- anorexia, nausea, vomiting, swallowing difficulties
- (less common) bradycardia, hypotension, convulsions, psychoses, arrhythmias, methaemoglobinaemia, respiratory and/or cardiac arrest

Interactions

- serum levels may increase if given with cimetidine, fluvoxamine, propranolol and metoprolol, increasing the risk of lidocaine (lignocaine) toxicity
- lidocaine (lignocaine) and phenytoin have synergistic cardiac effects
- cardiac effects may be potentiated if given with other antiarrhythmic agents
- caution if given with amiodarone as it may decrease lidocaine (lignocaine) clearance

- caution if given with muscle relaxants (e.g. suxamethonium) because excessive neuromuscular blockade may occur
- may decrease serum levels of inhalational anaesthetics (e.g. nitrous oxide)
- metabolism may be increased by phenytoin, phenobarbital (phenobarbitone), primidone and carbamazepine
- prolonged half-life may occur if given during acute, severe alcohol intoxication
- caution if used with other amide-type local anaesthetics
- may interfere with measurement of creatinine level using enzymatic methods

Nursing points/Cautions

- correct hypokalaemia, hypoxia and any acid–base imbalance before starting treatment
- monitor heart rate, blood pressure, plasma lidocaine (lignocaine) levels (especially for those in shock, on prolonged infusion (>24 hours) or with liver or cardiac failure) and ECG throughout IV administration
- IV infusion should be stopped as soon as cardiac rhythm stabilises or if signs of toxicity appear, including drowsiness, as this may be an early sign of high blood lidocaine (lignocaine) levels
- monitor IV infusion rate closely using an infusion pump
- IV dose should not exceed 100 mg in a single dose or 200–300 mg in a 1-hour period
- IV infusion should be started within 10 minutes of initial IV injection
- IV infusion duration is normally 2 or more days. Usually discontinued 24 hours after last signs of arrhythmia or at first signs of toxicity
- oral antiarrhythmic agent should replace IV therapy as soon as possible for maintenance
- have available diazepam (for convulsions), isoprenaline and atropine (reversing bradycardia, hypotension), facilities for cardiac monitoring, defibrillation and resuscitation (including oxygen therapy)
- caution if given to those with epilepsy, renal or liver failure, congestive cardiac failure, recent myocardial infarction, impaired cardiac conduction, severe digoxin toxicity, hypoxia or respiratory depression, hypovolaemia, severe shock, heart block or severe bradycardia, cardiac decompensation and hypotension, posterior diaphragmal infarction, acute porphyria, cardiac impairment or genetic predisposition to malignant hyperthermia
- contraindicated in those with Stokes–Adams syndrome, myasthenia gravis, severe shock, supraventricular arrhythmias, severe SA, AV or intraventricular block (without pacemaker) or in those with known hypersensitivity to amide-type local anaesthetics

Note

- (local anaesthetic) included in preparations (oral, dermatological, parenteral) to prevent local pain, itching or irritation

CLASS IC

- decrease rate of depolarisation and AV conduction time
- decreases contractility

FLECAINIDE ACETATE (Flecatab, Tambocor)

Available forms
Tablets: 50 mg, 100 mg; Ampoules: 10 mg/mL

Action
- structurally related to lidocaine (lignocaine)
- increases PR interval, QT interval and QRS duration
- does not alter HR, some increase in systolic and diastolic BP
- slight negative inotropic effect
- some local anaesthetic activity
- (oral) long half-life 12–27 hours that is slowed by alkaline urine
- therapeutic range 0.2–0.9 mg/L

Use
- suppression and prevention of supraventricular arrhythmias
- life-threatening ventricular arrhythmias (not controlled by other agents)

Dose
- (sustained ventricular tachycardia) 100 mg orally 12-hourly initially, increasing by 50 mg twice daily every 4 days (maximum 400 mg daily) **OR**
- (supraventricular arrhythmias) 50 mg orally 12-hourly initially, increasing by 50 mg twice daily every 4 days (maximum 300 mg daily) **OR**
- 2 mg/kg slowly IV over 10–15 minutes, or diluted with glucose 5% and given as a mini-infusion (maximum 150 mg)

Adverse effects
- dizziness, light-headedness, headache, fatigue, nervousness, tremor, paraesthesia, hypoaesthesia, asthenia
- ataxia
- blurred vision, diplopia, photophobia, visual field defects
- insomnia, somnolence
- nausea, vomiting, anorexia, diarrhoea, constipation, abdominal pain, dry mouth
- urinary retention and frequency, polyuria, dysuria
- increased sweating, flushing, fever
- palpitations, chest pain, congestive heart failure (new or worsening), (serious) ventricular arrhythmias (new or exacerbated), second/third degree AV block, bradycardia, sinus pause, sinus arrest, angina, conduction disorders, tachycardia, oedema
- dyspnoea, coughing
- rash, pruritus
- tinnitus
- arthralgia, myalgia
- (rare) blood dyscrasias, pulmonary fibrosis, pneumonitis, interstitial lung disease

Interactions
- serum levels may be increased by cimetidine
- alkaline urine decreases elimination
- not recommended with other antiarrhythmic agents
- may increase serum levels of digoxin

Nursing points/Cautions
- any electrolyte imbalance (especially potassium) should be corrected before starting therapy
- IV therapy should only be conducted where cardiac monitoring and defibrillation are readily available
- have available isoprenaline, dopamine or dobutamine, mechanical ventilator and facilities for cardiac monitoring and defibrillation
- dilute with glucose 5% only
- IV infusion should not continue for more than 24 hours

- once arrhythmia is controlled, dose should be reduced to lessen the risk of adverse effects
- (tablets) dose adjustments should not occur more frequently than every 4 days because of long half-life
- if changing from another antiarrhythmic agent, at least 2 half-lives should be allowed to elapse before starting flecainide. If withdrawal of antiarrhythmic agent is likely to produce a life-threatening arrhythmia, hospitalisation of the patient is strongly recommended
- caution if used in those with recent myocardial infarction, severe cardiomyopathy, congestive heart failure, sinus node disease, sick sinus syndrome, electrolyte imbalance, alkaline urine, kidney impairment or permanent pacemaker or temporary pacing electrodes in situ
- extreme caution if used in those with structural heart disease, especially if left ventricular ejection fraction ≤ 40%
- not recommended in those with chronic atrial fibrillation or arrhythmias due to digoxin toxicity
- contraindicated in those with severe liver or kidney impairment
- contraindicated in those with second/third degree AV block (without pacemaker), right bundle branch block (without pacemaker), cardiogenic shock, severe renal/hepatic impairment, asymptomatic premature ventricular contractions, advanced sinus node disease, non-programmable pacemaker (unless pacing rescue is available) or asymptomatic non-sustained ventricular tachycardia with a history of myocardial infarction

Patient teaching and advice

- patient should be warned not to drive or operate heavy machinery if dizziness, light-headedness or visual disturbances occur
- warn patient that dry mouth and/or taste disturbance may occur
- advise patient to immediately report any:
  - rapid or irregular heartbeat, chest pain
  - difficulty breathing
- see General Patient teaching and advice (p. xxvii)

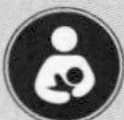

not used in pregnancy unless the expected benefit outweighs any potential risk

not recommended during breastfeeding

can be dispersed in 10–20 mL of water or crushed and given with spoonful of yoghurt or apple puree

CLASS II

- inhibit effects of sympathetic nervous system (beta adrenergic blockade, e.g. atenolol, esmolol, metoprolol), therefore are effective for arrhythmias induced by excessive sympathetic stimulation
- slow conduction at atria and AV node, increasing refractory period
- shown to reduce mortality post myocardial infarction
- see beta-adrenoceptor blocking agents in Antihypertensive agents (p. 508)

CLASS III

- prolong the duration of action potential (increase refractory period)
- decrease AV conduction

AMIODARONE HYDROCHLORIDE (Amdarone, Aratac, Cordarone X, Rithmik)

Available forms

Tablets: 100 mg, 200 mg; Ampoule: 150 mg/3 mL

Action

- prolongs action potential duration and hence refractory period of atrial, nodal and ventricular tissues
- increases coronary blood flow by vasodilation
- blocks sodium, calcium and potassium channels
- reduces cardiac oxygen requirement
- suppresses 'ectopic pacemakers'
- onset of action is 3–7 hours; half-life is about 14–59 days (with chronic dosing)
- active metabolite has longer half-life (60–90 days) (chronic dosing) than parent compound
- therapeutic range 1–2.5 mg/L (1.6–4 micromol/L)

Use

- ventricular fibrillation
- atrial flutter and fibrillation
- supraventricular, nodal and ventricular tachycardia refractory to other antiarrhythmic drugs
- severe tachyarrhythmias (e.g. Wolf-Parkinson-White syndrome)

Dose

- 200 mg orally 3 times daily for 1 week, then reduce to 200 mg orally twice daily for 1 week, then reduce to 200 mg daily or less (maintenance) **OR**
- 5 mg/kg IV diluted in 250 mL glucose 5% and given over 20 minutes to 2 hours at a rate less than 30 mg/min and repeated if needed (daily maximum 1.2 g) **OR**
- (emergency) 150–300 mg in 10–20 mL glucose 5% IV over 3 minutes

Adverse effects

- severe bradycardia, atypical ventricular arrhythmia, exacerbation of cardiac failure, cardiac arrest
- reversible benign yellowish-brown corneal micro-deposits
- skin photosensitivity and, rarely, discolouration of exposed areas such as face (slate grey/purple)
- peripheral neuropathy (long-term high dosage above 400 mg/day), myopathy
- insomnia, sleep disorders, vivid dreams and nightmares
- headache, tremor, dizziness, fatigue, vertigo, anxiety
- liver dysfunction, including elevated liver enzymes
- hyperthyroidism, hypothyroidism, weight gain/loss
- gait abnormalities, paraesthesia, muscle weakness, ataxia
- nausea, and, rarely, anorexia; constipation; salty, metallic taste, vomiting
- hair loss, rash, facial flushing
- fever
- (IV, rapid) severe hypotension, transient hot flushes, sweating, nausea
- pneumonitis, pulmonary fibrosis (rare and usually reversible, but potentially fatal), cough
- (injection site) inflammation, pain, erythema, urticaria, oedema, induration, phlebitis, cellulitis, pigmentation changes, extravasation, necrosis
- (rare) optic neuritis, optic neuropathy, cardiac failure, cardiac arrest

Interactions

- contraindicated with MAOIs
- contraindicated when given concurrently with other drugs that may

prolong QT interval or induce 'torsades de pointes' (see Glossary), including disopyramide, flecainide, TCAs, antihistamines, fluoroquinolones (e.g. moxifloxacin), antipsychotic agents, sotalol, erythromycin IV, pentamidine IV, or agents that may cause hypokalaemia or hypomagnesaemia, such as diuretics, stimulant laxatives, amphotericin B (amphotericin), corticosteroids
- increased risk of life-threatening bradycardia and heart block if given with anti-viral agents such as sofosbuvir, ledipasavir and daclatasvir
- may increase serum levels of digoxin, phenytoin, flecainide and ciclosporin, increasing the toxicity risk, therefore serum levels should be closely monitored
- may increase serum levels of warfarin significantly, increasing the risk of bleeding, therefore INR time should be closely monitored, especially when starting or stopping therapy
- not recommended with calcium channel blockers or beta-adrenoceptor blocking agents due to increased bradycardia and risk of conduction disorders
- give cautiously with general anaesthetics and oxygen therapy
- may increase effects of fentanyl, increasing the risk of toxicity
- increased risk of bleeding if given with dabigatran
- increased serum levels may occur if given with grapefruit juice
- increased risk of myopathy and rhabdomyolysis if given with statins (sim-vastatin, atorvastatin)
- may alter results of thyroid function tests

Nursing points/Cautions

- initial treatment closely monitored in hospital
- IV injection given only in a unit where facilities for monitoring and treating serious arrhythmias are available
- any electrolyte imbalance (especially potassium) should be corrected before starting therapy
- repeated or prolonged IV infusions are preferably given via a central venous catheter (CVC) to avoid thrombophlebitis
- before starting treatment, patients should have a thyroid function test (ultrasensitive TSH), serum potassium level measurement and an ECG. Liver and thyroid function tests, chest X-ray, ophthalmological examination and ECG should be monitored regularly throughout therapy and for several months after stopping therapy
- any hypersensitivity to iodine should be established before starting therapy because amiodarone structurally contains iodine molecules
- oral therapy should replace IV infusion as soon as possible (with up to 2-day overlap to maintain plasma levels)
- functioning of pacemakers or implantable defibrillators should be checked before starting, and regularly during therapy
- should only be diluted in glucose 5% as amiodarone is incompatible with sodium chloride 0.9%
- administer alone
- IV injections are not recommended as there is a high risk of hypotension, circulatory collapse and thrombophlebitis and therefore only recommended in extreme emergency situations with patient monitored continuously in a setting such as ICU
- IV injection should not be repeated within 15 minutes of initial injection
- infusion rate should not exceed 2 mg/mL unless a CVC is in situ
- should be infused using a volumetric pump

- (IV) not compatible with heparin or aminophylline
- prepare infusion solution immediately before use in either a glass or a rigid PVC container and use within 12 hours to reduce adsorption into PVC infusion bags and administration sets
- if surgery is planned, anaesthetist should be made aware of therapy with amiodarone
- caution if used in those with liver disease/dysfunction or heart failure as it may be exacerbated
- contraindicated in patients with or history of thyroid dysfunction, sinus bradycardia, sino-atrial heart block, AV block, sick sinus syndrome (risk of sinus arrest), severe AV conduction disorders (without pacemaker or pacing), cardiomyopathy, circulatory collapse, heart failure, hypotension, severe arterial hypotension and respiratory failure, or in those with iodine hypersensitivity
- (IV) contraindicated in neonates due to benzyl alcohol content

Patient teaching and advice

- advise patient to avoid skin exposure to direct sunlight and ensure protective clothing, hat and sunscreen (SPF 30+) is worn
- if patient is also taking hepatitis C antiviral medications, instruct to immediately seek medical advice if any slowed heart rate, shortness of breath, light headedness, fainting or palpitations occur
- warn patient against driving or operating machinery if dizziness or vertigo occur
- patient should be advised to avoid grapefruit or grapefruit juice during therapy
- patient should be instructed to report any of the following:
  - blurred or decreased vision
  - skin colour changes (blue tinge on exposed areas such as face)
  - numbness or tingling of feet or hands in glove/sock pattern
  - nausea, vomiting, yellowing of eyes/skin, upper abdominal pain, tiredness or dark urine
  - difficulty breathing or shortness of breath, cough
  - skin rashes with blisters
  - weight loss, increased appetite, restlessness, heat intolerance, increased sweating, tremor, rapid heartbeat, swelling in neck (goiter) (overactive thyroid symptoms)
  - weight gain, cold intolerance, slowed heartbeat, reduced activity, dry and flaky skin, hair loss, deep/husky voice, muscle weakness/cramps (underactive thyroid signs and symptoms)
- female patient of childbearing potential should be counselled to use adequate contraception during therapy, including 3 months before conception
- see also General Patient teaching and advice (p. xxvii)

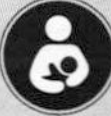

contraindicated in pregnancy and for 3 months before. If exposure is unavoidable, thyroid function of newborn infant should be assessed immediately

contraindicated during breastfeeding

tablets may be crushed and given with water or spoonful of yoghurt or apple puree

SOTALOL HYDROCHLORIDE (Cardol, Cardol 80 mg, Solavert, Sotacor)

Available forms

Tablets: 80 mg, 160 mg

Action

- prolongs atrial, ventricular and accessory pathway refractory periods and QT interval

- decreases heart rate, reduces cardiac work and myocardial oxygen demand
- inhibits renin release (at rest and during exercise)
- does not undergo any first pass metabolism in the liver, therefore bioavailability is 100%. However, this is reduced if given with food, especially milk
- onset of action 2–3 hours, half-life 12–14 hours
- non-selective beta-adrenergic receptor blocker

Use
- prevention and treatment of supraventricular and ventricular arrhythmias

Dose
- initially 80 mg orally twice daily 1–2 hours before food, increasing at 2–3-day intervals to 240–320 mg daily as needed

Adverse effects
- cardiac arrhythmias (including 'torsades de pointes' (see Glossary) and serious ventricular arrhythmias), bradycardia, hypotension, chest pain, palpitations, exacerbation of Prinzmetal's (variant) angina
- cold extremities
- oedema
- fatigue, asthenia, dizziness, headache, drowsiness, light-headedness, sleep disturbance, weakness, tiredness, lethargy, vertigo
- paraesthesia
- anxiety, depression, mood changes
- fever
- dyspnoea
- muscle cramps
- changes in plasma lipid levels
- rash, worsening of pre-existing psoriasis
- diarrhoea, nausea, vomiting, flatulence, dyspepsia, abdominal pain, taste disturbance
- eye irritation, blurred vision, photophobia, eyesight deterioration
- hearing disturbance
- sexual dysfunction

Interactions
- contraindicated with concurrent use of other drugs that may prolong QT interval and induce 'torsades de pointes' (see Glossary), including disopyramide, TCAs, calcium-channel blockers, clonidine, amiodarone, erythromycin IV or pentamidine IV, some quinolone antibiotics or agents which cause hypokalaemia or hypomagnesaemia, such as diuretics, stimulant laxatives, corticosteroids, amphotericin B (amphotericin)
- not recommended with clonidine, calcium-channel blockers, other beta-adrenoceptor agents
- contraindicated with anaesthetic agents (e.g. ether, cyclopropane, chloroform) as myocardial depression may occur
- clearance may be decreased by alcohol
- may prolong hypoglycaemic action of insulin and/or oral hypoglycaemic agents
- may require increased doses of beta-receptor stimulants (e.g. isoprenaline, salbutamol, terbutaline)

Nursing points/Cautions

- should not be withdrawn preoperatively unless there is a clear indication to do so
- serum electrolytes should be measured before and during therapy and any imbalance (especially potassium) corrected
- pulse rate, haemodynamic and ECG monitoring is recommended (especially during initial therapy and with dose increases as arrhythmias may occur)
- dose adjustments should be gradual, allowing 2–3 days to reach steady state
- medication withdrawal should be gradual over 8–14 days, especially in those with coronary artery disease

- atropine can be used to correct any excessive bradycardia (without/with hypotension)
- those with phaeochromocytoma should be pre-treated with phenoxybenzamine to avoid exacerbation of hypertension
- caution if used in those with congestive heart failure, psoriasis or hyperthyroidism
- caution if used in those with peripheral vascular disease as symptoms may be worsened
- caution if used in those with diabetes as signs of hypoglycaemia (e.g. tachycardia) may be masked
- caution if used in those with history of anaphylactic reaction due to increased risk of reaction
- caution if used in those with hyperthyroidism already managed with beta-adrenergic blocking agents. Abrupt withdrawal should be avoided to prevent exacerbation of symptoms including thyroid storm
- not recommended in those with recent myocardial infarction with left ventricular fraction ≤ 40%
- not recommended if QT interval > 450 milliseconds
- not recommended in those with Prinzmetal's (variant) angina due to the risk of exacerbated coronary artery spasm
- contraindicated in those with bronchial asthma, chronic obstructive airways disease, allergies (suggestive of bronchospasm), right ventricular failure (secondary to pulmonary hypertension), right ventricular hypertrophy, bradycardia (< 45–50 beats/min), second/third degree AV block, sick sinus syndrome (without pacemaker), cardiogenic or hypovolemic shock, uncontrolled congestive heart failure, kidney impairment (creatinine clearance < 10 mL/min) or congenital/acquired long QT syndromes

Patient teaching and advice

- patient should be advised not to drive or operate machinery if dizzy, fatigued, light-headed, drowsy or experiencing visual disturbances
- warn patient not to drink alcohol during therapy
- advise patient to take medication 1–2 hours before food to maximise absorption
- those with diabetes should be instructed to monitor blood glucose levels during therapy as hypoglycaemic actions of insulin and/or oral hypoglycaemic agent may be prolonged
- patient should be advised not to stop medication abruptly
- instruct patient to seek medical advice immediately if any of the following occur:
  - very slow heartbeat
  - very fast or irregular heartbeat, chest pain
  - shortness of breath
- see General Patient teaching and advice (p. xxvii)

permitted in sport subject to certain restrictions, routes, urinary thresholds or prohibited in some sports, not others

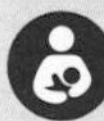

crosses placental barrier and causes bradycardia in the fetus and newborn, therefore should only be given during pregnancy (especially late stages) after weighing up the mother's needs versus those of the fetus/newborn

not recommended during breastfeeding

tablet can be crushed and mixed with water or given with spoonful of yoghurt or apple puree

CLASS IV

- decrease action potential duration
- decrease AV conduction
- decrease contractility
- see calcium-channel blockers in Antihypertensive agents (p. 520)

ATYPICAL ANTIARRHYTHMIC AGENTS

ADENOSINE (Adenocor, Adenoscan, Adenosine Juno Solution, Adenosine Mylan Injection)

Available forms

Ampoule: 6 mg/2 mL, 30 mg/10 mL (for cardiac scanning)

Action

- adenosine is a naturally occurring molecule that results from breakdown of ATP
- a number of adenosine receptors (A_1, A_{2A}, A_{2B}, A_3) exist throughout the CNS and peripheral tissue, including heart, liver, kidney, GI tract, adipose tissue, lung and blood vessels
- in the heart, binds to A1 receptors, opening potassium channels leading to hyperpolarisation, inhibiting calcium entry into cells
- at SA node, inhibits pacemaker activity decreasing spontaneous firing rate
- slows conduction through the AV node and re-establishes normal sinus rhythm
- no systemic haemodynamic effects
- produces peripheral vasodilation by A_2-receptor agonism
- rapid onset of action (less than 2 minutes), very short half-life (10 seconds)

Use

- paroxysmal supraventricular tachycardia (including those associated with accessory pathways such as Wolff-Parkinson-White syndrome)
- (diagnostic adjunct) diagnosis of broad and narrow QRS supraventricular tachycardias (Adenoscan)

Dose

- initially 3 mg rapid IV bolus over 2 seconds; if ineffective within 1–2 minutes, 6 mg may be given and, if necessary, 12 mg after a further 1–2 minutes **OR**
- (diagnostic adjunct) 140 microgram/kg/min IV over 6 minutes via infusion pump, followed by injection of radionuclide

Adverse effects

- flushing of face, head and body, heat sensation, burning sensation
- headache, light-headedness, dizziness, apprehension
- paraesthesia
- nausea
- chest pressure/pain/discomfort, severe bradycardia, ventricular excitability, transient increase or decrease in BP, sinus pause, skipped beats, atrial extrasystole, AV block, hypotension
- dyspnoea or urge to breathe deeply
- (diagnostic adjunct) abdominal discomfort, dry mouth
- (rare) injection site reaction, bronchospasm

Interactions

- may be antagonised by caffeine, aminophylline and theophylline and these should therefore be stopped for 24 hours before administration

- contraindicated with dipyridamole
- heart block may be potentiated if given with carbamazepine

Nursing points/Cautions

- given by rapid IV injection over 2 seconds, followed by rapid sodium chloride 0.9%
- treatment requires close monitoring
- have cardiorespiratory resuscitation equipment available for immediate use
- ineffective when given as an infusion rather than as a rapid IV bolus
- dipyridamole should be stopped for 24 hours before administration
- coffee, cola, chocolate and other caffeine-containing drinks/food should be stopped for 12 hours before administration
- repeat doses should not be given if patient develops second or third degree AV block during administration
- (diagnostic adjunct) administered undiluted
- (diagnostic adjunct) HR and BP recorded at 1-minute intervals with continuous ECG monitoring. BP should be measured in opposite arm to infusion
- caution if used in those with history of seizures
- caution if used in those with prolonged atrial fibrillation or flutter (with accessory pathway), recent heart transplantation (within 12 months), left main coronary stenosis, uncorrected hypovolaemia, left to right shunt, pericarditis, pericardial effusion, autonomic dysfunction, stenotic carotid artery disease with cerebrovascular insufficiency, recent myocardial infarction, heart failure, first degree AV block, bundle branch block
- contraindicated in those with chronic obstructive lung disease (including asthma), sick sinus syndrome (without pacemaker) or with second/third degree AV block (without pacemaker), long QT syndrome, severe hypotension and decompensated heart failure

Patient teaching and advice

- patient should be warned of 'feeling of impending doom', which occurs transiently after injection

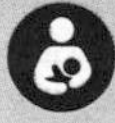

should only be used in pregnancy and breastfeeding if benefits outweigh risks

ANTIASTHMA AGENTS, BRONCHODILATORS AND RESPIRATORY AGENTS

Asthma prevalence in Australia is approximately 11%, equating to just over 2.7 million people, with Indigenous Australians almost twice as likely to report having asthma than the non-Indigenous population (AIHW 2019b). Health expenditure on asthma accounts for approximately 0.7% of the total healthcare budget (about $770 million). Furthermore, asthma accounted for 441 deaths in 2017, with those aged 5–34 being at the greatest risk (AIHW 2019b).

In susceptible people, asthma may be triggered by a number of allergens; however, the common cold is the most likely trigger. Some triggers are avoidable (e.g. cigarette smoke), while others are not. Asthma triggers include animal allergens (e.g. pets, animals in workplace), house dust mites, pollen, moulds, airborne or environmental irritants (e.g. cold or dry air, household aerosols, industrial or traffic pollution, perfumes/scents, smoke (e.g. bushfire, indoor wood fires, and more recently, thunderstorms). In addition, some medications can trigger asthma, including aspirin, non-steroidal anti-inflammatory drugs (NSAIDs), beta-adrenoceptor blocking agents (beta blockers), dietary triggers (food chemicals or additives, if the person is intolerant), thermal effects (e.g. cold drinks). Other triggers include physiological (e.g. exercise) and psychological changes (e.g. extreme emotions, hormonal changes (including pregnancy, sexual activity) and co-morbid medical conditions (e.g. obesity, allergic rhinitis, nasal polyposis) (National Asthma Council Australia 2017).

During an asthma attack bronchospasm causes wheezing, coughing, breathing difficulties, mucosal oedema and the formation of mucus. The asthma process is thought to be caused in part by IgE antibodies attaching to mast cells, causing degranulation and the production and release of inflammatory mediators (histamine, leukotrienes, cytokines, eosinophil and neutrophil chemotactic factors), leading to hyperresponsiveness of the bronchioles. Antihistamines are not useful in asthma management, suggesting that histamine plays a minor role (Bryant et al 2019).

The goal of asthma management is to relieve and control symptoms, prevent acute asthma and death, and maintain best lung function and quality of life for the person with asthma. It therefore involves the use of both symptomatic and prophylactic treatment. Antiasthma drugs can be divided into symptom relievers, symptom controllers and symptom preventers.

Symptom relievers (bronchodilators)

- short-acting beta-2 adrenoceptor agonists (e.g. salbutamol, terbutaline)
- anticholinergic (antimuscarinic) agents (e.g. ipratropium)
- xanthines (e.g. theophylline)

Symptom controllers (bronchodilators)

- longer acting beta-2 adrenoceptor agonists (e.g. salmeterol, formoterol)

Symptom preventers (prophylactic and anti-inflammatory drugs)

- mast cell stabilisers (e.g. sodium cromoglycate, nedocromil sodium)
- inhaled corticosteroids (anti-inflammatory) (e.g. budesonide, fluticasone)
- leukotriene-receptor antagonists (anti-inflammatory) (e.g. montelukast)
- oral or parenteral corticosteroids (anti-inflammatory)

The patient should develop a written *asthma action plan* in collaboration with a GP or respiratory doctor. The plan should outline the usual asthma (and allergy) medications, instructions on how to change medications if needed (e.g. if asthma worsens), when and how to get medical care (especially in the event of an emergency), and the name of the person preparing the plan with a date. This plan should be updated regularly (National Asthma Council Australia 2019). In 2017–18, 31% of people across all age groups had a written asthma plan; 67% of children (14 years and under) had written plans, but this number fell to 24% in those 15 years and over (AIHW 2019b).

A study by Roman-Rodriguez and colleagues (2019) found that poor asthma control and exacerbations could, in part, be related to poor inhaler technique resulting in no or insufficient medication reaching the lungs. Given that many of the agents used to manage asthma (both preventers and relievers) are delivered via some sort of inhaler device, it would appear to be of critical importance to optimise inhaler technique. The authors identified a number of issues including poor coordination between actuation and inhalation of the medication when using a metered dose inhaler, incomplete inspiration or failing to hold breath adequately, after inspiration and being prescribed multiple inhaled medications, leading to confusion. The authors concluded that two critical points in improving asthma control were correct device selection and sufficient education (including practice using the device) (Roman-Rodriguez et al 2019).

General Patient teaching and advice for antiasthma agents and bronchodilators

- before instructing any patient on correct techniques for monitoring and management of their asthma, it is important to ascertain that the person understands what asthma is (including its seriousness) and any avoidable triggers are identified
- instruct patient in correct technique for:
  - regularly monitoring peak flow using a peak flow meter
  - using metered dose aerosol inhalers, nebulisers, accuhalers, spacers

or other inhalation devices (there are a number of 'how to' videos on correct inhaler technique available from National Asthma Council Australia)
  - the importance of carrying a short-acting beta-2 agonist (e.g. salbutamol) for use when acute symptom relief is necessary
- long-acting bronchodilators are for maintenance, not acute episodes, and should be used regularly to keep asthma controlled
- ensure that patient is aware of his/her triggers and knows how to avoid or manage them (e.g. using medication before known exposure)
- wear a MedicAlert bracelet or pendant in case of respiratory emergencies, especially if using inhaled or oral corticosteroids
- seek medical advice promptly if symptoms worsen or medication does not provide its normal relief. Asthma can be a life-threatening condition
- advise patient against overuse of inhalers containing propellants as both propellant and active substance can be hazardous in large quantities
- warn patient against driving or operating machinery if dizziness, fatigue, blurred vision or other visual problems occur
- asthma control is important for both maternal and fetal health
- see also General Patient teaching and advice (p. xxvii)

Spacer device

- a spacer device may be useful for those with poor inhalation technique or to decrease adverse effects related to the amount of powder directly reaching the mouth and throat
- the patient should be informed that changing brands of spacer device may alter the amount of medication delivered to the lungs
- instruct patient in the correct technique for using their inhaler in conjunction with a spacer device. The inhaler is actuated into the spacer; the patient should then breathe in slowly and as far as possible. Breath is then held for as long as possible before breathing out slowly. If multiple inhalations are required, time in between should be minimised
- spacer device should be washed with warm water and detergent before first use and then at least monthly. It should be allowed to air dry. A cloth should not be used to dry spacer device as this produces static electricity which causes the medication to stick to the sides of the device, thereby reducing the amount available to reach the lungs
- it is important to note that some medication is lost in the spacer due to electrostatic attraction between the plastic spacer device and the medication

Nebuliser

- no substances other than the prescribed diluent should be added to the nebuliser solution (sodium chloride 0.9% or distilled water or propylene glycol spray diluent)
- nebuliser solution may be delivered undiluted, but is usually diluted to allow efficient operation of the nebuliser
- most nebulisers deliver 1 mL of solution over 3 minutes and 2 mL over 8–10 minutes. If given using medical oxygen or medical air rather than via compression pump, rate should be $>$ 6 L/min

- a small compressed air pump can be used at home to provide pressure for nebulisation
- any solution remaining in the nebuliser after therapy should be discarded. Chamber and mask should be rinsed after use and allowed to air dry to prevent build-up of medication
- solution remaining after the stock bottle has been opened for 3 months should be discarded

Aerolizer

- ensure patient knows manufacturer's instruction leaflet is in Aerolizer packet
- instruct patient in correct use of Aerolizer, including:
  1. pull cap off inhalation device
  2. to open device, hold base and turn mouthpiece in the direction of the arrow
  3. ensuring fingers/hands are dry, remove capsule from foil pack immediately before use
  4. place capsule in capsule-shaped slot, ensuring that it is on the bottom and lying flat
  5. twist mouthpiece until a 'click' is heard. Mouthpiece is now closed
  6. hold Aerolizer upright, firmly squeeze two blue buttons at the same time and then release. This will pierce the capsule – only do this once (piercing more often may release gelatin from capsule shell, which can then be inhaled into mouth or throat)
  7. while holding Aerolizer upright, open mouthpiece and ensure capsule is loose so that it can spin on inhalation; close mouthpiece
  8. breathe out as far as possible
  9. place mouthpiece well into the mouth, with lips closed firmly around it and the head tilted back slightly. Breathe in quickly and evenly and as deeply as possible (a whirring sound should be heard as the capsule spins)
  10. hold breath for as long as possible. Remove Aerolizer and breathe out through nose
  11. check Aerolizer to see if any powder is left. If there is, repeat steps 8 to 10
  12. remove empty capsule and wipe mouthpiece and capsule slot with dry cloth. Do not use water to clean Aerolizer
  13. close the mouthpiece and put cap on

BRONCHODILATORS (BETA-2 ADRENOCEPTOR AGONISTS (ALSO CALLED BETA-2 AGONISTS))

General Adverse effects of beta-2 adrenoceptor agonists

Common effects

- fine skeletal muscle tremor (due to beta effects), especially in the hands, palpitations, increased heart rate/tachycardia (beta effects), nervousness, headache

Less common

- dizziness, insomnia
- anxiety, agitation
- bad taste
- muscle cramps, myalgia
- (inhalation) cough, mouth and throat irritation, hoarse voice, dry mouth, increase in asthma symptoms, dyspnoea

- (rare) hyperglycaemia, paradoxical bronchospasm, hypokalaemia, rash, arrhythmias, exacerbation of existing arrhythmias, hypersensitivity reaction
- (rare, high dose) cardionecrosis, lactic acidosis

General Interactions of beta-2 adrenoceptor agonists

- theophylline, other xanthines, corticosteroids and potassium-losing diuretics, and hypoxia may increase the risk of hypokalaemia if given with beta-2 adrenoreceptor agonists
- hypoxia may aggravate effect of hypokalaemia on cardiac rhythm, increasing risk of arrhythmia
- increased risk of cardiac arrhythmias if given to those with hypokalaemia induced by salbutamol or other beta-2 agonist
- not recommended with sympathomimetic agents
- caution if given with anaesthetic agents, as these may sensitise the myocardium to catecholamines
- increased risk of hypokalaemia and hyperglycaemia when given with glucocorticoids (corticosteroids)
- bronchodilator effect may be inhibited by beta-adrenoceptor blocking agents (including ophthalmic preparations), which are therefore not recommended together
- increased risk of arrhythmias if given with digoxin or other cardiac glycosides because of salbutamol or other beta-2 agonist-induced hypokalaemia

FORMOTEROL (EFORMOTEROL) FUMARATE DIHYDRATE (Foradile, Oxis Turbuhaler)

Available forms

Capsules: 12 microgram (for Aerolizer device); metered dose Turbuhaler: 6 microgram/inhalation, 12 microgram/inhalation

Action

- potent, long-acting selective beta-2 adrenoceptor agonist
- inhibits histamine and leukotriene release
- some anti-inflammatory properties
- onset 1–3 minutes, peak effect 1–2 hours, duration 12 hours
- symptom controller for maintenance

Use

- long-term regular treatment of reversible airway obstruction associated with asthma in patients having concurrent corticosteroid therapy, including exercise-induced asthma, nocturnal asthma
- prophylaxis and treatment of bronchoconstriction associated with reversible/irreversible chronic obstructive pulmonary disease (COPD)

Dose

- (asthma) 1–2 inhalations (12–24 microgram) twice daily (daily maximum 48 microgram) (Foradile) **OR**
- (asthma) 6–12 microgram twice daily, up to 24 microgram twice daily if necessary (daily maximum 48 microgram) (Oxis) **OR**
- (COPD) 1 inhalation (12 microgram) twice daily (Foradile)

Adverse effects

- exacerbation of asthma
- (rare) prolongation of QT interval
- see also General Adverse effects of beta-2 adrenoreceptor agonists (p. 98)

Interactions

- increased risk of prolonged QT interval and arrhythmias if given with other agents known to prolong QT interval such as MAOIs, TCAs, erythromycin, disopyramide, phenothiazines or antihistamines
- not recommended with other long-acting beta-2 adrenoreceptor agonists
- see also General Interactions of beta-2 adrenoceptor agonists (p. 99)

Nursing points/Cautions

- should only be used as adjunct to inhaled corticosteroid therapy in those with asthma
- therapy should not be started in those with unstable or acutely deteriorating asthma
- once symptoms are controlled, consideration should be given to reducing dose
- not recommended in those under 5 years
- not recommended in those whose asthma can be managed with short-acting beta-2 agonists
- can increase blood glucose levels, therefore caution if used in those with diabetes mellitus
- caution if used in those with ischaemic heart disease, arrhythmias or severe heart failure as they are more likely to experience cardiovascular side-effects
- caution if used in those with idiopathic subvalvular aortic stenosis, hypertrophic obstructive cardiomyopathy, acquired/congenital QT interval prolongation, thyrotoxicosis or inadequately controlled hyperthyroidism, severe hypertension, phaeochromocytoma, aneurysm or severe cardiac decompensation
- contraindicated in those with rare hereditary galactose intolerance, Lapp lactase deficiency or glucose–galactose malabsorption as capsules contain lactose

Patient teaching and advice

- ensure patient understands that this medication is not recommended for use during an acute asthma episode
- patient should be advised to continue concurrent corticosteroid therapy, even if symptoms are improved
- warn the patient that tremor and palpitations may be experienced
- those with diabetes should be instructed to monitor blood glucose levels, especially when starting therapy
- if patient has underlying heart disease, advise him/her to seek medical advice immediately if chest pain or signs of worsening heart disease including shortness of breath occur during therapy
- ensure that patient understands capsules are for use with the Aerolizer, not to be taken orally
- instruct patient on correct use of Aerolizer (p. 98) or Turbuhaler (p. 108)
- see also General Patient teaching and advice for antiasthma agents and bronchodilators (p. 96)

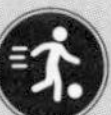
use in sport is subject to conditions

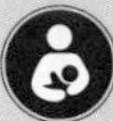
may inhibit labour due to relaxant effects on uterine smooth muscle

not recommended during breastfeeding unless benefits outweigh risks

Note

- combined with budesonide in Symbicort and DuoResp Spiromax, with fluticasone propionate in Flutiform and with aclidinium in Brimica Genuair

INDACATEROL (Onbrez Breezhaler)

Available form

Powder for inhalation: 150 microgram, 300 microgram

Action

- ultra-long-acting beta-2 adrenergic agonist
- rapid onset within 5 minutes, peak effect 2–4 hours, long duration of action

Use

- treatment of airflow limitation in those with chronic obstructive pulmonary disease (COPD)

Dose

- 150 microgram once daily by inhalation via Breezhaler, increasing to 300 microgram if needed

Adverse effects

- nasopharyngitis, cough, upper respiratory tract infection, sinusitis, oropharyngeal pain, rhinorrhoea
- headache
- muscle spasm, myalgia
- dry mouth
- hypokalaemia
- hyperglycaemia
- peripheral oedema, chest pain
- (rare) hypersensitivity (breathing or swallowing difficulties, tongue, lips or face swelling, urticaria, rash), paradoxical bronchospasm, prolongation of QT interval

Interactions

- increased risk of prolonged QT interval and arrhythmias if given with other agents known to prolong QT interval, such as MAOIs, TCAs, erythromycin, disopyramide, phenothiazines or antihistamines
- not recommended with other beta-2 adrenoceptor agonists
- see also General Interactions of beta-2 adrenoceptor agonists (p. 99)

Nursing points/Cautions

- should not be used in those with asthma or mixed airways disease; should be excluded before starting therapy
- not recommended for initial treatment of acute symptomatic COPD exacerbations
- if COPD worsens despite treatment, the patient should be re-evaluated
- not recommended in those < 18 years
- beta-2 adrenoreceptor agonists can increase blood glucose levels, therefore caution if used in those with diabetes mellitus
- caution if used in those with coronary artery disease, acute myocardial infarction, cardiac arrhythmia, hypertension, epilepsy, thyrotoxicosis or if patient is known to be unresponsive to beta-2 adrenergic agonist therapy
- contraindicated in those with rare hereditary galactose intolerance, Lapp lactase deficiency or glucose–galactose malabsorption as capsules contain lactose

Patient teaching and advice

- advise patient to continue long-term inhaled corticosteroids with indacaterol therapy
- instruct patient to seek medical advice if difficulty breathing or swallowing, or swelling of tongue, lips or face occurs
- ensure patient understands that indacaterol should not be used to relieve acute attack of breathlessness or wheezing
- if patient has underlying heart disease, advise him/her to seek medical advice immediately if chest pain or signs of worsening heart disease, including shortness of breath, occur during therapy
- those with diabetes should be instructed to monitor blood glucose levels, especially when starting therapy
- instruct patient that:
    - capsules are for use with Breezhaler and should not be taken orally
    - it should be administered at same time each day
    - capsules should be stored in blister and only removed just before use

- correct use of Breezhaler (inhalation device supplied) is important to ensure whole dose is administered, including:
  1. remove cap and open mouthpiece
  2. after removing capsule from blister pack, place in chamber and close mouthpiece (until click is heard)
  3. do not shake, but press side buttons in once and then release
  4. breathe out gently (away from inhaler) and then place mouth over mouthpiece (without biting) to form a good seal
  5. breathe in quickly and steadily (capsule should vibrate)
  6. hold breath for as long as is comfortable (or at least 5 seconds)
  7. while holding breath, remove inhaler from mouth and breathe out gently (away from inhaler)
  8. open mouthpiece and remove used capsule
  9. if other doses are required, repeat steps 3–8
  10. close mouthpiece and cap
- see also General Patient teaching and advice for antiasthma agents and bronchodilators (p. 96)

banned in sport

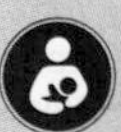

may inhibit labour due to relaxant effects on uterine smooth muscle

not recommended during breastfeeding unless benefits outweigh risks

Note

- contained in Ultibro Breezhaler 110/50 with glycopyrronium

SALBUTAMOL SULFATE (known as albuterol in the USA) (Airomir Autohaler and Inhaler, Asmol CFC-free Inhaler, Ventolin preparations, Ventolin Obstetric Injection)

Available forms

Inhaler/Autohaler: 100 microgram/metered dose; Nebules/Sterinebs/Ampoules (for inhalation): 2.5 mg/2.5 mL, 5 mg/2.5 mL; Syrup (sugar free): 2 mg/5 mL; Rotacap capsules: 200 microgram; Injection: 500 microgram/mL, 1 mg/mL

Action

- selective beta-2 adrenoreceptor stimulant causing bronchodilation mainly by stimulating pulmonary receptors
- relaxes uterine and blood vessel smooth muscle
- some cardiac stimulation
- onset of action 5–15 minutes, duration of action 3–6 hours
- symptom reliever

Use

- prevention of relief-reversible bronchospasm in asthma or chronic obstructive pulmonary disease (COPD)
- acute prophylaxis against exercise-induced asthma (or other known triggers)
- management of uncomplicated premature labour (24–33 weeks' gestation) (see Pregnancy, childbirth and breastfeeding, p. 1407)

Dose

- 2–4 mg (5–10 mL) orally 3–4 times daily **OR**
- 5 mg via nebuliser 4- to 6-hourly **OR**
- 1–2 inhalations (100–200 microgram) 4-hourly as required (if 2 inhalations are required, allow a 1-minute interval) (daily maximum 16 inhalations (8 treatments) (metered dose aerosol inhaler /Autohaler) **OR**

- 1–2 Rotacaps (200–400 microgram) inhaled 3–4 times daily (if 2 inhalations are required, allow a 5-minute interval) (daily maximum 12 Rotacaps) (Rotahaler) **OR**
- 500 microgram SC or IM 3–4-hourly **OR**
- 200–300 microgram over 1 minute IV, repeated after 15 minutes if required **OR**
- 200 microgram IV over 1 minute (loading dose), then 5–20 microgram/minute as IV infusion

Adverse effects
- (IM, SC, IM) stinging, pain
- see also General Adverse effects of beta-2 adrenoreceptor agonists (p. 98)

Interactions
- see General Interactions of beta-2 adrenoceptor agonists (p. 99)
- combination of nebulised salbutamol and ipratropium may result in closed-angle glaucoma

Nursing points/Cautions

- monitor vital signs, noting that an elevation of heart rate may be a side-effect and a reduced heart rate a sign of improvement
- before increasing dose, patient inhaler techniques should be checked
- symptoms of overdose are eased by rest and reassurance
- note and report any cardiac arrhythmias, especially in patients receiving digoxin, as these may result from salbutamol-induced hypokalaemia
- patient may also be prescribed an inhaled corticosteroid (e.g. fluticasone), in which case it is taken about 10 minutes after the salbutamol. Salbutamol promotes bronchodilation maximising inhalation of the corticosteroid
- excessive inhalation of the aerosol should be avoided to prevent overdose of the active therapeutic agent, reduce the risk of hazards from the propellant, and reduce the risk of worsening hypoxaemia
- parenteral salbutamol (IM, IV) is only used in cases of severe bronchospasm or status asthmaticus, in conjunction with glucocorticoids and oxygen therapy
- adverse effects are more common when salbutamol is given IV or IM
- if used IV in those with diabetes mellitus, solution should only be diluted using sodium chloride 0.9%
- if given by injection, IM is the route of choice
- (nebuliser) most nebulisers deliver 1 mL over 3 minutes or 2 mL over 8–10 minutes
- (nebuliser) fresh dilution should be prepared for each inhalation, any residue discarded and nebuliser cleaned
- can increase blood glucose levels, therefore caution if used in those with diabetes mellitus
- caution if used in those with liver or kidney dysfunction as lower doses may be required
- caution if used in those who have hypertension, coronary artery disease, congestive cardiac failure, phaeochromocytoma, diabetes mellitus, recent myocardial infarction, hyperthyroidism or thyrotoxicosis
- (dry powder inhaler formulation) contraindicated in patients with severe milk protein allergy

Patient teaching and advice

- see General Patient teaching and advice for antiasthma agents and bronchodilators (p. 96)
- instruct patient that exercise-induced bronchospasm may be prevented by 2 inhalations (200 microgram) 15 minutes before exertion

- advise the patient of the benefit of a small dose early in an attack before bronchospasm becomes too severe
- counsel patient that in an emergency, 6 puffs are taken immediately then 1 puff every 5 minutes while seeking medical attention
- warn patient against overuse of inhaled salbutamol as it may lead to worsening of hypoxaemia
- overdose may be avoided by instructing the patient thoroughly in the correct use of the metered dose aerosol inhaler, other inhaler devices and nebuliser, and ensuring that the inhaler is not used if the patient is receiving salbutamol by other means
- warn patient that tremor and palpitations are commonly experienced
- instruct patient to seek medical advice immediately if not obtaining adequate relief (i.e. if effect of each dose lasts for less than 3 hours)
- warn patient to avoid mist contacting eyes (e.g. ensuring nebulising mask fits correctly), especially if person is predisposed to glaucoma
- patient with diabetes should be advised to closely monitor blood glucose levels during therapy
- instruct patient that oral syrup may be diluted with purified water only. Diluted mixture should be used within 28 days and protected from light
- patients should be advised not to drive or operate machinery if they experience adverse effects
- if patient has underlying heart disease, advise him/her to seek medical advice immediately if experiencing chest pain or signs of worsening heart disease, including shortness of breath, occur during therapy

Metered dose aerosol inhaler

- advise patient that manufacturer's instruction leaflet is in inhaler packet and should be referred to
- instruct patient in correct technique for metered dose aerosol inhaler:
  1. inhaler is loaded with salbutamol canister
  2. remove mouthpiece cap and shake inhaler well
  3. prime inhaler by activating the aerosol 2 or 3 times into the air to ensure spray is even
  4. hold inhaler vertically with mouthpiece at the bottom and breathe out slowly and fully
  5. place mouthpiece well into the mouth, with lips closed firmly around it and the head tilted back slightly
  6. inhale rapidly and deeply through mouthpiece, at the same time administering a metered dose by pressing canister downwards
  7. release pressure on the canister and remove inhaler while holding breath for as long as possible (10 seconds)
  8. breathe out slowly through the mouth and replace mouthpiece cap
- if two inhalations required, allow a 5-minute interval before taking the second to enable better assessment of the first inhalation and deeper penetration of the second inhalation
- patient can practise with placebo inhaler (contains air)
- warn patient that the pressurised container should be kept intact and away from heat
- canister is about ¼ full if it floats at about 45° on the surface of a bowl of water (i.e. need to obtain new canister)
- children can usually manage a metered dose aerosol inhaler from about 7 years of age, but should be supervised by a responsible adult until competent
- CFC-free inhaler needs to be primed before first use or if unused for 5 days or more

- canisters should be protected from frost as cold temperatures may decrease therapeutic effect
- inhaler should be cleaned at least once a week by removing the metal canister from plastic casing as well as mouthpiece cover. Actuator should be rinsed under warm running water and then dried inside and out. Metal canister and mouthpiece cover should then be replaced. Metal canister should not be put into water

Rotahaler

- Rotahaler is a breath-actuated device that breaks the Rotacap in half, while airflow through the device during inspiration disperses the powder in the inspired air
- suitable for children aged from 3 to 6 years and others unable to coordinate the use of the metered dose aerosol inhaler, and in severe asthma with low inspiratory flow rate
- ensure patient understands that Rotacaps are not for oral use
- instruct patient in correct technique for Rotahaler:
    1. remove Rotahaler from container and hold vertically by dark blue mouthpiece with light blue body uppermost
    2. turn light blue body of Rotahaler as far as it will go in either direction
    3. push Rotacap, clear end first, firmly into the square hole, forcing any previously used Rotacap shell into Rotahaler
    4. holding Rotahaler horizontally to prevent Rotacap contents from falling out, turn the light blue body as far as it will go in the opposite direction to open Rotacap
    5. breathe out slowly and, keeping Rotahaler completely level, grip mouthpiece between the teeth, with lips closed firmly around it and head tilted back slightly
    6. inhale rapidly and deeply through the mouthpiece
    7. remove Rotahaler, hold breath as long as possible, then breathe out slowly through the mouth
    8. after each use, pull the two halves of the Rotahaler apart and remove loose Rotacap shells
    9. reassemble and store in container
- Rotahaler may be cleaned once every 2 weeks by rinsing both halves in warm water and drying thoroughly (removing empty shells first)
- protect Rotahaler from heat and from dirt and damage by keeping it in its container
- Rotacaps are designed to be used with Rotahaler for patients unable to satisfactorily use a metered dose aerosol inhaler, including children. Children's use should be supervised by a responsible adult

Autohaler

- advise patient that manufacturer's instruction leaflet is in Autohaler packet
- instruct patient in correct technique for Autohaler:
    1. if Autohaler is new or unused for 2 weeks, release 4 puffs into the air (away from face)
    2. remove mouthpiece cover by unclipping from back. Check that it is clean
    3. hold Autohaler upright and shake vigorously
    4. continue holding Autohaler upright (without blocking vents in base) and push lever up
    5. breathe out as far as possible and close lips around the mouthpiece
    6. breathe in slowly and deeply and continue to do so when you hear a click and feel the puff in mouth
    7. hold breath for as long as comfortable (or at least 10 seconds) and then breathe out slowly

8. after each puff, return lever to the down position while keeping Autohaler upright
9. push lever up before each puff and gently back down afterwards, keeping the Autohaler upright. Lever should be left down between treatments
10. if more than 1 dose is required, steps 4–8 should be repeated

- Autohaler should be cleaned weekly by wiping the mouthpiece only with a clean dry cloth. Other parts of the Autohaler should not be cleaned
- to check if Autohaler is empty, remove mouthpiece cover by unclipping from the back. Shake Autohaler and holding it upright with mouthpiece away from you, push lever up and release a puff by pushing the dose-release slide on the bottom of the Autohaler in the direction of the arrow. To release a second puff, first return lever to down position and repeat. Repeat this 4 times in total. If Autohaler is empty, you will not feel or hear a puff being discharged
- the dose-release slide is for testing the Autohaler ONLY; it should not be used to deliver medication

(IV, oral) banned in sport

(inhalers, nebulising solution) use in sport subject to conditions

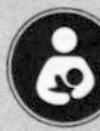

should not be used in pregnancy unless benefits outweigh risks. However, is used IV to treat premature labour (uncomplicated), but should not be used during first or second trimester to treat threatened abortion. IV administration is contraindicated in antepartum haemorrhage – salbutamol crosses the placental barrier and causes fetal tachycardia. If used immediately before childbirth, it may inhibit contractions

not recommended during breastfeeding unless potential benefits outweigh risks

SALMETEROL XINAFOATE (Serevent)

Available form

Accuhaler: 50 microgram/blister

Action

- selective long-acting beta-2 adrenoceptor agonist
- onset of action within 10–30 minutes, peak effect 3–4 hours, duration 12 hours
- symptom controller

Use

- long-term management of reversible airways obstruction in asthma or chronic obstructive pulmonary disease (COPD) (with concurrent corticosteroid therapy)

Dose

- 50–100 microgram (1–2 blisters) twice daily via Accuhaler

Adverse effects

- see General Adverse effects of beta-2 adrenoreceptor agonists (p. 98)

Interactions

- see General Interactions of beta-2 adrenoceptor agonists (p. 99)
- not recommended with itraconazole, clarithromycin, indinavir, ritonavir, saquinavir, nelfinavir or atazanavir

Nursing points/Cautions

- therapy should not be started if asthma is unstable or significantly deteriorating
- has slow onset of action, therefore a faster acting beta-2 agonist should be used if rapid bronchodilation is needed
- can increase blood glucose levels, therefore caution required if used in those with diabetes mellitus
- caution if used in those with pre-existing cardiovascular disease or predisposition to low serum potassium levels

Patient teaching and advice

- patient should be advised not to stop or reduce dose of corticosteroids without medical advice
- ensure patient understands that salmeterol is long acting and should not be used in the event of an acute asthma episode
- instruct patient that use before exercise is not appropriate because of slow onset of action (10–30 minutes) and full effect requires repeated doses
- instruct patient on correct technique for using Accuhaler (p. 133)
- see also General Patient teaching and advice for antiasthma agents and bronchodilators (p. 96)

use in sport subject to conditions

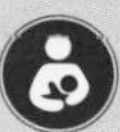

not recommended during pregnancy or breastfeeding unless potential benefits outweigh risks

Note

- combined with fluticasone in Seretide, Fluticasone, Seroflo and Salmeterol Cipla, Pavtide and Salplus F

TERBUTALINE SULFATE (Bricanyl)

Available forms

Elixir: 0.3 mg/mL; Injection: 0.5 mg/mL; Turbuhaler: 500 microgram/inhalation

Action

- direct-acting sympathomimetic agent with some selective beta-2 adrenoreceptor stimulant activity in the lungs
- also improves mucociliary clearance
- onset of action 30 minutes (SC), 1 hour (inhalation), duration 4–5 hours
- symptom reliever

Use

- relief of bronchospasm associated with asthma and chronic obstructive pulmonary disease (COPD)
- prophylaxis of exercise-induced asthma or other bronchospasm-inducing situation

Dose

- 1 inhalation (500 microgram) 4–6-hourly as required (may require up to 3 inhalations in severe cases, but should not exceed 12 inhalations in 24 hours)

OR

- 250 microgram SC 6-hourly as required

Adverse effects

- nausea, vomiting, diarrhoea
- sweating
- rash, urticaria
- see also General Adverse effects of beta-2 adrenoreceptor agonists (p. 98)

Interactions

- see General Interactions of beta-2 adrenoreceptor agonists (p. 99)

Nursing points/Cautions

- SC administration is for acute management only
- caution if used in those with thyrotoxicosis, hypertension, coronary artery disease, arrhythmias or diabetes mellitus
- contraindicated in those with hypersensitivity to other sympathomimetic agents

Patient teaching and advice

- see General Patient teaching and advice for antiasthma agents and bronchodilators (p. 96)
- ensure patient understands that this should not be used in emergency or acute situations
- advise patient to continue oral or inhaled corticosteroids or leukotriene antagonists

- patients with diabetes should be advised to closely monitor blood glucose levels during therapy
- if patient has underlying heart disease, advise him/her to seek medical advice immediately if experiencing chest pain or signs of worsening heart disease, including shortness of breath, occur during therapy

Turbuhaler

- manufacturer's instruction leaflet is in the packet
- breath-actuated multiple dose inhaler device that allows dispersion of the very fine propellant-free powder in the inspired air
- suitable for children aged from 3–4 years and others unable to coordinate the use of the metered dose aerosol inhaler, and in severe asthma with low inspiratory flow rate, and in patients sensitive to freon propellants
- instruct patient in correct Turbuhaler technique:
  1. unscrew cap and lift it off
  2. hold Turbuhaler upright and twist coloured base to the right as far as it will go, then twist it back to the left until it clicks
  3. breathe out slowly, put mouthpiece fully between the lips and inhale deeply through the mouth without covering air vents
  4. remove Turbuhaler, hold breath as long as possible, then breathe out slowly through mouth
- Turbuhaler has a dose indicator window in which a red mark appears when there are 20 doses remaining
- Turbuhaler should be cleaned 2–3 times per week by removing the mouthpiece and gently wiping away any particles that have collected inside the mouthpiece with a dry tissue or cloth (do not wash the mouthpiece with water)

banned in sport

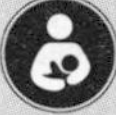
caution if used during the first trimester of pregnancy

transient hypoglycaemia may occur in breastfed preterm newborns

ANTICHOLINERGIC (ANTIMUSCARINIC) AGENTS

General Adverse effects of anticholinergic agents

- (local) irritated throat, cough, dry mouth, hoarseness
- dry mouth, dysphagia, thirst, constipation, nausea, vomiting, taste alteration, dyspepsia
- headache, nervousness, insomnia, confusion, drowsiness, dizziness
- urinary urgency, difficulty and retention
- impotence
- flushing and dryness of skin, decreased sweating
- tachycardia, palpitations, arrhythmias
- mydriasis, photophobia, cycloplegia, blurred vision, eye pain
- (less common) raised intraocular pressure, glaucoma, angina, heat intolerance, hypersensitivity, hyperpyrexia
- (rare) paradoxical bronchoconstriction

General Nursing points/Cautions for anticholinergic agents

- caution if used in those with unstable angina, myocardial infarction (in

last 6 months), newly diagnosed arrhythmia (in last 3 months), or hospitalised for heart failure (class III or IV) (last 12 months)
- caution if used in those with symptomatic prostatic hyperplasia, bladder neck obstruction or narrow-angle glaucoma
- contraindicated in those with hypersensitivity to atropine and related substances

General Patient teaching and advice for anticholinergic agents

- advise patient not to drive or operate machinery if dizziness, drowsiness, confusion or blurred vision occur
- warn patient that persistent dry mouth can lead to dental caries, therefore it is important to maintain good mouth and dental hygiene
- if patient has poor metered dose inhaler technique, suggest using a spacer device (p. 97)
- instruct patient to seek medical advice if any of the following occur:
  - difficulty passing urine, painful urination
  - any eye pain/discomfort, blurred vision, visual halos, coloured images and/or red eyes
  - rapid or irregular heartbeat

ACLIDIUNIUM BROMIDE (Bretaris Genuair)

Available form

Powder for inhalation: 322 microgram/dose

Action

- anticholinergic (antimuscarinic agent) that acts on M3 receptors in airway smooth muscle to induce bronchodilation
- onset of action within 5–15 minutes, half-life 2–3 hours

Use

- long-term bronchodilator maintenance treatment for chronic obstructive pulmonary disease (COPD)

Dose

- 322 microgram (1 inhalation) twice daily

Adverse effects

- diarrhoea, toothache, abdominal discomfort
- nasopharyngitis, sinusitis, rhinitis
- see General Adverse effects of anticholinergic agents (p. 108)

Interactions

- not recommended with other anticholinergic agents due to additive effects

Nursing points/Cautions

- not recommended in those with asthma
- not recommended in those under 18 years
- contains lactose and is therefore contraindicated in those with rare hereditary problems of galactose intolerance, Lapp lactase deficiency or glucose–galactose malabsorption
- see also General Nursing points/Cautions for anticholinergic agents (p. 108)

Patient teaching and advice

- advise patient that aclidinium should not be used for acute episodes of bronchospasm
- instruct patient in correct use of Genuair inhaler device:
  1. check dose counter (taking care not to shake device)
  2. remove green protective cap by squeezing arrows on each side and pulling outwards
  3. hold with green button facing upwards (not tilted)

4. press and release green button while breathing out completely away from inhaler (do not continue to hold green button down)
5. make sure control window is showing green. If window shows red, repeat above steps
6. place lips tightly around mouthpiece and breathe in strongly and deeply through inhaler (you should hear a click; continue to breathe in after this has occurred)
7. remove inhaler from mouth and hold breath for as long as comfortable, then breathe out slowly through nose
8. control window should return to red (to show dose has been administered). If control window is still green, continue inhaling through mouthpiece
9. replace green protective cap after use
10. when red stripes appear in dose indicator window, new prescription should be obtained

- see also General Patient teaching and advice for antiasthmatic agents and bronchodilators (p. 96) and anticholinergic agents (p. 109)

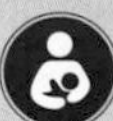

not recommended during pregnancy or breastfeeding unless benefits outweigh risks

Note

- contained in Bretaris Genuair 340/12 with formoterol (eformoterol) fumarate dihydrate

GLYCOPYRRONIUM (GLYCOPYRROLATE) (Seebri Breezhaler)

Available form

Inhalation powder capsules: 50 microgram

Action

- long-acting anticholinergic (antimuscarinic) agent
- onset of action 5 minutes, half-life 33–57 hours (inhalation)

Use

- long-term bronchodilator maintenance treatment for chronic obstructive pulmonary disease (COPD)

Dose

- 50 microgram via Breezhaler once daily

Adverse effects

- gastroenteritis, dyspepsia
- (uncommon) musculoskeletal pain, pain in extremity, rash, fatigue, asthenia, productive cough, congested sinus, throat irritation, blood nose, rhinitis
- see General Adverse effects of anticholinergic agents (p. 108)

Interactions

- not recommended with other anticholinergic agents due to additive effects

Nursing points/Cautions

- caution if used in those with severe kidney impairment
- contains lactose and is therefore contraindicated in those with rare hereditary problems of galactose intolerance, Lapp lactase deficiency or glucose–galactose malabsorption
- see also General Nursing points/Cautions for anticholinergic agents (p. 108)

Patient teaching and advice

- advise patient that glycopyrronium should not be used for acute episodes of bronchospasm
- ensure patient understands that capsules are not to be taken orally and are only for use with inhaler device

- instruct patient in correct use of Breezhaler, including:
  1. remove cap and flip mouthpiece to open
  2. remove capsule from blister pack and insert into chamber
  3. close mouthpiece (click should be heard)
  4. press side buttons in once and then release (taking care not to shake device)
  5. breathe out gently (away from device), then place mouthpiece between teeth and close lips to form tight seal
  6. breathe in quickly and steadily (capsule should vibrate) and then hold breath for 5 seconds, or as long as comfortable
  7. while holding breath, remove device from mouth
  8. breathe out gently (away from device)
  9. open device to remove capsule and repeat process if more than 1 dose is required
  10. close mouthpiece and cap
- see also General Patient teaching and advice for antiasthmatic agents and bronchodilators (p. 98) and anticholinergic agents (p. 109)

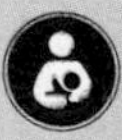

should only be used during pregnancy or breastfeeding if benefits outweigh risks

Note

- contained in Enerzair Breezhaler with indacaterol and mometasone, Trimbow solution for inhalation with beclometasone and formoterol, and Ultibro Breezhaler 110/50 with indacaterol

IPRATROPIUM BROMIDE (Aeron, Apoven, Atrovent preparations, Ipratrin Uni-Dose)

Available forms

Metered dose aerosol: 21 microgram/inhalation; Nebuliser solution: 250 microgram/mL, 500 microgram/mL; Nasal spray: 22 microgram/dose, 44 microgram/dose

Action

- anticholinergic (antimuscarinic) agent
- causes bronchodilation by blocking vagal reflexes
- (nasal spray) inhibits secretions from serous and seromucous glands lining nasal mucosa without altering any physiological nasal functions such as smell
- (inhalation) onset of action 3–5 minutes, peak response at 1.5–2 hours, duration of 4–6 hours, half-life 1.5–4 hours
- (asthma) symptom reliever

Use

- chronic asthma, moderate asthma attack, chronic obstructive bronchitis with bronchospasm
- bronchospasm during/after surgery, during ventilation with respirator
- rhinorrhoea associated with allergic or non-allergic rhinitis and common cold (nasal spray)

Dose

- 42–84 microgram (2–4 puffs) 3–4 times daily (metered dose aerosol) **OR**
- 250–500 microgram (1–2 mL) diluted to 2–3 mL with sodium chloride 0.9% and given 6-hourly via nebuliser until entire volume is inhaled (may be repeated after 2 hours as required) (daily maximum 2 mg) **OR**
- (rhinorrhoea associated with allergic/non-allergic rhinitis) 44–88 microgram into each nostril 2–3 times daily, decreasing dose/frequency when rhinorrhoea improves (nasal spray) **OR**
- (rhinorrhoea associated with cold) 88 microgram into each nostril 3–4 times daily decreasing dose when rhinorrhea improves (for up to 4 days) (nasal spray)

Adverse effects

- (local, nasal spray) nose bleed, nasal discomfort, irritation and dryness, headache, blood-tinged mucus, pharyngitis, nausea
- mild, reversible visual disturbances (blurred vision, eye pain, halo vision) if accidentally enters eyes
- hypersensitivity (skin rash, angio-edema of tongue, lips and face, urticaria, laryngospasm)
- see General Adverse effects of anticholinergic agents (p. 108)

Interactions

- not recommended with other anticholinergic agents due to additive effects
- bronchodilation may be enhanced if used with xanthines and beta-2 adrenoceptor agonists
- increased risk of glaucoma (in those with history of narrow angle glaucoma) if given simultaneously with beta-2 adrenoceptor agonists

Nursing points/Cautions

- (asthma) may be used alone or in combination with other bronchodilator agents and corticosteroids
- (common cold, nasal spray) treatment should be limited to 4 days
- if using wall oxygen/air with nebuliser, 6–8 L/min is the recommended flow rate
- (nasal spray) contains benzalkonium chloride, which may cause irritation of nasal mucosa
- caution if used in those with cystic fibrosis as they have an increased risk of gastrointestinal motility disturbance
- see also General Nursing points/Cautions for anticholinergic agents (p. 108)

Patient teaching and advice

- instruct patient on correct use of metered dose aerosol inhaler (p. 104)
- warn patient to avoid mist contacting eyes (e.g. ensuring nebulising mask fits correctly), especially if person is predisposed to glaucoma
- instruct patient in correct use of nasal spray, including:
  1. when taking nasal spray from foil pouch for first time, write expiry date (4 months) on space provided on nasal spray bottle. This should be checked each time nasal spray is used. Discard after this date
  2. do not spray near or in eyes
  3. do not attempt to pierce or enlarge hole in nozzle
  4. do not shake pump spray
  5. before first use, prime spray pump by activating spray 5–7 times until an even spray is released. If pump is unused for 24 hours, it should be re-primed by spraying once or until a fine mist appears
  6. blow nose before nasal administration
  7. insert spray adapter into nostril and administer spray while breathing gently through nose. Repeat for required number of sprays. Repeat in other nostril if required
  8. replace protective cap and store upright
  9. if nasal tip becomes clogged, run under warm running water for about 60 seconds, then dry tip and re-prime before replacing protective cap
- see also General Patient teaching and advice for antiasthma agents and bronchodilators (p. 96) and anticholinergic agents (p. 109)

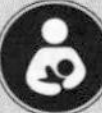

use with caution during first trimester of pregnancy

should only be used during breastfeeding if benefits are thought to outweigh risks

TIOTROPIUM BROMIDE (Braltus, Spiriva, Spiriva Respimat)

Available forms

Capsule (for inhalation device): 13 microgram, 18 microgram; Solution for inhalation: 2.5 microgram/actuation

Action

- long-acting anticholinergic (antimuscarinic) agent
- relaxes bronchial smooth muscle by inhibiting muscarinic receptors (M3)
- long duration of action (about 24 hours), allowing once-daily administration

Use

- prophylaxis and maintenance treatment of bronchospasm and dyspnoea associated with chronic obstructive pulmonary disease (COPD)
- maintenance treatment for moderate to severe asthma

Dose

- (COPD) 18 microgram (1 capsule) via inhalation once daily via HandiHaler or Zonda device **OR**
- (COPD, asthma) 5 microgram (2 puffs) daily via Respimat inhalation device

Adverse effects

- hypersensitivity reaction
- see also General Adverse effects of anticholinergic agents (p. 108)

Interactions

- not recommended with other anticholinergic agents due to additive effects

Nursing points/Cautions

- not first-line treatment in asthma management
- (capsules) contains 5.5 mg lactose/capsule, therefore use with caution; not recommended in those with rare hereditary problems of galactose intolerance, Lapp lactase deficiency or glucose–galactose malabsorption
- caution if used in those with moderate-to-severe kidney impairment (creatinine clearance ≤ 50 mL/minute)
- see also General Nursing points/Cautions for anticholinergic agents (p. 108)

Patient teaching and advice

- ensure patient understands that tiotropium should not be used for treatment of acute episodes of bronchospasm or relief of acute symptoms. A rapid beta-2 agonist is recommended to treat an acute attack
- avoid contact with eyes, especially if person is predisposed to glaucoma
- ensure patient understands that capsules should not be taken orally and are for use in an inhaler device
- instruct patient in correct technique for Respimat inhaler, Handi-Haler and Zonda devices (instructions below)

HandiHaler

- advise patient that manufacturer's instruction leaflet is in the packet
- instruct patient in correct technique for HandiHaler, including:
  1. open dust cap by pulling upwards and then open mouthpiece
  2. remove capsule gently from blister pack immediately before use
  3. place capsule in centre chamber and close mouthpiece firmly until click is heard (leaving dust cap open)
  4. hold device with mouthpiece upwards; press green button completely (once) and release (this pierces capsule, releasing powder for inhalation)
  5. breathe out fully away from inhaler
  6. close lips tightly around mouthpiece and breathe in slowly and

deeply, at a rate that causes the capsule to vibrate
7. hold breath for as long as comfortable, remove device from mouth and resume normal breathing
8. repeat steps 5 to 7
9. open mouthpiece and remove used capsule

- to clean HandiHaler, open dust cap and mouthpiece. Then open the base by lifting the piercing button, rinse with warm water and allow to air dry (this may take 24 hours)
- capsules should be used within 5 days of opening blister strip

Zonda device

- advise patient that manufacturer's instruction leaflet is in the packet
- instruct patient in correct technique for Zonda device, including:
    1. pull cap upwards
    2. firmly hold base of inhaler and pull mouthpiece upwards to open
    3. remove Braltus capsule from bottle and place it in capsule-shaped compartment at bottom of inhaler (ensure lid of bottle is closed tightly after capsule is removed)
    4. close mouthpiece (click should be heard) leaving cap open
    5. hold inhaler with mouthpiece upwards, press piercing button once only and release button
    6. breathe out fully (away from inhaler)
    7. place mouthpiece in mouth closing lips around it to form a tight seal then breathe in deeply and steadily (capsule should vibrate)
    8. hold breath for as long as possible, then breathe out normally
    9. repeat last two steps to ensure capsule is empty
    10. empty capsule from mouthpiece
    11. Zonda device should be discarded after 30 uses
- see also General Patient teaching for antiasthma agents and bronchodilators (p. 96) and anticholinergic agents (p. 109)

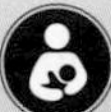

should only be used during pregnancy or breastfeeding if benefits are thought to outweigh risks

Note

- contained in Spiolto Respimat with olodaterol

UMECLIDINIUM (Incruse Ellipta)

Available form

Powder for inhalation: 62.5 microgram/dose

Action

- long-acting anticholinergic (antimuscarinic) agent
- onset of action 15 minutes, duration of action 24 hours, half-life 19 hours

Use

- long-term bronchodilator maintenance treatment for chronic obstructive pulmonary disease (COPD)

Dose

- 62.5 microgram once daily via inhaler

Adverse effects

- upper respiratory tract infection, sinusitis, nasopharyngitis
- urinary tract infection
- arthralgia
- see also General Adverse effects of anticholinergic agents (p. 108)

Interactions

- not recommended with other anticholinergic agents due to additive effects

Nursing points/Cautions

- therapy should not be started in those with acutely deteriorating COPD
- not recommended in those with asthma

- contains lactose and is therefore contraindicated in those with rare hereditary problems of galactose intolerance, Lapp lactase deficiency or glucose–galactose malabsorption
- contraindicated in those with severe milk protein allergy
- see also General Nursing points/Cautions for anticholinergic agents (p. 108)

Patient teaching and advice

- warn patient that umeclidinium is not for use if symptoms are acute
- advise patient to only use inhaler once per day
- instruct patient in correct use of Ellipta inhaler, including:
  1. inhaler should not be removed from sealed container/tray until patient is ready to inhale medication
  2. ensure inhaler is in 'closed' position. If the cover is opened and then closed without inhaling the dose will be lost and held inside device
  3. do not shake inhaler at any time
  4. slide cover down until you hear a click (the dose counter should also count down). If there is no click, the device may be faulty and needs to be returned to pharmacy
  5. holding inhaler away from mouth, breathe out as far as is comfortable and then put mouthpiece between lips. Close lips firmly around mouthpiece, taking care not to block air vents with fingers
  6. take a long steady deep breath in and hold for 3–4 seconds (or as long as is comfortable)
  7. remove inhaler from mouth and breathe out slowly (away from mouthpiece)
  8. you may or may not taste or feel medication when inhaling
  9. mouthpiece can be cleaned using dry tissue, then close cover
  10. when less than 10 doses remain in inhaler, half of the dose counter will show red. Inhaler is empty when 0 appears on dose counter which will appear red
  11. should be discarded 6 weeks after opening container/tray
- see also General Patient teaching and advice for antiasthmatic agents and bronchodilators (p. 96) and anticholinergic agents (p. 109)

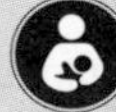

only used during pregnancy or breastfeeding if benefits outweigh risks

Note

- contained in Anora Ellipta with vilanterol (a long-acting beta-2 adrenoceptor agonist) and Trelegy Ellipta with vilanterol and fluticasone furoate

XANTHINES

AMINOPHYLLINE (DBL Aminophylline Injection)

Available form

Ampoule: 250 mg/10 mL

Action

- aminophylline dissociates to theophylline in biological tissue (1 mg aminophylline = 0.8 mg theophylline)
- see Action of theophylline (p. 118)
- narrow therapeutic index
- symptom reliever

Use

- reversible bronchospasm associated with chronic bronchitis, emphysema, bronchial asthma and chronic obstructive pulmonary disease (COPD)

- paroxysmal dyspnoea associated with left-sided heart failure

Dose

- (bronchospasm not currently undergoing theophylline therapy, cor pulmonale or congestive heart failure) 6 mg/kg IV over 20–30 minutes (loading dose), then 0.5–1 mg/kg IV infusion for 12 hours, then reduced to 0.1–0.8 mg/kg IV infusion **OR**
- (currently undergoing theophylline therapy and unable to obtain serum concentration) 3 mg/kg IV over 20–30 minutes (loading dose), then 0.5–1 mg/kg IV infusion for 12 hours, then reduced to 0.1–0.8 mg/kg IV infusion

Adverse effects

- (rapid administration) anxiety, headache, nausea, vomiting, severe hypotension, profound bradycardia, flushing, faintness, praecordial pain
- see also Adverse effects of theophylline (p. 119)

Interactions

- contraindicated with other xanthines due to risk of additive toxicity
- aminophylline should be withheld for 36 hours before myocardial perfusion studies as it reverses the effects of dipyridamole
- inhibition of bronchodilatory effect may occur if given with beta-adrenoceptor blocking agents (beta blockers), including ophthalmic preparations
- cardiotoxicity and hypoglycaemia may occur if given with beta-adrenergic agonists
- may reduce or reverse sedative effects of benzodiazepines
- may antagonise non-depolarising neuromuscular blocking agents
- may cause toxicity if given with cardiac glycosides
- may produce false positive on serum uric acid test (using Bittner or colourmetric methods)
- see also Interactions of theophylline (p. 119)

Nursing points/Cautions

- dosage is calculated on lean body mass and highly individualised, preferably on the basis of serum theophylline monitoring, to achieve a therapeutic concentration of 5–20 microgram/mL (27.5–110 micromol/L)
- coagulation time should be monitored regularly during therapy
- maintenance dose is dependent on patient's age, heart, liver or lung function, and/or smoking status
- if patient is already taking theophylline, dose may depend on serum theophylline concentration (aminophylline is converted to theophylline in the body)
- monitor vital signs during IV administration, which should be at a rate not greater than 20–25 mg/minute. Rapid administration should be avoided as it may result in anxiety, headache, nausea, vomiting, severe hypotension, dizziness, faintness, light-headedness, palpitations, syncope, flushing, bradycardia or cardiac arrest
- IV therapy should be replaced by oral theophylline as soon as possible
- if it is necessary to prepare an IV admixture, consult a compatibility chart, manufacturer's literature, a pharmacist or drug information centre, because aminophylline is chemically or physically incompatible with an extensive list of drugs
- precipitates in acidic solutions (see previous comment about compatibility)
- not given IM because of intense pain and tissue sloughing
- not used if solution contains crystals
- chronic overdose symptoms and toxicity can occur at lower serum concentration (40 microgram/mL) than acute overdosage (90 microgram/mL).

Management of overdose should be symptomatic and supportive

- caution if used in those with epilepsy as seizure threshold may be lowered
- caution if used in the elderly or those with decreased liver or kidney function, congestive cardiac failure, cor pulmonale, chronic alcohol use, chronic obstructive pulmonary disease (COPD), acute pulmonary oedema, hypothyroidism, acute febrile state and viral infection (including pneumonia, influenza or influenza immunisation) as clearance may be decreased thus increasing risk of toxicity
- caution if used in those with compromised cardiac or circulatory function, hypertension, tachyarrhythmias, angina or acute myocardial injury where cardiac effects may be harmful
- caution if used in those with hyperthyroidism, diabetes mellitus, or glaucoma as there may be an exacerbation of the conditions
- caution if used in those with gastric ulceration or gastro-oesophageal reflux disease (GORD) because of an increase in gastric acid secretion
- contraindicated in those with hypersensitivity to xanthines or ethylenediamine, or with coronary artery disease or bronchiolitis

Patient teaching and advice

- warn patient not to take other xanthine derivatives or excessive amounts of caffeine-containing beverages such as coffee, tea, cola or energy drinks (e.g. Red Bull) concurrently

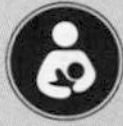

not to be used during pregnancy unless the expected benefit outweighs any potential risk. If used, serum theophylline levels should be monitored regularly

excreted in breastmilk, so dosage to mother minimised to avoid irritability and restlessness in infant

CAFFEINE CITRATE (Cafnea)

Available forms

Vial: 40 mg/2 mL; Oral solution: 25 mg/5 mL

Action

- methylxanthine related to theophylline and aminophylline
- centrally acting respiratory stimulant that increases respiratory rate significantly in premature infants, as well as decreasing apnoea attacks
- direct effect on myocardium increasing heart rate
- reduces pulmonary resistance and increases lung compliance with a reduction in amount of inspired oxygen required
- may also increase cerebral blood flow (but this has not been conclusively proven)
- poorly metabolised in preterm infants
- half-life in neonates is 65–102 hours, prolonged to 80–120 hours in preterm infants (28–32 weeks)

Use

- short-term management of apnoea in premature infants (gestational age 28 – < 33 weeks)

Dose

- 20 mg/kg IV over 30 minutes using syringe infusion pump (loading dose), followed by 5 mg/kg daily IV over 10 minutes or orally and further increased to 10 mg/kg once daily if apnoea persists (maintenance)

Adverse effects

- injection site reaction
- irritability, restlessness, jitteriness
- tachycardia, increased left ventricular output, increased stroke volume
- feeding intolerance, increased gastric aspirate
- vomiting, constipation, gastro-oesophageal reflux, dilated loops of bowel
- hypoglycaemia, hyperglycaemia

- anaemia
- hyponatraemia, increased calcium excretion, increased urine flow, increased creatinine clearance
- rash
- necrotising enterocolitis

Interactions

- increased serum levels may occur if given with artemisinin, cimetidine, fluvoxamine, fluconazole and verapamil
- decreased serum levels may occur if given with phenytoin
- may antagonise effects of benzodiazepines
- increases both endogenous and oral melatonin
- increases serum levels of clozapine
- may reduce bioavailability of fluvoxamine
- half-life increased and clearance decreased by ciprofloxacin and norfloxacin
- not recommended with aminophylline or theophylline

Nursing points/Cautions

- other causes of apnoea (e.g. CNS disorders, primary lung disease, anaemia, sepsis, metabolic or cardiovascular disturbances, obstructive apnoea) should be evaluated and/or treated before starting therapy
- baseline serum caffeine levels should be measured if mothers have consumed caffeine-containing fluids before delivery (caffeine crosses placenta)
- maintenance dose should be adjusted weekly according to changes in body weight
- maintenance dose begins 24 hours after loading dose and may be given IV over 10 minutes or orally if baby is tolerating full enteral feeds
- if baby shows signs of caffeine toxicity (e.g. tachycardia, tachypnoea, jitteriness, tremors, unexplained seizures and vomiting), dose can be reduced or withheld
- therapy should be stopped when apnoea ceases or therapy is no longer required
- infant should be closely monitored for any signs of necrotising enterocolitis which occurs commonly in preterm or low birthweight babies. Symptoms include abdominal distention, tenderness, blood in stool, bilious vomiting/drainage from enteral feeding tube, unstable temperature, apnoea, bradycardia, hypotension, acidosis and lethargy
- caution if used in infants with cardiovascular disease as caffeine may increase heart rate, left ventricular output and stroke volume
- caution if used in infants with seizure disorders or impaired kidney or liver function
- contraindicated in those with known sensitivity to caffeine or citrate

THEOPHYLLINE (Nuelin Syrup, Nuelin SR)

Available forms

Tablets (sustained-release): 200 mg, 250 mg, 300 mg; Syrup: 133.3 mg/25 mL

Action

- smooth muscle relaxation especially bronchial muscle and pulmonary blood vessels
- stimulant effect on myocardium (increasing heart rate and contractility), CNS and respiration (via medullary respiratory centre)
- decreases peripheral resistance by increasing pulmonary vasodilation
- diuresis (transient)
- increases gastric secretion
- active metabolite (less activity than theophylline)
- narrow therapeutic range

- therapeutic level 10–20 microgram/mL (doses above linked to adverse effects)
- half-life (3–12 hours) and clearance are affected by age, heart, liver and lung disease, viral infection, fever, some medications and smoking
- symptom reliever

Use

- relief and prophylaxis of reversible bronchospasm in asthma, chronic bronchitis, emphysema and related conditions

Dose

- 25 mL (133.3 mg) orally 6-hourly before meals (syrup) **OR**
- 200–300 mg orally 12-hourly, gradually increasing/decreasing dose by 100–150 mg if needed to achieve desired effects with minimal side-effects (sustained-release tablets)

Adverse effects

- anorexia, nausea, vomiting, epigastric pain, diarrhoea, abdominal cramps
- insomnia, headache, tremor, nervousness, restlessness, dizziness, anxiety, light-headedness
- palpitations, tachycardia, hypotension, cardiac arrhythmias
- tachypnoea
- increased urination, albuminuria, haematuria
- hyperglycaemia, hypokalaemia
- flushing
- rash
- alopecia
- reactivation of peptic ulcer or gastro-oesophageal reflux disease (GORD), haematemesis
- (high dose) inappropriate ADH secretion
- (early signs of toxicity) nausea, anorexia, vomiting, headache, irritability, agitation, anxiety, insomnia, hypotension, tachycardia, palpitations
- (late signs of toxicity) delirium, extreme thirst, sensory disturbance, confusion, delirium, hyperthermia, ventricular arrhythmias, convulsions

Interactions

- not recommended with other xanthine derivatives or concurrent excessive amounts of caffeine-containing products such as coffee, tea, cola and some energy drinks
- clearance may be decreased, increasing serum levels and risk of adverse effects and toxicity by alcohol, allopurinol (high dose > 600 mg/day), beta-adrenergic blocking agents, cimetidine, ciprofloxacin, clarithromycin, diltiazem, disulfiram, erythromycin, methotrexate, norfloxacin, oral contraceptives, propranolol, recombinant alpha interferons, thyroid hormones, ticlopidine, verapamil
- clearance may be increased, decreasing serum levels by barbiturates, carbamazepine, isoprenaline, phenytoin, phenobarbital (phenobarbitone), primidone, rifampicin, St John's wort, tobacco or marijuana smoking
- additive effect (e.g. increased nausea, insomnia, nervousness) when given with sympathomimetic agents, therefore caution if given together
- may decrease seizure threshold if given with ketamine
- may antagonise cardiovascular effects of adenosine
- may increase excretion of lithium causing decreased serum concentrations, therefore serum levels should be closely monitored

Nursing points/Cautions

- dosage should be highly individualised, preferably on the basis of serum theophylline concentration monitoring
- monitor serum concentrations by sampling blood immediately before

morning dose (trough level), then 1–2 hours after dose (5–10 hours if SR) for peak concentration, provided that therapy has been established for 48 hours and no excess drug has been given or doses missed
- serum concentrations should be regularly monitored if daily dose is greater than 1 g in adults (or 24 mg/kg in children)
- xanthine/caffeine-containing beverages (e.g. tea, coffee, cola, cocoa, energy drinks) may interfere with the theophylline assay
- caution if used in those with decreased liver function, congestive cardiac failure, chronic obstructive pulmonary disease, acute pulmonary oedema), severe hypoxia, decreased thyroid function, acute febrile state and viral infection (including pneumonia, influenza or influenza immunisation) as clearance may be decreased, increasing risk of toxicity
- caution if used in those with arrhythmias, coronary artery disease, unstable angina, cardiomyopathy and severe hypertension where cardiac effects may be harmful
- caution if used in those with gastric ulceration or GORD because of an increase in gastric acid secretion
- contraindicated in those with hypersensitivity to xanthines

Patient teaching and advice

- SR tablets may be broken along score line, but are not to be crushed or chewed
- patient should be advised that SR theophylline should not be used in acute asthma
- warn patient not to take other xanthine derivatives or excessive amounts of caffeine-containing products, such as coffee, tea, cola or energy drinks
- advise patient not to drive or operate machinery if dizziness persists
- serum concentrations are affected by smoking, therefore patient should be instructed to advise doctor if starting/stopping smoking
- theophylline has interactions with many other medications. Patient should be instructed to discuss taking any other medications with doctor or pharmacist
- (syrup) advise patient to take syrup 1 hour before meals with glass of water; however, if GI irritation is a problem, may be taken with or just after food

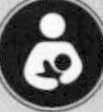

not to be used during pregnancy unless the expected benefit outweighs any potential risk. Crosses placental barrier, therefore if given near delivery neonate should be closely monitored for any adverse effects

theophylline is excreted in breastmilk, therefore, minimise dosage to mother to avoid irritability and restlessness in infant

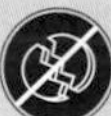

available as a syrup. Sustained-release tablets should not be crushed or chewed

PROPHYLACTIC AND ANTI-INFLAMMATORY DRUGS

MAST CELL STABILISERS

NEDOCROMIL SODIUM (Tilade CFC-free)

Available form

Metered dose inhaler: 2 mg/inhalation

Action

- inhibits release of inflammatory mediators from cells in the respiratory tract
- half-life 1.5–2 hours
- symptom preventer

Use

- prophylaxis of mild to moderate asthma
- prevention of bronchospasm (due to known irritants such as exercise, cold air and inhaled allergens)

Dose

- (asthma prophylaxis) 4 mg (2 inhalations) from metered dose aerosol inhaler 4 times daily, then reducing to twice daily if asthma is stable **OR**
- (bronchospasm prophylaxis) 4 mg (2 inhalations) a few minutes before exposure to trigger

Adverse effects

- headache
- nausea, vomiting, abdominal pain, dyspepsia, unpleasant or unusual taste
- cough, pharyngitis, bronchospasm

Nursing point/Cautions

- inhaler may be used with spacer device in those with poor inhalational technique or to prevent adverse effects
- should not be used in preference to corticosteroids in severe rapidly worsening asthma
- inhaler contains propellant (apaflurane)

Patient teaching and advice

- see p. 104 for instructions on metered dose aerosol inhaler technique
- patient should be advised that regular use is important and not to stop therapy suddenly as asthma control may deteriorate
- patient should understand that nedocromil sodium is not used for acute bronchospasm
- see also General Patient teaching and advice for antiasthma agents and bronchodilators (p. 96)

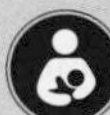

should be used with caution during pregnancy, especially first trimester

not recommended during breastfeeding unless benefits are thought to outweigh risks

OMALIZUMAB (rch) (Xolair)

Available forms

Vial: 150 mg; Prefilled syringe: 75 mg/0.5 mL, 150 mg/mL

Action

- recombinant monoclonal antibody that selectively binds to IgE, which is thought to be responsible for degranulation of mast cells releasing histamines, leukotrienes, cytokines and other mediators

Use

- moderate to severe asthma (in those who have raised IgE concentrations (> 30 IU/mL) and concurrent inhaled steroid therapy)
- chronic spontaneous urticaria (CSU) as an adjunct to antihistamine therapy where symptoms are not controlled

Dose

- (asthma, adults > 50 kg) 150–750 mg SC every 2 or 4 weeks **OR**
- (CSU) 150–300 mg SC every 4 weeks (with antihistamine therapy)

Adverse effects

- (injection site) pain, swelling, itching, redness
- headache, fatigue and less commonly, dizziness and somnolence
- fever
- weight gain, nausea, upper abdominal pain, diarrhoea
- urticaria, rash
- cough, pharyngitis, nasopharyngitis, sinusitis, upper respiratory tract infection (viral)
- myalgia, arthralgia, back pain
- decreased platelet count (asymptomatic)
- allergic reactions (immediate or delayed)
- (rare) arterial thromboembolic events, Churg-Strauss syndrome, hypereosinophilic syndrome, development of antibodies

Interactions

- may interfere with skin prick test, patch testing and RAST testing for hypersensitivity to potential allergens, therefore caution is recommended when interpreting test results

Nursing points/Cautions

- allergic reactions can occur after first and subsequent dose, often within the first 2 hours (but sometimes delayed); adrenaline (epinephrine) and resuscitation equipment should be readily available
- dose and frequency are determined by body weight and IgE concentrations and given every 2 or 4 weeks
- doses greater than 750 mg are not recommended
- if patient gains weight, dose will need to be adjusted
- IgE concentrations are usually only measured before starting therapy and if therapy has been stopped for 12 months or more. If therapy is stopped for less than 1 year, the dose should be based on IgE level before the initial dose. IgE remain elevated for up to 12 months after therapy is stopped
- platelet count is recommended before starting and then regularly during therapy
- patient's response to therapy should be assessed after 16 weeks. If patient's asthma is well controlled, withdrawal of inhaled corticosteroids may be attempted (with medical supervision)
- administered SC only
- SC sites should be rotated
- (vial) add 1.4 mL water for injections to vial (held upright) and swirl contents for 1 minute to wet powder, but do not shake. Continue swirling for 5–10 seconds every 5 minutes to dissolve powder (process usually requires 15–30 minutes). Invert vial for 15 seconds to allow solution to drain towards stopper. Using a new 3 mL syringe and large-bore needle (18 gauge), insert needle tip into vial (bottom of solution) and withdraw solution. Replace needle with 25 gauge for SC administration
- (vial) reconstituted solution should be clear and slightly opaque to pale brown-yellow in colour with no gel-like particles present. There may be small bubbles or foam around vial edge
- (vial) reconstituted solution is viscous in nature, therefore care should be taken that entire dose is retrieved when withdrawing solution from vial
- (vial) because of viscosity of solution, it may take 5–10 seconds to administer
- (prefilled syringe) patient may be taught to self-administer, but first 3 doses should be given under supervision
- (prefilled syringe) doses greater than 150 mg should be given into more than one site
- (prefilled syringe) contains latex and should not be handled by those with latex sensitivity
- (prefilled syringe) allow to come to room temperature for about 20 minutes before administration. Syringe should not be kept at room temperature for longer than 4 hours
- caution if used in those with (or a history of) thrombocytopenia
- caution if used in those with liver or kidney impairment
- caution if used in those with history of anaphylaxis as they are at increased risk of allergic reaction

Patient teaching and advice

- as allergic reactions can be delayed (1–5 days after injection or more), advise patient to seek medical attention immediately if an allergic reaction occurs (including rash, fever, swollen glands, joint pain, stiffness)

- warn patient against driving or operating machinery if fatigue, dizziness or somnolence are problematic
- (prefilled syringe) instruct patient in correct administration technique, including importance of rotation of SC sites, injection techniques, correct storage and disposal of used syringes

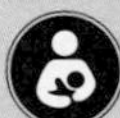

caution if used during pregnancy or breastfeeding

SODIUM CROMOGLYCATE (known as cromolyn sodium in the USA) (Chromo-Fresh Eye Drops, Intal CFC-Free, Intal Forte CFC-Free, Opticrom, Rynacrom Metered Dose Nasal Spray)

Available forms

Metered dose inhaler: 1 mg/inhalation, 5 mg/inhalation; Eye drops: 2% w/v; Nasal metered dose spray: 2% w/v

Action

- thought to inhibit the release of inflammatory mediators of type I allergic reaction from sensitised mast cells
- also inhibits type III (late allergic) reaction to some degree
- local effect in lung, nasal mucosa and eyes
- (asthma) symptom preventer

Use

- prophylactic treatment of asthma and exercise-induced bronchospasm
- allergic rhinitis
- treatment of keratoconjunctivitis and allergic conjunctivitis, prophylaxis of seasonal allergic symptoms

Dose

Asthma prophylaxis

- 2 inhalations (2 mg) from metered dose inhaler 4 times daily at 4- to 6-hourly interval (Intal CFC-free) **OR**
- 2 inhalations (10 mg) from metered dose inhaler twice daily, increasing to 4 times daily if necessary (Intal Forte CFC-free)

Exercise-induced asthma (or exposure to other triggers)

- 2–4 inhalations (10–20 mg) from metered-dose aerosol inhaler 5–10 minutes before exercise (Intal Forte CFC free)

Allergic rhinitis

- 1 spray (2.6 mg) into each nostril 2–4 times daily, increasing to 6 times daily if needed during times of high antigen challenge (e.g. high pollen) (nasal spray)

Keratoconjunctivitis, seasonal allergic conjunctivitis

- 1 or 2 drops into each eye 4–6 times daily (eye drops)

Adverse effects

- paradoxical bronchospasm
- (inhalation) cough, throat irritation, transient bronchospasm, pharyngitis, nausea
- (nasal spray) occasional irritation of nasal mucosa
- (eye drops) transient stinging and burning, swelling of the eyelids or conjunctiva (because of hypersensitivity to the preservative, benzalkonium)
- (rare) eosinophilic pneumonia, hypersensitivity

Nursing points/Cautions

- treatment with sodium cromoglycate may reduce the need for corticosteroids. Sodium cromoglycate should not be stopped until corticosteroid cover has been restarted or dose adjusted accordingly
- withdrawal should be gradual over a week
- caution if used in those with kidney or liver dysfunction
- (nasal spray, eye drops) contraindicated in those with sensitivity to benzalkonium chloride

Patient teaching and advice

- see General Patient teaching and advice for antiasthma agents and bronchodilators (p. 96)
- (eye drops) may be started in week before expected allergy season
- (eye drops) if patient wears contact lenses, instruct him/her to not apply eye drops with contact lens in eyes. Patient should be further instructed to wait 20–30 minutes before reinserting lenses
- (eye drops) advise patient to write opening date on container and discard 28 days after opening
- (nasal spray) instruct patient in correct technique for nasal spray use (p. 112)

Asthma

- it is essential the patient understands that sodium cromoglycate is not a bronchodilator and needs to be used regularly to be effective and is not suitable for treatment of acute asthma
- inhaler mouthpiece should be washed regularly to prevent blockage
- inhaler may be used with spacer device in those with poor inhalational technique or to prevent adverse effects
- Intal Forte CFC-free inhaler requires priming with 4 actuations before first use or if non-use of more than 7 days, and with 1–2 actuations if inhaler has not been used for 3–7 days
- advise patient that drug therapy is best withdrawn over several days unless there is an urgent need to stop abruptly

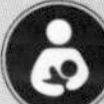

has been used during pregnancy with no increase in harmful effects on fetus; however, not recommended during first trimester

not to be used during breastfeeding unless the expected benefit outweighs any potential risk

CORTICOSTEROIDS

BECLOMETASONE (BECLOMETHASONE) (BECLOFOETALHASONE) DIPROPIONATE (Beconase Allergy & Hayfever 12 hour, Qvar)

Available forms

Metered dose inhaler: 50 microgram/inhalation, 100 microgram/inhalation; Autohaler: 50 microgram/inhalation, 100 microgram/inhalation; Nasal spray: 50 microgram/inhalation

Action

- inhibits inflammatory cells and prevents release of inflammatory mediators
- has an active metabolite, resulting in some systemic activity
- (asthma) symptom preventer

Use

- prophylaxis of symptoms of asthma (Qvar)
- prophylaxis and treatment of allergic rhinitis for up to 6 months (Beconase)

Dose

- (mild-to-moderate asthma) 50–200 microgram twice daily (daily maximum 800 microgram) (metered dose inhaler) **OR**
- (severe asthma) up to 400 microgram twice daily (daily maximum 800 microgram) (metered dose inhaler) **OR**

- (allergic rhinitis) initially 100 microgram (2 sprays) twice daily to each nostril, then reducing to 50 microgram (1 spray) twice daily to each nostril when symptoms are controlled (maximum 400 microgram (8 sprays/day)) (nasal spray)

Adverse effects

- hoarseness, pharyngitis
- taste sensation
- (nasal spray) stinging sensation, sneezing, bleeding, unpleasant taste and smell, dryness/irritation to nose and throat
- (rare) oral candidiasis, paradoxical bronchospasm, Cushing's syndrome, Cushingoid features, anxiety, sleeping disorders, hypersensitivity, cataract formation, elevated intraocular pressure, visual disturbances

Nursing points /Cautions

- not recommended for acute asthma episode or status asthmaticus
- asthma should be stable before adding inhaled corticosteroid to usual asthma maintenance regime
- discontinuation of oral corticosteroids may cause exacerbation of pre-existing allergic diseases such as atopic eczema which can be treated symptomatically
- if patient experiences any visual disturbances, referral to ophthalmologist is recommended
- if patient has been on oral corticosteroids, these may need to be restarted rapidly in times of stress or when there is airway obstruction or mucus that compromises inhaled route
- (nasal spray) if therapy is prolonged, twice-yearly examination of nasal mucosa is recommended
- Autohaler is breath-actuated and automatically releases medication during inhalation, therefore is suitable for those with poor inhaler technique
- canister does not require shaking before use, test firing if unused for a period of time or waiting between actuations
- (allergic rhinitis) any respiratory, nasal passage or paranasal sinus infection should be treated promptly with antibiotics
- (nasal spray) if used for several months, nasal mucosa should be examined regularly for any signs of mucosal damage
- (Qvar) contains propellant hydrofluoroalkane (norflurane)
- caution if used in those with active or latent tuberculosis (TB)
- (nasal spray) not recommended in those with nasal septal ulcers or recent nasal injury or surgery until healing has occurred
- (nasal spray) contraindicated if severe nasal infection is present or if patient has bleeding disorder or history of recurrent nasal bleeding

Patient teaching and advice

- patient should be advised not to exceed the recommended dose
- instruct patient to rinse mouth with water after using metered dose inhaler
- (allergic rhinitis) warn patient that benefits of therapy may take at least a week to become apparent and therapy should be continued as prescribed
- advise patient to report any blurred vision or other visual disturbances
- instruct patient in correct technique for using a metered dose inhaler (p. 104), Autohaler (p. 105) and nasal spray (p. 112)
- see also Patient teaching and advice for antiasthma agents and bronchodilators (p. 96)

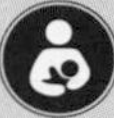

not recommended during pregnancy or breastfeeding unless benefits outweigh risks

BUDESONIDE (Budamax, Budenofalk, Budenofalk Foam Enema, Cortiment, Entocort, Jorveza Pulmicort, Rhinocort, Rhinocort Hayfever & Allergy)

Available forms

Nebulising solution (respules): 0.5 mg/2 mL, 1 mg/2 mL; Turbuhaler: 100 microgram/inhalation, 200 microgram/inhalation, 400 microgram/inhalation; Nasal spray: 32 microgram/dose, 64 microgram/dose; Capsules: 3 mg; Enema: 2 mg; Tablet (prolonged-release): 9 mg

Action

- glucocorticoid related to hydroxyprednisolone, with fewer systemic effects than beclometasone, although twice as potent
- lower influence on hypothalamo-pituitary-adrenal axis
- (Crohn's) anti-inflammatory with local action on intestinal mucosa
- (oral) half-life 3–4 hours
- (asthma) symptom preventer

Use

- treatment and prophylaxis of asthma (Pulmicort)
- laryngotracheobronchitis (croup) (Pulmicort)
- treatment and prophylaxis of allergic rhinitis (seasonal, perennial), nasal polyps (Budamax, Rhinocort)
- Crohn's disease (Budenofalk, Entocort)
- ulcerative colitis (active rectal and rectosigmoid disease) (Budenofalk Foam Enema)
- induction of remission in mild-to-moderate ulcerative colitis where mesalazine was insufficient or not tolerated (Cortiment)

Dose

- (mild asthma) 400–800 microgram daily in divided doses (metered dose aerosol inhaler, Turbuhaler) **OR**
- (when starting therapy, during severe asthma or reducing oral corticosteroid dose) 400–2400 microgram daily in 2–4 divided doses, reducing to lowest dose (100–400 microgram daily) to maintain the patient symptom-free (metered dose aerosol inhaler, Turbuhaler) **OR**
- (when starting therapy, during severe asthma or reducing oral corticosteroid dose) 1–2 mg twice daily, reducing to 0.5–1 mg twice daily via nebuliser **OR**
- (acute laryngotracheobronchitis) 2 mg via nebuliser **OR**
- (allergic rhinitis) initially 128 microgram in each nostril daily (morning) **OR**
- (allergic rhinitis) initially 64 microgram twice daily in each nostril morning and evening **OR**
- (allergic rhinitis, maintenance) reducing to 32–64 microgram in each nostril daily **OR**
- (nasal polyps) 64 microgram twice daily into each nostril morning and evening **OR**
- (acute Crohn's disease) 9 mg orally 30 minutes before food in the morning, for up to 12 weeks with dose being tapered over the last 2–4 weeks (sustained-release capsules) **OR**
- (acute Crohn's disease) 3 mg orally 30 minutes before food 3 times daily (morning, noon, evening) for no more than 8 weeks **OR**
- (active ulcerative colitis) 2 mg enema once daily (morning or evening) for 6–8 weeks **OR**
- (induction of remission of ulcerative colitis) 9 mg orally daily (morning) for up to 8 weeks

Adverse effects

- (oral) nausea, abdominal pain, dyspepsia, dry mouth, loose stools, diarrhoea, muscle/joint pain, headache, fatigue, insomnia, altered mood, depression, irritability, euphoria

- (inhalation) hoarseness, sore throat, cough, dry mouth, irritation of throat, tongue and mouth, oral candidiasis (thrush)
- (enema) rectal burning sensation and pain, headache, abdominal pain, diarrhoea, acne, depression, irritability, euphoria, muscle/joint pain, muscle weakness, osteoporosis
- (nasal spray) stinging, sneezing, dry/irritated nose, larynx and throat, unpleasant or strong smell and taste, dry mouth, nasal crust, increased sputum, sinusitis, epistaxis, headache, dizziness, tiredness, cough, dyspnoea, rhinitis, fever, rash
- (high dose, prolonged therapy) corticosteroid systemic effects (see Corticosteroids, p. 932), including increased risk of infection
- (nasal spray, prolonged use) nasal atrophy and perforation
- (inhalation, rare) paradoxical bronchospasm with wheezing
- (rare) hypersensitivity reaction, visual disturbances, cataract formation

Interactions

- (oral) increased serum levels may occur if given with itraconazole, ritonavir, clarithromycin and grapefruit juice
- (oral) decreased serum levels may occur if given with carbamazepine and rifampicin
- (oral) not recommended with live attenuated virus vaccines
- (oral) absorption may be decreased if given with colestyramine or antacids
- (oral) may cause increased potassium excretion which may potentiate effects of digoxin
- (oral) may cause false results on ACTH stimulation test for diagnosing pituitary or adrenal insufficiency

Nursing points/Cautions

- (asthma, non-oral corticosteroid dependent) if patient has large amounts of mucus, short course (2 weeks) of oral corticosteroids may be recommended in addition to inhaled corticosteroid
- (asthma) therapy should be started when patient's asthma is stable
- (ulcerative colitis) therapy is for active rectal or rectosigmoid disease only, not maintenance
- (ulcerative colitis, Cortiment) prolonged release formulation may result in lower corticosteroid levels than conventional (immediate release formulation) oral glucocorticoid therapy. Signs of adrenocortical suppression may be seen when the patient is transferred from immediate-release formulations with higher systemic effects
- (oral) discontinuation should be tapered
- if patient experiences any visual disturbances, referral to ophthalmologist is recommended
- (nasal spray) if patient has severe nasal obstruction/congestion, treatment with local decongestant can be used for 2–3 days
- (nasal spray) if therapy is prolonged, twice-yearly examination of nasal mucosa is recommended
- (allergic rhinitis, nasal polyposis) any respiratory, nasal passage or paranasal sinus infection should be treated promptly with antibiotics
- long-term use in children is not recommended because of potential growth suppression
- (asthma) caution if used in those transferring from oral to inhaled steroid therapy as there is an increased risk of adrenal impairment
- caution if given to those with active/latent tuberculosis, respiratory tract infection or severe liver impairment
- caution if used in those with hypertension, diabetes mellitus (or family history of), osteoporosis, peptic ulceration, glaucoma (or family history

of) or cataracts where corticosteroid therapy may have undesired effects
- (Crohn's disease) enteric-coated capsules are not recommended in those with upper GI Crohn's disease or extra-intestinal symptoms (e.g. skin, eyes, joints) as therapy appears to be ineffective
- (enteric-coated capsules) contain lactose and sucrose and are therefore not recommended in those with rare hereditary problems of galactose or fructose intolerance, glucose–galactose malabsorption, sucrose isomaltase insufficiency, Lapp lactase deficiency or congenital lactase deficiency
- (inhaled therapy) not recommended for bronchospasm relief or as sole therapy for acute asthma episode or status asthmaticus
- (nasal spray) not recommended in those with nasal septal ulcers or recent nasal injury or surgery until healing has occurred
- (nasal spray) contraindicated if severe nasal infection is present or if patient has bleeding disorder or history of recurrent nasal bleeding
- (prolonged-release tablets) contraindicated in those with rare hereditary galactose intolerance, Lapp lactase deficiency or glucose–galactose malabsorption as capsules contain lactose. Tablets also contain lecithin (of soya origin) and are therefore contraindicated in those with known lecithin sensitivity
- contraindicated in those with cirrhosis of the liver

Patient teaching and advice

- warn patient not to drive or operate machinery if visual disturbances or dizziness occur
- patient should be advised to seek medical advice if blurred vision or other visual disturbances occur

Asthma

- see also General Patient teaching and advice for antiasthma agents and bronchodilators (p. 96)
- patient should have full understanding of effects (i.e. it is not suitable for rapid relief of bronchospasm during acute asthma attack and is taken prophylactically regularly and should be continued even when patient is asymptomatic)
- patient should be instructed in correct use of metered dose inhalers (p. 104)
- patient using nebulised solution should be encouraged to wash face after use to reduce risk of facial irritation
- incidence of oral candidiasis and hoarseness may be reduced by encouraging patient to rinse mouth with water after each inhalation
- if patient requires 400 microgram or less for asthma treatment, may be given as a single daily dose (either morning or evening)
- if patient is also on bronchodilators, they should be taken several minutes before the budesonide to allow adequate penetration into the bronchial tree and bronchial dilation
- Turbuhaler is breath actuated, therefore is suitable for those with poor inhaler technique
- advise patient that nebulised solution may be diluted to 2 mL if necessary
- warn patient that the pressurised container should be kept intact and away from heat
- canisters should be protected from frost as cold temperatures may decrease therapeutic effect

Allergic rhinitis

- (allergic rhinitis) warn patient that full effects may not be seen for 2–3 days (and rarely, up to 2 weeks)
- (allergic rhinitis) advise patient to start therapy before exposure to allergen

- (nasal spray) if using decongestant for severe nasal congestion, it should be used 2–3 minutes before nasal spray

Crohn's disease, ulcerative colitis

- (oral) Instruct patient to avoid grapefruit juice during therapy
- (oral) patient should be advised to seek medical advice if any of the following occurs:
  - feeling unwell in a non-specific way (e.g. muscle or joint pain)
  - tiredness, headache, nausea and vomiting (may be signs of insufficient corticosteroid effect)
- (Crohn's disease, ulcerative colitis) advise patient to avoid close personal contact with chicken pox, herpes zoster and measles as minor illness can be fatal in those who are immunocompromised. If contact occurs, instruct patient to seek medical advice immediately
- (oral, sustained-release capsules) advise patient to swallow capsules whole, not chewed, crushed or broken. However, if patient has problems swallowing, capsules may be opened and contents swallowed whole (not chewed or crushed) with water
- (oral, prolonged-release tablets) instruct patient to swallow tablets whole, not broken, crushed or chewed
- (oral) if patient is also taking antacids and/or colestyramine, they should be separated by at least 2 hours from budesonide capsules
- (foam enema) instruct patient in correct use of foam enema, including:
  1. ensure enema is at room temperature before use
  2. warn patient that burning sensation or pain on using enema is normal feeling
  3. empty bowel (if possible) before insertion of enema
  4. wash hands with soap and water
  5. fit applicator onto spray can spout and shake for 15 seconds to mix contents
  6. remove safety tab under pump dome and twist dome until semicircular gap is in line with nozzle
  7. place finger on top of pump dome and turn spray can upside down (must be pointing down)
  8. insert applicator into rectum (as far as comfortable) and push pump dome fully once, holding for 5 seconds and release. Wait for 15 seconds for foam to be delivered and withdraw applicator from rectum
  9. remove applicator from spray can and dispose of safely
  10. wash hands with soap and water
  11. try not to open bowels for as long as possible (despite feeling of urgency to empty bowel – this is normal)
- (foam enema) instruct patient that enema should not be used after 4 weeks of opening container

(capsules, enema) banned in sport

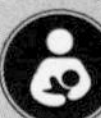

inhaled corticosteroids are preferred during pregnancy because of their lesser degree of systemic effects (including growth retardation and cleft palate development in animal studies)

capsule can be opened and granules dispersed in water or apple/orange juice but granules should not be chewed

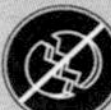

capsule/tablet should not be crushed

Note

- contained in Symbicort and DuoResp Spiromax with formoterol (eformoterol) fumarate dihydrate

CICLESONIDE (Alvesco, Omnaris Nasal Spray)

Available forms

Metered dose inhaler: 80 microgram/ inhalation, 160 microgram/inhalation; Metered dose nasal spray: 50 microgram/ spray

Action

- non-halogenated glucocorticosteroid that acts on the lungs without significant systemic effects
- prodrug, converted to active metabolite in the lung
- half-life about 1 hour (and 2.8 hours for metabolite)
- (asthma) symptom preventer

Use

- prophylactic management of asthma (metered dose inhaler)
- treatment of seasonal or perennial allergic rhinitis (nasal spray)

Dose

- (asthma) 80–320 microgram via metered dose inhaler daily (dose dependent on severity of asthma) **OR**
- (allergic rhinitis) 100 microgram (2 sprays) per nostril daily (daily total 200 microgram)

Adverse effects

- (metered dose inhaler) hoarseness, cough, pharyngeal pain, headache, bronchitis, nasopharyngitis, influenza, sinusitis, upper respiratory tract infection, back pain
- (nasal spray) stinging, sneezing, dry/ irritated nose and throat, unpleasant taste, dry mouth, dyspepsia, headache, epistaxis, nasopharyngitis, pharyngolayngeal pain, ear pain
- (nasal spray, prolonged use) nasal atrophy and nasal septum perforation
- (rare) hypersensitivity reactions, paradoxical bronchospasm, visual disturbances

Interactions

- not recommended with itraconazole, ritonavir or nelfinavir

Nursing points/Cautions

- (asthma) for mild asthma, dose should start at 160 microgram, moderate asthma 160–320 microgram, severe asthma 320 microgram
- if paradoxical bronchospasm with wheezing occurs after dose is given, an inhaled short-acting bronchodilator should be used. If ineffective and large number of inhalations are needed, medical advice should be sought
- if changing from oral corticosteroid to inhaled ciclesonide, patient should be stable. High doses of ciclesonide should be given with oral corticosteroid for about 10 days, then gradually reduce oral corticosteroid to lowest dose possible
- higher dosage may be required if patient was previously on an inhaled corticosteroid
- if patient experiences any visual disturbances, referral to ophthalmologist is recommended
- when transferring from oral corticosteroids, pre-existing allergic conditions (e.g. allergic rhinitis, eczema) may be unmasked
- (nasal spray) not recommended in those with nasal septal ulcers or recent nasal injury or surgery until healing has occurred
- caution if given to those with active/ latent tuberculosis or respiratory tract infection or liver impairment

Patient teaching and advice

- (asthma) patient should have full understanding of effects (i.e. it is not suitable for rapid relief of bronchospasm during acute asthma attack and is taken prophylactically regularly and should be continued even when patient is asymptomatic)

- advise patient to seek medical advice if any blurred vision or visual disturbances occur
- patient should be warned not to drive or operate machinery if any blurred vision or visual disturbances occur
- (asthma) patient should be advised not to stop therapy suddenly
- (asthma) instruct patient in correct use of metered dose inhaler (p. 104)
- instruct patient in correct technique for using nasal spray (p. 112) with the following exceptions:
    - shake bottle gently before removing cap
    - re-priming is only required if nasal spray has not been used for 4 days
- see General Patient teaching and advice for antiasthma agents and bronchodilators (p. 96)

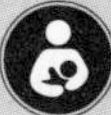

not recommended during pregnancy but if used, newborn should be observed for hypoadrenalism

should not be used during breastfeeding unless benefits outweigh risks

FLUTICASONE PROPIONATE (Axotide, Flixonase Allergy & Hayfever 24 hr, Flixonase Nasule Drops, Flixotide)

FLUTICASONE FUROATE (Arnuity Ellipta, Avamys)

Available forms

Accuhaler blister: 100 microgram/inhalation, 250 microgram/inhalation, 500 microgram/inhalation; Ellita inhaler: 100 microgram/inhalation; 200 microgram/inhalation; Metered dose inhaler (CFC free): 50 microgram/inhalation, 125 microgram/inhalation, 250 microgram/inhalation; Nasal spray: 27.5 microgram/spray, 50 microgram/spray; Nasal suspension (drops): 400 microgram/400 microlitre; Nebuliser solution (nebules): 0.5 mg/2 mL, 2 mg/2 mL

Action

- corticosteroid that acts on the lungs without significant systemic effects
- (asthma) symptom preventer

Use

- prophylactic management of asthma
- mild-to-moderate nasal polyps
- allergic rhinitis (seasonal, perennial) (short-term treatment, 3–6 months)

Dose

- (asthma) 100–200 microgram via inhalation once daily (Arnuity Ellipta) **OR**
- (mild asthma) 100–250 microgram via inhalation twice daily, then reducing to lowest dose to control symptoms (Flixotide) **OR**
- (moderate asthma) 250–500 microgram via inhalation twice daily, then reducing to lowest dose to control symptoms (Flixotide) **OR**
- (severe asthma) 500–1000 microgram via inhalation twice daily, then reducing to lowest dose to control symptoms (Flixotide) **OR**
- (severe asthma) 2 mg via nebuliser twice daily (Flixotide Nebules) **OR**
- (allergic rhinitis) initially 2 sprays (55 microgram) per nostril daily, decreasing to 1 spray (27.5 microgram) per nostril daily (nasal spray) (Avamys) **OR**
- (allergic rhinitis) initially 2 sprays (100 microgram) per nostril daily, decreasing to 1 spray (50 microgram) per nostril daily (nasal spray) (Flixonase) **OR**
- (nasal polyps) 400 microgram 1–2 times daily divided evenly between two nostrils (nasal drops) (Flixonase Nasule Drops)

Adverse effects

- (nasal spray/drops) stinging, sneezing, dry/irritated nose and throat,

unpleasant or strong smell and taste, dry mouth, nasal crust, headache, nosebleed, nasal ulceration
- (inhalation) mouth or throat candidiasis, lower/upper respiratory tract infection, influenza, hoarseness, bronchitis, nasopharyngitis, pharyngitis, sinusitis, headache, toothache, oropharyngeal pain, cough, back pain
- (inhalation, rare) paradoxical bronchospasm
- (rare, nasal spray, prolonged use) nasal atrophy and nasal septal perforation
- (rare) hypersensitivity reaction, impaired wound healing, glaucoma, increased intraocular pressure, cataract formation
- (long-term use) decreased bone mineral density

Interactions

- not recommended with ritonavir
- caution if used with itraconazole
- (nasal spray) caution if used with other formulations of corticosteroids due to increased risk of adverse effects

Nursing points/Cautions

- Accuhaler is breath-actuated and is suitable for anyone with difficulties using metered dose aerosol inhaler
- (allergic rhinitis) if prophylaxis is required, nasal spray should be administered before exposure to allergen
- (nasal spray) if therapy is prolonged, twice-yearly examination of nasal mucosa is recommended
- if patient experiences any visual disturbances, referral to ophthalmologist is recommended
- (nebules) can be diluted with sodium chloride if needed
- (nasal spray) caution if used in children as growth may be retarded
- caution if used in those with risk factors for reduced body mass (e.g. prolonged immobilisation, family history of osteoporosis or chronic use of agents that decrease body mass)
- (inhalation) caution if used in those with liver impairment. For those with moderate-to-severe liver impairment, maximum daily dose of 100 microgram is recommended
- (nasal spray) not recommended in those with nasal septal ulcers or recent nasal injury or surgery until healing has occurred
- (Arnuity Ellipta) contraindicated in those with severe milk-protein allergy or hypersensitivity to lactose
- contraindicated in those with hypersensitivity to other corticosteroids

Patient teaching and advice

- patient should be advised that fluticasone is not recommended for acute asthma episodes or status asthmaticus
- warn patient not to drive or operate machinery if blurred vision or visual disturbances occur
- (Arnuity Ellipta) instruct patient that inhalation should be used at the same time every day (either morning or night)
- if using nebuliser with mask, advise patient to wash face thoroughly after therapy
- ensure that patient is aware of detailed instructions for using both metered dose aerosol inhaler (p. 104), Ellipta inhaler (see p. 133) and Accuhaler (see p. 133). Extension tubes (spacers) are designed for attachment to the mouthpiece to increase lung deposition of inhaled drug if the patient is unable to master inhaler technique
- (allergic rhinitis) warn patient that it may take several days for full effect to be evident
- (allergic rhinitis) instruct patient to seek medical advice if there is not improvement in symptoms in 7 days

- (nasal drops) instruct patient in correct use of nasal drops, including:
  1. gently blow nose to clear both nostrils before using drops
  2. one nasule is sufficient for both nostrils
  3. flick/shake container several times to ensure solution is well mixed
  4. hold top of container and flick downwards in one quick motion to remove any solution from neck of container
  5. twist and remove top
  6. to instil drops, patient should lie on back with head supported
  7. squeeze container to insert 6 drops (half container/dose) into one nostril, then repeat in other nostril
  8. keep head in position for at least 1 minute
  9. avoid contact with eyes; however, if contact occurs, rinse eyes well with water
  10. drops should be protected from light and not frozen
- (Accuhaler) instruct patient in correct use of Accuhaler device, including:
  1. before starting, check dose counter and then open cover using thumb grip
  2. hold device horizontally and load dose by sliding lever until click is heard
  3. breathe out gently (away from inhaler) and place mouth around mouthpiece (closing lips to form good seal and keeping device horizontal)
  4. breathe in deeply and steadily, and then hold breath for as long as comfortable (at least 5 seconds)
  5. remove inhaler from mouth (while still holding breath)
  6. breathe out gently (away from inhaler)
  7. if another dose is needed, repeat steps 3–6
  8. close cover and click shut
  9. rinse mouth with water after use
- (Ellipta inhaler) instruct patient in correct use of Ellipta device, including:
  1. opening and closing device cover without inhaling medication results in loss of dose
  2. check dose counter. New device will show 30 doses. When fewer than 10 doses are left, half dose cover will be red. When last dose has been used, dose counter will show 0
  3. do not shake device but slide cover down until click is heard
  4. breathe out gently (away from inhaler), then place mouth over mouthpiece to form good seal, but taking care not to cover air vent
  5. breathe in deeply and steadily and then hold breath for as long as comfortable (or at least 5 seconds) and remove inhaler
  6. breathe out gently (away from inhaler)
  7. slide cover upwards as far as it will go to cover mouthpiece
  8. rinse mouth with water after use
- (nasal spray) instruct patient in correct use of nasal spray (see p.112) with the following exceptions:
  - shake bottle well before use
  - when finished, clean nozzle carefully with tissue and replace cap
  - therapy can be continued for up to 6 months
  - nasal spray should be discarded 12 weeks from first use or after expiry date
- see also General Patient teaching and advice for antiasthma agents and bronchodilators (p. 96)

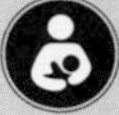

should only be used during pregnancy or breastfeeding if benefits outweigh risks

Note
- contained in Pavtide, Salplus F, Seroflo and Seretide with salmeterol, Dymista with azelastine, Flutiform with formoterol (eformoterol) fumarate dehydrate, Breo Ellipta with vilanterol and Trelegy Ellipta with vilanterol and umeclidium

LEUKOTRIENE RECEPTOR ANTAGONISTS

MONTELUKAST SODIUM (Lukair, Montelair, Singulair, Respikast)

Available forms
Tablets (chewable): 4 mg, 5 mg; Tablets: 10 mg

Action
- selective leukotriene receptor antagonist that specifically inhibits the leukotrienes LTC4, LTD4 and LTE4 that are potent pro-asthmatic mediators (leukotrienes mediate bronchoconstriction, mucus secretion, vascular permeability and eosinophil recruitment)
- symptom preventer
- bronchodilation within 2 hours

Use
- prophylaxis and treatment of chronic asthma
- symptomatic treatment of seasonal allergic rhinitis

Dose
- 10 mg orally (at night for asthma, individualised time for allergic rhinitis)

Adverse effects
- fever
- headache, dizziness, fatigue, asthenia
- agitation, anxiety, aggression, insomnia, abnormal dreams, sleep walking, depression, tremor, hallucinations, disorientation, hostility
- dyspepsia, abdominal pain, diarrhoea
- dental pain
- cough, nasal congestion
- rash
- elevated liver enzymes
- (rare) vasculitis, vasculitic rash, eosinophilia, Churg-Strauss syndrome, suicidal ideation, worsening lung condition

Nursing points/Cautions
- not used for relief of acute asthma attack
- chewable tablets (4 and 5 mg) contain aspartame, therefore caution if used in those with phenylketonuria

Patient teaching and advice
- patient should be warned not to drive or operate machinery if dizziness or fatigue are ongoing
- advise patient to keep taking medication regardless of their asthma status (i.e. whether stable or during an acute attack)
- can be given with inhaled corticosteroids. Corticosteroid dose may be reduced during therapy, but patient should understand that montelukast is not an inhaled steroid therapy substitute
- instruct patient (or carer) to seek medical advice if any of the following occur:
  - insomnia, sleep disturbance, sleep walking, abnormal dreams, hostility, aggression, restlessness, irritability, depression, tremor or hallucinations
  - any thoughts of self-harm, depressed mood or suicidal thoughts
- see General Patient teaching and advice for antiasthma agents and bronchodilators (p. 96)

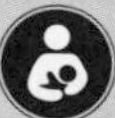

should not be used during pregnancy unless benefits outweigh risks

caution if used during breastfeeding

chewable and plain tablets can be crushed and mixed with spoonful of yoghurt or apple puree

OTHER RESPIRATORY AGENTS

BENRALIZUMAB (Fasenra)

Available form

Prefilled syringe: 30 mg/mL

Action

- antibody that binds to interleukin-5 receptor (IL-5Rα) (IL-5 receptor is expressed on surface of eosinophils and basophils)
- reduces eosinophilic inflammation which is an important component in asthma pathogenesis

Use

- severe eosinophilic asthma (eosinophil count ≥ 300 cells/microL or ≥ 150 cells/microL if on oral corticosteroid therapy)

Dose

- 30 mg SC every 4 weeks for 3 doses, then every 8 weeks

Adverse effects

- headache
- pharyngitis, cough
- arthralgia
- fever
- injection site reaction
- hypersensitivity

Nursing points/ Cautions

- before starting therapy, treatment with high-dose inhaled corticosteroids and long-acting beta agonists should be optimised
- any helminth infection should be treated before starting therapy. If infestation occurs during therapy and does not respond to antihelminth therapy, benralizumab should be stopped until infestation is treated successfully
- corticosteroid therapy can be gradually decreased if appropriate, but should not be stopped abruptly
- patient should be closely monitored for hypersensitivity reaction, which can occur within hours of administration (but can also be delayed)
- patient can be instructed in SC administration

Patient education and advice

- ensure patient understands that benralizumab should not be used to treat acute asthma exacerbation
- patient should be instructed to seek medical advice immediately if:
  - asthma remains uncontrolled or worsens after starting therapy
  - any signs of delayed hypersensitivity (e.g. urticaria, rash) occur
- ensure patient understands administration instructions (see Mepolizumab Patient teaching and advice p. 143)

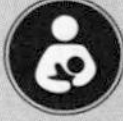

not recommended during pregnancy or breastfeeding unless benefits outweigh risks

BERACTANT (Survanta)

Available form

Vial: 25 mg/mL

Action

- pulmonary surfactant that lowers surface tension on alveolar surfaces during respiration and stabilises

alveoli against collapse at resting transpulmonary pressures
- deficiency of surfactant causes respiratory distress syndrome (hyaline membrane disease) in premature infants

Use
- prevention of respiratory distress syndrome (RDS) in premature infants weighing less than 1250 g or with evidence of surfactant deficiency (preferably within 15 minutes of birth)
- treatment of confirmed RDS in infants requiring mechanical ventilation (as soon as possible, preferably within 8 hours of birth)

Dose
- 100 mg/kg (4 mL/kg) via intratracheal administration 4 times in first 48 hours of life administered no more frequently than 6-hourly

Adverse effects
- transient bradycardia, hypotension, hypertension
- oxygen desaturation, hypercarbia, hypocarbia, apnoea
- endotracheal tube reflux, endotracheal blockage
- pallor, vasoconstriction
- increased risk of post-treatment nosocomial sepsis

Nursing points/Cautions
- should only be used in neonatal intensive care settings where infants can be frequently monitored with arterial or transcutaneous measurement of systemic oxygen and carbon dioxide
- oxygenation may improve markedly within minutes of administration, therefore infant should be frequently observed and monitored
- if transient bradycardia and desaturation occurs, procedure should be stopped and symptoms treated accordingly
- endotracheal suctioning is generally not required after administration unless airway obstruction occurs. Rales and moist breath sounds occur transiently after administration
- for intratracheal administration only
- solution is off-white to light brown in colour
- if solution has settled during storage, it should be swirled gently (not shaken) to redisperse
- allow to warm to room temperature for at least 20 minutes before administration. Alternatively, it can be warmed in the hand for at least 8 minutes
- artificial warming methods should not be used
- there are three different methods of administration involving end-hole catheter and disconnection of ventilator, instillation through secondary lumen of double lumen of endotracheal tube with no disconnection from ventilator, and third method being a combination of both. Consult manufacturer's instructions or institutional policies for administration details
- repeat doses are administered according to infant's birthweight and are determined by ongoing respiratory distress
- repeat doses should not be given within 6 hours of previous dose
- if given for prophylaxis, repeat doses should only be given after X-ray confirmation of RDS
- manual hand-bag ventilation should not be used to administer repeat doses. Ventilator settings may be changed to maintain appropriate oxygenation and ventilation
- unopened, unused vials that have been warmed to room temperature can be returned to refrigerator within 8 hours; however, this should only occur once

- not recommended in infants weighing < 600 g or > 1750 g

DORNASE ALFA (Pulmozyme)

Available form
Inhalation solution: 1 mg/mL

Action
- mucolytic
- produced by genetically modified Chinese hamster ovary cells containing DNA that codes for DNase. Recombinant DNase is similar to the human enzyme that hydrolyses DNA in accumulated neutrophils in sputum, reducing viscosity of purulent lung secretions
- those with cystic fibrosis produce infected sputum that contains large amounts of mucus glycoproteins and extracellular DNA
- half-life 3–4 hours

Use
- respiratory complications in those with cystic fibrosis

Dose
- 2.5 mg nebulised once daily (may increase to twice daily if needed in those > 21 years)

Adverse effects
- pharyngitis, hoarse voice, laryngitis, rhinitis, dyspnoea, decreased lung function
- rash, urticaria
- dyspepsia
- fever
- conjunctivitis
- non-cardiac chest pain

Nursing points/Cautions
- therapy continuation should be based on clinical response and lung function tests (if possible)
- ultrasonic nebulisers should not be used for administration
- (children < 5 years) administration should be via tight-fitting mask
- contraindicated in those with hypersensitivity to Chinese hamster ovary cell products

Patient teaching and advice
- advise the patient of the following:
  - nebulise using compressed air at 6–8 L/minute
  - do not dilute or mix with other drugs
  - may be used safely in conjunction with other standard treatments for cystic fibrosis
  - unused portion of opened ampoules should be discarded
  - should not be used if solution is cloudy or discoloured
  - normal chest physiotherapy should continue as normal
  - patient should be advised not to stop medication suddenly

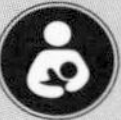

not recommended during pregnancy unless benefits outweigh potential risks

IVACAFTOR (Kalydeco)

Available forms
Tablet: 150 mg; Granules: 50 mg, 75 mg

Action
- selective potentiator of cystic fibrosis (CF) transmembrane conductance regulator (CFTR) protein, thought to enhance chloride transport; however, exact mechanism of action is not completely understood
- active metabolite
- half-life about 12 hours

Use
- treatment of CF in those ≥ 12 months who have G551D or other gating (class III) mutation in the CFTR gene

Dose
- (≥ 25 kg) 150 mg orally twice daily (tablet) **OR**
- (≥ 7 kg – < 14 kg) 50 mg orally twice daily (granules) **OR**
- (>14 kg – < 25 kg) 75 mg orally twice daily (granules)

Adverse effects
- dizziness, headache
- abdominal pain, diarrhoea, nausea, vomiting
- rash
- fever
- productive cough, upper respiratory tract infection, nasal congestion, pharyngeal erythema, oropharyngeal pain, rhinitis, sinus congestion, nasopharyngitis
- ear pain, ear discomfort, tinnitus, vestibular disorder, ear congestion
- bacteria in sputum
- (uncommon) elevated liver enzymes
- (rare) congenital lens opacities (cataract) (without vision impact)

Interactions
- serum levels may be increased by itraconazole, posaconazole, voriconazole, clarithromycin, fluconazole and erythromycin
- serum levels may be decreased by grapefruit juice, Seville oranges, rifampicin, rifabutin, dexamethasone, prednisolone (high dose), phenobarbital (phenobarbitone), carbamazepine, phenytoin and St John's wort
- may increase serum levels of midazolam, alprazolam, triazolam and diazepam, increasing risk of adverse effects
- may increase serum levels of digoxin, ciclosporin and tacrolimus, increasing risk of adverse effects, therefore serum levels should be monitored during therapy
- caution if given with warfarin, therefore INR should be closely monitored, especially when starting or stopping therapy

Nursing points/Cautions

- patient should only receive therapy if accurate and validated genotyping has been performed to confirm presence of gating (class III) mutation in at least one allele of CFTR gene
- baseline and regular ophthalmological examinations are recommended
- liver function tests are recommended before starting, 3-monthly during first year, then yearly during therapy. Therapy should be interrupted if AST or ALT are greater than 5 times upper normal limit
- contains lactose and are therefore not recommended in those with rare hereditary problems of galactose intolerance, Lapp lactase deficiency or glucose–galactose malabsorption
- caution if used in those with severe kidney impairment (creatinine clearance ≤ 30 mL/minute) or end-stage kidney disease
- not recommended in those with severe liver impairment
- not recommended in transplant patients
- not recommended in those with CF who are homozygous for F508del mutation in CFTR gene

Patient/Carer teaching and advice

- instruct patient to swallow tablets whole, not crushed, chewed, broken or dissolved
- patient should be advised to take medication with fat-containing snack or meal, including those prepared with oil or butter, containing eggs, cheeses, nuts, avocado, whole milk, full-fat yoghurt or meats
- advise patient to avoid food containing grapefruit juice or Seville oranges during therapy
- warn patient to avoid driving or operating machinery if dizziness occurs
- (granules) sachet should be mixed with teaspoon (5 mL) of age-appropriate soft food/liquid (e.g.

pureed fruits/vegetables, milk, yoghurt, water, juice) and should be ingested within 1 hour of mixing
- (granules) food/liquid should be at room temperature or lower when mixing with granules

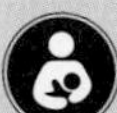

only used during pregnancy and breastfeeding if benefits outweigh risks

granules can be dispersed in 5 mL of water, milk or juice or mixed with spoonful of pureed fruit or vegetables. Tablet can be crushed and mixed with milk or spoonful of full-fat yoghurt

Note
- contained in Orkambi with lumacaftor and Symdeko with tezacaftor

MANNITOL (Aridol, Bronchitol)

Available forms
Powder for inhalation: 40 mg; Diagnostic kit containing capsules (0 mg, 5 mg, 10 mg, 20 mg, 40 mg) and inhalation device

Action
- when inhaled, increases osmolarity in airways in a similar way to other bronchial provocation tests causing a release of mediators from airway inflammatory cells that result in bronchoconstriction
- (diagnostic) response is greater in patient with asthma or exercise-induced asthma
- airway response is measured using forced expiratory volume in 1 second (FEV_1)
- (treatment) mannitol is spray-dried and delivered to lungs using a specific inhaler device to improve lung hygiene by correcting impaired mucociliary clearance
- (treatment) thought to change visco-elastic properties of mucus, but exact action is unknown

Use
- treatment of cystic fibrosis, either as adjunctive therapy with dornase alfa (p. 137) or in those intolerant to or with inadequate response to dornase alfa (Bronchitol)
- identifying bronchial hyperresponsiveness to help in diagnosis of asthma (Aridol)

Dose
- cumulative dose of 635 mg given (or until positive response is achieved) (Aridol) **OR**
- 400 mg via inhaler device twice daily (morning and 2–3 hours before bedtime) (after initiation dose assessment has been completed) (Bronchitol)

Adverse effects
- bronchospasm (chest tightness, cough or wheezing)
- cough, pharyngolaryngeal pain, rhinorrhea, haemoptysis, dyspnoea, nasopharyngitis, sinusitis
- eye pruritus
- nausea, vomiting, diarrhoea, upper abdominal pain, decreased appetite
- back pain, arthralgia, musculoskeletal pain
- headache, dizziness, fatigue, insomnia, sinus headache
- chest discomfort/tightness
- throat irritation, tonsillitis
- epistaxis
- flu-like illness
- rash
- fever

Interactions
- inhaled corticosteroids will reduce response and should be withheld before procedure

Nursing points/Cautions
- given by inhalation only

Diagnostic procedure
- patient must be supervised at all times during procedure

- medication to treat severe bronchospasm, bronchodilators and oxygen must be present in testing area
- spirometry should be performed before challenge to determine resting FEV_1
- seat patient comfortably and encourage him/her to maintain good posture during procedure to achieve effective delivery into lungs
- apply nose clip and direct patient to breathe through mouth
- place capsule (0 mg) in inhalation device and puncture it by depressing buttons on side of device slowly (capsule should only be punctured once to prevent fragmenting occurring)
- advise patient to exhale completely, then inhale from device in a controlled rapid deep inspiration. Sixty (60) second timer should be set and patient asked to hold breath for 5 seconds, then exhale and remove nose clip. At the end of 60 seconds, FEV_1 should be measured twice (this is the baseline). Procedure is then repeated using 5 mg, 10 mg, 20 mg, 40 mg until a cumulative dose of 635 mg has been given or patient has a positive response
- positive response is achieved when FEV_1 is 15% less than baseline (0 mg dose) or there is 10% incremental fall in FEV_1 between doses. A beta-2 agonist may be given to accelerate recovery and patients should be monitored until FEV_1 is within 5% of baseline levels
- there should be minimal delay between FEV_1 measurement and next dose
- at least 2 repeatable FEV_1 measurements should be obtained after each dose
- 80 mg and 160 mg doses are given in multiples of 40 mg capsules (e.g. 2 × 40 mg) with no interval between doses (i.e. one capsule should be followed immediately by next capsule until total dose has been inhaled)
- new inhalation device should be used for each test (not cleaned during test)
- a number of agents may interfere with response and should be withheld, including:
  - smoking (at least 6 hours)
  - vigorous exercise (not performed on day of testing)
  - significant amounts of coffee, tea and other caffeine-containing foods and drinks (day of testing)
  - inhaled non-steroidal anti-inflammatory agents (e.g. sodium cromoglycate, nedocromil sodium (6–8 hours)
  - short-acting beta-2 agonists (e.g. salbutamol) (8 hours)
  - inhaled corticosteroids, ipratropium (12 hours)
  - inhaled corticosteroids plus long-acting beta-2 agonists, theophylline (24 hours)
  - tiotropium bromide, antihistamines (72 hours)
  - leukotriene receptor antagonists (4 days)
- if 0 mg capsule induces a FEV_1 fall $>$ 10% or patient experiences spirometry-induced asthma, further testing should not be done and patient should be administered bronchodilator
- pharyngolaryngeal pain may be reduced by rinsing mouth after testing
- caution if patient has ventilatory impairment (resting FEV_1 $<$ 70% normal predicted value or absolute value of 1.5 L in adults), spirometry-induced bronchoconstriction, haemoptysis (of unknown origin), pneumothorax, recent abdominal, thoracic or eye surgery, unstable angina, inability to perform spirometry of suitable quality or respiratory

tract infection (upper or lower) in previous 2 weeks

- contraindicated in those where conditions may be compromised by induced bronchospasm or repeated blowing manoeuvres (e.g. aortic or cerebral aneurysms, myocardial infarction, uncontrolled hypertension or stroke in previous 6 months)

Treatment

- an initiation dose assessment for bronchial hyperresponsiveness should be conducted under supervision before staring therapy. Assessment requires measurement of oxygen saturation (SpO_2) and performing spirometry. Drugs and equipment for management of acute bronchospasm should be readily available in the event of an emergency
- initiation dose assessment:
  - patient should be instructed in correct inhaler technique
  - baseline FEV_1 and SpO_2 are measured
  - patient premedicated with bronchodilator 5–15 minutes before dose
  - all subsequent FEV_1 and SpO_2 measurements should be performed 1 minute after dose
  - patient inhales 40 mg then SpO_2 is monitored
  - patient inhales 80 mg then SpO_2 is monitored
  - patient inhales 120 mg, then FEV_1 is measured, SpO_2 is monitored
  - patient inhales 160 mg, then FEV_1 is measured, SpO_2 is monitored
  - FEV_1 is measured 15 minutes after last dose
- patient is considered hyperresponsive if:
  - SpO_2 falls $\geq$ 10% at any stage of the assessment
  - FEV_1 fall $\geq$ 20% at the cumulative 240 mg dose
  - FEV_1 fall $\geq$ 20% (from baseline) at the end of assessment and does not return to within $\leq$ 20% of baseline within 15 minutes
  - FEV_1 fall $\geq$ 50% (from baseline) at the end of assessment
- patient should be closely monitored to ensure FEV_1 returns to baseline level after assessment is complete
- patient should be monitored carefully for any signs of significant haemoptysis and therapy stopped if massive/severe haemoptysis (> 240 mL/24 hours or recurrent bleeding $\geq$ 100 mL over several days) occurs
- patient should be reviewed after 6 weeks of therapy for any signs of drug-induced bronchospasm. If any uncertainty exists, the initiation assessment should be repeated
- caution if used in those with history of asthma
- not recommended in those who are unable to complete spirometry or complete the initiation dose assessment
- not recommended in those with history of significant haemoptysis (> 60 mL) in previous 12 weeks, impaired lung function (FEV_1 < 30%), liver or kidney impairment or non-cystic fibrosis bronchiectasis
- contraindicated in those with hypersensitivity or with bronchial hyperresponsiveness to mannitol (either pre-existing or determined by initiation dose assessment)

Patient education and advice

- (Bronchitol) instruct patient:
  - correct inhaler technique (each capsule is loaded separately into device, capsules are inhaled using inhaler device with one or two breaths, then empty capsule discarded before inserting next capsule into device)
  - to replace inhaler device weekly
- if needed, inhaler device can be washed with warm water and

allowed to completely dry before re-use
- use bronchodilator 5–15 minutes before mannitol
- normal physiotherapy and dornase alfa therapy (if used) should be completed as normal after mannitol
- patient should be advised to report any persistent cough when using mannitol therapy

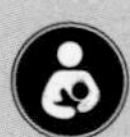

not recommended during pregnancy

caution if used during breastfeeding

Note
- also available as Osmitrol Intravenous Infusion for use as an osmotic diuretic (see Diuretics, p. 1031)

MEPOLIZUMAB (Nucala)

Available forms

Vial: 100 mg; Prefilled syringe/pen: 100 mg/mL

Action
- humanised monoclonal antibody (IgG1, kappa) that targets human interleukin-5 (IL-5) responsible for growth, differentiation, recruitment, activation and survival of eosinophils
- half-life 16–22 days

Use
- adjunctive therapy for severe refractory eosinophilic asthma (EA)
- relapsed or refractory eosinophilic granulomatosis with polyangiitis (EGPA)

Dose
- (severe EA) 100 mg SC once every 4 weeks **OR**
- (relapsed or refractory EGPA) 300 mg SC every 4 weeks

Adverse effects
- headache, fatigue
- pruritus, eczema
- abdominal pain, nausea, vomiting, diarrhoea
- back pain, muscle spasm, arthralgia
- dyspnoea, nasal congestion, nasopharyngitis, pharyngitis
- bronchitis, allergic rhinitis, exacerbation of asthma, viral respiratory infection, sinusitis, upper respiratory tract infection
- herpes zoster, influenza, urinary tract infection
- hypersensitivity (urticaria, angioedema, rash, bronchospasm, hypotension)
- development of neutralising antibodies
- (injection site) pain, redness, swelling, itching, burning sensation

Nursing points/Cautions
- patient should be monitored for any signs of hypersensitivity after SC administration
- any helminth infection should be treated before starting therapy. If helminth infection occurs during therapy, patient should be treated. However, if patient is unresponsive to helminth therapy, mepolizumab therapy should be interrupted
- rotate SC administration sites (upper arm, thigh or abdomen)
- patient may be taught to self-administer using prefilled syringe/pen
- to reconstitute vial, add 1.2 mL water for injections vertically onto centre of powder and gently swirl in circular motion for 10 seconds, then allow vial to rest for further 5 seconds until powder is dissolved avoiding any foaming or frothing
- reconstituted solution may be colourless to pale yellow or pale brown in colour
- do not shake reconstituted solution before administration to prevent foaming or precipitation

- caution if used in patients with pre-existing helminth infestation
- not recommended in children < 12 years

Patient teaching and advice

- advise patient that this should not be used for management of acute asthma episodes
- patient should be instructed to seek medical advice immediately if asthma remains uncontrolled or symptoms worsen after starting therapy
- advise patient to continue with corticosteroid therapy and not to stop this abruptly
- warn patient that hypersensitivity reaction (urticaria, angioedema, rash, bronchospasm, hypotension) may be delayed and occur days after starting therapy. If this occurs, patient should seek medical advice immediately
- ensure patient understands administration using prefilled syringe/pen, including:
  1. pen/syringe should not be shaken or used if pen/syringe is damaged or has been dropped on hard surface
  2. needle cap should not be removed until ready to use
  3. pen/syringe should be removed from fridge, pack opened and allowed to stand at room temperature for 30 minutes before administration (should not be warmed using hot water, direct sunlight or microwave)
  4. check expiry date and solution (not cloudy or containing particles). Solution should be colourless to pale yellow to pale brown
  5. choose injection site (abdomen or, if carer is administering injection, upper arm) and allow 5 cm between injection sites if more than one injection is needed. Injection site should be at least 5 cm from navel
  6. injection site should be free of scarring, bruising, redness or tenderness
  7. hands should be washed with soap and water
  8. injection site cleaned with alcohol wipe and area allowed to dry

Pen instructions

1. remove cap from pen but do not touch yellow needle guard
2. place pen on injection site with yellow needle guard against skin. Push pen down at 90° angle until first click is heard (injection started). Pen should be kept in place until second click is heard. Continue holding pen against skin while counting to 5 and then lift pen from skin (this ensures full dose is given)

Syringe instructions

1. remove needle cap (pulling firmly away from needle)
2. do not touch needle or plunger or expel any air bubbles from syringe
3. skin at injection site should be pinched up and needle inserted into pinched skin at 45° angle
4. slowly push plunger down to inject full dose (using thumb on plunger) until stopper reaches bottom of syringe
5. lift thumb slowly to allow plunger to come up and needle retract into syringe
6. release pinched skin
7. needle should not be recapped
   - if small drop of blood appears at injection site, press cotton wool ball or gauze against site for a few seconds
   - injection site should not be rubbed
   - used pen/syringe should be disposed of appropriately and safely in sharps container
   - prefilled pen/syringe can be removed from fridge and kept in

unopened pack for up to 7 days at room temperature (below 30°C and protected from light)
- should be administered within 8 hours of opening pack
- discard if more than 8 hours has passed after opening pack
- prefilled pen/syringe should be stored in fridge at 2–8°C but not frozen

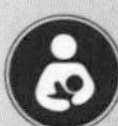
should only be used during pregnancy and breastfeeding if benefits outweigh risks

PORACTANT ALFA (Curosurf)

Available forms
Vial: 120 mg/1.5 mL, 240 mg/3 mL

Action
- pulmonary surfactant that reduces surface tension at air–liquid interface on the alveoli during ventilation
- stabilises alveoli against collapse at resting transpulmonary pressures
- lack of surfactant in preterm infants results in respiratory distress syndrome with poor lung expansion, inadequate gas exchange and gradual lung collapse (atelectasis)

Use
- treatment for respiratory distress syndrome (RDS) in preterm infants
- prophylaxis for infants at risk of RDS

Dose
- (treatment for RDS) 200 mg/kg (2.5 mL/kg) intratracheal as soon as RDS is diagnosed, followed by up to 2 further doses of 100 mg/kg (1.25 mL/kg) at 12-hour intervals if needed (maximum total dose (400 mg/kg) 5 mL/kg) **OR**
- (prophylaxis of RDS) 100–200 mg/kg as a single dose within 15 minutes of birth, with further doses of 100 mg/kg given 6–12 hours after initial dose, then 12 hours later in babies who have persistent symptoms of RDS and are ventilator dependent (maximum total dose 300–400 mg/kg)

Adverse effects
- bradycardia, hypotension
- endotracheal tube blockage
- oxygen desaturation

Nursing points/Cautions
- should only be administered in neonatal intensive care setting
- any acidosis, hypotension, anaemia, hypoglycaemia and hypothermia should be treated before starting therapy
- infants receiving therapy should be frequently monitored as medication can affect oxygenation and lung compliance rapidly requiring modification to oxygen and ventilator support
- if transient adverse effects occur (e.g. bradycardia, hypotension, endotracheal tube blockage, oxygen desaturation), therapy should be stopped and adverse effects treated
- for intratracheal administration only
- administered via 5 French end-hole catheter while briefly disconnecting endotracheal tube from ventilator or via secondary lumen of a dual lumen endotracheal tube without interrupting mechanical ventilation
- before instillation, proper position and patency of endotracheal tube should be established. If needed, endotracheal tube may be suctioned, but infant should be allowed to stabilise before instillation of therapy
- for endotracheal tube instillation with 5 French end-hole catheter: contents of vial should be withdrawn into 3 or 5 mL syringe through large gauge ($\geq$ 20 gauge) needle and then syringe attached to precut 8 cm 5 end-hole

French catheter. Catheter should be filled with solution and then excess solution discarded (through catheter), leaving the exact dose in the syringe. Before administration, change the infant's ventilator settings to 40–60 breaths/minute, inspiratory time 0.5 seconds and supplemental oxygen sufficient to maintain oxygen saturation (SaO_2) $>$ 92%. With infant in neutral position (head and body aligned with no inclination), disconnect the endotracheal tube from the ventilator. Precut 5 French catheter should be inserted into the endotracheal tube and 1.25 mL/kg instilled, and the infant positioned on either the right or left side. Remove the catheter and manually ventilate the infant with 100% oxygen for 1 minute at 40–60 breaths/minute. When the infant is stable, repeat the procedure on the other side with the remaining solution. Suctioning should not occur within 1 hour of instillation unless significant airway obstruction occurs. Ventilator management should return to pre-instillation settings

- for instillation via secondary lumen of dual lumen endotracheal tube: withdraw contents into 3 or 5 mL syringe through large gauge ($\geq$ 20 gauge) needle. Infant should be in neutral position (with head and body aligned and no inclination). Administer solution via secondary lumen as a single dose without interrupting ventilation. After dosing, some transient increase in ventilatory management may be required
- solution should be white to creamy white and allowed to come to room temperature slowly before administration
- vial should be slowly inverted (but not shaken) to ensure uniform distribution of solution
- unopened, unused vials that have been warmed to room temperature can be returned to fridge within 24 hours for storage; however, this should not occur more than once

ANTIBACTERIAL AGENTS

Organisms which can produce infection in humans include bacteria, mycoplasma, spirochaetes, fungi and viruses. Agents used to treat bacterial infections (antibacterial agents) will be discussed in this section, while antiviral agents, antifungal agents and antimycobacterial agents are discussed in other sections.

The 'ideal' antibacterial drug is one that is harmful to the invading organism without being harmful to the host (known as 'selective' toxicity) (Bryant et al 2019). Antibacterial agents exploit the differences between the host and the invading organism, and generally act in one of the following general ways:

- inhibiting bacterial cell wall synthesis (e.g. penicillins, cephalosporins, monobactams and carbapenems, glycopeptides)
- inhibiting bacterial protein synthesis (e.g. aminoglycosides, tetracyclines, chloramphenicol, macrolides, lincosamides, oxazolidinones, streptogramins)
- inhibiting synthesis of bacterial DNA (e.g. quinolones)
- disrupting bacterial cell membrane (e.g. colistimethate)
- interfering with metabolic processes such as bacterial nucleic acid synthesis or folate metabolism (e.g. sulfonamides, trimethoprim) (Bryant et al 2019).

Bactericidal drugs kill susceptible microorganisms, whereas *bacteriostatic* drugs inhibit their growth but do not kill the organisms. Whether a drug is bacteriostatic or bactericidal may be dependent on the dose given and the concentration achieved at the site of action. Because bacteriostatic drugs slow the growth of the organisms, they give the body's immune system time to become activated and rid itself of the invading organisms. Whether or not an antibacterial agent is successful or not in destroying or suppressing bacterial growth is dependent on factors such as bacterial load (concentration of bacteria present), phase of bacterial growth, ability to achieve an adequate drug concentration at the site of the infection and the minimum inhibitory concentration of the antibacterial agent (this is the lowest amount of drug needed to prevent visible bacterial growth and this is dependent on the antibacterial agent, the organism and the person being affected) (Bryant et al 2019).

Antibacterial agents are often overused for many reasons, including doctors prescribing multiple antibiotics when one is sufficient, prescribing long courses unnecessarily, prescribing for self-limiting illnesses that don't require antibiotics, overuse as prophylaxis before surgery, over-the-counter (OTC) sales in some countries (encouraging inappropriate and/or indiscriminate use), and use in animal feeds to promote growth and prevent infection (Levison 2014). One outcome of this overuse is the development of resistance, resulting in less agents being effective in treating infection. Some organisms have innate (or intrinsic) resistance to some antimicrobial agents (i.e. they have always been resistant to them), while others have acquired resistance (i.e. the organism changes its genetic make-up or acquires new DNA) (Bryant et al 2019). Antibacterial resistance has developed through the following processes:

- the antibacterial agent is unable to reach the target site because some organisms may form a protective membrane (e.g. glycocalyx or biofilm) that stops the antibacterial from reaching the bacterial cell wall. Gram-negative bacteria produce porins (outer membrane proteins) which allow diffusion of molecules (including antibacterials) into cytoplasm; however, mutations to porins impede antibacterial access (e.g. tobramycin-resistant *Pseudomonas aeruginosa*)
- developing enzymes that inactivate the drug (e.g. beta-lactamase is an enzyme produced by staphylococci that inactivates the penicillins and many of the cephalosporins). Extended spectrum beta-lactamases have developed which have led to bacteria having cross-resistance to penicillin and cephalosporins, as well as being resistant to other classes of antibacterial agents
- the antibacterial target site is altered so the drug can no longer bind to the site. Penicillin-binding proteins (PBP) are membrane-associated enzymes present in the cell wall of peptidoglycan-containing organisms. Changes to PBP can result in resistance occurring (e.g. *Staphylococcus aureus* resistance to beta-lactam antibiotics results from the development of highly resistant PBP)
- the antibacterial agent is pumped out by an efflux pump found in both Gram-positive and Gram-negative organisms (e.g. tetracycline-resistant *S. aureus*); development of bypass pathways that compensate for loss of function due to antibacterial agents (e.g. resistance to sulfonamides) (Brenner & Stevens 2017; Bryant et al 2019).

Many resistant strains of bacteria exist in Australia, including methicillin-resistant *S. aureus* (MRSA) and vancomycin-resistant *Enterococcus faecium* (VRE). Other issues include the emergence of multi-drug-resistant HIV and *Mycobacterium tuberculosis* (Bryant & Knights 2015). From a clinical perspective, it is this acquired resistance that has become a serious problem as it has reduced the number of drugs available to treat infection, potentially resulting in increased hospitalisation, longer lengths of stay in hospital and increased mortality (Bryant et al 2019). A number of programs are in place that attempt to combat this drug resistance, including limiting the availability of some antibacterial agents (e.g. vancomycin, teicoplanin, imipenem) unless they are specifically required, using combinations rather than single agents in certain circumstances (e.g. mixed infections), or using them in rotation, as well as ensuring that the lowest effective dose is used (Bryant et al 2019). It is therefore important that antibacterial agents are only used to treat bacterial infections (not viral or other types of infections), and that the organism is identified, along with its susceptibility or resistance (however, if the infection is life-threatening, treatment should be started immediately) (Bryant et al 2019). Use a dose that is high enough to be efficacious with minimal toxicity, but has the narrowest spectrum of that organism and is used for the shortest duration possible (unless there is evidence to suggest that longer is possible/advantageous) (Bryant et al 2019).

General Nursing points/Cautions for antibacterial agents

- appropriate culture and sensitivity testing should be done to isolate and identify the organism(s) and determine susceptibility to antibacterial agents
- careful routine history is taken to exclude previous reactions to antibacterial agents (e.g. penicillin, cephalosporin), other allergens or severe asthma in order to avoid anaphylaxis
- all relevant medical staff must be informed of any antibiotic allergy, and medical history, medication chart and patient suitably labelled (e.g. patient identification label) (as per workplace guidelines)
- after administration of drugs (especially penicillins and cephalosporins), observe patient closely for bronchospasm, urticarial rash, signs of cardiovascular collapse or angioneurotic oedema (anaphylactoid reactions can occur with the first dose)
- ensure hand-washing occurs after patient contact by all staff to prevent cross-infection with organisms
- mild- to life-threatening antibiotic-associated pseudomembranous colitis (caused by *Clostridium difficile* toxin; see Glossary) may occur weeks after finishing a course of antibiotics. The condition may be worsened or prolonged if peristalsis-delaying drugs are given (e.g. opioid analgesics)
- note and report gastrointestinal (GI) disturbances, especially diarrhoea
- note and report signs of superinfection, such as stomatitis, 'black tongue', vaginal and/or oral moniliasis. Superinfection occurs because of an overgrowth by non-susceptible microorganisms (e.g. *Candida albicans*) during therapy
- ensure administration at regular (and prescribed) intervals to maintain adequate plasma drug levels
- lidocaine (lignocaine) toxicity may occur in patients with hepatic disease if lidocaine (lignocaine) is used repeatedly as a diluent to reduce the pain of IM injection. Lidocaine (lignocaine) should not be used for IV administration and is contraindicated in anyone with a known hypersensitivity to lidocaine (lignocaine) or other amide-type local anaesthetics, or in those with non-paced heart block, severe heart failure or infants less than 30 months
- IM injections should be given into large muscle mass, ensuring that injection sites are rotated
- when giving IM, avoid intravascular injection by aspirating syringe plunger

prior to administration and checking for blood

- ensure that IV drugs are handled carefully to avoid spillage and spraying into the air during reconstitution and/or administration
- reconstitute drugs according to the manufacturer's instructions. Dry powders are generally reconstituted with water for injections (and then diluted with appropriate and compatible infusion fluid (e.g. sodium chloride 0.9%) if necessary). It is especially important to consult the manufacturer's product information if the antibacterial agent can be given both IM and IV as the amount of diluent required may vary according to the route of administration
- if the recommended method of administration is by slow infusion, dilute the reconstituted drug in 50–100 mL of compatible infusion fluid and infuse over 30–60 minutes via a burette (some drugs are infused over 1–6 hours)
- if a slow bolus injection is necessary, the drug should be reconstituted with or diluted in 10–20 mL water for injections and injected over 1–10 minutes into side arm (injection port) of flowing administration set or through three-way tap, followed by flush with sodium chloride 0.9%. Slow bolus means **slow** – this prevents irritation to the vein and reduces pain and some adverse reactions related to administration
- maintain asepsis during administration of IV antibacterial agents
- maintain activity of drug by correct storage conditions (especially if not administered immediately)
- have adrenaline (epinephrine), IV corticosteroids, oxygen and resuscitation equipment available in the event of anaphylaxis

General Patient teaching and advice for antibacterial agents

- the patient should be advised to obtain a MedicAlert bracelet or pendant if they have an allergy to antibacterial agent (or other drugs, foods, dyes or preservatives)
- instruct the patient to inform any medical or nursing personnel of allergy, especially when antibacterial agent is being administered
- emphasise the importance of completing the entire course of the prescribed antibacterial agent, even if the patient feels better quickly. Discourage keeping any antibacterial agents and self-medicating if symptoms recur
- instruct the patient to immediately seek medical advice if any of the following occurs:
  - diarrhoea (especially if severe, watery or bloody), severe stomach cramps and/or fever during therapy or up to several weeks after stopping antibacterial agents. It is essential to stress the importance of not taking any medication to stop the diarrhoea as this may worsen the condition
  - skin rash or hives, blistering or peeling of skin, swelling to face, lips, mouth or throat making it difficult to breathe or swallow or any breathing difficulty, including wheezing
- advise patient to seek medical advice (but not an emergency) if vaginal itching or discharge (vaginal thrush)

or white, sore, furry tongue and mouth (oral thrush) occurs
- ensure patient understands when to take oral preparations in relation to food (e.g. before or after meals) and other medications such as antacids
- instruct patient to keep any antibacterial mixtures/suspensions/syrups in the refrigerator (not freezer) and discard as advised by pharmacist
- advise patient not to drive or operate machinery if they experience dizziness, lethargy, tiredness, blurred vision or other similar side-effects which may impair judgement or driving ability
- as many antibacterial agents have been implicated in reducing the effectiveness of oral contraceptives, women are advised to check with the prescriber to ascertain whether additional contraceptive precautions (e.g. barrier method) are required during therapy
- with female patients of childbearing potential, the importance of seeking medical advice if she becomes pregnant or plans to breastfeed during therapy must be discussed
- see also General Patient teaching and advice (p. xxvii)

INHIBITORS OF BACTERIAL CELL WALL SYNTHESIS

Penicillins, cephalosporins, monobactams and carbapenems all contain a beta-lactam ring, which relates them structurally. It is this ring that is essential for antibacterial activity. Many bacteria produce beta-lactamase (penicillinase), an enzyme that breaks the beta-lactam ring, thereby rendering the antibacterial agent ineffective against that bacterial strain. It is now possible to add beta-lactamase inhibitors to penicillins, making them active against previously resistant strains; however, this does increase the cost (Bryant et al 2019). These inhibitors include clavulanic acid and tazobactam. Furthermore, some Gram-negative organisms have a phospholipid membrane that prevents some of the penicillins from entering the cell, making those organisms resistant to penicillin.

PENICILLINS

General Actions of penicillins

- selectively inhibit formation of a rigid bacterial cell wall
- bactericidal
- Gram-negative bacilli are generally resistant to penicillins
- classified as:
  - narrow spectrum (e.g. benzylpenicillin, phenoxymethylpenicillin)
  - narrow spectrum, penicillinase resistant (e.g. dicloxacillin)
  - moderate spectrum beta-lactamase sensitive aminopenicillins (e.g. amoxicillin, ampicillin)
  - broad and extended spectrum (e.g. piperacillin, ticarcillin)

General Uses of penicillins

- infections where the organisms are not resistant to penicillins, including:
  - upper and lower respiratory tract infections

- skin and skin structure infections
- bone and joint infections
- urinary tract infections
- gynaecological infections
- septicaemia, bacteraemia
- intra-abdominal infections
- sexually transmitted infections (e.g. gonorrhoea, syphilis, yaws, bejel, pinta)
- scarlet fever
- meningitis
- fusospirochaetosis (Vincent's gingivitis and pharyngitis)
- Group A streptococci infection without bacteraemia
- surgical (including obstetric and colorectal) prophylaxis (where there is significant risk of post-operative infection)
- prophylaxis of rheumatic fever, rheumatic heart disease and acute glomerulonephritis
- prophylaxis of subacute bacterial endocarditis (SBE)

General Adverse effects of penicillins

- hypersensitivity reaction, including urticaria, exfoliative dermatitis, maculopapular rash, rash, pruritus
- anaemia, leucopenia, thrombocytopenia, agranulocytosis, purpura and, rarely, prolongation of bleeding time and prothrombin time
- headache
- glossitis, stomatitis, black hairy tongue
- diarrhoea, nausea, vomiting, abdominal pain, taste/smell disturbance
- fever
- superinfection (vaginal and/or oral moniliasis), pseudomembranous colitis, serum sickness-like reaction (chills, fever, oedema, arthralgia), allergic reaction
- (high doses, rare) interstitial nephropathy
- (rare) hepatitis, cholestatic jaundice
- (rare, high doses) convulsions, dizziness, confusion, encephalopathy
- (rare) anaphylactic shock, anaphylactoid reaction, severe skin reactions
- (rapid IV) convulsions
- (IV) phlebitis, pain, burning, erythema, swelling
- (IM) pain
- (rare, repeated IM injection) quadriceps femoris fibrosis and atrophy

General Interactions of penicillins

- aminoglycosides and penicillins are physically and/or chemically incompatible
- increased risk of aminoglycoside-associated nephrotoxicity if aminoglycosides and penicillins are given together, especially in those with renal impairment. If given together, renal function should be closely monitored
- penicillins may affect the stability of anticoagulant control, therefore prothrombin time should be carefully monitored, especially when starting and stopping therapy
- increased risk of bleeding if given in high-dose IV with antiplatelet agents. If given together, patient should be closely monitored for any signs of bleeding
- probenecid increases and prolongs serum penicillin levels
- effect of penicillins may be reduced by the bacteriostatic agents chloramphenicol, erythromycin and tetracycline, therefore therapeutic response should be closely monitored
- some penicillins may cause failure of combined oral contraceptives, which may be due to increased oestrogen metabolism or decreased oestrogen reabsorption in the gut

- may decrease clearance of methotrexate, potentially resulting in methotrexate toxicity. If given together, methotrexate levels should be closely monitored
- lidocaine (lignocaine) toxicity may occur in patients with liver disease or reduced liver blood flow if lidocaine (lignocaine) is used repeatedly as a diluent to reduce the pain of IM injection
- increased risk of pseudomembranous colitis if given with peristalsis-delaying agents such as opioid analgesics or atropine/diphenoxylate combination
- absorption may be decreased by antacids
- may cause false-positive result on urine glucose testing with some reagents

General Nursing points/Cautions for penicillins

- see General Nursing points/ Cautions for antibacterial agents (p. 148)
- (meningitis) blood–brain barrier permeability is increased with inflammation, leading to an increased risk of encephalopathy occurring at a lower dose, therefore patients should be closely monitored
- probenecid 1 g may be given orally 30 minutes before injection to increase and prolong the serum penicillin level
- penicillin should be handled carefully by staff to prevent self-sensitisation
- when only part of a vial's contents is required (e.g. 750 mg from a 1 g vial), reconstitution should be according to dilution table found in the manufacturer's information; discard any remaining solution
- needle blockage is less likely if a small-bore syringe and 20-gauge needle are used
- if giving IM with lidocaine (lignocaine) (without adrenaline (epinephrine)), it is important to ensure patient does not have a hypersensitivity to lidocaine (lignocaine)
- treatment should continue 48–72 hours after symptoms have abated
- treatment should generally not exceed 14 days
- if treatment is prolonged, blood counts, and liver and renal function should be monitored
- IV injection should be given over at least 3–5 minutes to prevent pain and convulsions
- if single-dose therapy is used for urinary tract infection, urine should be cultured post therapy – if organisms are still present, a longer or higher dose treatment regimen is recommended
- if treating streptococcal disease, cultures should be taken at the end of therapy to ensure total eradication of organism
- all patients with gonorrhoea should also have serological testing for syphilis at time of diagnosis and then monthly for at least 4 months
- electrolyte monitoring is recommended if given in high doses and/or for prolonged therapy in some patients (e.g. those with heart or renal disease) for whom sodium intake may have an impact
- care should be taken if the person is on a salt-restricted diet as many parenteral preparations have a high sodium content that may worsen cardiac failure
- oxygen, adrenaline, IV corticosteroids and intubation equipment should be

readily available in the case of a severe hypersensitivity reaction occurring

- caution if used in those with a history of GI diseases (especially colitis), mononucleosis, bleeding disorders, cardiac disease, cystic fibrosis, impaired renal or liver function
- caution if used in those with allergic tendencies
- contraindicated in those with known hypersensitivity to beta-lactam antibiotics (penicillins and cephalosporins)
- (with lidocaine (lignocaine)) contraindicated in those with amide-type local anaesthetic hypersensitivity

General Patient teaching and advice for penicillins

- instruct patient that oral preparations are taken 1 hour before or 2 hours after meals (except amoxicillin) to avoid delayed absorption by food and to reduce destruction by gastric acid
- if antacids are used, patient should be instructed to separate by at least 2 hours from oral penicillins
- warn patient to avoid taking oral preparations with acidic fruit juices or liquids because these may accelerate drug decomposition
- advise patient to seek medical advice immediately if any of the following occur:
  - severe skin reaction
  - yellowing of skin or eyes, loss of appetite, nausea, upper abdominal pain, itchy skin, dark urine, pale stools (even if these occur weeks after stopping therapy)
- see also General Patient teaching and advice for antibacterial agents (p. 149)

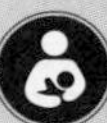

penicillins are thought to be safe to use during pregnancy

penicillins are excreted in breastmilk and could potentially sensitise the newborn infant, therefore risks versus benefits must be carefully considered before use

AMOXICILLIN SODIUM (Amoxil Parenteral, Fisamox, Ibiamox)

AMOXICILLIN TRIHYDRATE (Alphamox, Amiloxyn, Amoxil, Amoxycillin, Cilamox, Maxamox, Ranmoxy)

Available forms

Capsules: 250 mg, 500 mg; Tablets: 1 g; Vial: 500 mg, 1 g; Syrup/suspension: 125 mg/5 mL, 250 mg/5 mL, 500 mg/5 mL; Paediatric drops: 100 mg/mL

Action

- broad spectrum, acid-stable aminopenicillin that is not penicillinase resistant
- activity spectrum is the same as for ampicillin
- active against broader range of Gram-negative organisms than benzylpenicillin but not Gram-positive organisms
- half-life about 1 hour
- see also General Actions of penicillins (p. 150)

Use

- see General Uses of penicillins (p. 150)

Dose

- (upper respiratory tract infection, genitourinary tract infection, skin and soft tissue infections) 250 mg IM, by IV infusion over 30–60 minutes or IV bolus over 3–4 minutes 6–8-hourly **OR**

- (upper respiratory tract infection, genitourinary tract infection, skin and soft tissue infections) 250 mg orally 8-hourly **OR**
- (lower respiratory tract infections) 500 mg orally, IM, by IV infusion over 30–60 minutes or IV bolus over 3–4 minutes 8-hourly **OR**
- (acute uncomplicated urinary tract infection, urethritis, gonorrhoea) 3 g as single oral dose **OR**
- (bacterial septicaemia) 1 g 6-hourly by slow IV injection over 3–4 minutes or IV infusion over 30–60 minutes **OR**
- (prophylaxis – subacute bacterial endocarditis (SBE) after dental procedures, no anaesthetic and no penicillin taken in the past month) 3 g orally 1 hour before the procedure, followed by 3 g 6 hours later if necessary **OR**
- (prophylaxis – SBE, no penicillin taken in the past month, dental procedures with a general anaesthetic, oral antibiotics are not appropriate) 1 g IM immediately before induction, followed by 500 mg orally 6 hours later **OR**
- (prophylaxis – SBE after dental procedure; patient has taken penicillin in the past month and the patient needs general anaesthetic or has prosthetic valve replacements and needs general anaesthetic or has had one or more attacks of SBE) 1 g IM with 120 mg gentamicin IM immediately before induction or 15 minutes before dental procedure, followed by 500 mg orally 6 hours later **OR**
- (prophylaxis – SBE for genitourinary surgery/procedure under general anaesthesia) 1 g IM with 120 mg gentamicin IM immediately before induction, followed by 500 mg orally or IM 6 hours later **OR**
- (prophylaxis – SBE for genitourinary surgery/procedure under general anaesthesia) 1 g IM with 120 mg gentamicin IM immediately before induction, followed by 500 mg orally or IM 6 hours later **OR**
- (prophylaxis – SBE for obstetric and gynaecological procedures or GI procedures with prosthetic valve replacement) 1 g IM with 120 mg gentamicin IM immediately before induction, followed by 500 mg IM 6 hours later **OR**
- (prophylaxis – SBE for upper respiratory tract surgery/procedure in patient without prosthetic valve replacement) 1 g IM immediately before induction, followed by 500 mg IM 6 hours later

Adverse effects

- (rare) crystalluria, superficial tooth discolouration in children
- see also General Adverse effects of penicillins (p. 151)

Interactions

- increased risk of skin rashes if given with allopurinol, therefore not recommended together. If given together, patient should be monitored for appearance of any rash
- see also General Interactions of penicillins (p. 151)

Nursing points/Cautions

- doses greater than 500 mg not given as single IM injection
- ensure patient is adequately hydrated to maintain high urinary output during therapy with amoxicillin
- if patient has IDC in situ, regularly monitor for any crystalluria as high levels of amoxicillin may precipitate out at room temperature
- (SBE) dental procedures include tooth extraction, scaling or surgery involving gingival tissue
- (SBE) if given with gentamicin, should not be mixed in same syringe
- (acute lower urinary tract infection) urine should be cultured after single

dose is given. If culture is positive, longer or larger course may be required
- may be given by IV infusion run over 30–40 minutes or slow IV injection over 3–5 minutes (to prevent convulsions)
- harmless, transient pink colouration or slight cloudiness may appear during reconstitution of IM or IV solution may be diluted with lidocaine (lignocaine) 1% or procaine 0.5% to reduce pain IM
- parenteral solution contains 2.6–3.3 mmol sodium per 1 g amoxicillin, which may be a consideration in those with a sodium restriction
- (syrup/paediatric drops) contain aspartame and therefore not recommended in those with phenylketonuria
- (syrup/paediatric drops) contain benzoates, therefore may cause reaction in those with hypersensitivity
- not recommended for sore throat or pharyngitis because of increased risk of skin rash if amoxicillin is given to those with infectious mononucleosis (glandular fever)
- increased risk of rash if given to those with lymphatic leukaemia, therefore should be given with caution and patient closely monitored
- see also General Nursing points/Cautions for penicillins (p. 152)

Patient teaching and advice

- if parent is going to administer paediatric syrup to child, the following instructions should be given:
  - shake bottle well before use
  - use syringe adapter (provided to withdraw required dose)
  - rinse syringe well after use
  - refrigerate but do not freeze
  - discard 14 days after opening
- see also General Patient teaching and advice for penicillins (p. 153)

syrup/suspension is available. Tablet can be crushed or capsule opened and mixed with water or spoonful of yoghurt or apple puree

Note

- contained in Augmentin preparations, AlphaClav, Amclovax Duo, AmoxyClav, Clamohexal Duo preparations, Clavam, Curam preparations, and Moxiclav preparations with clavulanic acid
- contained in Nexium Hp7 with clarithromycin and esomeprazole, for the eradication of *Helicobacter pylori*

AMOXICILLIN TRIHYDRATE WITH CLAVULANIC ACID (AlphaClav Duo, AlphaClav Duo Forte, Amoxiclav, Amclovax Duo, AmoxyClav, Augmentin preparations, Clavam, Curam preparations, Moxiclav preparations)

Available forms

Vial: 500 mg amoxicillin/100 mg clavulanic acid, 1000 mg amoxicillin/200 mg clavulanic acid, 2000 mg amoxicillin/200 mg clavulanic acid; Tablets: 500 mg amoxicillin/125 mg clavulanic acid, 875 mg amoxicillin/125 mg clavulanic acid; Syrup/suspension: 125 mg amoxicillin/31.25 mg clavulanic acid/5 mL, 400 mg amoxicillin/57 mg clavulanic acid/5 mL

Action

- clavulanic acid is a potent inhibitor of beta-lactamase (penicillinase), and is added to some penicillins to enhance their activity against many previously resistant strains
- active against a range of Gram-positive and Gram-negative aerobic organisms
- see also General Actions of penicillins (p. 150)

Use

- see General Uses of penicillins (p. 150)

Dose

- 1000 mg amoxicillin/200 mg clavulanic acid by slow IV over 3–4 minutes or IV infusion over 30–40 minutes 6- to 8-hourly **OR**
- (serious infection) 2000 mg amoxicillin/200 mg clavulanic acid by slow IV over 3–4 minutes or IV infusion over 30–40 minutes 6- to 8-hourly **OR**
- (surgical prophylaxis) 1000 mg amoxicillin/200 mg clavulanic acid – 2000 mg amoxicillin/200 mg clavulanic acid by slow IV over 3–4 minutes at induction, then repeated after 2 hours if needed **OR**
- 500 mg amoxicillin/125 mg clavulanic acid 12-hourly orally immediately before food or with first mouthful **OR**
- (severe infections) 875 mg amoxicillin/125 mg clavulanic acid orally 12-hourly immediately before food or with first mouthful **OR**
- (syrup) 250 mg amoxicillin/62.5 mg clavulanic acid – 500 mg amoxicillin/125 mg clavulanic acid (5–10 mL) 8-hourly immediately before food or with first mouthful

Adverse effects

- see General Adverse effects of penicillins (p. 151)

Interactions

- amoxicillin increases risk of skin rashes if given with allopurinol, therefore not recommended together
- see General Interactions of penicillins (p. 151)

Nursing points/Cautions

- (parenteral) not given IM
- (parenteral) reconstitute using 10 mL water for injections for 600 mg vial or 20 mL for 1.2 or 2.2 mg vial and then further dilute using 50–100 mL for IV infusion
- (tablets) each preparation is different and the dose is based on the amoxicillin content and therefore correct preparation should be selected (clavulanic acid content is the same in tablet preparation (125 mg) but varies in the syrup/suspension)
- 400 mg amoxicillin/57 mg clavulanic acid oral suspension/syrup is intended for paediatric use and dose is based on child's weight. If child weighs ≥ 40 kg, dose should be according to adult guidelines
- (suspension) contains aspartame and is therefore not recommended in those with phenylketonuria
- (parenteral) vials contain 31.4–125.9 mg sodium, which may need to be considered if patient has salt restriction
- (parenteral) vials contain 19.6–39.3 mg potassium, which may need to be considered if patient has reduced kidney function or requires potassium-controlled diet
- (parenteral) less stable in solutions containing glucose, dextran or bicarbonate
- (parenteral) should not be mixed with blood products, protein hydrolysates or IV lipid emulsions
- not recommended in those with moderate to severe kidney impairment (creatinine clearance ≤ 30 mL/min)
- contraindicated in those with previous history of amoxicillin/clavulanic acid-associated jaundice or liver dysfunction
- see also Nursing points/Cautions for amoxicillin (p. 154) and General Nursing points/Cautions for penicillins (p. 152)

Patient teaching and advice

- advise patient/parent/carer to check discarding information carefully as some oral suspensions should be discarded 14 days after opening while others after 7 days

- instruct patient not to substitute tablets (e.g. 2 Augmentin for Augmentin Duo Forte, as they are not equivalent)
- see Patient teaching and advice for amoxicillin (p. 155) and General Patient teaching and advice for penicillins (p. 153)

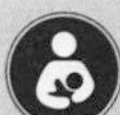

should only be used during pregnancy if benefits outweigh risks. May increase risk of necrotising enterocolitis in neonates

tablet can be crushed and mixed with water or spoonful of yoghurt or apple puree

AMPICILLIN SODIUM (Ampicyn, Austrapen, Ibimycin)

Available forms

Vial: 500 mg, 1 g

Action

- broad spectrum, acid-stable aminopenicillin
- not penicillinase resistant
- similar to benzylpenicillin, but more active against some Gram-negative bacilli and some *Enterobacteriaceae*
- half-life 1 hour (prolonged up to 20 hours in those with kidney impairment)
- see also General Actions of penicillins (p. 150)

Use

- see General Uses of penicillins (p. 150)

Dose

- (respiratory tract infection) 250–500 mg IM, IV injection over 3–5 minutes or IV infusion over 30–40 minutes 6-hourly **OR**
- (chronic bronchitis) 0.5–1 g IM, IV injection over 3–5 minutes or IV infusion over 30–40 minutes 6-hourly **OR**
- (urinary tract infection) 500 mg IM, IV injection over 3–5 minutes or IV infusion over 30–40 minutes 6-hourly **OR**
- (GI infections) 500–750 mg IM, IV injection over 3–5 minutes or IV infusion over 30–40 minutes 6-hourly **OR**
- (bacterial meningitis, septicaemia) 200 mg/kg daily IV in divided doses 4–6-hourly (daily maximum 12 g)

Adverse effects

- (rare) crystalluria
- see also General Adverse effects of penicillins (p. 151)

Interactions

- increased risk of skin rashes if given with allopurinol
- may decrease effectiveness of combined oral contraceptives
- see also General Interactions of penicillins (p. 151)

Nursing points/Cautions/Patient teaching and advice

- ensure patient is adequately hydrated to maintain high urinary output during therapy with ampicillin
- if patient has IDC in situ, regular monitoring for crystalluria is recommended as high levels of ampicillin may precipitate out at room temperature
- may be given IM, by IV infusion run over 30–40 minutes or slow IV injection over 3–5 minutes (to prevent convulsions)
- should be administered immediately after being reconstituted with diluents
- may also be given by intraperitoneal, intrapleural or intra-articular injection
- contains 2.7 mmol sodium per g ampicillin, which may need to be considered if patient has salt restriction
- not recommended intrathecally
- not recommended for sore throat or pharyngitis because of increased risk of skin rash if ampicillin is given to those with infectious mononucleosis (glandular fever)

- increased risk of rash if given to those with lymphatic leukaemia
- see General Nursing points/Cautions for penicillins (p. 152) and General Patient teaching and advice for penicillins (p. 153)

BENZATHINE PENICILLIN (Bicillin LA)

Available forms

Prefilled syringe: 600,000 units/1.17 mL, 1,200,000 units/2.3 mL

Action

- slowly absorbed and converted to benzylpenicillin, resulting in lower but more prolonged blood levels than other parenteral penicillins
- see also General Actions of penicillins (p. 150)

Use

- see General Uses of penicillins (p. 150)

Dose

- (venereal disease – primary, secondary and latent syphilis) 2,400,000 units as single IM injection **OR**
- (venereal disease – tertiary syphilis with neurosyphilis) 2,400,000 IM weekly for 3 weeks (total 3 doses) **OR**
- (venereal disease – yaws, bejel, pinta) 1,200,000 units as single IM injection **OR**
- (rheumatic fever, glomerulonephritis prophylaxis) 1,200,000 units IM monthly **OR**
- (rheumatic fever, glomerulonephritis prophylaxis) 600,000 units IM every 2 weeks **OR**
- (streptococcal (group A) upper respiratory tract infection) 1,200,000 units as a single IM injection

Adverse effects

- (syphilis) Jarisch–Herxheimer reaction (malaise, fever, chills, sore throat, myalgia, headache, tachycardia)
- severe agitation, confusion, visual/auditory hallucinations, fear of impending death
- see also General Adverse effects of penicillins (p. 151)

Interactions/Nursing points/Cautions/Patient teaching and advice

- given as deep IM injection
- administer alone
- before administration, the syringe should be rolled between the palms of the hands to resuspend contents
- administer at a slow and steady rate to prevent needle blockage
- contains hydroxybenzoates which may cause allergic reaction in hypersensitive individuals
- NEVER give IV as neurovascular damage may occur or into/near nerves
- see General Nursing points/Cautions for penicillins (p. 152)

BENZYLPENICILLIN SODIUM (crystalline penicillin, penicillin G) (BenPen)

Available forms

Vial: 600 mg, 1.2 g, 3 g

Action

- narrow spectrum penicillin
- active against most Gram-positive organisms (e.g. streptococci, pneumococci, non-beta-lactamase-producing staphylococci, clostridia) and some Gram-negative organisms (e.g. gonococci and meningococci and also some spirochaetes)
- reaches high blood levels quickly, which prevents resistance
- drug of choice for streptococcal pneumonia
- see also General Actions of penicillins (p. 150)

Use

- see General Uses of penicillins (p. 150)

Dose

- 300 mg IM or IV 6-hourly (increasing dose/frequency in more serious infections) **OR**

- (severe infections) 4–24 g/24 hours in 4–6 divided doses IM or IV **OR**
- (prophylaxis – surgery) 600 mg IV immediately before surgery, then 4–8-hourly for duration of procedure if necessary **OR**
- (treatment of SBE) not less than 1.2 g IV daily in divided doses for 4–6 weeks **OR**
- (treatment of SBE *Streptococci viridans*) 6–12 g IV daily in divided doses for 4–6 weeks **OR**
- (clostridial infection) 1.2 g IV 6-hourly for 48 hours **OR**
- (meningococcal meningitis (children)) initially 600 mg IM, then 300 mg IM 4–6-hourly **OR**
- (pneumococcal meningitis (children)) at least 300 mg IM 4-hourly for 2 weeks, then 6-hourly for 7 days

Adverse effects

- (syphilis) Jarisch–Herxheimer reaction (malaise, fever, chills, sore throat, myalgia, headache, tachycardia)
- see also General Adverse effects of penicillins (p. 151)

Interactions

- actions antagonised by chloramphenicol, erythromycin and tetracyclines
- see also General Interactions of penicillins (p. 151)

Nursing points and Cautions/ Patient teaching and advice

- should not be added to IV infusions as unstable at room temperature
- incompatible with some antihistamines, some antibacterial agents, noradrenaline, metaraminol, thiopentone and phenytoin
- must be used immediately after reconstitution with water for injections
- (IM) doses of 600 mg should be reconstituted using 1.6 mL water for injections. For doses > 600 mg, see manufacturer's table for reconstitution volumes
- (IV) recommended concentration is 60 mg/mL
- contains 3.0 mmol sodium per 1 g benzylpenicillin, therefore electrolyte monitoring is recommended if given in high doses, for prolonged therapy and/or in those with heart failure
- see General Nursing points/Cautions for penicillins (p. 152)

DICLOXACILLIN SODIUM (Distaph)

Available forms

Capsules: 250 mg, 500 mg

Action

- narrow spectrum antibiotic active against *Streptococcus pyogenes*, *S. viridans*, *S. pneumoniae* and penicillinase-producing staphylococci
- see also General Actions of penicillins (p. 150)

Use

- see General Uses of penicillins (p. 150)

Dose

- 250–500 mg orally 6-hourly 1–2 hours before food

Adverse effects

- (over 55 years, prolonged therapy) hepatitis, cholestatic jaundice
- (rare) oesophageal burning, oesophagitis, oesophageal ulceration
- see also General Adverse effects of penicillins (p. 151)

Interactions

- may decrease phenytoin and warfarin levels, therefore levels should be carefully monitored during therapy
- see also General Interactions of penicillins (p. 151)

Nursing points/Cautions

- white blood cell count and differential cell count should be measured before starting therapy, and then

weekly during therapy. Urinalysis, serum urea, creatinine and liver enzymes should also be monitored
- not recommended in patients over 55 years unless clearly indicated because of the risk of cholestatic hepatitis
- see also General Nursing points/Cautions for penicillins (p. 152)

Patient teaching and advice

- patient should be instructed to take capsules with a large glass of water and not to lie down immediately after (therefore should not be taken at bedtime)
- advise patient (especially if over 55) to immediately report any yellowing of eyes or skin or darkening of urine during therapy or weeks after therapy has stopped
- see also General Patient teaching and advice for penicillins (p. 153)

Capsule can be opened and dispersed in water or mixed with spoonful of yoghurt or apple puree

FLUCLOXACILLIN SODIUM MONOHYDRATE (FLUCLOXACILLIN SODIUM) (DBL Flopen, Flubiclox, Flucil, Flucloxacillin Sodium Powder for Injection, Staphylex)

Available forms

Vial: 500 mg, 1 g; Capsules: 250 mg, 500 mg; Syrup: 125 mg/5 mL, 250 mg/5 mL

Action

- acid stable and penicillinase resistant
- narrow spectrum antibiotic active against *S. pyogenes* or *S. pneumoniae*, and beta-lactamase producing and penicillin-sensitive *Staphylococcus aureus*
- not active against Gram-negative bacilli, *Streptococcus faecalis* or MRSA
- see also General Actions of penicillins (p. 150)

Use

- see General Uses of penicillins (p. 150)

Dose

- 250 mg orally 6-hourly 30–60 minutes before meals **OR**
- 250 mg IM 6-hourly **OR**
- 250–1000 mg 6-hourly by IV bolus or infusion over 3–4 minutes

Adverse effects

- (over 55 years or prolonged therapy) severe hepatitis, cholestatic jaundice
- see also General Adverse effects of penicillins (p. 151)

Interactions

- increased risk of metabolic acidosis if given with paracetamol
- see also General Interactions of penicillins (p. 151)

Nursing points/Cautions

- IV bolus may cause pain and irritation at injection site
- may also be given by intrapleural or intra-articular injection
- (IV) reconstitute 1 g in 15–20 mL water for injections
- (IM) reconstitute 1 g in 2.5 mL water for injections
- (parenteral) contains 2 mmol sodium per 1 g flucloxacillin
- (IV) should not be mixed with blood or protein-containing products
- (IV) incompatible with aminoglycosides, amiodarone, atropine, buprenorphine, calcium gluconate, chlorpromazine, ciprofloxacin, diazepam, dobutamine, erythromycin, metoclopramide, morphine, pethidine, prochlorperazine and verapamil
- (syrup) contains benzoates which may cause hypersensitivity reaction in sensitive individuals
- not recommended for those over 55 years because of increased risk of severe hepatitis and cholestatic jaundice

- contraindicated in those with flucloxacillin associated jaundice or liver dysfunction or for use in the eye (locally or conjunctivally)
- see also General Nursing points/Cautions for penicillins (p. 152)

Patient teaching and advice

- advise patient (especially if over 55) to immediately report any yellowing of eyes or skin or darkening of urine during therapy or weeks after therapy has stopped
- (syrup) instruct patient to shake bottle well before use and discard 14 days after opening
- see also General Patient teaching and advice for penicillins (p. 153)

syrup/suspension is available. Capsule can be opened and mixed with water or spoonful of yoghurt or apple puree

PHENOXYMETHYLPENICILLIN BENZATHINE (PENICILLIN V) (Cilicaine V)

PHENOXYMETHYLPENICILLIN POTASSIUM (Aspecillin, Aspecillin VK, Cilicaine VK, LPV, Phenoxymethylpenicillin AFT)

Available forms

Tablets: 250 mg, 500 mg; Capsules: 250 mg, 500 mg: Suspension: 125 mg/5 mL, 150 mg/5 mL, 250 mg/5 mL

Action

- narrow spectrum penicillin, less active than benzylpenicillin
- acid stable but not penicillinase resistant
- see also General Actions of penicillins (p. 150)

Use

- see General Uses of penicillins (p. 150)

Dose

- (mild-to-moderately severe streptococcal infections, including scarlet fever) 125–250 mg orally 6–8-hourly 1 hour before meals for 10 days **OR**
- (mild-to-moderately severe pneumococcal infections, otitis media) 250–500 mg orally 4–6-hourly 1 hour before meals until patient has been afebrile for 2 days **OR**
- (mild-to-moderately severe fusospirochaetosis of oropharynx) 250–500 mg orally 6–8-hourly 1 hour before meals **OR**
- (prevent recurrence of rheumatic fever and/or chorea) 125–250 mg orally twice daily 1 hour before meals **OR**
- (prophylaxis – SBE) 2 g orally 30 minutes before procedure, then 500 mg orally 1 hour before meals 6-hourly for 8 doses

Adverse effects/Interactions

- see General Adverse effects and Interactions of penicillins (p. 151)

Nursing points/Cautions/Patient teaching and advice

- (streptococcal infection) therapy should be continued for at least 10 days
- (suspension) contains hydroxybenzoates which may cause hypersensitivity reaction in sensitive individual
- not recommended for severe pneumonia, empyema, bacteraemia, pericarditis or arthritis during acute phase of illness
- see also General Nursing points/Caution and Patient teaching and advice for penicillins (p. 152)

syrup/suspension is available. Tablet can be crushed or capsule opened and mixed with water or spoonful of yoghurt or apple puree

PIPERACILLIN SODIUM WITH TAZOBACTAM SODIUM (PiperTaz, Piptaz, Tazocin EF, Tazopip)

Available form
Vial: 4 g piperacillin/0.5 g tazobactam

Action
- piperacillin is broad spectrum
- tazobactam is a beta-lactamase inhibitor
- active against a broad spectrum of both Gram-negative and Gram-positive beta-lactamase and non-beta-lactamase-producing organisms
- half-life 0.7–1.2 hours
- see also General Actions of penicillins (p. 150)

Use
- see General Uses of penicillins (p. 150)

Dose
- 4 g piperacillin/0.5 g tazobactam by slow IV infusion over 20–30 minutes, 6–8-hourly

Adverse effects
- increase in liver enzymes and serum creatinine
- (rare) hypokalaemia (in those with liver disease or receiving diuretic or cytotoxic therapy)
- see also General Adverse effects of penicillins (p. 151)

Interactions
- may prolong neuromuscular blockade of vecuronium, therefore caution if given with neuromuscular blocking agents
- increased risk of hypokalaemia if given in high doses with diuretics or cytotoxic therapy
- increased risk of kidney damage if given with vancomycin
- see also General Interactions of penicillins (p. 151)

Nursing points and Cautions/ Patient teaching and advice
- monitoring of liver and renal function and blood counts is recommended if therapy is longer than 21 days or patient has liver or kidney impairment
- potassium levels should be monitored in those at risk of hypokalaemia
- treatment usually 5 days minimum and continued for 48 hours after fever or symptoms abate (14 days maximum)
- administer alone
- reconstitute with 20 mL water for injections. Can be further diluted with 50 mL of sodium chloride 0.9% or glucose 5%
- not recommended with blood products including albumin
- not recommended with solutions containing lactated Ringer's solution, sodium bicarbonate or having basic pH
- contains 54 mg sodium per g piperacillin and should be used cautiously in those with heart failure or requiring sodium restriction
- increased risk of rash or fever if given to patients with cystic fibrosis
- not recommended for meningitis or brain abscesses because of poor penetration into CSF
- see General Nursing points/Cautions for penicillins (p. 152)

PROCAINE BENZYLPENICILLIN (PROCAINE PENICILLIN) (Cilicaine Syringe)

Available form
Syringe: 1.5 g

Action
- as for benzylpenicillin, but for moderately severe infections
- procaine salt has low solubility, therefore particles dissolve slowly allowing administration 1–2 times daily only

- see also General Actions of penicillins (p. 150)

Use

- see General Uses of penicillins (p. 150)

Dose

- 1.5 g IM daily for 2–5 days **OR**
- (gonorrhoea) 4.8 g as single IM dose with oral probenecid **OR**
- (gonorrhoea) 1 g IM daily for 7–14 days **OR**
- (syphilis) 1 g IM daily for 10–14 days

Adverse effects

- (syphilis) Jarisch–Herxheimer reaction (malaise, fever, chills, sore throat, myalgia, headache, tachycardia)
- extreme anxiety, sensation of impending death (thought to be caused by procaine; self-limiting and generally subsides after 15–30 minutes)
- see also General Adverse effects of penicillins (p. 151)

Interactions

- see also General Interactions of penicillins (p. 151)

Nursing points/Cautions/Patient teaching and advice

- only given IM
- NEVER given IV as neurovascular damage may occur
- may cause permanent neurological damage if given into or near nerves
- slowly absorbed and maintains antibacterial blood levels for up to 24 hours, but concentration achieved is lower than for benzylpenicillin
- not recommended in those with Brugada syndrome (due to procaine content) (potentially life-threatening cardiac rhythm disorder) or known cardiac conduction abnormalities
- contraindicated in those with known hypersensitivity to procaine
- see General Nursing points/Cautions and General Patient teaching and advice for penicillins (p. 153)

TICARCILLIN SODIUM WITH CLAVULANIC ACID (Timentin)

Available form

Vial: 3 g ticarcillin/0.1 g clavulanic acid

Action

- ticarcillin is a broad spectrum penicillin used primarily in Gram-negative infections, but also with Gram-positive and anaerobic bacteria
- clavulanic acid (potassium clavulanate) is a potent inhibitor of beta-lactamase (penicillinase), and is added to some penicillins to enhance their activity against many previously resistant strains
- half-life 68 minutes (ticarcillin) and 64 minutes (clavulanic acid)
- see also General Actions of penicillins (p. 150)

Use

- see General Uses of penicillins (p. 150)

Dose

- 3.1 g by IV infusion over 30 minutes 4–6-hourly (or 8-hourly for urinary tract infections) **OR**
- (patients weighing less than 60 kg) 200–300 mg/kg/day in divided doses 4–6-hourly by IV infusion over 30 minutes **OR**
- (prophylaxis – caesarean section) 3.1 g by IV infusion over 30 minutes when umbilical cord is clamped, followed by 3.1 g 4-hourly from first dose for 2 doses (total 9.3 g in 3 doses) **OR**
- (prophylaxis – abdominal hysterectomy) 3.1 g by IV infusion over 30 minutes 30–60 minutes before first incision, followed by 3.1 g 4-hourly for 2 doses (total 9.3 g in 3 doses) **OR**
- (prophylaxis – elective colorectal surgery) 3.1 g by IV infusion over 30 minutes, 30–60 minutes before first incision, followed by 3.1 g 8-hourly for 2 doses (total 9.3 g in 3 doses) **OR**

- (prophylaxis – elective colorectal surgery) 3.1 g by IV infusion over 30 minutes, 15 minutes before anaesthetic induction, followed by 3.1 g 2 hours later

Adverse effects

- abnormal coagulation (especially in those with renal impairment)
- elevated liver enzymes and serum creatinine, decreased uric acid, hypernatraemia
- (rare) hypokalaemia
- see also General Adverse effects of penicillins (p. 151)

Interactions

- not recommended with probenecid
- may cause false positive Coombs' test and false positive urinary protein (depending on the test)
- see also General Interactions of penicillins (p. 151)

Nursing points/Cautions/Patient teaching and advice

- daily maximum is 18 g (ticarcillin)
- duration of therapy is dependent on severity of infection. Should be continued for at least 2 days after signs and symptoms have disappeared. Usual duration is 10–14 days
- contains 20 mg potassium per vial and therefore serum potassium levels should be monitored during therapy
- reconstitute with 13 mL water for injections or sodium chloride 0.9% and then further dilute for IV administration
- incompatible with sodium bicarbonate
- contains 360 mg sodium per 3 g ticarcillin which may need to be considered if salt restriction exists
- caution if used in those with cardiac disease as cardiac failure may be exacerbated
- not recommended in those with hypersensitivity to clavulanic acid
- see General Nursing points/Cautions and General Patient teaching and advice for penicillins (p. 153)

CEPHALOSPORINS

General Actions of cephalosporins

- selectively interfere with bacterial cell wall synthesis, as with penicillin
- bactericidal
- broad spectrum, often second line of treatment in many infections
- divided into first, second, third and fourth generation
- some of the newer generation of cephalosporins resist the action of beta-lactamase (penicillinase)
- *S. aureus* (MRSA), *C. difficile*, *P. aeruginosa* and *Enterococcus faecalis* are resistant to the cephalosporins

General Uses of cephalosporins

- infections where the organisms are not resistant to cephalosporins, including:
  - upper and lower respiratory tract infections
  - skin and skin structure infections
  - bone and joint infections
  - urinary tract infection (complicated or uncomplicated)
  - intra-abdominal infections, including biliary tract infections
  - gynaecological infections
  - septicaemia, endocarditis

- febrile neutropenia
- meningitis
- gonorrhoea
- ear, nose and throat infections
- surgical prophylaxis

General Adverse effects of cephalosporins

- nausea, vomiting, dyspepsia, bad taste, abdominal pain/cramps, diarrhoea
- rash, urticaria, fever, pruritus
- dizziness, headache, insomnia, somnolence, malaise
- hypoprothrombinaemia
- superinfection (oral and/or vaginal moniliasis)
- granulocytopenia, leucopenia, neutropenia, eosinophilia
- anaphylactic shock, anaphylactoid reaction (rare), serum sickness-like reaction (rash, arthritis/arthralgia, fever), hypersensitivity
- (transient) elevation in liver enzymes and, rarely, hepatitis, cholestatic jaundice
- (high dose) reversible encephalopathy, neurotoxicity, seizures
- (rare) reversible nephritis, elevated serum creatinine and blood urea nitrogen levels, interstitial nephritis
- (rare) haemolytic anaemia, agranulocytosis
- (rare) severe skin reactions
- (rare but often fatal) pseudomembranous colitis (see Glossary)
- (IM) pain, induration, tenderness
- (IV) pain, inflammation, phlebitis, thrombophlebitis

General Interactions of cephalosporins

- cephalosporins may affect stability of warfarin, therefore prothrombin time should be closely monitored especially when starting and stopping therapy
- probenecid increases and prolongs serum levels of most cephalosporins by inhibiting excretion (not ceftriaxone or ceftazidime)
- increased risk of renal damage if used with other potentially nephrotoxic agents such as colistin, gentamicin, tobramycin, etacrynic acid (large doses) and furosemide (frusemide) (large doses) and therefore renal function should be monitored regularly
- absorption decreased by aluminium- and magnesium-containing antacids and therefore administration should be spaced 2 hours apart
- physical/chemical incompatibility with aminoglycosides
- lidocaine (lignocaine) toxicity may occur in those with liver disease if lidocaine (lignocaine) is used repeatedly as diluent to reduce pain of IM injection
- increased risk of GI ulceration and bleeding if given with NSAIDs, salicylates or sulfinpyrazone
- increased risk of hypoprothrombinaemia if given in high doses with high doses of salicylates
- if active against *Salmonella typhi* organisms, may interfere with live typhoid vaccine if given within 24 hours of last dose
- increased risk of pseudomembranous colitis if given with peristalsis-delaying agents such as opioid analgesics or atropine/diphenoxylate combination
- may cause false-positive Coombs' test and false-positive glucose test (urine)
- false high creatinine levels may occur using Jaffe technique, therefore blood samples for creatinine levels should not be drawn within 2 hours of drug administration

General Nursing points/Cautions for cephalosporins

- see General Nursing points/Cautions for antibacterial agents (p. 148)
- penicillin is the usual drug of choice for treatment and prophylaxis of streptococcal infections including rheumatic fever prevention
- serum sickness-like reaction often occurs after second (or subsequent) dose and occurs more frequently in children than in adults
- white blood cell monitoring is recommended if therapy > 7 days
- liver and/or renal function monitoring is recommended if liver or renal insufficiency exists
- all patients with gonorrhoea should also have serological testing for syphilis at time of diagnosis and then 3 months later
- therapy should be continued for 2 days after signs and symptoms have resolved unless treating a group A beta-haemolytic streptococci infection. Therapy should be given for at least 10 days to decrease risk of rheumatic fever or glomerulonephritis
- when reconstituting powders for injection, it is important to note the amount of diluent required for the specific route (e.g. IM cefepime 500 mg requires 1.5 mL of diluent, whereas IV it needs 5 mL of diluent to give the required level)
- reconstituted solution may darken on storage, but efficacy is not affected
- do not mix with other drugs in the same syringe or IV infusion container as a precipitate will form
- if cephalosporins are being administered by a Y-line infusion method, the primary or main infusion is stopped to avoid incompatibility
- incompatible with aminoglycosides and vancomycin as precipitation will occur if given together. Lines should be flushed between administration if given one after the other
- the amount of sodium should be noted as this may be important for those with cardiac disease or if a sodium restriction is required
- caution if used in those with allergic tendencies including asthma
- caution if given to those with a history of GI diseases (especially colitis or enteritis), impaired kidney or liver function or those with impaired or low vitamin K synthesis because of the increased risk of bleeding
- caution if used in those with history of bleeding disorders
- caution if used in those with pre-existing seizure disorders
- contraindicated in those with a history of anaphylaxis to penicillins, penicillin derivatives, penicillamine or cephalosporin-related bleeding disorder
- (with lidocaine (lignocaine)) contraindicated in those with amide-type local anaesthetic hypersensitivity

General Patient teaching and advice for cephalosporins

- instruct patient to seek medical advice immediately if any of the following occurs:
  - signs of frequent infection including fever, sore throat, swollen glands or mouth ulcers
  - unusual bleeding or bruising under skin
  - tiredness, headache, dizziness, paleness, shortness of breath
  - yellowing of skin or eyes
- see General Patient teaching and advice for antibacterial agents (p. 149)

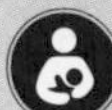

cephalexin and cefalotin are considered to be safe for use during pregnancy. Caution needs to be taken with the remainder of the cephalosporins as they have not been adequately studied in both humans and animals

generally low excretion rate in breastmilk; however, caution should be used with ceftriaxone as it is known to upset the normal GI flora of the newborn infant

CEFACLOR MONOHYDRATE (Aclor, Ceclor, Ceclor CD, Karlor CD, Keflor, Keflor CD)

Available forms

Tablets (sustained-release): 375 mg; Suspension: 125 mg/5 mL, 250 mg/5 mL

Action

- see General Actions of cephalosporins (p. 164)
- *Pseudomonas* spp., *Acinetobacter calcoaceticus*, enterococci, *Enterobacter* spp., indole-positive *Proteus* and *Serratia* spp. are resistant to cefaclor
- second generation cephalosporin
- half-life 40–60 minutes (increased to 2.3–2.8 hours in those with anuria)

Use

- see General Uses of cephalosporins (p. 164)

Dose

- (bronchitis, pneumonia) 250 mg orally 8-hourly (daily maximum 2 g) **OR**
- (severe infection) 500 mg orally 8-hourly (daily maximum 2 g) **OR**
- (skin or skin structure infection) 250 mg orally 8–12-hourly (daily maximum 2 g) **OR**
- 375 mg orally twice daily with food (SR preparation) **OR**
- (pneumonia, acute bacterial sinusitis) 750 mg orally twice daily with food (SR preparation) **OR**
- (lower urinary tract infection) 500 mg orally daily with food (SR preparation)

Adverse effects/Interactions

- see General Adverse effects and Interactions for cephalosporins (p. 165)

Nursing points/Cautions

- therapy should be continued for 10 days for acute bacterial sinusitis
- daily dose of 2 g should not be exceeded
- see also General Nursing points/Cautions for cephalosporins (p. 166)

Patient teaching and advice

- advise patient that tablets (sustained-release) should be swallowed whole and not chewed or crushed and taken with food to improve absorption
- if taking suspension, instruct patient to shake bottle well before use and discard 14 days after opening
- see also General Patient teaching and advice for cephalosporins (p. 166)

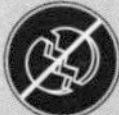

syrup/suspension is available. Tablet should not be crushed

CEFALEXIN MONOHYDRATE (Cephalex, Cephalexin, Ialex, Ibilex, Keflex)

Available forms

Capsules: 250 mg, 500 mg; Suspension: 125 mg/5 mL, 250 mg/5 mL

Action

- see General Actions of cephalosporins (p. 164)
- not active against most strains of enterococci, some strains of staphylococci, most strains of *Enterobacter* spp., *Morganella morganii*, *Proteus vulgaris*, *Pseudomonas* spp., *Acinetobacter calcoaceticus*
- first generation cephalosporin

Use

- see General Uses of cephalosporins (p. 164)

Dose

- 1–4 g orally in divided doses **OR**
- (streptococcal pharyngitis, tonsillitis, urinary tract infection, skin or skin structure infection) 500 mg orally twice daily

Adverse effects

- see General Adverse effects of cephalosporins (p. 165)

Interactions

- may decrease clearance of metformin
- see also General Interactions of cephalosporins (p. 165)

Nursing points/Cautions

- if daily dose is greater than 4 g, parenteral cephalosporin therapy should be considered
- twice daily dosing is not recommended when doses are greater than 1 g daily
- not recommended for bacterial infections of brain or spinal column
- see also General Nursing points/Cautions for cephalosporins (p. 166)

Patient teaching and advice

- (suspension) advise patient to shake suspension well before use, refrigerate solution and discard 14 days after opening
- see General Patient teaching and advice for cephalosporins (p. 166)

syrup/suspension is available. Capsule can be opened and contents mixed with water or spoonful of yoghurt or apple puree. Patient should be warned of bitter taste

CEFALOTIN (CEPHALOTHIN) SODIUM (DBL Cephalothin Sodium for Injection)

Available form

Vial: 1 g

Action

- see General Actions of cephalosporins (p. 164)
- not active against most strains of enterococci, *Pseudomonas* spp., indole-producing *Proteus* spp., methicillin-resistant staphylococci and motile *Enterobacter* spp.
- first generation
- half-life 30–50 minutes

Use

- see General Uses of cephalosporins (p. 164)

Dose

- (uncomplicated infection (pneumonia, furunculosis, urinary tract infection)) 500 mg IM, IV bolus over 3–5 minutes or IV infusion 6-hourly **OR**
- (severe infection) 1–2 g by IV bolus over 3–5 minutes or IV infusion 4-hourly **OR**
- (prophylaxis – surgery) 2 g by IV bolus over 3–5 minutes or IV infusion 30–60 minutes before surgery, 2 g during surgery and 2 g 6-hourly for 24 hours

Adverse effects

- see General Adverse effects of cephalosporins (p. 165)

Interactions

- efficacy of methotrexate may be reduced if given with cefalotin and hydrocortisone together
- may interfere with theophylline estimation
- may cause false positive on urinary steroid estimation (using Zimmerman colour reaction) or urine protein test
- see General Interactions of cephalosporins (p. 165)

Nursing points/Cautions

- (prophylaxis) continued for 72 hours after heart valve replacement and arthroplasty
- IV is the preferred route in severe or life-threatening infections (e.g.

septicaemia) or if co-morbidities such as diabetes, heart failure, malignancy, shock or malnourishment exist
- IM injection is very painful
- (IM) reconstitute with 4 mL water for injections per g of cefalotin
- increased risk of thrombophlebitis if greater than 6 g per day is given for more than 3 days. This can be lessened by adding 10–25 mg hydrocortisone to IV solution; use of large veins is recommended
- solution may precipitate if refrigerated. Precipitate can be re-dissolved by warming to room temperature with constant agitation
- concentrated solution may darken at room temperature
- contains 63 mg sodium per g cephalothin
- not recommended for the treatment of meningitis or GI disorders where anaerobic organisms prevail
- see also General Nursing points/ Cautions for cephalosporins (p. 166)

Patient teaching and advice

- see General Patient teaching and advice for cephalosporins (p. 166)

CEFAZOLIN (CEPHAZOLIN) SODIUM (Kefzol)

Available forms

Vial: 500 mg, 1 g, 2 g

Action

- see General Actions of cephalosporins (p. 164)
- not active against many strains of enterococci, *Enterobacter cloacae*, indole-producing *Proteus* spp., *Serratia* spp., *Pseudomonas* spp., methicillin-resistant staphylococci and *Acinetobacter calcoaceticus*

Use

- see General Uses of cephalosporins (p. 164)

Dose

- (mild infections) 250–500 mg IM or by IV bolus over 3–5 minutes or IV infusion 12-hourly **OR**
- (moderate-to-severe infections) 0.5–1 g IM or by IV bolus over 3–5 minutes or IV infusion 6- to 8-hourly **OR**
- (serious infection (e.g. endocarditis) 6 g IM or by IV bolus over 3–5 minutes or IV infusion daily in divided doses

Adverse effects/Interactions

- see General Adverse effects and Interactions for cephalosporins (p. 165)

Nursing points and Cautions/ Patient teaching and advice

- must not be given intrathecally, as convulsions may occur
- (IM) reconstitute using sodium chloride 0.9%, glucose 5% or
- not recommended via intraventricular route
- contains 43.3 mg sodium per 1 g cefazolin sodium
- see also General Nursing points/ Cautions and Patient teaching and advice for cephalosporins (p. 166)

CEFEPIME HYDROCHLORIDE (Cefepime Powder for Injection)

Available forms

Vial: 1 g, 2 g

Action

- see General Actions of cephalosporins (p. 164)
- not active against *C. difficile*, *Stenotrophomonas*, most strains of enterococci and some strains of *Enterobacter*
- fourth generation cephalosporin

Use

- see General Uses of cephalosporins (p. 164)

Dose

- (mild-to-moderate urinary tract infection) 0.5–1 g IM or by IV bolus over

3–5 minutes or IV infusion over 30 minutes 12-hourly **OR**
- (mild-to-moderate infections) 1 g IM or by IV bolus over 3–5 minutes or IV infusion over 30 minutes 12-hourly **OR**
- (severe infections) 2 g by IV bolus over 3–5 minutes or IV infusion over 30 minutes 12-hourly **OR**
- (very severe or life-threatening infections) 2 g by IV bolus over 3–5 minutes or IV infusion over 30 minutes 8-hourly **OR**
- (prophylaxis – surgery) 2 g stat by IV infusion over 30 minutes, given 60 minutes before first surgical incision (with metronidazole 500 mg IV when cefepime infusion is finished). If surgical procedure lasts for longer than 12 hours, a second dose of cefepime and metronidazole should be given 12 hours after the initial dose

Adverse effects/Interactions
- see General Adverse effects and Interactions for cephalosporins (p. 165)

Nursing points/Cautions/Patient teaching and advice
- reconstitute carefully according to manufacturer's instructions as the amount of diluent required varies with the size of the vial and the administration route
- when given for surgical prophylaxis with metronidazole, ensure line is flushed in between cefepime and metronidazole to prevent precipitation occurring
- not compatible with gentamicin, metronidazole, vancomycin or tobramycin
- contraindicated in those with hypersensitivity to l-arginine
- see also General Nursing points/Cautions and Patient teaching and advice for cephalosporins (p. 166)

CEFOTAXIME SODIUM (Cefotaxime Powder for Injection)

Available forms
Vial: 500 mg, 1 g, 2 g

Action
- see General Actions of cephalosporins (p. 164)
- not active against methicillin-resistant staphylococci, *Clostridium perfringens*, *Enterococcus faecalis* and *Enterobacter cloacae*
- third generation cephalosporin

Use
- see General Uses of cephalosporins (p. 164)

Dose
- (urinary tract infection) 1 g IM or IV bolus over 3–5 minutes or IV infusion over 30 minutes 12-hourly **OR**
- (other infections) 1 g IM or IV bolus over 3–5 minutes or IV infusion over 30 minutes 12-hourly, increasing to 3, 4 or 6 g daily if necessary **OR**
- (gonorrhoea – non-beta-lactamase-producing organism) 1 g as a single IM dose **OR**
- (gonorrhoea – beta-lactamase-producing organism) 0.5 g as single IM dose plus probenecid, 1 g orally, taken 1 hour earlier **OR**
- (prophylaxis – biliary surgery) 1 g as IV bolus over 3–5 minutes or IV infusion over 30 minutes at induction **OR**
- (prophylaxis – caesarean section) 1 g IV bolus over 3–5 minutes or IV infusion over 30 minutes after umbilical cord is clamped, followed by 1 g at 6 and 12 hours from first dose (total 3 doses) **OR**
- (prophylaxis – vaginal or abdominal hysterectomy) 1 g IM 30–60 minutes before incision, 1 g on completion of surgery, then 1 g 8-hourly for a total of 24 hours

Adverse effects
- (rare, rapid IV via CVC line) arrhythmias
- Jarisch–Herxheimer reaction (malaise, fever, chills, sore throat, myalgia, headache, tachycardia)
- see also General Adverse effects of cephalosporins (p. 165)

Interactions
- may decrease effectiveness of oral contraceptives
- not recommended with tetracycline, erythromycin or chloramphenicol
- see also General Interactions of cephalosporins (p. 165)

Nursing points/Cautions
- if patient is treated for more than 7 days, WBC count monitoring is recommended
- incompatible with sodium bicarbonate and aminoglycosides
- 0.5% lidocaine (lignocaine) (without adrenaline (epinephrine)) may be added to reduce pain at IM site
- not more than 4 mL given into single IM injection site
- if daily dose > 2 g or if frequency is more than twice daily, IV route is preferred
- contains 48.2 mg sodium per 1 g cefotaxime
- contraindicated in those with severe heart failure or non-paced heart block or infants less than 30 months
- see also General Nursing points/Cautions for cephalosporins (p. 166)

Patient teaching and advice
- warn female patients of childbearing potential that they require an alternative birth contraceptive during therapy as effectiveness of oral contraceptive may be reduced leading to pregnancy
- see also General Patient teaching and advice for cephalosporins (p. 166)

CEFOXITIN SODIUM (Cefoxitin Powder for Injection)

Available form
Vial: 1 g

Action
- see General Actions of cephalosporins (p. 164)
- not active against *Pseudomonas* spp., most strains of enterococci, methicillin-resistant staphylococci and many strains of *Enterobacter cloacae*
- second generation cephalosporin

Use
- see General Uses of cephalosporins (p. 164)

Dose
- (uncomplicated infection) 1 g IM or by IV bolus over 3–5 minutes or IV infusion 6 to 8-hourly **OR**
- (moderate to severe infection) 2 g IM or by IV bolus over 3–5 minutes or IV infusion 6–8-hourly **OR**
- (severe infections) 2–3 g IM or by IV bolus over 3–5 mins or IV infusion 4–6-hourly (daily maximum 12 g) **OR**
- (gonorrhoea) 2 g as a single IM dose plus probenecid, 1 g orally, taken immediately or 1 hour earlier **OR**
- (prophylaxis – surgery) 2 g IM 1 hour before surgery or by IV bolus over 3–5 minutes or IV infusion just before surgery, then 2 g IM or IV at 6 and 12 hours after first dose **OR**
- (prophylaxis – caesarean section) 2 g after umbilical cord is clamped, then 2 g IM or by IV bolus over 3–5 minutes or IV infusion at 4 and 8 hours after first dose

Adverse effects
- see General Adverse effects of cephalosporins (p. 165)

Interactions
- may interfere with measurement of urine corticosteroids

- see also General Interactions of cephalosporins (p. 165)

Nursing points/Cautions/Patient teaching and advice

- contains 51.2 mg sodium per 1 g cefoxitin
- 0.5% or 1% lidocaine (lignocaine) without adrenaline (epinephrine) may be added to reduce pain at IM site
- reconstitute carefully according to manufacturer's instructions as the amount of diluent required varies with the size of the vial and the administration route
- not recommended for treatment of meningitis or brain abscesses
- see also general Nursing points/ Cautions and Patient teaching and advice for cephalosporins (p. 166)

CEFTAROLINE FOSAMIL (Zinforo)

Available form
Vial: 600 mg

Action
- see General Actions of cephalosporins (p. 164)
- ceftaroline fosamil is a prodrug converted to active ceftaroline
- active against Gram-positive and Gram-negative bacteria including methicillin resistant *S. aureus* (MRSA) and penicillin non-susceptible *S. pneumoniae*
- half-life 2.5 hours

Use
- see General Uses of cephalosporins (p. 164)

Dose
- 600 mg by IV infusion over 60 minutes twice daily

Adverse effects
- see General Adverse effects for cephalosporins (p. 165)

Nursing points/Cautions/Patient teaching and advice

- (complicated skin and soft tissue infection) duration 5–14 days
- (community-acquired pneumonia) duration 5–7 days
- reconstitute using 20 mL water for injections and then dilute further for IV infusion
- caution if used in those with epilepsy or moderate to severe kidney impairment
- contraindicated in those with hypersensitivity to l-arginine
- see also General Nursing points/ Cautions and Patient teaching and advice for cephalosporins (p. 166)

CEFTAZIDIME (Ceftazidime Powder for Injection, Fortum)

Available forms
Vial: 1 g, 2 g

Action
- see General Actions of cephalosporins (p. 164)
- not active against *S. faecalis*, many other enterococci, methicillin-resistant staphylococci, *Listeria monocytogenes*, *Campylobacter* spp. or *C. difficile*
- third generation cephalosporin with antipseudomonal activity

Use
- see General Uses of cephalosporins (p. 164)

Dose
- (urinary tract or less serious infections) 0.5–1 g IM, by IV bolus over 3–5 minutes or IV infusion over 30 minutes 12-hourly **OR**
- (other infections) 1–2 g IM, by IV bolus over 3–5 minutes or IV infusion over 30 minutes 8–12-hourly **OR**
- (serious infections) 2 g by IV bolus over 3–5 minutes or IV infusion over 30 minutes 8–12-hourly

Adverse effects

- see General Adverse effects of cephalosporins (p. 165)

Interactions

- not recommended with chloramphenicol
- see also General Interactions of cephalosporins (p. 165)

Nursing points/Cautions/Patient teaching and advice

- doses greater than 1 g should be given IV
- vials supplied are under reduced pressure and, as the product dissolves, carbon dioxide is released, causing effervescence and a positive pressure develops
- amount of diluent required depends on dose and route of administration (e.g. 1 g IM requires 3 mL whereas 2 g IV requires 10 mL). Manufacturer's instructions should be consulted
- colour of solution may vary from pale yellow to amber
- to preserve sterility a gas relief needle should not be inserted until product has completely dissolved
- 0.5% lidocaine (lignocaine) (without adrenaline (epinephrine)) may be added to reduce pain at the IM site, but stable for only half the time compared with addition of water for injections
- solution contains 52 mg sodium per 1 g ceftazidime
- not recommended to treat CNS infections such as meningitis or brain abscess
- see General Nursing points/Cautions and Patient teaching and advice for cephalosporins (p. 166)

CEFTAZIDIME WITH AVIBACTAM (Zavicefta)

Available form

Vial: 2 g ceftazidime/0.5 g avibactam

Action

- cephalosporin with avibactam (beta-lactamase inhibitor)
- ceftazidime has little or no activity against most Gram-positive organisms or anaerobes
- avibactam does not inhibit class B enzymes (metallo-beta-lactamases) or class D enzymes
- half-life of both ceftazidime and avibactam is about 2 hours
- see General Actions of cephalosporins (p. 164)

Use

- complicated intra-abdominal infection (with metronidazole)
- complicated urinary tract infection, including pyelonephritis
- hospital-acquired pneumonia including ventilator-associated pneumonia

Dose

- (complicated intra-abdominal infection) 2 g ceftazidime/0.5 g avibactam by IV infusion over 2 hours 8-hourly for 5–14 days (with metronidazole) **OR**
- (complicated urinary tract infection, pyelonephritis) 2 g ceftazidime/0.5 g avibactam by IV infusion over 2 hours 8-hourly for 5–10 days **OR**
- (hospital-acquired pneumonia) 2 g ceftazidime/0.5 g avibactam by IV infusion over 2 hours 8-hourly for 7–14 days

Adverse effects

- hypokalaemia
- tachycardia, hypotension, hypertension
- pleural effusion, dyspnoea, cough
- peripheral oedema
- see also General Adverse effects for cephalosporins (p. 165)

Interactions

- caution if given with other nephrotoxic agents or potent diuretics due to risk of nephrotoxicity
- not recommended with probenecid

- not recommended with chloramphenicol
- may cause false-positive Coombs' test

Nursing points/Cautions

- (complicated urinary tract infection, pyelonephritis) if patient has bacteraemia, therapy can be extended to 14 days
- reconstitute powder using 10 mL water for injections, shake vial to dissolve powder then further dilute for IV infusion
- to preserve product sterility, gas relief needle should not be inserted before product is dissolved
- vial contains 148 mg sodium
- reconstituted solution is clear and colourless to yellow solution
- contraindicated in those with hypersensitivity to cephalosporins, other beta-lactam antibacterial agents or avibactam
- see also General Nursing points/Cautions for cephalosporins (p. 166)

Patient teaching and advice

- see General Patient teaching and advice for cephalosporins (p. 166)

CEFTOLOZANE WITH TAZOBACTAM (Zerbaxa)

Available forms

Vial: 1 g ceftolozane/0.5 g tazobactam

Action

- cephalosporin with tazobactam (beta-lactamase inhibitor)
- see General Actions of cephalosporins (p. 164)
- half-life of ceftolozane 3 hours, tazobactam 1 hour

Use

- see General Uses of cephalosporins (p. 164)

Dose

- (complicated intra-abdominal infection) 1 g ceftolozane/0.5 g tazobactam by IV infusion over 60 minutes 8-hourly for 4–14 days (with metronidazole 500 mg IV 8-hourly) **OR**
- (complicated urinary tract infections including pyelonephritis) 1 g ceftolozane/0.5 g tazobactam by IV infusion over 60 minutes 8-hourly for 7 days

Adverse effects

- hypokalaemia
- atrial fibrillation, hypotensions
- see also General Adverse effects of cephalosporins (p. 165)

Interactions

- increased serum levels may occur if given with probenecid, diclofenac or cimetidine

Nursing points/Cautions/Patient teaching and advice

- reconstitute using 10 mL water for injections or sodium chloride 0.9%, shaking gently to dissolve
- reconstituted solution is clear to slightly yellow
- for IV infusion, reconstituted solution should be added to 100 mL sodium chloride 0.9% or glucose 5% and infused over 60 minutes
- administer alone
- caution if used in those who are severely immunocompromised, receiving immunosuppressive therapy or with severe neutropenia
- contraindicated in those with hypersensitivity to tazobactam or piperacillin/tazobactam
- see also General Nursing points/Cautions/Patient teaching and advice for cephalosporins (p. 166)

CEFTRIAXONE SODIUM (Ceftriaxone Powder for Injection)

Available forms

Vial: 500 mg, 1 g, 2 g

Action
- see General Actions of cephalosporins (p. 164)
- active against some species of *Pseudomonas aeruginosa* but other *Pseudomonas* spp. are resistant. Most species of group D Streptococci, including *S. faecalis* and *S. faecium*, are resistant
- third generation cephalosporin
- half-life 5.8–8.7 hours

Use
- see General Uses of cephalosporins (p. 164)

Dose
- 1–2 g IM or by IV bolus over 2–4 minutes or by IV infusion over 30 minutes daily or in equally divided doses 12-hourly **OR**
- (uncomplicated gonorrhoea) 250 mg as single IM dose **OR**
- (prophylaxis – surgery) 1 g IM or IV 0.5–2 hours before surgery

Adverse effects
- (rare) pancreatitis, precipitations in gallbladder (not gall stones)
- (rare, neonates) lung and kidney precipitates (if given with calcium containing solutions)
- see General Adverse effects of cephalosporins (p. 165)

Interactions
- probenecid does not alter elimination of ceftriaxone
- (neonates) not recommended with or within 48 hours of calcium-containing solutions

Nursing points/Cautions/Patient teaching and advice
- contains 83 mg sodium per g
- incompatible with vancomycin, fluconazole, aminoglycosides, amsacrine or calcium-containing fluids (e.g. Hartmann's solution, Ringer's solution)
- 1% lidocaine (lignocaine) (without adrenaline (epinephrine)) may be added to reduce pain at IM site
- no more than 1 g injected IM into one site
- reconstituted solutions have a harmless yellowish tinge and may have a slight cloudiness
- caution if used in those with risk factors for biliary stasis or biliary sludge as this increases the risk of pancreatitis
- see General Nursing points/Cautions and General Patient teaching and advice for cephalosporins (p. 166)

CEFUROXIME AXETIL (Zinnat, Zinnat Suspension)

Available forms

Tablets: 250 mg; Suspension: 125 mg/5 mL

Action
- see General Actions of cephalosporins (p. 164)
- prodrug which is hydrolysed to active cefuroxime
- not active against *C. difficile*, *Pseudomonas* spp., *Campylobacter* spp., *Acinetobacter calcoaceticus*, *Proteus vulgaris*, *Morganella morganii*, *Serratia* spp., *Listeria monocytogenes*, *Bacteroides fragilis*, *Enterococcus faecalis*, *Enterobacter* spp., methicillin-resistant staphylococci or *Citrobacter* spp.
- second generation cephalosporin

Use
- see General Uses of cephalosporins (p. 164)

Dose
- (acute or chronic bronchitis) 250–500 mg twice daily after a light meal (for 5–7 days) **OR**
- (uncomplicated gonorrhoea) 1 g as single oral dose after a light meal **OR**
- (other infections) 250 mg twice daily after a light meal (for 7–10 days)

Adverse effects
- see General Adverse effects of cephalosporins (p. 165)

Interactions

- bioavailability may be decreased if given with ranitidine
- may decrease efficacy of oral contraceptives containing oestrogen
- see General Interactions of cephalosporins (p. 165)

Nursing points/Cautions

- tablets and suspension are not bioequivalent and should not be substituted
- suspension is recommended for paediatric use
- daily dose should not exceed 500 mg in those with kidney impairment
- (suspension) contains aspartame and is therefore not recommended in those with phenylketonuria
- (suspension) contains 3 g sucrose per dose (125 mg/5 mL) which may need to be considered if patient has diabetes mellitus
- see General Nursing points/Cautions for cephalosporins (p. 166)

Patient teaching and advice

- (suspension) advise parent/carer to shake bottle well before administering dose to child
- (suspension) instruct parent/carer to store bottle in fridge and discard 10 days after opening
- warn female patients using oestrogen-containing contraceptives that efficacy may be affected during therapy and an extra form of contraception should be used to prevent pregnancy occurring
- see General Patient teaching and advice for cephalosporins (p. 166)

syrup/suspension is available. Tablet can be dispersed in 40–60 mL orange, grape or apple juice or chocolate milk, or tablet can be crushed and mixed with water or spoonful of yoghurt, apple puree or icecream

MONOBACTAMS AND CARBAPENEMS

General Uses of monobactams and carbapenems

- moderate-to-serious infections of the lower respiratory tract, intra-abdominal infections, gynaecological infection, bacterial septicaemia, endocarditis, skin, bone and joint infections, including multi-bacterial infections
- diabetic foot infections (in those unable to tolerate other antibiotics or with resistant organisms)
- Gram-negative infections (e.g. gonorrhoea, urinary tract)
- meningitis (*Haemophilus influenzae*, *Neisseria meningitidis*) with other antibacterial agents
- *Pseudomonas* spp. infections (with aminoglycosides)

General Adverse effects of monobactams and carbapenems

- nausea, vomiting, altered taste, diarrhoea, abdominal pain/cramps, mouth ulcers
- increase in liver enzymes
- rash, urticaria, pruritus, fever, flushing, sweating
- headache, dizziness
- encephalopathy (confusion, impaired consciousness, seizures, movement disorders)
- superinfection

- pseudomembranous colitis
- hypersensitivity, anaphylaxis, anaphylactoid reaction
- haematological disorders (eosinophilia, neutropenia, thrombocytopenia), positive direct or indirect Coombs' test
- (rare) convulsions, severe skin reactions, jaundice, liver failure
- (IV site) phlebitis, thrombophlebitis, pain/discomfort, erythema, induration
- (IM) pain

General Interactions for monobactams and carbapenems

- increased serum levels may occur if given with probenecid
- increased risk of pseudomembranous colitis if given with peristalsis-delaying agents, such as opioid analgesics or diphenoxylate/atropine combination

General Nursing points/Cautions for monobactams and carbapenems

- see General Nursing points/Cautions for antibacterial agents (p. 148)
- cross-sensitivity can exist between penicillins, cephalosporins, imipenem, aztreonam and meropenem, so patients sensitive to one of these agents may also be sensitive to the others
- renal, liver and haematological function should be monitored regularly with prolonged therapy
- administer alone, ensuring IV line is adequately flushed before and after administration
- amount of diluent required for reconstitution is dependent on route of administration (IM or IV), therefore manufacturer's instructions should be consulted before reconstitution
- adrenaline (epinephrine), IV corticosteroids, oxygen and resuscitation equipment should be available in the event of anaphylaxis
- caution if used in those with kidney impairment
- caution if used in those with liver impairment. If used, liver function should be closely monitored during therapy
- contraindicated in those with hypersensitivity to monobactams or carbapenems or beta-lactams

General Patient teaching and advice for monobactams and carbapenems

- warn patient against driving or operating heavy machinery if dizziness, somnolence or seizures occur
- see General Patient teaching and advice for antibacterial agents (p. 149)

AZTREONAM (Azactam)

Available form

Vial: 1 g

Action

- synthetic monocyclic beta-lactam (monobactam) that binds to penicillin-binding proteins resulting in bacterial cell wall synthesis inhibition
- bactericidal against most aerobic Gram-negative bacteria
- resists the action of beta-lactamase (penicillinase, cephalosporinase)
- not well absorbed orally
- half-life 1.4–2.2 hours (normal renal function)

Use

- reserved for Gram-negative infections where other antibacterial agents are inappropriate or contraindicated

Dose

- (moderately severe infections) 1–2 g 8–12-hourly IM, by slow IV injection over 3–5 minutes or IV infusion over 30 minutes (daily maximum 8 g) **OR**

- (severe infections) 2 g 6–8-hourly by slow IV injection over 3–5 minutes or IV infusion over 30 minutes (daily maximum 8 g) **OR**
- (urinary tract infection) 0.5–1 g 8–12-hourly IM, by slow IV injection over 3–5 minutes or IV infusion over 30 minutes (daily maximum 8 g) **OR**
- (uncomplicated gonorrhoea, acute cystitis) 1 g as a single deep IM dose

Adverse effects

- see General Adverse effects of monobactams and carbapenems (p. 176)

Interactions

- increased serum levels may occur if given with furosemide (frusemide)
- see also General Interactions of monobactams and carbapenems (p. 177)

Nursing points/Cautions

- not used as monotherapy for management of meningitis
- (meningitis) therapy should be continued for 7–10 days (*N. meningitidis*) and 10–14 days (*H. influenzae*)
- IV route is recommended for single doses over 1 g or in those with septicaemia, intra-abdominal abscess, peritonitis or severe systemic/life-threatening infections
- (IV infusion) reconstitute the powder with water for injections or sodium chloride 0.9% and shake contents immediately and vigorously then dilute further for IV infusion with at least 50 mL compatible fluid per gram aztreonam
- (IV bolus) reconstitute with 6–10 mL water for injections
- (IM) reconstitute with at least 3 mL water for injections per gram of aztreonam
- colour of reconstituted IV solution may vary from colourless to pale yellow with a slight pink tint on standing
- IM injection is usually well tolerated and local anaesthetic is not required
- not recommended for gynaecological infections or other sites where aerobic Gram-negative organisms are not common
- see General Nursing points/Cautions for monobactams and carbapenems (p. 177)

Patient teaching and advice

- see General Patient teaching and advice for monobactams and carbapenems (p. 177)

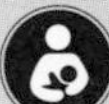

crosses placenta and enters fetal circulation, therefore should only be used during pregnancy if clearly needed

not recommended during breastfeeding

ERTAPENEM SODIUM (Invanz)

Available form

Vial: 1 g

Action

- carbapenem which inhibits bacterial wall synthesis
- wide activity against Gram-positive and Gram-negative aerobic and some anaerobic organisms
- carbapenems are related to beta-lactam antibiotics (penicillins, cephalosporins), but are structurally different
- half-life about 4 hours

Use

- see General Uses of monobactams and carbapenems (p. 176)

Dose

- (moderate to severe infections, diabetic foot infections) 1 g daily IM or by IV infusion over 30 minutes for 3–14 days

Adverse effects

- see General Adverse effects of monobactams and carbapenems (p. 176)

Interactions
- may decrease serum levels of valproic acid (sodium valproate) reducing seizure control, therefore levels should be monitored throughout therapy
- see also General Interactions of monobactams and carbapenems (p. 177)

Nursing points/Cautions/Patient teaching and advice
- not recommended with glucose-containing diluents
- reconstitute using 10 mL water for injections or sodium chloride 0.9%, then dilute to 50 mL using sodium chloride 0.9% for IV infusion
- for IM use, may be diluted using 3.2 mL lidocaine (lignocaine) (without adrenaline (epinephrine)) to reduce pain
- caution if used in those with CNS disorders (e.g. brain abscess, epilepsy, history of seizures) and/or liver impairment due to increased risk of seizures
- not recommended for meningitis or other CNS infections in children due to increased risk of seizures
- contraindicated in those with hypersensitivity to lidocaine (lignocaine) or amide-type local anaesthetics or with severe shock or heart block (if diluted using lidocaine (lignocaine))
- see General Nursing points/Cautions and Patient teaching and advice for monobactams and carbapenems (p. 177)

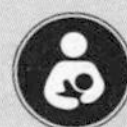

not recommended during pregnancy or breastfeeding unless benefits outweigh risks

IMIPENEM (with cilastatin sodium) (Primaxin)

Available forms
Vial: imipenem 500 mg/cilastatin 500 mg

Action
- imipenem is a carbapenem resistant to beta-lactamases, but is inactivated by a renal dihydropeptidase, therefore it is formulated in combination with cilastatin sodium, the specific inhibitor of the renal enzyme
- bactericidal against most aerobic and anaerobic Gram-negative and Gram-positive microorganisms
- carbapenems are related to beta-lactam antibiotics (penicillins, cephalosporins), but are structurally different

Use
- see General Uses of monobactams and carbapenems (p. 176)

Dose
- 0.5–1 g 6–8-hourly by IV infusion over 20–60 minutes (daily maximum 4 g or 50 mg/kg)

Adverse effects
- hypotension, somnolence
- (uncommon/rare) tremor, confusion, vertigo
- see General Adverse effects of monobactams and carbapenems (p. 176)

Interactions
- increased risk of seizures if given with ganciclovir, therefore these agents are not recommended together
- may decrease serum levels of valproic acid (sodium valproate), reducing seizure control, therefore levels should be monitored throughout therapy
- see also General Interactions of monobactams and carbapenems (p. 177)

Nursing points/Cautions/Patient teaching and advice
- dosages greater than 2 g per day are associated with increased risk of CNS-adverse effects (especially in those with renal impairment)
- for doses of 250–500 mg, infusion should be over 20–30 minutes, for 1 g dose, infusion over 40–60 minutes is recommended

- if patient develops nausea, slow the rate of IV infusion
- do not mix with other drugs in the same syringe or IV container
- reconstitute with 10 mL water for injections and dilute to 100 mL with compatible infusion fluid, mixing solution well until clear, then infuse over 30 minutes via burette (1 g infused over 40–60 minutes; 500 mg infused over 20–30 minutes)
- harmless pale yellow colour may occur
- contains 37.5 mg sodium per 500 mg imipenem, which may need to be considered if patient is on a salt restriction diet
- incompatible with lactate
- not recommended for meningitis because of increased risk of seizures
- see General Nursing points/Cautions and Patient teaching and advice for monobactams and carbapenems (p. 177)

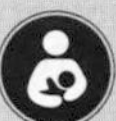

only used during pregnancy if benefits outweigh risks

not recommended during breastfeeding

MEROPENEM TRIHYDRATE (Meropenem Powder for Injection, Merrem)

Available forms
Vial: 500 mg, 1 g

Action
- carbapenem active against Gram-positive aerobes, Gram-negative aerobes and some anaerobic bacteria
- *Enterococcus faecium*, *Stenotrophomonas maltophilia* and methicillin-resistant *Staphylococcus aureus* (MRSA) are resistant to meropenem
- carbapenems are related to beta-lactam antibiotics (penicillins, cephalosporins), but are structurally different
- half-life about 1 hour

Use
- see General Uses of monobactams and carbapenems (p. 176)

Dose
- 0.5–1 g by IV bolus over 5 minutes or IV infusion over 15–30 minutes 8-hourly **OR**
- (febrile neutropenia) 1 g by IV bolus over 5 minutes or IV infusion over 15–30 minutes 8-hourly **OR**
- (meningitis) 2 g by IV bolus over 5 minutes or IV infusion over 15–30 minutes 8-hourly

Adverse effects
- see General Adverse effects of monobactams and carbapenems (p. 176)

Interactions
- may decrease serum sodium valproate levels, reducing seizure control, therefore serum levels should be monitored
- see also General Interactions of monobactams and carbapenems (p. 177)

Nursing points/Cautions/Patient teaching and advice
- administer alone
- reconstitute using water for injections (10 mL/500 mg meropenem) and then further dilute to 50–200 mL for IV infusion
- reconstituted solution may be clear to pale yellow
- see General Nursing points/Cautions and Patient teaching and advice for monobactams and carbapenems (p. 177)

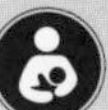

only used during pregnancy or breastfeeding if benefits outweigh risks

GLYCOPEPTIDES

General Actions of glycopeptides

- inhibit bacterial wall synthesis, but at a different site to beta-lactam antibacterials
- may be bactericidal or bacteriostatic depending on the organism
- primarily active against Gram-positive organisms
- growing resistance

General Adverse effects of glycopeptides

- nausea, vomiting, diarrhoea
- hearing loss, tinnitus, vertigo, vestibular disorders
- dizziness, headache
- eosinophilia, leucopenia, neutropenia, thrombocytopenia and rarely, agranulocytosis
- increase in liver enzymes
- increased creatinine and urea, kidney failure
- (IV site) redness, pain, phlebitis, abscess formation, thrombophlebitis
- (rapid IV infusion) 'red neck' or 'red man' syndrome (chills, fever, tachycardia, pruritus, and flushing to face, neck, upper body, back and arms)
- superinfection, pseudomembranous colitis
- (rare) hypersensitivity reactions, anaphylactoid reaction (hypotension, palpitations, substernal pressure, tachycardia), severe cutaneous reactions
- (rare) ototoxicity

General Nursing points/Cautions for glycopeptides

- see also General Nursing points/Cautions for antibacterial agents (p. 148)
- serial audiograms are recommended with prolonged therapy (especially in those over 60 years, if renal impairment is present or if given with other ototoxic agents such as aminoglycosides)
- blood tests, renal and liver function studies should be carried out regularly during prolonged therapy or in patients with renal insufficiency
- slowing or stopping infusion may stop 'red man' syndrome; it usually resolves within 20 minutes but may last several hours
- patient should be closely monitored for any signs of rash with blisters or oral lesions and therapy stopped if they occur
- contraindicated in those with glycopeptide hypersensitivity, deafness, hearing loss or kidney disease

General Patient teaching and advice for glycopeptides

- see also General Patient teaching and advice for antibacterial agents (p. 149)
- patients should be advised to immediately seek medical advice if any of the following occur:
  - ringing in the ears or changes to hearing
  - blistering or peeling of skin
- warn patient to avoid driving or operating machinery if dizziness or vertigo occurs

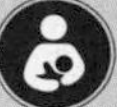

not recommended during pregnancy or breastfeeding unless the benefits outweigh the risks

TEICOPLANIN (Targocid, Teicoplanin Sandoz)

Available form
Vial: 400 mg

Action
- see General Actions of glycopeptides (p. 181)
- very long elimination half-life (70–100 hours)
- cross-sensitivity is possible between vancomycin and teicoplanin
- no cross-resistance with beta-lactams, macrolides, aminoglycosides, tetracycline, rifampicin or chloramphenicol

Use
- staphylococcal or streptococcal infection that cannot be treated using other antibiotics
- osteomyelitis, septic arthritis, septicaemia, non-cardiac bacteraemia

Dose
- (septicaemia/bacteraemia, acute/chronic osteomyelitis) initially 6–12 mg/kg as an IV bolus over 5 minutes or IV infusion over 30 minutes 12-hourly for 3 doses, then 6 mg/kg IM or IV daily for 2–4 weeks (bacteraemia) or 3–6 weeks (osteomyelitis) **OR**
- (septic arthritis) initially 12 mg/kg as an IV bolus over 5 minutes or IV infusion over 30 minutes 12-hourly for 3 doses, then 12 mg/kg IM or IV daily for 3–6 weeks

Adverse effects
- fever, rigors
- rash, pruritus
- see General Adverse effects of glycopeptides (p. 181)

Interactions
- use with caution if given with other nephrotoxic or ototoxic drugs (e.g. amphotericin B (amphotericin), aminoglycosides, furosemide (frusemide), ciclosporin, etacrynic acid). If given together, blood, liver and kidney function should be closely monitored

Nursing points/Cautions
- teicoplanin is well tolerated when administered by IV infusion
- (IM) should not exceed 400 mg (3 mL) at a single site
- loading dose of 12 mg/mL at 12-hourly intervals is given to achieve rapid steady state plasma levels. Creatinine levels should be closely monitored in addition to blood, liver and kidney function
- reconstitute by adding all of the supplied diluent slowly down the side of the vial, gently rolling between the palms of the hands until the powder is dissolved, taking care to avoid foaming. The vial should not be shaken. If foamy, allow to stand for 15 minutes until foam subsides. May be further diluted for IV infusion with sodium chloride 0.9%, glucose 5%, sodium chloride 0.18% or lactated Ringer's solution
- incompatible with aminoglycosides as precipitate will form
- caution is used in those with known hypersensitivity to vancomycin (however, history of 'red man' syndrome is not a contraindication in itself)
- see General Adverse effects and Nursing points/Cautions for glycopeptides (p. 181)

Patient teaching and advice
- see General Patient teaching and advice for glycopeptides (p. 181)

VANCOMYCIN HYDROCHLORIDE (DBL Vancomycin Hydrochloride for Intravenous Infusion, Vancocin, Vancocin CP, Vancomycin Powder for Infusion)

Available forms
Capsules: 125 mg, 250 mg; Vial: 500 mg, 1 g

Action

- see General Actions of glycopeptides (p. 181)
- also alters bacterial wall permeability and RNA synthesis
- elimination half-life 4–6 hours
- cross sensitivity is possible between vancomycin and teicoplanin
- active against Gram-positive organisms, with Gram-negative, mycobacteria and fungi resistant
- poorly absorbed orally
- not removed by haemodialysis or peritoneal dialysis
- resistance emerging, therefore recommendations/guidelines have been developed regarding usage and should be followed closely

Use

- life-threatening infections caused by beta-lactam resistant Gram-positive organisms or in patients who have serious allergies to beta-lactam antibacterial agents
- prophylaxis for endocarditis before some procedures in those at high risk of endocarditis
- surgical prophylaxis for major procedures involving prostheses or device implantation where risk of MRSA or MRSE is high
- life-threatening *C. difficile* associated disease (relapse or unresponsive to metronidazole)
- (oral route) only recommended for treatment of staphylococcal enterocolitis or antibiotic-induced pseudomembranous colitis

Dose

- 500 mg IV 6-hourly or 1 g IV 12-hourly by infusion over at least 60 minutes **OR**
- (antibiotic-associated pseudomembranous colitis) 0.5–2 g orally daily in 3–4 divided doses for 7–10 days **OR**
- (antibiotic-associated pseudomembranous colitis) 250 mg orally 6-hourly for 5–10 days

Adverse effects

- (rapid IV infusion) rash, generalised pruritus, chills, fever, severe hypotension and (rarely) cardiac arrest
- chills
- (oral) nausea, vomiting, diarrhoea, indigestion, stomach ache
- see also General Adverse effects of glycopeptides (p. 181)

Interactions

- concurrent or sequential use of vancomycin and other neurotoxic and/or nephrotoxic agents (e.g. amphotericin B (amphotericin), aminoglycosides, colistin, cisplatin) is not recommended and should be very carefully monitored
- serum levels may be altered if given with furosemide (frusemide), therefore close monitoring is recommended especially when starting or stopping therapy
- increased risk of infusion-related events (e.g. hypotension, flushing, pruritus, urticaria) if given with anaesthetic agents, therefore vancomycin infusion should be completed before anaesthetic induction
- caution if given with other agents known to cause neutropenia
- not recommended with other agents known to cause ototoxicity (e.g. etacrynic acid)
- may increase neuromuscular blockage if given with vecuronium or suxamethonium
- (oral) absorption decreased by colestyramine

Nursing points/Cautions

- should be used for 48–72 hours after fever and symptoms have resolved
- not given IM
- for IV infusion, reconstitute drug with 10 mL water for injections (for 500 mg) or 20 mL for 1 g, then dilute with 100 mL of fluid for 500 mg or 200 mL for 1 g. This should minimise risk of thrombophlebitis

- given by slow IV infusion (500 mg over 1 hour, 1 g over 2 hours) to decrease risk of hypersensitivity reaction and severe hypotension
- not recommended as an IV bolus (risk of hypotension and shock) or IM (risk of tissue irritation/necrosis)
- incompatible with beta-lactams (penicillins, cephalosporins) as precipitation may occur. IV lines should be carefully flushed before and after administration
- poorly absorbed orally, but is used in the treatment of antibiotic-associated pseudomembranous colitis
- for oral (or nasogastric) administration, 500 mg is reconstituted with 30 mL distilled or de-ionised water and then flavoured to improve taste (extremely unpalatable); however, capsules may eliminate the need to do this
- renal function monitoring is recommended if given with aminoglycosides
- adrenaline (epinephrine), IV corticosteroids and oxygen should be available to treat anaphylactic/anaphylactoid reaction
- (oral) caution if given to those with GI inflammatory disorders, which may increase absorption and the risk of systemic adverse effects
- caution if used in those with known hypersensitivity to teicoplanin
- caution if used in those with kidney impairment. If used, dose and/or dose intervals should be adjusted and kidney function carefully monitored
- see General Nursing points/Cautions for glycopeptides (p. 181)

Patient teaching and advice

- advise patient to swallow capsules whole with full glass of water
- (oral) if taking colestyramine as well, instruct patient to separate by at least 2 hours from vancomycin
- see General Patient teaching and advice for glycopeptides (p. 181)

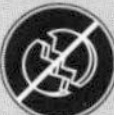
capsules should not be opened

INHIBITORS OF BACTERIAL PROTEIN SYNTHESIS

AMINOGLYCOSIDES

General Actions of aminoglycosides

- interfere with bacterial protein synthesis by binding irreversibly to ribosomal (30S) subunits of susceptible organisms
- bactericidal
- inhibit a wide range of Gram-negative and some Gram-positive organisms
- *Streptococcus pneumoniae* and the aerobic organisms *Bacteroides* and *Clostridium* spp. have shown resistance to aminoglycosides
- poorly absorbed from GI tract

General Uses of aminoglycosides

- serious or life-threatening infection where other antibacterial agents are contraindicated or ineffective

General Adverse effects of aminoglycosides

- ototoxicity (auditory and vestibular, including tinnitus, vertigo, dizziness) (hearing loss may be permanent)

- nephrotoxicity, increased or decreased urinary frequency, decreased creatinine clearance, azotaemia, increase in serum urea
- neurotoxicity (including ataxia, dizziness, peripheral neuritis, paraesthesia, tremor)
- nausea, vomiting, diarrhoea
- rash, pruritus, urticaria
- superinfection, pseudomembranous colitis
- drug fever
- (rare) blood dyscrasias
- (IM) pain
- (IV) thrombophlebitis

General Interactions of aminoglycosides

- nephrotoxicity and ototoxicity of aminoglycosides are increased when given with etacrynic acid, furosemide (frusemide) or other potent diuretics
- not recommended concurrently or sequentially with other neurotoxic or nephrotoxic agents (e.g. other aminoglycosides, amphotericin B (amphotericin), bacitracin, colistin, cisplatin, clindamycin, vancomycin)
- inactivated by solutions containing beta-lactam antibiotics (penicillins and cephalosporins)
- enhanced neuromuscular blockade (including respiratory paralysis) may occur intraoperatively or postoperatively if given with anaesthetics, neuromuscular blocking agents, other medications with neuromuscular activity or massive transfusions with citrated, anticoagulated blood
- increased risk of nephrotoxicity and enhanced neuromuscular blockade if given with methoxyflurane
- increased serum level may occur if given with NSAIDs (as NSAIDs may decrease renal function). If given together, drug level and renal function should be closely monitored

General Nursing points/Cautions for aminoglycosides

- see General Nursing points/Cautions for antibacterial agents (p. 148)
- baseline renal function should be measured before starting therapy and then regularly throughout course of treatment, especially in those with known or suspected renal impairment
- once-daily administration has proven to be as efficacious, safe and less costly than divided dose administration and is recommended in those with normal renal function
- urine should be monitored for specific gravity, protein, cells and casts to monitor for renal irritation
- if possible, serial audiograms are recommended before starting and throughout therapy, especially in those with renal impairment
- blood urea nitrogen, serum creatinine, calcium, magnesium and sodium and creatinine clearance should be monitored regularly throughout therapy
- note and report oliguria as therapy may need to be stopped if urine output decreases
- patients should be well hydrated during therapy to avoid nephrotoxicity and hydration should be increased if any signs of renal irritation occur
- monitoring for blood levels is not required if duration of therapy is < 48 hours. If therapy duration is > 48 hours, blood level monitoring is recommended in addition to other testing previously discussed. Blood for trough level is sampled immediately before the next IM or IV dose;

blood for peak level is obtained approximately 1 hour after IM or IV injection and 30 minutes after completion of a 30-minute IV infusion or at the completion of a 1-hour IV infusion; levels should be remeasured every 72 hours. The goal is to avoid excessive peak and/or trough level as this increases risk of ototoxicity and nephrotoxicity

- do not mix with other drugs in the same syringe or IV infusion container
- dilute and give by IV infusion according to manufacturer's instructions
- IV injection to be given very slowly over 2–3 minutes
- caution if used in those with muscular disorders, such as Parkinsonism, as muscle weakness may be aggravated
- caution if used in those with extensive burns as serum levels may be lowered. Serum levels should be monitored closely to ensure adequate concentrations are reached
- caution if used in those with known hearing impairment, fever, low haematocrit, advanced age, or renal damage/impairment as risk of ototoxicity is increased
- caution if used in the elderly as there may be pre-existing kidney and/or hearing impairments present
- contraindicated in those with myasthenia gravis
- contraindicated in those with known hypersensitivity to aminoglycosides or with subclinical renal or eighth nerve damage caused by nephrotoxic or ototoxic agents

General Patient teaching and advice for aminoglycosides

- see General Patient teaching and advice for antibacterial agents (p. 149)
- patient should be advised to immediately seek medical advice if any of the following occur:
  - headache, dizziness, nausea, vomiting, ataxia, nystagmus, vertigo, tinnitus (buzzing or ringing in the ears), hearing loss or roaring in the ears (signs of ototoxicity)
  - numbness, skin tingling, muscle twitching or convulsions (signs of neurotoxicity), even after therapy has stopped as damage can occur after drug has been discontinued
- female patients of childbearing potential should be counselled to use adequate contraception during therapy to avoid pregnancy

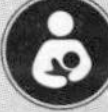

contraindicated during pregnancy. Aminoglycosides cross the placenta and may damage the eighth cranial nerve in the developing fetus. All aminoglycosides should be considered potentially nephrotoxic and ototoxic to the fetus regardless of maternal therapeutic blood levels

not recommended during breastfeeding

AMIKACIN (DBL Amikacin Injection)

Available form

Ampoules: 500 mg/2 mL

Action

- derivative of kanamycin used for treatment of many Gram-negative organisms that are resistant to gentamicin or tobramycin
- half-life 2–3 hours (but greatly prolonged in severe renal failure to 30–86 hours)
- desirable serum levels: peak 15–30 microgram/mL and trough 5–10 microgram/mL

- see General Actions of aminoglycosides (p. 184)

Use

- second-line treatment of serious staphylococcal infections or neonatal sepsis not responsive to other aminoglycosides
- see General Uses of aminoglycosides (p. 184)

Dose

- 15 mg/kg/day IM or by IV infusion over 30–60 minutes in 2–3 divided doses **OR**
- (non-pseudomonal urinary tract infections) 250 mg IM or by IV infusion over 30–60 minutes 12-hourly

Adverse effects

- (rare) increased liver enzymes, hepatotoxicity, hepatomegaly
- see also General Adverse effects of aminoglycosides (p. 184)

Interactions

- see General Interactions for aminoglycosides (p. 185)

Nursing points/Cautions

- some response to treatment should be seen in 24–48 hours. If no clinical response is seen in 72–120 hours bacterial sensitivities should be rechecked
- treatment should be limited to 10 days. If treatment is greater than 10 days, daily renal and auditory function monitoring is recommended
- IM is the preferred route of administration with IV used if IM is unavailable or infection is life threatening
- prolonged peak serum levels $>$ 30–35 microgram/mL increases risk of toxicity
- total treatment dose $>$ 15 g increases risk of nephrotoxicity and ototoxicity
- contains sodium bisulfite, which may cause allergy reactions in susceptible people (e.g. those with asthma)
- see also General Interactions/Nursing points/Cautions for aminoglycosides (p. 185)

Patient teaching and advice

- see General Patient teaching and advice for aminoglycosides (p. 186)

FRAMYCETIN SULFATE (Soframycin Ear, Soframycin Eye Drops)

Available forms

Ear drops: 5 mg/mL (0.5%); Eye drops: 5 mg/mL (0.5%)

Action

- aminoglycoside used to treat Gram-positive and Gram-negative infections

Use

- otitis externa
- infected corneal ulcer (bacterial keratitis), bacterial conjunctivitis, post-removal of foreign bodies, blepharitic corneal abrasions and burns

Dose

- (ear infection) 2–3 drops into the affected ear(s) 3 times daily **OR**
- (eye infection) 2 drops into the affected eye(s) 1–2-hourly, then 2–3 drops 3 times daily

Adverse effects

- (eye drops) redness, discharge, irritation, pain, oedema,
- (rare) hypersensitivity (eyelid swelling and irritation)

Nursing points/Cautions

- drops may also be applied to a wick and inserted into external auditory meatus
- caution if used in those with known hypersensitivity to neomycin because cross-sensitivity may exist
- (ear drops) contraindicated if there is perforation of tympanic membrane

Patient teaching and advice

Eye drops

- ensure patient has instructions on correct instillation of eye drops (see p. 189)

Ear drops

- instruct patient in correct instillation technique for ear drops, including:
  1. check expiry date
  2. if the ear drops are new, break safety cap and open
  3. wash hands thoroughly with soap and water
  4. hold bottle upside down in one hand (between thumb and middle finger)
  5. tilt head to one side with affected ear facing up (it may be easier in sitting or lying position)
  6. place dropper tip close to (but not touching) ear and gently tap or press base of container to release drops
  7. continue holding head in same position for one minute to allow drops to reach deeper into the ear
  8. repeat for other ear if needed
  9. replace cap on bottle and close tightly
  10. wash hands to remove any residue
- warn patient that feeling of drops flowing deeper into ear may be unpleasant
- advise patient that a bad taste in the mouth may occur after using ear drops
- patient should be advised to note opening date and discard after that date (e.g. 28 days)

Note

- contained in Otodex (Ear Drops) and Sofradex Ear Drops

GENTAMICIN SULFATE (Genoptic, Gentamicin Injection BP, Septopal)

Available forms

Ampoules: 80 mg/2 mL; Eye drops: 3 mg/mL; Beads (for surgical implantation): 30 beads on surgical wire (7.5 mg/bead)

Action

- aminoglycoside which is active against *Pseudomonas aeruginosa*, *Proteus*, *Salmonella*, *Shigella*, *Klebsiella*, *Enterobacter* and *Serratia* spp., and *Staphylococcus* spp.
- not active against anaerobic organisms
- half-life about 2 hours
- see General Actions of aminoglycosides (p. 184)

Use

- first-line treatment for Gram-negative sepsis
- (eye drops) infections of external eye (including corneal ulcer, keratitis), bacterial conjunctivitis, keratoconjunctivitis, blepharitis)
- (surgical beads) treatment or prophylaxis of bone or soft tissue infection
- see also General Uses of aminoglycosides (p. 184)

Dose

- (severe infections) 3 mg/kg/day IM or by IV infusion over at least 30 minutes in 3 divided doses 8-hourly for 7–10 days **OR**
- (life-threatening infections) initially 5 mg/kg/day IM or by IV infusion over at least 30 minutes in 3–4 divided doses 6–8 hourly, reducing to 3 mg/kg/day as soon as possible for total of 7–10 days **OR**
- (treatment and prophylaxis of bone or soft tissue infection) 10–90 acrylic beads containing gentamicin threaded onto surgical wire (chain) and implanted to treat bone infections after area has been cleaned and any necrotic tissue/foreign body removed (Septopal)
- (eye infection) 1–2 drops into affected eye(s) 4-hourly **OR**
- (severe eye infection) 2 drops into affected eye(s) hourly

Adverse effects

- (eye drops) redness, discharge, irritation, pain, oedema, hypersensitivity (eyelid swelling and irritation)

- see General Adverse effects of aminoglycosides (p. 184)

Interactions

- may inhibit actions of IV vitamin K
- added nephrotoxicity and ototoxicity may occur if given with cisplatin
- see also General Interactions of aminoglycosides (p. 185)

Nursing points/Cautions

- (IV) dose should never exceed 5 mg/kg/day without serum levels being closely monitored
- IM is the preferred route with IV being used if IM route is not available or infection is life threatening
- peak levels above 12 microgram/mL or trough levels above 2 microgram/mL should be avoided
- (IV) administer alone
- (IV) treatment should not exceed 10–14 days
- (IV) dilute in 100–200 mL sodium chloride 0.9% or glucose 5% and then infuse over at least 30 minutes at a rate not exceeding 1 mg/mL
- when given as an IV bolus, serum levels initially rise into the toxic range but rapidly fall. However, the safety of this administration method has not been established
- (bone infection) wire chain should be removed after 10–14 days (short-term management of chronic recurrent osteomyelitis) or after 3 months (long-term management of chronic recurrent osteomyelitis where bone grafting is intended)
- (soft tissue infection) wire chain should be removed after 7–10 days
- (surgical beads) contraindicated in those with known hypersensitivity to disodium edetate or nickel
- (eye drops) should not be administered directly into anterior chamber of the eye
- (eye drops) contraindicated in those with hypersensitivity to benzalkonium chloride (preservative)
- see General Nursing points/Cautions for aminoglycosides (p. 185)

Patient teaching and advice

- (eye infection) instruct patient not to wear contact lenses if there are any signs and symptoms of bacterial ocular infection present

Eye drops

- advise patient that eye drops should not be instilled if soft or gas-permeable contact lenses are in situ. Lenses should be removed before instillation and reinserted after at least a 15-minute interval
- warn patient that eye drops contain benzalkonium chloride (preservative), which can cause irritation and also discolour soft contact lenses
- instruct patient to write the expiry date on eye preparations and discard accordingly (usually 28 days)
- instruct patient in correct technique for instilling eye drops, including:
  1 not allowing tip of dispensing container to touch the eye as may cause injury and/or contaminate the eye drops
  2 if the container is new, remove protective seal, otherwise it is important to check expiry date
  3 wash hands thoroughly with soap and water
  4 remove lid/cap and hold container upside down in one hand between thumb and forefinger or index finger
  5 using other hand, gently pull down on lower eyelid to form a pouch/pocket and tilt head back looking up
  6 place tip of container close to lower eyelid (taking care not to make contact between tip and eye). Squeezing bottle gently, release one drop into pouch/pocket formed between eye and eyelid, taking care not to allow tip to touch eye

7 gently close eye but do not blink or rub eye
8 while eye is closed, place index finger against inside corner of eye and press against nose for about 2 minutes (this stops medicine from draining through tear duct into nose and throat)
9 blot any excess solution from around the eye with a tissue
10 replace lid/cap tightly
11 wash hands again to remove any residue

- see General Patient teaching and advice for aminoglycosides (p. 186)

TOBRAMYCIN (Tobi, Tobramycin Injection, Tobramycin Solution for Inhalation, Tobrex)

TOBRAMYCIN SULFATE (TobraDay, Tobramycin PF)

Available forms

Ampoules: 80 mg/2 mL, 500 mg/5 mL; Eye drops: 0.3%; Eye ointment: 0.3%; Solution for inhalation: 300 mg/5 mL; Powder for inhalation: 28 mg

Action

- aminoglycoside active against *Pseudomonas aeruginosa*, *Proteus*, *Salmonella*, *Shigella*, *Klebsiella*, *Enterobacter* and *Serratia* spp., *Escherichia coli*, *Citrobacter* spp., *Providencia* spp. and *Staphylococcus* spp. and low order activity against Gram-positive organisms
- half-life 2–3 hours (prolongs to 5–70 hours in those with kidney impairment)
- see General Actions of aminoglycosides (p. 184)

Use

- acute lung exacerbation including *Pseudomonas aeruginosa* infection in cystic fibrosis
- eye infection
- see General Uses of aminoglycosides (p. 184)

Dose

- (mild-to-moderate urinary tract infection) 2–3 mg/kg/day IM or by IV infusion over 20–60 minutes in 2–3 divided doses 8–12-hourly for 7–10 days **OR**
- (severe infections) 3 mg/kg/day IM or by IV infusion over 20–60 minutes in 3 equal divided doses 8-hourly **OR**
- (life-threatening infections) up to 5 mg/kg/day IM or by IV infusion over 20–60 minutes in 3–4 divided doses, reducing to 3 mg/kg/day as soon as possible **OR**
- (cystic fibrosis) initially 10 mg/kg/day by IV infusion over 30–60 minutes, adjusting dose according to serum levels, renal function and patient response, for 10–14 days (500 mg/5 mL) **OR**
- (cystic fibrosis) 300 mg via nebuliser over 10–15 minutes twice daily for 28 days, repeated after drug-free 28-day interval **OR**
- (cystic fibrosis) 112 mg (4 capsules) twice daily by inhalation via Tobi Podhaler **OR**
- (eye infection) 1–2 drops into affected eye(s) 4-hourly or 2 drops hourly (if severe) until improvement **OR**
- (eye infection) 1–1.5 cm ointment 2–3 times daily or 3–4-hourly (if severe) until improvement

Adverse effects

- (rare) neurotoxicity
- (inhalation) bronchospasm, cough, haemoptysis, voice alteration, tinnitus (transient), dizziness, pharyngitis, dyspnoea, oropharyngeal pain, increased serum creatinine
- see General Adverse effects of aminoglycosides (p. 184)

Interactions

- (IV) activity may be decreased by calcium and magnesium ions
- see General Interactions of aminoglycosides (p. 185)

Nursing points/Cautions

- (IV) if duration of treatment is > 10 days, renal and auditory monitoring is recommended. IV therapy should not exceed 10–14 days
- serum potassium, calcium, sodium, magnesium and urea levels should be monitored throughout therapy
- IV vial should be diluted with 50–100 mL sodium chloride 0.9% or glucose 5% and infused over 20–60 minutes
- (inhalation) first dose should be given under supervision with FEV_1 measured before and after inhalation administration to detect bronchospasm. Bronchodilator therapy may be required
- (inhalation) caution if concurrent tobramycin therapy is given (e.g. IV and inhalation) as there is a risk of cumulative toxicity
- (Podhaler) children 10 years and under should be supervised using Podhaler to ensure correct use
- (IV) contains sodium metabisulfite, therefore should be given with caution in susceptible people (e.g. those with asthma)
- caution if used in those with malignant disease as complex metabolic syndrome (hypocalcaemia, hypomagnesaemia, hypokalaemia, hypoalbuminaemia, hypophosphateaemia, hypouricaemia) may occur 2–8 weeks after finishing therapy
- see also General Nursing points/Cautions for aminoglycosides (p. 185)

Patient teaching and advice

- see General Patient teaching and advice for aminoglycosides (p. 186)

Inhaled therapy

- advise patient that inhalation therapy should be 12 hours apart if possible, but not less than 6-hour interval
- if patient is taking multiple inhaled medications, tobramycin inhalation should be taken last
- patient should know that therapy is a 28-day drug cycle followed by 28-day drug-free interval
- if using nebuliser solution, patient should be aware that it should not be mixed with other medications in the nebuliser
- ensure that patient knows that Tobi Podhaler capsules are for use in the Podhaler only and should not be taken orally
- ensure patient has instructions on correct use of Podhaler, including:
  1. remove Podhaler from case holding base and twisting top off case (counter clockwise direction)
  2. holding body of inhaler, unscrew and remove mouthpiece (set mouthpiece aside)
  3. peel back foil from capsule card to reveal capsule and remove
  4. insert capsule into inhaler chamber and replace mouthpiece, screwing on firmly until it stops (but don't over-tighten)
  5. to puncture capsule, hold inhaler with mouthpiece down, press button firmly with thumb (as far as goes) and release
  6. exhale fully, and place inhaler mouth over mouthpiece to make tight seal
  7. inhale fully with a single continuous inhalation
  8. remove inhaler and hold breath for about 5 seconds, then exhale normally after a few normal breaths, perform second inhalation from same capsule
  9. unscrew mouthpiece, remove capsule and inspect used capsule to ensure it is punctured and empty
  10. if capsule is punctured but is not empty, replace in chamber (with punctured side inserted first), replace mouthpiece and take 2 more inhalations, then reinspect capsule
  11. if capsule is unpunctured, place back in chamber, replace

mouthpiece and press button firmly (as far as it goes) and take 2 more inhalations. If capsule remains full, replace inhaler device and repeat steps 4–10
12. repeat for 3 remaining capsules to administer full dose
13. replace mouthpiece and screw it firmly until it stops
14. when 4 capsules have been administered, wipe mouthpiece with a clean dry cloth
15. store inhaler in storage case
16. inhaler should not be washed with water
17. Podhaler should be discarded after 7 days and a new Podhaler used for subsequent inhalations

Eye infections

- ensure patient has instructions on correct instillation of eye drops (see p. 189)
- ensure patient has instructions on correct instillation of eye ointment, including:
  1. check expiry date
  2. wash hands thoroughly before applying eye ointment
  3. tilt head back gently and gently pull lower eyelid down
  4. squeeze 1.5 cm of eye ointment inside lower eyelid (however not allowing tip of tube to touch eye, eyelid or lashes)
  5. release eyelid slowly and close eyes gently for 1–2 minutes or blink a few times to help spread the ointment over the eye
  6. blot any excessive ointment from around the eye with a tissue
  7. wash hands thoroughly after finishing applying eye ointment

TETRACYCLINES

General Actions of tetracyclines

- interfere with bacterial protein synthesis by blocking 30S ribosomal subunit
- bacteriostatic
- broad spectrum
- concentrate in developing teeth and bone
- not the drug of choice in staphylococcal infections
- oral tetracyclines are well absorbed and distribute in most body fluids

General Uses of tetracyclines

- infections due to susceptible strains of *E. coli*, *Enterobacter* spp., *H. influenzae*, *Klebsiella* spp., *Proteus* spp., *S. pyogenes*, *S. faecalis*

General Adverse effects of tetracyclines

- anorexia, dysphagia, nausea, vomiting, dyspepsia, diarrhoea, abdominal pain, glossitis, black hairy tongue, inflammatory lesions of the anogenital region
- (rare) oesophagitis, oesophageal ulceration
- dizziness, headache, tinnitus, vertigo, light-headedness, asthenia
- increase in serum urea, elevated liver enzymes
- tooth and nail discolouration (if given during pregnancy or to children under 8 years), tooth discolouration in adults
- urticaria, rash

- photosensitivity
- benign intracranial hypertension (pseudotumor celebri) (symptoms include headache and blurred vision), bulging fontanelles in infants
- enterocolitis, pseudomembranous colitis, superinfection
- (prolonged therapy) microscopic discolouration (black/brown) of thyroid gland (but thyroid function not affected)
- (rare) blood dyscrasias, acute renal failure, aggravated pre-existing kidney failure
- (rare) cholestatic hepatitis, fatty liver degeneration, severe skin reactions, hypersensitivity
- (IV) phlebitis

General Interactions of tetracyclines

- contraindicated with methoxyflurane because it increases the risk of fatal renal toxicity
- increased intracranial pressure (benign) may occur if given with oral retinoids (acitretin, isotretinoin) or vitamin A and is therefore contraindicated
- absorption may be reduced by milk, food, sodium bicarbonate, colestipol, colestyramine, oral iron, calcium, magnesium and aluminium salts (and any supplements or antacids containing these), sucralfate
- may reduce activity of penicillins and therefore should not be given together
- may affect the stability of oral anticoagulant control, therefore prothrombin time should be closely monitored, especially when starting and stopping therapy
- may cause failure of oral oestrogen-containing contraceptives
- increased risk of pseudomembranous colitis if given with agents that delay peristalsis, such as opioid analgesics and diphenoxylate/atropine combination
- anti-anabolic action and increased serum urea levels may occur if given with diuretics
- may give false-positive result on urinary catecholamine assay

General Nursing points/Cautions for tetracyclines

- see General Nursing points/Cautions for antibacterial agents (p. 148)
- therapy should be continued for 24–48 hours after fever and symptoms have resolved. If treating group A beta-haemolytic streptococcal infection, therapy should continue for 10 days
- if patient has prolonged therapy with tetracyclines, blood counts and renal and liver function should be monitored regularly
- all patients with gonorrhoea should also have serological testing for syphilis at time of diagnosis and monthly for at least 4 months
- see manufacturer's instructions for information about reconstituting solutions and stability
- avoid using out-of-date or deteriorated tetracyclines because degraded products cause reversible Fanconi's syndrome
- not recommended in those with renal impairment (except doxycycline)
- contraindicated in those with known hypersensitivity to tetracyclines, severe renal impairment or SLE

General Patient teaching and advice for tetracyclines

- see General Patient teaching and advice for antibacterial agents (p. 149)

- warn patients to avoid sunlamps or sunbeds or direct exposure to sunlight and if this cannot be avoided, they should wear protective clothing and sunscreen with high sun protection factor (SPF 30+) due to increased risk of photosensitivity. Reaction may be immediate or up to 3 days after sun exposure
- instruct patient not to take oral preparations while lying down (especially doxycycline). Tablets/capsules should be taken with at least 100 mL of fluid and the patient advised to remain upright for 30 minutes after ingestion to reduce risk of oesophageal ulceration
- patients should be advised to seek medical advice immediately if any of the following occur:
  - headache with any of the following – nausea, vomiting, dizziness and/or blurred vision
  - severe sunburn (redness, itching, swelling, blistering) occurring more quickly than usual
  - any diarrhoea or colitis (even if the antibacterial agent was ceased some weeks ago)
- warn patients to avoid driving or using heavy machinery if dizziness, headache, tinnitus, visual disturbances or light-headedness are ongoing problems
- advise patients to separate tetracycline administration from antacids or iron supplements by at least 2 hours to achieve maximum effect
- female patients should be counselled to use barrier method contraception in addition to oral contraceptives during therapy with tetracyclines and for 7 days after completion of course to avoid unwanted pregnancy

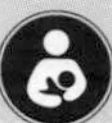

not recommended during pregnancy (after 18 weeks), breastfeeding or in the first 8 years of life because tetracyclines accumulate in the growing skeleton and may induce hypoplasia of enamel and permanent discolouration of teeth

DOXYCYCLINE HYCLATE (HYDROCHLORIDE) (Doryx, Doxsig, Doxylin)

DOXYCYCLINE MONOHYDRATE (Frakas)

Available forms

Tablets: 50 mg, 100 mg; Capsules: 50 mg, 100 mg

Action

- long half-life (10–24 hours), which enables once-daily administration
- see General Actions of tetracyclines (p. 192)

Use

- see General Uses of tetracyclines (p. 192)
- malaria prophylaxis

Dose

- 100 mg orally 12-hourly on the first day, then 100 mg as a single daily dose or 50 mg (or 100 mg for severe infections) 12-hourly **OR**
- (treatment for louse-borne or scrub typhus) 100–200 mg orally as a single dose **OR**
- (prevention of scrub typhus) 200 mg orally as single dose **OR**
- (gonococcal infection) 100 mg orally twice daily for 5–7 days **OR**
- (syphilis) 150 mg orally twice daily for at least 10 days **OR**
- (malaria prophylaxis) 100 mg orally daily starting 2 days before entering a malarial area, continued while in the area and 2 weeks after departure **OR**
- (severe acne) 50 mg orally daily for 12 weeks

Adverse effects
- see General Adverse effects for tetracyclines (p. 192)

Interactions
- plasma levels may be reduced by alcohol, barbiturates, phenytoin, carbamazepine, sodium bicarbonate, sodium lactate and acetazolamide
- increased risk of ergot toxicity if given with ergometrine or methysergide
- see General Interactions for tetracyclines (p. 193)

Nursing points/Cautions
- (malaria prophylaxis) maximum 100 mg daily for 8 weeks is recommended
- not recommended late at night due to increased risk of oesophageal ulceration
- see General Nursing points/Cautions for tetracyclines (p. 193)

Patient teaching and advice
- instruct patient that tablets/capsules may be given with meals and a glass of water or milk to reduce gastric irritation
- see General Patient teaching and advice for tetracyclines (p. 193)

tablet should be softened in 20 mL water, then crushed and mixed with milk, apple juice, chocolate pudding, yoghurt or apple puree. Capsules can be opened and contents given with yoghurt or apple puree but pellets must not be chewed

MINOCYCLINE HYDROCHLORIDE (Akamin, Minomycin)

Available forms
Tablets: 50 mg; Capsules: 100 mg

Action
- semi-synthetic derivative of tetracycline
- active against *S. aureus* organisms
- half-life about 13 hours
- see General Actions of tetracyclines (p. 192)

Use
- see General Uses of tetracyclines (p. 192)
- may be used for tetracycline-resistant acne

Dose
- initially 200 mg orally, then 100 mg 12-hourly (continued for 24–48 hours after fever and symptoms have resolved) **OR**
- (tetracycline-resistant acne) 50 mg orally twice daily (for up to 12 weeks)

Adverse effects
- blue-black cutaneous and mucous membrane hyperpigmentation (especially with prolonged use)
- decreased hearing
- (rare) hepatoxicity
- see also General Adverse effects of tetracyclines (p. 192)

Interactions
- caution if used with hepatotoxic agents
- see also General Interactions of tetracyclines (p. 193)

Nursing points/Cautions
- food and milk do not influence absorption so may be taken at any time
- acne usually resolves in 12 weeks
- caution if used in those with acne vulgaris, rheumatoid arthritis, pemphigus and pemphigoid as risk of blue-black hyperpigmentation is increased
- caution if used in those with liver dysfunction
- see also General Nursing points/Cautions of tetracyclines (p. 193)

Patient teaching and advice

- advise patient that blue-black discolouration usually resolves when minocycline is stopped; however, it may take months to years to resolve completely
- see also Patient teaching and advice for tetracyclines (p. 193)

tablet can be crushed or capsule opened and mixed with water or spoonful of yoghurt or apple puree

TIGECYCLINE (Tygacil)

Available form

Vial: 50 mg

Action

- glycylcycline tetracycline structurally related to minocycline but with expanded spectrum of activity against tetracycline-resistant organisms (e.g. penicillin-resistant *S. pneumonieae*, MRSA, MRSE, VRE)
- some resistance documented
- see General Actions of tetracyclines (p. 192)

Use

- see General Uses of tetracyclines (p. 192)

Dose

- initially 100 mg by IV infusion over 30–60 minutes, then 50 mg 12-hourly for 5–14 days

Adverse effects

- (IV site) phlebitis, pain, inflammation, swelling
- increased bilirubin, hypoproteinaemia
- (uncommon) pancreatitis
- see also General Adverse effects of tetracyclines (p. 192)

Interactions

- see General Interactions for tetracyclines (p. 193)

Nursing points/Cautions

- bolus IV administration is not recommended
- reconstitute using 5.3 mL of sodium chloride 0.9% or glucose 5%, swirl gently to dissolve powder, further dilute according to manufacturer's instructions and administer over 30–60 minutes
- reconstituted solution should be yellow to orange. If this does not occur, solution should be discarded
- administer alone
- incompatible with amphotericin B (amphotericin), chlorpromazine, diazepam, esomeprazole, methylprednisolone, omeprazole and voriconazole
- caution if used to treat complicated intra-abdominal infections secondary to intestinal perforation
- caution if used in those with liver impairment
- not recommended for hospital- or community-acquired pneumonia or diabetic foot infections
- see Nursing points/Cautions for tetracyclines (p. 193)

Patient teaching and advice

- advise patient to seek medical advice immediately if any signs of pancreatitis occur including nausea, vomiting, tender abdomen, abdominal pain that radiates to back, upper abdominal pain, abdominal pain that is worse after eating, rapid pulse and fever
- see also General Patient teaching and advice for tetracyclines (p. 193)

MACROLIDES

General Actions of macrolides

- contain a common macrocyclic lactone ring with attached sugars
- bind to bacterial ribosomal subunit 50S, inhibiting RNA-dependent protein synthesis
- bacteriostatic in low levels
- bactericidal in high levels (selected organisms)
- wide spectrum of action against Gram-positive and Gram-negative aerobic organisms and some anaerobes
- most strains of methicillin-resistant *S. aureus* (MRSA), Enterobacteriaceae, *Pseudomonas* and *Acinetobacter* spp. show resistance to macrolides and *S. pneumoniae* is showing increasing resistance
- cross-resistance may exist between clarithromycin, erythromycin and other macrolides as well as lincomycin and clindamycin

General Uses of macrolides

- community-acquired pneumonia, upper and lower respiratory tract infections (including Legionnaire's disease and pharyngitis)
- uncomplicated skin or skin structure infections
- disseminated or localised mycobacterial infection (including prevention of *M. avium* complex (MAC) infections in HIV-infected adults with other antimycobacterial agents)
- sinusitis, otitis media
- diphtheria (adjunct to antitoxin)
- non-gonococcal urethritis
- chlamydial infections, gonorrhoea, syphilis, acute pelvic inflammation (due to *Neisseria gonorrhoeae*)
- prophylaxis of SBE in penicillin-resistant patients
- combination therapy for peptic ulcer treatment associated with *H. pylori* infection

General Adverse effects of macrolides

- decreased appetite, nausea, vomiting, diarrhoea, abdominal pain, dyspepsia, constipation
- dizziness, headache, asthenia
- fever
- rash, pruritus, urticaria
- reversible hearing loss (high dose, prolonged therapy)
- dyspnoea
- altered liver enzymes, cholestatic jaundice, hepatic dysfunction
- pseudomembranous colitis, superinfection
- (uncommon) taste alteration, flatulence, depression, flushing, increased prothrombin time, photophobia
- (rare) hypersensitivity, angioedema, anaphylaxis, photosensitivity, tongue discolouration, severe skin reactions
- (rare) cardiac arrhythmia, prolongation of QT interval, palpitations, chest pain
- (rapid IV) arrhythmias, hypotension
- (IV site) pain, inflammation

General Interactions of macrolides

- contraindicated with statins (HMG-CoA reductase inhibitors) due to risk of myopathy and/or rhabdomyolysis
- may cause peripheral vasospasm and dysaesthesia (ergot toxicity) if given with ergot alkaloids such as ergotamine or dihydroergotamine;

therefore, contraindicated with these agents

- caution if given with agents known to prolong QT interval such as class IA and III antiarrhythmic agents, antipsychotics, antidepressants, antifungals, fluoroquinolones or agents that cause electrolyte disturbance (e.g. diuretics) especially hypokalaemia and hypomagnesaemia
- may enhance effects of alprazolam, midazolam and triazolam, causing increased and prolonged sedation, so should be used with caution (and avoid altogether with erythromycin)
- may increase serum digoxin levels increasing the risk of toxicity, therefore digoxin serum levels should be monitored carefully during therapy
- increased risk of neurotoxicity if given with carbamazepine (not azithromycin)
- caution if given with agents that delay peristalsis, such as opioid analgesics or diphenoxylate/atropine combination, because of the increased risk of antibiotic-associated pseudomembranous colitis
- may increase serum levels of phosphodiesterase inhibitors (sildenafil, tadalafil, vardenafil) increasing risk of adverse effects and toxicity
- may increase serum levels of alprazolam, carbamazepine, cilostazol, ciclosporin, disopyramide, ibrutinib, midazolam, methylprednisolone, phenytoin, quetiapine, rifabutin, sildenafil, sodium valproate, tacrolimus, tadalafil, theophylline, triazolam, vardenafil, vinblastine and warfarin, thereby increasing the risk of toxicity; serum levels should be closely monitored during therapy
- effects may be increased by protease inhibitors such as ritonavir
- increased risk of nephrotoxicity and/or neurotoxicity if given with ciclosporin or tacrolimus
- may increase the anticoagulant effects of warfarin, therefore INR should be closely monitored, especially when starting or stopping therapy

General Nursing points/Cautions for macrolides

- see General Nursing points/Cautions for antibacterial agents (p. 148)
- any electrolyte imbalance (especially hypokalaemia or hypomagnesaemia) should be corrected before starting therapy
- sensitivity checking is recommended for community-acquired pneumonia or moderate to severe skin and soft tissue infections due to emerging resistance to macrolides
- 5–10 days of treatment for streptococcal throat infection or 20 days for non-gonococcal genital infections
- caution if used in those with myasthenia gravis as disease exacerbation may occur
- caution or not recommended in those with predisposition to prolongation of the QT interval, bradycardia, cardiac arrhythmias or cardiac insufficiency
- caution if used in those with severe liver impairment
- contraindicated in those with known hypersensitivity to other macrolides

General Patient teaching and advice for macrolides

- see General Patient teaching and advice for antibacterial agents (p. 149)

- patient should be advised to avoid driving or operating machinery if dizziness occurs
- warn patients to seek medical advice immediately if any of the following occur:
  - unexplained muscle pain or weakness, dark-coloured urine
  - hearing difficulties
  - severe skin reactions, including blistering and peeling
  - yellowing of skin or eyes, loss of appetite, nausea, upper abdominal pain, itchy skin, dark urine, pale stools (even if these occur weeks after stopping therapy)
  - rapid or irregular heart beat

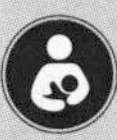

only used during pregnancy or breast-feeding when benefits outweigh potential risks and no other alternatives are available

AZITHROMYCIN (Azith, Zedd, Zithro, Zithromax IV)

AZITHROMYCIN DIHYDRATE (Zithromax)

Available forms

Tablets: 500 mg, 600 mg; Oral suspension: 200 mg/5 mL; Vial: 500 mg

Action

- see General Actions of macrolides (p. 197)
- shows cross-resistance with erythromycin-resistant Gram-positive organisms and Gram-negative *P. aeruginosa*
- long half-life (68 hours)

Use

- see General Uses of macrolides (p. 197)

Dose

- (chlamydial infections) 1 g orally as single dose 1 hour before or 2 hours after food **OR**
- (chlamydial infections) 500 mg orally daily 1 hour before or 2 hours after food for 3 days **OR**
- (other infections) initially 500 mg orally daily (day 1) 1 hour before or 2 hours after food, then 250 mg daily (days 2–5) **OR**
- (other infections) 500 mg orally daily 1 hour before or 2 hours after food for 3 days **OR**
- (conjunctivitis due to *Chlamydia trachomatis*) 1 g orally 1 hour before or 2 hours after food as either a single dose or weekly for up to 3 weeks **OR**
- (prevention of disseminated *Mycobacterium avium* complex (MAC)) 1.2 g orally 1 hour before or 2 hours after food weekly alone or with rifabutin **OR**
- (community-acquired pneumonia) 500 mg daily as IV infusion over 60 minutes for 2 days, followed by 500 mg orally 1 hour before or 2 hours after food daily (total course 7–10 days)

Adverse effects

- see General Adverse effects of macrolides (p. 197)

Interactions

- see General Interactions of macrolides (p. 197)
- should not be given with magnesium or aluminium-containing antacids

Nursing points/Cautions

- because of long half-life, allergic symptoms may continue after therapy has been ceased
- should not be given IM or as an IV bolus
- IV infusion rate should not exceed 2 mg/mL (administered over 1 hour) to avoid local site reactions

- reconstitute using 4.8 mL water for injections, then dilute further and infuse over 60 minutes
- administer alone IV
- (suspension) contains 3.87 g sucrose/ 5 mL and is therefore not recommended in those with fructose intolerance, glucose–galactose malabsorption or sucrase–isomaltase deficiency and should be used with caution in those with diabetes
- see General Nursing points/Cautions for macrolides (p. 198)

Patient teaching and advice

- see General Patient teaching and advice for macrolides (p. 198)
- advise patient to separate tablet or oral suspension by at least 2 hours from magnesium or aluminium-containing antacids
- instruct patient that capsules should be taken 1 hour before or 2 hours after meals but oral suspension can be taken with meals
- advise patient to discard suspension 10 days after opening
- if patient taking suspension has diabetes mellitus, they should be warned of the sucrose content

syrup/suspension is available. Tablet can be crushed or capsule opened and mixed with water or spoonful of yoghurt or apple puree

CLARITHROMYCIN (Clarithro, Kalixocin, Klacid)

Available forms

Tablets: 250 mg, 500 mg; Oral suspension: 250 mg/5 mL

Action

- see General Actions of macrolides (p. 197)
- not active against *Pseudomonas* spp., *Enterobacteriaceae* or *Mycobacterium tuberculosis*
- more potent than erythromycin against atypical mycobacteria
- metabolite has antibacterial properties
- half-life about 7 hours

Use

- see General Uses of macrolides (p. 197)

Dose

- (non-mycobacterial infections) 250–500 mg orally twice daily for 7–14 days **OR**
- (Legionnaire's disease) 500 mg orally twice daily for 4 weeks **OR**
- (treatment of mycobacterial infection) 500 mg orally twice daily, increasing to 1 g twice daily if there is no clinical response after 3–4 weeks **OR**
- (prophylaxis of mycobacterial infection (MAC) in HIV-infected adults) 500 mg orally twice daily **OR**
- (*H. pylori* eradication) 500 mg orally twice daily for 7–10 days (with amoxicillin 1 g twice daily and omeprazole 20 mg daily)

Adverse effects

- (immunocompromised patient) rash, dyspnoea, altered taste
- see also General Adverse effects of macrolides (p. 197)

Interactions

- contraindicated with colchicine, midazolam and ticagrelor
- not recommended in daily doses > 1 g with HIV protease inhibitors
- simultaneous administration of clarithromycin tablets and zidovudine in patients with HIV infection may lead to decreased absorption of zidovudine
- serum levels may be increased by fluoxetine, fluconazole and ritonavir
- serum levels may be decreased by carbamazepine, efavirenz, etravirine, nevirapine, phenytoin, phenobarbital

(phenobarbitone), St John's wort, tolterodine, rifabutin and rifampicin
- may increase serum levels of rifabutin, tolterodine and colchicine
- increased risk of hypotension, lactic acidosis and bradyarrhythmias if given with verapamil
- if given with itraconazole, serum levels of both agents may be raised, increasing risk of toxicity
- caution if given with calcium-channel blocker due to the risk of acute kidney injury and hypotension
- significant hypoglycaemia may occur if given with insulin and/or oral hypoglycaemic agents including repaglinide
- caution if used with ototoxic agents such as aminoglycosides. Vestibular and auditory function should be monitored during and after therapy if given together
- see General Interactions of macrolides (p. 197)

Nursing points/Cautions

- (MAC prophylaxis) some authorities recommend delaying therapy until CD4 cell count < 50 cells/mm^3
- (suspension) contains sucrose, therefore not recommended in those with rare hereditary problems of fructose intolerance, glucose–galactose malabsorption or sucrase–isomaltase insufficiency and should be taken into consideration if patient has diabetes mellitus
- caution if used in those with severe kidney impairment
- see also General Nursing points/Cautions for macrolides (p. 198)

Patient teaching and advice

- advise patient that oral doses of clarithromycin should be separated from zidovudine by at least 2 hours to prevent decreased absorption of zidovudine
- if patient taking suspension has diabetes mellitus, they should be advised to monitor blood glucose levels due to sucrose levels
- see General Patient teaching and advice for macrolides (p. 198)

syrup/suspension is available. Tablet can be dispersed in 20 mL water or crushed and mixed with spoonful of yoghurt or apple puree

Note

- contained in Nexium HP7 for the eradication of *H. pylori*

ERYTHROMYCIN (Eryc)

ERYTHROMYCIN ETHYL SUCCINATE (EMycin)

ERYTHOMYCIN LACTOBIONATE (Erythrocin IV)

Available forms

Tablets: 400 mg; Capsules: 250 mg; Oral suspension: 200 mg/5 mL, 400 mg/5 mL; Vial: 1 g

Action/Use

- see General Actions and Uses of macrolides (p. 197)
- not active against strains of *Haemophilus influenzae* and staphylococci
- half-life 1.4 hours (prolonged in anuric patient to 6 hours)

Dose

- 250–400 mg orally 6-hourly 1 hour before meals or 500–800 mg 12-hourly 1 hour before meals (daily maximum 4 g) **OR**
- (severe infections) 15–20 mg/kg/day IV in divided doses (up to 4 g/day) **OR**
- (Legionnaire's disease) 0.8–1.6 g orally 6-hourly 1 hour before meals for 14 days **OR**

- (Legionnaire's disease) 1–4 g IV daily in divided doses **OR**
- (chlamydial or mycoplasma infection) 500 mg orally 8-hourly 1 hour before meals for 10 days, 800 mg orally 6-hourly for 7 days or 400 mg 6-hourly for 14 days **OR**
- (primary syphilis) total dose of 30–64 g orally given over 10–15 days in divided doses 1 hour before meals **OR**
- (streptococcal prophylaxis) 250–400 mg orally 1 hour before meals twice daily for 10 days **OR**
- (prophylaxis – endocarditis prophylaxis) 1–1.6 g orally 90 minutes–2 hours before dental or surgical procedure, then 500–800 mg 6-hourly 1 hour before meals for 6–8 doses **OR**
- (acute pelvic inflammatory disease) 500 mg IV 6-hourly for 3 days, then 250–400 mg orally 6-hourly 1 hour before meals for 7 days **OR**
- (acne vulgaris) 250–400 mg orally 1 hour before meals 4 times daily for 2 weeks, continued for 3 months, adjusting dose 4–6-weekly as necessary

Adverse effects

- visual impairment
- (rare) infantile hypertrophic pyloric stenosis
- see General Adverse effects of macrolides (p. 197)

Interactions

- may decrease clearance of zopiclone, increasing the sedative/hypnotic effects
- may antagonise effects of clindamycin, lincomycin, chloramphenicol, streptomycin, tetracyclines, colistin, penicillins and cephalosporins
- may interfere with urinary catecholamine determination
- see General Interactions of macrolides (p. 197)

Nursing points/Cautions

- transfer from IV route to oral as soon as possible
- (IV) reconstitute with 20 mL water for injections only and then dilute further with sodium chloride 0.9% or lactated Ringer's solution for IV administration at a rate of 1–5 mg/mL over 60 minutes
- administer alone
- should not be given as IV bolus to prevent high serum levels and risk of QT prolongation
- see also General Nursing points/Cautions for macrolides (p. 198)

Patient teaching and advice

- instruct patient that most oral preparations are taken 1 hour before or 2 hours after food to improve absorption; however, some preparations can be given before or with food so pharmacist should be consulted
- advise patient to swallow capsules and tablets whole, not broken, crushed or chewed
- instruct patient to seek medical advice immediately if any changes to vision occur
- (suspension) instruct patient to discard suspension 10 days after opening
- see General Patient teaching and advice for macrolides (p. 198)

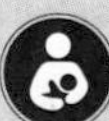

thought to be safe during pregnancy, but should only be used when needed

appears in breastmilk, therefore should be used with caution during breastfeeding

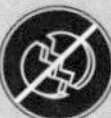

syrup/suspension is available. Tablet can be crushed or capsule opened and mixed with water or spoonful of yoghurt or apple puree; however, contents of capsule must not be chewed

ROXITHROMYCIN (Biaxsig, Roxar, Roximycin, Rulide, Rulide D)

Available forms

Tablets: 150 mg, 300 mg; Tablets (for suspension): 50 mg

Action

- see General Actions of macrolides (p. 197)
- shows activity against *H. influenzae* and *S. aureus* (not methicillin-resistant)
- long half-life (12 hours) (prolonged in the elderly or those with liver or kidney impairment)

Use

- see General Uses of macrolides (p. 197)

Dose

- 300 mg orally daily 1 hour before or 3 hours after food for 5–10 days **OR**
- (atypical pneumonia) 150 mg orally twice daily 1 hour before or 3 hours after food for 5–10 days

Adverse effects

- see General Adverse effects of macrolides (p. 197)

Interactions

- may increase serum levels of disopyramide, therefore ECG monitoring is recommended
- see General Interactions of macrolides (p. 197)

Nursing points/Cautions

- contraindicated in those with severe liver impairment
- see General Nursing points/Cautions for macrolides (p. 198)

Patient teaching and advice

- advise patient that tablets should be swallowed whole with fluid
- instruct parent/carer that Rulide D tablets:
  - are designed for use in children < 40 kg
  - should be added to 1–2 spoonfuls of water and allowed to dissolve for 30–40 seconds and then given to child to drink, followed by glass of water
- see General Patient teaching and advice for macrolides (p. 198)

available as tablet to make suspension (Rulide D) or other tablets can be crushed and mixed with spoonful of yoghurt or apple puree

LINCOSAMIDES

General Actions of lincosamides

- bind to bacterial ribosomal subunit 50S, inhibiting protein synthesis
- bacteriostatic but bactericidal at high doses with selected organisms

General Uses of lincosamides

- serious infections caused by streptococci, staphylococci, pneumococci and anaerobic bacteria, including infections of the bone and joints, pelvis, intra-abdominal area, skin and soft tissue, pneumonia, septicaemia
- reserved for infections where penicillin is inappropriate

General Adverse effects of lincosamides

- nausea, vomiting, diarrhoea, abdominal discomfort

- rash, urticaria, pruritus
- abnormal liver function
- eosinophilia
- pseudomembranous colitis,
- superinfection
- (rare) anaphylactoid reaction, thrombocytopenia, agranulocytosis, polyarthritis, jaundice, severe skin reactions
- (rapid IV administration) cardiac arrest, hypotension
- (IM site) pain, sterile abscess, induration, irritation
- (IV site) thrombophlebitis

General Interactions of lincosamides

- may enhance the action of neuromuscular blocking agents and therefore should not be given together
- use with erythromycin or chloramphenicol is not recommended
- increased risk of pseudomembranous colitis if given with peristalsis-delaying agents such as opioid analgesics and diphenoxylate/atropine combination

General Nursing points/Cautions for lincosamides

- cross-resistance exists between clindamycin, erythromycin and lincomycin, therefore a careful history is taken on admission to ascertain any previous allergic reactions
- blood counts, kidney and liver function should be monitored during prolonged therapy
- not to be given as an IV bolus because hypotension and cardiac arrest may occur
- not recommended for treatment of meningitis or non-bacterial infections
- caution if used in those with GI diseases (especially colitis, ulcerative colitis or regional enteritis) or severe kidney or liver impairment
- contraindicated in those with known hypersensitivity to lincomycin or clindamycin
- see also General Nursing points/Cautions for antibacterial agents (p. 148)

General Patient teaching and advice for lincosamides

- warn patients to seek medical advice immediately if any of the following occur:
  - unusual tiredness or weakness, bleeding or bruising easily
  - joint pains
  - severe skin reactions, including blistering and peeling
  - yellowing of skin or eyes, loss of appetite, nausea, upper abdominal pain, itchy skin, dark urine, pale stools (even if these occur weeks after stopping therapy)
- see General Patient teaching and advice for antibacterial agents (p. 149)

CLINDAMYCIN HYDROCHLORIDE (Calindamin, Clindamyk, ClindaTech, Dalacin C Capsules)

CLINDAMYCIN PHOSPHATE (Dalacin C Phosphate Injection, Dalacin T Topical Lotion, Dalacin V Cream 2%)

Available forms

Ampoules: 300 mg/2 mL, 600 mg/4 mL; Capsules: 150 mg; Topical solution: 10 mg/mL (1%); Vaginal cream: 20 mg/1 g (2%)

Action

- see General Actions of lincosamides (p. 203)

- semisynthetic derivative of lincomycin, therefore some cross-resistance between clindamycin and lincomycin but more effective
- clindamycin phosphate is hydrolysed in the skin to active clindamycin
- resistance to *P. acnes* has emerged
- half-life 2–3 hours

Use

- see General Uses of lincosamides (p. 203)
- acne vulgaris (where comedomes, papules and pustules predominate)
- bacterial vaginosis

Dose

- 150–450 mg orally 6-hourly **OR**
- (serious or complicated infections, intra-abdominal or female pelvic infection) 1.2–2.7 g IM in 2, 3 or 4 equally divided daily doses **OR**
- (serious or complicated infections, intra-abdominal or female pelvic infection) 1.2–2.7 g in 2, 3 or 4 equally divided daily doses infused IV at a rate not exceeding 30 mg/minute (over 10–60 minutes) **OR**
- (uncomplicated infections) 600–1200 mg IM or IV in 3–4 equally divided daily doses
- (bacterial vaginosis) 1 applicatorful (5 g) intravaginally nightly for 7 consecutive days **OR**
- (acne) apply thin film (using applicator if supplied) 1–2 times daily

Adverse effects

- (topical lotion) irritation, dry skin, peeling, pruritus, erythema, warm sensation, burning, dermatitis, diarrhoea
- (vaginal cream) irritation, itching, discharge
- eye irritation
- see also General Adverse effects of lincosamides (p. 203)

Interactions

- decreased serum levels may occur if given with rifampicin
- see also General Interactions of lincosamides (p. 204)

Nursing points/Cautions

- see General Nursing points/Cautions for lincosamides (p. 204)
- for beta-haemolytic streptococcal infections, treatment can be continued for 10 days minimum
- not more than 600 mg is given at a single IM site or not more than 1.2 g in a single 1-hour infusion
- (IV) should be diluted to concentration not greater than 12 mg/mL and infused at a rate not exceeding 30 mg/min
- (acne) therapy should be reviewed after 6–8 weeks for effectiveness
- (IV) incompatible with ampicillin, clindamycin, phenytoin, barbiturates, aminophylline, calcium gluconate, magnesium sulfate, ceftriaxone and ciprofloxacin
- caution if used in atopic individuals
- (topical) not recommended with other topical anti-acne preparations or topical preparations containing alcohol
- not recommended for meningitis as it does not diffuse adequately into CSF
- not recommended for severe and deep nodulocystic acne

Patient teaching and advice

- capsules should be given with a full glass of water to prevent oesophageal ulceration
- (acne) patient should be given the following instructions:
  - avoid contact with eyes, eyelids, mucous membranes, nasal folds or abraded skin or near mouth due to unpleasant taste
  - instruct patient to wash face with warm water and pH neutral soap, rinse and pat dry, ensuring all cosmetics are removed. Shave if necessary

  - after washing and shaving, wait 15 minutes before applying lotion
  - shake bottle well before use
  - apply lotion to face (using applicator if provided)
  - do not use lotion more than 1–2 times daily (as per instructions). Greater use does not improve outcome and causes skin drying
  - wash hands well after application
  - acne may initially worsen when starting treatment and take 8–12 weeks before full improvement is seen. Advise patient to seek medical advice if there is no improvement in 6 weeks
- patient should be instructed in the correct technique for insertion of intravaginal cream, including:
  1. wash hands before and after application
  2. remove cap from cream and screw applicator to tube, squeeze cream from base of tube to force cream into applicator
  3. choose comfortable position for insertion, remembering that cream should be inserted as high as possible into vagina
  4. part lips of vagina with finger of one hand and grasp applicator between thumb and middle finger of other hand. Insert (open end first) into vagina as deeply as possible
  5. slowly push plunger in until it stops and then carefully withdraw applicator
  6. use new applicator (disposable) for each dose
- (vaginal cream) counsel patient not to use condom or vaginal contraceptive device with or within 72 hours of finishing therapy because cream may weaken latex or rubber
- (vaginosis) advise patient to avoid vaginal intercourse or use vaginal products (such as tampons) during therapy
- see General Patient teaching and advice for lincosamides (p. 204)

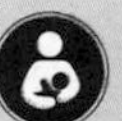

use during pregnancy only if potential benefits outweigh risks

not recommended during breastfeeding

capsules can be opened and mixed with 10 mL water or contents mixed with spoonful of yoghurt or apple puree

Note

- contained in Duac Once Daily Gel with benzoyl peroxide and Acnatac topical gel with tretinoin

LINCOMYCIN HYDROCHLORIDE MONOHYDRATE (LINCOMYCIN HYDROCHLORIDE) (Lincocin)

Available form

Ampoules: 300 mg/mL

Action

- see General Actions of lincosamides (p. 203)
- not active against most strains of *Enterococcus faecalis*, *N. gonorrhoeae*, *N. meningitides*, *H. influenza* or other Gram-negative organisms
- half-life 4.4–6.4 hours

Use

- see General Uses of lincosamides (p. 203)

Dose

- 600 mg IM daily (or 12-hourly for more serious infections) **OR**
- 600 mg–1 g by IV infusion over at least 1 hour 8–12-hourly

Adverse effects/Interactions/Nursing points/Cautions/Patient teaching and advice

- see General Adverse effects/Interaction/Nursing points/Cautions/Patient

teaching and advice for lincosamides (pp. 203–04)
- maximum recommended daily dose 8 g
- for beta-haemolytic streptococcal infections, therapy should be continued for at least 10 days to decrease risk of subsequent rheumatic fever or glomerulonephritis
- (IV) diluted with 100–400 mL or more of glucose 5% or sodium chloride 0.9% and infuse over 1–4 hours (depending on dose)
- incompatible with erythromycin and phenytoin
- contains benzyl alcohol, therefore contraindicated in newborns

OTHER MISCELLANEOUS INHIBITORS OF BACTERIAL PROTEIN SYNTHESIS

CHLORAMPHENICOL (Chloromycetin Ear Drops, Eye Drops and Eye Ointment, Chloromycetin Succinate, Chlorsig, Minims Chloramphenicol 0.5% Eye Drops)

Available forms

Vial: 1 g; Ear/Eye drops: 0.5%; Eye ointment: 1%

Action

- potent inhibitor of protein synthesis by binding to bacterial 50S ribosomal subunit
- bacteriostatic
- broad spectrum antibacterial and anti-rickettsial antibiotic
- chloramphenicol succinate is hydrolysed to active chloramphenicol in the liver
- half-life 1.6–3.3 hours
- development of resistance appears to be low

Use

- serious infections (e.g. bacterial meningitis, typhoid fever, rickettsial infections, septicaemia)
- intraocular infections, bacterial conjunctivitis
- otitis externa, chronic suppurative otitis media

Dose

- (serious infections) 50 mg/kg/day IV or IM divided into 6-hourly doses, increasing to 100 mg/kg/day for septicaemia, meningitis or infections due to resistant organisms **OR**
- (intraocular infections, bacterial conjunctivitis) 1–2 drops to affected eye(s) 2–6-hourly for 2–3 days **OR**
- (intraocular infections, bacterial conjunctivitis) 1.5 cm ointment to affected eye(s) 3-hourly, or 1.5 cm nightly if used concurrently with drops **OR**
- (otitis externa, chronic suppurative otitis media) 4 drops to affected ear(s) 4 times daily

Adverse effects

- bone marrow depression, blood dyscrasias, aplastic anaemia
- fever
- delirium, confusion, depression
- nausea, vomiting, glossitis, stomatitis, diarrhoea
- rash, urticaria, angioedema
- peripheral neuritis, optic neuritis
- pseudomembranous colitis, superinfection
- (ear drops) itching, burning sensation

- (eye drops, ointment) redness, itching, swelling, burning sensation, delayed corneal ulcer healing

Interactions

- not recommended during active immunisation
- not recommended with other agents that cause bone marrow depression or aplastic anaemia
- not recommended with agents that delay peristalsis due to the risk of pseudomembranous colitis
- caution if used with erythromycin, lincomycin or clindamycin
- may decrease clearance and prolong duration of action of alfentanil if chloramphenicol is used preoperatively or perioperatively
- may reduce efficacy of oral contraceptive containing oestrogen
- metabolism may be increased by rifampicin and phenobarbitone
- may increase serum level of tacrolimus increasing risk of toxicity

Nursing points/Cautions

- blood counts should be measured before starting and regularly throughout therapy
- plasma chloramphenicol levels should be monitored in those with severe kidney impairment or premature/full term neonates with immature metabolic processes
- (IV) not recommended for prophylaxis
- (IV) to reconstitute, add 2.5–10 mL of water for injections, sodium chloride 0.9% or glucose 5% (see manufacturer's instructions) to vial and swirl gently to dissolve
- (IV) prolonged use may cause haemolytic anaemia in those with glucose-6-phosphate dehydrogenase (G6PD) deficiency and should only be used with great caution
- eye drops should be continued for 2 days after symptoms resolve, but therapy duration should not be longer than 5 days
- caution if used in those with chronic suppurative otitis media
- caution if used in those with pre-existing haematological disorders
- (ear drops) contraindicated if patient has perforated tympanic membrane
- (eye preparations) not recommended in those with photophobia, severe eye pain or swelling, decreased or blurred vision, restricted eye movement, cloudy cornea, copious purulent discharge, eye injury (including after recent welding without eye protection), abnormal pupils, eye surgery or laser treatment in last 6 months, glaucoma, dry eyes or suspected foreign body present. Patient should be advised to see doctor or ophthalmologist
- not recommended in neonates due to risk of 'grey baby syndrome' (see glossary)
- contraindicated if hypersensitivity to chloramphenicol exists

Patient teaching and advice

- patient should be advised to immediately seek medical advice if any of the following occur:
  - diarrhoea
  - unusual tiredness, weakness, bleeding or bruising more easily than normal
  - eye pain, blurred vision or blind spots
  - numbness, tingling or weakness in the extremities
- instruct patient to discard ear drops, eye drops and ointment 4 weeks after opening
- ensure patient has instructions on correct technique for instilling eye drops (p. 189), eye ointment (p. 192) and ear drops (p. 188)
- (eye infection) advise patient to seek medical advice immediately if

symptoms worsen or if symptoms have not improved in 48 hours and not to use drops for longer than 5 days
- (eye infection) if patient wears contact lenses, advise patient to not insert lenses during or for 24 hours after stopping therapy
- female patients of childbearing potential should be warned that oral contraceptives containing oestrogen may lose their efficacy during therapy with chloramphenicol and another form of contraception should be used to prevent pregnancy
- see also General Patient teaching and advice for antibacterial agents (p. 149)

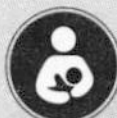

not recommended in week before birth is expected due to risk of 'grey baby syndrome' (see Glossary) which includes hypothermia and cyanosis

not recommended during breastfeeding

FUSIDIC ACID HEMIHYDRATE (SODIUM FUSIDATE) (Fucidin, Fucidin Topical)

Available form
Tablets: 250 mg; Topical ointment: 2%

Action
- inhibits protein synthesis by preventing translocation on ribosome
- bactericidal
- no activity against Gram-negative organisms or fungi

Use
- staphylococcal infections, including skin lesions (e.g. boils, impetigo, folliculitis)

Dose
- 250–500 mg orally 2–3 times daily for 5–10 days **OR**
- (skin lesions) apply thin film 2–3 times daily (without dressing) or daily if covered with protective dressing for 7 days

Adverse effects
- nausea, vomiting, dyspepsia, diarrhoea, flatulence, abdominal pain
- headache, lethargy, fatigue, asthenia
- urticaria
- (uncommon) elevated liver enzymes
- (topical) mild irritation, burning sensation, rash, urticaria, pruritus, redness
- (rare) jaundice, hypersensitivity, rash, pruritus, blood dyscrasias, serious skin reactions

Interactions
- contraindicated with or within 7 days of statins (lipid-lowering agents) due to increased risk of rhabdomyolysis, muscle weakness and pain
- caution if given with saquinavir, ritonavir or other HIV protease inhibitors due to risk of hepatoxicity

Nursing points/Cautions
- regular liver function tests are recommended for prolonged or high-dose therapy or in patients with pre-existing liver disease
- caution if used in those with liver impairment or biliary disease/obstruction
- tablets contain lactose, therefore are not recommended in those with rare hereditary problems of galactose intolerance, Lapp lactase deficiency or glucose–galactose malabsorption
- see also General Nursing points/Cautions for antibacterial agents (p. 148)

Patient teaching and advice
- patients should be warned to avoid driving or operating machinery if dizziness or blurred vision are ongoing problems

- (topical) warn patient to avoid contact with eyes
- see also General Patient teaching and advice for antibacterial agents (p. 149)

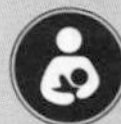

may cause neonatal kernicterus by displacing bilirubin from plasma albumin, therefore should be avoided during last weeks of pregnancy

secreted in breastmilk, therefore should be used with great caution during breastfeeding

tablet can be crushed and mixed with water or spoonful of yoghurt or apple puree

LINEZOLID (Linevox, Zyvox)

Available forms

Infusion solution: 2 mg/mL; Tablets: 600 mg; Oral suspension: 20 mg/mL

Action

- oxazolidinone which selectively inhibits bacterial protein synthesis by binding to a different ribosomal subunit (proximal to 50S subunit) than other antibacterial agents. Because site of action is different to other antibacterial agents, likelihood of cross-resistance is decreased
- active against Gram-positive aerobic and some anaerobic organisms, and some Gram-negative organisms
- not active against *Haemophilus influenzae*, *Neisseria* spp., *Enterobacteriaceae* or *Pseudomonas aeruginosa*
- combination therapy may be necessary if there is a concurrent Gram-negative organism
- well absorbed orally
- half-life 5–7 hours

Use

- serious infections due to Gram-positive organisms where other antibacterial agents are contraindicated or not appropriate because of resistance

Dose

- (community-acquired pneumonia, nosocomial pneumonia) 600 mg orally or IV infusion twice daily for 10–14 days **OR**
- (skin and soft tissue infections) 400–600 mg orally or 600 mg IV infusion twice daily for 10–14 days **OR**
- (enterococcal infections) 600 mg IV infusion or orally twice daily for 14–28 days

Adverse effects

- headache
- diarrhoea, nausea, vomiting, altered taste
- abnormal liver function
- myelosuppression, including thrombocytopenia, anaemia, leucopenia, neutropenia, eosinophilia
- superinfection
- pseudomembranous colitis
- (rare) peripheral and optic neuropathy, convulsions, lactic acidosis, tongue and/or tooth discolouration

Interactions

- contraindicated with or within 2 weeks of MAO inhibitors A or B
- caution if given with other myelosuppressive agents
- increased risk of pseudomembranous colitis if given with peristalsis-delaying agents, such as opioid analgesics or diphenoxylate/atropine combination
- not recommended with directly or indirectly acting sympathomimetic agents (e.g. pseudoephedrine), vasopressor agents (e.g. adrenaline (epinephrine), noradrenaline) or dopaminergic agents (e.g. dopamine, dobutamine)
- not recommended with serotonergic agents (e.g. SSRIs, TCAs, pethidine,

5HT1 receptor agonists) because of risk of serotonin syndrome

Nursing points/Cautions

- blood pressure should be monitored regularly throughout therapy
- visual function (e.g. visual acuity, colour vision, visual field) should be monitored if therapy is prolonged (greater than 12 weeks)
- monitoring of blood counts weekly is recommended if therapy extends beyond 14 days (especially in those with pre-existing myelosuppression, taking other myelosuppressive agents or have chronic previously treated infection)
- therapy duration should not exceed 28 days
- (IV) administer alone
- IV infusion over 30–120 minutes
- infusion should be kept in foil wrapping and carton until just before use
- discoloured or hazy solution should be discarded
- reconstituted oral suspension should be stored in outer container and gently inverted (not shaken) before use
- IV solution is incompatible with amphotericin B (amphotericin), chlorpromazine, sulfamethoxazole/trimethoprim, pentamidine, diazepam, erythromycin, phenytoin and ceftriaxone
- not recommended for treatment of CVC-related bloodstream infections
- not recommended in those with uncontrolled hypertension, phaeochromocytoma or thyrotoxicosis unless blood pressure can be carefully monitored during therapy
- caution if given to those with pre-existing myelosuppression, GI disorders (especially colitis), epilepsy, kidney and liver insufficiency
- see also General Nursing points/Cautions for antibacterial agents (p. 148)

Patient teaching and advice

- instruct patient to seek medical advice immediately if any of the following occurs:
  - any visual impairment, such as blurred vision or changes to colour vision
  - recurrent nausea and vomiting (may be first signs of lactic acidosis)
  - tiredness, paleness, headache, shortness of breath on exercising
  - fever, chills, sore throat, mouth ulcers
  - unusual bleeding or bruising
  - numbness, weakness or tingling in extremities
  - extreme fever, shivering, lack of coordination, dizziness, confusion
  - changes to colour of teeth or tongue
- (oral suspension) instruct patient not to shake bottle. To mix suspension before use, advise patient to invert bottle gently several times
- see also General Patient teaching and advice for antibacterial agents (p. 149)

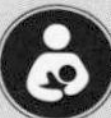

recommended during pregnancy or breastfeeding only if clearly needed and potential benefits outweigh risks

syrup/suspension is available. Tablet can be crushed and mixed with water or spoonful of yoghurt or apple puree

MUPIROCIN CALCIUM (Bactroban, Bactroban Nasal Ointment)

Available forms

Cream: 20 mg/g; Ointment: 20 mg/g; Nasal ointment: 20 mg/g

Action
- inhibits bacterial protein synthesis by binding to bacterial transfer RNA synthetase
- mainly active against Gram-positive aerobes, including *Staphylococcus* spp. and *Streptococcus* spp.
- no cross-resistance with other antibacterial agents

Use
- topical treatment of mild impetigo (ointment) and infected skin lesions (cream)
- elimination of nasal carriage of *Staphylococcus*, including MRSA

Dose
- apply to affected area 3 times daily (cover with gauze dressing if desired) for up to 10 days **OR**
- apply to inside of each nostril 2–3 times daily for no more than 10 days

Adverse effects
- (nasal) irritation, tingling, burning, itching, rhinitis, stinging, soreness, pain over the maxilla, post-nasal drip, sinusitis, conjunctivitis
- itching, burning, erythema, stinging, pain, swelling, dryness
- nausea, headache, diarrhoea
- (rare) superinfection, anaphylaxis, hypersensitivity

Interaction
- not recommended with other topical preparations

Nursing points/Cautions
- not suitable for application to cannulation site
- not suitable for eyes or other mucous membranes
- (Bactroban) not recommended for application to large surface areas because of polyethylene glycol (preservative) content (especially in those with moderate-to-severe kidney impairment)

Patient teaching and advice
- advise patient to avoid contact with eyes and mucous membranes and wash area well with water if contact occurs
- instruct patient that only specially formulated nasal ointment should be put into the nose
- instruct patient that an amount of nasal ointment the size of a match head should be placed on a swab or on the little finger and applied to the inside of each nostril and spread by pressing the sides of the nose together

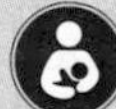

only used during pregnancy if clearly needed

if used on cracked nipples during breastfeeding, nipples should be washed well before breastfeeding

INHIBITORS OF DNA SYNTHESIS

QUINOLONES (ALSO KNOWN AS FLUOROQUINOLONES)

General Actions of quinolones
- inhibit bacterial DNA synthesis by interfering with enzymes involved in supercoiling DNA needed for duplication, transcription and repair of bacterial DNA
- bactericidal
- increasing bacterial resistance with cross-resistance existing between quinolones

General Uses of quinolones

- respiratory tract infections, including mild-to-moderate community-acquired pneumonia, acute exacerbation of chronic bronchitis, acute sinusitis, Legionnaire's disease
- severe complicated skin and skin structure infections, bone and joint infections
- complicated urinary tract infections, gonorrhoeal urethritis and cervicitis, chronic bacterial prostatitis, epididymo-orchitis
- shigellosis, traveller's diarrhoea, gastroenteritis
- septicaemia
- post-exposure inhalation anthrax

General Adverse effects of quinolones

- nausea, vomiting, diarrhoea, bad taste, dyspepsia, gastric irritation, abdominal pain, flatulence, dry mouth
- headache, dizziness, weakness, fatigue, drowsiness, nervousness, tremor, restlessness, light-headedness, agitation, insomnia, somnolence, depression
- rash, pruritus, urticaria
- fever
- photosensitivity
- eosinophilia
- pain, inflammation or rupture of tendon
- transient increase in liver enzymes, increased bilirubin
- crystalluria
- visual disturbances
- (IV) thrombophlebitis, burning pain, pruritus, erythema
- (rare) pseudomembranous colitis, hypersensitivity, superinfection, anaphylaxis, anaphylactoid reaction
- (rare) hallucinations, confusion, seizures, psychoses, suicidal ideation
- (rare) interstitial nephritis, blood dyscrasias, haemolytic anaemia, QT prolongation, peripheral neuropathy

General Interactions of quinolones

- caution if given with agents known to prolong QT interval, such as class IA and III antiarrhythmic agents, antipsychotics, antidepressants, antifungals, fluoroquinolones or agents that cause electrolyte disturbance (e.g. diuretics), especially hypokalaemia and hypomagnesaemia
- may increase theophylline levels, thereby increasing risk of theophylline toxicity
- renal clearance may be decreased if given with probenecid
- may prolong half-life of caffeine
- may enhance effects of warfarin, therefore INR should be closely monitored especially when starting or stopping therapy
- metoclopramide may accelerate absorption of quinolones
- quinolones (high dose) and some NSAIDs (not aspirin) may increase risk of CNS stimulation and seizures if given together
- iron, sucralfate, highly buffered drugs (e.g. antiretroviral agents) and antacids containing magnesium, aluminium or calcium interfere with quinolone absorption
- increased risk of pseudomembranous colitis if given with peristaltic-delaying agents such as opioid analgesics and diphenoxylate/atropine combination
- increased risk of tendon rupture if given with corticosteroids
- if given with ciclosporin, may cause a transient increase in serum creatinine

General Nursing points/Cautions for quinolones

- see General Nursing points/cautions for antibacterial agents (p. 148)
- before starting therapy, a careful history should be taken to exclude hypokalaemia or any family history of QT prolongation
- patient should be well hydrated and have good urine output throughout therapy to prevent crystalluria
- blood counts, renal and liver function should be monitored during prolonged therapy
- anaphylactoid reactions have occurred with quinolones (sometimes after the first dose), therefore patients should be closely observed, even if there is no known history of allergy
- all patients with gonorrhoea should also have serological testing for syphilis at time of diagnosis and then monthly for 4 months
- IV solution should be administered alone
- caution if used in those with epilepsy (as seizure threshold may be lowered), reduced brain flow, altered brain structure or stroke
- used with great caution in patients with myasthenia gravis because symptoms may be exacerbated
- caution if used in those with positive family history of aneurysm disease, or those with pre-existing aortic aneurysms and/or dissection, or with risk factors for aortic aneurysm and dissection
- caution if used in those with glucose-6-phosphate dehydrogenase (G6PD) deficiency because of increased risk of haemolytic anaemia
- caution if used in those with liver or renal impairment
- caution if used in those who have experienced quinolone-associated tendon rupture, are over 60 years of age and/or taking corticosteroids concurrently as there is an increased risk of tendon rupture. Young athletes undertaking extensive training are also at increased risk
- contraindicated in those with known hypersensitivity to quinolones

General Patient teaching and advice for quinolones

- see also General Patient teaching and advice for antibacterial agents (p. 149)
- advise patient that oral doses should be given 2 hours before or 2 hours after dietary supplements containing zinc, magnesium and iron or iron sulfate, and 2 hours before or 4 hours after antacids containing calcium, aluminium or magnesium
- instruct patient to drink sufficient fluids to maintain adequate hydration and urinary output to avoid crystalluria
- warn patient to avoid exposure to direct sunlight, wear protective clothing while outdoors and use a suitable sunscreen
- caution patients against driving or working in situations requiring mental alertness and coordination or operating machinery if any adverse effects such as dizziness, drowsiness or confusion occur
- patients should be advised to seek medical advice if any of the following occur:
  - pain, inflammation or suspected rupture of a tendon which may

occur within 48 hours of starting or up to 6 months after stopping therapy. Patient should also be advised to rest, refrain from exercising and stop therapy
  - pain, weakness, burning, tingling or numbness
  - rapid or irregular heart rate
  - fitting
  - depression, changes in mood, self-harming behaviours
- women using oral contraceptives should be counselled to use a barrier method during quinolone therapy and for 7 days thereafter

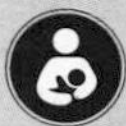

not recommended during pregnancy or breastfeeding

CIPROFLOXACIN HYDROCHLORIDE (CFlox, Cifran, CiloQuin, Ciloxan, Ciloxan Ear Drops, Ciprol)

CIPROFLOXACIN LACTATE (Aspen Ciprofloxacin Injection for Intravenous Infusion)

Available forms

Infusion solution: 100 mg/50 mL, 200 mg/100 mL, 400 mg/200 mL; Tablets: 250 mg, 500 mg, 750 mg; Eye/Ear drops: 0.3% (3 mg/mL)

Action

- see General Actions of quinolones (p. 212)
- Gram-negative organisms are more sensitive to ciprofloxacin than Gram-positive organisms
- resistance to ciprofloxacin occurs in a significant number of those with cystic fibrosis who have *P. aeruginosa* infections. This can occur after a single course
- metabolites have some antibacterial activity
- half-life about 4 hours

Use

- infected corneal ulcer (bacterial keratitis), bacterial conjunctivitis
- chronic suppurative otitis media
- see General Uses of quinolones (p. 213)

Dose

- (severe or complicated urinary tract, moderate lower respiratory tract infection) 200 mg by IV infusion over 60 minutes 12-hourly **OR**
- (severe lower respiratory tract infection; skin, skin structure, blood, bone or joint infection) 300 mg by IV infusion over 60 minutes 12-hourly **OR**
- (post-exposure to inhalation of anthrax) 400 mg by IV infusion over 60 minutes 12-hourly for 60 days, starting as soon as possible after exposure **OR**
- (post-exposure to inhalation of anthrax) 500 mg orally 12-hourly for 60 days, starting as soon as possible after exposure **OR**
- (bronchial, skin, bone or joint infection) 500–750 mg orally 12-hourly **OR**
- (chronic bacterial prostatitis) 250–500 mg orally 12-hourly for 14–28 days **OR**
- (urinary tract infection) 250–500 mg orally 12-hourly **OR**
- (acute uncomplicated gonorrhoeal urethritis) 250 mg as single oral dose **OR**
- (gastroenteritis) 500 mg orally 12-hourly for 5 days
- (corneal ulcers) 2 drops to affected eye(s) every 15 minutes for 6 hours, then 2 drops every 30 minutes for remainder of day 1, then 2 drops hourly for day 2, then 2 drops 4-hourly days 3–14 **OR**

- (bacterial conjunctivitis) 1 drop into conjunctival sac(s) 2-hourly for 2 days (while awake), then 1 drop 4-hourly for next 5 days **OR**
- 5 drops to affected ear(s) twice daily for 9 days

Adverse effects

- (ear drops) ear pain, stinging, ear pruritis, bitter taste, transient dizziness, headache, vertigo
- (eye drops) discomfort, foreign body sensation, white precipitate, itching, redness, bitter taste
- see also General Adverse effects of quinolones (p. 213)

Interactions

- hypoglycaemia may occur when given with sulfonylureas (e.g. glibenclamide)
- serum levels may be decreased by omeprazole
- may increase or decrease serum levels of phenytoin, therefore levels should be monitored during therapy with ciprofloxacin
- may increase serum levels of methotrexate increasing risk of toxicity, therefore close monitoring is recommended
- may increase serum levels of sildenafil leading to adverse effects
- may increase serum levels of agomelatine and zolpidem and are therefore not recommended together
- may decrease clearance of lidocaine (lignocaine)
- may increase serum levels of duloxetine, clozapine, olanzapine and ropinirole
- may interfere with *Mycobacterium* spp. culture causing false-negative result
- see also General Interactions of quinolones (p. 213)

Nursing points/Cautions

- patient should be well hydrated before starting IV therapy and alkaline urine should be avoided to decrease likelihood of crystalluria occurring
- treatment is usually for 7–14 days, continued for 2 days after fever and symptoms have resolved; bone/joint infections may require 4–6 weeks treatment and chronic bacterial prostatitis 14–28 days
- IV route should only be used when oral route is contraindicated. Changing from IV to oral is recommended as soon as practicable to avoid toxicity
- IV cannula should not be positioned in small veins of the hand to avoid local site reactions
- (IV) incompatible with alkaline solutions, penicillins and heparin
- IV solution will precipitate at cool temperatures and therefore should not be refrigerated. Precipitate will dissolve at room temperature
- (Ciproxin IV, Ciprofloxacin Alphapharm) because of sodium content (154 mmol sodium/L), caution if used in those where sodium load may be important (e.g. congestive cardiac failure, renal failure)
- (Aspen Ciprofloxacin Injection) contains 55 mg glucose/mL which may impact on blood glucose levels of patients with diabetes mellitus
- not recommended for pneumococcal infections
- not recommended in prepubertal children (except for post-exposure of anthrax inhalation) due to risk of cartilage erosion in weight-bearing joints
- see General Nursing points/Cautions for quinolones (p. 214)

Patient teaching and advice

- instruct patient on correct technique for insertion of ear drops (p. 188)
- (ear drops) if ear drops are cold, advise patient to warm in hands for 1–2 minutes before instillation
- instruct patient on correct technique for insertion of eye drops (p. 189)

- (eye drops) advise patient to discard eye drops 14 days after opening
- (eye drops) if patient wears soft contact lenses, warn him/her not to insert lenses during therapy as eye drops contain benzalkonium chloride (preservative) which discolour soft contact lenses and can cause eye reaction
- see General Patient teaching and advice for quinolones (p. 214)

tablet can be crushed and mixed with water or spoonful of apple puree. Should not be given with yoghurt or milk-based products

Note

- contained with hydrocortisone in Ciproxin HC Ear Drops

MOXIFLOXACIN HYDROCHLORIDE (Avelox)

Available forms

Tablets: 400 mg; IV solution: 400 mg/250 mL

Action

- see General Actions of quinolones (p. 212)

Use

- see General Uses of quinolones (p. 213)

Dose

- (acute sinusitis) 400 mg orally daily for 10 days **OR**
- (acute bacterial exacerbation of chronic bronchitis) 400 mg orally or IV infusion over 60 minutes for 5 days **OR**
- (community-acquired pneumonia) 400 mg orally or IV infusion over 60 minutes for 10 days (oral) or 7–14 days (sequential IV and oral therapy) **OR**
- (major skin or skin structure infection) 400 mg (sequential IV and oral therapy) for 7–21 days

Adverse effects

- see General Adverse effects of quinolones (p. 213)

Interactions

- see General Interactions of quinolones (p. 213)

Nursing points/Cautions

- IV infusion should be given over 60 minutes and NEVER as a bolus injection
- administer alone
- do not refrigerate IV solution as precipitate will occur
- because of sodium content (34 mmol sodium per 250 mL) caution if used in those where sodium load may be important (e.g. congestive cardiac failure, renal failure)
- no dose adjustment is necessary when changing from IV to oral
- incompatible with sodium chloride 10% or 20% or sodium hydrogen carbonate 4.2% or 8.4%
- see General Nursing points/Cautions for quinolones (p. 214)

Patient teaching and advice

- instruct patient to swallow tablets whole
- see also General Patient teaching and advice for quinolones (p. 214)

tablet can be crushed (very bitter taste) and mixed with water or spoonful of yoghurt or apple puree

NORFLOXACIN (Nufloxib, Roxin)

Available form

Tablets: 400 mg

Action
- see General Actions of quinolones (p. 212)
- broad spectrum
- active metabolites have less antibacterial activity than norfloxacin
- half-life 3–4 hours

Use
- see General Uses of quinolones (p. 213)

Dose
- (urinary tract infection) 400 mg orally twice daily 1 hour before or 2 hours after food for 7–10 days or 3 days (uncomplicated urinary tract infection) **OR**
- (suppression of chronic recurrent urinary tract infection) 400 mg orally twice daily 1 hour before or 2 hours after food for 4–12 weeks **OR**
- (shigellosis, traveller's diarrhoea) 400 mg orally twice daily 1 hour before or 2 hours after food for 5 days

Interactions
- antibacterial action may be antagonised by nitrofurantoin and therefore should not be given together

Adverse effects/Nursing points/Cautions/Patient teaching and advice
- see General Adverse effects/Nursing points/Cautions/Patient teaching and advice for quinolones (pp. 213–14)

tablet can be crushed (very bitter taste) and mixed with water or apple puree. Should not be given with yoghurt or milk-based products

OFLOXACIN (Ocuflox)

Available form
Eye drops: 3 mg/mL (0.3%)

Action
- see General Actions of quinolones (p. 212)

Use
- infected corneal ulcer (bacterial keratitis), bacterial conjunctivitis

Dose
- (corneal ulcers) 1–2 drops to affected eye(s) every 30 minutes while awake and 1–2 drops 4 hours after going to bed and again 2 hours later (days 1–2), 1–2 drops hourly while awake (days 3–7) and then 1–2 drops 4 times daily until ulcer has healed (usually 21 days) **OR**
- (bacterial conjunctivitis) 1 drop 4-hourly to affected eye(s) for 2 days, then 1 drop 6-hourly for up to 8 days

Adverse effects
- corneal precipitates and perforation (in those with pre-existing corneal ulcer or defect)
- burning, stinging, tearing, itching, foreign body sensation, photophobia, blurred vision, eye pain, dry eyes, eye/periorbital/facial oedema
- nausea
- dizziness

Nursing points/Cautions/Patient teaching and advice
- instruct patient on correct technique for insertion of eye drops (p. 189)
- (eye drops) advise patient to discard eye drops 14 days after opening
- (eye drops) if patient wears soft contact lenses, warn him/her not to insert lenses during therapy as eye drops contain benzalkonium chloride (preservative) which discolour soft contact lenses and can cause eye reaction

DISRUPTING BACTERIAL CELL MEMBRANE

COLISTIMETHATE SODIUM (Polymyxin E, also called Colistin) (Colistin Link, Tadim)

Available form

Vial: 150 mg; Powder (for nebulisation): 1 million IU

Action

- polypeptide that attaches to the bacterial cell membranes altering its permeability causing disruption and lysis
- bactericidal
- not recommended for infections due to *Proteus* spp. or *Neisseria* spp.
- half-life 1.5 hours (IV), prolonged to 2–4.8 hours in those with cystic fibrosis
- 1 million IU = 80 mg

Use

- infections (acute or chronic) due to *Acinetobacter* spp., *Klebsiella* spp., *Escherichia coli*, and *Pseudomonas aeruginosa*
- colonisation and lung infection due to *P. aeruginosa* in those with cystic fibrosis

Dose

- 2.5–5 mg/kg daily IM in 2–4 divided doses **OR**
- 1/2 of total daily dose (2.5–5 mg/kg/day) slowly IV over 3–5 minutes 12-hourly **OR**
- 1/2 of total daily dose (2.5–5 mg/kg/day) slowly IV over 3–5 minutes, then 1–2 hours later, remaining 1/2 of total daily dose by IV infusion at 5–6 mg/hour **OR**
- (cystic fibrosis – initial colonisation) 2 million IU via nebuliser twice daily for 3 weeks (with oral/parental antibiotics) **OR**
- (cystic fibrosis – frequent, recurrent infections) up to 2 million IU via nebuliser 3 times daily for up to 12 weeks (with oral/parental antibiotics) **OR**
- (cystic fibrosis – chronic colonisation) 1–2 million IU via nebuliser twice daily (with oral/parental antibiotics for acute exacerbations)

Adverse effects

- (transient neurological disturbance) paraesthesia or numbness, vertigo, slurring of speech, tingling or formication of extremities, dizziness, visual disturbances, confusion, psychoses
- generalised pruritus, itching, urticaria
- oliguria, increased serum creatinine, increased blood urea nitrogen (signs of nephrotoxicity)
- (nebulisation) coughing, bronchospasm, chest tightness, sore mouth and/or throat
- (IM) respiratory arrest
- (rare) hypersensitivity, superinfection

Interactions

- neuromuscular blockade may be potentiated if given with non-depolarising muscle relaxants and should be used with extreme caution
- use with neomycin, polymyxin, streptomycin and kanamycin is not recommended due to increased risk of interference of nerve transmission at the neuromuscular junction
- caution if used with other nephrotoxic or neurotoxic agents
- increased risk of nephrotoxicity if given with cefalotin

Nursing points/Cautions

- patients should be carefully monitored for any signs of decreasing renal function (e.g. decreased urine output, increasing serum creatinine, increasing blood urea nitrogen)

- decreasing dose may alleviate symptoms of transient neurological disturbance
- (IV) 150 mg vial reconstituted with 2 mL of water for injections, giving a concentration of 75 mg/mL
- (IV) swirl gently to avoid frothing during reconstitution
- IV dose should not exceed 5 mg/kg/day
- (IV infusion) solution can be diluted with sodium chloride 0.9%, glucose 5%, lactated Ringer's solution or glucose 5% in sodium chloride 0.45%
- (cystic fibrosis) sputum cultures to confirm colonisation with sensitive *P. aeruginosa* is recommended before starting therapy
- (cystic fibrosis) first dose should be administered via nebuliser under medical supervision observing for bronchospasm or bronchial hyperactivity by measuring FEV1 before and after dose
- (cystic fibrosis) I-neb AAD system is recommended for efficient nebulisation
- (cystic fibrosis) pre-dosing with bronchodilator is recommended
- (cystic fibrosis) if used with other therapies, should be used after physiotherapy and any other inhaled therapies
- (nebulisation) reconstitute powder with water for injections
- caution if used in those with impaired renal function or porphyria
- not recommended in those with myasthenia gravis

Patient teaching and advice

- caution patient against driving or operating machinery if dizziness, vertigo or visual disturbances occur
- advise patients to seek medical advice immediately if any of the following occur:
  - slurred speech, numbness, weakness or tingling of extremities, vertigo, dizziness
  - decreased urine output
- (cystic fibrosis) instruct patient to complete chest physiotherapy and/or inhaled therapy before using colistimethate
- see General Patient teaching and advice for antibacterial agents (p. 149)

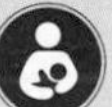

safety during pregnancy has not been established, therefore should be used with caution

not recommended during breastfeeding

OTHER ANTIBACTERIAL AGENTS

CO-TRIMOXAZOLE (TRIMETHOPRIM WITH SULFAMETHOXAZOLE) (Bactrim DS, Resprim, Resprim Forte, Septrin Forte, Septrin Sugar Free Oral Suspension)

Available forms

Ampoules: 400 mg sulfamethoxazole/80 mg trimethoprim/5 mL; Tablets (DS/Forte): 800 mg sulfamethoxazole/160 mg trimethoprim; Tablets: 400 mg sulfamethoxazole/80 mg trimethoprim; Oral suspension: 200 mg sulfamethoxazole/40 mg trimethoprim/5 mL

Action

- combination is bactericidal because it blocks two consecutive steps in bacterial folate metabolism, resulting in an inability to synthesise nucleic acids

- sulfamethoxazole and other sulfonamides block the conversion of para-aminobenzoic acid (PABA) to the co-enzyme dihydrofolic acid, whereas trimethoprim inhibits the enzyme dihydrofolate reductase, which converts dihydrofolic acid to tetrahydrofolic acid
- combination should not be used if organism is sensitive to trimethoprim but not sensitive to sulfamethoxazole
- trimethoprim has an active metabolite
- half-life 10 hours (trimethoprim) and 11 hours (sulfamethaxole)

Use

- respiratory tract infections (upper and lower), renal and urinary tract infections, genital tract infections, GI infections, skin and wound infections, septicaemia

Dose

- (800 mg sulfamethoxazole/160 mg trimethoprim) ½ – 1½ tablets orally twice daily after meals for 5 days or until symptom-free for 48 hours (DS or Forte tablets) **OR**
- (400 mg sulfamethoxazole/80 mg trimethoprim) 2 tablets orally twice daily, increasing to 3 tablets twice daily for severe infections after meals for 5 days or until symptom-free for 48 hours **OR**
- (*Pneumocystis carinii* pneumonitis) trimethoprim 20 mg/kg and sulfamethoxazole 100 mg/kg/day orally or by IV infusion in 4 divided doses for 14 days **OR**
- 800 mg sulfamethoxazole/160 mg trimethoprim (10 mL) by IV infusion twice daily **OR**
- (severe infection) 1200 mg sulfamethoxazole/240 mg trimethoprim (15 mL) by IV infusion twice daily

Adverse effects

- nausea, vomiting, anorexia
- rash, pruritus, urticaria
- photosensitivity reactions
- arthralgia, myalgia
- fever, symptoms resembling serum sickness
- crystalluria, oliguria, anuria, impaired kidney function
- aplastic anaemia, agranulocytosis, thrombocytopenia, leucopenia, bone marrow depression
- ataxia, convulsions, confusion, depression, apathy, hallucinations, nervousness
- vertigo, tinnitus
- peripheral and optic neuropathy
- headache, fatigue, insomnia
- hyperkalaemia, hyponatraemia
- increased liver enzymes and bilirubin, hepatitis
- hypersensitivity, allergic reactions
- pseudomembranous colitis, superinfection
- Stevens–Johnson syndrome (rare but possibly fatal) (see Glossary)
- (rare) diuresis, hypoglycaemia, haemolytic anaemia (associated with G6PD deficiency), aseptic meningitis, rhabdomyolysis
- (IV) pain, inflammation, thrombophlebitis

Interactions

- may decrease effectiveness of TCAs
- not recommended with amiodarone, paclitaxel and clozapine
- increased risk of delirium and myoclonus if given with amantadine or memantine
- increased risk of haematological adverse effects if given with pyrimethamine, azathioprine, zidovudine or mercaptopurine, therefore blood counts should be closely monitored if given together
- increased antibacterial activity may occur if given with polymyxin
- may increase serum levels of digoxin increasing risk of toxicity
- may increase serum levels of methotrexate, increasing the risk of bone marrow depression

- may increase serum levels of phenytoin, thereby increasing their risk of toxicity, therefore levels should be closely monitored, especially when starting or stopping therapy
- may enhance the effect of sulfonylurea hypoglycaemic agents, therefore blood glucose levels should be closely monitored
- increased risk of pseudomembranous colitis if given with peristalsis-delaying agents such as opioid analgesics and diphenoxylate/atropine combination
- not recommended with local anaesthetics (PABA derivatives such as procaine) as antibacterial activity may be antagonised
- increased risk of thrombocytopenia if given with thiazide diuretics in the elderly
- may decrease serum levels of ciclosporin
- caution if given with other agents that may cause hyperkalaemia
- increased risk of methaemoglobinaemia if given with dapsone
- may potentiate effects of warfarin, therefore INR should be closely monitored, especially when starting or stopping therapy
- rifampicin may decrease half-life of trimethoprim
- caution if given with ACE inhibitors or angiotensin receptor blockers
- may interfere with a number of laboratory tests including *Lactobacillus casei* serum folate assay and *Lactobacillus leishmania* serum cyanocobalamin (57Co) (vitamin B_{12}) assay

Nursing points/Cautions

- see also General Nursing points/Cautions for antibacterial agents (p. 148)
- blood cell counts should be monitored during prolonged therapy (greater than 14 days) (especially in those with predisposition to folate deficiency) or in those with malnutrition or treatment with antiepileptic agents
- urinalysis (with microscopic examination), renal function tests and serum potassium and sodium are recommended during prolonged therapy greater than 14 days
- patient should be well hydrated and have an adequate fluid intake during therapy
- urinary output should be monitored and kept above 1500 mL/day to reduce crystalluria and stone formation
- alkalinisation may be necessary to increase solubility of some sulfonamides and reduce the risk of crystalluria
- therapy should be discontinued if rash appears
- patients with AIDS who are being treated for PCP (*Pneumocystis jirovecii*, previously called *Pneumocystis carinii*) may show a higher incidence of rash, fever and leucopenia and should be carefully monitored during therapy
- cross-sensitivity may occur with other sulfonamides such as some antithyroid drugs, acetazolamide, thiazide diuretics and oral hypoglycaemic agents
- IV route is only recommended when oral route is unavailable
- (high dose) serum potassium and kidney function should be closely monitored during therapy
- (oral) therapy should continue for at least 5 days or until patient has been symptom-free for 48 hours
- should not be given undiluted or as an IV bolus
- dilute ampoule before administration according to manufacturer's instructions in 125–500 mL of IV fluid and mix well
- IV infusion should be completed within 90 minutes
- IV therapy should be limited to 3 days or less

- IV ampoule solution may precipitate if stored at low temperatures. If this occurs, solution should be discarded
- (IV) contains sodium metabisulfite which may cause allergic reaction in sensitive individuals
- (suspension) contains hydroxybenzoates, polysorbate and sorbitol
- caution if used in those with liver or kidney impairment, urinary obstruction, blood dyscrasias, asthma, allergies, porphyria or thyroid dysfunction
- not recommended in those with serious haematological disorders
- caution if used in those with folate deficiency, hypoglycaemia and electrolyte imbalance (especially hyperkalaemia)
- caution if used in those with malnutrition due to increased risk of crystalluria
- caution if used in the elderly due to increased risk of adverse effects
- caution if used in those with oedema of cardiac origin as sulfonamides may induce diuresis
- not recommended in those with G6PD deficiency due to risk of haemolytic anaemia
- not recommended in patients receiving peritoneal dialysis
- not recommended in infants under 12 weeks
- contraindicated in newborns during first 6 weeks of life or premature infants
- contraindicated for streptococcal pharyngitis
- contraindicated in those with known hypersensitivity to sulfonamides or trimethoprim or blood dyscrasias, bone marrow depression, parenchymal liver damage or severe renal impairment (creatinine clearance < 15 mL/minute)
- see also Nursing points/Cautions for antibacterial agents (p. 148)

Patient teaching and advice

- see General Patient teaching and advice for antibacterial agents (p. 149)
- patients with diabetes taking sulfonylurea hypoglycaemics should be advised that blood glucose control may be altered during therapy
- warn patients to avoid sunlamps or sunbeds or direct exposure to sunlight and if this cannot be avoided, should wear protective clothing and sunscreen with high sun protection factor (SPF 30+)
- instruct patient to seek medical advice immediately if any of the following occur:
  - rash, sore throat, fever, bleeding, painful joints
  - cough, shortness of breath, pallor
  - bleeding under skin
  - yellowing of skin or whites of the eyes
- patient should be advised to avoid driving or operating machinery if dizziness, drowsiness, confusion, insomnia, vertigo or fatigue are ongoing problems
- advise patient to increase fluid intake by drinking extra glasses of water during the day unless told not to do so by doctor
- advise patient to shake suspension well before use

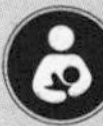

sulfonamides should not be given to women before delivery because they may cause jaundice and/or haemolytic anaemia in the newborn and are contraindicated in late pregnancy

animal studies have shown trimethoprim causes birth defects because of interference to folic acid metabolism and therefore folic acid supplements should be given if trimethoprim or trimethoprim–sulfonamide combination must be used during pregnancy

sulfonamides are contraindicated during breastfeeding of infants under 2 months or if infant has G6PD deficiency

trimethoprim is not recommended during breastfeeding

syrup/suspension is available. Tablet can be crushed and mixed with water or spoonful of yoghurt or apple puree

DAPTOMYCIN (Cubicin)

Available form
Vial: 350 mg, 500 mg

Action
- cyclic lipopeptide
- binds to bacterial membrane, causing depolarisation of membrane potential in growing and stationary phase cells, inhibition of protein, DNA and RNA synthesis
- active against Gram-positive organisms only

Use
- complicated skin and skin structure infections (where other antibacterial agents are ineffective or inappropriate)
- bacteraemia (due to *S. aureus*), including right-sided valve infective endocarditis

Dose
- (complicated skin and skin structure infection) 4 mg/kg daily as IV bolus over 2 minutes or infusion over 30 minutes for 7–14 days or until infection has resolved **OR**
- (bacteraemia, right-sided endocarditis) 6 mg/kg daily as IV bolus over 2 minutes or infusion over 30 minutes for 2–6 weeks

Adverse effects
- fungal infection, urinary tract infection
- anaemia
- anxiety, insomnia
- dizziness, headache
- hypertension, hypotension
- GI/abdominal pain, diarrhoea, nausea, vomiting, flatulence, bloating, distension, constipation
- rash, pruritus
- fever, asthenia
- increased creatine phosphokinase (CPK), muscle pain, (uncommon) weakness, rhabdomyolysis
- abnormal liver function
- eosinophilic pneumonia (fever, dyspnoea, hypoxic respiratory insufficiency, diffuse pulmonary infiltrates)
- hypersensitivity, pseudomembranous colitis, superinfection
- peripheral neuropathy
- (IV site) infusion site reaction

Interactions
- caution if used with other agents associated with myopathy and rhabdomyolysis (e.g. statins (HMG CoA reductase inhibitors), fibrates, ciclosporin)
- may cause false prolongation of prothrombin time and elevation of INR

Nursing points/Cautions
- plasma CPK should be measured before starting therapy and then weekly during therapy
- kidney function and plasma CPK should be measured regularly (> once per week) in anyone with pre-existing kidney impairment
- closely monitor patients for any muscle pain or weakness (especially in extremities)
- if infection persists or relapses, repeat blood cultures are recommended. Appropriate surgical intervention such as debridement or removal of prosthetic devices, should also be considered
- add 7 mL sodium chloride 0.9% to 350 mg vial (or 10 mL to 500 mg vial) and gently rotate, taking care to avoid foaming. The vial should not

be shaken. Allow vial to stand for 10 minutes and then swirl gently for several minutes to ensure powder is reconstituted

- if administering as an IV infusion over 30 minutes, further dilution with sodium chloride 0.9% is required
- not compatible with glucose-containing diluents or solutions
- administer alone
- not indicated for pneumonia or left-sided endocarditis
- caution if used in those with kidney impairment. If creatine clearance is < 30 mL/minute, dosing interval should be lengthened to 48 hours and kidney function closely monitored
- not recommended in children < 12 months
- see also General Nursing points/Cautions for antibacterial agents (p. 148)

Patient teaching and advice

- advise patient to seek medical advice if any of the following occur:
  - tender or aching muscles, muscle weakness
  - unusual tingling or numbness in feet or hands, loss of feeling, difficulty moving
  - new or worsening fever, cough or difficulty breathing
- see also General Patient teaching and advice for antibacterial agents (p. 149)

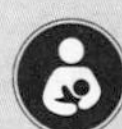

only used during pregnancy if benefits outweigh the risks

caution if used during breastfeeding

FIDAXOMICIN (Dificid)

Available form

Tablets: 200 mg

Action

- macrocycle
- inhibits RNA synthesis by RNA polymerases at a site different from the rifamycins
- active metabolite
- half-life 7–16 hours
- bactericidal against *C. difficile*

Use

- confirmed infection with *C. difficile*

Dose

- 200 mg orally twice daily for 10 days

Adverse effects

- nausea, constipation, vomiting, abdominal pain, diarrhoea
- headache, dizziness, fatigue, insomnia
- pruritus
- fever, chills
- peripheral oedema
- hypotension
- dyspnoea
- increased liver enzymes
- urinary tract infection, pneumonia
- hypokalaemia, hyperkalaemia, hypomagnesaemia
- anaemia
- back pain
- (rare) hypersensitivity

Nursing points/Cautions

- caution if used in those with severe kidney or liver insufficiency
- not recommended for systemic infections
- caution if used in those with known hypersensitivity to macrolides
- see General Nursing points/Cautions for antibacterial agents (p. 148)

Patient teaching and advice

- see General Patient teaching and advice for antibacterial agents (p. 149)

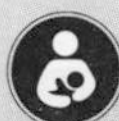

only used during pregnancy if clearly needed

caution if used during breastfeeding

tablet can be crushed and mixed with water or spoonful of apple puree

FOSFOMYCIN (Monurol)

Available form
Granules: 3 g/sachet

Actions
- inhibits first stage of bacterial wall synthesis
- bactericidal
- also reduces bacterial adhesion to bladder mucosa
- not metabolised and is excreted unchanged via kidneys
- half-life 4 hours

Use
- treatment of uncomplicated lower urinary tract infections (acute cystitis) in females due to *Enterobacteriaceae* spp. (including *Escherichia coli*) and *Enterococcus faecalis*

Dose
- 3 g orally as single dose on empty stomach or 2–3 hours after meals, preferably before bedtime

Adverse effects
- vulvovaginitis
- headache, dizziness
- diarrhoea, nausea, dyspepsia
- hypersensitivity, pseudomembranous colitis

Interactions
- may increase or decrease prothrombin time, therefore close monitoring of INR is recommended if patient is taking warfarin
- not recommended with metoclopramide as decreased serum levels of fosfomycin may occur
- not recommended with urinary alkalinisers

Nursing points/Cautions
- culture and susceptibility studies should be performed to identify causative organism and sensitivity. Therapy can be started before results are known
- only one dose should be used per single episode of acute cystitis. Repeated doses are not recommended as clinical outcomes are not improved but risk of adverse events increases
- contains sucrose, therefore not recommended in those with hereditary problems of fructose intolerance, glucose–galactose malabsorption or sucrase–isomaltase insufficiency
- not recommended for treatment of pyelonephritis or perinephric abscess or if resistance is likely (as indicated by previous treatment failure)
- not recommended in male patients
- contraindicated in those with severe kidney insufficiency (creatinine clearance < 10 mL/min) or undergoing haemofiltration, haemodialysis or peritoneal dialysis
- see also General Nursing points/Cautions for antibacterial agents (p. 148)

Patient teaching and advice
- advise patient to:
  - take on an empty stomach or at least 2–3 hours after meals, preferably before bedtime after emptying bladder
  - dissolve granules in glass of water and take immediately
  - hot water should not be used to dissolve granules
  - dry granules should not be ingested
- see also General Patient teaching and advice for antibacterial agents (p. 149)

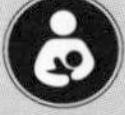

not recommended during pregnancy or breastfeeding

granules can be dispersed in 120–150 mL water or dissolved in 5 mL water and then mixed with spoonful of yoghurt or apple puree

METHENAMINE (HEXAMINE) HIPPURATE (Hiprex)

Available form
Tablets: 1 g

Action
- broad spectrum antibacterial agent that is active against both Gram-negative and Gram-positive organisms
- antibacterial action occurs when it is excreted in the urine where it dissociates to hippuric acid (bacteriostatic) and methenamine (which is further hydrolysed to ammonia and formaldehyde (bacteriostatic))
- takes 30 minutes to 2 hours to reach peak urinary formaldehyde level

Use
- long-term treatment of chronic or recurrent urinary tract infections

Dose
- 1 g orally twice daily

Adverse effects
- (occasionally) nausea, upset stomach, rash, dysuria, stomatitis

Interactions
- crystalluria may occur if administered with sulfonamides

Nursing points and Cautions/ Patient teaching and advice
- ensure patient is adequately hydrated before starting therapy
- only active if urinary pH is less than 5.5, therefore check pH frequently and do not alkalinise urine
- restrict alkalinising foods (e.g. vegetarian diet)
- additional urine acidification may be achieved by administration of ascorbic acid 2 g daily in divided doses
- contraindicated in those with kidney or liver insufficiency, metabolic acidosis, severe dehydration or parenchymal infection (as monotherapy)
- see also General Nursing points/ Cautions/Patient teaching and advice for antibacterial agents (pp. 148–149)

NITROFURANTOIN (Macrodantin)

Available forms
Capsules: 50 mg, 100 mg

Action
- nitrofuran antibiotic thought to interfere with several bacterial enzyme systems
- bacteriostatic in low levels, bactericidal in high levels
- active against both Gram-positive and Gram-negative urinary tract pathogens
- half-life 20 minutes

Use
- urinary tract infections (prophylactically and long-term suppressive therapy)

Dose
- (treatment) 50–100 mg orally 4 times daily with or after food for at least 1 week (daily maximum 400 mg) **OR**
- (prophylaxis) 50 or 100 mg orally nightly with or after food

Adverse effects
- anorexia, nausea, vomiting, diarrhoea, abdominal pain, dyspepsia, flatulence, constipation
- headache, drowsiness, dizziness, nystagmus, vertigo, depression, asthenia, confusion, amblyopia
- peripheral neuropathy, including optic neuritis
- eosinophilia, anaemia
- elevated liver enzymes
- rash, urticaria, pruritus, dermatitis, transient alopecia

- superinfection, hypersensitivity
- (rare) pulmonary hypersensitivity (acute, allergic pneumonitis, chronic interstitial pulmonary fibrosis), hepatitis, pseudomembranous colitis, psychosis, benign intracranial hypertension, blood dyscrasias including haemolytic anaemia, severe skin reactions

Interactions

- action may be inhibited by phenobarbital (phenobarbitone)
- excretion is decreased by acidifying drugs and increased by alkalising drugs
- antacids reduce effectiveness
- increased serum levels may result if given with probenecid or sulfinpyrazone, increasing the risk of toxicity
- increased risk of pseudomembranous colitis if given with peristalsis-delaying agents such as opioid analgesics and diphenoxylate/atropine combination
- interferes with some laboratory tests (e.g. serum bilirubin, urinary glucose, urine creatinine, serum urea)

Nursing points/Cautions

- pulmonary function (including X-ray examination) should be monitored 6-monthly during prolonged therapy
- liver function should be monitored regularly during prolonged therapy
- treatment should be continued for at least 3 days after clear urine culture has been obtained
- note and report muscle weakness, numbness and tingling (peripheral neuritis) because this necessitates ceasing therapy
- caution if used in those with G6PD deficiency
- caution if used in those with GI disorders, especially colitis because of increased risk of developing pseudomembranous colitis
- increased risk of peripheral neuropathy if given to those with renal impairment, anaemia, diabetes mellitus, electrolyte imbalance or vitamin B deficiency
- risk of pulmonary hypersensitivity is increased with prolonged therapy > 6 months
- caution if used in those with kidney impairment or acidosis. If therapy is prolonged, blood pH, CO_2 content, urea nitrogen and non-protein nitrogen should be monitored
- contraindicated in those with hypersensitivity to furan derivatives or with renal impairment (creatinine clearance < 60 mL/min or elevated serum creatinine), anuria or oliguria
- see also General Nursing points/Cautions for antibacterial agents (p. 148)

Patient teaching and advice

- instruct patient that GI side-effects can be lessened if given with food or milk
- patient should be advised to seek medical advice immediately if any of the following occur:
    - fever, chills, cough, chest pain, rash or shortness of breath (as these may indicate acute pneumonitis)
    - malaise, shortness of breath on exertion, cough, blue tinge to lips or fingernails (chronic interstitial pulmonary fibrosis)
    - yellowing of eyes or skin, loss of appetite, nausea, upper abdominal pain, dark urine (jaundice/hepatitis)
    - numbness or tingling of feet or hands (peripheral neuropathy)
- advise patients to take antacids 2 hours apart from nitrofurantoin
- warn patients that urine may become harmless brown colour
- patient should be warned to avoid driving or operating machinery if

dizziness, drowsiness or vertigo are ongoing problems
- male patients should be counselled regarding decreased sperm count that may occur during therapy
- see also General Patient teaching and advice for antibacterial agents (p. 149)

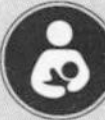

may cause haemolytic anaemia in newborn infants with G6PD deficiency, therefore it is contraindicated during labour or delivery, if labour is imminent, or during breastfeeding

capsule can be opened and mixed with water or spoonful of yoghurt or apple puree

PROPAMIDINE ISETHIONATE (Brolene)

Available form
Eye drops: 1 mg/mL (0.1%)

Action
- antibacterial activity against mainly Gram-positive organisms and acanthamoeba

Use
- mild acute conjunctivitis, acanthamoeba keratitis

Dose
- 1–2 drops 3–4 times daily for up to 1 week

Adverse effects
- pain, irritation (burning/stinging)
- (rare) hypersensitivity

Nursing points/Cautions/Patient teaching and advice
- patient should be advised to seek medical advice if there is no improvement within 7 days or if vision is disturbed or condition worsens. Improvement in condition should be noticeable within 2 days
- instruct patient on correct technique for insertion of eye drops (p. 189)
- (eye drops) advise patient to discard eye drops 14 days after opening
- (eye drops) if patient wears soft contact lenses, warn him/her not to insert lenses during therapy as eye drops contain benzalkonium chloride (preservative) which discolours soft contact lenses and can cause eye reaction

RIFAXIMIN (Xifaxan)

Available forms
Tablet: 200 mg, 550 mg

Action
- non-aminoglycoside, semisynthetic, non-systemic antibiotic derived from rifamycin
- binds to beta subunit of bacterial DNA dependent RNA polymerase, resulting in inhibition of bacterial RNA synthesis
- broad spectrum
- active against Gram-positive, Gram-negative, aerobic and anaerobic organisms causing intestinal infection
- (recurrent hepatic encephalopathy) thought to affect GI flora

Use
- traveller's diarrhoea caused by non-invasive strains of *Escherichia coli*
- prevention of hepatic encephalopathy (HE) (where other treatment is inappropriate)

Dose
- (traveller's diarrhoea) 200 mg orally 3 times daily for 3 days (total 9 doses)

OR
- (hepatic encephalopathy) 550 mg orally twice daily

Adverse effects
- nausea, vomiting, flatulence, abdominal pain, constipation, rectal tenesmus, defecation urgency
- fever
- headache

- (HE) anaemia, peripheral oedema, muscle spasm, back pain, dizziness, rash, pruritus, dyspnoea
- (rare) hypersensitivity, pseudomembranous colitis

Interactions

- charcoal may decrease absorption
- caution if given with ciclosporin
- may increase or decrease INR, therefore caution if given with warfarin. INR should be closely monitored especially when starting or stopping therapy

Nursing points/Cautions

- (HE) caution if used in those with severe liver impairment
- (traveller's diarrhoea) repeat course is not recommended
- (traveller's diarrhoea) not effective for traveller's diarrhoea caused by *Campylobacter* spp., *Salmonella* spp. or *Shigella* spp. which produce dysentery-like diarrhoea (with blood in stool, fever and high stool frequency)
- (traveller's diarrhoea) not recommended in those with diarrhoea complicated with fever and/or blood in stools, or diarrhoea caused by pathogens other than *E. coli*, therefore should only be used for areas where there is a low incidence of *Campylobacter* and not for travel in South-East Asia
- not recommended in children under 12 years
- contraindicated in those with intestinal obstruction or with hypersensitivity to rifamycins
- see also General Nursing points/ Cautions for antibacterial agents (p. 148)

Patient teaching and advice

- (traveller's diarrhoea) advise patient that if symptoms worsen, therapy should be stopped and medical advice sought immediately
- see also General Patient teaching and advice for antibacterial agents (p. 149)

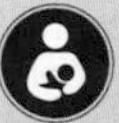

caution if used during pregnancy

only used during breastfeeding if benefits outweigh risks

SILVER SULFADIAZINE (Flamazine)

Available form

Cream: 1%

Action

- sulfonamide combined with silver
- structurally similar to para-aminobenzoic acid (PABA) and blocks conversion of PABA to dihydrofolic acid (reduced form of folic acid), therefore bacteria are deprived of folic acid because of incomplete synthesis and so cease to multiply
- active against both Gram-negative and Gram-positive organisms
- silver is reported to have some antibacterial properties of its own

Use

- prevention and treatment of infection in severe burns
- treatment of infections in leg ulcers and pressure injuries
- conservative management of fingertip injuries (where pulp, nail loss and/ or partial loss of distal phalanx has occurred)

Dose

- applied with a sterile spatula or gloved hand in a layer 3–5 mm thick and changed at least daily

Adverse effects

- systemic effects (in those with more than 20% burns), including nausea and vomiting

- (local reactions) pain, burning, itching, rash, contact dermatitis/eczema, pruritus
- (rare) skin discolouration (argyria) (due to silver), systemic absorption, transient leucopenia

Interactions

- may inactivate enzymatic debriding agents
- (large burns) caution if given with phenytoin or oral hypoglycaemic agents
- (large burns) increased risk of leucopenia if given with cimetidine

Nursing points/Cautions/Patient teaching and advice

- (long-term therapy) blood count monitoring is recommended
- (extensive burns) kidney function and serum sulfonamide levels should be monitored. Urine should also be checked for sulfonamide crystals
- may alter appearance of burn wound and/or delay separation of burn eschar
- non-ulcerated areas should be avoided to prevent skin maceration
- each jar or tube is for single patient use only; any remaining cream should be discarded after completion of treatment
- (fingertip injury) after haemostasis has been achieved, finger dressing can be applied over cream and changed every 2–3 days
- (leg ulcers/pressure injuries) cream should fill ulcer cavity, then be covered with absorbent pad/dressing and covered with compression bandaging (leg ulcers) if needed
- (hand burn) after applying cream, whole hand can be enclosed in glove or clear plastic bag, then closed at the wrist. Patient should be encouraged to move fingers and hand
- not recommended for leg ulcers or pressure injuries with high levels of exudate
- contraindicated in those with known hypersensitivity to sulfonamides, silver, cetyl alcohol or propylene glycol

TRIMETHOPRIM (Alprim, Triprim)

Available form

Tablets: 300 mg

Action

- selectively interferes with bacterial synthesis of nucleic acids and proteins by binding to bacterial dihydrofolate reductase enzyme
- half-life 8–12 hours
- not active against *Pseudomonas* spp.

Use

- treatment of acute urinary tract infection (not caused by *Pseudomonas* spp.)

Dose

- 300 mg orally nightly with food for 7 days (preferably before bedtime to maximise urinary concentration)

Adverse effects

- rash, pruritus, exfoliative dermatitis
- nausea, vomiting, epigastric pain, glossitis
- blood dyscrasias
- fever
- elevated liver enzymes, bilirubin and serum creatinine
- hyperkalaemia, hyponatraemia
- (rare) severe skin reactions, hypersensitivity

Interactions

- may potentiate anticoagulant action of warfarin, therefore INR should be closely monitored, especially when starting or stopping therapy
- folate supplements may be required if given with other antifolate drugs such as methotrexate
- serum levels may be decreased by rifampicin
- increased risk of nephrotoxicity if given with ciclosporin

- hyponatraemia may occur if given with diuretics
- increased risk of myelosuppression and megaloblastic anaemia if given with methotrexate or pyrimethamine
- may increase serum level of dapsone while having own serum level increased by dapsone
- increased risk of severe hyperkalaemia if given with ACE inhibitors, prednisolone, potassium sparing diuretics and zalcitabine
- may increase serum levels of phenytoin, digoxin and procainamide
- may decrease excretion and therefore increase serum levels of zidovudine and lamivudine increasing risk of haematological toxicity
- may interfere with assay for creatinine (produces overestimation) and serum methotrexate assay

Nursing point/Cautions

- any folate deficiency should be corrected before starting therapy with trimethoprim
- monthly blood counts are recommended if trimethoprim therapy is long term
- serum potassium should be monitored during therapy (especially in those with kidney insufficiency or taking agents that increase potassium levels)
- therapy should be stopped if any rash appears
- caution if used in the elderly or in those with blood dyscrasias, actual/potential folate deficiency or impaired liver or kidney function
- not recommended in those with porphyria
- contraindicated in those with severe kidney impairment (creatinine clearance less than 10 mL/minute unless plasma trimethoprim levels can be monitored regularly during therapy), severe haematological disorders or megaloblastic anaemia due to folate deficiency, or trimethoprim hypersensitivity
- see General Nursing points/Cautions for antibacterial agents (p. 148)

Patient teaching and advice

- patient should be advised to immediately seek medical advice if any of the following occur:
  - rash (especially if there is any blistering or peeling)
  - sore throat, mouth ulcers, fever, chills
  - advise patient to take tablets with food to minimise gastric irritation
- see also General Patient teaching and advice for antibacterial agents (p. 149)

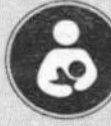

animal studies have shown birth defects because of interference to folic acid metabolism and therefore folic acid supplements should be given if trimethoprim or trimethoprim–sulfonamide combination must be used during pregnancy

not recommended during breastfeeding

tablet can be dispersed in water or crushed and mixed with spoonful of yoghurt or apple puree

ANTICOAGULANTS AND ANTITHROMBOTIC AGENTS

Normally blood vessels are kept free of thrombi by maintaining a balance between deposition of fibrinogen and its breakdown (fibrinolysis). When this balance is shifted towards fibrinogen deposition the result is the formation of a blood clot (thrombus), which may then threaten to occlude the vessel. Arterial thrombi usually form as a result of damage to the endothelial layer of the vessel wall, whereas venous thrombi are caused by venous stasis, which allows platelets and fibrin to build up. Arterial thrombi are composed mainly of platelets with little fibrin, so antiplatelet agents (p. 753) are more appropriate treatments because they are able to prevent platelet aggregation and clot formation. Venous thrombi are composed mainly of fibrin with fewer platelets and are amenable to treatment with anticoagulants (Bryant et al 2019; Hogg & Weitz 2018).

Anticoagulants are used in the prophylaxis and treatment of thromboembolic disorders, including the prevention of fibrin deposition and extension of existing thrombus, although they do not dissolve existing clots or restore tissue ischaemic injury caused by clot occlusion of blood vessel. Anticoagulant agents are divided into:

- heparin and the low molecular weight heparins (e.g. dalteparin, enoxaparin, danaparoid, nadroparin) (these are the drugs of choice for rapid anticoagulation)
- vitamin K antagonists (e.g. warfarin)
- anti-thrombin III-dependent anticoagulant (e.g. fondaparinux)
- agents that directly inhibit thrombin (e.g. bivalirudin, dabigatran)
- direct inhibitors of factor Xa (e.g. rivaroxaban, apixaban) (Bryant et al 2019).

The main side-effect of anticoagulants is bleeding, which can range from mild to severe. Administering and maintaining the correct dosage within the therapeutic range is achieved by regular monitoring of blood concentrations. These blood tests use plasma in which clotting has been prevented by a calcium-sequestering agent (citrate or oxalate). Calcium and an activating agent are then added to the blood and the time for clot formation is measured (Bryant et al 2019). There are several tests that measure different parts of the clotting cascade, including:

- *prothrombin time* (PT) measures factor VII and the common pathway in the clotting cascade. Thromboplastin is used as the activating agent. Because the thromboplastin reagent varies in sensitivity with each new batch, the standard way to report PT is as a ratio of patient PT to control PT, raised to the power of the International Sensitivity Index (ISI), which is established for each new batch of thromboplastin. This ratio is called the International Normalised Ratio (INR) and is used to regulate warfarin dosage
- *activated partial thromboplastin time* (aPTT) measures the extent to which heparin inhibits thrombin, factor Xa and factor IXa. aPTT is used to monitor heparin therapy, although low-dose heparin therapy does not require monitoring (Bryant et al 2019).

General Patient teaching and advice for anticoagulants

- patient should be advised to seek medical advice immediately if there is:
  - any leg numbness/weakness or bowel/bladder problems (after epidural/spinal anaesthesia or other spinal injections)
  - any unexplained/prolonged bleeding, bruising or swelling
  - bleeding from gums when brushing teeth
  - unusual nosebleeds
  - oozing from wounds
  - coughing or vomiting blood
  - blood in urine or stool
  - unusual pain (especially in back or stomach)
- patient should be advised of the importance of wearing a MedicAlert or other medical alert-type bracelet or pendant informing others of the anticoagulant therapy (especially if the person is unconscious or unable to speak). This information can also be included on the patient's mobile phone under 'medical ID'
- advise patient to inform dentist of anticoagulant therapy if any dental procedure is planned because of the risk of local bleeding
- warn patient not to drive or operate machinery if dizziness occurs
- patient should be instructed to seek advice from doctor or pharmacist before taking OTC analgesics (including aspirin)
- see also General Patient teaching and advice (p. xxvii)

HEPARIN AND LOW MOLECULAR WEIGHT HEPARINS (LMWHs)

HEPARIN SODIUM (DBL Heparin Injection, Heparin Sodium Injection, Heparinised Saline)

Available forms

Vial: 35,000 IU/35 mL; Ampoules: 1000 IU/1 mL, 5000 IU/0.2 mL, 5000 IU/1 mL, 5000 IU/5 mL, 25,000 IU/5 mL

Action

- complex proteoglycan consisting of protein core with repeating disaccharide units attached, varying in molecular weight from 5000–40,000

- combines with antithrombin III (heparin co-factor) inactivating factor X and inhibiting conversion of prothrombin to thrombin
- if thrombus exists, heparin inhibits further coagulation by inactivating thrombin, preventing conversion of fibrinogen to fibrin
- prevents stable clot formation by inhibiting activation of fibrin stabilising factor
- sourced from pig mucosa
- onset of action is immediate (IV) or 20–60 minutes (SC), acts for 3–6 hours and trebles blood-clotting time to 15–30 minutes
- half-life is dose dependent and generally 1–6 hours
- not absorbed from GI tract, therefore ineffective if given orally
- prevents further clotting but has no effect on existing clot
- does not cross placenta or enter breastmilk
- prolonged aPTT in those over 60 years

Use

- prophylaxis and treatment of thromboembolic disorders (e.g. deep vein thrombosis (DVT), pulmonary embolus (PE) or thrombophlebitis)
- prophylaxis of thromboembolic complications arising from heart and vascular surgery
- anticoagulant in blood collected for transfusion or laboratory tests
- extracorporeal circulation (heart/lung and renal dialysis machines)
- patency of IV devices (heparinised saline)

Dose

- (DVT prophylaxis postoperatively) 5000 units by SC injection 2 hours before surgery then 8–12-hourly for 7–10 days or until patient is fully mobile **OR**
- (DVT/PE treatment) initially 5000 units by IV bolus, then 20,000–40,000 units in sodium chloride 0.9% 1 L over 24 hours by continuous IV infusion **OR**
- (DVT/PE treatment) initially 10,000 units (either as IV bolus or diluted in 50–100 mL sodium chloride 0.9%), followed by 5000–10,000 units 4–6-hourly (intermittent IV injection) **OR**
- (DVT/PE treatment) 5000 units IV, then 10,000 units by deep SC injection 8-hourly or 15,000 units by deep SC injection 12-hourly **OR**
- (heart and blood vessel surgery) initially not less than 150 units/kg (300 units/kg may be used for surgery duration < 60 minutes or 400 units/kg > 60 minutes) **OR**
- (IV device patency) 10–50 units 4-hourly

Adverse effects

- haemorrhage (ranging from mild ecchymosis to severe bleeding)
- thrombocytopenia
- (SC injection site) local irritation, erythema, mild pain, haematoma, ulceration
- osteoporosis (4–12 weeks after prolonged, high-dose heparin therapy)
- hyperkalaemia
- elevated liver enzymes
- (high dose, prolonged therapy) suppression of kidney function
- hypoaldosteronism (rare), rebound hyperlipidaemia (when heparin is stopped), reversible hypereosinophilia
- (rare) allergic reactions (e.g. pruritus, urticaria, chills, fever, headache), skin necrosis at injection site, alopecia (delayed, transient), priapism, heparin-induced thrombocytopenia (HIT), heparin-induced thrombocytopenia and thrombosis (HITT) (also called white clot syndrome), delayed HIT, delayed HITT

Interactions

- decreased anticoagulant effect when given with antihistamines, digoxin, ascorbic acid (vitamin C), nicotine or tetracyclines
- decreased prothrombin time may occur if given simultaneously with IV

glyceryl trinitrate, therefore should be given with caution, especially when starting or stopping therapy
- increased risk of hypoprothrombinaemia if given with large doses of aspirin
- increased anticoagulant effect and risk of bleeding when given with abciximab, alcohol (heavy use), alprostadil, alteplase, antiplatelet agents, asparaginase (colaspase), aspirin, clopidogrel, contrast media (some), corticosteroids (systemic), dextran, dipyridamole, epoprostenol, etacrynic acid, hydroxychloroquine, ibuprofen, indometacin, NSAIDs, penicillins (high dose), probenecid, propylthiouracil, reteplase, rivaroxaban, sodium valproate, tenecteplase, ticlopidine, tirofiban, warfarin or vitamin K antagonists
- hyperkalaemia may occur if given with ACE inhibitors, potassium-sparing diuretics or potassium supplements, therefore potassium levels should be monitored regularly, especially in those who are at risk of hyperkalaemia
- may antagonise effects of insulin, corticosteroids and ACTH
- may interfere with aminotransferase determination of myocardial infarction, pulmonary embolus or liver disease, therefore results should be interpreted with caution

Nursing points/Cautions

Subcutaneous injection technique

- use care with SC administration to avoid local haematoma formation and ensure uniform absorption
- use a tuberculin syringe and a short-gauge (25–26 gauge) needle
- injection site is the subcutaneous fat of the anterior abdominal wall or anterior thighs, given at an angle perpendicular to the skin surface
- inject slowly at the rate of 1 mL/minute to prevent pain
- do not rub site of injection
- rotate and document the injection sites regularly

General

- heparin sodium may be given IV or SC
- to prevent painful haematoma formation, avoid giving IM
- all unnecessary procedures which might cause vascular damage (except IV injections) should be avoided if possible
- patient should be closely monitored for signs of spinal haematoma (e.g. midline back pain, numbness, weakness, lower limb paralysis, bowel/bladder dysfunction) if they have a spinal puncture or insertion/removal of epidural/spinal needle/catheter. Risk of haematoma formation is increased if the patient is taking NSAIDs, antiplatelet agents or other anticoagulants, or if the procedure is repeated or traumatic
- be alert to the early signs of overdose by looking for bruising, and testing the urine daily for blood (therapeutic dose only)
- platelet counts, haematocrit and occult blood test should be measured before starting and regularly throughout therapy
- if platelet count $<100,000$ mm^3 or recurrent thrombosis occurs, therapy should be stopped and an alternate anticoagulant considered
- heparin dose is adjusted to keep the APTT at 1.5–2 times the control value (or whole blood-clotting time 2.5–3 times control value)
- oral anticoagulants may be started 3–5 days before gradually reducing then discontinuing heparin
- when given with warfarin, and prothrombin time is required, at least 5 hours from last IV dose or 24 hours from last SC heparin dose should elapse before blood is drawn

- there are two types of thrombocytopenia which can result from heparin therapy:
  - an acute mild form occurring within 1–4 days of starting heparin which usually resolves without stopping therapy
  - a more serious delayed onset form which occurs within 7–11 days of starting heparin and necessitates ceasing therapy
- heparin-induced thrombocytopenia (HIT) and thrombosis (HITT) (also referred to as 'white clot syndrome') starts as a heparin-induced antibody mediated reaction resulting from irreversible aggregation of platelets and progressing to new thrombus formation with thrombocytopenia induced. It may lead to thromboembolic complications such as skin necrosis, gangrene, DVT and pulmonary embolism. HIT and HITT can occur as a delayed reaction several weeks after heparin is stopped
- (heparinised saline) IV device should be flushed with sodium chloride 0.9% before and after administration of heparinised saline
- when preparing infusion bags, it is important to invert bag at least 6 times to ensure even distribution of heparin throughout IV fluid
- monitor IV infusion rate closely using an infusion pump
- heparin infusion should be administered alone as there are many incompatibilities
- heparin therapy should be continued for several days after therapeutic APTT level has been reached and then stopped (without tapering)
- dose should be reduced or stopped if the person is having an oral surgical (dental) procedure
- heparin overdose resulting in severe bleeding should be treated with protamine sulfate (a small basic protein that counteracts the anticoagulant effect of heparin by neutralising its acidic charge) (see Antidotes, antagonists and chelating agents, p. 356). Minor bleeding can be managed by stopping heparin
- derived from animal source, therefore should be used with caution in those with a history of allergy or asthma
- caution if used in those with diabetes mellitus or renal insufficiency due to increased risk of hyperkalaemia occurring
- caution if used in those with fever, thrombosis, thrombophlebitis, infection (with thrombosing tendencies), myocardial infarction, cancer, post-surgery or antithrombin III deficiency as there is an increased risk of heparin resistance occurring
- caution if used in those with continuous tube drainage of stomach/small intestine, mild to moderate liver/kidney disease, hypertension, history of ulcers (gastric or duodenal), retinal vascular disease, hereditary antithrombin III deficiency or if over the age of 60 years (particularly women)
- (heparinised saline) not recommended in neonates
- contraindicated in those with active or potential bleeding or bleeding disorders (e.g. haemophilia, vitamin C deficiency, bleeding haemorrhoids), threatened abortion, immediately postpartum, subacute/acute bacterial endocarditis, severe hypertension, GI ulcerative disorders (at risk of bleeding), advanced kidney/liver disease, during or immediately post-surgery/injury (especially to brain, eye or spinal cord and also including spinal puncture and spinal/epidural anaesthesia), shock, severe thrombocytopenia, previous heparin-induced thrombocytopenia, haemorrhagic stroke or if there are inadequate laboratory facilities to monitor blood clotting on a regular basis

- contraindicated in those with sensitivity to port products

Patient teaching and advice

- see General Patient teaching and advice for anticoagulants (p. 234)

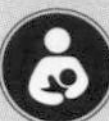

although heparin does not cause fetal malformations, there is an increased risk of fetal loss and prematurity associated with maternal haemorrhage if given in last trimester of pregnancy or the immediate postpartum period

LOW MOLECULAR WEIGHT HEPARINS

DALTEPARIN SODIUM (Fragmin)

Available forms

Fixed single dose syringe: 2500 IU/0.2 mL, 5000 IU/0.2 mL, 12,500 IU/0.5 mL, 15,000 IU/0.6 mL, 18,000 IU/0.72 mL; Graduated single-dose syringe: 7500 IU/0.75 mL, 10,000 IU/1 mL

Action

- low molecular weight heparin (smaller fragment of heparin prepared from unfractionated heparin using enzymatic or chemical methods, with a molecular weight about a third of heparin)
- increases neutralisation rate of factor Xa mainly, but also factor XIIa and kallikrein by antithrombin
- little effect on platelet function and adhesion compared to heparin
- some antithrombotic properties may be caused by an action on the vessel wall or fibrinolytic system
- half-life is 2 hours (IV) or 3–4 hours (SC)

Use

- prophylactically against thrombotic complications of haemodialysis
- treatment of acute DVT
- treatment of symptomatic venous thromboembolism (VTE) or reduce recurrence in those with solid tumour cancers
- treatment of unstable coronary artery disease (CAD) (e.g. unstable angina and non-Q wave myocardial infarction (also called non-ST elevation myocardial infarction (NSTEMI))
- prophylactically against thromboembolic complications during the perioperative and postoperative periods

Dose

Acute DVT treatment

- initially 100 IU/kg twice daily SC or 100 IU/kg over 12 hours by continuous IV infusion and then adjusted according to serum levels of prothrombin complex factors (factors II, VII and X), usually about 5 days

Treatment of symptomatic VTE in those with solid tumour cancers

- 200 IU/kg SC daily (month 1), then 150 IU/kg SC daily (months 2–6) (daily maximum 18,000 IU)

Anticoagulation for haemodialysis

- (haemodialysis > 4 hours, chronic renal failure, no bleeding risk) 30–40 IU/kg IV bolus followed by 10–15 IU/kg/hour IV infusion **OR**
- (haemodialysis of 4 hours maximum, chronic renal failure) as above or 5000 IU IV bolus only **OR**
- (haemodialysis, acute renal failure, high bleeding risk) 5–10 IU/kg IV bolus followed by 4–5 IU/kg/hour IV infusion

Thromboprophylaxis (surgery)

- 2500 IU SC 1–2 hours before surgery, followed by 2500 IU SC daily for 5–7 days until patient is mobile

Thromboprophylaxis (general surgery associated with high thrombosis risk)
- 5000 IU SC the evening before surgery, followed by 5000 IU SC the following evenings for 5–7 days until patient is mobile **OR**
- 2500 IU SC 1–2 hours before surgery, followed by 2500 IU SC 12 hours later, then 5000 IU SC each morning for 5–7 days until patient is mobile

Thromboprophylaxis (orthopaedic surgery e.g. hip replacement)
- 5000 IU SC the evening before surgery, followed by 5000 IU SC the following evenings for 5 weeks **OR**
- 2500 IU SC 1–2 hours before surgery, followed by 2500 IU SC 8–12 hours later, then 5000 IU SC each morning for 5 weeks

Unstable CAD
- 120 IU/kg SC twice daily for 6 days (maximum 10,000 IU/12 hours) with low-dose aspirin

Adverse effects
- bleeding tendency (especially at high doses), mild thrombocytopenia
- transient elevation of liver transaminases
- hyperkalaemia
- (uncommon) allergic reactions, rash, urticaria, pruritus
- (long term) osteoporosis
- (injection site) subcutaneous haemorrhage or haematoma, pain

Interactions
- anticoagulant effect increased by aspirin, cytostatic agents, dextran, dipyridamole, etacrynic acid, fibrinolytic agents, NSAIDs, probenecid, vitamin K antagonists
- anticoagulant effect decreased by antihistamines, digoxin, tetracyclines and ascorbic acid
- increased risk of hyperkalaemia if given with potassium-sparing agents, potassium supplements or ACE inhibitors, therefore potassium levels should be monitored during therapy

Nursing points/Cautions
- not interchangeable with heparin or other low molecular weight heparins
- should not be given IM
- doses above 5000 IU increase bleeding tendency
- new patients undergoing haemodialysis should have anti-Xa concentrations monitored during first few weeks
- routine monitoring of anti-Xa is not required (unless patient has cancer, kidney or liver failure, is very thin/morbidly obese, pregnant or at increased risk of bleeding), but platelet concentrations should be measured before starting therapy and regularly throughout, for the early detection of thrombocytopenia
- patient should be closely monitored for signs of spinal haematoma (e.g. midline back pain, numbness, weakness, lower limb paralysis, bowel/bladder dysfunction) if they have a spinal puncture or insertion/removal of epidural/spinal needle/catheter. Risk of haematoma formation is increased if the patient is taking NSAIDs, antiplatelet agents or other anticoagulants, or if the procedure is repeated or traumatic. Insertion/removal of epidural or spinal catheter should be delayed 10–24 hours (depending on dose) after last administration
- overdose treated with protamine sulfate at a dose of 1 mg protamine for 100 anti-Xa IU dalteparin. If aPTT remains prolonged 2–4 hours after first protamine infusion, second infusion (0.5 mg protamine/100 anti-Xa IU) can be given
- (high dose) caution if used in those who have undergone recent surgery
- caution if used in those with history of osteoporosis or spontaneous fractures

- caution if used in those with uncontrolled hypertension, hypertensive or diabetic retinopathy, primary or metastatic brain tumours, severe liver/kidney insufficiency, osteoporosis or spontaneous fractures, recent surgery, patients with cancer, high risk of bleeding, platelet disorder, thrombocytopenia or hereditary antithrombin III deficiency
- caution if used in those with diabetes mellitus, chronic renal failure or pre-existing metabolic acidosis due to increased risk of hyperkalaemia
- not recommended for prosthetic heart valve prophylaxis
- contraindicated in those with hypersensitivity to heparin or other low molecular weight heparins or pork products
- contraindicated in those with a history of heparin-induced thrombocytopenia, cerebral haemorrhage, GI ulceration, ulcerative colitis, severe coagulation disorder, acute/subacute bacterial endocarditis, sympathetic block, spinal/epidural puncture (not contraindicated in doses less than 5000 IU), surgery (brain, spinal cord, eyes, ears), haemorrhagic stroke or severe hypertension

Patient teaching and advice

- see General Patient teaching and advice for anticoagulants (p. 234)

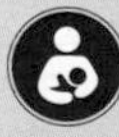

although heparin (and therefore dalteparin) does not cause fetal malformations, there is an increased risk of fetal loss and prematurity associated with maternal haemorrhage

not recommended during breastfeeding

DANAPAROID SODIUM (Orgaran)

Available forms

Ampoule: 750 antifactor Xa units/0.6 mL

Action

- heparinoids (not a low molecular weight heparin)
- inhibits thrombus formation
- little effect on platelet function and adhesion
- peak activity 4–5 hours, half-life 25 hours (SC) or 7 hours (IV)

Use

- prophylaxis of venous thromboembolism after surgery (general or orthopaedic)

Dose

- 750 anti-Xa units SC twice daily for 7–10 days

Adverse effects

- bleeding
- hypersensitivity (occasionally)
- (rare) thrombocytopenia, changes in liver enzymes
- (injection site) bruising and/or pain

Interactions

- caution when used with other anticoagulants, antiplatelet agents, NSAIDs or corticosteroids
- prolonged bleeding time may occur if given with aspirin
- may cause unreliable results if blood is taken within 5 hours of administration for prothrombin monitoring

Nursing points/Cautions

- low molecular weight heparins and danaparoid are not interchangeable
- should not be given IM
- rotate SC injection sites
- routine clotting assays are not suitable if anticoagulant monitoring is required
- if given preoperatively, last dose should be 1–4 hours before procedure
- patient should be closely monitored for signs of spinal haematoma (e.g. midline back pain, numbness, weakness, lower limb paralysis, bowel/bladder dysfunction) if they have a

spinal puncture or insertion/removal of epidural/spinal needle/catheter. Risk of haematoma formation is increased if the patient is taking NSAIDs, antiplatelet agents or other anticoagulants, or if the procedure is repeated or traumatic
- platelet count should be monitored before starting and during therapy for the early detection of thrombocytopenia
- caution if used in those with moderate kidney or liver impairment (with impaired haemostasis), GI tract lesions or other organs/sites at risk of bleeding
- contains sulfite, therefore is contraindicated in those with known hypersensitivity to sulfites
- contraindicated in those with diabetic retinopathy, acute/subacute bacterial endocarditis, severe hypertension, severe kidney or liver insufficiency, history of heparin-induced thrombocytopenia, uncontrolled active bleeding, severe gastric or duodenal ulceration (unless this is the reason for surgery), haemophilia or other bleeding disorders

Patient teaching and advice

- see General Patient teaching and advice for anticoagulants (p. 234)

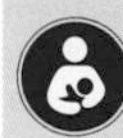

not recommended during pregnancy unless benefits are thought to outweigh risks

ENOXAPARIN SODIUM (Clexane, Clexane Forte)

Available forms

Prefilled syringe: 20 mg/0.2 mL, 40 mg/0.4 mL, 60 mg/0.6 mL, 80 mg/0.8 mL, 100 mg/mL, 120 mg/0.8 mL, 150 mg/mL; Ampoule: 40 mg/0.4 mL

Action

- low molecular weight heparin (smaller fragment of heparin prepared from unfractionated heparin using enzymatic or chemical methods, with a molecular weight about a third of heparin)
- binds to and accelerates antithrombin III action
- inactivates factor Xa and factor IIa (thrombin) leading to decreased thrombin formation preventing fibrin clot formation
- has four times the effect on factor Xa compared to factor IIa
- minimal effect on bleeding

Use

- prophylaxis of venous thromboembolism after surgery (general, orthopedic) or bedridden acutely ill patients
- prevention of thrombosis in extracorporeal circulation during haemodialysis
- treatment of established DVT
- unstable angina and non-Q wave myocardial infarction (with aspirin)
- treatment of acute ST segment elevation myocardial infarction (STEMI) (adjunct with fibrinolytics)

Dose

- (prophylaxis of venous thrombosis – high risk) 40 mg SC once daily for 7–10 days, initial dose 12 hours before surgery **OR**
- (prophylaxis of venous thrombosis – medium risk) 20 mg SC once daily for 7–10 days, initial dose 2 hours before surgery **OR**
- (prophylaxis of venous thrombosis – medical patient) 40 mg SC once daily for 6–14 days or until patient is fully mobile **OR**
- (prolonged thromboembolic prophylaxis e.g. total hip replacement) 40 mg SC once daily for 30 days postoperatively **OR**
- (treatment of DVT) 1 mg/kg SC twice daily or 1.5 mg/kg SC once daily for at least 5 days **OR**

- (haemodialysis) 1 mg/kg into the arterial line of the dialysis unit at start of session, with 0.5–1 mg/kg fresh addition if fibrin rings form and depending on time before end of dialysis **OR**
- (haemodialysis, high risk of haemorrhage) 0.5 mg/kg (double vascular access) or 0.75 mg/kg (single vascular access) **OR**
- (unstable angina and non-Q wave myocardial infarction) 1 mg/kg SC 12-hourly (with aspirin 100–325 mg daily) for 2–8 days **OR**
- (treatment of STEMI) 30 mg as IV bolus along with 1 mg/kg SC, then 1 mg/kg SC 12-hourly (with fibrinolytic therapy) for 8 days or until hospital discharge

Adverse effects

- haemorrhage, anaemia, mild transient thrombocytopenia
- nausea, diarrhoea
- fever
- peripheral oedema
- urticaria, pruritus, erythema
- elevated liver enzymes
- confusion, headache
- (uncommon) allergic reaction
- (injection site) haematoma, pain, swelling, bleeding
- (rare) hyperkalaemia, alopecia
- (prolonged therapy) osteoporosis

Interactions

- other drugs (e.g. anticoagulants, fibrinolytics, NSAIDs, aspirin, aspirin-containing preparations, ticlopidine, dextran, antiplatelet agents, clopidogrel, corticosteroids) affecting haemostasis should be withdrawn before starting therapy
- increased risk of hyperkalaemia if given with potassium-sparing agents, potassium supplements or ACE inhibitors, therefore potassium levels should be monitored during therapy

Nursing points/Cautions

- low molecular weight heparins are not interchangeable
- should not be given IM
- (IV) administer alone ensuring IV lines are well flushed with sodium chloride 0.9% or dextrose 5% before and after administration
- if patient has percutaneous coronary revascularisation procedure, 0.3 mg/kg IV bolus should be given if last enoxaparin dose was > 8 hours before balloon inflation. If closure device is used, sheath should be removed immediately. If manual compression is used to achieve haemostasis, sheath should be removed 6 hours after last dose. Enoxaparin should not be administered within 6–8 hours of sheath removal. Site should be closely monitored for any signs of bleeding or haematoma formation
- (acute STEMI treatment) enoxaparin should be given between 15 minutes before and 30 minutes after the start of fibrinolytic therapy. Aspirin (100–300 mg) should also be started (unless contraindicated)
- therapy should be ceased for 12–24 hours (depending on dose) before the insertion/removal of epidural/spinal needle/catheter and next dose given at least 4 hours after the procedure. If blood was present during needle/catheter placement, next dose should be delayed by 24 hours. Site should be closely monitored for any signs of spinal haematoma. Patient should be advised to immediately report any numbness/weakness of lower limbs, back pain or bowel/bladder dysfunction
- patient should be closely monitored for signs of spinal haematoma (e.g. midline back pain, numbness, weakness, lower limb paralysis, bowel/bladder dysfunction) if they have a spinal puncture or

insertion/removal of epidural/spinal needle/catheter. Risk of haematoma formation is increased if the patient is taking NSAIDs, antiplatelet agents or other anticoagulants, or if the procedure is repeated or traumatic

- (DVT treatment) therapy with warfarin should be started within 72 hours of commencing enoxaparin and continued for at least 5 days and until INR is 2.0–3.0
- should not be mixed with other injections or infusions
- platelet count should be monitored before starting and throughout therapy. If counts fall to 30–50% of pre-therapy level or below 100,000/mm^3, drug should be withdrawn
- when therapy is for DVT, warfarin is usually started 72 hours after enoxaparin and the two continued until the INR is 2.0–3.0
- routine monitoring of blood clotting is generally not required
- SC injection sites should be rotated
- SC injection site should not be rubbed after administration
- entire length of needle should be injected at 90 degrees to the skin which has been gently pinched between thumb and finger and held throughout injection
- prefilled syringe needles are coated with silicone to enhance ease of skin penetration. Needles should not be wiped or enoxaparin allowed to crystallise as this will damage the silicone coating
- air bubble should not be expelled from prefilled syringe before injection
- if overdosage occurs, it may be neutralised using protamine sulfate as IV infusion (1 mg protamine sulfate will neutralise 1 mg enoxaparin) if enoxaparin was given in previous 8 hours. If > 8 hours, 0.5 mg protamine sulfate is used for each 1 mg enoxaparin. If > 12 hours, protamine may not be necessary (depending on clinical circumstances)
- close monitoring for thromboembolism is recommended if patient has BMI > 30 kg/m^2
- caution if used in women weighing less than 45 kg or men weighing less than 57 kg due to increased risk of bleeding
- caution if used in those with diabetes, chronic kidney failure or pre-existing metabolic acidosis due to increased risk of hyperkalaemia
- caution if used in those with bacterial endocarditis, congenital/acquired bleeding disorders, active ulceration, GI disease, haemorrhagic stroke, recent surgery (brain, eye, spine), uncontrolled hypertension, bleeding disorders, liver impairment, diabetic retinopathy, recent ischaemic stroke or impaired haemostasis
- caution if used in those with kidney impairment as clearance is decreased resulting in increased risk of bleeding
- not recommended for thromboembolism prophylaxis in those with prosthetic heart valves
- contraindicated in those with hypersensitivity to heparin or other low molecular weight heparins
- contraindicated in those with a history of heparin-induced thrombocytopenia (within last 10 years or with antibodies present), thrombocytopenia (with antibodies), cerebral haemorrhage, gastric ulcer, ulcerative colitis, severe coagulation/bleeding disorders, acute/subacute bacterial endocarditis, spinal/epidural puncture, surgery (brain, spinal cord, eyes, ears), conditions with bleeding tendencies, haemorrhagic stroke or severe hypertension

Patient teaching and advice

- see General Patient teaching and advice for anticoagulants (p. 234)

- instruct patient in self-administration. This should include injection technique (under the skin and not into muscle), rotation of injection sites, not rubbing site after injection, correct storage and disposal of used syringes information

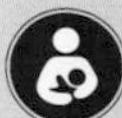

should only be used during pregnancy if the benefits to the mother outweigh the risks to the fetus

not recommended during breastfeeding

NADROPARIN CALCIUM (Fraxiparine, Fraxiparine Forte)

Available forms

Ungraduated prefilled syringe: 1900 IU anti-Xa/0.2 mL, 2850 IU anti-Xa/0.3 mL, 3800 IU anti-Xa/0.4 mL; Graduated prefilled syringe: 5700 IU anti-Xa/0.6 mL, 7600 IU anti-Xa/0.8 mL, 9500 IU anti-Xa/mL, 11,400 IU anti-Xa/0.6 mL, 15,200 IU anti-Xa/0.8 mL, 19,000 anti-Xa/mL

Action

- low molecular weight heparin with a high ratio of anti-Xa activity to anti-IIa compared to unfractionated heparin
- has both immediate and prolonged antithrombotic actions
- high affinity for antithrombin III leading to a rapid inhibition of factor Xa (and also factor IIa to a lesser extent) contributing to antithrombotic activity
- also activates fibrinolysis via release of tissue plasminogen activator, decreases blood viscosity and increases platelet and granulocyte membrane fluidity

Use

- prophylaxis and treatment of DVT associated with general and orthopaedic surgery
- prophylaxis of venous thromboembolism in at-risk medical patients
- prevention of clotting during haemodialysis

Dose

- (DVT treatment) dose is weight dependent and based on 171 anti-Xa IU/kg SC once daily for 10 days (Fraxiparine Forte) **OR**
- (DVT prophylaxis – general surgery) 2850 anti-Xa IU/0.3 mL SC 2–4 hours before surgery, then daily on subsequent days for at least 7 days until patient is ambulant (Fraxiparine) **OR**
- (DVT prophylaxis – orthopaedic surgery) dose is weight dependent and based on 38 anti-Xa IU/kg SC starting 12 hours before and after surgery, then once daily to third postoperative day, then increasing dose by 50% from fourth post-operative day for at least 10 days and until patient is ambulant (Fraxiparine) **OR**
- (DVT treatment) dose is weight dependent and based on 86 anti-Xa IU/kg SC twice daily for 10 days (Fraxiparine) **OR**
- (prevention of clotting during haemodialysis) 2850 anti-Xa IU/0.3 mL (weight $<$ 50 kg), 3800 anti-Xa IU/0.4 mL (weight 50–69 kg) or 5700 anti-Xa IU/0.6 mL (weight $\geq$ 70 kg) injected into arterial line at start of dialysis (for sessions up to 4 hours). If session $>$ 4 hours, an additional smaller dose may be given (Fraxiparine) **OR**
- (thromboembolism prophylaxis in medical patients) 3800 anti-Xa IU/0.4 mL (weight $\leq$ 70 kg) or 5700 anti-Xa IU/0.6 mL (weight $>$ 70 kg) started within 12–24 hours of admission and continued for up to 28 days

Adverse effects

- bleeding, anaemia
- transient elevated transaminases
- (rare) thrombocytopenia, rash, urticaria, erythema, pruritus

- (very rare) cutaneous necrosis (preceded by purpura and painful erythematous blotches), reversible hyperkalaemia, hypersensitivity
- (injection site) haematoma, reaction

Interactions

- not recommended with aspirin, other salicylates, NSAIDs, ticlopidine or other antiplatelet agents due to increased risk of bleeding
- caution if given with dextrans or systemic corticosteroids
- if used with warfarin, nadroparin calcium should be continued until INR is stabilised at target level
- increased risk of hyperkalaemia if given with potassium-sparing agents, potassium supplements or ACE inhibitors, therefore potassium levels should be monitored during therapy

Nursing points/Cautions

- low molecular weight heparins are not interchangeable
- should not be given IM
- platelet count should be monitored before starting and throughout therapy
- (medical patients) therapy should only be started if immobility/bed rest is expected to last longer than 3 days
- (DVT treatment) oral anticoagulant should be started as soon as possible (unless contraindicated), but nadroparin calcium should not be stopped until INR target level is reached and stabilised
- SC injection sites should be rotated (abdomen and thigh are recommended sites)
- (Fraxiparine ungraduated syringe) entire dose is injected
- (Fraxiparine ungraduated syringe) air bubble in syringe does not have to be removed before administration
- (Fraxiparine, Fraxiparine Forte graduated syringe) hold vertically with needle uppermost and air bubble at top of syringe. Plunger should be advanced to volume/dose required expelling air bubble and any excess
- SC injection site should not be rubbed after administration
- prefilled syringe may contain dry natural latex rubber which can cause allergic reactions in those with latex hypersensitivity
- patient should be closely monitored for signs of spinal haematoma (e.g. midline back pain, numbness, weakness, lower limb paralysis, bowel/bladder dysfunction) if they have a spinal puncture or insertion/removal of epidural/spinal needle/catheter. Risk of haematoma formation is increased if the patient is taking NSAIDs, antiplatelet agents or other anticoagulants, or if the procedure is repeated or traumatic. A minimum of 12–24 hours (depending on dose) should elapse before insertion/removal of spinal/epidural catheter
- increased risk of hyperkalaemia if used in those with pre-existing raised plasma potassium, diabetes mellitus, chronic renal failure, pre-existing metabolic acidosis or taking agents that cause hyperkalaemia (e.g. ACE inhibitors, NSAIDs). Potassium levels should be closely monitored
- in the event of serious overdosage, protamine sulfate can be given by slow IV injection (6 mg protamine sulfate neutralises about 950 IU anti-Xa (about 0.1 mL)), taking into account time elapsed from nadroparin injection. Fresh frozen plasma can be used if transfusion is needed
- caution if used in those at increased risk of bleeding, including kidney impairment, liver insufficiency, liver failure, severe arterial hypertension, history of peptic ulceration or other lesion likely to bleed, vascular disorder of chorio-retina, postoperatively after brain, eye or spinal cord surgery

- caution if used in those with history of heparin-induced thrombocytopaenia and should only be used if necessary. If used, patient should be carefully monitored included daily platelet count assessment as there is an increased risk of thrombocytopenia occurring
- not recommended in those under 18 years
- contraindicated in those with a history of nadroparin-induced thrombocytopaenia, increased risk of haemorrhage (including bleeding disorders), active bleeding or organic lesions likely to bleed (e.g. active peptic ulceration), infective endocarditis, haemorrhagic cerebrovascular accident or with severe kidney failure (creatinine clearance < 30 mL/min) receiving treatment for DVT

Patient teaching and advice

- see General Patient teaching and advice for anticoagulants (p. 234)

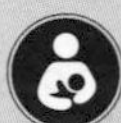

not recommended during pregnancy or breastfeeding unless benefits outweigh risks

VITAMIN K ANTAGONISTS

WARFARIN SODIUM (Coumadin, Marevan)

Available forms

Tablets: 1 mg, 2 mg, 3 mg, 5 mg

Action

- long-acting coumarin derivative
- interferes with vitamin K-dependent synthesis of prothrombin (factor II) and factors VII, IX and X in the liver, preventing the extension of established clot or formation of new clot(s)
- also decreases synthesis of protein C and S (vitamin K-dependent anticoagulant proteins)
- onset of action 24–48 hours, duration of action 2–5 days
- half-life 25–60 hours (average 40 hours)
- narrow therapeutic index
- some genetic variation in response and some patients may have a hereditary resistance to warfarin
- anticoagulant effect influenced by diet, drugs and disease states

Use

- prevention and management of venous thrombosis (e.g. DVT, pulmonary embolism)
- prevention and management of thromboembolism in atrial fibrillation, myocardial infarction or those with prosthetic heart valves
- adjunct in treatment of coronary occlusion

Dose

- initially 10 mg orally daily for 2–4 days then maintenance dose of 2–10 mg daily based on INR

Adverse effects

- haemorrhage (mild, severe or life threatening, affecting any tissue or organ)
- nausea, vomiting, diarrhoea, flatulence/bloating, taste alteration, abdominal pain
- pruritus, rash, urticaria
- fatigue, lethargy, malaise, asthenia
- headache, dizziness
- alopecia
- elevated liver enzymes, hepatitis
- fever, chills, cold intolerance, paraesthesia
- (rare) systemic cholesterol microemboli, purple toe syndrome (see Glossary), skin (or tissue) necrosis, hypersensitivity reaction, calciphylaxis

- (long-term therapy, rare) tracheal or tracheo-bronchial calcification

Interactions

- alcohol (acute intoxication), allopurinol, alteplase, amiodarone, amoxicillin, aspirin, azithromycin, bivalirudin, cefazolin, cefoxitin, ceftriaxone, celecoxib, chloramphenicol, cimetidine, ciprofloxacin, clarithromycin, clofibrate, clopidogrel, danazol, dextran, diazoxide, diclofenac, diflunisal, disopyramide, disulfiram, doxycycline, efavirenz, etacrynic acid, erythromycin, fenofibrate, fluconazole, fluorouracil, fluvastatin, gefitinib, gemcitabine, glucagon (high dose), heparin, ibuprofen, ifosfamide, indometacin, influenza virus vaccine, interferons, isoniazid, itraconazole, ketorolac, ketoprofen, levothyroxine, liothyronine, lovastatin, mefenamic acid, mefloquine, mesterolone, methylprednisolone, methyl salicylate ointment (topical), metronidazole, miconazole, nadroparin, nandrolone, naproxen, neomycin, norfloxacin, olsalazine, omeprazole, oxandrolone, pentoxifylline (oxpentifylline), paracetamol, piroxicam, posaconazole, prednisolone, prednisone, propranolol, quinine, ranitidine, rosuvastatin, roxithromycin, simvastatin, sodium valproate, sulfamethoxazole, sulindac, tamoxifen, testosterone, tetracyclines, ticlopidine, tramadol, trimethoprim/sulfamethoxazole, vitamin E and voriconazole enhance the activity of oral anticoagulants, which may lead to bleeding episodes
- activity reduced by chronic abuse of alcohol, aminoglutamide, aprepitant, ascorbic acid (vitamin C) (high dose), azathioprine, bosentan, carbamazepine, carbimazole, colestyramine, dicloxacillin, flucloxacillin, griseofulvin, isotretinoin, mercaptopurine, phenobarbital (phenobarbitone), primidone, propylthiouracil, ribavirin, rifabutin, rifampicin, spironolactone, sucralfate, vitamin K, vitamin K-rich diet
- extra caution if used with aspirin or NSAIDs as inhibition of platelet aggregation will occur in addition to the increased risk of GI bleeding, peptic ulceration and/or perforation
- may enhance hypoglycaemic effects of hypoglycaemic agents
- increased risk of bleeding if given with SSRIs and SNRIs
- if given with phenytoin, there may be a transient increase in anticoagulant effect, followed by a decrease in anticoagulant effect
- may increase serum levels of phenytoin
- caution if given with ciclosporin, cyclophosphamide, oestrogens, mesalazine or corticotropin as effects are unpredictable
- increased activity if given with glucosamine
- increased anticoagulant effect may occur if used with garlic, ginkgo or curcumin
- warfarin metabolism may be increased by St John's wort, ginseng and co-enzyme 10 leading to decreased INR

Nursing points/Cautions

- Coumadin and Marevan should not be interchanged as bioequivalence has not been established
- large loading doses (e.g. 30 mg) are not recommended because of the increased risk of bleeding and complications
- patient should be assessed for any risk factors for bleeding, including INR $>$ 4.0. age $\geq$ 75 years, highly variable INRs and long duration of warfarin therapy
- bleeding can occur within therapeutic range and may be due to the unmasking of a lesion such as a tumour

- if large daily doses are required to maintain INR with normal therapeutic range, acquired or inherited warfarin resistance should be considered as a cause
- signs of bleeding are dependent on location and extent of bleeding
- avoid IM injections, and any SC injection sites should be observed for haematoma
- if IM injections cannot be avoided, they should be restricted to upper extremities where manual compression, application of pressure bandage and easy observation of site is possible
- observe for early signs of overdose such as bleeding, especially from the gums
- urine is not routinely tested daily for blood
- oral therapy is usually initiated at the same time or soon after starting heparin or low molecular weight heparins; heparin/low molecular weight heparin is stopped gradually once the effect of oral anticoagulant is apparent, usually in 36–48 hours
- when heparin and warfarin are given together, blood for prothrombin activity is taken 5 hours after last IV heparin bolus dose, 4 hours after stopping IV heparin infusion or 24 hours after last SC heparin injection
- optimal dose is highly individual and dose is adjusted by monitoring the prothrombin activity of the blood, usually measured as INR (see p. 234); however, after dose adjustment, response is usually not apparent for 2–3 days
- baseline INR should be measured before starting therapy, then daily for first 5 days. When there are two consecutive INRs in target range, INR monitoring interval can be increased
- additional monitoring is recommended when other medications are started, stopped or dosages are changed, if the patient's medical condition alters (e.g. alcohol intake, dehydration, diarrhoea, oedema, poor nutrition), and/or if there are changes to other conditions such as diet and environment
- INR is maintained at 2.0–2.5 (prophylaxis of DVT), 2.0–3.0 (treatment of DVT, pulmonary embolism and atrial fibrillation), 2.5–3.5 (recurrent DVT and pulmonary embolism, myocardial infarction, arterial grafts, cardiac prosthetic valves and grafts)
- duration of therapy is dependent on reason for use (e.g. DVT or PE prophylaxis – usually at least 3 months, mitral stenosis – indefinite, rheumatic mitral valve disease – long term)
- (atrial fibrillation non-valvular) treatment is usually continued for at least 1 month after normal sinus rhythm has been established (unless contraindicated)
- oral anticoagulants are withdrawn gradually over 3–4 weeks
- therapy should be stopped 5 days before procedures with moderate-to-high risk of bleeding to allow INR to normalise. If patient is at high risk of thrombosis (e.g. prosthetic heart valve) low molecular weight heparin can be used for 12–24 hours before procedure
- patient should be educated before discharge (see p. 249 for list of teaching considerations)
- treatment of overdose is dependent on the extent of the bleeding. Severe life-threatening bleeding should be managed by stopping warfarin therapy, administration of phytomenadione (vitamin K) IV 5–10 mg over 30 seconds with fresh frozen plasma or prothrombin complex concentrate. Prothrombin time should be measured 3 hours later and a further dose given if response is inadequate

- caution if used in those over 70 years as there is an increased risk of bleeding, especially for females
- caution if used in those with congenital/acquired protein S or protein C deficiency due to increased risk of skin necrosis
- caution if given to those with severe-to-moderate liver/kidney insufficiency, moderate-to-severe hypertension, infectious diseases, disturbance to GI flora (including antibacterial therapy), trauma which may result in internal bleeding, surgery/trauma resulting in extensive wounds, indwelling catheters, bacterial endocarditis, pericarditis, pericardial effusion, cerebral aneurysm, dissecting aorta, known/suspected deficiency or protein C mediated anticoagulation response, warfarin resistance (inherited or acquired), polycythaemia vera, vasculitis or severe diabetes
- caution if used in those with congestive cardiac failure as a greater response may be seen, requiring more frequent INR monitoring
- contraindicated in those with active bleeding or bleeding tendency (with or without active ulceration), blood dyscrasias, threatened abortion, eclampsia or pre-eclampsia, alcoholism, psychosis, spinal puncture or regional lumbar block anaesthesia, malignant hypertension, recent (or planned) surgery of CNS or eyes or resulting in extensive surgical wounds, lack of patient cooperation (including those with dementia with no supervision) or if there are inadequate laboratory facilities available

Patient teaching and advice

- see General Patient teaching and advice for anticoagulants (p. 234)
- emphasise the importance of carrying the Anticoagulant handbook/booklet because it includes laboratory test results and daily anticoagulant dose
- advise the patient of the importance of attending doctor's visits and having regular blood tests as these determine the dose to be taken
- advise patient that tablets are to be taken whole, not chewed or crushed and taken at the same time every day (in the evening). The patient should be further instructed not to take a 'make up' dose (e.g. double dose) if the dose is missed and to seek advice from doctor or pharmacist if this occurs
- instruct patient to seek medical advice immediately if any of the following occur:
  - unusual or prolonged bleeding or bruising
  - increased menstrual flow or vaginal bleeding
  - unusual nosebleeds
  - bleeding gums when brushing teeth
  - vomiting or coughing up blood
  - red or dark brown urine
  - stools are tarry (black or dark brown) or red
  - well-demarcated red skin lesions (thighs, buttocks, toes, breast) occurring 2–5 days after starting therapy where the centre of the lesion becomes necrotic
  - blackness in tissue at extremities such as fingers, toes or penis
  - toes that become dark purple or mottled in colour, blanch with moderate pressure and fades with elevation, painful or tender (usually occurring 3–10 weeks after starting therapy)
  - intense pain in leg, foot or toes
  - new foot ulcers or severe skin wounds
  - abdominal, joint, chest, back or flank pain

  - fever, headache, dizziness or weakness
  - painful swelling or discomfort
  - swollen ankles
  - persistent diarrhoea
- instruct patient to avoid any activity that could result in traumatic injury
- advise patient of importance of seeking medical advice immediately if any serious fall or injury occurs
- warn patient to avoid alcohol during therapy
- emphasise the importance of notifying others (e.g. dentist or surgeon) of the anticoagulant therapy before any procedure
- warn patient that effects last for 2–5 days after warfarin has been stopped
- patient should not stop warfarin therapy abruptly or stop/start any other medication (including OTC medications such as aspirin and other analgesics, herbal or vitamin preparations) without first seeking medical advice (doctor, pharmacist) as *many* preparations interact with warfarin
- discuss the importance of maintaining a balanced diet and avoid large increases in vegetables containing vitamin K (e.g. green leafy vegetables)
- seek medical advice if travel is planned or if person becomes unwell (e.g. prolonged diarrhoea), which might also result in dietary change or exposure to prolonged hot weather (i.e. possibility of dehydration) as these are all factors that can affect the individual's response to warfarin
- women of childbearing years should be counselled to use effective contraception to avoid pregnancy while taking warfarin and should seek medical advice if pregnancy should occur
- see also General Patient teaching and advice (p. xxvii)

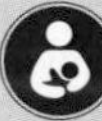

warfarin is contraindicated during pregnancy as it crosses the placenta and fetal blood concentrations are similar to those of mother. Warfarin use has been associated with fetal haemorrhage, birth malformations, increased risk of spontaneous abortion and perinatal bleeding

warfarin can be used safely during breastfeeding

tablet can be crushed and mixed with spoonful of yoghurt or apple puree

ANTITHROMBIN III-DEPENDENT ANTICOAGULANTS

FONDAPARINUX SODIUM (Arixtra)

Available form

Prefilled syringe: 2.5 mg/0.5 mL

Action

- synthetically produced selective inhibitor of factor Xa
- inhibits both thrombin formation and development of thrombus
- has no effect on platelet aggregation or thrombin
- not neutralised by protamine sulfate
- half-life is about 17 hours (prolonged to about 20 hours in the elderly)

Use

- prophylaxis of venous thromboembolism associated with major orthopaedic (hip, knee) or abdominal surgery
- treatment of acute deep vein thrombosis (DVT) or pulmonary embolus (PE)
- treatment of unstable angina or non-ST segment elevation myocardial infarction (UA/NSTEMI) in patients

where urgent invasive management is not indicated
- treatment of ST-segment elevation myocardial infarction (STEMI) in patients managed without any initial reperfusion therapy

Dose
- (prophylaxis of venous thromboembolism, < 75 years, no kidney or liver impairment, mild kidney impairment) 2.5 mg SC daily, starting 6 hours after surgical closure, for 5–9 days or as long as thromboembolic risk exists (maximum 31 days) **OR**
- (treatment of acute DVT or PE) 7.5 mg (5 mg if patient weight < 50 kg, 10 mg if patient weight >100 kg) SC daily for at least 5 days and until INR range is within 2–3 (until oral anticoagulant therapy is established) **OR**
- (UA/NSTEMI treatment) 2.5 mg SC once daily for up to 8 days or hospital discharge if earlier **OR**
- (STEMI treatment) initially 2.5 mg IV, then 2.5 mg SC once daily for up to 8 days or hospital discharge if earlier

Adverse effects
- bleeding, anaemia, purpura
- hypokalaemia
- insomnia, headache, dizziness, confusion
- hypotension, hypertension
- nausea, vomiting, diarrhoea, dyspepsia, constipation
- increase in liver enzymes
- rash, bullous eruption
- urinary retention, urinary tract infection
- fever
- oedema
- cough, pneumonia
- increased wound drainage
- pain, back pain
- (rare) angioedema, allergic reaction

Interactions
- agents increasing risk of bleeding should be stopped before starting fondaparinux. If this is not possible, closely monitor for bleeding

Nursing points/Cautions
- first dose should be given no earlier than 6 hours postsurgical closure and achievement of haemostasis
- should not be given IM
- platelet count should be monitored at the start and end of therapy
- (orthopedic patients) kidney function should be monitored regularly throughout therapy
- (STEMI, UA/NSTEMI) therapy should be stopped 24 hours before coronary artery bypass graft surgery and restarted after 48 hours
- if patient is to undergo percutaneous coronary intervention, therapy should not be restarted earlier than at least 2 hours (UA/NSTEMI) or 3 hours (STEMI) after sheath removal
- (IV, first dose, STEMI patients only) may be given as IV injection through existing line or via sodium chloride 0.9% mini bag (25–50 mL) and given over 1–2 minutes. IV line should be well flushed with sodium chloride 0.9% after administration
- SC injection sites should be rotated and documented
- to use the prefilled syringe the following instructions should be followed:
    - safety syringe is made up of needle guard, plunger, finger grip and security sleeve
    - needle guard should be removed by twisting and pulling it straight off and then discarding shield
    - air bubble should not be expelled before use
    - full length of needle should be inserted at 90 degrees into skin fold
    - after SC injection, needle will automatically withdraw into security sleeve to lock permanently

- discard used prefilled syringe into sharps disposal container
- patient should be closely monitored for signs of spinal haematoma (e.g. midline back pain, numbness, weakness, lower limb paralysis, bowel/bladder dysfunction) if they have a spinal puncture or insertion/removal of epidural/spinal needle/catheter. Risk of haematoma formation is increased if the patient is taking NSAIDs, antiplatelet agents or other anticoagulants, or if the procedure is repeated or traumatic
- for orthopaedic surgery where risk of venous thromboembolism persists, therapy may continue for up to 31 days
- patient can be taught self-administration
- (treatment of acute DVT or PE) oral anticoagulant should be started within 72 hours
- if switching to heparin or another LMWH, therapy should start one day after last fondaparinx injection
- needle guard may contain latex rubber which may cause allergic reaction in those with latex allergy
- caution if used in patients with history of heparin-induced thrombocytopenia
- caution if used in those weighing less than 50 kg, over 75 years of age, with renal impairment (creatinine clearance < 50 mL/min) or severe liver impairment
- caution if used in those at increased risk of bleeding, or with congenital/acquired bleeding disorders, active GI ulceration, recent surgery (brain, spinal, eye) or recent intracranial haemorrhage
- contraindicated in those with severe kidney impairment (creatinine clearance < 30 mL/min), acute bacterial endocarditis or major bleeding

Patient teaching and advice

- instruct patient in self-administration. This should include injection technique (under the skin and not into muscle), rotation of injection sites, not rubbing site after injection, correct storage and disposal of used syringes information
- see General Patient teaching and advice for anticoagulants (p. 234)

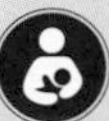

should only be used during pregnancy if benefits to the mother outweigh the risks to the fetus

not recommended during breastfeeding

DIRECT THROMBIN INHIBITORS

BIVALIRUDIN (Angiomax)

Available form

Vial: 250 mg

Action

- synthetic analogue of hirudin (anticoagulant found in leech saliva)
- reversible and specific thrombin inhibitor
- half-life 25 minutes

Use

- percutaneous coronary intervention (PCI) (with aspirin)
- treatment of moderate-to-high risk acute coronary syndrome (ACS) (e.g. unstable angina/non-ST segment elevation myocardial infarction) undergoing early invasive management

Dose

- (PCI) initially 0.75 mg/kg IV bolus, then 1.75 mg/kg/hour IV infusion for remainder of procedure or up to 4 hours post-procedure as needed (with 300–325 mg aspirin) **OR**
- (ACS) initially 0.1 mg/kg IV bolus, then 0.25 mg/kg/hour IV infusion for up to 72 hours (with aspirin 300–325 mg orally). If patient then has PCI, additional 0.5 mg/kg IV bolus should be given at the start of the procedure, then 1.75 mg/kg/hour IV infusion for remainder of procedure. When procedure is complete, IV infusion is decreased to 0.25 mg/kg/hour for 4–12 hours as needed

Adverse effects

- bleeding
- nausea, vomiting
- fever
- atrial fibrillation, hypotension, hypertension, angina, bradycardia
- back pain, chest pain
- headache, insomnia
- (IV site) pain, bleeding, haematoma
- (uncommon) hypersensitivity

Interactions

- heparin should be discontinued for 30 minutes before starting bivalirudin
- low molecular weight heparins should be discontinued for 8 hours before starting bivalirudin
- increased risk of bleeding if given with other anticoagulant or antiplatelet agents and should therefore be given with caution

Nursing points/Cautions

- not given IM
- (PCI) patient should be closely monitored for signs and symptoms of myocardial infarction throughout infusion
- (PCI) patient should be closely observed for at least 24 hours post-procedure as STEMI patients are at increased risk of acute stent thrombosis (especially in first 4 hours after procedure)
- therapy should be commenced just prior to PCI
- reconstitute using 5 mL water for injections, swirl gently until dissolved then dilute using sodium chloride 0.9% or glucose 5% for a total volume of 50 mL and concentration of 5 mg/mL
- incompatible with alteplase, amiodarone, amphotericin B (amphotericin), chlorpromazine, diazepam, prochlorperazine, reteplase and vancomycin as precipitation may occur. Other incompatibilities include dobutamine (4 mg/mL), haloperidol (0.2 mg/mL) and promethazine (2 mg/mL)
- not recommended during gamma brachytherapy (radiation therapy where the radiation source is placed in direct contact with tumour)
- caution if used in patients who are at risk of bleeding
- contraindicated in those with increased risk of active bleeding, irreversible coagulation disorders, severe uncontrolled hypertension, subacute bacterial endocarditis, severe kidney impairment (creatinine clearance < 30 mL/min) or dialysis dependent patients

Patient teaching and advice

- see General Patient teaching and advice for anticoagulants (p. 234)

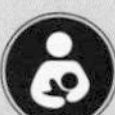

not recommended during pregnancy unless potential benefits outweigh risks

caution if used during breastfeeding

DABIGATRAN ETEXILATE (Pradaxa)

Available forms
Capsules: 75 mg, 110 mg, 150 mg

Action
- dabigatran etexilate is a prodrug which is converted to the active metabolite dabigatran
- dabigatran inhibits both free and clot-bound thrombin by binding specifically to the thrombin's active site
- half-life 8–10 hours (single dose) or 14–17 hours (multiple doses)

Use
- prophylaxis of venous thromboembolic event (VTE) after major orthopaedic surgery (total hip, knee replacement)
- prophylaxis of stroke and systemic embolism in those with non-valvular atrial fibrillation and at least one additional risk factor for stroke
- treatment of deep vein thrombosis (DVT) or pulmonary embolism (PE) and prevention of recurrent DVT or PE

Dose
- (prophylaxis of VTE after major orthopaedic surgery) initially 110 mg orally 1–4 hours after completed surgery, then 220 mg orally once daily for 10 days (knee replacement) or 28–35 days (hip replacement) **OR**
- (prophylaxis of stroke and systemic embolism in those with non-valvular atrial fibrillation) 150 mg orally twice daily **OR**
- (treatment of, or prevention of recurrent DVT or PE) 150 mg orally twice daily

Adverse effects
- bleeding, anaemia
- nausea, vomiting, dyspepsia, diarrhoea, constipation
- dizziness, headache, insomnia
- fever
- increased wound discharge/complication
- arthralgia, muscle spasm, extremity pain
- hypotension, syncope, atrial fibrillation, hypertension
- urinary tract infection, urinary retention
- rash, pruritus, erythema, blistering
- peripheral oedema
- hypokalaemia
- abnormal liver enzymes

Interactions
- contraindicated with verapamil (either starting verapamil and dabigatran simultaneously or adding verapamil to stable dabigatran therapy)
- contraindicated with glecaprevir/pibrentasvir combination
- not recommended with heparin, low molecular weight heparins, aspirin, antiplatelet agents, fondaparinux, fibrinolytic agents, ticagrelor, dextran or warfarin
- not recommended with itraconazole, tacrolimus, ciclosporin, ritonavir, nelfinavir, saquinavir
- increased risk of bleeding if given with SSRIs or SNRIs
- not recommended with P glycoprotein inducers such as carbamazepine, rifampicin, phenytoin and St John's wort as decreased serum level may occur
- increased serum levels may occur if given with P glycoprotein inhibitors such as amiodarone, clarithromycin, ritonavir and glecaprevir and should therefore be used with caution if at all
- increased risk of bleeding if given with NSAIDs (with half-life > 12 hours)
- may cause false positive INR elevation

Nursing points/Cautions
- liver and kidney function should be assessed before starting therapy

- (DVT/PE) treatment should be started with parenteral anticoagulant for at least 5 days before starting oral therapy with dabigatran
- dabigatran should be stopped 1–5 days preoperatively or pre-procedure to decrease risk of bleeding. The exact length of time is dependent on patient's risk of bleeding (high or standard), surgery type (e.g. major) and kidney function. If an acute intervention is required it should be delayed at least 12 hours after last dose to lessen risk of bleeding if possible
- (prophylaxis of VTE after major orthopaedic surgery) if treatment is not started on day of surgery, it should be started with 220 mg dose
- if switching from dabigatran etexilate to parenteral anticoagulant, 12–24 hours should be allowed to elapse from last oral dose to starting parenteral anticoagulant
- if switching from parenteral anticoagulant to dabigatran etexilate, dabigatran etexilate dose should be given up to 2 hours before next dose is due or if parenteral anticoagulant is being administered by continuous IV, dabigatran etexilate should be started when infusion is stopped
- if switching from dabigatran etexilate to warfarin, the starting time of warfarin should be based on creatinine clearance (CrC):
    - CrC > 50 mL/min, warfarin should be started 3 days before stopping dabigatran etexilate
    - CrC 31–50 mL/min, warfarin should be started 2 days before stopping dabigatran etexilate
    - CrC 15–30 mL/min, warfarin should be started 1 day before stopping dabigatran etexilate
- if switching from warfarin to dabigatran etexilate, warfarin should be stopped and dabigatran etexilate started when INR < 2.0
- patient should be closely monitored for signs of spinal haematoma (e.g. midline back pain, numbness, weakness, lower limb paralysis, bowel/bladder dysfunction) if they have a spinal puncture or insertion/removal of epidural/spinal needle/catheter. Risk of haematoma formation is increased if the patient is taking NSAIDs, antiplatelet agents or other anticoagulants, or if the procedure is repeated or traumatic
- INR should not be used for anticoagulation monitoring as it is unreliable and may produce false positive results
- if rapid reversal is required for emergency surgery/procedures or in the case of life-threatening bleeding, IV idarucizumab (see Antidotes, p. 350) can be used as it immediately reverses anticoagulant effects. A second dose may be required as dabigatran's anticoagulant actions may re-emerge up to 24 hours after first infusion
- dosage should be reduced in those aged ≥ 75 years or with moderate kidney impairment (CC 30–50 mL/min)
- capsules contain sunset yellow (FCF C/15985 (E110)), which is known to cause allergic reactions in some people
- not recommended in patients undergoing hip surgery, those with a PE and who are haemodynamically unstable, or who are eligible for fibrinolytic therapy or pulmonary embolectomy
- not recommended in those under 18 years
- caution if used in patients who are at risk of bleeding (including those with aPTT > 80 seconds), aged 75 years or older, congenital or acquired coagulation disorders, thrombocytopenia, functional platelet defect, recent biopsy, major trauma, recent intracranial haemorrhage, bacterial endocarditis or kidney impairment (creatinine clearance 30–50 mL/min)

- not recommended in those with history of thrombosis and antiphospholipid syndrome
- contraindicated in those with kidney impairment (creatinine clearance < 30 mL/min), increased risk of active bleeding, haemorrhagic stroke (within last 6 months), active peptic ulcer disease with recent bleeding, liver impairment/disease, history of intracranial, intraocular, spinal, retroperitoneal or atraumatic intra-articular bleeding, within 12 months of GI bleeding (unless permanently treated), prosthetic heart valves or within 2 hours of removal of indwelling spinal/epidural catheter, bleeding disorders, lesions or tumours at risk of bleeding, recent brain or spinal injury, recent brain or spinal surgery or injury, recent eye surgery, known or suspected oesophageal varices, arteriovenous malformations, vascular aneurysm, major intraspinal or intracerebral vascular abnormalities

Patient teaching and advice

- advise patient to swallow capsules whole, not chewed, broken or opened
- see also General Patient teaching and advice for anticoagulants (p. 234)

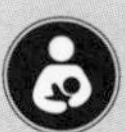

not recommended during pregnancy or breastfeeding

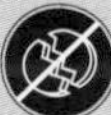

capsules should not be opened or crushed

DIRECT FACTOR XA INHIBITORS

General Action of direct factor Xa inhibitors

- highly selective and reversible inhibitor of factor Xa not requiring antithrombin III for its activity

General Adverse effects of direct factor Xa inhibitors

- bleeding, anaemia, bruising (contusion)
- nausea, vomiting, diarrhoea, constipation, dyspepsia, abdominal pain
- fever
- pain
- muscle spasm, arthralgia
- peripheral oedema
- wound discharge
- dizziness, somnolence, insomnia, headache
- hypotension, tachycardia, hypertension, chest pain
- cough, dyspnoea
- rash, pruritus, erythema, blistering
- jaundice, increased liver enzymes
- urinary retention, urinary tract infection

General Interactions of direct factor Xa inhibitors

- contraindicated with HIV protease inhibitors and azole antifungal agents
- contraindicated with heparin, low molecular weight heparins, fondaparinux and oral anticoagulants (except if switching from one agent to another)
- caution if given with NSAIDs, antiplatelet agents, aspirin, diltiazem, amiodarone, verapamil, SSRIs, SNRIs, and clarithromycin due to increased risk of bleeding
- decreased plasma levels may occur if given with phenytoin, carbamazepine, phenobarbital (phenobarbitone) or St John's wort

General Nursing points/Cautions of direct factor Xa inhibitors

- antiplatelet agents (except aspirin) should be stopped before surgical procedure and restarted as recommended. The risk of bleeding versus benefit (prevention of thrombotic risk) should occur for those patients requiring aspirin
- should be discontinued for at least 48 hours before elective surgery or invasive procedures with moderate-to-high risk of significant bleeding or 24 hours with low risk of bleeding
- patient should be closely monitored for signs of spinal haematoma (e.g. midline back pain, numbness, weakness, lower limb paralysis, bowel/bladder dysfunction) if they have a spinal puncture or insertion/removal of epidural/spinal needle/catheter
- not recommended as an alternative to heparin therapy as initial management of PE in those who are haemodynamically unstable or who may receive fibrinolytic therapy or pulmonary embolectomy
- caution in those with acute bacterial endocarditis, thrombocytopenia, platelet disorders, congenital or acquired bleeding disorders, history of haemorrhagic stroke, severe uncontrolled hypertension, > 75 years, bronchiectasis or history of lung bleeding
- not recommended for hip fracture surgery, prosthetic heart valves or antiphospholipid syndrome (with history of thrombosis)

APIXABAN (Eliquis)

Available forms

Tablet: 2.5 mg, 5 mg

Action

- see also General Action of direct factor Xa inhibitors, p. 256
- inhibits both free and clot-bound factor Xa and prothrombinase activity
- no direct effect of platelet aggregation
- half-life about 12 hours

Use

- prophylaxis of venous thromboembolism (VTE) after knee or hip replacement
- prophylaxis of stroke and systemic embolism in those with non-valvular atrial fibrillation with at least one other stroke factor
- treatment and prophylaxis of deep vein thrombosis (DVT) and pulmonary embolus (PE)

Dose

- (VTE prophylaxis after knee or hip surgery) 2.5 mg orally twice daily, starting 12–24 hours after surgery **OR**
- (prophylaxis of stroke and systemic embolism) 5 mg orally twice daily **OR**
- (treatment of DVT and PE) initially 10 mg orally twice daily for 7 days, then 5 mg orally twice daily **OR**
- (prophylaxis of DVT or PE) 2.5 mg orally twice daily for at least 6 months after treatment of DVT or PE (see above)

Adverse effects

- nasopharyngitis
- hypokalaemia
- see also General Adverse effects of direct factor Xa inhibitors, p. 256

Interactions

- see General Interactions of direct factor Xa inhibitors, p. 256

Nursing points/Cautions

- see also General Nursing points/Cautions of direct factor Xa inhibitors (above)
- duration of therapy depends on type of orthopaedic surgery: knee

replacement 10–14 days, hip replacement 32–38 days

- epidural catheter should not be removed within 20–30 hours of administration of apixaban and apixaban should not be started within 5 hours of epidural catheter removal
- (stroke prophylaxis) dose should be decreased to 2.5 mg twice daily if body weight ≤ 60 kg, serum creatinine ≥ 133 micromol/L or over 80 years of age
- if switching to or from parenteral anticoagulants, this should be done at next dose
- if switching from warfarin, warfarin should be stopped and apixaban started when INR < 2.0
- if switching to warfarin, apixaban should be continued for 48 hours. After first dose of warfarin, INR should be measured and both continued until INR ≥ 2.0
- can be started or continued during cardioversion procedure
- if patient has not previously received anticoagulant therapy, at least 5 doses of 5 mg apixaban (or 2.5 mg twice daily) should be given before procedure
- if procedure is required before 5 doses can be given, loading dose of 10 mg should be given at least 2 hours before procedure
- not recommended for haemodynamically significant rheumatic heart disease or mitral stenosis
- contraindicated in those with significant active bleeding, lesions at increased risk of bleeding, bleeding disorders or moderate-to-severe liver impairment (especially those associated with coagulopathy and risk of bleeding), recent surgery (brain, spinal, eyes), recent intracranial haemorrhage, known/suspected oesophageal varices, AV malformation, vascular aneurysm, major intraspinal/intracerebral vascular abnormalities, recent brain/spinal injury or severe kidney impairment (creatinine clearance < 25 mL/min)

Patient teaching and advice

- see General Patient teaching and advice for anticoagulants (p. 234)

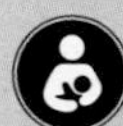

not recommended during pregnancy or while breastfeeding

tablet can be crushed and mixed with water, apple juice, apple puree or glucose 5%

RIVAROXABAN (Xarelto)

Available forms

Tablet: 10 mg, 15 mg, 20 mg

Action

- see also General Adverse effects of direct factor Xa inhibitors, p. 256
- half-life 5–9 hours (prolonged to 11–13 hours in the elderly)

Use

- prophylaxis of venous thromboembolism (VTE) after knee or hip replacement
- prophylaxis of stroke and systemic embolism in those with non-valvular atrial fibrillation with at least one other stroke factor
- treatment of deep vein thrombosis (DVT) and prophylaxis of recurrent DVT and pulmonary embolus (PE)
- prophylaxis of cardiovascular events in patients with coronary artery disease (CAD) and/or peripheral arterial disease (PAD) (with aspirin)

Dose

- (VTE prophylaxis for knee/hip surgery) 10 mg orally daily, starting 6–10 hours after surgery (when haemostasis has been established) **OR**

- (stroke and systemic embolism prophylaxis) 20 mg orally daily (or 15 mg orally if creatinine clearance is 30–49 mL/min) **OR**
- (treatment of DVT and prophylaxis of recurrent DVT and PE) initially 15 mg orally twice daily for 3 weeks, then 20 mg orally daily (while risk of VTE exists) **OR**
- prophylaxis of cardiovascular events in patients with CAD and/or PAD) 2.5 mg orally twice daily (with aspirin 100 mg orally daily)

Adverse effects

- see General Adverse effects of direct factor Xa inhibitors, p. 256

Interactions

- contraindicated with HIV protease inhibitors and azole antifungal agents (except fluconazole)
- caution if given with fluconazole
- see also General Interactions of direct factor Xa inhibitors, p. 256

Nursing points/Cautions

- see General Nursing points/Cautions of direct factor Xa inhibitors, p. 257
- duration of therapy depends on type of orthopaedic surgery: knee replacement 2 weeks, hip replacement 5 weeks
- epidural catheter should not be removed within 18 hours of rivaroxaban or longer if the puncture was traumatic, and rivaroxaban should be started within 6 hours of epidural catheter removal
- therapy can be started or continued with cardioversion procedure. Therapy should be started at least 4 hours before procedure in patients not previously receiving anticoagulant therapy
- if switching from parenteral anticoagulant, rivaroxaban should be given up to 2 hours before next parenteral dose is due or when continuous IV therapy is stopped
- if switching from warfarin, warfarin should be stopped and rivaroxaban started when INR $\leq$ 3.0 (for stroke/systemic embolism prophylaxis) or INR $\leq$ 2.5 (for DVT treatment or prophylaxis of recurrent DVT/PE)
- (recurrent DVT/PE prophylaxis) risk of recurrent DVT or PE should be reassessed after 6–12 months of therapy. Dose reduction to 10 mg daily may be considered
- (prophylaxis of cardiovascular event in those with CAD and/or PAD) caution if used in those $>$ 75 years because of increased risk of bleeding
- caution if used in those at risk of ulcerative GI disease. Prophylactic therapy is recommended
- (prophylaxis of cardiovascular event in those with CAD and/or PAD) not recommended in those who are within 4 weeks of experiencing an ischaemic, non-lacunar stroke
- not recommended for hip fracture surgery or prosthetic heart valves
- tablets contain lactose and are not recommended in those with galactose intolerance, Lapp lactase deficiency or glucose–galactose malabsorption
- caution in those with bronchiectasis or history of pulmonary bleeding
- contraindicated in those with significant active bleeding, lesions at increased risk of bleeding, bleeding disorders or moderate-to-severe liver impairment associated with coagulopathy, undergoing dialysis or severe kidney impairment (creatinine clearance $<$ 30 mL/min for 15–20 mg tablets or creatinine clearance $<$ 15 mL/min for 10 mg tablets)

Patient teaching and advice

- see General Patient teaching and advice for anticoagulants (p. 234)

- advise patient that 15 mg or 20 mg tablets should be taken with food
- women of childbearing years should be counselled to use adequate contraception during therapy to prevent pregnancy

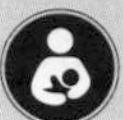

contraindicated during pregnancy and breastfeeding

tablet can be crushed and mixed with water or spoonful of apple puree

OTHER THROMBOTIC AGENTS

PROTEIN C (Ceprotin)

Available forms
Vial: 500 IU, 1000 IU

Action

- normally synthesised in the liver as a vitamin K-dependent plasma protein which is converted by thrombin-thrombomodulin complex on endothelial surface to activated protein C, which is a protease with anticoagulant activity, especially with cofactor protein S
- activated protein C inhibits activated forms of factors V and VIII resulting in decreased thrombin formation
- half-life 4.4–15.8 hours, but is shortened in conditions with acute thrombosis such as purpura fulminans and skin necrosis

Use

- purpura fulminans (intravascular thrombosis and haemorrhagic skin infarction)
- coumarin-induced skin necrosis in those with severe congenital protein C deficiency

Dose

- initially 60–80 IU/kg IV (to achieve protein C activity level of 100%), then adjusting dose based on protein C activity (maintained at above 25%)

Adverse effects

- (injection site) reaction, burning, stinging
- dizziness, restlessness, headache
- nausea, vomiting
- chest tightness, wheezing
- fever, sweating
- bleeding, thrombosis
- hypotension, tachycardia, cardiac arrhythmias, chest pain
- rash, urticaria, pruritus, skin ulceration
- bleeding, thrombosis
- hypersensitivity reaction, heparin-induced thrombocytopenia, protein C antibody development

Interactions

- transient hypercoagulable state may occur if given with vitamin K antagonist anticoagulants (e.g. warfarin) before anticoagulant effect becomes evident

Nursing points/Cautions

- should only be administered where protein C monitoring is available
- protein C activity should be estimated using protein C specific chromogenic substrates and measured before starting therapy, every 6 hours until patient is stabilised, then twice daily and always before next injection
- patient being treated during acute phase of disease may display lower increase in protein C activity
- resuscitation should be readily available in the case of acute allergic-type hypersensitivity occurring
- if patient is switched to permanent oral anticoagulant prophylaxis, protein C

should only be stopped when anticoagulation has stabilised. Anticoagulation should be started at low dose and slowly increased

- reconstitute using water for injections, gently rotating vial to dissolve powder. Reconstituted solution should then be withdrawn using sterile filter needle and then administered immediately via IV route. A separate sterile filter needle should be used for each individual vial used
- administration rate should not exceed 2 mL/minute (except for children under 10 kg where rate should not be greater than 0.2 mL/kg/minute)
- derived from human plasma, therefore carries a risk of transmission of infectious diseases. Vaccination against hepatitis A and B should be considered if patient is likely to receive regular or repeated doses
- may contain trace amount of heparin which may cause heparin-induced allergic reactions including heparin-induced thrombocytopenia. Heparin-induced thrombocytopenia (HIT) starts as a heparin-induced antibody mediated reaction resulting from irreversible aggregation of platelets and progressing to new thrombus formation with thrombocytopenia induced. If HIT is suspected, platelet count should be determined and therapy stopped if needed
- contains sodium and daily dose may exceed 200 mg which may be of importance in those on a sodium-controlled diet
- not recommended in those with combined severe congenital protein C deficiency and activated protein C resistance
- contraindicated in those with hypersensitivity to mouse protein or heparin (except in life-threatening thrombotic complications) including any previous heparin-induced thrombocytopenia

Patient teaching and advice

- instruct patient to immediately report any signs of allergy including hives, tightness in chest or wheezing

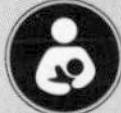

should only be used during pregnancy if benefits are thought to outweigh risks

safety during breastfeeding has not been established

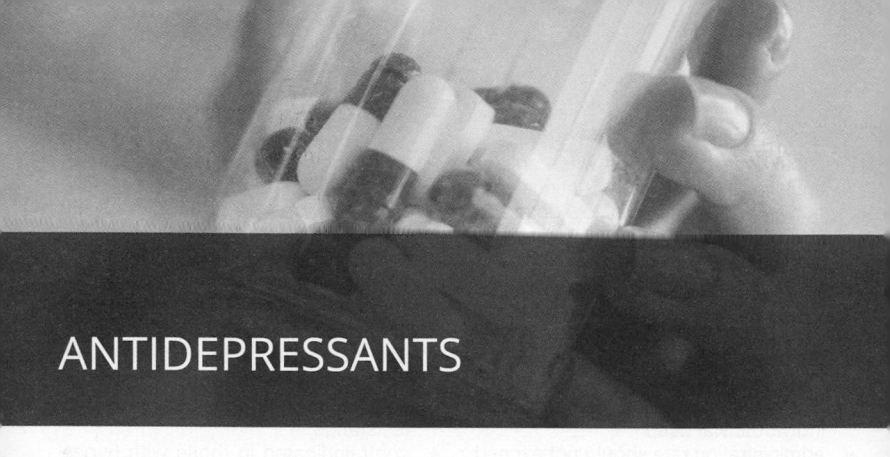

ANTIDEPRESSANTS

In 2017–18, 4.8 million Australians (or 20.1% of the population) reported experiencing mental or behavioural conditions, up from 4 million in 2014–15. Of these, one in 10 (10.4%) reported depression and 13.1% (3.2 million) reported anxiety, while 6.1% (or 1.5 million) had both anxiety and depression. Females reported feelings of depression at a higher rate than males (10.6% compared to 9.1%) (ABS 2019). Depression occurs throughout the life span, peaking in youth, early adulthood and early old age, with mean age of onset being 27 years, but 40% have had their first episode by the time they are 20 (Mahli et al 2018).

There are a number of risk factors for depression, including family history (e.g. high risk in families with history of depression or alcoholism), life events (e.g. recent negative experiences such as death, relationship break-up, health changes), childhood experiences (e.g. significant loss or disruptive/hostile environment), postpartum, personality traits (e.g. insecure, introverted, stress-sensitive, obsessive) or lack of social networks (Mahli et al 2018). Causes of depression can include some medications, substances of abuse (including alcohol), neurological diseases (e.g. dementias, Huntington's disease, multiple sclerosis), infectious diseases (e.g. HIV, tuberculosis, infectious hepatitis), cancers, metabolic and endocrine disorders (e.g. diabetes, thyroid disorders), collagen-vascular conditions (e.g. rheumatoid arthritis), cardiovascular disease (e.g. post-myocardial infarction, chronic heart disease) and postpartum (Loosen & Shelton 2019).

Symptoms of depression can vary from person to person and can be quite subtle, meaning that people often don't seek help until they become more marked. Symptoms include depressed or irritable/angry mood, lack of interest in activities that would normally please or decreased ability to feel pleasure, problems with memory and concentration, thoughts involving helplessness or hopelessness, changes in weight or appetite, insomnia or hypersomnia, low energy/fatigue, feelings of worthlessness or guilt and/or suicidal ideation (Mahli et al 2018). Treatment should be tailored to the individual and the type of depression (psychotic, manic, melancholic, reactive). Major depressive disorder is the most common presentation in the community with the aims of treatment being complete remission of symptoms with full recovery to premorbid functioning, reduction of associated morbidity, and limiting disability and risk of self-harm or fatality while focusing on the person's strengths in order to develop skills and resilience to prevent recurrence (Mahli et al 2018).

Pharmacotherapy is only one part of a treatment plan, which could also involve psychological therapies (e.g. cognitive behaviour therapy, interpersonal psychotherapy, mindfulness-based cognitive therapy) and general psychosocial interventions (e.g. self-help literature, drug and alcohol support groups) (Mahli et al 2018).

The decision to use antidepressants is very much based on clinical judgement of the doctor in collaboration with the patient. The first antidepressant (imipramine) became available in the 1950s and the range of agents used to treat depression has expanded since then to include:

- tricyclic antidepressants (tricyclics, TCAs) and related agents
- monoamine oxidase inhibitors (MAO inhibitors or MAOIs)
- reversible inhibitors of monoamine oxidase (RIMAs)
- selective serotonin reuptake inhibitors (SSRIs)
- serotonin and noradrenaline reuptake inhibitors (SNRIs)
- atypical antidepressants.

Antidepressants should be trialled for a minimum of 3 weeks at therapeutic dose in order to determine clinical response. It can take 2–4 weeks to determine effectiveness, therefore regular follow-up is necessary, not only to determine clinical response, but also adverse effects, including the potential of some antidepressants to produce suicidal thoughts and behaviours (especially in young adults or adolescents) (Mahli et al 2018).

Serotonin syndrome occurs when there is excessive serotonin acting on the CNS, resulting in effects that range from mild to life threatening. It is often the result of a drug interaction, commonly involving SSRIs. Other drugs implicated in serotonin syndrome are lithium, St John's wort, amphetamines (including recreational drugs), cocaine, anorectics, LSD, tramadol, pethidine, MAOIs, moclobemide, atypical antidepressants, TCAs, sumatriptan and tryptophan. They act by blocking serotonin reuptake, inhibiting its metabolism or being a serotonin agonist, precursor or releaser. Clinical symptoms of serotonin syndrome include agitation, confusion, hypomania, hyperactivity, restlessness, hyperthermia, sweating, tachycardia, hypertension, flushing, shivering, clonus, hyperreflexia, hypertonia, ataxia and tremor. Hyperreflexia and clonus are the main diagnostic symptoms of serotonin syndrome. Treatment should include ceasing the drug, ensuring adequate hydration and urine output, monitoring of vital signs, and may involve aggressive measures to treat hyperthermia. Serotonin antagonists such as cyproheptadine may also be useful.

General Nursing points/Cautions for all antidepressants

- patients should be screened carefully before starting therapy to determine the risk for bipolar disorders, including detailed psychiatric history and family history of depression, suicide and bipolar disorder
- all patients should be carefully monitored during initial stages of therapy or when the dosage is changed,

because the risk of suicide remains high. Family members/carers should be alerted to this possibility. Prescriptions are usually written for the smallest quantity to decrease the risk of overdose
- observe for a beneficial elevation in mood (although this may take weeks to become apparent)
- maintenance therapy should continue for at least 6–12 months after depressive symptoms have abated to avoid relapse
- observe for mania, hypomania, hallucinations, delusions and suicidal tendencies, which will necessitate discontinuation of therapy (especially those with pre-existing schizophrenia, bipolar disorder or paranoid delusions)
- when stopping therapy, the dose should be slowly tapered to prevent withdrawal symptoms, which include dizziness, paraesthesia, tremor, anxiety, nausea and palpitations. The risk of withdrawal symptoms is dependent on dose, duration of therapy and the slowness of the tapering regimen
- a washout period may be necessary when switching from one antidepressant to another and is based on the drug's half-life – the longer the half-life, the longer the washout period
- caution if used in those with unstable epilepsy or history of seizures due to risk of increased seizure activity
- caution if used to treat depression in those with schizophrenia as psychotic symptoms may be intensified; in manic depression there may be a shift towards mania; and paranoid delusion may be aggravated
- caution if used in those with kidney or liver impairment. Liver and kidney function should be monitored regularly during therapy

General Patient teaching and advice for all antidepressants

- patient should be advised that antidepressant effects are usually seen after 7–10 days and progress over 2–4 weeks, whereas a sedative effect is seen almost immediately and disappears with time
- patient (or carer) should be advised to seek medical advice immediately if any of the following occur:
  - thoughts/talk about self-harm, harm to others, suicide or death or recent attempts at self-harm or increase in aggression or hostility
  - change in mood, abnormal thinking or hallucinations
  - worsening of depression
- warn patient against driving a vehicle or operating machinery if dizziness, drowsiness, visual disturbances or concentration is impaired, especially during the initial period of treatment when sedation is common, and if dose is being increased
- advise patient that dizziness, lightheadedness and/or fainting (due to hypotension) can be avoided by moving gradually to a sitting or standing position, especially after sleep. Warn patient that postural hypotension is made worse by prolonged standing, hot baths or showers, hot weather, physical exertion, large meals and drinking alcohol
- warn patient to avoid alcohol during therapy
- advise patient against abruptly stopping therapy
- see also General Patient teaching and advice (p. xxvii)

TRICYCLIC AND RELATED ANTIDEPRESSANTS (TCAs)

General Actions of TCAs

- prevent reuptake of noradrenalinc (norepinephrine) and serotonin (5HT), prolonging their actions at the receptors
- histamine (H_1) receptor antagonist
- marked anticholinergic and sedative effects
- not used as first-line treatment because of potentially serious adverse effects

General Adverse effects of TCAs

- nausea, vomiting, anorexia, peculiar taste, diarrhoea, epigastric distress, black tongue, changes in appetite, weight gain
- dental caries
- elevated liver enzymes
- tinnitus
- slurred speech
- yawning
- hot flushes
- dizziness, headache, fatigue, drowsiness
- numbness, tingling and paraesthesia of extremities, ataxia
- disturbed concentration and memory, tremor, delirium, weakness, sedation, somnolence, insomnia, nightmares, confusion, anxiety, agitation, disorientation, hallucinations, excitement, restlessness, aggression
- tachycardia, palpitations, postural hypotension, occasionally hypertension, altered conduction, arrhythmias, heart block and non-specific ECG changes
- (anticholinergic effects) dry mouth, blurred vision, constipation, urinary retention/difficulty with micturition, sweating, hyperpyrexia, increased intraocular pressure, paralytic ileus
- testicular swelling, gynaecomastia, impotence, erectile dysfunction, changes to libido (males)
- breast enlargement, galactorrhoea, changes to libido (females)
- allergic reaction (oedema of face/tongue, rash, urticaria, photosensitivity)
- withdrawal syndrome (nausea, headache, malaise, vomiting, diarrhoea, abdominal pain, anxiety, dizziness, sleep and dream disturbance, restlessness, nervousness, irritability)
- (rare) blood dyscrasias, hepatitis, syndrome of inappropriate antidiuretic hormone secretion (SIADH), hyponatraemia, glaucoma, paralytic ileus, peripheral neuropathy, neuroleptic malignant syndrome, serotonin syndrome (see p. 263), suicidal ideation, seizures, glaucoma, alopecia, altered blood glucose levels
- (overdose) initially urinary retention, dry mucous membranes, decreased bowel motility, then temporary confusion, disturbed concentration, transient visual hallucinations, agitation, hyperactive reflexes, muscle rigidity, vomiting, drowsiness, hypothermia, tachycardia and other arrhythmias, dilated pupils, metabolic acidosis, hypokalaemia, hyponatraemia, convulsions, severe hypotension, stupor, coma

General Interactions of TCAs

- contraindicated with or within 14 days of MAOIs because this combination may cause coma, hyperpyrexia, convulsions and death
- when substituting a TCA for an MAOI, allow 14 days to elapse after discontinuing MAOI therapy
- serotonin toxicity may occur if given with moclobemide (reversible MAOI), which is therefore contraindicated with TCAs
- increased risk of agranulocytosis if given with carbimazole or propylthiouracil
- (ECT) hazards may be increased when ECT and TCAs are used together
- increased risk of toxicity (including cardiac arrhythmias) and therapeutic effects of both agents if TCAs and thyroid hormones are given together
- high doses may cause conduction defects and arrhythmias, therefore contraindicated with agents known to prolong QT interval such as antiarrhythmic agents and SSRIs
- may potentiate cardiovascular effects of sympathomimetic agents such as adrenaline (epinephrine), noradrenaline (norepinephrine) or amphetamines
- if given with phenothiazines, serum levels of both agents may be increased, increasing the risk of seizures and neuroleptic malignant syndrome
- CNS depressant effects may be enhanced by alcohol, barbiturates, benzodiazepines or general anaesthetic agents
- may precipitate hyperpyrexia, delirium and/or paralytic ileus if given with antihistamines, antiparkinsonian (anticholinergic) drugs, atropine, biperiden, phenothiazines (with anticholinergic effects) or anticholinergic drugs
- hyperpyrexia may occur if given with antipsychotic (neuroleptic) drugs, especially during hot weather
- increased risk of convulsions if given with tramadol
- delirium may occur if TCAs are given with disulfiram
- serum levels may be decreased by barbiturates, carbamazepine, colestyramine, colestipol, phenobarbital (phenobarbitone), phenytoin, St John's wort, rifampicin or nicotine (including smoking)
- serum levels may be increased by alprazolam, cimetidine, disulfiram, methylphenidate, phenothiazines, fluoxetine, fluvoxamine, paroxetine, sertraline or sodium valproate
- serotonin syndrome may occur if TCAs are given with serotonin-enhancing agents such as SSRIs (e.g. citalopram, fluoxetine, fluvoxamine, paroxetine, sertraline), SNRIs or lithium and are therefore not recommended together
- not recommended within 14–21 days of fluoxetine (as washout period is required)
- TCAs decrease hypotensive effects of clonidine and methyldopa sesquihydrate
- hypokalaemia (or use of potassium-losing diuretics) may increase risk of prolonged QT interval and associated arrhythmias and are therefore not recommended together
- may potentiate effects of oral anticoagulants, therefore INR should be carefully monitored throughout therapy, especially when starting or stopping therapy

- TCAs may increase serum levels of phenytoin or carbamazepine, increasing risk of toxicity
- increased risk of bone fracture if given with SSRIs in those over 50 years

General Nursing points/Cautions for TCAs

- see General Nursing points and Cautions for all antidepressant agents (p. 263)
- blood pressure should be measured before starting therapy
- any hypokalaemia should be corrected before starting therapy
- blood counts and ECG should be regularly monitored during therapy
- liver enzymes and renal function should be regularly monitored during therapy in those with pre-existing liver and kidney disease
- dosage should be started at a low level and increased gradually; however, higher doses may be used in severely depressed, hospitalised patients
- entire daily dose may be given in the morning, at night, or in divided doses, depending on requirements
- should be withdrawn before surgery as TCAs may increase the risk of arrhythmias if given with general anaesthetics
- caution if used in those with narrow angle glaucoma, raised intraocular pressure, urinary retention, chronic constipation and prostatic hyperplasia because symptoms may be exacerbated by anticholinergic actions of TCAs
- caution if used in those with hyperthyroidism, tumours of the adrenal medulla (may provoke hypertensive crisis), liver or kidney impairment, or cardiovascular disorders (including tachycardia, conduction disorders, arrhythmias and cardiac insufficiency)
- (depression) not recommended in those under 18 years
- contraindicated in those with or recovering from myocardial infarction, congenital long QT syndrome, epilepsy or with low seizure threshold (e.g. due to brain damage) or liver failure
- contraindicated in those with known hypersensitivity to other TCAs as cross-sensitivity is possible

General Patient teaching and advice for TCAs

- see General Patient teaching and advice for all antidepressant agents (p. 264)
- patient (or carer) should be advised to seek medical advice immediately if any of the following occur:
  - difficulty passing urine
  - increase in breast size, changes in libido (in both men and women)
  - numbness or tingling in feet or hands
  - fever, chills, mouth ulcers, unusual tiredness or sore throat, swollen glands
  - ringing in the ears
  - fast or irregular heart beat
  - unusual bruising or bleeding
- patient should have regular dental checks and maintain good dental hygiene throughout therapy as TCAs are known to increase the incidence of dental caries
- contact lens wearers should be warned about the potential for damage to the corneal epithelium from

decreased lacrimation and accumulation of mucoid secretions

- regular ophthalmological examination is recommended for all patients
- warn patient to avoid alcohol and OTC drugs that contain pseudoephedrine or phenylephrine (especially cough and cold preparations, antihistamines and weight-reduction tablets) during and for 2 weeks after stopping therapy
- if insomnia is a troublesome symptom, dose may be divided so that a higher amount is taken as the evening dose
- if patient is a smoker, he/she should be warned not to suddenly stop smoking as serum levels of TCA will be altered. Patient should stop smoking under medical supervision
- instruct patient that constipation may be treated with increased fluid intake, added dietary roughage or a laxative
- patient should be warned to avoid exposing skin to direct sunlight. When outdoors, patient should wear protective clothing, hat and sunscreen (with SPF 30+ or greater)

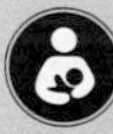

if used during pregnancy, benefits to the mother should be weighed against potential risks to the newborn infant as some have shown withdrawal symptoms when mothers have had prolonged therapy with TCAs. Gradual withdrawal before delivery date is recommended

AMITRIPTYLINE HYDROCHLORIDE (Endep, Entrip)

Available forms

Tablets: 10 mg, 25 mg, 50 mg

Action

- see General Actions of TCAs (p. 265)
- active metabolite (nortriptyline) (half-life 26 hours)
- half-life about 22 hours

Use

- major depression
- nocturnal enuresis (after organic causes have been excluded)

Dose

Depression

- (outpatient) initially 75 mg orally daily in divided doses, increasing gradually to a daily total of 150 mg if needed **OR**
- (outpatient) initially 50–100 mg orally at night, increasing by 25–50 mg to a daily total of 150 mg if needed **OR**
- (hospitalised patients) initially 100 mg orally daily, increasing gradually to 200–300 mg daily if needed **OR**
- (maintenance) 50–100 mg orally daily

Enuresis

- (11–16 years) 25–50 mg orally at night **OR**
- (6–10 years) 10–20 mg orally at night OR
- (less than 6 years) 10 mg orally at night

Adverse effects

- (enuresis) (common) drowsiness, anticholinergic effects (but less frequent than for depression)
- see also General Adverse effects/Interactions of TCAs (pp. 265–66)

Interactions

- see General Interactions of TCAs (p. 266)

Nursing points/Cautions

- 50 mg tablets are recommended for maintenance therapy only. Should not be used in those who are acutely ill and/or at risk of suicide
- (enuresis) response is usually seen within a few days but continued treatment is required

- see also General Nursing points/Cautions for TCAs (p. 267)

Patient teaching and advice

- see General Patient teaching and advice for TCAs (p. 267)
- tablets are not scored and patient should be advised to use a pill cutter for smaller dose (to ensure the tablet is evenly divided)
- warn patient that crushed tablet has a bitter/burning taste and may cause numbness to mouth. Patient should be advised to rinse mouth well and avoid hot drinks and food immediately after to avoid the possibility of burning mouth

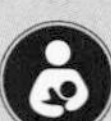
contraindicated during breastfeeding

tablets can be crushed and mixed with spoonful of yoghurt or apple puree

CLOMIPRAMINE HYDROCHLORIDE (Anafranil, Placil)

Available form

Tablets: 25 mg

Action

- see General Actions of TCAs (p. 265)
- derivative of imipramine
- active metabolite (half-life 13–25 hours)
- half-life 12–36 hours

Use

- major depression
- cataplexy associated with narcolepsy
- obsessive compulsive disorder (OCD)
- phobias

Dose

- (OCD, phobias, depression) initially 25 mg orally 2–3 times daily, increasing by 25 mg every 3–4 days to 100–150 mg daily in 2–3 divided doses, then 50–100 mg daily maintenance in 2–3 divided doses **OR**
- (catalepsy) 25–75 mg daily orally

Adverse effects

- see General Adverse effects of TCAs (p. 265)

Interactions

- serum levels may be increased by grapefruit, grapefruit juice or cranberry juice
- see also General Interactions of TCAs (p. 266)

Nursing points/Cautions

- tablets contain lactose and sucrose and therefore should not be used in those with galactose intolerance, fructose intolerance, sucrase–isomaltase insufficiency or glucose–galactose malabsorption
- nocturnal medication should only be given in cases where clomipramine does not exacerbate insomnia (cataplexy associated with narcolepsy)
- see also General Nursing points/Cautions for TCAs (p. 267)

Patient teaching and advice

- advise patient to avoid grapefruit, grapefruit juice or cranberry juice during therapy
- patients with panic disorders should be advised that intensified anxiety may occur at the start of therapy, but subsides within 2 weeks
- see also General Patient teaching and advice for TCAs (p. 267)

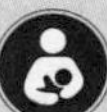
not recommended during breastfeeding

tablet can be dispersed in 10–20 mL of water (although Tofranil brand does not disperse easily). Tablet can be crushed (sugar coating may be hard to crush) and then mixed with water, or spoonful of yoghurt or apple puree

DOSULEPIN (DOTHIEPIN) HYDROCHLORIDE (Dothep)

Available forms

Capsules: 25 mg; Tablets: 75 mg

Action

- see General Actions of TCAs (p. 265)
- equivalent to amitriptyline but less potent than imipramine
- active metabolite
- biphasic elimination: phase one 15–18 hours, whole-body elimination 51 hours
- narrow therapeutic range, with onset of toxicity within 4–6 hours

Use

- major depression

Dose

- (depression) initially 25 mg orally 3 times daily for 7–14 days, then increasing daily dose by 25–50 mg after 1–2 weeks if needed (daily maximum 200 mg) (up to 150 mg of daily dose may be given as single nightly dose)

Adverse effects/Interactions/Nursing points/Cautions/Patient teaching and advice

- 75 mg tablets are recommended for maintenance therapy only. Should not be used in those who are acutely ill and/or at risk of suicide
- see General Adverse effects/Interactions/Nursing points/Cautions/Patient teaching and advice for TCAs (pp. 265–67)

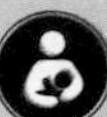

is secreted in breastmilk, therefore should only be used during breastfeeding if benefits outweigh risks

capsules can be opened and contents dispersed in water or mixed with spoonful of yoghurt or apple puree

DOXEPIN (Deptran)

Available forms

Capsules: 10 mg, 25 mg; Tablets: 50 mg

Action

- see General Actions of TCAs (p. 265)
- active metabolite (half-life is longer than parent compound)
- half-life 8–24 hours, extended in overdose

Use

- major depression

Dose

- (mild depression) initially 30 mg orally daily in 3 divided doses, increasing to 50 mg daily if needed **OR**
- (moderate–severe depression) initially 75 mg orally daily in 3 divided doses, increasing up to 300 mg daily if necessary and dose may be reduced once a satisfactory therapeutic response has been achieved

Adverse effects/Interactions/Nursing points/Cautions

- initial dose is dependent on severity of presenting symptoms
- 50 mg tablets are recommended for maintenance therapy only
- if insomnia is a problem, up to 150 mg of the dose can be given in the evening
- see also General Adverse effects/Interactions/Nursing points/Cautions/Patient teaching and advice for TCAs (pp. 265–67)

Patient teaching and advice

- warn patient that mouth numbing may occur if capsules are opened or tablets crushed. Patient should be advised to rinse mouth well after dose and avoid hot drinks or food immediately after dose to prevent burning mouth
- see also General Patient teaching and advice for TCAs (p. 267)

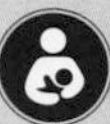
not recommended during breastfeeding

capsules can be opened and contents dispersed in water or mixed with spoonful of yoghurt or apple puree. Tablets can be crushed and mixed with water or spoonful of yoghurt or apple puree

IMIPRAMINE HYDROCHLORIDE (Tofranil)

Available forms
Tablets: 10 mg, 25 mg

Action
- see General Actions of TCAs (p. 265)
- active metabolite (desmethylimipramine)
- half-life 20 hours

Use
- major depression
- nocturnal enuresis (after organic causes have been excluded)

Dose
Depression
- (ambulant patient) initially 25 mg orally 3 times daily, increasing gradually to 150–200 mg by the end of the first week and maintained until there is improvement in condition, then reduced to 50–100 mg daily as maintenance **OR**
- (hospitalised patient) initially 25 mg orally 3 times daily increasing by 25 mg increments to 200 mg until condition improves, then reduced to 100 mg daily as maintenance

Enuresis
- (over 12 years) 25–75 mg orally at night **OR**
- (9–12 years) 25–50 mg orally at night **OR**
- (5–8 years) 20–30 mg orally at night

Interactions
- serum levels may be increased by verapamil, diltiazem, labetalol and propranolol
- see also General Interactions of TCAs (p. 266)

Adverse effects/ Nursing points/ Cautions

- tablets contain lactose and sucrose and therefore should not be used in those with galactose intolerance, fructose intolerance, severe lactase insufficiency, sucrase–isomaltase insufficiency or glucose–galactose malabsorption
- see also General Adverse effects (p. 265), General Nursing points/ Cautions (p. 267)

Patient teaching and advice

- warn patient that mouth numbing may occur if tablets are crushed. Patient should be advised to rinse mouth well after dose and avoid hot drinks or food immediately after dose to prevent burning mouth
- see also General Patient teaching and advice for TCAs (p. 267)

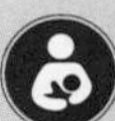
not recommended during breastfeeding

tablets can be crushed and mixed with water or spoonful of yoghurt or apple puree

NORTRIPTYLINE (Allegron, NortriTABS)

Available forms
Tablets: 10 mg, 25 mg

Action
- see General Actions of TCAs (p. 265)

Use
- major depression

Dose
- (depression) 25 mg orally 3–4 times daily increasing gradually if needed (daily maximum 100 mg)

Adverse effects/Interactions/Nursing points/Cautions/Patient teaching and advice
- see General Adverse effects/Interactions/Nursing points/Cautions/Patient teaching and advice for TCAs (pp. 265–67)

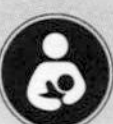
should only be used during breastfeeding if benefits outweigh risks

tablets can be dispersed in water or crushed and mixed with spoonful of yoghurt or apple puree

MONOAMINE OXIDASE INHIBITORS (MAOIs)

General Actions of MAOIs
- monoamine oxidase (MAO) is a mitochondrial enzyme that inactivates the biogenic amines (adrenaline (epinephrine), noradrenaline (norepinephrine), dopamine and serotonin). By inhibiting this enzyme, the level of the biogenic amines is allowed to increase
- two types of MAO enzymes exist in the body. MAO-A is located throughout the body and metabolises adrenaline (epinephrine), noradrenaline (norepinephrine), dopamine and serotonin producing diverse effects. MAO-B is found in human platelets
- long delay in mood improvement
- metabolism is via acetylation, therefore rate is dependent on whether the person is a slow or rapid acetylator
- when therapy is stopped, MAO activity usually recovers in 3–5 days, but may take up to 2 weeks
- considered second- or third-line treatment of depression if other antidepressants have been ineffective or inappropriate

General Uses of MAOIs
- major depression (not first-line treatment because of adverse effects and dietary restrictions where other antidepressants have been ineffective or inappropriate)

General Adverse effects of MAOIs
- drowsiness, dizziness, weakness, fatigue, headache, disturbed sleep, tremors, twitching, hyperreflexia, myoclonic movements
- postural hypotension, oedema
- palpitations, tachycardia
- impotence, ejaculation disorders
- dry mouth, constipation, weight gain, nausea, diarrhoea, abdominal pain, anorexia

- elevated liver enzymes
- (uncommon) urinary retention, blurred vision, glaucoma, pruritus, rash, sweating, chills
- (rare) blood dyscrasias, hypomania and agitation (high dose, prolonged therapy), hepatitis, suicidal ideation, syndrome of inappropriate anti-diuretic hormone secretion (SIADH)
- (severe, possibly fatal) hypertensive crisis

General Interactions of MAOIs

- contraindicated with pethidine (or related opioids) (due to risk of respiratory depression) and dextromethorphan (risk of psychosis)
- contraindicated with other MAOIs
- should not be given within 10 days of stopping therapy with another MAOI or other antidepressants
- contraindicated with or within 21 days of TCAs as combination may cause hyperpyrexia, diffuse intravascular coagulation and status epilepticus
- contraindicated with SSRIs or SNRIs
- contraindicated with carbamazepine due to risk of hyperpyrexia, hypertensive crises and/or convulsions. MAOI should be stopped for at least 2 weeks before starting carbamazepine
- contraindicated with sympathomimetic agents, local anaesthetics or cocaine with added adrenaline (epinephrine), amphetamines, dopamine, fenfluramine, methylphenidate, adrenaline (epinephrine), noradrenaline (norepinephrine), ephedrine, levodopa, l-tyrosine, methyldopa sesquihydrate, phenylalanine or tryptophan
- contraindicated with tyramine-containing foods and drinks as they cause a 'cheese reaction' (see Glossary)
- contraindicated with or within 14 days of bupropion
- not recommended with or within 10 days of buspirone hydrochloride due to risk of hypertension
- not recommended with alcohol or dextropropoxyphene due to increased CNS depression
- not recommended with high doses of caffeine or caffeine-containing drinks or food
- effects may be potentiated/prolonged if given with barbiturates. Barbiturates should be given at a reduced dose
- exaggerated hypotension may occur if given with antihypertensive agents, including thiazide diuretics
- increased hypotension and CNS depression may occur if given with inhalation anaesthetics
- increased risk of serotonin syndrome if sumatriptan is given with or within 14 days of MAOIs, therefore this should be avoided
- may cause profuse sweating, tremors and hyperpyrexia if given with anti-Parkinson's agents
- may potentiate hypoglycaemic agents or alter glucose metabolism
- may lower convulsive threshold by antagonising antiepileptic agents

General Nursing points/Cautions for MAOIs

- see General Nursing points and Cautions for all antidepressant agents (p. 263)
- blood pressure should be measured before starting and regularly throughout therapy
- may suppress anginal pain, which acts as a warning of myocardial ischaemia

- may cause excessive stimulation in schizophrenic patients or swing from depression to mania in those with bipolar disorder
- observe for hypoglycaemia in patients with diabetes
- TCAs and SSRIs generally should not be given within 10–14 days of MAOIs (allow 5 weeks if giving with fluoxetine)
- should be discontinued at least 10–14 days before elective surgery or other procedures requiring general anaesthetic or local anaesthetics containing adrenaline (epinephrine)
- treatment of hypertensive crisis includes discontinuing MAOI, giving phentolamine 5 mg slowly IV (to lower blood pressure) and treating hyperpyrexia symptomatically
- caution if used in those with epilepsy, diabetes, hyperthyroidism, impaired kidney function or angina
- not recommended in those over 60 years
- contraindicated in those with phaeochromocytoma, porphyria, liver disease (or with abnormal liver function), congestive cardiac failure, cerebrovascular disease, recurrent/frequent headaches or blood dyscrasias

General Patient teaching and advice for MAOIs

- see General Patient teaching and advice for all antidepressant agents (p. 264)
- patient must seek medical advice before taking any other preparations with MAOIs (including OTC preparations)
- warn patient to avoid alcohol and OTC products (including cough and cold preparations with dextromethorphan, nasal decongestants (tablets, drops, sprays), hay fever/sinus preparations, asthma inhalants, anti-appetite/weight-reduction preparations or tryptophan-containing products) during and for 2 weeks after stopping therapy, unless advised by the doctor
- patient should be instructed to avoid tyramine-containing foods and drinks because these may cause a severe hypertensive crisis (including nausea, headache, rapid heartbeat and fainting). Foods include cheeses (especially matured/aged such as blue, brie, parmesan, stilton, gruyere), aged, cured and pickled meats and fish (e.g. game, caviar, herring, sausages (kabana, pepperoni, salami, hot-dogs), corned beef, bacon), vegetables (e.g. over-ripe avocado, broad beans, pickled vegetables (e.g. sauerkraut), soy products such as soy sauce), fruits (e.g. over-ripe figs, bananas, raisins or pineapples), meat or yeast extracts (e.g. Bonox, Vegemite, stock cubes, packet soups) and alcoholic beverages (e.g. red wine (especially Chianti), sherry, beer, liqueurs). These foods should also be avoided for 14 days after stopping therapy with MAOIs. Medical advice should be sought immediately if patient eats tyramine-containing food
- if patient stops taking MAOI (under medical supervision), a normal diet (with tyramine-containing foods and drink) should not be resumed for 2 weeks after discontinuation

- advise patient about the need to continue therapy and to keep follow-up appointments
- patient should be warned to avoid large intakes of caffeine (including tea, coffee, cola and chocolate) during therapy
- instruct patient to immediately report any headache (which may radiate frontally), rapid or slowed heart rate, nausea, vomiting, neck stiffness or soreness, photophobia, dilated pupils, sweating (sometimes with fever and cold/clammy skin) and constricting chest pain
- if insomnia is a problem, patient can be advised to take last dose before 3 pm
- if patient has diabetes, they should be instructed to monitor blood glucose levels closely during therapy

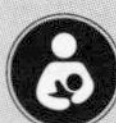

use with caution during pregnancy and only if benefits outweigh risks to fetus

caution if used during breastfeeding

PHENELZINE (Phenelzine Sulphate USP)

Available form

Tablets: 15 mg

Action

- see General Action for MAOIs (p. 272)
- two metabolites, although it is unknown if they are clinically active
- short half-life (1.2 hours)

Dose

- (depression) initially 15 mg orally 3 times daily, increasing to 60–90 mg daily for at least 4 weeks, then reduced slowly to as low as 15 mg daily or every second day (maintenance)

Action/Use/Adverse effects/Interactions/Nursing points/Cautions/Patient teaching and advice

- see General Use/Adverse effects/Interactions/Nursing points/Cautions/Patient teaching and advice for MAOIs (pp. 272–74)

tablet can be crushed and mixed with water or spoonful of yoghurt or apple puree

TRANYLCYPROMINE (Parnate)

Available form

Tablets: 10 mg

Dose

- (depression) initially 20 mg orally daily (given as 10 mg morning and 10 mg evening); if ineffective after 2 weeks, add a further 10 mg at midday; when response is established, dose may be reduced to 10–20 mg daily (daily maximum 30 mg) **OR**
- (treatment in combination with ECT) 10 mg orally twice daily during ECT therapy, then 10 mg daily

Interactions

- not recommended with or within 14 days of moclobemide
- see General Interactions for MAOIs (p. 273)

Action/Use/Adverse effects/Nursing points/Cautions/Patient teaching and advice

- see General Action/Use/Adverse effects/Nursing points/Cautions/Patient teaching and advice for MAOIs (pp. 272–74)

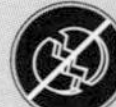

tablets contain sucrose and are therefore not recommended in those with rare hereditary problem of fructose intolerance, glucose–galactose malabsorption or sucrase–isomaltase insufficiency

tablet can be crushed and mixed with water or spoonful of yoghurt or apple puree

REVERSIBLE INHIBITORS OF MONOAMINE OXIDASE TYPE A (RIMAs)

MOCLOBEMIDE (Amira, Aurorix, Clobemix)

Available forms
Tablets: 150 mg, 300 mg

Action
- selectively inhibits monoamine oxidase A (MAO A) over MAO B in a ratio of 4:1
- causes an increase in extracellular levels of noradrenaline (norepinephrine), dopamine and serotonin, which results in an increase in mood and psychomotor activity, relieving symptoms such as dysphoria, poor concentration, exhaustion and lack of drive
- MAO activity restored within 1–2 days of stopping therapy
- increases total sleep time while not impairing alertness or reaction time
- half-life 2 hours

Use
- major depression

Dose
- initially 300–450 mg orally daily in 2 divided doses after meals, increasing after at least a week if needed to 300–600 mg in 2 divided doses (maintenance)

Adverse effects
- nausea, diarrhoea, constipation, dry mouth
- dizziness, headache, restlessness, anxiety, agitation, irritability
- insomnia
- paraesthesia
- hypotension
- rash
- (rare) suicidal ideation, serotonin syndrome (see p. 263)

Interactions
- contraindicated with TCAs, SSRIs or SNRIs because of increased risk of serotonin syndrome
- contraindicated with selegiline, clomipramine, pethidine, tramadol, triptans, bupropion, linezolid and dextromethorphan
- may increase pressor effect if given with sympathomimetic agents at high doses
- serum levels may be affected by concurrent use of cimetidine. If cimetidine is started first, dose of moclobemide should be started at lowest possible dose. If cimetidine is added to existing moclobemide therapy, moclobemide dose will need to be reduced to ⅓ to ½ dose
- may increase effects of opioids and therefore should be used with caution
- may increase serum levels of proton pump inhibitors
- not recommended with dextropropoxyphene
- not recommended with St John's wort due to increased risk of serotonin syndrome
- caution if used with venlafaxine

Nursing points/Cautions
- see General Nursing points/Cautions for all antidepressant agents (p. 263)
- allow the correct amount of time to elapse between stopping SSRIs and

starting moclobemide (5 weeks after stopping fluoxetine; 2 weeks after stopping paroxetine; 1 week after stopping citalopram or fluvoxamine)
- may theoretically precipitate hypertensive crisis in patients with thyrotoxlcosis or phaeochromocytoma, therefore caution if used
- caution if used in those with liver or kidney impairment
- not recommended in those with rare hereditary problems of galactose intolerance, Lapp lactase deficiency or glucose–galactose malabsorption
- not recommended in those under 18 years
- contraindicated in those with acute confusion

Patient teaching and advice

- see General Patient teaching and advice for all antidepressant agents (p. 264)
- advise patient to take tablets after meals
- restriction of tyramine-rich foods is not as stringent as for MAOIs; however, some people may be sensitive to tyramine and therefore ingesting large amounts of tyramine-rich food should be discouraged (see 'cheese reaction', see Glossary)
- hypertensive patients should be advised to avoid tyramine-rich foods
- warn patient to avoid alcohol and OTC products (including cough and cold preparations with dextromethorphan)

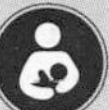

use in pregnancy is not recommended unless benefits outweigh the risks

not recommended during breastfeeding

tablet can be crushed and mixed with water or spoonful of yoghurt or apple puree

SELECTIVE SEROTONIN REUPTAKE INHIBITORS (SSRIS)

General Actions of SSRIs

- selectively inhibit reuptake of serotonin (5 hydroxytryptamine, 5HT) prolonging serotonin action
- anxiolytic action
- increases prolactin levels
- suppresses rapid eye movement (REM) sleep and increases deep slow-wave sleep

General Adverse effects of SSRIs

- palpitations, tachycardia, hypotension (including postural hypotension)
- dizziness, tremor, headache, migraine, asthenia, twitching, amnesia, apathy, anxiety, nervousness, aggravated depression, fatigue, agitation, paraesthesia, impaired concentration, confusion
- anorexia, nausea, vomiting, abdominal pain, diarrhoea, altered taste, dry mouth, flatulence, increased appetite, increased/decreased weight, dyspepsia, increased saliva, constipation
- hot flushes, increased sweating, chills, fever

- insomnia, somnolence, abnormal dreams
- yawning
- decreased libido/impotence, ejaculation disorders
- amenorrhoea, menstrual disorders
- myalgia, arthralgia, back pain
- cough, pharyngitis, rhinitis, sinusitis
- rash, pruritus, urticaria
- polyuria, urinary frequency
- blurred vision
- tinnitus
- bleeding disorders (purpura, haematoma, epistaxis, GI and vaginal bleeding)
- (rare) hyponatraemia, syndrome of inappropriate antidiuretic hormone secretion (SIADH), akathisia/psychomotor restlessness, increased risk of bone fractures, seizures, suicidal ideation, suicidal behaviours, mania, serotonin syndrome (see p. 263), prolongation of QT interval
- withdrawal symptoms (nausea, vomiting, diarrhoea, headache, dizziness, paraesthesia, insomnia, nightmares, disturbed dreams, visual disturbances, palpitations, emotional instability, anxiety, agitation, tremor, confusion, sweating)

General Interactions of SSRIs

- contraindicated with or within 14 days of stopping MAOIs or linezolid because of increased risk of serotonin syndrome
- contraindicated with or within 1 day of stopping moclobemide
- moclobemide should not be started within 14 days of stopping SSRIs
- not recommended with 5HT agonists (serotonergic agents) (e.g. sumatriptan, tramadol, tryptophan, fentanyl, lithium, St John's wort) as risk of serotonin syndrome is increased
- use with alcohol should be avoided
- not recommended with SNRIs due to risk of serotonin syndrome and increased serum levels and toxicity of SNRIs
- not recommended with TCAs or antipsychotic agents
- not recommended with other agents known to prolong QT interval
- prothrombin time should be carefully monitored if given with warfarin (not citalopram)
- caution if given with agents that lower seizure threshold, such as other SSRIs, TCAs, antipsychotic agents, tramadol, bupropion or mefloquine
- caution if given with other centrally acting agents
- caution if used with ECT
- may prolong action of neuromuscular blocking agents such as suxamethonium and mivacurium
- increased effects may occur if given with tryptophan
- increased serum levels may result if given with cimetidine or omeprazole
- caution if given with lithium
- increased risk of bleeding if given with aspirin, NSAIDs, antiplatelet agents, anticoagulants, TCAs or other agents affecting coagulation
- glycaemic control may be affected, therefore blood glucose levels should be closely monitored and antidiabetic agent dose adjusted accordingly
- may increase serum levels (and therefore associated adverse effects/toxicity) of phenytoin, carbamazepine, flecainide, metoprolol (when used for cardiac failure), clomipramine,

nortriptyline, imipramine, risperidone, theophylline, methadone, clozapine, ciclosporin, tacrine or haloperidol

General Nursing points/Cautions for SSRIs

- see General Nursing points/Cautions for all antidepressant agents (p. 263)
- any hypokalaemia and/or hypomagnesaemia should be corrected before starting and potassium and magnesium levels should be monitored regularly throughout therapy
- treatment should be over at least 6 months to prevent relapse
- electrolytes should be monitored at the start of therapy in the elderly because of the increased risk of hyponatraemia
- ECG monitoring is recommended for patients with any risk factors for QT interval prolongation
- not recommended in those with unstable heart disease or recent history of myocardial infarction
- not recommended in those under 18 years
- caution if used in those with a history of bleeding disorders or taking drugs affecting platelet function, with epilepsy or history of seizures, impaired kidney or liver function, diabetes, acute narrow angle glaucoma or raised intraocular pressure
- caution if used in those at risk of QT interval prolongation such as congestive cardiac failure, bradyarrhythmias or predisposition to hypokalaemia or hypomagnesaemia
- contraindicated in those with congenital long QT syndrome

General Patient teaching and advice for SSRIs

- see General Patient teaching and advice for all antidepressant agents (p. 264)
- if patient has diabetes, instruct them to carefully monitor blood glucose levels as glucose tolerance may be disrupted
- patients should be advised to seek medical advice immediately if any of the following occur:
  - unusual bleeding or bruising
  - change in heart rate (fast, irregular) and/or fainting
  - unpleasant or distressing restlessness, inability to sit or stand still
  - dizziness when first standing up

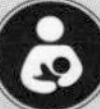

crosses the placental barrier and may produce withdrawal symptoms in the newborn. Furthermore, if used in the third trimester, may lead to neonatal complications, including prolonged hospitalisation, respiratory support and tube feeding. However, SSRIs should not be abruptly stopped during pregnancy. Newborn should be closely monitored if mother has taken SSRI during pregnancy

excreted in breastmilk, therefore breastfeeding is not recommended

CITALOPRAM (Celapram, Celica, Cipramil, Talam)

Available forms

Tablets: 10 mg, 20 mg, 40 mg

Action

- see General Actions of SSRIs (p. 277)

- active metabolites have SSRI properties but less than citalopram itself
- half-life 36 hours

Use
- major depression

Dose
- initially 20 mg orally daily, increasing by 10 mg at 2–3-weekly intervals to 40 mg daily maximum if necessary

Adverse effects/Interactions/Nursing points/Cautions/Patient teaching and advice
- tablets contain lactose and therefore should not be used in those with galactose intolerance, Lapp lactase insufficiency or glucose–galactose malabsorption
- see also General Adverse effects, Interactions and Nursing points/Cautions/Patient teaching and advice for SSRIs (pp. 277–79)

tablets can be dispersed in water (stir for 5 minutes) or crushed and given with spoonful of yoghurt or apple puree

ESCITALOPRAM (Cilopam-S, Escicor, Esipram, Lexam, Lexapro, Loxalate)

Available forms

Tablets: 10 mg, 20 mg; Oral solution: 20 mg/mL

Action
- see General Actions of SSRIs (p. 277)
- long half-life (30 hours) (extended in those with mild-to-moderate liver impairment or over 65 years)

Use
- major depression
- social anxiety disorder (social phobia), generalised anxiety disorder
- obsessive compulsive disorder (OCD)

Dose
- (major depression, social or generalised anxiety disorder, OCD) initially 10 mg orally daily, increasing gradually to a daily maximum of 20 mg

Adverse effects/Interactions/Nursing points/Cautions
- contraindicated in those with hypersensitivity to citalopram
- see also General Adverse effects, Interactions and Nursing points/Cautions for SSRIs (pp. 277–79)

Patient teaching and advice
- warn patient that crushed tablet has bitter taste

Oral solution
- instruct patient to turn bottle upside down completely. If no drops come out, tap bottle lightly to start flow
- advise patient that 10 mg = 10 drops of the 20 mg/mL solution
- drops should be added to drink (water, apple or orange juice but no other fluids), stirred and drunk
- oral solution should be stored below 25°C and discarded after 2 months after opening
- see also General Patient teaching and advice for SSRIs (p. 279)

oral solution is available. Tablet can be dispersed in water (some brands are slow to disperse) or crushed and mixed with spoonful of yoghurt or apple puree

FLUOXETINE (Fluotex, Lovan, Prozac, Zactin Tabs)

Available forms

Capsules: 20 mg; Tablets (dispersible): 20 mg

Action

- see General Actions of SSRIs (p. 277)
- active metabolite norfluoxetine (long half-life 9–16 days)
- half-life is 1–3 days (acute administration), which is extended to 4–6 days with chronic administration

Use

- major depression
- obsessive–compulsive disorder (OCD)
- premenstrual dysphoric disorder (PMDD)

Dose

- (depression, OCD) initially 20 mg orally morning, increasing to twice-daily dosage (morning, noon) after several weeks if no clinical improvement is noted (daily maximum 80 mg) **OR**
- (PMDD) 20 mg orally daily **OR**
- (PMDD) 20 mg orally daily starting 14 days before anticipated onset of menstruation, continuing until first day of menses, repeating for each menstrual cycle

Adverse effects

- (common) rash, urticaria
- (rare) allergy, anaphylactic events
- see also General Adverse effects of SSRIs (p. 277)

Interactions

- may increase serum levels of diazepam, alprazolam and imipramine
- may decrease efficacy of tamoxifen
- may alter lithium levels
- see also General Interactions of SSRIs (p. 278)

Nursing points/Cautions/Patient teaching and advice

- patient should be advised to immediately seek medical advice if any rash or hives occur
- advise patient to swallow capsule whole or dissolve tablets in 100 mL water
- see also General Nursing points/Cautions/Patient teaching and advice for SSRIs (p. 279)

dispersible tablets available. Capsule can be opened and contents mixed with yoghurt or apple puree

FLUVOXAMINE MALEATE (Faverin, Luvox, Movox)

Available form

Tablets: 50 mg, 100 mg

Action

- see General Actions of SSRIs (p. 277)
- half-life is 12–13 hours (single dose) or 22 hours (repeated dosing)

Use

- major depression
- obsessive–compulsive disorder (OCD)

Dose

- (depression) initially 50 mg orally at night for 7 days, increasing gradually by 50 mg/week if needed (daily maximum 300 mg) **OR**
- (OCD) initially 50 mg orally daily for 3–4 days, then increasing by 50 mg every 4–6 days until effective (daily maximum 300 mg)

Interactions

- may increase serum levels of caffeine, propranolol, triazolam, midazolam, haloperidol, ropinirole, alprazolam and diazepam
- serum levels may be decreased by smoking
- see also General Interactions of SSRIs (p. 278)

Adverse effects/Nursing points/Cautions

- doses greater than 150 mg should be given in 2–3 doses

- see also General Adverse effects/Nursing points/Cautions for SSRIs (pp. 277, 279)

Patient teaching and advice

- instruct patient that tablets should be swallowed whole, not chewed or crushed
- patient should be advised to avoid large doses of caffeine including tea, coffee, cola and chocolate
- warn patient not to suddenly stop smoking without first seeking medical advice
- see also General Patient teaching and advice for SSRIs (p. 279)

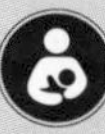

contraindicated during breastfeeding

tablet is difficult to crush. If crushed, crush finely and mix with spoonful of yoghurt or apple puree

PAROXETINE (Aropax, Extine, Paxtine, Roxtine 20)

Available form

Tablets: 20 mg

Action

- see General Actions of SSRIs (p. 277)
- half-life about 24 hours

Use

- major depression
- obsessive–compulsive disorder (OCD)
- social anxiety disorder (social phobia), generalised anxiety disorder
- post-traumatic stress disorder (PTSD)

Dose

- (depression) initially 20 mg orally daily, increasing by 10 mg at weekly intervals if needed (daily maximum 50 mg) **OR**
- (OCD) initially 20 mg orally daily, increasing by 10 mg at weekly intervals if needed (daily maximum 60 mg) **OR**
- (panic disorder) initially 10 mg orally daily, increasing by 10 mg at weekly intervals if needed (daily maximum 60 mg) **OR**
- (social anxiety disorder/social disorder, anxiety, PTSD) initially 20 mg orally daily, increasing by 10 mg at weekly intervals if needed (daily maximum 50 mg)

Interactions

- decreased serum levels may occur if given with ritonavir/fosamprenavir
- may decrease efficacy of tamoxifen
- see also General Interactions of SSRIs (p. 278)

Adverse effects/Nursing points/Cautions/Patient teaching and advice

- advise patient that tablets should be swallowed whole, not chewed
- see also General Actions/Adverse effects/Nursing points/Cautions/Patient teaching and advice for SSRIs (pp. 277–79)

tablet does not disperse in water but can be crushed and mixed with spoonful of yoghurt or apple puree

SERTRALINE (Eleva, Sertra, Setrona, Zoloft)

Available forms

Tablets: 50 mg, 100 mg

Action

- see General Actions of SSRIs (p. 277)
- half-life about 24 hours

Use
- major depression
- obsessive–compulsive disorder (OCD)
- panic disorder
- premenstrual dysphoric disorder (PMDD)
- social anxiety disorder (social phobia), generalised anxiety disorder

Dose
- (major depression, OCD) initially 50 mg orally daily, increasing at weekly intervals if needed (daily maximum 200 mg) **OR**
- (panic disorder, social phobia) initially 25 mg orally daily, increasing to 50 mg daily after 1 week **OR**
- (PMDD) 50 mg orally daily, increasing by 50 mg per menstrual cycle if needed (daily maximum 150 mg) **OR**
- (PMDD) 50 mg orally daily for 14 days before anticipated menstruation continued until first day of menses, repeated each menstrual cycle. Dose can be increased by 50 mg per menstrual cycle if needed (daily maximum 100 mg)

Adverse effects/Interactions/Nursing points/Cautions/Patient teaching and advice
- increases serum levels of diazepam
- see also General Adverse effects, Interactions and Nursing points/Cautions/Patient teaching and advice for SSRIs (pp. 277–79)

tablet can be dispersed in water or crushed and mixed with spoonful of yoghurt or apple puree

SEROTONIN AND NORADRENALINE REUPTAKE INHIBITORS (SNRIs)

General Actions of SNRIs
- selective serotonin and noradrenaline reuptake inhibitor that prolongs action of serotonin and noradrenaline at receptor sites

General Adverse effects of SNRIs
- nausea, vomiting, diarrhoea, constipation, dry mouth, anorexia, decreased/increased weight, dyspepsia, abdominal pain, altered taste
- headache, fatigue, asthenia, dizziness, somnolence, insomnia, disturbed dreams, tremor, paraesthesia, anxiety, altered concentration, irritability, agitation, feeling jittery, nervousness
- ecchymosis, haematoma, epistaxis, petechiae
- yawning
- tinnitus, vertigo
- sweating, hot flushes
- pruritus, rash
- palpitations, tachycardia, increased BP, postural hypotension, syncope
- (males) abnormal ejaculation, erectile dysfunction, impotence, decreased libido, testicular pain
- (females) abnormal orgasm, menorrhagia
- dysuria, urinary retention, urinary hesitancy, proteinuria
- blurred vision, mydriasis
- chills
- increased serum cholesterol and triglycerides, elevated liver enzymes, altered glycaemic control
- withdrawal symptoms (nausea, vomiting, fatigue, dizziness, headache, lethargy, agitation, anxiety,

confusion, irritability, vertigo, somnolence, insomnia, vivid nightmares, sweating, paraesthesia, seizures)
- (rare) hyponatraemia, suicide ideation, seizures, syndrome of inappropriate antidiuretic hormone secretion (SIADH), akathisia/psychomotor restlessness, hypomania/mania, serotonin syndrome (see p. 263), neuroleptic malignant syndrome

General Interactions of SNRIs

- contraindicated with or within 14 days of stopping MAOIs
- should be stopped for at least 7 days before starting an MAOI
- contraindicated with reversible MAOIs (RIMAs) (e.g. moclobemide, linezolid, IV methylene blue)
- increased risk of serotonin syndrome if given with SSRIs, other SNRIs, TCAs, amphetamine, lithium, sibutramine, fentanyl, methadone, St John's wort, triptans, tramadol, pethidine or tryptophan
- caution if used with other CNS active agents
- SNRIs may inhibit metabolism of TCAs, increasing serum levels and anticholinergic effects
- INR should be monitored if given with warfarin, especially when starting, stopping or adjusting dose
- not recommended with tryptophan supplements
- not recommended with alcohol
- increases risk of bleeding if given with NSAIDs, aspirin, warfarin or other agents
- increased risk of hyponatraemia if given with diuretics (especially in the elderly)

General Nursing points/Cautions for SNRIs

- see General Nursing points/Cautions for all antidepressant agents (p. 263)
- any dehydration, hypovolemia or pre-existing hypertension should be corrected before starting therapy
- BP monitoring is recommended (especially in those with hypertension or cardiac disease). If BP remains elevated, the dose should be reduced or therapy stopped
- liver function (including serum lipids and cholesterol) should be monitored regularly during therapy
- those at risk of narrow angle glaucoma should be closely monitored throughout therapy
- caution if used in those with pre-existing or uncontrolled hypertension, history of bleeding disorders, unstable heart disease, hyperthyroidism, heart failure, recent myocardial infarction, cerebrovascular disease, raised serum cholesterol or triglycerides, dehydration, hypovolaemia, history of seizures or mania, raised intraocular pressure, at risk of narrow angle glaucoma, urinary retention, prostatic hypertrophy or over 65 years with hypertension and/or other cardiac disease

General Patient teaching and advice for SNRIs

- see General Patient teaching and advice for all antidepressant agents (p. 264)
- patients with diabetes should be instructed to monitor blood glucose levels closely during therapy
- advise patient to seek medical advice if any of the following occur:
  - rash or hives (allergy)
  - unpleasant or distressing restlessness, inability to sit or stand

still (akathisia/psychomotor restlessness)
  - headache, difficulty concentrating, impaired memory, confusion, weakness, unsteadiness (hyponatraemia)
- women should be advised to discuss pregnancy with their doctor and are recommended to use adequate contraception throughout therapy

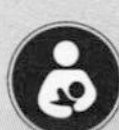

should only be used during pregnancy if benefits outweigh potential risks to the fetus. Increased risk of postpartum haemorrhage if taken during last month of pregnancy. Withdrawal symptoms or other adverse effects may occur in the newborn if given during third trimester

not recommended during breastfeeding. If used, infant should be closely observed

DESVENLAFAXINE (Desfax, Desven, Desvenlafaxine GH XR, Pristiq)

Available forms

Tablets (extended-release): 50 mg, 100 mg

Action

- see General Actions of SNRIs (p. 283)
- active metabolite of venlafaxine
- half-life 11 hours (prolonged in those with kidney impairment)

Use

- major depression

Dose

- initially 50 mg orally daily, increasing dose gradually at 1-week intervals (daily maximum 200 mg)

Interactions

- not recommended with venlafaxine
- caution if used with midazolam due to risk of increased sedation
- may cause false positive results on urine immunoassay screening for amphetamine and phencyclidine (PCP) for up to several days after therapy is stopped
- see also General Interactions of SNRIs (p. 284)

Adverse effects/Nursing points/ Cautions

- contraindicated in those with hypersensitivity to venlafaxine
- see also General Adverse effects/ Nursing points/Cautions for SNRIs (pp. 283–84)

Patient teaching and advice

- patient should be advised to take tablets whole, not crushed or chewed
- warn patient that inert tablet matrix/ shell may be noticed when defecating or via colostomy. Active medication has already been absorbed
- see also General Patient teaching and advice for SNRIs (p. 284)

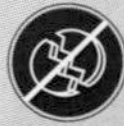

tablets should not be dispersed, crushed or chewed

DULOXETINE (Cymbalta, Depreta, Duloxecor, Dytrex, Tixol)

Available forms

Capsules (enteric-coated): 30 mg, 60 mg

Action

- see General Actions of SNRIs (p. 283)
- half-life is about 12 hours with no difference between males and females

Use

- major depression
- generalised anxiety disorder
- diabetic neuropathic pain

Dose

- (depression, diabetic neuropathic pain) 60 mg orally daily **OR**
- (generalised anxiety disorder) initially 30 mg orally daily, increasing at 30 mg increments if needed (daily maximum 120 mg)

Interactions

- contraindicated with fluvoxamine
- may decrease efficacy of tamoxifen
- may increase serum levels of flecainide and risperidone
- clearance may be decreased by paroxetine or other SSRIs increasing serum levels
- caution if used with agents which may slow motility or increase gastric pH
- see also General Interactions of SNRIs (p. 284)

Adverse effects/Nursing points/Cautions/Patient teaching and advice

- not recommended in those with acute or chronic liver disease (including those who consume large amounts of alcohol)
- contraindicated in those with liver impairment
- also General Adverse effects/Nursing points/Cautions/Patient teaching and advice for SNRIs (pp. 283–84)

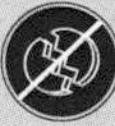

capsules should not be crushed. Capsules can be opened and pellets dispersed in apple juice or sprinkled on apple juice. Pellets should not be chewed

MILNACIPRAN HYDROCHLORIDE (Joncia)

Available form

Capsules: 25 mg, 50 mg, 100 mg

Action

- see General Actions of SNRIs (p. 283)
- inhibits noradrenaline uptake greater than serotonin uptake
- half-life is about 8 hours

Use

- management of fibromyalgia

Dose

- initially 25 mg orally at night (day 1–2), then 25 mg orally twice daily morning and evening (days 3–7), increasing to 50 mg orally twice daily morning and evening

Adverse effects

- see General Adverse effects of SNRIs (p. 283)

Interactions

- contraindicated with adrenaline (epinephrine) and noradrenaline (norepinephrine). If required as part of subcutaneous or gingival injection (i.e. with local anaesthetic), amount of adrenaline should be limited to 0.1 mg in 10 minutes or 0.3 mg in an hour
- may inhibit antihypertensive effect of clonidine
- caution if given with IV digoxin due to increased risk of potentiated haemodynamic effects
- see also General Interactions of SNRIs (p. 284)

Nursing points/Cautions/ Patient teaching and advice

- see General Nursing points/Cautions/Patient teaching and advice for SNRIs (p. 284)
- patient should be reassessed after 12 weeks to determine effectiveness of therapy
- not recommended in patients with chronic kidney disease stage 5
- contraindicated in patients with uncontrolled narrow angle glaucoma, severe cardiac function impairment, high risk of serious cardia arrhythmias, uncontrolled hypertension, severe or unstable coronary disease or conditions compromised by increases in BP and HR

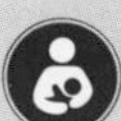

contraindicated during breastfeeding

capsules can be opened and contents dispersed in water or mixed with spoonful of yoghurt or apple puree

REBOXETINE (Edronax)

Available form

Tablets: 4 mg

Action

- see General Actions of SNRIs (p. 263)
- weakly inhibits serotonin uptake
- half-life is about 12 hours

Use

- major depression

Dose

- initially 4 mg orally twice daily, increasing after 3 weeks, up to 10 mg daily if needed

Adverse effects

- see General Adverse effects of SNRIs (p. 283)

Interactions

- contraindicated with or within 14 days of MAOIs
- serum levels may be decreased by carbamazepine or phenobarbital (phenobarbitone)
- caution if used with antihypertensive agents as orthostatic hypotension may be exacerbated
- use with ergot alkaloids may increase hypertension, therefore BP should be closely monitored during therapy
- increased serum levels may occur if given with azole antifungal agents, macrolide antibiotics (e.g. erythromycin) and fluvoxamine
- caution if given with lithium

Nursing points/Cautions/Patient teaching and advice

- see General Nursing points/Cautions/Patient teaching and advice for SNRIs (p. 264)

tablets can be dispersed in water or crushed and given with spoonful of yoghurt or apple puree

VENLAFAXINE HYDROCHLORIDE (Efexor XR, Elaxine SR, Enlafax-XR)

Available forms

Capsules (modified-release): 37.5 mg, 75 mg, 150 mg

Action

- see General Actions of SNRIs (p. 283)
- active metabolite

Use

- major depression
- generalised anxiety disorder, social anxiety disorder
- panic disorder

Dose

- (panic disorder) initially 37.5 mg orally daily with food for 4–7 days, then increasing to 75 mg daily. If needed, dose can be increased at 2-week intervals at 75 mg increments (daily maximum 225 mg) **OR**
- (depression, generalised or social anxiety disorder) initially 75 mg orally daily with food, increasing after 2 weeks to 150 mg daily, then gradually to 225 mg if necessary

Adverse effects

- sustained hypertension
- (uncommon) rash, pruritus
- (rare) prolongation of QTc interval, stress cardiomyopathy

- see also General Adverse effects of SNRIs (p. 283)

Interactions

- may increase serum levels of clozapine, haloperidol, lithium and risperidone with its associated toxicity/ adverse effects
- increased serum levels may occur if given with cimetidine (in the elderly with liver impairment)
- increased serum levels may occur if given with erythromycin, fluconazole or grapefruit juice
- caution if given with metoprolol as antihypertensive effect may be reduced
- caution if given with other agents that prolong QTc interval
- may decrease serum levels of indinavir
- see also General Interactions of SNRIs (p. 284)

Nursing points/Cautions

- caution if used in those at risk of QTc prolongation
- see General Nursing points/Cautions for SNRIs (p. 284)

Patient teaching and advice

- patient should be advised to seek medical advice if any of the following occur:
  - rash, hives or other skin condition develops
  - heart rate becomes rapid or irregular
- advise patient that tablets should be swallowed whole and not chewed or crushed
- instruct patient to avoid grapefruit juice during therapy
- see General Patient teaching and advice for SNRIs (p. 284)

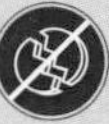

capsules and contents should not crushed. Efexor XR (only) – capsules can be opened and contents given with spoonful of apple puree

ATYPICAL ANTIDEPRESSANT AGENTS

AGOMELATINE (Domion, Valdoxan)

Available form

Tablets: 25 mg

Action

- melatonin receptor (MT_1 and MT_2) agonist and $5HT_{2C}$ receptor antagonist
- increases noradrenaline and dopamine in prefrontal cortex specifically thereby decreasing GI, sexual function and cardiovascular adverse effects
- improves sleep
- rapid half-life (1–2 hours)

Use

- major depression (including prevention of relapse)

Dose

- initially 25 mg orally at night (bedtime) for 2 weeks, increasing to 50 mg orally if needed

Adverse effects

- elevated liver enzymes
- nausea, vomiting, dry mouth, diarrhoea, abdominal pain, dyspepsia
- headache, migraine, dizziness, somnolence, insomnia, abnormal dreams, tremor, anxiety, fatigue
- sweating
- back pain
- (rare) hepatitis, suicidal ideation, urinary retention

Interactions

- contraindicated with fluvoxamine and ciprofloxacin

- caution if given with oestrogens (oral contraceptives), propranolol and rifampicin
- not recommended with alcohol

Nursing points/Cautions

- see General Nursing points/Cautions for all antidepressant agents (p. 263)
- before starting therapy, patient should be assessed for any risk factors for liver injury including alcohol use, substantial alcohol intake, non-alcoholic liver disease, diabetes, being overweight or obese
- liver function tests are recommended before starting therapy, at 3, 6, 12 and 24 weeks and then regularly or if increasing dose to 50 mg
- if liver enzymes become elevated, liver function test should be repeated within 48 hours
- if liver transaminases are more than 3 times normal upper limits or if patient has signs of liver injury, therapy should be stopped
- dose does not need to be tapered when discontinuing therapy
- tablets contain lactose and therefore should not be used in those with galactose intolerance, Lapp lactase insufficiency or glucose–galactose malabsorption
- caution if used in those with elevated liver enzymes or at risk of liver impairment (e.g. obese, overweight, non-alcoholic fatty liver, substantial alcohol use, concurrent use of hepatotoxic medications)
- not recommended for major depression in patients with dementia or those over 75 years
- contraindicated in those with liver impairment including cirrhosis and active liver disease or with liver transaminases more than 3 times upper normal limit

Patient teaching and advice

- see General Patient teaching and advice for all antidepressant agents (p. 264)
- advise patient to immediately report any abdominal pain, tiredness, yellowing of skin or eyes or dark urine

not recommended during pregnancy and breastfeeding

tablets can be crushed and mixed with water or spoonful of yoghurt or apple puree

MIANSERIN HYDROCHLORIDE (Lumin)

Available forms

Tablets: 10 mg, 20 mg

Action

- tetracyclic antidepressant (chemically unrelated to TCAs) that blocks noradrenaline uptake
- also acts on serotonin (5HT) receptors on CNS
- anxiolytic, promotes sleep
- long half-life (21–61 hours)

Use

- major depression

Dose

- initially 30 mg orally daily as 3 divided doses or single at night (bedtime) dose, slowly increasing at weekly intervals to a maintenance dose of 30–90 mg daily if needed (daily maximum 120 mg)

Adverse effects

- tiredness, lethargy, drowsiness, sedation, headache, tremor, dizziness, faintness, weakness, vertigo
- dry mouth, constipation
- (rare) altered glucose tolerance, hypotension

- (very rare) convulsions, bone marrow depression (neutropenia, thrombocytopenia, agranulocytosis), jaundice, hypomania, bradycardia, QT prolongation, cardiac arrest

Interactions

- contraindicated with or within 2 weeks of MAOIs
- MAOIs should not be commenced within 2 weeks of stopping mianserin
- may have unpredictable effects on warfarin serum levels, therefore INR levels should be closely monitored, especially when starting or stopping therapy, or adjusting dose
- CNS depressant effects enhanced by alcohol, barbiturates and benzodiazepines
- not recommended with alcohol
- BP monitoring is recommended if given with antihypertensive agents
- caution if given with other agents that prolong QTc interval
- serum levels may be decreased by phenytoin and carbamazepine

Nursing points/Cautions

- see General Nursing points/Cautions for all antidepressant agents (p. 263)
- any hypokalaemia or hypomagnesaemia should be corrected before starting therapy
- blood glucose levels should be carefully monitored in those with diabetes because glucose tolerance may be altered
- full blood count is recommended if patient complains of sore throat, malaise, mouth ulcers, flu-like symptoms or infection
- caution if used in elderly with a history of white cell disorders, or those with narrow angle glaucoma, diabetes, prostatic hypertrophy, epilepsy, liver/renal impairment, female or aged 65 years and over
- caution if used in those with cardiac impairment (including recent myocardial infarction, heart block or unstable heart disease), structural heart disease, left ventricular dysfunction or those at risk of QT prolongation including long QT syndrome
- not recommended in those under 18 years
- contraindicated in those with mania or severe liver disease

Patient teaching and advice

- see General Patient teaching and advice for all antidepressant agents (p. 264)
- advise patient to swallow tablet whole between meals
- if patient has diabetes, instruct him/her to carefully monitor blood glucose levels as glucose tolerance may be disrupted
- instruct patient that daily dose should be divided or may be taken as a single dose at night
- patients should be advised to seek medical advice immediately if any of the following occur:
  - sore throat, fever, chills, mouth ulcers, malaise, flu-like symptoms or signs of infection
  - unusual bleeding or bruising
  - change in heart rate (fast, irregular) and/or fainting

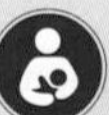

should only be used during pregnancy if benefits outweigh risks

not recommended during breastfeeding

tablet can be dispersed in water (2–5 minutes) or crushed and given with spoonful of yoghurt or apple puree

MIRTAZAPINE (Avanza, Axit, Mirtanza, Remeron Sol Tab)

Available forms

Tablets: 15 mg, 30 mg, 45 mg; Tablets (dissolvable): 15 mg, 30 mg, 45 mg

Action

- tetracyclic antidepressant that is an analogue of mianserin but unrelated to TCAs, SSRIs or MAOIs
- increases release of noradrenaline and serotonin (5HT)
- blocks $5HT_2$ and $5HT_3$ receptors, allowing serotonin to act on $5HT_1$ receptors
- weak anticholinergic properties
- sedative properties
- half-life (20–40 hours) with shorter half-life noted in young men

Use

- major depression

Dose

- initially 15 mg orally at night, increasing gradually to 30–45 mg if no response in 2–4 weeks (daily maximum 60 mg)

Adverse effects

- drowsiness, sedation (during first weeks of treatment)
- oedema (local or generalised)
- increased appetite, weight gain
- (uncommon) dizziness, headache
- (rare) bone marrow depression, postural hypotension, hyponatraemia, seizures, serotonin syndrome (see p. 263), suicidal ideation, akathisia/psychomotor restlessness

Interactions

- contraindicated with or within 2 weeks of MAOIs
- caution if given with agents that prolong QTc interval
- INR should be closely monitored if given with warfarin, especially when stopping or starting therapy, or adjusting dose
- may potentiate effects of alcohol, antipsychotics, antihistamines, opioids, sedatives and benzodiazepines
- risk of serotonin syndrome is increased if given with other serotonergic agents, including SSRIs, lithium, tramadol, linezolid, triptans, L-tryptophan, St John's wort, SNRIs or methylene blue
- serum levels may be decreased if given with carbamazepine, rifampicin or phenytoin
- caution if used with azole antifungal agents, HIV protease inhibitors, cimetidine or erythromycin as serum levels may be increased
- not recommended with alcohol

Nursing points/Cautions

- see General Nursing points and cautions for all antidepressant agents (p. 263)
- any dehydration, hypovolaemia or electrolyte imbalance should be corrected before starting therapy
- liver function and blood counts should be measured before starting therapy and regularly throughout
- not recommended in those under 18 years
- (dissolvable tablets) contain aspartame and are therefore not recommended in those with phenylketonuria
- tablets contain lactose/sucrose and therefore should not be used in those with galactose intolerance, Lapp lactase insufficiency, fructose intolerance or glucose–galactose malabsorption
- caution if used in those with epilepsy, organic brain syndrome, liver/kidney impairment, hypotension, dehydration, hypovolaemia, prostate hypertrophy, raised intraocular pressure, narrow angle glaucoma, recent myocardial infarction, angina or diabetes mellitus

Patient teaching and advice

- see General Patient teaching and advice for all antidepressant agents (p. 261)
- advise patient that tablets should be swallowed whole, without chewing
- instruct patient that dose may be divided into morning and evening doses
- if patient has diabetes, instruct him/her to carefully monitor blood glucose levels as glucose tolerance may be disrupted
- if patient is taking dissolvable tablets, the following instructions should be given:
  - take care not to crush tablets when removing from foil
  - carefully peel off foil lid starting at corner indicated by arrow
  - ensure hands/fingers are dry
  - place dissolvable tablet on tongue, then swallow when dissolved (with or without water)
- patient should be advised to seek medical advice immediately if any of the following occur:
  - sore throat, fever, chills, mouth ulcers, malaise, flu-like symptoms or signs of infection
  - seizures (fits)
  - feeling sick, weak, confused, exhausted, muscle weakness or cramping (signs of low sodium level)
  - unpleasant or distressing restlessness, inability to sit or stand still

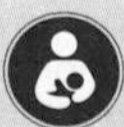

should only be used during pregnancy if benefits clearly outweigh potential risks to the fetus

not recommended during breastfeeding

available as an orally dissolving tablet which can be dissolved on the tongue with or without water

VORTIOXETINE (Brintellix)

Available forms

Tablets: 5 mg, 10 mg, 15 mg, 20 mg

Action

- serotonin receptor activity modulator, 5HT transporter reuptake inhibitor
- half-life 66 hours

Use

- major depression (including prevention of relapse)

Dose

- initially 10 mg orally daily, increasing to 20 mg or decreasing to 5 mg daily if needed

Adverse effects

- headache, dizziness, somnolence, sedation, fatigue, asthenia, insomnia
- sweating, pruritus
- decreased appetite, nausea, vomiting, dry mouth, dyspepsia, abdominal discomfort
- back pain, arthralgia
- nasopharyngitis, flu-syndrome
- sexual dysfunction
- (rare) seizure, serotonin syndrome (see p. 263), neuroleptic malignant syndrome, abnormal bleeding (ecchymoses, purpura and GI haemorrhage), hyponatraemia, mania/hypomania

Interactions

- contraindicated with or within 2 weeks of MAOIs, including irreversible nonselective MAOI (e.g. selegiline, rasagiline), reversible MAO-A (e.g. moclobemide), reversible nonselective MAOI (e.g. linezolid)
- increased risk of serotonin syndrome if given with serotonergic agents (e.g. tramadol, SSRIs, sumatriptan and other triptans)
- increased risk of adverse effects and serotonin syndrome if given with St John's wort

- increased risk of seizures if given with agents that lower seizure threshold such as SSRIs, SNRIs, phenothiazines, thioxanthenes, butyrophenones, mefloquine, bupropion and tramadol
- decreased serum levels may occur if given with rifampicin
- increased serum levels and therefore risk of adverse effects may occur if given with bupropion
- may increase serum levels of TCAs increasing risk of toxicity and serotonin syndrome
- caution if given with anticoagulants or other agents that affect platelet function due to risk of bleeding
- caution if used with other agents that cause hyponatraemia
- caution if used with ECT

Nursing points/Cautions

- see General Nursing points/Cautions for all antidepressants (p. 263)
- unlike many other antidepressants, may be stopped without gradual reduction
- dose should be started at 5 mg in those 65 years and over
- not recommended in those under 18 years

Patient teaching and advice

- see General Patient teaching and advice for all antidepressants (p. 264)

only used during pregnancy if benefits outweigh risks

not recommended during breastfeeding

tablet can be crushed and mixed with water or spoonful of yoghurt or apple puree

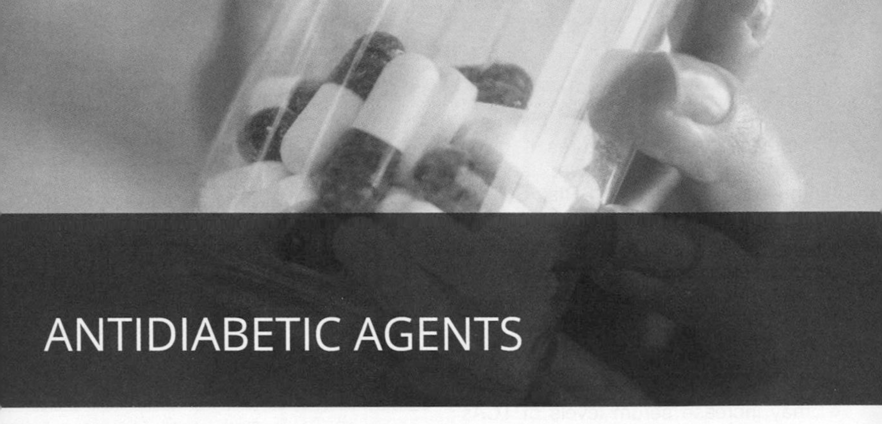

ANTIDIABETIC AGENTS

Diabetes mellitus is classified according to the process that leads to hyperglycaemia. Earlier classification used criteria such as age of onset (e.g. juvenile onset diabetes) or type of therapy (e.g. insulin dependent, non-insulin dependent). However, both of these are now outdated as it is now recognised that diabetes can develop at any age and those who start as non-insulin dependent may become insulin dependent as the disease progresses (Powers 2019). The two main categories of diabetes are type 1 and type 2, but there are other forms of diabetes that share characteristics of type 1 and/or type 2 (Powers et al 2019).

Worldwide, the prevalence of diabetes has been estimated at 415 million in 2017 (Powers 2019). Australian data estimates that in 2017–18, 1.2 million people (or 6% of Australian adults) had diabetes, with the prevalence of type 2 rising more rapidly than type 1 and thought to be due in part to the rising prevalence of obesity in the community (AIHW 2019d). In 2016–17, diabetes was the principal and/or additional diagnosis for 10% of all hospital admissions, as well as contributing to 11% of recorded deaths (17,000) in 2017. The diabetes-related death rate is three times higher in Aboriginal and Torres Strait Islanders compared to non-Indigenous Australians (AIHW 2019d).

Normally, beta cells in the islets of Langerhans in the pancreas release *insulin* to regulate blood glucose levels, keeping them between 5 and 8 mmol/L. Insulin is made up of 51 amino acids arranged in A and B chains joined by disulfide bonds (Powers 2019). It has a short half-life (3–5 minutes) and is mainly metabolised in the liver, but also in the kidney and muscles. After a meal, blood glucose levels rise and insulin is released. Insulin has a number of functions, including:

- stimulating the storage of glucose in the liver as glycogen and in adipose tissue as triglycerides
- stimulating the storage of amino acids in muscle as protein
- inhibiting the breakdown of triglycerides, glycogen and protein and conversion of amino acids to glucose (Powers 2019).

Types of diabetes include:

- *type 1*, which accounts for about 15% of diabetes overall and results from complete or near-complete insulin deficiency and can occur at any age, although commonly before

20 years of age. The insulin deficiency is due to autoimmune destruction of the pancreatic beta cells, while other pancreatic cells (e.g. alpha, delta) remain intact and function normally (Bryant et al 2019; Powers 2019)

- *type 2*, a heterogeneous group of disorders characterised by degrees of insulin resistance, impaired insulin secretion and increased glucose production. Risk factors for developing type 2 diabetes include family history, obesity (especially central and visceral fat), physical inactivity, race/ethnicity, history of gestational diabetes mellitus, hypertension, elevated HDL cholesterol and triglycerides, polycystic ovary syndrome, and history of cardiovascular disease (Powers 2019)
- *gestational diabetes mellitus*, which occurs in some women during pregnancy. Blood glucose levels generally return to normal after delivery; however, these women have a substantial risk (35–60%) of developing type 2 diabetes in later life. In 2016–17, one in seven pregnant women in Australia had gestational diabetes with incidence increasing with age. Over half (56%) of these women were able to manage their diabetes with diet and lifestyle modifications and the remainder required oral hypoglycaemic agents, insulin or both (AIHW 2019e).

Monitoring blood glucose levels (BGLs) is an important part of diabetes management in order to decrease microvascular complications such as neuropathy, retinopathy and nephropathy, and other cardiovascular complications. The diabetes educator or doctor will recommend the frequency of blood glucose testing, which is generally done before meals and at bedtime, but this may change if the person is unwell, exercising or having hypoglycaemic episodes or has changed antidiabetic agent and/or dosage. This simple test, using a drop of blood from a finger prick, indicates what is happening to the blood glucose level at that moment. Glycated haemoglobin (HbA1c) is a blood test that looks at the long-term diabetes management. HbA1c measures the average blood glucose level over the previous 3 months, but doesn't reflect any variations that may have occurred during that time (e.g. highs and/or lows). Persistently elevated blood glucose levels correlate with diabetes-related complications (Bryant et al 2019).

Patient education is an important part of the management plan and the newly diagnosed person should receive education about nutrition, exercise, care of diabetes during illness, how and when to monitor blood glucose levels, medication (how and when to administer), how to look after themselves generally to prevent complications (e.g. the importance of correct footwear, regular inspection of feet, ophthalmology review and podiatry visits), as well as managing associated conditions such as dyslipidaemia, hypertension, cardiovascular disease and obesity (Powers et al 2019). It is important that regular reviews are scheduled and attended. Education should not be a once-off occurrence, but should be ongoing, especially if there are any changes or problems (e.g. changing from an oral hypoglycaemic agent to insulin; hypoglycaemia occurring frequently; eyesight problems changing a person's ability to manage his or her own insulin injection; a change from one type of device to another, such as from a syringe to an insulin prefilled pen). Many of these issues are considered below in more detail.

INSULINS

Early insulin preparations were from beef (bovine) or pork (porcine) pancreas. Currently, insulin with an amino acid sequence identical to that of human insulin is obtained by either enzymatic modification of purified pork insulin (emp) (semisynthetic) or recombinant DNA techniques using bacteria (crb, prb) or yeast (pyr) (biosynthetic). Human insulins are less likely to cause antigen reactions than beef insulins, which are no longer commonly used in Australia.

Insulins are classified according to onset, peak and duration of action (e.g. ultra-short, short, intermediate and long acting). Insulins are also available in a pre-mixed combination (e.g. short acting plus intermediate, or ultra-short plus long acting).

Available forms

- vial, prefilled/cartridge pens
- 100 U/mL, 300 U/mL
- formulations include ultra-short-acting, short-acting, intermediate acting or long-acting insulins (see Table, pp. 302–03)
- premixed (or biphasic) insulins – include both short-acting and long-acting insulins in same formulation

General Actions of insulins

- see Introduction (p. 294)
- duration of action is dependent on dose, formulation, site of injection, blood supply to the area, temperature and physical activity

General Use of insulins

- type 1 diabetes
- type 2 diabetes not adequately controlled by diet and/or oral hypoglycaemic agents, or at times of increased or unusual stress such as pregnancy, infection, illness, trauma or surgery
- gestational diabetes mellitus
- emergency management of diabetic ketoacidosis (regular insulin)
- hyperglycaemic (hyperosmolar), non-ketotic coma

Dose

- no standard dose
- dose is individual and determined in consultation with the medical practitioner, and is dependent on BGLs, as well as the person's weight, diet, lifestyle, exercise levels, stress, illness, pregnancy, type of insulin and regimen in order to avoid fluctuation in BGLs and hypo- or hyperglycaemia
- generally given SC

General Adverse effects of insulins

- hypoglycaemia (timing is dependent on action profile of particular insulin; signs and symptoms include cold sweats, cool pale skin, tremor, nervousness, anxiety, tiredness, weakness, confusion, altered concentration, drowsiness, excessive hunger, visual disturbance, headache, nausea and palpitations. Severe hypoglycaemia can lead to unconsciousness, brain impairment and death). Some patient groups (e.g. elderly people, those with long-standing diabetes or markedly improved glycaemic control or on concurrent medications which interact with insulin) may not experience the typical early warning symptoms of a hypoglycaemic reaction

- (initially) sodium retention, oedema, visual impairment, including refraction anomalies, acute reversible painful neuropathy
- (injection site reaction) erythema, pain, swelling, hives or itching
- nasopharyngitis, sinusitis, rhinitis
- nausea, upper abdominal pain, gastroenteritis
- back pain, arthralgia
- fatigue, dizziness, headache
- (uncommon) lipodystrophy (lipoatrophy or lipohypertrophy) at injection site, which disappears slowly if site is changed. Lipodystrophy will delay insulin absorption from that site
- (rare) (general allergic reaction) urticaria, pruritus, angioedema, bronchospasm, hypotension, generalised skin reaction
- (rare) insulin resistance (requiring a change to purified porcine or human insulin), antibody development
- peripheral neuropathy

General Interactions of insulins

- alcohol, clonidine, lithium, isoniazid, interferons, oestrogen-containing oral contraceptives and beta-adrenoceptor blocking agents can produce variable effects (either increasing or decreasing actions of insulin)
- insulin requirements may be increased if given with beta-2 stimulants (e.g. salbutamol), clozapine, corticosteroids, danazol, diazoxide, glucagon, growth hormone, lanreotide, octreotide, olanzapine, phenothiazines, progestogens, somatotrophin, sympathomimetic agents, thiazide diuretics and thyroid hormones
- insulin requirements may be decreased if given with ACE inhibitors (captopril, enalapril), alcohol, alpha-adrenoceptor blocking agents (e.g. prazosin), beta-adrenoceptor blocking agents (non-selective), anabolic steroids (except danazol and oxymetholone), fibrates, fluoxetine, MAOIs, octreotide, pentoxifylline (oxpentifylline), oral hypoglycaemic agents, perhexiline, quinine, salicylates and sulfonamides
- increased risk of hypoglycaemia if given with oral hypoglycaemic agents
- caution if given with protease inhibitors as hyperglycaemia may occur
- extreme caution if given with disopyramide due to additive hypoglycaemia risk (especially in the elderly or those with malnutrition, kidney or cardiac impairment)
- if given with pentamidine, there is an increased risk of hypoglycaemia, which may be followed by hyperglycaemia
- beta-adrenoceptor blocking agents may mask the symptoms and delay recovery from hypoglycaemia by blocking gluconeogenesis
- decreased insulin requirements may be required in those with renal or liver impairment

- increased risk of congestive cardiac failure if given with thiazolidinediones (rosiglitazone, pioglitazone)

General Nursing points/Cautions for insulins

- it is important to review patient education and injection technique regularly, especially if the person has an increase in the frequency of hypo- or hyperglycaemic episodes or uncontrolled BGLs
- hypoglycaemia is likely if BGL is less than 3 mmol/L; convulsions may occur if it is less than 2 mmol/L
- changes between types, brand or species of insulin should be done with caution and careful monitoring
- have available 50% glucose and glucagon (glucagon is injected to increase the BGL temporarily to treat any severe hypoglycaemic reaction when the person cannot or will not swallow or is unconscious; see Antidotes, antagonists and chelating agents, p. 348). Glucagon can be given IM or SC, but glucose must be given IV by a medical professional if the person has not responded to glucagon in 10–15 minutes
- (Lantus) should not be diluted or mixed with other insulins or solutions
- (Levemir) not for use in insulin-infusion pumps
- (Fiasp) must not be diluted or mixed with other products except infusion fluids (glucose 5% or sodium chloride 0.9%)
- caution in those using protamine-containing insulin if protamine is used to reverse heparinisation after cardiac catheterisation as a severe anaphylactic-type reaction is possible
- caution if used in those who have had recent surgery or trauma or who have liver or kidney impairment, fever, severe infection, hyperthyroidism, adrenal or pituitary disorders (not adequately controlled), diarrhoea, intestinal obstruction or vomiting
- insulin is contraindicated in those with hypoglycaemia or with hypersensitivity to insulin preparations

Short-acting insulin

- includes very short-acting (aspart, lispro, glulisine) and short-acting (neutral) preparations
- clear solution, usually given SC, but may be given IV or IM in emergencies such as diabetic ketoacidosis, pre-coma and coma
- when given IM, onset of action is more rapid than SC but duration is shorter
- usually given 15–30 minutes before meals
- cloudy solutions should be discarded
- injection should be followed by carbohydrate-containing snack/meal within 15–30 minutes (depending on the very short-acting or short-acting insulin)

Long-acting insulin

- appears white and cloudy
- contains zinc or protamine, allowing slow release of insulin, so prolonging the duration of action
- used in people with stabilised insulin-sensitive diabetes
- given SC, never IM or IV or in an emergency
- should be gently shaken or agitated by rolling in the palms of the hands to evenly distribute insulin throughout solution before using (should not be vigorously shaken)

- newer formulations (e.g. insulin detemir, insulin glargine) should not be mixed

Storage

- store unopened insulin (vials/cartridges/prefilled pens) at 2–8°C, but do not freeze and do not store next to freezer compartment or freezer packs
- before first use, insulin should be allowed to come to room temperature for 1–2 hours as injecting cold insulin is painful
- insulin in use can be stored at room temperature provided that the room temperature does not exceed 25°C; mark date of opening on label and discard after 28 days
- avoid overexposure to light or heat
- insulin should be discarded if it has been frozen or exposed to high temperatures (as the protein becomes denatured), if discoloured or if any lumps or flakes are present
- do not store cartridge pens (that are in use) in the refrigerator

Preparation

- select correct preparation
- porcine insulin should not be given to those of Islamic or Jewish faith
- not mixed with other drugs
- keep insulin at room temperature for at least 1–2 hours before use to reduce pain
- check expiry date
- suspensions are rotated gently (not vigorously shaken) and inverted several times to ensure full dispersion and prevent frothing
- insulin of one brand should not be mixed with insulin of another brand
- model and brand of syringe or needle should not be changed without consulting the doctor
- when mixing insulins, use the same procedure every time for accuracy and constant effect
- short-acting insulin is drawn up first to prevent its contamination in the vial by the long-acting insulin (containing zinc or protamine), which binds soluble insulin, thereby reducing the amount of soluble insulin available for immediate effect. Mixture should be injected immediately after mixing
- majority of insulins are available in 100 units/mL vials, together with a standard insulin syringe marked in units for U100 insulin (dose ranges from 10 to 100 or more units depending on the severity of the diabetes and is adjusted according to blood glucose level). The exception to this is glargine insulin (Toujeo), which is available as 300 units/mL
- incompatible with agents containing thiols or sulfites

Administration

- ineffective if given orally
- usually given SC; avoid IV injection by withdrawing syringe plunger before injecting
- area should not be massaged after injection because this may speed up absorption
- given usually 30 minutes before breakfast (however, some of the ultra rapid insulins can be given just before or with a meal) or if twice daily, give second injection before the evening meal
- injection sites include the upper arms, thighs and abdomen; however, because absorption rates vary so much it is advisable to rotate injection sites within the same anatomical location, preferably the abdomen,

which has the most rapid absorption rate

- injection sites are rotated so that the same site is not injected more than once per month to prevent thickening and dimpling of the site (lipodystrophy), which may result in decreased insulin absorption
- instructions enclosed with the injection pen and cartridge vial must be followed carefully to ensure correct dose is administered

General Patient teaching and advice for insulins

After diagnosis, patient education should begin at least several days before discharge from hospital, giving the person the opportunity to ask questions and practise skills such as blood glucose monitoring and insulin injection. Education should be lifelong.

Points for consideration include:

- importance of exercise, maintaining a healthy weight range and correct diet (referral to a dietitian may be necessary)
- advising the patient about the temporary changes to vision that can occur at the start of treatment with insulin, which can impact on ability to drive or operate machinery
- type of insulin to be used (e.g. short-acting, long-acting) and an understanding of why it is being used
- monitoring of BGLs, including technique, when to monitor, recording of information
- understanding how to manage BGL if fasting for diagnostic or surgical procedures
- choice of appropriate insulin devices, depending on:
  - the person's vision and ability to see the dose (e.g. some devices have an audible click when insulin doses are dialled up and this may maintain a visually impaired person's independence)
  - fine motor skills (e.g. some devices require the person to load a cartridge and dial up the dose, while others are preloaded)
  - ability to manage the actual device itself, including loading cartridges, performing safety test (if needed), cleaning, knowing when the device has malfunctioned and what to do if there is a problem
- emphasise importance of checking insulin label (on cartridge, reusable pen or vial) before each injection to ensure correct insulin is being used. This is especially important if the person uses more than one formulation type. Insulin should also be checked for any cloudiness or particles and not used if they are present and the insulin solution is not clear
- injection technique (with opportunity to practise skills), including not rubbing area after injection
- importance of rotating injection sites (e.g. not using the same site more than once per month) including abdomen, thigh, buttock and upper arm
- if injection pen is damaged or not working, it should not be used
- disposal of sharps into a sharps container, including not reusing needles and not sharing needles or devices with others
- correct storage of insulin (both unopened and opened; with or without needles attached)
- importance of following injection with carbohydrate-containing meal or snack

- significance of carrying some form of oral glucose at all times (e.g. jellybeans, barley sugar) to prevent hypoglycaemia
- if using an infusion pump, understanding importance of having an alternative delivery device in case of pump failure (e.g. SC therapy) and understanding pump use and changing of infusion set. Person should understand that pump malfunction may lead to fast onset of hypoglyaemia and ketosis and what to do if any of these occur
- symptoms of hypoglycaemia (e.g. cool pale skin, fatigue, drowsiness, unusual tiredness, sweating, shaking, anxiety, crying, vomiting, headache, excessive hunger, visual changes, palpitations and confusion). However, it is important to emphasise that symptoms vary between people, with some experiencing only a few symptoms and others many. It is essential that the person knows what his/her individual symptoms are and acts immediately
- anticipating when hypoglycaemia is likely to occur (e.g. increased exercise) and working out a snack or meal pattern to prevent or overcome it
- understanding that hypoglycaemia causes slower reaction time (important when driving or operating machinery)
- symptoms of hyperglycaemia include loss of appetite, drowsiness, flushed dry skin, dry mouth, increased thirst, blurred vision, passing large amounts of urine and 'fruity' breath
- patient/carer needs to understand that hyperglycaemia is a potentially life-threatening situation
- benefits of obtaining and wearing a MedicAlert bracelet or pendant (especially in the event of confusion or loss of consciousness)
- need for extra food requirements before or during increased activity such as sport or, alternatively, that the insulin dose may require adjustment. If the patient exercises regularly, a doctor should be consulted regarding food intake and insulin requirements to ensure that hypoglycaemia is prevented
- patient should be instructed to seek advice from a doctor/diabetes educator when travelling overseas and crossing time zones, as these may affect administration times of insulin, increasing risk of unstable BGLs. It is also important for the person to carry a letter from the doctor explaining why he/she has injecting pens and needles
- advise patient that if feeling ill (including cold and flu, or vomiting), he/she should continue to use insulin, take food in liquid form as replacement and consult a doctor if unable to eat a normal diet or if blood or urine tests become positive for glucose and/or ketones. Infection and fever often increase insulin requirements
- changes in insulin strength, brand, type and/or species should be done under medical supervision as requirements may change. Early warning symptoms of hypoglycaemia may also be altered when changing from an animal source insulin to another type
- a relative, friend, colleague or teacher should be alerted that the person has diabetes and instructed on how to identify and deal with hypoglycaemia

or hyperglycaemia, including recognising symptoms and what to do if the person loses consciousness (e.g. place on side, get medical assistance, do not give the person who is unconscious anything to eat or drink as they may choke; he or she may be instructed in injecting glucagon if the person has hypoglycaemia)
- if the person wears glasses and is currently experiencing uncontrolled blood glucose levels, they should be advised to postpone obtaining new corrective lenses until BGLs have stabilised for 3–6 weeks, as it can take this length of time for visual disturbances to stabilise
- warn patient of the dangers of drinking alcohol (especially excessive amounts) as it can affect the actions of insulin and may lead to hypoglycaemia occurring. Alcohol may also predispose person to hyperglycaemia on the morning following alcohol intake
- female patients should be advised to inform doctor if they become pregnant or are planning pregnancy
- advise patient about organisations such as Diabetes Australia and Diabetes New Zealand, that are able to provide further information about diabetes and management
- see also General Patient teaching and advice (p. xxvii)

insulin preparations are banned in sport

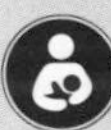

insulin requirements usually fall in the first trimester and increase during the second and third trimesters of pregnancy. Insulin requirements fall to pre-pregnancy levels within 6 weeks of delivery. BGLs should be monitored closely post-delivery to prevent hypoglycaemia from occurring as insulin requirements may decrease 24–72 hours after delivery

if breastfeeding, insulin requirements, diet or both may need to be adjusted

CHARACTERISTICS OF DIFFERENT INSULIN PREPARATIONS

Preparation	Examples	Onset	Peak	Duration
Ultra short-acting (rapid)				
Insulin glulisine	Apidra	15 minutes	1 hour	
Insulin lispro	Humalog	15 minutes	1–3 hours	3–5 hours
Insulin aspart	Fiaso NovoRapid	15 minutes	1–3 hours	3–5 hours
Short-acting				
Neutral (regular, soluble) insulin	Actrapid Humulin R	30 minutes	2–5 hours	6–8 hours

CHARACTERISTICS OF DIFFERENT INSULIN PREPARATIONS—CONT'D

Preparation	Examples	Onset	Peak	Duration
Intermediate-acting				
Isophane insulin (with protamine)	Humulin NPH Hypurin Isophane Protaphane	1–2.5 hours	4–10 hours	16–24 hours
Long-acting (basal)				
Insulin glargine	Lantus Semglee Optisulin Toujeo	1–2 hours	Steady state	24 hours (does not peak)
Insulin detemir	Levemir	3–4 hours	3–14 hours	12–24 hours
Biphasic/combination				
30/70 or 50/50 mixtures of short-acting plus intermediate-acting insulin; or ultra-short plus long-acting insulin	Humalog Mix (insulin lispro + insulin lispro protamine) Humulin 30/70 (insulin isophane human + insulin neutral human) Mixtard (insulin isophane human + insulin neutral human) NovoMix (insulin aspart +insulin aspart protamine) Ryzodeg 70/30 (insulin aspart + insulin degludec)	0.5–1 hour	2–12 hours	16–24 hours

ORAL HYPOGLYCAEMIC AGENTS

The oral hypoglycaemic agents are divided into a number of classes:

- sulfonylureas (e.g. glibenclamide)
- biguanides (e.g. metformin hydrochloride)
- alpha glucosidase inhibitors (e.g. acarbose)
- thiazolidinediones (e.g. rosiglitazone)
- dipeptidyl peptidase 4 (DPP-4) inhibitors (e.g. linagliptin)

- glucagon-like peptide-1 (GLP-1) analogues (e.g. exenatide)
- sodium-glucose cotransporter 2 inhibitors (SGLT2 inhibitors) (e.g. canagliflozin)

General Nursing points/Cautions for oral hypoglycaemic agents

- caution if using these agents in those who are elderly, malnourished and/or debilitated
- contraindicated in those with type 1 diabetes mellitus, diabetic ketoacidosis, diabetic coma or pre-coma or severe kidney/liver impairment/dysfunction

General Patient teaching and advice for oral hypoglycaemic agents

- it is important that the patient understands and adheres to managing their diet and weight, personal hygiene and physical exercise, as well as identifying and managing any cardiovascular risk factors, including hypertension and dyslipidaemia
- ensure the patient understands the need to avoid infection and report to the doctor if any signs of illness occur
- instruct the patient how oral hypoglycaemic agents work and the importance of not stopping medication if BGLs appear stable
- the patient should be educated on how to monitor BGLs and the importance of regular medical checks, especially if blood glucose control is not optimal or if he/she is changing antidiabetic agents
- the patient should be aware not to increase the dose if a dose is missed. It is important to discuss what to do if a dose or meal is missed and understand the consequences of skipping a meal after the oral hypoglycaemic agent has been taken
- the patient needs to be educated in the identification of the symptoms of hypoglycaemia, which include weakness, listlessness, sweating, hunger, nausea, vomiting, trembling/shaking, restlessness, sleep disturbance, impaired concentration, alertness and/or reactions, light-headedness, irritability, numbness around lips/tongue, headache, palpitations and confusion. This list is not extensive and varies from person to person
- the patient should know how to treat hypoglycaemia and the importance of having carbohydrates readily available. For example, eating 5–7 jelly beans, 3 teaspoons of sugar/honey, drinking 1/2 can of non-diet soft drink, 2–3 glucose tablets or a tube of glucose gel, followed up by extra carbohydrates such as plain biscuits, fruit or milk if next meal is not within next 10 to 15 minutes
- the patient needs to anticipate when hypoglycaemia is likely to occur and work out a snack or meal pattern to prevent or overcome it. Risk factors for hypoglycaemia include not understanding directions for medication use (e.g. taking too much), the need to monitor BGLs, malnutrition, irregular meal intake (including skipping meals or fasting), dietary changes, imbalance between exercise and carbohydrate intake and physical problems (e.g. kidney or liver impairment)
- warn the patient to take care when driving or operating machinery, because hypoglycaemia causes slow reaction time, or decreased alertness

- hypoglycaemia may occur during the first month of therapy because sulfonylureas also cause insulin to be released from the pancreas
- ensure that the patient knows the symptoms of hyperglycaemia, including nausea, vomiting, drowsiness, dry mouth, flushed dry skin, polyuria, polydipsia, decreased appetite and acetone ('fruity') breath
- warn patient that hyperglycaemia is a potentially life-threatening situation
- the patient should be closely monitored during times of unusual stress, such as infection, fever, surgery and trauma, as this predisposes them to hyperglycaemia and ketosis; the patient may require insulin during this time. Other causes of hyperglycaemia include eating more carbohydrates than usual, too little hypoglycaemic agent, too little exercise (depending on usual level) and other medications
- ensure that the patient understands there is a reduced tolerance to alcohol, which may also affect blood levels of oral hypoglycaemic agents, and therefore is best to be avoided altogether. If alcohol is consumed, it is important to warn the patient to immediately report any flushing, headache, problems with breathing, rapid heart rate, stomach pain, feeling nauseous and/or vomiting (possible disulfiram-like reaction) (see Glossary)
- a relative, friend, colleague or teacher needs to know how to identify and deal with hypoglycaemia and hyperglycaemia
- advise the patient to wear a Medic-Alert bracelet or pendant
- instruct the patient to immediately tell the doctor of the return of any symptoms, such as lethargy, tiredness, headache, thirst, blurred vision or passing large amounts of urine, or if BGLs are unstable/fluctuating, as this may indicate the particular oral hypoglycaemic agent is no longer effective at lowering BGLs
- see General Patient teaching and advice (p. xxvii)

SULFONYLUREAS

General Actions of sulfonylureas

- orally active sulfonylurea (sulfonamide derivative) agents that stimulate insulin release from functioning pancreatic cells
- improve sensitivity of beta cells of the pancreas to glucose stimulus, leading to insulin secretion
- enhance peripheral sensitivity to insulin
- reduce basal glucose production by the liver

General Uses of sulfonylureas

- type 2 diabetes (unresponsive to diet alone and in whom other antidiabetic agents have been ineffective)

General Adverse effects of sulfonylureas

- hypoglycaemia and, rarely, severe or prolonged and fatal hypoglycaemia
- anorexia, nausea, vomiting, epigastric fullness/pressure, abdominal pain, constipation, diarrhoea, dyspepsia, heartburn

- rash, pruritus, erythema, urticaria, photosensitivity
- blurred vision, changes to accommodation, diplopia (transient, at start of therapy)
- abnormal liver enzymes and function, (rare) cholestatic jaundice, hepatitis, pancreatitis
- (rare) hyponatraemia, syndrome of inappropriate antidiuretic hormone secretion (SIADH)
- (rare) anaemia, leucopenia, thrombocytopenia, agranulocytosis

General Interactions of sulfonylureas

- hypoglycaemic action enhanced by ACE inhibitors, alcohol (acute intake), anabolic steroids, antidiabetic agents (oral), aspirin, beta-adrenoceptor blocking agents, biguanides, chloramphenicol, clarithromycin, clonidine, cyclophosphamide, disopyramide, fibrates, fluconazole, fluoxetine, gemfibrozil, heparin, ifosfamide, insulin, MAOIs, miconazole, NSAIDs, pentoxifylline (oxpentifylline) (high dose, IV), phosphamides, probenecid, fluoroquinolone antibacterial agents, ranitidine, salicylates, sulfonamides, testosterone, tetracyclines and voriconazole, which may result in loss of blood glucose control
- hypoglycaemic effects reduced by acetazolamide, barbiturates, chronic alcohol use, calcium-channel blockers, cimetidine, clonidine, corticosteroids, diazoxide, furosemide (frusemide), glucagon, isoniazid, laxatives (prolonged use), nicotinic acid (high dose), oral contraceptives, oestrogens, phenothiazines, phenytoin, progestogens, rifampicin, sympathomimetics, thiazide diuretics or thyroid hormones
- may either increase or decrease warfarin effects and therefore should be given with caution and INR closely monitored
- may increase serum levels of ciclosporin, increasing the risk of toxicity, therefore levels should be closely monitored, especially if starting or stopping sulfonylureas
- (rare) when combined with alcohol, may cause a disulfiram-like reaction (see Glossary)
- beta-adrenoceptor blocking agents, clonidine, H_2-receptor antagonists (e.g. cimetidine) may prolong or mask the symptoms of hypoglycaemia
- increased hypoglycaemia may occur if given to those with acute alcohol intoxication
- decreased duration of action may occur in those who ingest alcohol chronically

General Nursing points/Cautions for sulfonylureas

- when first starting therapy, clinical status should be checked after 4–8 weeks and then regularly to ascertain that the dosage is correct to maintain BGLs within normal range
- patient should be closely monitored if changing from one sulfonylurea to another sulfonylurea/other hypoglycaemic agent
- sulfonylureas are not oral insulins, but are capable of increasing circulating insulin in a person with a functioning pancreas
- any hypersensitivity reaction requires prompt discontinuation
- caution if used in those with alcoholism, insulinoma, or adrenal, thyroid or pituitary insufficiency because they may have increased sensitivity to sulfonylureas

- caution if used in those with porphyria as the condition may be exacerbated
- there is an increased risk of hypoglycaemia if the person is undertaking intense or prolonged exercise, drinks alcohol, has a decreased food intake, is taking multiple antidiabetic agents, has severe endocrine disorders or adrenal/pituitary insufficiency or the person is elderly, debilitated, malnourished or has liver or kidney impairment
- not recommended in those with G6PD deficiency as haemolytic anaemia may occur
- contraindicated in those with type 1 diabetes, diabetes complicated with ketosis, diabetic ketoacidosis, serious metabolic decompensation with acidosis (especially pre-coma or coma), severe kidney or liver dysfunction or impairment
- contraindicated if given to those with sensitivity to another sulfonamide or thiazide diuretic because cross-sensitivity may be possible
- see General Nursing points/Cautions for oral hypoglycaemic agents (p. 304)

General Patient teaching and advice for sulfonylureas

- patient should be instructed to protect skin by using protective clothing and sunscreen with high protective factor (SPF 30+) as skin may be more sensitive to sunlight
- advise patient to ensure meal has adequate amount of carbohydrates to prevent hypoglycaemia occurring
- advise patient to seek medical advice immediately if any of the following occur:
  - yellowing of skin and/or eyes, tiredness, loss of appetite, nausea, vomiting, upper abdominal pain, dark urine, pale stools
  - unexplained bleeding or bruising
  - pale appearance, tiredness, shortness of breath during exercise or exertion
  - rash, hives, skin redness, itching
- see also General Patient teaching and advice for oral hypoglycaemic agents (p. 304)

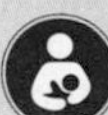

animal studies have shown sulfonylureas to be embryotoxic and cause fetal abnormalities and are therefore contraindicated during pregnancy. May also cause neonatal hypoglycaemia. Oral hypoglycaemics should be replaced with insulin during pregnancy

contraindicated during breastfeeding

GLIBENCLAMIDE (Daonil)

Available form

Tablets: 5 mg

Action/Use

- see General Actions and Uses of sulfonylureas (p. 305)
- inhibits glucagon-producing alpha cells and increases release of somatostatin from delta cells in the pancreas
- has a mild diuretic action
- peak effect 2–6 hours, half-life 2–10 hours

Dose

- initially 2.5 mg orally daily before breakfast, increasing by 2.5 mg at 7-day intervals if needed (daily maximum 20 mg)

Adverse effects

- see General Adverse effects of sulfonylureas (p. 305)

Interactions

- contraindicated with bosentan because of the increased risk of

hepatotoxicity. In addition, serum levels of both agents can be significantly decreased if given together
- see General Interactions of sulfonylureas (p. 306)

Nursing points/Cautions/Patient teaching and advice

- if the patient has only a light breakfast, the first dose should be delayed until lunchtime
- if the patient is changed from insulin to glibenclamide, test urine for ketones and glucose 3 times daily during changeover period. For patients receiving up to 40 units/day, insulin can be stopped gradually and glibenclamide started (2.5 mg for < 20 units or 5 mg for 20–40 unit). Dose can be increased in increments of 1.25–2.5 mg/day at intervals of 2–10 days, depending on patient response and tolerance
- if changing from another oral antidiabetic agent, dose should be started at 2.5–5 mg
- doses up to 10 mg can be given as a single daily dose. Amounts in excess of 10 mg can be given with the evening meal
- caution if used in those with coronary artery disease due to increased risk of cardiovascular mortality
- see Nursing points/Cautions/Patient teaching and advice for sulfonylureas (pp. 306–07)

Note

- contained in Glucovance with metformin hydrochloride

tablets can be crushed and mixed with water or spoonful of yoghurt or apple puree

GLICLAZIDE (Ardix Gliclazide MR, Diamicron 60 mg MR, Glyade, Glyade MR, Nidem)

Available forms

Tablets: 80 mg; Tablets (modified-release): 30 mg, 60 mg

Action/Use

- see General Actions and Uses of sulfonylureas (p. 305)
- also reduces platelet adhesiveness and aggregation, increases vascular endothelial fibrinolytic activity and has some antioxidant properties
- peak effect 4–6 hours, half-life 12 hours

Dose

- initially 40 mg daily, increasing up to 320 mg if necessary **OR**
- initially 30 mg daily, increasing by 30 mg every 14 days if needed (up to 120 mg daily) (modified-release tablets)

Adverse effects

- see General Adverse effects of sulfonylureas (p. 305)

Interactions

- caution if used with fluoroquinolones as BGL may become disturbed
- efficacy may be decreased if given with St John's wort
- caution if given with chlorpromazine (high dose)
- contraindicated with miconazole
- not recommended with danazol
- see also General Interactions of sulfonylureas (p. 306)

Nursing points/Cautions

- (tablets) up to 160 mg as a single dose at the same time every morning; amounts in excess of 160 mg should be taken in divided doses morning and evening
- transferring from insulin is not recommended

- tablets contain lactose and therefore are not recommended in those with galactose intolerance, glucose–galactose malabsorption or Lapp lactose deficiency
- see General Nursing points/Cautions for sulfonylureas (p. 306)

Patient teaching and advice

- suggest to patient that dose should be taken at breakfast
- (modified-release tablets) patient should be advised to swallow tablets whole, not chewed or crushed; however, tablet has a break line if half-dose is required
- see also General Patient teaching and advice for sulfonylureas (p. 307)

modified-release tablets should not be crushed

immediate-release tablets can be dispersed in 10–20 mL water or crushed and mixed with spoonful of yoghurt or apple puree.

GLIMEPIRIDE (Amaryl, Diapride, Dimirel)

Available forms

Tablets: 1 mg, 2 mg, 3 mg, 4 mg

Action/Use

- see General Actions and Uses of sulfonylureas (p. 305)
- peak effect 2.5 hours, half-life 5–8 hours, duration of action 24 hours

Dose

- initially 1 mg orally daily before breakfast. If needed, may be increased by 1 mg at 1–2 week intervals according to response, 1–4 mg daily (maintenance)

Adverse effects/Interactions/Nursing points/Cautions/Patient teaching and advice

- if the patient has only a light breakfast, the first dose should be delayed until lunchtime
- see General Adverse effects/Interactions/Nursing points/Cautions/Patient teaching and advice for sulfonylureas (pp. 305–07)

tablet can be dispersed in water or crushed and mixed with spoonful of yoghurt or apple puree

GLIPIZIDE (Melizide, Minidiab)

Available form

Tablets: 5 mg

Action/Use

- see General Actions and Uses of sulfonylureas (p. 305)
- peak action 1–2 hours, half-life 2–4 hours

Dose

- initially 2.5–5 mg orally daily 30 minutes before breakfast, increasing gradually in increments of 2.5–5 mg if needed (maximum total daily dose is 40 mg)

Adverse effects

- dizziness, drowsiness, vertigo, headache
- see also General Adverse effects of sulfonylureas (p. 305)

Interactions/Nursing points/Cautions/Patient teaching and advice

- amounts in excess of 15 mg should be divided and given before meals
- if single dose is not effective, dosage may be divided and given twice daily
- contraindicated in those with severe thyroid dysfunction, severe trauma, infections, febrile conditions, major surgical procedures or gangrene
- see also General Interactions/Nursing points/Cautions/Patient teaching and advice for sulfonylureas (pp. 306–07)

tablet can be dispersed in water or crushed and mixed with spoonful of yoghurt or apple puree

BIGUANIDES

METFORMIN HYDROCHLORIDE (Diabex, Diabex XR, Diaformin, Diaformin XR, Formet, Glucobete, Metex XR)

Available forms

Tablets: 500 mg, 850 mg, 1000 mg; Tablets (extended-release): 500 mg, 1000 mg

Action

- orally active biguanide derivative
- does not stimulate insulin release, but does require insulin to be present to be effective
- inhibits gluconeogenesis in the liver and glucose absorption from the GI tract, and increases peripheral uptake and utilisation in muscle by increasing insulin sensitivity
- increases insulin sensitivity via increasing number of receptors and affinity for receptors
- decreases risk of diabetes-related complications or mortality
- affects lipid metabolism by reducing total cholesterol, low density lipoprotein cholesterol and triglycerides
- considered first-line treatment for type 2 diabetes mellitus
- peak effect 2–3 hours, half-life 3 hours

Use

- type 2 diabetes (unresponsive to diet and exercise alone as monotherapy, with insulin or with other oral hypoglycaemic agents)

Dose

- initially 500 mg orally 1–2 times daily with meals, increasing slowly to 1 g 3 times daily if needed (daily maximum 2 g) **OR**
- initially 500–750 mg orally with evening meal, increasing dose by 500–750 mg every 10–15 days if needed (daily maximum 2 g) (extended-release tablets)

Adverse effects

- (mild, transient) diarrhoea, nausea, vomiting, metallic taste, anorexia, abdominal pain
- (very rare) mild erythema, pruritus, urticaria
- (uncommon) decreased vitamin B_{12} absorption, decreased vitamin B_{12} levels
- (very rare) serious and often fatal lactic acidosis (nausea, vomiting, abdominal pain, diarrhoea, malaise, myalgia, somnolence, hyperventilation, decreased blood pH), liver function abnormalities, hepatitis

Interactions

- risk of lactic acidosis may be increased if given with alcohol or diuretics (especially loop diuretics, acetazolamide, topiramate), in cases of renal impairment or with doses greater than 2 g per day
- alcohol may delay and/or mask the symptoms of hypoglycaemia and also increase the risk of lactic acidosis and therefore are not recommended together
- ACE inhibitors and calcium-channel blockers may affect blood glucose control, therefore should be given with caution and dose adjustment of metformin may be required according to BGLs
- beta-adrenoceptor blocking agents may mask signs of hypoglycaemia (e.g. tachycardia)
- contraindicated with contrast media (containing iodine) used for radiological examination due to risk of altered kidney function and lactic acidosis. Must be discontinued for 48 hours before examination
- increased plasma levels may occur if given with cimetidine or nifedipine
- may increase elimination time of vitamin K antagonists, therefore prothrombin time should be monitored

when starting, stopping or changing doses
- clearance may be decreased if given with cimetidine, dolutegravir, triamterene and trimethoprim
- if given with agents that intrinsically elevate BGLs (e.g. glucocorticoids, tetracosactides, danazol, chlorpromazine (doses > 100 mg/day), thyroid hormones and diuretics) more frequent monitoring of BGLs is recommended, especially when starting or stopping therapy or adjusting doses of either agent
- caution if used with other agents which may impair kidney function (e.g. NSAIDs, thiazide diuretics, antihypertensive agents)
- efficacy may be decreased if given with verapamil
- efficacy and GI absorption may be increased if given with rifampician

Nursing points/Cautions

- creatinine clearance (CC) and/or serum creatinine should be assessed before starting therapy and then yearly (if patient has normal kidney function) or 2–4 times yearly (if patient is elderly or has serum creatinine levels at the upper side of normal levels)
- regular monitoring of liver and cardiovascular function is also recommended, especially if patient has pre-existing heart failure
- vitamin B_{12} levels should be measured before starting therapy, at 6 months then yearly if therapy is continuous
- should be stopped before and for at least 48 hours after radiological examination using IV iodinated contrast medium or surgery. Should only be restarted after renal function is evaluated and found to be normal
- does not normally cause hypoglycaemia when given as monotherapy
- switching to extended-release tablets is not recommended in patients managed on immediate-release metformin dose > 2000 mg/day
- caution if given to the elderly, those with kidney impairment or in doses over 2 g/day because of increased risk of life-threatening lactic acidosis
- contraindicated in those with type 1 diabetes mellitus, diabetes mellitus (controlled by diet alone), during/after surgery where insulin is needed, diabetic ketoacidosis, lactic acidosis, diabetic pre-coma, kidney dysfunction/failure (CC < 60 mL/min), other conditions that could affect kidney function (e.g. shock, dehydration, severe infection, IV administration of iodinated contrast agents), severe liver insufficiency, alcoholism, acute alcohol intoxication, acute/chronic disease causing tissue hypoxia (e.g. recent myocardial infarction, cardiac/respiratory failure, sepsis), pulmonary embolism, gangrene or pancreatitis
- see also Nursing points/Cautions for oral hypoglycaemic agents (p. 304)

Patient teaching and advice

- patient should be advised to avoid alcohol during therapy
- instruct patient that GI adverse effects may be avoided if metformin is taken with food and dose is increased slowly
- advise the patient to swallow extended-release tablets whole, not broken, crushed or chewed
- warn patient that tablet shell may appear in the faeces (and this is normal)
- patient should be advised that BGL control usually takes about 2 weeks to achieve
- ensure that patient understands that lactic acidosis is a medical emergency and can be life threatening. The patient should be therefore advised to immediately report any of the following:
  - abdominal cramps
  - muscle pain or cramping
  - nausea, vomiting, loss of appetite, diarrhoea

- feeling generally unwell, unusually tired or sleepy
- weakness
- shivering, feeling extremely cold
- fast, shallow breathing
- see also General Patient teaching and advice for oral hypoglycaemic agents (p. 304)

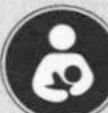

oral hypoglycaemics should be replaced with insulin during pregnancy

contraindicated if used during breastfeeding as animal studies have shown metformin to be secreted in breastmilk

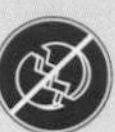

modified-release tablets should not be crushed

immediate-release tablets can be crushed and mixed with water or spoonful of yoghurt or apple puree.

Note

- contained in Galvumet with vildagliptin, Glucovance with glibenclamide, Janumet and Janumet XR with sitagliptin, KombiglyzeXR with saxagliptin, NesinaMet with alogliptin, Trajentamet with linagliptin, XigduoXR with dapagliflozin, Segluromet with ertugliflozin, and Jardiamet with empagliflozin

ALPHA GLUCOSIDASE INHIBITORS

ACARBOSE (Glucobay, Glybosay)

Available forms

Tablets: 50 mg, 100 mg

Action

- complex oligosaccharide with action on GI tract
- inhibits intestinal alpha glucosidase involved in the breakdown of disaccharides, oligosaccharides and polysaccharides, but not monosaccharides, leading to delayed digestion
- monosaccharides are absorbed more slowly into the blood, reducing the fluctuation in BGLs throughout the day related to food ingestion
- does not induce hypoglycaemia
- no effect on the pancreas
- active metabolite
- half-life about 2 hours

Use

- type 2 diabetes (when diet alone or diet and other oral hypoglycaemic agents have been ineffective)

Dose

- initially 50 mg orally daily for the first week, increasing to 50 mg orally twice daily in the second week, 50 mg orally 3 times daily in the third week, increasing further after 4–8 weeks if necessary (daily maximum 600 mg)

Adverse effects

- (very common) flatulence
- (common) diarrhoea, abdominal pain
- (uncommon) nausea, vomiting, dyspepsia, distension, bloating, increased serum transaminases (transient, reversible)
- (rare) hepatitis, jaundice, oedema

Interactions

- use with thiazide diuretics, furosemide (frusemide), corticosteroids, phenothiazines, oestrogens, oral contraceptives, thyroid hormones, phenytoin, nicotinic acid, sympathomimetics and isoniazid may result in loss of blood glucose control
- if given concurrently with colestyramine, effects may be increased
- use with digoxin may require dose adjustment of digoxin
- use with charcoal or enzyme preparations is not recommended

- if hypoglycaemia occurs when given with sulfonylureas or metformin, dose of both agents should be reduced

Nursing points/Cautions

- hypoglycaemia should be treated using glucose/dextrose. Cane sugar/ sucrose should not be given to patients treated with acarbose alone or in combination with another hypoglycaemic agent because the breakdown of sucrose will be slowed and hypoglycaemia will persist
- if diarrhoea persists, patient should be closely monitored and dose decreased
- starting at a low dose helps to alleviate some of the adverse intestinal effects
- liver enzymes should be monitored monthly for the first 6–12 months and if changes occur the dose reduced or withdrawn and enzymes monitored weekly until normal
- contraindicated in those with severe renal impairment (creatinine clearance < 25 mL/min), malabsorption disorders, ulcerative colitis, Crohn's disease, predisposition to intestinal obstruction or ileus, partial bowel obstruction or conditions aggravated by intestinal gas formation or under 18 years of age
- see General Nursing points/Cautions for oral hypoglycaemic agents (p. 304)

Patient teaching and advice

- advise patient to swallow tablets whole before meals or chew with the first mouthful of the meal
- patient should be advised to avoid cane sugar (sucrose) or products containing cane sugar as they may cause stomach pains/discomfort and possibly diarrhoea
- warn patient that it is common for side-effects (flatulence/wind, stomach rumbling, feeling full, sometimes stomach cramps) to occur in the first few days of therapy, especially if foods containing sugar are eaten. If symptoms persist for longer than 2–3 days or are severe, the patient should seek medical advice
- if hypoglycaemia occurs, cane sugar/ sucrose should not be given in patients treated with acarbose alone or in combination with another hypoglycaemic agent because the breakdown of sucrose will be slowed and hypoglycaemia will persist. Glucose or dextrose should be used
- instruct patient to not use antacids to treat indigestion as they will be ineffective
- see also General Patient teaching and advice for oral hypoglycaemic agents (p. 304)

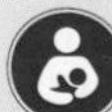

contraindicated during pregnancy and breastfeeding

tablet can be chewed with first mouthful of food. Tablet can be crushed and mixed with spoonful of yoghurt

THIAZOLIDINEDIONES

General Actions of thiazolidinediones

- improve insulin sensitivity in the liver, skeletal muscle and adipose tissue
- inhibit gluconeogenesis in the liver
- decrease insulin resistance
- decrease circulating free fatty acid levels
- require insulin to be present to be effective

- may take several weeks for full effect to become noticeable

General Uses of thiazolidinediones

- type 2 diabetes inadequately controlled by diet and exercise alone (as monotherapy, or with metformin, insulin or sulfonylurea)

General Adverse effects of thiazolidinediones

- increased incidence of bone fractures (upper arm, hand, foot) (women)
- hypoglycaemia (if given with insulin, metformin or sulfonylureas)
- peripheral oedema, fluid retention, new or worsening cardiac failure
- weight gain
- fatigue, headache
- back pain
- decreased haemoglobin (anaemia) and haematocrit
- upper respiratory tract infection, pharyngitis, sinusitis
- abnormal liver function test results, transient increase in creatine phosphokinase levels (CPK)
- (very rare) new/worsening diabetic macular oedema, decreased visual acuity

General Interactions of thiazolidinediones

- increased serum levels if given with gemfibrozil
- decreased serum levels may occur if given with rifampicin
- increased risk of hypoglycaemia if given with insulin and/or oral antidiabetic agent

General Nursing points/Cautions for thiazolidinediones

- liver function tests should be monitored every second month for the first year, and regularly thereafter
- blood tests (haemoglobin and haematocrit) should be monitored regularly throughout therapy
- patients should be closely monitored for any signs of cardiac failure during therapy, including excessive rapid weight gain, dyspnoea and/or oedema
- caution if used in those with pre-existing oedema
- contraindicated in those with class II, III or IV heart failure (New York Heart Association (NYHA) classification), type 1 diabetes mellitus or diabetic ketoacidosis

General Patient teaching and advice for thiazolidinediones

- warn patient that weight gain is a common side-effect
- patient should be advised to seek medical advice immediately if any of the following occur:
  - loss of appetite, nausea, vomiting, upper abdominal pain, dark urine, pale stools, fatigue or yellowing of skin and/or eyes
  - excessive rapid weight gain, difficulty breathing, swelling of ankles, feet and hands
  - eye problems, including blurred or double vision
- may result in resumption of ovulation, increasing the risk of pregnancy in anovulatory pre-menopausal women with insulin resistance (e.g. polycystic ovary syndrome) and therefore they should be counselled regarding the use of adequate contraception if pregnancy is unwanted
- see also General Patient teaching and advice for oral hypoglycaemic agents (p. 304)

PIOGLITAZONE (Acpio, Actaze, Actos, Vexazone)

Available forms
Tablets: 15 mg, 30 mg, 45 mg

Action/Use
- see General Actions and Uses of thiazolidinediones (pp. 313–14)
- 3 active metabolites
- peak effect 2–4 hours, half-life 5–23 hours (parent and metabolites)

Dose
- (monotherapy) initially 15–30 mg orally daily, increasing after 4 weeks to 45 mg daily if necessary (daily maximum 45 mg) **OR**
- (double therapy) 15–30 mg orally daily (with insulin, metformin or sulfonylurea) **OR**
- (triple therapy) 30 mg orally daily, increasing to 45 mg if needed (with metformin and sulfonylureas)

Adverse effects
- asthenia, malaise
- myalgia, leg cramps
- upper abdominal pain, diarrhoea
- tooth disorder
- abnormal vision
- urinary tract infection
- (female) increased risk of oedema, resumption of ovulation
- (rare) bladder cancer with prolonged use
- see also General Adverse effects of thiazolidinediones (p. 314)

Interactions
- may decrease effectiveness of oral contraceptives
- see also General Interactions of thiazolidinediones (p. 314)

Nursing points/Cautions
- (female patient) dose should be started at 15 mg and increased gradually monitoring for any oedema
- (double therapy) if patient is using insulin, pioglitazone should be started at 15 mg once daily
- not recommended in those with history of bladder cancer, active liver disease or liver transaminases > 2.5 times upper normal limit
- see also General Nursing points/Cautions for oral hypoglycaemic agents (p. 304)

Patient teaching and advice
- warn patient to seek medical advice if there is blood, pain and burning when passing urine (as these could be symptoms of bladder cancer)
- female patients should be counselled regarding the need to use additional contraceptive methods to protect against unwanted pregnancy
- see General Patient teaching and advice for thiazolidinediones (p. 314)

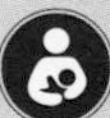

only used during pregnancy if benefits outweigh risks

not recommended during breastfeeding

tablets can be crushed and mixed with water or spoonful of yoghurt or apple puree

DIPEPTIDYL PEPTIDASE-4 (DPP-4) INHIBITORS

General Actions of DPP-4 inhibitors

- dipeptidyl peptidase 4 (DPP-4) enzyme inhibitor that enhances levels of incretin hormones (glucagon-like peptide 1 (GLP1) and glucose-dependent insulinotropic polypeptide (GIP)), which are released by the intestine in response to a meal and are involved in the regulation of glucose homeostasis
- improves pancreatic beta cell responsiveness to glucose, as well as increasing insulin synthesis and release
- reduces glucagon secretion from pancreatic alpha cells, decreasing liver glucose

General Uses of DPP-4 inhibitors

- type 2 diabetes (inadequately controlled by diet and exercise alone) in combination with metformin, sulfonylurea and/or thiazolidinedione

General Adverse effects

- nasopharyngitis, sinusitis, upper respiratory tract infection
- headache
- pancreatitis
- hypoglycaemia (when combined with sulfonylurea)
- hypersensitivity (urticaria, angioedema, localised skin reaction, bronchial hyperreactivity)
- (rare) arthralgia, bullous pemphigoid

General Nursing points/Cautions for DPP-4 inhibitors

- not recommended in those with type 1 diabetes or diabetic ketoacidosis
- see General Nursing points/Cautions for oral hypoglycaemic agents (p. 304)

General Patient teaching and advice for DPP-4 inhibitors

- advise patient to seek medical advice immediately if any of the following occur:
  - any allergic reactions such as shortness of breath, wheezing, difficulty breathing, face/lips/tongue swelling, skin rash, itching or hives
  - any persistent abdominal pain, especially if associated with nausea and/or vomiting (as these may be signs of pancreatitis)
  - exacerbation of joint pain
  - skin blistering or ulceration
- ensure patient is aware of increased risk of hypoglycaemia if he/she is also taking insulin (with or without metformin) or combination of metformin with pioglitazone

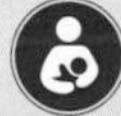

not recommended during pregnancy or breastfeeding

ALOGLIPTIN (Nesina)

Available form

Tablets: 6.25 mg, 12.5 mg, 25 mg

Action/Use

- see General Actions and Uses of DPP-4 inhibitors (p. 316)
- peak activity 1–2 hours, half-life 21 hours

Dose

- 25 mg orally daily

Adverse effects

- abdominal pain, gastroesophageal reflux disease, rash, pruritus
- (rare) liver damage, pancreatitis

- see also General Adverse effects of DPP-4 inhibitors (p. 316)

Nursing points/Cautions

- if patient has any signs of liver injury, liver function tests should be conducted immediately
- dose should be reduced if given with insulin or sulphonylurea to decrease risk of hypoglycaemia
- dose reduction and monitoring of kidney function is recommended if used in those with kidney impairment
- caution if used in those with congestive cardiac failure
- not recommended for those with severe liver impairment
- see also General Nursing points/Cautions for DPP-4 inhibitors (p. 316)

Patient teaching and advice

- advise patient to seek medical advice immediately if any of the following occur:
  - yellowing of eyes/skin, loss of appetite, nausea, vomiting, upper abdominal pain, dark urine or pale stools
- see also General Patient and teaching for DPP-4 inhibitors (p. 316)

tablets can be crushed and mixed with water or spoonful of yoghurt or apple puree

Note

- contained in NesinaMet with metformin hydrochloride

LINAGLIPTIN (Trajenta)

Available form

Tablets: 5 mg

Action/Use

- see General Actions and Uses for DPP-4 inhibitors (p. 316)
- peak effect 1.5 hours, triphasic half-life

Dose

- 5 mg orally daily

Adverse effects

- increased uric acid levels
- (uncommon) cough, constipation
- see also General Adverse effects of DPP-4 inhibitors (p. 316)

Nursing points/Cautions/Patient teaching and advice

- see General Nursing points/Cautions/Patient teaching and advice for DPP-4 inhibitors (p. 316)

tablets can be crushed and mixed with water or spoonful of yoghurt and apple puree

Note

- contained in Trajentamet with metformin hydrochloride and Glyxambi with linagliptin

SAXAGLIPTIN (Onglyza)

Available form

Tablets: 2.5 mg, 5 mg

Action/Use

- see General Actions and Uses for DPP-4 inhibitors (p. 316)
- active metabolite (half as potent as saxagliptin) (half-life 3.1 hours)
- peak effect 2 hours, duration of action 24 hours, half-life 2.5 hours

Dose

- 5 mg orally daily

Adverse effects

- urinary tract infection
- see also General Adverse effects of DPP-4 inhibitors (p. 316)

Nursing points/Cautions

- kidney function should be assessed before starting therapy and then monitored regularly during therapy
- dose should be decreased if given with sulfonylurea to decrease risk of hypoglycaemia

- caution if used in those with moderate-to-severe kidney impairment or cardiac failure
- not recommended in those with end-stage kidney disease on haemodialysis
- see General Nursing points/Cautions for DPP-4 inhibitors (p. 316)

Patient teaching and advice

- advise patient that tablets should be swallowed whole, not broken or divided
- see General Patient teaching and advice for DPP-4 inhibitors (p. 316)

tablets can be crushed and mixed with water or spoonful of yoghurt or apple puree; however, do not disperse readily in water and are hard to crush

Note

- contained in Kombiglyze XR with metformin hydrochloride and Qtern with dapaglifozin

SITAGLIPTIN (Januvia)

Available forms

Tablets: 25 mg, 50 mg, 100 mg

Action/Use

- see General Actions and Uses for DPP-4 enzyme inhibitors (p. 316)
- peak effect 1–4 hours, half-life 12.4 hours

Dose

- 100 mg orally daily (as monotherapy or in combination with metformin, sulfonylurea, thiazolidinedione or insulin)

Adverse effects

- diarrhoea, constipation
- hypertension
- back ache, osteoarthritis, pain in extremities
- see also General Adverse effects of DPP-4 inhibitors (p. 316)

Nursing points and Cautions/ Patient teaching and advice

- dose should be decreased for those with renal insufficiency and is dependent on creatinine clearance. Kidney function should be monitored before starting and regularly throughout therapy
- see General Nursing points/Cautions/ Patient teaching and advice for DPP-4 inhibitors (p. 316)

tablets can be crushed and mixed with water or spoonful of yoghurt or apple puree; however, does not disperse readily in water and difficult to crush

Note

- contained in Janumet and Janumet XR with metformin hydrochloride, and Steglujan with ertugliflozin

VILDAGLIPTIN (Galvus)

Available form

Tablets: 50 mg

Action/Use

- see General Actions and Uses for DPP-4 inhibitors (p. 316)
- peak effect 1.75 hours, half-life 2–3 hours

Dose

- (combination therapy) 50–100 mg orally daily **OR**
- (monotherapy) 50 mg orally twice daily

Adverse effects

- peripheral oedema
- headache, dizziness
- constipation
- (rare) changes in liver enzymes, liver dysfunction, hepatitis
- see also General Adverse effects of DPP-4 inhibitors (p. 316)

Nursing points/Cautions

- liver and kidney function should be assessed before starting therapy and then monitored 3-monthly during therapy

- tablets contain lactose and therefore are not recommended in those with galactose intolerance, glucose-galactose malabsorption or Lapp lactose deficiency
- not recommended in those with moderate-to-severe kidney impairment, end-stage kidney disease on haemodialysis or those with liver impairment (ALT or AST 2.5 times > upper normal limit) or cardiac failure (NYHA functional class IV)
- see General Nursing points/Cautions for DPP-4 inhibitors (p. 316)

Patient teaching and advice

- advise patient to seek medical advice if any loss of appetite, nausea, vomiting, upper abdominal pain, lethargy, dark urine or pale stools occurs
- warn patient not to drive or operate machinery if dizziness is an ongoing problem
- see General Patient teaching and advice for DPP-4 inhibitors (p. 316)

tablets can be crushed and mixed with water or spoonful of yoghurt or apple puree

Note

- combined with metformin hydrochloride in Galvumet

GLUCAGON-LIKE PEPTIDE-1 (GLP-1) ANALOGUES

General Actions of GLP-1 analogues

- binds to and activates glucagon-like peptide-1 (GLP-1) receptors mimicking incretin, leading to increase in synthesis and secretion of insulin by the pancreas
- suppresses glucagon secretion in those with type 2 diabetes leading to decreased glucose output by the liver
- does not impair normal glucagon response to hypoglycaemia
- slows gastric emptying

General Uses of GLP-1 analogues

- type 2 diabetes (with metformin, sulfonylurea or both where glycaemic control has not been achieved)

General Adverse effects of GLP-1 analogues

- nausea, vomiting, decreased appetite, anorexia, diarrhoea, constipation dyspepsia, abdominal pain and distension, GI reflux disease
- headache
- upper respiratory tract infection
- hypoglycaemia (if given with sulfonylurea)
- (injection site) pruritus, redness, pain, haematoma, induration and rarely, abscess formation, cellulitis, ulceration, necrosis
- (rare) acute renal failure, pancreatitis, kidney impairment, worsening of chronic kidney failure

General Interactions of GLP-1 analogues

- caution if given with agents that require rapid GI absorption (e.g. bisphosphonates) because of the delay in GI emptying, or that can cause GI irritation (e.g. tetracyclines)
- increased risk of hypoglycaemia if given with sulfonylureas (in those with type 2 diabetes)

General Nursing points/Cautions for GLP-1 analogues

- not given IV or IM
- dose of sulfonylurea may be reduced to lessen risk of hypoglycaemia
- administer alone
- caution if used in those with history of pancreatitis, gallstones, alcoholism and severe hypertriglyceridaemia
- not recommended in those with diabetes mellitus type 1 or diabetic ketoacidosis or history of pancreatitis
- contraindicated in those with history of GLP-1 analogue-associated pancreatitis
- see also General Nursing points/ Cautions for oral hypoglycaemic agents (p. 304)

General Patient teaching and advice for GLP-1 analogues

- patient should be instructed to seek medical advice immediately if the following occur:
  - any persistent severe abdominal pain, especially if accompanied by diarrhoea, nausea and/or vomiting
- see also General Patient teaching and advice for oral hypoglycaemic agents (p. 304)

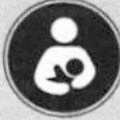

not recommended during pregnancy or breastfeeding. Insulin is recommended during pregnancy

DULAGLUTIDE (Trulicity)

Available forms

Prefilled pen: 1.5 mg/0.5 mL

Action/Use

- see General Actions and Uses for GLP-1 analogues (p. 319)
- half-life 4.7 days

Dose

- 1.5 mg weekly SC

Adverse effects

- fatique
- sinus tachycardia
- elevated pancreatic enzymes
- hypersensitivity
- see also General Adverse effects for GLP-1 analogues (p. 319)

Interactions

- see General Interactions of GLP-1 analogues (p. 319)

Nursing points/Cautions

- not recommended in those with end-stage kidney disease
- see also General Nursing points/ Cautions for GLP-1 analogues (p. 320)

Patient teaching and advice

- advise patient that gastrointestinal adverse effects usually peak in first 2 weeks and then decline over next 4 weeks
- patient should be educated:
  - in correct use of pen (see also General Patient teaching and advice for insulins (p. 300))
  - on the importance of rotating injection sites to include upper arms, thighs and abdomen
  - to inject into skin (not into veins or muscle)
  - not to use solution if cloudy, coloured or if it contains particles, or if expiry date has passed
  - to store pen in fridge, but should not be frozen. Pen should be discarded if it becomes frozen
  - in safe disposal of used pens/ syringe
  - if dose is missed and there is less than 3 days before next dose, dose should not be given, but administered on next scheduled day
- see General Patient teaching and advice for GLP-1 analogues (p. 320)

EXENATIDE (Bydureon, Byetta)

Available forms

Prefilled pen: 5 microgram/20 microL, 10 microgram/40 microL; 2 mg (extended-release formulation)

Action/Use

- see General Actions and Uses for GLP-1 analogues (p. 319)
- may alter LDL-C or total cholesterol
- (Byetta) peak effect 2 hours, half-life 2.4 hours
- (Bydureon) formulated with biodegradable polyglactin microspheres to extend release into circulation

Dose

- initially 5 microgram SC twice daily up to 1 hour before meal, increasing after 4 weeks to 10 microgram if needed (Byetta) **OR**
- 2 mg SC weekly (Bydureon)

Adverse effects

- weight loss
- dizziness, depression, insomnia, anxiety
- gastroenteritis
- hypokalaemia
- hypertension
- nasopharyngitis, sinusitis, cough, oropharyngeal pain
- urinary tract infection
- erectile dysfunction
- back pain, arthralgia, muscle spasm
- development of antibodies
- see also General Adverse effects for GLP-1 analogues (p. 319)

Interactions

- not recommended with other GLP-1 receptor agonists
- delays gastric emptying decreasing absorption of hydrocortisone and paracetamol and should be given 1 hour before or 4 hours after exenatide
- caution when given with other agents which stimulate insulin release (e.g. sulfonylureas)
- not recommended with insulin or thiazolidinedione
- caution if given with warfarin. INR should be closely monitored during therapy
- see also General Interactions of GLP-1 analogues (p. 319)

Nursing points/Cautions

- blood lipids should be monitored regularly during therapy
- worsening or failure to achieve target glycaemic control may be due to antibody development
- if switching from 10 microgram twice daily to 2 mg weekly once weekly, transient increase in BGLs may occur during first 2 weeks of therapy
- (Bydureon) use diluent provided in prefilled syringe to reconstitute powder
- (immediate-release formulation) caution if increasing dose from 5 microgram to 10 microgram in those over 70 years
- caution if used in those with mild-to-moderate kidney impairment
- not recommended in those under 18 years
- not recommended in those with GI disease such as gastroparesis or dumping syndrome or history of pancreatitis
- caution if used in those with nausea, vomiting, diarrhoea or dehydration as risk of renal impairment and failure is increased
- contraindicated in those with known hypersensitivity to metacresol (Byetta only), end-stage kidney disease or severe kidney impairment (with creatinine clearance <30 mL/minute)
- see also General Nursing points/Cautions for GLP-1 analogues (p. 320)

Patient teaching and advice

- advise patient not to drive or operate machinery if dizziness is problematic
- patient should be instructed to seek medical advice immediately if they

experience rapid weight loss (more than 1.5 kg/week)

- (Byetta) patient should be educated:
  - in correct use of pen (see also General Patient teaching and advice for insulins (p. 300))
  - on the importance of rotating injection sites to include upper arms, thighs and abdomen
  - to inject into skin (not into veins or muscle)
  - not to use solution if cloudy, coloured or if it contains particles
  - to use a new needle for each injection
  - to store pen in fridge (but not with needle attached). If solution freezes it should be discarded
  - to discard pen after 30 days (even if there is some solution remaining)
  - in safe disposal of used needles
  - if also using insulin, should be given as two separate injections
- (Byetta) advise patient to separate twice-daily doses by at least 6 hours up to 1 hour before meals
- (Byetta) instruct patient that drug is not to be used after meals and if dose is missed, injection should be given before next mealtime
- (Byetta) advise patient to use the following medications either an hour before or 4 hours after exenatide injection: hydrocortisone and paracetamol
- (Bydureon) patient should be instructed in:
  - correct reconstitution of powder using provided diluent in prefilled syringe
  - correct SC administration technique
  - correct storage and disposal of vial, prefilled syringe with diluent and needles
  - if changing day of administration, allow an interval of at least 3 days between injections
- (Bydureon) if switching from 10 microgram twice daily to 2 mg once weekly, transient increase in BGLs may occur during first 2 weeks of therapy, therefore close monitoring should be advised
- see General Patient teaching and advice for GLP-1 analogues (p. 320)

LIRAGUTIDE (Saxenda, Victoza)

Available form

Prefilled pen: 6 mg/mL

Action

- see General Actions of GLP-1 analogues (p. 319)
- protracted release is due to self-association (resulting in slow absorption), binding to albumin and enzymatic stability, resulting in long plasma half-life
- physiological regulator of appetite and calorie intake as GLP-1 receptors are present in the brain in areas involved in appetite regulation, as well as being present in the intestine
- increases fullness and satiety and decreases hunger signals
- decreases plasma triglycerides, total cholesterol, LDL and VDL while increasing HDL, but does not reduce size of any existing plaques
- peak effect 8–12 hours, duration of action 24 hours, half-life about 13 hours

Use

- see General Uses of GLP-1 analogues (p. 319)
- chronic weight management in those with BMI ≥ 30 kg/m^2 (obese) or ≥ 27 kg/m^2 and < 30 kg/m^2 (overweight) with ≥ one weight-related co-morbidity (e.g. dyslipidaemia, hypertension, obstructive sleep apnoea) (adjunct to reduced calorie diet and increased physical activity)

Dose

- (type 2 diabetes) initially 0.6 mg SC once daily, then increasing to 1.2 mg after 7 or more days, increasing to

1.8 mg after a further 7 days if needed **OR**
- (weight management) initially 0.6 mg SC once daily, increasing by 0.6 mg increments at 7-day intervals to 3 mg (as maintenance)

Adverse effects
- gastritis, flatulence, altered taste, dry mouth, eructation
- increased heart rate, hypotension
- insomnia (especially in first 12 weeks of therapy), fatigue, asthenia, dizziness
- (uncommon) rash, urticaria, pruritus
- cholelithiasis, cholecystitis, elevated liver enzymes
- (uncommon) dehydration
- (rare) increased blood calcitonin, goitre, thyroid adenomas/carcinomas, allergic reactions, depression, suicidal ideation
- injection site reactions
- see also General Adverse effects for GLP-1 analogues (p. 319)

Interactions
- not recommended with insulin
- caution if used with other agents that increase heart rate such as sympathomimetic agents
- not recommended with other agents containing GLP-1 analogues
- see General Interactions of GLP-1 analogues (p. 319)

Nursing points/Cautions
- (weight management) if there has not been a weight loss of at least 5% of initial body weight on 3 mg daily dose, therapy should be stopped
- heart rate should be monitored regularly during therapy
- should not be used as substitute for insulin
- (weight management) intervals of at least 7 days are needed to improve GI tolerability. If increasing dose to next level is not tolerated for 2 consecutive weeks, stopping treatment should be considered
- (weight management) therapy should be reviewed each time prescription is written and at least annually
- caution if used in those with pre-existing thyroid disease
- (weight management) not recommended in those with obesity secondary to endocrinological issues or eating disorders
- caution if used in those with kidney impairment, especially end-stage kidney failure or liver insufficiency
- (weight management) not recommended with other agents for weight loss (including over-the-counter or complementary/herbal medicines)
- not recommended in those with inflammatory bowel disease or diabetic gastroparesis
- increased risk of GI adverse effects in those > 65 years
- not recommended in those > 75 years
- not recommended in those with history of major depression or other psychiatric illnesses
- see also General Nursing points/Cautions for GLP-1 analogues (p. 320)

Patient teaching and advice
- patient should be advised to avoid dehydration during therapy, especially if nausea, vomiting and/or diarrhoea occur
- warn patient not to drive or operate machinery if dizziness is ongoing
- advise patient to seek medical advice if any of the following occur:
  - palpitations, feelings of racing heartbeat while at rest
  - upper right-sided abdominal pain, yellowing of eyes or skin
  - lump or swelling in neck, hoarseness, difficulty swallowing, shortness of breath
  - sadness, depression, change in mood, ideas of self-harm

- patient should be educated in the following:
  - correct use of pen (see also General Patient teaching and advice for insulins, p. 300)
  - importance of rotating injection sites to include upper arms, thighs and abdomen
  - injecting into skin (subcutaneously) (not into veins or muscle)
  - not to use solution if cloudy, coloured or if it contains particles
  - to use a new needle for each injection
  - after first use, pen can be kept at room temperature (not > 30° C)
  - if solution freezes, it should be discarded
  - store pen without injection needle attached to prevent contamination, infection and leakage
  - pen cap should be kept on to protect from light when pen is not in use
  - to discard pen after 30 days (even if there is some solution remaining)
  - safe disposal of used needles
- see General Patient teaching and advice for GLP-1 analogues (p. 320)

SODIUM-GLUCOSE COTRANSPORTER 2 INHIBITORS (SGLT2 INHIBITORS)

General Actions of SGLT2 inhibitors

- reversibly inhibits sodium-glucose cotransporter 2 (SGLT2) in the proximal renal tubules. Normally SGLT2 is responsible for most of the reabsorption of filtered glucose from renal tubular lumen. Those with diabetes have raised renal glucose reabsorption which adds to persistently elevated BGLs. SGLT2 is inhibited, reducing reabsorption of filtered glucose lowering renal glucose threshold, increasing glucose excretion, resulting in decreased BGLs
- blood glucose excretion leads to osmotic diuresis (and therefore decreased fluid load), caloric loss and subsequent weight reduction
- do not depend on insulin secretion or sensitivity

General Uses of SGLT2 inhibitors

- type 2 diabetes mellitus with diet and exercise (as monotherapy when metformin is not tolerated or inappropriate or as combination therapy with other antidiabetic agents)

General Nursing points/Cautions for SGLT2 inhibitors

- any volume deficit should be corrected before starting therapy. Volume status should be assessed using physical examination, BP measurements and laboratory tests (including haematocrit)
- kidney function should be monitored before starting and yearly during therapy. If any medications are added that impair kidney function, test should be conducted again and if the patient has moderate kidney impairment, kidney function tests should be 2–4 times yearly
- lower doses of insulin or sulfonylurea may be needed if used as combination therapy to decrease risk of hypoglycaemia
- therapy should be stopped prior to major surgery and restarted when

patient's condition has stabilised and oral intake is normal
- not recommended in those with diabetes mellitus type 1 or diabetic ketoacidosis
- not recommended in patients receiving loop diuretics, are volume depleted or have a history of hypotension or dehydration when receiving diuretics
- contraindicated in those with moderate-to-severe kidney or liver impairment

General Patient teaching and advice for SGLT2 inhibitors

- patient should be instructed to seek medical advice immediately if any of the following occurs:
  - feeling dizzy or light-headed
  - vomiting or diarrhoea, severe thirst, urinating less than normal
  - increased urination, urgent need to urinate, cloudy urine, strong odour, burning sensation on urination, passing frequent small amounts of urine
  - rash or redness in the vagina or penis
- advise patient to take care in going from lying or sitting position to standing as light-headedness, dizziness or fainting may occur
- see also General Patient teaching and advice for oral hypoglycaemic agents (p. 304)

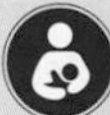

contraindicated during pregnancy and breastfeeding

DAPAGLIFLOZIN (Forxiga)

Available form

Tablets: 10 mg

Action/Use

- see General Actions and Uses for SGLT2 inhibitors (p. 324)
- peak activity within 2 hours, half-life 13 hours

Dose

- 10 mg orally once daily (as mono or combination therapy)

Adverse effects

- hypotension, dehydration, hypovolemia
- polyuria, renal impairment, decreased creatinine clearance
- urinary tract infection, genital infection (vulvovaginal, balanitis)
- back pain
- (uncommon) pyelonephritis, urosepsis
- hypoglycaemia (when given with insulin or sulfonylurea)
- (rare) Fournier's gangrene

Interactions

- not recommended with pioglitazone due to an increased risk of bladder cancer

Nursing points/Cautions

- patient should be monitored for any signs and symptoms of urinary tract infection during therapy
- therapy should be interrupted if patient develops pyelonephritis or urosepsis
- caution if used in the elderly or those with cardiovascular disease, on antihypertensive therapy or history of hypotension where a fall in blood pressure could be risky
- not recommended in those > 75 years or with severe liver impairment
- see also General Nursing points/Cautions for SGLT2 inhibitors (p. 324)

Patient teaching and advice

- instruct patient to take adequate fluids to avoid dehydration especially during infection, illness (especially GI with vomiting and/or diarrhoea) or during hot conditions

- advise patient to seek medical advice immediately if any pain/tenderness, redness or swelling in genital/perineal area, fever or malaise occurs
- see also General Patient teaching and advice for SGLT2 inhibitors (p. 325)

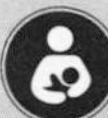

not recommended during second or third trimester of pregnancy or during breastfeeding

tablet can be crushed and mixed with water or spoonful of yoghurt or apple puree

Note

- contained in Xigduo XR with metformin hydrochloride or Qtern with saxagliptin

EMPAGLIFLOZIN (Jardiance)

Available form

Tablets: 10 mg, 25 mg

Action/Use

- see General Actions and Uses for SGLT2 inhibitors (p. 324)
- peak activity 1.5 hours, half-life 12.4 hours

Dose

- initially 10 mg orally once daily, increasing to 25 mg if additional glycaemic control is needed

Adverse effects

- urinary tract infections, genital infections
- thirst
- hypotension, dehydration, hypovolaemia, syncope
- increased serum lipids, decreased haematocrit
- increased urination
- hypoglycaemia (if given with insulin or sulfonylureas)

Interactions

- not recommended with GLP-1 analogues
- may cause positive glucose result on urine test
- increased risk of dehydration and hypotension if given with thiazide and loop diuretics

Nursing points/Cautions

- renal function should be assessed before starting and then yearly during therapy. It should be reassessed regularly if medications which impair renal function are used concurrently. Therapy should be stopped if creatinine clearance is persistently < 45 mL/min
- therapy should be interrupted if pyelonephritis or urosepsis occurs
- tablets contain lactose and are therefore not recommended in those with galactose intolerance, Lapp lactase deficiency or glucose–galactose malabsorption
- caution if used in the elderly (> 75 years) or those with cardiovascular disease, on antihypertensive therapy or history of hypotension where a fall in blood pressure could be risky
- contraindicated in those with severe kidney impairment including those on dialysis (creatinine clearance < 30 mL/min)
- see also General Nursing points/Cautions for SGLT2 inhibitors (p. 324)

Patient teaching and advice

- see General Patient teaching and advice for SGLT2 inhibitors (p. 325)

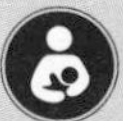

not recommended during pregnancy or breastfeeding

Note

- contained in Jardiamet with metformin hydrochloride and Glyxambi with linagliptin

ERTUGLIFLOZIN (Steglatro)

Available form

Tablets: 5 mg, 15 mg

Action/Use

- see General Actions and Uses for SGLT2 inhibitors (p. 324)
- half-life 16.6 hours

Dose

- initially 5 mg orally once daily mane, increasing to 15 mg if additional glycaemic control is needed

Adverse effects

- urinary tract infections, mycotic genital infections
- vulvovaginal pruritus
- thirst
- increased serum lipids, increased haemoglobin, increased serum phosphate, increased serum creatinine, decreased kidney impairment
- increased urination
- hypoglycaemia (if given with insulin or sulfonylureas)
- (rare) Fournier's gangrene, lower limb amputation (mainly toe)

Interactions

- not recommended with GLP-1 analogues

Nursing points/Cautions

- renal function should be assessed before starting and then yearly during therapy. It should be reassessed regularly if medications that impair renal function are used concurrently. Therapy should be stopped if creatinine clearance is persistently < 45 mL/min
- therapy should be interrupted if pyelonephritis or urosepsis occurs
- caution if used in those with increased risk of genital infections (e.g. recurrent or pre-existing urogenital infections, obesity, immunosuppression, smoking, alcohol abuse, end-stage kidney or liver failure, or elevated glycated haemoglobin (HbA1c > 10%))
- see also General Nursing points/Cautions for SGLT2 inhibitors (p. 324)

Patient teaching and advice

- advise patient to seek medical advice immediately if any pain/tenderness, redness or swelling in genital/perineal area, fever or malaise occurs
- see also General Patient teaching and advice for SGLT2 inhibitors (p. 325)

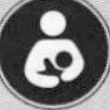

not recommended during pregnancy or breastfeeding

tablets can be crushed and mixed with water or spoonful of yoghurt or apple puree

Note

- contained in Steglujan with sitagliptin and Segluromet with metformin hydrochloride

ANTIDIARRHOEAL AGENTS

Diarrhoea can be defined as frequent passage of loose (liquid or unformed) stools and may be acute (lasting < 2 weeks), persistent (2–4 weeks) or chronic (lasting > 4 weeks). For most people, diarrhoea is self-limiting and does not require any intervention; however, acute infectious diarrhoea is still one of the most common causes of mortality (especially in infants) in developing countries (Camilleri & Murray 2018).

Acute diarrhoea is primarily caused by infectious agents and often accompanied by vomiting, fever and abdominal pain, while a smaller proportion may be due to medication (e.g. antibiotics, NSAIDs, some antidepressants), ischaemia, toxins, food-related and other conditions. Those most at risk of developing acute diarrhoea include travellers (especially to Asia, Africa and Latin America), immunodeficient individuals, those in institutions such as hospitals and long-term care facilities, children attending daycare and their family members, and consumers of some foods (e.g. *Listeria* from uncooked foods or soft cheeses, *Salmonella* from eggs, seafood, cream, mayonnaise) (Camilleri & Murray 2018).

Management of severe acute diarrhoea should include:

- investigating the underlying cause (e.g. a stool sample may be collected to isolate an organism), recommended if patient has diarrhoea that is profuse with dehydration, grossly bloody stools, fever $\geq 38.5°C$, lasting longer than 48 hours without improvement, recent antibiotic use, associated with abdominal pain (especially if over 70 years), immunocompromised and if there is a current community outbreak (Camilleri & Murray 2018). Caution should be used if diarrhoea is thought to be a result of antibiotic-induced colitis or pseudomembranous colitis
- preventing/treating fluid and electrolyte imbalance, especially in the elderly and very young, because dehydration can occur very quickly
- use of antibacterial agents (if appropriate), which may reduce the severity and duration of the diarrhoea depending on the causative organism
- antimotility and antisecretory agents (e.g. loperamide) can be useful in controlling symptoms in moderately

severe non-febrile and non-bloody diarrhoea (Camilleri & Murray 2018).

Chronic diarrhoea is generally non-infectious and should be investigated to rule out serious underlying pathology. Causes of chronic diarrhoea include chronic alcohol intake, decreased absorption due to bowel resection, disease or fistula, lactase deficiency, gluten intolerance, idiopathic inflammatory bowel disease (e.g. Crohn's, ulcerative colitis), irritable bowel syndrome, eating disorders (with laxative abuse), ileal resection and radiation enterocolitis. Management of chronic diarrhoea is dependent on identification and management of the underlying cause if possible, as this will result in control of the diarrhoea (Camilleri & Murray 2018).

General Nursing points/Cautions for antidiarrhoeal agents

- agents that delay or inhibit intestinal motility may induce toxic megacolon in patients with Crohn's disease or ulcerative colitis and therefore should be stopped at the first signs of abdominal distension or other untoward symptoms
- it may not always be appropriate to slow the motility of the bowel (e.g. if the cause is infectious), because this may allow time for the organism to replicate further or the toxin to accumulate

General Patient teaching and advice for antidiarrhoeal agents

- patient should be warned against driving or operating machinery if drowsiness, dizziness or confusion occur
- advise patient to avoid alcohol while taking medication
- instruct patient to stop taking medication when bowel motions return to normal
- advise patient to seek medical advice if diarrhoea persists for more than 2 days or if there is blood present in diarrhoea
- instruct patient to drink plenty of liquids (such as rehydration solution) to prevent becoming dehydrated. Milk, dairy products, fatty or fried foods, chocolate, fruit, acidic vegetables and alcohol should be avoided as these may make the diarrhoea worse. Food intake should be restricted during first few days to unbuttered toast, plain crackers, boiled potatoes, rice or pasta. Normal diet can be restarted when diarrhoea stops
- see General Patient teaching and advice (p. xxvii)

DIPHENOXYLATE HYDROCHLORIDE

Available forms

Tablets

Action

- pethidine-related drug that reduces peristalsis
- half-life is 2.5 hours
- active metabolite

Use

- treatment of acute and chronic diarrhoea (adjunctive therapy)

Adverse effects

- drowsiness, sedation, headache, confusion, dizziness, restlessness, euphoria, malaise, lethargy
- numbness of extremities
- anorexia, nausea, vomiting, abdominal discomfort
- anaphylaxis, urticaria, rash, pruritus
- gum swelling

- paralytic ileus, toxic megacolon
- (atropine) tachycardia, dry mouth and skin, flushing, hyperthermia, urinary retention
- (high dose) addiction/dependency

Interactions

- may precipitate hypertensive crisis if given with MAOIs
- may have additive effect when given with alcohol and other CNS depressants

Nursing points/Cautions

- patient should be assessed for cause of diarrhoea
- patient should be closely monitored for any signs of fluid and/or electrolyte imbalance, and treated if it occurs
- combined with small amount of atropine to discourage excessive self-medication and misuse
- may induce toxic megacolon if given to patients with ulcerative colitis
- respiratory depression may occur up to 30 hours after overdose, therefore patients should be monitored for at least 48 hours if overdose does occur. Respiratory depression should be treated with naloxone (IV) initially, then given SC or IM for more prolonged effect if respiratory depression does not improve. Repeated doses may be required since naloxone has a short duration of action
- caution if used in those with abnormal liver function or hepatorenal disease as hepatic coma can occur
- caution if used in those with a history of drug addiction or currently taking drugs which may be addictive as diphenoxylate hydrochloride has the potential to be addictive
- caution (because of atropine content) if used in those with Down syndrome
- contraindicated in those with jaundice, bacterial/amoebic colitis, diarrhoea associated with pseudomembranous enterocolitis or inflammatory bowel disease (e.g. Crohn's disease, ulcerative colitis) and in children under 12 years
- see also General Nursing points/Cautions for antidiarrhoeal agents (p. 329)

Patient teaching and advice

- warn patient to not take more than 8 tablets per 24 hours
- see General Patient teaching and advice for antidiarrhoeal agents (p. 329)

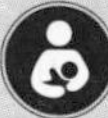

chemically related to pethidine and may cause respiratory depression in the newborn; therefore should not be given at or near term

not recommended during breastfeeding

tablets can be crushed and mixed with water (does not readily disperse) or given with spoonful of yoghurt or apple puree

Note

- contained in Lofenoxal and Lomotil with atropine sulfate

LOPERAMIDE HYDROCHLORIDE (Diareze, Gastrex, GastroStop, Harmonise, Imodium, Pharmacy Action Diarrhoea Relief, StopIt)

Available forms

Tablets: 2 mg; Capsules: 2 mg; Dissolvable tablets (melts): 2 mg

Action

- binds to opiate receptors in the gut wall, reducing peristalsis by suppressing intestinal motility through direct action on circular and longitudinal muscles of the intestinal wall
- may also increase anal sphincter tone, decreasing urgency and incontinence

- no analgesic properties
- more potent as an antidiarrhoeal agent than diphenoxylate hydrochloride (3 times) and codeine phosphate (25 times)
- onset of action (symptomatic improvement) in 1–3 hours, half-life 9–14 hours

Use

- relief of acute non-specific diarrhoea
- to reduce the volume of discharge in patients with ileostomies and colostomies, chronic diarrhoea

Dose

- (acute diarrhoea) initially 4 mg orally, then 2 mg after each unformed stool, up to 16 mg/day **OR**
- (chronic diarrhoea or reduce volume of ileostomy/colostomy discharge) initially 4 mg orally, then 2 mg after each unformed stool, then maintained on 4–8 mg daily as a single or divided dose

Adverse effects

- nausea, abdominal pain/cramps, constipation, flatulence, abdominal distension
- (very rare) dizziness, drowsiness
- (melts) burning, prickling sensation on tongue

Interactions

- caution if used with alcohol
- increased plasma levels may occur if given with ritonavir
- action may be potentiated by MAOIs

Nursing points/Cautions

- patient should be carefully assessed for cause of diarrhoea
- patient should be closely monitored for any signs of fluid and/or electrolyte imbalance, and treated if it occurs
- improvement usually seen in 48 hours
- therapy should be stopped if constipation, abdominal distension or ileus develops
- sublingual tablets (melts) are recommended for those with swallowing difficulties
- may induce toxic megacolon if given to patients with ulcerative colitis or Crohn's disease
- caution if used in those with AIDS due to risk of toxic megacolon
- caution if used in those with urinary retention, glaucoma, pyloric obstruction, gastric retention or intestinal stasis
- caution if used in those with liver dysfunction as CNS toxicity may occur
- contraindicated in those with constipation, conditions where constipation should be avoided, high fever, blood in stools of unknown origin, acute dysentery, inflammatory bowel disease, bacterial enterocolitis, antibiotic-induced pseudomembranous colitis, megacolon, toxic megacolon or in children under 12 years
- see also General Nursing points/Cautions for antidiarrhoeal agents (p. 329)

Patient teaching and advice

- (melt tablets) advise patient to place tablet on tongue and allow to melt, then swallow with saliva
- see General Patient teaching and advice for antidiarrhoeal agents (p. 329)

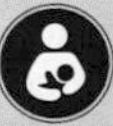

not recommended during pregnancy or breastfeeding unless the expected benefit outweighs any potential risk

capsules can be opened and contents dispersed in water or sprinkled on apple puree. Tablets can be crushed and mixed with water or spoonful of apple puree

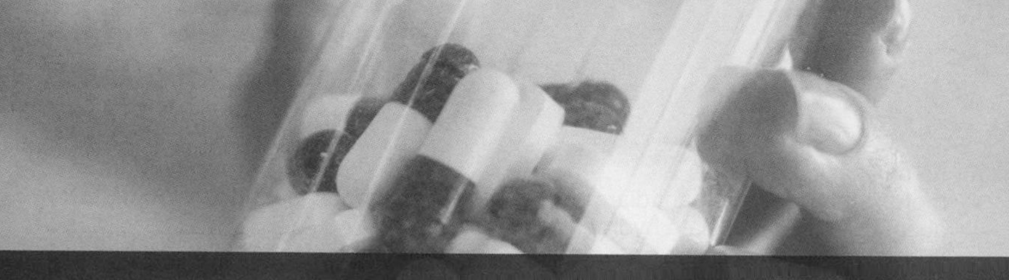

ANTIDOTES, ANTAGONISTS AND CHELATING AGENTS

Chelating agents, antidotes and antagonists are used to counter the toxic effects of exogenous and endogenous substances in the body (e.g. iron overload) and manage poisoning and overdosage (e.g. cyanide, opioids, paracetamol).

ACETYLCYSTEINE (Acetadote Concentrated Injection, DBL Acetylcysteine Injection Concentrate)

Available forms

Ampoules: 200 mg/mL, 6 g/30 mL

Action

- the liver normally converts paracetamol to a toxic alkylating intermediate metabolite that is inactivated by conjugation with glutathione to form non-toxic derivatives. With hepatotoxic doses/overdosage of paracetamol, glutathione levels are rapidly depleted and excess toxic metabolite is formed, causing liver damage and necrosis. Hepatic necrosis can be seen at 6 g and death at 15 g of paracetamol
- IV administration of acetylcysteine, a sulfhydryl donor, within 10 hours of paracetamol ingestion prevents severe liver damage, primarily by restoring glutathione levels

Use

- antidote for paracetamol poisoning to protect against liver toxicity

Dose

- initially 150 mg/kg IV in 200 mL glucose 5% over 15–60 minutes (loading dose), followed by continuous infusion of 50 mg/kg in 500 mL over 4 hours, followed by 100 mg/kg in 1 L over 16 hours (total dose 300 mg/kg in 20 hours)

Adverse effects

- rash, urticaria, flushing, sweating
- fever
- blurred vision, eye pain
- cyanosis
- facial pain, facial and periorbital oedema
- arthralgia
- hypokalaemia, acidosis, decreased liver function
- nausea, vomiting
- hypotension/hypertension, tachycardia, bradycardia, chest pain, ECG changes
- anxiety, malaise, rigors
- bronchospasm, coughing, stridor, dyspnea, angioedema
- injection site reaction

- (rare) anaphylactoid reaction, seizures, thrombocytopenia

Interactions

- hepatotoxicity may occur at lower paracetamol doses if taken with rifampicin, isoniazid, phenytoin, carbamazepine, primidone, phenobarbital (phenobarbitone) or sodium valproate, or with chronic alcohol intake
- false positive for urinary ketones may occur with dipstick testing

Nursing points/Cautions

- urea, electrolytes (including potassium to monitor for hypokalaemia), Hb, WBC count, platelets, blood glucose, urea and bilirubin, liver function, ECG, blood gases and prothrombin should be monitored on admission and then daily for coagulation disorders, hepatic encephalopathy, renal failure and cardiac toxicity
- general management for paracetamol overdose should include tests as above, airway management, cardiac monitoring and then infusion of acetylcysteine
- if patient is conscious and within 1 hour of paracetamol ingestion, activated charcoal (1–2 g/kg (maximum 50 g)) should be given
- liver damage may not be apparent (biochemically) for 24–48 hours and patient may appear well, but hepatic necrosis is preventable if treatment can be instituted within 10–12 hours of ingestion
- obtain urgent serum paracetamol levels (but no earlier than 4 hours after ingestion as they may be unreliable) and ascertain the degree of potential liver damage from the semi-logarithmic graph of serum paracetamol levels plotted against hours since ingestion (for single ingestion). The graph may not be useful in determining acetylcysteine requirements if there was multiple or chronic ingestion or if sustained preparations were taken
- the decision to give acetylcysteine is made on the basis of the amount of paracetamol ingested and should not be delayed pending laboratory results. If the time of ingestion is unknown, paracetamol levels should be measured immediately
- may be used 15 hours after paracetamol overdose, but should be discussed first with doctors experienced in the treatment of paracetamol poisoning for use in high-risk patients, as effectiveness has not been proven
- dose/volume may need to be adjusted if the patient weighs less than 40 kg or if on a fluid restriction to decrease risk of hyponatraemia and seizures
- anaphylactic-like reactions (bronchospasm, dyspnoea, hypotension, tachycardia, shock, urticaria) occur most commonly during or after loading dose has been administered. Patient should be closely monitored during this time
- dilute in glucose 5% or sodium chloride 0.9% before administration
- slight colour change (pink/purple) may occur when stopper is punctured; however, this does not indicate any loss of activity
- not compatible with rubber and some metals (iron, copper, nickel)
- caution if used in those with asthma or bronchospasm, or oesophageal varices or peptic ulceration (because of increased risk of bleeding with associated vomiting) or in those with known liver/kidney impairment
- caution if used in those with a history of chronic alcohol use or taking medications such as antiepileptics, isoniazid or rifampicin as there is an increased risk of hepatotoxicity due to paracetamol overdose

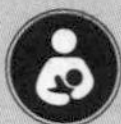

safety of acetylcysteine during pregnancy has not been established

not recommended during breastfeeding

CALCIUM FOLINATE (Leucovorin Calcium Injection and Tablets)

Available forms

Tablets: 15 mg; Vial: 50 mg/5 mL; Ampoules: 15 mg/2 mL

Action

- also known as folinic acid, which is the active form of folic acid
- member of the water soluble vitamin B group
- neutralises folic acid antagonists
- active metabolite

Use

- administered a few hours after folic acid antagonists (e.g. methotrexate) to 'rescue' the normal cells of the host preferentially, after the drug has been bound within tumour cells
- impaired elimination or overdose of methotrexate
- megaloblastic anaemia (not vitamin B_{12} deficiency)
- pyrimethamine overdose

Dose

- (folinic acid rescue) 15 mg IV, IM or orally 6-hourly starting 24 hours after beginning methotrexate administration for 10 doses or until methotrexate serum level decreases and then dose and interval altered accordingly **OR**
- (impaired methotrexate elimination or overdose) 10 mg/m^2 IV, IM or orally 6-hourly until methotrexate serum levels are less than 10^{-8} M. Dose may be increased to 100 mg/m^2 IV 3-hourly if creatinine is 50% over baseline or methotrexate level is 5×10^{-6} M (at 24 hours) or 9×10^{-7} M or greater (at 48 hours) **OR**
- (megaloblastic anaemia) up to 1 mg IM daily **OR**
- (megaloblastic anaemia) 5–15 mg orally daily **OR**
- (pyrimethamine overdose) 3–9 mg/day IM for 3 days or until platelet and leucocyte counts have returned to acceptable limits

Adverse effects

- fever, rash, pruritus
- leukocytosis, thrombocytopenia
- (high dose) nausea, vomiting and rarely, insomnia, agitation, depression
- (rare) seizures, syncope, urticaria, allergic reaction, severe skin reaction

Interactions

- high doses may counteract antiepileptic action of phenytoin, primidone and phenobarbital (phenobarbitone)
- high doses may reduce efficacy of intrathecal methotrexate or other folic acid antagonists if given together
- may enhance toxicity (enterocolitis, diarrhoea, dehydration) of fluorouracil
- incompatible with droperidol and foscarnet

Nursing points/Cautions

- should be administered as soon as possible after methotrexate overdose to ensure effectiveness
- serum methotrexate and creatinine are monitored daily to determine dose and duration of therapy. Blood leucocyte and thrombocyte counts and serum electrolytes should also be closely monitored
- parenteral route is recommended for doses greater than 25 mg or if the patient is vomiting or at risk of not absorbing oral dose
- not administered intrathecally
- may be diluted to 1 L with sodium chloride 0.9% or glucose 5% for IV administration
- injection rate should be no greater than 160 mg/minute (because of calcium content)

- (folinic acid rescue) hydration (3 L/day), urinary alkalisation (pH ≥7) and therapy with calcium folinate should be continued until methotrexate level is less than 5×10^{-8} M
- caution if used in those with CNS metastases due to increased risk of seizures and/or syncope
- contraindicated in those with pernicious anaemia or vitamin B_{12} deficiency anaemias

Patient teaching and advice

- instruct patient to take oral doses on an empty stomach
- advise patient to seek medical advice immediately if any of the following occur:
  - fitting
  - fever, rash, itching, hives, swelling (face, lips, tongue, other body parts), shortness of breath or difficulty breathing
- see General Patient teaching and advice (p. xxvii)

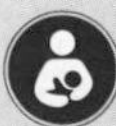

caution if used during breastfeeding

tablets can be dispersed in water and crushed and mixed with spoonful of yoghurt or apple sauce

CHARCOAL, ACTIVATED (Carbosorb X)

Available form

Oral suspension: 0.2 g/mL

Action

- physically adsorbs drugs and toxic agents onto its surface (including aspirin, barbiturates, phenytoin, TCAs, digoxin, quinine, amphetamine, morphine, cocaine, paracetamol and phenothiazines) in the GIT, thereby reducing or preventing systemic absorption

Use

- poisoning and drug overdose by oral ingestion

Dose

- 1 g/kg orally or via nasogastric/orogastric tube as soon as possible after ingestion or suspected ingestion of the potential poison or after induced emesis or stomach washout (may be repeated 2–6-hourly until first black stool has been passed (maximum dose 50 g))

Adverse effects

- vomiting, constipation, black-coloured faeces
- (multiple doses) electrolyte imbalance, intestinal obstruction
- (rare) aspiration pneumonia

Interactions

- not recommended with agents that reduce gut motility (including supportive agents such as atropine and verapamil) as this may result in repeated doses of activated charcoal being given, increasing risk of intestinal obstruction
- not recommended at same time as emetics
- should not be given with specific oral antidotes because they may become inactivated

Nursing points/Cautions

- should be given within 1 hour of ingestion to absorb maximum amount of poison/drug from GI tract
- patient should be closely monitored for any signs of vomiting because of risk of aspiration pneumonia
- if specific antidote is available, it should be given in preference to activated charcoal
- for nasogastric/orogastric administration, should be diluted with water (ratio 0.25 parts water to 1 part activated charcoal) and administered via nasogastric tube

- shake container well before administration
- given after emptying stomach contents by emesis or washout. However, if patient is drowsy (or likely to become drowsy within 30 minutes of receiving emetic), unconscious or fitting, induced emesis is not recommended due to the risk of aspiration
- other medication should preferably be given parenterally
- monitor for fluid and electrolyte changes (especially if multiple doses are administered in children) because activated charcoal can absorb vitamins, minerals and amino acids from the GIT
- contains sucrose (0.33 g/mL) and should be used with care in those with diabetes mellitus
- use with great caution if person has diminished or no bowel sounds, has taken large quantity of agent that reduces gut motility (such as opioid) or is at risk of GI haemorrhage or perforation
- contraindicated if poisoning is caused by strong acids or alkalis or iron salts, cyanides, sulfonylureas, malathion, lithium, ethanol, methanol, ethylene glycol or hydrocarbons as adsorptive capacity is too low
- contraindicated if patient has unprotected airway (due to risk of aspiration) or GIT is not intact (e.g. recent surgery)

Note

- potency of activated charcoal is enhanced when combined with the osmotic laxative sorbitol (in Carbosorb XS); however, it is contraindicated in children < 1 year
- also used in tablet and capsule form as a GI adsorbent to reduce symptoms of bloating and flatulence from intestinal gas (Charcocaps, Charcotabs)
- Charcotrace is used in addition to stereotactic or ultrasonic localisation of small impalpable breast lesions for later surgical incision
- may be used locally as a deodorant in ostomy pouches, wounds and ulcers

DEFERASIROX (Jadenu)

Available forms

Tablets: 90 mg, 180 mg, 360 mg

Action

- chelates iron and promotes excretion, mainly in the faeces
- low affinity for zinc and copper
- half-life 8–16 hours

Use

- chronic iron overload due to blood transfusion (transfusion haemosiderosis)
- chronic iron overload in children 2–5 years (when desferrioxamine is inappropriate or ineffective)
- chronic iron overload in those with non-transfusion-dependent thalassemia syndrome

Dose

Chronic iron overload due to blood transfusion

- (adult, receiving > 4 units of blood/month) 21 mg/kg body weight orally daily **OR**
- (adult, receiving < 2 units of blood/month) 7 mg/kg body weight orally daily **OR**
- initially ⅓ dose of desferrioxamine orally daily 30 minutes before food **OR**
- (maintenance) 3.5–7 mg/kg/day, adjusting dose at 3–6-month intervals according to serum ferritin levels (up to 28 mg/kg/day)

Non-transfusion-dependent thalassemia syndrome

- initially 7 mg/kg orally daily, then adjusted every 3–6 months if needed, by increments of 3.5–7 mg/kg (up to 14 mg/kg)

Adverse effects

- nausea, vomiting, diarrhoea, abdominal pain/distension, dyspepsia, constipation
- headache, fatigue
- fever, flu-like syndrome
- cough, pharyngitis, nasopharyngitis, nasopharyngeal pain
- arthralgia
- increased serum creatinine, elevated liver enzymes
- proteinuria
- rash, pruritus
- (uncommon) loss of hearing, lens opacities, cataract formation, increased intraocular pressure, retinal disorders
- (uncommon) GI ulceration and/or haemorrhage
- (rare) neutropenia, thrombocytopenia, hypersensitivity, severe skin reaction

Interactions

- not recommended with other iron chelating agent or aluminium-containing antacids
- increased risk of GI ulceration/haemorrhage if given with other ulcerogenic agents (e.g. NSAIDs, corticosteroids, oral bisphosphonates) and therefore not recommended together
- may decrease serum levels of midazolam, ciclosporin, simvastatin, colestyramine and oral contraceptives
- decreased serum levels may occur if given with rifampicin, phenytoin, ritonavir and phenobarbital (phenobarbitone)
- may increase serum levels of theophylline, clozapine, imipramine, haloperidol, fluvoxamine, naproxen, olanzapine and zolmitriptan, increasing risk of toxicity and are therefore not recommended together
- caution if given with busulfan. Busulfan levels should be closely monitored if given together
- blood glucose levels should be closely monitored if given with repaglinide

Nursing points/Cautions

- therapy should be started after about 20 units of blood have been transfused (100 mL/kg) or when serum ferritin > 1000 microgram/L
- dose should be rounded to nearest whole tablet size
- ensure patient is adequately hydrated before starting therapy (especially if diarrhoea or vomiting occurs)
- serum ferritin should be measured monthly and dose adjusted every 3–6 months if needed on that basis. If level falls consistently below 500 microgram/L, therapy interruption may be considered
- serum creatinine and/or creatinine clearance should be measured before starting therapy and then monthly (weekly monitoring for the first month is recommended in those with kidney impairment or if taking medication which may depress kidney function)
- blood counts and urine (for protein) should be monitored monthly
- liver function should be measured before starting therapy, every second week for 4 weeks, then monthly. If liver enzymes increase due to therapy (other causes ruled out), therapy should be stopped until they return to normal and then restarted slowly at a lower dose
- vision and hearing should be checked before starting, then yearly during treatment (disturbances of vision or

hearing are reversible if the drug is stopped early)

- (non-transfusion-dependent thalassemia syndrome) therapy should be started when liver iron concentration (LIC) ≥ 5 mg iron/g dry weight or serum ferritin is consistently > 800 microgram/L
- (non-transfusion-dependent thalassemia syndrome) doses > 14 mg/kg are not recommended
- (non-transfusion-dependent thalassemia syndrome) if LIC is not assessed and serum ferritin ≤ 2000 microgram/L, dose should not be greater than 7 mg/kg
- (non-transfusion-dependent thalassemia syndrome) once LIC is satisfactory (< 3 mg/g dry weight or serum ferritin < 300 microgram/L), therapy should be interrupted and resumed if chronic iron overload recurs
- body weight and longitudinal growth should be measured regularly in children
- caution if used in the elderly who are at increased risk of adverse effects, those with pre-existing kidney conditions or using agents that suppress renal function or if creatinine clearance between 40 and 90 mL/min
- dispersible tablets contain lactose and therefore are not recommended in those with galactose intolerance, Lapp lactase deficiency or glucose–galactose malabsorption
- not recommended in those with severe liver impairment and dose should be reduced in those with moderate liver impairment
- contraindicated in those with creatinine clearance < 40 mL/min, serum creatinine more than twice age-appropriate upper normal limit or if platelet count is less than 50×10^9/L, in those at high risk of myelodysplastic syndrome or other haematological/non-haematological disorders where chelation therapy would not be beneficial

Patient teaching and advice

- instruct patient to take tablets on empty stomach or with a light meal (not high fat content)
- patient should be advised to seek medical advice if any of the following occur:
  - hearing difficulties
  - blurry or loss of vision
  - vomiting with blood and/or black stools
  - upper abdominal pain, yellowing of skin or eyes, dark urine and drowsiness (liver problem)
  - reduced urine output (kidney problem)
  - frequent heartburn or stomach pain, especially when taking medication or after eating
  - rash, severe skin reaction
- female patients should be counselled regarding the possibility of oral contraceptive failure and the need to use a non-hormonal contraceptive device (e.g. condom, diaphragm) to prevent an unwanted pregnancy from occurring
- see also General Patient teaching and advice (p. xxvii)

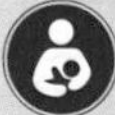

should only be used during pregnancy if benefits outweigh risks

not recommended during breastfeeding

tablets can be crushed and sprinkled on yoghurt or apple puree and taken immediately

DEFERIPRONE (Ferriprox)

Available forms

Tablets: 500 mg, 1 g; Oral solution: 100 mg/mL

Action

- chelates iron in a ratio of 3:1
- half-life 2–3 hours

Use

- iron overload in thalassaemia major (when desferrioxamine is inappropriate or ineffective)

Dose

- 25–33 mg/kg orally 3 times daily (daily total 75–100 mg/kg body weight)

Adverse effects

- abdominal pain/discomfort, nausea, vomiting, increased appetite, increased weight, dyspepsia, diarrhoea, anorexia
- headache
- arthralgia, back pain, joint swelling, pain in extremities
- neutropenia, agranulocytosis, thrombocytopenia
- increased liver enzymes, liver fibrosis
- red/brown urine
- peripheral oedema
- (rare) QT prolongation

Interactions

- not recommended with aluminium-based antacids
- not recommended with other agents known to cause neutropenia or agranulocytosis
- caution if used with vitamin C
- caution if used with agents known to prolong QT interval or cause electrolyte imbalance (e.g. diuretics)

Nursing points/Cautions

- neutrophil count should be measured before starting therapy, and therapy not commenced if patient is found to be neutropenic
- monitoring neutrophil count weekly is recommended. If patient develops neutropenia, therapy should be stopped and patient advised to avoid any potential risk of infection. Blood counts (including WBC, neutrophil and platelet counts) should be monitored daily until neutrophil count returns to normal, then weekly for 3 weeks to ensure complete recovery
- liver function tests are recommended in patients with hepatitis C
- therapy should be interrupted if patient develops infection. Neutrophil should be monitored more frequently. If neutropenia occurs, daily blood counts are recommended until neutrophil count recovers, then weekly for 3 consecutive weeks to ensure full recovery has occurred
- serum ferritin and plasma zinc levels should be monitored every 2–3 months during therapy; zinc supplementation may be required
- dose adjustment is dependent on serum ferritin levels and therapy interrupted if levels fall below 500 microgram/L
- daily doses greater than 100 mg/kg not recommended
- dose should be calculated to nearest half tablet or 2.5 mL
- (oral solution) contains yellow colouring agent (sunset yellow (E110)) which may cause an allergic reaction in sensitive individuals
- caution if used in those with liver or kidney impairment
- caution if used in those at risk of QT prolongation including those with bradycardia, congestive heart failure or cardiac hypertrophy or if taking agents that may cause electrolyte imbalance, especially hypokalaemia or hypomagnesaemia

- not recommended in immunocompromised patients, such as those with HIV
- contraindicated in those with recurrent neutropenia or history of agranulocytosis

Patient teaching and advice

- patient should be advised to seek medical advice immediately if any of the following occur:
  - any fever, sore throat or flu-like symptoms
  - palpitations, irregular heartbeat, dizziness, light-headedness, fainting
- warn patient that urine discolouration (reddish/brown) is normal
- instruct patient to separate medication by 2 hours from aluminium-based antacids and not to take vitamin C
- oral solution should be refrigerated and used within 35 days of opening
- women of childbearing years should be advised to use adequate contraception during therapy and to tell doctor if she plans to or becomes pregnant
- see also General Patient teaching and advice (p. xxvii)

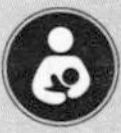

contraindicated during pregnancy or breastfeeding as deferiprone is embryotoxic and teratogenic

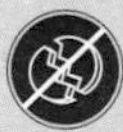

available as oral solution. If crushing tablets, mask and gloves should be worn. Mix with spoonful of yoghurt or apple puree

DESFERRIOXAMINE MESYLATE (DBL Desferrioxamine Mesylate for Injection BP)

Available forms

Vial: 500 mg, 2 g

Action

- chelating agent that forms ferrioxamine, a non-toxic stable complex (chelate) with iron
- parenteral desferrioxamine removes iron from various iron-containing proteins (ferritin, haemosiderin), but not from haemoglobin or iron-containing enzymes; the water-soluble chelate is excreted rapidly in urine and some in bile
- does not remove iron deposits from lungs
- chelates copper, aluminium, calcium and zinc
- suppresses lymphocytes
- neurotoxic (possibly due to chelation of copper or zinc)
- causes release of histamine (causing acute hypotension) with rapid IV administration
- 1 g desferrioxamine binds 85 mg ferric iron (500 mL transfusion of whole blood adds 250 mg iron to body); however, iron excretion is non-linear, therefore there is reduced efficiency when given at high doses

Use

- transfusion haemosiderosis (chronic iron overload from repeated transfusions in thalassaemia and other chronic anaemias)
- acute iron poisoning (as an adjunct to other measures)
- diagnosis of iron storage disease

Dose

Chronic iron overload

- 20–40 mg/kg SC or IV 3–7 times weekly (frequency depending on the extent of the iron overload) (daily maximum 80 mg/kg)

Acute iron poisoning (as adjunct to standard measures)

- (normotensive patient) 2 g deeply IM stat **OR**
- (hypotensive patient) 15 mg/kg/hour IV, reduced after 4–6 hours to a daily maximum of 80 mg/kg

Diagnostic desferrioxamine test

- 500 mg IM then collect urine for 6 hours to measure iron content

Treatment in terminal renal failure

- 1–4 g IM or IV weekly (patient on haemodialysis or haemofiltration)

Adverse effects

- (rapid IV or high dose) pain, induration, swelling, pruritus, erythema, weal formation
- (prolonged SC infusion, IV, IM) local irritation
- (rapid IV) flushing, urticaria, hypotension, shock
- nausea, vomiting, abdominal pain, black stools
- hypotension, tachycardia, shock
- fever
- transient bone pain, leg cramps
- dysuria, urine discolouration ('vin rose'), kidney failure, aggravation of pyelonephritis
- hypocalcaemia (transient), hyperparathyroidism
- growth retardation, bone changes (especially if given in first 3 years of life)
- headache, dizziness, reversible aphasia, convulsion
- (prolonged therapy, high dose) disturbances of vision and hearing (may be irreversible), pulmonary toxicity
- liver impairment
- (rare) rash, fever, oedema, anaphylactic shock
- (very rare) blood dyscrasias, fungal infection
- (dialysis patients) aluminium toxicity ('dialysis dementia'), renal impairment, aggravation of pyelonephritis

Interactions

- use with prochlorperazine may result in temporary but severe change in consciousness and are therefore not recommended together
- use with phenothiazines or methyldopa sesquihydrate may potentiate neuro-ophthalmic toxicity
- increased risk of cataract formation and impaired cardiac function if given long term with vitamin C (ascorbic acid)
- addition of oral vitamin C (ascorbic acid) (up to 200 mg) may increase excretion of formed iron complex (but should not be started until desferrioxamine therapy has been in progress for at least 1 week)

Nursing points/Cautions

- therapy should be started after 10–20 units of blood have been transfused or when serum ferritin = 1000 microgram/L
- dose should be estimated according to iron levels to prevent toxic effects. Expected iron excretion rate is 10–20 mg/day
- normal serum ferritin is less than 300 microgram/L
- patients with heavy iron load may require treatment 5–7 times weekly to prevent iron toxicity occurring. Regular doses > 50 mg/kg/day are not recommended unless intense chelation is required
- vision and hearing should be checked before starting, then at 3-monthly intervals during treatment (disturbances of vision or hearing are reversible if the drug is stopped early)
- urine output should be carefully measured and if oliguria or anuria occurs, peritoneal dialysis or haemodialysis may be necessary
- urinary iron is initially measured daily and dose adjusted by increments of 0.5 g daily until excretion reaches a plateau
- vitamin C (ascorbic acid) (150–250 mg daily) may be given as adjunctive therapy after initial 4 weeks of chelation therapy because it increases urinary excretion of iron and it should be given on same day as

desferrioxamine 1–2 hours after IV infusion has started
- cardiac function should be monitored if given with vitamin C (ascorbic acid)
- (children) height and weight should be measured 3-monthly and doses should be kept to a minimum
- IM administration is less effective than SC or IV. May also be added to dialysis fluid and given via intraperitoneal route
- if given IM reconstitute using ≥ 1.5 mL water for injections, diluted to a volume of at least 3 mL and then administered using more than one site (0.5–1.5 g per site) (per treatment) to reduce pain and ensure adequate dilution and distribution
- addition of 1–2 mg hydrocortisone and dilution reduces local reaction at IM site
- monitor IV infusion rate closely by using a burette or infusion pump and do not exceed 15 mg/kg/hour
- not given by IV bolus as rapid IV infusion may result in hypotension, flushing, tachycardia, urticaria and/or collapse
- caution if flushing IV line as this is the same as giving an IV bolus (see above point)
- continuous IV infusion is recommended in those unable to continue SC infusion or if patient has a cardiac problem related to iron overload
- (IV) reconstitute by adding water for injections (not sodium chloride), (5 mL for 500 mg vial, 20 mL for 2 g vial) making a 10% solution, which may then be further diluted with glucose 5%, sodium chloride 0.9% or Ringer's solution
- incompatible with heparin because precipitation or cloudiness may occur
- IV infusion can be administered at the same time as blood transfusion via Y-adapter
- SC needle should not be inserted too close to the skin
- continuous SC infusion is controlled by battery-operated syringe pump and can be given over 8–12 hours 5–6 nights/week (or 3–5 nights/week if iron load is low)
- (prolonged therapy, high dose, IV) patient should be closely monitored in first 32–72 hours for any signs of respiratory distress
- (acute poisoning) gastric lavage, emesis, control of shock and correction of any acid–base imbalance
- (acute poisoning) plasma/serum iron levels should be measured 3–4 hours after ingestion of iron products. After 4 hours, results may be an underestimate because iron may have bound to ferritin or been distributed into tissues
- (acute poisoning) if slow-release/enteric-coated tablets have been ingested, levels should be repeated 6–8 hours later as absorption may be erratic
- (acute poisoning) if serum iron is between 62 and 90 micromol/L, brief chelation therapy is indicated; 90–180 micromol/L, vigorous support and chelation therapy; greater than 180 micromol/L, vigorous support, chelation and possible transfusion and haemo/peritoneal dialysis is recommended
- (acute poisoning) if oliguria or anuria develops, peritoneal or haemodialysis may be needed
- (acute poisoning) end point of treatment is when 'vin rose' coloured urine disappears, when serum iron is less than 54 micromol/L or when symptoms have disappeared
- (desferrioxamine test) excretion of 1–1.5 mg over 6 hours is suggestive of iron overload; > 1.5 mg is considered pathological (if kidney function is normal)

- if used in those on haemodialysis without iron overload, may cause increase in plasma aluminium levels
- caution if used in those with severe kidney failure or pyelonephritis
- not recommended in those with primary haemochromastosis
- contraindicated if iron overload has not been proven

Patient teaching and advice

- patient should be advised to seek medical advice if any of the following occur:
  - high fever, painful inflamed sore throat, abdominal pain and/or severe diarrhoea
  - blurred vision or other problems with sight
  - hearing problems, ringing in ears
- reassure patient that reddish discolouration ('vin rose') in the urine is normal and indicates the iron is being removed from the body
- warn patient not to drive or operate machinery if dizziness or vision problems occur
- instruct patients (and carers) in the reconstitution of medication, insertion of SC needles, rotation of sites, operation and care of the SC pump, as well as correct storage of medication vials and disposal of used needles
- see also General Patient teaching and advice (p. xxvii)

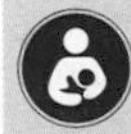

not used during pregnancy or breastfeeding unless the expected benefit outweighs any potential risks. Has been found to cause fetal damage in animal studies

DIGOXIN SPECIFIC IMMUNE ANTIGEN BINDING FRAGMENT (FAB) (DigiFab)

Available form

Vial: 40 mg

Action

- digoxin-binding antibody derived from immunised sheep that binds free (unbound) digoxin
- FAB fragment-digoxin complex is excreted from the kidneys, alleviating symptoms within 30 minutes of administration
- 38/40 mg digoxin immune FAB binds approximately 0.5 mg digoxin
- half-life 15–20 hours (normal kidney function)

Use

- digoxin overdose (life threatening)

Dose

- dose is dependent on the number of digoxin tablets ingested and is administered IV over 30 minutes. Half the estimated dose is given, and response monitored for 6–12 hours. Remainder may be given within 2 hours if no clinical response is evident or if toxicity recurs

Adverse effects

- (IV site) phlebitis
- hypokalaemia, hyperkalaemia
- headache, confusion, fatigue
- nausea, vomiting, diarrhoea, constipation, abdominal distension
- flu-like illness
- kidney failure
- exacerbation of cardiac failure, chest pain, hypotension, orthostatic hypotension
- hypersensitivity reaction (urticaria, pruritus, erythema, angioedema, bronchospasm with cough or stridor, laryngeal oedema, hypotension)

Interactions

- will interfere with digoxin immunoassay measurements, therefore standard serum digoxin concentration may be misleading until FAB is eliminated (several days to week depending on kidney function)

Nursing points/Cautions

- if overdose is intentional, toxic effects of other drugs or poisons should be considered if no response is seen
- serum digoxin levels should be established before starting therapy if possible, but at least 5–6 hours after ingestion
- any electrolyte, acid–base imbalance or hypoxia should be corrected and any cardiac arrhythmias treated
- serum potassium levels should be frequently monitored throughout therapy and treatment given with great caution (because potassium shifts in and out of cells leading to hyper- and hypokalaemia). Serum potassium may fall rapidly when therapy is discontinued
- temperature, BP and ECG (for deterioration of cardiac function) should be monitored during and after therapy and patient should be closely observed for any signs of hypersensitivity
- bolus injection is possible if cardiac arrest is imminent
- re-digitalisation should not occur until antibodies have been eliminated from the body (several days) or longer if patient has kidney impairment
- skin testing has not proven to be useful in predicting allergic response
- for reconstitution, gently add 4 mL water for injections to give a concentration of 9.5–10 mg/mL. May be further diluted with sodium chloride 0.9% and should be infused through membrane filter (0.22 micrometre)
- not recommended in those with known allergy to sheep protein or papaya extracts, or who have been previously treated with digoxin immune FAB

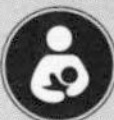
caution should be used in pregnancy or breastfeeding

DISODIUM EDETATE (Disodium Edetate 3 g + Sodium Ascorbate 5 g in 50 mL Solution)

Available form

Vial: Disodium Edetate 3 g + Sodium Ascorbate 5 g in 50 mL Solution)

Action

- disodium salt of EDTA (ethylenediamine tetra-acetic acid) dehydrate, which is a chelating agent that incorporates heavy metal ion into ring structure
- also removes iron, zinc, calcium, cadmium and lead
- sodium ascorbate is added as it acts synergistically as a weak chelating agent as well as having antioxidant activity, which is protective during metal mobilisation
- 3 g disodium edetate can remove about 324 mg of calcium ions, which can cause a rapid drop in serum calcium levels if given too rapidly IV
- lead poisoning can occur by ingestion or inhalation of lead dust or fumes. Signs and symptoms of poisoning include metallic taste, anorexia, irritability, apathy, abdominal colic, vomiting, diarrhoea, constipation, headache, leg cramps, black stools, oliguria, stupor, convulsions and coma
- chronic lead poisoning may involve central nervous system, blood forming organs and GIT
- diagnosis of lead poisoning includes blood lead levels, hair analysis, urine testing, 12-hour urine collection and X-rays of long bones and abdomen
- no recognised safe limits for lead poisoning

Use

- low level lead accumulation and lead poisoning (with or without hypercalcaemia)
- temporary reduction of serum calcium levels in hypercalcaemia

- management of severe digitalis arrhythmias where rapid response is needed
- elimination of some radioactive metals (e.g. calcium, strontium, radium, cobalt and plutonium)

Dose

- (removal of lead, lead poisoning, elimination of radioactive metals) 50 mg disodium edetate/kg IV over 3–4 hours daily (daily maximum 3 g disodium edetate) for 5 days, followed by 2-day drug-free interval. Cycle is repeated twice more **OR**
- (digitalis arrhythmia) 15–60 mg/kg/hour IV

Adverse effects

- nausea, vomiting, diarrhoea
- transient paraesthesia, numbness, headache
- transient drop in both diastolic and systolic BP
- febrile reaction
- hyperuricaemia
- anaemia
- exfoliating dermatitis, skin and mucous membrane reactions
- nephrotoxicity
- (excessive dose) damage to reticuloendotheilial system with haemorrhagic tendency
- thrombophlebitis

Interactions

- not recommended with other chelating agents
- may interfere with oxalate method of measuring serum calcium, therefore other methods should be used for accurate measurement

Nursing points/Cautions

- not recommended IM
- creatinine clearance should be measured at each infusion and therapy not given if there is a decreased creatinine clearance or elevated serum creatinine
- urine should be checked with each course of treatment for proteinuria and haematuria to monitor for any kidney damage; however, severe acute lead poisoning can also produce proteinuria and haematuria. If protelnuria worsens or there are large renal epithelial cells or an increasing number of red blood cells in the urine, therapy should be stopped
- urine flow should be established before administration of first dose using IV fluids if not clinically contraindicated. This is especially necessary if patient has been vomiting and is dehydrated. If urine flow stops, therapy should be stopped
- because minerals are chelated during therapy, it is recommended that:
  - the patient is monitored for any signs of hypocalcaemic tetany, convulsions and respiratory arrest
  - zinc supplementation should be considered after each treatment (as it is more prone to removal by edentates)
- ECG, BP and pulse should be monitored during therapy
- plasma calcium levels should be closely examined
- potassium may be added to IV solution if hypokalaemia is present
- magnesium may be added to infusion to reduce pain and venous wall spasm
- heparin (2000 U) may be added (if not contraindicated) to reduce clotting at injection site
- local anaesthetic (procaine hydrochloride) may be used to reduce injection site pain
- pH of solution should be between 7 and 7.4. If needed, sodium bicarbonate 8.4% may be added

- any additions to the IV solution (e.g. magnesium, potassium) should be added individually and mixed well before addition of next ingredient
- (removal of lead, lead poisoning) initial test dose of 20 mg disodium edetate/kg may be given to check patient sensitivity
- (lead encephalopathy) any acute increase in intracranial pressure (ICP) should be treated before starting therapy
- must be further diluted before administration 500 mL of sodium chloride 0.45% or glucose 5%
- ensure solution is isotonic before administration
- caution if used in those with congestive cardiac failure, history or seizures/ epilepsy or on anticoagulant therapy
- caution if used in those with hypertension and/or previous history of kidney. If given, dose should be adjusted
- contraindicated in those with inadequate kidney function, active liver disease, history of tuberculosis or hypocalcaemia

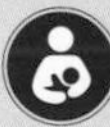
only recommended during pregnancy if benefits outweigh risks

FLUMAZENIL (Anexate, DBL Flumazenil Injection, Flumazenil for Injection)

Available form
Ampoules: 0.5 mg/5 mL

Action
- benzodiazepine antagonist that acts competitively at CNS benzodiazepine receptors reversing sedative effects
- has some weak antiepileptic action
- hypnotic/sedative effects reversed after 1–2 minutes (IV), but may return (depending on half-life of benzodiazepine)
- half-life 53 minutes, prolonged in those with moderate to severe liver impairment

Use
- reverse acute benzodiazepine effects (in hospitalised patients)

Dose
- (reversal of benzodiazepine effects at therapeutic doses) 200 microgram IV over 15 seconds, followed at 1-minute intervals by further doses of 100 microgram if necessary (up to a total dose of 1 mg) **OR**
- (known or suspected overdose of benzodiazepines) 300 microgram IV over 15 seconds followed at 1-minute intervals by further doses of 300 microgram until the patient wakes up or up to a total dose of 2 mg; if drowsiness recurs, an IV infusion of 100–400 microgram/hour may be commenced

Adverse effects
- nausea, vomiting
- withdrawal symptoms (agitation, anxiety, emotional lability, mild confusion, sensory distortion)
- panic attacks (in patients with panic disturbances)
- seizures (in patients with epilepsy or liver impairment)
- convulsions, cardiac arrhythmias (mixed drug overdose including TCAs)
- (infrequent) dizziness, vertigo, anxiety, fearfulness, depression, tearfulness, agitation, palpitations
- (rare) hypersensitivity

Interactions
- (anaesthesia) should not be used until neuromuscular blocking agent effects have been reversed
- withdrawal may precipitate convulsions or withdrawal symptoms
- antagonises non-benzodiazepines (e.g. zopiclone)

Nursing points/Cautions

- may be diluted with glucose 5% or sodium chloride 0.9%
- administered by an anaesthetist or experienced doctor
- patient should be closely monitored for signs of respiratory depression or re-sedation or withdrawal symptoms (e.g. agitation, anxiety, mild confusion, sensory distortion and/or emotional lability)
- should not be used to treat benzodiazepine dependence
- not recommended in those with epilepsy especially in those treated with benzodiazepines for prolonged time
- caution should be taken when used in mixed drug overdose (because some of the toxic effects of other drugs may emerge with the benzodiazepine reversal), or in those with benzodiazepine dependence, or if large doses have been taken recently (before overdose) as withdrawal symptoms or convulsions may be provoked
- caution if used in those with head injuries as it may cause raised intracranial pressure and/or altered cerebral blood flow
- caution if used in those with liver impairment or panic disorders
- contraindicated if benzodiazepine has been used to control status epilepticus or intracranial pressure or in mixed drug overdose containing TCAs

Patient teaching and advice

- warn patient against driving a vehicle or operating machinery within 24 hours of reversal as sedation and dizziness may occur
- see also General Patient teaching and advice (p. xxvii)

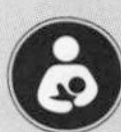

should only be used in pregnancy or breastfeeding if benefits are thought to outweigh risks

FOMEPIZOLE (Antizol Concentrated Injection)

Available form

Vial: 1 g/mL

Action

- competitive inhibitor of alcohol dehydrogenase (which catalyses oxidation of ethanol to acetaldehyde, as well as the initial steps in ethylene glycol and methanol metabolism to toxic metabolites)
- ethylene glycol (main component of antifreeze and coolant) is metabolised to glycolaldehyde and oxalate, which are responsible for metabolic acidosis and kidney damage in poisoning (lethal dose of ethylene glycol is 1.4 mL/kg)
- methanol (main component of windshield wiper fluid) is slowly metabolised via alcohol dehydrogenase to formic acids which is responsible for metabolic acidosis and visual disturbances in methanol poisoning (lethal dose of methanol is about 1–2 mL/kg)
- lack of treatment leads to accumulation of toxic metabolites
- half-life varies with dose

Use

- treatment of ethylene glycol or methanol poisoning

Dose

- 15 mg/kg IV over 30 minutes (loading dose), followed by 10 mg/kg 12-hourly for 4 doses, then 15 mg/kg 12-hourly until concentration of ethylene glycol or methanol are either undetectable or reduced below 20 mg/dl and patient is asymptomatic with normal pH

Adverse effects

- fever
- facial flushing
- headache, feeling drunk, agitation, seizures, anxiety, drowsiness, toxic encephalopathy, dizziness, lightheadedness

- abdominal pain or tenderness, vomiting, nausea, haematemesis, diarrhoea, metallic/bad taste
- abnormal smell
- transient blurred vision
- hypotension, bradycardia, hypertension, collapse
- backache
- anuria, worsening acute kidney failure
- anaemia, lymphangitis, disseminated intravascular coagulation (DIC), eosinophilia
- hypocalcaemia
- pulmonary oedema, pharyngitis, sinusitis, rhinitis
- (IV site) bleeding, burning/tingling
- (rare) allergic reaction (major and minor)

Interactions

- ineffective in treatment of ethanol intoxication and would prolong intoxication if given together
- ethanol decreases rate of elimination

Nursing points/Cautions

- therapy should be started on suspicion of ethylene glycol or methanol poisoning, based on patient history, anion gap metabolic acidosis, increased osmolar gap, visual disturbances or oxalate crystals in urine or documented levels of ethylene glycol or methanol > 20 mg/dl
- patient should be managed for metabolic acidosis, acute kidney failure (ethylene glycol), adult respiratory syndrome, visual disturbances (methanol) and hypocalcaemia. Supportive therapy should include fluids and sodium bicarbonate, in addition to oxygen, and potassium and calcium supplements. If patient is anuric or has severe metabolic acidosis or azotemia, haemodialysis is recommended
- ECG, liver enzymes, WBC, blood gases, pH, serum electrolytes, creatinine and urea, and urinalysis should be monitored regularly
- should not be given undiluted or by bolus injection
- if solution has solidified in vial, it can be liquefied by running vial under warm water or holding in hand. This does not affect stability
- to dilute, add calculated dose from vial to 100 mL sodium chloride 0.9% or glucose 5% and mix well. Administer by infusion over 30 minutes
- patient should be closely monitored for signs of allergic reaction
- contraindicated in patients with ethanol intoxication, other poisons alone or in combination with ethylene glycol or methanol
- contraindicated in those with hypersensitivity to other pyrazoles

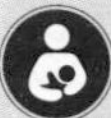

not recommended during pregnancy unless benefit outweighs risk

caution if used during breastfeeding

GLUCAGON HYDROCHLORIDE (GlucaGen HypoKit)

Available form

Vial: 1 mg

Action

- polypeptide hormone, synthesised from yeast cells, which is identical to human hormone
- increases blood glucose level by mobilising liver glycogen (but not muscle glycogen)
- stimulates secretion of insulin from beta cells in the pancreas, as well as catecholamines
- reduces tone and motility of the GIT
- onset of action is 5–15 minutes (IM) or 1 minute (IV) and duration of action is 10–40 minutes (IM) or 5–20 minutes (IV)

- when treating hypoglycaemia, action on blood glucose is within 10 minutes
- short half-life (3–6 minutes)

Use

- treatment of severe hypoglycaemia
- as an aid in radiological examination of the GIT to inhibit motility

Dose

- (hypoglycaemia) 0.5–1 mg SC, IM or IV **OR**
- (endoscopy and radiography) 0.2–2 mg IM or IV

Adverse effects

- nausea, vomiting, abdominal pain
- secondary hypoglycaemia
- (diagnostic procedure, fasting) nausea, hypoglycaemia, BP changes

Interactions

- may increase effects of warfarin when given in high doses
- has positive inotropic effects, which can reverse cardiac depression caused by beta blockade, therefore should be given with caution in those taking beta-adrenoceptor blocking agents
- antagonises insulin
- unpredictable effects if given with indometacin

Nursing points/Cautions

- no effect will be seen if patient is fasting, has chronic hypoglycaemia, adrenal insufficiency or alcohol-induced hypoglycaemia
- not given as IV infusion
- reconstitute with accompanying diluent (in prefilled syringe) and use immediately
- when patient responds (usually within 10 minutes) or at the end of diagnostic procedure (especially if patient has been fasting), supplemental oral carbohydrate should be given to prevent secondary hypoglycaemia by restoring liver glycogen
- IV glucose must be given if patient with hypoglycaemia fails to respond to glucagon. IV glucose is preferred if hypoglycaemia has been induced by sulfonylureas. If glucagon is used alone, secondary hypoglycaemia may occur. Blood glucose levels should be closely monitored
- (diagnostic procedure) onset of action if given IV is within 1 minute with a duration of 5–20 minutes (depending on the organ being examined). If given IM, onset is 5–15 minutes with a duration of 10–40 minutes (depending on organ being examined)
- (diagnostic procedure) caution if used in the elderly with cardiac disease or in patients with diabetes undergoing radiological procedures using glucagon
- contraindicated in those with insulinoma, glucagonoma or phaeochromocytoma (as acute hypertensive crisis may be provoked)

Patient/Carer teaching and advice

- although an emergency drug, the patient, a relative, friend, colleague or teacher may be educated in its use (SC or IM in thigh, buttock or upper arm). Person should be aware that if patient does not wake within 10 minutes, medical assistance must be sought immediately. It is important the doctor is aware that glucagon has been used as it may impact on subsequent management of hypoglycaemia
- patient should be advised not to drive after diagnostic procedure until he/she has eaten carbohydrate-containing food to prevent potential hypoglycaemia from occurring
- see also General Patient teaching and advice (p. xxvii)

IDARUCIZUMAB (Praxbind)

Available form

Vial: 50 mg/mL

Action

- monoclonal antibody fragment that binds to dabigatran and its metabolites with high affinity neutralising anticoagulant effect
- degraded to smaller molecules such as peptides and amino acids, which are then reabsorbed and used for protein synthesis
- does not reverse effects of other anticoagulants

Use

- specific reversal agent for dabigatran when rapid anticoagulant reversal is needed (e.g. emergency surgery, urgent procedures, life-threatening or uncontrolled bleeding)

Dose

- 5 g IV as either bolus dose or 2 consecutive infusions (2 × 2.5 g/50 mL) over 5–10 minutes each

Adverse effects

- headache
- nasopharyngitis
- diarrhoea
- back pain, musculoskeletal stiffness
- skin irritation
- transient proteinuria (not indicative of renal damage)
- pain at catheter site
- (uncommon) recurrence of elevated coagulation parameters up to 24 hours after administration
- thrombotic events
- hypersensitivity

Nursing points/Cautions

- anticoagulant therapy should be resumed as soon as medically appropriate to reduce risk of thromboembolic events. Anticoagulation therapy with dabigatran can be started after 24 hours of administration of idarucizumab
- second dose may be required if there is a recurrence of clinically relevant bleeding with prolonged clotting times or if the patient requires second emergency surgery or urgent procedure and has prolonged clotting times
- administer alone
- flushing IV line with sodium chloride 0.9% before and after administration is recommended
- contains sorbitol (4 g), therefore benefits versus risks should be considered if emergency situation arises in patient with hereditary fructose intolerance
- contains 50 mg sodium per dose which may need to be considered if patient is on controlled sodium diet

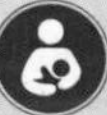

should only be used during pregnancy if benefits outweigh risks

LANTHANUM (Fosrenol)

Available forms

Tablets (chewable): 500 mg, 750 mg, 1000 mg

Action

- dietary phosphate binder that forms insoluble complex that is then excreted

Use

- hyperphosphataemia (in those with chronic renal failure on haemodialysis or peritoneal dialysis)

Dose

- (serum phosphate 1.8–2.4 mmol/L) initially 250 mg orally 3 times daily with food **OR**
- (serum phosphate 2.4–2.9 mmol/L) initially 500 mg orally 3 times daily with food **OR**

- (serum phosphate > 2.9 mmol/L) initially 750 mg orally 3 times daily with food **OR**
- (maintenance) dose adjusted every 2–3 weeks depending on serum phosphate levels

Adverse effects

- nausea, vomiting, diarrhoea, abdominal pain, dyspepsia, flatulence, constipation, taste alteration
- bronchitis, rhinitis
- headache, dizziness, vertigo
- hypocalcaemia, hypercalcaemia
- hypotension
- dialysis graft occlusion/complication

Interactions

- activity may be affected by agents which alter gastric pH (e.g. proton pump inhibitors)
- may increase gastric pH and affect absorption of hydroxychloroquine, thyroid hormones and fluoroquinolone antibiotics
- may impact on results of abdominal X-rays causing a radio opaque appearance

Nursing points/Cautions

- serum phosphate and calcium should be monitored regularly throughout therapy. Calcium supplements may be required
- liver function monitoring is recommended in those with reduction in bile flow
- caution if used in those with biliary atresia or other causes of reduced bile flow as this may result in higher serum levels and deposition in tissue
- caution if used in those with predisposition of bowel obstruction (such as GI surgery, diverticular disease, GI cancer or ulceration, Crohn's disease or ulcerative colitis) or hypomotility disorders (e.g. constipation, diabetic gastroparesis)
- caution if used in those with renal insufficiency as hypocalcaemia may occur
- contraindicated in those with hypophosphataemia

Patient teaching and advice

- patient should be advised to immediately report any abdominal distention or constipation
- instruct patient to continue recommended diet to control phosphate and fluids
- advise patient to chew tablets completely, not swallow them whole
- if patient has dentures and is unable to chew tablets, he/she should be advised to crush tablets
- instruct patient to separate lanthanum by 2 hours from hydroxychloroquine, thyroid hormones, some antibiotics (e.g. tetracyclines)
- if patient is also prescribed norfloxacin or ciprofloxacin, he/she should be instructed to take it either 2 hours before or 4 hours after lanthanum
- warn patient against driving or operating machinery if dizziness or vertigo occurs
- see also General Patient teaching and advice (p. xxvii)

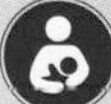

should only be used during pregnancy and breastfeeding if benefits outweigh potential risks

tablets are chewable or can be crushed and mixed with water or spoonful of yoghurt or apple puree

METHYLENE BLUE TRIHYDRATE (Methylene Blue Injection, Proveblue Solution for Injection)

Available form

Vial: 50 mg/5 mL

Action

- thiazide dye able to stain tissue
- in methaemoglobinaemia, methylene blue lowers levels in RBCs by activating a normally dormant reductase enzyme system which reduces methylene blue to leucomethylene blue, which then reduces methaemoglobin to haemoglobin
- monoamine oxidase inhibitor properties
- weak antiseptic and bacteriological staining properties
- binds irreversibly to viral nucleic acid, causing disruption of virus molecule on light exposure

Use

- treatment of drug-induced or idiopathic methaemoglobinaemia
- bacteriological stain
- diagnostic stain (e.g. to detect fistula)
- delineation of some body tissues during surgery

Dose

- (methaemoglobinaemia) 1–2 mg/kg by IV injection over 5 minutes, may be repeated after 1 hour if needed (maximum dose 7 mg/kg) **OR**
- (parathyroid gland staining) 5 mg/kg diluted in 500 mL glucose 5% and given as IV infusion over 60 minutes **OR**
- 5–10 mL diluted in 100–200 mL water for injections and taken orally immediately after dilution

Adverse effects

- nausea, vomiting, abdominal pain, unusual or metallic taste
- headache, dizziness, anxiety, tremor, fever, aphasia, confusion, agitation, parasthaesia
- hypertension, hypotension, arrhythmias, chest pain, tachycardia
- dyspnoea, tachypnoea, hypoxia
- pain in extremities
- mydriasis
- profuse sweating, photosensitivity
- rash (blue macules, severe burning pain)
- skin, urine, faeces and saliva coloured bluc
- (high dose) haemolysis, methaemoglobinaemia, thrombophlebitis
- (injection site) pain
- anaphylaxis

Interactions

- not recommended with SSRIs, SNRIs, MAOIs or other serotonergic agents as serotonin syndrome may occur
- may cause false positive result on phenolsulfonphthalein excretion test or interfere with bispectral index (BIS)
- may cause underestimation of oxygen saturation using pulse oximetry

Nursing points/Cautions

- IV route is recommended for management of methaemoglobinaemia
- blood pressure and ECG monitoring is recommended during therapy to monitor for hypotension and/or arrhythmias
- full blood count (including reticulocyte count, haemoglobin and methaemoglobin levels) should be monitored throughout therapy to ensure anaemia or haemolysis has not occurred
- slow injection rate is recommended to prevent high concentration as necrotic abscess may result if extravasation occurs
- should not be diluted with sodium chloride 0.9% as precipitation will occur
- ensure solution is adequately diluted (not more than 350 mg methylene blue in 500 mL) to prevent thrombophlebitis
- any skin discolouration can be removed with hypochlorite solution

- incompatible with caustic alkalis, iodides and dichromates and oxidising and reducing substances
- cumulative dose of 4 mg/kg should not be exceeded in those with dapsone-induced methaemoglobinaemia
- caution if used in those with mild-to-moderate kidney impairment
- caution if used in those with hyperglycaemia or diabetes mellitus if diluting using glucose 5%
- caution if used to treat aniline-induced methaemoglobinaemia as Heinz body formation and haemolytic anaemia may be exacerbated. Lower doses are recommended
- not recommended in infants < 4 months
- contraindicated SC or by intrathecal administration
- contraindicated in those with known hypersensitivity of other thiazide dyes, severe kidney impairment or if methaemoglobinaemia is due to chlorate or cyanide poisoning
- contraindicated in those with G6PD deficiency as there is a reduced capacity to convert methylene blue to leucomethylene blue, as well as being susceptible to haemolytic anaemia induced by methylene blue

Patient teaching and advice

- warn patient about blue-green colouring that may occur to saliva, skin, urine or faeces
- patient should be advised to avoid or take protective measures against exposure to strong light sources

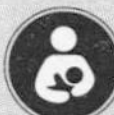

not recommended during pregnancy as ileal abnormalities including fetal intestinal atresia has occurred

not recommended during breastfeeding

NALOXONE HYDROCHLORIDE DIHYDRATE (NALOXONE HYDROCHLORIDE) (Junalox, Naloxone Hydrochloride Injection, Narcan, Nyxoid, Prenoxad)

Available forms

Ampoule: 400 microgram/mL, 1 mg/mL; Nasal spray: 1.8 mg/100 microL

Action

- antagonises effects of opioids (narcotics) by competing for the same receptor sites
- acts on mu, kappa and sigma opioid receptors in CNS
- prevents or reverses opioid effects, including respiratory depression, sedation and hypotension
- also reverses effects of partial agonists or mixed agonist/antagonists but requires higher doses and may be incomplete
- reverses analgesic effects of opioids
- no pharmacological effect in the absence of opioids or opioid agonists
- does not reverse respiratory depression caused by non-opioid agents
- onset of action 1–2 minutes (IV), duration 1–4 hours, half-life 60–90 minutes

Use

- reversal of opioid-induced depression, including respiratory depression, sedation or hypotension
- (nasal spray) reversal of opioid-induced depression, including respiratory depression, sedation or hypotension in home or other non-medical setting
- diagnosis and treatment of suspected acute opioid overdose

Dose

- (postoperative opioid-induced depression) 0.1–0.2 mg IV over 1 minute repeated every 2–3 minutes depending on response. Additional doses may be needed at 1–2-hour intervals **OR**

- (opioid overdose – known or suspected) 0.4–2 mg IV over 1 minute repeated every 2–3 minutes up to 10 mg (if no response at 10 mg, question diagnosis) **OR**
- (opioid overdose) 1 spray into nostril. If no response after 2–3 minutes or if respiratory depression relapse occurs, readminister to other nostril using new container

Adverse effects

- nausea, vomiting
- headache, dizziness
- tachycardia, hypotension, hypertension
- (opioid overdose reversal) nausea, vomiting, sweating, tachycardia, hypertension, tremulousness, seizures, ventricular tachycardia and fibrillation, pulmonary oedema, cardiac arrest
- withdrawal syndrome

Interactions

- antagonises analgesic and respiratory depressant effects of opioids and opioid agonists
- caution if used with agents with cardiovascular effects such as hypotension, ventricular tachycardia or fibrillation or pulmonary oedema

Nursing points/Cautions

- IV administration is recommended in emergencies, but can be given SC or IM if IV route is not available
- when used to reverse opioid-induced depression or opioid overdose, patient can wake up violently, in extreme pain or angry
- may be diluted with glucose 5% or sodium chloride 0.9% (2 mg in 500 mL) to give solution 4 microgram/mL and given IV
- cardiopulmonary resuscitative measures may be required, so resuscitation equipment including vasopressors should be readily available
- observe respiration, heart rate and BP, and for signs of reversal of analgesia such as nausea, vomiting, sweating, tachycardia and raised BP and also any recurrence of respiratory depression (if opioid is long acting)
- (nasal spray) nasal spray device should not be tested before use as this device is then no longer usable
- administer with caution if there is known or suspected physical dependence on opioids, or if large doses of opioids have been taken, as acute withdrawal syndrome may be precipitated
- signs and symptoms of withdrawal include nausea, vomiting, diarrhoea, abdominal cramps, sneezing, yawning, sweating, tearing, stuffy or runny nose, dysphoria, disrupted sleep, irritability, pupil dilation, weakness, nervousness, restlessness, inability to concentrate or focus, piloerection (goose bumps), anxiety, shivering, feeling of skin crawling, fasciculations, fever, hypertension, tachycardia, muscle aches or cramps
- repeated doses may be necessary because the duration of action (short or long acting) of some opioids may exceed that of the antagonist
- (Narcan) contains 17.7 mg sodium/ 2 mg dose (5 mL), which may need to be taken into consideration in a sodium-restricted diet
- incompatible with preparations that contain sulfite or metasulfite, are alkaline or contain long chain or high molecular weight anions
- caution if used in those with cardiovascular disease (including those taking medications with cardiovascular effects), liver or kidney impairment
- caution if used in those with pre-existing lung disease as sudden worsening of disease may occur

Patient teaching and advice

- advise patient not to drive, operate machinery or engage in physically or mentally exerting activities for at least 24 hours after opioid reversal as opioid effect may recur, especially if long-acting opioid was used
- (nasal spray) the following instructions should be given to the person using the nasal spray device:
  - know the signs of overdose (breathing problems, severe sleepiness, not responding to loud noise or touch)
  - call an ambulance before administering nasal spray
  - person should be lying on their back with head allowed to tilt back supporting the neck
  - ensure nose is clear if possible
  - remove nasal spray device from blister pack
  - <u>do not</u> prime or test device before use (this will make it unusable)
  - place thumb on bottom of plunger with first and middle fingers on either side of nozzle
  - nozzle should be gently inserted into one nostril
  - press plunger firmly until it clicks to administer dose
  - remove from nostril
  - place person in recovery position on one side with mouth open pointing towards the ground
  - continue to observe person for improvement in breathing, alertness and response to noise and touch until ambulance arrives. If person starts breathing normally, no further dose is needed
  - if there is no improvement in 2–3 minutes and ambulance has not arrived, a second dose can be given into other nostril using a new device
- see General Patient teaching and advice (p. xxvii)

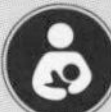

use in pregnancy and during breastfeeding should only occur if benefits outweigh risks. Withdrawal syndrome may be precipitated in newborns of opioid-dependent mothers, with symptoms including excessive crying, convulsions and hyperactive reflexes

Note

- contained in Suboxone with buprenorphine (for use in drug dependence) and in Targin with oxycodone (as an analgesic)

PATIROMER (Veltassa)

Available form

Powder for oral suspension: 8.4 g

Action

- a non-absorbed cation exchange polymer containing a calcium-sorbitol complex (as a counterion)
- increased faecal potassium excretion through potassium binding in GI tract lumen reducing concentration of free potassium thereby reducing serum potassium levels
- onset of action 4–7 hours after administration
- potassium levels may return to pre-treatment levels within 2 days of stopping therapy

Use

- treatment of hyperkalaemia in adults

Dose

- initially 8.4 g orally once daily, adjusting daily dose at weekly intervals of 8.4 g increments according to serum potassium levels (daily maximum 25.2 g)

Adverse effects

- hypomagnesaemia, hypokalaemia
- constipation, diarrhoea, abdominal pain, flatulence, nausea, vomiting

Interactions

- should be separated by at least 3 hours from oral medications as it may decrease GI absorption and efficacy
- may reduce bioavailability of ciprofloxacin, levothyroxine and metformin
- caution if given with thiamine and quinidine
- if given with agents with narrow therapeutic index, close monitoring is recommended

Nursing points/Cautions

- reversible causes of hyperkalaemia should be excluded before starting therapy
- serum potassium levels should be monitored throughout therapy including after any changes to other agents affecting serum potassium or when dose is titrated
- serum magnesium should be monitored for at least 4 weeks after starting therapy and continued if there is a decrease in magnesium levels. If low magnesium levels occur, supplementation should be considered
- serum calcium levels should be monitored in those at risk of hypercalcaemia. Calcium is part of the counterion complex and is partially released which may lead to absorption
- when therapy is stopped, potassium levels return to pre-treatment levels. Therapy should not be stopped without consulting doctor
- should not be used as the sole emergency treatment of hyperkalaemia
- caution if used in those at risk of hypercalcaemia
- caution if used in those with a history of bowel obstruction or major GI surgery, severe GI disorders or swallowing problems because of increased risk of GI ischaemia, necrosis and/or intestinal perforation (reported with other potassium binders)

Patient teaching and advice

- ensure patient understands the following:
  - powder should initially be mixed with 40 mL of water and then stirred. Another 40 mL of water is then added and solution mixed thoroughly
  - powder does not dissolve and solution looks cloudy. More water can be added
  - mixture should be drunk immediately. If powder remains in the glass, water should be added, stirred and drunk. This should be repeated until no powder remains in the glass
  - apple juice or cranberry juice can be used instead of water
  - other fluids containing high levels of potassium should not be used (e.g. juices from oranges, tomatoes, prunes, apricot and grapefruit)
  - solution should not be heated or added to hot food or liquids
  - dry form should not be taken
  - solution should be taken after food at the same time every day
  - solution should be taken at least 3 hours apart from any other oral medications
  - therapy should not be stopped suddenly without first consulting doctor

PROTAMINE SULFATE (Protamine Sulphate Injection BP)

Available form

Ampoules: 10 mg/mL

Action

- basic protein that combines with acidic heparin to form a stable inactive complex

Use
- neutralises anticoagulant action of heparin (e.g. before surgery, if excessive bleeding occurs after overdose)

Dose
- based on 1 mg neutralising approximately 100 units of mucous heparin or 80 mg of lung heparin; given slowly by IV injection over 10 minutes and repeated depending on the whole blood clotting time or plasma APTT

Adverse effects
- sudden drop in BP, bradycardia, pulmonary/systemic hypertension
- nausea, vomiting
- weakness, exhaustion
- dyspnoea, non-cardiogenic pulmonary oedema
- transitory flushing, feeling of warmth,
- back pain
- (rapid administration) severe hypotension, anaphylactoid reaction, hypersensitivity
- (rare) thrombocytopenia, antibody formation

Nursing points/Cautions
- should not be administered rapidly as anaphylaxis and/or hypotension may occur
- resuscitation equipment should be readily available
- dose reduction is required if heparin was administered more than 15 minutes before
- vital signs monitored closely
- no more than 50 mg to be given at any one time
- if used in excess or in the absence of heparin, has an anticoagulant action
- ineffective in overdose of oral anticoagulants
- caution if used in those who may have an increased risk of allergic reaction (e.g. known allergy to fish, use of protamine insulin, previous exposure to protamine during procedures such as coronary angioplasty or cardiopulmonary bypass, infertile men or men having had vasectomy who may have protamine antibodies)
- caution if repeated doses are given as rebound bleeding may occur (up to 18 hours)

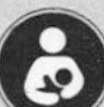
use in pregnancy and during breastfeeding should only occur if benefits outweigh risks

SEVELAMER HYDROCHLORIDE (Renagel)

Available form
Tablets: 800 mg

Action
- phosphate binder that lowers serum phosphate concentration (those with end-stage kidney disease retain phosphorus)
- also lowers low-density lipoprotein (LDL) and total serum cholesterol
- does not contain calcium, therefore decreased risk of hypercalcaemia compared to other phosphate-binding agents

Use
- hyperphosphataemia (stage 4/5 chronic renal disease)

Dose
- (no previous phosphate binder, serum phosphorus 1.78–2.42 mmol/L) initially 800 mg orally 3 times daily with food **OR**
- (no previous phosphate binder, serum phosphorus 2.42–2.91 mmol/L) initially 1600 mg orally 3 times daily with food **OR**
- (no previous phosphate binder, serum phosphorus $>$ 2.91 mmol/L) initially 1600 mg orally 3 times daily with food **OR**

- (previous calcium-based phosphate binder) initial equivalent dose orally daily **OR**
- (maintenance) dose adjusted at 2-week intervals depending on serum phosphorus levels

Adverse effects

- headache
- fever
- pain in limb, arthralgia, back pain
- hypertension
- nausea, vomiting, dyspepsia, diarrhoea, flatulence, abdominal pain, constipation
- cough, dyspnoea, nasopharyngitis, bronchitis, upper respiratory tract infection
- pruritus
- (rare) intestinal obstruction

Interactions

- may decrease bioavailability of ciprofloxacin
- caution if given with levothyroxine, therefore TSH levels should be monitored if given together
- caution if given with antiepileptic agents or antiarrhythmic agents
- if given with ciclosporin, mycophenolate mofetil or tacrolimus, serum levels should be monitored, especially when stopping therapy
- may increase phosphate levels if given with proton pump inhibitors

Nursing points/Cautions

- serum phosphorus is measured regularly and dose adjusted accordingly
- serum calcium, bicarbonate, chloride, vitamin A, D, E and K should be monitored throughout therapy and supplementation given if needed
- increased risk of hypocalcaemia or hypercalcaemia in those with renal insufficiency
- caution in those with GI disorders, swallowing problems, severe constipation, motility disorders or major GI surgery
- not recommended in those under 18 years or pre-dialysis patients
- contraindicated in those with hypophosphataemia or bowel obstruction

Patient teaching and advice

- patients should be advised to swallow tablets whole with water and not crushed, broken or chewed
- instruct patient to report any constipation as it may precede intestinal obstruction
- see also General Patient teaching and advice (p. xxvii)

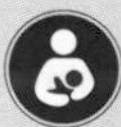

use in pregnancy and during breastfeeding should only occur if benefits outweigh risks

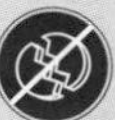

tablets <u>should not</u> be crushed, broken or dispersed in water

SODIUM NITRITE (DBL Sodium Nitrite Injection)

Available form

Vial: 300 mg/10 mL

Action

- cyanide poisoning is rapidly fatal in high doses. Low doses cause toxicity within minutes
- cyanide has affinity for ferric ions reacting with ferric ion in mitochondrial cytochrome oxidase
- reacts with haemoglobin to form methaemoglobin, to which cyanide will preferentially bind, thereby restoring cytochrome oxidase activity. Cyanide dissociates and is converted to thiocyanate (non-toxic)
- vasodilatory activity on smooth muscle
- peak effect within 30–70 minutes (IV)

Use

- antidote to cyanide poisoning (with sodium thiosulfate)

Dose
- 300 mg IV at 75–150 mg/minute (followed by sodium thiosulfate)

Adverse effects
- hypotension, syncope, tachycardia, methaemoglobinaemia
- headache, dizziness
- nausea, vomiting, abdominal pain
- cyanosis, dyspnoea, tachypnoea

Nursing points/Cautions
- should only be used in severe poisoning (e.g. loss of consciousness, decreasing vital signs)
- methaemoglobin levels should be monitored throughout therapy and not allowed to exceed 40%
- BP should be monitored throughout therapy and IV rate decreased if hypotension occurs
- if symptoms recur, half dose of sodium nitrite and sodium thiosulfate can be given after 30 minutes
- rapid administration should be avoided because hypotension may occur
- characteristic bitter almond smell usually occurs with cyanide poisoning; however, not everyone is able to detect its presence
- should be administered alone because it has a large number of incompatibilities
- incompatible with caffeine, citrate, chlorates, iodides, mercury salts, morphine, oxidising agents, permanganate, phenazone, sulfites and tannic acid
- caution if used in those with congenital/acquired methaemoglobinaemia (because the condition may be exacerbated) or with G6PD (due to risk of haemolysis)
- contraindicated in those who have asymptomatic poisoning or combined smoke inhalation, or combined carbon monoxide and cyanide poisoning (unless treated at the same time with hyperbaric oxygen)

SODIUM POLYSTYRENE SULFONATE HYDROGEN (POLYSTYRENE SULFONATE) (Resonium A)

Available form
Powder

Action
- cation exchange resin
- removes potassium ions from the body by exchanging sodium ions for potassium ions in the large intestine
- not selective for potassium and may remove other cations (e.g. magnesium, calcium)
- potassium exchange can be variable (about 1 mmol/g)

Use
- hyperkalaemia

Dose
- 15 g orally with sufficient water/syrup to make solution of 3–4 mL/g of resin 3–4 times daily **OR**
- 30–50 g mixed with glucose 10% and/or water up to 150 mL as a retention enema daily

Adverse effects
- anorexia, nausea, vomiting, gastric irritation and occasionally, diarrhoea
- (large dose, elderly patients) constipation, faecal impaction
- sodium retention, hypokalaemia, hypocalcaemia and sometimes, hypomagnesaemia
- (rare) aspiration pneumonia, ischaemic colitis, intestinal obstruction, gastrointestinal stenosis

Interactions
- may increase risk of toxicity if given with digoxin (if hypokalaemia develops)
- may decrease absorption of lithium or thyroxine
- increased risk of alkalosis if given with magnesium hydroxide
- not recommended with sorbitol because intestinal necrosis may occur

- should be separated by a 3-hour interval from oral medications
- may cause intestinal obstruction if given with aluminium hydroxide

Nursing points/Cautions

- if a rapid decrease in serum potassium is required, may be administered both orally and rectally. Dialysis may be required because therapy with sodium polystyrene sulfonate hydrogen may take hours to days to be effective
- in extreme hyperkalaemia, serum potassium level can be decreased temporarily by IV glucose and insulin or IV sodium bicarbonate
- electrolytes (especially potassium, magnesium and calcium) should be monitored daily during therapy. Serum potassium levels should be measured more frequently if patient is taking digoxin. Therapy should be stopped in all patients if potassium level falls below 5 mmol/L
- small amounts of magnesium and calcium ions can be lost during therapy together with potassium ions, therefore observe for features of electrolyte imbalance, including anorexia, nausea, vomiting, dry mouth, thirst, excessive diuresis, oliguria, weakness, lethargy, hypotension, tachycardia
- not given in fruit juices as many have a high potassium content
- mild laxative relieves constipation and avoids faecal impaction. If severe constipation occurs, therapy should be stopped and should only be restarted when normal bowel habits return
- magnesium containing laxatives should be avoided
- rectal administration should be used if patient is vomiting or has paralytic ileus
- patient should be encouraged to retain enema for at least 9 hours, followed by colonic irrigation to remove resin
- caution if used in those affected by increased sodium levels (even small amounts) (e.g. congestive cardiac failure, severe hypertension, severe oedema or kidney damage)
- contraindicated in those with obstructive bowel disease or if potassium levels are less than 5 mmol/L

Patient teaching and advice

- instruct patient to use spoon provided to accurately measure 15 g and to mix with water or syrup but not fruit juices (as these contain potassium)
- warn patient to avoid inhaling powder
- patient should be advised to report any constipation (especially if patient is elderly) as bowel obstruction may occur
- advise patient to separate by at least 3 hours from oral medications
- if patient has gastroparesis, advise to separate by at least 6 hours from oral medications

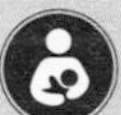
not used during pregnancy unless the expected benefit outweighs any potential risk

Note

- calcium polystyrene sulfonate hydrogen (Calcium Resonium) can be used at the same dosages with similar effects

SODIUM THIOSULFATE PENTAHYDRATE (SODIUM THIOSULFATE) (DBL Sodium Thiosulfate Injection)

Available form

Vial: 2.5 g/10 mL

Action
- combines with cyanide ions from cyanohaemoglobin to form the relatively harmless thiocyanate, which is excreted in the urine
- cytochrome oxidase is protected from the cyanide ions by an initial injection of sodium nitrite, which oxidises haemoglobin to methaemoglobin with which the cyanide ions combine preferentially, forming cyanohaemoglobin
- poorly absorbed orally

Use
- cyanide poisoning (in combination with sodium nitrite)
- prevention of sodium nitroprusside-induced cyanide toxicity

Dose
- (cyanide poisoning) 12.5 g slowly IV over 10 minutes at a rate of 5 mL/minute **OR**
- (prevention of sodium nitroprusside-induced cyanide toxicity) 5–10 times dose rate of sodium nitroprusside IV (with sodium nitroprusside)

Adverse effects
- hypotension
- headache, agitation, disorientation, delusions, hallucination
- diarrhoea, nausea, vomiting
- arthralgia, hyperreflexia, muscle cramps
- blurred vision, tinnitus
- diuresis, osmotic disturbances

Nursing points/Cautions
- if signs of toxicity are still present 0.5–2 hours after infusion, may be repeated at half dose (with sodium nitrite)
- if given with sodium nitrite, should be administered immediately after sodium nitrite infusion has been completed
- caution if used in those with hypertension, congestive cardiac failure, liver cirrhosis, renal impairment or toxaemia of pregnancy because symptoms may be exacerbated

SUCROFERRIC OXYHYDROXIDE (Velphoro)

Available form

Tablets (chewable): 2.5 g (equivalent 500 mg iron)

Action
- phosphate binder

Use
- control of serum phosphate in patients with chronic kidney disease on dialysis

Dose
- initially 3 tablets orally daily with meals, then titrating up or down in increments of 1 tablet, at 2–4-week intervals until serum phosphorus levels are acceptable (daily maximum 3 g iron = 6 tablets)

Adverse effects
- diarrhoea, discoloured faeces, nausea, vomiting, constipation, dyspepsia, abdominal pain, flatulence, abnormal taste, temporary discolouration of tongue and/or teeth
- hyperphosphataemia, hypophosphataemia, hyperkalaemia, hypocalcaemia, hypercalcaemia
- hypertension, hypotension
- dyspnoea
- nasopharyngitis
- fever
- muscle spasm
- headache
- anaemia

Interactions
- if used with agents known to interact with iron (e.g. alendronate, doxycycline, levothyronine), should be separated and given 1 hour before or 2 hours later

Nursing points/Cautions

- serum phosphate levels should be closely monitored during therapy
- contains sucrose (750 mg), starches and iron
- caution if used within 3 months of peritonitis, significant gastric or liver disorders or major GI surgery
- not recommended in those with rare hereditary problems of fructose intolerance, glucose–galactose malabsorption or sucrase–isomaltase insufficiency
- contraindicated in those with haemochromatosis and other iron accumulation disorders

Patient teaching and advice

- advise patient that tablets should be chewed, not swallowed whole and may be crushed if needed
- if taken with other agents that interact with iron (alendronate, cefalexin, doxycycline, thyroid hormone), instruct patient that tablets should be taken 1 hour before or 2 hours after other medications
- warn patient that discolouration of tongue and/or teeth is temporary and that faeces is coloured black
- see General Patient teaching and advice (p. xxvii)

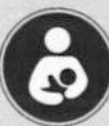

should only be used during pregnancy and breastfeeding if benefits outweigh risks

tablets are chewable or can be crushed and mixed with spoonful of yoghurt or apple puree

SUGAMMADEX SODIUM (Bridion)

Available forms

Vial: 200 mg/2 mL, 500 mg/5 mL

Action

- modified gamma cyclodextrin
- selective relaxant binding agent that forms a complex with neuromuscular blocking agents (vecuronium, rocuronium), reducing amount available to bind with receptors at neuromuscular junction
- result is reversal of neuromuscular blockade induced by vecuronium or rocuronium

Use

- reversal of neuromuscular blockade induced by vecuronium or rocuronium

Dose

- (routine reversal, rocuronium or vecuronium) 4.0 mg/kg IV if recovery has reached 1–2 post-tetanic counts (recovery time approx. 3 minutes) **OR**
- (routine reversal, rocuronium or vecuronium) 2.0 mg/kg IV if recovery is spontaneous (recovery time approx. 2 minutes) **OR**
- (immediate reversal of rocuronium) 16 mg/kg IV administered 3 minutes after bolus dose of rocuronium (1.2 mg/kg) (recovery time approx. 1.5 minutes)

Adverse effects

- procedural pain, anaesthetic complication (e.g. limb movement, coughing, grimacing, sucking endotracheal tube during surgery/anaesthetic procedure)
- nausea, vomiting, constipation, abdominal pain, diarrhoea
- hypotension, hypertension
- cough, oropharyngeal pain
- headache, dizziness, hypoaesthesia, insomnia
- fever, chills
- back pain, generalised pain
- prolonged aPTT and PT (INR)
- peripheral oedema
- recurrence of blockade (suboptimal dose)
- (rare) marked bradycardia, hypersensitivity

Interactions

- recovery time may be delayed if given with toremifene (on same day as operation/anaesthetic procedure) or fusidic acid
- may decrease efficacy of oral contraceptives
- may interfere with serum progesterone assay

Nursing points/Cautions

- all patients require ventilator support and respiratory function monitoring until spontaneous respiration is restored. Haemodynamic monitoring is also required during and after reversal of neuromuscular blockage
- coagulation (APTT, PT and INR) should be assessed before and after treatment
- suboptimal doses (< 2 mg/kg) are not recommended
- recurrence of neuromuscular blockade is possible (especially if suboptimal doses are administered)
- given rapidly as IV bolus over 10 seconds directly into vein or IV line
- if readministration is required after immediate reversal, a 24-hour interval should be allowed between doses
- not compatible with verapamil, ondansetron and ranitidine
- not recommended in patients with severe kidney impairment (creatinine clearance < 30 mL/min) or severe liver impairment (with or without coagulopathy)
- not recommended for reversal of other neuromuscular blocking agents other than rocuronium or vecuronium
- caution if used in those who are older, have cardiovascular disease, pre-existing coagulation disorders or oedema as longer recovery times may occur

Patient teaching and advice

- female patients should be counselled to use a non-hormonal contraceptive (e.g. condom) in addition to hormonal contraceptive for next 7 days to avoid unwanted pregnancy
- see General Patient teaching and advice (p. xxvii)

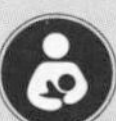

should only be used during pregnancy or breastfeeding if benefits are thought to outweigh risks

VITAMIN K (PHYTOMENADIONE) (VITAMIN K1) (Konakion, Konakion MM Paediatric)

Available form

Ampoules (adult): 10 mg/mL; (paediatric): 2 mg/0.2 mL

Action

- promotes hepatic biosynthesis of prothrombin (factor II) and coagulation factors VII, IX and X and coagulation inhibitors protein C and protein S
- antagonises the effects of indirect, orally acting anticoagulants

Use

- prothrombin deficiency
- prophylaxis and treatment of vitamin K deficiency bleeding in infants
- hypovitaminosis K
- reverse of oral anticoagulant overdose

Dose

Adults

- (severe life-threatening haemorrhage) 5–10 mg IV over 30 seconds with fresh frozen plasma (FFP) and prothrombin complex concentrate (PCC) **OR**
- (INR 5–9, with or without mild haemorrhage) 0.5–1 mg IV over 30 seconds, or 1–2.5 mg orally **OR**
- (INR > 9, with or without mild haemorrhage) 1 mg IV over 30 seconds, or 2.5–5.0 mg orally

Paediatrics

- (prophylaxis, healthy neonate) 1 mg IM at birth **OR**
- (prophylaxis, healthy neonate) 2 mg orally at birth, at 3–5 days and at 4 weeks **OR**
- (neonate with special risk factor) 1 mg IM at birth **OR**
- (neonate with special risk factors weighing < 1.5 kg) 0.5 mg IM at birth **OR**
- (treatment of vitamin K deficiency bleeding) initially 1 mg IV, with further doses based on coagulation status (with whole blood or coagulation factor transfusion)

Adverse effects

- facial flushing, sweating, unusual taste
- (IV site) local pain, phlebitis or irritation
- (IV rare) anaphylactoid reaction, thromboembolism

Interactions

- antagonises coumarin-type anticoagulants
- action may be impaired by antiepileptic agents
- effects inhibited by some cephalosporin antibiotics

Nursing points/Cautions

- (reversal of anticoagulant overdose) oral anticoagulant should be stopped
- should not be given IM
- ineffective in heparin or heparin-like (e.g. low molecular weight heparin) overdose
- prothrombin time should be estimated 3 hours after IV administration and may be repeated if necessary. Blood transfusion may also be necessary
- administer alone
- should not be diluted
- (adult oral administration) withdraw required amount from vial, remove needle and administer directly into patient's mouth, followed by fluid to wash down
- elderly patients are more sensitive to reversal of anticoagulation and should be prescribed lower doses
- (paediatric) if newborn is not breastfed (i.e. formula is used) last oral dose can be omitted
- (paediatric) special risk factors for decreased dose include prematurity, birth asphyxia, delay in establishing oral feeding, maternal use of anticoagulants, antiepileptic, antibiotic or antimycobacterial agents, prolonged use of antibiotics, liver dysfunction with obstructive jaundice or malabsorption
- (paediatric) dispenser delivers 2 mg at mark and should be placed directly into infant's mouth
- (paediatric) if infant spits oral dose out, vomits or has diarrhoea within 24 hours of administration, a repeat dose is recommended
- caution if used in those with severe liver impairment (INR should be monitored), biliary atresia, fat malabsorption syndromes or pancreatic insufficiency
- contraindicated in those with severe allergic predisposition

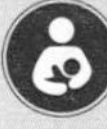

contraindicated during pregnancy

not recommended during breastfeeding as prophylaxis for neonatal haemorrhagic disease

Note

- vitamin K is contained in many multivitamin preparations in varying quantities, which may undermine control of warfarin

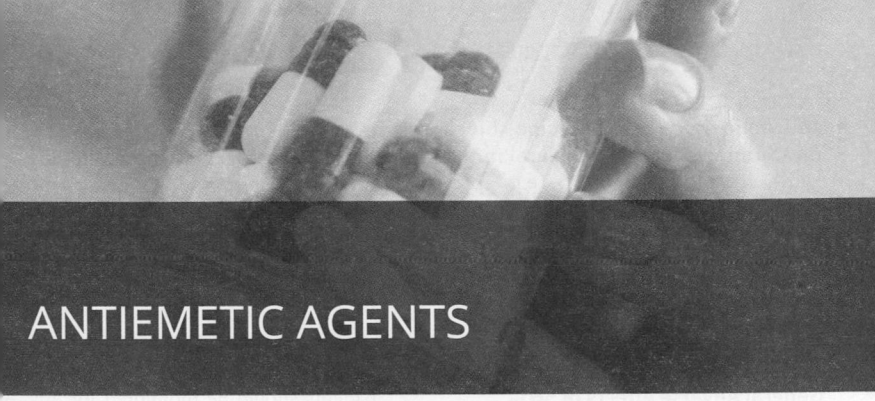

ANTIEMETIC AGENTS

The emetic centre (in the medulla) receives input from a number of other areas, including the chemoreceptor trigger zone (CTZ, located in the fourth ventricle), the vestibular apparatus, higher brain centres (relaying sensory input, such as pain, smell and sight), and organs such as the heart, testes and parts of the gastrointestinal tract (GIT). All of these areas have different densities of receptors (e.g. dopamine, serotonin, histamine, muscarinic, NK1). For example, the CTZ has high concentrations of all these receptors, while the vestibular apparatus is rich with muscarinic (M1) and histamine (H1) receptors (Bryant et al 2019; McQuaid 2018).

Because the CTZ sits outside the blood–brain barrier, it can be stimulated by blood-borne emetics (e.g. chemical and bacterial toxins, drugs), cerebrospinal fluid-borne emetics and 5-hydroxytryptamine (5HT, serotonin) released from the stomach and small intestine. The CTZ is activated by a number of triggers, including smells, strong or unpleasant emotions, severe pain, increased intracranial pressure, labyrinthine disturbances (motion sickness and inner ear disturbances), endocrine and metabolic disturbances (including pregnancy), toxic reactions to drugs, GIT disease (including obstruction and ischaemia), GIT inflammatory diseases, infection, radiation treatment and chemotherapy. The CTZ then relays messages via neurotransmitters to the emetic centre, which then sends messages via a number of pathways and neurotransmitters to the upper GIT, diaphragm and abdominal muscles, causing contraction, which results in vomiting (emesis). Neurotransmitters involved in the process include 5HT (serotonin), acetylcholine, dopamine, histamine and substance P (Bryant et al 2019; Hasler 2018).

Management of nausea and vomiting should include symptom control (usually with antiemetic agents), prevention or management of dehydration, resumption of normal oral intake and prevention of abnormal blood glucose levels, especially in those with diabetes (Hasler 2018).

Antiemetics act by blocking transmission of neurotransmitters. For example, dopamine antagonists (e.g. domperidone, metoclopramide, prochlorperazine) act to block dopamine receptors (D2) in the stomach and CTZ; $5HT_3$ receptor antagonists (e.g. granisetron, ondansetron, tropisetron) block $5HT_3$ receptors in the GIT, CTZ and vomiting centre;

anticholinergics (e.g. hyoscine) block muscarinic receptors; and neurokinin-1 (NK_1) receptor antagonists (e.g. aprepitant, fosaprepitant) block NK_1 receptors located in the CNS (Hasler 2018; McQuaid 2018).

Note

- highly emetogenic chemotherapy includes cisplatin
- less emetogenic chemotherapy includes carboplatin, cyclophosphamide, doxorubicin

5HT₃ RECEPTOR ANTAGONISTS

General Adverse effects of $5HT_3$ receptor antagonists

- headache, dizziness, fatigue
- diarrhoea, constipation, abdominal pain
- fever
- changes in liver enzymes
- insomnia, somnolence, drowsiness
- (uncommon) bradycardia, arrhythmias, hypotension, angina, ECG changes
- (rare) prolongs QT interval, torsade de pointes (see Glossary)
- (rare) seizures, extrapyramidal reactions, hypersensitivity, serotonin syndrome

General Interactions of $5HT_3$ receptor antagonists

- caution if given with other agents known to prolong QT interval, cause arrhythmias or cause electrolyte imbalances
- serotonin syndrome may occur if given with other serotonergic agents such as SSRIs

General Nursing points/Cautions for $5HT_3$ receptor antagonists

- any electrolyte imbalance such as hypo- or hyperkalaemia should be corrected before starting therapy
- pulse and ECG should be monitored during therapy
- patients should be monitored for any signs of subacute intestinal obstruction
- patient should be carefully observed for any signs of serotonin syndrome if given with other serotonergic agents. Clinical symptoms of serotonin syndrome include agitation, confusion, hypomania, hyperactivity, restlessness, hyperthermia, sweating, tachycardia, hypertension, flushing, shivering, clonus, hyperreflexia, hypertonia, ataxia and tremor
- not recommended in those with congenital QT syndrome
- caution in those who have or may develop QT prolongation, cardiac rhythm or conduction disturbances, with electrolyte disturbance or receiving cardiotoxic chemotherapy
- caution if used in those with subacute intestinal obstruction as stimulation of gastric motility may be dangerous
- caution if used in those with hypersensitivity to other $5HT_3$ antagonists as cross-sensitisation may occur

General Patient teaching and advice for $5HT_3$ receptor antagonists

- patient should be advised not to drive or operate machinery if dizziness, fatigue or insomnia occur
- instruct patient to seek medical advice if any chest pain or changes to

heart rate (such as palpitations or pounding heart) are felt

- see also General Patient teaching and advice (p. xxvii)

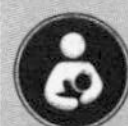

not used during pregnancy unless the expected benefit outweighs any potential risk

not recommended during breastfeeding

GRANISETRON (Granisetron-AFT, Granisetron Kabi, Kytril)

Available forms

Tablets: 2 mg; Ampoules: 1 mg/1 mL, 3 mg/3 mL

Action

- $5HT_3$ receptor antagonist
- (oral) half-life 9 hours

Use

- prevention of nausea and vomiting associated with chemotherapy, radiotherapy
- postoperative nausea and vomiting

Dose

- (prophylaxis of nausea and vomiting associated with chemotherapy) 2 mg orally daily up to 7 days following chemotherapy, with first dose given 1 hour before the start of chemotherapy **OR**
- (prophylaxis of nausea and vomiting associated with chemotherapy) 3 mg by IV infusion over 5 minutes, starting 30 minutes before and completed just prior to chemotherapy **OR**
- (treatment of established nausea and vomiting associated with chemotherapy) 1 mg by IV infusion over 5 minutes, repeated at 10-minute intervals if needed (daily maximum 9 mg) **OR**
- (prophylaxis of nausea and vomiting associated with radiotherapy) 3 mg by IV infusion over 5 minutes before start of radiotherapy **OR**
- (prophylaxis of postoperative nausea and vomiting) 1 mg IV over 30 seconds before induction of anaesthesia **OR**
- (treatment of established postoperative nausea and vomiting) 1 mg IV over 30 seconds as a single dose

Adverse effects

- see General Adverse effects of $5HT_3$ antagonists (p. 366)
- asthenia
- agitation, anxiety, CNS stimulation
- alopecia
- anaemia, thrombocytopenia, leucopenia
- hypertension
- anorexia, altered taste

Interactions

- see General Interactions of $5HT_3$ receptor antagonists (p. 366)

Nursing points/Cautions

- see General Nursing points/Cautions for $5HT_3$ receptor antagonists (p. 366)
- efficacy is increased by adding corticosteroid (e.g. dexamethasone 8–20 mg IV) just before chemotherapy
- solution should be diluted with 20–50 mL of infusion fluid before IV administration
- dilution fluids include glucose 5%, sodium chloride 0.9%, mannitol 10%, Hartmann's solution, sodium chloride 0.18%/glucose 4%, or compound sodium lactate
- should be administered alone, but may be mixed with dexamethasone
- tablets not recommended in those with hereditary problems of galactose intolerance, Lapp lactase deficiency or glucose–galactose malabsorption

Patient teaching and advice

- see also General Patient teaching and advice for $5HT_3$ receptor antagonists (p. 366)

tablets can be crushed and mixed with water, or spoonful of yoghurt or apple puree

ONDANSETRON (Ondansetron Injection, Onsetron, Zofran, Zoten)

Available forms

Tablets: 4 mg, 8 mg; Wafers: 4 mg, 8 mg; Syrup: 4 mg/5 mL; Ampoules: 4 mg/2 mL (IM or IV), 8 mg/4 mL (IV)

Action

- serotonin antagonist highly selective against $5HT_3$ receptors

Use

- prevention and treatment of nausea and vomiting induced by radiotherapy or chemotherapy
- prevention and treatment of postoperative nausea and vomiting

Dose

Highly emetogenic chemotherapy

- 8 mg by slow IV injection or IV infusion over 15 minutes immediately before chemotherapy, followed by further IV doses if necessary (daily maximum 32 mg)

Radiotherapy or less emetogenic chemotherapy

- 8 mg by slow IV injection or IV infusion over 15 minutes immediately before chemotherapy or radiotherapy, then 8 mg orally 12-hourly or 16 mg rectally daily for up to 5 days **OR**
- 8 mg orally 2 hours before chemotherapy or radiotherapy, then 8 mg orally 12-hourly or 16 mg PR daily for up to 5 days

Postoperative nausea and vomiting

- (prevention) 4 mg IM or slow IV at induction of anaesthesia **OR**
- (treatment) 4–8 mg IM or slow IV **OR**
- (prevention) 16 mg orally 1 hour before anaesthesia

Adverse effects

- see General Adverse effects of $5HT_3$ receptor antagonists (p. 366)
- sensation of flushing or warmth
- anxiety
- dry mouth
- (uncommon) hiccups
- (IV) local reaction, shivering
- (rapid IV administration) transient visual disturbances (including blurred vision or blindness), dizziness

Interactions

- may decrease analgesic effect of tramadol
- increased clearance and decreased antiemetic effect may occur if given with phenytoin, carbamazepine and rifampicin
- contraindicated with apomorphine
- see General Interactions of $5HT_3$ receptor antagonists (p. 366)

Nursing points/Cautions

- see General Nursing points/Cautions for $5HT_3$ receptor antagonists (p. 366)
- do not administer any other drug in the same syringe or infusion
- see manufacturer's instructions for dilution and compatibility with other drugs
- diluted solutions that are hazy, discoloured or contain visible particulate matter must be discarded
- IV doses over 8 mg should be given as an IV infusion over 15 minutes
- should not be given rapidly as visual disturbances may occur. Transient blindness should resolve within 20 minutes
- single dose of IV dexamethasone (20 mg) administered before first ondansetron dose will potentiate the

antiemetic effect in patients receiving highly emetogenic chemotherapy
- wafers contain aspartame and should be used with caution in those with phenylketonuria
- wafers should be placed on tongue, allowed to dissolve and then swallowed

Patient teaching and advice

- advise patient to place wafer on tongue and allow to dissolve before swallowing
- see also General Patient teaching and advice for $5HT_3$ receptor antagonists (p. 366)

wafers should be used if patient has swallowing difficulties

PALONOSETRON HYDROCHLORIDE (Aloxi)

Available form

Vial: 250 microgram/5 mL

Action

- selective $5HT_3$ receptor antagonist
- half-life about 40 hours

Use

- prevention of nausea and vomiting induced by cytotoxic therapy
- prevention of nausea and vomiting postoperatively for up to 24 hours

Dose

- 250 microgram IV over 30 seconds given 30 minutes before start of cytotoxic therapy **OR**
- (postoperatively) 75 microgram IV as a single dose before induction of anaesthesia

Adverse effects

- see General Adverse effects of $5HT_3$ receptor antagonists (p. 366)
- weakness, asthenia, anxiety
- hyperkalaemia
- (IV site) burning, pain, discomfort, induration

Interactions

- see General Interactions of $5HT_3$ receptor antagonists (p. 366)

Nursing points/Cautions

- see General Nursing points/Cautions for $5HT_3$ receptor antagonists (p. 366)
- IV line should be flushed with 0.9% sodium chloride before and after administration of palonosetron
- administer alone

Patient teaching and advice

- patient should be advised not to drive or operate machinery if dizziness, fatigue or insomnia are ongoing
- see also General Patient teaching and advice (p. xxvii)

Note

- contained in Akynzeo with netupitant (a substance P neurokinin-1 receptor antagonist)

TROPISETRON (Tropisetron-AFT, Tropisetron-MYX)

Available forms

Ampoules: 2 mg/2 mL, 5 mg/5 mL

Action

- selective $5HT_3$ receptor antagonist
- long duration of action (24 hours)

Use

- prevention of nausea and vomiting induced by cytotoxic therapy (5 mg/5 mL ampoule only)
- treatment and prevention of postoperative nausea and vomiting (2 mg/2 mL ampoule only)

Dose

Prevention of nausea and vomiting induced by cytotoxic therapy

- 5 mg IV infusion over 15 minutes or slow IV injection over at least 60 seconds immediately before chemotherapy (day 1), then

- days 2–6: 5 mg orally in the morning 1 hour before food

Postoperative nausea and vomiting

- 2 mg by slow IV injection over at least 30 seconds or infusion just before induction of anaesthesia

Adverse effects

- see General Adverse effects of $5HT_3$ receptor antagonists (p. 366)
- (rare) collapse, syncope

Interactions

- rifampicin and phenobarbital (phenobarbitone) may reduce serum levels of tropisetron
- see General Interactions of $5HT_3$ receptor antagonists (p. 366)

Nursing points/Cautions

- see General Nursing points/Cautions for $5HT_3$ receptor antagonists (p. 366)
- for IV use, ampoule may be diluted to 100 mL with sodium chloride 0.9%, glucose 5%, mannitol 10% or Ringer's solution
- should be avoided in doses of 10 mg or greater in patients with uncontrolled hypertension
- antiemetic effect may be enhanced if given with dexamethasone

Patient teaching and advice

- see also General Patient teaching and advice for $5HT_3$ receptor antagonists (p. 366)

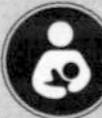
contraindicated during pregnancy and breastfeeding

NEUROKININ-1 (NK_1) RECEPTOR ANTAGONISTS

APREPITANT (Emend)

Available forms

Capsules: 80 mg, 125 mg, 165 mg

Action

- neurokinin-1 (NK_1) receptor antagonist which blocks substance P
- half-life 9–13 hours

Use

- prevention of acute and delayed nausea and vomiting associated with moderately or highly emetogenic chemotherapy (e.g. cisplatin) (with ondansetron and dexamethasone)
- prevention of postoperative nausea and vomiting

Dose

Chemotherapy-induced nausea and vomiting (highly emetogenic)

- 165 mg orally 1 hour before chemotherapy (with dexamethasone 12 mg orally and ondansetron 32 mg IV 30 minutes before chemotherapy) (day 1), followed by dexamethasone 8 mg orally mane (day 2), then dexamethasone 8 mg orally BD (days 3 and 4) **OR**
- 125 mg orally 1 hour before chemotherapy (with dexamethasone 12 mg orally and ondansetron 32 mg IV 30 minutes before chemotherapy) (day 1), then 80 mg orally mane (with dexamethasone 8 mg orally) (days 2 and 3), then dexamethasone 8 mg orally mane (day 4)

Chemotherapy-induced nausea and vomiting (moderately emetogenic)

- 165 mg orally 1 hour before chemotherapy (with dexamethasone 12 mg orally and ondansetron 32 mg IV 30 minutes before chemotherapy) **OR**
- 125 mg orally 1 hour before chemotherapy (with dexamethasone 12 mg

orally and ondansetron 32 mg IV 30 minutes before chemotherapy) (day 1), then 80 mg orally mane (days 2 and 3)

Prevention of postoperative nausea and vomiting

- 40 mg orally within 3 hours of anaesthetic induction

Adverse effects

- asthenia, fatigue, dizziness, insomnia, somnolence, anxiety
- fever
- anorexia, nausea, burping, abdominal pain, flatulence, constipation or diarrhoea, dyspepsia, reflux
- headache
- anaemia, febrile neutropenia
- hiccups
- increase in liver enzymes
- pruritus, rash, urticaria
- hypotension, bradycardia

Interactions

- may result in decreased prothrombin time if given with warfarin, therefore INR should be closely monitored for 14 days following therapy
- may decrease efficacy of oral contraceptives during and for 28 days following therapy
- caution if given with ciclosporin, tacrolimus or sirolimus
- may decrease serum levels of phenytoin and warfarin
- may increase serum levels of dexamethasone, methylprednisolone, midazolam, alprazolam, triazolam
- decreased plasma levels may result if given with rifampicin and paroxetine
- not recommended with St John's wort
- caution if given with ifosfamide as neurotoxicity may occur

Nursing points/ Cautions

- tablets not recommended for those with fructose intolerance, glucose–galactose malabsorption or sucrase–isomaltase insufficiency

Patient teaching and advice

- patient should be advised not to drive or operate machinery if they experience fatigue or dizziness
- female patients using hormonal contraceptives should be instructed to use alternative or extra contraception methods during therapy and for 1 month after last dose
- (165 mg capsule) advise patient to take either with a light meal or on an empty stomach
- see General Patient teaching and advice (p. xxvii)

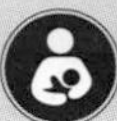

not recommended during pregnancy or breastfeeding unless benefits outweigh potential risks

capsules can be opened and contents dispersed in water or sprinkled on spoonful of yoghurt or apple puree

FOSAPREPITANT (Emend IV)

Available form

Vial: 150 mg

Action

- prodrug of aprepitant (neurokinin-1 (NK_1) receptor antagonist which blocks substance P)
- conversion to aprepitant occurs within 30 minutes of IV infusion being completed

Use

- prevention of acute and delayed nausea and vomiting associated with moderate to highly emetogenic chemotherapy (e.g. cisplatin) (with ondansetron and dexamethasone)

Dose

- (highly emetogenic chemotherapy) 150 mg IV over 20–30 minutes

30 minutes before chemotherapy (dexamethasone 12 mg orally and ondansetron 30 minutes before chemotherapy) (day 1), then dexamethasone 8 mg orally mane (day 2), then dexamethasone 8 mg orally twice daily (days 3 and 4) **OR**
- (moderately emetogenic chemotherapy) 150 mg IV over 20–30 minutes 30 minutes before chemotherapy (dexamethasone 12 mg orally and ondansetron 30 minutes before chemotherapy)

Adverse effects
- see Adverse effects for Aprepitant (p. 371)
- IV site reaction
- (high dose) thrombosis
- (rare) hypersensitivity reaction

Interactions
- see Interactions for Aprepitant (p. 371)

Nursing points/Cautions
- should not be given as bolus injection or IM or SC
- to reconstitute powder, inject sodium chloride 5 mL gently into vial and swirl gently to avoid foaming
- inject reconstituted solution into sodium chloride infusion bag (for 150 mg IV infusion, volume of infusion bag should be 145 mL; for 115 mg IV infusion, volume of infusion bag should be 110 mL (extra sodium chloride will need to be added to infusion bags to make up correct volume)
- invert infusion bag gently 2–3 times to ensure even mixing
- IV infusion given over 20–30 minutes
- administer alone
- incompatible with solutions containing divalent cations (e.g. Mg^{2+}, Ca^{2+}), including Hartmann's solution and lactated Ringer's solution
- contraindicated in those with hypersensitivity to aprepitant or polysorbate 80
- see also Nursing points/Cautions for Aprepitant (p. 371)

Patient teaching and advice
- see also Patient teaching and advice for Aprepitant (p. 371)

DOPAMINE ANTAGONISTS

DOMPERIDONE (Motilium)

Available form

Tablets: 10 mg

Action
- prokinetic agent
- dopamine antagonist that seldom causes extrapyramidal reactions because it does not cross the blood–brain barrier
- antiemetic action thought to be caused by peripheral effects, as well as antagonism of central dopamine receptors in CTZ
- half-life 7–9 hours

Use
- intractable nausea and vomiting
- treatment (short term) of diabetic gastroparesis symptoms

Dose
- 10 mg orally, 3 times daily 15–30 minutes before meals and before retiring if needed (daily maximum 30 mg)

Adverse effects
- mild abdominal cramps, diarrhoea, dry mouth
- headache, somnolence, akathisia, asthenia, depression, anxiety
- endocrine disturbance (including breast enlargement, breast tenderness

or pain, irregular menstruation, amenorrhoea), decreased libido
- (uncommon) increase in prolactin levels, thirst, nervousness, insomnia, dizziness, lethargy, irritability
- (rare) extrapyramidal symptoms, QT prolongation, arrhythmias, sudden cardiac death

Interactions

- contraindicated with erythromycin, fluconazole, voriconazole, clarithromycin and amiodarone because of QT interval prolongation
- antacids and antisecretory drugs (e.g. cimetidine, ranitidine) reduce bioavailability of domperidone and block absorption
- effects decreased if given with anticholinergic agents. If given before atropine, may decrease relaxation on lower oesophageal sphincter
- plasma levels may be increased by azole antifungal agents, macrolide antibiotics, HIV protease inhibitors, calcium-channel blockers, amiodarone and aprepitant and are therefore not recommended together
- may affect the absorption of enteric-coated or SR preparations
- caution if used with agents that cause electrolyte disturbance as it may increase risk of QT prolongation

Nursing points/Cautions

- any electrolyte disturbance should be corrected before starting therapy
- (acute nausea and vomiting) therapy should be continued for more than 7 days
- contains lactose and therefore is not recommended in those with lactose intolerance, galactosaemia or glucose–galactose malabsorption
- (diabetic gastroparesis) once diabetic control has been established (either by diet or insulin or both), domperidone should be stopped
- may lead to increased serum prolactin levels with prolonged use, therefore it should be used with caution in those with a history of breast cancer as some are prolactin dependent
- caution if used in those over 60 years or in patients with diabetes or cardiac disease due to increased risk of cardiac death
- not recommended in children or if patient weighs < 35 kg
- not recommended in those with liver or kidney impairment
- contraindicated in those with moderate-to-severe liver impairment, or with prolactin-releasing pituitary tumours (prolactinoma), where stimulation of gastric motility may be dangerous such as GIT haemorrhage or obstruction, or in those with QT prolongation, cardiac disease or significant electrolyte disturbance

Patient teaching and advice

- advise patient to take domperidone 2 hours apart from any antacid or antisecretory preparation
- warn patients not to drive or operate machinery if they experience dizziness or somnolence
- instruct patient to seek medical advice immediately if any of the following occur:
  - uncontrollable face, leg or arm movements, excessive trembling, unusual muscle stiffness or spasm
  - fast or irregular heart rate
  - swelling of hands, ankles or feet
  - unusual milk secretion from breast, breast enlargement, breast tenderness or pain, irregular or absent menstruation, decreased sex drive
- see also General Patient teaching and advice (p. xxvii)

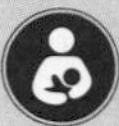

not used during pregnancy or breastfeeding unless the expected benefit outweighs any potential risk

tablets can be dispersed in water or crushed and mixed with water, or spoonful of yoghurt or apple puree

METOCLOPRAMIDE HYDROCHLORIDE MONOHYDRATE (METOCLOPRAMIDE HYDROCHLORIDE) (Emexlon, Maxolon, Metoclopramide Injection, Pramin)

Available forms

Tablets: 10 mg; Ampoules: 10 mg/2 mL

Action

- prokinetic agent with dopamine antagonistic actions
- stimulates the motility of the upper GIT without affecting gastric, biliary or pancreatic secretions
- increases rate of gastric emptying by enhancing peristalsis, thereby accelerating intestinal transit time
- increases resting tone of lower oesophageal sphincter
- little or no effect on colon or gallbladder activity
- increases prolactin secretion and circulating aldosterone levels (transient)
- effective within 1–3 minutes (IV), 10–15 minutes (IM) or 30–60 minutes (oral); duration 1–2 hours, half-life 2.5–5 hours (increased to about 15 hours in those with kidney impairment)

Use

- controls nausea and vomiting in most cases, except for motion sickness or other labyrinth disturbances
- adjunct to radiological examination of stomach and duodenum
- facilitates and accelerates introduction of tubes or biopsy capsules into small intestine
- enhances absorption of a range of drugs, including aspirin in a migraine attack (given IM 10 minutes before aspirin)
- after gastric surgery for gastric retention
- assists with intestinal intubation
- mild-to-moderate diabetic gastroparesis

Dose

- (nausea/vomiting) 10 mg orally, slow IV over 1–2 minutes or IM 1–3 times daily **OR**
- (diagnostic purpose) 10–20 mg slow IV over 1–2 minutes or IM 5–10 minutes before examination

Adverse effects

- restlessness, drowsiness, lassitude, fatigue, insomnia, headache, dizziness
- nausea, constipation or diarrhoea
- extrapyramidal reactions (e.g. dystonic type, such as facial muscle spasm, trismus, oculogyric crises, increase in muscle tone, hyperextension/spasticity of head, neck and back) (dystonic reactions are more common in children and young adults)
- tardive dyskinesia (especially in the elderly on long-term therapy)
- hypertensive crisis (if patient has phaeochromocytoma)
- raised prolactin levels, galactorrhoea, breast enlargement
- (rare) Parkinsonian symptoms (new or exacerbated, including tremor, rigidity, akinesia, bradykinesia), methaemoglobinaemia
- (very rare) neuroleptic malignant syndrome, acute depression, hypersensitivity, bradycardia, heart block
- (rapid IV) anxiety, agitation, restlessness, drowsiness

Interactions

- contraindicated or use with great caution with other agents known to cause extrapyramidal reactions such as phenothiazines
- not recommended with MAO inhibitors
- may prolong recovery time if given with suxamethonium
- may increase absorption of paracetamol, tetracyclines, alcohol, levodopa and controlled-release preparations of morphine
- may decrease absorption of digoxin, bromocriptine, cimetidine and penicillin
- may potentiate action of other CNS depressants, such as alcohol, barbiturates, anaesthetics, sedatives, hypnotics, opioid analgesics or tranquillisers
- effects on GI motility are antagonised by anticholinergic agents and opioid analgesics
- may increase bioavailability of ciclosporin, therefore ciclosporin blood levels should be closely monitored to prevent toxicity
- increased risk of neuroleptic malignant syndrome and extrapyramidal symptoms if given with phenothiazines
- increased risk of neurotoxicity if given with lithium
- may increase plasma levels of diazepam
- diabetic control may be affected because the rate of food absorption will be altered, necessitating an adjustment in dose and/or time of insulin

Nursing points/Cautions

- cause of vomiting should be identified before treatment. If vomiting persists despite therapy, patient should be reassessed to exclude underlying causes, such as cerebral irritation
- treatment should not be longer than 5 days
- should be withheld for 3–4 days post GI surgery (e.g. pyloroplasty, anastomosis) as wound healing may be inhibited by vigorous muscular contraction
- extrapyramidal reaction (see Glossary) may not develop if drug is stopped when the early sign of fine vermicular (worm-like) movements of the tongue occurs
- extrapyramidal reactions usually occur within 36 hours of starting and cease within 24 hours of stopping therapy. Patient should be closely observed if this occurs
- acute dystonic reactions may occur after a single dose, especially in children and young adults
- tardive dyskinesia may occur after therapy has been stopped and risk is greatest in elderly females on high-dose therapy
- compatible with morphine or pethidine when mixed in the same syringe, if the resultant solution is used within 15 minutes and there is no precipitation
- see manufacturer's instructions for compatibility with cytotoxic and other agents
- slow IV administration over 1–2 minutes is advised to prevent intense feeling of anxiety, restlessness and drowsiness (transient)
- if given as IV infusion, should be diluted in 50 mL and administered over 15 minutes. Suitable fluids include glucose 5%, sodium chloride 0.9%, Hartmann's solution and Ringer's solution
- discard any ampoules showing yellow discolouration
- caution if used in those with prior history of depression, breast cancer, impaired kidney or liver function or Parkinson's disease
- caution if used in those with hypertension

- not recommended in those under 20 (because of increased risk of dystonic reactions), except for severe intractable vomiting of known cause, to aid with GI intubation or vomiting associated with radiotherapy and intolerance to cytotoxic agents
- contraindicated in those with phaeochromocytoma (due to risk of hypertensive crisis), where increase in GI motility may be dangerous (e.g. obstructed or perforated bowel), in those with epilepsy or porphyria or in those with known sensitivity to procaine due to possible cross-sensitivity

Patient teaching and advice

- warn patient against driving a vehicle or operating machinery if drowsy or dizzy
- patient should be instructed to seek medical advice promptly if any of the following occur:
  - nausea and vomiting persist despite therapy
  - fast heartbeat
  - uncontrolled or repeated movements (such as darting tongue, chewing movement, uncontrolled movement of legs or arms), muscle spasm, upturned eyes, locked jaw or shuffling walk
  - sudden increase in body temperature
- advise patient to avoid using alcohol during therapy
- see also General Patient teaching and advice (p. xxvii)

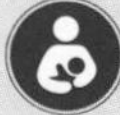

not recommended during pregnancy or breastfeeding unless the expected benefit outweighs any potential risk

tablets can be crushed and mixed with water, or spoonful of yoghurt or apple puree

Note

- contained in Anagraine and Metomax with paracetamol for migraine treatment

PROCHLORPERAZINE (Stemetil suppository)

PROCHLORPERAZINE MALEATE (Nausetil, Nausrelief, Procalm, Stemetil, Stemzine)

PROCHLORPERAZINE MESILATE (Stemetil Solution for Injection)

Available forms

Tablets: 5 mg; Suppositories: 5 mg, 25 mg; Ampoules: 12.5 mg/mL

Action

- centrally acting phenothiazine that has antidopamine actions, antagonises alpha-adrenoreceptors, blocks noradrenaline reuptake and has weak anticholinergic, antihistamine and antiserotonin actions
- has an effect on temperature control and blocks conditioned avoidance response
- less sedating than chlorpromazine
- half-life about 24 hours

Use

- nausea and vomiting
- vertigo, labyrinthitis

Dose

- (nausea and vomiting) 12.5 mg deep IM or 25 mg rectal suppository, then 6 hours later 5–10 mg orally 2–3 times daily if required **OR**
- (nausea and vomiting) 5–10 mg orally 2–3 times daily **OR**
- (acute nausea) 20 mg orally, followed by 10 mg 2 hours later if necessary **OR**
- (vertigo) 5–10 mg orally 3–4 times daily reduced gradually over several weeks to 5–10 mg daily

Adverse effects

- constipation, dry mouth
- drowsiness, akathisia, extrapyramidal reactions (Parkinsonian type), blurred vision, tardive dyskinesia
- urinary retention/hesitancy
- endocrine disturbances (including breast enlargement, breast tenderness or pain, irregular menstruation, amenorrhoea), decreased libido
- very serious acute dystonic reactions in children
- (IV) hypotension
- (IM) postural hypotension with tachycardia, local pain, nodule formation
- (rare) neuroleptic malignant syndrome, prolongation of QT interval, ECG changes, photosensitivity, hyperglycaemia, blood dyscrasias

Interactions

- caution if used with other agents known to prolong QT interval, induce bradycardia or cause hypokalaemia
- may increase hypotensive effects of most antihypertensive agents, especially alpha-adrenergic blocking agents
- high dose may decrease response to hypoglycaemic agents
- may increase serum levels of amitriptyline increasing risk of adverse effects
- may lower convulsive threshold, therefore antiepileptic dose may need adjustment
- use with propranolol may result in increased serum levels of both drugs
- may induce transient metabolic encephalopathy (loss of consciousness for 48–72 hours) when given simultaneously with desferrioxamine
- thiazide diuretics may accentuate orthostatic hypotension
- not recommended with levodopa, clonidine, adrenaline or neuroleptic agents
- CNS depressant effects are enhanced by alcohol and other depressant drugs
- may potentiate anticholinergic effects of TCAs and atropine-like drugs
- use with procarbazine may result in the potentiation of extrapyramidal side-effects
- may result in increased and/or impaired phenytoin metabolism if given together, therefore phenytoin levels should be closely monitored during therapy
- may diminish effects of oral anticoagulants, therefore INR should be closely monitored
- caution if used with other antipsychotic agents
- absorption may be decreased if given with lithium, anti-Parkinson's agents and antacids
- increased risk of neurotoxicity if given with lithium
- increased risk of agranulocytosis if given with carbamazepine or myelosuppressive agents

Nursing points/Cautions

- blood counts should be monitored regularly during prolonged therapy
- acute dystonic reactions should be managed with benztropine IM immediately
- extrapyramidal reaction (see Glossary) may not develop if drug is stopped when the early sign of fine vermicular (worm-like) movements of the tongue occurs
- should be stopped immediately if tardive dyskinesia symptoms occur
- do not use darkened solution (more than pale yellow)
- not normally mixed in the same syringe with other drugs, but is compatible with morphine or pethidine when mixed in the same syringe, if the resultant solution is used within 15 minutes and there is no precipitation
- (solution) avoid contact with skin to prevent sensitisation occurring

- response may be delayed in those with schizophrenia
- not given to children aged under 2 years or weighing less than 10 kg as they are at greater risk of extrapyramidal symptoms
- caution if used in the elderly due to risk of hypotension, sedation and/or extrapyramidal reactions
- caution if used with spinal anaesthesia because hypotension may occur
- caution if used in those with liver impairment, epilepsy or history of seizures, urinary dysfunction, constipation or acute narrow angle glaucoma
- caution if used in those with hypoparathyroidism because of increased risk of dystonic reactions
- caution if used in those with congenital or acquired prolongation of QT interval
- caution if used in those with risk factors for stroke or thromboembolism
- not recommended in those with history of agranulocytosis or narrow angle glaucoma
- not recommended in those with kidney impairment, hypothyroidism, Parkinson's disease, dementia, phaeochromocytoma, prostatic hypertrophy, cardiac failure or myasthenia gravis
- contraindicated in those with CNS depression (e.g. coma, drug intoxication), circulatory collapse, bone marrow depression or previous hypersensitivity to other phenothiazines due to the possibility of cross-sensitivity

Patient teaching and advice

- advise patient to take antacids 2 hours apart from therapy
- warn patient against driving a vehicle or operating machinery if blurred vision, drowsiness, dizziness or light-headedness occur
- if patient has diabetes mellitus, careful monitoring of blood glucose levels should be suggested as they may become erratic
- advise patient to avoid alcohol during therapy as dizziness or light-headedness may worsen
- instruct patient to avoid exposure to sun or wear long-sleeved garments and SPF 30+ sunscreen during therapy as skin may be more sensitive to sun
- warn patient to keep cool in hot weather and warm in cool weather and avoid swimming in cold water as temperature regulation may be affected
- instruct patient in correct suppository insertion technique (see General Patient teaching and advice for NSAIDs, p. 14)
- advise patient to immediately seek medical advice if any of the following occur:
  - muscle spasm or unusual trembling, uncontrolled movements of tongue, face, mouth and jaw, rigid posture, twitching or restlessness
  - sudden increase in body temperature
  - unexplained fever or infection
  - fitting (seizures)
  - unusual milk secretion from breast, breast enlargement, breast tenderness or pain, irregular or absent menstruation, decreased libido

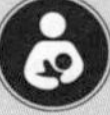

high doses of phenothiazines used late in pregnancy may cause jaundice, hyperreflexia, hyporeflexia or prolonged extrapyramidal symptoms in the newborn, therefore not used during pregnancy or breastfeeding unless the expected benefit outweighs any potential risk

tablets can be dispersed in water or crushed and mixed with water, or spoonful of yoghurt or apple puree

OTHER ANTIEMETIC AGENTS

CYCLIZINE HYDROCHLORIDE (Nausicalm)

CYCLIZINE LACTATE (Valoid)

Available forms

Ampoule: 50 mg/mL; Tablets: 50 mg

Action

- piperazine antihistamine (H_1 receptor antagonist) with anticholinergic and antiemetic actions
- half-life about 14 hours

Use

- postoperative nausea and vomiting
- prevention and treatment of motion sickness

Dose

- (treatment of postoperative nausea and vomiting) 50 mg IV up to 3 times daily (for up to 48 hours) **OR**
- (prevention of postoperative nausea and vomiting) 50 mg IV 20 minutes before end of surgery **OR**
- (prevention and treatment of motion sickness) 50 mg orally 6–8-hourly starting 1–2 hours before anticipated travel (daily maximum 150 mg)

Adverse effects

- (anticholinergic side-effects) dry mouth, nose and throat, constipation, urinary retention, blurred vision, tachycardia, asthenia, somnolence, headache, drowsiness, oculogyric crisis
- extrapyramidal symptoms
- (IV site) erythema, pain, thrombophlebitis and (rarely) chills, pruritus, heavy sensation
- (rare) transient paralysis, decreased consciousness, blood dyscrasias, liver dysfunction, jaundice

Interactions

- may increase effects of alcohol and CNS depressants such as hypnotics, opioid analgesics, anaesthetics and tranquillisers
- may enhance side-effects of other anticholinergic agents if given together
- antiemetic effect may be decreased if given with atropine
- caution if given with aminoglycosides due to risk of masking ototoxicity

Nursing points/Cautions

- should be given within 24 hours of surgery for best effect. For prophylaxis, first dose should be given 20 minutes before anticipated end of surgery
- patient should be carefully observed for any signs of limb paralysis which may occur within minutes of administration and usually resolves within hours of stopping medication
- (motion sickness) not recommended for longer than 48 hours
- (motion sickness) not recommended in children under 12 years
- caution if used in those with neuromuscular disorders, asthma, chronic obstructive pulmonary disease, urinary retention or obstruction, prostatic hypertrophy, closed angle glaucoma, untreated intra-ocular hypertension, uncontrolled open angle glaucoma, GI obstructive disorder, phaeochromocytoma, liver disease, hypertension or epilepsy
- not recommended in those with porphyria
- contraindicated in those with sensitivity to other piperazines or with severe heart failure, acute myocardial infarction or acute alcohol intoxication

Patient teaching and advice

- advise patient to avoid alcohol during therapy

- patient should be advised to be careful when getting out of bed or going from bed to chair to prevent dizziness occurring
- patient should be warned not to drive or operate machinery if somnolence or drowsiness occur
- (motion sickness) patient should be advised to take tablet 1–2 hours before anticipated travel
- see General Patient teaching and advice (p. xxvii)

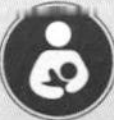

not recommended during pregnancy and breastfeeding

tablet is difficult to crush and does not disperse in water. If crushed, can be given with spoonful of yoghurt or apple puree

ANTIEPILEPTICS

A *seizure* is a 'transient alteration of behaviour due to the disordered synchronous and rhythmic firing of populations of brain neurons' while *epilepsy* is considered to be a condition in which a person has recurrent seizures due to a chronic underlying aetiology, suggesting that a single seizure or recurrent seizures due to correctable causes (e.g. induced by medication or biochemical abnormalities) does not mean the person has epilepsy (Lowenstein 2019; Ropper et al 2019).

Seizures are classified as:

- *generalised*, and include absence (either typical or atypical), tonic–clonic (grand mal), clonic, tonic, atonic or myoclonic seizures. Generalised seizures involve both hemispheres and may result from cellular, biochemical or structural abnormalities of the brain (Lowenstein 2019).
- *focal* (previously known as partial) seizures start at a particular focus and do not spread beyond one hemisphere and may be associated with structural brain abnormalities. Focal seizures can further be described as having intact or impaired awareness, motor or non-motor onset and can develop into a generalised seizure (Lowenstein 2019).
- *unclassifiable* or *unknown onset* seizures are those that cannot easily be classified as generalised or focal (Lowenstein 2019).
- *status epilepticus* is a life-threatening medical emergency in which there is no regaining of consciousness between seizures (i.e. the seizures are continuous for at least 30 minutes) and may be caused by non-adherence with antiepileptic medications, cerebral irritation, CNS tumours or infection, trauma, hypoglycaemia or low blood levels of calcium. First-line treatment is usually fast-acting benzodiazepines (e.g. diazepam, clonazepam, midazolam), followed by long-acting antiepileptic (e.g. phenytoin, phenobarbital (phenobarbitone), sodium valproate) (Bryant et al 2019).

Antiepileptics (also known as anticonvulsants) are required to control primary recurrent seizures. The ideal antiepileptic agent is one that is highly effective, with low toxicity; is inexpensive; controls a number of seizure types without adverse effects, such as sedation; does not interact with other medications; is long acting and does not result in the development of tolerance. Unfortunately, such an agent does not exist, with current antiepileptic agents failing to control seizures completely or having adverse effects that range from unwanted (e.g. drowsiness, nausea) to severe (e.g. liver failure, blood dyscrasias) (Bryant et al 2019).

Selection of a particular antiepileptic medication is generally determined by the type of seizure. For example, phenytoin and carbamazepine are considered first-line drugs for generalised tonic–clonic seizures, whereas sodium valproate is used for myoclonic seizures. Other factors which may need to be considered in choosing an epileptic agent include age, sex, other medications, other medical or psychiatric conditions, and kidney and liver function (Lowenstein 2019; Ropper et al 2019). Therapy usually commences as a single drug (monotherapy), the dose of which is increased gradually until seizure activity is controlled or adverse reactions become unacceptable to the patient. Combination therapy (consisting of two or more antiepileptic drugs) is required in people who are refractory to treatment or who have two or more types of seizures (Lowenstein 2019; Ropper et al 2019). It is important that plasma drug concentrations are measured at the start of therapy, when doses are adjusted, if therapeutic effect is not achieved or toxic adverse effects appear or if multiple drug therapy is initiated (Bryant et al 2019).

Antiepileptic therapy is usually continued until a person has been seizure-free for 2–3 years (Bryant et al 2019); however, some patients continue to have seizures despite treatment due to pharmacoresistance (defined as failure to control seizure despite adequate doses of two antiepileptic agents). In some patients, seizures may recur after ceasing antiepileptic agents. Risk factors for recurrence include age of seizure onset (i.e. after 12 years of age), family history, abnormal EEG despite therapy, total number of seizures, taking 2–6 years to achieve seizure control or presence of mental retardation or organic neurological disorder/s (Bryant et al 2019).

General Adverse effects of antiepileptics

- drowsiness, dizziness, headache, fatigue, somnolence, insomnia, asthenia, vertigo
- ataxia, gait or balance disturbance, muscle weakness
- nausea, vomiting
- rash
- diplopia, blurred vision, nystagmus
- confusion, hostility, irritation, nervousness, anxiety, tremor, aggressiveness, hyperactivity, inability to concentrate, memory impairment, depression, sleep disturbances including night terrors, disorientation, transient amnesia
- increased seizure activity
- (rare) suicidal ideation

General Nursing points/Cautions for antiepileptics

- changing from one antiepileptic agent to another should be done gradually because sudden withdrawal may precipitate seizures
- some antiepileptic agents require regular monitoring of blood levels. This is especially recommended if there is any increase in seizure activity, during pregnancy, in children or adolescents, if there is a suspected malabsorption disorder, or if the patient's adherence to therapy is questionable
- many antiepileptics increase the risk of suicidal thoughts or behaviours, and patients should therefore be

closely monitored for any signs of depression, suicidal thoughts or behaviour, or any changes in mood or behaviour
- tolerance, physical and psychological dependence may occur with barbiturates
- drug withdrawal should be gradual to prevent provoking withdrawal seizure and patients should be cautioned about abruptly stopping medication
- patients may be discontinued from antiepileptics if they have been seizure-free for 2–3 years
- long-term antiepileptic therapy has been associated with decreased folate levels, therefore folic acid supplements (5 mg daily) are recommended 4 weeks before and for the first 12 weeks of pregnancy to decrease the risk of spina bifida in the fetus

General Patient teaching and advice for antiepileptics

- instruct patients to immediately report any changes in seizure activity (either frequency or severity). Encourage patient to keep a diary documenting seizure activity, including triggers and medication
- patient should be advised to be aware of and try to avoid (if possible) seizure triggers, such as poor nutrition, lack of sleep, excess alcohol, fever, stress, bright lights (especially flashing and strobe), or changes in levels of fluids, electrolytes and hormones. Some drugs are also known to provoke seizures or reduce the seizure threshold
- many antiepileptic agents cause drowsiness, dizziness, vertigo, blurred or double vision and impaired concentration. Patients should therefore be advised of the dangers of driving or operating machinery while these adverse effects are occurring. Many of these adverse effects are transient and occur at the start of therapy
- advise patient that fatigue, amnesia and muscle weakness are transient and generally disappear with ongoing therapy
- warn patient about reduced tolerance to alcohol. Alcohol intake can also result in increased/decreased serum antiepileptic agent levels (depending on acute or chronic intake) and should therefore be avoided during therapy
- many antiepileptic agents interact with other medications (prescription and non-prescription), therefore it is important that the patient is advised not to start or stop any medication without first consulting his/her doctor
- instruct patients to continue therapy and not stop medication abruptly (as this may provoke withdrawal symptoms, including increased seizure activity). Non-adherence to medications may be a particular issue with adolescent patients who may be struggling with having a chronic condition requiring ongoing medications (and wanting to appear normal in the eyes of their peers)
- ensure the patient understands the importance of keeping follow-up appointments, blood tests and any other examinations required during therapy
- it is important that the person discusses driving with his/her doctor so that they have a full understanding

of the requirements to hold a driver's licence, including the need for an annual medical review. Requirements vary depending on the type of seizure/epilepsy the person has and whether the person requires a private or commercial licence. For example, a conditional licence may be granted to a person who is treated for the first time with antiepileptics if he/she has been treated for at least 6 months, with no seizure for the preceding 6 months or if a seizure occurred after the start of therapy only in the first 6 months and not in the last 6 months (Austroads 2017)
- emphasise the importance of seeking medical advice if any of the following occur:
  - rash or skin reactions
  - changes in mood or behaviour, including aggression, hostility, anger, anxiety or nervousness
  - sleep disturbances
  - signs of depression, thoughts of self-harm or harm to others, or thoughts of suicide. This should also be discussed with family members, carers or significant others
- many antiepileptic agents interact with hormonal contraceptives. Female patients should be warned that breakthrough bleeding can occur and an alternative method of contraception should be used
- advise female patients that seizure activity may increase during menstruation
- women of childbearing potential should be counselled regarding the risks of using antiepileptic agents when pregnant versus the risks to the fetus of uncontrolled epilepsy. This pregnancy counselling and planning should occur on diagnosis (in an adult). Uncontrolled epilepsy is a greater danger to both mother and fetus than is the risk of having an abnormal child as a result of taking antiepileptic agents. The risk of fetal abnormalities in a mother taking antiepileptics is about three times that of the general population (Lander 2008). Taking more than one antiepileptic agent increases the risk of fetal abnormalities, therefore monotherapy at the lowest dose to control seizure activity is recommended. Fetal malformations due to the older antiepileptic agents, such as phenytoin, carbamazepine and sodium valproate, are well documented. However, long-term studies involving the newer agents have not been carried out and therefore the longer term risks are not well known (e.g. those adverse effects which might emerge in childhood) (Bryant et al 2019)
- supplementation with folic acid is advised if a woman is planning pregnancy, with 5 mg daily recommended 4–12 weeks before conception and for first 12 weeks of pregnancy to reduce the risk of spina bifida
- see General Patient teaching and advice (p. xxvii)

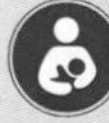

some antiepileptic agents have been associated with coagulation defects, with haemorrhage risk in the fetus and newborn, which may be prevented by giving vitamin K prophylactically to the mother before delivery

most antiepileptic agents are excreted in breastmilk, but at low levels (except phenobarbital (phenobarbitone)); therefore breastfeeding is not recommended

ACETAZOLAMIDE (Diamox, Glaumox Powder for Injection)

Available forms
Tablets: 250 mg; Vial: 500 mg

Action
- non-bacterial sulfonamide derivative that inhibits the action of carbonic anhydrase
- appears to retard abnormal, paroxysmal excessive discharge from CNS neurons
- decreases secretion of aqueous humour, thereby reducing intraocular pressure
- increases bicarbonate excretion in the renal tubules and consequently sodium, potassium and water excretion, resulting in an alkaline diuresis

Use
- some types of epilepsy (absence (petit mal) and unlocalised seizures)
- adjunctive treatment in chronic simple (open angle) glaucoma, secondary glaucoma and preoperatively in acute closed-angle glaucoma (see Antiglaucoma agents, p. 455)
- cardiac and drug-induced oedema, oedema associated with altitude sickness (see Diuretics, p. 1012)

Dose
- (epilepsy) 250–1000 mg orally or IV daily in divided doses (alone or with other antiepileptic agents)

Adverse effects
- (IV site) pain
- see Adverse effects of acetazolamide in Diuretics (p. 1012)

Interactions
- not recommended with other carbonic anhydrase inhibitors
- see also Interactions of acetazolamide in Diuretics (p. 1012)

Nursing points/Cautions
- if used with other antiepileptic agents, dose should be started at 250 mg daily and increased slowly
- reconstitute powder using at least 5 mL of water for injections and administer IV
- IV route should only be used short term until oral route is available
- see also Nursing points/Cautions for acetazolamide in Diuretics (p. 1013)

Patient teaching and advice
- see General Patient teaching and advice for antiepileptics (p. 383)

banned in sport

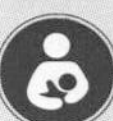

not recommended during pregnancy, especially during first trimester

caution if used during breastfeeding

tablet can be crushed and mixed with water or spoonful of yoghurt or apple puree. Chocolate syrup can be used to mask bitter taste

BRIVARACETAM (Brivact)

Available forms
Vial: 50 mg/5 mL; Tablets: 25 mg, 50 mg, 75 mg, 100 mg; Oral solution: 10 mg/mL

Action
- antiepileptic action unclear, but thought to be related to selective affinity for synaptic vesicle protein 2A in the brain
- half-life 9 hours

Use
- as adjunctive therapy of partial-onset seizures (with or without secondary generalisation) in those aged 4 years and over

Dose
- initially 50 mg orally or IV twice daily, increasing in increments of 50 mg per day every 2 weeks if needed (dose range 50–200 mg daily)

Adverse effects

- diarrhoea, constipation, upper abdominal pain, toothache, decreased appetite, weight increase/decrease
- hyponatraemia
- myalgia, back pain, pain in extremities
- nasopharyngitis, upper respiratory tract infection, flu-like symptoms, cough, dyspnoea
- paraesthesia
- pruritus, eczema
- (IV) infusion site pain
- (rare) hypersensitivity (bronchospasm and angioedema)
- see also General Adverse effects of antiepileptic agents (p. 382)

Interactions

- serum levels may be decreased if given with rifampicin
- may increase serum levels of carbamazepine epoxide (active metabolite of carbamazepine)
- may decrease serum levels of carbamazepine, phenobarbital and phenytoin
- may increase effects of alcohol and are therefore not recommended together

Nursing points/Cautions

- (IV) may be administered as an IV bolus undiluted or diluted with sodium chloride 0.9% or glucose 5% and given over 15 minutes
- not recommended in those with end-stage kidney disease undergoing dialysis
- caution if used in those with liver impairment. Daily dose should not exceed 150 mg in two divided doses
- see also General Nursing points/Cautions for antiepileptics (p. 382)

Patient teaching and advice

- (IV) warn patient that bitter taste may be experienced after IV administration
- (oral solution) ensure patient understands how to use adaptor/syringe for oral solution, including:
  1. press cap down and turn it clockwise to open bottle
  2. separate adapter from the syringe (both provided with oral solution)
  3. adaptor should be inserted into neck of bottle, ensuring it is well fitted
  4. insert syringe into adaptor opening and turn bottle upside down
  5. fill syringe with a small amount of solution by pulling piston down, then push piston upwards to remove any air bubbles
  6. pull piston down to graduation mark that corresponds to dose in mL (as prescribed by doctor)
  7. turn bottle right way up and remove syringe from adaptor
  8. empty contents of syringe into glass of water and drink immediately
  9. close solution bottle with cap
  10. wash syringe with water only
  11. store at less than 30°C
- advise patient to seek medical advice if any of the following occur:
  - wheezing or difficulty breathing
  - swelling of face, lips, tongue or other body parts
  - rash, itching or hives on the skin
- see also General Patient teaching and advice for antiepileptics (p. 383)

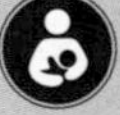

not recommended during pregnancy or breastfeeding unless benefit outweighs risk

oral solution available. Tablet can be crushed and mixed with water or spoonful of yoghurt or apple puree

CARBAMAZEPINE (Tegretol)

Available forms

Tablets: 100 mg, 200 mg; Tablets (controlled-release): 200 mg, 400 mg; Suspension: 100 mg/5 mL

Action

- antiepileptic, neurotrophic, psychotropic
- stabilises hyperexcited nerve membranes
- inhibits repetitive neuronal discharge
- reduces propagation of excitatory impulse
- anticholinergic, antidiuretic activity
- decreases turnover of dopamine and noradrenaline (psychotrophic (antimania) effects)
- active metabolite (carbamazepine-epoxide) (half-life 6 hours)
- half-life 16–24 hours (with repeated dosing)

Use

- generalised tonic–clonic (grand mal) epilepsy
- partial seizures (complex or simple) (with or without generalisation)
- mixed seizures (tonic–clonic and partial)
- trigeminal neuralgia, glossopharyngeal neuralgia
- mania, bipolar disorder (see Antipsychotic and mood stabilising agents, p. 780)

Dose

- (epilepsy) initially 100–200 mg orally once or twice daily with or after food, increasing gradually until optimal response is achieved (usually 400 mg 2–3 times daily) **OR**
- (neuralgia) initially 100–200 mg orally twice daily with or after food, increasing gradually for several days until pain is controlled, then reduced to a minimum effective level (maximum daily dose 1200 mg)

Adverse effects

- see General Adverse effects of antiepileptics (p. 382)
- dry mouth
- urticaria, allergic dermatitis
- leucopenia, thrombocytopenia, eosinophilia
- elevated liver enzymes
- oedema, fluid retention, increased weight, hyponatraemia, decreased blood osmolarity
- (rare) lens opacities, conjunctivitis, urinary frequency and retention, cholestatic hepatitis, folate deficiency
- (very rare) serious dermatological reactions, blood dyscrasias, hypersensitivity

Interactions

- contraindicated with or within 2 weeks of stopping MAOIs
- if given with aripiprazole, haloperidol, lithium, metoclopramide may lead to neurotoxicity
- may reduce tolerance to alcohol
- may decrease serum levels of albendazole, alprazolam, amitriptyline, apixaban, aprepitant, atorvastatin, buprenorphine, bupropion, citalopram, clobazam, clomipramine, clonazepam, clozapine, cyclophosphamide, ciclosporin, dabigatran, dexamethasone, digoxin, doxycycline, ethosuximide, everolimus, felodipine, haloperidol, imatinib, imipramine, indinavir, itraconazole, ivabradine, lapatinib, lamotrigine, levothyroxine, lovastatin, methadone, mianserin, midazolam, nortriptyline, olanzapine, oral contraceptives, oxcarbazepine, paliperidone, paracetamol, phenytoin, praziquantel, prednisolone, primidone, progesterone-containing products, quetiapine, rifabutin, risperidone, ritonavir, saquinavir, sertraline, simvastatin, sirolimus, sodium valproate, tacrolimus, tadalafil, theophylline, tiagabine, topiramate, tramadol, voriconazole, warfarin and ziprasidone

- serum levels may be increased by acetazolamide, antiviral protease inhibitors, clarithromycin, cimetidine, ciprofloxacin, dantrolene, danazol, dextropropoxyphene, diltiazem, erythromycin, fluconazole, fluoxetine, fluvoxamine, grapefruit juice, ibuprofen, isoniazid, itraconazole, loratadine, nicotinamide (high dose), olanzapine, omeprazole, oxybutynin, paroxetine, primidone, quetiapine, ritonavir, sodium valproate, ticlopidine, TCAs, verapamil, vigabatrin and voriconazole, resulting in adverse reactions
- serum levels may be decreased by aminophylline, barbiturates, cisplatin, clonazepam, doxorubicin, isotretinoin, oxcarbazepine, phenobarbital (phenobarbitone), phenytoin, primidone, rifampicin, sodium valproate, St John's wort and theophylline
- use with lamotrigine may result in carbamazepine toxicity, as well as decreasing serum levels of lamotrigine
- increased risk of toxicity if given with levetiracetam
- may decrease serum levels of hormonal contraceptives, increasing risk of bleeding
- hepatotoxicity may occur if given with isoniazid
- may increase metabolism of paracetamol, reducing its analgesic effects as well as increasing risk of hepatotoxicity due to increase in levels of hepatoxic metabolite
- may reduce serum levels of isotretinoin and other retinoids by increasing clearance
- may antagonise non-depolarising muscle relaxants (e.g. pancuronium)
- hyponatraemia may result if given with frusemide or hydrochlorothiazide. If given together, serum sodium levels should be measured before starting, after 2 weeks and monthly for 12 weeks during therapy
- may cause serotonin syndrome (see Glossary) if given with SSRI antidepressants
- may interfere with some serological tests

Nursing points/Cautions

- elderly patients may become confused or agitated and so will require close supervision
- full blood count (including serum iron) is recommended before starting therapy, then weekly for the first month, then monthly for the first year
- baseline and regular ophthalmological and liver function tests (especially in the elderly or those with liver impairment), complete urinalysis and blood urea nitrogen (BUN) are recommended
- absorption of suspension is faster than for tablets
- if change occurs from tablets to suspension, dose should remain the same, but frequency should be increased
- (neuralgia) large doses should be given as 3–4 divided doses
- (neuralgia) attempts to discontinue should be at intervals not more than 12 weeks as there may be periods of remission from the neuralgia
- caution if used in the elderly or others at risk of confusion, agitation or psychosis
- caution if used in those with pre-existing kidney conditions associated with low sodium or in those treated with sodium-lowering medications (e.g. diuretics). Sodium levels should be measured before starting therapy, after 2 weeks, then monthly for 3 months
- caution if used in those with glaucoma, urinary retention or prostatism (because of anticholinergic adverse effects)
- caution if used in those with mixed seizures as seizure activity may be exacerbated

- caution if used in those with history of cardiac, liver or kidney damage, previous interrupted course of carbamazepine or those who have had previous haematological reactions to other drugs
- caution if used in those with hypothyroidism as thyroid replacement therapy may need to be increased. Regular thyroid function monitoring is also recommended
- caution if used in those with genetic risk of severe dermatological reactions, including those from Japan, Southern India, Indigenous Americans, Asia (Philippines, Thailand, Malaysia, Hong Kong, Taiwan, North China), or of Hispanic or Arabic descent. Genetic testing for specific gene is recommended (if available) and not recommended in those with HLA-A*3101 or HLA-B*1502 allele positive
- suspension contains parahydroxybenzoates, which can cause allergic reactions, and also sorbitol, and therefore should not be given to those with hereditary fructose intolerance
- cross-hypersensitivity can occur with primidone, phenobarbital, phenytoin, oxcarbazepine and carbamazepine
- contraindicated in those with systemic lupus erythematosus (SLE), porphyria, bone marrow depression or liver failure
- see General Nursing points/Cautions for antiepileptics (p. 382)

Patient teaching and advice

- sustained/controlled-release tablets should be swallowed whole (not crushed or chewed), but those which are scored may be halved
- advise patient to shake suspension well before administration
- patient should be warned to avoid grapefruit and grapefruit juice during therapy
- advise patient against taking paracetamol for a prolonged period during therapy
- patient should be advised to seek medical advice immediately if any of the following occur:
  - flu-like symptoms (e.g. fever, sore throat, swollen glands, aching joints, lack of energy)
  - frequent infections including fever, chills, sore throat or mouth ulcers
  - persistent nausea and vomiting, loss of appetite, generally feeling unwell
  - easy bruising or bleeding
  - lethargy, vomiting, headache, confusion
  - rash or other skin lesions
- patient should be advised to have regular ophthalmological examinations
- see General Patient teaching and advice for antiepileptics (p. 383)

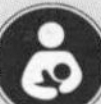

associated with spina bifida, hypospadias, craniofacial defects, cardiovascular malformations, fingernail hypoplasia and developmental disability. May also cause coagulation defects leading to the risk of fetal haemorrhage, which may be prevented by prophylactic administration of vitamin K to the mother before delivery. May also cause neonatal withdrawal syndrome (vomiting, diarrhoea and/or reduced feeding), as well as seizures and/or respiratory depression

secreted in breastmilk, therefore use with great caution and observe the newborn for skin reaction, including jaundice or excessive sleepiness

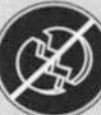

Controlled-release tablets should not be crushed, chewed or broken

oral liquid available. Plain tablet can be dispersed in water or crushed and mixed with flavoured syrup.

CLONAZEPAM (Paxam, Rivotril)

Available forms

Tablets: 0.5 mg, 2 mg; Suspension: 2.5 mg/mL; Ampoule: 1 mg/mL

Action

- benzodiazepine closely related to nitrazepam, with antiepileptic, sedative and muscle relaxant properties
- long half-life (31–47 hours)
- tolerance may occur after 4–24 weeks, leading to increase in seizure frequency

Use

- status epilepticus (IV)
- generalised epilepsy (myoclonic, akinetic, tonic, tonic–clonic)
- partial epilepsy (including psychomotor seizures)

Dose

- initially 0.5 mg orally twice daily, then 4–8 mg in 3–4 divided doses as maintenance (daily maximum 20 mg) **OR**
- (status epilepticus) 1 mg by slow IV injection over 2–4 minutes or IV infusion at 0.25–0.5 mg/min, repeated IV or IV infusion until status is controlled (maximum 10 mg)

Adverse effects

- see General Adverse effects of antiepileptics (p. 382)
- ankle/face oedema
- dyspepsia, increased appetite, constipation, dysphagia
- hirsutism
- leucopenia, eosinophilia, anaemia
- dysuria, nocturia, enuresis, urinary retention
- double vision (high dose or long-term therapy)
- shortness of breath, respiratory depression
- transient amnesia
- hypersalivation (especially in infants and children)
- bronchial hypersecretions
- (IV) respiratory depression, tachycardia, palpitations
- (IV) thrombophlebitis
- dependence, tolerance, withdrawal syndrome on stopping therapy suddenly, abuse potential
- (rare) paradoxical reactions (agitation, nervousness, hostility, anxiety, sleep and dream disturbance, rage, excitement), hypotension, cardiac failure, thrombocytopenia

Interactions

- CNS depressant effects enhanced by alcohol
- may enhance effects of other CNS depressant drugs such as other antiepileptic agents, barbiturates, antipsychotic agents, anaesthetics, sedatives, hypnotics, lithium, TCAs, antihistamines, opioid analgesics, MAOIs
- serum levels may be decreased by phenytoin, phenobarbital (phenobarbitone), sodium valproate, lamotrigine and carbamazepine
- serum levels may be increased by cimetidine and disulfiram
- may decrease serum levels of carbamazepine
- may increase or decrease serum levels of phenytoin
- may increase anticholinergic effects of antihistamines, some antidepressants and atropine-like drugs
- if given with sodium valproate may produce absence seizures

Nursing points/Cautions

- clonazepam can be absorbed by PVC, therefore glass containers should be used, or if PVC infusion bags are used, the mixture should be infused immediately at greater than 60 mL/hour and short tubing used
- BP and respiratory rate should be monitored continually during IV administration

- blood counts and liver function should be monitored if therapy is longer than 4 weeks
- only large vessels should be used for IV administration to avoid thrombophlebitis
- contents of ampoule to be mixed thoroughly with supplied diluent
- IV infusion prepared by diluting 3 mg in 250 mL of sodium chloride 0.9%, glucose 5% or 10% or sodium chloride 0.45% plus glucose 2.5%
- not compatible with sodium bicarbonate as precipitation will occur
- regular blood counts and liver function tests are recommended in those with impaired liver or kidney function
- changes in behaviour (e.g. agitation, hostility, anxiety) suggestive of paradoxical reaction may require withdrawal of drug
- tablets contain lactose and are therefore not recommended in those with rare hereditary problems of galactose intolerance, Lapp lactase deficiency or glucose–galactose malabsorption
- ampoules contain benzyl alcohol and may lead to irreversible brain damage in newborn infants, so should be avoided unless no alternative is available
- in the case of overdosage, flumazenil should be given with extreme caution as it may provoke seizures
- suspension contains lactose and therefore not recommended in those with galactose intolerance
- caution if used in those with mild-to-moderate liver impairment. Lowest dose possible should be prescribed
- caution if used in the elderly (because of the increased risk of falls) or those with a predisposition to hypotension, glaucoma, myasthenia gravis, respiratory depression, ataxia, blood dyscrasias, kidney impairment or porphyria
- not recommended in those with pre-existing depression, psychosis, schizophrenia, spinal or cerebellar ataxia or sleep apnoea
- contraindicated in those with hypersensitivity to benzodiazepines, alcohol/drug dependency (or history), COPD (with developing respiratory failure) or severe liver impairment
- see General Nursing points/Cautions for antiepileptics (p. 382)

Patient teaching and advice

- see General Patient teaching and advice for antiepileptics (p. 383)
- advise patient that tablet is scored if half or quarter tablet is required
- (suspension) suspension is recommended for infants
- suspension is delivered via dropper (1 drop = 0.1 mg clonazepam). Instruct patient (or parent/carer) to use supplied dropper to measure dose and deliver onto spoon (not directly into mouth)

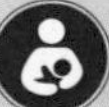

clonazepam is a benzodiazepine and if given during pregnancy may result in hypotonia, respiratory depression and hypothermia of the newborn. The newborn may also display signs of withdrawal symptoms

not recommended during breastfeeding as it may cause drowsiness and feeding difficulties

suspension available. Tablet can be dispersed in 5–20 mL water or crushed and mixed with spoonful of apple puree

ETHOSUXIMIDE (Zarontin)

Available forms

Capsules: 250 mg; Suspension: 250 mg/5 mL

Action

- succinimide that may depress the motor cortex and elevate convulsive threshold, reducing frequency of seizures

Use
- simple partial (petit mal) epilepsy

Dose
- initially 20–30 mg/kg orally given in 2 divided doses, increasing by 250 mg every 4–7 days until control is achieved with minimal side-effects (daily maximum 1.5 g)

Adverse effects
- see General Adverse effects of antiepileptics (p. 382)
- anorexia, cramps, diarrhoea, epigastric pain, upper abdominal pain, weight loss, gum hypertrophy, tongue swelling
- hiccups
- urticaria
- blood dyscrasias
- (rare) SLE, myopia, vaginal bleeding, hirsutism, hypersensitivity, serious skin reactions, haematuria, psychosis, increased libido, liver and kidney impairment

Interactions
- serum levels may be altered if given with sodium valproate
- may increase phenytoin serum levels

Nursing points/Cautions
- doses greater than 1.5 g/ day in divided doses only administered under strict medical supervision
- be aware of the possibility of increased frequency of tonic–clonic (grand mal) seizures when ethosuximide is used alone in mixed types of epilepsy
- full blood count weekly for the first month, then monthly for the first year
- regular urinalysis and liver function tests are recommended during therapy
- caution if used in those with blood dyscrasias, liver or kidney impairment
- contraindicated in those with hypersensitivity to succinimides
- see General Nursing points/Cautions for antiepileptics (p. 382)

Patient teaching and advice
- advise patient to seek medical advice immediately if any of the following occurs:
  - rash, blistering, fever, swollen glands (especially in first 28 days of therapy)
  - flu-like symptoms (e.g. fever, sore throat, swollen glands, aching joints, lack of energy)
  - frequent infections, including fever, chills, sore throat or mouth ulcers
  - easy bruising or bleeding
- see General Patient teaching and advice for antiepileptics (p. 383)

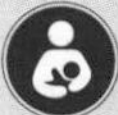

not recommended during pregnancy as birth defects may occur

not recommended during breastfeeding unless benefits outweigh risks

oral suspension is available. Contents of capsule cannot be extracted easily

GABAPENTIN (Gabacor, Gabaran, Gantin, Gapentin, Neurontin, Nupentin)

Available forms

Tablets: 600 mg, 800 mg; Capsules: 100 mg, 300 mg, 400 mg

Action
- structurally related to the neurotransmitter GABA, but its exact antiepileptic action is unknown, although it is not thought to interact with the sodium channels
- half-life 5–7 hours

Use

- as adjunct therapy for partial seizures, including generalised tonic–clonic seizures in patients who have not achieved control with standard antiepileptic drugs
- neuropathic pain

Dose

- (epilepsy) 300 mg on day 1 (at night to minimise adverse effects), 300 mg twice daily (day 2), and 300 mg 3 times daily (day 3), increasing dose further if needed (up to 2.4 g) **OR**
- (neuropathic pain) initially 300 mg orally 3 times daily, increasing if necessary (daily maximum 3.6 g)

Adverse effects

- see General Adverse effects of antiepileptics (p. 382)
- abdominal pain, increased appetite, weight increase, dyspepsia, dry mouth, constipation, diarrhoea, dental abnormalities
- impotence
- rhinitis, pharyngitis, coughing
- pruritus, acne
- myalgia, back pain
- peripheral oedema
- leucopenia
- fever
- (rare) drug rash with eosinophilia and systemic symptoms (DRESS), anaphylaxis, abuse and dependence, respiratory depression

Interactions

- cimetidine may decrease renal excretion
- bioavailability may be decreased by antacids
- increased risk of CNS depression if given with morphine
- may produce false positive reading on urinary protein test

Nursing points/Cautions

- caution in those with mixed epilepsy that includes absence seizures because gabapentin may exacerbate absence seizures
- caution if used in those with kidney insufficiency or on dialysis or history of drug abuse
- see General Nursing points/Cautions for antiepileptics (p. 382)

Patient teaching and advice

- patient should be advised not to allow more than 12 hours between doses. If a dose is missed by less than 4 hours it may be taken. If more than 4 hours, the dose should be missed and the next dose taken at the usual time
- may be taken with or without food
- advise patient not to take antacids for heartburn or reflux within 2 hours of gabapentin
- instruct patient to seek medical advice immediately if any of the following occur:
  - fever, swollen glands or rash
  - breathing difficulty, swelling of lips, throat or tongue, feeling light-headed
- see General Patient teaching and advice for antiepileptics (p. 383)

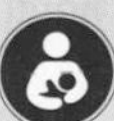

only used during pregnancy or breastfeeding if benefits outweigh risks

capsules can be opened and contents dispersed in water or orange juice. Tablet can be crushed and mixed with water or orange juice or spoonful of apple puree or chocolate pudding (Note: tablet is very hard to crush)

LACOSAMIDE (Vimpat)

Available forms

Tablets: 50 mg, 100 mg, 150 mg, 200 mg; Oral liquid: 10 mg/mL; Ampoule: 200 mg/20 mL

Action

- appears to selectively enhance slow inactivation of voltage-gated sodium channels reducing hyperexcitability of neuronal membranes
- half-life about 13 hours

Use

- therapy for partial seizures, with or without secondary generalisation (in patients over 16 years) as monotherapy or adjunct therapy

Dose

- (monotherapy) 200 mg orally or IV infusion over 15–60 minutes (loading dose), then 50 mg twice daily, increasing dose at weekly intervals if needed to maximum daily dose 600 mg

OR

- (adjunctive therapy) 200 mg orally or IV infusion over 15–60 minutes (loading dose), then 50 mg twice daily, increasing dose at weekly intervals if needed to maximum daily dose 400 mg

Adverse effects

- see General Adverse effects of antiepileptics (p. 382)
- tinnitus
- muscle spasm
- constipation, flatulence, dry mouth, dyspepsia, diarrhoea
- pruritus
- nasopharyngitis
- (rare) PR interval prolongation, elevated liver enzymes, hepatitis
- (IV) pain, discomfort, irritation, erythema

Interactions

- caution if used with other agents known to prolong PR interval or class I antiarrhythmic agents

Nursing points/Cautions

- IV route is recommended where oral route is not feasible
- if loading dose is not required, dose should be started at 50 mg twice daily
- (IV) can be given undiluted or as diluted solution with sodium chloride 0.9%, glucose 5% or lactated Ringer's solution
- IV infusion should be given over 15–60 minutes
- conversion from IV to oral dosage can be done without titrations
- if converting to monotherapy from other antiepileptic agents, other agents should be withdrawn over at least 6 weeks
- ECG is recommended before starting therapy
- when discontinuing therapy, gradual withdrawal at a rate of 200 mg per week is recommended
- dose reduction is recommended in those with severe kidney impairment
- caution if used in those with severe liver impairment
- caution if used in those with known conduction problems (e.g. sick sinus syndrome without pacemaker, marked first degree AV block), severe cardiovascular disease, diabetic neuropathy
- contraindicated in those with second or third degree AV block
- see General Nursing points/Cautions for antiepileptics (p. 382)

Patient teaching and advice

- see General Patient teaching and advice for antiepileptics (p. 383)
- advise patient that oral solution can be diluted in water if needed
- patient should be advised to seek medical advice immediately if any of the following occur:
    - light-headedness and/or fainting
    - slow or irregular pulse
    - shortness of breath or palpitations

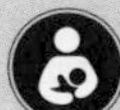

only recommended during pregnancy if benefits to mother clearly outweigh risks to fetus

oral solution available. Tablet can be dispersed in water or crushed and mixed with spoonful of yoghurt or apple puree

LAMOTRIGINE (Lamictal, Lamidus, Lamitan, Lamotrust, Logem, Reedos, Torlemo DT)

Available forms

Tablets (dispersible/chewable): 2 mg, 5 mg, 25 mg, 50 mg, 100 mg, 200 mg

Action

- phenyltriazine compound
- exact mechanism of action unknown, but thought to inhibit voltage-gated sodium channels and decrease release of glutamate and aspartate (excitatory amino acids)
- half-life 29 hours

Use

- partial and generalised seizures, as both monotherapy and adjunct therapy
- prevention of depressive episodes in patients with bipolar disorder

Dose

- (epilepsy, monotherapy) initially 25 mg orally daily for 2 weeks, increased to 50 mg (weeks 3 and 4), then increasing by 50–100 mg every 1–2 weeks until optimum dose is achieved, and then maintained on 100–200 mg orally daily or in 2 divided doses **OR**
- (epilepsy, with sodium valproate) initially 25 mg orally on alternate days for 2 weeks, increased to 25 mg daily (weeks 3 and 4), then increasing by 25–50 mg every 1–2 weeks until optimum dose is achieved, and then maintained on 100–200 mg daily or in 2 divided doses **OR**
- (epilepsy, with other antiepileptic agents) initially 25–50 mg orally for 2 weeks, then increased by 50–100 mg every 1–2 weeks, and then maintained on 100–400 mg daily in divided doses **OR**
- (bipolar disorder, adjunct therapy) initially 25 mg orally on alternate days for 2 weeks, then 25 mg orally daily (weeks 3 and 4), then 50 orally (as either single daily or divided dose) (week 5), increasing to 100 mg (as either single daily or divided dose) (daily maximum 200 mg)

Adverse effects

- see General Adverse effects of antiepileptics (p. 382)
- maculopapular rash, Stevens–Johnson syndrome (see Glossary), toxic epidermal necrolysis
- pharyngitis
- elevated liver enzymes, diarrhoea
- (bipolar disorder) worsening of symptoms or appearance of new symptoms of bipolar disorder
- (uncommon) transient haematological abnormalities, hypersensitivity
- (rare) liver dysfunction, aseptic meningitis, worsening of parkinsonian symptoms, haemophagocytic lymphohistiocytosis

Interactions

- metabolism may be increased by phenytoin, carbamazepine, phenobarbital (phenobarbitone), primidone, rifampicin, ritonavir and combined oral contraceptives
- serum levels may be increased by sodium valproate, increasing risk of severe rash
- serum levels may be decreased by oral contraceptives, therefore caution when starting or stopping therapy
- not recommended with other lamotrigine-containing preparations

- CNS adverse effects may be increased by carbamazepine

Nursing points/Cautions

- skin rash usually appears within 8 weeks of starting therapy and disappears on withdrawal
- dose adjustments are required for those with liver or kidney impairment, the elderly or women taking hormonal contraceptives
- caution if used in those with Parkinson's disease, kidney or liver failure
- caution if used in those with history of allergy or antiepileptic-induced rash as risk of severe skin reactions is increased
- caution if used in those with bipolar disorder or history of suicidal thoughts or behaviours
- (epilepsy) not recommended as monotherapy in newly diagnosed children
- (bipolar disorder) not recommended in those under 18 years
- see also General Nursing points/Cautions for antiepileptics (p. 382)

Patient teaching and advice

- advise patient that dispersible/chewable tablets can be swallowed whole, chewed or dispersed in a small amount of water
- warn parents that children have a higher risk of serious skin reactions
- patient/carer should be advised to seek medical advice immediately if any of the following occur:
  - rash or skin reaction
  - fever, rash, swollen glands (especially if they occur 8–24 days after starting therapy)
- (bipolar disorder) patient/carer should be warned to immediately report any change in mood, depression, thoughts of self-harm or suicide
- see General Patient teaching and advice for antiepileptics (p. 383)

may cause cleft palate if used during pregnancy, therefore should be avoided unless benefits outweigh risks

only used during breastfeeding if benefits outweigh risks

tablets can be dispersed in 2.5 mL water and then mixed with spoonful of yoghurt or apple puree.

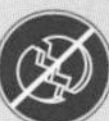

Pregnant staff should not disperse tablets

LEVETIRACETAM (Hospira Levetiracetam Concentrate for IV Infusion, Keppra Oral, Kerron, Kevtam, Levactam, Levecetam, Levi, Levitam, Noumed)

Available forms

Vial: 500 mg/5 mL; Tablets: 250 mg, 500 mg, 1000 mg; Suspension: 100 mg/mL

Action

- unknown antiepileptic action although thought to interact with specific binding site in CNS
- active metabolite
- half-life about 6–8 hours

Use

- as monotherapy or adjunct therapy in partial seizures (with or without secondary generalisation), myoclonic seizures in those with juvenile myoclonic epilepsy, or primary generalised tonic–clonic seizures in those with idiopathic generalised epilepsy

Dose

- (monotherapy) initially 250 mg orally or by IV infusion twice daily for 2 weeks, then increasing to 500 mg twice daily for 2 weeks; further increases of 250 mg increments twice daily at 2-week intervals may be

necessary, depending on clinical response (daily maximum 1500 mg twice daily) **OR**
- (adjunct therapy) initially 500 mg orally or by IV infusion twice daily, increasing by 500 mg twice daily increments at 2–4-week intervals if necessary (daily maximum 1500 mg twice daily)

Adverse effects
- see General Adverse effects of antiepileptics (p. 382)
- upper respiratory tract infection, flu-like syndrome, increased cough, pharyngitis, rhinitis, sinusitis, nasopharyngitis, bronchitis
- fever
- eczema, pruritus
- anorexia, gastroenteritis, gingivitis, tooth disorders, weight gain, abdominal pain
- ecchymosis, thrombocytopenia
- myalgia, back pain

Interactions
- probenecid inhibits renal clearance of metabolite but not levetiracetam

Nursing points/Cautions
- should not be given as a direct IV injection or rapid infusion
- dilute IV concentrate with at least 100 mL of sodium chloride 0.9%, glucose 5% or lactated Ringer's solution
- IV infusion given over 15 minutes
- (IV) not compatible with IV phenytoin
- (IV) administer alone
- not suitable for status epilepticus
- (oral solution) contains hydroxybenzoates which may cause allergic reactions in susceptible individual
- (oral solution) contains glycerol and is not recommended in those with fructose intolerance
- caution if used in those with kidney impairment as dose adjustment is required
- contraindicated in those with hypersensitivity of pyrrolidine derivatives
- see General Nursing points/Cautions for antiepileptics (p. 382)

Patient teaching and advice
- advise patient that oral suspension may be diluted with water
- warn patient that bitter taste may be experienced after oral administration
- see also General Patient teaching and advice for antiepileptics (p. 383)

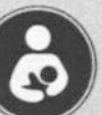

only used during pregnancy if benefits outweigh risks

secreted in breastmilk, therefore not recommended during breastfeeding

available as an oral liquid. Tablet can be crushed and mixed with water or spoonful of yoghurt or apple puree

OXCARBAZEPINE (Trileptal)

Available forms
Tablets: 150 mg, 300 mg, 600 mg; Oral suspension: 60 mg/mL

Action
- analogue of carbamazepine
- inhibits voltage-sensitive sodium channels, stabilising hyperexcited neural membrane, inhibiting repetitive neural firing and decreasing synaptic impulse propagation
- increases potassium conductance and modulates high-voltage activated calcium channels
- activity due to active metabolite
- half-life 1.3–2.3 hours, metabolite half-life 7.5–11 hours

Use
- partial or generalised tonic–clonic seizures in adults or children as either monotherapy or adjunctive therapy

Dose
- initially 300 mg orally twice daily, increasing by 600 mg per day at weekly intervals if required (maximum daily dose 2400 mg)

Adverse effects

- see General Adverse effects of antiepileptics (p. 382)
- abdominal pain, constipation, diarrhoea, weight increase
- asymptomatic hyponatraemia
- alopecia, acne
- (rare) hypersensitivity, anaphylaxis, angioedema, multi-organ hypersensitivity
- (very rare) Stevens–Johnson syndrome (see Glossary), toxic epidermal necrolysis, erythema multiforme, hypothyroidism, blood dyscrasias

Interactions

- caution if used with St John's wort
- serum levels may be increased by phenobarbital (phenobarbitone)
- may increase serum levels of amitriptyline, citalopram, clomipramine, cyclophosphamide, diazepam, imipramine, lansoprazole, omeprazole, pantoprazole, phenobarbital (phenobarbitone), phenytoin, progesterone, proguanil, propranolol and sodium valproate
- serum levels may be lowered by phenytoin
- serum levels may be increased by ciclosporin
- may increase hyponatraemic effects of drugs that lower serum sodium levels
- may decrease serum levels of felodipine and carbamazepine
- may decrease effectiveness of combined oral contraceptives containing progestogens
- may increase sedative effects of alcohol

Nursing points/Cautions

- doses of oral suspension and tablets are bioequivalent
- regular weight measurement is recommended in those with cardiac insufficiency/failure to detect any fluid retention. Serum sodium levels should be measured if fluid retention occurs
- serum sodium levels should be measured before starting, after 2 weeks then monthly throughout therapy, especially in those who have low sodium levels (due to either medical conditions or sodium-lowering agents or the elderly)
- thyroid function should be monitored in children starting therapy
- (oral suspension) contains parabens, which can cause allergic reaction in susceptible individuals
- (oral suspension) contains sorbitol which is converted to fructose and may be problematic for those with fructose intolerance
- caution if used in those with genetic risk of severe dermatological reactions, including those from Japan, Southern India, Indigenous Americans, Asia (Philippines, Thailand, Malaysia, Hong Kong, Taiwan, North China), or of Hispanic or Arabic descent. Genetic testing for specific gene is recommended (if available) and not recommended in those with HLA-A*3101 or HLA-B*1502 allele positive
- cross-hypersensitivity can occur with phenytoin, oxcarbazepine and carbamazepine
- caution if used in those with AV block, arrhythmias or other conduction disorders
- caution in those with liver or kidney impairment
- see also General Nursing points/Cautions for antiepileptics (p. 382)

Patient teaching and advice

- patient should be advised to seek medical advice immediately if any of the following occur:
  - rash or skin reactions
  - headache, lethargy, dizziness, nausea, vomiting or confusion (may be signs of hyponatraemia)

- shake suspension well before administration
- patient should be advised to use supplied dosing syringe for administration
- oral suspension may be taken directly from syringe or mixed with water and taken immediately
- female patients should be warned of potential decrease in effectiveness of oral contraceptives during therapy and advised to use a barrier form of contraception
- see also General Patient teaching and advice for antiepileptics (p. 383)

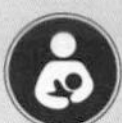

not recommended during pregnancy or breastfeeding. Related to carbamazepine, which is teratogenic

oral suspension is available. Tablet can be crushed and mixed with water or spoonful of yoghurt or apple puree. Tablet is hard to crush and should be crushed in a closed tablet crusher.

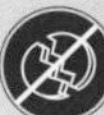

staff should wear gown and gloves if crushing tablets

PERAMPANEL (Fycompa)

Available forms

Tablets: 2 mg, 4 mg, 6 mg, 8 mg, 10 mg, 12 mg

Action

- AMPA glutamate receptor antagonist (glutamate is a CNS excitatory neurotransmitter thought to be involved in neurological disorders involving neuronal overexcitation)
- half-life 25 hours
- decreased clearance in females

Use

- adjunctive treatment of partial-onset seizures (with or without generalised seizures) in patients over 12 years
- adjunctive treatment of primary generalised tonic–clonic seizures in adults and those over 12 years with idiopathic generalised epilepsy

Dose

- initially 2 mg orally at night, increasing in increments of 2 mg/day at 1–2-weekly intervals to daily maintenance of 4–8 mg (depending on response and tolerance to a daily maximum 12 mg)

Adverse effects

- see General Adverse effects of antiepileptics (p. 382)
- arthralgia, myalgia, musculoskeletal pain, back pain
- constipation, weight gain
- cough

Interactions

- may decrease efficacy of combined oral contraceptives
- decreased plasma levels may occur if given with carbamazepine, phenytoin, oxcarbazepine, rifampicin, St John's wort
- caution if given with alcohol or other CNS depressants

Nursing points/Cautions

- see General Nursing points/Cautions for antiepileptics (p. 382)
- dose should not exceed 8 mg in those with mild-to-moderate liver impairment
- tablets contain lactose and should not be used in those with rare hereditary problems of galactose intolerance, Lapp lactase deficiency or glucose–galactose malabsorption
- caution if used in the elderly due to increased risk of dizziness and falls
- caution if used in those with history of substance abuse
- not recommended in children under 12 years
- not recommended as monotherapy

Patient teaching and advice

- see General Patient teaching and advice for antiepileptics (p. 383)

- women of childbearing potential taking combined oral contraceptives should be counselled to use additional non-hormonal contraceptive methods (e.g. condom, intrauterine advice) during therapy to avoid the risk of pregnancy

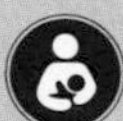

not recommended during pregnancy or breastfeeding unless benefits are thought to outweigh risks

tablets can be dispersed in water or crushed and mixed with spoonful of yoghurt or apple puree

PHENOBARBITAL (PHENOBARBITONE) (Orion Phenobarbital Elixir, Phenobarbital Injection, Phenobarb)

Available forms

Tablets: 30 mg; Ampoules: 200 mg/mL; Suspension: 15 mg/5 mL

Action

- long-acting barbiturate with sedative, hypnotic and antiepileptic properties
- thought to mimic or enhance actions of GABA
- depresses synaptic transmission and increases threshold for electrical stimulation in motor cortex
- long half-life (90–100 hours)
- therapeutic serum level 15–40 microgram/mL (65–170 microM/L)

Use

- epilepsy (grand mal and psychomotor)
- status epilepticus
- sedation

Dose

- (epilepsy) 60–240 mg orally in 2–3 divided doses daily **OR**
- (epilepsy) 100–300 mg IM, repeated if necessary (daily maximum 600 mg) **OR**
- (status epilepticus) 10–20 mg/kg IM or slow IV injection, repeated after 20 minutes if necessary (maximum daily total 1–2 g) **OR**
- (sedative) 30–120 mg orally daily in 2–3 divided doses **OR**
- (sedative) 30–120 mg IM daily in 2–3 divided doses

Adverse effects

- sedation, disorientation, dizziness, depression, drowsiness, lethargy, hangover effect, confusion, restlessness, irritability, excitement, memory impairment, mood changes
- rash, bullae (skin blisters)
- dependence (physical and psychological), tolerance, withdrawal syndrome (including status epilepticus) if abruptly stopped
- (uncommon) folate deficiency, hypocalcaemia, megaloblastic anaemia, injection site reactions, nausea, vomiting, diarrhoea, vitamin D deficiency
- (rare) rickets, osteomalacia, exacerbated hyperthyroid symptoms, fibromas, Dupuytren's contracture, frozen shoulder, joint pain

Interactions

- CNS depressant effects may be increased by other CNS depressants, including alcohol, MAOIs, benzodiazepines, antihistamines, phenothiazines, anaesthetics and opioid analgesics
- hypotension, respiratory depression and prolonged recovery time may occur if given with ketamine
- not recommended with MAOI tranylcypromine due to increased CNS depressant effects
- may impair absorption of griseofulvin
- may decrease effects of warfarin by increasing metabolism, therefore prothrombin time should be closely

monitored, especially when starting, stopping and changing doses
- may increase metabolism of paracetamol, increasing level of toxic metabolite and risk of hepatotoxicity
- absorption may be decreased by amphetamines
- effects may be reduced by folic acid (high dose) or alkalinising the urine
- serum levels may be decreased by St John's wort. Serum levels should be monitored when starting or stopping therapy
- serum levels may be increased by sodium valproate, disulfiram, methylphenidate, flu vaccine, chloramphenicol and dextropropoxyphene
- may decrease effectiveness of oral contraceptives by increasing metabolism of both oestrogen and progestogen components
- increased risk of hepatotoxicity if given with halothane or enflurane
- may increase metabolism of opioid analgesics leading to withdrawal symptoms
- may potentiate hepatotoxicity of sodium valproate
- may alter levels (unpredictable) of phenytoin, therefore serum levels should be closely monitored
- phenytoin may alter serum levels of phenobarbital (phenobarbitone), therefore serum levels should be closely monitored
- may increase metabolism (and therefore decrease serum levels and effectiveness) of antiarrhythmics, carbamazepine, chloramphenicol, chlorpromazine, corticosteroids, corticotrophin, ciclosporin, digoxin, disopyramide, doxycycline, etoposide, haloperidol, itraconazole, lamotrigine, metronidazole, nifedipine, paracetamol, phenothiazines, propranolol, ritonavir, tacrolimus, theophylline, SSRIs and TCAs. Serum level monitoring is recommended
- increased risk of hypothermia if given with other hypothermia-producing agents
- increased risk of nephrotoxicity if given with methoxyflurane (even several weeks after phenobarbital has been stopped)
- increased risk of respiratory depression may occur if given with TCAs
- increased risk of osteopenia if given with carbonic anhydrase inhibitors such as acetazolamide
- may decrease effects of vitamin D by increasing metabolism, increasing risk of osteomalacia with long-term therapy
- may interfere with a number of laboratory tests

Nursing points/Cautions

- blood counts should be monitored at the start and regularly throughout long-term therapy
- therapeutic serum levels should be monitored regularly if therapy is ongoing
- calcium and vitamin D supplements are recommended during long-term therapy
- regular bone mineral density monitoring is recommended with long-term therapy
- physical dependency and tolerance may develop, therefore therapy should not be discontinued suddenly to prevent withdrawal symptoms occurring
- hypotension and vasodilation may occur if given by rapid IV administration
- highly alkaline, may cause tissue necrosis if extravasation occurs
- not given SC or intra-arterially due to risk of tissue necrosis
- (IV) dilute solution 1 in 10 with water for injections and administer at a rate less than 60 mg/minute
- oxygen, vasopressor agents and resuscitation equipment should be

readily available when given IV due to risk of overdose and CNS depression (including respiratory depression) occurring
- injection given deep IM (not greater than 5 mL per site)
- caution if used in the elderly (as confusion, depression or excitement may occur) or those with asthma, urticaria, angioedema, hypotension, hypoadrenalism, hyperthyroidism, history of haematological disorders, cardiovascular or respiratory disease or kidney or liver dysfunction
- contraindicated if used in those with acute or chronic pain (especially if uncontrolled) as paradoxical excitement may occur or other symptoms may be masked
- contraindicated in those with hypersensitivity to barbiturates, severe folate-deficiency anaemia, porphyria, severe depression, suicidal tendencies, severe respiratory, kidney or liver impairment, sleep apnoea, past addiction to sedatives/hypnotics or alcohol, nephritis, premonitory signs of hepatic coma, asthma, diabetes mellitus or in the elderly if nocturnal confusion/restlessness from sedatives or hypnotics has occurred
- see also General Nursing points/ Cautions for antiepileptics (p. 382)

Patient teaching and advice

- patient should be advised to seek medical advice if any of the following occur:
  - sore throat, fever, bruising or bleeding (sign of blood dyscrasias)
  - nosebleeds
  - signs of infection
  - rash or other skin reactions, severe itching
- encourage patients to have adequate sunlight exposure (or take vitamin D supplement) and regular weightbearing exercise
- advise female patient using oral contraceptives that additional forms of contraception are required to prevent pregnancy occurring
- see also General Patient teaching and advice for antiepileptics (p. 383)

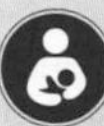

barbiturates distribute throughout fetal tissue, especially liver and brain and may be associated with minor craniofacial defects, fingernail hypoplasia, developmental disability and brain tumours. Barbiturate withdrawal may be seen in newborns up to 2 weeks after birth

CNS depression and withdrawal symptoms may be seen in breastfed babies. Infant serum levels should be closely monitored

available as oral liquid. Tablets can be crushed and mixed with water or fruit juice or spoonful of yoghurt or apple puree

PHENYTOIN SODIUM (Dilantin, DBL Phenytoin Injection BP)

Available forms

Tablets (chewable): 50 mg; Capsules: 30 mg, 100 mg; Ampoules: 100 mg/2 mL, 250 mg/5 mL; Suspension: 30 mg/5 mL

Action

- hydantoin
- acts by preventing the spread of seizure activity across the motor cortex (promotes efflux of sodium ions from neurons), stabilises excitability threshold
- antiarrhythmic actions (positive inotropic effect and enhances AV conduction, decreases automaticity, shortens refractory period, shortens QT interval and duration of action potential)
- not effective for absence (petit mal) seizures
- (oral) absorption is slow and variable, especially in neonates

- onset of action 30–60 minutes (IV), duration of action up to 24 hours
- half-life 7–42 hours (average 24 hours); however, this is dependent on dose and serum levels

Use
- psychomotor seizures
- tonic–clonic (grand mal) epilepsy
- status epilepticus
- prophylactic control of seizures during and after neurosurgery or after severe head trauma
- arrhythmias not responding to other antiarrhythmic agents or cardioversion

Dose
- (epilepsy) initially 4–5 mg/kg orally daily in 2–3 divided doses, adjusting dose at 2-week intervals according to plasma levels (daily maximum 600 mg) **OR**
- (status epilepticus) 10–15 mg/kg slowly IV (loading dose), then 100 mg IV or orally 6–8-hourly given with a short-acting IV benzodiazepine to rapidly control seizure **OR**
- (neurosurgery prophylaxis) 250 mg slowly IV 6–12-hourly until oral administration is possible **OR**
- (cardiac arrhythmias) 3–5 mg/kg slow IV injection initially, at a rate not exceeding 50 mg/minute and repeated if necessary

Adverse effects
- see General Adverse effects of antiepileptics (p. 382)
- constipation, altered taste, epigastric pain, weight loss
- hyperplasia of gums and gum bleeding, lip enlargement,
- coarsened facial features
- acne
- abnormal thyroid function
- lymphadenopathy, anaemia, thrombocytopenia, agranulocytosis, megaloblastic anaemia, leucopenia, pancytopenia
- hirsutism, hypertrichosis
- (rapid IV infusion) hypotension, cardiac arrhythmias, impaired cardiac conduction, CNS depression, respiratory depression
- (long-term therapy > 10 years) osteomalacia, bone fractures
- (IV) irritation, thrombophlebitis, inflammation, pain, tissue necrosis
- (rare) hypersensitivity, toxic hepatitis, liver damage, phenytoin-induced dyskinesia, anticonvulsant hypersensitivity syndrome, angioedema, hyperglycaemia (patients with diabetes)
- (phenytoin toxicity) lateral gaze/nystagmus, ataxia, dysarthria, followed by tremor, hyperreflexia, dizziness, somnolence, drowsiness, lethargy, slurred speech, blurred or double vision, hypotension, confusion, hallucinations, clumsiness, nausea and vomiting, and, in severe poisoning or overdose, respiratory depression, bradycardia and heart block

Interactions
- serum levels may be increased or decreased (unpredictable effect) by benzodiazepines, carbamazepine, ciprofloxacin, phenobarbital (phenobarbitone), phenothiazines, primidone, sodium valproate and theophylline; therefore, serum levels should be closely monitored
- serum levels may be increased by acute alcohol intake, amiodarone, amphotericin B (amphotericin), capecitabine, chloramphenicol, cimetidine, clopidogrel, diazepam, diltiazem, disulfiram, erythromycin, ethosuximide, fluconazole, fluorouracil (5FU), fluvastatin, fluvoxamine, fluoxetine, gabapentin, halothane, isoniazid, itraconazole, methylphenidate, miconazole, nifedipine, oestrogens, omeprazole, oxcarbamazine, phenothiazines, ranitidine, salicylates, sertraline, SSRIs, sodium

valproate, sulfonamides, tacrolimus, ticlopidine, topiramate, voriconazole and warfarin
- serum levels may be decreased by chronic alcohol abuse, aminophylline, bleomycin, calcium folinate, carboplatin, carmustine, ciprofloxacin, cisplatin, diazoxide, folic acid, HIV protease inhibitors, methotrexate, oral contraceptives, rifabutin, rifampicin, sucralfate, St John's wort, theophylline, vigabatrin, vinblastine
- absorption is interfered with by calcium ions, therefore administration of antacids containing calcium should be staggered
- TCAs, haloperidol, tramadol, antipsychotic agents and MAOIs may precipitate seizures in susceptible patients by lowering convulsive threshold
- reduces efficacy of aminophylline, amiodarone, amlodipine, azole antifungal agents, carbamazepine, clozapine, corticosteroids, ciclosporin, digoxin, doxycycline, felodipine, frusemide, ivabradine, lamotrigine, lercanidipine, methadone, nifedipine, nimodipine, oestrogens, combined oral contraceptives, perampanel, praziquantel, progestogens, teniposide, theophylline, verapamil, vinca alkaloids
- caution if given with other highly protein-bound drugs such as nifedepine and verapamil
- may decrease serum levels of topiramate and increase serum levels of phenytoin if given together
- large doses may increase serum glucose levels, increasing insulin and/or oral hypoglycaemic agent requirements
- caution if given with warfarin as effects may be unpredictable, therefore drug levels and INR should be monitored during therapy
- food and enteral feeding may affect phenytoin absorption
- seizure control may be decreased if given with folic acid due to increased phenytoin metabolism
- may increase metabolism of vitamin D, increasing risk of osteoporosis and bone fractures
- if combined with cranial irradiation and gradual decreasing doses of corticosteroids, may result in severe skin reactions
- caution if used with pancuronium as recovery time from neuromuscular blockade may be faster
- chronic phenytoin therapy may result in resistance to vecuronium-induced neuromuscular blockage requiring higher dose
- (IV) additive cardiac depressive effects may occur if given with lidocaine (lignocaine) or beta-adrenergic blocking agents
- (IV) bradycardia and hypotension may occur if given with dopamine
- may interfere with thyroid function, folic acid, calcium, dexamethasone and metyrapone tests

Nursing points/Cautions

- any hypoalbuminaemia should be corrected immediately because it may lead to toxicity (due to increased levels of unbound phenytoin)
- serum levels should be measured 7–10 days after starting therapy, if dose is altered, if adding or subtracting another antiepileptic agent or when switching from one formulation to another or at first signs of toxicity, as prolonged high phenytoin levels may lead to encephalopathy and/or confusional state
- regular blood count monitoring is recommended for long-term therapy
- long-term therapy requires adequate vitamin D and folic acid intake in diet or supplements. Bone density should also be measured regularly

- IV administration should not exceed 50 mg/minute to prevent cardiac arrhythmias and/or hypotension. Patient requires constant heart rate, blood pressure and ECG monitoring and observation for respiratory depression
- injectable solutions are strongly alkaline, so avoid mixing with other drugs or IV solutions as crystallisation/precipitation may occur
- SC or IM administration is not recommended. IM absorption is also slow and erratic
- (IV) contains propylene glycol, which can cause toxicity if used for a prolonged period
- (IV) not for dilution
- IV lines should be flushed with sodium chloride 0.9% before and after administration of phenytoin
- (IV) if solution is refrigerated, precipitate may form. This will dissolve at room temperature with no adverse effects on solution
- (IV) avoid extravasation as tissue necrosis may occur
- (suspension) it is suggested that phenytoin should not be administered with continuous enteral feeds. Phenytoin should be administered 2 hours after an intermittent feed and a 2-hour interval allowed before the next feed is commenced
- suspension should be diluted before administration via feeding tube. Tube should be flushed well after administration
- caution if used in the elderly or those with porphyria, liver or kidney impairment, (IV) hypotension or severe myocardial insufficiency or diabetes (as hyperglycaemia may be increased)
- caution if used in those who have experienced or have a family history of anticonvulsant hypersensitivity syndrome previously (to phenytoin or other antiepileptic agents) or are immunosuppressed
- caution if used in those of Chinese heritage as there is an increased risk of severe skin reactions
- extreme caution if combined with cranial irradiation as gradual decreasing doses of corticosteroids may result in severe skin reactions
- contraindicated in those with hypersensitivity to hydantoins, sinus bradycardia, SA block, second/third degree AV block or Stokes–Adams syndrome
- see also General Nursing points/Cautions for antiepileptics (p. 382)

Patient teaching and advice

- advise patients to take tablets with at least half a glass of water before meals, but, if there is a tendency to nausea, take with or after food (always taken in the same relation to food for consistent absorption)
- if gastric irritation is a problem, splitting dose into 3 is recommended
- advise patient (or carer) to shake suspension well before use
- instruct patient to seek medical advice immediately if any of the following occur:
  - fever or sore throat (early signs of bone marrow depression)
  - any rash or skin reaction including blisters or itching
  - joint or muscle pain, fever, chills, yellowing of skin or eyes, fatigue, itching, nausea, vomiting, loss of appetite, abdominal pain
- advise about good oral hygiene (e.g. frequent brushing, gum massage) to reduce gingival (gum) hyperplasia
- if patient has diabetes, he/she should be advised to monitor blood glucose more frequently due to the risk of hyperglycaemia
- see also General Patient teaching and advice for antiepileptics (p. 383)

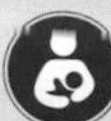

has been associated with fetal hydantoin syndrome (craniofacial defects, fingernail hypoplasia, developmental disability, growth retardation and, less often, oral clefts and cardiac anomalies). May also cause coagulation defects, with haemorrhage risk in the fetus and newborn, which may be prevented by giving vitamin K prophylactically to the mother before delivery

not recommended during breastfeeding

oral suspension available. Capsules can be opened and contents dispersed in water. Tablets can be crushed and mixed with water.

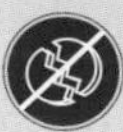

if opening capsules or crushing tablets, mask and gloves should be worn

PREGABALIN (Lypralin, Lyrica, Lyzalon, Neuroccord, Prebalin)

Available forms

Capsules: 25 mg, 50 mg, 75 mg, 100 mg, 150 mg, 200 mg, 225 mg, 300 mg

Action

- analogue of GABA with analgesic and antiepileptic properties
- binds to protein subunit of voltage-gated calcium channels in CNS
- reduces release of glutamate, noradrenaline and substance P although the significance of this is currently unknown
- half-life 6.3 hours

Use

- adjunct therapy in partial seizures with or without secondary generalisation
- neuropathic pain

Dose

- (epilepsy, neuropathic pain) initially 75 mg orally twice daily, increasing to 150 mg twice daily after 3–7 days. After a further 7-day interval, this can be increased to 300 mg twice daily if needed

Adverse effects

- see also General Adverse effects of antiepileptics (p. 382)
- flatulence, dry mouth, diarrhoea, bloating, increased appetite, weight gain
- peripheral oedema, generalised oedema
- decreased libido and uncommonly, erectile dysfunction, sexual dysfunction, dysmenorrhoea
- muscle cramp, back pain, arthralgia, limb pain
- nasopharyngitis
- elevated creatine kinase levels
- (rare) myopathy, rhabdomyolysis, hypersensitivity

Interactions

- may enhance effects of alcohol, oxycodone and lorazepam
- increased risk of CNS depression if used with opioid analgesics

Nursing points/Cautions

- therapy should be stopped if creatine kinase levels are markedly elevated or if there are any signs of myopathy
- if patient has diabetes, kidney function should be measured before starting therapy and dose adjusted if needed
- (neuropathic pain) if pain is not adequately controlled in 12 weeks, risk versus benefit to patient should be assessed before continuing therapy
- (epilepsy) not recommended as monotherapy
- caution if used in those with congestive cardiac failure or kidney impairment
- not recommended in those with hereditary problems of galactose intolerance, lactase deficiency or glucose–galactose malabsorption
- see also General Nursing points/Cautions for antiepileptics (p. 382)

Patient teaching and advice

- patient should be advised of weight gain and counselled regarding healthy eating options, especially if the person also has diabetes; added weight may require dose adjustment of hypoglycaemic agents
- warn patient to immediately seek medical advice if any swelling of face, lips or upper airway occurs
- see also General Patient teaching and advice for antiepileptics (p. 383)

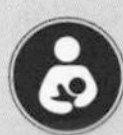

not recommended during pregnancy or breastfeeding unless benefits are thought to outweigh risks

capsules can be opened and contents dispersed in 120 mL water or mixed with spoonful of yoghurt or apple puree

PRIMIDONE (Mysoline)

Available form

Tablets: 250 mg

Action

- barbiturate
- reduces sensitivity to stimuli that might provoke seizure activity
- active metabolites include phenobarbital (phenobarbitone) and phenylethylmalonamide

Use

- tonic–clonic (grand mal) epilepsy
- temporal lobe (psychomotor) epilepsy
- partial (focal) epileptic seizures
- myoclonic jerks, akinetic attacks

Dose

- initially 125 mg orally at night, gradually increasing by increments of 125 mg every 3 days until 500 mg is reached, then increasing by increments of 250 mg every 3 days until control is achieved (750–1500 mg daily in 2 divided doses, morning and evening)

Adverse effects

- see General Adverse effects of antiepileptics (p. 382)
- severe skin eruptions
- tolerance, dependence, withdrawal syndrome
- (rare) megaloblastic anaemia, Dupuytren's contracture, arthralgia, osteomalacia

Interactions

- may alter serum levels of other antiepileptic agents or warfarin
- may reduce effectiveness of oral contraceptives
- may enhance effects of alcohol and other CNS depressants
- affects metabolism of vitamin D

Nursing points/Cautions

- it is advisable to give the larger part of the dose when the seizures are known to be more frequent (e.g. if the seizures are nocturnal, most of the dose is given in the evening)
- bone mineral density should be measured regularly with long-term use
- vitamin D supplements are recommended with long-term therapy
- caution if used in the elderly or those with kidney, liver or respiratory impairment
- contraindicated in those with porphyria
- see General Nursing points/Cautions for antiepileptics (p. 382)

Patient teaching and advice

- female patients should be counselled to use other methods of contraception to avoid pregnancy occurring as oral contraceptives may be ineffective during therapy
- see General Patient teaching and advice for antiepileptics (p. 383)

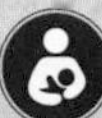

barbiturates distribute throughout fetal tissue, especially liver and brain and may be associated with minor craniofacial defects, fingernail hypoplasia, developmental disability and brain tumours. Barbiturate withdrawal may be seen in newborns up to 2 weeks after birth

CNS depression and withdrawal symptoms may be seen in breastfed babies. Infant serum levels should be closely monitored

Tablet can be dispersed in water or crushed and mixed with spoonful of yoghurt or apple puree

RUFINAMIDE (Inovelon)

Available form
Tablets: 100 mg, 200 mg, 400 mg

Action
- modulates sodium channel activity prolonging inactive state
- half-life 6–10 hours

Use
- adjunct therapy to seizures associated with Lennox–Gastaut syndrome in patients 4 years and older. (Lennox–Gastaut syndrome is a rare, complex and severe epilepsy which starts in childhood (usually between 3 and 5 years), and can persist into adulthood. It is characterised by multiple and concurrent seizure types)

Dose
- (adults, adolescents and children > 4 years and > 30 kg, not receiving sodium valproate) initially 200 mg orally twice daily, increasing by increments of 400 mg daily if needed (daily maximum 1.8 g–3.2 g depending on patient weight) **OR**
- (adults, adolescents and children > 4 years and > 30 kg, receiving sodium valproate) initially 200 mg orally twice daily, increasing by increments of 400 mg daily if needed (daily maximum 1.2 g–2.2 g depending on patient weight) **OR**
- (children > 4 years and < 30 kg, not receiving sodium valproate) initially 100 mg orally twice daily, increasing at 3-day intervals of 200 mg daily increments if needed (daily maximum 600 mg) **OR**
- (children > 4 years and < 30 kg, receiving sodium valproate) initially 100 mg orally twice daily, increasing at 2-day intervals of 200 mg daily increments if needed (daily maximum 1 g)

Adverse effects
- pneumonia, flu-like symptoms, nasopharyngitis, sinusitis, rhinitis
- ear infection
- back pain
- oligomenorrhoea
- decreased appetite, anorexia, upper abdominal pain, constipation, dyspepsia, diarrhoea, weight change
- (rare) hypersensitivity reaction, increased liver enzymes, decrease in QTc interval
- see General Adverse effects for antiepileptics (p. 382)

Interactions
- serum levels increased by sodium valproate
- decreased serum levels may occur if given with primidone, phenobarbital, carbamazepine or vigabatrin
- may decrease efficacy of oral contraceptives
- caution if given with triazolam
- caution if used with amiodarone, aprepitant, atorvastatin, carbamazepine, ciclosporin, felodipine, hydrocortisone, HIV protease inhibitors (e.g. saquinavir), simvastatin, tacrolimus, tyrosine kinase inhibitors (e.g. axitinib), verapamil, zolpidem. Patients should be closely monitored for 2 weeks at the start, end or dose adjustment if given with rufinamide

- caution if given with warfarin or digoxin. Serum levels should be closely monitored if given together

Nursing points/Cautions

- treatment should be started by paediatrician or neurologist specialised in management of epilepsy
- caution if used in those with or family history of congenital short QT syndrome
- caution if used in patients with mild-to-moderate liver impairment. Careful dose titration is recommended
- not recommended in patients with severe liver impairment
- tablets contain lactose and are therefore not recommended in those with rare hereditary problems of galactose intolerance, Lapp lactase deficiency or glucose–galactose malabsorption
- see also General Nursing points/Cautions for antiepileptics (p. 382)

Patient teaching and advice

- see General Patient teaching and advice for antiepileptics (p. 383)

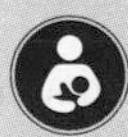

not recommended during pregnancy or breastfeeding unless benefits are thought to outweigh risks

tablet can be crushed and mixed with water

SODIUM VALPROATE (Epilim, Epilim IV, Valprease, Valpro)

Available forms

Tablets (sustained-release): 200 mg, 500 mg; Tablets (crushable): 100 mg; Suspension: 200 mg/5 mL; Vial: 400 mg

Action

- anticonvulsant, antipsychotic
- thought to raise brain levels of the inhibitory synaptic transmitter GABA, as well as blocking voltage-dependent sodium channels
- half-life 8–12 hours

Use

- simple partial (petit mal) epilepsy
- tonic–clonic (grand mal) epilepsy
- myoclonic epilepsy
- mono or adjuvant therapy in partial (focal) epilepsy
- mania (see Antipsychotic and mood stabilising agents, p. 802) (where other agents are inadequate or inappropriate)

Dose

- initially 600 mg orally daily with or after food, increasing by 200 mg daily at 3-day intervals until control is reached (1000–2000 mg). If control is not reached after 2 weeks, dosage may be increased to a maximum of 2500 mg daily or another antiepileptic agent may be added **OR**
- initially 400–800 mg (up to 10 mg/kg) IV over 3–5 minutes or by IV infusion, then 1–2 mg/kg/hr (daily maximum 2.5 g or another antiepileptic agent may be added)

Adverse effects

- see General Adverse effects of antiepileptics (p. 382)
- anorexia, diarrhoea, abdominal cramps, increased appetite, weight gain
- transient hair loss, nail/nailbed disorder
- gingival hyperplasia
- elevated liver enzymes, hyponatraemia
- dysmenorrhoea
- urinary incontinence
- prolonged bleeding time (reversible), thrombocytopenia
- (rare) liver damage/failure, pancreatitis, vasculitis, hyperammonaemia (with or without symptoms, including lethargy, coma, vomiting, ataxia, clouded consciousness), hypersensitivity
- (IV) pain, discomfort, erythema, inflammation

Interactions

- not recommended with carbapenem antibiotics
- increased risk of liver damage if given with salicylates, including aspirin
- increased risk of neutropenia/leucopenia if given with quetiapine
- use with clozapine may result in increased serum levels of either clozapine or sodium valproate
- may increase serum levels of midazolam, primidone, nimodipine and zidovudine, increasing the risk of adverse effects
- may decrease renal clearance of lorazepam
- may inhibit metabolism of TCAs, therefore serum levels should be monitored
- may increase serum levels of diazepam and inhibit its metabolism, increasing the risk of sedation
- use with clonazepam may result in absence seizures
- use with aspirin may result in increased sodium valproate serum levels by displacement from receptor site, as well as inhibiting its metabolism
- may increase or decrease serum phenytoin levels, therefore close monitoring of serum levels is recommended
- may inhibit metabolism of carbamazepine (and its metabolite), lamotrigine, phenobarbital (phenobarbitone) and ethosuximide increasing risk of toxicity, therefore monitoring serum levels is recommended
- may decrease serum levels of olanzapine and propofol
- increased risk of encephalopathy and/or hyperammonaemia if given with topiramate or acetazolamide
- use with antidepressants may decrease seizure threshold in patients whose seizures have not been stabilised
- may potentiate CNS effects of alcohol, antidepressants, antipsychotics, benzodiazepines, phenobarbital (phenobarbitone) and MAOIs
- serum levels decreased by phenytoin, phenobarbital (phenobarbitone), carbamazepine, colestyramine, protease inhibitors (e.g. ritonavir), imipenem, rifampicin or meropenem
- serum levels increased by erythromycin, cimetidine, fluoxetine, chlorpromazine, felbamate, MAOIs, TCAs and SSRIs
- seizures may occur if given with mefloquine
- caution if given with warfarin as serum levels of warfarin may be increased, therefore INR should be closely monitored especially when starting or stopping therapy
- may give false positive result to ketone bodies in urine testing in those with diabetes (ketone bodies are produced from elimination of sodium valproate by the kidneys). May also alter thyroid function tests

Nursing points/Cautions

- may take 2–6 weeks for optimal seizure control to be achieved
- risk of urea cycle disorders should be evaluated before starting therapy (including those with unexplained encephalopathy or coma, encephalopathy associated with protein, pregnancy or postpartum, cyclical vomiting and lethargy, extreme irritability, ataxia, low blood nitrogen urea (BUN) or protein avoidance)
- liver function is assessed before starting therapy then monitored monthly for 6 months, then less frequently
- blood counts (including prothrombin time, serum fibrinogen and albumin) and platelet counts should be monitored before and regularly throughout therapy and especially before

surgery (because bleeding time may be prolonged)
- pregnancy should be excluded before starting therapy
- enteric-coated tablets are recommended for those requiring higher doses
- not recommended IM due to risk of tissue necrosis
- (IV) administer alone
- (IV) reconstitute using 4 mL of provided diluent
- (IV) administer by slow IV injection or infusion
- (IV) patient should be transferred to oral therapy as soon as practicable
- if patient requires surgery, platelet function should be closely monitored
- increased risk of rhabdomyolysis if given to those with carnitine palmitoyltransferase (CPT) type II deficiency
- caution if used in those with ornithine transcarbamylase deficiency due to the risk of hyperammonaemia
- caution if used in those with pancreatitis, impaired kidney or liver function or SLE
- contraindicated in those with liver dysfunction (including family history of hepatitis), porphyria or known urea cycle disorders or some mitochondrial disorders
- see also General Nursing points/Cautions for antiepileptics (p. 382)

Patient teaching and advice

- patient should be advised to take with or after food to reduce GI adverse effects, but avoid taking with carbonated water
- warn patient that gastrointestinal symptoms are usually transient at the start of therapy and usually disappear within a few days
- patient should be warned about hair loss as a common adverse effect. Hair usually grows back but may be curly
- instruct patient to take regular dosage at least 3 times daily to avoid excessive fluctuations in serum and brain drug levels
- advise patient to take with milk to avoid unpleasant taste
- warn patient not to remove tablets from foil until ready to ingest as they absorb water
- care should be taken when using Epilim syrup in patients with diabetes because it contains 3.6 g sucrose/5 mL. Sugar-free syrup is available as an alternative
- syrup should be shaken well before use
- normal syrup may be diluted but used within 14 days; sugar-free syrup should not be diluted
- patient should be advised to seek medical advice immediately if any of the following occur:
    - sudden bruising or bleeding (signs of blood dyscrasias)
    - nausea, vomiting, anorexia and/or abdominal pain (signs of pancreatitis)
    - ongoing lethargy, vomiting or changes in mental state (hyperammonaemia)
    - signs of liver dysfunction (malaise, weakness, lethargy, facial oedema, anorexia, vomiting, abdominal pain, drowsiness, yellowing of skin or eye whites, darkened urine)
- warn patient against using aspirin for pain or as an antipyretic
- counsel patient about possible weight gain and suitable diet
- female patients of childbearing potential should be counselled regarding the need to use two reliable forms of contraception (including a barrier method) during therapy and the need to seek medical advice if pregnancy occurs
- see also General Patient teaching and advice for antiepileptics (p. 383)

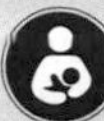

contraindicated during pregnancy due to increased risk of neural tube defects if taken during first trimester. Pregnant women taking sodium valproate should be encouraged to consider ultrasound and amniocentesis for diagnosis of possible abnormalities. A haemorrhagic syndrome related to hypofibrinaemia in neonates has also been seen (decreased coagulation factors). It is recommended that fibrinogen serum levels, platelet count and coagulation should be monitored carefully in the neonate

secreted in breastmilk, therefore mothers are advised against breastfeeding

available as a syrup or crushable tablet. Crushable tablets can be crushed and mixed with water or spoonful of yoghurt or apple puree

STIRIPENTOL (Diacomit)

Available forms

Capsules: 250 mg, 500 mg; Sachets: 250 mg, 500 mg

Action

- potentiates GABA transmission both presynaptically (increasing GABA release from nerve terminals) and postsynaptically, increasing brain levels of GABA
- half-life 4–13 hours (dose dependent)

Use

- adjunctive therapy in treatment of generalised tonic–clonic seizures associated with severe myoclonic epilepsy in infancy (known as Dravet syndrome) in those not adequately controlled with a benzodiazepine (usually clobazam) and sodium valproate

Dose

- dose is calculated on mg/kg of body weight and then divided into 2 or 3 daily doses
- initially 20 mg/kg/day (for first week), then increasing to 30 mg/kg/day (for second week), then increasing according to child's age (recommended daily dose is 50 mg/kg/day)

Adverse effects

- anorexia, loss of appetite, weight loss, nausea, vomiting
- insomnia, aggressiveness, irritability, behaviour disorders, opposing behaviour, hyperexcitability, sleep disorders
- drowsiness, ataxia, hypotonia, dystonia, hyperactivity, inability to concentrate
- neutropenia
- elevated liver enzymes
- (uncommon) photosensitivity, rash, urticaria
- (rare) thrombocytopenia

Interactions

- not recommended with carbamazepine, phenytoin or phenobarbital (phenobarbitone)
- not recommended with tacrolimus, ciclosporin or sirolimus as serum levels and risk of adverse effects and toxicity are increased
- increased risk of adverse effects such as rhabdomyolysis if given with statins and are therefore not recommended together
- caution if used with macrolide antibacterial agents or azole antifungals
- caution if used with citalopram, omeprazole, HIV protease inhibitors, antihistamines, calcium-channel blockers, statins, codeine and oral contraceptives. Plasma levels should be monitored if given together
- not recommended with caffeine or theophylline or agents with narrow therapeutic index
- increased action if given with other agents that enhance GABA activity such as benzodiazepines, barbiturates and bromides

Nursing points/Cautions

- starting therapy should be done slowly with dose escalation depending on child's age. During 3rd week:
  - (child < 6 years) an additional 20 mg/kg/day (to recommended dose of 50 mg/kg/day)
  - (child > 6 years but < 12 years) an additional 10 mg/kg/day each week, achieving recommended daily dose of 50 mg/kg/day in 4 weeks
  - (child > 12 years, adolescent) an additional 5 mg/kg/day each week until optimum dose is achieved
- formulations are not bioequivalent, therefore switching from one formulation to the other should be done under medical supervision
- blood count and liver function tests are recommended before starting therapy and then 6-monthly
- growth rate in children should be closely monitored during therapy (especially if the combination therapy causes gastrointestinal side-effects including anorexia, loss of appetite, nausea and vomiting)
- not recommended in those with any liver or kidney impairment
- contraindicated in those with history of psychoses or delirium

Patient teaching and advice

- parents/carers should be instructed not to switch formulations without seeking medical advice
- advise patient/parent/carer that capsules should be swallowed whole with glass of water during meal. If using sachet, powder should be mixed in glass of water and taken with meal
- instruct patient/parent/carer that medication should not be taken with milk or dairy products (including yoghurt, ice cream, soft cream cheese), carbonated drinks, fruit juice or foods/drinks which contain caffeine (e.g. cola drinks, energy drinks) or theophylline (e.g. chocolate)
- advise patient/parent/carer to seek medical advice if any of the following occur:
  - drowsiness or excessive sleepiness
  - depressed mood, self-harming behaviours, suicidal thoughts

SULTHIAME (Ospolot)

Available forms

Tablets: 50 mg, 200 mg

Action

- sulfonamide derivative with no antibacterial actions
- carbonic anhydrase inhibitor

Use

- temporal lobe epilepsy
- myoclonic seizures
- tonic–clonic (grand mal) epilepsy
- partial motor (Jacksonian) seizures
- hyperkinetic behaviour

Dose

- initially 100 mg orally twice daily with fluids after meals, increasing gradually to 200 mg 3 times daily (maintenance) **OR**
- initially 50 mg orally 3 times daily with fluids after meals, increasing gradually to 200 mg 3 times daily (maintenance)

Adverse effects

- see General Adverse effects of antiepileptics (p. 382)
- paraesthesia of face and extremities
- hyperpnoea, dyspnoea, tachypnoea
- anorexia, weight loss
- angina
- hiccups
- (rare) calcium and vitamin D metabolism disturbance

Interactions
- use with primidone may lead to severe adverse effects, including psychosis
- increased serum levels of phenytoin may occur when added to established phenytoin therapy, therefore phenytoin serum levels should be closely monitored
- may lead to increased phenobarbital (phenobarbitone) serum levels
- use with alcohol is not recommended
- may increase lamotrigine serum levels if given together
- caution if used with carbonic anhydrase inhibitors such as topiramate and acetazolamide
- may interfere with barbiturate estimation test

Nursing points/Cautions
- kidney function should be closely monitored during therapy
- caution if used in those with kidney or liver impairment
- not recommended in those with psychiatric history
- not recommended in those with rare hereditary problems of galactose intolerance, lactase deficiency or glucose–galactose malabsorption
- contraindicated in those with hypersensitivity to sulfonamides, acute porphyria, hyperthyroidism or arterial hypertension
- see also General Nursing points/ Cautions for antiepileptics (p. 382)

Patient teaching and advice
- patient should be advised to report any shortness of breath, rapid or difficulty breathing
- ensure patient understands the importance of not consuming alcohol during therapy due to risk of severe reaction, including severe flushing, pulsating headache, decreased breathing, nausea, vomiting, low BP and racing heart
- see also General Patient teaching and advice for antiepileptics (p. 383)

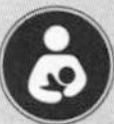

not recommended during pregnancy and breastfeeding

tablets can be dispersed in water or crushed and mixed with spoonful of yoghurt or apple puree

TIAGABINE HYDROCHLORIDE (Gabitril)

Available forms
Tablets: 5 mg, 10 mg, 15 mg

Action
- selectively inhibits uptake of GABA in neurons and glial cells
- half-life 7–9 hours

Use
- partial seizures (as adjunct therapy where epilepsy is not controlled by other antiepileptics)

Dose
- initially 2.5–5 mg orally 3 times daily with food, increasing at weekly intervals by 5–15 mg weekly until optimal response is achieved, 30–50 mg daily (maintenance) (daily maximum 70 mg)

Adverse effects
- see General Adverse effects of antiepileptics (p. 382)
- diarrhoea, abdominal pain
- pharyngitis, rhinitis, flu syndrome
- (rare) visual field defects, bleeding, serious skin reactions

Interactions
- contraindicated with St John's wort
- metabolism enhanced by phenytoin, carbamazepine, phenobarbital (phenobarbitone) and primidone, therefore serum levels should be closely monitored

Nursing points/Cautions

- if visual symptoms occur, patient should be referred to ophthalmologist
- caution if used in those with history of behavioural problems including anxiety and depression or mild-to-moderate liver impairment
- not recommended in those under 12 years
- contraindicated in those with severe liver impairment
- see also General Nursing points/Cautions for antiepileptics (p. 382)

Patient teaching and advice

- instruct patient to seek medical advice immediately if any of the following occur:
  - bruising or bleeding
  - visual changes
  - rash or blistering
- warn patient that tablets should not be refrigerated
- see also General Patient teaching and advice for antiepileptics (p. 383)

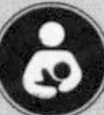

caution if used during pregnancy as animal studies have demonstrated some fetal abnormalities

should only be used during breastfeeding if benefits are thought to outweigh risks

tablet can be crushed and mixed with water or spoonful of yoghurt or apple puree

TOPIRAMATE (Epiramax, Tamate, Topamax)

Available forms

Tablets: 25 mg, 50 mg, 100 mg, 200 mg; Sprinkle capsules: 15 mg, 25 mg, 50 mg

Action

- reduces frequency of neuronal action potential generation
- enhances activity of GABA by an action different to that of barbiturates
- antagonises ability of kainate to activate glutamate receptors
- has weak carbonic anhydrase inhibitor activity (less than acetazolamide)
- antimigraine action is unknown
- half-life 21 hours

Use

- newly diagnosed epilepsy (monotherapy)
- primary generalised tonic–clonic seizures
- partial seizures with or without secondary generalised seizures (adjunct therapy)
- drop attacks associated with Lennox-Gastaut syndrome
- migraine prophylaxis

Dose

- (epilepsy – monotherapy) initially 25 mg orally at night for 7 days or longer, increasing by 25–50 mg daily at weekly or longer intervals until clinical response is achieved (daily maximum 500–1000 mg) **OR**
- (epilepsy – add-on therapy) initially 25–50 mg orally at night or in divided doses for 7 days or longer, increasing by 25–100 mg daily at weekly or longer intervals until clinical response is achieved (daily maximum 1000 mg) **OR**
- (migraine prophylaxis) initially 25 mg orally at night for 7 days, increasing by 25 mg per day at weekly intervals to 100 mg daily in 2 divided doses

Adverse effects

- see General Adverse effects of antiepileptics (p. 382)
- myalgia, muscle spasm, arthralgia
- anorexia, weight loss, alteration to taste, dyspepsia, dry mouth, diarrhoea, abdominal pain

- leucopenia, bleeding (mild to severe), anaemia
- paraesthesia, hypoaesthesia
- ear pain, tinnitus
- dyspnoea
- (rare) renal calculi, oligohidrosis, hyperthermia, eye pain, dry eyes, acute myopia, decreased visual acuity, redness, increased intra-ocular pressure, decreased serum sodium bicarbonate, metabolic acidosis, hyperammonaemia, dysuria, nephrolithiasis

Interactions

- may increase serum levels of phenytoin and lithium, increasing risk of toxicity
- may decrease digoxin serum levels, therefore levels should be closely monitored especially when starting or stopping therapy
- not recommended with alcohol or other CNS-depressant drugs
- may decrease efficacy of combined oral contraceptives
- serum levels may be decreased by phenytoin and carbamazepine
- serum levels may be increased by hydrochlorothiazide
- increased risk of hypokalaemia if given with hydrochlorothiazide
- may alter serum levels of metformin, glibenclamide and pioglitazone, therefore blood glucose levels should be closely monitored
- caution if used with carbonic anhydrase inhibitors as these may increase risk of oligohidrosis and hyperthermia
- risk of nephrolithiasis increased if given with other agents that predispose to it
- increased risk of hyperammonaemia (with or without encephalopathy) if given with sodium valproate
- caution if given with warfarin. INR should be closely monitored during therapy

Nursing points/Cautions

- any dehydration should be corrected before starting therapy
- patient should be closely monitored for any decreased sweating and/or increase in body temperature
- sodium bicarbonate levels should be monitored during therapy
- caution if used in those with psychiatric history, kidney or liver impairment or prior kidney stone formation or hypercalciuria
- see also General Nursing points/Cautions for antiepileptics (p. 382)

Patient teaching and advice

- patient should be advised to maintain good hydration throughout therapy (especially if exercising or exposed to warm conditions) to decrease the risk of renal calculi formation
- advise patient to seek medical advice immediately if any of the following occur:
  - eye pain or changes in vision
  - fatigue, anorexia or hyperventilation
  - numbness or tingling of hands or feet
  - decreased sweating
  - kidney or flank pain
  - changes to consciousness, lethargy, confusion
- women taking oral contraceptives should be counselled to report any changes in bleeding patterns and use alternative contraceptive methods (e.g. barrier) to avoid pregnancy occurring during therapy
- warn patient that if sprinkle capsules are used in food, food should not be stored
- (migraine prophylaxis) advise patient that medication should not be used for acute attack
- see also General Patient teaching and advice for antiepileptics (p. 383)

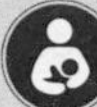

increased risk of cleft palate, hypospadias and body anomalies if given during pregnancy, therefore only used if benefits outweigh risks. Folic acid supplementation is recommended to decrease risk of spina bifida

not recommended during breastfeeding

capsules can be opened and mixed with yoghurt or apple puree. Tablet can be dispersed in water (has bitter taste) or mixed with spoonful of yoghurt or apple puree

VIGABATRIN (Sabril)

Available forms

Tablets: 500 mg; Powder: 500 mg

Action

- inhibitor of GABA, leading to an increase in GABA levels which leads to reduced neuronal activity
- half-life 5–8 hours

Use

- epilepsy (unresponsive to other drugs)

Dose

- initially 2 g orally daily in 1–2 doses, increasing or decreasing as necessary at weekly (or more) increments of 1 g (daily maximum 4 g)

Adverse effects

- see General Adverse effects of antiepileptics (p. 382)
- weight gain
- abdominal pain
- oedema
- alopecia
- anaemia
- arthralgia
- visual field defects

Interactions

- may decrease serum level of phenytoin
- contraindicated with retinotoxic agents
- caution if used with clonazepam due to increased sedation

Nursing points/Cautions

- visual fields should be monitored before starting and every 6 months throughout therapy
- therapy is usually started as add-on therapy to other antiepileptic agents
- not recommended in those with pre-existing significant visual field defects
- caution if used in those with a psychiatric history or kidney impairment (creatinine clearance < 60 mL/min)
- see also General Nursing points/Cautions for antiepileptics (p. 382)

Patient teaching and advice

- patient should be advised to seek medical advice immediately if any changes to vision occur
- advise patient that granules should be dissolved in water or soft drink just before administration
- see also General Patient teaching and advice for antiepileptics (p. 383)

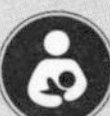

not recommended during pregnancy or breastfeeding unless benefits outweigh risks

powder can be dissolved in 100 mL water or soft drink. Tablet can be dispersed in water or crushed and mixed with spoonful of yoghurt or apple puree

ZONISAMIDE (Zonegran)

Available form

Capsules: 25 mg, 50 mg, 100 mg

Action

- benzisoxazole unrelated to other antiepileptic agents that preferentially acts on seizures coming from the cortex
- acts on sodium and calcium channels

- enables dopaminergic and serotonergic neurotransmission
- effective against tonic (not clonic) seizure types
- raises generalised seizure threshold
- shortens seizure duration
- inhibits carbonic anhydrase
- half-life about 60 hours

Use
- (monotherapy) adults with partial seizures (with or without secondary generalisation) (newly diagnosed, intolerant to other agents or where other agents are contraindicated)
- (adjunctive therapy) adults with partial seizures (with or without secondary generalisation)

Dose
- (monotherapy) 100 mg orally daily (weeks 1 and 2), increasing to 200 mg orally daily (weeks 3 and 4), increasing to 300 mg orally (weeks 5 and 6), then 300 mg orally daily as maintenance. If higher dose is needed, dose can be increased at 100 mg increments at 2-weekly intervals to a maximum of 500 mg **OR**
- (adjunctive therapy with carbamazepine, phenytoin, phenobarbital (phenobarbitone)) 25 mg orally twice daily (week 1), increasing to 50 mg orally twice daily (week 2), then increasing at weekly intervals of 100 mg (weeks 3 to 5) with maintenance of 300–500 mg (once daily or in divided doses) **OR**
- (adjunctive therapy, or in those with renal/liver impairment) 25 mg orally twice daily (weeks 1 and 2), increasing to 50 mg orally twice daily (weeks 3 and 4), then increasing at 2-weekly intervals of up to 100 mg (weeks 5 to 10), with maintenance of 300–500 mg (once daily or in divided dose)

Adverse effects
- see General Adverse effects of antiepileptics (p. 382)
- abdominal pain, anorexia, constipation, diarrhoea, dry mouth, dyspepsia, altered taste, weight loss
- ecchymosis, leucopenia
- arthralgia, myasthenia
- otitis media, tinnitus
- urinary tract infection, nephrolithiasis,
- metabolic acidosis, decreased bicarbonate, osteomalacia, osteoporosis, decreased serum phosphorus
- acne, oligohidrosis, hyperthermia
- increased cough, pharyngitis, rhinitis, sinusitis
- pancreatitis
- (rare) allergic reaction, flu-like syndrome, hypersensitivity, serious skin reaction, acute myopia and secondary angle closure glaucoma

Interactions
- not recommended with carbonic anhydrase inhibitors (e.g. topiramate) due to increased risk of metabolic acidosis and nephrolithiasis
- caution if given with bicarbonate-lowering drugs such acetazolamide due to increased risk of metabolic acidosis
- increased risk of kidney stone development if given with other agents that cause urolithiasis
- caution if given with phenytoin, carbamazepine, phenobarbital (phenobarbitone) and rifampicin

Nursing points/Cautions
- see General Nursing points/Cautions for antiepileptics (p. 382)
- patient should be monitored for signs of metabolic acidosis, which can occur at any dose, although more commonly at high doses, and early in treatment. If metabolic acidosis occurs, dose should be decreased or drug discontinued
- monitor patient for any signs of muscle weakness or muscle pain. If they occur, creatine phosphokinase should be measured

- serum bicarbonate levels should be measured before starting therapy, when reaching maintenance dose, if doses are increased, if other anti-epileptic agents are added to the regimen and then 6-monthly
- 100 mg capsules contain yellow colouring (sunset yellow), which may cause allergic reaction
- caution if used in those with low body weight (<40 kg)
- caution if used in younger patients as metabolic acidosis occurs more frequently and more severely
- caution if given to those with predisposition to metabolic acidosis, such as kidney disease, respiratory disorders, status epilepticus, diarrhoea, surgery, ketogenic diet or if taking bicarbonate-lowering drugs
- caution if used in those with risk factors for nephrolithiasis, including previous kidney stone formation, family history of nephrolithiasis and hypercalciuria
- caution if used in those with history of eye disorders due to risk of acute myopia
- not recommended in those under 18 years
- contraindicated in those with hypersensitivity to sulfonamides

Patient teaching and advice

- see General Patient teaching and advice for antiepileptics (p. 383)
- advise patients (especially children) to avoid exposure to high temperatures and maintain hydration in order to avoid heat stroke as medication can decrease sweating and raise body temperature
- patient should be instructed to increase fluid intake during therapy to decrease risk of kidney stones forming
- warn patient to avoid ketogenic diet during therapy due to increased risk of metabolic acidosis
- instruct patient to seek medical advice immediately if any of the following occur:
  - rash or skin blistering
  - significant weight loss
  - loss of appetite, fatigue, rapid breathing
  - nausea, vomiting, fever, chills, abdominal pain radiating to back, pale fatty stools
  - eye pain, changes to vision
  - kidney or flank pain
  - muscle pain or weakness
- women of childbearing potential should be counselled to use reliable contraception during and for 4 weeks after therapy is discontinued

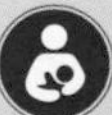

teratogenic in animal studies, therefore should only be used in pregnancy if benefits are thought to outweigh risks

breastfeeding is not recommended during or for 4 weeks after therapy is discontinued

capsules can be opened and contents dispersed in water or mixed with spoonful of yoghurt or apple puree

ANTIFUNGAL AGENTS

Fungal infections (termed mycoses) are usually caused by:

- moulds (which grow in filamentous forms (hyphae) at room temperature and in invaded tissue; e.g. dermatophytes such as *Tinea* spp., which cause 'athlete's foot', and *Aspergillus*)
- yeasts (rounded, single cells or budding organisms; e.g. *Cryptococcus* (the cause of cryptococcal meningitis), *Candida* spp. (oral and vaginal thrush))
- dimorphic fungus (these grow as yeasts but are filamentous at room temperature in the environment in which they occur; e.g. blastomycosis, histoplasmosis) (Edwards 2018).

Fungal infections can be superficial (e.g. skin, nails) or systemic (e.g. organs, deeper tissue) with deep organ infections causing severe illness and, at times, becoming fatal (Edwards 2018). *Endemic* fungal infections are acquired from environmental sources (and most commonly inhaled), while *opportunistic* fungal infections occur when normally occurring human flora overgrow due to suppression of the immune system (Edwards 2018). For example, *Candida albicans* is a yeast-like fungus that normally resides in the gastrointestinal tract (GIT) and vagina, and is usually kept under control by the normal bacteria that also reside in those areas. When a person is treated with antibacterial agents, corticosteroids, monoclonal antibodies or antineoplastic agents, the fungus is no longer under control and overgrowth occurs (Edwards 2018).

Antifungal agents are used topically, orally or parenterally to treat infections and have no activity against other organisms such as bacteria or viruses. Classes of antifungal agents include azoles (e.g. fluconazole, voriconazole), echinocandins (e.g. caspofungin, anidulafungin) and other agents which have similar modes of action.

AMOROLFINE (Aporyl, Loceryl, MycoNail, Sandoz Nail Repair)

Available form

Nail lacquer: 5%

Action

- alters fungal cell membrane targeting ergosterol, changing cell permeability and causing leakage of cell contents
- broad spectrum
- penetrates and diffuses through nail plate effectively

Use

- onychomycoses caused by dermatophytes, yeasts and moulds

Dose

- apply nail lacquer to affected finger(s) or toe(s) 1–2 times weekly

Adverse effects

- itching, pruritus, erythema, periungual scaling
- (rare) nail discolouration, brittle/ broken nails, transient burning sensation, contact dermatitis

Nursing points/Cautions

- should not be used in those who have shown previous hypersensitivity reaction

Patient teaching and advice

- instruct patient that affected finger/ toenails should be cut short to allow better penetration of the antifungal agent
- patient should be advised to:
    - file and clean nails (using supplied nail file and cleansing pad) before applying or reapplying lacquer
    - avoid applying lotion to skin surrounding nail
    - allow nails to dry (3–5 minutes) after entire surface of affected nail has been coated using supplied reusable spatula, taking care not to apply lacquer to surrounding healthy tissue
    - discard nail file after use and do not reuse it because of reinfection risk
    - clean neck of bottle and spatula with supplied cleansing pad after each use
    - ensure bottle is tightly closed immediately after use
- treatment should be continued uninterrupted for 6 months (fingernails) or longer (toenails) until nail has regrown and area is cured
- patient should be advised not to use cosmetic nail polish, artificial nails, other topical medications or occlusive dressings on the nail(s) being treated with amorolfine
- warn patient to wear impermeable gloves if working with solvents such as paint thinners to protect nail lacquer

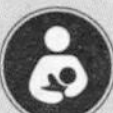

should be avoided during pregnancy and breastfeeding

AMPHOTERICIN B (AMPHOTERICIN) (AmBisome, Fungilin)

Available forms

Vial: 50 mg; Lozenges: 10 mg

Action

- binds to ergosterol leading to membrane permeability and leakage of cell contents causing potassium loss
- fungistatic or fungicidal (depending on concentration and/or susceptibility of organisms)
- lipid formulations have been developed to overcome nephrotoxicity and infusion reactions. The liposomal vesicles stay intact during prolonged circulation until they selectively bind to the fungal cell membrane and release the amphotericin B (amphotericin)
- not absorbed from GIT
- (IV) elimination half-life 26–32 hours (depending on dose)

Use

- oral and perioral candidiasis
- prophylaxis and treatment of potentially fatal systemic fungal infections (in liver transplant patients)
- presumed fungal infection in those with febrile neutropenia (where fever has not responded to broad spectrum antibiotics)

- visceral leishmaniasis due to *Leishmania infantum*

Dose

Oral candidiasis

- 10 mg orally (1 lozenge) sucked and allowed to dissolve slowly, 4 times daily after meals and nightly for 7–14 days

Systemic fungal infections

- (systemic mycoses) initially 1 mg/kg daily by IV infusion over 30–60 minutes, increasing gradually to 5 mg/kg if needed **OR**
- (prophylaxis of fungal infection in liver transplantation) 1 mg/kg daily by IV infusion over 30–60 minutes for 5 days following transplantation **OR**
- (HIV-associated disseminated cryptococcosis) 3 mg/kg daily by IV infusion over 30–60 minutes for up to 42 days **OR**
- (visceral leishmaniasis, immunocompromised patient) 1–1.5 mg/kg daily by IV infusion over 30–60 minutes for 21 days **OR**
- (visceral leishmaniasis, immunocompetent patient) as for immunocompromised patient or 3.0 mg/kg daily by IV infusion over 30–60 minutes for 10 days **OR**
- (febrile neutropenia with presumed fungal infection) 1–3 mg/kg by IV infusion over 30–60 minutes, adjusting dose according to clinical condition

Adverse effects

- (oral) mild nausea, vomiting, diarrhoea, transient yellowing of teeth
- (infusion reaction) chills, fever, rigors, back pain (usually within minutes of infusion starting)
- nausea, vomiting, abdominal pain, diarrhoea
- headache, tremor
- back pain
- hypotension, tachycardia, vasodilation, flushing, chest pain
- dyspnoea, cough
- rash, pruritus
- abnormal liver/kidney function, hypokalaemia, hyperglycaemia, hyponatraemia, hypomagnesaemia, hypocalcaemia, hyperbilirubinaemia, increased creatinine and blood urea
- toxic nephropathy
- (rare) anaphylactoid reactions, anaphylaxis

Interactions

- contraindicated with cidofovir. Amphotericin should be discontinued for at least 7 days before starting cidofovir
- risk of digitalis toxicity is increased in the presence of amphotericin-induced hypokalaemia when given with digoxin, therefore serum potassium and digoxin levels should be closely monitored
- not recommended with azole antifungal agents due to antagonistic effect reducing antifungal activity
- increased risk of pulmonary toxicity if given with or near to leucocyte transfusion so should be separated for the longest possible time period. Lung function should be monitored
- increased risk of myelotoxicity and nephrotoxicity if given with zidovudine
- effects of skeletal muscle relaxants may be potentiated in the presence of amphotericin-induced hypokalaemia. Patient should be monitored for any enhanced neuromuscular blockade if given together
- increases nephrotoxicity of ciclosporin, nephrotoxic antibiotics (e.g. aminoglycosides), other nephrotoxic agents and parenteral pentamidine, therefore renal function should be closely monitored if given together
- increased risk of nephrotoxicity, bronchospasm and hypotension if given with antineoplastic agents such as cisplatin and nitrogen mustard compounds
- corticosteroids and corticotropin may increase amphotericin-induced

hypokalaemia, predisposing to cardiac arrhythmias, therefore serum potassium level and cardiac function should be closely monitored if given together
- increased risk of toxicity if given with flucytosine
- caution if used with loop diuretics. If given together, serum potassium and kidney function should be monitored

Nursing points/Cautions

- should not be used for superficial infections
- (lozenge) should not be used to treat systemic infections
- blood counts, serum electrolytes, kidney and liver function should be monitored at least weekly during prolonged therapy (especially if receiving concurrent nephrotoxic agent). Potassium supplements may be required
- slowing infusion rate may decrease infusion-related reaction symptoms
- resuscitation equipment should be readily available during IV administration
- reconstitute using water for injections only and shake solution until any yellow sediment has dissolved, withdraw required amount from vial(s), discard needle and replace with 5 micron high-flow filter needle (supplied) and inject into glucose 5% solution
- administer alone using separated IV line or ensure existing IV line is adequately flushed with glucose 5% before administration
- in-line filter (1 micron or greater) may be used for IV infusion
- leucocyte transfusion should be separated for the longest possible period to avoid risk of acute lung toxicity. Lung function should be closely monitored
- if patient is having renal dialysis, amphotericin B (amphotericin) should not be administered until dialysis is completed. Monitoring of serum potassium and magnesium is recommended
- should not be mixed with solutions containing sodium chloride or potassium
- contains 900 mg sucrose per vial and therefore blood glucose levels should be closely monitored if patient has diabetes mellitus
- should only be used after dialysis has been completed in those with kidney impairment

Patient teaching and advice

- (lozenge) advise patient that dentures should be removed while sucking lozenges and then thoroughly cleaned
- (lozenge) patient should be warned that any yellowing of teeth is from sucking lozenges and is temporary. It can be removed by brushing teeth

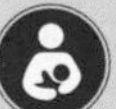

not recommended during pregnancy and breastfeeding unless benefits outweigh risks

ANIDULAFUNGIN (Eraxis)

Available form

Vial: 100 mg

Action

- echinocandin that inhibits glucan synthesis in the fungal wall (which is not present in human cells)
- fungicidal for *Candida* and *Aspergillus* species
- elimination half-life 20 hours

Use

- invasive candidiasis, including candidaemia

Dose

- initially 200 mg IV over 180 minutes (day 1, loading dose), then 100 mg daily over 90 minutes continued for at least 14 days after last positive culture (but not exceeding 28 days)

Adverse effects

- thrombocytopenia, coagulopathy, decreased platelet count
- hyperkalaemia, hypokalaemia, hypomagnesaemia
- increase in liver enzymes, elevated bilirubin and creatinine
- headache, flushing
- diarrhoea
- rash, pruritus
- seizures
- prolonged QT interval
- (rare) anaphylactic reaction
- (infusion reaction) rash, pruritus, flushing, urticaria, dyspnoea, bronchospasm, hypotension

Nursing points/Cautions

- fungal culture and histopathology should be performed on specimen to identify species before starting therapy
- liver function, FBC, ECG and electrolytes should be monitored during therapy
- not recommended as IV bolus
- reconstitute using 30 mL water for injections and then dilute with either sodium chloride 0.9% or glucose 5% (to give concentration of 0.77 mf/mL)
- infusion rate should not be greater than 1.1 mg/minute
- not recommended in those under 18 years
- contraindicated in those with hypersensitivity to echinocandins

Patient teaching and advice

- advise patient to seek medical advice if any of the following occur:
  - increased heart rate
  - fever, infection
  - unexplained bleeding or bruising
  - seizures (fitting)
- female patients of childbearing potential should be counselled to use adequate and effective contraception during therapy

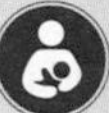

not recommended during pregnancy or breastfeeding

BIFONAZOLE (Canesten Once Daily Bifonazole Cream 1%, Mycospor)

Available form

Topical cream: 1%

Action

- imidazole antifungal agent that inhibits ergosterol synthesis in fungal cell membrane
- fungicidal against dermatophytes, fungistatic against yeasts

Use

- mycoses of skin caused by dermatophytes and yeasts
- pityriasis versicolor caused by *Malassezia furfur*

Dose

- applied thinly to affected area and rubbed gently into skin once daily before sleeping

Adverse effects

- burning, pruritus, irritation, erythema, scaling
- (less frequent) contact dermatitis

Nursing points/Cautions

- not recommended for fungal infections of the mucous membranes or eyes

Patient teaching and advice

- patient should be advised to complete the course of treatment, which may continue for days/weeks after symptoms have resolved. If there is no resolution of the symptoms after the treatment period, the diagnosis should be reassessed or the likelihood of resistance to the agent used should be considered

- warn patient that superficial fungal infections can be highly contagious
- advise patient not to share clothing or personal linen (e.g. face washers, towels)
- patient should be advised to continue treatment uninterrupted for the following times:
  - 3 weeks for tinea pedis, tinea pedis interdigitalis
  - 2–3 weeks for tinea corporis, tinea cruris, tinea manuum
  - 2 weeks for pityriasis versicolor
  - 2–4 weeks for superficial candidiasis of the skin
- patient being treated for tinea pedis should be encouraged to wash and dry the feet (especially between toes) carefully each day and apply antifungal powder. They should also be advised to wear shoes or sandals that are well ventilated (if possible), wear waterproof sandals in public showers, change hosiery (preferably cotton socks) daily and dust shoes inside with powder
- instruct patient not to use cream for fungal infection of other areas of the body, particularly vagina or mouth

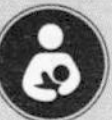

safety during pregnancy has not been established; animal studies have shown bifonazole to be embryotoxic

caution if used during breastfeeding

Note

- contained in Canesten Fungal Nail Treatment with urea for treatment of onychomycosis

CASPOFUNGIN ACETATE (Cancidas)

Available forms

Vial: 50 mg, 70 mg

Action

- echinocandin that inhibits glucan synthesis in the fungal wall (which is not present in human cells)
- fungicidal for *Candida*, fungistatic for *Aspergillus*

Use

- invasive candidiasis (including candidaemia)
- oesophageal candidiasis
- invasive aspergillosis (when other treatment was ineffective or inappropriate)
- fungal infection in febrile neutropenia patient (when fever has failed to respond to other treatments)

Dose

- (invasive candidiasis, invasive aspergillosis, febrile neutropenia) initially 70 mg by slow IV infusion over 1 hour (day 1, loading dose), then 35–50 mg daily IV (maintenance) **OR**
- (oesophageal candidiasis) 35–50 mg daily by slow IV infusion over 1 hour

Adverse effects

- myalgia
- diarrhoea, nausea, vomiting, abdominal pain
- fever, chills, sweating, flushing
- dyspnoea
- rash, pruritus, erythema
- tremor, insomnia
- headache
- tachycardia, hypertension
- increased liver enzymes, hypokalaemia, hypomagnesaemia, increased creatinine and bilirubin
- (hypersensitivity reaction) rash, pruritus, facial swelling, bronchospasm, flushing sensation
- (IV site) phlebitis, thrombophlebitis, pain

Interactions
- not recommended with ciclosporin because of increased risk of liver toxicity. If given together, liver function should be closely monitored
- may decrease serum levels of tacrolimus, therefore blood levels should be monitored
- serum levels decreased if given with rifampicin (if added to already existing rifampicin therapy), efavirenz, nevirapine, phenytoin, dexamethasone and carbamazepine

Nursing points/Cautions
- treatment should continue for a minimum of 14 days and at least 28 days after neutropenia and clinical symptoms have resolved
- not compatible with glucose
- administer alone
- allow vial to come to room temperature, then reconstitute using water for injections or sodium chloride 0.9% (10.5 mL) and mix gently. When solution clears, inspect for particulate matter or discolouration, then dilute with sodium chloride 0.9% infusion bag (100–250 mL) and infuse over 1 hour
- caution if used in those with moderate liver impairment or with a history of allergic skin reactions

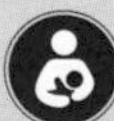

not recommended during pregnancy or breastfeeding unless benefits outweigh risks

CICLOPIROX (Rejuvenail)

Available form
Solution: 80 mg/g

Action
- pyridone antifungal agent with some anti-inflammatory activity

Use
- mild-to-moderate onchomycoses (without lunar involvement) due to dermatophytes, yeasts or moulds

Dose
- apply to infected nail(s) at night until healthy nail has regrown

Adverse effects
- pain, irritation, redness, burning, tenderness, ingrown nail

Patient teaching and advice
- patient should be advised to:
  - wash and dry infected nail
  - apply thin layer to within 5 mm of surrounding skin and under nail if possible
  - allow to dry for 30 seconds
  - area should not be washed for 6 hours
  - fingernails may require up to 6 months of treatment, toenails 9–12 months

CLOTRIMAZOLE (Canesten preparations, Clonea, Clonea Clotrimazole Thrush Treatment 3 Day Cream, Clonea Clotrimazole Thrush Treatment 6 Day Cream, Clozole Topical Cream, Clozole Vaginal Cream 10 mg/g & 20 mg/g, Trust Fem V)

Available forms
Topical cream: 10 mg/g; Solution: 10 mg/mL (1%); Vaginal cream: 10 mg/g, 20 mg/g; Vaginal pessaries: 100 mg

Action
- imidazole antifungal agent that inhibits ergosterol synthesis in fungal cell membrane

Use
- dermatophytes (e.g. tinea pedis, tinea cruris, tinea corporis, pityriasis versicolor)

- onychia, paronychia
- candidiasis, cutaneous candidiasis, vaginal and vulvovaginal candidiasis

Dose

Cutaneous candidiasis, dermatophytes

- gently massage cream into affected and surrounding skin areas 2–3 times daily for at least 2 weeks after symptoms have resolved **OR**
- apply cream or solution 2–3 times daily sparingly to affected areas

Vaginal, vulvovaginal candidiasis

- 5 g (1 applicator full) inserted nightly as deeply as possible into the vagina for 6 successive days (vaginal cream 1%) or 3 doses (vaginal cream 2%) or 1 dose (vaginal cream 10%) **OR**
- 100 mg nightly inserted as deeply as possible into the vagina for 6 successive days (vaginal tablet/pessary) or 2 × 100 mg tablets for 3 doses or 1 × 500 mg (vaginal tablet/pessary) as a single dose

Adverse effects

- (cream/solution) erythema, oedema, pruritus, urticaria, stinging/burning, blistering, peeling, general irritation of skin
- (pessaries/vaginal tablets) (uncommon) mild burning, skin rash, lower abdominal pain

Interactions

- vaginal cream may reduce effectiveness of latex products (e.g. condoms, diaphragms)

Nursing points/Cautions

- (skin conditions) treatment time depends on the location of the infection:
  - dermatomycoses: 2–4 weeks
  - onychia and paronychia: 4–8 weeks
  - tinea pedis, corporis: 4 weeks
  - tinea cruris: 2 weeks
  - cutaneous candidiasis: 2 weeks
- if no improvement in 4 weeks, diagnosis should be reviewed
- vaginal cream and pessaries can be used together to manage vulvovaginitis or perianal infection
- caution if used in those with sensitivity to another azole

Patient teaching and advice

- patient should be advised to complete the course of treatment, which may continue for days/weeks after symptoms have resolved. If there is no resolution of the symptoms after the treatment period, the diagnosis should be reassessed or the likelihood of resistance to the agent used considered
- warn patient that superficial fungal infections can be highly contagious
- advise patient not to share clothing or personal linen (e.g. face washers, towels)
- patient being treated for tinea pedis should be encouraged to wash and dry the feet (especially between toes) carefully each day and apply antifungal powder. They should also be advised to wear shoes or sandals that are well ventilated (if possible), wear waterproof sandals in public showers, change hosiery (preferably cotton socks) daily and dust shoes inside with powder

Vaginal/Vulvovaginal candidiasis

- ensure patient understands correct insertion technique for vaginal cream, pessaries and tablets
- advise patient that a second course of treatment may be required if first course was unsuccessful
- treatment should be timed to avoid menstruation or to be complete before its onset or should be continued if menstruation occurs
- warn patient that vaginal cream/pessaries may decrease the effectiveness and safety of condoms and diaphragms

- for prevention of reinfection, the partner(s) should be treated locally at the same time with application of cream to the glans penis
- if patient is pregnant and in second or third trimester, digital insertion of tablets/pessaries is recommended rather than plastic applicator
- instruct women being treated for vaginal infection that they should refrain from sexual intercourse or encourage partner to use a condom. Sexual partner(s) should also be treated to prevent reinfection. Perineal pads (or panty liners) will prevent staining of underwear or clothing when vaginal tablets or creams are used. Wearing cotton underwear and pantyhose with a cotton gusset is also recommended (especially if infection recurs). Use of tampons or douching between doses of vaginal medications is not recommended

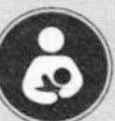

intravaginal preparations are not recommended during first trimester of pregnancy unless benefits outweigh risks

Note

- contained in Candacort, Extra Clotrimazole and Hydrocortisone Cream, Hydrozole Cream with hydrocortisone, Afeme Duo, Canesoral Duo and Femazole Duo (oral fluconazole tablet with clotrimazole cream)

ECONAZOLE NITRATE (Pevaryl Antifungal Cream, Pevaryl Foaming Solution)

Available forms

Foaming solution: 1%; Cream 1%

Action

- imidazole antifungal agent that inhibits ergosterol synthesis in fungal cell membrane

Use

- tinea pedis, tinea cruris, tinea corporis, tinea versicolor (pityriasis versicolor)

Dose

- apply foaming solution to wet body (skin and scalp) after showering nightly. Rub in well for 3–5 minutes and then allow to dry, rinse off the following morning and repeat for 3 consecutive evenings **OR**
- apply cream to affected area 2–3 times daily for up to 14 days until symptoms disappear, to prevent relapse

Adverse effects

- (foaming solution) tightening of facial skin

Nursing points/Cautions

- course should be repeated after 4 weeks and again at 12 weeks after initial treatment to prevent recurrence
- caution if used in those with sensitivity to another azole

Patient teaching and advice

- patient should be advised to complete the course of treatment, which may continue for days/weeks after symptoms have resolved. If there is no resolution of the symptoms after the treatment period, the diagnosis should be reassessed or the likelihood of resistance to the agent used should be considered
- warn patient that superficial fungal infections can be highly contagious
- advise patient not to share clothing or personal linen (e.g. face washers, towels)
- patient should be advised to avoid contact with eyes
- patient being treated for tinea pedis should be encouraged to wash and dry the feet (especially between toes) carefully each day and apply antifungal powder. They should also be advised to wear shoes or sandals that are well ventilated (if possible), wear

waterproof sandals in public showers, change hosiery (preferably cotton socks) daily and dust shoes inside with powder

FLUCONAZOLE (Canesoral, Diflucan, Diflucan One, Dizole, Dizole One, Femazole One, Femrelief One, Fluconazole Injection for Intravenous Infusion, Flufeme, Fluzole, Ozole, Ozole 150 mg)

Available forms

Capsules: 50 mg, 100 mg, 150 mg, 200 mg; Powder (for oral suspension): 50 mg/5 mL; Infusion bags: 100 mg/50 mL, 200 mg/100 mL, 400 mg/200 mL

Action

- triazole (similar to the imidazoles) which shows good penetration into body fluids including ocular fluid and CSF
- inhibits ergosterol synthesis in fungal cell membrane
- (oral, IV) half-life about 30 hours, prolonged in those with impaired kidney function (98–125 hours)

Use

- treatment and prophylaxis of cryptococcal meningitis (in those unable to tolerate amphotericin B (amphotericin) or prevent relapse in patients with AIDS)
- serious or life-threatening *Candida* infections (in patients unable to tolerate amphotericin B (amphotericin))
- oropharyngeal or oesophageal candidiasis
- vaginal candidiasis (where topical therapy has failed)
- extensive tinea infection (in immunocompromised patients where topical treatment has failed or is not practicable)

Dose

- (cryptococcal meningitis) 400 mg orally or IV on first day, then 200–400 mg orally or IV daily and continue for 10–12 weeks after CSF becomes culture negative **OR**
- (prevention of relapse of cryptococcal meningitis in patient with AIDS) 100–200 mg orally or IV daily after full course of primary treatment **OR**
- (oropharyngeal candidiasis) 100 mg orally or IV on first day, then 50 mg orally or IV daily for 2–3 weeks **OR**
- (oesophageal candidiasis) 200 mg on first day, then 100 mg daily for 2–3 weeks **OR**
- (secondary prophylaxis against oropharyngeal candidiasis in HIV patients) 150 mg as single weekly oral or IV dose **OR**
- (serious candidiasis where amphotericin B (amphotericin) unable to be used) 400 mg orally or IV on first day, then 200–400 mg orally or IV daily for a minimum of 4 weeks and at least 2 weeks after symptoms have resolved **OR**
- (failed topical treatment of vaginal candidiasis) 150 mg as single oral dose **OR**
- (extensive tinea infection) 150 mg as single weekly dose for 4 weeks

Adverse effects

- nausea, vomiting, abdominal pain, diarrhoea, dyspepsia
- headache, dizziness
- rash, acne
- elevated liver enzymes
- (rare) anaphylaxis, prolonged QT interval, hepatotoxicity, serious cutaneous reactions, leucopenia

Interactions

- contraindicated with agents known to prolong QT interval such as erythromycin
- not recommended with voriconazole

- serum levels may be decreased by rifampicin
- increased risk of uveitis if given with rifabutin
- may enhance anticoagulant effect of warfarin, therefore prothrombin time should be closely monitored during therapy, especially when starting or stopping therapy
- may increase serum levels of alfentanil, amitriptyline, carbamazepine, ciclosporin, calcium-channel blockers (nifedipine, amlodipine, verapamil, felodipine), celecoxib, methadone, midazolam, nortriptyline, NSAIDs, phenytoin, rifabutin, saquinavir, sirolimus, tacrolimus, theophylline and triazolam, increasing risk of adverse effects and toxicity. Patients receiving concurrent therapy should be closely observed and serum levels monitored if appropriate
- may increase serum levels of sulfonylureas and risk of hypoglycaemia
- serum levels may increase when given with hydrochlorothiazide
- may decrease metabolism of zidovudine leading to increased serum levels increasing the risk of adverse effects
- may decrease antihypertensive effect of losartan
- increased risk of myopathy and rhabdomyolysis if given with HMG-CoA reductase inhibitors (statins)
- if given long term with prednisolone, patient should be monitored for adrenal cortex insufficiency when fluconazole is stopped
- may increase respiratory depression if given with fentanyl
- may increase serum bilirubin and creatinine if given with cyclophosphamide
- increased risk of neurotoxicity if given with vinca alkaloids
- increased risk of CNS adverse effects if given with vitamin A
- not recommended with amphotericin B (amphotericin) as it reduces antifungal activity

Nursing points/Cautions

- IV fluconazole should only be given when oral administration is not possible
- monitor liver function frequently during therapy
- (cryptococcal meningitis) if no response after 60 days, alternative therapy should be considered
- IV rate not to exceed 200 mg/hour
- should not be mixed with other IV drugs
- compatible with Ringer's solution and sodium chloride 0.9%
- IV solution contains 15 mmol sodium chloride/100 mL which may need to be considered if patient has a sodium restriction
- development of rash in immunocompromised patients may require withdrawal of drug
- oral suspension contains sucrose and capsules contain lactose and are therefore not recommended in those with rare hereditary problems of galactose intolerance, Lapp lactase deficiency or glucose–galactose malabsorption
- caution if used in those with known cardiac arrhythmias, structural heart disease, electrolyte imbalance or if given with other agents that are known to prolong QT interval
- caution if used in patients with HIV or AIDS infection as there is an increased likelihood of adverse effects occurring
- caution if used in those with kidney impairment
- contraindicated in those with sensitivity to another azole

Patient teaching and advice

- if patient has diabetes treated with sulfonylureas, he/she should be advised to monitor blood glucose levels carefully as there is a risk of hypoglycaemia occurring
- if patient has HIV infection or is immunocompromised, he/she should be instructed to immediately report any rash as this may require stopping fluconazole
- warn patient against driving or operating machinery if dizziness occurs
- advise patient to seek medical advice if any of the following occur:
  - yellowing of eyes or skin, loss of appetite, lethargy or tiredness, upper abdominal pain, dark urine, pale stools
  - fast or irregular heart rate
  - sudden severe itching, hives or rash
- patient should be advised to swallow capsules whole and take with water
- instruct patient to shake oral suspension well before measuring and discard after 14 days
- patients being treated for tinea pedis should be encouraged to wash and dry the feet (especially between toes) carefully each day and apply antifungal powder. They should also be advised to wear shoes or sandals that are well ventilated (if possible), wear waterproof sandals in public showers, change hosiery (preferably cotton socks) daily and dust shoes inside with powder
- women of childbearing potential should be advised to use adequate contraception throughout therapy to avoid pregnancy

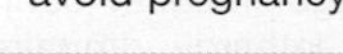

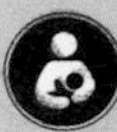

should be avoided during pregnancy except in situations where life-threatening fungal infection exists and benefits are thought to outweigh risks to the fetus

not recommended during breastfeeding

available as oral solution. Capsules can be opened and contents dispersed in water or mixed with spoonful of yoghurt or apple puree

Note

- contained in Afeme Duo, Canesoral Duo and Femazole Duo (combination pack with clotrimazole)

FLUCYTOSINE (Ancotil)

Available form

Infusion solution: 2.5 g/250 mL

Action

- fluorinated pyramidine that is converted in the fungal cell to 5 fluorouracil, which inhibits nucleic acid and protein synthesis
- some resistance has developed, therefore monotherapy is not recommended
- good penetration of CSF
- half-life 3–6 hours (prolonged in those with impaired kidney function)

Use

- generalised candidiasis, cryptococcosis, chromoblastomycosis

Dose

- 37.5–50 mg/kg IV infusion over 20–40 minutes, 6–24-hourly (depending on renal function)

Adverse effects

- nausea, vomiting, diarrhoea
- rash
- leucopenia, neutropenia, thrombocytopenia, agranulocytosis, aplastic anaemia and rarely, bone marrow toxicity
- increased liver enzymes, hepatitis, hepatic necrosis
- (rare) allergy, seizures, headache, sedation, vertigo, myocardial toxicity, ventricular dysfunction

Interactions

- may increase serum levels of phenytoin, thereby increasing risk of toxicity
- increased risk of leucopenia if given with antineoplastic agents, therefore daily blood counts are recommended if given together
- half-life may be increased if given with agents that inhibit glomerular filtration. If given together, creatinine clearance should be closely monitored
- antifungal action may be inhibited by cytosine arabinoside
- caution if used with cytarabine
- increased risk of GI bleeding if given with corticosteroids or amphotericin

Nursing points/Cautions

- monitor blood count, kidney and liver function before starting and throughout therapy
- frequency of administration is dependent on creatinine clearance. Creatinine clearance > 40 mL/min 6-hourly; 20–40 mL/min 12-hourly; 10–20 mL/min daily
- precipitate may occur if solution stands for a prolonged time at below 15°C. This can be dissolved by heating to less than 80°C for up to 30 minutes. If stored at >25°C, 5-fluorouracil formation may occur
- increased risk of toxicity in those with dihydropyrimidine dehydrogenase (DPD) deficiency
- extreme caution if used in those with known bone marrow depression or blood dyscrasias

Patient teaching and advice

- advise patient to seek medical advice immediately if any of the following occur:
  - skin inflammation that leads to blistering
  - changes in heartbeat
  - fitting (seizures)

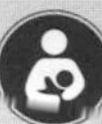

safety during pregnancy has not been established; animal studies have shown some teratogenic effects, therefore should only be used if benefits outweigh potential risks

not recommended during breastfeeding

GRISEOFULVIN (Grisovin)

Available forms

Tablets: 125 mg, 500 mg

Action

- derived from *Penicillium* species and inhibits fungal mitosis
- deposited in the keratin precursor cells, mainly in the diseased tissue, causing the new keratin to become highly resistant to fungal invasion, allowing uninfected new growth to replace older infected structures
- has no antibacterial action and is therefore unlikely to upset GI flora
- absorption is variable and incomplete (fatty food will increase rate and extent of absorption)
- half-life 9–21 hours

Use

- fungal infections of skin, scalp, hair and nails (where topical therapy has failed or is inappropriate)

Dose

- 500–1000 mg orally once daily after meals

Adverse effects

- nausea, vomiting, diarrhoea, thirst, flatulence, dyspepsia, GI bleeding, oral thrush
- headache (sometimes severe), drowsiness, vertigo, fatigue, confusion, insomnia, lethargy, impaired performance
- peripheral neuritis
- rash, urticaria, erythema, photosensitivity
- leucopenia, neutropenia
- albuminuria

- (rare) SLE-like syndrome, exacerbation of existing SLE, hepatotoxicity, proteinuria, menstrual irregularities, nephrosis, serum sickness, angio-edema

Interactions

- may enhance effects of alcohol
- absorption and effectiveness may be decreased by barbiturates
- reduces effectiveness of oral contraceptives
- warfarin effects may be reduced, therefore prothrombin time should be closely monitored especially when starting or stopping therapy
- blood levels and effectiveness may be decreased by sedatives and hypnotics

Nursing points/Cautions

- contraindicated for prophylaxis
- treatment may last for at least 4 weeks (hair and skin) and extend to 12 months for some nail infections and should continue for at least 2 weeks after symptoms have disappeared
- monitor blood cell count weekly for 4 weeks and then regularly during therapy. Kidney and liver function should also be monitored periodically (especially if therapy is prolonged)
- contraindicated in those with porphyria, systemic lupus erythematosus (SLE), severe liver failure or hepatocellular failure

Patient teaching and advice

- instruct patient to take tablets after meals (which include some fat) to help with absorption
- advise patient to immediately seek medical advice if any of the following occur:
  - menstrual irregularities
  - confusion
  - numbness, tingling, pain or weakness in hands or feet
  - sore throat, fever
  - yellowing of skin or eyes
- warn patient to avoid skin exposure to direct or intense sunlight (real or artificial) and the need to wear sunscreen (at least SPF 30+), protective clothing, hat and sunglasses when outside
- advise patient not to drive or operate machinery if drowsy or dizzy
- patient should be warned that the effects of alcohol may be enhanced and should be avoided during therapy. If patient has alcohol, and rapid heartbeat, flushing, redness in the face and/or increased sweating occurs (disulfiram–alcohol reaction) (see Glossary), he/she should seek medical advice immediately
- female patient should be counselled regarding the need to consider additional non-hormonal contraceptive precautions (such as condoms) during and for 1 month after treatment because of the possibility that oral contraceptive containing oestrogen may fail
- women and men should be advised to use adequate contraception during therapy and for 4 weeks (women) or 24 weeks (men) after ceasing therapy as griseofulvin can cause birth defects

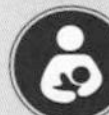

teratogenic in animal studies, therefore contraindicated during pregnancy or breastfeeding. Women should be advised not to become pregnant within 4 weeks of taking griseofulvin

men should allow 6 months after treatment before fathering children because griseofulvin may cause abnormal segregation of chromosomes after cell division

tablet can be crushed and mixed with water or milk, or spoonful of yoghurt

ISAVUCONAZOLE SULFATE (Cresemba)

Available forms

Vial: 200 mg; Capsules: 100 mg

Action

- triazole (similar to the imidazoles)
- inhibits ergosterol synthesis in fungal cell membrane
- isavuconazole sulfate is a prodrug converted to active isavuconazole

Use

- treatment of invasive aspergillosis and mucormycosis in patients where amphotericin B is inappropriate

Dose

- 200 mg orally or IV infusion over 1 hour 8-hourly for 6 doses (loading dose), followed by 200 mg orally or IV infusion over 1 hour once daily

Adverse effects

- elevated liver enzymes
- decreased appetite, nausea, vomiting, abdominal pain, diarrhoea
- dyspnoea, acute respiratory failure
- headache, confusion, delirium, somnolence, fatigue
- chest pain
- rash, pruritus
- hypokalaemia
- kidney failure
- infusion-related reaction
- injection site reaction, thrombophlebitis
- (rare) severe skin reactions, hypersensitivity

Interactions

- contraindicated with high-dose ritonavir (> 200 mg every 12 hours), rifampicin, rifabutin, carbamazepine, long-acting barbiturates (e.g. phenobarbital), phenytoin, St John's wort, efavirenz and etravirine
- caution if used with agents known to decrease QT interval
- increased plasma levels may occur if given with clarithromycin, indinavir and other protease inhibitors, therefore should be given with caution
- decreased plasma levels may occur if given with aprepitant or pioglitazone
- caution if given with mycophenolate mofetil, ciclosporin, sirolimus and tacrolimus. If given together, plasma levels should be closely monitored
- not recommended with prednisolone
- may increase plasma levels of midazolam, colchicine, dabigratran, metformin, vincristine, vinblastine, daunorubicin, doxorubicin irinotecan or topotecan leading to adverse effects
- may decrease plasma level of bupropion, cyclophosphamide, amprenavir or nelfinavir
- digoxin plasma levels should be closely monitored if given together

Nursing points/Cautions

- liver enzymes should be measured before starting therapy and monitored regularly throughout therapy
- duration of treatment is determined by clinical response; however, if therapy is longer than 6 months, risk versus benefit should be considered
- IV infusion should be stopped if infusion-related reaction (hypotension, dyspnoea, dizziness, paraesthesia, nausea, headache) occur
- to reconstitute, add 5 mL water for injections to vial, shake well to dissolve, then further dilute by adding to 250 mL infusion bag of either glucose 5% or sodium chloride 0.9% and inverting bag gently several times to minimise particulate formation. Diluted solution may contain fine white-to-translucent particulates which can be removed by administration through in-line filter
- must be administered using in-line filter (0.2–1.2 micrometre pore size) made of polyether sulfone (PES)

- administer alone
- infuse over at least 1 hour to reduce risk of infusion-related reactions
- IV infusion should be completed within 6 hours of reconstitution and dilution
- caution if used in patients with hypersensitivity to other azole antifungals
- not recommended in those with severe liver impairment or in those under 18 years
- contraindicated in patient with family history of short QT syndrome

Patient teaching and advice

- instruct patient that capsules should be swallowed whole and not chewed, crushed, opened or dissolved
- advise patient not to drive or operate machinery if any confusion, dizziness, somnolence or syncope occur

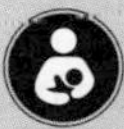

not recommended during pregnancy unless fungal infection is severe or life threatening

not recommended during breastfeeding

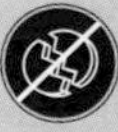

capsules should not be opened, crushed or chewed

ITRACONAZOLE (Itracap, Itranox, Lozanoc, Sporanox Capsules, Sporanox Oral Solution)

Available forms

Capsules: 50 mg, 100 mg; Oral solution: 10 mg/mL

Action

- triazole (similar to the imidazoles) which has poor penetration into CSF
- inhibits ergosterol synthesis in fungal cell membrane
- variable oral absorption although this improves if taken with food
- metabolite has equal antifungal activity

Use

- oral and oesophageal candidiasis (when other treatment has been ineffective or inappropriate)
- vaginal candidiasis (not responding to topical treatment)
- pityriasis versicolor (tinea versicolor) (not responding to treatment)
- systemic mycoses, aspergillosis, histoplasmosis, sporotrichosis
- fungal keratitis (not responding to treatment, progressing or threatening sight)
- superficial dermatomycosis (tinea corporis, tinea cruris, tinea pedis, tinea manus, tinea unguium) (not responding to topical treatment)
- onychomycosis (caused by dermatomycoses)
- disseminated/chronic histoplasmosis in patient with AIDS (treatment and maintenance)
- non-invasive candidiasis (non-neutropenic patient not responding to other treatments)
- prophylaxis of fungal infection (neutropenic patient)

Dose

- (superficial dermatomycosis) 100 mg orally daily for 2–4 weeks **OR**
- (superficial dermatomycosis) 50 mg orally daily for 2–4 weeks (Lozanoc) **OR**
- (onychomycosis) 200 mg orally daily for 3 months **OR**
- (onychomycosis) 100 mg orally daily for 3 months (Lozanoc) **OR**
- (onychomycosis – pulsed) 200 mg orally twice daily for 7 days, followed by drug-free 21 days, repeated for fingernails (2 pulses) or repeated twice more (3 pulses) for toenails **OR**
- (onychomycosis – pulsed) 100 mg orally twice daily for 7 days, followed by drug-free 21 days, repeated for

fingernails (2 pulses) or repeated twice more (3 pulses) for toenails (Lozanoc) **OR**

- (vulvovaginal candidiasis) 200 mg orally twice daily for 1 day, or 200 mg daily for 3 days **OR**
- (vulvovaginal candidiasis) 100 mg orally twice daily for 1 day, or 100 mg daily for 3 days (Lozanoc) **OR**
- (fungal keratitis) 200 mg orally daily for 3 weeks **OR**
- (fungal keratitis) 100 mg orally daily for 3 weeks (Lozanoc) **OR**
- (pityriasis versicolor) 200 mg orally daily for 1 week **OR**
- (pityriasis versicolor) 100 mg orally daily for 1 week (Lozanoc) **OR**
- (oral candidiasis in immunosuppressed patients) 100–200 mg for 4 weeks **OR**
- (oral candidiasis in immunosuppressed patients) 50–100 mg for 4 weeks (Lozanoc) **OR**
- (oral/oesophageal candidiasis) 200 mg orally daily, or 100 mg twice daily for 1 week (may be repeated for a second week if no response) (Sporanox Oral Solution) **OR**
- (fluconazole-resistant oral/oesophageal candidiasis) 200 mg orally daily, or 100 mg twice daily for 2 weeks, increasing to 400 mg daily for a further 2 weeks if no response (Sporanox Oral Solution) **OR**
- (prophylaxis of fungal infection in neutropenic patient) 5 mg/kg orally daily as 2 divided doses until neutrophils recover (up to 8 weeks) (Sporanox Oral Solution) **OR**
- (aspergillosis) 200 mg orally daily for 2–5 months (increasing dose to 200 mg twice daily for invasive or disseminated disease) **OR**
- (aspergillosis) 100 mg orally daily for 2–5 months (increasing dose to 100 mg twice daily for invasive or disseminated disease) (Lozanoc) **OR**
- (candidiasis) 100–200 mg orally daily for 3 weeks to 7 months **OR**
- (candidiasis) 50–100 mg orally daily for 3 weeks to 7 months (increasing dose to 100 mg twice daily for invasive or disseminated disease) (Lozanoc) **OR**
- (histoplasmosis) 200 mg orally daily for 8 months, increasing dose to 200 mg twice daily if needed **OR**
- (histoplasmosis) 100 mg orally daily for 8 months, increasing dose to 100 mg twice daily if needed (Lozanoc) **OR**
- (sporotrichosis) 100 mg orally daily for 12 weeks, increasing dose to 200 mg daily if needed **OR**
- (sporotrichosis) 50 mg orally daily for 12 weeks, increasing dose to 100 mg daily if needed (Lozanoc)

Adverse effects

- abdominal pain, constipation, diarrhoea, dyspepsia, nausea, vomiting
- dizziness, headache
- increased hepatic enzymes (reversible)
- (rare) erectile dysfunction, menstrual disorders
- (rare) pruritus, rash, urticaria, angioedema, hepatitis (with prolonged therapy), hepatotoxicity, peripheral neuropathy, severe congestive cardiac failure, QT prolongation, transient or permanent hearing loss

Interactions

- contraindicated with disopyramide, domperidone, ergot alkaloids, felodipine, HMG-CoA reductase inhibitors (statins) (e.g. simvastatin, lovastatin), irinotecan, lercanidipine, methadone, midazolam, ticagrelor and triazolam
- contraindicated with colchicine, solifenacin and telithromycin in those with severe kidney impairment or moderate-to-severe liver impairment
- not recommended with apixaban, dabrafenib, darifenacin semprevir, sunitinib, telaprevir or tolvaptan

- may increase serum levels of sulfonylureas, leading to hypoglycaemia
- decreased plasma levels may occur when given with carbamazepine, isoniazid, phenobarbital (phenobarbitone), phenytoin, rifabutin or rifampicin, and are therefore not recommended together
- increased risk of toxicity when given with busulfan, docetaxel and vinca alkaloids (e.g. vincristine)
- may increase serum levels of alfentanil, alprazolam, atorvastatin, calcium-channel blockers, carbamazepine, cilostazol, ciclosporin, disopyramide, digoxin, eletriptan, fentanyl, glucocorticoids (budesonide, dexamethasone, fluticasone, methylprednisolone), imatinib, indinavir, midazolam (IV), norehisterone, phenytoin, reboxetine, rifabutin, ritonavir, saquinavir, sildenafil, sirolimus and tacrolimus, increasing the risk of toxicity/adverse effects, so serum levels should be closely monitored
- may increase activity of warfarin, increasing the risk of bleeding, so prothrombin time should be closely monitored
- absorption decreased by antacids, H_2-receptor antagonists and proton pump inhibitors (e.g. omeprazole), and therefore should not be given together
- increased serum levels may occur if given with clarithromycin, erythromycin, indinavir and ritonavir, increasing risk of adverse effects
- caution if given with calcium-channel blockers due to increased risk of oedema and chronic heart failure
- can inhibit metabolism of calcium-channel blockers
- not recommended with amphotericin B (amphotericin) as it reduces antifungal activity. May also affect liver function, therefore liver enzymes should be monitored during therapy

Nursing points/Cautions

- (disseminated mycoses) monitoring of itraconazole serum levels is recommended regularly throughout therapy
- (systemic candidiasis) sensitivity should be checked before starting therapy
- liver function monitoring is recommended throughout therapy
- oral availability may be decreased in those who are immunocompromised, requiring an increase in dosage
- capsules and oral solution are not interchangeable
- (Lozanoc) capsules have a higher bioavailability than other itraconazole formulations: 50 mg Lozanoc = 100 mg other itraconazole formulations and therefore are not interchangeable
- not recommended in patients with life-threatening systemic fungal infections
- not recommended for treatment of oral and/or oesophageal candidiasis in severely neutropenic patients
- caution if used in those with known sensitivity to another azole
- caution if used in those with impaired liver or kidney function
- caution if used in those with cystic fibrosis as therapeutic levels may vary and an alternative therapy may be considered if response is suboptimal
- contraindicated in those with congestive cardiac failure (or history of) unless infection is life threatening

Patient teaching and advice

- patient should be advised to complete the course of treatment, which may continue for days/weeks after symptoms have resolved. If there is no resolution of the symptoms after the treatment period, the diagnosis should be reassessed or the likelihood of resistance to the agent used considered

- warn patient that superficial fungal infections can be highly contagious
- advise patient not to share clothing or personal linen (e.g. face washers, towels)
- patient should be advised against driving or operating machinery if dizziness is a problem
- those with diabetes treated with sulfonylureas should be warned to monitor blood glucose levels closely throughout therapy because of the increased risk of hypoglycaemia
- instruct patient to take capsules with food
- (Sporanox Oral Solution) advise patient that oral solution should be taken at least 1 hour before food
- (Sporanox Oral Solution) advise patient to swish oral solution around the mouth for 20 seconds before swallowing when treating oral/oesophageal candidiasis. Patient should also be instructed not to rinse mouth after swallowing oral solution
- advise patient to take capsules 2 hours apart from antacids
- if patient has achlorhydria or is taking H_2-receptor antagonists (e.g. cimetidine) or proton pump inhibitors (e.g. omeprazole), advise taking capsules with an acidic drink (e.g. cola) because adequate gastric acidity is required for tablet dissolution
- warn patient to immediately seek medical advice if any of the following occur:
  - unusual fatigue, loss of appetite, nausea, vomiting, abdominal pain, yellowing of skin/eyes, dark urine or pale stools
  - numbness/tingling or weakness of feet/hands
  - hearing loss
  - skin disorder with peeling or blistering
  - swelling of hands or feet, shortness of breath, unusual fatigue, unexpected weight gain
- (vulvovaginal candidiasis) for prevention of reinfection, the partner(s) should be treated locally at the same time with application of antifungal cream to the glans penis
- counsel women of childbearing years to use adequate contraception during therapy and for one menstrual cycle after completion

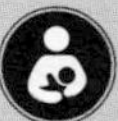

contraindicated during pregnancy except in the treatment of life-threatening systemic mycoses

not recommended during breastfeeding

available as oral solution. Capsules can be opened and contents dispersed in apple juice or cola, or mixed with spoonful of yoghurt or apple puree

KETOCONAZOLE (DaktaGOLD, Nizoral Cream and Anti-Dandruff Shampoo, Sebizole Shampoo)

Available forms

Cream: 20 mg/g; Shampoo: 10 mg/g (1%), 20 mg/g (2%)

Action

- inhibits ergosterol synthesis in fungal cell membrane
- action in seborrheic dermatitis is unknown

Use

- (shampoo) seborrhoeic dermatitis and dandruff (associated with fungal infection)
- cutaneous candidiasis, dermatophyte infections

Dose

- (dermatophyte and *Candida* infections) apply cream to affected area 1–2 times daily for 14 days after symptoms have disappeared **OR**
- (seborrhoeic dermatitis) apply cream to affected area twice daily for up to 4 weeks **OR**

- (seborrhoeic dermatitis, dandruff) shampoo twice weekly for up to 4 weeks

Adverse effects
- (cream) pruritus, burning sensation, dermatitis
- (shampoo) burning sensation, itchiness, oiliness/dryness of hair/scalp, rash, erythema, and rarely, discolouration of hair (grey or coloured)

Nursing points/Cautions
- has a high affinity for keratin and remains active in the skin 7–14 days after the last topical application
- (seborrhoeic dermatitis) if previously treated with topical corticosteroids, skin should be allowed to recover for at least 2 weeks before using ketoconazole cream to avoid skin sensitisation
- not indicated for nail or hair infections
- more resistant cases should be treated twice daily
- caution if used in those with sensitivity to another azole

Patient teaching and advice
- patient should be advised to continue treatment uninterrupted for the following times:
  - 4–6 weeks for tinea pedis
  - 3–4 weeks for tinea corporis
  - 2–4 weeks for tinea cruris
  - 2–3 weeks for pityriasis versicolor
  - 2–3 weeks for superficial candidiasis of the skin
- patient should be advised to complete the course of treatment, which may continue for days/weeks after symptoms have resolved. If there is no resolution of the symptoms after the treatment period, the diagnosis should be reassessed or the likelihood of resistance to the agent used should be considered
- warn patient that superficial fungal infections can be highly contagious
- advise patient not to share clothing or personal linen (e.g. face washers, towels)
- instruct patient to wet hair, add sufficient shampoo to lather, leave for 3–5 minutes and rinse thoroughly with water, avoiding contact with eyes. Eyes should be thoroughly washed with cold water if contact occurs
- patient should be instructed to allow a 4-week gap between consecutive courses of treatment with shampoo

MICAFUNGIN (Mycamine)

Available forms
Vial: 50 mg, 100 mg

Action
- echinocandin that non-competitively inhibits glucan, which is essential in fungal cells but not present in mammalian cells
- fungicidal against most *Candida* species and inhibits *Aspergillus* species
- cross-resistance with other echinocandins possible
- half-life 10–17 hours

Use
- treatment of invasive candidiasis
- treatment of oesophageal candidiasis in those over 16 years
- prophylaxis of *Candida* infection in those undergoing allogenic haematopoietic stem cell transplantation or are expected to have neutropenia (absolute neutrophil count (ANC) $<$ 500 cells/micromol) for 10 or more days

Dose

Invasive candidiasis
- (body weight $>$ 40 kg) 100 mg daily IV over 1 hour for a minimum of 14 days **OR**
- (body weight $\leq$ 40 kg) 2 mg/kg daily IV over 1 hour for a minimum of 14 days

Oesophageal candidiasis

- (body weight > 40 kg) 150 mg daily IV over 1 hour for a minimum of 7 days after symptoms have resolved **OR**
- (body weight ≤ 40 kg) 3 mg/kg daily IV over 1 hour for a minimum of 7 days after symptoms have resolved

Candida **infection prophylaxis**

- (body weight > 40 kg) 50 mg daily IV over 1 hour for a minimum of 7 days after neutrophil recovery **OR**
- (body weight ≤ 40 kg) 1 mg/kg daily IV over 1 hour for a minimum of 7 days after neutrophil recovery

Adverse effects

- anorexia, nausea, vomiting, abdominal pain, dyspepsia, diarrhoea, constipation, mucosal inflammation
- fever, rigors
- fatigue, headache, insomnia, anxiety
- peripheral oedema, fluid overload
- back pain, arthralgia
- tachycardia, atrial fibrillation, arrhythmia, hypotension
- hypokalaemia, hypomagnesaemia, hypocalcaemia, hyperglycaemia, hyponatraemia
- elevated liver enzymes
- rash, pruritus
- cough, dyspnoea, epistaxis
- hypotension, hypertension
- thrombocytopenia, neutropenia, anaemia
- bacteraemia, sepsis, pneumonia
- (rare) hypersensitivity, severe skin reaction, haemolysis, haemolytic anaemia, hepatotoxicity
- (IV site) phlebitis

Interactions

- caution if used with other hepatotoxic agents
- may increase serum levels of sirolimus, nifedipine and itraconazole increasing risk of toxicity

Nursing points/Cautions

- liver function should be monitored during therapy and stopped if there is any persistent and significant elevation of liver enzymes
- (invasive candidiasis) therapy should continue for at least 1 week after two sequential negative blood cultures have been obtained and symptoms have resolved
- to reconstitute add 5 mL sodium chloride 0.9% or glucose 5% slowly to vial to avoid foaming. Rotate vial gently (not shaking) to dissolve powder and then add to 100 mL infusion bag (final concentration between 0.5 mg/mL and 2 mg/mL depending on dose)
- administer alone
- caution if used in those with severe liver impairment, chronic liver disease or congenital enzyme defects
- contraindication in those with hypersensitivity to other echinocandins

Patient teaching and advice

- advise patient to immediately report any rash

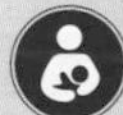

should only be used during pregnancy if benefit outweighs risk

caution if used during breastfeeding

MICONAZOLE (Daktarin Oral Gel, Daktarin Tincture, Decozol Oral Gel, Eulactol Antifungal Spray, Hair Science Anti-Dandruff Shampoo, Resolve Solution)

MICONAZOLE NITRATE (Daktarin preparations, Resolve preparations)

Available forms

Oral gel: 20 mg/mL; Topical cream: 2% (20 mg/g); Lotion/Solution: 2%; Powder: 2%; Spray powder: 2%; Tincture: 2%; Spray (liquid): 2%; Shampoo: 2%

Action

- imidazole which inhibits ergosterol synthesis in fungal cell membrane

Use

- candidiasis (cutaneous, oral)
- dermatophytosis, pityriasis versicolor
- seborrhoeic dermatitis (scalp)

Dose

- (dermatophytosis, pityriasis versicolor, cutaneous candidiasis) apply thin layer and rub well into skin daily (tinea versicolor (pityriasis versicolor)) or twice daily (tinea pedis, cruris or corporis, cutaneous candidiasis) **OR**
- (powder) apply powder directly to lesion twice daily and also dust inside articles of clothing in contact with affected areas until lesion is completely healed **OR**
- (tincture) apply tincture to affected nail and surrounding skin twice daily (after cutting very short) for at least 2 months or until new nail has grown **OR**
- (spray powder) apply spray twice daily to affected area, for at least 14 days after symptoms resolve **OR**
- (oral candidiasis) half of the supplied measuring spoon 4 times daily dropped on tongue and kept in mouth as long as possible before swallowing **OR**
- (seborrhoeic dermatitis) shampoo 2–3 times weekly for 4 weeks, then weekly

Adverse effects

- (oral) nausea, vomiting, regurgitation of food
- (topical cream, lotion) stinging, local irritation, pruritus, warmth at application site
- superinfection (prolonged therapy)
- (rare) anaphylaxis, angioedema, serious skin reactions

Interactions

Oral administration

- may increase serum levels of alfentanil, alprazolam, busulfan, calcium-channel blockers, carbamazepine, cilostazol, ciclosporin, disopyramide, docetaxel, methylprednisolone, midazolam (IV), phenytoin, reboxetine, rifabutin, saquinavir, sildenafil, sirolimus, tacrolimus and vinca alkaloids, increasing the risk of adverse effects
- increased risk of hypoglycaemia if given with sulfonylureas
- contraindicated with midazolam (oral) and triazolam (due to prolonged sedation), simvastatin and lovastatin (increased risk of rhabdomyolysis), and ergot alkaloids (risk of ergotism) and any agents known to prolong QT interval
- contraindicated with warfarin, as anticoagulant effects may be enhanced, increasing the risk of bleeding, so prothrombin time should be closely monitored
- antifungal action may be blocked by amphotericin B (amphotericin)

Nursing points/Cautions

- if patient is unresponsive to treatment, check for undiagnosed diabetes
- candida should be treated for not less than 2 weeks and dermatophytes not less than 4 weeks
- contraindicated in those with sensitivity to another azole
- (oral gel) contraindicated in those with liver impairment or infants under 6 months

Patient teaching and advice

- patient should be advised to complete the course of treatment, which may continue for days/weeks after symptoms have resolved. If there is no resolution of the symptoms after the treatment period, the diagnosis should be reassessed or the likelihood of resistance to the agent used should be considered
- warn patient that superficial fungal infections can be highly contagious

- advise patient not to share clothing or personal linen (e.g. face washers, towels)
- patient being treated for tinea pedis should be encouraged to wash and dry the feet (especially between toes) carefully each day and apply antifungal powder. They should also be advised to wear shoes or sandals that are well ventilated (if possible), wear waterproof sandals in public showers, change hosiery (preferably cotton socks) daily and dust shoes inside with powder

Oral gel

- advise patient (or carer) that gel should be placed on tongue and left for as long as possible before swallowing. Gel may be applied to dentures and left overnight. However, it should be washed off before reinsertion of dentures in the morning
- instruct patient/carer that gel should only be measured with supplied measuring spoon
- advise patient/carer to continue for at least 7 days after symptoms have subsided

Shampoo

- instruct patient to wet hair, add sufficient shampoo to lather, massage well and rinse. Repeat with larger amount of shampoo, leave for 3–5 minutes and rinse thoroughly with water
- warn patient to avoid contact with eyes

Spray powder

- advise patient to shake can well before use and hold about 15 cm from area to be treated
- warn patient to avoid contact with eyes

Topical cream

- instruct patient to cleanse skin using a soap alternative as normal soap may cause skin irritation
- warn patient to avoid contact with eyes

Tincture

- instruct patient to:
  - cut nails as short as possible before applying tincture. Apply under nail also if possible
  - continue treatment until new nail has grown and area is cured (8 weeks or more)
  - clean nail using acetone-based nail polish remover before reapplying tincture
- ensure patient understands that nail falling off is due to infection, not the treatment, which should not be interrupted
- warn patient that tincture contains alcohol and should not be applied to open lesions

Note

- contained in Daktozin and Resolve Nappy Rash (with zinc oxide) and Resolve Plus 0.5 and Resolve Plus 1.0 (with hydrocortisone)

NYSTATIN (Mycostatin Oral Drops, Mycostatin Topical, Nilstat Oral, Nilstat Oral Drops, Nilstat Vaginal)

Available forms

Tablets: 500,000 units; Capsules: 500,000 units; Oral drops: 100,000 units/mL; Topical cream: 100,000 units/g; Vaginal cream: 100,000 units/5 g

Action

- alters fungal cell membrane, targeting ergosterol, changing cell permeability and causing leakage of cell contents
- not absorbed from the GIT

Use

- prophylaxis and treatment of infections caused by *Candida* spp. (vulvovaginal, cutaneous, oral, intestinal)

Dose

- (cutaneous candidiasis) apply liberally to affected areas 2–3 times daily (topical cream) **OR**
- (intestinal candidiasis) 500,000–1,000,000 units (1–2 tablets or capsules) 3 times daily and continued for 48 hours after symptoms resolve **OR**
- (oral candidiasis) 100,000 units (1 mL) 4 times daily, swirled around mouth as long as possible before swallowing, and continued for 48 hours after symptoms have resolved (oral drops) **OR**
- (vaginal candidiasis) 1 full applicator (5 g) 1–2 times daily for 14 days (vaginal cream)

Adverse effects

- (oral, large doses, uncommon) nausea, vomiting, diarrhoea, oral irritation
- (rare, oral) urticaria, rash, angioedema
- (topical cream, uncommon) rash, burning, pruritus, dermatitis
- (vaginal cream, uncommon) irritation

Nursing points/Cautions

- not suitable for systemic fungal infections
- to prevent relapse, oral administration should continue for at least 48 hours after clinical cure
- smears or other diagnostic methods should be used to rule out other causes of infection and repeated if there is no response to therapy
- if symptoms persist or worsen after 14 weeks, alternate therapy should be considered
- (oral drops) caution if used in those with known hypersensitivity to hydroxybenzoates

Patient teaching and advice

- patient should be advised to complete the course of treatment, which may continue for days/weeks after symptoms have resolved. If there is no resolution of the symptoms after the treatment period, the diagnosis should be reassessed or the likelihood of resistance to the agent used should be considered
- warn patient that superficial fungal infections can be highly contagious
- advise patient not to share clothing or personal linen (e.g. face washers, towels)

Vaginal candidiasis

- instruct patient to continue treatment even if menstruation occurs
- ensure patient has instructions for correct insertion of vaginal cream and cleaning instructions for applicator (taking plunger and barrel apart and washing with warm water and mild soap)
- for prevention of reinfection, the partner(s) should be treated locally at the same time with application of cream to the glans penis
- patient should be advised that vaginal cream may decrease the effectiveness and safety of latex products such as condoms and diaphragms
- instruct women being treated for vaginal infection that they should refrain from sexual intercourse or encourage their partner to use a condom. Sexual partner(s) should also be treated to prevent reinfection. Perineal pads (or panty liners) will prevent staining of underwear or clothing when vaginal tablets or creams are used. Wearing cotton underwear and pantyhose with a cotton gusset is also recommended (especially if infection recurs). Use of tampons or douching between doses of vaginal medications is not recommended

Oral drops

- patient should be advised to avoid food or drink for 1 hour after oral drops

- instruct patient to:
  - shake bottle well before use
  - use graduated dropper to measure correct amount
  - keep drops in mouth as long as possible before swallowing
  - wash dropper with hot water after use
  - discard drops after expiry date

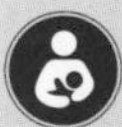

(oral) use during pregnancy only if clearly needed

available as oral drops. Capsules can be opened and contents dispersed in water or tablet crushed and mixed with water

Note
- contained in Kenacomb Ointment, Kenacomb Otic Ear (drops and ointment), Otocomb Otic Ear (drops and ointment)

POSACONAZOLE (Noxafil, Noxafil Concentrated Injection)

Available forms
Vial: 300 mg/16.7 mL; Oral suspension: 40 mg/mL; Modified-release tablets: 100 mg

Action
- broad spectrum triazole that inhibits ergosterol synthesis in fungal cell membrane
- effective against a number of species, including fluconazole-resistant *Candida* spp.
- half-life 20–66 hours (oral suspension) or 27 hours (IV)

Use
- invasive aspergillosis (where other agents are inappropriate or ineffective)
- fusariosis, zygomycosis, coccidioidomycosis, chromoblastomycosis and mycetoma (where other agents are inappropriate or ineffective)
- oropharyngeal candidiasis (in immunocompromised patients or those resistant to itraconazole or fluconazole)
- prophylaxis of invasive fungal infections (in patients at high risk)

Dose
- (refractory invasive fungal infection) 400 mg orally twice daily with food or nutritional supplement (oral suspension) **OR**
- (refractory invasive fungal infection) 200 mg orally 4 times daily with food or nutritional supplement (oral suspension) **OR**
- (refractory invasive fungal infection) 300 mg orally or IV infusion twice daily (day 1) then 300 mg daily (concentrated solution, modified-release tablets) **OR**
- (oral candidiasis refractory to itraconazole or fluconazole) 400 mg orally twice daily with food or nutritional supplement (oral suspension) **OR**
- (prophylaxis of invasive fungal infection) 200 mg orally 3 times daily with food or nutritional supplement (oral suspension) **OR**
- (prophylaxis of invasive fungal infection) 300 mg orally or IV infusion twice daily (day 1), then 300 mg daily (concentrated solution, modified-release tablets) **OR**
- (oral candidiasis in immunocompromised patient) 200 mg orally daily (day 1) (loading dose), then 100 mg orally daily for 13 days (oral suspension)

Adverse effects
- neutropenia, anaemia, thrombocytopenia
- anorexia, dry mouth, nausea, vomiting, abdominal pain, diarrhoea, dyspepsia, flatulence, constipation, inflamed mucosa
- electrolyte imbalance (e.g. hypokalaemia, hypomagnesaemia), elevated liver function test, elevated liver enzymes and bilirubin

- dizziness, headache, somnolence
- paraesthesia
- rash, peticchiae
- asthenia, fatigue, fever, chills
- peripheral oedema
- hypertension
- cough, dyspnoea, epistaxis
- (rare) hepatitis, QT prolongation

Interactions

- contraindicated with any agents that prolong QT interval
- contraindicated with ergot alkaloids because of the risk of ergotism
- contraindicated with HMG-CoA reductase inhibitors (statins) due to increased risk of myopathy and rhabdomyolysis
- not recommended with phenytoin, rifabutin, H_2-receptor antagonists, cimetidine or efavirenz as decreased serum levels may occur
- may increase serum levels of atazanavir/ritonavir, calcium-channel blockers, ciclosporin, digoxin, fosamprenavir, rifabutin, sirolimus, tacrolimus and vinca alkaloids
- increased risk of hypoglycaemia if given with sulfonylureas
- not recommended with amphotericin B (amphotericin) as it reduces antifungal activity
- increased risk of prolonged sedation if given with benzodiazepines (e.g. alprazolam, midazolam, triazolam)
- increased risk of neurotoxicity and other serious adverse effects if given with vinca alkaloids

Nursing points/Cautions

- liver function and serum electrolytes should be monitored (especially potassium, magnesium and calcium) before starting and throughout therapy (especially if receiving concentrated solution). Any imbalance should be corrected before starting therapy
- tablets and oral suspension are not interchangeable
- ensure vial is at room temperature before dilution with 150–283 mL of suitable fluid to give a concentration of 1–2 mg/mL, and infused over 90 minutes via central venous catheter (CVC) or peripherally inserted central catheter (PICC)
- multiple infusions via peripheral venous line are not well tolerated. If used, infusion should be over 30 minutes
- should not be administered as an IV bolus
- concentrated solution should not be diluted with lactated Ringer's solution, 5% dextrose with lactated Ringer's or 4.2% sodium bicarbonate
- caution if used in those with sensitivity to another azole
- caution if used in those with liver impairment, known arrhythmias or at risk of QT prolongation
- (concentrated injection) not recommended in those with moderate-to-severe kidney impairment. If used, serum creatinine should be closely monitored

Patient teaching and advice

- if patient has diabetes and is treated using sulfonylureas, instruct to monitor blood glucose levels closely as hypoglycaemia may occur
- instruct patient to shake oral suspension well before use and use measuring spoon provided
- advise patient to take oral suspension with food or at least 240 mL of nutritional supplement
- warn patient that tablets should be swallowed whole, not chewed, crushed or divided
- warn patient not to drive or operate machinery if dizziness occurs

- patient should be advised to seek medical advice if any of the following occur:
  - tingling or numbness of hands or feet, muscle weakness
  - fatigue, loss of appetite, any yellowing of eyes or skin, upper abdominal pain, dark urine, pale stools
- women of childbearing potential should be counselled to use adequate contraception throughout and for at least 2 weeks after completing therapy

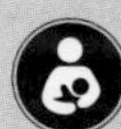
not recommended during pregnancy or breastfeeding unless benefits outweigh potential risks

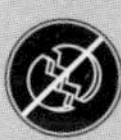
Modified-release tablets should not be crushed or broken

oral liquid available

TERBINAFINE (Jock Itch DermaGel, Lamisil DermGel, Lamisil Once, Lamisil Spray, Lamisil Tablets, Tamsil, Tinasil)

TERBINAFINE HYDROCHLORIDE (Lamisil Cream, SolvEasy Tinea Cream, Gel or Spray)

Available forms
Tablets: 250 mg; Solution/Gel/Cream/ Spray: 10 mg/g (1%)

Action
- allylamine (mainly active against dermatophytes) that prevents ergosterol (lipid) synthesis of fungal cell membrane, resulting in cell disruption and death
- (oral) concentrates in superficial tissues, including nails, hair and skin

Use
- (oral) *Tinea* infection (not responding to topical treatment)
- onychomycosis
- cutaneous candidiasis

Dose
- 250 mg orally daily **OR**
- apply to clean and dry affected area and surrounding skin and rub lightly daily (solution, cream, spray or gel) **OR**
- apply solution daily in a thin layer to BOTH feet around and between toes (even if there is no sign of infection), covering sole and sides of feet (1.5 cm) and allow to dry for 1–2 minutes

Adverse effects
- (oral) nausea, vomiting, anorexia, dyspepsia, gastritis, belching, diarrhoea, flatulence, abdominal discomfort and cramps, feeling of fullness, taste loss (ageusia)
- (oral) headache, depression, dizziness, light-headedness
- (oral) myalgia, arthralgia
- (oral) visual impairment
- (oral) rash, pruritus, urticaria, erythema and uncommonly, photosensitivity
- (cream/gel/solution) itching, stinging, redness and rarely, rash, pruritus, urticaria
- (oral) (rare) transient increase in liver enzymes, jaundice, blood dyscrasias, serious skin reactions

Interactions

Oral
- plasma clearance may be increased by rifampicin, leading to decreased serum levels
- may cause menstrual abnormalities in women taking oral contraceptives
- may inhibit metabolism of antiarrhythmic agents (class 1A, 1B, 1C), beta-adrenoceptor blocking agents, TCAs, SSRIs and MAOIs (type B)
- may affect prothrombin time if given with warfarin, therefore it should be closely monitored throughout therapy

- may decrease clearance of caffeine and theophylline, leading to increased serum levels
- may increase clearance of ciclosporin, leading to decreased serum levels
- serum levels may be increased, amiodarone, cimetidine and fluconazole
- may increase serum levels of dextromethorphan

Nursing points/Cautions

- (oral) liver function tests are recommended before starting and then every 4–6 weeks during therapy
- if therapy is longer than 6 weeks, blood counts should be monitored
- oral therapy is recommended when topical therapy is ineffective or site, severity or extent of infection warrants oral therapy
- length of administration depends on cause:
  - tinea pedis, tinea cruris, tinea corporis: oral treatment 2–6 weeks
  - tinea cruris, tinea corporis: oral treatment 2–4 weeks
  - onychomycosis: oral treatment 6 weeks–3 months, cream: 1–4 weeks)
- (oral) caution if used in those with psoriasis or lupus erythematosus as conditions may be precipitated and/or exacerbated
- (oral) not recommended in those with impaired kidney function (creatinine clearance $<$ 50 mL/min or serum creatinine $>$ 300 micromol/L)
- (oral) contraindicated in those with severe liver disease (chronic or active)

Patient teaching and advice

- if tablets cause upset stomach, patient should be instructed to take after a light meal
- patient should be advised to complete the course of treatment, which may continue for days/weeks after symptoms have resolved. If there is no resolution of the symptoms after the treatment period, the diagnosis should be reassessed or the likelihood of resistance to the agent used should be considered
- warn patient that superficial fungal infections can be highly contagious
- advise patient not to share clothing or personal linen (e.g. face washers, towels)
- advise patient to immediately seek medical advice if any of the following occur:
  - unusual fatigue or tiredness, loss of appetite, nausea, vomiting, right upper abdominal pain, yellowing of skin/eyes, dark urine or pale stools
  - fever, sore throat, mouth ulcers, chills, tiredness, swollen glands and aching joints
- warn patient not to drive or operate machinery if dizziness or lightheadedness occurs
- patient should be advised that loss of taste usually recovers within several weeks of discontinuing oral therapy
- instruct patient that both feet should be treated even if only one is symptomatic. Feet should be washed and dried before applying solution to one foot at a time. Solution should be applied between and all around toes, soles and 1.5 cm up sides of feet and then allowed to dry (not massaged into skin). Feet should not be washed for 24 hours after application of solution
- advise patient to wash hands thoroughly after using solution and avoid contacting eyes with solution
- for infections which are sub-breast, between digits, inguinal or intergluteal, gauze may be used to cover cream or gel, especially at night
- (solution) warn patient that solution should not be massaged into skin

and that treated area should not be washed for 24 hours after application
- advise patient to seek medical advice if there is no improvement in 7 days
- (oral) female patients taking tablets and oral contraceptives should be warned of the possibility of menstrual disorders

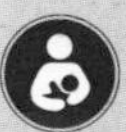
not recommended during pregnancy or breastfeeding unless benefits outweigh potential risks

TOLNAFTATE (Tinaderm)

Available forms
Powder spray: 0.9 mg/g; Powder: 10 mg/g

Action
- fungicidal

Use
- ringworm
- tinea pedis

Dose
- (ringworm, tinea) sprinkle or spray enough powder to cover affected area 2–3 times daily; powder should also be dusted into footwear **OR**
- (prevention of tinea) dust footwear and feet regularly

Adverse effects
- mild irritation

Nursing points/Cautions
- review diagnosis if there is no improvement after 4 weeks of treatment
- powder/spray powder are recommended as adjunctive treatment with other antifungal treatments

Patient teaching and advice
- patient should be advised to complete the course of treatment, which may continue for days/weeks after symptoms have resolved. If there is no resolution of the symptoms after the treatment period, the diagnosis should be reassessed or the likelihood of resistance to the agent used should be considered
- warn patient that superficial fungal infections can be highly contagious
- advise patient not to share clothing or personal linen (e.g. face washers, towels)
- warn patient to avoid contact with eyes or mucous membranes or inhaling powder preparations
- patient being treated for tinea pedis should be encouraged to wash and dry the feet (especially between toes) carefully each day and apply antifungal powder. They should also be advised to wear shoes or sandals that are well ventilated (if possible), wear waterproof sandals in public showers, change hosiery (preferably cotton socks) daily and dust shoes inside with powder
- (spray powder, liquid) shake can well before use

Note
- contained in Mycil Healthy Feet and Tinea Dusting Powder with chlorhexidine

VORICONAZOLE (Vfend, Vttack, Vzole, Zolfend)

Available forms
Vial: 200 mg; Tablets: 50 mg, 200 mg; Powder (for oral suspension): 40 mg/mL

Action
- broad spectrum triazole that inhibits ergosterol synthesis in fungal cell membrane
- active against *Candida* spp, *Aspergillus*, *Scedosporium* and *Fusarium*
- half-life about 6 hours

Use

- invasive aspergillosis (first-line treatment)
- serious *Candida* infections (including oesophageal and systemic candidiasis)
- serious infections caused by *Scedosporium* and *Fusarium* species
- other fungal infections (when other therapy has been ineffective or inappropriate)
- prophylaxis in high-risk patients

Dose

- initially 6 mg/kg 12-hourly by IV infusion for 24 hours (loading dose), then 3–4 mg/kg 12-hourly (maintenance) **OR**
- 200–400 mg orally either 1 hour before or after food, 12-hourly for 24 hours (loading dose), then 100–200 mg twice daily (maintenance) **OR**
- (prophylaxis) initially 6 mg/kg 12-hourly by IV infusion for 24 hours (loading dose), then 4 mg/kg 12-hourly (maintenance) **OR**
- (prophylaxis) 100–200 mg orally either 1 hour before or after food 12-hourly

Adverse effects

- dry mouth, nausea, vomiting, diarrhoea, abdominal pain, dyspepsia, cheilitis, gingivitis
- sinusitis, respiratory distress syndrome, pulmonary oedema
- fever, chills
- headache, dizziness, tremor, paraesthesia, somnolence, fainting
- confusion, depression, hallucinations, anxiety, agitation, insomnia, asthenia
- back pain
- hypotension
- chest pain, tachycardia, bradycardia, arrhythmia
- rash, pruritus, photosensitivity, alopecia, dermatitis, purpura
- oedema (peripheral, facial)
- visual disturbances (including blurred vision, changes in colour perception), photophobia, retinal haemorrhage
- hypokalaemia, hypoglycaemia, hyponatraemia
- elevated liver enzymes, jaundice, cholestatic jaundice
- elevated creatinine, acute kidney failure, haematuria
- agranulocytosis, anaemia, leucopenia, pancytopenia, thrombocytopenia
- (IV site) inflammation, phlebitis, thrombophlebitis, infusion-related reactions (e.g. chest tightness, dyspnoea, flushing, fever, nausea, pruritus, rash, sweating, tachycardia)
- (rare) optic neuritis, papilloedema, QT prolongation, periostitis, severe skin reactions

Interactions

- contraindicated with any agents that prolong QT interval or cause electrolyte imbalance
- contraindicated with ergot alkaloids (increased risk of ergotism), carbamazepine, rifabutin, rifampicin, sirolimus and long-acting barbiturates (e.g. phenobarbital (phenobarbitone)) (increased risk of toxicity), ritonavir (high dose, 800 mg daily) and efavirenz (daily doses > 400 mg) and St John's wort (decrease efficacy of voriconazole)
- not recommended with everolimus, fluconazole, phenytoin or ritonavir (low dose 200 mg daily)
- may decrease metabolism of HMG-CoA reductase inhibitors (statins), increasing serum levels and risk of rhabdomyolysis
- may increase serum levels of efavirenz, NSAIDs, tacrolimus, oxycodone and other long-acting opioids, and ciclosporin, increasing risk of adverse effects
- may increase prothrombin time if given with warfarin, therefore closely monitor throughout therapy

- may increase the risk of hypoglycaemia by increasing serum levels of sulfonylureas
- may prolong the sedative effect of midazolam, triazolam and alprazolam
- increased risk of respiratory depression if given with alfentanil, fentanyl or remifentanil
- increased risk of neurotoxicity if given with vinca alkaloids
- may increase serum levels of methadone increasing risk of toxicity and QT interval prolongation
- serum levels may be decreased by phenytoin, rifabutin and HIV protease inhibitors
- if therapy is added to already existing omeprazole, omeprazole dose should be halved
- increased risk of toxicity if given with HIV protease inhibitors
- may increase adverse effects if given with oral contraceptives containing norethisterone and ethylestradiol
- not recommended with amphotericin B (amphotericin) as it reduces antifungal activity

Nursing points/Cautions

- any hypokalaemia, hypomagnesaemia or hypocalcaemia should be corrected before starting therapy
- liver and kidney function (including serum creatinine and bilirubin) should be monitored weekly for first month and then monthly throughout therapy. Pancreatic function (amylase, lipase) monitoring is also recommended in those at risk of acute pancreatitis (e.g. recent chemotherapy)
- (long-term therapy) regular dermatological monitoring is recommended to detect any pre-malignant lesions
- (IV) patient should be carefully observed at start of infusion for any infusion-related reaction
- (IV) if response to 3 mg/kg is inadequate, dose should be increased to 4 mg/kg or if patient is intolerant to 4 mg/kg, dose can be reduced to 3 mg/kg
- reconstitute IV powder using 19 mL water for injections, shake thoroughly and further dilute with compatible fluid (e.g. sodium chloride 0.9%, glucose 5%, compounded lactate sodium IV infusion, glucose 5% and sodium chloride 0.45%)
- should not be given as an IV bolus
- recommended administration rate is 3 mg/kg/hour over 1–2 hours
- (IV) not compatible with blood products or concentrated electrolyte solutions. If infused with non-concentrated electrolyte solutions or total parenteral nutrition (TPN), infusion should be via separate lines
- (vial) contains 217.6 mg sodium, which should be considered if patient has sodium restriction
- (tablets) contain lactose and are not recommended in those with galactose intolerance, Lapp lactase deficiency or glucose–galactose malabsorption
- (oral powder) (used to make up suspension) contains sucrose and is not recommended in those with fructose intolerance, sucrase–isomaltase deficiency or glucose–galactose malabsorption
- if patient has creatinine clearance < 50 mL/minute (including those on dialysis), oral therapy (not IV) is recommended
- caution if used in those with risk factors for pancreatitis (e.g. chemotherapy, stem cell transplantation)
- use with great caution in patients who are at risk of QT prolongation, including those with existing symptomatic arrhythmias, congenital or acquired QT prolongation, sinus bradycardia, cardiomyopathy or if given

with other agents that may prolong QT interval, induce arrhythmias or cause electrolyte imbalance (e.g. hypokalaemia)

- caution if used in those with sensitivity to another azole
- (IV) not recommended for oesophageal candidiasis

Patient teaching and advice

- (IV) warn patient that mild visual disturbances (e.g. blurred vision, colour vision changes, photophobia) occur commonly and usually resolve within 60 minutes of infusion completion
- instruct patient to avoid direct sunlight during therapy and when outdoors to wear sunscreen (at least SPF 30+), protective clothing, hat and sunglasses
- if patient is receiving long-term therapy, advise to have regular skin checks by dermatologist
- patient should be advised not to drive or operate machinery if photophobia, visual problems (e.g. blurred vision, colour vision changes), hypotension, dizziness, confusion or hallucinations occur. Patient should be warned against driving at night
- warn patient to immediately seek medical advice if any of the following occur:
  - any rash or other skin condition such as skin flaking or blistering
  - any ongoing changes to vision or sensitivity to light
  - bone pain
  - any new or changing skin lesions
  - increased or irregular heart rate
  - yellowing of skin or eyes, lethargy, loss of appetite, upper abdominal pain, dark urine, pale stools
  - signs of frequent or worsening infections such as fever, chills, sore throat and/or mouth ulcers
  - face or limb swelling
  - blood in urine
- instruct patient to take tablets or oral suspension 1 hour before or 1 hour after meals
- patient should be advised to shake solution well before using and measured using supplied syringe and amount slowly squirted into mouth towards cheek. Oral suspension should not be mixed with any other medication or water. Syringe should be taken apart and rinsed with warm water each time it is used
- advise patient to discard oral suspension 14 days after opening
- female patients of childbearing years should be counselled to use effective contraception during therapy to prevent pregnancy occurring

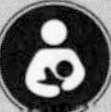

not recommended during pregnancy or breastfeeding unless infection is severe or life threatening

oral liquid is available. Tablet can be crushed and mixed with water or spoonful of yoghurt or apple puree

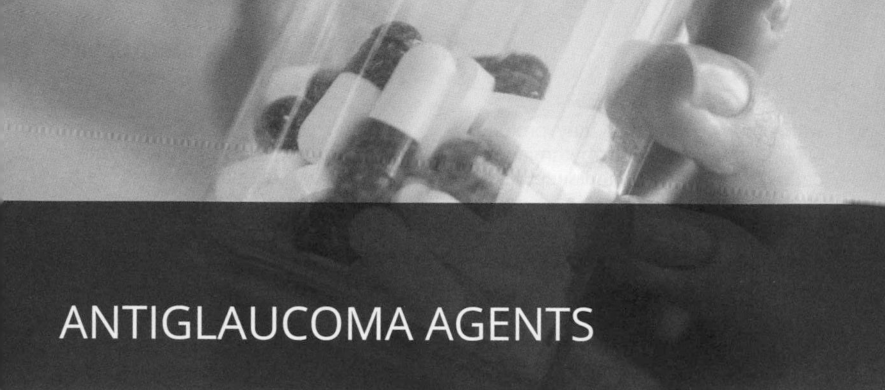

ANTIGLAUCOMA AGENTS

Glaucoma is an eye condition characterised by optic disk cupping and visual field loss, usually associated with a raised intraocular pressure; however, it can occur at normal or near-normal pressure. Although raised intraocular pressure may be symptomless in the early stages, damage to the optic nerve leads to loss of vision and when severe, is one of the leading causes of preventable blindness worldwide. Risk factors for glaucoma include family history, increasing age, high intraocular pressure, extreme short-sightedness, co-morbidities such as diabetes and hypertension, and some medications such as long-term corticosteroids (Salmon 2018).

The main types of glaucoma are open-angle glaucoma (caused by impaired aqueous outflow due to anterior chamber drainage system abnormalities), closed-angle glaucoma (impaired access to drainage system) and secondary glaucoma (related to other diseases, such as diabetes). Open-angle glaucoma is the most common type of glaucoma and is usually chronic, slow in developing and accounts for about 80% of people who have glaucoma (Salmon 2018).

Glaucoma management involves reducing the intraocular pressure by either decreasing production of aqueous humour or increasing aqueous outflow using either medical (medications), laser or surgical therapy (Salmon 2018). Medical management consists of:

- prostaglandins analogues (latanoprost, tafluprost, travoprost) (first-line management)
- beta-adrenoceptor blocking agents (betaxolol, timolol) (first-line management)
- carbonic anhydrase inhibitors (acetazolamide, brinzolamide, dorzolamide)
- alpha-adrenergic agonists/sympathomimetic agents (apraclonidine, brimonidine)
- parasympathomimetic agents (pilocarpine)
- prostamide analogue (bimatoprost)

General Actions of antiglaucoma agents

- decrease intraocular pressure (either by increasing aqueous output or reducing production) since sustained intraocular pressure and poor ocular perfusion result in damage to the head of the optic nerve and loss of visual field

- agents may be used alone or in combination to reduce intraocular pressure

General Ocular Adverse effects of antiglaucoma agents

- ocular pruritus, ocular ache or pain
- tearing, burning or stinging, blurring of vision, decreased visual acuity
- discomfort, foreign body sensation, eye irritation
- lid oedema or erythema, eyelid crusting
- ocular hyperaemia
- ocular allergic reaction
- conjunctivitis, conjunctival oedema, conjunctival follicles
- dry eyes
- discharge
- photophobia

General Adverse effects (uncommon) of antiglaucoma agents

- headache, asthenia, malaise, dizziness, nervousness, depression, insomnia, somnolence, fatigue, drowsiness, decreased coordination
- chest pain, palpitations, bradycardia, hypotension
- dry mouth, taste perversion
- dry nose, rhinitis
- dermatitis

General Nursing points/Cautions for antiglaucoma agents

- intraocular pressure should be monitored regularly throughout therapy, especially at the start of treatment as it may take some time to stabilise the pressure
- there may be diurnal variations in intraocular pressure, therefore it is recommended that it is measured at different times of the day
- some antiglaucoma agents (eye drops) contain benzalkonium chloride (preservative), which can cause irritation to the eye, as well as discolouration of soft contact lenses. Contact lenses should be removed before instilling eye drops and not replaced for at least 15 minutes
- responsiveness to agents may decrease with time
- patients with pre-existing depression should be closely monitored during therapy

General Patient teaching and advice for antiglaucoma agents

- encourage patients to continue using antiglaucoma agents as there is a high non-adherence rate with these agents. A study has found that only 15% of patients had good adherence with glaucoma medications over 4 years. Some 20–30% of patients never filled their first prescription for glaucoma medication and about 50% of patients did not persist with their medication after filling their first prescription. Another group of patients tried to use their medication; however, were unable to correctly instil the eye drops. All of these result in poor outcomes for patients with glaucoma progressing (Newman-Casey & Myers 2019)
- patient should be advised to avoid driving (especially at night) or operating machinery if visual disturbances, dizziness, fatigue or drowsiness occur
- instillation of any eye drops may cause transient vision blurring and the patient should be advised not to drive or operate machinery until their vision has cleared completely

- advise patient to seek medical advice immediately if any of the following occur:
  - other eye conditions (such as infection, surgery, trauma)
  - reactions after using eye drops, including conjunctivitis or lid reactions
- eye drops should not be instilled if soft or gas-permeable contact lenses are in situ. Lenses should be removed before instillation and reinserted after an interval of at least 15 minutes
- many eye preparations contain benzalkonium chloride (preservative), which can cause irritation and also discolours soft contact lenses
- ensure the patient understands the importance of attending appointments with an ophthalmologist
- patient should be escorted to and from an ophthalmological examination if cycloplegic mydriatic drops are used for retinoscopy, because accommodation is paralysed for several hours. They should be advised not to drive or operate machinery during this time
- instruct the patient to write the expiry date on eye preparations and discard accordingly (usually 28 days)
- warn patient not to use drops if they are cloudy or change colour
- advise patients that eye preparations are for one patient only
- patients should be warned not to stop treatment suddenly
- if patients are using more than one type of eye drop, they should be advised to wait at least 5 minutes before instillation to prevent washout of previous dose

Instillation of eye drops

- instruct patient in the correct technique for instilling eye drops, including:
  1. do not allow the tip of the dispensing container to touch the eye as it may cause injury and/or contaminate the eye drops
  2. if the container is new, remove the protective seal, otherwise it is important to check the expiry date
  3. wash hands thoroughly with soap and water
  4. remove lid/cap and hold container upside down in one hand between thumb and forefinger or index finger
  5. using the other hand, gently pull down on the lower eyelid to form a pouch/pocket and tilt the head back looking up
  6. place tip of container close to lower eyelid (taking care not to make contact between tip and eye). Squeezing bottle gently, release one drop into pouch/pocket formed between the eye and the eyelid taking care not to allow the tip to touch the eye
  7. gently close the eye, but do not blink or rub the eye
  8. while the eye is closed, place index finger against the inside corner of the eye and press against the nose for about 2 minutes (this stops the medicine from draining through the tear duct into the nose and throat)
  9. replace the lid/cap tightly
  10. wash hands again to remove any residue
- see also General Patient teaching and advice (p. xxvii)

ACETAZOLAMIDE (Diamox, Glaumox Powder for Injection)

Available forms
Tablets: 250 mg; Vial: 500 mg

Action
- non-bacteriostatic sulfonamide derivative
- inhibits the action of carbonic anhydrase in the ciliary process of the eye, inhibiting secretion of aqueous humour, so reducing intraocular pressure
- (tablets) onset of action 1–1.5 hours, peak effect 2–4 hours, duration of action 8–12 hours
- (IV) onset of action 2 minutes, peak effect 15 minutes, duration of action 4–5 hours

Use
- adjunctive treatment in chronic simple (open-angle) glaucoma, secondary glaucoma and preoperatively in acute closed-angle glaucoma (where delay in surgery is required to lower intraocular pressure)
- other uses (see Diuretics, p. 1012 and Antiepileptics, p. 385)

Dose
- (open-angle glaucoma) 250 mg orally or IV 1–4 times daily **OR**
- (secondary glaucoma and preoperatively in acute closed-angle glaucoma) 250 mg orally or IV 4-hourly **OR**
- (acute glaucoma) initially 500 mg orally or IV, then 125–250 mg 4-hourly

Adverse effects
- see General Adverse effects of acetazolamide in Diuretics (p. 1012)

Interactions
- see Interactions of acetazolamide in Diuretics (p. 1012)
- increased risk of chronic salicylism if given with aspirin

Nursing points/Cautions
- see also Nursing points/Cautions for acetazolamide in Diuretics (p. 1012)
- usually used as adjunctive therapy
- doses should be adjusted according to symptoms and intraocular pressure readings
- doses > 250 mg should be given as divided doses
- daily doses > 2 g show no increased effects
- IV route should be used when rapid relief from raised intraocular pressure is required
- IV administration should only be used when oral route is not available
- cross-sensitivity possible between acetazolamide and other sulfonamides
- contraindicated in those with hypersensitivity to sulfonamides or related products as long-term therapy in chronic non-congestive angle-closure glaucoma, severe liver or kidney impairment, hyperchloraemic acidosis, hypokalaemia, hyponatraemia or suprarenal failure

Patient teaching and advice
- see also Patient teaching and advice for acetazolamide in Diuretics (p. 1012)

banned in sport

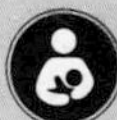

teratogenic in animal studies at high doses, therefore not recommended during pregnancy, especially first trimester

caution if used during breastfeeding

APRACLONIDINE HYDROCHLORIDE (Iopidine)

Available form
Eye drops: 5 mg/mL (0.5%)

Action
- alpha-2 adrenergic agonist
- onset of action 1 hour, peak effect 3–5 hours

Use
- control of intraocular pressure in patients with glaucoma who are on maximum tolerated therapy

Dose
- 1 drop to affected eye(s) 3 times daily

Adverse effects
- see General Ocular Adverse effects and General Adverse effects of antiglaucoma agents (p. 453)
- corneal changes
- (uncommon) depression

Interactions
- contraindicated with MAOIs, TCAs or systemic sympathomimetic agents
- caution if given with beta-adrenoceptor blocking agents (systemic or ophthalmic), antihypertensive agents, clonidine or cardiac glycosides
- may have additive CNS depressive effects if given with alcohol, barbiturates, opioids, sedatives and anaesthetics

Nursing points/Cautions

- if used with cardiovascular agents, heart rate and BP should be closely monitored
- if patient has severe cardiovascular disease, he/she should be closely monitored at start of therapy for vasovagal attack
- therapy should be limited to 3 months. Any decision to continue therapy beyond this time should be based on continued effectiveness of therapy and ophthalmological examination for any corneal changes
- caution if used in those with coronary or cerebral insufficiency, recent myocardial infarction, severe uncontrolled cardiac disease, Raynaud's disease or thromboangiitis obliterans, chronic renal failure, impaired liver function, hypertension, cerebrovascular disease, postural hypotension, depression or previous history of vasovagal attacks in patients with cardiovascular disease
- contraindicated in those with hypersensitivity to clonidine
- see also General Nursing points/Cautions for antiglaucoma agents (p. 453)

Patient teaching and advice

- advise patient to report any:
  - changes in mood or depression
  - chest pain or irregular heart beat
- see also General Patient teaching and advice for antiglaucoma agents (p. 453)

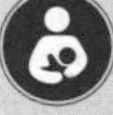

not recommended during pregnancy or breastfeeding

BETAXOLOL (Betoptic, Betoquin)

Available forms

Eye drops: 2.5 mg/mL (0.25%), 5 mg/mL (0.5%)

Action
- beta1-adrenoceptor blocking agent that decreases production of aqueous humour
- onset of action 30 minutes, peak effect 2 hours, duration of action 12–18 hours

Use
- chronic open-angle glaucoma
- ocular hypertension

Dose
- 1 drop in the affected eye(s) twice daily

Adverse effects

- (systemic) asthma, bradycardia, bronchospasm, congestive cardiac failure, dyspnoea, heart block, respiratory failure
- see also General Ocular Adverse effects and General Adverse effects of antiglaucoma agents (p. 453)

Interactions

- not recommended with other beta-adrenoceptor blocking agents, calcium-channel blockers or antiarrhythmic agents
- may prolong AV conduction time if given with digoxin and therefore not recommended together
- additive reduction in intraocular pressure may occur if given with IV acetazolamide or topical miotic agents
- caution if used with catecholamine depleting agents (e.g. adrenergic psychotropic drugs) due to risk of hypotension and/or bradycardia
- hypotension may occur if given with phenothiazines
- may decrease effectiveness of adrenaline (epinephrine)

Nursing points/Cautions

- Betoptic and Betoquin are solutions
- those with severe cardiac disease should be closely monitored at start of therapy for any cardiac-related adverse effects
- if used to treat angle-closure glaucoma, should be given with miotic agent
- should be stopped gradually 24–48 hours before surgery with a general anaesthetic
- because there may be systemic absorption and effects, caution if used in those with asthma, myasthenia gravis or thyrotoxicosis
- caution if used in those with diabetes mellitus as signs of hypoglycaemia (tachycardia) may be masked
- caution if used in those with thyrotoxicosis as thyroid storm may be provoked if withdrawal is abrupt
- caution if used in those with sick sinus syndrome, Prinzmetal's (variant) angina, hypotension, metabolic acidosis, first-degree heart block, hypotension, cerebrovascular insufficiency, phaeochromocytoma (untreated), hyperthyroidism, cardiac failure, severe COPD, asthma, severe peripheral circulatory insufficiency (e.g. Raynaud's disease), severe allergic rhinitis or bronchial hyperreactivity
- contraindicated in those with sinus bradycardia (greater than first-degree block), cardiac failure or cardiogenic shock
- see also General Nursing points/Cautions for antiglaucoma agents (p. 453)

Patient teaching and advice

- see General Patient teaching and advice for antiglaucoma agents (p. 453)

generally banned in sport, but may be permitted under certain circumstances or in some sports

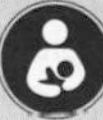

not recommended during pregnancy and breastfeeding. May cause bradycardia in fetus and newborn

BIMATOPROST (Bimprozt, Bimtop, Lumigan Eye Drops, Lumigan PF, Vizo-PF Bimatoprost)

Available form

Eye drops: 0.3 mg/mL (0.03%)

Action

- prostamide analogue that increases outflow of aqueous humour through trabecular meshwork and enhances uveoscleral outflow

- onset of action within 4 hours, peak effect in 8–12 hours, duration of action 24–36 hours

Use

- chronic open-angle glaucoma or ocular hypertension (as monotherapy or adjunctive therapy with beta-adrenoceptor blocking agents)

Dose

- 1 drop to affected eye(s) once daily, at night

Adverse effects

- see General Ocular Adverse effects and General Adverse effects of antiglaucoma agents (p. 453)
- increased iris pigmentation
- pigmentation of periocular and eyelid skin
- eyelash darkening, thickening, lengthening, increased number of lashes and misdirected growth
- macular oedema

Nursing points/Cautions

- caution if used in those with liver or kidney impairment, compromised lung function, aphakia (absence of lens in the eye) or with a torn posterior lens capsule, uncontrolled congestive cardiac failure, heart block (> first degree), predisposition to hypotension or low heart rate or those with risk factors for macular oedema (e.g. diabetic retinopathy, intraocular surgery) or active intraocular inflammation (e.g. uveitis) (as inflammation may be exacerbated)
- see also General Nursing points/Cautions for antiglaucoma agents (p. 453)

Patient teaching and advice

- warn patient that iris colour may darken, eyelashes darken, thicken and lengthen and eyelid skin and skin around eyes may also darken. If only one eye is being treated, this may cause a noticeable difference between the eyes
- advise patient to avoid allowing solution to run onto cheeks or other skin areas
- see also General Patient teaching and advice for antiglaucoma agents (p. 453)

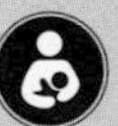

not recommended in pregnancy unless benefits outweigh risks

not recommended during breastfeeding

Note

- combined with timolol in Ganfort 0.3/5 and Ganfort PF 0.3/5

BRIMONIDINE TARTRATE (Alphagan Eye Drops, Alphagan P, Enidin)

Available forms

Eye drops: 1.5 mg/mL (0.15%), 2 mg/mL (0.2%)

Action

- alpha-2 adrenergic agonist that reduces aqueous humour production and increases uveoscleral outflow
- rapid onset of action, peak effect 2 hours, duration of action 8–12 hours

Use

- chronic open-angle glaucoma or ocular hypertension (monotherapy or adjunctive therapy)

Dose

- 1 drop in affected eye(s) twice daily (approximately 12-hourly) (alone or with beta-adrenoceptor blocking agent)

Adverse effects

- see General Ocular Adverse effects and General Adverse effects of antiglaucoma agents (p. 453)

Interactions

- contraindicated with MAOIs, TCAs or systemic sympathomimetic agents
- caution if given with beta-adrenoceptor blocking agents (systemic or ophthalmic), antihypertensive agents, clonidine or cardiac glycosides
- may have additive CNS depressive effects if given with alcohol, barbiturates, opioids, sedatives and anaesthetics

Nursing points/Cautions

- if used with cardiovascular agents, heart rate and BP should be closely monitored
- if patient has severe cardiovascular disease, he/she should be closely monitored at start of therapy for vasovagal attack
- therapy should be limited to 3 months. Any decision to continue therapy beyond this time should be based on continued effectiveness of therapy and ophthalmological examination for any corneal changes
- caution if used in those with coronary or cerebral insufficiency, recent myocardial infarction, severe uncontrolled cardiac disease, Raynaud's disease or thromboangiitis obliterans, chronic renal failure, hypertension, cerebrovascular disease, postural hypotension, depression or previous history of vasovagal attacks in patients with cardiovascular disease
- contraindicated in those with hypersensitivity to clonidine
- see also General Nursing points/Cautions for antiglaucoma agents (p. 453)

Patient teaching and advice

- see also General Patient teaching and advice for antiglaucoma agents (p. 453)

Note

- contained in Combigan with timolol maleate and Simbrinza with brinzolamide

BRINZOLAMIDE (Azopt Eye Drops 1%, BrinzoQuin Eye Drops 1%)

Available form

Eye drops: 10 mg/mL (1%)

Action

- carbonic anhydrase inhibitor which decreases production of aqueous humour
- duration of action 8–12 hours

Use

- chronic open-angle glaucoma
- ocular hypertension

Dose

- 1 drop in affected eye(s) twice daily

Adverse effects

- see General Ocular Adverse effects and General Adverse effects of antiglaucoma agents (p. 453)

Interactions

- not recommended with oral carbonic anhydrase inhibitors

Nursing points/Cautions

- if changing from another antiglaucoma agent, patient should be advised to use first agent on last day at usual dose, then next day start brinzolamide at recommended dose
- caution if used in those liver impairment, diabetes mellitus or corneal dystrophies
- contraindicated in those with hypersensitivity to sulfonamides, severe kidney impairment or hyperchloraemic acidosis
- see also General Nursing points/Cautions for antiglaucoma agents (p. 453)

Patient teaching and advice

- see also General Patient teaching and advice for antiglaucoma agents (p. 453)

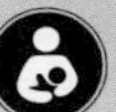

only used during pregnancy or breast-feeding if benefits outweigh risks

Note

- contained in Azarga with timolol maleate and Simbrinza with brimonidine tartrate

DORZOLAMIDE (Trusamide, Trusopt)

Available form

Eye drops: 20 mg/mL (2%)

Action

- non-bacteriostatic sulfonamide
- topical carbonic anhydrase inhibitor that decreases production of aqueous humour
- duration of action 8–12 hours

Use

- chronic open-angle glaucoma or ocular hypertension (monotherapy or adjunctive therapy with beta-adrenoceptor blocking agent)

Dose

- (monotherapy) 1 drop to the affected eye(s) 3 times daily **OR**
- (adjunct to beta-adrenoceptor antiglaucoma agents) 1 drop to affected eye(s) twice daily

Adverse effects

- transient bitter taste
- see also General Ocular Adverse effects and General Adverse effects of antiglaucoma agents (p. 453)

Interactions

- not recommended with oral carbonic anhydrase inhibitors

Nursing points/Cautions

- see also General Nursing points/Cautions for antiglaucoma agents (p. 453)
- not recommended in those with severe kidney or liver impairment or with sulfonamide sensitivity

Patient teaching and advice

- see General Patient teaching and advice for antiglaucoma agents (p. 453)

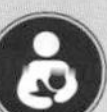

not recommended during pregnancy and breastfeeding

Note

- contained in Cosdor and Cosopt Eye Drops with timolol maleate

LATANOPROST (Lanpro, Xalaprost, Xalatan)

Available form

Eye drops: 50 microgram/mL

Action

- prostaglandin analogue (F_{2alpha})
- prodrug that is hydrolysed to active form in the aqueous humour
- increases outflow by secondary pathway (uveoscleral flow)
- onset of action 3–4 hours, peak action 8–12 hours, duration of action 24–36 hours

Use

- chronic open-angle glaucoma
- ocular hypertension

Dose

- 1 drop to affected eye(s) nightly

Adverse effects

- see General Ocular Adverse effects and General Adverse effects of antiglaucoma agents (p. 453)
- iris colour change
- pigmentation of periocular and eyelid skin
- eyelash darkening, thickening, lengthening, increased number of lashes and misdirected growth
- (rare) macular oedema

Interactions

- precipitation may occur if given with thiomersal containing eye drops, therefore should be separated by at least 5 minutes
- not recommended with other prostaglandin analogues

Nursing points/Cautions

- caution if used in those with aphakia (absence of lens in the eye), pseudoaphakia, or those with risk factors for macular oedema (e.g. diabetic retinopathy, intraocular surgery), inflammatory or neovascular glaucoma, inflammatory ocular conditions, congenital glaucoma, during perioperative cataract surgery, recurrent history of herpes simplex keratitis, with risk factors for iritis or uveitis
- see also General Nursing points/Cautions for antiglaucoma agents (p. 453)

Patient teaching and advice

- warn patient of possible change in eye colour, particularly in those with mixed eye colour (e.g. blue-brown, grey-brown) and which generally occurs within first 8 months of treatment
- patients should be advised that eyelashes may darken, thicken and lengthen and eyelid skin and skin around eyes may also darken
- see General Patient teaching and advice for antiglaucoma agents (p. 453)

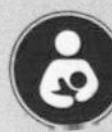

not recommended during pregnancy and breastfeeding

Note

- contained in Latanocom, Latanoprost/Timolol AN 50/5, Lantim 50/5, Xalacom, Xalamol 50/5 and Xanopan 50/5 with timolol maleate

PILOCARPINE (Isopto Carpine, Minims Pilocarpine)

Available forms

Eye drops: 10 mg/mL (1%), 20 mg/mL (2%), 40 mg/mL (4%)

Action

- parasympathomimetic agent (cholinergic)
- decreases intraocular pressure
- miotic
- action within 30 minutes, peak effect 1–1.25 hours, duration of action 4–12 hours

Use

- chronic open-angle glaucoma
- emergency management of acute narrow-angle glaucoma

Dose

- 1–2 drops to affected eye(s) 3–4 times daily **OR**
- (emergency management of acute narrow-angle glaucoma) 1 drop to affected eye(s) every 5 minutes until miosis is achieved

Adverse effects

- (uncommon) retinal tear
- (rare) retinal detachment, ciliate muscle spasm
- see also General Ocular Adverse effects and General Adverse effects of antiglaucoma agents (p. 453)

Interactions

- miotic effects may be reduced by belladonna alkaloids

Nursing points/Cautions

- available in a range of strengths, so select correct preparation
- may cause bronchospasm in susceptible individuals
- not recommended if there is acute inflammation of anterior chamber
- caution if used in those with cardiac failure, asthma, peptic ulcer, hyperthyroidism, GI spasm, recent myocardial infarction, Parkinson's disease, urinary tract obstruction and hypo/hypertension
- caution if used in those with corneal or conjunctival damage

- contraindicated where pupillary constriction is not desirable (e.g. acute iritis and uveitis, anterior uveitis), previous history of retinal detachment or conditions that predispose to retinal detachment
- see also General Nursing points/Cautions for antiglaucoma agents (p. 453)

Patient teaching and advice

- see also General Patient teaching and advice for antiglaucoma agents (p. 453)

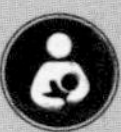

not recommended during pregnancy

only used during breastfeeding if benefits outweigh risks

TAFLUPROST (Saflutan)

Available form

Eye drops: 15 microgram/mL

Action

- prostaglandin F_{2alpha}
- active metabolite is tafluprost acid
- increases uveoscleral outflow of aqueous humour
- action within 2–4 hours of administration, peak effect 12 hours, duration of action 24 hours

Use

- (monotherapy or with beta-adrenergic blocking agents) open-angle glaucoma, ocular hypertension

Dose

- 1 drop to affected eye(s) nightly

Adverse effects

- see General Ocular Adverse effects of antiglaucoma agents (p. 453)
- iris colour change
- pigmentation of periocular and eyelid skin
- eyelash darkening, thickening, lengthening, increased number of lashes and misdirected growth
- macular oedema
- dyspnoea, asthma

Nursing points/Cautions

- caution if used in those at risk of macular oedema or iritis/uveitis
- caution if used in those with compromised lung function
- see also General Nursing points/Cautions for antiglaucoma agents (p. 453)

Patient teaching and advice

- warn patient of possible change in eye colour, particularly in those with mixed eye colour (e.g. blue-brown, grey-brown), which generally occurs within first 8 months of treatment
- patients should be advised that eyelashes may darken, thicken and lengthen and eyelid skin and skin around eyes may also darken. Advise patient to wipe off any excess solution from the skin to reduce risk of skin darkening
- women of childbearing potential should be counselled to use adequate contraception during therapy
- see also General Patient teaching and advice for antiglaucoma agents (p. 453)

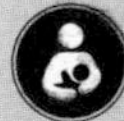

only recommended during pregnancy if benefits outweigh risks

caution if used during breastfeeding

TIMOLOL MALEATE (Timoptol, Timoptol XE)

Available forms

Eye drops: 2.5 mg/mL (0.25%), 5 mg/mL (0.5%)

Action

- non-selective beta-adrenoceptor blocking agent which reduces production of aqueous humour
- onset of action 20 minutes, peak effect 1–2 hours, duration of action 24 hours

Use

- chronic open-angle glaucoma
- ocular hypertension

Dose

- 1 drop of 0.25% ophthalmic solution to affected eye(s) 1–2 times daily until intraocular pressure at satisfactory level, then once daily (0.5% solution may be required if response is inadequate)

Adverse effects

- see General Ocular Adverse effects and General Adverse effects of antiglaucoma agents (p. 453)

Interactions

- not recommended with methoxyflurane
- increased risk of tachycardia and hypotension if given with anaesthetics
- decreased AV conduction and bradycardia may occur if given with digoxin
- increased risk of rebound hypertension if given with clonidine
- increased risk of hypotension if given with nifedipine
- increased risk of conduction disorders if given with verapamil or diltiazem
- decreased heart rate may occur if given with SSRIs
- may prolong QT interval if given with mefloquine
- caution if given with adrenaline (epinephrine) due to the risk of bradycardia and/or hypertensive crisis
- increased effect if given with oral beta-adrenoceptor blocking agents
- not recommended with other topical beta-adrenoceptor blocking agents
- increased serum levels may occur if given with cimetidine and hydralazine
- may mask signs of hypoglycaemia (tachycardia)
- may increase effects of insulin
- caution if given with amiodarone due to risk of bradycardia
- not recommended with lidocaine (lignocaine)

Nursing points/Cautions

- see also General Nursing/Cautions for antiglaucoma agents (p. 453)
- cardiac failure should be controlled before starting therapy
- intraocular pressure should be reassessed 2–4 weeks after starting therapy
- should be stopped gradually 24–48 hours before surgery with a general anaesthetic
- because there may be systemic absorption and effects, caution if used in those with asthma, myasthenia gravis or thyrotoxicosis
- caution if given to those with myasthenia gravis due to risk of increased muscle weakness
- caution if used in those with diabetes mellitus as signs of hypoglycaemia (tachycardia) may be masked
- caution if used in those with thyrotoxicosis as thyroid storm may be provoked if withdrawal is abrupt
- caution if used in those with metabolic acidosis, severe cardiac disease, cerebrovascular insufficiency or with a history of atopy or anaphylaxis
- caution if used in those with severe peripheral circulatory insufficiency (e.g. Raynaud's disease)
- contraindicated in those with severe COPD, asthma, reactive airway disease, bronchospasm, SA block, sinus bradycardia (greater than first degree), AV block (second- or third-degree block), cardiac failure, cardiogenic shock or hypersensitivity to timolol or other beta-adrenoceptor blocking agents

Patient teaching and advice

- see General Patient teaching and advice for antiglaucoma agents (p. 453)

generally banned in sport during competition, but may be permitted under certain circumstances. This also includes combination eyedrops that contain timolol maleate

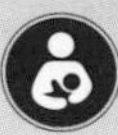

not recommended during pregnancy and breastfeeding

Note

- combined with brimonidine in Combigan, dorzolamide in Cosdor and Cosopt, travoprost in DuoTrav, latanoprost in Latanocom, Xalacom, Xalamol 50/5 and Xanopan 50/5, brinzolamide in Azarga; and with bimatoprost in Ganfort 0.3/5 and Ganfort 0.3/5

TRAVOPROST (Travatan Eye Drops)

Available form

Eye drops: 40 microgram/mL

Action

- prostaglandin analogue
- prodrug of prostaglandin F_2 alpha analogue which increases aqueous humour outflow
- onset of action 2 hours, peak effect 12 hours, duration of action 24–36 hours

Use

- chronic open-angle glaucoma
- ocular hypertension

Dose

- 1 drop into affected eye(s) daily, in the evening

Adverse effects

- see General Ocular Adverse effects for antiglaucoma agents (p. 453)
- iris colour change
- pigmentation of periocular and eyelid skin
- eyelash darkening, thickening, lengthening, increased number of lashes and misdirected growth
- macular oedema

Nursing points/Cautions

- caution if used in those with aphakia (absence of lens in the eye), pseudoaphakia, or those with risk factors for macular oedema (e.g. diabetic retinopathy, intraocular surgery), acute intraocular inflammation or risk factors for uveitis or iritis
- see also General Nursing points/Cautions for antiglaucoma agents (p. 453)

Patient teaching and advice

- warn patient of possible change in eye colour, particularly in those with mixed eye colour (e.g. blue-brown, grey-brown), which generally occurs within first 8 months of treatment
- patient should be advised that eyelashes may darken, thicken and lengthen and eyelid skin and skin around eyes may also darken. Advise patient to wipe off any excess solution from the skin to reduce risk of skin darkening
- women of childbearing potential should be counselled to use adequate contraception during therapy
- see also General Patient teaching and advice for antiglaucoma agents (p. 453)

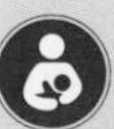

contraindicated during pregnancy or in those trying to become pregnant

not recommended during breastfeeding

Note

- contained in DuoTrav with timolol maleate

ANTIGOUT AND URICOLYTIC AGENTS

Gout is a metabolic disorder caused by excess uric acid (hyperuricaemia) in the blood that crystallises in the joints, commonly the big toe, but other joints such as wrists, fingers, elbows, toes, ankles and knees can also be affected. While the prevalence varies worldwide, gout occurs more commonly in developed countries compared to developing nations (AIHW 2017). In Australia, about 1% of the population has gout, with men four times more likely to be affected (AIHW 2017). Gout is often viewed as non-serious; however, it not only causes pain but impacts on a person's ability to function and work, with 7352 hospitalisations in 2015–16 having a diagnosis of gout (AIHW 2017). Furthermore, gout is associated with a number of co-morbidities, including hypertension, diabetes mellitus, ischaemic heart disease, obesity and kidney disease. Therefore, it is essential that when patients present with gout, they are also screened for these other conditions (Robinson & Stamp 2016).

Uric acid is produced in the body from purines (adenosine, guanine) via a number of steps catalysed by the enzyme xanthine oxidase. It is normally filtered by the kidneys, reabsorbed and then excreted in the urine. Conditions that may cause the uric acid to crystallise (the crystals are known as 'tophi') include an acid environment (such as in the kidney filtrate) or temperatures less than 37°C (such as body extremities). When the uric acid crystallises as urates in the joint spaces (usually toes and/or ankles) an inflammatory response is mediated, resulting in swelling, heat, inflammation and pain. Initially, one joint is affected; however, with subsequent attacks, other joints become involved. In the renal tubules, the crystals can lead to stone formation, and impaired renal function, which can proceed to renal failure. Early attacks usually subside without treatment in 3–10 days with no residual symptoms (Schumacher & Chen 2018).

The goal of therapy is to manage gout by reducing serum urate levels in order to reduce the gout flares (acute gouty attacks) and resolve tophi. The recommended target is < 0.36 mmol/L for those without tophi, or < 0.30 mmol/L for those with tophi. Patients should be aware that the gout flares may still occur for 12–18 months after the levels are below the target. However, these flares should be less frequent and should stop altogether if the target urate level is maintained (Robinson & Stamp 2016). Acute flares should be managed with NSAIDs or colchicine, with oral corticosteroids used in those who have contraindications or are intolerant to the other agents. NSAIDs and colchicine are also used for prophylaxis of gout flares for at least 6 months, or 3 months after achieving target urate levels in patients without tophi or 6 months in those with tophi (Robinson & Stamp 2016). Unfortunately, many patients do not adhere to the pharmacological management, possibly because of misconceptions about medications. It is important for patients to understand that the gout flares may still occur in the short term; however, the goal is to eliminate these in the longer term. Evidence surrounding the use of low-purine diets is scant; however, it has been shown that large intakes of sugar or sweetened soft drinks are a risk for gout and should be avoided (Robinson & Stamp 2016).

ALLOPURINOL (Allosig, Progout, Zyloprim)

Available forms

Tablets: 100 mg, 300 mg

Action

- reduces uric acid levels in both body fluids and urine by inhibiting xanthine oxidase which catalyses the conversion of hypoxanthine and xanthine to urate/uric acid
- active metabolite (oxypurinol)
- half-life of allopurinol 1–2 hours while active metabolite oxypurinol has a half-life of 15 hours

Use

- chronic gout (gouty arthritis, skin tophi)
- hyperuricaemia resulting from neoplastic disease or myeloproliferative disorders (with high cell turnover), antineoplastic or thiazide diuretic therapy or radiotherapy
- recurrent renal stones (mixed calcium oxalate) with hyperuricaemia (where other forms of management have failed) or enzyme disorders resulting in overproduction of urate

Dose

Gout

- (mild) 100–200 mg orally daily after food **OR**
- (moderately severe) 300–600 mg orally daily after food **OR**
- (severe) 700–900 mg orally daily after food

High urate turnover conditions

- dosage should be started at lower range (see mild gout above)

High urate turnover conditions (with renal impairment)

- initially 100 mg orally daily after food, increasing only if serum and/or urinary urate levels do not respond

Adverse effects

- rash
- nausea, vomiting
- headache, fever, malaise, somnolence, vertigo, asthenia, ataxia
- (rare) hypersensitivity reaction (fever, arthralgia, eosinophilia, exfoliation), hepatotoxicity, bone marrow depression, ataxia

Interactions

- prolongs activity of azathioprine and mercaptopurine, therefore lower doses of both agents are recommended
- excretion of active metabolite (oxypurinol) may be increased when given with probenecid or high-dose salicylates
- may increase theophylline or ciclosporin plasma concentrations, requiring more frequent monitoring to decrease the risk of toxicity, especially

at start of therapy or when increasing dose of allopurinol
- may increase frequency of rash in patients receiving ampicillin or amoxicillin and are therefore not recommended together
- may increase risk of toxicity of ifosamide, pyrazinamide and cyclophosphamide if given with allopurinol
- increased risk of bone marrow depression if given with other agents which also depress bone marrow

Nursing points/Cautions

- should not be started until acute attack has subsided (otherwise further attacks may be precipitated)
- serum urate and urinary urate/uric acid levels should be measured regularly during therapy
- if dose is greater than 300 mg and gastric symptoms are present, dose may be divided
- if allopurinol is stopped because of rash, it can be restarted at a lower dose when the rash has totally disappeared and the dose gradually increased. However, if rash recurs therapy should be stopped immediately and not restarted as there is an increased risk of hypersensitivity
- dose is dependent on severity of gout
- colchicine or NSAIDs may also be given in the early stages of allopurinol therapy as prophylaxis for acute gout attacks
- (high urate turnover conditions) any hyperuricaemia and/or hyperuricosuria should be corrected before starting cytotoxic therapy. Adequate hydration is also required to ensure optimal diuresis to minimise kidney stone formation or deposition in the urinary tract
- (high urate turnover conditions with renal impairment) dose may be started at less than 100 mg per day or 100 mg at a longer interval (e.g. every second day)
- in those with pre-existing liver disease, regular liver function tests are recommended, especially early in therapy
- allopurinol is removed by renal dialysis, therefore alternate dose (300–400 mg orally immediately after dialysis) should be considered if dialysis is needed 2 to 3 times per week
- caution if used in those with liver or renal impairment as a lower dose is required
- caution if used in those with hypertension, cardiac insufficiency with renal impairment, haemochromatosis or abnormal iron storage conditions

Patient teaching and advice

- warn patient not to take allopurinol during an acute attack of gout
- patient should be warned that acute gout attacks may occur early in therapy due to mobilisation of urate from tissue and this is managed with NSAIDs or colchicine for at least 4 weeks
- advise patient to take with food or milk to minimise gastric irritation
- if not contraindicated, fluid intake should be increased to maintain a urinary output of at least 2 L/24 hours and urine made alkaline to minimise kidney stone formation or deposition in the urinary tract
- instruct patient to report rash, pruritus (itch), anorexia (loss of appetite) or weight loss immediately to doctor because this indicates the need to stop therapy
- warn patient against driving a vehicle or operating machinery if drowsy or experiencing vertigo or ataxia
- advise patient to avoid using aspirin, foods with high purine content such as organ meat (e.g. kidney, liver), sardines, anchovies, mackerel, herring, minced meat, shrimp, broth, consommé, gravies and yeast, limiting the use of alcohol and fructose-containing foods and drinks

- see also General Patient teaching and advice (p. xxvii)

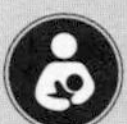

only use in pregnancy if benefits outweigh potential risks

use during breastfeeding with caution if doses are high or therapy is long term

tablet can be broken in half and dispersed with water or crushed and mixed with water or spoonful of yoghurt or apple puree

COLCHICINE (Colgout, Lengout)

Available form

Tablets: 500 microgram

Action

- inhibits leucocyte migration and phagocytosis in gouty joints, counteracting the inflammatory response to urate crystals
- decreases deposition of urate crystals, although it has no effect on production or excretion of uric acid
- has no analgesic properties, but does have prophylactic, suppressive effects reducing the incidence of acute attacks
- half-life 4.4 hours, which increases to 18.8 hours in kidney dysfunction

Use

- acute gout (where NSAIDs are contraindicated or are ineffective)

Dose

- initially 1 mg orally, followed 6-hourly by 0.5 mg until relief is obtained (up to a total of 2.5 mg in first 24 hours) (total dose should not exceed 6 mg over 96 hours)

Adverse effects

- nausea, vomiting, diarrhoea, abdominal pain
- rash, urticaria, purpura, dermatitis
- delayed or impaired corneal wound healing
- reversible azoospermia and oligospermia, decreased sperm motility
- anuria, bladder spasm, oliguria
- increased alkaline phosphatase
- muscle weakness, myopathy
- (long-term or prolonged therapy or overdose) blood dyscrasias, hair loss (body and scalp), anorexia, myopathy, peripheral neuropathy, rhabdomyolysis, vascular damage, malabsorption syndrome, hypersensitivity
- (toxic dose) haemorrhagic diarrhoea, dehydration, metabolic acidosis, hypotension, shock, haematuria, oliguria, renal damage

Interactions

- increased risk of myopathy and/or rhabdomyolysis if used with ciclosporin, especially if kidney impairment is also present
- toxicity may occur if given with erythromycin and clarithromycin (especially if liver/kidney impairment exists or in the elderly)
- increased serum levels, and therefore risk of toxicity may occur if given with clarithromycin, erythromycin, atazanavir, indinavir, ritonavir, saquinavir and itraconazole
- inhibited by acidifying agents such as ammonium chloride and ascorbic acid
- potentiated by alkalinising agents such as sodium bicarbonate and potassium citrate
- may increase sensitivity to CNS depressants (e.g. opioids, sedatives, hypnotics, alcohol, benzodiazepines)
- increased risk of GI toxicity if given with alcohol
- alcohol increases blood uric acid levels thereby decreasing prophylactic actions of colchicine
- increased risk of GI bleeding/ulceration if given with NSAIDs
- increased risk of bone marrow depression if given with radiation treatment and/or cytolytic antineoplastic agents

- increased risk of bleeding if given with other agents that impair blood clotting or cause haemorrhage
- may cause reversible malabsorption of vitamin B_{12}
- leucopenic and/or thrombocytopenic effects may be increased if given with myelotoxic agents (i.e. those with bone marrow depressing effects or those causing blood dyscrasias)
- action may be decreased if given with antineoplastic agents which cause rapid cell turnover
- may affect a number of laboratory tests

Nursing points/Cautions

- treatment continued during acute attack until relief, or if nausea and diarrhoea occur (even if acute attack has not subsided). Patient should be advised to note the cumulative dose at which GI symptoms occurred and remain below this with subsequent treatments
- additional treatment should not occur within 3 days of completing course
- therapy should be stopped before any eye surgery because of delayed or impaired corneal wound healing
- complete blood counts are recommended if therapy is prolonged or long term
- any dental work should be delayed if leucopenia or thrombocytopenia occur due to increased risk of gum bleeding, delayed healing and infection
- overdose symptoms may be delayed 2–12 hours after ingestion, therefore it is recommended the patient is monitored for at least 12 hours after overdose or acute poisoning
- caution if used in the elderly (especially if under 50 kg) or debilitated, or those with heart, kidney or GI disease
- contraindicated in those with kidney and/or liver disease/impairment, severe GI or cardiac disorders and blood dyscrasias

Patient teaching and advice

- warn patient to avoid alcohol during therapy
- patient should be advised to avoid vitamin C preparations because they acidify the urine, leading to the possibility of renal stone formation
- instruct patients to continue therapy until relief occurs or abdominal pain, diarrhoea, nausea or vomiting appear. These symptoms usually occur within 8–12 hours of starting therapy (especially if maximum dose is given). Patient should also be asked to take a note of the total dose taken when the symptoms occurred and seek medical advice immediately
- warn patient to not take colchicine again within 3 days of stopping treatment or abdominal pain, diarrhoea, nausea or vomiting occurring
- advise patient to avoid using aspirin, and foods with high purine content, such as organ meat (e.g. kidney, liver), sardines, anchovies, mackerel, herring, minced meat, shrimp, broth, consommé, gravies and yeast, limiting the use of alcohol and fructose-containing foods and drinks
- patient should be instructed to seek medical advice immediately if any of the following occur:
  - burning sensation in throat or stomach
  - severe stomach pain, nausea or vomiting
  - severe diarrhoea with bloody or black stools
  - difficulty passing urine or urine contains blood
  - muscle weakness
  - numbness in fingers or toes
- see also General Patient teaching and advice (p. xxvii)

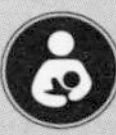

not recommended during pregnancy or breastfeeding.

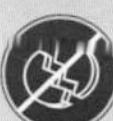

tablets should not be crushed or dispersed by women who are pregnant

tablets can be dispersed in water or crushed and given with water or spoonful of yoghurt or apple puree

FEBUXOSTAT (Adenuric)

Available form

Tablets: 80 mg

Action

- nonpurine selective xanthine oxidase inhibitor
- active metabolites
- half-life 5–8 hours

Use

- gouty arthritis and/or tophus formation

Dose

- initially 40 mg orally daily, increasing to 80 mg daily after 2–4 weeks if serum uric acid levels are greater than 357 micromol/L (6 mg/dL)

Adverse effects

- gout flares (acute gouty attacks)
- liver function abnormalities
- diarrhoea, nausea
- headache
- rash
- oedema
- (uncommon) dizziness, somnolence, paraesthesia, blurred vision, altered taste
- (rare) severe hypersensitivity reaction

Interactions

- not recommended with mercaptopurine or azathioprine due to increased risk of toxicity
- caution if given with theophylline as there may be an increase in levels of theophylline's metabolite
- metabolism may be increased by phenytoin. Serum uric acid should be monitored 12 weeks after starting therapy if given together
- may increase serum levels of tacrolimus

Nursing points/Cautions

- therapy should not be started until acute gout has subsided
- gout flares (acute gouty attacks) commonly occur soon after start of therapy and during first 6 months of therapy due to mobilisation of urate from tissue deposits resulting in changing serum uric acid levels. Gout flares can be prevented by concurrent therapy with colchicine or NSAIDs for up to 6 months
- liver function tests are recommended before starting and regularly throughout therapy. If patient experiences symptoms of liver dysfunction, liver function tests should be completed immediately and therapy stopped if ALT is three times greater than normal levels
- patient should be carefully monitored for signs and symptoms of stroke or myocardial infarction during therapy
- tablets contain lactose and therefore are not recommended in those with hereditary problems of galactose intolerance, Lapp lactase deficiency or glucose–galactose malabsorption
- caution if used in those with thyroid dysfunction, liver or kidney impairment
- not recommended in those with ischaemic heart disease, congestive heart failure or organ transplant recipients
- not recommended in those with an increased rate of urate formation such as during treatment for malignancy or those with Lesch Nyhan syndrome

Patient teaching and advice

- warn patient that gout flares may occur more frequently during the first 6 months of therapy due to changes in serum uric acid levels, but will decrease in both frequency and intensity. Febuxostat should be continued during these gout flares
- patient should be advised not to drive or operate machinery if somnolence, dizziness, blurred vision or numbness occur

- advise patient to seek medical advice immediately if any of the following occur:
  - rash, itchiness, breathing difficulties, limb/face swelling
  - skin/eyes yellowing, dark urine, fatigue, loss of appetite, pain in right upper abdomen
  - increase in gout symptoms
- see also General Patient teaching and advice (p. xxvii)

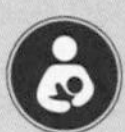

not recommended during pregnancy or breastfeeding

tablet may be crushed and mixed with water or spoonful of yoghurt or apply puree

PROBENECID (Pro-Cid)

Available form

Tablets: 500 mg

Action

- promotes uric acid excretion by inhibiting its renal tubular absorption (uricosuric)
- reduces renal tubular excretion of some anti-infective agents, thereby prolonging and increasing their plasma concentrations by 2–4 times
- half-life 6–12 hours

Use

- chronic gout
- adjuvant to therapy with penicillins and most cephalosporins (beta lactam antibacterial agents)
- reduce nephrotoxicity risk of cidofovir

Dose

- (gout) 250 mg orally twice daily for 1 week, then increased to 500 mg twice daily. If needed, dose may be further increased by 500 mg every 4 weeks (maximum daily dose 2 g) **OR**
- (beta lactam co-therapy) 500 mg orally 4 times daily **OR**
- (uncomplicated gonorrhoea) 1 g orally as a single dose taken with a single high dose of oral ampicillin, IM procaine benzylpenicillin (procaine penicillin) or IM cefoxitin sodium **OR**
- (with cidofovir) 2 g orally 3 hours before dose of cidofovir, then 1 g orally 2 and 8 hours after cidofovir infusion (total 4 g)

Adverse effects

- headache, dizziness
- flushing, dermatitis, alopecia
- sore gums
- anorexia, nausea, vomiting
- urinary frequency, renal colic, renal stones (with or without haematuria)
- hypersensitivity reaction, including skin reactions
- exacerbation of gout
- anaemia, haemolytic anaemia

Interactions

- contraindicated with aspirin or other salicylates as they antagonise uricosuric action
- may prolong action of sulfonylureas, increasing risk of hypoglycaemia
- may decrease excretion of sulfonamides
- may increase plasma concentrations of penicillins, dapsone, some cephalosporins, midazolam, nitrazepam, methotrexate, paracetamol, rifampicin, NSAIDs, antiviral agents, lorazepam, ketorolac, ciprofloxacin, famotidine
- increased plasma concentrations of both if given with allopurinol
- may increase plasma concentrations of methotrexate leading to toxicity, therefore plasma concentrations should be closely monitored and dose adjusted as needed
- may potentiate effects of thiazide diuretics
- may increase and prolong anaesthetic effect of ketamine and thiopental
- may decrease dose needed for induction using thiopental

- may cause false positive test for glycosuria using reagents strips containing copper sulfate

Nursing points/Cautions

- therapy should not be started until acute attack has subsided. If acute gout is precipitated, probenecid should be continued with colchicine, indometacin or other agents to control acute attack
- gastric symptoms (anorexia, nausea and vomiting) may indicate overdose, and dose may be reduced without losing clinical response
- alkaline urine can be achieved by taking sodium bicarbonate (3–7.5 g/day) or potassium citrate (7.5 g/day) and this should be continued until serum uric acid levels return to normal and tophi have disappeared. Acid–base balance should be closely monitored during this time
- if patient has been free of acute attacks for 6 months and serum uric acid levels are normal, dose may be reduced
- blood glucose levels (BGLs) should be monitored frequently in patients with diabetes who are treated concurrently with sulfonylureas and probenecid
- when used in gonorrhoea, oral ampicillin is given at the same time, whereas IM penicillin or cefoxitin should be given 30 minutes after probenecid
- not effective if patient has chronic renal insufficiency and glomerular filtration rate is less than 30 mL/min
- caution if used in those with GI disease (e.g. peptic ulcer) or chronic kidney insufficiency
- contraindicated in those with blood dyscrasias or uric acid stones

Patient teaching and advice

- patient should be warned not to start therapy until acute attack has settled
- patient should be advised to take paracetamol instead of aspirin for pain relief
- instruct patient to report any loss of appetite, nausea and/or vomiting to doctor immediately
- if patient is involved in elite sport, he/she should be advised that probenecid is banned in sport both in and out of competition
- if patient has diabetes and is managed using sulfonylureas, he/she should be warned that there is an increased risk of hypoglycaemia occurring
- warn patient against driving a vehicle or operating machinery if experiencing dizziness
- if patient has diabetes, he/she should be advised that false positive test results may occur if the test involves copper sulfate
- instruct patient to drink plenty of water while taking probenecid to prevent kidney stones from forming
- advise patient to seek medical advice if blood appears in the urine, severe/sharp pain occurs in the side or lower back, fever, infection, increased bruising or bleeding, unusual hair loss or painful swollen joints occurs
- advise patient to avoid aspirin, foods with high purine content such as organ meat (e.g. kidney, liver), sardines, anchovies, mackerel, herring, minced meat, shrimp, broth, consommé, gravies and yeast, limiting the use of alcohol and fructose-containing foods and drinks
- see also General Patient teaching and advice (p. xxvii)

banned in sport (in and out of competition)

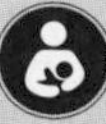

crosses placental barrier and should only be used in pregnancy if benefits outweigh risks

caution if used during breastfeeding

can be dispersed in water or crushed and given in water or spoonful of yoghurt or apple puree

RASBURICASE RYS (Fasturtec)

Available forms

Vial: 1.5 mg, 7.5 mg

Action

- recombinant urate oxidase
- catalyses oxidation of uric acid to allantoin, which is water soluble and therefore more easily excreted by the kidney
- produces hydrogen peroxide as a byproduct
- half-life 19 hours

Use

- prophylaxis and treatment of acute hyperuricaemia (caused by malignancy with high risk of rapid tumour lysis)

Dose

- 0.20 mg/kg/day IV infusion over 30 minutes once daily for 5–7 days

Adverse effects

- fever
- nausea, vomiting
- rash, urticaria
- (uncommon) bronchospasm, allergic reaction, antibody formation, haemolytic anaemia, methaemoglobinaemia, headache, diarrhoea, hypotension
- (rare) anaphylaxis

Nursing points/Cautions

- patient should be carefully monitored during therapy for any signs of allergy including skin reactions and bronchospasm
- if patient is already hyperuricaemic, chemotherapy should be administered within 48 hours of rasburicase rys
- if patient is not hyperuricaemic, chemotherapy should be administered within 24 hours of rasburicase rys
- patient should be monitored for hyperphosphataemia, hyperkalaemia and hypocalcaemia, as these can also arise from rapid tumour lysis
- when reconstituting solution, it should be swirled gently and not shaken
- after reconstitution, solution should be further diluted using sodium chloride 0.9% to make up a total infusion of 50 mL
- reconstituted solution should be inspected for any particulate matter
- inline filter should not be used
- solution should be infused over 30 minutes
- infusion should be via a separate IV line to that used for chemotherapy. If separate IV line is not available, IV should be flushed with sodium chloride between chemotherapy and rasburicase rys
- if blood is needed for uric acid concentrations it should be collected into pre-chilled tubes (with heparin to prevent coagulation), samples placed in ice/water bath, centrifuged in a pre-cooled centrifuge, plasma kept in ice/water bath and analysed within 4 hours of collection
- physically incompatible with glucose
- caution if used in those with history of atopic allergies because of the increased risk of hypersensitivity reactions
- contraindicated in those with G6PD deficiency or other metabolic disorders because of the hydrogen peroxide by-product, which is known to induce haemolytic anaemia in susceptible individuals or with uricase hypersensitivity

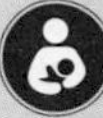

not recommended during pregnancy or breastfeeding unless benefits to the mother are thought to outweigh risks to fetus

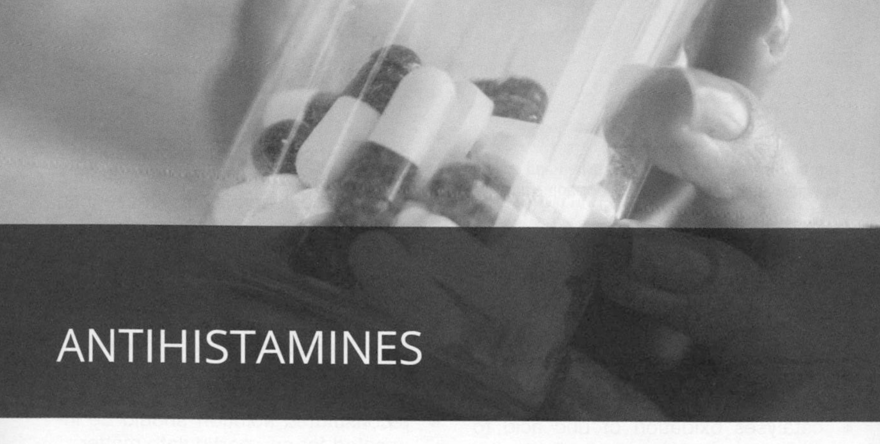

ANTIHISTAMINES

Histamine is a naturally occurring amine that is stored in mast cells or in circulating basophils and is the major mediator of inflammation, anaphylaxis and gastric acid secretion. Mast cells are found in large numbers in bronchial smooth muscle and small blood vessels, which may account for some of the immediate hypersensitivity and allergic responses. Histamine has also been found stored in the GI mucosa, epidermis and the CNS. It should be noted that some medications act directly, causing mast cells to release histamine, leading to adverse effects (Skidgel 2018).

There are four types of histamine receptors:

- H_1 receptors are widely distributed in the periphery and CNS involved in type 1 hypersensitivity reactions (see Glossary). These reactions range from mild (e.g. urticaria) to life threatening (e.g. anaphylactoid reaction). Histamine is responsible for capillary and venous dilation, increased vascular permeability (and resultant oedema) and constriction of smooth muscle (including bronchial and GI), resulting in a fall in blood pressure, dyspnoea and airway obstruction. Histamine may cause flush, flare, itch, secretion from nasal mucosa and weals of the skin (Skidgel 2018).
- H_2 receptors are involved in the regulation of gastric acid secretion. Histamine is released from enterochromaffin-like cells found in the stomach, adjacent to the parietal cells. H_2-receptor antagonists are used in the treatment of gastric and duodenal ulcers (Skidgel 2018) (see Antiulcer agents, p. 806).
- H_3 receptors are found in the CNS, especially the basal ganglia, hippocampus and cortex. H_3 agonists promote sleep while H_3 antagonists promote wakefulness (Skidgel 2018).
- H_4 receptors are similar to H_3 receptors and are found on eosinophils, dendritic cells, mast cells, monocytes, basophils and T cells, as well as in the GI tract, dermal fibroblasts and CNS. It has been postulated that H_4-receptor antagonists will be useful for the treatment of allergy and inflammation (Skidgel 2018).

H_1-receptor antagonists are commonly referred to as 'antihistamines' and are used in the treatment of allergic disorders, including seasonal allergic rhinitis (hay fever), allergic skin reactions, including rash, pruritus and insect stings, and also with adrenaline (epinephrine) in the management of anaphylaxis or severe angioedema. The older style antihistamines (e.g. promethazine, chlorpheniramine) have also been used as mild hypnotic agents because they cross the blood–brain barrier and cause sedation, and also as antiemetics, especially in the treatment of motion sickness (Skidgel 2018).

General Actions of antihistamines

- block main actions of histamine at H_1 receptors

General Adverse effects of antihistamines

- sedation, decreased motor skills and coordination, fatigue, dizziness, headache, somnolence, insomnia, confusion, anxiety, hallucinations
- (anticholinergic effects) dry eyes, nose and mouth, blurred vision, urinary hesitancy/retention, constipation, tachycardia
- nausea, vomiting, diarrhoea, dyspepsia
- tinnitus, vertigo
- pruritus, rash, urticaria, allergic dermatitis
- (rare) blood dyscrasias

General Interactions of antihistamines

- may enhance CNS depressant effects of alcohol and other CNS depressing agents, such as barbiturates, hypnotics, sedatives, anticholinergics, antipsychotics and opioid analgesics

General Nursing points/Cautions for antihistamines

- should be discontinued 48–72 hours before skin testing for allergies is performed
- caution if used in those with epilepsy (especially in children), liver or kidney impairment
- caution if used in the elderly as they are more prone to adverse effects, such as confusion, dizziness, sedation and hypotension, which increases the risk of falls
- caution/contraindicated if used in those with cardiovascular disease, hypertension, narrow-angle glaucoma, predisposed to urinary retention (e.g. prostatic hypertrophy, spinal cord lesion), bladder neck obstruction, pyloroduodenal obstruction, stenosing peptic ulcer, thyroid disease or raised intra-ocular pressure

General Patient teaching and advice for antihistamines

- counsel patient to avoid contact with allergen (if possible) and to take antihistamine before start of exposure (e.g. at the beginning of hay fever season)
- ensure patient understands that antihistamine does not protect against allergic reactions
- advise patient against driving a vehicle or operating machinery if drowsy, dizzy or experiencing any other CNS adverse effects
- warn patient about reduced tolerance to alcohol and the need to avoid it during therapy with antihistamine
- see General Patient teaching and advice (p. xxvii)

Nasal spray instillation

- if using a nasal spray, instruct the patient to:
  1. ensure nasal spray is primed for use, if new, dust cover has been left off or device has been unused for some time (priming instructions vary from nasal spray to nasal

spray, but essentially involves vigorously shaking container (with cap on) for 10 seconds and then priming by releasing 6–7 sprays until spray is uniform)
2 blow nose
3 insert spray adapter/nozzle into nostril while closing other nostril
4 tilt head slightly forwards, keeping nasal spray container upright
5 avoid tilting head back as this will result in bitter smell/taste
6 depress pump while breathing gently and slowly through the nostril
7 repeat procedure in same nostril if second spray per nostril is required
8 remove adapter/nozzle from nostril and repeat in other nostril
9 after prescribed amount has been delivered, remove adapter/nozzle from nostril and wipe with tissue
10 wash spray adapter/nozzle regularly with warm water
11 re-prime with 2 sprays after cleaning
12 if nozzle/adapter becomes blocked, pins or other sharp devices should not be used to unblock device as it may become damaged and not deliver required amount of nasal spray
13 replace dust cap after each use

Eye drop instillation

- instruct patient in correct technique for instilling eye drops, including:
  1 removal of contact lenses before using eye drops and not replacing lenses for at least 15 minutes (eye drops contain preservative benzalkonium chloride which discolours contact lenses)
  2 not allowing tip of dispensing container to touch eye as it may cause injury and/or contaminate eye drops
  3 if container is new, remove protective seal, otherwise it is important to check expiry date
  4 when opening for first time, container should be dated and discarded 28 days after opening
  5 wash hands thoroughly with soap and water
  6 remove lid/cap and hold container upside down in one hand between thumb and forefinger or index finger
  7 using other hand, gently pull down on lower eyelid to form a pouch/pocket and tilt head back, looking up
  8 place tip of container close to lower eyelid (taking care not to make contact between tip and eye). Squeezing the bottle gently, release one drop into pouch/pocket formed between eye and eyelid, taking care not to allow tip to touch eye
  9 gently close eye, but do not blink or rub eye
  10 while eye is closed, place index finger against inside corner of eye and press against nose for about 2 minutes (this stops medicine from draining through tear duct into nose and throat)
  11 blot any excess solution from around the eye with a tissue
  12 replace lid/cap tightly
  13 wash hands again to remove any residue

AZELASTINE HYDROCHLORIDE (Azep Nasal Spray, Eyezep)

Available forms

Metered dose nasal spray: 137 microgram/0.137 mL; Eye drops: 0.5 mg/mL

Action

- see General Actions of antihistamines (p. 475)
- active metabolite (half-life 56 hours)
- half-life 22 hours
- (nasal spray) onset of action 15 minutes, duration up to 12 hours

Use

- seasonal or perennial allergic rhinitis, seasonal/non-seasonal (perennial) allergic conjunctivitis

Dose

- (nasal spray) 1 spray to each nostril twice daily **OR**
- (eye drops) 1 drop per eye twice daily, increasing to 4 times daily if needed

Adverse effects

- (nasal spray) nasal stinging, itching, sneezing, rhinitis, bitter taste, nausea, epistaxis, headache
- (eye drops) mild transient burning or stinging, and uncommonly, bitter taste

Interactions

- see General Interactions of antihistamines (p. 475)

Nursing points/Cautions

- (perennial allergic rhinitis) treatment should not exceed 6 weeks
- (non-seasonal conjunctivitis) treatment should not exceed 6 months
- (eye drops) not recommended in those with eye infections
- (eye drops) contains benzalkonium chloride (preservative) which can cause irritation and discolouration of soft contact lenses
- see also General Nursing points/Cautions for antihistamines (p. 475)

Patient teaching and advice

- (nasal spray) prime 2–3 times before first use, and again if not used for > 3 days until spray is even
- (eye drops) if allergen exposure is anticipated, should be instilled before exposure
- see General Patient teaching and advice for antihistamines (including instillation instructions for nasal spray and eye drops) (pp. 475–76)

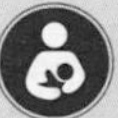

not recommended during pregnancy unless benefits are thought to outweigh risks

caution if used during breastfeeding

Note

- contained in Dymista 125/50 with fluticasone propionate

CETIRIZINE HYDROCHLORIDE (Alzene, Little Allergies for Children, Zilarex, Zyrtec)

Available forms

Tablets: 10 mg; Oral solution: 1 mg/mL; Oral drops: 10 mg/mL (2.5 mg/5 drops)

Action

- non-sedation antihistamine
- half-life 8 hours
- see also General Actions of antihistamines (p. 475)

Use

- seasonal or perennial allergic rhinitis
- chronic idiopathic urticaria

Dose

- (adult, children > 12 years) initially 10 mg orally daily, increasing to 20 mg if necessary

Adverse effects

- (rare) severe skin reactions
- see also General Adverse effects for antihistamines (p. 475)

Interactions

- see General Interactions for antihistamines (p. 475)

Nursing points/Cautions

- (oral drops) not recommended in children < 1 year

- (oral solution) not recommended in children < 2 years as sorbitol may cause diarrhoea
- (tablets) not recommended in children < 6 years
- (Zyrtec) tablets are not recommended in those with galactose intolerance, Lapp lactase deficiency or glucose–galactose malabsorption
- (oral solution) not recommended in those with fructose intolerance
- contraindicated in those with hypersensitivity to hydroxyzine or piperazine derivatives or severe kidney impairment (creatinine clearance < 10 mL/minute)
- see also General Nursing points/Cautions for antihistamines (p. 475)

Patient teaching and advice

- patient should be advised to seek medical advice immediately if any pustules with fever occur within first 2 days of treatment (especially in skin folds, trunk or upper extremity)
- see also General Patient teaching and advice for antihistamines (p. 475)

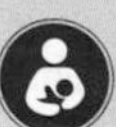

only used during pregnancy if benefits outweigh risks

not recommended during breastfeeding

available as oral solution. Tablet can be crushed and mixed with water or spoonful of yoghurt or apple puree

CYPROHEPTADINE HYDROCHLORIDE SESQUIHYDRATE (CYPROHEPTADINE HYDROCHLORIDE) (Periactin)

Available form

Tablets: 4 mg

Action

- serotonin and histamine antagonist with anticholinergic and sedative actions

Use

- acute and chronic allergies, pruritus
- anaphylactic reaction (with adrenaline (epinephrine) after acute manifestations have subsided)
- prophylaxis and treatment of migraine and vascular headache

Dose

- (allergy, pruritus) initially 4 mg orally 3 times daily, then dose adjusted according to response (not exceeding 32 mg daily) **OR**
- (prophylaxis and treatment of migraine/headache) initially 4 mg orally, repeated in 30 minutes if necessary, then 4 mg every 4–6 hours if needed (not exceeding 8 mg in any 4–6-hour period)

Adverse effects

- see General Adverse effects of antihistamines (p. 475)

Interactions

- contraindicated with MAOIs because anticholinergic effects may be prolonged and intensified
- may interfere with SSRIs
- may cause false positive on urine drug screen for TCAs
- see also General Interactions of antihistamines (p. 475)

Nursing points/Cautions

- caution if used in those with hyperthyroidism, cardiovascular disease, hypertension, history of asthma or raised intra-ocular pressure due to atropine-like actions
- contraindicated in those with acute asthma attack or lower respiratory tract symptoms
- see also General Nursing points/Cautions for antihistamines (p. 475)

Patient teaching and advice

- see General Patient teaching and advice for antihistamines (p. 475)

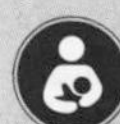

not recommended during pregnancy unless benefits are thought to outweigh risks

contraindicated during breastfeeding

tablet can be dispersed in 10–20 mL of water and settles quickly, so should be mixed well before use. Tablet can be crushed and mixed with spoonful of yoghurt or apple puree

DESLORATADINE (Aerius)

Available forms

Tablets: 5 mg; Syrup: 0.5 mg/mL

Action

- long-acting, non-sedating antihistamine
- peak effect 3 hours
- half-life 27 hours
- see also General Actions of antihistamines (p. 475)

Use

- seasonal or perennial allergic rhinitis

Dose

- 5 mg orally daily

Adverse effects/Interactions

- see General Adverse effects and Interactions for antihistamines (p. 475)

Nursing points/Cautions

- tablets are not recommended for those under 12 years
- contraindicated in those with hypersensitivity to loratadine
- see also General Nursing points/Cautions for antihistamines (p. 475)

Patient teaching and advice

- see General Patient teaching and advice for antihistamines (p. 475)

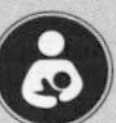

not recommended during pregnancy and breastfeeding

available as liquid. Tablet can be crushed and mixed with spoonful of yoghurt or apple puree

DEXCHLORPHENIRAMINE MALEATE (Polaramine)

Available forms

Tablets: 2 mg; Oral suspension: 2 mg/5 mL

Action

- sedating antihistamine with no anti-emetic actions
- onset of action 30–60 minutes, peak effect hours, duration of action 4–8 hours
- see also General Actions of antihistamines (p. 475)

Use

- seasonal allergic rhinitis, vasomotor rhinitis, allergic conjunctivitis, mild skin manifestations of urticaria and angioedema
- relief of itch associated with allergic eczema, pruritus ani/vulvae and atopic/contact dermatitis, insect bites and drug reactions

Dose

- 2 mg orally 6-hourly (tablet or syrup)

Adverse effects

- (children) paradoxical excitation
- photosensitivity
- see also General Adverse effects of antihistamines (p. 475)

Interactions

- contraindicated with MAOIs because anticholinergic effects may be prolonged and intensified
- may decrease effects of anticoagulants
- see also General Interactions of antihistamines (p. 475)

Nursing points/Cautions

- (tablets) not recommended in children < 12 years
- oral suspension contains sorbitol which may cause diarrhoea
- see also general Nursing points/ Cautions for antihistamines (p. 475)

Patient teaching and advice

- instruct patient to wear sun protection (sunscreen (SPF 30+ or greater), hat, protective clothing) when outdoors
- see also General Patient teaching and advice for antihistamines (p. 475)

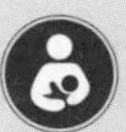

not recommended during third trimester of pregnancy

caution if used during breastfeeding

suspension is available. Tablets can be crushed and mixed with spoonful of yoghurt or apple puree

DIPHENHYDRAMINE HYDROCHLORIDE (Snuzaid Tabs, Unisom Sleepgels)

Available forms

Capsules: 50 mg; Tablets: 50 mg

Action

- see General Actions of antihistamines (p. 475)
- crosses blood–brain barrier causing sedation
- peak effect 1–4 hours, half-life 2.4–9.3 hours

Use

- insomnia (short-term management)

Dose

- (insomnia) 50 mg orally at night, 20–30 minutes before retiring (capsules, tablets, oral liquid)

Adverse effects

- see General Adverse effects of antihistamines (p. 475)

Interactions

- contraindicated with MAOIs and TCAs or with other products containing diphenhydramine hydrochloride (see Note below)
- see also General Interactions of antihistamines (p. 475)

Nursing points/Cautions

- not recommended in children <12 years
- see also General Nursing points/ Cautions for antihistamines (p. 475)

Patient teaching and advice

- patient should be advised to seek medical advice if insomnia lasts for > 10 days
- see also General Patient teaching and advice for antihistamines (p. 475)

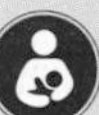

not recommended during pregnancy unless benefits are thought to outweigh risks

contraindicated during breastfeeding

tablets can be crushed and mixed with water or spoonful of yoghurt or apple puree

Note

- contained in Benadryl Original Oral Liquid, Children's Paedamin Decongestant and Antihistamine Oral Liquid, MersynoNight Night Time Pain Relief, Panadol Night

DOXYLAMINE SUCCINATE (Dozile, Restavit)

Available forms

Capsules: 25 mg; Tablets: 25 mg

Action

- sedating antihistamine with anticholinergic actions

- peak activity 2–3 hours, half-life 10 hours
- see also General Actions of antihistamines (p. 475)

Use

- temporary insomnia

Dose

- (insomnia) 25–50 mg orally, 20–30 minutes before bed

Adverse effects

- (high dose) nervousness, tremor, insomnia, agitation, irritability
- see also General Adverse effects of antihistamines (p. 475)

Interactions

- contraindicated with MAOIs and TCAs because of prolonged and intensified anticholinergic and CNS effects
- see also General Interactions of antihistamines (p. 475)

Nursing points/Cautions

- not recommended in children < 12 years
- see General Nursing points/Cautions for antihistamines (p. 475)

Patient teaching and advice

- patient should be advised to seek medical advice if insomnia lasts for >10 days
- see also General Patient teaching and advice for antihistamines (p. 475)

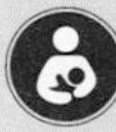

not recommended during pregnancy and breastfeeding

tablet can be crushed and mixed with water or spoonful of yoghurt or apple puree

Note

- contained in Dimetapp Cough, Cold & Flu Night Relief Liquid Caps, Dimetapp PSE Cough Cold & Flu Day & Night Relief, Dimetapp PSE Cough Cold & Flu Day & Night, Dolased Analgesic-Calmative, Dolased Forte, Maxydol, Mersyndol, Mersyndol Forte, Mevadol Forte, Sandoz/Trust Analgesic/Calmative

FEXOFENADINE HYDROCHLORIDE (Fexit, Fexotabs, Telfast, Xergic)

Available forms

Tablets: 30 mg, 60 mg, 120 mg, 180 mg; Oral suspension: 6 mg/mL

Action

- non-sedating antihistamine with no anticholinergic actions
- half-life 14–15 hours
- see also General Actions of antihistamines (p. 475)

Use

- seasonal allergic rhinitis, urticaria

Dose

- (allergic rhinitis) 60 mg orally twice daily **OR**
- (seasonal allergic rhinitis) 120–180 mg orally daily **OR**
- (urticaria) 180 mg orally daily

Adverse effects

- see General Adverse effects of antihistamines (p. 475)

Interactions

- serum levels may be increased by erythromycin
- bioavailability reduced by magnesium or aluminium-containing antacids
- see also General Interactions of antihistamines (p. 475)

Nursing points/Cautions

- see General Nursing points/Cautions for antihistamines (p. 475)
- 30 mg tablets are recommended for children 6–11 years and oral suspension for children > 6 months
- (oral suspension) contains hydroxybenzoates, which may cause hypersensitivity reaction in sensitive individuals

Patient teaching and advice

- advise patient that magnesium or aluminium-containing antacids should be taken 2 hours before or after fexofenadine
- see General Patient teaching and advice for antihistamines (p. 475)

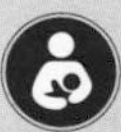

not recommended during pregnancy and breastfeeding

available as oral suspension. Tablets can be dispersed in 10–20 mL of water (Telfast). Tablets can be crushed and mixed with spoonful of yoghurt or apple puree

Note

- contained in Telfast Decongestant (with pseudoephedrine) (these should not be crushed)

LEVOCABASTINE HYDROCHLORIDE (Livostin Eye Drops, Livostin Nasal Spray, Zyrtec Eye Drops, Zyrtec Nasal Spray)

Available forms

Eye drops: 0.5 mg/mL; Nasal spray: 0.5 mg/mL

Action

- see General Actions of antihistamines (p. 475)
- (eye drops) immediate action, duration of action several hours
- half-life 33 hours

Use

- allergic conjunctivitis (eye drops)
- seasonal or perennial allergic rhinitis (nasal spray)

Dose

- (eye drops) 1 drop to each eye twice daily, may be increased to 3–4 times daily if needed (for up to 8 weeks) **OR**
- (nasal spray) 2 sprays to each nostril twice daily, increasing to 3–4 times if needed (up to 8 weeks)

Adverse effects

- headache, somnolence, fatigue, dizziness
- (nasal spray) epistaxis, nasal irritation, sinusitis, nausea, pharyngolaryngeal pain, epistaxis, cough
- (eye drops) eye irritation

Interactions

- oxymetazoline may transiently decrease absorption of nasal spray

Nursing points /Cautions

- (eye drops) contains benzalkonium chloride (preservative), which can cause irritation and discolouration of soft contact lenses
- use should be limited to 8 weeks
- (nasal spray) caution if used in those with kidney impairment, especially if therapy is prolonged
- see also General Nursing points/ Cautions for antihistamines (p. 475)

Patient teaching and advice

- patient should be advised not to drive or operate machinery if fatigue or somnolence occurs
- see also General Patient teaching and advice for antihistamines (including instillation instructions for nasal spray and eye drops) (pp. 475–76)

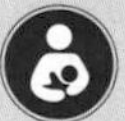

not recommended during pregnancy and breastfeeding

LORATADINE (Allereze, Children's Claratyne Chewable Tablets, Children's Claratyne Syrup, Claratyne, Claratyne Reditabs, Lorano, Lorapaed)

Available forms

Capsules: 10 mg; Tablets: 10 mg; Tablets (effervescent/disintegrating): 10 mg;

Tablets (chewable): 5 mg; Oral suspension/syrup: 1 mg/mL

Action

- long-acting, non-sedating antihistamine
- active metabolite (desloratadine) (half-life 20 hours)
- rapid onset 1 hour, half-life 12 hours
- see also General Actions of antihistamines (p. 475)

Use

- seasonal and perennial allergic rhinitis, chronic urticaria

Dose

- 10 mg orally daily

Adverse effects/Interactions

- see General Adverse effects and Interactions of antihistamines (p. 475)

Nursing points/Cautions

- (syrup, grape flavoured) contains sorbitol and maltitol, which may cause diarrhoea
- (chewable tablets) contain phenylalanine and are not recommended in those with phenylketonuria
- contraindicated in those with hypersensitivity to desloratadine or sodium benzoate (oral suspension)
- see also General Nursing points/Cautions for antihistamines (p. 475)

Patient teaching and advice

- advise patient that effervescent tablets should be dissolved in a glass of water
- instruct patient (or parent/carer) that chewable tablets for children should be chewed before swallowing
- see also General Patient teaching and advice for antihistamines (p. 475)

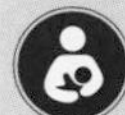

only used during pregnancy if benefits outweigh risks

not recommended during breastfeeding

available as oral liquid, chewable and effervescent tablets

Note

- contained in Claratyne D with Decongestant Repetabs with pseudoephedrine (should not be crushed)

OLOPATADINE HYDROCHLORIDE (Paladopt, Patanol)

Available form

Eye drops: 1 mg/mL (0.1%)

Action

- antihistamine
- inhibits pro-inflammatory mediator release from conjunctival mast and epithelial cells
- half-life 8–12 hours

Use

- seasonal allergic conjunctivitis

Dose

- 1–2 drops into affected eye(s) twice daily for up to 14 weeks

Adverse effects

- headache, asthenia
- blurred vision
- burning, stinging, dry eye(s), foreign body sensation, lid oedema, hyperaemia
- pharyngitis, rhinitis, sinusitis
- pruritus
- altered taste, nausea
- hypersensitivity

Nursing points/Cautions

- not for injection or oral ingestion
- contains benzalkonium chloride (preservative), which can cause irritation and discolouration of soft contact lenses
- see General Nursing points/Cautions for antihistamines (p. 475)

Patient teaching and advice

- advise patient that blurred vision may occur just after instillation of eye drops and should wait until this has resolved before driving or operating heavy machinery
- see General Patient teaching and advice for antihistamines (including instillation instructions for eye drops) (pp. 475–76)

PHENIRAMINE MALEATE

Available form

Tablets: 45.3 mg

Action

- antihistamine with sedating properties
- onset of action within 15–30 minutes with full effect within 1 hour
- half-life 16–19 hours
- see also General Actions of antihistamines (p. 475)

Use

- allergic conditions
- respiratory conditions with increased secretions (e.g. vasomotor rhinitis)
- prevention and treatment of motion sickness
- prevention of nausea, vomiting and vertigo associated with Ménière's disease and other labyrinthine disorders
- itching skin conditions (e.g. eczema, chronic urticaria)

Dose

- initially 22.65 mg (1/2 tablet) orally with food, up to 3 times daily, increasing to 45.3 mg (1 tablet) 3 times daily if needed

Adverse effects

- see General Adverse effects of antihistamines (p. 475)

Interactions

- contraindicated with MAOIs because anticholinergic effects may be prolonged and intensified
- anticholinergic effects may be enhanced by atropine and related agents
- see also General Interactions of antihistamines (p. 475)

Nursing points/Cautions

- daily maximum dose of 3 mg/kg should not be exceeded
- antiemetic action may mask other conditions
- contraindicated in those with hypersensitivity to pheniramine derivatives or with sensitivity to hydroxybenzoate
- see also General Nursing points/Cautions for antihistamines (p. 475)

Patient teaching and advice

- instruct patient that if usesd for motion sickness, tablets should be taken 30 minutes before travelling
- warn patient not to take on an empty stomach
- see also General Patient teaching and advice for antihistamines (p. 475)

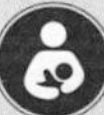

only used in pregnancy and breastfeeding if needed

tablets can be crushed and mixed with water or spoonful of yoghurt or apple puree

Note

- contained in Naphcon A and Visine Allergy with Antihistamine

PROMETHAZINE HYDROCHLORIDE (Allersoothe, DBL Promethazine Hydrochloride Injection, Phenergan, Sandoz Fenezal)

Available forms

Tablets: 10 mg, 25 mg; Ampoules: 50 mg/2 mL; Oral suspension: 1 mg/mL

Action

- long-acting sedating phenothiazine derivative antihistamine with mild anticholinergic and antiserotonin actions
- other actions due to CNS effects include antiemetic, antivertigo, anti-motion sickness, hypnotic and tranquilliser
- antihistamine action lasts 4–12 hours, sedative effect 2–8 hours, half-life 5–14 hours
- onset of action 3–5 minutes (IV) or 20 minutes (IM)

Use

- motion sickness
- nausea and vomiting, or where avoiding vomiting is essential (e.g. after neuro or eye surgery)
- allergic conditions (e.g. drug, insect bites and stings, urticaria, contact dermatitis)
- relief from excessive upper respiratory tract secretions (e.g. hay fever, allergic rhinitis)
- sedation (short-term management)
- pre-anaesthetic medication

Dose

- (allergy) 10–20 mg orally 2–3 times daily **OR**
- (allergy, sedation) 25–75 mg orally at night **OR**
- (allergy) 25–50 mg deep IM or slow IV, may be repeated after 2 hours if needed (daily maximum 150 mg) **OR**
- (motion sickness) 25 mg orally the night before travel and repeated 6–8 hours on following day if needed (for long journey) **OR**
- (motion sickness) 25 mg orally 1–2 hours before short journey **OR**
- (nausea and vomiting) 25 mg orally 4–6-hourly (daily maximum 100 mg) **OR**
- (nausea and vomiting, not related to motion sickness) 12.5–25 mg deep IM or slow IV 4-hourly as needed **OR**
- (preoperative or postoperative sedation, hypnotic) 25–50 mg deep IM or slow IV 1–2 hours before surgery (usually with pethidine and atropine) **OR**
- (sedation, hypnotic) 25–50 mg deep IM or slow IV **OR**
- (obstetric sedation, early labour) 50 mg deep IM **OR**
- (obstetric sedation, established labour) 25–75 mg deep IM or slow IV (with reduced dose of opioid analgesic), may be repeated 1–2 times at 4-hourly intervals (daily maximum 100 mg)

Adverse effects

- marked irregular respiration
- jaundice
- photosensitisation
- angioneurotic oedema
- oculogyric crisis, seizures, extrapyramidal symptoms, tardive dyskinesia, hysteria, catatonic state
- (rare) paralytic ileus (if given with anticholinergic agents)
- (rare) neuroleptic malignant syndrome, cardiac arrhythmias, QT prolongation
- (IV site) venous thrombosis
- (rapid IV) transient hypotension
- (high dose, IV) extrapyramidal reactions
- see also General Adverse effects of antihistamines (p. 475)

Interactions

- contraindicated after large doses of other CNS depressants, including alcohol
- QT prolongation is possible with phenothiazines, therefore not recommended with other agents known to prolong QT interval

- effects potentiated if given with anticholinergic agents, increasing risk of adverse effects such as constipation, paralytic ileus and heat stroke
- may lower seizure threshold, therefore antiepileptic dose may require adjustment during therapy
- if given with propranolol may result in increased plasma levels of both agents, resulting in increased hypotension, irreversible retinopathy, cardiac arrhythmias and tardive dyskinesia
- may increase serum prolactin levels, interfering with effects of bromocriptine
- may block action of levodopa
- increased severity and frequency of extrapyramidal effects may occur if given with other phenothiazines
- may block actions of adrenaline (epinephrine), resulting in severe hypotension and tachycardia and should not be used for phenothiazine overdose
- may decrease pressor response to ephedrine and metaraminol
- may block effects of centrally acting appetite suppressants and amphetamines
- increased risk of hypotension, extrapyramidal and anticholinergic effects if given with TCAs
- increased risk of hepatotoxicity if given with other hepatotoxic agents
- may increase hypotension caused by antihypertensive agents
- may mask tinnitus and dizziness caused by ototoxic agents such as aminoglycosides
- may enhance the CNS depressant effects of alcohol and other CNS depressing agents, such as barbiturates, hypnotics, sedatives, antipsychotics and opioid analgesics
- not recommended with MAOIs or TCAs because anticholinergic and CNS depressant effects may be prolonged and intensified
- may interfere with pregnancy test and glucose tolerance test

Nursing points/Cautions

- see General Nursing points/Cautions for antihistamines (p. 475)
- (IV) very long list of incompatibilities and should usually be administered alone
- preferably given by deep IM
- slow IV injection is only recommended if benefits outweigh risks (e.g. emergency situations, where IM route is contraindicated)
- large vessels should be used IV. Wrist and hand veins are not recommended
- IV site should be carefully monitored for extravasation and/or any signs of burning, pain, phlebitis, swelling or blistering, as these may be early signs of tissue injury
- contraindicated SC or intra-arterially to avoid tissue damage and necrosis
- (IV) should be diluted 1 in 10 with water for injections or given into tubing of free-flowing infusion
- transient fall in BP and increased risk of tissue damage may occur if given rapidly IV
- IV rate should not exceed 25 mg/min
- caution if used in those with eczema or rheumatoid conditions (increased risk of solar dermatitis) or epilepsy (may increase severity of convulsions)
- caution if used in children due to increased risk of central and obstructive apnoea and decreased arousal. Excessive doses can cause hallucinations, convulsions and sudden death in children
- caution if used in those with acute or chronic respiratory impairment
- caution if used in those at risk of QT prolongation
- (25 mg tablets) not recommended for children 12 years and under
- not recommended in children or adolescents with signs of Reye's syndrome (see Glossary)

- not recommended in anyone experiencing hypertensive crisis
- (IV, IM) contains sodium metabisulfite, sodium sulfite or sodium benzoate and is therefore contraindicated in those with known hypersensitivity
- contraindicated in those with history of phenothiazine-induced jaundice or hypersensitivity to phenothiazines
- contraindicated in children under 2 years due to risk of respiratory depression
- contraindicated in comatose patients

Patient teaching and advice

- instruct patient that tablets should not be taken for more than 10 days. If symptoms persist, patient should seek medical advice
- warn patient that taken for sedation at bedtime, 'hangover' effect can exist in the morning, increasing risk of accidents and/or falls. Patient should be further advised not to drive or operate machinery while this exists
- patient should be advised to immediately seek medical advice if any of the following occur:
  - any abdominal pain, cramping and/or distension with failure to pass wind or stools
  - high fever, sweating, muscle cramps or stiffness, dizziness, very bad headache, fast heart rate, confusion, agitation, hallucinations
  - irregular heart rate
  - yellowing of eyes or skin
  - fits
  - twitching or jerking movements
- instruct patient to wear sun protection (sunscreen (SPF 30+ or greater), hat, protective clothing) when outdoors (especially if patient has eczema or rheumatism, due to risk of solar dermatitis)
- see General Patient teaching and advice for antihistamines (p. 475)

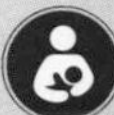

may cause prolonged extrapyramidal disturbances in newborn if given in high doses late in pregnancy

contraindicated during breastfeeding

available as suspension. Tablet can be dispersed in water or crushed and mixed with spoonful of yoghurt or apple puree

Note

- contained in Painstop Night Time Pain Relief (with paracetamol and codeine)

ANTIHYPERTENSIVE AGENTS

Figures for 2017–18 show that 10.6% of Australians (2.6 million people) have hypertension, with a similar prevalence between males and females. These numbers have remained relatively stable over the last 10 years. The proportion of the population with hypertension increases with age, especially over 35 years, with the highest proportion being those aged 75 years and over (41.5%) (ABS 2019).

Normal adult blood pressure (BP) is considered to be 120–129 mmHg systolic and 80–84 mmHg diastolic. Although definitions vary, one definition of mild hypertension is an elevation of systolic BP between 140 and 159 mmHg, diastolic BP above 90–99 mmHg, or both based on measurement taken on several separate occasions (National Heart Foundation of Australia 2016). Lowering of elevated BP by even 1–2 mmHg reduces absolute cardiovascular disease risk (i.e. risk of having stroke or myocardial infarction). Modifiable risk factors include smoking status, BP, serum lipids, waist circumference and body mass index (BMI), nutrition, physical activity level and alcohol intake, while non-modifiable risk factors are age, sex, family history of premature cardiovascular disease and social history (e.g. cultural identity, ethnicity, socioeconomic status). Related conditions include diabetes, chronic kidney disease (with albuminuria), familial hypercholesterolaemia and/or evidence of atrial fibrillation (National Vascular Disease Prevention Alliance (NVDPA) 2012).

Management of hypertension should begin with modification of lifestyle factors, such as weight and alcohol reduction, smoking cessation, increasing physical daily activity to 30 minutes if possible and limiting salt intake (Bryant et al 2019). If this is not successful in lowering blood pressure, an antihypertensive medication needs to be considered.

Antihypertensive medication is usually recommended in individuals with persistently elevated BP ≥ 160/100 mmHg (at least two measurements of seated BP on separate occasions). It should also be noted that ambulatory BP measurement is a better predictor of outcomes than clinical BP measurement and should be used to monitor BP-lowering therapy (National Heart Foundation of Australia 2016). The decision of which antihypertensive agent to use is based on the patient's age, any co-morbidities that may determine target BP (e.g. < 140/90 mmHg for adults with diabetes), potential interactions with other medications, implications for adherence and cost with the overall aim being blood pressure control with minimal adverse effects (National Heart Foundation of Australia 2016).

Major drugs used in the treatment of hypertension are:

- alpha-adrenoceptor blocking agents (e.g. prazosin)
- angiotensin-converting enzyme (ACE) inhibitors (e.g. captopril) (first-line management)
- angiotensin II receptor antagonists (e.g. irbesartan) (first-line management)
- beta-adrenoceptor blocking agents (e.g. propranolol) (no longer used as first-line management)
- calcium-channel blockers (e.g. diltiazem) (first-line management)
- centrally acting agents (e.g. clonidine)
- direct acting vasodilators (e.g. hydralazine)
- Thiazide diuretics (usually for patients > 65 years) (see Diuretics, p. 1020).

Therapy is usually begun with a single agent, starting at a small to moderate dose of a first-line drug. If the target is not achieved after 3 months, a second antihypertensive from a different class is usually added to the patient's regimen, rather than increasing the dose of the first agent. After 3 months, if the target is still not reached but the patient is tolerating both drugs, the dose of one agent is usually increased. It is important to also assess any non-adherence issues, possible hypertensive effects of other medications, and any undisclosed alcohol or recreational drug use or high salt intake, which may all be contributing to the antihypertensives not managing the high blood pressure (National Heart Foundation of Australia 2016).

Some manufacturers have produced 'fixed dose combination' medications (e.g. ACE inhibitor plus calcium-channel blocker; thiazide diuretic plus beta-adrenoceptor blocking agent), which decreases the number of tablets needed, potentially increasing patient adherence.

General Patient teaching and advice for antihypertensive agents

- ensure the patient understands the risks and benefits of therapy and especially the risks of not treating hypertension. It is important to stress the importance of having prescriptions filled and taking the antihypertensive medications. Studies have shown that many (50%) patients stop taking antihypertensives after about 2 years, while 19% do not get a second prescription filled (National Heart Foundation of Australia 2016).
- advise patient that postural hypotension can be avoided by moving gradually to a standing or sitting position, especially after sleep and it is made worse by prolonged standing, hot baths or showers, hot weather, physical exertion, large meals or alcohol ingestion. If the patient feels dizzy or faint, he/she should be advised to sit or lie down
- patient should be warned against driving a vehicle or operating machinery if drowsiness or dizziness is a problem
- advise patient to avoid alcohol during therapy
- patient should be advised to avoid stopping therapy suddenly or missing doses as rebound hypertension may occur

- reinforce lifestyle modification strategies
- see General Patient teaching and advice (p. xxvii)

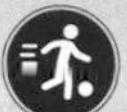

it should also be noted that those antihypertensive combinations with diuretics are generally banned in sport

ALPHA-ADRENOCEPTOR BLOCKING AGENTS

General Adverse effects of alpha-adrenoceptor blocking agents

- 'first dose' effect (see General Nursing points, below)
- postural hypotension, palpitations, tachycardia, syncope, oedema
- headache, drowsiness, dizziness, light-headedness, asthenia, drowsiness, weakness, fatigue, nervousness, depression
- dyspnoea
- blurred vision, miosis
- nasal congestion
- abnormal ejaculation, impotence, increased frequency, incontinence
- dry mouth, nausea, vomiting, diarrhoea, constipation
- rash, pruritus
- intraoperative floppy iris syndrome (during cataract surgery)
- (uncommon) angina
- (rare) priapism

General Nursing points/Cautions for alpha-adrenoceptor blocking agents

- 'first dose' effect may occur with the first dose, an increase in dosage or if there is an interruption to the regimen. Symptoms, including marked hypotension (especially in the upright position), dizziness and syncope usually occur within 30–90 minutes of initial dose
- both supine and standing systolic and diastolic BP should be monitored (especially when starting therapy or when adjusting dose) in all patients, regardless of the indication for use
- caution if used in those with ischaemic heart disease, angina (because angina may be exacerbated), cerebral or coronary arteriosclerosis, marked renal impairment or where a fall in BP or tachycardia is not desirable (e.g. recovery period after acute myocardial infection (AMI))
- not recommended in those with congestive heart failure caused by aortic or mitral valve stenosis, pulmonary embolism or restrictive pericardial disease
- contraindicated in those with any hypersensitivity to alpha-adrenoceptor blocking agents

General Patient teaching and advice for alpha-adrenoceptor blocking agents

- advise patient to take the first dose (and any increase in dosage) before sleep, to reduce the 'first dose' effect
- warn patient to avoid driving or operating machinery or other hazardous activities for 12 hours after initial dose, when the dose is increased or after an interruption to the therapy and the medication is resumed, or if dizziness, drowsiness, blurred vision or light-headedness continues

- male patient should be instructed to seek medical advice immediately if prolonged (lasting > 4 hours) painful penile erection occurs
- see General Patient teaching and advice for antihypertensive agents (p. 490)

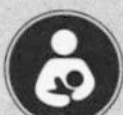

only used during pregnancy or breast-feeding if benefits outweigh potential risks

PHENOXYBENZAMINE HYDROCHLORIDE (Dibenyline)

Available form
Capsules: 10 mg

Action
- long-acting
- irreversible non-selective alpha-1 and alpha-2 adrenoceptor antagonists
- blocks uptake of amines, potentiating effects of noradrenaline and adrenaline (epinephrine) on beta-adrenergic receptors
- non-competitive block of histamine, serotonin and muscarinic (acetylcholine) receptors
- increases blood flow to skin, mucosa and abdominal viscera, lowering both standing and supine BP
- blocks alpha receptors on distal urethral sphincter and smooth muscle of bladder neck, resulting in decreased bladder outflow resistance, improving urinary flow and reducing bladder urine volume
- does not block beta-adrenoceptor receptors
- oral absorption variable

Use
- hypertension associated with pheochromocytoma
- urinary retention due to neuropathic bladder

Dose
- (hypertension associated with pheochromocytoma) initially 10 mg orally twice daily, increasing gradually at 4-day intervals to 20–60 mg in 2 divided doses as required **OR**
- (urinary retention) 10 mg orally twice daily

Adverse effects
- see General Adverse effects of alpha-adrenoceptor blocking agents (p. 490)

Interactions
- may block noradrenaline-induced hyperthermia
- not recommended with sympathomimetic agents (e.g. adrenaline (epinephrine)) as exacerbated hypotension and reflex tachycardia will occur

Nursing points/Cautions/Patient teaching and advice
- may require beta-adrenoceptor blocking agents to control tachycardia and arrhythmias in pheochromocytoma with the alpha-adrenoceptor blocking agent started first
- (pheochromocytoma) a 4-day interval should be allowed after each dose increase to observe patient response
- (urinary retention) if therapy is not effective in 2–3 weeks it should be discontinued
- caution if used in those with respiratory infection as symptoms may be exacerbated
- contraindicated in those where a fall in BP is undesirable (e.g. cerebral vascular accident (CVA), recovery period after AMI)
- see also General Nursing points/Cautions/Patient teaching and advice for alpha-adrenoceptor blocking agents (p. 490) and antihypertensive agents (p. 489)

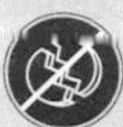

if opening capsule, mask and gloves should be worn (do not open capsules if pregnant)

contents can be dispersed in water or mixed with spoonful of yoghurt or apple puree

PRAZOSIN HYDROCHLORIDE (Minipress)

Available forms

Tablets: 1 mg, 2 mg, 5 mg

Action

- quinazoline derivative
- high affinity for alpha-1A, alpha-1B and alpha-1D receptors, with little affinity for alpha-2 receptors resulting in peripheral vasodilation with no reflex tachycardia
- BP is lowered in both supine and standing positions with diastolic effect more pronounced
- no rebound hypertension when therapy is stopped
- blocks alpha receptors on distal urethral sphincter and smooth muscle of bladder neck, resulting in decreased bladder outflow resistance, improving urinary flow and reducing bladder urine volume
- increased plasma renin activity (in those with congestive cardiac failure)
- peak concentration in 1–3 hours, half-life 2.5–3.5 hours (6–8 hours in heart failure)

Use

- hypertension
- congestive heart failure (CCF) (refractory to cardiac glycosides and diuretic therapy)
- Raynaud's disease, Raynaud's phenomenon
- benign prostatic hyperplasia

Dose

- (hypertension) initially 0.5 mg orally twice daily for 3 days, then increased to 1 mg 2–3 times daily for a further 3 days, then 2 mg 2–3 times daily, then up to 20 mg in divided doses if needed **OR**
- (congestive heart failure) initially 0.5 mg orally daily, increasing to 4–20 mg daily in 2–3 divided doses **OR**
- (Raynaud's disease/phenomenon) initially 0.5 mg orally twice daily for 3–7 days, increasing to 1–2 mg twice daily if needed **OR**
- (benign prostatic hyperplasia) 0.5 mg orally twice daily for 3–7 days, increasing to 2–4 mg twice daily if needed

Adverse effects

- see General Adverse effects of alpha-adrenoceptor blocking agents (p. 490)

Interactions

- hypotension may be increased if given with beta-adrenoceptor blocking agents, diuretics and calcium-channel blockers
- caution if used with phosphodiesterase-5 (PDE-5) inhibitors due to increased risk of hypotension
- may cause false positive in screening test for pheochromocytoma

Nursing points/Cautions/Patient teaching and advice

- (hypertension) response should be seen within 14 days, although optimal response may require 6 weeks
- (Raynaud's disease) BP should be monitored during initial administration and dose titrated accordingly
- (benign prostatic hypertrophy) prostatic carcinoma should be excluded before starting therapy
- if given with other antihypertensive agents, other agent dose should be reduced when starting prazosin
- diuretic may be added to therapy for hypertension to increase efficacy (usually started when patient is at 2 mg dose)

- caution if used in those with liver impairment as dose may need to be reduced
- caution if used in those with ischaemic heart disease as angina may be exacerbated
- contraindicated in those with any hypersensitivity to alpha-adrenoceptor blocking agents or quinazolines
- see also General Nursing points/ Cautions/ Patient teaching and advice for alpha-adrenoceptor blocking agents (p. 490) and general points for antihypertensive agents (p. 489)

tablets can be dispersed in water or crushed and mixed with spoonful of yoghurt or apple puree

ANGIOTENSIN CONVERTING ENZYME (ACE) INHIBITORS

General Actions of ACE inhibitors

- prevent conversion of angiotensin I to angiotensin II (which is a powerful vasoconstrictor) by inhibiting ACE, resulting in reduced peripheral vascular resistance and therefore decreased BP
- decreases aldosterone production (from the adrenal cortex), thereby reducing sodium and water reabsorption, which also plays a role in BP reduction
- increase plasma renin levels by negative feedback
- inhibits degradation of bradykinin leading to accumulation of both bradykinin and substance P sensitising airways and producing cough
- most ACE inhibitors are prodrugs that are converted in the body to an active form after oral ingestion (except captopril and lisinopril)
- most ACE inhibitors (except captopril) have a long duration of action, allowing once-daily administration

General Adverse effects of ACE inhibitors

- hypotension, palpitations, tachycardia, chest pain
- dizziness, vertigo, fatigue, headache, weakness, asthenia
- abdominal pain, nausea, anorexia, diarrhoea, dry mouth, taste disturbances (including decreased taste or metallic taste)
- persistent, dry, non-productive cough (may require discontinuance of therapy), dyspnoea
- rash (with or without fever/arthralgia), pruritus and uncommonly, photosensitivity
- elevated potassium levels, hyperkalaemia, hyponatraemia
- hypoglycaemia (in patients with diabetes)
- raised liver enzyme levels
- proteinuria, nephrotic syndrome
- neutropenia, agranulocytosis
- (rare) angioedema (head and neck) with or without urticaria (may be delayed for weeks to months), intestinal angioedema
- (rare) anaphylactoid reaction
- (rare) cholestatic jaundice, hepatitis, renal impairment
- (rare) loss of libido, impotence, insomnia, somnolence, syndrome of inappropriate antidiuretic hormone (SIADH)

General Interactions of ACE inhibitors

- contraindicated with or within 36 hours of sacubitril (nepilysin inhibitor) because of risk of angioedema
- significant hypotension may occur if given with other antihypertensive

agents, diuretics, alpha-adrenoceptor blocking agents, TCAs, antipsychotics and some anaesthetic agents
- antihypertensive effect may be decreased if given with sympathomimetic agents
- hyperkalaemia may occur when given potassium-sparing diuretics, potassium supplements or agents that increase potassium levels
- increased risk of hyperkalaemia if given with trimethoprim/sulfamethoxazole combination
- increased risk of hyperkalaemia and decreased hypotensive effect if given with NSAIDs and therefore not recommended together
- increased risk of renal impairment if given concurrently with combination of NSAIDs and thiazide diuretics
- may increase serum concentrations of lithium, increasing the risk of lithium toxicity; risk is further increased if there is also a concurrent diuretic. Lithium levels and renal function should be closely monitored if given together
- increased risk of 'first dose hypotension' if given with loop diuretic (e.g. frusemide) in patient with hypovolaemia or hyponatraemia
- increased risk of hypokalaemia and renal impairment if given with loop diuretic
- may cause facial flushing, nausea, vomiting and hypotension if given with sodium aurothiomalate (gold)
- effects of alcohol may be potentiated
- bioavailability may be decreased if given with antacids and therefore should be given 2 hours apart
- increased risk of hypoglycaemia if given with insulin and oral hypoglycaemic agents
- may decrease absorption of tetracyclines
- increased risk of angioedema if given with mTOR inhibitors (e.g. temsirolimus, sirolimus, everolimus) or DPP-IV inhibitors (e.g. vildagliptin)

General Nursing points/Cautions for ACE inhibitors

- before starting an ACE inhibitor, diuretic therapy should be stopped for at least 3 days to prevent 'first dose hypotension'. If diuretic cannot be stopped, initial dose of ACE inhibitor should be as low as possible and patient carefully monitored for several hours post-administration
- any volume or salt depletion should be corrected before starting therapy
- check for urinary protein before treatment, then monthly for the first 8 months and periodically thereafter in those with renal disease
- BP is recorded every 15 minutes for 1 hour after the initial dose and, if a hypotensive response occurs, place the patient in a supine position
- medical supervision should be maintained for at least 1 hour after the initial dose
- transient hypotension may be minimised by giving the initial dose at night
- regular monitoring of serum potassium, sodium and urea is recommended (especially if taking diuretics concurrently)
- WBC count monitoring (with differential) is recommended before starting and regularly throughout therapy in those with diseases affecting bone marrow function, collagen diseases, pre-existing neutropenia or if taking medication that is associated with bone marrow depression
- persistent non-productive cough appears more frequently in women and worsens on lying down. If cough

becomes intolerable, switching to another ACE inhibitor or another class of antihypertensives is recommended
- angioedema may be fatal if associated with laryngeal oedema
- (congestive heart failure) BP and renal function should be monitored before starting and regularly during therapy
- (myocardial infarction) therapy can be started within 1–3 days of myocardial infarction and usually in combination with aspirin, beta-adrenoceptor blocking agent and fibrinolytic (thrombolytic) agent
- anaphylactoid reaction may occur during exposure to the high-flux dialysis/lipoprotein apheresis membrane
- should be withheld while patient is undergoing desensitisation to hymenoptera (ant, honey bee, wasp) venom
- should be stopped for 24 hours before surgery or anaesthesia to decrease risk of excessive hypotension
- low-density lipoprotein (LDL) apheresis with dextran or haemodialysis using high-flux polyacrylonitrite (AN 69) membranes is not recommended during ACE therapy as there is an increased risk of anaphylactoid reactions
- caution if used in those of African origin as risk of angioedema is higher
- caution if used in those with liver impairment as most ACE inhibitors are converted to active form in the liver
- caution if used in those with renal failure, aortic stenosis, hypertrophic cardiomyopathy, SLE, scleroderma, bone marrow depression, cerebrovascular or cardiac insufficiency
- contraindicated in those with known hypersensitivity to ACE inhibitors, hyperkalaemia, renal transplant or impairment, severe renal artery stenosis or history of hereditary/idiopathic angioedema or ACE inhibitor-induced angioedema

General Patient teaching and advice for ACE inhibitors

- patients should be advised to avoid driving or operating machinery or other hazardous activity for 12 hours after initial dose, when the dose is increased or after an interruption to the therapy and the medication is resumed or if dizziness continues
- patient should be advised to seek medical advice immediately if any of the following occur:
  - rash, fever or sore throat (early signs of neutropenia)
  - rash, with or without urticaria (red patches and weals on skin)
  - persistent non-productive cough
  - swelling of the face, lips, tongue, throat, hands or feet (signs of facial angioedema)
  - unusual abdominal pain (with or without nausea or vomiting), especially if accompanied by facial angioedema (as described in previous point)
  - yellowing of eyes or skin, itching, upper abdominal pain, nausea, vomiting, tiredness, dark urine (signs of liver impairment)
- warn patient to avoid dehydration and excessive perspiration as it may lead to a greater fall in BP, increasing the risk of fainting, therefore patient should maintain hydration within prescribed limits (e.g. there may be a fluid restriction for those with cardiac failure). Excessive vomiting or diarrhoea may also cause dehydration and increase the risk of fainting

- instruct patient against taking over-the-counter NSAIDs as these interact with ACE inhibitors
- patient should be advised that loss of taste or metallic taste often occurs with ACE inhibitors and this usually lasts for 2–3 months
- warn patient that rash may occur in first 4 weeks of therapy and often resolves without need for any intervention. However, antihistamines may be used if pruritus (itchiness) exists as well as rash
- advise patient that brief, mild light-headedness may be experienced after the first few days of therapy. If fainting occurs, this should be reported immediately to doctor
- instruct patient that a low salt diet may be beneficial in reducing BP. However, potassium-containing salt substitutes are not recommended because of the increased risk of hyperkalaemia
- patients with diabetes mellitus should be advised to carefully monitor blood glucose levels during therapy (especially first month)
- women of childbearing potential should be counselled to avoid pregnancy during therapy by using adequate contraception, and if pregnancy occurs, to immediately report to doctor. Pregnancy should be excluded before starting therapy
- see General Patient teaching and advice for antihypertensive agents (p. 489)

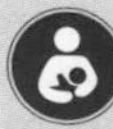

contraindicated during pregnancy because of the association with abnormalities such as renal dysfunction, skull hypoplasia and decreased amniotic fluid, and also because of increased risk of fetal death in utero

not recommended during breastfeeding

CAPTOPRIL (Capoten, Zedace)

Available forms

Tablets: 12.5 mg, 25 mg, 50 mg; Oral Solution: 5 mg/mL

Action

- see General Actions of ACE inhibitors (p. 493)
- onset of action 15–60 minutes, duration of effect 6–12 hours

Use

- hypertension
- congestive cardiac failure (with diuretic and/or digoxin)
- myocardial infarction (to reduce risk of heart failure)
- diabetic nephropathy (studies have shown ACE inhibitors decrease progression of renal impairment)

Dose

- (hypertension) initially 12.5 mg orally daily 1 hour before meals, then increased to 25 mg twice daily. If satisfactory BP decrease has not occurred in 2–4 weeks then increase to 50 mg twice daily. If BP is still not satisfactory after a further 2 weeks, a thiazide diuretic may be added (daily maximum 50 mg) **OR**
- (severe refractory hypertension or high-dose diuretics/low salt diet or dialysis) initially 6.25–12.5 mg orally daily 1 hour before meals, then titrated to 25–50 mg twice daily **OR**
- (severe hypertension) up to 75 mg twice daily 1 hour before meals **OR**
- (congestive heart failure) initially 6.25 mg (2.5 mg in sodium-depleted patients or with high doses of diuretics) orally 3 times daily 1 hour before meals, increasing gradually at 2-week intervals to 25–75 mg twice daily (maximum daily dose 150 mg) **OR**
- (myocardial infarction) initially 6.25 mg orally daily 1 hour before meals, increasing to 25 mg 3 times daily during next 2–3 days, then increasing gradually over several weeks to 50 mg orally 3 times daily **OR**

- (diabetic nephropathy) 75–100 mg orally daily in 3 divided doses 1 hour before meals

Adverse effects

- see General Adverse effects of ACE inhibitors (p. 493)

Interactions

- glyceryl trinitrate and other nitrates should be discontinued when starting captopril and if recommenced, should be started at a lower dose
- may cause false positive on acetone urine test
- see General Interactions of ACE inhibitors (p. 493)

Nursing points/Cautions

- (hypertension) if possible, any other antihypertensive agent should be stopped before starting therapy
- if the patient is receiving diuretics or has renal damage, the first dose may cause a precipitous fall in BP, so give a test dose of 6.25 mg
- if patient has renal disease or daily dose > 150 mg, urine protein estimation (using first morning urine sample) is recommended before starting and regularly during therapy
- (myocardial infarction) usually started 3 days post infarction for best effect
- (diabetic neuropathy) if patient has microalbuminuria, BP and blood glucose levels should be optimised to prevent progression to proteinuria
- (oral solution) contains sodium benzoate which may cause hypersensitivity in sensitive individuals
- see General Nursing points/Cautions for ACE inhibitors (p. 494)

Patient teaching and advice

- advise patient that tablets should be taken 1 hour before meals for best effect
- oral solution is available for a smaller initial dose, which can be made up to 100 mL with water, fruit juice, tea, coffee or cola and drunk immediately
- instruct patient to discard oral solution 28 days after opening
- see general points for ACE inhibitors (p. 493)

available as an oral liquid. Tablet can be dispersed in water or crushed and mixed with spoonful of yoghurt or apple puree

ENALAPRIL MALEATE (Acetec, Malean, Renitec)

Available forms

Tablets: 5 mg, 10 mg, 20 mg

Action

- see General Actions of ACE inhibitors (p. 493)
- enalapril (prodrug) is converted to active enalaprilat
- onset of action 60 minutes, duration of effect 24 hours

Use

- mild-to-moderate hypertension
- congestive heart failure (with diuretic and/or digoxin)
- renovascular hypertension
- left ventricular dysfunction without heart failure

Dose

- (essential hypertension) initially 5 mg orally daily (2.5 mg if in renal failure or if patient is receiving a diuretic), increasing gradually to 10–40 mg orally daily as a single or 2 divided doses **OR**
- (renovascular hypertension) initially 5 mg orally daily, increasing gradually to 20 mg daily **OR**
- (congestive heart failure) initially 2.5 mg orally daily, increasing gradually at 2–4-week intervals to 10–20 mg as a single or 2 divided doses **OR**
- (left ventricular dysfunction without heart failure) initially 2.5 mg orally twice daily, then increasing gradually at 2–4-week intervals to 10 mg twice daily

Adverse effects/Interactions/ Nursing points/Cautions/Patient teaching and advice

- see general points for ACE inhibitors (p. 493)

tablet can be crushed and mixed with water or spoonful of yoghurt or apple puree

Note

- contained in Renitec Plus 20/6 and Enalapril/HCT Sandoz with hydrochlorothiazide, and in Zan-Extra with lercanidipine

FOSINOPRIL SODIUM (Monace, Monopril)

Available forms

Tablets: 10 mg, 20 mg

Action

- see General Actions of ACE inhibitors (p. 493)
- fosinopril (prodrug) is converted to active fosinopril diacid
- onset of action less than 60 minutes, duration of action 24 hours

Use

- mild-to-moderate hypertension
- congestive heart failure (with diuretic and/or digoxin)

Dose

- (hypertension, heart failure) initially 10 mg orally daily, increasing gradually to 40 mg daily

Interactions

- decreased absorption may occur if given with antacids, therefore should be separated by 2 hours
- may cause false low serum digoxin levels if charcoal absorption method is used for estimation
- should be discontinued for 2 days before parathyroid function test
- see General Interactions of ACE inhibitors (p. 493)

Adverse effects/Nursing points/ Cautions/Patient teaching and advice

- see general points for ACE inhibitors (p. 493)

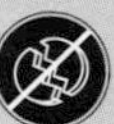

tablet should not be crushed or dispersed by pregnant staff

tablet can be crushed and mixed with water, or mixed with spoonful of yoghurt or apple puree

Note

- contained in APO Fosinopril HCTZ and Fosetic 20/12.5 with hydrochlorothiazide

LISINOPRIL DIHYDRATE (Fibsol, Zestril, Zinopril)

Available forms

Tablets: 5 mg, 10 mg, 20 mg

Action

- see General Actions of ACE inhibitors (p. 493)
- onset of action 60 minutes, duration of action 24 hours

Use

- mild-to-moderate hypertension
- congestive heart failure (with diuretic and/or digoxin)
- acute myocardial infarction (within 24 hours of symptom onset)

Dose

- (hypertension) initially 5–10 mg orally daily (2.5 mg for diuretic-treated or salt/volume-depleted patients), increasing gradually at 2–4-week intervals to 10–20 g daily (maximum daily dose 40 mg) **OR**
- (congestive cardiac failure) initially 2.5 mg orally daily, increasing

gradually at increments ≤ 10 mg at 2-week intervals to 5–20 mg daily **OR**
- (acute myocardial infarction (AMI), within 24 hours of onset of symptoms) initially 5 mg (2.5 mg if systolic BP is less than 120 mmHg or if within 72 hours of AMI) orally daily, 5 mg 24 hours later, 10 mg after 48 hours, then 10 mg orally daily for 6 weeks

Adverse effects/Interactions/Nursing points/Cautions/Patient teaching and advice

- may be started within 24 hours of symptoms of acute myocardial infarction; however, should not be started until patient is haemodynamically stable. If systolic BP < 90 mmHg for more than 60 minutes, therapy should be stopped or if systolic BP ≤ 100 mmHg maintenance dose of 5 mg is recommended
- if patient with acute myocardial infarction develops heart failure, therapy should be continued beyond 6 weeks
- see general points for ACE inhibitors (p. 493)

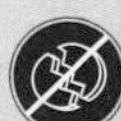

tablet should not be crushed or dispersed by pregnant staff

tablet can be crushed and mixed with water, or mixed with spoonful of yoghurt or apple puree

PERINDOPRIL ARGININE (Coversyl, Prexum)

PERINDOPRIL ERBUMINE (Idaprex, Indosyl Mono, Ozapace, Perindo)

Available forms

Tablets: 2 mg, 2.5 mg, 4 mg, 5 mg, 8 mg, 10 mg

Action

- see General Actions of ACE inhibitors (p. 493)
- perindopril (prodrug) is converted to active perindoprilat
- less 'first dose' hypotension when compared to enalapril or captopril in those with congestive cardiac failure
- onset of action 3–6 hours, duration of action 24 hours

Use

- mild-to-moderate hypertension
- congestive heart failure (with diuretic and/or digoxin)
- reduction of cardiovascular event risk in those with stable coronary artery disease

Dose

- (mild-to-moderate hypertension) initially 4–5 mg orally daily (2–2.5 mg for renovascular hypertension or salt/volume-depleted patients) 1 hour before meals, increasing gradually to daily maximum of 8–10 mg **OR**
- (congestive cardiac failure) initially 2–2.5 mg orally daily 1 hour before meals, increasing gradually to 4–5 mg daily **OR**
- (reduction of risk of cardiovascular event) initially 4–5 mg orally daily 1 hour before meals for 14 days, then increasing to 8–10 mg daily (depending on tolerance and/or renal function)

Adverse effects

- visual disturbances
- discomfort on exertion
- muscle cramps
- tinnitus
- epistaxis
- constipation
- see General Adverse effects of ACE inhibitors (p. 493)

Interactions

- caution if given with baclofen as antihypertensive effect may be increased

- see General Interactions of ACE inhibitors (p. 493)

Nursing points/Cautions

- if patient has episode of angina during first 4 weeks of therapy, risk analysis should be conducted to determine benefits of continuing therapy
- tablets contain lactose and should not be used in those with rare hereditary problems of galactose intolerance, Lapp lactase deficiency or glucose–galactose malabsorption
- see General Nursing points/Cautions for ACE inhibitors (p. 494)

Patient teaching and advice

- advise patient to take tablets 1 hour before food
- see General Patient teaching and advice for ACE inhibitors (p. 495)

tablet should not be crushed or dispersed by pregnant staff

tablet can be crushed and mixed with water, or mixed with spoonful of yoghurt or apple puree

Note

- contained with indapamide in Coversyl Plus, Idaprex Combi 4/1.25, Indosyl Combi 4/1.25, Perindo Combi, Prexum Combi 5/1.25
- contained with amlodipine in Coveram and Reaptan

QUINAPRIL (Accupril, Acquin, Quinapril)

Available forms

Tablets: 5 mg, 10 mg, 20 mg

Action

- see General Actions of ACE inhibitors (p. 493)
- quinapril (prodrug) is converted to active quinaprilat
- onset of action ≤ 60 minutes, duration of action ≤ 24 hours

Use

- mild-to-moderate hypertension
- congestive heart failure (with diuretic and/or digoxin)

Dose

- (mild-to-moderate hypertension) initially 5–10 mg orally daily (2.5–5 mg for diuretic-treated patients) 1 hour before meals, increasing gradually at 4-week intervals to 10–40 mg daily or in 2 divided doses **OR**
- (congestive heart failure) initially 5 mg orally daily 1 hour before meals, increasing at weekly intervals gradually to 20–40 mg daily in 2 divided doses

Interactions

- serum potassium may increase if given with heparin
- see General Interactions of ACE inhibitors (p. 493)

Adverse effects/Nursing points/Cautions/Patient teaching and advice

- advise patient not to drink alcohol during therapy
- see general points for ACE inhibitors (p. 493)

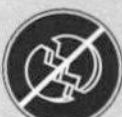

tablets should not be crushed or dispersed in water

Note

- contained in Accuretic with hydrochlorothiazide

RAMIPRIL (Prilace, Ramace, Tritace, Tryzan, Vascalace)

Available forms

Tablets: 1.25 mg, 2.5 mg, 5 mg; Capsules: 1.25 mg, 2.5 mg, 5 mg, 10 mg

Action
- see General Actions of ACE inhibitors (p. 493)
- ramipril (prodrug) is converted to active ramiprilat
- onset of action 1–2 hours, duration of action 24 hours

Use
- hypertension
- myocardial infarction
- reduction of risk of myocardial infarction, stroke, cardiovascular death or revascularisation procedure in those ≥ 55 years with clinical evidence of coronary artery disease, stroke or peripheral vascular disease
- reduction of risk of myocardial infarction, stroke, cardiovascular death or revascularisation procedure in those with diabetes ≥ 55 years with one or more risk factors (e.g. systolic BP > 160 mmHg, diastolic BP > 90 mmHg, total cholesterol > 5.2 mmol/L, HDL cholesterol < 0.9 mmol/L, current smoker, evidence of peripheral vascular disease or known microalbuminaemia)
- prevention of progressive renal failure in patients with persistent proteinuria > 1 g/day

Dose
- (hypertension) initially 2.5 mg orally daily (1.25 mg for diuretic-treated or salt/volume-depleted patients), increasing gradually at 2–3-week intervals to 5–10 mg daily **OR**
- (after myocardial infarction) initially 1.25–2.5 mg orally twice daily, increasing gradually at 1–3-day intervals to 5 mg twice daily, starting 2–10 days after infarction **OR**
- (reducing risk of cardiovascular event) initially 2.5 mg orally daily, doubling dose after 1 week, then increasing to 10 mg daily after 3 weeks **OR**
- (prevention of progressive renal failure in patients with persistent proteinuria > 1 g/day) initially 1.25 mg orally daily, then doubling dose at 2–3-week intervals to 5 mg daily

Adverse effects
- muscle spasm/cramps, myalgia
- see General Adverse effects of ACE inhibitors (p. 493)

Interactions
- contraindicated with angiotensin II receptor antagonists in patients with diabetic nephropathy and not recommended in other patients taking angiotensin II receptor antagonists
- serum potassium may increase if given with heparin
- see General Interactions of ACE inhibitors (p. 493)

Nursing points/Cautions/Patient teaching and advice

- increased risk of hypotension post myocardial infarction if patient has impaired renal function
- treatment for myocardial infarction should be reviewed after 15 months
- if patient has creatinine clearance of 20–50 mL/minute, dose should be started at 1.25 mg daily and increased at 2–3-day intervals as tolerated
- see general points for ACE inhibitors (p. 493)

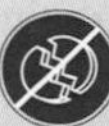

tablet should not be crushed or dispersed by pregnant staff.

tablet can be crushed and mixed with water, or mixed with spoonful of yoghurt or apple puree. Capsule can be opened and contents dispersed in water or apple juice, or mixed with spoonful of apple puree

Note
- contained in Triasyn with felodipine

TRANDOLAPRIL (Dolapril, Gopten, Tranalpha)

Available forms

Capsules: 0.5 mg, 1 mg, 2 mg, 4 mg

Action

- see General Actions of ACE inhibitors (p. 493)
- prodrug trandolapril is converted to active trandolaprilat
- onset of action 30 minutes, duration of action 48 hours

Use

- hypertension
- left ventricular dysfunction after myocardial infarction

Dose

- (hypertension) initially 1 mg orally daily (0.5 mg for diuretic-treated, renally impaired or salt-depleted patients), increasing gradually to 2–4 mg daily **OR**
- (left ventricular dysfunction after myocardial infarction) after 0.5 mg test dose, 1 mg orally daily for 3 days, then increased to 2 mg for 4 weeks, then further increased to 4 mg daily

Adverse effects/Interactions/Nursing points/Cautions/Patient teaching and advice

- patient should be advised to take medication at the same time every day (i.e. 24-hour interval) and as a single (not divided) dose
- response should be seen in 2–4 weeks
- see general points for ACE inhibitors (p. 493)

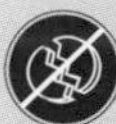

tablet or capsule should not be crushed or dispersed by pregnant staff

capsule can be opened and contents mixed with water, or mixed with spoonful of yoghurt or apple puree

Note

- contained in Tarka with verapamil

ANGIOTENSIN II RECEPTOR ANTAGONISTS

General Actions of angiotensin II receptor antagonists

- antagonise angiotensin II receptors (AT1 subtype) on vascular smooth muscle and adrenal cortex (angiotensin II is responsible for vasoconstriction, stimulation of aldosterone, regulation of salt and water homeostasis and cell growth stimulation)
- increases renal blood flow and maintains/increases glomerular filtration rate while decreasing renal vascular resistance
- no inhibition of angiotensin converting enzyme (ACE), therefore no potentiation of bradykinin and substance P activity (which are thought to be responsible for non-productive cough associated with ACE inhibitors)
- some angiotensin II receptor antagonists are prodrugs, which are converted to active form
- antihypertensive effect may be slightly less in those of African origin
- also known as sartans

General Adverse effects of angiotensin II receptor antagonists

- hypotension, palpitations, tachycardia, chest pain
- dizziness, headache, depression, fatigue, tiredness, asthenia
- back pain, myalgia, arthralgia
- nausea, vomiting, abdominal pain, diarrhoea, dyspepsia

- flu-like symptoms, upper respiratory tract infection, rhinitis, pharyngitis, dyspnoea, cough
- urinary tract infection
- hypertriglyceridaemia, hyperkalaemia
- decreased haematocrit, decreased haemoglobin
- raised liver enzymes
- (rare) angioedema

General Interactions of angiotensin II receptor antagonists

- risk of hyperkalaemia is increased if given with potassium-sparing diuretics or potassium supplements, salt substitutes containing potassium, other agents that raise potassium levels such as heparin or trimethoprim/sulfamethoxazole
- not recommended with ACE inhibitors in those with diabetic neuropathy
- may increase serum lithium levels, increasing the risk of toxicity, therefore levels should be closely monitored, especially when starting, stopping or adjusting dose
- increased hypotension may occur if given with other antihypertensive agents or diuretics
- increased risk of renal impairment if given in combination with NSAIDs and diuretics (especially in the elderly or those with pre-existing renal impairment)
- efficacy decreased by NSAIDs especially indometacin

General Nursing points/Cautions for angiotensin II receptor antagonists

- any sodium or intravascular volume depletion should be corrected before initiating therapy
- if changing from a beta-adrenoceptor blocking agent, dose should be gradually decreased over 8–14 days before starting the angiotensin II receptor antagonist
- serum potassium and creatinine levels should be regularly monitored if used for heart failure or in those also taking ACE inhibitors and/or potassium-sparing diuretics
- thiazide diuretic or another antihypertensive agent may be added to regimen if BP is not adequately controlled by angiotensin II receptor antagonist alone
- caution if used in patients undergoing haemodialysis
- caution if used during anaesthesia and surgery due to increased risk of hypotension
- not recommended in those with primary hyperaldosteronism or with heart failure
- caution if used in those with volume/sodium depletion, severe congestive heart failure or renal disease (e.g. renal artery stenosis), aortic or mitral valve stenosis, obstructive hypertrophic cardiomyopathy, mild-to-moderate liver impairment or renal impairment
- contraindicated in those with known hypersensitivity to angiotensin II receptor antagonists or who have haemodynamically significant bilateral renovascular disease or severe stenosis of solitary functioning kidney

General Patient teaching and advice for angiotensin II receptor antagonists

- patients should be advised to avoid potassium-based salt substitutes
- women of childbearing potential should be counselled to avoid pregnancy during therapy and immediately report pregnancy if it occurs
- see General Patient teaching and advice for antihypertensive agents (p. 489)

contraindicated during pregnancy because of the association with abnormalities such as renal dysfunction, skull hypoplasia and decreased amniotic fluid, and also because of increased risk of fetal death in utero

not recommended/contraindicated during breastfeeding

CANDESARTAN CILEXETIL (Adesan, Atacand, Candesan)

Available forms
Tablets: 4 mg, 8 mg, 16 mg, 32 mg

Action
- see General Actions of angiotensin II receptor antagonists (p. 502)
- prodrug (candesartan cilexetil) is converted to active candesartan in the GI tract
- time to peak effect 6–8 hours, half-life 5–10 hours

Use
- hypertension
- heart failure (as adjunct to ACE inhibitors or where ACE inhibitors are not tolerated)

Dose
- (hypertension) 8–16 mg orally daily, increasing to 32 mg daily if needed **OR**
- (heart failure) initially 4 mg orally daily, increasing at 2-week intervals to 32 mg

Adverse effects/Interactions/ Nursing points/Cautions/Patient teaching and advice
- may take 4 weeks for effective BP control to be achieved
- (heart failure) may be given with ACE inhibitors, beta-adrenergic blocking agents, diuretics or digoxin (or combination)
- contraindicated in those with sever livor impairment and/or cholestasis
- see general points for angiotensin II receptor antagonists (p. 502)

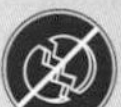

tablet should not be crushed or dispersed by pregnant staff

tablet can be crushed and mixed with water, or mixed with spoonful of yoghurt or apple puree

Note
- contained in Adesan HCT, Atacand Plus, APO-Candesartan HCTZ, Auro-Candesartan HCT, Candesan Combi, Candesartan HCT, Candesartan HCTZ with hydrochlorothiazide

EPROSARTAN MESILATE (EPROSARTAN MESYLATE) (Teveten)

Available forms
Tablets: 400 mg, 600 mg

Action
- see General Actions of angiotensin II receptor antagonists (p. 502)
- time to peak effect 1–2 hours, half-life 5–9 hours

Use
- hypertension

Dose
- (hypertension) initially 600 mg orally daily (400 mg in sodium- or volume-depleted patients or those with liver or renal impairment), increasing to 800 mg daily if necessary

Adverse effects/Interactions/ Nursing points/Cautions/Patient teaching and advice
- may take 2–3 weeks for effective BP control to be achieved
- contains lactose, therefore not recommended in those with galactose

intolerance, Lapp lactase deficiency or glucose–galactose malabsorption
- see general points for angiotensin II receptor antagonists (p. 502)

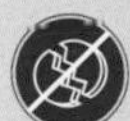

tablet should not be crushed or dispersed by pregnant staff

tablet is very hard to crush but can be mixed with water, or mixed with spoonful of yoghurt or apple puree

Note
- contained in Teveten Plus with hydrochlorothiazide

IRBESARTAN (Abisart, Avapro, Avsartan, Irprestan, Karbesart, Karvea)

Available forms
Tablets: 75 mg, 150 mg, 300 mg

Action
- see General Actions of angiotensin II receptor antagonists (p. 502)
- time to peak effect 3–6 hours, half-life 11–15 hours

Use
- hypertension
- delaying progression of renal disease in those with type 2 diabetes and persistent microalbuminaemia (> 30 mg/day) or urinary protein (> 900 mg/day)

Dose
- (hypertension) initially 150 mg orally daily (75 mg daily for volume- or salt-depleted patients), increasing to 300 mg if needed **OR**
- (hypertension and type II diabetic renal disease) 300 mg orally daily

Interactions
- contraindicated with ACE inhibitors in those with diabetic nephropathy
- not recommended with ACE inhibitors
- see General Interactions of angiotensin II receptor antagonists (p. 503)

Adverse effects/Nursing points/Cautions/Patient teaching and advice
- caution if used in those with psoriasis as condition may be exacerbated
- see general points for angiotensin II receptor antagonists (p. 502)

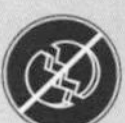

tablet should not be crushed or dispersed by pregnant staff

tablet can be crushed and mixed with water, or mixed with spoonful of yoghurt or apple puree

Note
- contained with hydrochlorothiazide in Abisart HCTZ, APO-Irbesartan HCTZ, Arsartan HCT, Avapro HCT, Irbesartan HCT and Karvezide

LOSARTAN POTASSIUM (Cozaar, Cozavan)

Available forms
Tablets: 25 mg, 50 mg

Action
- see General Actions of angiotensin II receptor antagonists (p. 502)
- active metabolite (half-life 4–9 hours)
- time to peak effect 6 hours, half-life 1.5–2 hours

Use
- hypertension
- delaying progression of renal disease in those with type II diabetes and persistent microalbuminaemia (> 30 mg/day) or urinary protein (> 900 mg/day)

Dose
- initially 50 mg orally daily (25 mg daily for volume- or salt-depleted patients). If BP is not adequately controlled, then 25 mg orally twice daily, increasing to 100 mg orally daily if necessary

Adverse effects/Interactions/Nursing points/Cautions/Patient teaching and advice

- maximum BP effect in 3–6 weeks after starting therapy
- see general points for angiotensin II receptor antagonists (p. 502)

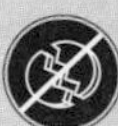
tablet should not be crushed or dispersed by pregnant staff

tablet can be crushed and mixed with water, or mixed with spoonful of yoghurt or apple puree

OLMESARTAN MEDOXOMIL (Olmertan, Olmesartan MYL, Olmetec)

Available forms
Tablets: 10 mg, 20 mg, 40 mg

Action
- see General Actions of angiotensin II receptor antagonists (p. 502)
- olmesartan medoxomil (prodrug) is hydrolysed to olmesartan in the GI tract
- time to peak effect 1.4–2.8 hours, half-life 12–18 hours

Use
- hypertension

Dose
- (hypertension) initially 20 mg orally daily (10 mg for volume-depleted patients or impaired renal function), increasing to 40 mg daily if needed

Adverse effects
- sprue-like enteropathy (severe chronic diarrhoea with substantial weight loss, occurring months to years after therapy has started)
- haematuria
- see General Adverse effects of angiotensin II receptor antagonists (p. 502)

Interactions
- bioavailability may be reduced if given with antacids
- see General Interactions for angiotensin II receptor antagonists (p. 503)

Nursing points/Cautions
- contraindicated in those with severe kidney impairment (creatinine clearance < 30 mL/minute), biliary obstruction or severe liver impairment
- see General Nursing points/Cautions for angiotensin II receptor antagonists (p. 503)

Patient teaching and advice
- patient should be advised to seek medical attention if severe chronic diarrhoea with weight loss occurs
- see General Patient teaching and advice for angiotensin II receptor antagonists (p. 503)

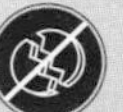
tablet should not be crushed or dispersed by pregnant staff

tablet can be crushed and mixed with water, or mixed with spoonful of yoghurt or apple puree

Note
- contained in Olmesartan/HCTZ, Olmesartan HCT-MYL, Olmetec Plus and Olmertan Combi with hydrochlorothiazide
- contained in Olmekar, Olmesartan/Amlodipine, Olmesartan/Amlodipine-MYL and Sevikar with amlodipine
- contained in Olmesartan/Amlodipine/HCTZ and Sevikar HCT with hydrochlorothiazide and amlodipine

TELMISARTAN (Micardis, Mizart, Teltartan)

Available forms
Tablets: 40 mg, 80 mg

Action
- see General Actions of angiotensin II receptor antagonists (p. 502)
- peak effect 0.5–1 hour, half-life 24 hours

Use
- hypertension
- prevention of cardiovascular morbidity or mortality in those ≥ 55 years, with coronary artery disease, peripheral arterial disease, previous stroke, transient ischaemic attacks, high-risk diabetes with evidence of end organ damage

Dose
- (hypertension) initially 40 mg orally daily, increasing to 80 mg daily if needed **OR**
- (prevention of cardiovascular morbidity/mortality) 80 mg orally daily

Adverse effects
- see General Adverse effects of angiotensin II receptor antagonists (p. 502)

Interactions
- may increase serum levels of digoxin, increasing the risk of toxicity, therefore digoxin levels should be closely monitored, especially when starting or stopping therapy or adjusting dose
- systemic corticosteroids may decrease antihypertensive effects
- see General Interactions of angiotensin II receptor antagonists (p. 503)

Nursing points/Cautions
- (prevention of cardiovascular morbidity/mortality) BP should be closely monitored during therapy
- contains sorbitol (338 mg), therefore not recommended in those with hereditary fructose intolerance
- may take 4–8 weeks for effective BP control to be achieved
- caution if used in those with diabetes due to risk of undiagnosed cardiac disease
- caution if used in those with mild-to-moderate liver impairment. Dose should not exceed 40 mg
- contraindicated in those with biliary obstructive disorder or severe liver impairment
- see General Nursing points/Cautions for angiotensin II receptor antagonists (p. 503)

Patient teaching and advice
- see General Patient teaching and advice for angiotensin II receptor antagonists (p. 503)

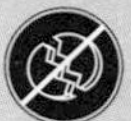

tablet should not be crushed or dispersed by pregnant staff

tablet can be crushed and mixed with water, or mixed with spoonful of yoghurt or apple puree

Note
- contained in APO Telmisartan HCTZ, Micardis Plus, Mizart HCT, Telmisartan HCT and Teltartan with hydrochlorothiazide
- contained in APO-Telmisartan/Amlodipine, Pritor/Amlodipine and Twynsta with amlodipine

VALSARTAN (Dilart, Diovan)

Available forms
Tablets: 40 mg, 80 mg, 160 mg, 320 mg

Action
- see General Actions of angiotensin II receptor antagonists (p. 502)
- peak effect in 2 hours, half-life 6–9 hours

Use
- hypertension
- heart failure (with diuretic and/or digoxin in those intolerant to ACE inhibitors)
- post myocardial infarction

Dose
- (hypertension) initially 80 mg orally daily, increasing to 160 mg daily after

4 weeks if BP control is not achieved (daily maximum 320 mg) **OR**
- (heart failure) initially 40 mg orally twice daily, increasing to 80–160 mg twice daily if needed **OR**
- (post myocardial infarction) initially 20 mg orally twice daily, increasing to 40 mg twice daily, then 80 mg twice daily, to 160 mg twice daily, over a number of weeks as tolerated by the patient

Adverse effects
- neutropenia
- see General Adverse effects of angiotensin II receptor antagonists (p. 502)

Interactions
- caution if given with rifampicin, ciclosporin and ritonavir
- not recommended with ACE inhibitors
- see General Interactions of angiotensin II receptor antagonists (p. 503)

Nursing points/Cautions/Patient teaching and advice
- (hypertension) maximum effect is usually seen after 4 weeks. If further BP reduction is needed, diuretic may be added or dose may be increased to 320 mg daily
- (myocardial infarction) therapy can be started within 12 hours of myocardial infarction
- (heart failure, post myocardial infarction) renal function should be monitored regularly during therapy
- (post myocardial infarction) dose may be reduced if patient becomes hypotensive or if renal function declines
- contraindicated in those with severe liver impairment, biliary cirrhosis and cholestasis
- see general points for angiotensin II receptor antagonists (p. 502)

tablet should not be crushed or dispersed by pregnant staff

tablet can be crushed and mixed with water, or mixed with spoonful of yoghurt or apple puree

Note
- contained in APO-Valsartan HCTZ, Co-Diovan and Dilart HCT with hydrochlorothiazide, Exforge with amlodipine, Exforge Plus HCT with amlodipine and hydrochlorothiazide
- contained in Entresto with sacubitril for the management of chronic heart failure (with reduced ejection fraction)

BETA-ADRENOCEPTOR BLOCKING AGENTS

General Actions of beta-adrenoceptor blocking agents
- also known as 'beta-adrenoceptor antagonists', 'beta blockers' or b-blockers
- competitively inhibit beta-adrenoceptors (sympathetic nervous system), thereby reducing some of the body's responses to adrenaline (epinephrine), noradrenaline and isoprenaline. Beta receptors are found in the heart, bronchi smooth muscle, blood vessel smooth muscle, kidneys, pancreas, uterus, brain and liver
- some agents have equal affinity for both beta-1 (heart) and beta-2 (lung) receptors (i.e. non-cardioselective; oxprenolol, propranolol, pindolol, timolol), whereas others have more affinity for beta-1 receptors (i.e. cardioselective; atenolol, bisoprolol, betaxolol, esmolol, metoprolol,

nebivolol). Selectivity reduces with high doses
- reduce rate of impulses through the cardiac conducting system
- reduce cardiac rate and force of contraction
- reduce cardiac output and myocardial oxygen demand
- reduce BP by decreasing cardiac output
- inhibits exercise-induced tachycardia
- bronchospasm
- inhibition of renin release from the kidneys
- inhibition of catecholamine-induced lipid and carbohydrate metabolism
- decreases melatonin release via blockage of central beta1 adrenoreceptors (possibly contributing to sleep disturbances
- (non-selective) increases plasma levels of triglycerides and lowers HDL
- reduction of elevated, as well as normal, intra-ocular pressure, probably by reducing aqueous humour formation (see Antiglaucoma agents p. 452)

General Adverse effects of beta-adrenoceptor blocking agents

- bronchospasm (uncommon but serious), dyspnoea on exertion, coughing, wheezing, asthma, nasal congestion (including topical beta blockers), exacerbation of allergic conditions (e.g. allergic rhinitis (hay fever) during pollen season)
- bradycardia, heart block, hypotension, postural hypotension, arrhythmias, development of or worsening of heart failure, exacerbation of angina, tachycardia
- nausea, vomiting, diarrhoea, constipation, abdominal pain, indigestion, dry mouth
- cold extremities, exacerbation of Raynaud's phenomenon or other circulation disorders such as intermittent claudication
- fatigue, dizziness, headache, malaise, asthenia
- sleep disturbances, including vivid dreams and nightmares, insomnia
- oedema (generalised, leg and/or dependent)
- impotence, decreased libido
- blurred vision, dry eyes/decreased lacrimation
- rash, pruritus, reversible alopecia, exacerbation of psoriasis
- increase in free thyroxine (T4) levels
- hypoglycaemia, elevated triglyceride levels
- (uncommon) depression, confusion, mood changes, hallucinations
- (rarely) thrombocytopenia, purpura, elevated liver enzymes, urea and creatinine levels, hepatic toxicity

General Interactions of beta-adrenoceptor blocking agents

- may cause bradycardia, hypotension and asystole when given with verapamil (and diltiazem to a lesser degree), therefore not recommended if used together
- caution if used with dihydropyridine calcium-channel blockers (e.g. felodipine, amlodipine) due to increased risk of increased hypotension and deterioration of ventricular pump function
- may enhance effects of other antihypertensive agents
- careful monitoring is required if given with other beta-adrenoceptor blocking agents (including eye drops) and generally not recommended together
- not recommended with Class I antiarrhythmic agents
- caution if given with amiodarone due to prolongation of AV conduction time

- may cause loss of diabetic control and delayed recovery from hypoglycaemia requiring adjustment of insulin and/or oral hypoglycaemic agents
- use with clonidine may result in severe withdrawal symptoms (rebound hypertension and arrhythmias) and is not recommended. If used together, beta-adrenoceptor blocking agent should be withdrawn first, at least 3 days before clonidine, which is then gradually stopped
- may cause excessive bradycardia if given with digoxin in the treatment of digoxin toxicity and therefore heart rate should be closely monitored
- hypotensive effect may be decreased if given with prostaglandin-synthesis blocking NSAIDs (e.g. ibuprofen, indometacin)
- increased hypotension may occur if given with phenothiazines, barbiturates and TCAs
- effects may be counteracted if given with sympathomimetic agents (e.g. adrenaline (epinephrine))
- peripheral circulation disturbance may be exacerbated if given with ergot alkaloids
- decreased serum levels may occur if given with rifampicin
- caution if given with amisulpride due to increased bradycardia
- not recommended with MAOIs due to increased risk of bradycardia and hypotension and also risk of hypertensive crisis

General Nursing points/Cautions for beta-adrenoceptor blocking agents

- before giving the drug, note bradycardia (especially if heart rate, 50 beats/minute), hypotension, dyspnoea, cyanosis and circulation in the extremities
- during therapy, if heart rate , 50–55 beats/minute at rest or patient has signs of bradycardia, dose should be decreased or stopped gradually
- check weight and keep a fluid chart to detect fluid retention
- early signs of acute hypoglycaemia (e.g. tachycardia) may be masked, pain also masked
- (surgery) anaesthetist must be informed that the patient is taking beta-adrenoceptor blocking agents
- if patient has atrial fibrillation post myocardial infarction, digitalisation with digoxin is recommended before starting therapy
- (congestive heart failure) patient should be monitored closely for any signs of bradycardia, vasodilation or worsening heart failure before increasing dose. Any symptoms should be stabilised before increasing dose
- (coronary artery disease) should not be stopped abruptly as exacerbation of angina, myocardial infarction and cardiac arrhythmias may occur. Discontinuation should be over 8–14 days
- may precipitate cardiac failure in patients with undiagnosed heart failure. If this occurs, patient should be treated with digoxin and/or ACE inhibitors or vasodilator and/or diuretic. Therapy should be stopped if heart failure continues despite added therapy
- may exaggerate allergic reactions and should be avoided if there is a risk or history of bronchospasm or anaphylaxis
- may exacerbate peripheral vascular disease (e.g. Raynaud's disease/syndrome, intermittent claudication)
- may aggravate psoriasis and should be given with caution

- ensure alpha-receptor blockade before beta-receptor blockade in phaeochromocytoma to avoid exacerbation of hypertension
- overdosage should be treated with atropine or isoprenaline (for bradycardia); noradrenaline or glucagon (for hypotension); salbutamol and/or aminophylline (for bronchospasm); digoxin, diuretics and oxygen (for acute heart failure). Blood glucose levels should also be monitored
- caution if used in those with hyperthyroidism (clinical signs may be masked), diabetes mellitus or history of spontaneous hypoglycaemia (signs of hypoglycaemia such as tachycardia and palpitations may be masked) or cardiac failure (patient should be stabilised and digitalised and/or receiving ACE inhibitor with/without diuretic), heart block (first degree) or impaired kidney or liver function
- not recommended in those with variant (Prinzmetal's) angina as coronary artery spasm may be exacerbated
- not recommended in those with Raynaud's disease/syndrome
- not recommended in those with systolic BP < 120 mmHg with first degree heart block
- contraindicated in untreated pheochromocytoma
- contraindicated in those with hypersensitivity to beta-adrenoceptor blocking agents as cross-sensitivity may occur
- contraindicated in allergic disorders, asthma, chronic obstructive pulmonary disease, bronchospasm or other conditions involving airway obstruction as life-threatening bronchoconstriction may occur
- contraindicated in AV heart block (second or third degree) (without pacemaker), hypotension, sinus bradycardia (< 45–50 beats/minute), cardiogenic or hypovolaemic shock, congestive heart failure, severe hypotension, right ventricular failure secondary to pulmonary hypertension, significant right ventricular hypertrophy, sick sinus syndrome, severe untreated peripheral arterial circulatory disturbance and metabolic acidosis

General Patient teaching and advice for beta-adrenoceptor blocking agents

- see general points for antihypertensive agents (p. 488)
- advise patient not to stop the drug abruptly to decrease the risk of angina pectoris, acute myocardial infarction or cardiac arrhythmias
- contact lens users should be advised that dry eyes due to decreased lacrimation may occur
- warn patient with diabetes mellitus regarding:
  - masked signs (e.g. tachycardia, palpitations) of hypoglycaemia
  - prolonged recovery from hypoglycaemia
  - need to monitor blood glucose levels vigilantly due to potential loss of diabetic control, necessitating adjustment of insulin and/or hypoglycaemic agent dose
- advise patient to seek medical advice immediately if any of the following occur:
  - slowed heart rate
  - dizziness, fainting
  - tingling, pins and needles
  - sexual problems
  - skin rash, itchiness
  - dry eyes

  - increase in cramp-like pain in one or both legs when walking
- counsel female patient of childbearing potential to use adequate contraception to avoid pregnancy during therapy
- see General Patient teaching and advice for antihypertensive agents (p. 489)

beta-adrenoceptor blocking agents are banned in sport, but may be allowed in some circumstances, or banned in some sports but not others

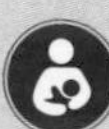

crosses placental barrier; fetal levels reach similar levels to maternal ones. May decrease placental perfusion and cause bradycardia and hypoglycaemia in the fetus and newborn. Prolonged therapy during pregnancy may cause intrauterine growth retardation. If used, lowest possible dose should be given and discontinued at least 2–3 days before delivery to avoid uterine contractility and effects on newborn, including bradycardia and hypoglycaemia. Should only be given if benefits to mother outweigh risks to fetus

not recommended during breastfeeding as may cause bradycardia in the infant

ATENOLOL (Noten, Tenolten, Tenormin, Tensig)

Available forms

Tablets: 50 mg; Oral liquid: 50 mg/mL

Action

- see General Actions of beta-adrenoceptor blocking agents (p. 508)
- cardioselective
- decreases size of infarction and incidence of ventricular dysrhythmia, decreases mortality in first 7 days post infarction
- antiarrhythmic action due to antisympathetic effect depressing both sinus and AV node function and prolonging atrial refractory period
- less airway constriction than non-selective beta-adrenoceptor blocking agents
- slightly less effective in those of Afro-Caribbean origin
- half-life 7–9 hours

Use

- hypotension
- angina pectoris (without heart failure)
- cardiac arrhythmias
- myocardial infarction, late intervention with patient presenting 12 hours after onset of chest pain

Dose

- (hypertension) initially 50 mg orally daily, increasing weekly by 50 mg, then up to 200 mg if necessary **OR**
- (angina pectoris) initially 50 mg orally daily, increasing to 100 mg daily as a single or 2 divided doses if needed **OR**
- (cardiac arrhythmias) controlled with other IV agents initially, then 50–100 mg orally daily (maintenance) **OR**
- (myocardial infarction, late intervention with patient presenting 12 hours after onset of chest pain) 50 mg orally daily for 1–3 years

Adverse effects/Interactions/ Nursing points/Cautions/Patient teaching and advice

- oral doses of 50–100 mg are given once daily, doses greater than 100 mg should be divided
- (myocardial infarction) most beneficial if given in first 48 hours post myocardial infarction
- absorption reduced by apple juice
- (oral liquid) contains hydroxybenzoates and propylene glycol, which may cause hypersensitivity reaction in sensitive individuals
- see general points for beta-adrenoceptor blocking agents (p. 508)

available as oral liquid. Tablet can be crushed and mixed with spoonful of yoghurt (but not apple puree)

BISOPROLOL FUMARATE (Bicard, Bicor, Bispro)

Available forms
Tablets: 1.25 mg (starter pack), 2.5 mg, 5 mg, 10 mg

Action
- see General Actions of beta-adrenoceptor blocking agents (p. 508)
- cardioselective
- half-life 10–12 hours

Use
- stable, chronic moderate-to-severe heart failure

Dose
- (stable chronic moderate-to-severe heart failure) initially 1.25 mg orally daily for 1 week, then (if tolerated) 2.5 mg for 1 week, then 3.75 mg for 1 week, then 5 mg for 4 weeks, then 7.5 mg for 4 weeks, then 10 mg daily (maintenance) (with ACE inhibitor, diuretic +/– digoxin)

Interactions
- AV conduction and risk of bradycardia may be increased if given with cholinergic (parasympathomimetic) agents
- increased risk of bradycardia if given with mefloquine
- may decrease effects of dobutamine or isoprenaline
- slight decrease in half-life if given with rifampicin
- see General Interactions of beta-adrenoceptor blocking agents (p. 509)

Adverse effects/Nursing points/Cautions/Patient teaching and advice
- patient should be in stable condition after heart failure (without any acute failure in previous 6 weeks) and stabilised on therapy for previous 2 weeks before starting bisoprolol
- heart rate, BP, ECG and any signs of worsening heart failure should be monitored during dose titration. If heart rate ≤ 50–55 beats/minute, dose should be decreased gradually
- each increase should be monitored for any signs of intolerance
- transient worsening of heart failure, hypotension and/or bradycardia may occur during titration period
- contraindicated in those with acute heart failure
- see general points for beta-adrenoceptor blocking agents (p. 508)

tablets can be dispersed in water or crushed and mixed with spoonful of yoghurt or apple puree

CARVEDILOL (Carvidol, Dicarz, Dilatrend, Vedilol, Volirop)

Available forms
Tablets: 3.125 mg, 6.25 mg, 12.5 mg, 25 mg

Action
- see General Actions of beta-adrenoceptor blocking agents (p. 508)
- non-selective
- also blocks alpha1 adrenoceptors
- half-life 6–10 hours

Use
- hypertension
- mild-to-severe heart failure

Dose
- (hypertension) initially 12.5 mg orally daily for 2 days, then increasing at 2-week intervals to 25 mg daily and, if necessary, increasing to 50 mg daily if needed **OR**
- (congestive heart failure) initially 3.125 mg orally twice daily with food for 2 weeks, then doubling of dose at 2-week intervals if tolerated (daily maximum 50 mg (if < 85 kg or with severe heart failure), 100 mg (if > 85 kg) in 2 divided doses)

Adverse effects
- increased sweating
- arthralgia, myalgia, back pain
- see also General Adverse effects of beta-adrenoceptor blocking agents (p. 509)

Interactions

- may increase serum levels of ciclosporin and digoxin, increasing risk of adverse effects and therefore serum levels should be closely monitored during therapy
- caution if given with fluoxetine if patient is clinically unstable
- serum levels may be increased by grapefruit juice
- see also General Interactions of beta-adrenoceptor blocking agents (p. 509)

Nursing points/Cautions

- (severe congestive heart failure) patient should be assessed for any signs of peripheral oedema, systolic BP $\geq$ 85 mmHg and other therapies (digoxin, diuretics, ACE inhibitors) should be stabilised first before introducing carvedilol
- (congestive heart failure) patient should be monitored for any symptoms of worsening heart failure, vasodilation or bradycardia before each dose increase
- (congestive heart failure) if pulse rate $<$ 55 beats/minute, dose should be reduced
- caution if used in those with labile or secondary hypertension
- not recommended in those with significant liver disease
- see General Nursing points/Cautions for beta-adrenoceptor blocking agents (p. 510)

Patient teaching and advice

- instruct patient to avoid grapefruit juice during therapy
- see General Patient teaching and advice for beta-adrenoceptor blocking agents (p. 511)

tablets can be dispersed in water or crushed and mixed with spoonful of yoghurt or apple puree

ESMOLOL HYDROCHLORIDE (Brevibloc)

Available form

Vial: 100 mg/10 mL

Action

- see General Actions of beta-adrenoceptor blocking agents (p. 508)
- cardioselective
- rapid onset, short duration of action, half-life 5–23 minutes
- active metabolite (half-life 3.7 hours, which is prolonged tenfold in those with severe kidney disease)

Use

- supraventricular tachycardia

Dose

- (supraventricular tachycardia) initially 500 microgram/kg/minute IV over 1 minute (loading dose), then 50 microgram/kg/minute for 4 minutes
- if satisfactory response, then 50 microgram/kg/minute by IV infusion (maintenance)
- if unsatisfactory response, repeat initial loading dose of 500 microgram/kg/minute IV over 1 minute, followed by 100 microgram/kg/minute for 4 minutes. This may be repeated, increasing the maintenance dose by 50 microgram/kg/minute until response is satisfactory. As satisfactory heart rate or BP is approached, infusion rate should be decreased

Adverse effects

- symptomatic hypotension with sweating and dizziness, asymptomatic hypotension
- dizziness, somnolence, confusion, headache, agitation, fatigue, paraesthesia, asthenia
- nausea, vomiting
- sweating
- (IV site) inflammation, induration, swelling, redness, skin discolouration, thrombophlebitis and rarely, skin necrosis (from extravasation)

Interactions
- plasma level may be increased by IV morphine
- may prolong suxamethonium's neuromuscular blockade
- not recommended with dopamine, adrenaline (epinephrine) or noradrenaline to slow heart rate due to risk of blocking contraction
- contraindicated within 48 hours of discontinuing verapamil
- increased risk of hypotension if given with nifedipine and amlodipine
- increased serum level may occur if given with warfarin or digoxin
- increased AV conduction time may occur if given with disopyramide or amiodarone
- may decrease serum levels of digoxin
- see General Interactions of beta-adrenoceptor blocking agents (p. 509)

Nursing points/Cautions/Patient teaching and advice

- ECG, heart rate and BP should be monitored continuously during therapy. If pulse falls to less than 50–55 beats/minute with symptoms of bradycardia, dose should be reduced
- therapy should be limited to 24 hours
- infusion into small veins or at levels greater than 10 mg/mL is not recommended
- butterfly needles are not recommended
- intervals may be increased from 5 to 10 minutes if necessary
- avoid extravasation and monitor IV site regularly to prevent venous irritation and/or tissue necrosis
- 100 mg vial is pre-diluted and ready to administer
- incompatible with sodium bicarbonate, furosemide, diazepam and thiopentone
- maintenance dose should not exceed 200 microgram/kg/minutes due to risk of increased hypotension
- contains about 20% alcohol and this should be considered if this is administered to young children of those who have suffered from alcoholism
- therapy should be discontinued gradually once arrhythmia has been controlled, patient is stable and alternative antiarrhythmic agent has been started
- caution if used to control ventricular rate
- caution if used in those with impaired kidney function as acid metabolite elimination may be prolonged tenfold
- contraindicated if patient requires inotropic agents and/or vasodilators to maintain systemic BP and cardiac output
- see general points for beta-adrenoceptor blocking agents (p. 508)

LABETALOL HYDROCHLORIDE (Presolol, Trandate)

Available forms
Tablets: 100 mg, 200 mg

Action
- see General Actions of beta-adrenoceptor blocking agents (p. 508)
- antagonises both alpha and beta receptors
- beta blockade is non-selective, whereas alpha-receptor antagonism is mainly on peripheral arterioles, resulting in a reduction of peripheral resistance
- beta blockade on the heart causes reflex peripheral vasodilation, reducing BP without cardiac stimulation
- half-life 6–8 hours (however, hypotensive effect may last for up to 11 hours after administration)

Use
- hypertension

Dose
- (hypertension) initially 100–200 mg orally twice daily after meals,

increasing at weekly intervals up to 2400 mg daily in 3–4 divided doses if needed

Adverse effects/Interactions/Nursing points/Cautions/Patient teaching and advice

- increased serum levels may occur if given with cimetidine
- may interfere with some laboratory tests including assays using fluorimetric or photometric methods
- may also produce false positive result using urine screening for amphetamines
- see general points for beta-adrenoceptor blocking agents (p. 508)

tablets can be dispersed in water or crushed and mixed with spoonful of yoghurt or apple puree

METOPROLOL SUCCINATE (Metrol-XL, Minax-XL, Toprol-XL)

METOPROLOL TARTRATE (Betaloc, Lopresor, Metatar, Metrol, Metoprolol IV Mylan, Minax, Mistrom)

Available forms

Tablets: 50 mg, 100 mg; Tablets (controlled-release): 23.75 mg, 47.5 mg, 95 mg, 190 mg; Ampoules: 5 mg/5 mL

Action

- see General Actions of beta-adrenoceptor blocking agents (p. 508)
- cardioselective
- half-life 3–5 hours

Use

- mild-to-severe hypertension
- angina pectoris prophylaxis
- myocardial infarction (definite or suspected)
- migraine prophylaxis
- cardiac arrhythmias (IV)
- stable chronic heart failure

Dose

- (mild hypertension) 50–100 mg orally daily **OR**
- (severe hypertension) 50–100 mg orally twice daily **OR**
- (angina pectoris) 50–100 mg orally 2–3 times daily **OR**
- (myocardial infarction) initially 50 mg orally twice daily for 48 hours, then 100 mg twice daily **OR**
- (migraine prophylaxis) 100–150 mg orally daily in 2 divided doses **OR**
- (cardiac arrhythmias, particularly supraventricular tachyarrhythmias) 5 mg IV at 1–2 mg/minute repeated at 5-minute intervals as required, up to a dose of 15 mg **OR**
- (heart failure) initially 11.875–23.75 mg (1/2–1 tablet) orally once daily for 2 weeks, then 47.5 mg daily for 2 weeks, then 95 mg daily for 2 weeks, then 190 mg daily or the highest tolerated dose once daily (maintenance) (controlled-release tablets)

Interactions

- plasma levels may be increased by alcohol, cimetidine, diphenhydramine, fluoxetine, hydralazine, sertraline and paroxetine
- caution if given with hydroxychloroquine or diphenhydramine
- caution if given with warfarin as increased anticoagulation may occur. INR should be monitored during therapy
- plasma levels may be decreased by rifampicin
- see General Interactions of beta-adrenoceptor blocking agents (p. 509)

Adverse effects/Nursing points/Cautions

- parenteral administration is only conducted in a unit where suitable

monitoring and resuscitation equipment is available
- (IV) BP and ECG should be monitored throughout therapy
- (IV) caution if systolic BP < 100 mmHg as further significant decrease in BP can occur
- no equivalence has been shown between controlled-release tablets and immediate-release formulations
- controlled-release tablets should only be used for chronic heart failure
- if dose ≤ 150 mg, it may be given as a single daily dose
- caution if used in those with liver cirrhosis as clearance may be decreased, leading to elevated serum levels
- see general points for beta-adrenoceptor blocking agents (p. 508)

Patient teaching and advice

- patient should be advised to avoid alcohol during therapy
- advise patient that controlled-release tablets may be halved
- patient should be instructed that controlled-release tablets should be swallowed whole (or halved if tablets are scored), not chewed or crushed
- see General Patient teaching and advice for beta-adrenoceptor blocking agents (p. 511)

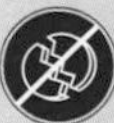

controlled-release tablets should not be chewed or crushed

plain tablets can be dispersed in water or crushed and mixed with spoonful of yoghurt or apple puree

NEBIVOLOL (Nebilet)

Available forms

Tablets: 1.25 mg, 5 mg, 10 mg

Action

- see General Actions of beta-adrenoceptor blocking agents (p. 508)
- cardio-selective with very high affinity for beta1-adrenoceptors
- causes vasodilation through release of nitrous oxide in endothelial cells
- active metabolite
- half-life about 10 hours

Use

- hypertension (monotherapy or with diuretic)
- stable chronic heart failure (adjunct therapy in those > 70 years with diuretic and/or digoxin and/or ACE inhibitor and/or angiotensin II antagonist)

Dose

- (hypertension) 5 mg orally daily **OR**
- (chronic heart failure) initially 1.25 mg orally daily increasing at 1–2-week intervals to 2.5 mg daily, then 5 mg daily and up to 10 mg daily

Adverse effects

- paraesthesia, hypoaesthesia
- nervousness
- myalgia, back pain
- increased sweating
- chest pain
- see General Adverse effects of beta-adrenoceptor blocking agents (p. 509)

Interactions

- increased serum levels may occur if given with paroxetine and fluoxetine increasing risk of excessive adverse effects including bradycardia
- increased hypotension may occur if given with baclofen or amifostine
- see General Interactions of beta-adrenoceptor blocking agents (p. 509)

Nursing points/Cautions

- (hypertension) effects should be seen in 2 weeks; however, may take 4 weeks in some patients
- (chronic heart failure) condition should be stable with acute heart failure in last 6 weeks before starting therapy

- (chronic heart failure) other drug therapy (diuretic, digoxin, ACE inhibitor and/or angiotensin II antagonist) should be stabilised in 2 weeks before starting nebivolol
- (chronic heart failure) therapy should be started under medical supervision over at least 2 hours to monitor BP, heart rate, ECG, signs of worsening heart failure to ensure clinical condition remains stable
- (chronic heart failure) should not be stopped abruptly to prevent worsening heart failure
- tablets contain lactose and are therefore not recommended in those with rare hereditary problems of galactose intolerance, Lapp lactase deficiency or glucose–galactose malabsorption
- contraindicated in those with liver insufficiency or impairment
- see General Nursing points/Cautions for beta-adrenoceptor blocking agents (p. 510)

Patient teaching and advice

- advise patient to take tablets whole, not chew or crush them
- see General Patient teaching and advice for beta-adrenoceptor blocking agents (p. 511)

tablets can be dispersed in water or crushed and mixed with spoonful of yoghurt or apple puree

PINDOLOL (Barbloc)

Available forms

Tablets: 5 mg, 15 mg

Action

- see General Actions of beta-adrenoceptor blocking agents (p. 508)
- non-selective
- half-life 3–4 hours

Use

- hypertension
- angina pectoris prophylaxis
- cardiac arrhythmias
- functional hyperadrenergic cardiac disturbances

Dose

- (hypertension) 10–30 mg orally daily **OR**
- (angina pectoris) 7.5–20 mg orally daily in 3 divided doses **OR**
- (cardiac arrhythmias) 15–30 mg orally daily in 3 divided doses **OR**
- (functional hyperadrenergic cardiac disturbances) 10–20 mg orally daily

Adverse effects/Interactions/Nursing points/Cautions/Patient teaching and advice

- given in 2–3 divided doses if more than 15 mg
- serum levels may be increased if given with cimetidine
- see general points for beta-adrenoceptor blocking agents (p. 508)

tablets can be dispersed in water or crushed and mixed with spoonful of yoghurt or apple puree

PROPRANOLOL HYDROCHLORIDE (Deralin, Inderal)

Available forms

Tablets: 10 mg, 40 mg, 160 mg

Action

- see General Actions of beta-adrenoceptor blocking agents (p. 508)
- non-selective
- active metabolite
- half-life 3–6 hours

Use
- hypertension
- angina pectoris
- essential tremor
- migraine prophylaxis
- myocardial infarction
- preoperatively for pheochromocytoma
- cardiac dysrhythmia (including anxiety tachycardia, drug-induced dysrhythmia)
- Fallot's tetralogy (relief of right ventricular outflow tract shutdown)

Dose
- (hypertension) initially 40 mg orally twice daily, increasing at weekly intervals according to response to 60–160 mg twice (daily maximum 320 mg) **OR**
- (angina pectoris) 40 mg orally 2–3 times daily, increasing at weekly intervals according to response up to 60–160 mg twice daily **OR**
- (essential tremor) 40 mg orally 2–3 times daily, increasing at weekly intervals according to response to 40–80 mg twice daily **OR**
- (migraine prophylaxis) 40 mg orally twice daily, increasing to 40–80 mg twice daily **OR**
- (myocardial infarction) initially 40 mg orally 4 times daily for 2–3 days, then 80 mg twice daily **OR**
- (preoperatively for pheochromocytoma) 60 mg orally daily for 3 days in divided doses, then 30 mg daily in divided doses (maintenance) (with alpha receptor blockade) **OR**
- (cardiac dysrhythmias) 10–40 mg orally 3–4 times daily **OR**
- (Fallot's tetralogy – children) up to 1 mg/kg orally 3–4 times daily

Adverse effects
- (rare) hearing loss, tinnitus
- see also General Adverse effects of beta-adrenoceptor blocking agents (p. 509)

Interactions
- not recommended with lidocaine (lignocaine) as may increase lidocaine (lignocaine) serum levels
- may increase serum levels of rizatriptan
- increased serum levels may occur if given with alcohol, cimetidine and hydralazine
- propranolol and chlorpromazine given together may result in increased plasma levels of both drugs
- see General Interactions of beta-adrenoceptor blocking agents (p. 509)

Adverse effects/Nursing points/Cautions/Patient teaching and advice
- advise patient to avoid alcohol during therapy
- (migraine prophylaxis) response generally seen in 12 weeks. If significant reduction in frequency of migraine is seen, therapy may be gradually stopped
- increased risk of hepatic encephalopathy
- caution if used in those with liver impairment including decompensated cirrhosis and portal hypertension
- see general points for beta-adrenoceptor blocking agents (p. 508)

tablets can be dispersed in water or crushed and mixed with spoonful of yoghurt or apple puree

CALCIUM-CHANNEL BLOCKERS

General Actions of calcium-channel blockers

- also known as calcium antagonists
- impede the influx of calcium ions through slow channels of cell membrane during depolarisation of cardiac and vascular smooth muscle improving myocardial oxygen supply and cardiac output and reducing myocardial work by reducing afterload
- dilate coronary artery decreasing resistance, improving oxygen supply to ischaemic area, as well as improving blood flow to collateral vessels
- dilate peripheral arteries and arterioles reducing peripheral vascular resistance and therefore BP
- negative inotropic effect
- half-life increased in the elderly (amlodipine, diltiazem, felodipine, verapamil)
- subdivided into:
  - phenylalkylamine type (e.g. verapamil)
  - benzothiazepine type (e.g. diltiazem)
  - dihydropyridine type (e.g. amlodipine, felodipine, nifedipine, nimodipine, lercanidipine)

General Adverse effects of calcium-channel blockers

- headache, dizziness/vertigo, flushing (feeling of warmth), light-headedness, fatigue, somnolence, asthenia/weakness, malaise
- nausea, vomiting, dyspepsia, constipation, abdominal pain, flatulence, dry mouth
- gingivitis, gingival hyperplasia
- rash, pruritus, urticaria
- AV block, palpitations, tachycardia, peripheral oedema, hypotension, exacerbation of angina
- (rare) elevated liver enzymes, severe skin reactions, hyperglycaemia, impotence, gynaecomastia, bronchospasm, asthma aggravation

General Interactions of calcium-channel blockers

- serum levels may be increased by grapefruit juice (especially immediate-release formulations)
- great caution if used with beta-adrenoceptor blocking agents as may result in profound (potentially life threatening) bradycardia, heart block and hypotension
- may enhance hypotensive effect of antihypertensives, diuretics and other calcium-channel antagonists
- excessive cardiovascular depression may occur if given with inhalation anaesthetics
- increased vasodilation (hypotension and faintness) may occur if given with nitrates

General Nursing points/Cautions for calcium-channel blockers

- gingival enlargement can be avoided or reversed by attention to dental hygiene
- ER (extended-release) or SR (slow- or sustained-release) are not bioequivalent to immediate-release tablets and should not be substituted
- (sustained-release preparation) caution if used in those with previous history of severe gastrointestinal

narrowing or obstruction due to increased risk of bowel obstruction because of non-conformable nature of sustained-release formulation

- caution if used in those with short bowel syndrome, Crohn's disease, ulcerative colitis or other conditions with chronic diarrhoea as transit time is shortened, resulting in inadequate serum levels
- caution if used in those with bronchial hyperreactivity, including asthma, as bronchospasm may occur
- caution if used in those with diabetes mellitus
- caution if used in those with aortic stenosis, heart failure, liver or kidney impairment, bradycardia or first-degree AV block
- contraindicated in those with sick sinus syndrome (without pacemaker), second- or third-degree AV block (without pacemaker), severe bradycardia (< 40 beats/minute), hypotension (< 90 mmHg systolic), severe uncompensated heart failure, cardiogenic shock, unstable angina, within 4–8 weeks of acute myocardial infarction or left ventricular failure with pulmonary congestion
- contraindicated in those with hypersensitivity to calcium-channel blockers

General Patient teaching and advice for calcium-channel blockers

- patient should be advised that ER (extended-release) or SR (slow- or sustained-release) tablets should be swallowed whole (not divided, crushed or chewed)
- instruct patient to maintain good dental hygiene (e.g. brush teeth twice daily, floss daily) and attend regular professional teeth cleaning to decrease gingival hyperplasia
- warn patient to immediately report any
  - skin reaction (e.g. red, painful or itchy spots, blisters, skin peeling) that persists
  - wheezing or difficulty breathing
- advise patient not to stop therapy suddenly as severe angina may occur
- patient should be warned to avoid grapefruit or grapefruit juice during therapy
- patients with diabetes should be instructed to monitor blood glucose levels closely during therapy
- see General Patient teaching and advice for antihypertensive agents (p. 489)

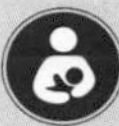

not recommended/contraindicated during pregnancy as these agents have the potential to produce fetal hypoxia associated with maternal hypotension

not recommended during breastfeeding

AMLODIPINE (Amlo, Nordip, Norvasc)

Available forms

Tablets: 5 mg, 10 mg

Action

- see General Actions of calcium-channel blockers (p. 520)
- dihydropyridine
- peak effect 6–12 hours, half-life 35–50 hours

Use

- chronic stable angina (as monotherapy or with other antianginal agents)
- hypertension

Dose

- (hypertension, angina) 2.5–5 mg orally daily, increasing at 7–14-day intervals to a daily maximum of 10 mg if needed

Interactions

- increased risk of hypotension if given with clarithromycin

- caution if given with simvastatin
- serum levels may be increased if given with erythromycin, itraconazole or ritonavir
- decreased serum levels may occur if given with rifampicin or St John's wort
- may increase serum levels of tacrolimus

Adverse effects/Nursing points/ Cautions/Patient teaching and advice

- dose titration should occur over 7–14 days to assess patient response to dose changes
- 5 mg tablets are scored and can be divided for smaller dose
- see general points for calcium-channel blockers (p. 520)
- see General Patient teaching and advice for antihypertensive agents (p. 489)
- see General Patient teaching and advice for antianginal agents (p. 61)

tablet can be dispersed in water or crushed and mixed with spoonful of yoghurt or apple puree. Crushed tablet has a bitter taste

Note

- contained in Caduet, Cadivast with atorvastatin, Coveram and Reaptan with perindopril, Exforge with valsartan, Exforge HCT with valsartan and hydrochlorothiazide, Reaptan with perindopril arginine, Sevikar with olmesartan, Sevikar HCT with olmesartan and hydrochlorothiazide, Twynsta and Pritor/Amlodipine with telmisartan

CLEVIDIPINE (Cleviprex)

Available form

Vial: 0.5 mg/mL

Action

- dihydropyridine calcium-channel blocker
- see General Actions of calcium-channel blockers (p. 520)

Use

- short-term hypertension management when oral therapy is not feasible or desirable

Dose

- initially 1–2 mg/hour, doubling dose every 90 seconds until BP is approaching target level, then dose adjustments should be every 5–10 minutes until desired target is reached (maximum 32 mg/hour)

Adverse effects

- atrial fibrillation, tachycardia, ventricular tachycardia, supraventricular extrasystoles
- hypotension
- peripheral oedema
- headache, dizziness
- fever, feeling hot, flushing
- polyuria
- atelectasis, pulmonary oedema, wheezing, dyspnoea, pneumonia
- anxiety, restlessness, disorientation, insomnia
- renal insufficiency, acute renal failure
- nausea, vomiting, constipation
- pruritus
- (rare) congestive cardiac failure, hypersensitivity, decreased oxygen saturation

Interactions

- beta-adrenoceptor blocking agents should not be used to treat any clevidipine-induced tachycardia

Nursing points/Cautions

- BP and heart rate should be monitored continuously during therapy until vital signs are stable
- dose should be decreased if hypotension and reflex tachycardia occur with worsening clinical outcome
- when transitioning to oral antihypertensive agent, clevidipine should be titrated downwards or stopped and BP should continue to be monitored
- if patient is not being transitioned to oral antihypertensive agent, BP and heart rate should continue to be monitored for at least 8 hours after stopping infusion as rebound hypertension may occur
- no more than 1000 mL or an average of 21 mg/mL is recommended per 24 hours
- vial should be inverted gently before infusion to ensure emulsion is evenly distributed
- should not be diluted
- administer alone
- should be used within 12 hours and any remaining solution discarded after this time
- contains 0.2 g lipid/mL (2.0 kcal) which may need to be considered if patient has lipid load restrictions
- caution if used in elderly patients. Patients should be closely monitored and titration of dose started at low end of dose range
- caution if used in those with heart failure, as negative inotropic effects can exacerbate heart failure. If used, patient should be closely monitored during therapy
- not recommended in children or adolescents
- not recommended in those with defective lipid metabolism (e.g. pathologic hyperlipidaemia, lipoid nephrosis, acute pancreatitis with hyperlipidaemic) or severe aortic stenosis
- contraindicated in those with known allergies to soybeans, soy products, eggs or egg products

DILTIAZEM HYDROCHLORIDE (Cardizem, Cardizem CD, Diltiazem AN, Dilzem, Vasocardol, Vasocardol CD)

Available forms

Tablets: 60 mg; Capsules (extended-release): 180 mg, 240 mg, 360 mg

Action

- see General Actions of calcium-channel blockers (p. 520)
- decreases conduction through SA and AV node
- inhibits coronary artery spasm
- onset of action 30 minutes (immediate-release), 30–60 minutes (controlled-release)
- peak effect 2–3 hours (immediate-release) or 6–11 hours (controlled-release)
- duration of action 4–8 hours (immediate-release) or 12 hours (controlled-release)
- half-life about 3.5 hours (single or chronic dosing)

Use

- chronic stable angina pectoris
- hypertension

Dose

- (hypertension) initially 180–240 mg orally daily, increasing at 2-week intervals to 240–360 mg daily if needed (extended-release capsules) **OR**

- (angina) initially 30 mg orally 4 times daily before meals and at night, increasing at 1–2-day intervals until response is achieved (usually 180–240 mg) (daily maximum 360 mg) (immediate-release tablets) **OR**
- (angina) initially 180 mg orally daily, increasing gradually over 7–14 days if needed to 360 mg daily (controlled-release capsules)

Adverse effects

- mood changes, depression
- see General Adverse effects of calcium-channel blockers (p. 520)

Interactions

- contraindicated with dantrolene and ivabradine
- may decrease clearance of some beta-adrenoceptor blocking agents increasing serum levels
- increased risk of bradycardia if given with amiodarone
- increased hypotension may occur if given with alpha-adrenoceptor blocking agents
- not recommended with antiarrhythmic agents
- serum levels may be increased by cimetidine or ranitidine
- may increase serum levels of digoxin, theophylline, ciclosporin, cilostazol, methylprednisolone, midazolam, triazolam, phenytoin and carbamazepine, increasing the risk of toxicity, therefore serum levels should be closely monitored especially when starting or stopping therapy
- serum levels may be decreased by diazepam and rifampicin
- increased risk of neurotoxicity if given with lithium
- caution if given with statins as there is an increased risk of myalgia and rhabdomyolysis due to increased serum levels
- caution if given with aspirin, other salicylates or antiplatelets due to increased risk of bleeding
- increased risk of depression if given with beta-adrenoceptor blocking agents
- caution if given with X-ray contrast media due to increased risk of hypotension
- see General Interactions of calcium-channel blockers (p. 520)

Nursing points/Cautions

- immediate-release tablets are only used as antianginal agents not antihypertensives
- sustained-release preparations are only recommended for chronic stable angina (not variant angina)
- see General Nursing points/Cautions for calcium-channel blockers (p. 521)

Patient teaching and advice

- advise patient to seek medical advice if low mood or depression occurs
- see General Patient teaching and advice for antianginal agents (p. 61)
- see General Patient teaching and advice for calcium-channel blockers (p. 521) and antihypertensive agents (p. 489)

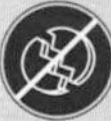

tablet can be crushed and mixed with spoonful of yoghurt or apple puree. Capsule can be opened and pellets mixed with yoghurt but pellets should not be crushed, broken or chewed

FELODIPINE (Felodil XR, Felodur ER, Plendil ER)

Available forms

Tablets (extended-release): 2.5 mg, 5 mg, 10 mg

Action

- see General Actions of calcium-channel blockers (p. 520)
- dihydropyridine
- mild natriuretic and diuretic effect
- no effect of conduction or contractility
- onset of action 120–300 minutes, peak effect 2.5–5 hours, duration of action 24 hours, biphasic half-life (4 hours, 24 hours)

Use

- hypertension

Dose

- (hypertension) initially 2.5–5.0 mg orally daily, increasing gradually to 5–10 mg orally daily (daily maximum 20 mg) (extended-release tablets)

Interactions

- serum levels may be reduced by carbamazepine, phenobarbital (phenobarbitone), rifampicin, phenytoin and St John's wort
- serum levels may be increased if given with grapefruit juice, itraconazole, cimetidine or erythromycin
- may increase serum levels of tacrolimus, increasing the risk of toxicity
- see General Interactions of calcium-channel blockers (p. 520)

Adverse effects

- mood changes, depression
- see General Adverse effects for calcium-channel blockers (p. 520)

Nursing points/Cautions/Patient teaching and advice

- see general points for calcium-channel blockers (p. 520)
- (Felodur ER) contains lactose and is not recommended in those with hereditary galactose intolerance or glucose–galactose malabsorption
- advise patient that extended-release tablets should be swallowed whole, not chewed, broken or divided
- patient should be warned to seek medical advice if low mood or depression occurs

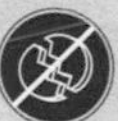

extended-release tablets should not be broken, chewed or crushed

Note

- contained in Triasyn with ramipril

LERCANIDIPINE HYDROCHLORIDE (Lercadip, Lercan, Zanidip, Zircol)

Available forms

Tablets: 10 mg, 20 mg

Action

- see General Actions of calcium-channel blockers (p. 520)
- dihydropyridine
- peak effect 1.5–3 hours, duration of action 24 hours

Use

- hypertension

Dose

- (hypertension) initially 10 mg orally daily at least 15 minutes before food, increasing after 2 weeks to 20 mg if necessary

Interactions

- not recommended with alcohol because of potentiation of vasodilation
- increased serum levels may occur if given with erythromycin, ritonavir, itraconazole and fluoxetine
- decreased serum levels may occur if given with phenytoin, metoprolol, carbamazepine and rifampicin resulting in decreased hypertensive effect
- caution if given with amiodarone or other antiarrhythmic agents
- may increase serum levels of simvastatin

- contraindicated with ciclosporin
- see General Interactions of calcium-channel blockers (p. 520)

Adverse effects/Nursing points/ Cautions

- if given in patients undergoing peritoneal dialysis, peritoneal effluent may become cloudy which can be mistaken for infection
- contraindicated in those with severe renal (creatinine clearance < 12 mL/ minute) or liver impairment
- see general points for calcium-channel blockers (p. 520)

Patient teaching and advice

- patients should be advised to avoid alcohol
- instruct patient to take tablets at least 15 minutes before meals
- if patient is taking simvastatin concurrently, advise taking lercanidipine in the morning and simvastatin in the evening
- see General Patient teaching and advice for calcium-channel blockers (p. 521) and antihypertensive agents (p. 489)

tablet can be crushed and mixed with water or spoonful of yoghurt or apple puree

Note

- contained in Zan-Extra with enalapril

NIFEDIPINE (Adalat, Addos XR, Adefin XL)

Available forms

Tablets: 10 mg, 20 mg; Tablets (controlled-/ modified-release): 20 mg, 30 mg, 60 mg

Action

- see General Actions of calcium-channel blockers (p. 520)
- dihydropyridine
- inhibits coronary artery spasm
- decreases myocardial oxygen consumption at rest, during exercise and during episodes of coronary artery spasm
- onset of action 15 minutes, peak effect 0.5–1 hour, duration of action 4–8 hours
- elimination may be decreased in South Asian patients

Use

- prophylaxis of chronic angina pectoris and variant (Prinzmetal's) angina
- mild-to-moderate hypertension

Dose

- (hypertension) initially 10–20 mg orally twice daily, increasing to 20–40 mg twice daily if needed (daily maximum 80 mg) **OR**
- (hypertension) initially 30 mg orally daily, increasing (or decreasing) at 7–14-day intervals if necessary to 120 mg daily (controlled-/modified-release tablets) **OR**
- (variant angina) initially 10–20 mg orally twice daily, increasing to 40 mg twice daily if needed (daily maximum 80 mg) **OR**
- (chronic stable angina) initially 30 mg orally once daily, increasing gradually to 90 mg if needed (controlled-/ modified-release tablets)

Interactions

- serum levels may be increased if given with cimetidine, sodium valproate, fluoxetine, erythromycin, HIV protease inhibitors (e.g. ritonavir) or diltiazem
- contraindicated with rifampicin
- may potentiate effects of salbutamol and terbutaline
- may increase hypotensive effect of candesartan or irbesartan
- may increase serum levels of digoxin increasing the risk of toxicity
- may alter (increase or decrease) serum levels of theophylline, therefore should be given together with caution

- serum levels may be decreased if given with carbamazepine, phenytoin or phenobarbital (phenobarbitone)
- may increase serum level of tacrolimus, increasing risk of toxicity
- may cause false positive result on barium contrast X-ray
- see General Interactions of calcium-channel blockers (p. 520)

Adverse effects/Nursing points/ Cautions

- see general points for calcium-channel blockers (p. 520)
- tablets and controlled-/modified-release preparations are not bio-equivalent
- controlled-/modified-release preparations are only recommended for prevention of stable chronic angina
- (Adefin) contain lactose and therefore not recommended in those with hereditary galactose intolerance or glucose–galactose malabsorption
- contraindicated within 8 days of acute myocardial infarction or in those with cardiogenic shock or ileostomy after proctocolectomy (Kock pouch)

Patient teaching and advice

- see General Patient teaching and advice for calcium-channel blockers (p. 521)
- see General Patient teaching and advice for antianginal agents (p. 61)

NIMODIPINE (Nimotop)

Available forms

Tablets: 30 mg; Infusion solution: 10 mg/50 mL

Action

- dihydropyridine calcium-channel blocker that preferentially dilates cerebral vessels, increasing cerebral perfusion especially in areas of early damage or restricted circulation
- onset of action 15 minutes, peak effect 1–1.5 hours, half-life 1.2–1.8 hours (IV) or 5–10 hours (oral)

Use

- prophylaxis and treatment of ischaemic neurological deficits caused by cerebral vasospasm after subarachnoid haemorrhage caused by ruptured intracranial aneurysm

Dose

- 1 mg/hour by IV infusion for 2 hours, then 2 mg/hour, provided there is no marked decrease in BP **OR**
- initially up to 0.5 mg/hour by IV infusion (if patient $<$ 70 kg or has unstable BP) **OR**
- 60 mg orally every 4 hours for 7 days (following parenteral administration) **OR**
- 60 mg orally every 4 hours for 10–14 days (oral administration only)

Adverse effects

- hypotension, tachycardia, flushing
- nausea, vomiting
- headache
- rash
- thrombocytopenia
- (IV) infusion site reaction, thrombophlebitis
- (rare) paralytic ileus, bradycardia, abnormal liver function, sweating, pruritus

Interactions

- (oral) contraindicated with rifampicin, phenytoin, phenobarbital (phenobarbitone) and carbamazepine
- (IV) not recommended with other calcium-channel blockers or antihypertensive agents
- increased serum levels may occur if given within 4 days of grapefruit juice ingestion
- increased serum levels may occur if given with erythromycin, clarithromycin, ritonavir, fluoxetine, cimetidine and sodium valproate, therefore not recommended together

- (IV) increased risk of nephrotoxicity if given with aminoglycosides, cephalosporins, furosemide or other potentially nephrotoxic agents and renal function monitoring is recommended
- caution if given with doxorubicin or vincristine
- slightly decreased serum levels may occur if given with nortriptyline
- (IV) may decrease clearance of IV zidovudine
- see General Interactions of calcium-channel blockers (p. 520)

Nursing points/Cautions

- BP should be monitored throughout therapy
- start within 4 days of onset of symptoms and continue for at least 7 days (maximum 14 days)
- decreased dose is recommended if patient weighs < 70 kg or has labile BP
- IV should be continued for at least 5 days post aneurysm clipping
- renal function monitoring is recommended if given IV in those with renal disease
- IV solution is light sensitive, although no protective measures are required if used in artificial or diffuse light
- PVC tubing should not be used because it absorbs nimodipine
- administered via a 'bypass' (3-way stop cock) into a running IV infusion (20 mL/hour initially, increasing to 40 mL/hour with increase in nimodipine) using an infusion pump via a central catheter (CVC). Suitable IV fluids include sodium chloride 0.9%, glucose 5%, Hartmann's solution/lactated Ringer's solution, lactated Ringer's solution with magnesium, Dextran 40, mannitol 10%, human albumin and blood
- administer alone
- all infusion tubing should be changed 24-hourly
- IV solution contains 23.7% alcohol (50 g/daily dose) and therefore should be used with caution in those with alcoholism or impaired alcohol metabolism, impaired liver function, epilepsy, during pregnancy or breastfeeding
- caution if used in those with known raised intracranial pressure, cerebral oedema, kidney and liver dysfunction or in those with hypotension (systolic BP < 100 mmHg)
- caution if used in those with unstable angina or within 28 days of acute myocardial infarction
- see General Nursing points/Cautions for calcium-channel blockers (p. 521)

Patient teaching and advice

- advise patient to swallow tablets whole
- patient should be instructed to seek medical advice immediately if any of the following occur:
  - lack of bowel motions, stomach pain or cramping
  - irregular heart rate
- see General Patient teaching and advice for calcium-channel blockers (p. 521) and antihypertensive agents (p. 489)

VERAPAMIL HYDROCHLORIDE (Anpec, Cordilox SR, Isoptin, Isoptin SR)

Available forms

Tablets: 40 mg, 80 mg, 120 mg, 160 mg; Tablets (sustained-release): 180 mg, 240 mg; Ampoules: 5 mg/2 mL

Action

- see General Actions of calcium-channel blockers (p. 520)
- class IV antiarrhythmic agent
- increases AV node refractory period and prolongs conduction time
- dilates coronary arteries and arterioles, inhibits coronary artery spasm
- onset of action 1–5 minutes (IV), 1–2 hours (oral)

- peak effect 1–2 hours (oral)
- duration of action 2 hours (IV), 8–10 hours (oral), 24 hours (controlled-release formulation)
- half-life 2.8–7.4 hours (single dose) increasing to 4.5–12 hours (chronic dosing)

Use

- management of unstable angina pectoris or variant (Prinzmetal's) angina
- prophylaxis and management of arrhythmias (e.g. supraventricular arrhythmias)
- hypertension, hypertensive crises

Dose

- (hypertension) initially 80 mg orally 2–3 times daily, increasing to 160 mg 2–3 times daily if needed **OR**
- (hypertension) 120–240 mg orally once daily, increasing dose if needed (SR tablets) **OR**
- (arrhythmias, hypertensive crisis) 5 mg IV bolus over 2–3 minutes, repeated 5–10 minutes later if necessary, then 5–10 mg/hour by IV infusion (up to 100 mg/day) **OR**
- (tachyarrhythmias) initially 80 mg orally 2 to 3 times daily, increasing to 160 mg 2–3 times daily if needed (immediate-release tablets) **OR**
- (angina) initially 80 mg orally 2–3 times daily, increasing to 160 mg 2–3 times daily if needed **OR**
- (angina) 180–240 mg orally once daily, increasing dose to obtain a response if necessary (sustained-release) (daily maximum 480 mg as 2 divided doses)

Adverse effects

- dyspnoea
- (IV, rare) second- to third-degree AV block, bradycardia, transient asystole
- see General Adverse effects of calcium-channel blockers (p. 520)

Interactions

- contraindicated IV with beta-adrenoceptor blocking agents (unless in ICU setting)
- contraindicated with dabigatran etexilate
- may decrease serum lithium levels if verapamil is introduced to stable lithium therapy, therefore serum levels should be closely monitored
- may increase serum levels of buspirone, digoxin, carbamazepine, everolimus, sirolimus, tacrolimus, midazolam, doxorubicin, imipramine, theophylline, atorvastatin, simvastatin, ciclosporin, glibenclamide and benzodiazepines increasing risk of adverse effects and/or toxicity
- increased serum levels may result if given with cimetidine, erythromycin, clarithromycin, ritonavir, indinavir and saquinavir
- added cardiac depressant effects may result if given with class 1c antiarrhythmic agents (e.g. flecainide). Cardiac monitoring is recommended if given together
- disopyramide should be discontinued 48 hours before starting therapy and not restarted within 24 hours of stopping verapamil
- may potentiate effects of neuromuscular blocking agents
- may decrease metabolism of alcohol prolonging its effects
- increased bleeding may occur if given with aspirin
- not recommended with colchicine
- not recommended with quinidine in patients with hypertrophic cardiomyopathy
- may increase serum levels of digoxin which may result in excessive bradycardia or AV block
- excessive cardiac depression may occur if given with inhalation anaesthetics, therefore combination should be given with extreme caution
- phenobarbital (phenobarbitone) and phenytoin may decrease serum verapamil levels
- has an additive effect with other antihypertensives, diuretics, vasodilators or antiarrhythmic medications

- antihypertensive effects may be reduced if given with rifampicin or sulfinpyrazone
- hyperkalaemia and myocardial depression may occur if given with IV dantrolene
- if starting simvastatin or atorvastatin with verapamil, lowest dose should be used in the first instance. If adding verapamil to already existing simvastatin or atorvastatin, statin dose should be reduced
- see General Interactions of calcium-channel blockers (p. 520)

Nursing points/Cautions

- given by slow IV over 2 minutes with continuous BP and ECG monitoring during IV therapy and if severe hypotension occurs, verapamil should be stopped
- liver enzymes should be monitored regularly throughout therapy
- sustained-release preparations are not considered interchangeable
- have noradrenaline, isoprenaline, atropine (reversing bradycardia, hypotension), dopamine, digoxin and calcium gluconate monohydrate 10% solution available
- may require digoxin pretreatment in the presence of existing congestive cardiac failure
- ensure that correct formulation of tablets is selected because verapamil is available in sustained-release formulation as well as immediate-release formulation
- caution if given to those with supratentorial tumour as increased intracranial pressure may occur during anaesthetic induction
- caution if used in those with advanced Duchenne's muscular dystrophy or decreased neuromuscular transmission (e.g. myasthenia gravis) due to decrease in neuromuscular transmission. Can precipitate respiratory muscle failure in patients with progressive muscular dystrophy
- contraindicated in those with atrial flutter or fibrillation with accessory bypass tracts (e.g. Wolff-Parkinson-White syndrome), ventricular tachycardia or decreased liver function
- see Nursing points/Cautions for calcium-channel blockers (p. 521)

Patient teaching and advice

- see for General Patient teaching and advice for antianginal agents (p. 61)
- see Patient teaching and advice for calcium-channel blockers (p. 521) and antihypertensive agents (p. 489)

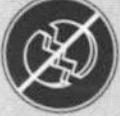

modified-release tablets should not be chewed, broken or crushed

plain tablets can be crushed and mixed with spoonful of yoghurt or apple puree

Note

- contained in Tarka with trandolapril

CENTRALLY ACTING AGENTS

General Actions of centrally acting agents

- central action by stimulating alpha-2 adrenoceptors, causing a reduction in sympathetic tone, resulting in reduced heart rate, peripheral vascular resistance and BP
- decrease both supine and standing BP

CLONIDINE HYDROCHLORIDE (Catapres)

Available forms

Tablets: 100 microgram, 150 microgram; Ampoules: 150 microgram/mL

Action

- see General Actions of centrally acting agents (above)

- thought to modify the response of peripheral blood vessels to vasoconstricting and vasodilating stimuli (e.g. noradrenaline, isoprenaline, angiotensin)
- (oral) onset of action 0.5–1 hour, peak effect 2–4 hours, duration of action 6–12 hours, half-life 9–26 hours

Use

- hypertension
- acute hypertensive crisis (parenteral)
- prophylaxis of migraine or recurrent vascular headache (more than one headache/month)
- menopausal flushing

Dose

- (hypertension) initially 75 microgram orally 2–3 times daily, then increasing gradually by 75 microgram increments to 150–300 microgram orally 3 times daily if needed (daily maximum 900 microgram) (150 microgram tablets) OR
- (hypertension) initially 50–100 microgram orally 2–3 times daily, increasing gradually to daily maximum of 600 microgram in divided doses (100 microgram tablets) OR
- (hypertensive crisis) 150–300 microgram IM, may be repeated at 3–6-hour intervals if needed OR
- (hypertensive crisis) 150–300 microgram diluted in 10 mL sodium chloride 0.9% given slowly IV over 5 minutes, may be repeated at 3–6-hour intervals if needed OR
- (migraine prophylaxis, menopausal flushing) initially 25 microgram orally each morning and night. If necessary, increasing dose to 50 microgram twice daily after 2 weeks, and then to 75 microgram twice daily

Adverse effects

- depression, sleep disturbance, dizziness, sedation, headache, fatigue, anxiety, weakness
- erectile dysfunction
- hypotension
- dry mouth, constipation, nausea, vomiting, anorexia, salivary gland pain
- (uncommon) reduced lacrimal flow, increased blood glucose levels, bradycardia, nasal dryness, blurred vision, pruritus, rash, urticaria, Raynaud's phenomenon

Interactions

- increased risk of QT prolongation and arrhythmias when IV clonidine is given with high-dose IV haloperidol
- bradycardia may be caused or potentiated if given with cardiac glycosides or beta-adrenoceptor blocking agents
- if given with beta-adrenoceptor blocking agents and therapy is interrupted, beta-adrenoceptor blocking agents should be stopped first, followed by clonidine
- antihypertensive activity may be reduced by TCAs and some antipsychotic agents (with alpha receptor blocking effects)
- not recommended with NSAIDs because they decrease the effects of clonidine
- effects decreased if given with alpha-2 adrenoceptor blocking agents (e.g. phentolamine)
- caution if used with other antihypertensive agents
- may potentiate effects of alcohol, sedatives, hypnotics and other centrally acting agents
- increased risk of bradycardia if given with digoxin or beta-adrenoceptor blocking agents

Nursing points/Cautions

- IM injection should be given while patient is supine
- there may be a transient hypertensive response of 5–10 mmHg lasting for about 5 minutes after IV injection (reduced by slower IV administration)

- withdrawal from oral therapy should be gradual over 7 days or more to avoid rebound hypertension, especially if taking high doses
- regular ophthalmological examination is recommended if therapy is prolonged
- score and carefully divide tablet for doses under 100 mg
- (migraine) if frequency of attacks decreases significantly, dose should be reduced and gradually stopped
- tablets contain lactose and are not recommended in those with galactose intolerance
- ampoule contains 3.3 mg sodium per ampoule
- should only be used for one indication at a time (e.g. if used for migraine, should not be used as antihypertensive concurrently)
- caution if used in the elderly or those with history of depression, advanced cerebrovascular disease, diabetes mellitus, mild-to-moderate bradyarrhythmias, cerebral or peripheral perfusion disorders, polyneuropathy, history of constipation, recent myocardial infarction or renal insufficiency
- contraindicated in those with sick sinus syndrome, second- or third-degree AV block, severe coronary disease or heart failure

Patient teaching and advice

- patient wearing contact lenses should be warned about reduced lacrimal flow
- patient should be advised to avoid driving or operating machinery if dizziness or blurred vision are ongoing problems
- those with diabetes mellitus should be instructed to closely monitor blood glucose levels during therapy
- patient should be warned to avoid alcohol during therapy
- see also General Patient teaching and advice for antihypertensive agents (p. 489)

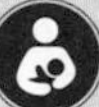

may cause fetal bradycardia and also elevated blood glucose in the newborn, therefore only used during pregnancy if benefits outweigh risks. Should not be used IV during pregnancy

not recommended during breastfeeding

tablet can be dispersed in water or crushed and mixed with spoonful of yoghurt or apple puree (has bitter taste)

METHYLDOPA SESQUIHYDRATE (METHYLDOPA) (Aldomet, Hydopa)

Available form

Tablets: 250 mg

Action

- see General Actions of centrally acting agents (p. 530)
- active metabolite thought to stimulate central alpha-2 receptors reducing sympathetic outflow to heart, kidneys and peripheral blood vessels
- no direct action on cardiac function, with little effect on kidney function
- may decrease renin activity
- peak effect 4–6 hours (single dose) or 48–72 hours (multiple dosing), duration of action 12–24 hours (single dose) or 24–48 hours (multiple dosing)

Use

- hypertension

Dose

- (hypertension) initially 250 mg orally 2–3 times daily for 2 days, then increased/decreased gradually at 2-day intervals as required (daily maximum 3 g)

Adverse effects

- transient drowsiness/sedation, headache, weakness/asthenia, dizziness, light-headedness, impaired mental acuity
- postural hypotension, oedema and associated weight gain
- bradycardia, carotid sinus hypersensitivity, aggravation of angina, AV block
- depression, mild reversible psychoses, nightmares, anxiety
- nausea, vomiting, dry mouth, sore or 'black' tongue, flatulence, abdominal distension, constipation or diarrhoea, colitis
- fever (usually in first 3 weeks of therapy)
- rash, eczema
- nasal stuffiness
- impotence, decreased libido
- mild arthralgia (with or without joint swelling), myalgia
- abnormal liver function tests, jaundice (with or without fever), hepatitis
- breast enlargement, gynaecomastia, lactation, hyperprolactinaemia, amenorrhoea
- (prolonged therapy) positive Coombs' test
- (rare, but serious requiring prompt discontinuation) haemolytic anaemia, leucopenia, thrombocytopenia, bone marrow depression, hepatic necrosis

Interactions

- enhanced hypotension when given with thiazide diuretics and antihypertensive agents
- contraindicated with MAOIs
- bioavailability may be reduced if given with oral iron (or multivitamin preparations containing iron)
- may increase serum lithium levels, increasing the risk of lithium toxicity, therefore serum levels should be closely monitored, especially when starting or stopping therapy or adjusting dose
- antihypertensive effect may be reduced if given with TCAs
- reduced doses of anaesthetic agents may be needed if given together
- may cause fluorescence in urine samples, therefore will interfere with diagnosis of pheochromocytoma

Nursing points/Cautions

- urine may darken on exposure to air
- differential blood counts and liver function tests should be monitored for first 6–12 weeks of therapy or if patient has unexplained fever
- if dose increase is required and patient has previously experienced sedation, evening dose should be first increased
- if patient requires blood transfusion and has had positive Coombs' test, retesting using indirect Coombs' test is recommended to prevent possibility of incompatible blood transfusion occurring
- hypertension returns within 48 hours of stopping therapy
- caution if used in those with impaired kidney or liver function or history of depression
- contraindicated in those with active cirrhosis, acute hepatitis, porphyria, pheochromocytoma or paraganglioma, haemolytic anaemia, sulfite sensitivity or methyldopa-induced liver disorder

Patient teaching and advice

- advise patient that sedation usually lasts 2–3 days when therapy is started or dose is increased
- patient should be warned that fever commonly occurs in first 3 weeks of therapy

- patient should be instructed to seek medical advice immediately if any of the following occur:
  - any fever (especially in first 12 weeks of therapy)
  - yellowing of eyes or skin, tiredness, loss of appetite, upper abdominal pain, dark urine, pale stools
  - fever, chills, sore throat, mouth ulcers
  - tiredness, pallor, shortness of breath
  - feelings of lowered mood or depression
- instruct patient to separate any iron supplements or vitamins (containing iron) by at least 2 hours from therapy
- see also General Patient teaching and advice for antihypertensive agents (p. 489)

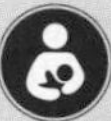

only used during pregnancy if benefits are thought to outweigh risks

caution if used during breastfeeding

tablet can be dispersed in water or crushed and mixed with spoonful of yoghurt or apple puree

MOXONIDINE (Moxotens, Physiotens)

Available forms

Tablets: 0.2 mg, 0.4 mg

Action

- centrally acting antihypertensive, which differs from others in this class because it has a low affinity for alpha-2 adrenoreceptors
- also binds to I_1-imidazoline receptors decreasing sympathetic tone
- decreases systemic vascular resistance reducing arterial BP
- heart rate, cardiac output and stroke volume are unaffected
- half-life 2.2–2.8 hours

Use

- hypertension

Dose

- initially 0.2 mg orally mane, increasing after a 2-week interval to 0.4 mg (single or divided dose, morning and evening). If unsatisfactory response after 2 weeks, dose increased to 0.6 mg (as a divided dose) (single dose maximum 0.4 g or daily maximum as divided dose 0.6 g)

Adverse effects

- asthenia, headache, dizziness, somnolence, sleep disturbance
- anxiety
- vertigo
- dry mouth, diarrhoea, nausea
- (uncommon) sedation, insomnia, rash, pruritus, urticaria, peripheral oedema
- (rare) hypotension, postural hypotension, angioedema

Interactions

- hypotensive effect enhanced if given with other antihypertensive agents
- may intensify effects of sedative, hypnotics and benzodiazepines
- not recommended with TCAs or alcohol

Nursing points/Cautions

- if therapy is concurrent with beta-adrenoceptor blocking agent and stopping is required, beta-adrenoceptor blocking agent should be stopped first, followed by monoxidine several days later to prevent rebound hypertension. Blood pressure should be closely monitored during this time
- tablets contain lactose and are therefore not recommended in those with rare hereditary problems of galactose intolerance, Lapp lactase deficiency or glucose–galactose malabsorption
- caution if used in those with history of angioneurotic oedema, severe coronary artery disease, unstable angina, predisposition to AV block (including those with first-degree AV block)

- caution if used in those with moderate kidney impairment (GFR > 30 < 60 mL/min, serum creatinine > 105 < 160 micromol/L). Dose should not exceed 0.4 g as daily divided dose or 0.2 g as single daily dose
- not recommended in those with intermittent claudication, Raynaud's disease/syndrome, Parkinson's disease, epilepsy, depression or glaucoma
- contraindicated in those over 75 years or with heart failure, bradycardia (< 50 beats/min), severe bradyarrhythmias (e.g. sick sinus syndrome), AV block (second or third degree), malignant arrhythmias or severe kidney impairment (GFR < 30 mL/min or serum creatinine > 160 micromol/L)

Patient teaching and advice

- patient should be instructed to immediately seek medical advice if any unusual swelling of face, eyes, lips, inside nose, mouth or throat or shortness of breath or breathing difficulties occur
- see General Patient teaching and advice for antihypertensive agents (p. 489)

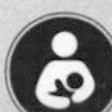

only used during pregnancy or breastfeeding if benefits are thought to outweigh risks

tablet can be dispersed in water or crushed and mixed with spoonful of yoghurt or apple puree

DIRECT ACTING VASODILATORS

DIAZOXIDE (Diazoxide Injection BP)

Available form

Ampoules: 300 mg/20 mL

Action

- reduces elevated BP by activation of potassium channels resulting in relaxation of constricted smooth muscle in the peripheral arterioles (vasodilation), which reduces peripheral resistance
- reflex increase in heart rate and cardiac output
- increases blood glucose levels
- onset of action 1 minute, peak effect 2–5 minutes, duration 2–12 hours, long elimination half-life (28 hours)

Use

- hypertensive crises (e.g. acute glomerular nephritis)
- malignant hypertension (emergency management)
- reduce danger of haemorrhage in hypertensive patients undergoing renal biopsy or arteriography
- control of chronic hypertension before starting oral antihypertensive therapy

Dose

- 1–3 mg/kg as an IV bolus over 30 seconds (up to a maximum of 150 mg), may be repeated at 5–15-minute intervals if required **OR**
- 300 mg as an IV bolus over 30 seconds, may be repeated at 5–15-minute intervals if required

Adverse effects

- transient nausea, vomiting, abdominal cramps
- transient hyperglycaemia

- sodium and water retention (and therefore weight gain, oedema and possibly congestive cardiac failure)
- headache, sensation of warmth, flushing, sweating, light-headedness, transient weakness, burning/itching, dizziness
- (local) pain, sensation of warmth along vein
- (rare) rash, fever, leucopenia, thrombocytopenia, severe hypotension

Interactions

- may potentiate antihypertensive effect of other antihypertensive agents
- diuretics may enhance hyperglycaemic, hyperuricaemic and hypotensive effects of diazoxide
- hyperglycaemic effect may be potentiated if hypokalaemia is present

Nursing points/ Cautions

- must be given undiluted IV rapidly over 30 seconds for maximum effect as slow administration may reduce effectiveness
- may be repeated at 4–24-hour intervals for up to 5 days if needed, then replaced with oral antihypertensive agent
- avoid extravasation
- not given SC or IM because of high alkalinity
- patient should remain recumbent during and for 30 minutes after IV bolus
- BP is recorded before and at 1-minute intervals after IV bolus for the first 5 minutes, then at 5-minute intervals until BP has stabilised, then hourly
- if patient is ambulant, final BP should be measured while patient is standing
- blood counts are recommended if therapy is prolonged
- serum uric acid should be monitored if patient has a history of hyperuricaemia or gout
- monitor blood glucose levels daily
- diuretic may be necessary if sodium and water retention occur
- has a very long half-life (28 hours), therefore patient should be observed carefully for a longer period if overdosage occurs
- incompatible with hydralazine, lidocaine (lignocaine) and propranolol
- caution if used in those with renal insufficiency, impaired carbohydrate metabolism (including diabetes mellitus), impaired cardiac or cerebral circulation or uraemia (e.g. gout)
- contraindicated in those with hypersensitivity to diazoxide or other thiazide derivatives or with hypertension caused by mechanical obstruction (e.g. aortic coarctation)

Patient teaching and advice

- see General Patient teaching and advice for antihypertensive agents (p. 489)

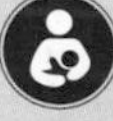

may inhibit uterine contractions if given during labour. Also, enters fetal circulation and may cause fetal bradycardia and hyperglycaemia in the newborn

HYDRALAZINE HYDROCHLORIDE (Alphapress, Apresoline)

Available forms

Tablets: 25 mg, 50 mg; Ampoule: 20 mg

Action

- causes direct relaxation of arteriolar smooth muscle reducing peripheral vascular resistance (little effect on veins)
- reflex increase in heart rate, stroke volume and cardiac output
- causes sodium and fluid retention
- increase renal blood flow and plasma renin activity

- maintains cerebral blood flow
- increased risk of toxicity due to decreased metabolism in some Caucasians and Asians
- onset of action 45 minutes (oral), 10–20 minutes (IV)
- peak effect 1 hour (oral), 15–30 minutes (IV)
- duration of action 3–8 hours, half-life 3–7 hours

Use

- moderate-to-severe drug resistant hypertension (with other antihypertensive agents)
- hypertensive crises (especially in pre-eclampsia and eclampsia) (see Pregnancy, childbirth and breastfeeding, p. 1389)

Dose

- (hypertension) initially 25 mg orally twice daily, increasing over several weeks, maintenance 50–200 mg in 2 divided doses

Adverse effects

- tachycardia, palpitations, flushing, hypotension, angina, ECG changes
- headache
- arthralgia, myalgia, joint swelling
- stuffy nose
- rash
- peripheral neuritis
- diarrhoea, nausea, vomiting, anorexia
- (prolonged therapy, daily dose > 100 mg) SLE-like syndrome (fever, rash, arthralgia, anaemia)
- (uncommon) proteinuria, anaemia, leucopenia, purpura, agranulocytosis, dizziness, increased lacrimation

Interactions

- caution if given with MAOIs as severe hypotension may occur
- hypotensive effect may be enhanced if given with other antihypertensive agents, vasodilators, diuretics, TCAs, antipsychotic agents and alcohol
- may increase bioavailability of beta-adrenoceptor blocking agents
- enhanced cardiac effects if given with adrenaline (epinephrine)
- hypotensive effect may be antagonised by NSAIDs or oestrogens
- increased hypotension may occur if given just before or after diazoxide

Nursing points/Cautions

- daily dose >100 mg should be avoided to decrease risk of SLE-like syndrome
- (long-term therapy) urinalysis, FBE and antinuclear factor (ANF) should be monitored 6-monthly. Microhaematuria and/or proteinuria with positive ANF titres may indicate early SLE-like syndrome
- may cause hypotension during surgery, which should not be corrected with adrenaline (epinephrine) due to increased heart rate effects
- women are at greater risk of SLE-like syndrome
- not recommended in those with kidney or liver impairment, heart failure or until post-infarction stabilisation has occurred
- caution if used in those with coronary artery disease (beta-adrenoceptor blocking agent should be started at least 3 days before hydralazine) or angina
- caution if used in those with cerebrovascular disease as ischaemia may occur
- contraindicated in those with SLE or related diseases, severe tachycardia, heart failure with high cardiac output (e.g. thyrotoxicosis), myocardial insufficiency with aortic/mitral valve stenosis, constrictive pericarditis, dissecting aortic aneurysm, cor pulmonale, porphyria, dissecting aortic aneurysm or hypersensitivity to dihydrazine

Patient teaching and advice

- advise patient to avoid alcohol during therapy
- patient should be instructed to immediately report any:
  - joint pain, fever and skin rash
  - chest pain
- see General Patient teaching and advice for antihypertensive agents (p. 489)

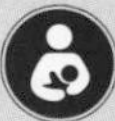

may cause fetal distress and arrhythmias if given during third trimester and should only be used if benefits are thought to outweigh risks

not recommended during breastfeeding unless benefits are thought to outweigh risks

tablet can be dispersed in water or crushed and mixed with spoonful of yoghurt or apple puree

MINOXIDIL (Hair A-Gain, Loniten, Regaine)

Available forms

Tablets: 10 mg; Topical solution: 20 mg/mL, 50 mg/mL; Foam: 50 mg/mL

Action

- selectively relaxes arteriolar smooth muscle reducing peripheral vascular resistance lowering BP (little effect on veins)
- reflex mediated increase in cardiac output
- increases plasma renin activity
- onset of action 30 minutes, peak effect 2–3 hours, half-life 4–4.5 hours, hypotensive action lasts 24 hours

Use

- as adjunctive therapy with beta-adrenoceptor blocking drugs and diuretics in adults with severe refractory hypertension (Loniten)
- alopecia androgenetica (hereditary or common baldness) (Hair A-Gain, Regaine) (see Minoxidil in Dermatological agents, p. 965)

Dose

- (hypertension) initially 5 mg orally daily, increasing by 5–10 mg at 3-day intervals to 50 mg, then increasing at 25 mg daily increments to 100 mg as a single or divided dose if needed (daily maximum 100 mg)

Adverse effects

- fluid and salt retention, oedema, weight gain
- nausea, vomiting, anorexia
- reversible hypertrichosis, hair colour changes
- pericarditis, tachycardia, pericardial effusion, ECG changes, cardiac tamponade
- (rare) rash, leucopenia, thrombocytopenia, pleural effusion, breast tenderness

Interactions

- hypotensive effects may be enhanced by other antihypertensive agents
- must be given with a diuretic to avoid fluid retention and a beta-adrenoceptor blocking agent to control reflex cardiovascular effects (or methyldopa sesquihydrate or clonidine if beta-adrenoceptor blocking agent is contraindicated)

Nursing points/Cautions

- (heart failure) weight, fluid and electrolyte balance should be carefully monitored and diuretic given if fluid retention occurs. Diuretic therapy +/– salt restriction may be recommended if fluid retention occurs
- not recommended for labile or mild hypertension or for extended time in those with hypertension improved by surgery or with myocardial infarction until post infarction stabilisation has occurred

- caution if used in those with unstable or recently diagnosed angina pectoris, pulmonary hypertension with mitral valve regurgitation or those with symptomatic heart failure as deterioration may occur
- caution if used in those with symptomatic heart failure as fluid retention may cause worsening
- contraindicated in those with pheochromocytoma and pulmonary hypertension caused by mitral valve stenosis

Patient teaching and advice

- warn patient of unusual growth, thickening and darkening of fine body hair (face, arms and back), which usually occurs within 3–6 weeks of starting therapy and disappears within 1–3 months of stopping. Hair may also show colour change
- patient should be advised that excessive salt and water retention reduce effectiveness, therefore restrict dietary salt and take diuretic if prescribed
- advise patient to immediately report any:
  - puffiness or swelling of face, eyes, ankles, hands or feet
  - weight gain (especially if > 2 kg)
  - increase in heart rate or chest pain
- see also General Patient teaching and advice for antihypertensive agents (p. 489)

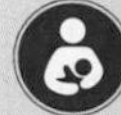

not recommended during pregnancy or breastfeeding. Minoxidil has been associated with abnormal amount of hair growth in the newborn when used during pregnancy

tablet can be dispersed in water or crushed and mixed with spoonful of yoghurt or apple puree

SODIUM NITROPRUSSIDE (DBL Sodium Nitroprusside Concentrated Injection)

Available form

Vial: 50 mg/2 mL

Action

- potent short-acting IV agent that relaxes vascular smooth muscle, producing peripheral vasodilation by a direct action on vascular smooth muscle, more active on veins than arteries
- decreases preload and afterload, improving cardiac output
- metabolised to cyanide and cyanmethaemoglobin. Ordinarily, the body deals with cyanide by combining it with thiosulfate to produce thiocyanate, which is excreted in the urine. Cyanide also binds to erythrocytic methaemoglobin and mitochondrial cytochromes. However, when the mitochondrial cytochromes become saturated, there is a switch from aerobic to anaerobic metabolism producing lactic acid
- onset of action/peak effect within minutes, half-life 2 minutes, half-life of thiosulfate 3 days (prolonged if kidney failure exists)
- duration of effect 1–10 minutes after stopping infusion

Use

- hypertensive crises
- elective hypotension to reduce surgical haemorrhage
- short-term management of cardiac failure

Dose

- initially 0.3 microgram/kg/minute by IV infusion, then titrated upwards to a maximum of 10 microgram/kg/minute if needed

Adverse effects

- (if too rapid reduction in BP) nausea, vomiting/retching, abdominal pain,

flushing, sweating, muscle twitching, anxiety, agitation, restlessness, dizziness, headache, palpitations
- excessive postural hypotension, tachycardia, bradycardia, ECG changes
- rash, flushing, skin irritation
- ileus
- methaemoglobinaemia
- (prolonged administration or excessive dose) thiocyanate toxicity (tinnitus, miosis, hyperreflexia, blurred vision, ataxia, headache, nausea, vomiting, shortness of breath, delirium, psychosis, confusion, coma)
- cyanide toxicity (hypotension, metabolic acidosis, pink colour (skin, mucous membranes), shallow breathing, decreased reflexes, widely dilated pupils, coma)
- signs of hypothyroidism
- decreased platelet aggregation
- increased intracranial pressure
- (IV site) reddened, venous streaking

Interactions

- hypotensive action enhanced by other antihypertensive agents, inhalation anaesthetics, negative inotropes and most other circulatory depressants
- hypertension and pretreatment with antihypertensive agents may sensitise patient to the effects of sodium nitroprusside and therefore risk of cyanide poisoning
- thiocyanate interferes with iodine uptake in thyroid gland

Nursing points/Cautions

- BP should be monitored continuously during therapy as hypotensive effect can occur rapidly. BP should not be allowed to drop rapidly (systolic BP should not be less than 60 mmHg). Venous oxygen level and acid–base balance should be measured frequently. Patient should also be monitored closely for any signs of air hunger, confusion or metabolic (lactic) acidosis, which is indicative of cyanide poisoning. However, acidosis is not a reliable indication of cyanide poisoning because it is a late sign appearing about 1 hour after dangerous cyanide levels have been reached. Patient should also be monitored for retching or vomiting, muscular twitching, sweating and/or agitation as these are signs of a rapid drop in BP
- patient should remain recumbent during infusion to avoid severe postural hypotensive effects
- if severe hypotension occurs, infusion should be stopped and patient placed in a head-down (Trendelenburg) position to maximise venous return
- if BP is not controlled within 10 minutes at maximum infusion rate, therapy should be stopped immediately
- (elective hypotension for surgery) any pre-existing anaemia and/or hypovolaemia should be corrected before starting therapy
- (acute congestive heart failure) infusion rate should be titrated to haemodynamic monitoring results and urine output. Oral therapy should be commenced as soon as possible
- BP returns to pretreatment levels within 1–10 minutes of infusion being stopped or slowed
- if patient is receiving maximum rate (10 microgram/kg/min) and has impaired oxygen delivery, methaemoglobin levels should be closely monitored
- dilute concentrated solution in 500 mL glucose 5% (100 microgram/mL) or 1000 mL glucose 5% (50 microgram/mL), depending on the desired concentration
- no other drugs to be added as solution becomes highly coloured (blue, green, dark red), even if small

quantities of organic or inorganic substances are mixed with IV solution. If colour occurs, solution should be discarded
- protect from light by wrapping immediately in aluminium foil, black plastic sheeting or some other opaque material. However, it is not necessary to protect drip chamber
- burette, infusion pump or micro-drip regulator should be used to deliver the IV solution
- infusion rate should not exceed 2 microgram/kg/minute as this will lead to accumulation of cyanide ions
- avoid extravasation
- when infusion is stopped, IV tubing should be changed to prevent any extra administration from residual solution in tubing
- simultaneous infusion of sodium thiosulfate pentahydrate (rate 5–10 times rate of sodium nitroprusside infusion) should prevent cyanide poisoning from occurring
- cyanide toxicity may be treated with sodium nitrite (4–6 mg/kg), followed by sodium thiosulfate pentahydrate (150–200 mg/kg). This may be repeated after a 2-hour interval at half the previous dose if needed
- if haemodialysis is used in overdose, it does not remove cyanide, but does remove thiocyanate
- caution if used in the elderly (because of increased sensitivity to hypotension), those with known raised intracranial pressure, hypothyroidism, severe renal or liver dysfunction or hypothermia
- not recommended for compensatory hypertension due to arteriovenous shunt or coarctation of the aorta
- contraindicated in those with acute congestive heart failure associated with decreased peripheral vascular resistance, arteriovenous shunt or coarctation of the aorta, uncorrected anaemia or hypovolaemia, inadequate cerebral circulation, severe renal disease, congenital optic atrophy or tobacco amblyopia or vitamin B_{12} deficiency disorder

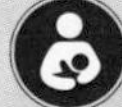

not used in pregnancy or breastfeeding unless the expected benefits outweigh any potential risks

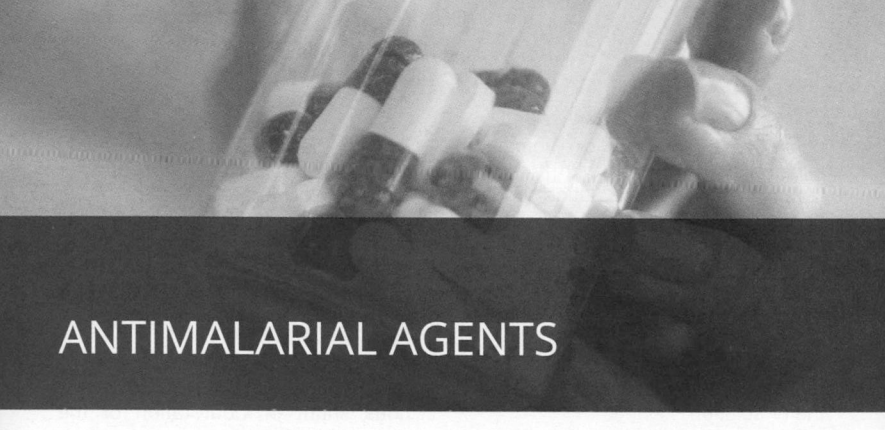

ANTIMALARIAL AGENTS

Malaria is the major parasitic illness in tropical and subtropical countries, with an estimated 219 million cases spread across 87 countries in 2017. Figures show that there were about 435,000 deaths in 2017, with an estimate of one child dying every 2 minutes from malaria. In 2017, Africa had disproportionally high numbers, accounting for 92% of all cases and 93% of all deaths from malaria (WHO 2019c).

Malaria is spread by *Plasmodium* parasites, transmitted through the bites of infected female *Anopheles* mosquitoes (referred to as malaria vectors). There are five species known to cause malaria in humans (*Plasmodium vivax*, *P. ovule*, *P. falciparum* or *P. malariae*, *P. knowlesi*). *P. vivax* and *P. falciparum* pose the greatest threat, with *P. falciparum* being responsible for the most malaria-related deaths worldwide, being most prevalent in Africa (White & Ashley 2018; WHO 2019c).

Initial symptoms of malaria begin 10 to 15 days after the infected mosquito bite and include headache, fatigue, muscle and joint aches, abdominal discomfort and lethargy (similar to symptoms of any simple viral illness), followed by fever, chills, sweating, anorexia, vomiting and worsening malaise. Infections with *P. vivax* or *P. ovule* have cycles of fever spikes, chills and rigors that occur at regular intervals, weeks to months after the first infection. If left untreated or treated ineffectively, the parasites continue to replicate and severe disease may result (especially if due to *P. falciparum*), which may be fatal (White & Ashley 2018; WHO 2019c).

The malarial life cycle

The infected mosquito feeds on a human and, in doing so, injects sporozoites into the bloodstream. The sporozoites enter the liver's hepatocytes where they multiply and develop into exo-erythrocytic (pre-erythrocytic or tissue) schizonts. Schizonts of *P. vivax* and *P. ovule* may lie dormant in the liver and are responsible for relapses (primaquine acts at this point) (White & Ashley 2018).

After 5–16 days, tissue schizonts rupture, releasing merozoites into the bloodstream, where they invade erythrocytes (blood, or erythrocytic, stage) (quinine, mefloquine and proguanil act at this point). Merozoites multiply asexually and mature, causing the erythrocytes to rupture, releasing the matured asexual merozoites (after 48–72 hours), which then invade more erythrocytes and continue the multiplying, maturing and rupturing cycle (this produces the clinical symptoms of slowly rising temperature, shaking chills, rapidly rising temperature and profuse sweating). Within these infected erythrocytes, some merozoites also develop into male and female gametocytes (White & Ashley 2018).

A non-infected mosquito then feeds on the infected human, ingesting male and female gametocytes, which then multiply sexually and develop into sporozoites. Some of these sporozoites migrate to the mosquito's salivary glands and will subsequently infect the next person the mosquito feeds on (the mosquito life cycle is 8–35 days, depending on the species of parasite and temperature) (White & Ashley 2018).

Treatment

Before starting any treatment, it is essential that malaria is confirmed using a diagnostic test (e.g. thick and thin blood smears), rather than relying on symptoms alone. Repeat blood smears every 12–24 hours for 48 hours if the first smears are negative, but malaria is strongly suspected (White & Ashley 2018; WHO 2019c).

Many of the original treatments for malaria were herbal-based (such as quinine, extracted from tree bark). Unfortunately, *P. falciparum* developed resistance to chloroquine in the 1950s and since then multiple drug resistance has made prophylaxis and treatment very difficult in many areas of the world. The choice of antimalarial should therefore be based on sensitivity of the infecting parasite, with chloroquine being considered first-line treatment for non-*falciparum* malarias, except in areas (such as Indonesia and Papua New Guinea) where high levels of resistance in *P. vivax* are present (White & Ashley 2018).

First-line treatment of uncomplicated falciparum malaria has changed and is now based on artemisinin-based combination therapy. This treatment is also suitable for other malarias. However, some resistance to artemisinin combination therapy has emerged in parts of South-east Asia, including Vietnam, Cambodia and Thailand, increasing the risk that this multi-drug resistance could spread to other regions (WHO 2019c).

Prevention

Malaria transmission can be prevented by controlling the vector (mosquito). Successful programs have included the use of insecticide-treated nets for sleeping and spraying indoors with insecticides. In 2015, the World Health Organization (WHO) recommended a large clinical trial be carried out to evaluate a vaccine (RTS, S) against *P. falciparum*, which is currently being piloted in three African countries with promising results including preventing about 4 in 10 cases of malaria in children over a 4-year period (WHO 2019c).

Other agents used for prevention and treatment include doxycycline (see Antibacterial agents, p. 194) and hydroxychloroquine (see Disease-modifying antirheumatic drugs (DMARDS), p. 977).

General Patient teaching and advice for people travelling in malarial areas

- prophylactic antimalarial therapy may not always prevent malaria
- travellers should purchase their prophylactic antimalarials from a reputable source before going into a

malarious country as there have been issues with counterfeit and substandard drugs in some countries
- prophylactic antimalarial therapy should be started 2 days to 2 weeks (depending on the drug) before departure and generally continued for 4 weeks after leaving the endemic area (except for atovaquone-proguanil or primaquine, which can be stopped 1 week after leaving the endemic area). Starting the prophylactic antimalarial therapy before departure will allow a therapeutic blood concentration to build up before entering the endemic area, as well as detecting any adverse effects
- avoid being out at dusk or in the early night hours when mosquitoes feed
- wear long sleeves and long pants and avoid dark colours
- avoid using colognes and perfumes because these may attract mosquitoes
- use a recommended insect repellent containing up to 10–35% diethyltoluamide (commonly known as DEET); however, it is not recommended for young children. Insect repellent containing 7% picaridin can also be used
- use mosquito nets, ensuring that the nets have no holes and are tucked into mattresses
- close windows and doors at night if they do not have screens
- if possible, use pyrethroid mosquito coils at night
- seek medical advice promptly if fever, malaise, headache, backache, muscle ache and/or weakness, vomiting, diarrhoea or cough develop within 1 week of entering a known malarial area.

Malaria and pregnancy

Pregnant women are advised to avoid travelling to malarial areas if possible. Malaria can result in miscarriage and low birth weight, as well as increasing the risk of maternal death (White & Ashley 2019b).

ARTEMETHER AND LUMEFANTRINE (Riamet)

Available forms

Tablets and Tablets (dispersible): artemether 20 mg/lumefantrine 120 mg

Action

- schizonticide
- both drugs inhibit the conversion of haem (toxic) to haemozoin (non-toxic) and also inhibit nucleic acid synthesis in the parasite
- lumefantrine interferes with polymerisation step
- artemether is a derivative of artemisinin and produces reactive metabolites
- ratio is 1:6 (artemether:lumefantrine)
- artemether has an active metabolite
- antimalarial effect of combination is greater than either substance alone. Clears gametocytes from blood in less than a week and more rapidly than non-artemisinin antimalarial agents
- lumefantrine half-life 2–3 days, artemether half-life 2 hours

Use

- treatment of acute uncomplicated malaria caused by *P. falciparum* in adults, children and infants ≥ 5 kg
- (dispersible tablets) as above in infants and children between 5 and 35 kg

Dose

- 4 tablets orally with food at 0 (time of diagnosis), 8, 24, 36, 48 and 60 hours (total of 24 tablets) **OR**

- (infants, children 3 months–12 years, 5 kg < 15 kg) initially 1 tablet orally, then 1 tablet after 8 hours, followed by 1 tablet twice daily (morning and evening) for 2 days (total 6 tablets) (dispersible tablets) **OR**
- (children 3 months–12 years, 15 kg–< 25 kg) initially 2 tablets orally, then 2 tablets after 8 hours, followed by 2 tablets twice daily (morning and evening) for 2 days (total 12 tablets) (dispersible tablets) **OR**
- (children 3 months–12 years, 25 kg–< 35 kg) initially 3 tablets orally, then 3 tablets after 8 hours, followed by 3 tablets twice daily (morning and evening) for 2 days (total 18 tablets) (dispersible tablets)

Adverse effects

- headache, dizziness, sleep disturbance
- palpitations
- decreased appetite, anorexia, abdominal pain, nausea, vomiting, dyspepsia, diarrhoea
- infection
- myalgia, arthralgia, back pain
- fever, asthenia, fatigue, rigors
- pharyngitis, coughing
- anaemia
- increased liver function tests, splenomegaly
- pruritus, rash, urticaria
- (rare) QT interval prolongation, hypersensitivity including angioedema

Interactions

- contraindicated with any other agents known to prolong QT interval (such as macrolides, azole antifungals, antipsychotics, some antidepressants, fluoroquinolones and antiarrhythmic agents class IA or III) or cause electrolyte disturbance, especially hypokalaemia or hypomagnesaemia
- contraindicated with other agents metabolised by cytochrome enzyme CYP2D6 (e.g. metoprolol, flecainide, imipramine, amitriptyline, clomipramine)
- contraindicated with rifampicin, carbamazepine, phenytoin and St John's wort
- food (including milk) enhances absorption
- not recommended with other antimalarial agents (as some prolong QT interval)
- caution if used with protease inhibitor antiretroviral agents
- not recommended with grapefruit juice
- may decrease effectiveness of hormonal contraceptives

Nursing points/Cautions

- not recommended for malaria prophylaxis or treatment of malaria due to other causes, including complicated malaria (e.g. cerebral malaria)
- a second course may be given for new infection or recurrence
- tablets and dispersible tablets are not bioequivalent
- ECG and blood potassium monitoring are recommended for those with cardiac, renal or hepatic impairment
- caution should be used if given to those with a cardiac history (e.g. bradycardia, congestive heart failure, electrolyte disturbances (low potassium or magnesium), cardiac arrhythmias, pre-existing QT interval prolongation) or those taking drugs that are known to prolong the QT interval. ECG and potassium monitoring should occur in such patients before starting and regularly throughout therapy
- caution if used in those with severe liver impairment
- contraindicated in those with severe malaria (WHO definition), with known or family history of prolonged QT interval (or sudden death) or other

condition which may prolong QT interval or those with an electrolyte imbalance (e.g. hypokalaemia, hypomagnesaemia)

Patient teaching and advice

- patient should be advised to take tablets whole with food or fluids as food increases bioavailability, especially those rich in fat such as milk
- instruct patient that dispersible tablets should be dissolved in water (about 10 mL per tablet), gently stirred and taken immediately. Glass should be rinsed with small amount of water and taken to ensure total dose is administered
- if patient vomits within 1 hour of taking tablets, dose should be readministered
- warn patient not to drive or operate machinery if dizziness, fatigue or asthenia occur
- advise patient to avoid grapefruit juice during therapy
- instruct patient to seek medical advice immediately if any of the following occur:
  - feeling too unwell to eat or drink
  - unexplained persistent nausea and vomiting
  - irregular or fast heart beat
  - yellowing of skin/eyes, dark urine, tiredness, upper right-sided abdominal pain
- women of childbearing potential should be counselled to use effective forms of contraception during therapy to prevent pregnancy occurring. Two methods (hormonal and non-hormonal) are recommended
- see General Patient teaching and advice for people travelling in malarial areas (p. 543), and General Patient teaching and advice (p. xxvii)

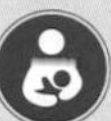

contraindicated during the first trimester of pregnancy and should be used during trimester 2 or 3 only if benefits outweigh potential risks to the fetus

not recommended during breastfeeding. Breastfeeding should not recommence within 4 weeks of last dose

tablets are dispersible in water

ATOVAQUONE AND PROGUANIL HYDROCHLORIDE (Malarone Tablets 250/100, Malarone Junior Tablets 62.5/25, Promozio 250/100)

Available forms

Tablets: atovaquone 62.5 mg/proguanil hydrochloride 25 mg, atovaquone 250 mg/ proguanil hydrochloride 100 mg

Action

- interferes with two different pathways in biosynthesis of pyrimidines needed for nucleic acid replication
- combined activity is synergistic
- half-life of atovaquone is 2–3 days in adults and 1–2 days in children
- half-life of proguanil and active metabolite is 12–15 hours in both adults and children
- proguanil has active metabolites which have antimalarial actions

Use

- prophylaxis and treatment of *P. falciparum* malaria

Dose

Prophylaxis

- (adults, children weighing > 40 kg) 1 tablet (250/100) orally daily starting 1–2 days before entering malaria endemic area and continued for 7 days after leaving area **OR**

- (children weighing 11–20 kg) 1 tablet (62.5/25) orally daily starting 1–2 days before entering malaria endemic area and continued for 7 days after leaving area **OR**
- (children weighing 21–30 kg) 2 tablets (62.5/25) orally daily starting 1–2 days before entering malaria endemic area and continued for 7 days after leaving area **OR**
- (children weighing 31–40 kg) 3 tablets (62.5/25) orally daily starting 1–2 days before entering malaria endemic area and continued for 7 days after leaving area

Treatment

- (adults, children weighing $>$ 40 kg) 4 tablets (250/100) orally as a single dose for 3 consecutive days **OR**
- (children weighing 11–20 kg) 1 tablet (250/100) orally as a single dose for 3 consecutive days **OR**
- (children weighing 21–30 kg) 2 tablets (250/100) orally as a single dose for 3 consecutive days **OR**
- (children weighing 31–40 kg) 3 tablets (250/100) orally as a single dose for 3 consecutive days

Adverse effects

- diarrhoea, dyspepsia, gastritis, vomiting, abdominal pain, mouth ulcers, anorexia, constipation
- hepatomegaly, elevated liver function tests
- pruritus, hair loss, rash
- fever
- headache, dreams, insomnia
- dizziness, lethargy, asthenia
- backache, myalgia
- visual impairment
- cough
- postural hypotension, palpitations
- anaemia, neutropenia

Interactions

- not recommended with rifampicin, rifabutin, tetracycline or metoclopramide as they decrease atovaquone plasma levels reducing antimalarial activity
- if given with metoclopramide or tetracycline, parasitaemia should be closely monitored
- proguanil may potentiate warfarin, therefore INR should be closely monitored especially when starting or stopping therapy
- may decrease serum levels of indinavir
- serum levels may be decreased if given with efavirenz
- serum levels may be decreased by paracetamol, benzodiazepines, aciclovir, opioids, cephalosporins, antidiarrhoeals and laxatives

Nursing points/Cautions

- if recurrent infection or treatment fails, a different antimalarial agent should be used
- not recommended for treatment of cerebral malaria or other severe manifestations of complicated malaria (e.g. hyperparasitaemia, pulmonary oedema or renal failure)
- not recommended for prophylaxis or treatment of malaria in paediatric patients weighing $<$ 11 kg
- not recommended in those with severe liver impairment
- contraindicated in those with known sensitivity to atovaquone or proguanil or for prophylaxis in those with severe renal impairment (creatinine clearance $<$ 30 mL/minute)

Patient teaching and advice

- instruct patient to swallow tablet whole at same time every day with food or a milky drink
- warn patient that tablet has a bitter taste
- if children have problems swallowing the tablet whole, advise parent to crush tablet and add to small amount of milk, which should be taken immediately

- advise patient that if he/she vomits within 1 hour of dosing, a repeat dose should be taken. If diarrhoea occurs, normal dosing should occur
- (prophylaxis) patient should be advised to start tablets 1 to 2 days before entering malaria endemic area and continue for 7 days after leaving area
- see General Patient teaching and advice for people travelling in malarial areas (p. 543), and General Patient teaching and advice (p. xxvii)

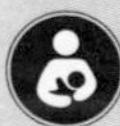

should only be used during pregnancy if benefits are thought to outweigh risks

not recommended during breastfeeding

tablet can be crushed and mixed with small amount of milk or yoghurt

MEFLOQUINE HYDROCHLORIDE (Lariam)

Available form

Tablets: 250 mg

Action

- quinoline-methanol antimalarial
- structurally related to quinine
- blood schizonticide that destroys asexual erythrocytic form of *P. vivax* and *P. malariae* and most strains of *P. falciparum*, although some resistance has been reported in South-east Asia
- no effect on gametocytes of *P. falciparum*
- half-life about 21 days

Use

- (treatment) acute attack of *P. falciparum* malaria resistant to conventional antimalarial drugs
- (prophylaxis) multi-drug-resistant *P. falciparum* in those considered at high risk of malaria

Dose (adults and children more than 45 kg

- (treatment) initially 750 mg orally, followed by 500 mg 6–8 hours later (total 1250 mg) **OR**
- (prophylaxis) 250 mg orally as a single weekly dose starting 1 week before exposure and continuing for 2 weeks after leaving the malarial area

Adverse effects

- anorexia, nausea, vomiting, diarrhoea, abdominal pain, mouth ulcers
- tinnitus
- rash, pruritus
- hair loss
- myalgia
- fever, chills
- dizziness, dream disturbances, insomnia, fatigue, headache, vertigo, fuzzy thinking
- visual disturbances
- palpitations, cardiac conduction alterations, bradycardia
- anxiety, depression
- (uncommon) mood changes, confusion, agitation, hallucinations, paranoia, psychosis, seizures
- (rare) aplastic anaemia, agranulocytosis, hypersensitivity

Interactions

- not recommended with quinine because ECG abnormalities or convulsions may occur
- may decrease serum levels of antiepileptic agents and therefore decrease seizure control
- immunisation with live typhoid vaccine should be completed at least 3 days before starting mefloquine
- not recommended with any other agents that are known to prolong the QT interval (e.g. antiarrhythmic agents, beta-adrenergic blocking agents, calcium-channel blockers, antihistamines, phenothiazines, tricyclic antidepressants, H_1 receptor blocking agents)
- serum levels may be reduced by rifampicin

Nursing points/Cautions

- not recommended for malaria prophylaxis in patients with epilepsy because the risk of seizures is increased
- not recommended in children under 14 years or those adults with cardiac disease
- caution if used in those with impaired liver function as clearance may be prolonged, increasing risk of adverse effects
- contraindicated in those with active or history of depression, psychosis, anxiety disorders, schizophrenia or other major psychiatric disorders, epilepsy, severe liver or kidney impairment, or known hypersensitivity to related compounds (e.g. quinine)

Patient teaching and advice

- advise patient to immediately seek medical advice if any of the following occur:
  - signs of anxiety, depression, confusion, hallucinations, paranoia or restlessness (these signs may signal more serious psychiatric problems)
  - any visual disturbances or eye problems
  - difficulty sleeping or abnormal/strange dreams
  - seizures (fits)
  - chest pain, irregular heart beat
- patient should be instructed that malaria prophylaxis with mefloquine be started at least 1 week before travel commences as acute psychiatric adverse effects usually occur at the start of therapy
- instruct patient that tablet should be swallowed whole with plenty of liquid and taken always on the same day of the week. If patient vomits within 30 minutes of tablet ingestion, a second full dose should be taken. If vomiting occurs between 30 and 60 minutes, half dose should be taken
- advise patient that because of the long half-life, adverse effects may continue after medication has been withdrawn
- warn patient against driving a vehicle or operating machinery if dizziness, loss of balance or confusion are a problem
- women of childbearing potential should be counselled to use effective contraceptive throughout therapy and for at least 3 months after taking mefloquine because it may cause fetal abnormalities
- see General Patient teaching and advice for people travelling in malarial areas (p. 543), and General Patient teaching and advice (p. xxvii)

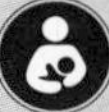

use in treatment of malaria is acceptable because small risk to fetus is outweighed by benefits to mother and fetus

should not be used during breastfeeding

tablet can be crushed and mixed with juice or water or spoonful of yoghurt, apple puree, jam or honey

PRIMAQUINE PHOSPHATE (Primacin)

Available form

Tablets: 7.5 mg

Action

- aminoquinoline
- schizontocide active against exo-erythrocytic forms of *P. vivax* and *P. ovule* and primary exo-erythrocytic stage of *P. falciparum*
- prevents transmission of *P. falciparum* by eliminating reservoir
- more active against tissue form and gametes than asexual blood form

- active metabolite longer half-life than parent
- half-life 4.3–7.4 days

Use

- (radical cure) prevention of relapse of *P. vivax* and *P. ovale* infection
- adjunct treatment for *P. falciparum* infection (gametocytes)

Dose

- (radical treatment) 15 mg orally daily with food for 14 days, increasing to 30 mg for malaria-resistant strains or where treatment has failed at 15 mg **OR**
- (radical treatment in those with G6PD deficiency) up to 45 mg once weekly for 8 weeks (with monitoring for haemolysis) **OR**
- (reduction of *P. falciparum* gametocyte numbers) 45 mg orally with food as a single dose

Adverse effects

- nausea, vomiting, abdominal cramps/pain
- headache, dizziness
- rash, pruritus
- cardiac arrhythmia, QT interval prolongation
- haemolytic anaemia (at high doses or those with G6PD deficiency) methaemoglobinaemia
- (high dose) leucopenia, agranulocytosis, neutropenia

Interactions

- contraindicated with drugs that suppress bone marrow or cause haemolysis
- caution if used with other agents known to prolong QT interval or cause electrolyte imbalance

Nursing points/Cautions

- testing for G6PD is recommended before starting therapy and not commenced if deficiency is found to be severe
- frequent blood cell counts and haemoglobin estimations should be done during therapy for early detection of haemolysis
- ECG monitoring is recommended in those with cardiac disease, history of arrhythmias, bradycardia, long QT syndrome or uncorrected hypokalaemia or hypomagnesaemia
- tablets contain lactose and should be used with caution in lactose-intolerant individuals
- caution if used in those with family or personal history of favism due to increased risk of haemolytic anaemia
- caution if used in those with nicotinamide adenine dinucleotide (NADH) methaemoglobin reductase deficiency as methaemoglobinaemia may occur
- contraindicated in acutely ill patients with tendency to granulocytopenia (e.g. rheumatoid arthritis, SLE)
- contraindicated in those with severe G6PD deficiency because haemolytic anaemia may occur. If used in those with moderate G6PD deficiency, close blood monitoring of haemoglobin and haematocrit is recommended
- contraindicated in those with known hypersensitivity to hydroxyquinolines

Patient teaching and advice

- patient should be advised not to drive or operate machinery if dizziness occurs
- advise patient to immediately seek medical advice if any of the following occur:
  - loss of appetite, back, leg or abdominal pain, reddening or darkening of the urine, pale skin, weakness, fever (haemolytic anaemia)
  - bluish tint to skin, gums, fingernails or around mouth, dizziness, breathing difficulties, weakness (methaemoglobinaemia)
  - rapid or irregular heart beats

- see General Patient teaching and advice for people travelling in malarial areas (p. 543), and General Patient teaching and advice (p. xxvii)

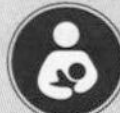

contraindicated during pregnancy

caution if used during breastfeeding

tablet can be crushed and mixed with water or spoonful of yoghurt or apple puree

QUININE BISULFATE HEPTAHYDRATE (QUININE BISULFATE) (Quinbisul)

QUININE DIHYDROCHLORIDE (Quinine Dihydrochloride 6% Sterile Concentrate)

QUININE SULFATE DIHYDRATE (QUININE SULFATE) (Quinate)

Available forms

Tablets: 300 mg; Vial: 600 mg/10 mL

Action

- antimalarial thought to interfere with plasmodial DNA inhibiting replication
- also leads to accumulation of haem during erythrocytic stages of infection
- no action on liver stages
- half-life 16 hours (in those with malaria), 11 hours (healthy people)
- half-life prolonged in those with hepatitis or moderate chronic liver disease

Use

- effective against *P. falciparum* that is resistant to other antimalarial drugs (chloroquine and related 4 aminoquinolines)
- (IV) severe *P. falciparum* malaria
- (IV) can also be used in the treatment of Babesiosis (malaria-like parasitic disease) (with clindamycin)

Dose

- initially 20 mg/kg by IV infusion over 4 hours (up to 1400 mg) (loading dose), then 10 mg/kg (up to 700 mg) 8–12-hourly after loading dose and repeated 8–12-hourly if needed
- 600 mg orally 3 times daily after meals for 7–14 days (with pyrimethamine 75 mg and sulfadoxine 1.5 g orally on day 2 of therapy)

Adverse effects

- headache
- fever
- nausea, vomiting, epigastric pain
- (hypersensitivity reaction) rash, urticaria, pruritus, skin flushing, fever, facial oedema, sweating, dyspnoea, tinnitus, GI distress
- blood dyscrasias, thrombocytopenia, acute haemolysis
- reversible visual disturbances (including photophobia, blurred vision, diplopia, scotomata, disturbed colour vision)
- vertigo, tinnitus, deafness
- apprehension, restlessness, confusion
- syncope
- anuria, uraemia, haemoglobinuria
- hypoglycaemia
- hypoprothrombinaemia
- cardiac rhythm disturbance including ventricular tachycardia, angina
- hepatotoxicity
- cinchonism: initially tinnitus, dizziness, rash and abdominal pain/cramping, followed by (at higher doses) headache, fever, vomiting, apprehension, confusion and convulsions

Interactions

- may increase serum digoxin levels, increasing the risk of toxicity, therefore serum levels should be monitored regularly throughout therapy

- risk of toxicity may be increased if given with pyrimethamine
- may enhance effects of anticoagulants, therefore prothrombin time should be monitored regularly especially when starting or stopping quinine
- clearance may be reduced if given with cimetidine increasing serum levels and risk of toxicity
- absorption may be decreased by aluminium-containing antacids
- beverages containing quinine (e.g. tonic water) should be avoided in excess amounts because the risk of adverse effects and toxicity is increased
- may potentiate effects of neuromuscular blocking agents increasing risk of respiratory difficulties
- HIV protease inhibitors may have an unpredictable effect on quinine, therefore are not recommended together
- may inhibit HMG-CoA reductase inhibitor (statins) metabolism, increasing risk of toxicity including rhabdomyolysis
- decreased serum levels may result if given with rifampicin and are therefore not recommended together
- serum levels may be increased by acetazolamide and sodium bicarbonate (urinary alkalisers), increasing the risk of toxicity
- may potentiate effects of depolarising and non-depolarising muscle relaxants
- excretion may be increased if given with urinary acidifiers, resulting in decreased serum levels

Nursing points/Cautions

- before administering, patient should be asked about any known sensitivities to quinine or quinidine
- if the patient has atrial fibrillation, digitalisation should be completed before starting quinine
- therapy should be changed from IV to oral as soon as practical
- during IV administration, pulse, BP and blood glucose should be closely monitored
- IV loading dose is not required if antimalarial agents have been taken in previous 24 hours
- (IV) diluted in 500 mL glucose 5% or sodium chloride 0.9% and infused slowly over 4 hours
- if IV therapy is required for longer than 48 hours, maintenance dose should be reduced to 5 mg/kg to avoid accumulation. Serum levels should also be monitored
- not recommended by IM route due to being highly irritant causing pain, necrosis and abscess formation. However, if IV route is not available, IM can be used as last resort
- (IV) incompatible with amiodarone, pancuronium, suxamethonium, rocuronium, atracuronium, mivacurium, vecuronium, mannitol, ketamine, diuretics especially furosemide (frusemide) and heparin
- discontinue immediately if any haemolytic or hypersensitivity reaction occurs
- solution should be protected from light
- caution if used in those with atrial fibrillation or impaired hepatic or renal function
- contraindicated in those with haemolysis, history of blackwater fever (dengue fever), diabetes, G6PD deficiency, tinnitus, myasthenia gravis, optic neuritis, hypersensitivity to quinine or quinidine or previous quinine-induced thrombocytopenia or uraemic syndrome

Patient teaching and advice

- warn patient about bitter taste of tablets
- patients should be advised to seek medical advice immediately if any of the following occur:
  - flushing, itching, rash, fever, facial swelling, shortness of breath
  - ringing in the ears
  - changes to vision
  - increased heart rate
  - persistent diarrhoea or cramping
  - loss of appetite, back, leg or abdominal pain, reddening or darkening of the urine, pale skin, weakness, fever
- advise patient that aluminium-containing antacids should be avoided or spaced at least 2 hours apart from quinine
- warn patient not to drink excess amounts of quinine-containing drinks (e.g. tonic water, bitter lemon)
- see General Patient teaching and advice for people travelling in malarial areas (p. 543), and General Patient teaching and advice (p. xxvii)

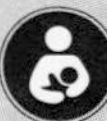

in high doses, quinine may cause deafness, disturbed development and/or cranial and extremity malformation in the fetus, as well as inducing uterine contractions, increasing the risk of abortion

the use of antimalarial agents in the treatment of malaria during pregnancy is an acceptable risk because the benefits to the mother and fetus outweigh the risks to the fetus

use with caution during breastfeeding because quinine is secreted in breastmilk

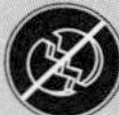

tablets should not be crushed by pregnant women

tablet can be crushed and mixed with orange juice or spoonful of yoghurt or apple puree

Note

- sulfate and bisulfate salts are used interchangeably

TAFENOQUINE SUCCINATE (Kodatef, Kozenis)

Available form

Tablets: 100 mg, 150 mg

Action

- aminoquinoline
- exact mechanism of action unknown, but kills developing asexual, developing exoerythrocytic and latent hypnozoites
- long half-life 17 days

Use

- malaria prophylaxis (for up to 6 months) (Kodatef)
- radical cure (prevention of relapse) of *P. vivax* malaria in patients aged 16 years and over (Kozenis)

Dose

- 200 mg orally once daily for 3 days before travelling to malarial area (loading dose), then 200 mg orally weekly starting 7 days after last loading dose (maintenance dose) while in malarial area, then 200 mg orally in last week following exit from malarial area 7 days after last maintenance dose (terminal/final dose) (Kodatef) **OR**
- 300 mg orally as single dose on day 1 or 2 of 3-day chloroquine therapy (Kozenis)

Adverse effects

- diarrhoea, nausea, vomiting, gastrointestinal reflux disorder
- headache, migraine, tension headache, dizziness, motion sickness
- back pain
- insomnia, abnormal dreams, nightmares, sleep disorder, depression, depressed mood, anxiety
- vortex keratopathy (corneal deposits)

- increased/abnormal liver enzymes
- (rare) haemolytic anaemia, methaemoglobinaemia, anaemia
- (rare) hypersensitivity (can be delayed in onset and/or duration), neurosis, agitation

Interactions

- caution if given with procainamide
- caution if used with metformin due to increased risk of lactic acidosis
- caution if used with other agents such as dapsone which may cause haemolysis

Nursing points/Cautions

- all patients should be screened for glucose-6-phosphate dehydrogenase (G6PD) deficiency before starting therapy because of the risk of haemolytic anaemia
- therapy should only be continued for up to 6 months continuously (Kodatef)
- recommended in those 18 years and over (Kodatef)
- contraindicated in those with current or history of psychosis, delusions or hallucinations
- contraindicated in those with G6PD deficiency or if G6PD status is unknown
- contraindicated in those with known hypersensitivity to other aminoquinolines

Patient teaching and advice

- advise patient to swallow tablets whole, not chewed or broken apart
- if patient vomits within 60 minutes, dose can be readministered (but only once) (Kozenis)
- if gastrointestinal disturbances occur, suggest tablets are taken with food
- patients are advised to seek medical attention immediately if any of the following occur:
  - pale skin, weakness, dizziness, confusion, dark coloured urine
  - headache, shortness of breath, fatigue, lethargy, confusion, nausea, rapid heart beat
  - changes in mood, depression
- females of reproductive capacity should be counselled to use effective contraception during and for 12 weeks after stopping therapy
- see General Patient teaching and advice for people travelling in malarial areas (p. 543), and General Patient teaching and advice (p. xxvii)

contraindicated during pregnancy and breastfeeding

ANTIMIGRAINE AGENTS

Migraine is a common neurological condition affecting about 20.5% of Australians (4.9 million). Women are more than twice as likely to experience migraine than men, with females aged 25 to 29 having the highest prevalence of chronic migraine ($\geq$ 15 migraine days/month), and those aged 35 to 39 having the highest rate of episodic migraine. The economic cost of migraine in Australia in 2018 was estimated to be $35.7 billion, made up of health system costs, costs due to lost productivity and other costs (Deloitte Access Economics 2018). However, this does not take into account the impact of migraine on the wellbeing and quality of life of the person experiencing migraine.

The International Headache Society has the following criteria for migraine which include: attacks being episodic; the duration of an attack being 4 to 72 hours in length (untreated or unsuccessfully treated); headache being unilateral, throbbing and/or aggravated by movement or routine activity (e.g. walking, climbing stairs); moderate-to-severe in intensity; causing either nausea/vomiting or both photophobia and phonophobia (International Headache Society 2019). Not all headache disorders respond to the same medication, therefore correct diagnosis is essential in ensuring migraine is promptly treated while other causes of headache are ruled out.

The premonitory phase (predrome) of migraine is defined as non-painful symptoms that precede hours to days before the headache onset and are predictive of impending migraine. These symptoms can include neck stiffness, photophobia, phonophobia, osmophobia, nausea, yawning, sleep disturbance, thirst, food craving, fatigue, memory impairment, difficulty with concentration, depression and irritability. These premonitory symptoms can also exist during the headache, as well as postdrome, once the headache has resolved (Karsan et al 2018).

Every person diagnosed with migraine should have an action plan for management of an acute attack. The plan should be individualised to include individual differences, such as the presence of nausea or vomiting and time to peak severity. First-line treatment usually involves paracetamol, NSAIDs (e.g. aspirin, diclofenac, naproxen) and triptans. It is important that patients understand the importance of optimising treatment by taking medication early. Furthermore, it is also important that the clinician assesses response to treatment by determining factors, such as whether the person was pain-free within 2 hours of taking medication, whether one dose of medication relieved headache and kept it away for at least 24 hours, and whether taking the medication led to the patient feeling in control of the migraine with minimal to no disruption of daily activities. Not meeting patient expectations on factors such as these leads to non-adherence and dissatisfaction with the management plan (Vargas 2018).

Prevention of migraine involves a multi-pronged attack, including modification of lifestyle (e.g. regular sleep/wake cycle, regular meals, exercising, reducing stress), identification and avoidance of triggers and risk factors (e.g. excessive caffeine, sleep disorders, obesity), and if needed, the use of preventative medication. The goal of this combined approach is to reduce migraine attack frequency and duration, as well as reducing the severity of symptoms and migraine-related disability. Behavioural therapies, such as relaxation and cognitive behavioural therapy, should also be considered in the overall management plan. It is important to ensure the patient is engaged in any preventative plan (especially pharmacological agents) as the rate of adherence has been shown to be low (Schwedt 2018).

Medication overuse can lead to the development of chronic headaches ('medication overuse headache') in some people, resulting in refractory headaches that are unresponsive to treatment and occur more frequently (daily or almost daily). The definition of 'overuse' is dependent on the medication used. For example, overuse of simple analgesics is considered if taken for 15 or more days per month, whereas antimigraine medications or combination analgesics are considered overused when taken 10 or more days per month (Schwedt 2018).

ELETRIPTAN HYDROBROMIDE (Relpax)

Available forms

Tablets: 40 mg, 80 mg

Action

- potent and selective $5HT_{1B/1D}$ agonist
- $5HT_{1B}$ receptors are thought to mediate intracranial blood vessel constriction
- half-life about 4 hours

Use

- acute migraine (with or without aura)

Dose

- initially 20–80 mg orally, with second dose after $>$ 2 hours if migraine recurs (maximum dose 160 mg in 24-hour period)

Adverse effects

- paraesthesia, dizziness, somnolence, headache, asthenia, hypoaesthesia, vertigo
- pharyngitis, throat tightness
- chest tightness/pain/pressure, palpitations, tachycardia
- abdominal discomfort/pain/cramps, dry mouth, dyspepsia, dysphagia, nausea, vomiting
- chills, sensation of warmth/flushing, sweating
- back pain, myalgia, myasthenia, hypertonia
- medication overuse headache (see introduction, above)

Interactions

- contraindicated with or within 24 hours of ergot alkaloids
- contraindicated with or within 48 hours of macrolide antibiotics (erythromycin, clarithromycin), antifungal agents (itraconazole) or protease inhibitors (ritonavir, indinavir or saquinavir)

- contraindicated with other $5HT_1$ receptor agonist
- caution if used with SSRIs, SNRIs or triptans due to risk of serotonin syndrome
- caution if given with St John's wort

Nursing points/Cautions

- a clear diagnosis of migraine should be established and other neurological conditions ruled out before starting therapy in those with no previous history of migraine
- cardiovascular assessment is recommended for those who are at risk of coronary artery disease
- caution if used in postmenopausal women, males > 40 years, or those with other risks for coronary artery disease
- not recommended for hemiplegic, ophthalmoplegic or basilar migraine or atypical headaches where cerebrovascular vasoconstriction could be harmful
- not recommended for those with heart failure
- contraindicated in those with severe liver impairment, uncontrolled hypertension, coronary artery disease, angina, previous myocardial infarction, ischaemic heart disease, variant (Prinzmetal's) angina, peripheral vascular disease, CVA, transient ischaemic attack

Patient teaching and advice

- patient should be advised to take medication early in onset of symptoms during acute migraine attack, although still effective if taken later in attack
- instruct patient to swallow tablets whole with water
- advise patient that if first dose is not effective, second dose is unlikely to relieve migraine during same attack. However, if migraine recurs after initial relief, second dose can be administered after 2 hours of initial dose (daily maximum 160 mg)
- patient should be warned against driving or operating machinery if dizziness or drowsiness occur
- see General Patient teaching and advice (p. xxvii)

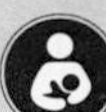

only used during pregnancy if benefits outweigh risks

caution if used during breastfeeding. Not recommended within 24 hours of therapy

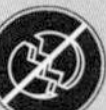

tablet should not be crushed, but can be dispersed in water

ERENUMAB (Aimovig)

Available form

Prefilled pen (Autoinjector): 70 mg/mL

Actions

- human immunoglobulin G2 (IgG2) (monoclonal antibody) with a high affinity for CGRP receptor (CGRP is a neuropeptide that modulates nociceptive signalling and a vasodilator whose levels increase during migraine and return to normal with headache relief)
- half-life 28 days

Use

- prevention of migraine

Dose

- 70 mg SC monthly, increasing to 140 mg if needed

Adverse effects

- constipation
- fatigue
- pruritus
- sinusitis, bronchitis, flu-like symptoms
- (injection site) pain, redness, pruritus
- antibody development
- (rare) hypersensitivity

Nursing points /Cautions

- initial therapy should be started by neurologist or migraine specialist
- therapy should be evaluated after 8–12 weeks, then 3–6-monthly
- if patient is receiving 140 mg, given as two consecutive SC injections
- first injection should be under medical supervision
- name and batch number should be recorded in patient history
- needle cover contains latex and may cause allergic reaction in those with latex sensitivity

Patient teaching and advice

- instruct patient that medication has no effect during an acute attack
- patient should be instructed in correct administration technique, including:
    - check expiry date and do not use if expired
    - pen should be at room temperature for 30 minutes before administration
    - pen should be protected from direct sunlight and not warmed using heat source (e.g. microwave, hot water)
    - pens should not be returned to fridge once they have reached room temperature
    - SC injections into abdomen (not within 5 cm of navel), thigh or upper arm
    - injection sites should be rotated and area not used if skin is broken, reddened, bruised or tender
    - inspect pen before use and do not use if cloudy, discoloured or contains flakes/particles, or if the pen is cracked, broken or has been dropped or white cap is missing
    - site should be cleaned with alcohol wipe and allowed to dry
    - remove white cap from pen (do not recap) and inject within 5 minutes to prevent solution drying out
    - stretch or pinch skin to make firm surface, place pen on skin at 90 degrees and firmly push pen down until it stops moving. When ready to inject, press purple start button and click should be heard. Keep pushing down on skin (should take about 15 seconds) until window turns yellow showing injection is complete
    - do not rub injection site. If there is small sign of blood, adhesive plaster (e.g. Band-Aid) can be applied
    - if 140 mg is required, a second injection will be required using the above steps
    - needle should automatically be covered with green safety guard when removed from skin
    - pen and white cap should be disposed of safely in a sharps container (not in household waste)
    - pen should not be reused or recycled
    - pens should be stored in original carton in refrigerator (2–8°C) and protected from sunlight
    - if removed from fridge, can be kept at room temperature for up to 14 days but must be discarded after that time if not used
    - pen should not be frozen or shaken

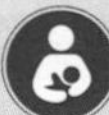

not recommended during pregnancy or breastfeeding unless benefits outweigh risks

FREMANEZUMAB (Ajovy)

Available form

Prefilled syringe: 150 mg/mL

Actions

- humanised monoclonal antibody (IgG4) with a high affinity for CGRP receptor (CGRP is a neuropeptide

that modulates nociceptive signalling and a vasodilator whose levels increase during migraine and return to normal with headache relief)
- derived from recombinant DNA technology using Chinese hamster ovary
- half-life 31 days

Use
- prevention of migraine

Dose
- 225 mg SC once-monthly **OR**
- 675 mg SC 3-monthly

Adverse effects
- (injection site) pain, induration, erythema, pruritus
- development of neutralising antibodies
- (uncommon) rash
- (rare) hypersensitivity

Nursing points/Cautions
- initial therapy should be started by neurologist or migraine specialist
- therapy should be evaluated after 8–12 weeks, then 3–6-monthly
- patient can be taught to self-administer
- first self-administered injection should be under medical supervision
- if changing from one dosing regimen to the other, dose should be given on next scheduled administration date
- name and batch number should be recorded in patient history
- contraindicated in those with hypersensitivity to Chinese hamster ovary protein

Patient teaching and advice
- instruct patient that medication has no effect during an acute attack
- advise patient that injection site reactions usually occur within 1 day of injection and resolve within 5 days
- patient should be instructed to seek medical advice if any signs of allergy occur, including swelling of lips/tongue/face, trouble breathing, shortness of breath, wheezing, rash, hives or itching
- see Galcanezumab Patient Teaching and advice for self-administration instructions (p. 560)
- for multiple injections (3-monthly dosing), same injection site should not be used
- do not administer at same injection site with any other injectable agents

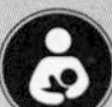
not recommended during pregnancy or breastfeeding unless benefits outweigh risks

GALCANEZUMAB (Emgality)

Available form
Prefilled pen (Autoinjector)/prefilled syringe: 120 mg/mL

Actions
- humanised monoclonal antibody (IgG4) with a high affinity for CGRP receptor (CGRP is a neuropeptide that modulates nociceptive signalling and a vasodilator whose levels increase during migraine and return to normal with headache relief)
- derived from recombinant DNA technology using Chinese hamster ovary
- half-life 27 days

Use
- prevention of migraine

Dose
- initially 240 mg SC (loading dose), then 120 mg monthly

Adverse effects
- vertigo
- constipation
- pruritus, rash
- (injection site) redness, pruritus, bruising, swelling
- (rare) anaphylaxis, angioedema, urticaria
- antibody development

Nursing points/Cautions

- initial therapy should be started by neurologist or migraine specialist
- therapy should be evaluated after 8–12 weeks, then 3–6-monthly
- for loading dose of 240 mg, given as two consecutive SC injections
- first injection should be under medical supervision
- name and batch number should be recorded in patient history
- contraindicated in those with hypersensitivity to Chinese hamster ovary protein

Patient teaching and advice

- instruct patient that medication has no effect during an acute attack
- advise patient that injection site reactions usually occur within 1 day of injection and resolve within 5 days
- patient should be instructed to seek medical advice if any signs of allergy occur including swelling of lips/tongue/face, trouble breathing, shortness of breath, wheezing, rash, hives or itching
- patient should be instructed in correct administration technique, including:
    - check expiry date and do not use if expired
    - pen/syringe should be at room temperature for 30 minutes before administration
    - pen/syringe should be protected from direct sunlight and not warmed using heat source (e.g. microwave, hot water)
    - pen/syringe should not be returned to fridge once they have reached room temperature
    - SC injections into abdomen (not within 5 cm of navel), thigh or upper arm
    - injection sites should be rotated and area not used if skin is broken, reddened, bruised or tender
    - do not administer at same injection site with any other injectable agents
    - inspect pen/syringe before use and do not use if cloudy, discoloured or contains flakes/particles or if pen/syringe is damaged in any way
    - pen/syringe should not be reused or recycled
    - pen/syringe should be stored in original carton in refrigerator (2–8°C) and protected from sunlight
    - if removed from fridge, syringe can be kept at room temperature for up to 7 days, but must be discarded after that time if not used
    - pen/syringe should not be frozen or shaken
    - dispose of used pen/syringe safely in a sharps container (not in household waste)

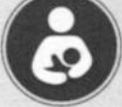

not recommended during pregnancy or breastfeeding unless benefits outweigh risks

NARATRIPTAN HYDROCHLORIDE (Naramig)

Available form

Tablets: 2.5 mg

Action

- selective serotonin agonist ($5HT_1$ receptors are found mainly in the cerebral and dural vessels) with little or no effect on other serotonin receptors
- half-life 6 hours

Use

- treatment of acute migraine attack (with or without aura)

Dose

- 2.5 mg orally and, if symptoms recur, a further 2.5 mg may be given after 4 hours (daily maximum 5 mg)

Adverse effects

- palpitations, chest pain/discomfort, chest pressure/heaviness
- warm sensation, feeling of heaviness, numbness
- nausea, vomiting, hyposalivation
- muscle pain, stiffness and tightness
- dizziness, drowsiness, malaise, fatigue, vertigo, headache
- medication overuse headache (see introduction, p. 556)
- (rare) severe cardiac events, ischaemic colitis, somnolence, hypersensitivity, peripheral vascular ischaemia, long-term ophthalmological effects

Interactions

- contraindicated with other $5HT_1$ receptor agonists or other triptans
- side-effects may be increased if given with St John's wort, therefore not recommended together
- not recommended with SSRIs or SNRIs due to risk of serotonin syndrome

Nursing points/Cautions

- a clear diagnosis of migraine should be established and other neurological conditions ruled out before starting therapy in those with no previous history of migraine
- cardiovascular assessment is recommended for those who are at risk of coronary artery disease
- caution if used in postmenopausal women, males > 40 years, or those with other risks for coronary artery disease
- not recommended for hemiplegic, basilar or ophthalmoplegic migraine
- not recommended in those <12 or >65 years
- contains sulfonamide, therefore is contraindicated in those with known hypersensitivity to any sulfonamide
- contraindicated in those with a history of myocardial infarction, ischaemic heart disease, variant (Prinzmetal's) angina, history of CVA or transient ischaemic attacks, peripheral vascular disease, uncontrolled hypertension or severe impaired kidney (creatinine clearance < 15 mL/minute) or liver function

Patient teaching and advice

- ensure that patient understands therapy is for management of acute migraine, not prevention
- instruct patient to take early in onset of headache for best effect
- patient should be advised that if dose is not effective, second dose is unlikely to work during same attack
- advise patient to take tablets whole with water
- patient should be warned not to drive or operate machinery if they experience dizziness, vertigo or drowsiness
- advise patient to report any pain or purple discolouration of fingers, toes, ears, nose or jaw (peripheral vascular ischaemia)
- see General Patient teaching and advice (p. xxvii)

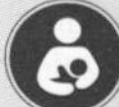

not recommended during pregnancy unless benefits outweigh the risks

breastfeeding should be discontinued for 24 hours after taking naratriptan

tablet can be dispersed in water or crushed and mixed with spoonful of yoghurt or apple puree

PIZOTIFEN MALEATE (Sandomigran)

Available form

Tablets: 0.5 mg

Action

- serotonin antagonist with anti-bradykinin and antihistamine actions, as well as weak anticholinergic (muscarinic) actions

- action not fully understood but thought to inhibit reuptake of serotonin by platelets preventing loss of tone in extracranial blood vessels
- half-life 23 hours

Use

- prophylactically against recurrent typical or atypical migraine, vascular, vasomotor and cluster headaches (Horton's syndrome)

Dose

- initially 0.5 mg orally daily then increasing to 1.5 mg orally daily in single (nightly) or divided doses **OR**
- (refractory cases) 3–4.5 mg orally daily in 2–3 divided doses

Adverse effects

- sedation, dizziness, somnolence, fatigue
- dry mouth, nausea,
- increased appetite, increased weight
- medication overuse headache (see introduction, p. 556)
- (rare) seizures, insomnia, anxiety, hypersensitivity reaction, paraesthesia
- (withdrawal symptoms) depression, tremor, nausea, anxiety, malaise, dizziness, sleep disorder, decreased weight

Interactions

- CNS effects may be enhanced if given with alcohol, antihistamines (including common cold preparations), sedatives and hypnotics
- not recommended with MAOIs because of prolonged and intensified anticholinergic effects

Nursing points/Cautions

- abrupt cessation should be avoided to prevent withdrawal symptoms
- tablets contain lactose, therefore are not recommended in those with severe lactase deficiency, rare hereditary problems of galactose intolerance or glucose–galactose malabsorption
- caution if given to those with narrow-angle glaucoma, prostatic hypertrophy or urinary retention because of anticholinergic effects
- caution in those with epilepsy
- caution if used in those with kidney or liver impairment

Patient teaching and advice

- instruct patient that medication has no effect during an acute attack
- patient should be advised not to drink alcohol or use common cold preparations
- warn patient against driving or using machinery if dizziness and sedation are problems
- advise patient to avoid stopping therapy suddenly
- see General Patient teaching and advice (p. xxvii)

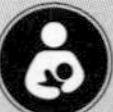

not recommended during pregnancy or breastfeeding unless benefits outweigh risks

tablet can be crushed and mixed with water or spoonful of yoghurt or apple puree

RIZATRIPTAN BENZOATE (Maxalt, Maxatan, Rixalt)

Available form

Wafer: 10 mg

Action

- $5HT_{1B/1D}$ agonist that causes selective constriction of extracerebral, intracranial arteries (which have been dilated during migraine attack)
- onset of action 30 minutes, half-life is 2–3 hours

Use

- acute migraine attack (with or without aura)

Dose

- 10 mg orally, dose can be repeated within 2 hours (maximum dose 30 mg in 24-hour period)

Adverse effects

- chest pain, palpitations, tachycardia
- dry mouth, nausea, vomiting, abdominal pain, diarrhoea, dyspepsia, thirst
- muscle heaviness, muscle pain, neck pain and stiffness, muscle weakness
- dizziness, headache, somnolence, paraesthesia, insomnia, tremor, ataxia, nervousness, vertigo, disorientation, asthenia, fatigue, decreased mental acuity
- flushing, pruritus, sweating
- blurred vision
- pharyngeal discomfort, dyspnoea
- medication overuse headache (see introduction, p. 556)

Interactions

- contraindicated with or within 2 weeks of MAOIs
- not recommended with other $5HT_{1B/1D}$ agonists
- not recommended within 6 hours of ergot alkaloids
- increased risk of serotonin syndrome if given with SSRIs, SNRIs and triptans
- increased serum levels may occur if given with propranolol
- caution if used with St John's wort

Nursing points/Cautions

- a clear diagnosis of migraine should be established and other neurological conditions ruled out before starting therapy in those with no previous history of migraine
- cardiovascular assessment is recommended for those who are at risk of coronary artery disease
- not recommended in those with basilar or hemiplegic migraine or atypical headaches
- tablets contain phenylalanine and therefore are not recommended in those with phenylketonuria
- contraindicated in those with uncontrolled hypertension, coronary artery disease, angina, variant (Prinzmetal's) angina, history of myocardial infarction, ischaemic heart disease, history of stroke or transient ischaemic attacks or peripheral vascular disease, including ischaemic bowel disease

Patient teaching and advice

- ensure that patient understands therapy is for management of acute migraine, not prevention
- patient should be advised that if first dose is ineffective in relieving migraine, second dose is unlikely to be effective
- if migraine recurs within 24 hours, dose can be repeated as long as there is a 2-hour separation from last dose and 30 mg daily maximum is not exceeded
- instruct patient to handle wafer with dry fingers and place on the tongue, allow to dissolve, and swallow with saliva
- see General Patient teaching and advice (p. xxvii)

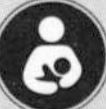

only recommended during pregnancy or breastfeeding if benefits outweigh risks

wafers can be dissolved on the tongue

SUMATRIPTAN (Clustran, Imigran, Imigran FDT, Imigran Mk II injection, Iptam, Sumatran)

Available forms

Tablets: 50 mg, 100 mg; Tablets (fast disintegrating): 50 mg, 100 mg; Nasal spray: 10 mg/0.1 mL, 20 mg/0.1 mL; Prefilled syringe/Autoinjector: 6 mg/0.5 mL

Action

- $5HT_1$ receptor agonist that selectively constricts cranial blood vessels
- response in 10–15 minutes (SC), 30 minutes (oral)

Use

- acute migraine attack (with or without aura)
- cluster headaches

Dose

- (migraine, cluster headache) 6 mg SC, followed by a further 6 mg SC at least 1 hour later if symptoms recur (maximum dose 12 mg in 24-hour period) **OR**
- (migraine) 50–100 mg orally, may be repeated after a 2-hour interval if symptoms recur (maximum dose 300 mg in 24-hour period) **OR**
- (migraine) 20 mg nasal spray into one nostril, may be repeated after a 2-hour interval if symptoms recur (maximum dose 40 mg in 24-hour period by nasal spray)

Adverse effects

- (injection site) transient pain, stinging, burning, erythema, bruising, bleeding, swelling
- transient (and possibly intense) tingling, heaviness, heat/cold, pain or pressure/tightness in any part of the body
- flushing, dizziness, weakness, fatigue, drowsiness, paraesthesia, hypoaesthesia
- dyspnoea
- nausea, vomiting, taste disturbance
- transient increase in BP
- medication overuse headache (see introduction, p. 556)
- (nasal spray) irritation and burning sensation in nose or throat, epistaxis
- (rare) severe cardiac events, seizures

Interactions

- contraindicated with or within 24 hours of ergot alkaloids
- contraindicated with or within 2 weeks of stopping MAOIs
- not recommended with or within 24 hours of other $5HT_1$ receptor agonists or St John's wort
- caution and monitoring are recommended if given with SSRIs or SNRIs due to risk of serotonin syndrome

Nursing points/Cautions

- a clear diagnosis of migraine should be established and other neurological conditions ruled out before starting therapy in those with no previous history of migraine
- cardiovascular assessment is recommended for those who are at risk of coronary artery disease
- tablets and fast-disintegrating tablets are bioequivalent
- not given IV, only SC
- first SC dose should be given by medical personnel
- nasal spray is recommended in those with nausea and vomiting associated with migraine or if rapid onset of action is required
- allergic reaction may occur in those with a hypersensitivity to sulfonamides
- (nasal spray) caution if used in those with asthma
- (nasal spray) caution if used in those with a rubber or latex allergy because of the rubber stopper
- caution if used in those with epilepsy, liver or kidney impairment, or controlled hypertension
- caution if used in those with risk factors for cardiovascular disease (e.g. hypertension, smoking, obesity, diabetes, males > 40 years, menopausal females, hypercholesterolaemia)
- not recommended in those over 65 years
- contraindicated in those with hemiplegic, basilar or ophthalmoplegic migraine

- contraindicated in those with a history of myocardial infarction, peripheral vascular disease, ischaemic heart disease, variant (Prinzmetal's) angina, uncontrolled hypertension, CVA, transient ischaemic attacks or severe liver impairment

Patient teaching and advice

- ensure that patient understands therapy is for management of acute migraine, not prevention
- patient should be adequately educated in the use of the autoinjector and nasal spray, including correct disposal of needles and syringes
- patient should be advised to use medication when first symptoms occur
- advise patient that if first dose is ineffective in relieving migraine, second dose is unlikely to be effective. However, if migraine recurs, further dose may be taken (24-hour maximum dose and interval, see Dose, p. 564)
- advise patient that tablets should be swallowed whole with water and tablets have a bitter taste
- patient should be warned against driving or using machinery if dizziness and sedation are problems
- instruct patient not to take multiple forms of sumatriptan during acute migraine attack
- advise patient to seek medical advice immediately if any of the following occur:
  - pain in lower stomach, bloody diarrhoea
  - irregular heart rate
  - heaviness, pressure or tightness in any part of the body including throat and heart
- see General Patient teaching and advice (p. xxvii)

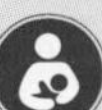

only used during pregnancy if benefits outweigh risks to the fetus

secreted in breastmilk, therefore avoid breastfeeding within 24 hours of last dose

fast-disintegrating tablets can be dispersed in water

ZOLMITRIPTAN (Zoltrip, Zomig)

Available form
Tablets: 2.5 mg

Action
- selective serotonin ($5HT_{1B/1D}$) agonist
- onset of action within 1 hour, half-life 4.7 hours (prolonged in those with liver impairment)
- active metabolite (half-life 5.7 hours)

Use
- acute migraine (with or without aura)

Dose
- initially 2.5 mg orally and, if symptoms persist or recur, a further 2.5 mg may be taken 2 hours after first dose (maximum dose 10 mg in 24-hour period)

Adverse effects
- nausea, vomiting, dry mouth, abdominal pain, dysphagia, taste disturbance
- dizziness, somnolence, headache, warm/cold sensation, hyperaesthesia, paraesthesia
- asthenia, heaviness/tightness/pain/pressure in throat, neck, limbs or chest
- myalgia, muscle weakness
- palpitations
- (uncommon) transient increase in BP
- (very rare) arrhythmias, myocardial infarction, angina, ischaemic colitis
- medication overuse headache (see introduction, p. 556)

Interactions

- contraindicated with and within 24 hours of ergot alkaloids
- serum levels may increase if given with quinolone antibacterial agents (e.g. ciprofloxacin) and cimetidine
- not recommended with or within 24 hours of MAOIs (selective or non-selective)
- caution and monitoring recommended if given with SSRIs or SNRIs due to risk of serotonin syndrome, especially at start of therapy
- contraindicated with or within 12 hours of other $5HT_{1D}$ receptor agonists
- caution if given with St John's wort

Nursing points/Cautions

- a clear diagnosis of migraine should be established and other neurological conditions ruled out before starting therapy in those with no previous history of migraine
- cardiovascular assessment is recommended for those who are at risk of coronary artery disease
- if 2.5 mg dose is ineffective, dose can be increased to 5 mg for subsequent migraine attacks
- tablets contain phenylalanine and therefore are not recommended in those with phenylketonuria
- not recommended in those with hemiplegic or basilar migraines or atypical headaches
- not recommended in those aged > 65 years or < 12 years
- contraindicated in those with myocardial infarction, arrhythmias or accessory pathway disorders, ischaemic heart disease, variant (Prinzmetal's) angina, peripheral vascular disease, moderate-to-severe controlled hypertension, uncontrolled mild hypertension, stroke or transient ischaemic attacks or kidney impairment (creatinine clearance < 15 mL/min)

Patient teaching and advice

- ensure that patient understands therapy is for management of acute migraine, not prevention
- instruct patient to take medication early in onset of headache for best effect
- advise patient that if first dose is not effective, second dose is unlikely to relieve migraine during same attack
- advise patient to swallow tablets whole
- patient should be advised against driving and using machinery if dizziness is a problem
- see General Patient teaching and advice (p. xxvii)

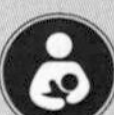

should only be given during pregnancy if benefits outweigh risks to fetus

secreted in breastmilk, therefore should be used with great caution during breastfeeding

tablet can be dispersed in water (3–5 minutes) or crushed and mixed with spoonful of yoghurt or apple puree

ANTIMYCOBACTERIAL AGENTS

Mycobacteria are a group of slow-growing acid-fast bacilli which are quite different from other Gram-positive or Gram-negative bacteria, with over 150 different species identified (Holland 2015). Antimycobacterial agents are a group of antibacterial drugs used in the treatment of tuberculosis (caused by *Mycobacterium tuberculosis*), leprosy (or Hansen's disease, caused by *M. leprae*) and other mycobacterial infections (referred to as nontuberculous mycobacterial infections), including *M. avium* complex (MAC) and *M. ulcerans* (Buruli ulcer). MAC organisms commonly cause illness in humans, especially those who are immunocompromised and have concurrent lung disease, such as bronchiectasis or chronic obstructive pulmonary disease (COPD). Prolonged multi-drug therapy is recommended for MAC infection (Holland 2018; Reddy & O'Donnell 2018).

In 2017, 1.6 million people died of tuberculosis (TB); however, it should be noted that TB is preventable and curable. Those people who are HIV positive are 20 to 30 times more likely to develop active TB compared to those without HIV (WHO 2018). Tuberculosis commonly occurs in the lungs (pulmonary TB), although it may also be found in bone, meninges, lymph glands, GI tract, pericardium, kidneys and urinary tract (extrapulmonary TB). Interestingly, TB of the upper airways, or pleura, is considered extrapulmonary TB (Raviglione 2018). People with active pulmonary TB are symptomatic (e.g. cough lasting longer than 2 weeks, chest pain, coughing up sputum or blood, weakness, chills, fever, night sweats, weight loss, anorexia) and the disease is contagious by aerosol spread. If a person has latent TB, the disease is not contagious and the bacteria do not cause disease. It has been estimated that one-quarter of the world's population has latent TB (WHO 2018). The disease may become activated in the future if the person's immune system becomes weakened, including by the use of immunosuppressive agents (Raviglione 2018).

First-line drugs (isoniazid, rifampicin and ethambutol) are used successfully in most patients with tuberculosis. Second-line drugs are used when the first-line drugs cannot be used, because of either the adverse effects of, or resistance to, the first-line agents. Second-line drugs include some of the newer macrolide antibacterial agents and also the fluoroquinolones. Before starting any treatment it is important to take cultures and establish the susceptibility of the organism to the drug(s). Patient education is an important part of treatment to prevent microbial resistance occurring when courses of therapy are not completed, as well as ensuring patients are aware of drug and alcohol interactions and possible adverse effects. Because of the increase in multi-drug resistant organisms (MDR-TB) worldwide (resistant to both rifampicin and isoniazid), the antimycobacterial agents are not given as monotherapy but as part of a multi-drug regimen (generally a 6-month course of four agents) (Reddy & O'Donnell 2018). A test (Xpert MTB/RIF®) is available to detect TB and resistance to rifampicin within 2 hours, with other tests also being developed to test resistance to other first- and second-line TB drugs. Extensively or extreme drug-resistant TB (XDR-TB) now exists in about 58 countries worldwide and occurs when organisms are resistant to second-line drugs in addition to the first-line drugs, with sporadic cases also appearing in Australia (Traver & Cheng 2016; WHO 2018).

With the first case documented in 600 BC, leprosy is a condition that has been recognised since biblical times (WHO 2019b). Although numbers have decreased globally, leprosy is still found in endemic numbers in pockets of developing countries, with Africa having the highest prevalence, but Asia having the greatest numbers (WHO 2019b). While rarely acquired in Australia, Aboriginal and Torres Strait Islanders living in remote areas of Australia (such as in the Northern Territory or Far North Queensland), have the greatest burden of disease with 20 cases diagnosed between 1989 and 2018 (Hempenstall et al 2019). Droplet transmission, contact with contaminated soil or insect vectors have all been implicated as likely routes of transmission. The disease has a very long incubation period (average 5 years). It generally affects skin, peripheral nerves and mucous membranes (eyes and upper respiratory tract) to varying degrees and other organs can be involved (WHO 2019b). Long-term complications include neuropathy, nerve damage (which can lead to paresis, paralysis and muscle atrophy), ulceration, foot drop, destruction of nose cartilage, blindness, impotency and infertility in males, and nerve abscesses (Gelber 2018).

First-line drug treatment for leprosy is with a multi-drug regimen, including rifampicin, clofazimine, dapsone and minocycline; thalidomide is used as a second-line drug. No resistance has developed to treatment when used as part of multi-drug therapy (WHO 2019b). Because it is a known teratogen, thalidomide is only used when other treatment options have been exhausted. Leprosy reactional states (Lepra reaction, see Glossary) may occur before diagnosis and treatment have begun or after the commencement of treatment, which may result in patients losing confidence in the treatment regimen as it is perceived to be ineffective (Gelber 2018).

DAPSONE

Available forms

Tablets: 25 mg, 100 mg

Action

- sulfone with actions similar to sulfonamide
- active against a wide range of bacteria which inhibit folic acid synthesis

- bacteriostatic against *M. leprae*
- active against *Plasmodium* spp and *Pneumocystis carinii*
- active metabolite
- half-life of 10–80 hours

Use
- leprosy (as part of a multi-drug regimen)
- dermatitis herpetiformis
- actinomycotic mycetoma

Dose
- (dermatitis herpetiformis) 50–100 mg orally daily with food **OR**
- (leprosy) 100 mg (1–2 mg/kg) orally daily with food (with rifampicin) **OR**
- (actinomycotic mycetoma) 100 mg orally twice daily with food, continued for 2–3 months after symptoms have abated (with streptomycin for first and alternate months)

Adverse effects
- muscle weakness, peripheral neuropathy, reversible sensory impairment
- leprosy reactional states (type 1 and type 2 reactions) (see Glossary)
- nausea, vomiting, abdominal pain
- blurred vision, tinnitus, vertigo
- insomnia, headache
- fever
- psychosis
- haemolysis
- phototoxicity
- (rare) dapsone syndrome (rash, fever, jaundice, eosinophilia)
- (rare) agranulocytosis, severe cutaneous reaction, decrease in liver function, jaundice, toxic hepatitis
- (very rare) aplastic anaemia

Interactions
- great caution if given with other agents that can cause blood dyscrasias or liver impairment, such as folic acid antagonists (e.g. pyrimethamine)
- plasma levels may be increased if given with probenecid and amprenavir, increasing risk of toxicity
- plasma levels may be decreased if given with rifampicin
- increased risk of methaemoglobinaemia if given with rifampicin because of the increase in active metabolite concentration
- increased serum levels of both dapsone and trimethoprim may occur if given together, increasing risk of dapsone toxicity
- increased risk of haemotoxicity if given with cimetidine due to increased levels of active metabolite
- anti-inflammatory action of clofazimine may be inhibited by dapsone

Nursing points/Cautions
- any anaemia should be treated before starting therapy
- regular blood count throughout therapy is recommended (weekly for first month, monthly for 6 months, then twice-yearly or more regularly if given with other agents that can cause haematological reactions)
- baseline liver function test is recommended, as well as regular monitoring throughout therapy
- patients should be monitored for ‘dapsone reaction’ in first 6 weeks of therapy (persistent rash, fever, jaundice and eosinophilia)
- therapy should be stopped if any blood disorder or dermatological reaction occurs
- caution if given to those with G6PD deficiency or methaemoglobin reductase deficiency
- caution if used in those with cardiac, hepatic, renal or pulmonary disease
- not recommended in those with porphyria because acute attack may be induced
- contraindicated in those with hypersensitivity to sulfonamides

Patient teaching and advice

- patient should be advised to take tablets whole (not split), with or after food
- instruct patient to immediately report any of the following:
  - sore throat, fever, pallor, bruises, bleeding under the skin
  - yellowing of eyes or skin, dark urine, pale stools, lethargy, nausea, upper abdominal pain
  - muscle weakness, unusual tiredness
  - severe skin rash
  - tingling, pain, burning sensation, numbness or weakness in hands and/or feet, bluish fingernails, lips or skin
- warn patients not to drive or operate machinery if dizziness or blurred vision occur
- female patients of childbearing potential should be counselled to use adequate contraception to avoid pregnancy during therapy
- see General Patient teaching and advice (p. xxvii)

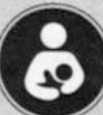

contraindicated during pregnancy

excreted in substantial amounts in breastmilk and may cause haemolytic reaction in infants with G6PD deficiency

tablets can be dispersed in 10–20 mL of water or crushed and mixed with spoonful of yoghurt or apple puree

ETHAMBUTOL HYDROCHLORIDE (Myambutol)

Available forms

Tablets: 100 mg, 400 mg

Action

- impairs cell metabolism, stops multiplication and causes cell death
- effective against *Mycobacterium* spp

Use

- first line drug in treatment of primary and extrapulmonary TB (as part of a multi-drug regimen, the exact combination depending on previous treatment and the development of any microbial resistance)

Dose

- (no previous treatment) 15 mg/kg orally daily **OR**
- (retreatment) initially 25 mg/kg orally daily decreasing to 15 mg/kg after 60 days **OR**
- (intermittent therapy) initially 15–25 mg/kg orally daily for 2 months (or longer depending on type and extent of disease, and at least one negative sputum sample) then 50 mg/kg orally twice weekly

Adverse effects

- reduced visual acuity, colour vision disturbances (usually reversible) (unilateral or bilateral), visual defects, scotoma
- rash, pruritus, dermatitis
- fever, joint pains
- nausea, vomiting, anorexia, abdominal pain
- malaise, headache, dizziness, confusion, disorientation
- elevated serum uric acid, precipitation of gout
- transient liver function impairment
- anaphylactoid reaction
- (rare) peripheral neuritis, hallucinations, severe skin reactions

Nursing points/Cautions

- should only be used as part of multidrug regimen (not monotherapy)
- ophthalmological examinations (including colour discrimination) are recommended before and during therapy (monthly if dose is greater than 15 mg/kg/day)
- blood counts, kidney and liver function monitored regularly throughout therapy

- maintenance intermittent dose is lower if given with isoniazid
- use with caution in those with gout because it may be exacerbated by elevated uric acid concentrations
- contraindicated in those with optic neuritis (unless benefits of treatment are thought to outweigh risks)

Patient teaching and advice

- patients with diabetes should be advised to monitor blood glucose levels closely during therapy
- warn patient to report immediately and seek medical advice if any of the following occur:
  - visual disturbances such as blurred vision (reversible if the drug is stopped early; however, recovery may take weeks to months after drug is stopped)
  - any weakness, burning sensation, numbness or tingling in hands and/or feet
- advise patient not to drive or operate machinery if visual problems, dizziness, confusion or disorientation occur
- see General Patient teaching and advice (p. xxvii)

tablets can be crushed and mixed with water, apple juice or spoonful of apple puree, chocolate pudding, peanut butter or jelly if bitter taste is unpalatable

ISONIAZID

Available form

Tablets: 100 mg

Action

- bacteriostatic against mycobacteria only
- resistance may develop in only a few weeks if given alone
- half-life 1–4 hours (this is influenced by whether patient is fast or slow acetylator, which influences the rate of drug metabolism)

Use

- first-line drug in the treatment of pulmonary and extrapulmonary TB (as part of a multi-drug regimen)

Dose

- (treatment) 4–5 mg/kg orally in divided daily doses (300 mg maximum) **OR**
- (tuberculosis meningitis) up to 10 mg/kg orally daily for first 1–2 weeks

Adverse effects

- peripheral neuropathy, optic neuritis, convulsions, memory impairment, toxic encephalopathy, toxic psychosis
- nausea, vomiting, epigastric distress, anorexia
- fever, skin eruptions, lymphadenopathy, vasculitis
- fatigue, malaise, weakness
- elevated liver enzymes and bilirubin, jaundice, severe hepatitis
- pyridoxine deficiency, pellagra, metabolic acidosis,
- hyperglycaemia
- gynaecomastia
- pancreatitis
- haemolytic, aplastic or sideroblastic anaemia, agranulocytosis, thrombocytopenia, eosinophilia
- rheumatic syndrome, SLE-like syndrome

Interactions

- not recommended with hepatotoxic agents
- increased risk of CNS adverse effects if given with disulfiram
- may potentiate anticoagulant activity of warfarin, therefore prothrombin time should be closely monitored, especially when starting or stopping therapy
- may decrease excretion of phenytoin, increasing the risk of phenytoin toxicity, therefore blood levels should be monitored throughout therapy
- not recommended with carbamazepine because of the increased risk of isoniazid-induced hepatotoxicity

- may increase serum levels of carbamazepine increasing risk of toxicity
- may increase metabolism of paracetamol to hepatotoxic metabolites
- increased risk of hepatotoxicity if given with rifabutin or rifampicin as part of a multi-drug regimen
- increased risk of peripheral neuropathies and liver damage if used with alcohol
- may cause false positive on urine glucose determination using Benedict's reagent or Clinitest

Nursing points/Cautions

- risk of peripheral neuritis is greatest in those with poor nutrition, alcohol abuse, uraemia or diabetes or if they are slow acetylators
- liver function should be monitored monthly throughout therapy
- changes in liver enzymes usually occur in first 4–6 months of therapy
- ophthalmological examination is recommended before starting and regularly throughout therapy
- pyridoxine (vitamin B_6) is often given concurrently to prevent isoniazid-induced peripheral neuropathy or if there is already existing peripheral neuritis
- may be given concurrently with ethambutol or rifampicin to reduce the development of resistance. If used with rifampicin, liver function tests and vitamin D levels should be monitored regularly
- caution if used in those aged 50 or over (increased risk of hepatitis), if drinking alcohol on a daily basis, with diabetes or kidney impairment
- caution if used in those with liver disorders including hepatitis B and C, alcoholic hepatitis, cirrhosis or use alcohol regularly
- contraindicated in those with previous adverse reactions during isoniazid therapy or acute liver damage or severe hypersensitivity reactions

Patient teaching and advice

- advise patient to take isoniazid 1 hour before aluminium-containing antacids
- patient should be advised to avoid alcohol during therapy
- warn patient to seek medical advice immediately if any of the following occur:
  - visual disturbances
  - numbness or tingling in the hands or feet
  - fatigue, weakness, malaise, anorexia, nausea or vomiting
- counsel patients to avoid driving or operating machinery if visual disturbances or fatigue occur
- see General Patient teaching and advice (p. xxvii)

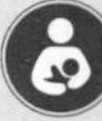

should only be used during pregnancy if benefits outweigh potential risks. However, preventative therapy should be started soon after childbirth because there is an increased risk of reactivated TB in the new mother

secreted in breastmilk, so observe breastfed infants for adverse effects

can be dispersed in water or crushed and mixed with orange juice or spoonful of apple puree, chocolate pudding, jelly or peanut butter

RIFABUTIN (Mycobutin)

Available form

Capsules: 150 mg

Action

- ansamycin antibiotic similar to rifampicin, with a wide spectrum of activity
- active against atypical and multidrug resistant mycobacteria
- long half-life (45 hours)

Use
- pulmonary tuberculosis (as part of a multi-drug regimen)
- MAC prophylaxis in patients with advanced HIV (as part of a multi-drug regimen)
- treatment of MAC infections and other atypical mycobacterium infections

Dose
- (MAC prophylaxis) 300 mg orally daily **OR**
- (non-TB mycobacterium infection) 300–600 mg orally daily for up to 6 months after negative sputum culture **OR**
- (chronic, multi-drug resistant pulmonary TB) 300–450 mg orally daily for up to 6 months after negative sputum culture **OR**
- (newly diagnosed TB) 150–300 mg orally daily for 6 months

Adverse effects
- fever, rash, arthralgia, myalgia
- reversible uveitis (mild to severe), corneal deposits
- nausea, vomiting, jaundice, elevated liver enzymes
- leucopenia, anaemia, neutropenia
- discolouration (red-orange) of urine, skin and body secretions
- breakdown of vitamin K (during pregnancy)
- (rare) thrombocytopenia, antibiotic associated pseudomembranous colitis, hypersensitivity

Interactions
- contraindicated with ritonavir
- increased risk of uveitis if given with clarithromycin, other macrolide antibiotics or fluconazole or related compounds
- increases metabolism of oral contraceptives, reducing effectiveness
- increases metabolism and therefore decreases serum levels of atovaquone, benzodiazepines, calcium-channel blockers, clarithromycin, corticosteroids, ciclosporin, dapsone, erythromycin, fluconazole, indinavir, itraconazole, lidocaine (lignocaine), lovastatin, methadone, midazolam, nevirapine, oestrogens, opioid analgesics, phenytoin, posaconazole, ritonavir, saquinavir, sulfamethoxazole, tacrolimus, theophylline, triazolam, trimethoprim, warfarin and zidovudine
- plasma levels may be increased by ciprofloxacin, clarithromycin, erythromycin, fluconazole, indinavir, itraconazole, ritonavir, posaconazole and saquinavir
- caution if given with barbiturates, benzodiazepines, verapamil, beta-adrenergic blocking agents, disopyramide, chloramphenicol and antiepileptic agents

Nursing points/Cautions
- should only be given as part of multi-drug regimen
- liver function tests, WBC and platelet counts should be monitored regularly throughout therapy
- if given with indinavir, dose should be halved and indinavir dose increased
- if given with clarithromycin, dose should be decreased to 300 mg daily
- caution if used in those with progressing HIV disease due to altered gastric pH leading to malabsorption of some drugs
- caution if used in those with severe liver insufficiency or severe kidney impairment (creatinine clearance < 30 mL/min)
- contraindicated in those with known hypersensitivity to other rifamycins

Patient teaching and advice
- warn patient that urine and body secretions may be stained red-orange and that soft contact lenses may be permanently stained

- advise patient to seek medical advice immediately if any of the following occur:
  - any eye pain, red eyes, blurred vision or black floating spots
  - yellowing of eyes or skin, dark urine, pale stools, lethargy, nausea, upper abdominal pain
- female patients should be counselled to use other forms of contraception as efficacy of oral contraceptives may be compromised
- see General Patient teaching and advice (p. xxvii)

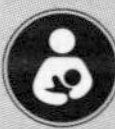

if used during the last weeks of pregnancy, vitamin K should be given to the mother and newborn to prevent bleeding. Should only be used during pregnancy if benefits outweigh potential risks

it is recommended to discontinue either the drug or breastfeeding

capsules can be opened and contents mixed with water or spoonful of apple puree

RIFAMPICIN (Rifadin, Rimycin)

Available forms

Capsules: 150 mg, 300 mg; Tablets: 600 mg; Suspension: 100 mg/5 mL; Vials: 600 mg

Action

- inhibits DNA dependent RNA polymerase activity
- half-life about 3 hours
- cross resistance to other rifamycins

Use

- first-line drug in the treatment of TB (as part of a multi-drug regimen)
- leprosy (as part of a multi-drug regimen)
- prophylaxis of meningococcal disease and *Haemophilus influenzae* type B

Dose

- (tuberculosis) 600 mg orally daily 30 minutes before or 2 hours after food **OR**
- (leprosy) 450–600 mg orally daily 30 minutes before or 2 hours after food **OR**
- (meningococcal disease prophylaxis) 600 mg orally daily 30 minutes before or 2 hours after food for 4 days **OR**
- (*H. influenzae* type B prophylaxis) 20 mg/kg orally daily 30 minutes before or 2 hours after food for 4 days (daily maximum 600 mg) **OR**
- 600 mg by IV infusion over 1–3 hours (if unable to take oral preparation)

Adverse effects

- dyspepsia, anorexia, nausea, vomiting, flatulence, diarrhoea, abdominal cramps, sore mouth/tongue
- headache, drowsiness, fatigue, dizziness, decreased concentration, confusion
- visual disturbances, conjunctivitis
- discolouration of sputum, urine, sweat, tears and/or teeth
- muscle weakness, myalgia, myopathy, pain in legs and feet, numbness, ataxia
- rash, fever, flushing, pruritus, urticaria, acne-like lesions
- purpura, eosinophilia, leucopenia, acute haemolytic anaemia
- vitamin K deficiency, hypoprothrombinaemia, vitamin K-dependent coagulopathy
- menstrual disturbances, postpartum haemorrhage, fetal maternal haemorrhage
- lepromatous reaction (when given for leprosy)
- (IV) thrombophlebitis
- (flu-like syndrome) fever, chills, headache, dizziness, bone pain (occurring during third and sixth month of therapy)
- (rare) antibiotic associated pseudomembranous colitis, liver dysfunction,

hepatitis, haemolytic anaemia, increased serum uric acid concentrations, thrombocytopenia (reversible if drug stopped early), kidney failure, severe hypersensitivity reactions (including drug reaction with eosinophilia and systemic systems (DRESS)), severe skin reactions, psychosis, cerebral haemorrhage

Interactions

- contraindicated with saquinavir/ritonavir combination
- not recommended with other hepatotoxic agents or hepatis C antiviral agents
- serum levels may be increased by probenecid and atovaquone
- may decrease efficacy of oral contraceptives
- not recommended with other antibacterial agents causing vitamin K dependent coagulopathy such as cephalosporins
- increased risk of hepatotoxicity if given with alcohol, isoniazid or halothane
- may decrease serum levels of atovaquone and enalaprilat (active metabolite of enalapril)
- increases metabolism, decreases serum levels and activity of antiarrhythmic agents, antiepileptic agents, antipsychotic agents, barbiturates, beta-adrenoceptor blocking agents, benzodiazepines, calcium-channel blockers, chloramphenicol, clarithromycin, clofibrate, corticosteroids, ciclosporin, digoxin, dapsone, disopyramide, doxycycline, efavirenz, fluconazole, fluoroquinolones, haloperidol, oral hypoglycaemic agents, indinavir, irinotecan, itraconazole, levothyroxine, losartan, methadone, oestrogens, ondansetron, opioid analgesics, phenytoin, progestins, quinine, rosiglitazone, saquinavir, statins, systemic hormonal contraceptives, tacrolimus, tamoxifen, theophylline, TCAs, verapamil, zidovudine, zolpidem and zopiclone
- absorption decreased by antacids
- may decrease serum levels of warfarin, therefore increased monitoring of prothrombin is recommended, especially when starting and stopping therapy
- blood glucose control may become disrupted because of decreased serum levels of oral hypoglycaemics (sulfonylureas) when given with rifampicin
- increases metabolism of vitamin D, thyroid hormones and adrenal hormones
- may interfere with some laboratory tests including false positive urine screening for opioids

Nursing points/Cautions

- patient should be reviewed monthly during therapy
- baseline liver function tests including liver enzymes, bilirubin, creatinine; full blood count and platelet count should be measured before starting therapy
- liver function tests every 2–4 weeks during therapy (in those who are malnourished, have liver disease or are taking hepatotoxic agents)
- vitamin K supplementation is recommended if vitamin K deficiency or hypoprothrombinaemia occur
- IV therapy is indicated for those unable to tolerate oral therapy
- (leprosy) should be used as part of multi-drug regimen to decrease risk of resistance
- (leprosy) patient should be assessed for concurrent TB and treated accordingly
- prothrombin time should be monitored daily if patient is also taking oral anticoagulants, or blood glucose in patients with diabetes taking oral hypoglycaemics

- IV preparation should not be administered IM or SC
- dissolve vial with water for injections and add to 500 mL of glucose 5% or sodium chloride 0.9% and infuse over 1–3 hours
- precipitate may occur if given with IV diltiazem
- (suspension) contains sodium metabisulfite, which can cause allergic reactions in some people, especially those with asthma or eczema
- use with caution in those with porphyria or pre-existing liver disease
- not recommended for treatment of meningococcal disease
- not recommended as intermittent therapy (less than 2–3 times per week) because of increased risk of immunological reactions or anaphylaxis
- contraindicated in those with known hypersensitivity to other rifamycins or with jaundice

Patient teaching and advice

- advise patient of the importance of continuous therapy (i.e. not stopping therapy) because intermittent therapy may result in hypersensitivity reaction. Rifampicin should not be used less than 2–3 times weekly
- patient should be warned that flu-like syndrome commonly occurs between third and sixth month of therapy
- warn patient that urine, faeces, sweat, sputum and tears may become a harmless red-orange colour and that soft contact lenses may become permanently stained
- advise patient to seek medical advice immediately if any of the following occur:
    - yellowing of eyes or skin, dark urine, pale stools, lethargy, nausea, upper abdominal pain
    - visual disturbances
    - rash, blistering or peeling of skin
    - fever, enlarged glands, rash
    - severe watery diarrhoea, abdominal cramping (even if it occurs several weeks after stopping therapy)
    - white furry, sore mouth or tongue (oral thrush)
    - sore/itchy vagina, discharge (vaginal thrush)
- patient should be instructed not to drive or operate machinery if drowsiness, dizziness, visual disturbances or decreased concentration occurs
- warn patient to avoid alcohol during therapy
- patient should be advised to tell doctor that he/she is taking rifampicin because of the long list of drug interactions that may occur
- suggest that patient take oral preparation 30 minutes before or 2 hours after a meal
- advise patient not to take antacids within 1 hour of taking rifampicin
- those with diabetes who use oral hypoglycaemics (sulfonylureas) should be advised to monitor blood glucose levels closely during therapy
- counsel women of childbearing potential taking oral contraceptives to use other forms of contraception (non-hormonal) during therapy to avoid pregnancy occurring
- see General Patient teaching and advice (p. xxvii)

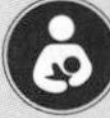

crosses placental barrier. If rifampicin is used during the last few weeks of pregnancy, vitamin K should be given to the mother and infant to reduce the risk of bleeding from hypoprothrombinaemia

appears in breastmilk, so not recommended during breastfeeding

available as a syrup. Capsules can be opened or tablets can be crushed and mixed with water or spoonful of apple puree

THALIDOMIDE (Thalomid)

Available forms

Capsules: 50 mg, 100 mg

Action

- exact mode of action is unknown
- (multiple myeloma) inhibits growth and survival of myeloma cells and bone marrow stromal cells, suppresses tumour necrosis factor (alpha) (TNF-α), inhibits leucocyte migration, shifts ratio of helper T cells to cytotoxic T cells and blocks growth of blood vessels from tumour
- (leprosy) appears to block fever and cutaneous symptoms by blocking TNF-α
- does not consistently decrease TNF-α in all disease states
- half-life 5–7 hours

Use

- multiple myeloma (as monotherapy when standard therapies have failed; in combination therapy for untreated multiple myeloma with melphalan and prednisolone in those over 65 years or ineligible for high-dose chemotherapy; or in combination with dexamethasone for induction therapy prior to high-dose chemotherapy with autologous stem cell rescue)
- treatment and maintenance of moderate-to-severe erythema nodosum leprosum (ENL) associated with leprosy

Dose

- (untreated multiple myeloma) 200 mg orally daily for a maximum of 12 cycles of 6 weeks (with prednisolone and melphalan) **OR**
- (untreated multiple myeloma) 200 mg orally daily for 4 cycles of 4 weeks (with dexamethasone) (induction) **OR**
- (multiple myeloma after failure of standard therapy) initially 200 mg orally daily 1 hour after food, increasing by 100 mg at weekly intervals if necessary (daily maximum 400 mg) **OR**
- (ENL associated with leprosy) initially 100 mg orally daily 1 hour after food, increasing by 100 mg at weekly intervals if symptoms remain uncontrolled (daily maximum 400 mg) (treatment) then dose reduced if possible to maintain active reaction control (maintenance)

Adverse effects

- teratogenic – severe birth defects
- leucopenia, neutropenia, anaemia, thrombocytopaenia
- peripheral neuropathy, paraesthesia, dysaesthesia
- bradycardia, cardiac failure
- orthostatic hypotension, syncope
- depression, confusion, lack of coordination
- drowsiness, dizziness, somnolence, sedation, fatigue, weakness
- fever, asthenia, malaise
- tremor
- nausea, vomiting, dry mouth, constipation
- peripheral oedema
- rash, dry skin, urticaria
- dyspnoea
- delayed wound healing
- (rare) hypothyroidism, seizures, severe skin reaction, tumour lysis syndrome, reactivation of hepatitis B
- (multiple myeloma) increased risk of deep vein thrombosis (DVT) and pulmonary embolus (PE)

Interactions

- caution if used with other agents that cause bradycardia such as beta-adrenoceptor blocking agents and anticholinesterases
- caution if used with other agents which increase the risk of thromboembolic events (e.g. erythropoietin, oestrogens)

- increased risk of neutropenia or thrombocytopenia if given with melphalan or prednisolone
- may increase sedative effects of barbiturates, alcohol and chlorpromazine
- may increase effects of morphine derivatives, benzodiazepines, antianxiety agents, hypnotics, sedatives, antidepressants, antihistamines with sedative properties, antipsychotics, baclofen and centrally acting antihypertensive agents
- increased risk of peripheral neuropathy if used with didanosine, zalcitabine and vincristine
- increased risk of thromboembolic events (e.g. DVT, PE) and/or thrombosis if used with doxorubicin, melphalan, prednisolone and dexamethasone

Nursing points/Cautions

- thalidomide can only be prescribed under a restricted distribution program
- if patient is over 75 years, starting dose should be 100 mg orally daily
- patient must receive counselling to ensure good understanding of the potential therapy risks and outcomes (as well as alternative therapies), including the contraceptive requirements associated with thalidomide to prevent pregnancy occurring before giving a full, informed and written consent prior to starting therapy. Patient's sexual partner should also receive counselling and information
- females who report having had a hysterectomy or being post-menopausal for more than 2 years should have status confirmed before starting therapy
- it is suggested that pregnancy testing, prescription issuing and dispensing all occur on the same day. If this is not possible, dispensing of thalidomide should occur within 7 days of pregnancy test
- it is recommended that women of childbearing potential have a medically supervised pregnancy test either at the time of consultation or 3 days before starting therapy. Pregnancy tests are then recommended weekly during first month and then monthly (if menstrual cycles are regular) or 2-weekly (if menstrual cycles are irregular) up to 4 weeks after therapy ends. Effective contraception should continue throughout and include the 4 weeks after therapy ends
- therapy should start on day 2 or 3 of menstrual cycle in those women who have regular cycles and have had a negative pregnancy test
- (ENL) corticosteroids are sometimes added as an adjunct to control moderate-to-severe leprosy-associated neuritis
- (ENL) when symptoms are controlled, therapy may be tapered by 50 mg every 2–4 weeks, with the aim of discontinuing therapy in 3–6 months
- patient should be monitored for bradycardia and/or syncope and dose reduced if symptoms occur
- thyroid function tests, WBC count and differential count should be monitored throughout therapy
- therapy should be stopped 7 days before surgery if wound healing may be affected
- if therapy is long term, sensory nerve action potential data should be collected before starting therapy, then 6-monthly. Clinical evaluation for peripheral neuropathy (numbness, tingling, pain) should occur monthly
- if patient is at increased risk of thromboembolic events (DVT, PE), concurrent therapy with warfarin or low molecular weight heparin is recommended

- if thromboembolic event occurs, thalidomide should be stopped and anticoagulation therapy started. Thalidomide may be restarted once anticoagulation therapy has stabilised
- (ENL) should not be used in anyone with neuritis unless benefits are thought to outweigh risks
- not recommended as monotherapy for ENL associated with leprosy
- caution in those with epilepsy or if other risk factors for seizures exist
- caution if used in those who may experience tumour lysis syndrome
- caution if used in those with hypothyroidism
- caution if used in those with risk factors for myocardial infarction including prior thrombosis, smoking, hypertension and hyperlipidaemia
- caution if used in those with neutropenia. If count is $< 0.75 \times 10^9$/L neutrophils, therapy should be withheld
- caution if used in those with malignant disease due to increased risk of thromboembolic events (DVT, PE) (risk is greatest in first 5 months of therapy)
- caution if used in combination with corticosteroids in those with previous hepatitis B infection as reactivation may occur
- contraindicated in those (males and females) who are unable or unwilling to comply with adequate contraception measures throughout therapy
- contraindicated in those under 12 years

Patient teaching and advice

- advise patient to swallow tablets whole (not crushed or chewed) with a full glass of water
- suggest to patient that dose could be taken in the evening to overcome drowsiness, sedation and somnolence, which may be problematic during the day
- warn patient not to drive or operate machinery if drowsiness, dizziness, somnolence, weakness or fatigue occurs
- instruct patient to avoid alcohol because it may increase drowsiness
- if dizziness or a spinning feeling in the head occurs when getting out of bed (low blood pressure), advise patient to sit up slowly before standing
- advise patient to seek medical advice immediately if any of the following occur:
  - any rash or blistering of skin
  - unusual bleeding or bruising, including vomiting blood or experiencing bloody diarrhoea, blood noses
  - seizures (fitting)
  - slow heart rate, fainting
  - blurred vision, severe headache
  - numbness, tingling, pain or abnormal coordination in hands or feet
  - sudden pain in chest or difficulty breathing, shortness of breath
  - pain or swelling in legs, especially lower legs or calves
  - fever, severe chills, sore throat, mouth ulcers, tiredness, flu-like symptoms, signs of infection
- instruct all patients not to donate blood during or for 4 weeks after stopping therapy
- counsel male patient not to donate semen during or within 4 weeks of stopping therapy
- male patients should be advised that thalidomide is present in semen and therefore they should not have unprotected sex. Adequate contraceptive methods (latex or polyurethane condoms) must always be used during sexual activity with women of childbearing potential (or who have not been menopausal for at least 1 year); condom use must continue for at least 4 weeks after stopping therapy

- if male patient is allergic to latex or polyurethane, at least one reliable contraceptive measure (as outlined below) should be utilised by female partner
- women of childbearing potential (who have not had a hysterectomy or are not post-menopausal for more than 1 year) must use one reliable contraceptive measure (e.g. intrauterine device, hormone contraception, tubal ligation, partner vasectomy) for 1 month before, during and 1 month after stopping therapy. In addition, a second contraceptive measure (e.g. diaphragm, cervical cap, condom) is also recommended during this period of time
- women using oral contraceptives and thalidomide should be advised that there are a number of other medications which reduce the effectiveness of oral contraceptive agents and another form of contraception should be used
- any woman (either taking thalidomide or whose partner is taking thalidomide) who is of childbearing potential and who experiences menstrual irregularities or suspects she is pregnant must seek medical advice immediately
- see General Patient teaching and advice (p. xxvii)

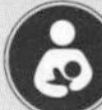

under no circumstances should thalidomide be used during pregnancy. It is a known human teratogen causing mortality at or just after birth and birth defects that include absence or shortness of limbs, external ear abnormalities, eye abnormalities, facial palsy, congenital heart defects and malformation of alimentary tract, urinary tract and/or genital tract. Birth defects have occurred after taking a single dose of thalidomide

contraindicated during breastfeeding

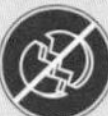

capsules should not be opened or crushed

ANTINEOPLASTIC AGENTS

The characteristics shared by most cancers include the differences between malignant and normal cells (e.g. different cell surface receptors), increased proliferation of the abnormal (or malignant) cells, infiltration of the surrounding tissue and a tendency to metastasise (or spread) to other sites.

In Australia in 2018, cancer represented four out of the top ten causes of death in males and three out of the top ten causes in women. However, the number of cancer-related deaths has fallen from 209 per 100,000 in 1982 to 150 per 100,000 in 2019 (AIHW 2020).

Treatment of cancer involves surgical removal, radiotherapy or chemotherapy, or a combination of these to remove the malignant cells and prevent more from proliferating, giving a person an overall 69% chance of surviving for 5 years, up from 51% in 1987–91. This number does vary, however, with the type of cancer, stage of diagnosis and/or treatment options (AIHW 2020).

Very toxic agents, termed antineoplastic agents (also called chemotherapy, cytotoxics or chemotherapeutic agents), are used to inhibit the growth of malignant cells by attacking them at different stages in the cell reproductive cycle. The ideal agent is one that destroys the malignant cells while doing minimal damage to the patient's normal cells. However, because all dividing cells, both malignant and normal, are affected, the use of these agents may be limited because of their effects on rapidly dividing normal cells (e.g. gastrointestinal tract cells, hair follicles, bone marrow cells). Some antineoplastic agents are effective during specific phases of the cell cycle (phase specific), whereas others act throughout the entire cycle (cycle specific) (Bryant et al 2019).

Antineoplastic agents can be divided into alkylating agents (e.g. cyclophosphamide), antimetabolites (e.g. methotrexate, mercaptopurine), cytotoxic antibiotics (e.g. doxorubicin), mitotic inhibitors (e.g. vincristine), topoisomerase inhibitors (e.g. etoposide), proteasome inhibitors (e.g. bortezomib), hormonal antineoplastics (e.g. flutamide, tamoxifen, goserilin), immunomodulatory drugs (e.g. check point inhibitors, interferons) and non-cytotoxic antineoplastics (e.g. monoclonal antibodies) (Bryant et al 2019). These agents may be given orally, intravenously, intrathecally or by regional perfusion, with the maximum tolerated doses being administered. Combinations of high doses of cytotoxic drugs are usually given intermittently (in cycles) to allow normal cells to recover. Because many of the antineoplastic agents are highly emetogenic, antiemetic agents are usually given concurrently to reduce the nausea and vomiting.

General Adverse effects of antineoplastic agents

- headache, migraine, asthenia, malaise, dizziness, depression, insomnia, somnolence, confusion
- loss of appetite, anorexia, nausea, vomiting, dyspepsia, diarrhoea, abdominal pain, flatulence, burping, mucositis, stomatitis, gastrointestinal ulceration and bleeding, weight loss
- anaemia, thrombocytopenia, ecchymosis, leucopenia, neutropenia, febrile neutropenia
- dyspnoea, rhinitis, cough, sinusitis, pneumonia, bronchitis, pharyngitis
- epistaxis
- rash, urticaria, pruritus, alopecia, sweating
- chest or back pain, arthralgia, myalgia, muscle cramps
- abnormal vision, double vision, amblyopia
- tinnitus
- (flu-like syndrome) fever, chills, rigors
- opportunistic infection (viral, bacterial, fungal)
- palpitations, arrhythmias, tachycardia, heart failure, angina, chest pain
- hypertension, hypotension
- dehydration
- peripheral oedema
- dysuria, haematuria, urinary tract infection
- elevated liver enzymes, hepatitis
- tumour lysis syndrome, hyperuricaemia
- secondary malignancy development
- (IV) extravasation, ulceration, soft tissue necrosis

General Interactions of antineoplastic agents

- use with live attenuated vaccines may potentiate replication of vaccine virus, increase the adverse effects of the vaccine virus, and/or may decrease the patient's antibody response to the vaccine and can be life threatening
- may decrease antibody response to killed vaccine virus
- it may take 3–12 months for the body to respond normally to vaccine
- close contacts should postpone immunisation with oral polio vaccine (because of viral shedding)
- caution if used with other agents known to cause bone marrow depression or blood dyscrasia, or with radiotherapy
- caution if used with other hepatotoxic, nephrotoxic, neurotoxic or cardiotoxic agents or those known to produce pulmonary toxicity

General Nursing points/Cautions for antineoplastic agents

- trade name and batch number should be recorded in patient medical history for traceability
- any dehydration or electrolyte imbalance should be corrected before starting therapy
- blood counts (including WBC with differential, platelet count) and haemoglobin should be measured before starting and then regularly throughout therapy to monitor bone marrow depression. Serum electrolytes, liver enzymes and creatinine clearance should also be monitored

- therapy should not be started if bone marrow function is markedly depressed
- if patient has a high tumour burden, blood uric acid, potassium, calcium phosphate and creatinine should be measured 3–4 times in first week to monitor for tumour lysis syndrome (lysis of a massive number of cells, resulting in the production of large amounts of uric acid from the breakdown of the nucleoproteins and hyperuricaemia)
- cardiac function should be assessed carefully when agents known to be cardiotoxic are to be used. Cardiotoxicity may be delayed and not manifest itself for months after treatment is completed. Depending on the agent, this may include ECG, echocardiogram or measurement of left ventricular ejection fraction
- audiograms are recommended before starting and regularly during therapy with agents known to be ototoxic
- an adequate interval should be left between cycles of therapy (including radiation therapy) to allow bone marrow to recover
- allopurinol and adequate hydration are used to prevent tumour lysis syndrome
- patient should be closely monitored if severe diarrhoea occurs to prevent dehydration and electrolyte imbalance occurring
- administer alone, ensuring lines are flushed well before and after administration
- prevent extravasation of cytotoxic drugs by ensuring that the IV cannula remains securely in position, thereby avoiding severe pain and tissue damage. If extravasation occurs, elevate limb and apply cold compress for 45 minutes
- observe closely for and report extravasation immediately
- protect patient from infection by maintaining strict asepsis, standard precautions and high standard of hygiene
- to reduce risk of infection, patient may be nursed in a positive-pressure room, if available
- observe closely for signs of infection, bleeding tendencies, paraesthesia, loss of reflexes, ataxia, mouth ulcers and alopecia
- staff should be aware of any concurrent therapy that may potentiate adverse effects (e.g. therapy with other drugs that are ototoxic, hepatotoxic, nephrotoxic or neurotoxic)
- caution if given within 14–21 days of surgery as wound healing may be impaired
- when handling any cytotoxic agents, staff should avoid inhaling or any contact with skin or eyes. If contact occurs, the area should be washed with copious quantities of water
- staff handling cytotoxics should be aware of hospital protocols or guidelines regarding preparation, administration, dealing with spillage, extravasation and disposal of used equipment and patients' body wastes
- pregnant staff should not handle antineoplastic agents
- depending on the patient's immune status, visitors (and staff) may need to be restricted if they display any signs of infections, especially influenza, measles or chicken pox
- staff should be aware of their own immunisation status and ensure that

it is up to date to protect immunocompromised patients
- (IV) some antineoplastic agents should be protected from light
- (IV) administer alone via dedicated line as many antineoplastic agents have incompatibilities. Lines should be flushed thoroughly after use
- caution if used in those who have had previous exposure to antineoplastic agents or radiotherapy
- caution or contraindicated if used in those with liver, kidney or cardiac impairment
- caution or contraindicated in those with current active infection, herpes zoster or recent chicken pox (including exposure), because severe generalised disease may result
- contraindicated in those with severe pre-existing bone marrow depression. Bone marrow should be allowed to recover before starting treatment

General Patient teaching and advice for antineoplastic agents

- reassure the patient that nausea and vomiting are transient and that drugs are available to counteract or prevent these adverse effects. Avoiding food for 4–6 hours before therapy may also reduce the severity of nausea and vomiting
- instruct the patient that tablets and capsules should be swallowed whole, not crushed, sucked, broken or chewed. If capsule/tablet is broken or opened, contact with powder should be avoided. If any contact is made with skin or eyes, area should be thoroughly washed with water. Hands should be washed well after handling tablets or capsules
- patient should be advised that any dental work should be completed before chemotherapy starts or deferred until blood counts return to normal. Good oral hygiene should be encouraged; however, patient should be advised to take care with toothbrush, dental floss or toothpicks as risk of gingival bleeding is increased
- warn patient against driving or handling heavy machinery if dizziness, drowsiness, extreme tiredness or lethargy, visual disturbances, headache or pain occurs
- advise patient that hair will regrow and that a wig may be worn in the meantime. Other options include hats and creative use of scarves. As hair may fall out unevenly (i.e. in clumps), some patients may prefer to shave their head at the start of the alopecia
- instruct the patient to seek medical advice immediately if any of the following occur:
  - fever, chills or other signs of infection
  - persistent bruising or unusual bleeding or black tarry stools
  - cough, hoarseness, side or lower back pain
  - blood in urine, difficulty with urination
  - yellowing of skin/eyes, unusual tiredness, loss of appetite, nausea, upper abdominal pain, dark urine, pale stools
  - unusual tiredness, pallor, shortness of breath on exertion
  - burning sensation in mouth and pharynx
- advise the patient to avoid contact with those with any infection

- instruct the patient to avoid contact sports or any other activities which may cause bruising or injury during therapy
- patient should be warned to take care using sharp objects such as nail cutters and razors that may result in bleeding
- symptoms of hand–foot syndrome can be reduced by advising patients to keep hands/feet cool (e.g. not wearing restricting gloves, socks or shoes; soaking hands/feet in cool water) starting 4–7 days after therapy. Other treatment may consist of pyridoxine (50–150 mg daily) and/or corticosteroids. Symptoms usually subside in 7–14 days
- during therapy and for 1 week after, patient should be instructed to:
  - flush toilet twice after use
  - wear gloves and use paper towels and bleach or a large quantity of water to wipe up any body spills
  - wash clothes or bed linen separately if contaminated
  - use a barrier method (e.g. condom) during sexual intercourse
- counsel men about the effects of drugs on sperm count and the possibility of sperm storage; use of a condom is also recommended during treatment period and in some instances for weeks to months after therapy (manufacturer's instructions should be consulted)
- women should be counselled that antineoplastic agents are not recommended or are contraindicated during pregnancy and it is therefore important to use reliable contraceptive methods (in some cases more than one method is recommended) while undergoing treatment and for a number of months post-therapy (time is dependent on the individual agents)
- counsel women to avoid breastfeeding during treatment as antineoplastic agents may be secreted into breastmilk, potentially causing severe adverse effects in the infant
- see also General Patient teaching and advice (p. xxvii)

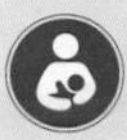

contraindicated or not recommended during pregnancy or breastfeeding

in general, antineoplastic capsules should not be opened or tablets crushed, chewed or broken

ABIRATERONE ACETATE (Zytiga)

Available forms

Tablets: 250 mg, 500 mg

Action

- hormonal antineoplastic (androgen biosynthesis inhibitor)

Use

- newly diagnosed metastatic hormone-sensitive prostate cancer (with androgen deprivation therapy)
- metastatic advanced prostate cancer (with prednisolone or prednisone) (asymptomatic, mildly symptomatic after failure of androgen deprivation therapy or previously treated with taxanes)

Dose

- 1 g orally daily 1 hour before or 2 hours after food (with 10 mg prednisolone or prednisone for metastatic castration-resistant cancer or 5 mg for hormone-sensitive cancer)

Adverse effects

- peripheral oedema
- cardiac failure, arrhythmias, atrial fibrillation, tachycardia, hypertension

- increased liver enzymes
- hypertriglyceridemia
- hypokalaemia

Interactions

- not recommended with spironolactone
- not recommended with phenytoin, carbamazepine, rifampicin, rifabutin, phenobarbital (phenobarbitone) as decreased serum levels may occur
- caution if used with agents that have a narrow therapeutic index
- combination with prednisolone/prednisone is contraindicated with radium 223 dichloride

Nursing points/Cautions

- BP, any fluid retention and serum potassium should be closely monitored during therapy
- liver enzymes should be measured before starting, second weekly for 12 weeks, then monthly throughout therapy
- if prednisolone or prednisone are withdrawn, the patient should be monitored for any signs of mineralocorticoid excess
- doses of prednisolone or prednisone may need to be increased if the patient undergoes severe stress
- caution if used in those affected by increases in BP, hypokalaemia or fluid retention (such as those with recent myocardial infarction or heart failure)
- contraindicated in those with severe liver impairment
- see also General Nursing points/Cautions for antineoplastic agents (p. 582)

Patient teaching and advice

- if the patient has diabetes, monitoring blood glucose levels should be advised as corticosteroids (prednisolone or prednisone) may cause hyperglycaemia
- see General Patient teaching and advice for antineoplastic agents (p. 584)

AFATINIB (Giotrif)

Available forms

Tablets: 20 mg, 30 mg, 40 mg, 50 mg

Action

- protein kinase inhibitor blocking epidermal growth factor receptors (EGFR) B1, B2, B3 and B4

Use

- treatment of locally advanced or metastatic non-squamous non-small cell carcinoma of the lung (either as first-line treatment or after failed cytotoxic treatment)
- locally advanced or metastatic squamous cell carcinoma (with disease progression or after platinum-based therapy)

Dose

- 40 mg orally daily either 3 hours before or 1 hour after food, increasing to 50 mg daily if well tolerated in first 3 weeks (daily maximum 50 mg) until disease progresses or it is no longer tolerated

Adverse effects

- eye inflammation, light sensitivity, lacrimation, eye pain, blurred vision, red eye and uncommonly, keratitis
- renal impairment
- hypokalaemia
- (rare) interstitial lung disease, liver impairment, severe dermatological reactions, pancreatitis, left ventricular dysfunction
- see also General Adverse effects of antineoplastic agents (p. 582)

Interactions

- may increase availability of rosuvastatin and sulfasalazine
- decreased serum levels may occur if given with carbamazepine, phenytoin,

phenobarbital (phenobarbitone), rifampicin and St John's wort
- increased serum levels may occur if given with ritonavir, ciclosporin, itraconazole, erythromycin, verapamil, tacrolimus, nelfinavir, amiodarone and saquinavir

Nursing points/Cautions

- EGFR mutation should be confirmed by robust method before starting therapy
- patient should be well hydrated during therapy
- antidiarrhoeal drugs (e.g. loperamide) should be given at the first sign of diarrhoea. If diarrhoea is severe, IV rehydration with fluid and electrolytes may be required
- therapy should be stopped if severe dermatological reactions occur
- if patient has any visual disturbance, urgent ophthalmology review is recommended
- tablets contain lactose and are therefore not recommended in those with rare hereditary conditions of galactose intolerance, Lapp lactase deficiency or glucose–galactose malabsorption
- caution if used in females, those of lower body weight or with kidney impairment as risk of diarrhoea, skin reactions and stomatitis is increased
- caution if used in those with history of keratitis, ulcerative keratitis or severe dry eye
- caution if used in those with abnormal left ventricular ejection fraction. Cardiac assessment is recommended before starting therapy if used
- not recommended in those with severe liver or kidney failure or on dialysis
- see also General Nursing points/Cautions for antineoplastic agents (p. 582)

Patient teaching and advice

- if patient is unable to swallow tablet, instruct them that it can be dissolved in 100 mL non-carbonated water only and allowed to dissolve, stirring occasionally over 15 minutes (tablet should not be crushed or broken). After drinking, the glass should be rinsed with another 100 mL and the remainder drunk
- instruct the patient to take antidiarrhoeal medication at the first sign of diarrhoea and continue until loose bowel motions have stopped for 12 hours. The patient should be advised to drink plenty of fluids to avoid becoming dehydrated
- advise the patient to seek medical advice immediately if any of the following occur:
  - diarrhoea not controlled after 48 hours of antidiarrhoeal medication or severe diarrhoea (4 or more bowel motions in 24 hours)
  - severe skin reaction such as peeling or blistering of skin
  - cough, shortness of breath, fever
  - blurred vision, eye pain, red eye, tearing, eye inflammation, sensitivity to light
- see General Patient teaching and advice for antineoplastic agents (p. 584)

ALEMTUZUMAB (Lemtrada, MabCampath)

Available forms

Vial: 12 mg/1.2 mL, 30 mg/mL

Action

- IgG_{1kappa} monoclonal antibody specific for cell surface glycoprotein (CD52)

Use

- B-cell chronic lymphocytic leukaemia (where two other therapies were ineffective) (MabCampath)

- treatment of relapsing multiple sclerosis (see Movement disorder agents p. 1310) (Lemtrada)

Dose

- initially 3 mg IV on day 1, 10 mg on day 2 and 30 mg on day 3 (if tolerated), then 30 mg IV 3 times weekly on alternate days for a maximum of 12 weeks (daily maximum 30 mg or weekly maximum 90 mg) (MabCampath)

Adverse effects

- infusion-related reaction (hypotension, chills, rigors, fever, shortness of breath, rash)
- opportunistic infection (fungal, viral, bacterial)
- hyponatraemia, hypocalcaemia
- conjunctivitis
- vasospasm, flushing
- bronchospasm, haemoptysis
- (IV site) pain, reaction
- (rare) haemophagocytic lymphohistiocytosis
- see General Adverse effects of antineoplastic agents (p. 582)

Interactions

- not recommended within 21 days of other antineoplastic agents
- not recommended with irradiated blood products
- vaccination with live vaccines is not recommended with or within 12 months of finishing therapy

Nursing points/Cautions

- premedication with antihistamines and analgesic is recommended 30 minutes before infusion
- patient should be closely monitored for any signs of infusion-related reaction
- BP should be measured during therapy as transient hypotension occurs commonly
- prophylaxis with antibacterial agent (e.g. trimethoprim/sulfamethoxazole) and/or antiviral agents (e.g. famciclovir) is recommended during and for 8 weeks after completion of therapy to decrease likelihood of opportunistic infection
- if adverse reactions occur at 3 mg or 10 mg doses, they should be repeated daily until well tolerated before moving on to next dose
- therapy should be stopped if there is no response
- if platelet count falls (< 25,000/ microL), therapy should be interrupted and restarted when platelet count recovers
- if therapy is withheld for ≥ 7 days, it should be restarted at 3 mg dose and gradually escalated
- if retreatment is considered, CD52 gene expression should be checked before starting
- dilute with 100 mL of sodium chloride 0.9% or glucose 5% before administration. Infusion bag should be inverted gently to avoid foaming and ensure even distribution
- given as IV infusion over 2 hours
- if infusion-related reaction occurs, infusion time can be extended to 8 hours
- contraindicated in those with hypersensitivity to murine proteins or other monoclonal antibodies, with HIV infection or if active secondary malignancies or active infection are present
- see also General Nursing points/ Cautions for antineoplastic agents (p. 582)

Patient teaching and advice

- see General Patient teaching and advice for antineoplastic agents (p. 584)

ANAGRELIDE (Agrylin)

Available form

Capsules: 0.5 mg

Action
- quinazoline derivative antineoplastic agent that reduces platelet count

Use
- essential thrombocytopenia

Dose
- initially 0.5 mg orally twice daily for ≥ 7 days, then adjusting dose to lowest effective dose (daily maximum 10 mg or dose maximum 2.5 mg)

Adverse effects
- abnormal vision, double vision, amblyopia
- (rare) QT prolongation, pulmonary hypertension
- see General Adverse effects of antineoplastic agents (p. 582)

Interactions
- caution if given with other agents known to cause QT prolongation or electrolyte imbalance (especially hypokalaemia or hypomagnesaemia)
- caution if used with heparin as anticoagulant effect may be increased
- may increase effects of milrinone or similar agents
- may inhibit clearance of theophylline, increasing risk of toxicity
- clearance may be inhibited by fluvoxamine and ciprofloxacin
- caution if used with omeprazole
- enhances antiplatelet effect of aspirin and should only be given with great caution because of haemorrhagic risk

Nursing points/Cautions
- cardiovascular examination should be conducted before starting therapy
- any hypokalaemia or hypomagnesaemia should be corrected before starting therapy
- platelet count should be monitored second daily for 7 days, then weekly. Platelet count usually responds to therapy in 7–14 days
- liver function tests, renal function test, electrolytes and full blood count are recommended before starting and regularly during therapy
- plasmapheresis may be more appropriate if immediate platelet reduction is required
- dose should not be increased by more than 0.5 mg weekly
- target platelet count 150–400 × 10^9/L
- increased risk of renal toxicity if serum creatinine ≥ 0.18 mmol/L
- increased risk of thromboembolic events if therapy is suddenly stopped
- caution if used in those with mild-to-moderate liver impairment (starting dose should be decreased to 0.5 mg daily)
- caution if used in those with congenital or acquired QT prolongation or electrolyte imbalance
- contraindicated in those with severe liver impairment
- see also General Nursing points/Cautions for antineoplastic agents (p. 582)

Patient teaching and advice
- advise patient to seek medical advice immediately if any of the following occur:
  - rapid or irregular heart rate
  - chest pain
- warn patient not to drive or operate machinery if visual disturbances occur
- see also General Patient teaching and advice for antineoplastic agents (p. 584)

ANASTROZOLE (Anastrol, Anzole, Arianna, Arimidex)

Available form
Tablets: 1 mg

Action
- highly selective non steroidal aromatase inhibitor that decreases serum estradiol (oestradiol) levels with no effect on formation of adrenal corticosteroids or aldosterone

Use
- early breast cancer (first-line treatment, post-menopausal, oestrogen/progesterone-positive tumour) (adjunctive treatment)
- advanced breast cancer (first-line treatment, post-menopausal, oestrogen/progesterone-positive tumour)
- advanced breast cancer (post-menopausal) (after tamoxifen failure)

Dose
- 1 mg orally daily for up to 5 years

Adverse effects
- hot flushes
- nausea, vomiting, diarrhoea, anorexia
- elevated liver enzymes, hypercholesterolaemia
- headache, asthenia, somnolence
- joint pain/stiffness, bone pain, myalgia
- rash, hair thinning
- vaginal dryness or bleeding
- (rare) osteoporosis, bone fractures, trigger finger

Interactions
- not recommended with tamoxifen, oestrogen-containing products or LHRH agonists

Nursing points/Cautions
- bone density should be measured before starting and regularly throughout therapy and treatment or prophylaxis therapy started if needed
- 2–3 years of tamoxifen therapy should be completed before switching to anastrozole
- caution if used in those with kidney or liver impairment
- not recommended in pre-menopausal women or in those with oestrogen/progesterone-negative tumour
- see also General Nursing points/Cautions for antineoplastic agents (p. 582)

Patient teaching and advice
- see also General Patient teaching and advice for antineoplastic agents (p. 584)

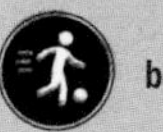

banned in sport

APALUTAMIDE (Erlyand)

Available form
Tablets: 60 mg

Action
- hormonal antineoplastic agent that blocks androgen receptor
- active metabolite has one-third the activity of apalutamide

Use
- treatment of non-metastatic castration-resistant prostate cancer

Dose
- 240 mg orally daily (with gonadotropin-releasing hormone (GnRH) analogue unless patient has had bilateral orchiectomy)

Adverse effects
- fatigue
- arthralgia
- hot flushes
- decreased appetite, decreased weight, nausea, diarrhoea, altered taste
- depression
- peripheral oedema
- haematuria
- rash
- osteopenia, osteoporosis, fractures, increased risk of falls
- anaemia, leukopenia, lymphopenia
- hypercholesterolaemia, hyperglycaemia, hypertriglyceridemia, hyperkalaemia

- hypothyroidism (in those receiving thyroid replacement therapy)
- hypertension, ischaemic heart disease, heart failure, QT interval prolongation
- (rare) seizures

Interactions

- caution if used with agents known to prolong QT interval
- decreased serum level may occur if given with gemfibrozil, itraconazole and rifampicin
- caution if given with warfarin. INR should be monitored closely if given together
- may decrease serum levels of fexofenadine and rosuvastatin
- may reduce effects of levothyroxine increasing risk of hypothyroidism

Nursing points/Cautions

- caution if used in those with pre-existing active cardiac disease or history of QT prolongation
- caution if used in those with history of seizures
- caution if used in those with history of thyroid dysfunction receiving thyroid replacement therapy or over 75 years
- contraindicated in women

Patient teaching and advice

- see General Patient teaching and advice for antineoplastic agents (p. 584)

ARSENIC TRIOXIDE (Phenasen)

Available form

Vial: 10 mg/10 mL

Action

- antineoplastic agent with unknown action that induces partial differentiation and apoptosis in leukaemic cells
- stored in bone marrow, lung, liver, kidney, heart, hair and nails with hair and nails showing increasing levels of arsenic during therapy

Use

- induction of remission and consolidation of acute promyelocytic leukaemia (APL) (refractory or relapsed from other therapy) or previously untreated APL (with retinoic acid and/or chemotherapy)

Dose

- (newly diagnosed APL) 0.15 mg/kg IV over 2 hours from days 9–28 days (cycle 1, induction), then after 3–4 weeks, 0.15 mg/kg from days 1–28 (cycle 2), then after 3–4 weeks, 0.15 mg/kg for 5 days, followed by 2 days off for 5 weeks (consolidation) (with tretinoin and/or chemotherapy) **OR**
- (refractory or relapsed APL) 0.15 mg/kg IV over 2 hours until bone marrow remission occurs (induction), then after 3–4 weeks, 0.15 mg/kg for 25 daily doses for up to 5 weeks (consolidation)

Adverse effects

- cardiac arrhythmia, QT interval prolongation
- APL differentiation syndrome (fever, dyspnoea, weight gain, pulmonary infiltrates, pleural/pericardial effusions (with or without leucocytosis))
- peripheral neuropathy
- see also General Adverse effects of antineoplastic agents (p. 582)

Interactions

- not recommended with agents known to prolong QT interval (e.g. amiodarone, disopyramide, clarithromycin, sotalol, methadone, ziprasidone) or cause electrolyte disturbances, especially hypokalaemia and hypomagnesaemia (e.g. diuretics, amphotericin B (amphotericin))

Nursing points/Cautions

- any electrolyte imbalance should be corrected before starting therapy

- 12-lead ECG is recommended before starting and then weekly during therapy
- serum electrolytes (especially potassium, calcium and magnesium), creatinine, blood counts and coagulation should be measured before starting and then regularly throughout therapy (more frequent if patient is unstable)
- (newly diagnosed APL) 1 mg/kg daily prednisolone/prednisone is recommended for at least 10 days during induction
- dilute with 100–250 mL sodium chloride 0.9% or glucose 5% for IV infusion
- if patient shows signs of APL differentiation syndrome, dexamethasone 10 mg IV twice daily should be administered for 3 or more days or until symptoms resolve
- (refractory/relapsed APL) therapy should be discontinued after 2 months if bone marrow remission does not occur
- caution if used in those with known congenital or acquired prolonged QT syndrome or electrolyte imbalance
- not recommended in those with congestive cardiac failure or in children under 5 years
- contraindicated in those with hypersensitivity to arsenic
- see also General Nursing points/Cautions for antineoplastic agents (p. 582)

Patient teaching and advice

- patient should be instructed to seek medical advice immediately if any of the following occur:
  - any fever, shortness of breath or weight gain (signs of APL differentiation syndrome)
  - rapid or irregular heart rate or fainting
  - numbness, weakness or tingling in hands or feet
- see also General Patient teaching and advice for antineoplastic agents (p. 584)

AVELUMAB (Bavencio)

Available form

Vial: 200 mg/10 mL

Action

- monoclonal antibody (IgG1) that blocks interaction between PD-L1 (expressed on tumour cells and/or tumour infiltrating immune cells) restoring anti-tumour T cell responses

Use

- treatment of metastatic Merkel cell carcinoma

Dose

- 10 mg/kg by IV infusion over 60 minutes every 2 weeks

Adverse effects

- infusion-related reactions (e.g. fever, chills, flushing, hypotension, dyspnoea, wheezing, back or abdominal pain, urticaria)
- pneumonitis
- hepatitis
- colitis
- thyroid disorders, adrenal insufficiency, hyperglycaemia, diabetes mellitus
- see also General Adverse effects for antineoplastic agents (p. 582)

Nursing points/Cautions

- premedication with antihistamine and paracetamol is recommended before first 4 infusions
- observe patient for any signs of infusion-related reactions (e.g. fever, chills, flushing, hypotension, dyspnoea, wheezing, back or abdominal pain, urticaria)
- dilute with either sodium chloride 0.45% or 0.9%
- use 0.2 micron inline or add-on filter

- see also General Nursing points/Cautions for antineoplastic agents (p. 582)

Patient teaching and advice

- advise patient to seek medical advice if any of the following occur:
  - fever, chills, shortness of breath, dizziness (which can occur up to several hours after the infusion as finished)
  - shortness of breath, chest pain, coughing
  - eye or skin yellowing, loss of appetite, nausea, vomiting, pain in right upper abdominal area, dark urine
  - increased number of bowel movements, diarrhoea, black stools, stools with blood or mucus, severe stomach pain or tenderness
  - increased hunger or thirst, needing to urinate more often, weight loss, increased tiredness
  - extreme tiredness, rapid heartrate, increased sweating, weight gain or loss, change in mood or behaviour (e.g. irritability forgetfulness), feeling cold
- see General Patient teaching and advice for antineoplastic agents (p. 584)

AXICABTAGENE CILOLEUCEL (Yescarta)

Available form

Suspension bag: 1–2.4 x 10^6 anti-CD19 CAR T-cells/kg suspension

Action

- CD19 directed genetically modified autologous T-cell immunotherapy prepared from patient's own T cells which have been harvested via leukapheresis and then genetically modified by retroviral transduction to express a chimeric antigen receptor (CAR)

Use

- relapsed or refractory diffuse large B-cell lymphoma (after two or more types of systemic therapy)
- primary mediastinal large or high grade B-cell lymphoma
- diffuse large B-cell lymphoma arising from follicular lymphoma

Dose

- single IV infusion for a target dose of 2×10^6 anti-CD19 CAR T cells/kg (range 1×10^6 to 2.4×10^6 cells/kg) (maximum 2 x 10^8 anti-CD19 CAR T cells)

Adverse effects

- cytokine-release syndrome
- neurologic toxicity (including encephalopathy, tremor, confusion, aphasia, somnolence)
- bacterial and viral infections, virus reactivation
- hypogammaglobinaemia
- tumour lysis syndrome
- see also General Adverse effects for antineoplastic agents (p. 582)

Interactions

- vaccination with live vaccines is not recommended for at least 6 weeks before lymphodepleting chemotherapy, during therapy and until immune recovery has occurred

Nursing points/Cautions

- before collecting cells for therapy, patient should be screened for hepatitis B and C and HIV
- after infusion, blood counts, uric acid and immunoglobulin levels should be monitored
- severe or life-threatening cytokine-release syndrome should be treated with tocilizumab (see DMARDs, p. 1003) or tocilizumab and corticosteroids. A minimum of 4 doses of tocilizumab must be readily available in case of cytokine-release syndrome, along with emergency equipment.

Treatment and supportive care (e.g. oxygen, fluids, vasopressor and, if life threatening, ventilator support, haemodialysis) must be instituted at first signs of cytokine-release syndrome
- pre-treatment involves lymphodepleting chemotherapy (cyclophosphamide 500 mg/m^2 IV and fludarabine 30 mg/m^2 IV on days 5, 4 and 3 before infusion). If patient has high uric acid levels or high tumour burden, allopurinol (or alternative prophylaxis) should be given before conditioning chemotherapy to reduce risk of tumour lysis syndrome
- premedication (500–1000 mg paracetamol orally with diphenhydramine 12.5 mg IV or orally (or equivalent)) is recommended 1 hour before infusion
- prophylactic systemic corticosteroids should not be used
- important to coordinate thaw and infusion timing so that infusion is thawed and available for infusion when the patient is ready
- patient identity must be confirmed (matching patient ID with patient identifiers on infusion cassette). When correctly identified, product bag is removed from cassette and inspected for any breaks or cracks before thawing. Infusion bag should then be placed in second sterile bag and then thawed, either in water bath or by dry thaw method until there is no visible ice in infusion bag. Bag should be gently mixed to disperse any cellular clumps. Solution should not be washed, spun down or re-suspended before infusion
- leukodepleting filter should not be used
- only given IV (with central venous line recommended)
- line should be primed with sodium chloride 0.9% before and after infusion
- infused via gravity or peristaltic infusion pump
- standard precautions for blood-borne pathogens should be adhered to and handling and disposal should be as per institution biosafety guidelines
- patient should be monitored for at least 7 days post-infusion for any signs of cytokine-release syndrome
- solution must not be irradiated
- contains dimethyl sulfoxide and residual gentamicin which may cause hypersensitivity reaction in sensitive individuals
- not recommended for primary central nervous system lymphoma
- not recommended in those with active systemic infections

Patient teaching and advice

- patient should be instructed to remain within close proximity of healthcare facility (< 2 hours) for at least 4 weeks post-infusion
- warn patient not to drive or operate machinery for at least 8 weeks after infusion due to the risk of fitting or other neurological issues
- ensure patient understands the importance of ongoing monitoring (at least 15 years) for secondary malignancies
- patient should be advised to immediately seek medical advice if any of the following occur:
  - fever, chills, low blood pressure which can lead to feeling lightheaded or dizzy, or rapid heart rate (signs of cytokine-release syndrome, which can be serious or life threatening)
  - headache, tremor, confusion, difficulty talking, sleepy or drowsiness
  - signs of infection, including fever, chills, swollen glands
  - fatigue, confusion, nausea, vomiting, diarrhoea, muscle weakness, cramps or spasms, tingling

around mouth or hands/feet, heart beats slower, faster or flutters, fitting (signs of tumour lysis syndrome)
- instruct patient not to donate blood, organs, tissue or cells for transplantation

AXITINIB (Inlyta)

Available forms
Tablets: 1 mg, 3 mg, 5 mg, 7 mg

Action
- tyrosine kinase receptor inhibitor (vascular endothelial growth factor (VEGF) receptor 1, 2, 3)
- receptors are thought to be responsible for tumour growth and metastatic spread

Use
- advanced renal cell carcinoma (where other therapy has failed)

Dose
- initially 5 mg orally twice daily, increasing or decreasing dose according to patient tolerance

Adverse effects
- hypertension
- elevated haemoglobin and haematocrit, increased risk of thromboembolic events
- gastrointestinal haemorrhage or perforation, fistula formation
- haemorrhagic events
- thyroid dysfunction
- thromboembolism
- impaired wound healing
- proteinuria
- hand–foot syndrome (hand/foot numbness, paraesthesia, tingling, erythema, pain, swelling and, at worst, ulceration, blistering or moist desquamation)
- (uncommon) reversible posterior leukoencephalopathy syndrome (RPLS)
- see also General Adverse effects of antineoplastic agents (p. 582)

Interactions
- increased serum levels may occur if given with grapefruit juice, itraconazole, clarithromycin, ritonavir, saquinavir, indinavir, nelfinavir and atazanavir
- decreased serum levels may occur if given with phenytoin, phenobarbital (phenobarbitone), carbamazepine, rifampicin, rifabutin, dexamethasone and St John's wort

Nursing points/Cautions
- patient should be monitored for any signs of cardiac failure
- urine should be checked for protein before starting and during therapy, and interrupted if moderate-to-severe proteinuria occurs
- any pre-existing hypertension should be controlled before starting therapy
- BP and thyroid function should be measured before starting and regularly during therapy
- increase in dose should only occur if there are no adverse effects and patient is not being treated with antihypertensive agents
- therapy should be stopped 24 hours before any surgical procedures
- tablets contain lactose and are therefore not recommended in those with rare hereditary problems of galactose intolerance, Lapp lactase deficiency or glucose–galactose malabsorption
- caution if used in those at risk for or having risk factors for thromboembolism (especially if patient has experienced event in last 6 months)
- not recommended in those with untreated brain metastases or recent active GI bleeding
- see also General Nursing points/Cautions for antineoplastic agents (p. 582)

Patient teaching and advice

- instruct patient that dose should not be readministered if dose is missed or patient vomits
- patient should be advised to avoid grapefruit and grapefruit juice during therapy
- advise patient to seek medical advice immediately if any of the following occur:
  - chest pain, coughing, shortness of breath, difficulty breathing
  - leg/calf swelling, pain or tenderness of leg/calf, warmth, redness
  - vomiting blood or coffee ground-like material, black sticky stools, abdominal pain
  - headache, altered mental state, visual disturbances or fitting (seizures)
- symptoms of hand–foot syndrome can be reduced by advising patients to keep hands/feet cool (e.g. not wearing restricting gloves, socks or shoes; soaking hands/feet in cool water) starting 4–7 days after therapy. Other treatment may consist of pyridoxine (50–150 mg daily) and/or corticosteroids. Symptoms usually subside in 7–14 days
- see also General Patient teaching advice for antineoplastic agents (p. 584)

AZACITIDINE (Azadine, Celazadine, Vidaza)

Available form

Vial: 100 mg

Action

- pyrimidine analogue antimetabolite that acts on DNA and also has direct cytotoxic action on abnormal haemopoietic cells in bone marrow

Use

- acute myeloid leukaemia (AML) (with 20–30% blasts and multilineage dysplasia, stem cell transplant is not recommended)
- chronic myelomonocytic leukaemia (CML) (with 10–29% blasts, no myeloproliferative disease)
- intermediate- to high-risk myelodysplastic syndrome (MDS)

Dose

- 75 mg/m^2 SC or IV over 10–40 minutes for 7 days followed by 21-day rest interval (cycle 1), repeated for ≥ 6 cycles (treatment may continue if benefit is noted)

Adverse effects

- (injection site) pain, redness, rash, inflammation, itching, bruising, induration
- eye/conjunctival haemorrhage
- (rare) hypersensitivity, interstitial lung disease
- see also General Adverse effects of antineoplastic agents (p. 582)

Nursing points/Cautions

- patient should be pre-medicated to prevent nausea and vomiting
- dose reduction is required if severe adverse effects occur
- (SC) reconstitute with 4 mL water for injections and use within 1 hour (if at room temperature). Can be refrigerated for up to 8 hours, but should be brought to room temperature for at least 30 minutes before SC administration
- (SC) if dose > 4 mL it should be divided and given into separate sites
- (SC) rotate SC injection sites avoiding any areas that are red, tender, hard or bruised. Injections should not be within 2.5 cm of previous injection site
- (IV) reconstitute with 10 mL water for injections, and dilute with sodium chloride 0.9% or lactated Ringer's solution (50–100 mL) and infuse over 10–40 minutes
- (IV) infusion should be completed within 45 minutes of reconstitution

- incompatible with glucose 5% and solutions containing bicarbonate
- contraindicated in those with advanced malignant liver tumours or severe kidney impairment (creatinine clearance < 30 mL/minute)
- see also General Nursing points/Cautions for antineoplastic agents (p. 582)

Patient teaching and advice

- see General Patient teaching and advice for antineoplastic agents (p. 584)

BCG (Non-Vaccine) (OncoTICE)

Available form

Vial: 2–8 × 10^8 CFU

Action

- immunostimulant that causes inflammatory response resulting in reduction or elimination of non-muscle cancerous lesions in the urinary bladder
- live attenuated *Mycobacterium bovis*

Use

- primary or recurrent bladder cancer (BC) in situ
- adjunct to transurethral resection of high grade and/or relapsing superficial papillary transitional cell bladder cancer (stage TA or T1)

Dose

- (in situ BC) 50 mL of reconstituted solution instilled into bladder and left in situ for 2 hours if possible weekly for 6 weeks, then monthly for 12 months **OR**
- (superficial papillary transitional cell bladder cancer) 50 mL of reconstituted solution instilled into bladder and left in situ for 2 hours if possible weekly for 6 weeks, repeated at week 8 and 12, then monthly for 4–12 months

Adverse effects

- dysuria, haematuria, urinary retention, urgency and frequency, bladder cramps/pain, contracted bladder
- cystitis, urinary tract infection
- nausea
- malaise, fatigue
- fever, chills, flu-like symptoms
- (rare) systemic disease, hypersensitivity

Interactions

- caution if used with immunosuppressive agents, bone marrow depressants or radiotherapy as they may interfere with immune response

Nursing points/Cautions

- patient should be assessed for active TB disease before starting therapy
- monitor patient for any signs of BCG infection and toxicity during therapy
- if patient develops signs of BCG disease, immediate evaluation is recommended as treatment with antimycobacterial agents may be required
- great care should be taken during reconstitution to avoid contact with or inhalation of powder. Person should wear adequate eye and face protection, gloves, mask and gown during procedure. Reconstitute powder with 1 mL of sodium chloride 0.9% and then dilute with 49 mL sodium chloride 0.9% (total volume 50 mL)
- do not shake solution during reconstitution
- incompatible with hypotonic or hypertonic solution
- if patient develops bacterial urinary tract infection (UTI), therapy should be withheld until UTI has totally resolved to decrease risk of adverse effects
- not given with IV, SC or IM
- therapy should be withheld if patient is being treated with antibiotics

- caution if used in those with small bladder capacity as greater irritation may occur
- contraindicated in those with urinary tract infection, febrile illness, gross haematuria, existing active tuberculosis, impaired immune response (including AIDS), taking corticosteroids or immunosuppressants (including radiotherapy)
- within 7–14 days of biopsy or traumatic catheterisation until mucosa has healed
- see also General Nursing points/ Cautions for antineoplastic agents (p. 582)

Patient teaching and advice

- patient should be instructed not to drink for 4 hours before instillation
- patient is asked to empty bladder, urethral catheter inserted, diluted solution instilled and catheter removed
- patient should rotate every 15 minutes from left, prone, right and supine for 1 hour
- after retaining solution for another 1 hour (if possible), patient is asked to void in seated position
- warn patient that he/she may experience burning sensation with first void after completion of therapy
- patient should be instructed to void in seated position in 6 hours following procedure, and add an equal volume of household chlorine bleach (e.g. White King) to the toilet. Urine and bleach should be allowed to stand in toilet for 15 minutes before flushing
- male patients should be advised to either refrain from sexual intercourse or wear a condom for 7 days after treatment

BENDAMUSTINE HYDROCHLORIDE (Ribomustin)

Available forms

Vial: 25 mg, 100 mg

Action

- alkylating agent (nitrogen mustard analogue) that impairs DNA synthesis and repair
- active against both quiescent and dividing cells

Use

- treatment of chronic lymphocytic leukaemia (CLL)
- previously untreated indolent CD20 positive non-Hodgkin lymphoma stage III or IV (with rituximab)
- previously untreated CD20 positive stage III–IV mantle cell lymphoma (with rituximab in those ineligible for stem cell transplantation)
- relapsed/refractory indolent non-Hodgkin lymphoma

Dose

- (CLL monotherapy) 100 mg/m^2 by IV infusion over 30–60 minutes on days 1 and 2, every 4 weeks for up to 6 cycles **OR**
- (non-Hodgkin lymphoma monotherapy) 120 mg/m^2 by IV infusion over 30–60 minutes on days 1 and 2, every 3 weeks for 6–8 cycles (maximum 8 cycles) **OR**
- (non-Hodgkin lymphoma, mantle cell lymphoma, combination therapy) 90 mg/m^2 by IV infusion over 30–60 minutes on days 1 and 2 of 4-week cycle for up to 6 cycles (with rituximab)

Adverse effects

- prolonged lymphocytopenia (for at least 7–9 months after treatment)
- hypokalaemia
- (infusion reaction) fever, chills, rash, itching

- (rare) severe skin reaction, anaphylaxis
- see also General Adverse effects of antineoplastic agents (p. 582)

Interactions

- contraindicated with yellow fever vaccination
- increased risk of myelosuppression if given with other myelosuppressive agents, including ciclosporin and tacrolimus
- caution if used with ciprofloxacin, fluvoxamine, aciclovir or cimetidine

Nursing points/Cautions

- patient should be tested for hepatitis B before starting therapy as reactivation may occur
- ensure patient is well hydrated during therapy
- (non-Hodgkin lymphoma, mantle cell lymphoma, combination therapy) therapy should be interrupted if leucocyte and/or platelet counts drops to $< 3 \times 10^9$/L or $< 75 \times 10^9$/L
- serum potassium should be closely monitored during therapy and potassium supplements administered if serum potassium < 3.5 mEq/L. ECG monitoring is also recommended
- reconstitute powder with 40 mL water for injections (for 100 mg vial) or 10 mL (for 25 mg vial) to given concentration of 2.5 mg/mL and then finally dilute further with sodium chloride 0.9% to a final volume of 500 mL
- contraindicated in those with severe liver impairment (bilirubin > 3 mg/dL), jaundice, severe marrow depression, within 30 days of major surgery or active infection
- see also General Nursing points/Cautions for antineoplastic agents (p. 582)

Patient teaching and advice

- advise patient to seek medical advice immediately if severe skin reaction, including peeling and blistering occurs
- warn patient that susceptibility to infection will exist for 7–9 months after therapy has stopped
- see also General Patient teaching and advice for antineoplastic agents (p. 584)

BEVACIZUMAB (Avastin)

Available forms

Vial: 100 mg/4 mL, 400 mg/16 mL

Action

- antivascular endothelial growth factor (VEGF) monoclonal antibody
- neutralises VEGF, reducing tumour vascularisation and inhibiting tumour growth

Use

- metastatic colorectal cancer
- local recurrent or metastatic breast cancer
- advanced and/or metastatic renal cell carcinoma
- grade IV glioma
- epithelial ovarian, fallopian tube or primary peritoneal cancer
- recurrent epithelial ovarian, fallopian tube or primary peritoneal cancer
- advanced, metastatic or recurrent non-squamous non-small cell lung (NSCLC) cancer
- cervical cancer

Dose

- (metastatic colorectal cancer – first-line treatment) 5 mg/kg IV once every 2 weeks or 7.5 mg/kg IV once every 3 weeks **OR**
- (metastatic colorectal cancer – second-line treatment) 10 mg/kg IV once every 2 weeks or 15 mg/kg IV once every 3 weeks **OR**

- (breast cancer) 10 mg/kg IV once every 2 weeks or 15 mg/kg IV every 3 weeks **OR**
- (NSCLC) 15 mg/kg IV once every 3 weeks (with carboplatin and paclitaxel) for up to 6 cycles, then as a single agent until disease progresses **OR**
- (renal cell cancer) 10 mg/kg IV once every 2 weeks (with interferon alfa 2a) **OR**
- (glioma) 10 mg/kg IV once every 2 weeks or 15 mg/kg IV once every 3 weeks **OR**
- (epithelial ovarian, fallopian tube or primary peritoneal cancer) 15 mg/kg IV once every 3 weeks (with carboplatin and paclitaxel) for up to 6 cycles, then as a single agent for 15 months or until disease progresses **OR**
- (recurrent epithelial ovarian, fallopian tube or primary peritoneal cancer) 15 mg/kg IV once every 3 weeks (with carboplatin and gemcitabine) for 6–10 cycles, then as a single agent until disease progresses **OR**
- (recurrent epithelial ovarian, fallopian tube or primary peritoneal cancer) 15 mg/kg IV once every 3 weeks (with carboplatin and paclitaxel) for 6–8 cycles, then as a single agent until disease progresses **OR**
- (cervical cancer) 15 mg/kg IV once every 3 weeks (with cisplatin and paclitaxel or paclitaxel and topotecan)

Adverse effects

- hypertension
- impaired wound healing
- thromboembolism
- proteinuria
- peripheral neuropathy
- infusion-related reactions
- (NSCLC) pulmonary haemorrhage, haemoptysis
- haemorrhage, epistaxis
- (uncommon) (GI and non-GI) fistulae formation and rarely, GI or gall bladder perforation
- (rare) hypersensitivity, posterior reversible encephalopathy syndrome (PRES), hand–foot syndrome (hand/foot numbness, paraesthesia, tingling, erythema, pain, swelling and, at worst, ulceration, blistering or moist desquamation)
- (rare) osteonecrosis of the jaw (generally occurring in those with cancer (especially those with bony metastases or multiple myeloma), existing periodontal disease, oral trauma, poor oral hygiene or being treated with antineoplastic agents, radiotherapy or corticosteroids. Most cases are associated with dental procedures (e.g. tooth extraction) and symptoms include jaw pain, toothache, altered sensation, recurrent infection (including osteomyelitis), non-healing sores of the mouth/jaw and/or exposed bone)
- (very rare) hypertensive encephalopathy
- see also General Adverse effects of antineoplastic agents (p. 582)

Interactions

- caution if given with sunitinib maleate due to increased risk of microangiopathic haemolytic anaemia
- increased risk of severe neutropenia if given with liposomal doxorubicin, platinum- or taxane-based therapy

Nursing points/Cautions

- any pre-existing hypertension should be controlled before starting therapy
- dental examination and any dental treatment should be completed before starting therapy
- BP should be monitored during therapy as hypertension commonly occurs

- patient should be closely monitored during infusion for any signs of infusion reaction
- therapy is not recommended within 28 days of surgery or until surgical wound has healed due to increased risk of wound-healing complications
- urine should be monitored for protein before and during therapy
- not recommended with dextrose or glucose solutions
- not given as IV push or bolus
- after dilution with sodium chloride 0.9%, given by IV infusion over 90 minutes (first dose) and if tolerated, next infusion is given over 60 minutes. If this is tolerated, next and subsequent infusions are given over 30 minutes
- increased risk of thromboembolic events if given to those $>$ 65 years with diabetes mellitus or previous history of thromboembolism
- caution if used in those with bleeding tendencies, congestive cardiac failure or cardiovascular disease
- caution if used in those with history or symptoms of bowel obstruction, abdominal fistulae or prior pelvic irradiation due to increased risk of fistulae formation
- contraindicated in those with hypersensitivity to Chinese hamster ovary cell products, other recombinant monoclonal antibodies or untreated CNS metastases
- see also General Nursing points/Cautions for antineoplastic agents (p. 582)

Patient teaching and advice

- advise patient to seek medical advice immediately if any of the following occur:
  - headache, altered mental state, visual disturbances or fitting (seizures)
  - cough or spitting blood
  - pain in gums or jaw, swelling or jaw numbness or heavy jaw feeling, loosening of teeth
  - leg/calf swelling, pain or tenderness of leg/calf, warmth, redness
- encourage patient to practise good dental hygiene, including brushing teeth and tongue after meals and before bed, daily flossing to remove plaque and using a mirror to check teeth and gums regularly for any sores or bleeding of the gums
- symptoms of hand–foot syndrome can be reduced by advising patients to keep hands/feet cool (e.g. not wearing restricting gloves, socks or shoes; soaking hands/feet in cool water) starting 4–7 days after therapy. Other treatment may consist of pyridoxine (50–150 mg daily) and/or corticosteroids. Symptoms usually subside in 7–14 days
- see also General Patient teaching and advice for antineoplastic agents (p. 584)

BICALUTAMIDE (Bicalox, Calutex, Cosamide, Cosudex 50, Cosudex 150)

Available form

Tablets: 50 mg

Action

- non-steroidal hormonal antineoplastic agent (anti-androgen)
- impairs growth of androgen-dependent tumour cells and regression of prostatic tumours

Use

- locally advanced prostate cancer (with LHRH agonist therapy)
- prevention of disease flare associated with LHRH agonists

Dose
- 50 mg orally daily (with LHRH agonist therapy)

Adverse effects
- breast tenderness, gynaecomastia
- decreased libido, erectile dysfunction, impotence
- nocturia, haematuria
- flushing
- (uncommon) interstitial lung disease
- (rare) photosensitivity, QT prolongation
- see also General Adverse effects of antineoplastic agents (p. 582)

Interactions
- contraindicated with midazolam
- may increase serum levels of ciclosporin, carbamazepine, calcium-channel blockers, HIV protease inhibitors and HMG-CoA reductase inhibitors (statins) and therefore given with caution
- may increase serum levels of warfarin, increasing the risk of bleeding, therefore INR should be closely monitored, especially when starting or stopping therapy
- caution if given with other agents known to prolong QT interval or cause electrolyte imbalance (especially hypokalaemia and hypomagnesaemia)

Nursing points/Cautions
- any electrolyte imbalance should be corrected before starting therapy
- blood glucose levels should be monitored regularly due to risk of glucose intolerance (when combined with LHRH)
- ECG, electrolyte and liver function monitoring are recommended regularly during therapy
- caution if used in those with moderate-to-severe liver impairment
- caution if used in those with congenital or acquired QT prolongation or electrolyte abnormalities
- not recommended in those with metastatic prostate cancer with LHRH analogues
- contraindicated in females and children
- see also General Nursing points/Cautions for antineoplastic agents (p. 582)

Patient teaching and advice
- advise patient to seek medical advice immediately if rapid or unusual heart rate occurs
- if patient has diabetes, recommend close monitoring of blood glucose levels during therapy
- see General Patient teaching and advice for antineoplastic agents (p. 584)

Note
- contained in ZolaCos CP with goserelin and BiEligard CP with leuprorelin

BLEOMYCIN SULFATE (Blenamax, Cipla Bleomycin 15K, DBL Bleomycin Sulfate for Injection)

Available form
Vial: 15,000 IU

Action
- cytotoxic antibiotic that causes breaks in DNA strands resulting in inhibition of DNA cell synthesis
- most effective during M and G_2 phases of cell division
- bone marrow sparing

Use
- squamous cell carcinoma of skin, neck, head, oesophagus, penis, larynx and cervix
- choriocarcinoma and embryonal testicular cancer
- advanced Hodgkin lymphoma, non-Hodgkin lymphoma
- mycosis fungoides
- malignant pleural effusion (sclerosing treatment)

Dose

- initially 10,000–20,000 IU/m^2 given 1–2 weekly IM, IV or SC **OR**
- 15,000 IU IM, IV or SC for 7 days, followed by 21 days treatment-free interval, repeated twice (total dose about 300,000 IU) **OR**
- 30,000–60,000 IU IA 1–2 times weekly until recommended total dose of 300,000 IU is reached
- (malignant pleural effusion) 60,000 IU as single intrapleural administration

Adverse effects

- (pulmonary toxicity) pneumonitis, interstitial fibrosis
- idiosyncratic reaction (similar to anaphylaxis) (hypotension, fever, chills, confusion, wheezing)
- hypoaesthesia, hyperaesthesia, urticaria, swelling, tenderness, pruritus, hyperpigmentation (in areas of pressure or friction including skin folds, nail cuticles, scars and IM injection sites), alopecia
- (IA) dermal lesions in area supplied by artery
- (injection site) pain, phlebitis
- (rare) cardiovascular toxicity (including myocardial infarction, haemolytic uraemic syndrome)
- see also General Adverse effects of antineoplastic agents (p. 582); however, it does not cause severe bone marrow toxicity

Interactions

- may decrease serum levels of digoxin and phenytoin

Nursing points/Cautions

- regular physical examination for cough, dyspnoea or basal rales is recommended to detect early signs of lung toxicity. In addition, patient monitoring should also include some of the following:
    - weekly X-rays are recommended, including 4 weeks after stopping therapy
    - lung function tests (including total lung volume, forced vital capacity)
    - baseline and monthly evaluation of carbon monoxide diffusion capacity
    - high-resolution computerised tomography (CT)
- (lymphoma) test dose of 1–5 units should be given for the first 2 treatments and patient should be observed for 4–6 hours. If no reaction (hypotension, fever, chills, wheezing, confusion) occurs, balance of dose should then be given
- patient should be closely observed after first and second dose for any idiosyncratic reaction (hypotension, fever, chills, wheezing, confusion)
- increased risk of acute adult respiratory distress syndrome if patient has surgery/anaesthetic within 6–12 months of therapy. If patient has surgery, percentage of oxygen should be kept as low as possible, crystalloid fluids restricted and patient carefully observed for any signs of pulmonary oedema
- more successful if given before irradiation
- note and report fever, dyspnoea and cough as bleomycin is pulmonary-toxic
- improvement in lymphoma and testicular cancer is usually seen quickly, while squamous cell cancers may take up to 3 weeks to respond to therapy
- if response is not seen after 150,000 IU cumulative dose, therapy should be re-evaluated
- if response is incomplete, repeat course may be considered after a treatment-free interval of at least 3–4 weeks and only if there are no signs of lung toxicity
- may be given by IV, IM, SC, IA or intrapleural administration
- IA administration is used when increased drug concentration at cancer site is required

- reconstitute using 1–5 mL water for injections (for IM or SC) or 5–10 mL (for IV or IA) and given slowly over 10 minutes
- (malignant pleural effusion) reconstitute using 50–100 mL sodium chloride 0.9% and administer via thoracostomy tube after drainage of any excess pleural fluid and lung expansion is complete. Tube should be clamped and patient moved from left and right lateral position over next 4 hours. Tube is then unclamped and suction reapplied
- pulmonary toxicity is more likely in those who receive total cumulative doses > 400,000 IU
- incompatible with amino acids, aminophylline, ascorbic acid, dexamethasone, furosemide, hyoscine and riboflavin
- caution if used in those aged over 70 years, with lung cancer, smokers or those with compromised lung function as there is an increased risk of pulmonary toxicity
- repeat course is contraindicated if pneumonitis occurs
- see also General Nursing points/Cautions for antineoplastic agents (p. 582)

Patient teaching and advice

- patient should be advised to seek medical advice immediately if any of the following occur:
  - cough, shortness of breath, difficulty breathing, chest pain related to breathing, wheezing
- see also General Patient teaching and advice for antineoplastic agents (p. 584)

BLINATUMOMAB (Blincyto)

Available form

Vial: 38.5 microgram

Action

- bispecific monoclonal antibody that binds to CD19 and CD3

Use

- treatment of relapsed or refractory B-cell precursor acute lymphocytic leukaemia (ALL)
- treatment of minimal residual disease (MRD) positive B-cell precursor ALL

Dose

- (relapsed or refractory B-cell precursor ALL, weight > 45 kg) 9 microgram IV daily for first 7 days, increasing to 28 microgram IV starting at week 2 through to week 4 (cycle 1), with 28 microgram IV for subsequent cycles **OR**
- (MRD positive B-cell positive ALL, weight > 45 kg) 28 microgram IV daily for days 1–28, followed by 14-day treatment-free interval

Adverse effects

- cytokine-release syndrome (fever, asthenia, headache, hypotension, nausea, increased bilirubin)
- neurological toxicity (encephalopathy, seizures, speech disorders, confusion, disorientation, disturbed consciousness, coordination and balance disorders)
- reactivation of John Cunningham (JC) virus, posterior reversible encephalopathy syndrome (PRES)
- see also General Adverse effects of antineoplastic agents (p. 582)

Interactions

- vaccination with live vaccine is not recommended for 2 weeks before and during therapy, and after until B lymphocyte recovery to normal range

Nursing points/Cautions

- each cycle is 4 weeks with a 2-week treatment-free interval between cycles
- hospitalisation is recommended for first 9 days of first cycle and first

2 days of second cycle (relapsed or refractory ALL) or minimum first 3 days of first cycle and first 2 days of second cycle (MRD positive B-cell positive ALL). Supervision or hospitalisation is also recommended for subsequent treatment cycles

- premedication with dexamethasone IV 20 mg 1 hour before the start of each cycle is recommended
- prophylactically intrathecal chemotherapy is additionally recommended before and during therapy to prevent CNS ALL relapse
- (relapsed or refractory B-cell precursor ALL) for patient with high tumour burden ($\geq$ 50% leukaemic blasts or $>$ 15,000 microL peripheral blood leukaemic blast cells), pre-phase treatment with dexamethasone (not exceeding 24 mg daily) is recommended
- infusion using dedicated lumen and infusion pump is recommended
- contraindicated in those with hypersensitivity to Chinese hamster ovary cell derived protein
- see also General Nursing points/ Cautions for antineoplastic agents (p. 582)

Patient teaching and advice

- see General Patient teaching and advice for antineoplastic agents (p. 584)

BORTEZOMIB (Velcade)

Available forms
Vial: 1 mg, 3 mg

Action

- reverse inhibitor of chymotrypsin-like activity of 26S proteasome preventing signalling cascades within cells resulting in tumour cell death

Use

- multiple myeloma (MM) (progressive disease where at least one therapy was ineffective) (with melphalan and prednisone)
- previously untreated multiple myeloma (with melphalan and prednisone) (unsuitable for high-dose chemotherapy)
- induction therapy in those with previous untreated multiple myeloma prior to high-dose chemotherapy and autologous stem cell rescue (< 65 years)
- untreated mantle cell lymphoma (with rituximab, cyclophosphamide, doxorubicin and prednisone)

Dose

- (previously untreated MM – transplant eligible) 1.3 mg/m^2 SC or IV bolus over 3–5 seconds on days 1, 4, 8 and 11 of 21-day cycle (with thalidomide and dexamethasone or dexamethasone only) for 3 cycles **OR**
- (previously untreated MM – transplant ineligible) 1.3 mg/m^2 SC or IV bolus over 3–5 seconds on days 1, 4, 8, 11, 22, 25, 29 and 32 of 6-week cycle for cycles 1–4, then days 1, 8, 22 and 29 of 6-week cycle for cycles 5–9 (with melphalan and prednisolone) **OR**
- (relapsed/refractory MM) 1.3 mg/m^2 SC or IV bolus over 3–5 seconds on days 1, 4, 8 and 11 of 2-week cycle followed by 10-day rest period, repeated for 2 additional cycles if response is confirmed **OR**
- (untreated mantle cell lymphoma) 1.3 mg/m^2 SC or IV bolus over 3–5 seconds on days 1, 4, 8 and 11, followed by 10-day drug-free interval (for 6 cycles) (with rituximab, cyclophosphamide, doxorubicin and prednisolone)

Adverse effects

- peripheral neuropathy
- hypotension
- hyperglycaemia
- new or exacerbation of cardiac failure
- (uncommon) seizure

- (rare) acute liver failure, pulmonary disorders, posterior reversible encephalopathy syndrome (PRES), thrombocytopenic purpura
- see also General Adverse effects of antineoplastic agents (p. 582)

Interactions

- caution if given with antihypertensive agents as excessive hypotension may occur
- increased risk of peripheral neuropathy if given with amiodarone, isoniazid, nitrofurantoin, antiviral agents and statins
- not recommended with rifampicin, carbamazepine, phenytoin, phenobarbital (phenobarbitone) and St John's wort
- increase serum levels may occur if given with ritonavir
- caution if used with oral antidiabetic agents. Blood glucose levels should be closely monitored during therapy

Nursing points/Cautions

- BP should be monitored during therapy as hypotension occurs commonly
- patient should be well hydrated during therapy
- (relapsed/refractory MM) a minimal 72-hour drug-free interval should be allowed between treatment doses
- (SC) rotate administration sites avoiding areas that are tender, bruised, broken or scarred and not within 2.5 cm of previous injection site
- (IV) reconstitute using 3.5 mL sodium chloride 0.9% (for 3.5 mg vial) or 1.0 mL sodium chloride 0.9% (for 1.0 mg vial) for final concentration of 1 mg/mL for IV bolus administration
- (SC) reconstitute using 1.4 mL sodium chloride 0.9% (for 3.5 mg vial) for final concentration of 2.5 mg/mL for SC administration
- caution if used in those with diabetes mellitus as blood glucose levels may become unstable (however, hyperglycaemia may occur in those without diabetes)
- caution if used in those with pre-existing epilepsy, neuropathy, history of syncope or hypotension, or dehydration
- contraindicated if patient has hypersensitivity to mannitol or boron
- see also General Nursing points/Cautions for antineoplastic agents (p. 582)

Patient teaching and advice

- patient should be advised to seek medical advice if any of the following occur:
  - new or worsening numbness, pain or burning sensations in hands or feet
  - light-headedness, dizziness, fainting
  - headache, altered mental state, visual disturbances or fitting (seizures)
  - cough, shortness of breath, breathing difficulties
  - excessive or easy bruising, superficial bleeding (pinpoint sized reddish-purple spots) into skin resembling rash (commonly on lower legs)
- if patient has diabetes, advise to monitor blood glucose levels closely as hyperglycaemia occurs with therapy
- see also General Patient teaching and advice for antineoplastic agents (p. 584)

BRENTUXIMAB VEDOTIN (Adcetris)

Available form

Vial: 50 mg

Action

- CD30-directed antibody-drug conjugate antineoplastic that disrupts microtubules resulting in death of CD30-expressing tumour cell

Use

- previously untreated CD30+ peripheral T-cell lymphoma (PTCL) (with cyclophosphamide, doxorubicin and prednisolone)
- treatment of relapsed or refractory CD30+ Hodgkin lymphoma (after autologous stem cell transplant or after ≥ 2 therapies when stem cell transplant is not an option)
- cutaneous T-cell CD30+ lymphoma (CTCL) after at least one other systemic treatment

Dose

- 1.8 mg/kg IV over 30 minutes every 3 weeks for 8–16 cycles (about 1 year) (maximum 180 mg)

Adverse effects

- infusion-related reaction (chills, nausea, cough, dyspnoea, pruritus)
- peripheral neuropathy
- hyperglycaemia
- (rare) progressive multifocal leukoencephalopathy, pulmonary toxicity, pancreatitis, severe skin reaction, GI complications
- see also General Adverse effects of antineoplastic agents (p. 582)

Interactions

- contraindicated with bleomycin due to increased risk of pulmonary toxicity

Nursing points/Cautions

- premedication with paracetamol, corticosteroid and antihistamine is recommended for those who experienced infusion-related reaction after first dose
- patient should be closely monitored during and after infusion
- if patient's weight > 100 kg dose should be calculated according to ideal weight
- liver function and blood glucose levels should be measured before and regularly during therapy
- (previously untreated PTCL) therapy should be started with G-CSF
- reconstitute with 10.5 mL water for injections to give concentration of 5 mg/mL and then further dilute with 150 mL sodium chloride 0.9%, glucose 5% or lactated Ringer's solution
- not given by IV push or bolus
- caution if used in those with pre-existing GI conditions due to increased risk of complications, including perforation
- see also General Nursing points/Cautions for antineoplastic agents (p. 582)

Patient teaching and advice

- advise patient to seek medical advice immediately if any of the following occur:
  - cough, shortness of breath
  - abdominal pain with or without nausea
  - burning sensation, numbness and/or tingling sensation, weakness
  - severe skin reactions including blistering or peeling
  - confusion, trouble thinking, memory loss, blurred vision, loss of vision, balance or walking problems, decreased strength in arms or legs
  - excessive thirst, increased frequency or volume of urination
- caution patient with diabetes mellitus to monitor blood glucose levels closely as hyperglycaemia may occur during therapy
- see also General Patient teaching and advice for antineoplastic agents (p. 584)

BRIGATINIB (Alunbrig)

Available forms

Tablets: 30 mg, 90 mg, 180 mg

Action

- tyrosine kinase inhibitor (including ALK, ROS1, insulin-like growth factor 1 receptor)

Use

- anaplastic lymphoma kinase positive advanced non-small cell lung cancer

Dose

- initially 90 mg orally daily for 7 days, then increasing to 180 mg daily

Adverse effects

- pneumonitis, interstitial lung disease
- hypertension, bradycardia
- visual disturbances
- elevated creatine phosphokinase and pancreatic enzymes, hyperglycaemia
- peripheral neuropathy
- see also General Adverse effects for antineoplastic agents (p. 582)

Interactions

- caution if used with other agents known to cause bradycardia. If given together, HR should be monitored more regularly
- not recommended with indinavir, nelfinavir, ritonavir, saquinavir, clarithromycin and voriconazole as serum levels of brigatinib may increase leading to toxicity
- not recommended with grapefruit or grapefruit juice
- serum levels may be decreased by rifampicin, carbamazepine, phenytoin, rifabutin, phenobarbital, St John's wort, efavirenz, modafinil, bosentan and etravirine and are not recommended together
- may increase serum levels of digoxin, dabigatran, colchicine, pravastatin, methotrexate, rosuvastatin and sulfasalazine increasing risk of adverse effects and toxicity

Nursing points/Cautions

- patient ALK-positive status should be confirmed using a validated test before starting therapy
- HR and BP should be monitored throughout therapy
- fasting blood glucose should be measured before starting therapy, then regularly throughout
- if therapy is stopped for 14 days or longer (not related to adverse effects), dose should be restarted at 90 mg daily for 7 days before increasing to previously tolerated dose
- increased risk of pneumonitis and interstitial lung disease if in those who are older or have received crizotinib within last 7 days
- see also General Nursing points/Cautions for antineoplastic agents (p. 582)

Patient teaching and advice

- advise patient to seek medical advice immediately if any of the following occur:
  - cough, shortness of breath, tight chest, loss of appetite, weight loss, fatigue, fever, chills
  - slowed heart rate
  - new or worsening visual disturbances
  - unexplained muscle pain, tenderness or weakness
  - numbness/tingling or altered sensation in hands or feet
- if patient has diabetes, advise close monitoring of blood glucose levels during therapy
- instruct patient to avoid grapefruit and grapefruit juice during therapy
- see also General Patient teaching and advice for antineoplastic agents (p. 584)

BUSULFAN (Busulfex, Myleran)

Available forms

Ampoules: 60 mg/10 mL; Tablets: 2 mg

Action

- non-phase specific bifunctional alkylating agent
- more selective than nitrogen mustard or folic acid antagonists on myeloid cells

Use
- chronic granulocytic leukaemia (CGL)
- polycythaemia vera, essential thrombocythaemia and myelofibrosis
- conditioning before stem cell transplantation (with other antineoplastic agents) (IV)

Dose
- (CGL) 0.06 mg/kg orally as a single dose (daily maximum 4 mg) (induction), then 0.5–2 mg orally (maintenance) **OR**
- (polycythaemia vera, essential thrombocythaemia) 4–6 mg orally daily (induction), then 2–3 mg (half induction dose) (maintenance) **OR**
- (myelofibrosis) initially 2–4 mg orally daily, then dose reduced for maintenance **OR**
- (conditioning treatment – myeloablative) 3.2 mg/kg IV over 3 hours for 4 days (total dose 12.8 mg/kg) **OR**
- (conditioning treatment – non-myeloablative) 0.8–6.4 mg/kg IV over 3 hours for 2–4 days

Adverse effects
- lung toxicity
- cardiac toxicity
- liver toxicity, hepatic veno-occlusive disease
- acute graft versus host disease, chronic graft versus host disease
- Fanconi's anaemia
- hyperuricaemia, uric acid nephropathy
- hyperpigmentation (especially in those with dark complexion)
- corneal thinning
- (high dose) seizures
- see also General Adverse effects of antineoplastic agents (p. 582)

Interactions
- not recommended with tioguanine (thioguanine) due to risk of nodular regenerative hyperplasia, portal hypertension and oesophageal varices
- increased risk of toxicity if given with itraconazole or metronidazole
- if given with or within 72 hours of paracetamol, may decrease busulfan clearance
- clearance may be increased if given with phenytoin
- increased risk of pulmonary toxicity if oxygen is given during surgery. Percentage of oxygen should be kept as low as possible
- (high dose) if given with cyclophosphamide, interval of > 24 hours should be allowed to decrease risk of toxicity
- decreased clearance may occur if given with iron chelating agents. They should be stopped before starting therapy with busulfan
- see also General Interactions of antineoplastic agents (p. 582)

Nursing points/Cautions
- (IV) premedication with antiepileptic agents (starting 12 hours before therapy and up to 24 hours after last dose) is recommended with high-dose therapy to decrease risk of seizures
- any hyperuricaemia and/or hyperuricosuria should be corrected before starting therapy
- (CGL) not useful once blast transformation has occurred
- (CGL maintenance therapy) aim to maintain WBC 10,000–15,000/mm^3
- (IV) daily liver function tests are recommended until transplant day 28
- (IV) therapeutic drug monitoring is recommended after first dose. Blood should not be sampled from same lumen as busulfan is being administered
- prolonged therapy may lead to pulmonary toxicity
- if surgery and anaesthesia are required, inspired oxygen concentration should be kept as low as possible
- (IV) if patient is obese, dose should be based on ideal body weight

- should not be administered via peripheral line. Central venous line is recommended
- not recommended by rapid IV bolus
- must be diluted with sodium chloride 0.9% or glucose 5% for IV infusion to concentration of 0.5 mg/mL
- IV infusion is given over 2–3 hours
- caution if used in those with epilepsy
- (IV) increased risk of liver toxicity if patient has received previous radiation therapy ($\geq$ 3 cycles of chemotherapy) or prior stem cell transplant
- increased risk of lung toxicity if used in those with history of lung or mediastinal radiation
- see also Nursing points/Cautions for antineoplastic agents (p. 582)

Patient teaching and advice

- warn patient to avoid paracetamol or paracetamol-containing preparations for at least 72 hours before and after therapy
- patient should be advised to report any new or worsening unproductive cough (which may be first sign of lung toxicity)
- patient (especially if dark complexion) should be warned about skin hyperpigmentation
- see also General Patient teaching and advice for antineoplastic agents (p. 584)

CABAZITAXEL (Jevtana)

Available form

Vial: 60 mg/1.5 mL

Action

- taxane antimetabolite that inhibits mitotic and cellular functions

Use

- hormone refractory metastatic castration-resistant prostate cancer (previously treated with docetaxel) (with prednisolone or prednisone)

Dose

- 20 mg/m^2 IV over 1 hour every 3 weeks (with prednisolone or prednisone 10 mg orally daily)

Adverse effects

- tachycardia, atrial fibrillation
- peripheral neuropathy
- urinary disorder
- pneumonitis, interstitial lung disorder, acute respiratory distress syndrome
- hypersensitivity
- see also General Adverse effects of antineoplastic agents (p. 582)

Interactions

- increased serum levels may result if given with itraconazole, clarithromycin, atazanavir, indinavir, ritonavir, saquinavir and voriconazole
- decreased serum levels may result if given with phenytoin, carbamazepine, rifampicin, rifabutin, phenobarbital (phenobarbitone) and St John's wort and are therefore not recommended together
- contraindicated with live or live attenuated vaccines

Nursing points/Cautions

- premedication with antihistamine, corticosteroid and H_2 antagonist is recommended 30 minutes before infusion. Antiemetic prophylaxis should also be considered at this time
- patient should be closely observed during first two doses for any signs of hypersensitivity
- ensure patient is well hydrated during therapy
- dilute powder using supplied diluent, taking care to minimise foaming. Allow solution to stand for 5 minutes before further diluting with sodium chloride 0.9% or glucose 5% to give a concentration of 0.10–0.26 mg/mL
- inline filter (0.22 microns) is recommended

- not recommended with PVC bags or bottles or polyurethane tubing, filters or pumps
- contraindicated in those with hypersensitivity to polysorbate 80 or previous reaction to cabazitaxel or neutrophil count ≤ 1500/mm^3 or severe liver impairment (total bilirubin > 3 upper limit of normal)
- see also General Nursing points/Cautions for antineoplastic agents (p. 582)

Patient teaching and advice

- advise patient to seek medical advice if any of the following occur:
  - pain, burning, tingling, numbness or weakness of hands or feet
  - rapid or irregular heart rate
  - difficulty breathing, tight chest, cough
- see also General Patient teaching and advice for antineoplastic agents (p. 584)

CAPECITABINE (Xelabine)

Available forms

Tablets: 150 mg, 500 mg

Action

- fluoropyrimidine antimetabolite that is activated by thymidine phosphorylase in tumours to cytotoxic metabolite fluorouracil (5FU)

Use

- locally advanced or metastatic breast cancer (not responding to taxanes or anthracycline-containing chemotherapy) (with docetaxel)
- advanced or metastatic colorectal cancer
- advanced oesophagogastric cancer (first-line treatment with platinum-based regimen)
- colon cancer (monotherapy or with cisplatin)

Dose

- (colon, colorectal, breast cancer – monotherapy) initially 1.25 g/m^2 orally twice daily within 30 minutes of meal for 2 weeks, followed by 2-week rest cycle, given as a 3-week cycle **OR**
- (breast cancer – combination therapy) 1.25 g/m^2 orally twice daily within 30 minutes of meal for 2 weeks (with docetaxel 75 mg/m^2 IV over 1 hour every 3 weeks) followed by a 7-day rest period **OR**
- (colorectal – combination therapy) 1.0 g/m^2 orally twice daily within 30 minutes of meal for 2 weeks followed by 7-day rest cycle (with oxaliplatin with or without bevacizumab) **OR**
- (colon cancer adjunct) 1.0 g/m^2 orally twice daily within 30 minutes of meal for 2 weeks followed by 7-day rest cycle (with oxaliplatin IV) **OR**
- (oesophagogastric cancer) 625 mg/m^2 orally twice daily within 30 minutes of meal continuously for 3-week cycle (with epirubicin and either cisplatin or oxaliplatin) **OR**
- (gastric cancer) 1.0 g/m^2 orally twice daily within 30 minutes of meal for 2 weeks followed by 7-day rest cycle (with cisplatin IV)

Adverse effects

- myocardial infarction, angina, arrhythmias, cardiac failure, cardiac arrest, ECG changes
- hand–foot syndrome (hand/foot numbness, paraesthesia, tingling, erythema, pain, swelling and, at worst, ulceration, blistering or moist desquamation)
- hyperbilirubinaemia
- see also General Adverse effects of antineoplastic agents (p. 582)

Interactions

- may increase serum levels of phenytoin, increasing the risk of toxicity

- may increase activity of warfarin, therefore INR should be closely monitored, especially when starting or stopping therapy. Changes in coagulation have been seen up to a month after stopping therapy
- increased risk of toxicity if given with folinic acid (calcium folinate)

Nursing points/Cautions

- patient should be well hydrated at the start and during therapy (especially if combined with cisplatin)
- (colorectal – combination therapy, colon cancer adjunct, gastric cancer) therapy should be started on day 1 evening and finished on day 15 morning of 21-day cycle
- for metastatic disease, therapy is ongoing
- as adjunct therapy, therapy is for 2 weeks
- caution if used in those with coronary artery disease as there is an increased risk of cardiac toxicity
- contraindicated in those with known hypersensitivity to fluorouracil or severe/unexpected reaction to fluoropyrimidine or those with dihydropyrimidine dehydrogenase (DPD) deficiency or severe kidney impairment (creatinine clearance < 30 mL/minute)
- see also General Nursing points/Cautions for antineoplastic agents (p. 582)

Patient teaching and advice

- instruct patient to swallow tablets whole within 30 minutes of completing meal
- advise patient to seek medical advice if any of the following occur:
  - painful swelling and redness of hands and/or feet
  - irregular heart rate or chest pain
- symptoms of hand–foot syndrome can be reduced by advising patients to keep hands/feet cool (e.g. not wearing restricting gloves, socks or shoes; soaking hands/feet in cool water) starting 4–7 days after therapy. Other treatment may consist of pyridoxine (vitamin B_6) (50–150 mg daily) and/or corticosteroids. Symptoms usually subside in 7–14 days. However, pyridoxine (vitamin B_6) is not recommended during combination therapy with cisplatin
- see also General Patient teaching and advice for antineoplastic agents (p. 584)

CARBOPLATIN (Carboplatin Solution for Injection, DBL Carboplatin Injection)

Available forms

Solution: 50 mg/5 mL, 150 mg/15 mL, 450 mg/45 mL

Action

- inorganic heavy metal (platinum) that interferes with DNA synthesis
- analogue of cisplatin

Use

- advanced ovarian cancer (epithelial origin)
- small cell lung cancer
- neuroblastoma
- head and neck cancer
- soft tissue sarcoma
- testicular cancer
- paediatric cerebral tumour

Dose

- 400 mg/m^2 IV over 15–60 minutes, with at least 4 weeks between infusions

Adverse effects

- peripheral neuropathy, paraesthesia, decreased deep tendon reflexes
- new or worsening hearing loss
- transient sight loss, cortical blindness
- see also General Adverse effects of antineoplastic agents (p. 582)

Interactions

- hepatotoxic, myelotoxic, neurotoxic and ototoxic, therefore should not be given with other drugs with similar adverse effects (e.g. aminoglycosides)
- increased risk of fatigue, myalgia and arthralgia if given with paclitaxel
- pain, asthenia and visual disturbance may occur if given with cyclophosphamide
- increased risk of neurotoxicity and ototoxicity in those previously treated with cisplatin
- not recommended with live or live attenuated vaccines
- may decrease phenytoin serum levels increasing risk of seizures

Nursing points/Cautions

- incidence and severity of nausea and vomiting can be reduced by premedicating with antiemetic (e.g. metoclopramide, ondansetron), administering as a continual infusion over 24 hours or as divided doses over 5 consecutive days, rather than a single infusion
- 4-week interval is recommended between treatment cycles
- may be diluted with glucose 5%
- reacts with aluminium (e.g. needles, IV administration sets) to form black precipitate
- contraindicated in those with known hypersensitivity to platinum-containing compounds or mannitol, severe bleeding tendency or myelodepression or severe renal impairment
- see also General Nursing points/Cautions for antineoplastic agents (p. 582)

Patient teaching and advice

- advise patient to seek medical advice if any of the following occur:
  - changes in vision
  - new or worsening hearing loss, ringing in ears (tinnitus)
  - pain, burning, tingling, numbness or weakness of hands or feet
- see also General Patient teaching and advice for antineoplastic agents (p. 584)

CARMUSTINE (BiCNU, Gliadel Implant)

Available forms

Surgical implant: 7.7 mg; Vial: 100 mg

Action

- alkylating agent (nitrosourea)
- (implant) designed to deliver and release carmustine into cavity created by surgical resection of tumour

Use

- high-grade malignant glioma (as adjunct to surgery and radiation)
- recurrent glioblastoma multiforme (as adjunct to surgery)
- multiple myeloma (MM) with prednisolone
- Hodgkin's disease or non-Hodgkin lymphomas (relapsed or failed to respond to primary therapy)

Dose

- (high-grade malignant glioma, recurrent glioblastoma multiforme) up to 8 implants in tumour resection cavity

OR

- (MM, Hodgkin's disease, non-Hodgkin lymphoma) (previously untreated) 200 mg/m^2 IV every 6 weeks (given as either a single dose or split into 2 doses given on successive days)

Adverse effects

- (IV) pulmonary infiltrates/fibrosis
- (implant) seizures, delay in wound healing
- brain oedema
- (rare) pulmonary toxicity
- (IV site) burning, swelling, pain, erythema, skin necrosis
- see also General Adverse effects of antineoplastic agents (p. 582)

Interactions

- (implant) radiation therapy is not recommended within 3 weeks of implant insertion
- (implant) hemotherapy should be withheld for 4–6 weeks before and 2 weeks after surgery for malignant glioma
- (IV) not recommended with other agents that affect lung function

Nursing points/Cautions

- (IV) lung function tests are recommended before starting and regularly throughout therapy
- after implant insertion via craniotomy patients should be closely monitored for any complications, including seizures, infection, oedema or impaired wound healing
- implant should only be inserted after pathology has been confirmed and haemostasis achieved
- implants should be handled with gloves (double gloved) to prevent severe burning and hyperpigmentation of exposed skin
- implants should be stored at –20°C and may be refrozen if unopened and at room temperature for not more than 6 hours
- no more than 8 implants should be used per surgical procedure
- (IV) should be allowed to come to room temperature before reconstitution. Reconstitute using 27 mL water for injections. May be further diluted using sodium chloride (0.9%) or glucose 5%
- (IV) given by slow IV infusion over 1–2 hours
- (IV) should not be given by rapid infusion
- (IV) dose should not be repeated in less than 6 weeks (until platelets > 100,000/mm^3 and leucocytes > 4000/mm^3)
- caution if used in those with pre-existing lung disease or thoracic irradiation
- see also General Nursing points/Cautions for antineoplastic agents (p. 582)

Patient teaching and advice

- warn patient that lung problems can occur years after therapy is stopped. Patient should be advised to seek medical advice if new or worsening breathing problems occur
- see also General Patient teaching and advice for antineoplastic agents (p. 584)

CETUXIMAB (RMC) (Erbitux)

Available forms

Vial: 100 mg/20 mL, 500 mg/100 mL

Action

- epidermal growth factor receptor (EGFR) monoclonal antibody whose activity results in decreased neovascularisation of tumours and metastasis
- overexpression of EGFR has been found in a number of human cancers, including rectal and colon
- retinoic acid syndrome (RAS) is a frequently activated family of oncogenes in human cancers

Use

- EGFR-expressing RAS wild type metastatic colorectal cancer (as monotherapy or as part of combination therapy)
- squamous cell cancer of the neck and head (with radiation (for locally advanced cancer) or platinum-based chemotherapy (for recurrent or metastatic disease))

Dose

- initially 400 mg/m^2 by IV infusion over 120 minutes once weekly, then reducing to 250 mg/m^2 by IV infusion over 60 minutes

Adverse effects

- infusion-related reactions
- severe hypomagnesaemia

- keratitis, ulcerative keratitis
- (rare) interstitial lung disease, severe skin reactions
- see also General Adverse effects of antineoplastic agents (p. 582)

Interactions

- not recommended with capecitabine and irinotecan to treat metastatic colorectal cancer
- increased risk of severe diarrhoea if given with capecitabine and oxaliplatin
- increased risk of leucopenia and neutropenia if given with platinum-based therapy
- caution if given with fluoropyrimidines due to increased risk of cardiac ischaemia (including myocardial infarction and congestive cardiac failure) and hand–foot syndrome
- may increase risk of local radiation side-effects (e.g. mucositis, radiation dermatitis) if radiation therapy to head and neck is given with cetuximab

Nursing points/Cautions

- (colorectal cancer) RAS mutational status must be evaluated using a validated test method before starting therapy
- cardiovascular assessment before starting therapy is recommended, especially in those > 65 years
- premedication with antihistamine and corticosteroid is recommended to prevent infusion-related reaction
- infusion-related reactions can occur hours after infusion has stopped. Patient should be closely observed for at least 1 hour after infusion
- first dose should be given over 2 hours at a rate of 5 mg/mL, then reduced to 60 minutes for next infusion if no reaction occurred (never greater than 10 mg/minute)
- (squamous cell neck and head cancer) therapy is started 1 week before and continued throughout course of radiation
- other chemotherapy is not recommended within an hour of completing infusion
- if dilution is required, use sodium chloride 0.9% only
- caution if used in those with history of keratitis, ulcerative keratitis or severe dry eyes
- not recommended in those with metastatic colorectal cancer with resectable liver metastases
- (combination therapy with oxaliplatin) contraindicated in those with mutant RAS metastatic colorectal cancer or in those whose status is unknown
- see also General Nursing points/Cautions for antineoplastic agents (p. 582)

Patient teaching and advice

- patient should be advised to seek medical advice immediately if any of the following occur:
  - skin reactions especially any skin peeling or blistering
  - persistent cough, shortness of breath
  - fever, chills, dizziness
  - eye disorders such as red, watery eyes, eye pain, blurring, dry eyes
- warn patient that acne-like rash occurs commonly
- see also General Patient teaching and advice for antineoplastic agents (p. 584)

CHLORAMBUCIL (Leukeran)

Available form

Tablets: 2 mg

Action

- alkylating agent (nitrogen mustard analogue) that interferes with cell replication

Use
- Hodgkin's disease, some forms of non-Hodgkin lymphoma
- chronic lymphocytic leukaemia (CLL)
- Waldenstrom's macroglobulinaemia (lymphoplasmacytic lymphoma)
- advanced ovarian adenocarcinoma
- breast cancer

Dose
- (Hodgkin's disease – monotherapy) 0.2 mg/kg orally 1 hour before or 3 hours after food daily for 4–8 weeks **OR**
- (non-Hodgkin lymphoma – monotherapy) 0.1–0.2 mg/kg orally 1 hour before or 3 hours after food daily for 4–8 weeks **OR**
- (CLL) 0.15 mg/kg orally 1 hour before or 3 hours after food daily until leucocytes ≤ 10,000/microL, then 0.1 mg/kg orally 1 hour before or 3 hours after food daily from 4 weeks after first course **OR**
- (Waldenstrom's macroglobulinaemia) 6–12 mg orally 1 hour before or 3 hours after food daily until leucopenia occurs, then 2–8 mg daily indefinitely **OR**
- (advanced ovarian cancer – monotherapy) initially 0.2 mg/kg orally 1 hour before or 3 hours after food daily for 4–6 weeks or 0.3 mg/kg orally 1 hour before or 3 hours after food daily until leucopenia occurs, then 0.2 mg/kg daily for 2–4 weeks with drug-free interval of 2–6 weeks **OR**
- (breast cancer – monotherapy) 0.2 mg/kg orally 1 hour before or 3 hours after food daily for 6 weeks

Adverse effects
- seizures
- (rare) interstitial lung fibrosis
- see also General Adverse effects of antineoplastic agents (p. 582)

Interactions
- caution if given with other agents that increase risk of seizures
- increased risk of toxicity if given with fludarabine and cladribine
- see General Interactions of antineoplastic agents (p. 582)

Nursing points/Cautions
- (breast cancer) may be given in combination therapy with prednisolone and either methotrexate or fluorouracil
- caution if used in those with history of epilepsy or head trauma, prescribed high-dose pulse regimens or children with nephrotic syndrome due to increased risk of seizure activity
- not recommended in those who have recently undergone radiation therapy or chemotherapy
- contraindicated in those with prior chlorambucil resistance
- see also General Nursing points/Cautions for antineoplastic agents (p. 582)

Patient teaching and advice
- advise patient to seek medical advice if persistent cough and/or shortness of breath occur
- see also General Patient teaching and advice for antineoplastic agents (p. 584)

CISPLATIN (Cisplatin Concentrate for Infusion, DBL Cisplatin Injection)

Available forms
Vial: 50 mg/50 mL, 100 mg/100 mL

Action
- inorganic heavy metal (platinum) that inhibits DNA synthesis (also RNA and protein synthesis to a lesser extent)
- properties similar to other alkylating agents

Use
- metastatic non-seminomatous germ cell carcinoma

- advanced refractory bladder or ovarian cancer
- refractory squamous cell carcinoma of the head and neck

Dose

- 50–100 mg/m^2 as single IV infusion over 1–2 hours every 3–4 weeks **OR**
- 15–20 mg/m^2 by IV infusion over 1–2 hours for 5 days every 3–4 weeks

Adverse effects

- nephrotoxicity
- neurotoxicity, including seizures
- peripheral neuropathy and vision loss
- hypertension, arrhythmias, congestive heart failure
- hearing loss, tinnitus
- hypomagnesaemia, secondary hypocalcaemia, hypokalaemia
- (rare) anaphylaxis
- see also General Adverse effects of antineoplastic agents (p. 582)

Interactions

- not recommended with nephrotoxic medication, especially aminoglycosides and loop diuretics
- contraindicated with live or live attenuated vaccines

Nursing points/Cautions

- before starting therapy, renal and liver function, neurological status, full blood count and electrolytes should be measured and repeated regularly during therapy
- any dehydration should be corrected before starting therapy
- risk of peripheral neuropathy is increased with prolonged therapy
- audiometric hearing tests should be performed before and during therapy
- to decrease nephrotoxicity, pre-treatment hydration with 2 L of glucose 4% in, ⅕ sodium chloride 0.18% or sodium chloride 0.9% over 2–4 hours and post-treatment hydration 2 L over 6–12 hours. During last 30 minutes of pre-treatment hydration, patient should also receive 375 mL mannitol 10%
- renal function must return to normal before any further doses are given
- infusion bag should be protected from light during therapy
- reacts with aluminium (e.g. needles, IV administration sets) to form black precipitate
- caution if used in those with history of atopy
- contraindicated in those with known hypersensitivity to platinum-containing compounds or mannitol, cisplatin-induced neuropathy, dehydration, hearing impairment or creatinine clearance > 0.2 mmol/L
- see also General Nursing points/Cautions for antineoplastic agents (p. 582)

Patient teaching and advice

- patient should be instructed to seek medical attention if any of the following occur:
  - decrease in hearing, ringing/buzzing in ears
  - numbness/tingling to feet or hands, burning sensation, weakness
  - fitting
  - blurred vision, altered colour perception
- see also General Patient teaching and advice for antineoplastic agents (p. 584)

CLADRIBINE (Leustatin, Litak, Mavenclad)

Available forms

Vial: 10 mg/5 mL, 10 mg/10 mL; Tablets: 10 mg

Action

- antimetabolite (purine nucleoside analogue)

Use

- hairy cell leukaemia
- Waldenstrom's macroglobulinaemia (lymphoplasmacytic lymphoma) (after failure of alkylating agents)

- B-cell chronic lymphocytic leukaemia (CLL) (after failure of alkylating agents)
- relapsing multiple sclerosis (see Movement disorder agents, p. 1312) (Mavenclad)

Dose
- (hairy cell leukaemia) 0.14 mg/kg as SC bolus for 5 days **OR**
- (hairy cell leukaemia) 0.10 mg/kg as IV infusion over 24 hours for 7 days (further courses may be needed) **OR**
- (Waldenstrom's macroglobulinaemia) 0.10 mg/kg as SC bolus for 5 days at monthly intervals **OR**
- (B-cell CLL) 0.12 mg/kg as IV infusion over 2 hours on days 1–5 of 28-day cycle

Adverse effects
- graft versus host disease
- see also General Adverse effects of antineoplastic agents (p. 582)

Interactions
- not recommended with antiviral agents
- increased risk of infection if given with corticosteroids and therefore not recommended together
- see also General Interactions of antineoplastic agents (p. 582)

Nursing points/Cautions
- may be given as SC bolus (with no dilution) or IV
- dilute with 100–500 mL sodium chloride 0.9% and administer by IV infusion over 2–24 hours (depending on use)
- dilution with glucose 5% is not recommended
- low temperatures may cause precipitate, which may redissolve if allowed to warm naturally and shaken vigorously; however, solution should not be heated or microwaved if frozen – allow to thaw at room temperature
- increased risk of graft versus host disease if patient receives transfusion of non-irradiated cellular blood product
- if patient becomes Coombs' positive, there is an increased risk of haemolysis, therefore patient should be closely monitored
- contraindicated in those under 18 years, or with moderate-to-severe renal impairment (creatine clearance ≤ 50 mL/min) or moderate-to-severe liver impairment
- see also General Nursing points/Cautions for antineoplastic agents (p. 582)

Patient teaching and advice
- see General Patient teaching and advice for antineoplastic agents (p. 584)

CLOFARABINE (Evoltra)

Available form
Vial: 20 mg/20 mL

Action
- purine nucleoside antimetabolite

Use
- acute lymphocytic leukaemia (ALL) in children (relapsed or refractory to at least 2 other regimens)

Dose
- 52 mg/kg by IV infusion over 2 hours for 5 consecutive days, cycle repeated after 2–6 weeks

Adverse effects
- haematuria
- tachycardia, pericardial effusion
- hand–foot syndrome (hand/foot numbness, paraesthesia, tingling, erythema, pain, swelling and, at worst, ulceration, blistering or moist desquamation)
- capillary leak syndrome, tumour lysis syndrome

- see also General Adverse effects of antineoplastic agents (p. 582)

Interactions

- not recommended within 5 days of known nephrotoxic agents
- not recommended with hepatotoxic agents
- see also General Interactions of antineoplastic agents (p. 582)

Nursing points/Cautions

- IV fluids are recommended with therapy to decrease risk of tumour lysis syndrome
- prophylactic corticosteroids may decrease risk of capillary leak syndrome
- response is usually seen after 1–2 cycles. If no response, use of therapy should be re-evaluated
- inline filter (0.22 micron) is recommended
- dilute with 100–200 mL sodium chloride 0.9% (volume is dependent on surface area of patient)
- if child weighs < 20 kg, infusion time should be increased to > 2 hours to reduce symptoms of anxiety and irritability
- increased risk of hepatotoxicity in those with history of haemopoietic stem cell transplant
- not recommended in those > 21 years
- contraindicated in those with severe kidney or liver impairment
- see also General Nursing points/ Cautions for antineoplastic agents (p. 582)

Patient teaching and advice

- patient/parent/carer should be advised to report any:
  - dizziness, light-headedness, fainting or decreased urine output (which may be suggestive of dehydration)
  - breathing problems
  - rapid heart rate
- see also General Patient teaching and advice for antineoplastic agents (p. 584)

COBIMETINIB (Cotellic)

Available form

Tablets: 20 mg

Action

- mitogen extracellular kinase (MEK) protein inhibitor (MEK 1 and MEK 2 kinases are thought to be involved in cell proliferation, cell cycle regulation, cell survival, angiogenesis and cell migration. MEK levels are often high in BRAF mutant tumours)
- half-life 23.1–69.6 hours

Use

- treatment of BRAF V600 mutation positive unresectable or metastatic melanoma (with vemurafenib)

Dose

- 60 mg orally once daily for 21 consecutive days in 28-day cycle, continued until benefits are no longer obtained or unacceptable toxicity occurs

Adverse effects

- chorioretinopathy, retinal detachment, blurred vision
- decreased left ventricular ejection fraction, hypertension
- photosensitivity, severe rash, skin reactions
- (rare) rhabdomyolysis
- see also General Adverse effects of antineoplastic agents (p. 582)

Interactions

- increased risk of bleeding if given with antiplatelet agents or anticoagulants
- increased serum levels may result if given with itraconazole, clarithromycin, atazanavir, indinavir, ritonavir,

saquinavir, voriconazole and grapefruit juice and are therefore not recommended together
- decreased serum levels may result if given with phenytoin, carbamazepine, rifampicin, rifabutin, phenobarbital (phenobarbitone) and St John's wort and are therefore not recommended together

Nursing points/Cautions

- BRAF V600 mutation should be confirmed before starting therapy
- left ventricular ejection fraction should be measured before starting, after first month, then 3-monthly until therapy is stopped
- creatine phosphokinase (CPK) levels should be monitored before starting and then regularly during therapy
- if patient experiences visual disturbances, prompt ophthalmological review is recommended
- caution if used in those with extra risk factors for bleeding such as brain metastases

Patient teaching and advice

- advise patient that if vomiting occurs, extra dose should not be taken. Treatment should be continued next day as prescribed
- patient should be warned to avoid sun exposure, wear protective clothing and use broad spectrum sunscreen and lip balm (SPF 30+) when outdoors
- patient should be advised to seek medical advice immediately if any of the following occur:
  - new or worsening visual disturbances, including eye pain and blurred vision
  - sensitivity to sun, including severe sunburn
  - rash or severe skin reactions including blistering
  - muscle pain or weakness, difficulty moving arms or legs, nausea, vomiting or abdominal pain
- see also General Patient teaching and advice for antineoplastic agents (p. 584)

CRIZOTINIB (Xalkori)

Available forms

Capsules: 200 mg, 250 mg

Action

- anaplastic lymphoma kinase (ALK) inhibitor
- also inhibits hepatocyte growth factor receptor

Use

- anaplastic lymphoma kinase (ALK) positive advanced non-small cell lung cancer
- ROS1-positive advanced non-small cell lung cancer

Dose

- 250 mg orally twice daily

Adverse effects

- bradycardia, QT interval prolongation
- pneumonitis
- hepatotoxicity
- vision loss
- GI perforation
- see also General Adverse effects of antineoplastic agents (p. 582)

Interactions

- caution if used with agents that prolong QT interval or cause electrolyte imbalance
- not recommended with other agents that cause bradycardia including beta-adrenoceptor blocking agents, digoxin, verapamil, diltiazem and clonidine
- not recommended with itraconazole, voriconazole, clarithromycin, ritonavir, saquinavir, atazanavir, indinavir and grapefruit or grapefruit juice due to increased serum levels

- may increase serum levels of midazolam
- decreased serum levels may occur if given with rifampicin, carbamazepine, phenytoin, rifabutin, rifampicin and St John's wort
- not recommended with alfentanil, ciclosporin, fentanyl, sirolimus and tacrolimus

Nursing points/Cautions

- ALK and ROS1-positive advanced non-small cell lung carcinoma should be confirmed before starting therapy
- monthly BP and pulse rate is recommended
- caution if used in those with congenital or acquired QT prolongation or electrolyte imbalance. ECG and electrolyte monitoring is recommended if used together
- see also General Nursing points/Cautions for antineoplastic agents (p. 582)

Patient teaching and advice

- instruct patient to avoid grapefruit and grapefruit juice during therapy
- advise patient to seek medical advice immediately if any of the following occur:
  - slow or irregular heart rate
  - cough, shortness of breath, difficulty breathing
  - yellowing of eyes/skin, decreased appetite, weight loss, nausea, upper abdominal pain, dark urine, pale stools
  - dizziness, fainting
  - changes to vision
- see also General Patient teaching and advice for antineoplastic agents (p. 584)

CYCLOPHOSPHAMIDE (Cyclonex, Endoxan)

Available forms

Vial: 500 mg, 1 g, 2 g; Tablets: 50 mg

Action

- nitrogen mustard analogue
- converted to active form in the liver that interferes with growth of susceptible cancers

Use

- (antineoplastic) treatment of stage III or IV malignant lymphomas, multiple myeloma, leukaemias, advanced mycosis fungoides; less useful in neuroblastoma, retinoblastoma and adenocarcinoma of the ovary, breast and lung cancer
- (immunosuppressive) treatment of autoimmune diseases resistant to other treatments; preventing transplantation rejection

Dose

- (antineoplastic-induction) initially 40–50 mg/kg IV in divided doses over 2–5 days (loading dose) **OR**
- (antineoplastic-induction) 1–5 mg/kg orally daily **OR**
- (antineoplastic-maintenance) 1–5 mg/kg orally, 10–15 mg/kg IV every 7–10 days or 3–5 mg/kg IV twice weekly **OR**
- (immunosuppressive) 1–3 mg/kg orally daily

Adverse effects

- cystitis, haemorrhagic cystitis, haematuria, bladder oedema
- skin hyperpigmentation, nail changes
- (high dose) inappropriate water retention, hyponatraemia, veno-occlusive disease
- see also General Adverse effects of antineoplastic agents (p. 582)

Interactions

- not recommended with grapefruit juice
- increased risk of bone marrow depression if given with allopurinol or hydrochlorothiazide
- increased metabolism may occur if given with high-dose phenobarbital (phenobarbitone)
- activation of cyclophosphamide may be inhibited by corticosteroids

- increased risk of toxicity if given with barbiturates, phenytoin or benzodiazepines
- decreased effects may occur if given with chloramphenicol, imipramine, phenothiazines, potassium iodide or vitamin A
- increased risk of arrhythmias if given with digoxin
- may potentiate effects of suxamethonium prolonging apnoea
- increased risk of hyponatraemia if given with indometacin
- may potentiate effects of insulin or oral hypoglycaemic agents
- increased risk of cardiotoxicity if given after radiotherapy of chest area or with anthracycline (such as doxorubicin)
- not recommended with alcohol
- increased risk of veno-occlusive disease if given with busulfan or whole body irradiation
- may cause false negative on skin tests for candida, mumps and tuberculin and false positive on Papanicolaou test
- see also General Interactions of antineoplastic agents (p. 582)

Nursing points/Cautions

- risk of cystitis and/or haemorrhagic cystitis is high, therefore high fluid intake (oral or IV) for 24 hours before, during and 24 hours after therapy is recommended. Frequent voiding is recommended
- urine should be tested for red cells (may precede haemorrhagic cystitis)
- in some oncology units, during bone marrow transplantation work-up, continuous bladder washouts are performed during therapy to prevent haemorrhagic cystitis
- mesna (see Antineoplastic support agents, p. 716) protects bladder from haemorrhagic cystitis
- caution if used in those with diabetes mellitus
- not recommended in those with porphyria
- contraindicated in those with active infection, depressed bone marrow function, cystitis, acute systemic or urinary infection, urinary outflow obstruction, drug or radiation-induced haemorrhagic cystitis or within 8 days of major surgery
- see also General Nursing points/Cautions for antineoplastic agents (p. 582)

Patient teaching and advice

- patient should be advised to void frequently in 24-hour period after therapy
- instruct patient to avoid grapefruit and grapefruit juice during therapy
- advise patient to avoid alcohol during therapy
- warn patient that darkening of skin or nails may occur during therapy
- if patient has diabetes, recommend blood glucose levels should be closely monitored
- patient should be advised to seek medical advice if any of the following occur:
    - painful urination, increased frequency of urination
    - blood in urine
    - sudden weight gain, build-up of fluid around abdomen
- see also General Patient teaching and advice for antineoplastic agents (p. 584)

CYTARABINE (Cytarabine Injection)

Available forms

Vial: 100 mg/5 mL, 1 g/10 mL, 2 g/20 mL

Action

- pyrimidine antimetabolite that appears to inhibit DNA synthesis

Use
- induction and maintenance of remission in acute myeloid leukaemia, acute lymphocytic leukaemia, chronic myeloid leukaemia (blast phase)
- non-Hodgkin lymphoma (children)
- meningeal leukaemia (intrathecally)

Dose
- (monotherapy) 200 mg/m^2 by continuous IV infusion over 24 hours for 5 days, repeated every 2 weeks (induction), then similar dose but longer intervals between cycles (maintenance) **OR**
- (meningeal leukaemia) 5–75 mg/m^2 intrathecally daily for 4 days once every 4 weeks or once every 4 days, until CSF is normal, then one additional treatment

Adverse effects
- pancreatitis
- cytarabine (ara-C) syndrome (fever, myalgia, bone pain, rash, malaise, chest pain, conjunctivitis) (within 6–12 hours of administration)
- anaphylaxis
- (intrathecal) nausea, vomiting, fever and rarely, paraplegia
- (IV) thrombophlebitis
- see also General Adverse effects of antineoplastic agents (p. 582)

Interactions
- (intrathecal) increased risk of severe neurological adverse effects if given with methotrexate
- may decrease effectiveness of methotrexate
- activity may be decreased by methotrexate
- (as part of multi-drug regimen) may decrease serum levels of digoxin, therefore digoxin levels should be closely monitored during therapy
- may antagonise effects of gentamicin
- may inhibit antifungal activity of flucytosine
- increased risk of spinal cord toxicity if given within a few days both intrathecally and IV
- see also General Interactions of antineoplastic agents (p. 582)

Nursing points/Cautions
- dilute with sodium chloride 0.9% or glucose 5%
- may also be given SC, IV infusion and occasionally, intrathecally
- if given SC, injection sites should be rotated
- 100 mg/mL solution is not suitable for intrathecal use
- intrathecal use may result in systemic toxicity so patient should be closely monitored
- corticosteroids are recommended to treat cytarabine (ara-C) syndrome
- incompatible with heparin, insulin, fluorouracil, penicillins and methylprednisolone
- if precipitate occurs as a result of low temperature, it may be redissolved by warming solution to 55°C for up to 30 minutes and shaking solution. Solution should be cooled before administration
- see also General Nursing points/Cautions for antineoplastic agents (p. 582)

Patient teaching and advice
- see also General Patient teaching and advice for antineoplastic agents (p. 584)

DABRAFENIB (Tafinlar)

Available forms

Capsules: 50 mg, 75 mg

Action
- protein kinase inhibitor that inhibits BRAF enzymes that have been identified in melanoma

Use

- treatment of BRAF V600 mutation positive unresectable stage III or IV (metastatic) melanoma (monotherapy)
- treatment of BRAF V600 mutation positive locally advanced or metastatic anaplastic thyroid cancer (with trametinib)
- adjunct treatment of BRAF V600 mutation positive melanoma with lymph node involvement (with trametinib)
- adjunct treatment of BRAF V600 mutation positive non-small cell lung cancer (with trametinib)

Dose

- 150 mg orally twice daily 1 hour before or 2 hours after meals (with or without trametinib) until disease progression or unacceptable toxicity occurs

Adverse effects

- cutaneous squamous cell carcinoma, melanoma
- uveitis, iritis
- hyperglycaemia
- renal failure
- (uncommon) QT interval prolongation, cardiomyopathy
- (rare) pancreatitis, retinal vein occlusion
- see also General Adverse effects of antineoplastic agents (p. 582)

Interactions

- caution if used with agents known to prolong QT interval or cause electrolyte imbalance
- caution if used with HMG-CoA reductase inhibitors (statins)
- caution if used with itraconazole, voriconazole, posaconazole, clarithromycin, saquinavir, ritonavir, atazanavir or gemfibrozil as increased serum levels may occur
- caution if used with rifampicin, rifabutin, phenytoin, phenobarbital (phenobarbitone), carbamazepine and St John's wort as decreased serum levels may occur
- bioavailability may be decreased if given with proton pump inhibitors, H_2-receptor inhibitors or antacids
- caution if given with warfarin, therefore INR should be closely monitored, especially when starting or stopping therapy
- may decrease efficacy of midazolam, digoxin, hormonal oral contraceptives, dexamethasone and antiretroviral agents

Nursing points/Cautions

- BRAF V600 mutation should be confirmed before starting therapy
- ECG, head, neck, oral mucosa and skin examinations, lymph node palpation and chest and abdominal CT are recommended before starting and regularly during therapy
- serum creatinine should be measured regularly during therapy
- caution if used in those with G6PD deficiency as haemolytic anaemia may occur
- caution if used in those with diabetes as hyperglycaemia may occur
- caution if used in those with known congenital or acquired QT interval prolongation or electrolyte imbalance (especially hypokalaemia and hypomagnesaemia)
- not recommended in those with BRAF wild type melanoma
- see also General Nursing points/Cautions for antineoplastic agents (p. 582)

Patient teaching and advice

- instruct patient to check skin regularly for any new or changing skin lesions
- patient should be advised to seek medical advice immediately if any of the following occur:
    - fever ≥ 38.5° C
    - any new skin lesions

- change of vision, photosensitivity, eye pain
- unexplained abdominal pain
- excessive thirst, increased frequency or volume of urination
- irregular heart rate
- caution patient with diabetes mellitus to monitor blood glucose levels closely as hyperglycaemia may occur during therapy
- see also General Patient teaching and advice for antineoplastic agents (p. 584)

DACARBAZINE (DBL Dacarbazine For Injection)

Available form
Vial: 200 mg

Action
- inhibits DNA synthesis
- has an active metabolite with alkylating properties similar to nitrogen mustard

Use
- metastatic malignant melanoma
- sarcomas

Dose
- 4.5 mg/kg IV over 1 minute daily for 10 days, repeated every 4 weeks if needed **OR**
- 250 mg/m^2 IV over 1 minute daily for 5 days, repeated every 3 weeks if needed

Adverse effects
- (rare) hepatotoxicity with hepatic vein thrombosis
- (injection site) severe pain along vein
- see also General Adverse effects of antineoplastic agents (p. 582)

Interactions
- may decrease response to levodopa
- may increase effects of azathioprine, allopurinol and mercaptopurine
- lung toxicity may occur if given before fotemustine
- see also General Interactions of antineoplastic agents (p. 582)

Nursing points/Cautions
- prophylactic antiemetic therapy with 5HT3 (e.g. ondansetron) or dexamethasone is recommended
- reconstitute with 19.7 mL water for injections and administer over 1 minute
- see also General Nursing points/Cautions for antineoplastic agents (p. 582)

Patient teaching and advice
- see General Patient teaching and advice for antineoplastic agents (p. 584)

DACTINOMYCIN (ACTINOMYCIN D) (Cosmegen)

Available form
Vial: 0.5 mg

Action
- cytotoxic antibiotic

Use
- Wilms' tumour
- rhabdomyosarcoma
- testicular and uterine cancer
- palliative therapy for Ewing's sarcoma and sarcoma botryoides

Dose
- 15 microgram/kg IV daily for 5 days, may be repeated after ≥ 3 weeks if no sign of toxicity **OR**
- 400–600 microgram/m^2 IV daily for 5 days, may be repeated after ≥ 3 weeks if no sign of toxicity **OR**
- (regional perfusion – lower extremity, pelvis) 50 microgram/kg **OR**
- (regional perfusion – upper extremity) 35 microgram/kg

Adverse effects
- liver veno-occlusive disease
- (perfusion technique) oedema, damage to soft tissue of perfused area

- see also General Adverse effects of antineoplastic agents (p. 582)

Interactions

- increased GI disturbance and bone marrow depression may occur if given with radiotherapy
- potentiates effects of radiation therapy, causing adverse effects at a lower dose of radiation
- radiation therapy potentiates effects of dactinomycin
- may interfere with assay for antibacterial drug levels
- see also General Interactions of antineoplastic agents (p. 582)

Nursing points/Cautions

- lower dose may be required if other chemotherapy or radiation is used at the same time or has been previously used
- may reactivate erythema from previous radiation therapy if given alone
- reconstitute using 1.1 mL of preservative-free water for injections. Should not be reconstituted using water for injections containing preservatives (benzyl alcohol or parabens) as precipitate may occur. Can be further diluted with glucose 5% or sodium chloride 0.9% to a concentration not less than 10 microgram/mL
- reconstituted solution is clear gold colour
- not recommended with or within 2 months of irradiation for Wilms' tumour unless benefits outweigh risks due to high risk of hepatotoxicity
- contraindicated at time of infection with chicken pox or herpes zoster as generalised disease may occur
- see also General Nursing points/Cautions for antineoplastic agents (p. 582)

Patient teaching and advice

- see General Patient teaching and advice for antineoplastic agents (p. 584)

DAROLUTAMIDE (Nubeqa)

Available form

Tablets: 300 mg

Action

- non-steroidal androgen receptor antagonist

Use

- treatment of non-metastatic castration-resistant prostate cancer

Dose

- 600 mg orally twice daily (with gonadotropin-releasing hormone (GnRH) analogue if patient has not had bilateral orchiectomy)

Adverse effects

- fatigue
- pain in extremities
- rash
- decreased neutrophils
- increased AST and bilirubin
- ischaemic heart disease

Interactions

- not recommended with rifampicin, carbamazepine, phenobarbital or St John's wort
- increased serum levels may occur if given with itraconazole
- may increase serum levels of rosuvastatin, methotrexate, sulfasalazine, fluvastatin and atorvastatin and are not recommended together

Nursing points/Cautions

- tablets contain 176.9 mg lactose and are therefore not recommended in those with rare hereditary conditions of galactose intolerance, Lapp lactase deficiency or glucose–galactose malabsorption
- caution if used in those with moderate liver impairment or severe kidney impairment (dose reduction required in both cases)
- caution if used in those with recent (within 6 months) cardiac events, including uncontrolled hypertension,

stroke, myocardial infarction, severe or unstable angina, coronary or peripheral artery bypass grafts or heart failure

Patient teaching and advice

- counsel patient to use effective contraception during therapy and for 12 weeks after last dose
- see General Patient teaching and advice for antineoplastic agents (p. 584)

DASATINIB (Sprycel)

Available forms

Tablets: 20 mg, 50 mg, 70 mg, 100 mg

Action

- tyrosine, serine/threonine kinase inhibitor which stops replication of tumour cells

Use

- newly diagnosed Philadelphia chromosome positive (Ph+) chronic myeloid leukaemia (CML) (in chronic phase)
- chronic myeloid leukaemia (CML) in chronic, accelerated or myeloid or lymphoid blast phase (resistant or intolerant to imatinib)
- Ph^+ acute lymphoblastic leukaemia (ALL) (resistant or intolerant to other therapies)

Dose

- (CML – chronic phase) 100 mg orally daily **OR**
- (CML – accelerated, myeloid or lymphoid blast phase) 140 mg orally daily **OR**
- (Ph+ ALL – newly diagnosed) 100 mg orally daily **OR**
- (Ph+ ALL – resistant or intolerant) 140 mg orally daily

Adverse effects

- prolongation of QT interval
- fluid retention, pleural or pericardial effusion
- pulmonary arterial hypertension
- severe skin reaction
- see General Adverse effects of antineoplastic agents (p. 582)

Interactions

- not recommended with proton pump inhibitors or histamine H_2-receptor antagonists
- not recommended with agents known to prolong QT interval (e.g. amiodarone, disopyramide, clarithromycin, sotalol, methadone) or cause electrolyte imbalance especially hypokalaemia and hypomagnesaemia
- increased serum levels may occur if given with itraconazole, erythromycin, ritonavir, clarithromycin, lopinavir, grapefruit juice and atazanavir and therefore not recommended together
- decreased serum levels may occur if given with dexamethasone, phenytoin, rifampicin, carbamazepine, phenobarbital (phenobarbitone) and St John's wort and therefore not recommended together
- absorption decreased by antacids
- may increase serum levels of simvastatin and ergot alkaloids
- see also General Interactions of antineoplastic agents (p. 582)

Nursing points/Cautions

- cardiopulmonary assessment is recommended before starting therapy
- any hypokalaemia or hypomagnesaemia should be corrected before starting therapy (as these may predispose to prolongation of QT interval)
- chest X-ray is recommended if shortness of breath or cough occurs
- tablets contain lactose and therefore not recommended in those with galactose intolerance, Lapp lactase insufficiency or glucose–galactose malabsorption
- caution if used in those with congenital or acquired prolongation of

QT interval or electrolyte imbalance (especially hypokalaemia and hypomagnesaemia)
- caution if used in those taking antiplatelet or anticoagulant medications
- caution if used in those > 65 years due to increased risk of pleural effusion, congestive cardiac failure, dyspnoea and gastrointestinal bleeding
- see also General Nursing points/Cautions for antineoplastic agents (p. 582)

Patient teaching and advice

- patient should be instructed to consistently take tablets at same time every day (e.g. always at night or always in the morning)
- patient should be advised to seek medical advice if any of the following occur:
  - any new or worsening shortness of breath (at rest or on exertion), dry cough or pleuritic chest pains
  - fatigue, shortness of breath
  - irregular heart rate
  - severe skin reaction, especially any peeling or blistering
- instruct patient to avoid antacids for 2 hours after taking tablets
- advise patient to avoid grapefruit and grapefruit juice during therapy
- see also General Patient teaching and advice for antineoplastic agents (p. 584)

DAUNORUBICIN (Daunorubicin Injection)

Available form
Vial: 2 mg/mL

Action
- antineoplastic (anthracycline) antibiotic structurally related to doxorubicin
- antibacterial and immunosuppressive properties
- active metabolite

Use
- acute lymphoblastic (lymphocytic) leukaemia (ALL) and acute myeloblastic leukaemia (AML) (alone or with other antineoplastic agents)
- disseminated neuroblastoma, rhabdomyosarcoma

Dose
- (ALL) 1 mg/kg IV, repeated at 1–4-day intervals if needed **OR**
- (AML) 2 mg/kg IV, repeated at 4–7-day intervals if needed

Adverse effects
- (acute cardiotoxicity) ECG changes, tachycardia; (delayed cardiotoxicity) cardiac failure, cardiomyopathy
- (IV site) phlebitis, thrombophlebitis, cellulitis, ulceration, necrosis
- see also General Adverse effects of antineoplastic agents (p. 582)

Interactions
- increased skin reaction and mucositis if given with radiation therapy
- increased cardiac toxicity may occur if given with cyclophosphamide
- may worsen cyclophosphamide-induced haemorrhagic cystitis
- any hyperuricaemia should be controlled with allopurinol, not other uricosuric agents due to risk of uric acid nephropathy
- not recommended with other cardiotoxic agents unless cardiac function can be closely monitored
- increased risk of cardiotoxicity if given with doxorubicin and should not be given if total cumulative dose of doxorubicin has been given
- not recommended with hepatotoxic agents
- see also General Interactions of antineoplastic agents (p. 582)

Nursing points/Cautions

- potentially cardiotoxic, therefore ECG and left ventricular ejection fraction should be measured before each

course of therapy. Baseline ECHO cardiogram is also recommended. Cardiotoxicity typically appears 1–6 months after starting therapy
- not given IM or SC or direct IV injection
- second and subsequent injections are dependent on response
- facial flushing and vein streaking will occur if given by rapid IV administration
- incompatible with heparin, dexamethasone, aluminium, aztreonam, allopurinol, fludarabine and piperacillin/tazobactam
- should be added to free-flowing IV infusion to reduce risk of local adverse effects
- increased risk of cardiotoxicity in those receiving total cumulative dose > 550 mg/m^2 or 400 mg/m^2 if patient has had chest irradiation (mediastinal or pericardial) or concurrently with cyclophosphamide
- contraindicated in those with hypersensitivity to anthracycline, having previously received full cumulative doses of doxorubicin and/or daunorubicin, cytotoxic radiotherapy, cardiac impairment including myocardial insufficiency, recent myocardial infarction or cardiac arrhythmias or severe liver or renal impairment (serum creatinine > 7.9 mg/dL)
- see also General Nursing points/Cautions for antineoplastic agents (p. 582)

Patient teaching and advice

- during administration, patient to be advised to immediately report any stinging or burning as this may indicate extravasation
- patient should be advised that urine may become harmless red colour 2–3 days after IV administration
- instruct patient to seek medical advice if any of the following occur:
- shortness of breath, cough, pink frothy sputum
- swelling of ankles, legs or abdomen
- decrease urine output
- see also General Patient teaching and advice (p. 584)

DEGARELIX (Firmagon)

Available forms
Vial: 80 mg, 120 mg

Action
- hormonal antineoplastic agent (third generation GnRH receptor blocker)
- forms depot from SC injections which form sustained-release formulation

Use
- prostate cancer (androgen deprivation therapy)

Dose
- initially 240 mg SC (given as two 120 mg injections), then after 4 weeks, 80 mg SC monthly

Adverse effects
- hot flushes, night sweats, chills
- insomnia, headache, dizziness, fatigue
- nausea, constipation
- weight increase
- hypertension
- back pain, arthralgia
- elevated liver enzymes
- (rare) prolongation of QT interval, decreased bone density, antibody development, hypersensitivity
- (injection site) pain, redness, swelling, induration, nodule formation

Interactions
- not recommended with agents known to prolong QT interval (e.g. amiodarone, sotalol) or cause electrolyte imbalance (especially hypokalaemia and hypomagnesaemia)

Nursing points/Cautions

- observe patient for at least 60 minutes after administration for any signs of hypersensitivity
- SC injection should not be rubbed or massaged after administration as this may alter release
- reconstitute with water for injections (4.2 mL for 80 mg, 3 mL for 120 mg) and avoid shaking or excessive foaming
- caution if used in those with congenital or acquired QT interval prolongation or electrolyte imbalance
- contraindicated in women and children
- see also General Nursing points/Cautions for antineoplastic agents (p. 582)

Patient teaching and advice

- advise patient to seek medical advice if any irregular heart rate occurs
- see also General Patient teaching and advice for antineoplastic agents (p. 584)

DENOSUMAB (Prolia, Xgeva)

Available forms

Prefilled syringe: 60 mg/mL; Vial: 120 mg/1.7 mL

Action

- monoclonal antibody with high affinity and specificity for RANK ligand (essential for formation, function and survival of osteoclast) inhibiting osteoclast formation, thereby decreasing bone resorption and increasing bone mass and strength, as well as decreasing cancer-induced bone destruction

Use

- treatment of osteoporosis in postmenopausal women (see Bone and calcium regulating agents, p. 902) (Prolia)
- prevention of skeletal events in those with multiple myeloma or bony metastases from solid tumours, giant cell tumour of bone (recurrent or unresectable), hypercalcaemia of malignancy (refractory to IV bisphosphonates) (Xgeva)

Dose

- (prevention of skeletal events) 120 mg SC monthly **OR**
- (giant cell bone tumour, hypercalcaemia of malignancy) 120 mg SC monthly with extra doses on day 8 and 15 of first month

Adverse effects

- hypocalcaemia
- dyspnoea, cough
- headache, insomnia, fatigue, asthenia
- back ache, arthralgia, bone pain, musculoskeletal pain
- anorexia, vomiting, abdominal pain, nausea, diarrhoea, constipation, weight loss
- fever
- peripheral oedema
- anaemia
- (rare) osteonecrosis of the jaw (generally occurring in those with cancer also being treated with antineoplastic agents and corticosteroids. Most cases are associated with dental procedures (e.g. tooth extraction) and symptoms include jaw pain, toothache, altered sensation, recurrent infection (including osteomyelitis), non-healing sores of the mouth/jaw and/or exposed bone)
- (rare) atypical femoral fractures, pancreatitis, vertebral fractures (after stopping therapy)

Interactions

- increased risk of osteonecrosis of the jaw if given with corticosteroids
- not recommended with bisphosphonates

Nursing points/Cautions

- any hypocalcaemia should be identified and treated before starting therapy
- calcium levels should be closely monitored during therapy, especially during first weeks of therapy
- supplementation with calcium 500 mg and vitamin D 400 IU orally is generally recommended (unless otherwise contraindicated)
- in those patients with risk factors (e.g. poor dental hygiene, chronic periodontal disease, head/neck radiotherapy as well as treatment with antineoplastic agents and corticosteroids), a dental examination and any necessary treatment should be carried out before starting therapy with bisphosphonate. Invasive dental procedures should be avoided if possible during therapy to prevent osteonecrosis of the jaw occurring
- should not be treated with both formulations concurrently
- should be allowed to come to room temperature for 20–30 minutes before administration
- caution if used in those with growing skeletons or after discontinuation of therapy for giant cell bone tumours as hypercalcaemia may occur weeks to months after stopping therapy
- not recommended in those with rare hereditary problems of fructose intolerance
- contraindicated in those with known sensitivity to Chinese hamster ovary proteins, severe untreated hypocalcaemia or unhealed dental or oral surgery lesions

Patient teaching and advice

- instruct patient to seek medical advice if any of the following occur:
    - jaw or dental pain
    - persistent or bleeding gums
    - non-healing sores in mouth or jaw
    - new or unusual thigh, hip or groin pain (even if it occurs months after finishing therapy)
- encourage patient to practise good dental hygiene including brushing teeth and tongue after meals and before bed, daily flossing to remove plaque and using a mirror to check teeth and gums regularly for any sores or bleeding of the gums
- warn patient not to stop therapy suddenly without seeking medical advice
- see also General Patient teaching and advice for antineoplastic agents (p. 584)

DOCETAXEL (Docetaxel Concentrated Injection)

Available forms

Vial: 20 mg/mL, 20 mg/2 mL, 80 mg/2 mL, 80 mg/8 mL, 160 mg/8 mL, 160 mg/16 mL

Action

- taxane antimetabolite

Use

- breast cancer (node positive) (adjunctive treatment)
- locally advanced or metastatic breast cancer (where other chemotherapy has failed)
- locally advanced or metastatic non-small cell lung cancer
- metastatic ovarian cancer (when first-line treatment has failed)
- hormone refractory (androgen independent) prostate cancer
- locally advanced squamous cell carcinoma of head and neck

Dose

- (metastatic breast cancer) 75–100 mg/m^2 IV over 60 minutes every 3 weeks (alone or with capecitabine or trastuzumab) **OR**
- (breast cancer – adjunctive) 75 mg/m^2 IV over 60 minutes on day 1 of 21-day cycle (in combination with cyclophosphamide) (for 4 cycles) **OR**

- (non-small cell lung cancer, ovarian cancer) 75–100 mg/m^2 IV over 60 minutes every 3 weeks **OR**
- (prostate cancer) 75–100 mg/m^2 IV over 60 minutes every 3 weeks (with prednisone or prednisolone 5 mg) **OR**
- (head and neck cancer) 75–100 mg/m^2 IV over 60 minutes every 3 weeks (with cisplatin, fluorouracil and radiotherapy or chemoradiotherapy)

Adverse effects

- fluid retention
- hypersensitivity
- eye disorders
- (rare) ototoxicity
- see also General Adverse effects of antineoplastic agents (p. 582)

Interactions

- caution if given with protease inhibitor such as ritonavir
- bioavailability increased by dexamethasone, clofibrate and phenobarbital (phenobarbitone)
- bioavailability may be decreased by ciclosporin and erythromycin

Nursing points/Cautions

- patients should be closely monitored during first and second doses for any signs of hypersensitivity which can occur at the start, during or just after infusion is stopped
- fluid retention and risk of hypersensitivity reaction may be reduced by administering dexamethasone (8 mg twice daily orally) for 3 days before starting therapy (or dexamethasone 8 mg 12 hours, 3 hours and 1 hour before infusion if treatment is for prostate cancer)
- reconstitute powder using diluent provided; avoid shaking and allow to stand for 5 minutes before further diluting
- further dilute reconstituted solution or concentrate for infusion with sodium chloride 0.9% or glucose 5%
- if dose > 200 mg, dilution volume should be greater than 250 mL for concentration of 0.74 mg/mL or less
- if crystallisation occurs, solution should be discarded
- caution if used in those with pleural effusion, pericardial effusion and ascites as fluid retention may worsen these conditions
- contraindicated in those with hypersensitivity to polysorbate 80, severe liver impairment or baseline neutrophil count $< 1.5 \times 10^9$ cells/L
- see also General Nursing points/Cautions for antineoplastic agents (p. 582)

Patient teaching and advice

- advise patient to seek medical advice if any changes to hearing occur
- see also General Patient teaching and advice for antineoplastic agents (p. 584)

DOXORUBICIN HYDROCHLORIDE (Adriamycin, Doxorubicin Hydrochloride Injection)

DOXORUBICIN HYDROCHLORIDE (LIPOSOMAL) (Caelyx, Liposomal Doxorubicin SUN)

Available forms

Solution: 10 mg/5 mL, 20 mg/10 mL, 50 mg/25 mL, 200 mg/100 mL

Action

- anthracycline antineoplastic antibiotic
- active metabolites which are cytotoxic
- pegylated liposomal formulation increases drug circulation time
- lifetime cumulative dose 550 mg/m^2 body surface area or if patient is 70 years or over, 450 mg/m^2

Use

- acute leukaemias, soft tissue and bone sarcoma, neuroblastomas,

hepatomas, Wilms' tumour, malignant carcinoma of breast, bladder, liver, lung, ovary and thyroid
- Hodgkin's lymphoma, non-Hodgkin lymphoma
- advanced epithelial ovarian cancer (after failed platinum therapy)
- metastatic breast cancer (alone)
- progressive multiple myeloma (MM) (with bortezomib in those who have had or are unsuitable for bone marrow transplant)
- AIDS-related Kaposi's sarcoma (AIDS KS) (low CD4 counts and extensive mucocutaneous or visceral disease)
- non-metastatic bladder cancer (intravesicular)

Dose
- (breast cancer, ovarian cancer) 50 mg/m^2 by IV infusion once every 4 weeks (liposomal formulation) **OR**
- (multiple myeloma) 30 mg/m^2 by IV infusion on day 4 of bortezomib 3-week cycle (liposomal formulation) **OR**
- (AIDS KS) 20 mg/m^2 by IV infusion over 30 minutes every 2–3 weeks (liposomal formulation) **OR**
- 60–75 mg/m^2 IV over 3–5 minutes at 21-day intervals **OR**
- 30 mg/m^2 IV over 3–5 minutes daily for 3 days every 4 weeks **OR**
- 45–100 mg/m^2 via intra-arterial infusion for 1–3 days **OR**
- (intravesicular) 80 mg/100 mL instilled into bladder monthly

Adverse effects
- cardiotoxicity including cardiac failure
- hyperpigmentation (hands, nails, buccal mucosa)
- discoloured urine (red)
- hand–foot syndrome (hand/foot numbness, paraesthesia, tingling, erythema, pain, swelling and, at worst, ulceration, blistering or moist desquamation)
- (intravesical administration) local transient reactions, including bladder contraction/cramp/pain, chemical cystitis, haematuria, painful micturition, frequency and urgency
- see also General Adverse effects of antineoplastic agents (p. 582)

Interactions
- increased risk of hepatotoxicity and haemorrhagic cystitis if given with 6-mercaptopurine in those with AIDS KS
- increased risk of hepatotoxicity if given with high-dose methotrexate
- cyclophosphamide, propranolol or mediastinal radiotherapy given with doxorubicin may increase cardiotoxicity
- may exacerbate cyclophosphamide-induced cystitis
- if given with cytarabine, colitis and necrosis may occur
- calcium-channel blockers may increase risk of cardiotoxicity
- cyclophosphamide, dactinomycin and mitomycin may sensitise heart to cardiac effects
- increased risk of cardiotoxicity if given within 7 months of stopping trastuzumab
- may decrease serum levels of phenytoin, phenobarbital (phenobarbitone) and St John's wort
- increased risk of mucositis if patient has previously received mucosal irradiation
- increased risk of hypersensitivity reaction if patient has recently received clindamycin
- increased serum levels and risk of congestive cardiac failure may occur if paclitaxel is given before doxorubicin
- increased risk of haematological toxicity, seizures and coma if given with ciclosporin
- total cumulative dose should be decreased if given with cyclophosphamide, daunorubicin, epirubicin or idarubicin
- see also General Interactions of antineoplastic agents (p. 582)

Nursing points/Cautions

- regular ECG monitoring or evaluation of left ventricular ejection fraction is recommended before starting and regularly throughout therapy
- two formulations of doxorubicin are not interchangeable and have different administration requirements
- (liposomal formulation) initial infusion should be given over 90 minutes as follows: 10 mL over 10 minutes, 20 mL over next 10 minutes, 40 mL over next 10 minutes and remainder of 60 minutes. If no reaction is observed, subsequent IV infusions can be given over 1 hour
- (non-liposomal formulation) IV administration should be given into freely running infusion at a rate ≥ 3–5 minutes. Patient facial flushing or local red streaking along vein is indicative that rate was too fast
- (non-liposomal formulation) IV push is not recommended due to risk of extravasation
- patient observed for infusion-related reaction which may occur within minutes of starting infusion (although usually occurs with subsequent doses)
- antihistamines, corticosteroids, oxygen and resuscitation equipment should be readily available
- (liposomal formulation) not recommended IM, SC, IV bolus or undiluted
- (liposomal formulation) dilute with glucose 5% for IV infusion (250 mL for doses < 90 mg or 500 mL for doses > 90 mg)
- (liposomal formulation) contains sucrose and is infused in glucose 5%, which may need to be taken into consideration if patient has diabetes
- (intravesical) dilute to concentration of 80 mg in 100 mL and instil via catheter
- incompatible with aminophylline, cefalotin, dexamethasone, diazepam, fluorouracil, frusemide, heparin, hydrocortisone and ganciclovir
- solution will change from red to purple if mixed with aminophylline or fluorouracil
- caution if used in those with impaired cardiac function, prior mediastinal radiation or concurrent cyclophosphamide therapy due to increased risk of cardiomyopathy
- (AIDS KS) therapy is not recommended in those who have had a splenectomy
- (non-liposomal formulation) caution if used in obese patients as clearance may be reduced
- (intravesicular) contraindicated in those with haematuria, urinary infection, inflamed bladder, invasive bladder tumours or bladder catheterisation because of large intravesical tumour
- contraindicated in those with known hypersensitivity to anthracyclines or anthracenediones, severe arrhythmias, recent myocardial infarction, myocardial insufficiency, persistent myelosuppression or previous severe stomatitis (induced by chemotherapy or radiotherapy) or in those having previously received full cumulative doses of doxorubicin and/or daunorubicin
- (liposomal formulation) contraindicated for AIDS-related Kaposi's sarcoma that could be effectively treated with alfa-interferon or local therapy
- see also General Nursing points/Cautions for antineoplastic agents (p. 582)

Patient teaching and advice

- for patient teaching and advice related to intravesicular instillation see BCG (non-vaccine) (p. 597)
- advise patient that hyperpigmentation of hands, nails and buccal mucosa may develop and does

not improve when therapy is terminated
- patient should be warned that urine may be red for 1–2 days after therapy
- symptoms of hand–foot syndrome can be reduced by advising patients to keep hands/feet cool (e.g. not wearing restricting gloves, socks or shoes; soaking hands/feet in cool water) starting 4–7 days after therapy. Other treatment may consist of pyridoxine (50–150 mg daily) and/or corticosteroids. Symptoms usually subside in 7–14 days
- instruct patient to seek medical advice if any of the following occur:
  - shortness of breath
  - swelling of ankles or legs
- see General Patient teaching and advice for antineoplastic agents (p. 584)

DURVALUMAB (Imfinzi)

Available forms
Vial: 120 mg/2.4 mL, 500 mg/10 mL

Action
- monoclonal antibody (IgG1 kappa) immune checkpoint inhibitor that blocks interaction between PD-L1 and PD-1 and CD80 leading to increased T-cell activation and decreased tumour size (in animal models)

Use
- treatment of locally advanced or metastatic urothelial cancer (with disease progression with or after platinum-containing chemotherapy, or with disease progression within 12 months of adjunct treatment with platinum-containing chemotherapy)
- treatment of locally advanced non-small cell lung cancer (NSCLC) (with locally advanced unresectable NSCLC that has not progressed following platinum-based chemoradiation therapy)

Dose
- (urothelial cancer) 10 mg/kg as IV infusion over 60 minutes every 2 weeks (for as long as there is clinical effectiveness or unacceptable toxicity) **OR**
- (locally advanced NSCLC) 10 mg/kg at IV infusion over 60 minutes every 2 weeks (for 1 year, disease progression or unacceptable toxicity)

Adverse effects
- infusion-related reaction
- pneumonitis
- hepatitis
- constipation, nausea, diarrhoea, colitis, abdominal pain, vomiting, decreased appetite
- musculoskeletal pain, arthralgia
- fatigue, insomnia
- dyspnoea, exertional dyspnoea, cough
- rash
- peripheral oedema
- fever
- liver injury
- urinary tract infection
- hypothyroidism, hyperthyroidism, adrenal insufficiency, diabetes mellitus, hypophysitis/hypopituitarism
- nephritis
- anaemia

Nursing points/Cautions
- premedication may be considered for prophylaxis of subsequent infusion reactions if infusion-related reaction occurs with first infusion
- dilute with sodium chloride 0.9% or glucose 5% to final concentration between 1–15 mg/mL
- solution should not be shaken
- use low protein binding inline filter (0.2–0.22 micron)
- see also General Nursing points/Cautions (p. 582)

Patient teaching and advice
- advise patient to seek medical advice if any of the following occur:
  - shortness of breath, chest pain, new or worsening cough

- eye or skin yellowing, loss of appetite, nausea, vomiting, pain in right upper abdominal area, dark urine
- increased number of bowel movements, diarrhoea, black stools, stools with blood or mucus, severe stomach pain or tenderness
- increased hunger or thirst, needing to urinate more often, weight loss, increased tiredness
- need to urinate more frequently or urgently, burning pain/sensation when urinating, bladder still feeling full after urinating, blood in urine, pain above pelvic bone
- changes to the amount or colour of urine, swelling of ankles, loss of appetite
- headache that doesn't go away or unusual headache, extreme tiredness, weight gain or loss, dizziness, feeling faint, feeling more thirsty or hungry than usual, hair loss, feeling cold, constipation, voice changes, nausea, vomiting, changes to mood, behaviour or sex drive
- rash, itching, skin blistering, mouth ulcers

- see General Patient teaching and advice for antineoplastic agents (p. 584)

ENZALUTAMIDE (Xtandi)

Available form
Capsules: 40 mg

Action
- antiandrogen that competitively inhibits androgen binding to androgen receptors
- active metabolites

Use
- castration-resistant metastatic prostate cancer (previously treated with docetaxel, following androgen deprivation therapy failure (chemotherapy not indicated))
- castration-resistant non-metastatic prostate cancer

Dose
- 160 mg orally once daily

Adverse effects
- bone loss, falls, falls-related injury
- hypertension
- QT interval prolongation
- (rare) seizures, posterior reversible encephalopathy syndrome (PRES)
- see also General Adverse effects of antineoplastic agents (p. 582)

Interactions
- caution if used with agents that lower seizure threshold
- caution if used with agents known to prolong QT interval or cause electrolyte imbalance (especially hypokalaemia and hypomagnesaemia)
- not recommended with rifampicin and gemfibrozil
- may decrease serum levels and is therefore not recommended with warfarin. If used, INR should be closely monitored, especially when starting or stopping therapy
- caution if used with agents with a narrow therapeutic index such as digoxin, colchicine and dabigatran
- may decrease serum levels of omeprazole
- increased risk of liver damage if given with paracetamol
- caution if given with atorvastatin, bisoprolol, cabazitaxel, carbamazepine, ciclosporin, clarithromycin, clonazepam, clopidogrel, dexamethasone, diazepam, digoxin, diltiazem, doxycycline, fentanyl, felodipine, haloperidol, indinavir, midazolam, nifedipine, phenytoin, prednisolone, primidone, propranolol, ritonavir, simvastatin, tacrolimus, thyroxine, tramadol, valproic acid, verapamil and zolpidem

Nursing points/Cautions

- monitor BP regularly during therapy
- caution if used in those with known congenital or acquired QT prolongation or electrolyte imbalance (especially hypokalaemia and hypomagnesaemia)
- not recommended in those with uncontrolled hypertension, recent myocardial infarction (within last 6 months), unstable angina (within last 3 months), class III or IV heart failure or bradycardia
- caution in those with history of seizures, epilepsy, head injury, stroke, primary brain tumours, brain metastases or alcoholism that may increase risk of seizures. If patient has seizure, therapy should be stopped
- contraindicated in women
- see also General Nursing points/Cautions for antineoplastic agents (p. 582)

Patient teaching and advice

- advise patient to seek medical advice immediately if any of the following occur:
  - confusion, trouble thinking, memory loss, blurred vision, loss of vision, balance or walking problems, decreased strength in arms or legs
  - irregular heart rate
  - fitting
- see also General Patient teaching and advice for antineoplastic agents (p. 584)

EPIRUBICIN HYDROCHLROIDE (DBL Epirubicin Hydrochloride, Pharmorubicin)

Available forms

Solution: 10 mg/5 mL, 20 mg/10 mL, 50 mg/25 mL, 100 mg/50 mL, 150 mg/75 mL, 200 mg/100 mL

Action

- antineoplastic antibiotic (anthracycline)

Use

- breast, ovarian, superficial bladder and gastric cancer, small cell lung cancer, soft tissue sarcomas (advanced metastatic), non-Hodgkin lymphoma
- prophylaxis of recurrence after transurethral resection of stage T1 papillary and stage Ta multifocal papillary cancers (grade 2 and 3)

Dose

- 75–90 mg/m^2 IV over 3–20 minutes at 21-day intervals **OR**
- (breast cancer) up to 135 mg/m^2 (alone) or 120 mg/m^2 (combination therapy) IV over 3–20 minutes every 3–4 weeks **OR**
- (early breast cancer, node positive, adjunctive therapy) 100–120 mg/m^2 IV over 3–20 minutes every 3–4 weeks **OR**
- (papillary transitional cell bladder cancer) 50 mg instilled into bladder every 8 weeks **OR**
- (prophylaxis after transurethral resection) 50 mg instilled into bladder weekly for 4 weeks, followed by monthly instillation for 11 months

Adverse effects

- ECG changes, cardiomyopathy, congestive cardiac failure, pericardial effusion
- (IV) thrombophlebitis
- (intravesical administration) local transient reactions, including bladder contraction/cramp/pain, chemical cystitis, haematuria, painful micturition, frequency and urgency
- see also General Adverse effects of antineoplastic agents (p. 582)

Interactions

- increased risk of cardiotoxicity if given with fluorouracil, cyclophosphamide, calcium-channel blockers, cisplatin,

trastuzumab, taxanes or propranolol. A 7-month interval is recommended between stopping trastuzumab and starting epirubicin
- concurrent mediastinal irradiation may potentiate cardiotoxicity
- serum levels may increase if given with cimetidine
- if paclitaxel is given before epirubicin, serum levels of epirubicin may increase
- see also General Interactions of antineoplastic agents (p. 582)

Nursing points/Cautions

- cardiac function should be measured before starting therapy
- cardiac monitoring (ECG, echocardiogram of measurement of left ventricular ejection fraction) is recommended before each cycle of therapy
- maximum lifetime cumulative dose 900 mg/m^2
- not given IM or SC
- IV push is not recommended and administration rate should be 3–20 minutes. Facial flushing and vein streaking will occur if given too rapidly
- incompatible with heparin and alkaline solutions
- solution may gel if refrigerated. Allow solution to remain at room temperature for at least 2 hours (maximum 4 hours) to come to infusible consistency
- contraindicated in those who have received full cumulative doses of doxorubicin, daunorubicin, mitozantrone or mitomycin hypersensitivity to other anthracyclines or anthracenediones, severe arrhythmias, myocardial insufficiency, recent myocardial infarction, unstable angina, persistent severe stomatitis or myelosuppression from other drug therapy or radiotherapy, or decreased liver function
- (intravesical) contraindicated in those with urinary infection, haematuria, inflamed bladder, invasive tumours penetration bladder wall or problems associated with catheterisation
- see also General Nursing points/Cautions for antineoplastic agents (p. 582)

Patient teaching and advice

- (bladder cancer) instruct patient not to drink fluids for 12 hours before bladder instillation
- patient should be warned that heart-related adverse effects may occur months after finishing treatment
- advise patient to seek medical advice if any of the following occur:
  - irregular heart rate, swelling of ankles, shortness of breath
  - (bladder administration) blood in urine, pain on urination, increased frequency or difficulty urinating
- warn patient that urine may be discoloured red for 1–2 days after treatment
- see BCG (non-vaccine) for intravesical instillation patient teaching and advice (p. 598)
- see also General Patient teaching and advice for antineoplastic agents (p. 584)

ERIBULIN MESILATE (Halaven)

Available form

Vial: 1 mg/2 mL

Action

- halichondrin antineoplastic

Use

- treatment of locally advanced or metastatic breast cancer (where anthracycline and taxane failure)
- unresectable liposarcoma (after chemotherapy for advanced metastatic disease)

Dose

- 1.4 mg/m^2 by IV bolus over 2–5 minutes on days 1 and 8 of 21-day cycle

Adverse effects

- peripheral neuropathy
- QT prolongation
- see also General Adverse effects of antineoplastic agents (p. 582)

Interactions

- caution if used with agents known to prolong QT interval and cause electrolyte imbalance (e.g. diuretics) (especially hypokalaemia and hypomagnesaemia)

Nursing points/Cautions

- premedication with antiemetic or corticosteroids is recommended
- may be used undiluted or diluted with 100 mL sodium chloride 0.9%
- should not be diluted with glucose 5%
- contains alcohol (100 mg/dose)
- dose should be delayed on day 1 or day 8 for up to 7 days if platelets $< 75 \times 10^9$/L or absolute neutrophil count (ANC) $< 1 \times 10^9$/L
- caution if used in those with pre-existing peripheral neuropathy
- not recommended in those with known congenital or acquired QT interval prolongation or electrolyte imbalance especially hypokalaemia and hypomagnesaemia
- see also General Nursing points/Cautions for antineoplastic agents (p. 582)

Patient teaching and advice

- advise patient to seek medical advice immediately if any of the following occur:
  - irregular heart rate
  - numbness/tingling in limbs, weakness, tingling or burning sensation
- see also General Patient teaching and advice for antineoplastic agents (p. 584)

ERLOTINIB HYDROCHLORIDE (Tarceva)

Available forms

Tablets: 25 mg, 100 mg, 150 mg

Action

- human growth factor receptor type 1/epidermal growth factor receptor (HER1/EGFR) tyrosine kinase inhibitor

Use

- locally advanced or metastatic non-small cell lung cancer (NSCLC) (with activating EGFR mutation)
- locally advanced, unresectable or metastatic pancreatic cancer (with gemcitabine)

Dose

- (NSCLC) 150 mg orally daily 1 hour before or 2 hours after food, reducing dose in 50 mg increments if needed **OR**
- (pancreatic cancer) 100 mg orally daily 1 hour before or 2 hours after food (with gemcitabine)

Adverse effects

- interstitial lung disease
- severe skin reactions
- gastrointestinal perforation
- (rare) ocular disorders including ulceration, corneal perforation, keratitis, conjunctivitis, abnormal eyelash growth, hypokalaemia, renal failure
- see also General Adverse effects of antineoplastic agents (p. 582)

Interactions

- increased serum levels may occur if given with atazanavir, clarithromycin, erythromycin, indinavir, itraconazole, ritonavir, saquinavir and voriconazole

- decreased serum levels may occur if given with rifampicin, rifabutin, phenytoin, carbamazepine, phenobarbital (phenobarbitone) and St John's wort
- caution if given with warfarin; INR should be closely monitored especially when starting or stopping therapy
- serum levels are decreased in smokers
- increased risk of gastric perforation if given with corticosteroids, NSAIDs and/or taxane-based agents
- solubility decreases as pH increases, therefore not recommended with agents that reduce gastric acid production (e.g. ranitidine or proton pump inhibitors)
- increased risk of myopathy and rhabdomyolysis if used with statins
- see also General Interactions of antineoplastic agents (p. 582)

Nursing points/Cautions

- EGFR mutation should be confirmed by valid and reliable testing before starting therapy
- tablets contain lactose and therefore not recommended in those with galactose intolerance, Lapp lactase insufficiency or glucose–galactose malabsorption
- caution if used in those with history of peptic ulceration or diverticular disease due to increased risk of gastric perforation
- see also General Nursing points/Cautions for antineoplastic agents (p. 582)

Patient teaching and advice

- advise patient to take tablets either 1 hour before or 2 hours after food for maximum absorption
- instruct patient to take erlotinib either 2 hours before or 10 hours after H_2 antagonist (e.g. ranitidine) or proton pump inhibitors (e.g. omeprazole)
- warn patient not to change smoking habits (i.e. stop smoking) without first consulting their doctor as this will affect serum levels
- advise patient to seek medical advice if any of the following occur:
  - new or worsening cough, shortness of breath and fever
  - severe skin reaction including any peeling or blistering
  - eye pain, abnormally growing eyelashes
  - severe abdominal pain, vomiting blood or coffee ground-like material, black tarry bowel motions, bloody diarrhoea
  - unusual muscle weakness, cramps or contractions, decreased muscle tone
- see General Patient teaching and advice for antineoplastic agents (p. 584)

ETOPOSIDE (Etopophos, Vepesid)

Available forms

Vial: 100 mg, 1 g; Solution: 100 mg/5 mL, 500 mg/25 mL; Capsules: 50 mg, 100 mg

Action

- etoposide phosphate (prodrug) is converted to etoposide (antineoplastic)
- synthetic derivative of podophyllotoxin that inhibits the cell cycle during late S and G_2 phases
- absorption from oral route is variable (50–55% of IV dose)

Use

- small cell lung carcinoma, acute monocytic and myeloblastic leukaemia, Hodgkin's disease, non-Hodgkin lymphoma, testicular tumour

Dose

- 100–200 mg/m^2 orally before food daily, days 1–5 **OR**

- 50–100 mg/m² by IV infusion over 30–60 minutes, days 1–5, every 3–4 weeks (with other antineoplastic agents) **OR**
- 100–150 mg/m² by IV infusion over 30–60 minutes, days 1, 3 and 5, every 3–4 weeks (with other antineoplastic agents)

Adverse effects
- injection site reactions
- anaphylaxis (including cardiac arrest)
- see also General Adverse effects of antineoplastic agents (p. 582)

Interactions
- increased serum levels occur if given orally with high-dose ciclosporin
- clearance may be decreased by cisplatin
- may increase INR if given with warfarin, therefore close monitoring is required especially when starting or stopping therapy
- efficacy may be decreased if given with phenytoin or other antiepileptic agents
- may increase risk of anthracycline-induced cardiomyopathy with given anthracyclines
- seizure control of antiepileptic agents may be decreased if given together
- see also General Interactions of antineoplastic agents (p. 582)

Nursing points/Cautions
- increased risk of toxicity if patient has low serum albumin
- not recommended as IV push or bolus, rapid infusion or by intra-cavity injection
- hypotension can be avoided by giving IV infusion over 30–60 minutes
- reconstitute powder with 5–10 mL of diluent for concentration of 10–20 mg/mL
- concentrate for solution must be diluted before administration, usually in 250 mL sodium chloride 0.9% or glucose 5%. Diluted solution should not be greater than 0.4 mg/mL to prevent precipitation occurring
- undiluted concentrate may cause hard plastic to crack and leak
- should not be mixed with alkaline solutions with pH greater than 8
- contraindicated in those with kidney impairment (creatinine clearance < 15 mL/minute) or WBC < 2000 cells/mm³ or platelet count $< 75,000$ cells/mm³ (not due to malignant disease)
- see also General Nursing points/Cautions for antineoplastic agents (p. 582)

Patient teaching and advice
- instruct patient that capsules should be taken with water either 2 hours before or 1 hour after food
- see also General Patient teaching and advice for antineoplastic agents (p. 584)

EXEMESTANE (Aromasin)

Available form
Tablets: 25 mg

Action
- hormonal antineoplastic agent (steroidal, aromatase inactivator)
- effective and selective treatment of hormone-dependent breast cancer in post-menopausal women

Use
- early breast cancer (oestrogen receptor positive, post-menopausal) after tamoxifen therapy
- advanced breast cancer (oestrogen receptor positive, post-menopausal after failure of anti-oestrogen therapy)

Dose
- 25 mg orally once daily with food (for 5 years or tumour relapse in early breast cancer; or in tumour progression in advanced breast cancer)

Adverse effects
- decreased bone density, osteoporosis, fractures
- hot flushes, increased sweating
- fatigue, headache, dizziness, insomnia, depression, asthenia
- anorexia, nausea, vomiting, abdominal pain, diarrhoea, constipation, dyspepsia
- hypertension
- vaginal haemorrhage
- increased weight
- hypercholesterolaemia, increased liver enzymes and bilirubin
- arthralgia, joint and musculoskeletal pain, back and limb pain, osteoarthritis, carpal tunnel syndrome
- peripheral oedema
- leukopenia
- rash, alopecia

Interactions
- actions antagonised if given with oestrogen-containing agents
- see also General Interactions of antineoplastic agents (p. 582)

Nursing points/Cautions
- post-menopausal status (such as LH, FSH and estradiol (oestradiol) levels) should be confirmed before starting therapy
- vitamin D levels should be monitored and supplements given if needed
- bone densitometry is recommended before starting and regularly throughout therapy in women who are at risk of osteoporosis. Treatment or prophylaxis for osteoporosis should be started if needed
- caution if used in women with osteoporosis
- not recommended in pre-menopausal women
- see also General Nursing points/Cautions for antineoplastic agents (p. 584)

Patient teaching and advice
- see General Patient teaching and advice for antineoplastic agents (p. 584)

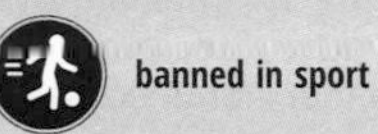

FLUDARABINE PHOSPHATE (Fludara, Fludarabine for Injection)

Available forms
Vial: 50 mg, 50 mg/2 mL; Tablets: 10 mg

Action
- antineoplastic antibiotic
- purine analogue antagonist that inhibits DNA synthesis

Use
- B-cell chronic lymphocytic leukaemia

Dose
- 25 mg/m^2 by IV injection or IV infusion over 30 minutes for 5 consecutive days every 28-day cycle (until complete or partial remission) **OR**
- 40 mg/m^2 orally daily for 5 consecutive days every 28-day cycle (until complete or partial remission)

Adverse effects
- autoimmune phenomena, haemolytic anaemia
- peripheral neuropathy
- neurotoxicity
- visual disturbances
- (rare) skin cancers
- see also General Adverse effects of antineoplastic agents (p. 582)

Interactions
- efficacy may be decreased if given with dipyridamole and other adenosine-uptake inhibitors
- may increase intracellular concentrations of cytarabine
- see also General Interactions of antineoplastic agents (p. 582)

Nursing points/Cautions
- (IV) reconstitute powder with 2 mL water for injections, then further

dilute with sodium chloride 0.9% for IV administration (10 mL for IV bolus injection or 100 mL for IV infusion over 30 minutes)
- patients receiving fludarabine should only receive irradiated blood transfusions to decrease risk of transfusion-related graft versus host disease
- may cause reversible worsening or flare up of pre-existing skin cancer lesions
- contraindicated in those with haemolytic anaemia or creatinine clearance < 30 mL/minute
- see also General Nursing points/Cautions for antineoplastic agents (p. 582)

Patient teaching and advice

- advise patient to seek medical advice if any of the following occur:
  - numbness, tingling or weakness in arms or legs
  - changes to skin or development of skin lesions
  - confusion, agitation, fitting, changes to vision
- see also General Patient teaching and advice for antineoplastic agents (p. 584)

FLUOROURACIL (APOC-5FU, DBL Fluorouracil Injection BP, Efudix)

Available forms

Vial: 500 mg/10 mL, 1 g/20 mL, 2.5 g/50 mL, 2.5 g/100 mL, 5 g/100 mL; Cream: 50 mg/g (5%)

Action

- uracil analogue that is converted to active metabolite which has antimetabolic properties, interfering with both DNA and RNA synthesis
- half-life 8–22 minutes and is dose dependent
- narrow margin of safety, highly toxic

Use

- breast, colon, rectal or stomach cancer (alone or as part of palliative treatment)
- treatment of gastric, pancreas, liver, uterine, cervical, ovarian or bladder cancer
- solar and senile keratosis, Bowen's disease (cream)

Dose

- 15 mg/kg by IV infusion over 4 hours daily until GI side-effects occur, then stop therapy until side-effects recede, then 5–10 mg/kg by IV injection weekly (daily maximum 1 g) **OR**
- 12 mg/kg by IV injection on 3 consecutive days, if no toxic side-effects, then 6 mg/kg on days 5, 7 and 9. If no toxic side-effects, then 5–10 mg/kg by IV injection weekly **OR**
- 5–7 mg/kg by intra-arterial infusion over 24 hours **OR**
- (cream) apply thin layer to lesion 1–2 times daily until erosive stage (3–4 weeks)

Adverse effects

- severe toxicity (can be life threatening)
- photosensitivity
- neurotoxicity
- hand–foot syndrome
- (cream) pain, pruritus, burning, hyperpigmentation, phototoxicity, rash, ulceration
- see also General Adverse effects of antineoplastic agents (p. 582)

Interactions

- caution if used with leucovorin (folinic acid) because of increased GI toxicity
- decreased bone marrow depression if given with allopurinol; however, increased gastrointestinal toxicity may occur if given together
- decreased clearance and increased serum levels may occur if given with cimetidine

- may increase serum levels of phenytoin, therefore serum levels should be closely monitored
- efficacy may be affected if given with methotrexate, metronidazole and folinic acid
- may potentiate necrosis caused by radiation
- myelotoxic effects may be potentiated if given with radiation
- increased risk of multifocal inflammatory leuko-encephalopathy (MILE) if given with levamisole
- caution if used with warfarin. INR should be closely monitored during therapy, especially when starting or stopping therapy
- may interfere with thyroid function test
- see also General Interactions of antineoplastic agents (p. 582)

Nursing points/Cautions

- IV dose should be reduced by one-third to half if patient has a poor nutritional status, within 30 days of major surgery, WBC $< 5000/mm^3$ or platelet $< 100{,}000/mm^3$ or impaired liver or kidney function
- (IV) dilute with 300–500 mL glucose 5% and infuse over 4 hours
- (IV) incompatible with acidic agents
- (cream) occlusive dressing is not recommended for senile or solar keratoses as it may increase penetration and inflammatory response of adjacent skin
- (cream) treatment area should not exceed 23 × 23 cm
- (cream) not recommended in those who work outdoors for prolonged periods
- caution if used in those who have received high-dose pelvic radiation or therapy with alkylating agents
- not recommended in those who have previously documented cardiovascular reaction (e.g. angina, arrhythmia, ST segment change) due to risk of sudden death
- contraindicated in those with poor nutritional state, debilitated or with dihydropyrimidine dehydrogenase (DPD) enzyme deficiency
- see also General Nursing points/Cautions for antineoplastic agents (p. 582)

Patient teaching and advice

- symptoms of hand–foot syndrome can be reduced by advising patients to keep hands/feet cool (e.g. not wearing restricting gloves, socks or shoes; soaking hands/feet in cool water) starting 4–7 days after therapy. Other treatment may consist of pyridoxine (50–150 mg daily) and/or corticosteroids. Symptoms usually subside in 7–14 days
- instruct patient to seek medical advice immediately if any of the following occur:
  - sore, red or ulcerated mouth or difficulty swallowing within 5–8 days of starting therapy (this can be early sign of severe toxicity)
  - disorientation, confusion, headache, slurred speech, dizziness, muscle weakness (which may persist after therapy has stopped)
- (cream) instruct patient that cream should be applied with gloves or non-metal applicator and application to normal skin, perioral area or nasolabial folds should be avoided
- (cream) advise patient that the normal sequence of events is for skin to redden (within 3–5 days), blister, peel and crack over 14 days. Redness may persist for some time after stopping therapy
- (cream) patient should be advised that cosmetics and skin preparations should not be applied to same area
- warn patient to avoid or minimise sun exposure during and immediately after therapy

- see also General Patient teaching and advice for antineoplastic agents (p. 584)

FOTEMUSTINE (Muphoran)

Available form

Vial: 208 mg

Action

- alkylating agent (nitrogen mustard analogue)

Use

- disseminated malignant melanoma (including cerebral metastases) (alone or as part of combination therapy)

Dose

- initially 100 mg/m^2 by IV infusion over 1 hour or intra-arterial infusion over 4 hours for 3 doses at weekly intervals (induction), followed by rest period of 4–5 weeks, then 100 mg/m^2 every 3 weeks (maintenance)

Adverse effects

- see General Adverse effects of antineoplastic agents (p. 582)

Interactions

- contraindicated with yellow fever vaccine
- caution if given with warfarin, INR should be closely monitored, especially when starting or stopping therapy
- not recommended concurrently with dacarbazine because of increased risk of pulmonary toxicity and at least a week interval should be allowed between administration of two agents
- not recommended with phenytoin due to increased risk of seizures as absorption of phenytoin may be impaired
- see also General Interactions of antineoplastic agents (p. 582)

Nursing points/Cautions

- regular ophthalmology examination is recommended before starting and regularly throughout therapy
- should not be given within 4 weeks of other chemotherapy or 6 weeks of nitrosoureas
- if given as part of combination therapy, induction phase can be omitted
- reconstitute using 4 mL of supplied diluent, then further dilute with glucose 5%
- IV solution should be protected from light during administration
- reconstituted solution contains equivalent of 2.7 g of 100% alcohol which may harmful if used in those with alcoholism, liver disease or epilepsy
- contraindicated in those with hypersensitivity to nitrosourea
- see also General Nursing points/Cautions for antineoplastic agents (p. 582)

Patient teaching and advice

- see General Patient teaching and advice for antineoplastic agents (p. 584)

FULVESTRANT (Faslodex)

Available form

Prefilled syringe: 250 mg/5 mL

Action

- hormonal antineoplastic agent (anti-oestrogen) which inhibits growth of some oestrogen-sensitive human breast cancer cells

Use

- locally advanced or metastatic breast cancer (hormone receptor-positive, post-menopausal) with disease progression (after tamoxifen therapy)

Dose

- initially 500 mg slowly IM (as two 250 mg injections in each buttock), then 500 mg after 2 weeks, followed by 500 mg at monthly intervals

Adverse effects

- hot flushes
- headache, asthenia

- anorexia, nausea, vomiting, diarrhoea
- rash
- joint and musculoskeletal pain
- hypersensitivity
- elevated liver enzymes and bilirubin
- injection site reaction
- urinary tract infection
- (uncommon) liver failure, hepatitis

Interactions
- may interfere with antibody-based oestradiol assay

Nursing points/Cautions
- not recommended in men
- caution if used in those with bleeding disorders or thrombocytopenia or on anticoagulant therapy due to risk of bleeding associated with IM administration
- see also General Nursing points/Cautions for antineoplastic agents (p. 582)

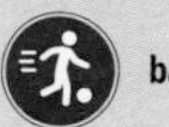
banned in sport

GEFITINIB (Iressa)

Available form
Tablets: 250 mg

Action
- inhibits epidermal growth factor receptor (EGFR) tyrosine kinase expressed in solid tumours of epithelial origin

Use
- locally advanced or metastatic non-small cell lung cancer (that express EGFR tyrosine kinase mutation)

Dose
- 250 mg orally daily

Adverse effects
- interstitial lung disease
- ulcerative keratitis, keratitis, conjunctivitis, dry eye
- gastrointestinal perforation
- see also General Adverse effects of antineoplastic agents (p. 582)

Interactions
- INR should be monitored if given with warfarin, especially when starting or stopping therapy
- increased serum levels may occur if given with itraconazole, clotrimazole or ritonavir
- efficacy may be reduced if given with agents that increase gastric pH above 5, such as ranitidine
- caution if used with corticosteroids or NSAIDs due to risk of gastrointestinal perforation
- decreased serum levels may occur if given with rifampicin, phenytoin, carbamazepine, barbiturates or St John's wort
- may increase serum levels of metoprolol
- increased neutropenia may occur if given with vinorelbine
- see also General Interactions of antineoplastic agents (p. 582)

Nursing points/Cautions
- EGFR mutation status of patient should be confirmed before starting therapy using a valid and reliable method
- may also be administered via nasogastric tube after dissolving as below
- caution if used in those with history of gastrointestinal ulceration, smoking or bowel metastases as risk of gastrointestinal perforation is increased
- see also General Nursing points/Cautions for antineoplastic agents (p. 582)

Patient teaching and advice
- instruct patient that tablets may be dispersed in non-carbonated water if swallowing is difficult. Whole tablet (must not be crushed) should be dropped into water and stirred until dissolved (about 10 minutes) and

drunk immediately. Glass should be rinsed and contents drunk

- advise patient to seek medical advice if any of the following occur:
  - new or worsening cough, shortness of breath or difficulty breathing
  - eye inflammation, tearing, blurred vision, eye pain, red eye, light sensitivity
  - severe abdominal pain, vomiting blood or coffee ground-like material, black tarry bowel motions, bloody diarrhoea
- see also General Patient teaching and advice for antineoplastic agents (p. 584)

GEMCITABINE (DBL Gemcitabine for Injection, DBL Gemcitabine Solution for Injection, Gemaccord, Gemplan)

Available forms

Vial: 200 mg, 1 g, 2 g, 200 mg/5.3 mL; 1 g/26.3 mL; 2 g/52.6 mL

Action

- pyrimidine analogue with antimetabolic activity
- cell phase specific (S phase)

Use

- locally advanced or metastatic non-small cell lung cancer (NSCLC)
- locally advanced or metastatic adenocarcinoma of the pancreas
- bladder cancer (alone or with cisplatin)
- recurrent epithelial ovarian carcinoma (relapsed more than 6 months after platinum-based treatment)
- unresectable, locally recurrent or metastatic breast cancer (who have relapsed) (with paclitaxel)
- refractory pancreatic cancer (where fluorouracil was ineffective)

Dose

- (NSCLC, monotherapy) 1 g/m^2 weekly IV over 30 minutes for 3 weeks of 4-week cycle **OR**
- (NSCLC, combination therapy) 1.25 g/m^2 IV over 30 minutes on days 1 and 8 of 21-day cycle (with cisplatin) **OR**
- (NSCLC, combination therapy) 1 g/m^2 IV over 30 minutes on days 1, 8 and 15 of 28-day cycle **OR**
- (pancreatic cancer) 1 g/m^2 weekly IV over 30 minutes for up to 7 weeks, with 1 week rest interval, then 1 g/m^2 weekly IV for 3 weeks of 4-week cycle **OR**
- (bladder cancer – monotherapy) 1.25 g/m^2 IV over 30 minutes on days 1, 8 and 15 of 28-day cycle **OR**
- (bladder cancer – combination therapy) 1 g/m^2 IV over 30 minutes on days 1, 8 and 15 of 28-day cycle (with cisplatin) **OR**
- (breast cancer – combination therapy) 1.25 g/m^2 IV over 30 minutes on days 1 and 8 of 21-day cycle (with paclitaxel) **OR**
- (ovarian cancer – combination therapy) 1 g/m^2 IV over 30 minutes on days 1 and 8 of 21-day cycle (with carboplatin)

Adverse effects

- (uncommon) interstitial pneumonitis with pulmonary infiltrates and rarely, pulmonary oedema and acute respiratory distress syndrome
- see also General Adverse effects of antineoplastic agents (p. 582)

Interactions

- increased risk of interstitial pneumonitis, colitis and oesophagitis if given with or within 7 days of radiotherapy
- see also General Interactions of antineoplastic agents (p. 582)

Nursing points/Cautions

- toxicity increased with prolonged infusion time and increased dosing frequency
- reconstitute using sodium chloride 0.9% (5 mL for 200 mg vial, 25 mL for 1 g vial, 50 mL for 2 g vial), which

can be further diluted with sodium chloride 0.9% for infusion
- caution if used in those with liver metastases, history of hepatitis, liver cirrhosis or alcoholism as liver insufficiency may be exacerbated
- see also General Nursing points/Cautions for antineoplastic agents (p. 582)

Patient teaching and advice

- advise patient to seek medical advice if any persistent cough, shortness of breath or fever occurs
- see also General Patient teaching and advice for antineoplastic agents (p. 584)

HYDROXYCARBAMIDE (HYDROXYUREA) (Hydrea)

Available form
Capsules: 500 mg

Action
- thought to inhibit DNA synthesis during S phase of cell cycle
- antimetabolite

Use
- chronic myelocytic leukaemia (CML) (resistant) (pre-treatment phase and palliative care)
- recurrent metastatic or inoperable ovarian cancer

Dose
- (solid tumours – intermittent therapy) 80 mg/kg orally every third day **OR**
- (solid tumours – continuous therapy) 20–30 mg/kg orally daily **OR**
- (head/neck cancer with radiotherapy) 80 mg/kg orally every third day starting at least 7 days before, during and after radiotherapy (depending on any adverse effects) **OR**
- (CML) 20–30 mg/kg orally daily

Adverse effects
- skin ulceration
- exacerbation of post-irradiation erythema
- see also General Adverse effects of antineoplastic agents (p. 582)

Interactions
- any uricosuric dose should be adjusted according to increases in the serum uric acid level
- increased risk of hepatotoxicity, pancreatitis and peripheral neuropathy if given to those with HIV infection treated concurrently with stavudine
- irradiation erythema and mucositis may be worsened by hydroxycarbamide (hydroxyurea)
- may cause falsely elevated results for determination of urea, uric acid and lactic acid
- see also General Interactions of antineoplastic agents (p. 582)

Nursing points/Cautions

- (CML) therapy should be reviewed after 6 weeks to assess effectiveness
- hydroxyurea-induced ulcers generally heal when therapy is stopped
- see also General Nursing points/Cautions for antineoplastic agents (p. 582)

Patient teaching and advice

- if capsules are difficult to swallow, instruct patient that contents can be emptied into water and drunk immediately. However, patient should be warned to avoid inhaling or making contact with powder. Hands should be washed thoroughly immediately after handling
- advise patient to seek medical advice if any skin ulcerations occur
- see also General Patient teaching and advice for antineoplastic agents (p. 584)

IBRUTINIB (Imbruvica)

Available form
Capsules: 140 mg

Action
- tyrosine kinase inhibitor

Use
- mantel cell lymphoma (MCL)
- previously untreated chronic lymphocytic leukaemia (CLL)/small lymphocytic lymphoma (SLL) (monotherapy or with obinutuzamab)
- chronic CLL/SLL (after ≥ 1 treatment) (as monotherapy or with bendamustine and rituximab)
- Waldenstrom's macroglobinaemia (WM) (after ≥ 1 treatment or as first-line therapy in those unsuitable for chemoimmunotherapy
- Waldenstrom's macroglobinaemia (WM) (with rituximab)

Dose
- (MCL) 560 mg orally daily **OR**
- (CLL/SLL, WM) 420 mg orally daily

Adverse effects
- atrial flutter, atrial fibrillation, arrhythmias
- bleeding
- (rare) progressive multifocal leukoencephalopathy, reactivation of hepatitis B, interstitial lung disease
- see also General Adverse effects of antineoplastic agents (p. 582)

Interactions
- contraindicated with St John's wort
- not recommended with warfarin or other vitamin K antagonists due to increased risk of bleeding
- not recommended with fish oil and vitamin E preparations
- not recommended with grapefruit, Seville oranges, amiodarone, aprepitant, atazanavir, ciprofloxacin, clarithromycin, cobicistat, crizotinib, diltiazem, erythromycin, fluconazole, imatinib, indinavir, itraconazole, nelfinavir, posaconazole, ritonavir, saquinavir, verapamil and voriconazole, due to increased serum levels
- not recommended with carbamazepine, phenytoin, phenobarbital (phenobarbitone), rifabutin, rifampicin and St John's wort due to decreased serum levels
- increased risk of bleeding if given with antiplatelet or anticoagulants agents
- caution if given with digoxin or methotrexate

Nursing points/Cautions
- patient should be monitored for any signs of atrial fibrillation or arrhythmias during therapy
- screen patient for hepatitis B before starting therapy
- should be withheld for 3–7 days before surgery
- not recommended in those with atrial fibrillation, acute infections or cardiac risk factors
- see also General Nursing points/Cautions for antineoplastic agents (p. 582)

Patient teaching and advice
- instruct patient to avoid grapefruit and Seville oranges during therapy
- advise patient to seek medical advice immediately if any of the following occur:
  - confusion, trouble thinking, memory loss, blurred vision, loss of vision, balance or walking problems, decreased strength in arms or legs
  - irregular heart rate, shortness of breath
- see also General Patient teaching and advice for antineoplastic agents (p. 584)

IDARUBICIN HYDROCHLORIDE (Idarubicin Concentrate for Infusion, Zavedos)

Available forms
Capsules: 5 mg; Solution: 5 mg/5 mL, 10 mg/10 mL

Action

- anthracyoline antibiotic analogue of doxorubicin, inhibits nucleic acid synthesis
- half-life 10–35 hours
- active metabolite with long half-life (33–60 hours)

Use

- remission and induction of acute myeloid leukaemia (AML) (untreated, relapsed or refractory patient)

Dose

- (monotherapy) 30 mg/m^2 orally daily for 3 days **OR**
- (combination therapy) 15–30 mg/m^2 orally daily for 3 days (with other antineoplastic agents) **OR**
- 12 mg/m^2 daily IV over 10–15 minutes for 3 days (with cytarabine (Ara-C) IV for 7 days)

Adverse effects

- ECG changes, tachycardia, arrhythmias, congestive cardiac failure, cardiomyopathy
- (rare) gastrointestinal perforation
- see also General Adverse effects of antineoplastic agents (p. 582)

Interactions

- added myelosuppressive effect if given with or within 14–21 days of radiation therapy
- caution if used with other cardiotoxic agents such as calcium-channel blockers and trastuzumab. If given after trastuzumab, a 7-month interval should be allowed before starting idarubicin
- see also General Interactions of antineoplastic agents (p. 582)

Nursing points/Cautions

- cardiac function should be assessed before starting and regularly throughout therapy
- (IV) injection given into freely running IV solution over 10–15 minutes
- IV solution is incompatible with heparin or with alkaline drugs
- (oral) not recommended in those who have previously experienced full body irradiation or bone marrow transplantation
- caution if used in those with pre-existing heart disease or previous irradiation to mediastinal area
- contraindicated in those with recent myocardial infarction, severe arrhythmias, severe myocardial insufficiency or previous treatment with maximum cumulative dose of idarubicin or other anthracyclines or anthracenediones
- see also General Nursing points/Cautions for antineoplastic agents (p. 582)

Patient teaching and advice

- patient should be advised that urine may appear harmless red colour for 1–2 days after therapy
- instruct patient to seek medical advice if any of the following occur:
  - shortness of breath, cough, pink frothy sputum
  - swelling of ankles, legs or abdomen
  - decreased urine output
  - rapid or abnormal heart rate
  - severe abdominal pain
- see also General Patient teaching and advice for antineoplastic agents (p. 584)

IDELALISIB (Zydelig)

Available forms

Tablets: 100 mg, 150 mg

Action

- phosphatidylinositol 3-kinase (PIK3 delta) inhibitor (PIK3 delta is hyperactive in B-cell malignancies)

Use

- chronic lymphocytic leukaemia (CLL)/small lymphocytic lymphoma

(SLL) (after relapse where chemoimmunotherapy is not suitable) (with rituximab or ofatumumab)
- refractory follicular lymphoma (who have received two prior therapies, including an alkylating agent and rituximab)

Dose
- 150 mg orally twice daily (until toxicity or disease progression)

Adverse effects
- serious infection
- colitis, intestinal perforation
- pneumonitis
- severe cutaneous reaction
- (rare) progressive multifocal leukoencephalopathy (PML)
- see also General Adverse effects of antineoplastic agents (p. 582)

Interactions
- not recommended with live or live attenuated vaccines
- serum levels may be decreased by carbamazepine, rifampicin, phenytoin and St John's wort and therefore not recommended together
- caution if given with sirolimus, tacrolimus, ciclosporin, fentanyl or alfentanil
- may increase serum levels of warfarin, midazolam, calcium-channel blockers, some antiarrhythmics, benzodiazepines, HMG-CoA reductase inhibitors (statins) and phosphodiesterase 5 (PDE-5) inhibitors increasing the risk of adverse effects

Nursing points/Cautions
- patient should be screened for hepatitis B and hepatitis C before starting therapy
- patient should be closely monitored for any signs of cytomegalovirus (CMV) infection
- antibiotic prophylaxis against *Pneumocystis jirovecii* is recommended during and for 2–6 months after last dose
- if patient presents with colitis, infection causes (e.g. *Clostridium difficile*) should be excluded
- caution if used in those with active hepatitis
- see also Nursing points/Cautions for antineoplastic agents (p. 582)

Patient teaching and advice
- advise patient that diarrhoea can occur months after starting therapy
- patient should be instructed to seek medical advice if any of the following occur:
  - any severe skin reaction including peeling or blistering
  - abdominal pain, diarrhoea
  - moderate-to-severe diarrhoea, new or worsening abdominal pain, chills, fever, nausea, vomiting
  - fever, chills, cough, shortness of breath, malaise
  - confusion, trouble thinking, memory loss, blurred vision, loss of vision, balance or walking problems, decreased strength in arms or legs
  - signs of CMV infection including fever, night sweats, sore throat, joint or muscle pain, loss of appetite and/or large mouth ulcers
- see also Patient teaching and advice for antineoplastic agents (p. 584)

IFOSFAMIDE (Holoxan)

Available forms

Vial: 500 mg, 1 g, 2 g

Action
- requires activation by microsomal liver enzymes to produce active metabolite, which is an alkylating agent (nitrogen mustard analogue)

Use
- ovarian and cervical tumours
- some response in lung and breast cancers

- sarcomas, lymphomas and germ cell tumours

Dose

- 8–10 g/m^2 divided into 5 equal doses and administered daily for 5 days given IV, and repeated at 2–4-week intervals **OR**
- 5–6 g/m^2 IV given over 24 hours (maximum 10 g), repeated at 3–4-week intervals

Adverse effects

- haematuria, haemorrhagic cystitis, tubular dysfunction
- encephalopathy, drowsiness
- see also General Adverse effects of antineoplastic agents (p. 582)

Interactions

- increased risk of bleeding if given with warfarin, therefore INR should be closely monitored when starting or stopping therapy
- hypoglycaemia may be increased if given with sulfonylureas
- increased myelosuppression if given with allopurinol or hydrochlorothiazide
- caution if given with agents acting on the CNS (e.g. antiemetics, opioid analgesics, antihistamines) especially in those with ifosfamide-induced encephalopathy
- efficacy may be decreased by grapefruit juice
- may potentiate muscle relaxant effects of suxamethonium
- effects and toxicity may be increased if given with liothyronine (triiodothyronine), chlorpromazine or disulfiram
- increased risk of nephrotoxicity, neurotoxicity or myelosuppression if given before or with cisplatin, aminoglycosides, aciclovir or amphotericin B (amphotericin)
- caution if given with bupropion, orphenadrine or cyclophosphamide
- may increase radiodermatitis
- see also General Interactions of antineoplastic agents (p. 582)

Nursing points/Cautions

- any electrolyte imbalance, cystitis, outflow disturbance or urinary tract infection should be identified and treated before starting therapy
- renal function, urinary status, urinary sediment and urinary output should be monitored regularly
- urinalysis should be performed before each course and if haematuria (> 10 RBCs/high power field) is present, therapy should be postponed until resolved
- haemorrhagic cystitis is a common side-effect, therefore ifosfamide is given with aggressive oral or parenteral hydration
- to prevent bladder toxicity, uroprotector mesna (see Antineoplastic support agents, p. 716) should be administered concurrently
- reconstitute with water for injections (13 mL for 500 mg, 25 mL for 1 g and 50 mL for 2 g) to give concentration of 40 mg/mL, then dilute further for IV infusion
- not recommended within 3 months of nephrectomy or caution if used in unilaterally nephrectomised patients
- caution if used in those who are older or with brain metastases, cerebral symptoms, history of alcohol abuse, obese, impaired renal function, pre-treated with nephrotoxic before nephrectomy, electrolyte imbalance, post-renal obstruction or are female, due to increased risk of encephalopathy
- caution if used in those with pre-existing cardiac disorders, those who have had previous irradiation to heart area and/or have been previously treated with anthracyclines
- contraindicated in those with urinary obstruction or bladder inflammation (cystitis)
- see also General Nursing points/Cautions for antineoplastic agents (p. 582)

Patient teaching and advice

- those with diabetes managed with sulfonylurea agents should be warned to monitor blood glucose levels closely during therapy
- patient should be advised to avoid grapefruit and grapefruit juice during therapy
- instruct patient to seek medical advice if any of the following occur:
  - blood in urine, bladder pain, difficulty passing urine
  - drowsiness, confusion, hallucinations, fitting (seizure) or loss of consciousness
  - fatigue, chest pain, palpitations, altered heart rate
- see General Patient teaching and advice for antineoplastic agents (p. 584)

IMATINIB (Gilmat, Glivec)

Available forms

Tablets: 100 mg, 400 mg

Action

- tyrosine kinase inhibitor
- inhibits activity of tyrosine kinase (TK), as well as several receptor TKs (KIT), receptor for stem cell factor (SCF) coded for by KIT oncogenes, platelet-derived growth factor receptor (PDGFR), colony-stimulating factor receptor (CSF-1R and others)
- KIT mutation and PDGFR activation have been implicated in a number of conditions including GIST, MDS/MPD, HES/CEL, DFSP and ASM (see below)

Use

- chronic myeloid leukaemia (CML)
- Philadelphia chromosome positive (Ph+) acute lymphoblastic leukaemia (ALL) (newly diagnosed, relapsed or refractory) (alone or with other agents)
- KIT (CD117) positive unresectable and/or metastatic malignant GI stromal tumours (GIST) (treatment or as adjuvant therapy post resection to prevent recurrence)
- unresectable, recurrent and/or metastatic dermatofibrosarcoma protuberans (DFSP)
- myelodysplastic/myeloproliferative disorder (MDS/MPD) with PDGFR rearrangement (where conventional therapy has failed)
- aggressive systemic mastocytosis (ASM) (where conventional therapy has failed)
- hypereosinophilic syndrome (HES) and/or chronic eosinophilic leukaemia (CEL)

Dose

- (CML – chronic phase) 400 mg orally daily, increasing to 600 mg if no adverse effects occur, and further 400 mg twice daily if no greater than mild toxicity occurs **OR**
- (CML – accelerated phase or blast crisis) 600 mg orally daily, increasing to 400 mg twice daily if no adverse effects occurred **OR**
- (Ph+ ALL) 600 mg orally daily **OR**
- (MDS/MPD) initially 400 mg orally daily, increasing to 600–800 mg if response is inadequate **OR**
- (ASM) initially 400 mg orally daily, increasing to 600–800 mg if response is inadequate **OR**
- (SM with eosinophilia) initially 100 mg orally daily, increasing to 400 mg if response is inadequate and no adverse effects have occurred **OR**
- (HES/CEL) initially 400 mg orally daily, increasing to 600–800 mg if response is inadequate **OR**
- (GIST) 400 mg orally daily, increasing to 800 mg if disease progression occurs during therapy at 400 mg **OR**
- (GIST – unresectable and/or metastases present) 600 mg orally daily **OR**
- (GIST, adjunctive) 400 mg orally daily (after resection) for up to 3 years **OR**
- (DFSP) 400 mg orally twice daily

Adverse effects

- fluid retention, oedema, pleural effusion, pericardial effusion, pulmonary oedema, ascites
- severe congestive cardiac failure, left ventricular dysfunction
- (HES) cardiogenic shock, left ventricular dysfunction
- hypothyroidism
- phototoxicity
- see also General Adverse effects of antineoplastic agents (p. 582)

Interactions

- increased serum levels may occur if given with erythromycin, clarithromycin, itraconazole, HIV protease inhibitors and grapefruit juice
- decreased serum levels may occur if given with dexamethasone, phenytoin, carbamazepine, rifampicin, phenobarbital (phenobarbitone) and St John's wort
- may increase serum levels of ciclosporin, some benzodiazepines, calcium-channel blockers and HMG-CoA reductase inhibitors (statins), increasing risk of adverse effects
- may inhibit metabolism of paracetamol
- if given with warfarin, prothrombin time should be closely monitored especially when starting or stopping therapy
- see also General Interactions of antineoplastic agents (p. 582)

Nursing points/Cautions

- before starting therapy, patient should be tested for hepatitis B as reactivation can occur
- patient should be weighed and monitored closely for any signs of fluid retention (which can be serious)
- before starting therapy, echocardiogram and serum troponin levels should be measured before starting therapy in those with high eosinophilia levels. If either is abnormal, prophylactic corticosteroids for 1–2 weeks should be considered to prevent hypereosinophilic-cardiac toxicity
- TSH levels should be monitored if patient is taking levothyroxine after thyroidectomy
- doses of 400–600 mg can be given as a single daily dose, 800 mg dose should be divided and given as 400 mg twice daily
- caution if used in those with pre-existing heart disease
- see also General Nursing points/Cautions for antineoplastic agents (p. 582)

Patient teaching and advice

- instruct patient to take tablets with a large glass of water and food to minimise GI disturbances
- warn patient to avoid or minimise exposure to direct sunlight by wearing protective clothing and high protection factor (30+) sunscreen. Sunlamps and tanning beds should be avoided
- patient should be advised to avoid grapefruit, grapefruit juice, paracetamol and paracetamol-containing preparations during therapy
- if tablets cannot be swallowed, advise patient that they may be dispersed in 50 mL (for 100 mg tablet) or 200 mL (for 400 mg tablet) of water or apple juice. Stir well to ensure tablets are dissolved and drink immediately
- advise patient to seek medical advice if any of the following occur:
    - rapid weight gain, swelling of ankles, calves or face
    - shortness of breath, difficulty breathing, chest pain, cough
- see also General Patient teaching and advice for antineoplastic agents (p. 584)

INOTUZUMAB OZOGAMICIN (Besponsa)

Available form

Vial: 1 mg

Action

- CD22 antibody-drug conjugate consists of three components – recombinant immunoglobulin (IgG4 kappa) (inotuzumab), semi-synthetic calicheamicin derivative that causes double-stranded DNA breaks and an acid-cleavable linker that joins inotuzumab with the calicheamicin derivative

Use

- relapsed or refractory CD22-positive B-cell precursor acute lymphoblastic leukaemia (ALL)

Dose

- initially 0.8 mg/m^2 (day 1), 0.5 mg/m^2 (day 8) and 0.5 mg/m^2 (day 15) of 21-day cycle (cycle 1) by IV infusion over 1 hour, then 0.5 mg/m^2 (days 1, 8 and 15) of 28-day cycle if patient has achieved complete remission or complete remission with incomplete haematologic recovery **OR**
- 0.8 mg/m^2 (day 1), 0.5 mg/m^2 (day 8) and 0.5 mg/m^2 (day 15) of 28-day cycle if patient has not achieved complete remission or complete remission with incomplete haematologic recovery

Adverse effects

- hepatotoxicity, hepatic venoocclusive disease
- infusion-related reactions
- QT prolongation
- increased amylase and lipase
- see also General Adverse effects for antineoplastic agents (p. 582)

Interactions

- not recommended with other agents known to prolong QT interval

Nursing points/Cautions

- liver function tests (e.g. ALT, AST, total bilirubin, alkaline phosphatase) and full blood counts should be monitored before and after each dose or more frequently if abnormal liver tests occur. For patients undergoing stem cell transplantation, liver function should be monitored closely for first month post-transplant, and regularly thereafter
- premedication with corticosteroid, antipyretic and antihistamine is recommended before infusion
- patient should be closely monitored during and for at least 1 hour post-infusion for any hypotension, hot flushes, rash or breathing difficulties
- before first dose, if patient has circulating lymphoblasts, cytoreduction with hydroxyurea, corticosteroids and/or vincristine is recommended to reduce blast count to $\leq$ 10,000/mm^3
- patient should be monitored during and for at least 1 hour post-infusion for any signs of infusion-related reactions
- if complete remission or complete remission with incomplete haematologic recovery does not occur within 3 cycles of treatment, therapy should be stopped
- if patient is not having haematopoietic stem cell transplant (HSCT), 6 cycles of therapy may be given, whereas only 2 cycles are recommended for those to have HSCT (however, a third cycle may be given if the patient has not achieved complete remission or complete remission with incomplete haematologic recovery)
- therapy interruption is recommended if patient experiences haematologic toxicity or non-haematolgic toxicity (e.g. liver toxicity, veno-occlusive disease, infusion-related reactions)
- not given as IV bolus or push

- solution is light sensitive and must be protected during reconstitution, dilution and administration using UV light-blocking cover such as aluminium foil or amber, dark brown or green bags. Infusion line does not need to be protected
- reconstitute using 4 mL water for injections and swirl gently (do not shake), then add to sodium chloride 0.9% for a total volume of 50 mL. Invert gently to mix
- infusion rate should be 50 mL/hour
- caution if used in those with mild-to-moderate liver disease or history of liver disease or hepatitis, have experienced mild-to-moderate venoocclusive liver disease or sinusoidal obstruction syndrome, are older or have undergone stem cell transplantation
- caution if used in those with history of QT interval prolongation or those with electrolyte disturbances. If used, ECG and electrolyte monitoring is recommended before start and regularly during treatment
- contraindicated in those with serious ongoing liver disease (e.g. cirrhosis, active hepatitis) or those who have experienced serious or ongoing veno-occlusive liver disease or sinusoidal obstruction syndrome
- see also general Nursing points/Cautions for antineoplastic agents (p. 584)

Patient teaching and advice

- advise patient to seek medical advice immediately if any of the following occur:
  - rapid weight gain, upper right abdominal pain, abdominal swelling
  - feeling dizzy or light-headed, abnormal heart rate
  - fever, chills, hot flushes, dizzy or light-headed, rash, trouble breathing during or shortly after infusion
- see General Patient teaching and advice for antineoplastic agents (p. 584)

IPILIMUMAB (Yervoy)

Available forms

Vial: 50 mg/10 mL, 200 mg/40 mL

Action

- recombinant monoclonal antibody that binds cytotoxic T lymphocyte associated antigen 4 (CTLA-4) (CTLA-4 is a key regulator of T cell activity that increase number of tumour-reactive T effector cells)
- also increases anti-tumour immune response

Use

- unresectable or metastatic melanoma (previous therapy failed or intolerable) (alone or with nivolumab)
- untreated advanced renal cell (RCC) carcinoma (with nivolumab)
- metastatic or recurrent non-small cell lung cancer (NSCLC) (with nivolumab and 2 cycles of platinum-double chemotherapy

Dose

- (unresectable or metastatic melanoma) 3 mg/kg IV over 90 minutes every 3 weeks for 4 doses or 16 weeks (induction, alone or with nivolumab), followed by single agent (nivolumab) therapy (maintenance) (until disease progression or unacceptable toxicity) **OR**
- (RCC) 1 mg/kg IV over 30 minutes every 3 weeks for 4 doses, then nivolumab alone **OR**
- (NSCLM) 1 mg/kg IV every 6 weeks (with nivolumab every 3 weeks and platinum therapy every 3 weeks)

Adverse effects

- severe and life-threatening immune-related adverse reactions (including enterocolitis, intestinal perforation, hepatitis, dermatitis, neuropathy, pneumonitis and endocrinopathies) (occurring weeks to months after last dose)

- see also General Adverse effects of antineoplastic agents (p. 582)

Interactions

- Immune-related adverse effects occur more commonly when therapy is combined with nivolumab
- not recommended with vemurafenib
- corticosteroids are not recommended before starting ipilimumab therapy; however, may be used to treat immune-related adverse effects. Corticosteroid therapy should be tapered over at least 1 month
- caution if used with anticoagulants due to increased risk of GI bleeding

Nursing points/Cautions

- electrolytes, liver and thyroid function should be measured before starting and before each dose
- patient should be closely monitored for any signs of immune-related adverse effects
- (melanoma) tumour response should be assessed after 4 doses
- (melanoma) if 4 doses are not completed within 16 weeks, therapy should be stopped
- (combination therapy) if given with nivolumab and/or chemotherapy, nivolumab should be administered first, then ipilimumab at least 30 minutes later and chemotherapy should be given last (if required)
- not given by IV push or bolus
- stand vial at room temperature for 5 minutes before administration
- may be used undiluted or dilute with sodium chloride 0.9% or glucose 5% to a concentration of 1–4 mg/mL
- low protein binding filter (0.2 micron) is recommended for IV administration
- regimen can be repeated if needed
- not recommended in those with severe active autoimmune disease where further immune activation could be life threatening
- contraindicated in those with hypersensitivity to polysorbate 80
- see also General Nursing points/Cautions for antineoplastic agents (p. 582)

Patient teaching and advice

- patient should be advised to seek medical advice immediately if any of the following occur:
  - any rash, itching, peeling or blistered skin
  - headache, fatigue, muscle weakness, decreased strength, difficulty walking, numbness/tingling in hands or feet, difficulty waking up, loss of consciousness
  - diarrhoea, abdominal pain or tenderness, increase in stool frequency, bloody or dark-coloured stools, constipation
  - yellowing of eyes or skin, fatigue, nausea, loss of appetite, upper abdominal pain, dark urine, pale stools
- advise patient that the adverse effects (listed on p. 655) may occur weeks to months after the last dose and should not be managed with over-the-counter preparations. The importance of seeking medical advice immediately should be emphasised due to the potentially life-threatening nature of the adverse effects
- see General Patient teaching and advice for antineoplastic agents (p. 584)

IRINOTECAN HYDROCHLORIDE TRIHYDRATE (IRINOTECAN HYDROCHLORIDE) (Camptosar, DBL Irinotecan Injection, Meditab Irinotecan)

IRINOTECAN (LIPOSOMAL) (Onivyde)

Available forms

Vial: 40 mg/2 mL, 100 mg/5 mL, 300 mg/15 mL, 500 mg/25 mL; Vial (liposomal): 43 mg/10 mL

Action

- camptothecin that binds to topoisomerase1 enzyme interfering with DNA synthesis
- active metabolite
- some cholinergic effects
- liposomal formulation prolongs activity at tumour site (Onivyde)

Use

- metastatic carcinoma of the rectum or colon (as first-line treatment or after disease recurrence or progression after initial therapy)
- metastatic pancreatic adenocarcinoma (previously treated with gemcitabine) (with folinic acid and 5FU (fluorouracil))

Dose

- (monotherapy) 125 mg/m^2 IV over 90 minutes on days 1, 8, 15 and 22 followed by 2-week rest interval (6-week cycle). Dose may be increased to 150 mg/m^2 or decreased to 50 mg/m^2 depending on patient tolerance **OR**
- (rectum or colon cancer – monotherapy) 350 mg/m^2 IV over 90 minutes once every 3 weeks, decreasing dose to 200 mg/m^2 in 50 mg increments if needed **OR**
- (rectum or colon cancer– combination therapy) 125 mg/m^2 IV over 90 minutes on days 1, 8, 15 and 22 followed by 2-week rest interval (with folinic acid and fluorouracil) (6-week cycle) **OR**
- (rectum or colon cancer– combination therapy) 180 mg/m^2 IV over 90 minutes on days 1, 15 and 29 followed by 2-week rest interval (with folinic acid and fluorouracil) (6-week cycle) **OR**
- (pancreatic adenocarcinoma) 70 mg/m^2 IV over 90 minutes every 2 weeks (with folinic acid and fluorouracil) (Onivyde)

Adverse effects

- (cholinergic effects, early, transient) diarrhoea, increased salivation and lacrimation, miosis, sweating, bradycardia, flushing and intestinal hyperperistalsis (causing abdominal cramping)
- colitis, paralytic ileus
- see also General Adverse effects of antineoplastic agents (p. 582)

Interactions

- not recommended with diuretics (especially during periods of active vomiting or diarrhoea) because of the increased risk of severe dehydration
- not recommended with atazanavir, clarithromycin, gemfibrozil, indinavir, itraconazole, lopinavir, nelfinavir, ritonavir, saquinavir, voriconazole and grapefruit juice as increased serum levels may occur. Should be stopped for at least 7 days before starting therapy with irinotecan
- may prolong neuromuscular blocking actions of suxamethonium
- may antagonise neuromuscular blockade of non-depolarising blocking agents
- not recommended with St John's wort, phenobarbital (phenobarbitone), phenytoin or carbamazepine as serum levels may increase. These should be stopped at least 14 days before starting therapy with irinotecan
- increased risk of myelosuppression and neutropenia if patient has previously received pelvic/abdominal irradiation
- increased incidence of akathisia if given with prochlorperazine
- increased risk of hyperglycaemia and lymphocytopenia if given with dexamethasone
- see also General Interactions of antineoplastic agents (p. 582)

Nursing points/Cautions

- liposomal and non-liposomal formulations are not interchangeable
- premedication with dexamethasone 10 mg and ondansetron or granisetron

is recommended starting 30 minutes before therapy
- not given as a bolus or undiluted
- IV or SC atropine (0.25–1 g) can be used prophylactically or to relieve cholinergic adverse effects
- (liposomal formulation) dilute to 500 mL with glucose 5% or sodium chloride 0.9%
- (non-liposomal formulation) must be diluted with glucose 5% or sodium chloride 0.9% before IV administration to concentration of 0.12–2.8 mg/mL
- (Onivyde) contains 3.31 mg sodium/mL which may need to be considered if patient has sodium restriction
- caution if used in those with asthma, cardiovascular disease, or urinary or GI obstruction due to cholinergic effects
- (non-liposomal formulation) not recommended in those with fructose intolerance
- see also General Nursing points/Cautions for antineoplastic agents (p. 582)

Patient teaching and advice

- advise patient to have loperamide readily available at first sign of poorly formed or loose stools
- patient should be instructed that delayed (or late) diarrhoea (more than 24 hours after treatment) should be treated promptly with loperamide (at first sign of loose stools) (initially 4 mg, then 2 mg 2-hourly (or 4 mg 4-hourly overnight) until diarrhoea-free for 12 hours) to prevent dehydration and electrolyte imbalance. Loperamide is not recommended for longer than 48 hours due to increased risk of paralytic ileus. Further, patient should be instructed to seek medical advice immediately if diarrhoea is not controlled in 24 hours using this regimen
- see also General Patient teaching and advice for antineoplastic agents (p. 584)

LAPATINIB DITOSILATE MONOHYDRATE (LAPATINIB DITOSYLATE MONOHYDRATE) (Tykerb)

Available form

Tablets: 250 mg

Action

- selective and potent tyrosine kinase inhibitor of both epidermal growth factor (ErbB1) and HER2 (ErbB2) receptors

Use

- hormone-receptor positive metastatic breast cancer in post-menopausal women (tumours overexpressing HER2 where hormonal therapy is indicated) (with aromatase inhibitor)
- advanced or metastatic breast cancer with tumours overexpressing HER2 (where tumours have progressed after treatment with anthracycline, taxane and trastuzumab) (with capecitabine)
- metastatic breast cancer with tumours overexpressing HER2 (where trastuzumab is inappropriate) (first-line treatment with paclitaxel)

Dose

- 1250 mg orally daily at least 1 hour before or after food (with capecitabine)

OR

- 1500 mg orally daily at least 1 hour before or after food (with paclitaxel or aromatase inhibitor)

Adverse effects

- decreased left ventricular fraction, QT interval prolongation
- interstitial lung disease, pneumonitis
- see also General Adverse effects of antineoplastic agents (p. 582)

Interactions

- increased serum levels may occur if given with grapefruit juice, clarithromycin, erythromycin, itraconazole and ritonavir and are therefore not recommended. Should be stopped at least 7 days before starting therapy with lapatinib

- decreased serum levels may occur if given with rifampicin, dexamethasone, phenytoin, carbamazepine, phenobarbital (phenobarbitone) and St John's wort and are therefore not recommended. Should be stopped at least 14 days before starting therapy with lapatinib
- absorption may be decreased by food and proton pump inhibitors
- caution if given with digoxin as digoxin toxicity may occur due to increased serum levels
- increased risk of diarrhoea and neutropenia if given with paclitaxel
- caution if given with agents known to prolong QT interval or cause electrolyte imbalance (especially hypokalaemia and hypomagnesaemia)
- see also General Interactions of antineoplastic agents (p. 582)

Nursing points/Cautions

- HER2 overexpression and/or HER2 gene amplification should be confirmed by valid and reliable testing before starting therapy
- any electrolyte imbalance (especially hypokalaemia and hypomagnesaemia) should be corrected before starting therapy
- left ventricular ejection fraction should be measured before starting therapy, then 8–12-weekly
- caution if used in those with known congenital or acquired prolongation of QT interval or electrolyte imbalance (especially hypokalaemia or hypomagnesaemia)
- see also General Nursing points/Cautions for antineoplastic agents (p. 582)

Patient teaching and advice

- patient should be advised to avoid food 1 hour before and 1 hour after taking tablets
- instruct patient to avoid grapefruit juice during therapy
- advise patient to seek medical advice if any of the following occur:
  - new or worsening cough, shortness of breath or difficulty breathing
  - abnormal or rapid heart rate
  - palpitations, shortness of breath, difficulty breathing, swelling of ankle or calf
- see also General Patient teaching and advice for antineoplastic agents (p. 584)

LETROZOLE (Femara, Femolet, Fera, Gynotril)

Available form

Tablets: 2.5 mg

Action

- non-steroidal aromatase inhibitor that blocks oestrogen-dependent tumour growth

Use

- hormone receptor-positive breast cancer (in post-menopausal women)

Dose

- 2.5 mg orally daily for 5 years or tumour response

Adverse effects

- hot flushes, sweating
- nausea, vomiting, diarrhoea, anorexia, abdominal pain, dyspepsia, increased weight
- hypercholesterolaemia
- hypertension, palpitations, chest pain
- depression
- peripheral oedema
- headache, asthenia, fatigue, malaise, dizziness, vertigo
- bone pain, myalgia, arthralgia, arthritis
- rash, alopecia, dry skin
- vaginal bleeding
- osteoporosis, falls, bone fractures

Interactions

- not recommended with tamoxifen, other anti-oestrogens or oestrogen-containing agents

- increased serum levels may occur if given with itraconazole, voriconazole, ritonavir and clarithromycin
- decreased serum levels may occur if given with phenytoin, rifampicin, carbamazepine, phenobarbital (phenobarbitone) and St John's wort
- may increase serum levels of phenytoin and clopidogrel increasing risk of adverse effects

Nursing points/Cautions

- if menopausal status is unclear, luteinising hormone (LH), follicle stimulating hormone (FSH) and/or estradiol (oestradiol) levels should be measured before starting therapy
- bone densitometry is recommended before starting and during therapy
- caution if used in those with severe liver insufficiency
- not recommended for hormone-negative breast cancer
- contraindicated in pre-menopausal women
- see also General Nursing points/Cautions (p. 582)

Patient teaching and advice

- see General Patient teaching and advice for antineoplastic agents (p. 584)

banned in sport

LOMUSTINE (CeeNU)

Available forms
Capsules: 10 mg, 40 mg, 100 mg

Action
- alkylating agent (nitrosourea)

Use
- palliative treatment of primary, metastatic brain tumours (with surgery and/or radiotherapy and/or chemotherapy)
- Hodgkin's disease (alternative therapy where other therapies were ineffective)

Dose
- 130 mg/m^2 orally 1 hour before or 1 hour after food once every 6 weeks

Adverse effects
- pulmonary fibrosis
- see also General Adverse effects of antineoplastic agents (p. 582)

Interactions
- see General Interactions of antineoplastic agents (p. 582)

Nursing points/Cautions

- lung function should be measured before starting and regularly throughout therapy
- pulmonary toxicity symptoms may occur months to years after stopping therapy
- see also General Nursing points/Cautions for antineoplastic agents (p. 582)

Patient teaching and advice

- ensure patient understands that capsules are taken only once every 6 weeks
- advise patient that nausea and vomiting are reduced if lomustine is taken on an empty stomach; however, if nausea and vomiting do occur, patient should ensure that capsule has not been vomited
- instruct patient to report any new or worsening cough, shortness of breath or difficulty breathing
- see also General Patient teaching and advice for antineoplastic agents (p. 584)

LORLATINIB (Lorviqua)

Available forms
Tablets: 25 mg, 100 mg

Action

- adenosine triphosphate competitive inhibitor of ALK and ROS1 tyrosine kinases that addresses mechanisms of resistance after prior treatment with ALK inhibitors

Use

- treatment of anaplastic lymphoma kinase (ALK)-positive advanced non-small cell lung cancer (that has progressed despite therapy with crizotinib and at least one other ALK inhibitor)

Dose

- 100 mg orally daily

Adverse effects

- hypercholesterolaemia, hypertriglyceridaemia
- oedema
- peripheral neuropathy
- hallucinations, changes in cognitive function, mood changes, altered mental status, speech difficulties
- (uncommon) PR interval prolongation, AV block
- elevated lipase and amylase
- interstitial lung disease, pneumonitis
- see also General Adverse effects of antineoplastic agents (p. 582)

Interactions

- contraindicated with carbamazepine, enzalutamide, phenytoin, rifampicin and St John's wort. A 3-week washout period should be allowed before starting therapy with lorlatinib
- not recommended with boceprevir, cobicistat, elvitegravir, indinavir, itraconazole, paritaprevir, lopinavir, posaconazole, ritonavir, saquinavir, telaprevir, voriconazole and grapefruit juice
- may decrease serum levels of hormonal contraceptives, alfentanil, ciclosporin, ergotamine, fentanyl, midazolam, sirolimus and tacrolimus, and are therefore not recommended together

Nursing points/Cautions

- ALK-positive status must be established using validated test before starting therapy
- serum lipids and cholesterol should be measured before starting, 8 weeks after and then regularly during therapy. Lipid-lowering agents may be required
- ECG and measurement of lipase and amylase is recommended before starting therapy and then monthly
- dose reduction may be required if severe adverse effects occur. If patient is unable to tolerate 50 mg, therapy should be stopped
- not recommended in those with moderate-to-severe liver impairment or severe kidney impairment (creatinine clearance < 30 mL/minute)
- see General Nursing points/Cautions for antineoplastic agents (p. 582)

Patient teaching and advice

- patient should be advised to seek medical advice immediately if any of the following occur:
  - shortness of breath, difficulty breathing, cough, fever
  - feeling confused, difficulty with speech, mood changes, hallucinations, memory problems
- advise patient to avoid grapefruit juice during therapy
- see also General Patient teaching and advice for antineoplastic agents (p. 584)

MELPHALAN (Alkeran, Melpha)

Available forms

Vial: 50 mg; Tablets: 2 mg

Action

- alkylating agent (nitrogen mustard derivative)

Use

- palliative treatment of multiple myeloma (MM) and advanced ovarian adenocarcinoma

- advanced breast cancer
- polycythaemia vera

Dose

- (MM) 0.15 mg/kg orally daily in divided doses (with prednisolone 40 mg orally) for 4 days, repeated every 6 weeks **OR**
- (MM) 16 mg/m^2 by IV infusion over 15–20 minutes every 2 weeks for 4 doses, then every 4 weeks **OR**
- (advanced ovarian cancer) 0.2 mg/kg orally daily in 3 divided doses for 5 days, repeated every 4–8 weeks **OR**
- (advanced breast cancer) 0.15 mg/kg or 5 mg/m^2 orally daily for 4–6 days, repeated every 6 weeks **OR**
- (polycythaemia vera) 6–10 mg orally daily for 5–7 days, followed by 2–4 mg daily until satisfactory control (remission induction), then 2–6 mg orally once weekly (maintenance)

Adverse effects

- (IV) hypersensitivity
- see also General Adverse effects of antineoplastic agents (p. 582)

Interactions

- increased risk of impaired renal function if given with ciclosporin or cisplatin
- may increase pulmonary toxicity if given with carmustine
- see also General Interactions of antineoplastic agents (p. 582)

Nursing points/Cautions

- (MM) IV therapy is indicated when oral therapy is not available or inappropriate
- after reconstitution with 10 mL of supplied diluent, dilute with sodium chloride 0.9% to concentration of ≤ 0.45 mg/mL
- should be completely administered within 60 minutes of reconstitution
- reconstituted solution should not be refrigerated as precipitate will form
- (MM) treatment beyond 12 months does not appear to improve results
- see also General Nursing points/Cautions antineoplastic agents (p. 582)

Patient teaching and advice

- see also General Patient teaching and advice antineoplastic agents (p. 584)

MERCAPTOPURINE MONOHYDRATE (Allmercap, Puri-Nethol)

Available forms

Tablets: 50 mg; Oral solution: 20 mg/mL

Action

- purine analogue antimetabolite that interferes with nucleic acid synthesis
- half-life 90 minutes
- active metabolites have longer life than parent agent

Use

- acute lymphoblastic and myelogenous leukaemia (remission induction and maintenance), chronic granulocytic leukaemia

Dose

- 2.5 mg/kg orally daily

Adverse effects

- macrophage activation syndrome (high non-abating fever, lymphadenopathy, hepatosplenomegaly, CNS dysfunction, bleeding)
- photosensitivity
- see also General Adverse effects of antineoplastic agents (p. 582)

Interactions

- may inhibit anticoagulant action of warfarin, therefore INR should be closely monitored, especially when starting and stopping therapy
- not recommended with ribavirin which may decrease efficacy and increase toxicity of mercaptopurine

- increased serum level may occur if given with allopurinol, therefore dose of mercaptopurine should be decreased to 25%
- onset of pancytopenia is slowed when taken with unregulated amounts of salicylates, sulfonamides or tranquillisers
- increased serum levels may occur if given with high-dose methotrexate
- caution if given with olsalazine, mesalazine or sulfasalazine (in those with inherited deficiency of thiopurine methyltransferase) due to risk of increased myelosuppression
- caution if given with infliximab
- see also General Interactions of antineoplastic agents (p. 582)

Nursing points/Cautions

- cross-resistance may exist between mercaptopurine and tioguanine (thioguanine)
- (oral solution) only recommended for paediatric use
- (oral solution) contains aspartame and hydroxybenzoates
- not recommended in those with Lesch-Nylan syndrome
- increased risk of toxicity if used in those with inherited mutated NUDT15 gene
- see also General Nursing points/ Cautions for antineoplastic agents (p. 582)

Patient teaching and advice

- instruct patient to limit exposure to sunlight and UV light by wearing long-sleeved clothing, hat and factor 30+ sunscreen if going outdoors
- if patient is taking oral suspension, instruct in the following:
  - take suspension 1 hour before or 2 hours after food or dairy products
  - shake bottle vigorously for at least 30 seconds before using
  - push bottle adapter firmly into top of bottle
  - two dosing syringes are provided: orange 5 mL syringe marked 1–5 mL should be used to measure amounts > 1 mL with each 0.2 mL = 4 mg; purple 1 mL syringe marked 0.1–1 mL should be used to measure amounts ≤ 1 mL with each 0.1 mL = 2 mg
  - put tip of correct dosing syringe into bottle adapter, turn bottle upside down and pull plunger back to point on scale that corresponds with dose
  - turn bottle right way up, withdraw syringe and gently put tip into mouth inside cheek. Gently squirt suspension into mouth (not forcefully) and swallow
  - drink a small amount of water to ensure suspension is not left in mouth
  - wash syringe with warm soapy water, rinse well and let dry completely before reusing
  - wash hands well after handling oral suspension and syringe
  - discard any unused suspension 8 weeks after opening
- see also General Patient and teaching for antineoplastic agents (p. 584)

METHOTREXATE (DBL Methotrexate Injection, Methoblastin, Methotrexate Ebewe, Trexject)

Available forms

Tablets: 2.5 mg, 10 mg; Vial: 5 mg/2 mL, 50 mg/2 mL, 500 mg/5 mL, 500 mg/20 mL, 1000 mg/10 mL, 5000 mg/50 mL; Prefilled syringe: 7.5 mg/0.3 mL, 10 mg/0.4 mL, 15 mg/0.6 mL, 20 mg/0.8 mL, 25 mg/mL

Action

- inhibits metabolism of folic acid, thereby interfering with DNA and RNA synthesis (cell replication) (especially in rapidly dividing cells such as dermal epithelial cells, buccal and intestinal cells)

Use

- (with other agents) palliative treatment of acute lymphoblastic leukaemia, Burkitt's lymphoma, advanced lymphosarcoma, advanced mycosis fungoides, prophylaxis and treatment of meningeal leukaemia
- breast cancer, choriocarcinoma, chorioadenoma destruens, hydatidiform mole
- high-dose therapy used for osteogenic sarcoma, acute leukaemias, bronchogenic carcinoma, head and neck epidermoid carcinoma (with calcium folinate)
- unresponsive disabling psoriasis, rheumatoid arthritis (see Disease modifying antirheumatic drugs (DMARDs), p. 982)

Dose

- (trophoblastic neoplasm, hydatidiform mole, chorioadenoma destruens) 15–30 mg IM or orally daily before food for 5 days, may be repeated ≥ 1 week rest interval for 3–5 cycles **OR**
- (lymphoblastic leukaemia) 3.3 mg/m^2 orally daily (with prednisolone) (remission induction) then 30 mg/m^2 orally twice weekly (maintenance) **OR**
- (lymphoblastic leukaemia) 30 mg/m^2 IM twice weekly or 2.5 mg/kg IV every 14 days (maintenance) **OR**
- (lymphoma) 10–25 mg orally daily for 4–8 days, repeated after 7–10 days if needed, repeated for several courses **OR**
- (mycosis fungoides) 2.5–10 mg orally daily for weeks to months **OR**
- (mycosis fungoides) 50 mg IM weekly or 25 mg IM twice weekly **OR**
- (breast cancer) 40 mg/m^2 IV on days 1 and 8 of cyclic chemotherapy (with cyclophosphamide and fluorouracil) **OR**
- (meningeal leukaemia) 12 mg intrathecally every 2–5 days until CSF cell count returns to normal, then one extra dose

Adverse effects

- interstitial lung disease, pulmonary fibrosis
- see also General Adverse effects of antineoplastic agents (p. 582)

Interactions

- (intrathecal) contraindicated with CNS radiotherapy
- contraindicated with acitretin or other retinoids
- contraindicated with alcohol and other hepatotoxic agents (e.g. retinoids, azathioprine, leflunomide, sulfasalazine)
- serum levels (and associated risk of toxicity) may be increased by chloramphenicol, omeprazole, pantoprazole, phenytoin, probenecid, penicillins, salicylates, sulfonamides, sulfonylureas, tetracyclines and aminobenzoic acid, and therefore not recommended together
- (high dose) not recommended with NSAIDs due to increased risk of myelosuppression and GI toxicity because half-life of methotrexate is prolonged. Caution should also be used with lower doses of methotrexate
- toxicity may be increased by folate deficiency
- increased risk of myelosuppression and decreased folate levels if given with triamterene
- serum levels may be decreased by colestyramine
- not recommended with vitamin supplements containing folic or folinic acid
- if used with nitrous oxide, may potentiate methotrexate's effects on folate metabolism
- increased risk of bone marrow depression if given with allopurinol,

trimethoprim, trimethoprim/sulfamethoxazole and pyrimethamine
- may decrease clearance of theophylline, thereby increasing risk of toxicity. Theophylline levels should be closely monitored during concurrent therapy
- increased risk of toxicity if given with transfusion of packed red blood cells
- absorption and metabolism may be decreased by tetracycline and non-absorbable broad-spectrum antibiotics
- may increase plasma levels of mercaptopurine
- increased risk of pancytopenia and interstitial pneumonitis if given with leflunomide
- increased risk of skin cancer if given with PUVA therapy
- may interfere with folic acid detection assay
- see also General Interactions of antineoplastic agents (p. 582)

Nursing points/Cautions

- folinic acid (leucovorin) is given to neutralise the toxic effects of methotrexate (folinic acid rescue). Folinic acid is given orally, IM or IV within 24 hours of methotrexate administration (10 doses 6-hourly) (see Antidotes, antagonists and chelating agents, p. 334)
- if dose $>$ 200 mg, patient should be encouraged to drink plenty of fluids for 2 days after dose, as well as keeping urine alkaline for $\geq$ 24 hours
- only preservative-free methotrexate should be used for intrathecal administration
- (prefilled syringe) used for management of psoriasis and rheumatoid arthritis only
- incompatible with cytarabine, fluorouracil and prednisolone
- see also General Nursing points/Cautions for antineoplastic agents (p. 582)

Patient teaching and advice

- instruct patient to seek medical advice immediately if any dry persistent non-productive cough occurs
- see also General Patient teaching and advice for antineoplastic agents (p. 584)

METHYL AMINOLEVULINATE HYDROCHLORIDE (Metvix)

Available form

Cream: 160 mg/g

Action

- sensitiser for photodynamic therapy
- after application to skin, photoactive porphyrins accumulate and after light activation, photochemical reaction destroys target cells

Use

- squamous cell carcinoma (SCC) in situ (Bowen's disease) (where surgery is inappropriate)
- superficial or nodular basal cell carcinoma (BCC) (where surgery is inappropriate)
- facial or scalp actinic keratoses (AK) that are thin or nonhyperkeratotic and nonpigmented (where other therapies are unacceptable)

Dose

- apply cream 1 mm thick to lesion and 5–10 mm surrounding skin and cover with occlusive dressing for 3 hours

Adverse effects

- pain, warm sensation, burning, tingling, stinging, erythema, itching, oedema, crusting, ulceration, exudates, blisters, peeling, hypo/hyperpigmentation, bleeding
- allergic contact dermatitis

Nursing points/Cautions

- any UV therapy should be discontinued before starting therapy

- (BCC) lesions should be assessed 3 months after treatment for response. If not complete, retreatment is recommended
- (AK) usually only require one treatment with photodynamic therapy with natural light or red LED light with suitable lamp
- (BCC, SCC) require two treatments with a week interval in between with red LED light with suitable lamp
- (AK) thick lesions should not be treated
- multiple lesions may be treated at the same time
- protective goggles should be worn by both the patient and the operator during photosensitisation procedure with red light
- (SCC/BCC) should only be used to treat primary lesions
- (SCC/BCC) should be reviewed at 6–12-month intervals to detect any recurrence
- contains hydroxybenzoates (which can cause hypersensitivity) and cetostearyl alcohol and arachis oil which can cause local skin reaction (e.g. contact dermatitis)
- caution if used in those with hypertension as pain associated with procedure may increase BP. BP should be closely monitored
- contraindicated in those with hypersensitivity to peanut oil, porphyria, invasive SCC or morpheaform BCC

Patient teaching and advice

- patient should be given the following instructions:
    - avoid getting cream in eyes
    - sun exposure should be avoided for 2–3 days after treatment
    - any crust or scale should be removed and lesion roughened (but not to bleeding stage) before application of cream (with spatula)
    - (BCC, SCC) after application of cream, occlusive dressing should be applied over lesion/s for 3 hours
    - before exposure to light source, cream should be removed and lesion and surrounding skin cleaned using saline
    - (BCC, SCC) goggles should be worn to protect eyes during exposure to red light source
    - if light source is natural sunlight (for scalp and facial actinic keratosis only), sunscreen (SPF 30+) (but not containing zinc oxide, titanium dioxide or iron oxide) should be applied to all exposed areas 15 minutes before preparation of lesion(s) (see second instruction) and application of cream. No occlusion is needed. Exposure to sunlight should occur within 30 minutes of applying cream and continue for 2 hours, during which time person should stay outside and carry out normal activities. After 2 hours, cream should be washed off and further sun exposure avoided for 2–3 days (see first instruction)
    - warn patient that burning sensation generally only lasts for a few hours after therapy
    - inform patient that healthy, untreated skin does not need to be protected during therapy

MIDOSTAURIN (Rydapt)

Available form

Capsules: 25 mg

Action

- tyrosine kinase inhibitor (including FLT3 and KIT kinase)
- also inhibits mast cell proliferation and survival, and histamine release

Use

- newly diagnosed acute myeloid leukaemia (AML) who are FLT3-mutation positive

- aggressive systemic mastocytosis (ASM), systemic mastocytosis with associated haematological neoplasms (SM-AHN)
- mast cell leukaemia

Dose

- (AML) 50 mg orally twice daily with food on days 8–21 of induction and consolidation cycles, then 50 mg orally twice daily with food (as single agent maintenance therapy) for up to 12 cycles of 28-day cycle or relapse **OR**
- (advanced SM) 100 mg orally twice daily with food continued while clinical response is evident or unacceptable toxicity occurs

Adverse effects

- decrease in left ventricular ejection fraction
- interstitial lung disease, pneumonitis
- see also General Adverse effects for antineoplastic agents (p. 582)

Interactions

- serum levels may increase if given with itraconazole, ritonavir, clarithromycin
- decreased serum levels may occur if given with carbamazepine, rifampicin, phenytoin and St John's wort

Nursing points/Cautions

- WBC should be monitored at start of and regularly during therapy
- dose interruption, reduction or discontinuation is recommended in patients that develop severe adverse effects
- pregnancy test is recommended within 7 days of starting therapy
- caution if used in those with congestive cardiac failure
- not recommended in women of childbearing potential not using contraception
- see also General Nursing points/Cautions for antineoplastic agents (p. 582)

Patient teaching and advice

- instruct patient that if vomiting occurs, additional dose should not be taken
- advise patient to seek medical advice immediately if any of the following occur:
  - chest pain/discomfort, lightheadedness, dizziness, blue discolouration of lips or extremities, shortness of breath, swelling of lower limbs
  - new or worsening cough, chest pain, shortness of breath, difficulty breathing

MITOZANTRONE (Mitozantrone Ebewe, Onkotrone)

Available forms

Vial: 20 mg/10 mL, 25 mg/12.5 mL

Action

- non-cell cycle specific antineoplastic antibiotic (anthracycline)

Use

- breast carcinoma (metastatic, locally advanced)
- non-Hodgkin lymphoma
- relapsed acute non-lymphocytic leukaemia
- blast crisis of chronic myelogenous leukaemia

Dose

- (breast cancer, non-Hodgkin lymphoma – monotherapy) 14 mg/m^2 IV over 3–5 minutes or by IV infusion over 15–30 minutes once every 3 weeks **OR**
- (leukaemia (patients with low marrow reserve) – monotherapy) 12 mg/m^2 IV over 3–5 minutes or by IV infusion over 15–30 minutes daily for 5 days, repeated if relapse occurs **OR**
- (leukaemia – combination therapy) 10–12 mg/m^2 IV over 3–5 minutes or by IV infusion over 15–30 minutes for 3 days with cytosine arabinoside for

7 days. If second course is required, mitozantrone is given for 2 days with cytosine arabinoside for 5 days **OR**
- (breast cancer, lymphoma-combination therapy) 2–4 mg/m² IV over 3–5 minutes or by IV infusion over 15–30 minutes (with other antineoplastic agents)

Adverse effects
- congestive cardiac failure, decreased left ventricular ejection fraction
- see also General Adverse effects of antineoplastic agents (p. 582)

Interactions
- (AML) clearance may be decreased if given with ciclosporin

Nursing points/Cautions
- cardiac monitoring is recommended before starting and during therapy
- dose should be reduced by 2–4 mg/m² if given as part of combination therapy
- may precipitate if given with heparin
- may cause skin staining. If contact occurs, area should be washed with copious amounts of water
- (Onkatrone) dilute to at least 50 mL with glucose 5% or sodium chloride 0.9% and infuse over 15–30 minutes or can be added to free-running IV solution
- increased risk of cardiac toxicity if used in those with pre-existing heart disorders, previous treatment with anthracyclines or prior mediastinal radiotherapy
- contraindicated in those with known hypersensitivity to anthracyclines or sulfite or if cardiac function is abnormal
- contraindicated by intrathecal, SC, IM or intra-arterially administration
- see also General Nursing points/Cautions for antineoplastic agents (p. 582)

Patient teaching and advice
- warn patient that blue/green discolouration of the urine can be expected for 24 hours after treatment and that bluish discolouration of the sclera may also occur
- advise patient to seek medical advice immediately if any shortness of breath, difficulty breathing or swelling of ankles occurs
- see General Patient teaching and advice for antineoplastic agents (p. 584)

NERATINIB (Nerlynx)

Available form

Tablets: 40 mg

Action
- irreversible inhibitor of three epidermal growth factor receptors, including HER2 receptor, thereby inhibiting tumour cell proliferation

Use
- adjunctive treatment of early stage HER2-overexpressed/amplified breast cancer

Dose
- 240 mg orally daily with food for 1 year after completion of trastuzumab therapy

Adverse effects
- diarrhoea, dehydration
- left ventricular dysfunction
- see also General Adverse effects for antineoplastic agents (p. 582)

Interactions
- contraindicated with carbamazepine, phenytoin, phenobarbital (phenobarbitone), rifampicin and St John's wort
- contraindicated with diltiazem, erythromycin, fluconazole and verapamil
- not recommended with proton pump inhibitors

- not recommended with atazanavir, clarithromycin, indinavir, itraconazole, nelfinavir, ritonavir, saquinavir, telithromycin and voriconazole
- not recommended with grapefruit, grapefruit juice, pomelos, star-fruit and Saville oranges as serum levels may increase
- caution if used with sulfasalazine or rosuvastatin
- caution if used with dabigatran, digoxin and fexofenadine. Serum levels should be closely monitored

Nursing points/Cautions

- liver function tests (including ALT, AST and total bilirubin) should be measured after 1 week, then monthly for 3 months, and then every 6 weeks or more frequently if needed
- anti-diarrhoeal prophylaxis (loperamide) is recommended with first dose and should be titrated to number of bowel motions per day (e.g. during days 1–14, 4 mg 3 times daily is recommended, days 57–365, 4 mg is recommended as needed). Additional antidiarrhoeal agents may be required if patient has loperamide-refractory diarrhoea
- caution if used in those with significant chronic gastrointestinal disorders with diarrhoea. If used, patient should be very closely monitored
- caution if used in those with cardiac risk factors. Cardiac monitoring with assessment of left ventricular ejection fraction recommended
- caution if used in those over 65 years due to increased risk of dehydration and renal insufficiency
- not recommended in those with severe renal impairment or receiving dialysis
- contraindicated in those with severe liver impairment
- see also General Nursing points/Cautions for antineoplastic agents (p. 582)

Patient teaching and advice

- warn patient that diarrhoea usually starts in first 1–2 weeks of therapy and is often recurrent
- ensure patient understands diarrhoea management, including use of anti-diarrhoeal agent (for first 1–2 months titrating dose to maintain 1–2 bowel motions a day, and then continued prophylactically), diet modification and need for at least 2 L of fluid daily to avoid dehydration
- advise patient to seek medical advice immediately if diarrhoea does not stop or patient feels dizzy or weak (which can be signs of dehydration)
- if antacids are used, advise patient that there should be a 3-hour interval between antacid and neratinib
- advise patient to avoid grapefruit, grapefruit juice, pomelos, star-fruit and Saville oranges during therapy
- see also General Patient teaching and advice for antineoplastic agents (p. 584)

NILOTINIB (Tasigna)

Available forms

Capsules: 150 mg, 200 mg

Action

- BCR-ABL tyrosine kinase inhibitor which stops replication of tumour cells

Use

- chronic myeloid leukaemia (CML) (Philadelphia chromosome positive (Ph+)) in chronic or accelerated phase (newly diagnosed or resistant or intolerant to other therapies)

Dose

- (newly diagnosed CML (Ph+), chronic phase) 300 mg orally twice daily 2 hours before or 1 hour after food **OR**

- (CML, resistant or intolerant to other therapies, chronic or accelerated phase) 400 mg orally twice daily 2 hours before or 1 hour after food

Adverse effects

- may prolong QT interval, ischaemic heart disease, peripheral arterial occlusive disease
- elevated blood glucose and cholesterol
- elevated serum lipase, pancreatitis
- see also General Adverse effects of antineoplastic agents (p. 582)

Interactions

- absorption may be increased by food
- absorption may be decreased by antacids and histamine H_2-receptor antagonists
- not recommended with other agents known to prolong QT interval (e.g. amiodarone, disopyramide, clarithromycin, sotalol, methadone) or cause electrolyte imbalance (especially hypokalaemia and hypomagnesaemia)
- increased serum levels may occur if given with grapefruit juice, clarithromycin, erythromycin, itraconazole, voriconazole and ritonavir and therefore not recommended together
- decreased serum levels may occur if given with rifampicin, dexamethasone, phenytoin, carbamazepine, phenobarbital (phenobarbitone) and St John's wort
- may increase serum levels of midazolam, ciclosporin, fentanyl, alfentanil, sirolimus, tacrolimus and ergot alkaloids
- INR should be measured for first 2 weeks of therapy if given with warfarin
- see also General Interactions of antineoplastic agents (p. 582)

Nursing points/Cautions

- any hypokalaemia or hypomagnesaemia should be corrected before starting therapy to decrease risk of QT prolongation
- ECG should be taken before starting and regularly throughout therapy
- blood lipids and serum lipases should be measured before starting therapy, 3 and 6 months after starting therapy and then yearly
- blood glucose should be measured before starting and then regularly throughout therapy
- hepatitis B status should be evaluated before starting therapy as reactivation can occur
- therapy may be discontinued after 3 years depending on BCR-ABL transcript levels and molecular response. If therapy is discontinued, patient should be closely monitored thereafter
- tablets contain lactose and are therefore not recommended in those with galactose intolerance, lactase insufficiency or glucose–galactose malabsorption
- caution if used in those with known congenital or acquired QT prolongation or electrolyte imbalance (especially hypokalaemia and hypomagnesaemia)
- caution if used in those with history of pancreatitis
- see also General Nursing points/Cautions for antineoplastic agents (p. 582)

Patient teaching and advice

- if taking antacids, advise patient to take either 2 hours before or after taking capsules
- instruct patient to take H_2-receptor antagonist (e.g. famotidine) 2 hours before or 10 hours after capsules
- if patient is unable to swallow capsule whole, suggest that contents of capsules can be sprinkled on teaspoon of applesauce and swallowed
- patient should be warned to avoid grapefruit and grapefruit juice during therapy

- instruct patient to seek medical advice immediately if any of the following occur:
  - rapid or irregular heart rate
  - pain or discomfort in chest, difficulty breathing, shortness of breath
  - abdominal pain
- see General Patient teaching and advice for antineoplastic agents (p. 584)

NINTEDANIB (Ofev)

Available forms

Capsules: 100 mg, 150 mg

Action

- tyrosine kinase inhibitor blocking vascular endothelial growth factor receptors, platelet-derived growth factor receptors and fibroblast growth factor receptors kinase activity

Use

- idiopathic pulmonary fibrosis (IPF)
- locally advanced metastatic or relapse non-small cell lung cancer (NSCLC) (after failure of first-line treatment)
- slowing rate of pulmonary function decline in those with sclerosis-associated interstitial lung disease (SSc-ILD)

Dose

- (NSCLC) 200 mg orally twice daily with food on days 2 to 21 of 21-day cycle (with docetaxel given on day 1) **OR**
- (IFP, SSc-ILD) 150 mg orally twice daily with food

Adverse effects

- gastrointestinal perforation
- hyperbilirubinaemia
- thromboembolic events
- peripheral neuropathy
- see also General Adverse effects of antineoplastic agents (p. 582)

Interactions

- decreased serum levels may occur if given with rifampicin, carbamazepine, phenytoin and St John's wort
- increased serum levels may occur if given with erythromycin

Nursing points/Cautions

- (NSCLC) nintedanib can be continued alone after starting docetaxel while clinical response is evident or toxicity occurs
- should not be started within 4 weeks of gastrointestinal surgery
- capsules contain soya lecithin
- caution if used in those who have had previous abdominal surgery due to the risk of gastrointestinal perforation
- caution if used in females, those of low body weight or of Asian race due to increased risk of elevated liver enzymes
- caution if used in those with brain metastases as there is increased risk of cerebral haemorrhage
- not recommended in those with an inherited predisposition to bleeding or receiving full dose of anticoagulant therapy
- not recommended in those who have had recent lung haemorrhage, centrally located tumours with invasion of major blood vessels or necrotic tumours
- contraindicated in those with hypersensitivity to nintedanib, peanut or soya
- see also General Nursing points/Cautions for antineoplastic agents (p. 582)

Patient teaching and advice

- patient should be instructed to seek medical advice if any of the following occur:
  - moderate-to-severe diarrhoea, new or worsening abdominal pain, chills, fever, nausea, vomiting

  - any tingling, numbness of hands or feet, burning sensation
  - leg/calf swelling, pain or tenderness of leg/calf, warmth, redness
- see also General Patient teaching and advice for antineoplastic agents (p. 584)

NIVOLUMAB (Opdivo)

Available forms
Vial: 40 mg/4 mL, 100 mg/10 mL

Action
- anti-PD-1 monoclonal antibody (human IgG4)

Use
- unresectable stage III or metastatic stage IV melanoma (MM) (monotherapy or with ipilimumab)
- adjunctive treatment of melanoma (with metastatic disease or lymph node involvement) after resection (monotherapy)
- locally advanced or metastatic squamous or non-squamous non-small cell lung cancer (NSCLC)
- intermediate/poor-risk, previously untreated, advanced renal cell carcinoma (RCC) (with ipilimumab)
- advanced clear cell RCC after anti-angiogenic therapy (monotherapy)
- relapsed or recurrent classical Hodgkin lymphoma (cHL) (after stem cell transplant and brentuximab vedotin) (monotherapy)
- recurrent or metastatic squamous cell carcinoma of head and neck (SCCHN) (progressing on or after platinum-based therapy) (monotherapy)
- locally advanced unresectable or metastatic urothelial carcinoma (UC) (after platinum-based therapy) (monotherapy)
- hepatocellular carcinoma (HCC) (after sorafenib) (monotherapy)

Dose
- (MM, NSCLC, RCC, cHL, HC, SCCHN) 3 mg/kg IV over 60 minutes every 2 weeks, 240 mg IV over 60 minutes every 2 weeks or 480 mg IV over 60 minutes over 8 weeks **OR**
- (combination therapy – metastatic or unresectable melanoma) 1 mg/kg IV over 30 minutes every 3 weeks for 4 doses (on same day as ipilimumab after nivolumab infusion is complete), followed by nivolumab alone **OR**
- (combination therapy – RCC) 3 mg/kg IV over 30 minutes every 3 weeks for 4 doses with ipilimumab, followed by nivolumab alone

Adverse effects
- immune-related adverse effects (all systems can be affected)
- see also General Adverse effects of antineoplastic agents (p. 582)

Interactions
- increased risk of immune-related adverse effects if given with ipilimumab
- use with corticosteroids is not recommended at start of therapy. If used to treat immune-related adverse effects, corticosteroids can be used and should be tapered slowly when discontinued

Nursing points/Cautions
- patient should be closely monitored for any signs of immune-related adverse effects
- when given as part of combination therapy, nivolumab should be given first, followed by ipilimumab at least 30 minutes later, followed by platinum-based therapy, if used
- not given as IV push or bolus
- may be used undiluted or dilute with sodium chloride 0.9% or glucose 5% for concentration of 1–10 mg/mL. If patient weight $<$ 40 kg, infusion volume should not be $>$ 4 mL/kg
- inline low protein binding 0.2–1.2 micron filter recommended

- contains sodium 2.5 mg/mL
- increased risk of solid organ rejection or severe graft versus host disease after stem cell transplant

Patient teaching and advice

- advise patient to carry patient alert card at all times
- patient should be instructed to seek medical advice if any of the following occur:
  - moderate-to-severe diarrhoea, new or worsening abdominal pain, chills, fever, nausea, vomiting
  - any tingling, numbness of hands or feet, burning sensation
  - cough, shortness of breath, difficulty breathing
- see also General Patient teaching and advice for antineoplastic agents (p. 584)

OBINUTUZUMAB (Gazyva)

Available form

Vial: 1000 mg/40 mL

Action

- anti-CD20 monoclonal antibody

Use

- previously untreated chronic lymphocytic leukaemia (CLL) (with chlorambucil)
- maintenance of previously untreated follicular lymphoma (FL) (with disease progression, unresponsive or progression after rituximab-containing regimen)

Dose

- (CLL) initially 1000 mg IV on days 1–2, 8 and 15 of 28-day cycle, followed by 1000 mg IV on day 1 only of subsequent cycles (cycles 2–6) (with chlorambucil) **OR**
- (FL) 1000 mg IV given on days 1, 8 and 15 of 21- or 28-day cycle (depending on combination therapy)

Adverse effects

- infusion-related reactions (IRR)
- progressive multifocal leukoencephalopathy (PML)
- worsening of pre-existing cardiac conditions
- reactivation of hepatitis B
- see also General Adverse effects of antineoplastic agents (p. 582)

Interactions

- see General Interactions of antineoplastic agents (p. 582)

Nursing points/Cautions

- all patients should be screened for hepatitis B before starting therapy. Therapy should be stopped if reactivation of hepatitis B occurs during therapy
- antihypertensive therapy should be withheld for 12 hours before, during and 1 hour after therapy to decrease risk of hypotension occurring
- for prophylaxis of infusion-related reactions (IRR), premedication with IV or oral corticosteroid (methylprednisolone or dexamethasone) at least 1 hour before and oral analgesic/antipyretic and antihistamine 30 minutes before infusion is recommended. If patient has no or low-grade IRR, corticosteroids can be omitted from premedication regime
- (previously untreated FL) can be given as 6 × 28-day cycles (with bendamustine), 6 × 21-day cycles (with CHOP regimen) plus 2 cycles of obinutuzumab alone, or 8 × 21-day cycles (with CVP regimen)
- not given as IV push or bolus
- dilute with sodium chloride 0.9% only
- infusion-related reactions occur most commonly during first 1000 mg dose
- patient must be closely monitored during infusion period. If mild-to-moderate reaction occurs, rate should be slowed and symptoms treated. If reaction is severe, infusion

should be stopped and symptoms treated. Infusion can be restarted at half the rate that caused the reaction once symptoms have been resolved and slowly increased. If second severe reaction occurs, infusion should be permanently stopped. If life-threatening reactions occur, therapy should be stopped and not restarted
- (CLL, day 1, cycle 1) 1000 mg should be prepared as two infusion bags (100 mg and 900 mg) by diluting 4 mL in 100 mL infusion bag and 36 mL in 250 mL infusion bag. Gently invert bags to ensure even distribution
- (CLL, day 1, cycle 1) administer 100 mg infusion at 25 mg/hour over 4 hours. If there are no modifications or interruptions to infusion due to infusion-related reactions, 900 mg infusion can be administered on same day (day 1) starting at a rate of 50 mg/hour for first 30 minutes. If no reaction, rate can be increased at 50 mg/hour increments every 30 minutes to a maximum of 400 mg/hour
- (CLL, day 1, cycle 1) if infusion-related reactions occur during 100 mg infusion, 900 mg infusion should be withheld until day 2 and commence at 50 mg/hour and proceed as outlined in above point
- (CLL, cycle 1, days 8 and 15; cycles 2–6, day 1) if there is no IRR during previous infusion and rate was ≥ 100 mg/hour, 1000 mg infusion can be started at 100 mg/hour and increased at increments of 100 mg/hour every 30 minutes to a maximum of 400 mg/hour, monitoring carefully for any infusion-related reactions
- (FL, cycle 1, day 1) 1000 mg IV given at 50 mg/hour and increasing in 50 mg/hour increments every 30 minutes to 400 mg/hour (maximum)
- (FL, cycle 1, days 8, 15 and cycles 2–6 or 28 as maintenance) if no IRR occurs and previous infusion rate ≥ 100 mg/hour, infusion can start at 100 mg/hour and increased at 30-minute intervals by 100 mg/hour increments to 400 mg/hour maximum. If patient experiences IRR, infusion should be started at 50 mg/hour and increased at 30-minute intervals at 50 mg/hour increment to 400 mg/hour (maximum)
- (FL) dilute 40 mL in 250 mL of sodium chloride 0.9% and infuse IV
- diluted solution should not be shaken or frozen
- caution if used in those with pre-existing cardiac or lung conditions due to increased risk of infusion-related reactions
- contraindicated in those with hypersensitivity to murine protein

Patient teaching and advice

- during infusion, instruct patient to immediately report any swelling of throat, tongue, lips or face, shortness of breath, difficulty breathing, wheezing, nausea or vomiting, diarrhoea, rash, hives or itching, cough or throat irritation, chest pain, abnormal or irregular heart rate, headache, dizziness or light-headedness
- patient should be instructed to seek medical advice immediately if any muscle weakness, sensory disturbances, paralysis, aphasia or visual disturbances occur
- also see General Patient teaching and advice for antineoplastic agents (p. 584)

OFATUMUMAB (Arzerra)

Available forms

Ampoule: 100 mg/5 mL, 1000 mg/50 mL

Action

- recombinant human anti-CD20 monoclonal antibody (IgG1)

Use

- chronic lymphocytic leukaemia (CLL) (as part of combination therapy in

those who have not been previously treated or where fludarabine is inappropriate)
- chronic lymphocytic leukaemia (CLL) (as monotherapy in patients who are refractory to fludarabine and alemtuzumab)

Dose
- (previously untreated CLL) 300 mg IV over 4.5 hours (day 1) then 1000 mg (day 8) (cycle 1), followed by 1000 mg IV over 4 hours (day 1) of subsequent cycles (every 28 days) (until best response or maximum of 12 cycles) **OR**
- (refractory CLL) 300 mg IV (day 1), followed by 2000 mg IV (day 1 of next 7 weeks) (total 8 weeks) followed 4–5 weeks later by monthly infusions for 4 weeks (12 infusions total)

Adverse effects
- infusion-related reactions
- bowel obstruction
- progressive multifocal leukoencephalopathy
- reactivation of hepatitis B
- severe skin reaction
- see also General Adverse effects of antineoplastic agents (p. 582)

Interactions
- see General Interactions of antineoplastic agents (p. 582)

Nursing points/Cautions
- all patients should be screened for hepatitis B and any current infection treated before starting therapy
- premedication with paracetamol (1 g orally), antihistamine (oral or IV) and corticosteroid (IV) 30 minutes to 2 hours before infusion
- first infusion rate should be 12 mL/hour, then doubled every 30 minutes. In no adverse reactions, subsequent infusion rate can be started at 25 mL/hour and then increased in increments to 400 mL/hour maximum
- (refractory CLL) initial infusion rate is 12 mL/hour (for first two infusions), doubling rate every 30 minutes to a maximum of 200 mg/hour. If there are no adverse reactions, remaining infusions can start at 25 mL/hour and be doubled every 30 minutes to a maximum of 400 mg/hour
- dilute to 1000 mL with sodium chloride 0.9%, invert gently to ensure even mixing, but do not shake
- not given as IV bolus or push
- contains 34.8 mg sodium per 300 mg and 232 mg sodium per 2 g dose, which may need to be considered if patient requires a sodium-controlled diet
- caution if used in those with decreased pulmonary function due to increased risk of infusion-related reactions
- see also General Nursing points/Cautions for antineoplastic agents (p. 582)

Patient teaching and advice
- advise patient to seek medical advice if any of the following occur:
  - abdominal pain
  - skin reactions especially any peeling or blistering
  - memory loss, trouble thinking, loss of vision, difficulty walking
- see also General Patient teaching and advice for antineoplastic agents (p. 584)

OLAPARIB (Lynparza)

Available forms

Capsules: 50 mg; Tablets: 100 mg, 150 mg

Action
- inhibitor of human poly (ADP ribose) polymerase enzymes (PARP enzymes)
- PARP enzymes are needed for efficient single-strand DNA repair

Use

- maintenance treatment of platinum-sensitive relapsed BRCA-mutated (germline or mutated) high-grade serous epithelial ovarian, breast, fallopian tube or peritoneal cancer (after ≥ 2 platinum courses)

Dose

- (capsules) 400 mg orally twice daily at least 1 hour after food until disease progression **OR**
- (tablets) 300 mg orally twice daily for up to 2 years or disease progression

Adverse effects

- pneumonitis
- see also General Adverse effects of antineoplastic agents (p. 582)

Interactions

- decreased serum levels may occur if given with rifampicin, rifabutin, carbamazepine, nevirapine, phenobarbital, phenytoin and St John's wort, and therefore not recommended together
- increased serum levels may occur if given with ciprofloxacin, clarithromycin, erythromycin, itraconazole, fluconazole, protease inhibitors boosted with ritonavir or cobicistat, indinavir, saquinavir, boceprevir, diltiazem, verapamil, grapefruit, Seville oranges and star fruit and are therefore not recommended together
- not recommended with statins
- caution if used with bosentan, efavirenz, modafinil and etravirine as serum levels may be decreased
- caution if used with simvastatin, pravastatin, ciclosporin, midazolam, sirolimus, tacrolimus, fentanyl, digoxin, colchicine or dabigatran

Nursing points/Cautions

- BRCA mutation status should be confirmed by valid and reliable test before starting therapy
- tablets and capsules are not interchangeable
- increased risk of pneumonitis in those with lung cancer, lung metastasis, underlying lung disease, smoking history, previous radiotherapy or chemotherapy
- see also General Nursing points/Cautions for antineoplastic agents (p. 582)

Patient teaching and advice

- advise patient to take capsules at least 1 hour after food and then refrain from eating for at least another 2 hours. Tablets can be taken with or without food
- warn patient to avoid grapefruit, Seville oranges and star fruit during therapy
- patient should be instructed to seek medical advice if any shortness of breath, cough and/or fever occurs
- see also General Patient teaching and advice for antineoplastic agents (p. 584)

OXALIPLATIN (DBL Oxaliplatin Concentrate, Oxalatin, Oxaliplatin)

Available forms

Vial (powder): 50 mg, 100 mg; Vial (concentrate solution): 50 mg/10 mL, 100 mg/20 mL, 200 mg/40 mL

Action

- platinum-containing analogue of cisplatin that inhibits DNA synthesis (also RNA and protein synthesis to a lesser extent)

Use

- colon cancer (Duke's C) (after resection) (with fluorouracil and folinic acid) (adjuvant)
- advanced colorectal cancer

Dose

- (advanced colorectal cancer or as adjunctive therapy) 85 mg/m^2 IV over 2–6 hours (before fluorouracil) every

2 weeks for 12 cycles (with fluorouracil and folinic acid)

Adverse effects

- peripheral neuropathy, laryngopharyngeal dysaesthesia, reversible posterior leukoencephalopathy
- QT prolongation
- rhabdomyolysis
- see also General Adverse effects of antineoplastic agents (p. 582)

Interactions

- may increase serum levels of fluorouracil (if given with weekly fluorouracil and 3-weekly oxaliplatin)
- caution if given with statins due to increased risk of rhabdomyolysis
- not recommended with agents known to prolong QT or cause electrolyte imbalance
- see also General Interactions of antineoplastic agents (p. 582)

Nursing points/Cautions

- neurological examination is recommended before each infusion
- if patient develops laryngopharyngeal dysaesthesia (e.g. dysphagia, dyspnoea, feeling of suffocation) within 48 hours of infusion, subsequent infusions should be given over 6 hours
- reconstitute powder with 10 mL (for 50 mg vial) or 20 mL (for 100 mg vial) water for injections or glucose 5% and then further dilute with 250–500 mL glucose 5%
- concentrate for infusion should be further diluted with 250–500 mL glucose 5%
- incompatible with chloride-containing solutions. Fluorouracil should not be given via same infusion line
- do not use with any material containing aluminium
- re-challenging is contraindicated if patient experiences an anaphylactic reaction
- contraindicated in those with a history of peripheral sensory neuropathy with functional impairment or hypersensitivity to platinum-containing preparations
- see also General Nursing points/Cautions for antineoplastic agents (p. 582)

Patient teaching and advice

- warn patient to avoid exposure to cold or ingesting cold food or drinks within 48 hours of therapy to decrease risk of laryngopharyngeal dysaesthesia (e.g. dysphagia, dyspnoea, feeling of suffocation) occurring
- patients should be advised to seek medical advice if any of the following occur:
  - weakness, tingling or numbness of arms or feet
  - difficulty swallowing, feeling of suffocation or difficulty breathing
  - headache, memory loss, trouble thinking, loss of vision or other visual disturbances, difficulty walking or muscle weakness
  - rapid or unusual heart rate
  - muscle weakness or pain, dark urine, decreased urination
- see General Patient teaching and advice for antineoplastic agents (p. 584)

PACLITAXEL (Abraxane, Anzatax Injection, Paclitaxel Concentrate, Paclitaxin)

Available forms

Vial: 100 mg, 30 mg/5 mL, 100 mg/16.7 mL, 150 mg/25 mL, 300 mg/50 mL

Action

- taxane antimetabolite
- (Abraxane) albumin nanoparticle form of paclitaxel

Use

- metastatic breast cancer (after anthracycline failure)

- metastatic breast cancer (with trastuzumab) (in those with tumours HER2 overexpression/no previous treatment)
- unresectable, locally recurrent or metastatic breast cancer (relapsed after adjunctive chemotherapy including an anthracycline) (with gemcitabine)
- metastatic ovarian cancer (after standard therapy failure)
- node-positive breast cancer (sequentially after doxorubicin and cyclophosphamide) (adjuvant)
- ovarian cancer (with platinum agent)
- non-small cell lung cancer (NSCLC) (with carboplatin when surgery and/or radiation are unsuitable)
- metastatic pancreatic adenocarcinoma (with gemcitabine)

Dose

- (metastatic breast cancer) 260 mg/m^2 IV over 30 minutes every 3 weeks (Abraxane) **OR**
- (node-positive breast cancer) 175 mg/m^2 IV over 3 hours every 3 weeks for 4 cycles (following doxorubicin cyclophosphamide combined therapy) **OR**
- (metastatic breast cancer) 175 mg/m^2 IV over 3 hours on day 1, with gemcitabine IV on days 1 and 8 of 21-day cycle **OR**
- (HER2 overexpressive breast cancer) 175 mg/m^2 IV over 3 hours every 3 weeks for 6 cycles (with trastuzumab) **OR**
- (NSCLC) 100 mg/m^2 IV over 30 minutes on days 1, 8 and 15 of 21-day cycle (with carboplatin) (Abraxane) **OR**
- (NSCLC, metastatic breast or ovarian cancer) 175 mg/m^2 IV over 3 hours every 3 weeks (up to 9 cycles for metastatic breast or ovarian cancer) **OR**
- (pancreatic adenocarcinoma) 125 mg/m^2 IV over 30 minutes on days 1, 8 and 15 of 28-day cycle (with gemcitabine) (Abraxane) **OR**
- (ovarian cancer) 175 mg/m^2 IV over 3 hours (with cisplatin) every 3 weeks **OR**
- (ovarian cancer) 135 mg/m^2 IV over 24 hours (with cisplatin) every 3 weeks

Adverse effects

- peripheral neuropathy
- see also General Adverse effects of antineoplastic agents (p. 582)

Interactions

- increased serum levels may occur if given with itraconazole, erythromycin, fluoxetine, imidazole antifungal agents, cimetidine, clopidogrel, gemfibrozil, ritonavir, saquinavir and indinavir
- decreased serum levels may occur if given with rifampicin, carbamazepine, phenytoin, efavirenz and nevirapine
- may increase serum levels of doxorubicin and its active metabolite
- if cisplatin is given before paclitaxel, clearance is decreased leading to increased myelosuppression. Combination also increases risk of renal failure
- arthralgia and myalgia may be increased if given with filgrastim
- see also General Interactions of antineoplastic agents (p. 582)

Nursing points/Cautions

- albumin form of paclitaxel is not interchangeable with other formulations
- should be given before platinum-containing therapy
- because of the possibility of hypersensitivity, patient may require premedication before each treatment with corticosteroid (e.g. dexamethasone 20 mg orally 12 hours and 6 hours before), antihistamine (e.g. promethazine 25–50 mg IV 30 minutes before paclitaxel) and H_2-receptor antagonist (e.g. cimetidine 300 mg or ranitidine 50 mg IV over 15 minutes

30 minutes before paclitaxel) (not Abraxane)
- patient should be closely observed during first 30 minutes of infusion for any signs of hypersensitivity (not Abraxane)
- ECG monitoring is recommended if given with doxorubicin or trastuzumab for metastatic breast cancer
- (Abraxane) reconstitute powder by injection 20 mL sodium chloride 0.9% down side of vial (not directly on powder to prevent foaming) and then allow to stand for 5 minutes, then swirl gently for at least 2 minutes to dissolve powder. If foaming occurs, allow vial to stand for at least 15 minutes to allow foam to subside. Reconstituted solution should be milky without visible particles. Dilute further if proteinaceous strands result, administer infusion via 15 micron filter
- inline filter less than 0.15 micron should not be used
- concentrate should be diluted with either glucose 5% or sodium chloride 0.9% to concentration of 0.3–1.2 mg/mL before administration
- IV administration only
- micropore filter (0.22 micron or less) is recommended
- (Abraxane) contains 85 mg sodium/vial when reconstituted with sodium chloride 0.9% which may need to be considered in sodium-restricted diet
- caution if used in those with pre-existing neuropathy
- contraindicated in those with hypersensitivity to PEG35 castor oil or with solid tumours and neutrophil count $< 1.5 \times 10^9$/L
- (Abraxane) contraindicated in those with hypersensitivity to albumin
- see also General Nursing points/Cautions for antineoplastic agents (p. 582)

Patient teaching and advice

- instruct patient to seek medical advice if any of the following occur:
  - numbness or tingling in hands or feet, muscle weakness
  - visual disturbances
- see also General Patient teaching and advice for antineoplastic agents (p. 584)

PANITUMUMAB (Vectibix)

Available forms
Vial: 100 mg/5 mL, 400 mg/20 mL

Action
- epidermal growth factor receptor (EGFR) monoclonal antibody

Use
- wild type RAS metastatic colorectal cancer (mCRC)

Dose
- 6 mg/kg IV once every 2 weeks (until disease progression or intolerance occurs)

Adverse effects
- infusion-related reactions
- interstitial lung disease
- phototoxicity
- deep vein thrombosis, pulmonary embolism
- see also General Adverse effects of antineoplastic agents (p. 582)

Nursing points/Cautions

- mutational status of RAS should be determined by valid and reliable testing before starting therapy
- dilute with 100 mL sodium chloride 0.9% to give concentration of 10 mg/mL
- gently invert (avoiding foaming) to ensure contents are evenly mixed
- given as IV infusion over 60 minutes (first infusion) increasing rate to infuse over 30–60 minutes for second

and subsequent infusions if first infusion was well tolerated
- for doses > 1000 mg, should be diluted with 150 mL and infused over 90 minutes
- 0.2–0.22 micron inline filter is recommended
- not recommended as IV bolus or push
- not recommended in those with history of pulmonary fibrosis or interstitial lung disease
- contraindicated with oxaliplatin-based therapy in those in whom RAS gene status is unknown or where mutant RAS mCRC exists
- see also General Nursing points/ Cautions for antineoplastic agents (p. 582)

Patient teaching and advice

- patient should be advised to limit exposure to sun during therapy (including wearing protective clothing, hats and sunscreen (SPF 30+)) as skin reactions may be worsened
- instruct patient to seek medical advice immediately if any of the following occur:
    - any new or worsening cough, difficulty breathing or shortness of breath
    - calf swelling with redness, warmth and pain
    - cough, chest pain, shortness of breath, difficulty breathing, coughing up blood
- see General Patient teaching and advice for antineoplastic agents (p. 584)

PAZOPANIB (Votrient)

Available forms
Tablets: 200 mg, 400 mg

Action
- multi-target tyrosine kinase inhibitor of vascular endothelial growth factor receptor (VEGFR)

Use
- advanced metastatic renal cell carcinoma (RCC)
- advanced metastatic unresectable soft tissue sarcoma (STS) (with prior chemotherapy)

Dose
- 800 mg orally once daily 1 hour before or 2 hours after food

Adverse effects
- prolongation of QT interval
- interstitial lung disease, pneumonitis
- hypertension, hypertensive crisis
- thromboembolism
- severe, fatal hepatotoxicity
- gastrointestinal perforation
- delayed wound healing
- hypothyroidism
- proteinuria, nephrotic syndrome
- hair depigmentation
- hand–foot syndrome (hand/foot numbness, paraesthesia, tingling, erythema, pain, swelling and, at worst, ulceration, blistering or moist desquamation)
- posterior reversible encephalopathy syndrome
- see also General Adverse effects of antineoplastic agents (p. 582)

Interactions
- not recommended with proton pump inhibitors or other agents that increase gastric pH
- caution if given with simvastatin as increased serum enzymes (ALT) may occur increasing risk of hepatotoxicity
- not recommended with agents known to prolong QT interval or cause electrolyte imbalance (especially hypokalaemia or hypomagnesaemia)
- increased serum levels may occur if given with atazanavir, clarithromycin, indinavir, itraconazole, lapatinib, ritonavir, saquinavir, voriconazole, and grapefruit juice, and therefore not recommended together
- decreased serum levels may occur if given with rifampicin

- may increase serum levels of dextromethorphan, irinotecan, midazolam, paclitaxel and rosuvastatin, increasing risk of adverse effects
- see also General Interactions of antineoplastic agents (p. 582)

Nursing points/Cautions

- liver function tests should be performed before starting, monthly for 4 months, then regularly throughout therapy
- BP monitoring is recommended starting during first week of therapy
- urinalysis should be performed regularly throughout therapy to monitor for protein (nephrotic syndrome)
- left ventricular ejection fraction should be monitored regularly in those with cardiac dysfunction
- thyroid function should be measured before starting and regularly during therapy
- urinalysis should be conducted before starting and regularly throughout therapy to detect any worsening proteinuria that may lead to nephrotic syndrome
- therapy should be stopped 7 days before surgery to decrease risk of wound-healing complications
- caution if used in those with history of congenital or acquired QT prolongation or electrolyte imbalance
- caution if used in those at risk of gastrointestinal perforation or fistula formation
- not recommended in those under 18 years
- see also General Nursing points/Cautions for antineoplastic agents (p. 582)

Patient teaching and advice

- warn patient that hair depigmentation occurs commonly during therapy
- instruct patient to avoid grapefruit and grapefruit juice during therapy
- advise patient to seek medical advice if any of the following occur:
  - irregular heart rate
  - headache, fitting (seizures), lethargy, confusion, visual disturbances
  - cough, shortness of breath, difficulty breathing
  - swollen tender hot calf, shortness of breath, difficulty breathing, chest pain, coughing, coughing up blood
  - chest pain
  - severe abdominal pain
  - yellowing of eyes or skin, loss of appetite, nausea, upper abdominal pain, dark urine, pale stools
- symptoms of hand–foot syndrome can be reduced by advising patients to keep hands/feet cool (e.g. not wearing restricting gloves, socks or shoes; soaking hands/feet in cool water) starting 4–7 days after therapy. Other treatment may consist of pyridoxine (50–150 mg daily) and/or corticosteroids. Symptoms usually subside in 7–14 days
- see also General Patient teaching and advice for antineoplastic agents (p. 584)

PEMBROLIZUMAB (Keytruda)

Available forms

Vial: 50 mg; Vial (concentrate): 100 mg/4 mL

Action

- recombinant monoclonal IgG4 kappa antibody

Use

- unresectable or metastatic malignant melanoma
- non-small cell lung cancer (NSCLC)
- urothelial carcinoma (UC)
- head and neck squamous cell cancer (HNSCC)
- classical Hodgkin lymphoma (cHL)
- primary mediastinal B-cell lymphoma (PMBCL)

- endometrial cancer (EC)
- renal cell carcinoma (RCC)
- colorectal or non-colorectal microsatellite instability-high cancer (MSI-H)

Dose

- (melanoma, NSCLC) 200 mg IV over 30 minutes every 3 weeks or 400 mg IV over 30 minutes every 6 weeks (monotherapy) **OR**
- (NSCLS, EC, RCC) 200 mg IV over 30 minutes every 3 weeks (as part of combination therapy) **OR**
- (HNSCC, cHL, PMBCL, UC, MSI-H) 200 mg IV over 30 minutes every 3 weeks (monotherapy)

Adverse effects

- infusion-related reactions
- immune-related adverse effects (including nephritis, pneumonitis, colitis, autoimmune hepatitis, adrenal insufficiency, hypophystitis, thyroid dysfunction)
- solid organ transplant rejection, graft versus host disease
- see also General Adverse effects of antineoplastic agents (p. 582)

Interactions

- not recommended with thalidomide-analogue and dexamethasone due to increased mortality if treated for multiple myeloma
- systemic corticosteroids or immunosuppressants should be avoided before starting therapy because they may interfere with activity and efficacy; however, can be used after starting therapy to treat immune-mediated adverse effects and tapered slowly, or as part of premedication regime

Nursing points/Cautions

- PD status should be assessed using validated testing before starting therapy
- liver and thyroid function, and blood glucose levels should be monitored before starting and regularly during therapy
- premedication with antihistamine and antipyretic should be considered to decrease infusion-related reactions
- initial increase in tumour size or appearance of new lesion is often seen in first month of therapy
- reconstitute powder with 2.3 mL water for injections or bring concentrate solution to room temperature and dilute further with sodium chloride 0.9% or glucose 5% to concentration of 1–10 mg/mL, taking care to avoid foaming or shaking vial
- low protein (0.2–0.5 micron) inline or add-on filter is recommended
- caution if used in those with HIV, hepatitis B or C, active infection or with previous history of severe immune-mediated adverse reactions
- contraindicated in those with sensitivity to Chinese hamster ovary protein
- see also General Nursing points/Cautions for antineoplastic agents (p. 582)

Patient teaching and advice

- patient should be advised to carry 'Patient Alert Card'
- advise patient to seek medical advice if any of the following occur:
  - cough, shortness of breath, chest pain
  - weight loss, increased sweating, weight gain, hair loss, feeling cold, constipation, voice getting deeper, muscle aches, dizziness, fainting, headache that doesn't go away or unusual headache
  - feeling more hungry or thirsty, needing to urinate more often
  - diarrhoea or more frequent stools, black tarry sticky stools, severe stomach pain or tenderness
  - yellowing of eyes or skin, loss of appetite, nausea, upper abdominal pain, dark urine, pale stools

- see also General Patient teaching and advice for antineoplastic agents (p. 584)

PEMETREXED DISODIUM (Alimta, DBL Pemetrexed)

Available forms
Vial: 100 mg, 500 mg

Action
- anti-folinic antimetabolite
- active potent metabolites which have longer half-life than parent

Use
- malignant pleural mesothelioma (with cisplatin)
- locally advanced or metastatic non-small cell lung cancer (as monotherapy before platinum-based therapy or with cisplatin)

Dose
- 500 mg/m^2 IV over 10 minutes (day 1 of 21-day cycle) (with cisplatin)

Adverse effects
- severe rash, radiation recall
- see also General Adverse effects of antineoplastic agents (p. 582)

Interactions
- NSAIDs should not be taken for 5 days before, during or for 2 days after therapy with pemetrexed in those with mild-to-moderate kidney insufficiency as renal clearance may be decreased
- caution if used with radiation before, during or after therapy due to risk of radiation-pneumonitis
- caution if used with nephrotoxic agents or those that are tubularly secreted as clearance is decreased increasing serum levels and risk of adverse effects
- see also General Interactions of antineoplastic agents (p. 582)

Nursing points/Cautions
- patient should be well hydrated before and during therapy to decrease risk of severe dehydration when given with cisplatin
- premedication with corticosteroids (e.g. dexamethasone 4 mg orally twice daily, starting day before, day of and day after therapy) lessens incidence and severity of rash
- reconstitute using sodium chloride 0.9% only (20 mL for 500 mg vial, 4.2 mL for 100 mg vial)
- dilute further with 100 mL sodium chloride 0.9%
- incompatible with calcium-containing diluents (including lactated Ringer's solution)
- caution if used in those with pre-existing cardiovascular risk factors
- see also General Nursing points/Cautions for antineoplastic agents (p. 582)

Patient teaching and advice
- patient should be advised to take prophylactic oral folic acid (350–1000 microgram) (at least 5 doses in 7 days before, during and 21 days after last dose) and IM vitamin B_{12} (one dose in week before first dose, then every 3 cycles) during therapy
- if patient has mild-to-moderate kidney insufficiency, advise to avoid taking NSAIDs for 5 days before and up to 2 days after therapy
- see General Patient teaching and advice for antineoplastic agents (p. 584)

PERTUZUMAB (Perjeta)

Available form
Vial: 420 mg/14 mL

Action
- antihuman epidermal growth factor receptor 2 (HER2) monoclonal antibody that inhibits proliferation of tumour cells
- activity improved when used with trastuzumab

Use

- HER2-positive inflammatory or locally advanced or early stage (either node positive or lesion ≥ 2 cm) breast cancer (with trastuzumab)
- HER2-positive metastatic breast cancer (with no prior anti-HER2 or chemotherapy) (with docetaxel, trastuzumab)

Dose

- initially 840 mg IV over 60 minutes, then 420 mg IV over 30–60 minutes every 3 weeks (with trastuzumab and docetaxel) (until disease progression or toxicity occurs (metastatic breast cancer), or 3–6 cycles (early breast cancer before surgery) or maximum 18 cycles, disease progression or toxicity occurs (early breast cancer after surgery))

Adverse effects

- infusion-related reactions, hypersensitivity, anaphylaxis
- decreased left ventricular ejection fraction
- see General Adverse effects of antineoplastic agents (p. 582)

Nursing points/Cautions

- positive HER2 gene overexpression should be verified using valid and reliable testing before starting therapy
- left ventricular ejection fraction (LVEF) should be measured before starting and then 3-monthly during therapy
- patient should be observed for 30–60 minutes after infusion for any signs of infusion-related reaction
- not given as IV push or bolus
- dilute with 250 mL with sodium chloride 0.9%, inverting bag gently to mix solution, but avoid foaming
- incompatible with glucose 5%
- during combination therapy, pertuzumab and trastuzumab can be given in any order. If docetaxel is also used, it should be given after pertuzumab and trastuzumab. If anthracycline-based therapy is used, pertuzumab and trastuzumab should be given after total anthracycline regimen is completed
- caution if used in those previously treated with anthracyclines or radiation to chest area due to increased risk of decreased LVEF
- caution if used in those with baseline LVEF ≤ 50%, history of cardiac failure, decreases in LVEF to < 50% during prior trastuzumab adjunct therapy, uncontrolled hypertension, recent myocardial infarction, serious cardiac arrhythmias requiring treatment or doxorubicin total cumulative dose > 360 mg/m^2
- contraindicated in those with hypersensitivity to Chinese hamster ovary protein
- see also General Nursing points/Cautions for antineoplastic agents (p. 582)

Patient teaching and advice

- advise patient to seek medical advice if any of the following occur:
  - shortness of breath or tiredness on light physical activity (such as walking)
  - shortness of breath at night, especially when lying flat
  - cough
  - irregular or abnormal heart rate
  - swelling of hands/feet (due to fluid build-up)
- see also General Patient teaching and advice for antineoplastic agents (p. 584)

PLITIDEPSIN (Aplidin)

Available form

Vial: 2 mg

Action

- interacts with eukaryotic elongation factor (eEF1A2) which is overexpressing in some tumour cells, including some multiple myeloma cells

Use

- relapsed and refractory multiple myeloma (who has received 2–3 previous treatments with or is intolerant to a proteasome inhibitor and immunomodulator) (with dexamethasone)

Dose

- 5 mg/m^2 IV over 3 hours on day 1 and 15 of 28-day cycle (with dexamethasone 40 mg orally 1 hour before infusion on days 1, 8, 15 and 22 of 28-day cycle)

Adverse effects

- infusion-related reactions
- muscle weakness, myalgia and uncommonly, myopathy
- (uncommon) bradycardia, QT interval prolongation, sinus tachycardia, orthostatic hypotension
- (injection site) pain, phlebitis, thrombosis
- see also General Adverse effects of antineoplastic agents (p. 582)

Interactions

- caution if used with other agents associated with rhabdomyolysis such as statins
- not recommended with clarithromycin, itraconazole, voriconazole and grapefruit juice. These should be discontinued for at least 1 week before starting therapy
- caution if used with aprepitant, diltiazem, erythromycin, fluconazole and verapamil
- not recommended with phenytoin, phenobarbital, carbamazepine, rifampicin, rifabutin and St John's wort. These should be discontinued for at least 2 weeks before starting therapy
- caution if given with bosentan and modafinil

Nursing points/Cautions

- premedication with ondansetron (8 mg IV) or granisetron (3 mg IV), diphenhydramine (25 mg IV) (or equivalent) and ranitidine (50 mg IV or equivalent) is recommended 30 minutes before infusion
- emergency equipment and oxygen should be readily available in event of severe or life-threatening infusion-related reactions
- CPK should be measured before each infusion (day 1 and 15) from cycle 1 to cycle 4
- use of infusion pump and low protein filter (0.2 micron) are recommended
- reconstitute using 4 mL diluent (provided) and dilute further with sodium chloride 0.9% or glucose 5% for total volume of 500 mL (peripheral line) or 250 mL (central venous line)
- caution if used in patient with risk factors for or existing heart disease. Regular ECG monitoring is recommended
- contraindicated in those with hypersensitivity to PEG-35 castor oil or ethanol
- see also General Nursing points/Cautions for antineoplastic agents (p. 582)

Patient teaching and advice

- patient should be advised to immediately seek medical advice if muscle weakness or muscle pain occurs
- see also General Patient teaching and advice for antineoplastic agents (p. 584)

POLATUZUMAB VEDOTIN (Polivy)

Available form

Vial: 140 mg

Action

- CD79b-targeted antibody-drug conjugate

Use
- treatment of diffuse large B-cell lymphoma (in those ineligible for haematopoietic stem cell transplant) (with bendamustine and rituximab)

Dose
- 1.8 mg/kg as IV infusion over 90 minutes every 21 days (with bendamustine and rituximab) for 6 cycles

Adverse effects
- peripheral neuropathy
- (rare) progressive multifocal leukoencephalopathy, tumour lysis syndrome
- see General Adverse effects of antineoplastic agents (p. 582)

Interactions
- caution if used with rifampicin, phenytoin, carbamazepine, phenobarbital (phenobarbitone) and St John's wort
- caution if used with clarithromycin, cobicistat, itraconazole, ritonavir, saquinavir and voriconazole as toxicity may occur

Nursing points/Cautions
- premedication with antihistamine and antipyretic is recommended 30 minutes before infusion
- patient should be monitored during and for 30 minutes after infusion for any infusion-related reactions
- if 90-minute infusion is well tolerated, subsequent infusions can be given over 30 minutes
- reconstitute with 7.2 mL water for injections and then dilute further with either glucose 5% or sodium chloride 0.45% or 0.9%
- 0.2–0.22 micron low-protein binding inline or add-on filter is recommended
- not given as IV push or bolus
- see also General Nursing points/Cautions for antineoplastic agents (p. 582)

Patient teaching and advice
- see General Patient teaching and advice for antineoplastic agents (p. 584)

PONATINIB (Iclusig)

Available forms
Tablets: 15 mg, 45 mg

Action
- tyrosine kinase inhibitor

Use
- chronic, accelerated or blast phase chronic myeloid leukaemia (CML) (resistant to or intolerant of ≥ 2 prior tyrosine kinase inhibitors) or with T3151 mutation
- Philadelphia chromosome positive acute lymphoblastic leukaemia (ALL) (resistant to or intolerant of dasatinib where subsequent imatinib not appropriate) or with T3151 mutation

Dose
- initially 45 mg orally daily

Adverse effects
- heart failure, arrhythmias
- fluid retention (including peripheral oedema, ascites, pleural effusion, pericardial effusion)
- new or worsening hypertension, hypertensive crisis
- thromboembolism, arterial occlusion, retinal arterial occlusion
- peripheral neuropathy
- pancreatitis, hepatotoxicity
- reactivation of hepatitis B
- see General Adverse effects of antineoplastic agents (p. 582)

Interactions
- may increase serum levels of digoxin, colchicine, dabigatran, pravastatin, methotrexate, sulfasalazine and rosuvastatin increasing risk of adverse effects
- not recommended with phenytoin, carbamazepine, phenobarbital (phenobarbitone), rifampicin, rifabutin and St John's wort, as decreased serum levels of ponatinib may occur
- increased serum levels may occur if given with atazanavir, clarithromycin, erythromycin, indinavir, itraconazole,

nelfinavir, ritonavir, voriconazole and grapefruit juice

Nursing points/Cautions

- cardiovascular status should be assessed before starting therapy and any identified risk factors managed
- hepatitis B status should be assessed before starting therapy as reactivation is possible
- BP should be monitored regularly during therapy
- tablets contain lactose, therefore not recommended in those with lactose intolerance
- caution if used in those with a history of pancreatitis or alcohol abuse
- not recommended in those with history of myocardial infarction, stroke or revascularisation unless benefits outweigh risks
- see also General Nursing points/Cautions for antineoplastic agents (p. 582)

Patient teaching and advice

- instruct patient to avoid grapefruit and grapefruit juice during therapy
- advise patient to seek medical advice immediately if any of the following occur:
    - shortness of breath, chest pain, weakness on one side of body, leg pain or swelling, decreased or blurred vision, speech problems
    - shortness of breath, chest pain, palpitations, fluid retention, dizziness or fainting
    - headache, dizziness, chest pain or shortness of breath
    - nausea, vomiting, abdominal tenderness or discomfort, loss of appetite, yellowing of skin or whites of the eyes
    - numbness or tingling of hands or feet
    - leg swelling, weight gain, shortness of breath
    - decreased or blurred vision
- see also General Patient teaching and advice for antineoplastic agents (p. 584)

PROCARBAZINE (Natulan)

Available form

Capsules: 50 mg

Action

- inhibits protein and nucleic acid synthesis
- some immunosuppressant action
- weak MAOI properties

Use

- Hodgkin's disease, lymphosarcoma, reticulosarcoma

Dose

- initially 50 mg orally daily, then increasing by 50 mg daily to daily maximum of 250–300 mg after 5–6 days (induction) and dose maintained for as long as possible, then 50–150 mg daily (maintenance) (to a total of 6 g)

Adverse effects

- severe skin reactions
- see also General Adverse effects of antineoplastic agents (p. 582)

Interactions

- may potentiate barbiturates, psychotropic and sympathomimetic agents due to MAOI (weak) properties
- decreases tolerance to alcohol
- see also General Interactions of antineoplastic agents (p. 582)

Nursing points/Cautions

- therapy should be stopped if severe allergic skin reaction occurs
- see also General Nursing points/Cautions for antineoplastic agents (p. 582)

Patient teaching and advice

- patient should be warned about eating certain foodstuffs (see Glossary for 'cheese reaction')

- advise patient to avoid alcohol during treatment
- see also General Patient teaching and advice for antineoplastic agents (p. 584)

RADIUM (223RA) DICHLORIDE (Xofigo)

Available form
Vial: 6.6 MBq/6 mL

Action
- alpha particle emitting radiopharmaceutical
- mimics calcium and selectively targets areas of bone metastases by forming complexes with bone mineral hydroxyapatite

Use
- treatment of castration-resistant prostate cancer with symptomatic bone metastases and no known visceral metastatic disease

Dose
- 55 kBq/kg by slow IV over at least 1 minute at 4-week intervals for 6 injections

Adverse effects
- thrombocytopenia, neutropenia, leucopenia, pancytopenia
- diarrhoea, vomiting, nausea
- bone fracture, osteoporosis
- injection site reaction (pain, redness, swelling)

Interactions
- contraindicated with abiraterone acetate and prednisolone/prednisone

Nursing points/Cautions
- full blood tests are recommended before starting and before each dose. Baseline blood counts should be absolute neutrophil count (ANC) $\geq 1.0 \times 10^9$/L, platelet count $\geq 100 \times 10^9$/L and haemoglobin $\geq$ 100 g/L. Blood counts should have recovered to ANC $\geq 1.0 \times 10^9$/L and platelet count $\geq 50 \times 10^9$/L before next dose is given. If there is no recovery within 6 weeks, therapy should only be continued if benefits outweigh risks
- dose contributes to patient's overall long-term cumulative radiation exposure
- patient risk for bone fractures (e.g. osteoporosis, low body weight, medications increasing risk) should be assessed and monitored for least 2 years. Prophylactic denosumab or bisphosphonates should be considered
- should only be received, used and administered by those authorised to handle radiopharmaceuticals
- receipt, storage, use, transfer and disposal are subject to license and regulation by the Australian Radiation Protection and Nuclear Safety Agency (ARPANSA)
- administration is associated with potential risks to others (including medical staff, care givers and patient's household contacts). Risks include radiation or contamination from body fluids (e.g. urine, faeces, vomit) and therefore the greatest care should be taken when cleaning up spills
- any unused product or material used in preparation should be treated as radioactive waste and disposed of according to ARPANSA Code of Practice for disposal of radioactive waste
- should not be diluted or mixed with other solution
- caution if used in those with Crohn's disease and ulcerative colitis
- caution if used in those with pre-existing compromised bone marrow reserve
- any untreated spinal cord compression (imminent or established) or bone fractures should be treated before starting or resuming therapy
- not recommended in women

Patient teaching and advice

- advise patient to
  - flush toilet twice and then wash hands after using bathroom
  - promptly wash clothes separately if soiled with bodily fluids
  - use gloves if handling bodily fluids and then wash hands

RALTITREXED (Tomudex)

Available form
Vial: 2 mg

Action
- folic acid analogue antimetabolite

Use
- palliative treatment of advanced colorectal cancer

Dose
- 3 mg/m^2 IV over 15 minutes, repeated every 3 weeks

Adverse effects
- see General Adverse effects of antineoplastic agents (p. 582)

Interactions
- should not be given with folinic acid or folic acid (or multivitamin preparations containing either substance) as effectiveness will be reduced
- see also General Interactions of antineoplastic agents (p. 582)

Nursing points/Cautions

- reconstitute with 4 mL water for injections then dilute further with 50–250 mL sodium chloride 0.9% or glucose 5% and gently invert to mix but prevent foaming
- see also General Nursing points/Cautions for antineoplastic agents (p. 582)

Patient teaching and advice

- advise patient to avoid multivitamin preparations containing folic acid during therapy
- see also General Patient teaching and advice for antineoplastic agents (p. 584)

RAMUCIRUMAB (Cyramza)

Available form
Vial: 100 mg/10 mL

Action
- recombinant IgG1 monoclonal antibody, vascular endothelial growth factor receptor 2 (VEGFR 2) inhibitor

Use
- treatment of advanced or metastatic gastric, gastro-oesophageal junction adenocarcinoma (with disease progression after prior platinum and fluoropyrimidine chemotherapy) as monotherapy or with paclitaxel if appropriate

Dose
- 8 mg/kg IV over 60 minutes every 2 weeks (as monotherapy) **OR**
- 8 mg/kg IV over 60 minutes on days 1 and 15 of 28-day cycle (before paclitaxel)

Adverse effects
- thromboembolic events (including myocardial infarction, cardiac arrest, cerebral vascular accident)
- gastrointestinal perforation
- infusion-related reactions (IRR)
- hypertension
- impaired wound healing
- proteinuria, nephrotic syndrome
- see also General Adverse effects of antineoplastic agents (p. 582)

Nursing points/Cautions

- premedication with IV antihistamine (e.g. promethazine) is recommended. If patient experiences IRR, dexamethasone should be added to subsequent premedication regimen
- patient should be closely monitored for any signs of infusion-related reaction especially first and second infusions

- BP should be measured regularly during therapy
- urine should be monitored for protein during therapy. If level ≥ 2+/24-hour urine collection is recommended and therapy should be temporarily stopped and resumed at a lower dose when protein level < 2 g/24 hours
- IV push or bolus not recommended
- add solution to sodium chloride 0.9% to final volume 250 mL
- therapy should be withheld for at least 4 weeks before major surgery
- glucose 5% should not be used as a diluent
- see also General Nursing points/ Cautions for antineoplastic agents (p. 582)

Patient teaching and advice

- advise patient to seek medical advice immediately if any of the following occur:
  - chest pain, chest heaviness
  - sudden numbness or weakness of arm, leg and face, feeling confused, difficulty speaking or understanding others, difficulty walking, loss of balance or coordination, sudden dizziness
  - severe abdominal pain, nausea, vomiting, fever and chills
- see also General Patient teaching and advice for antineoplastic agents (p. 584)

RITUXIMAB (MabThera, MabThera SC, Riximyo, Truxima)

Available forms

Solution: 100 mg/10 mL, 500 mg/50 mL, 1400 mg/11.7 mL

Action

- anti-CD20 monoclonal antibody

Use

- untreated CD20 positive stage III/IV follicular, B-cell non-Hodgkin lymphoma (NHL)
- relapsed or refractory CD20 positive low grade or follicular, B-cell non-Hodgkin lymphoma (NHL)
- CD20 positive diffuse large B-cell non-Hodgkin lymphoma (NHL)
- CD20 positive chronic lymphocytic leukaemia (CLL) (with chemotherapy)
- induction of remission of granulomatosis with polyangiitis (GPA) (Wegener's) and microscopic polyangiitis (MPA) (with corticosteroids)
- severe rheumatoid arthritis (with methotrexate) (see Disease modifying antirheumatic drugs (DMARDs), p. 981)

Dose

- (relapsed/refractory low-grade follicular NHL) 375 mg/m^2 IV weekly for 4 weeks (monotherapy) or on day 1 each cycle for up to 6 cycles (with CHOP chemotherapy) **OR**
- (relapsed/refractory low-grade follicular NHL) first dose is IV, as above, then 1400 mg SC over 5 minutes weekly per cycle (for 4 weeks total) (2nd and subsequent cycles) **OR**
- (relapsed/refractory low-grade follicular NHL – maintenance) 375 mg/m^2 IV once every 12 weeks **OR**
- (previously untreated stage III/IV follicular NHL) 375 mg/m^2 IV on day 1 of each chemotherapy cycle (for 8 cycles) **OR**
- (previously untreated stage III/IV follicular NHL) first dose is IV as above, then 1400 mg SC over 5 minutes on day 1 each cycle for up to 8 cycles (induction), then 1400 mg SC once every 12 weeks (until disease progression or 2 years) **OR**
- (previously untreated stage III/IV follicular NHL – maintenance) 375 mg/m^2 IV once every 8 weeks **OR**
- (diffuse large cell B-cell NHL) 375 mg/m^2 IV on day 1 of each chemotherapy cycle (for up to 8 cycles) (with CHOP chemotherapy) **OR**
- (diffuse large cell B-cell NHL) 1400 mg SC over 5 minutes on day 1 each

cycle for up to 8 cycles (with CHOP chemotherapy) **OR**

- (CLL) 375 mg/m^2 IV on day 1 of first cycle, then 500 mg/m^2 on day 1 of subsequent cycles for 6 cycles (with chemotherapy) **OR**
- (GPA/MPA) 375 mg/m^2 IV weekly for 4 weeks

Adverse effects

- infusion reactions (hypo/hypertension, nausea, rash, pruritus, urticaria, chills, fever, rhinitis, throat irritation, flushing)
- progressive multi-focal leukoencephalopathy
- (SC site) pain, induration, swelling, redness, rash, itch, bleeding
- see General Adverse effects of antineoplastic agents (p. 582)

Interactions

- see General Interactions of antineoplastic agents (p. 582)

Nursing points/Cautions

- product labels should be carefully checked to ensure correct formulation (IV or SC) is selected
- chemotherapy should always be administered after rituximab
- premedication with paracetamol/salicylate/NSAIDs, antihistamine and glucocorticoid (e.g. methylprednisolone 100 mg IV) is recommended 30–60 minutes before infusion (if chemotherapy regimen does not contain a glucocorticoid)
- SC administration is only recommended after a full cycle with IV rituximab has been tolerated
- rapid tumour lysis may occur (with symptoms of hyperkalaemia, hypocalcaemia and hyperuricaemia) within 1–2 hours of first infusion
- (IV) patient should be monitored during and at least 2 hours after first infusion for any signs of cytokine syndrome (dyspnoea, bronchospasm, hypoxia, chills, fever, rigors, urticaria and angioedema)
- if severe cytokine syndrome occurs, infusion should be stopped
- (GPA/MPA) severe vasculitis should be treated with IV methylprednisolone for 1–3 days, followed by prednisolone 1 mg/kg/day orally (up to 80 mg daily), then rapidly tapered when symptoms are controlled
- (SC) SC injections should only be administered into abdomen
- (IV) for first infusion, rate should be started at 50 mg/hour and the patient carefully monitored. If no hypersensitivity or infusion-related event occurs, rate may be increased by 50 mg/hour at 30-minute intervals to maximum of 400 mg/hour. If hypersensitivity reaction occurs, infusion rate should be halved. If no hypersensitivity occurs, subsequent infusions can be started at 100 mg/mL and increased at 100 mg increments at 30-minute intervals to 400 mg/hr maximum
- antibody development has been associated with worsening infusion or allergic reactions after second infusion
- any concurrent antihypertensive agent may need to be withheld for 12 hours before and during infusion because of added risk of severe hypotension occurring
- (IV) dilute further with sodium chloride 0.9% or glucose 5% to give a concentration of 1–4 mg/mL
- not given as IV push or bolus
- contraindicated in those with murine protein hypersensitivity
- see also General Nursing points/Cautions for antineoplastic agents (p. 582)

Patient teaching and advice

- warn patient that reactions (e.g. fever, chills, shivering) may occur after infusion (especially first 2 hours of first infusion) and are transient. They occur less frequently after first infusion

- advise patient or carer to seek medical advice immediately if any of the following occur:
  - headache, confusion, fitting (seizures), changes in thinking, walking or talking, decreased strength, blurred or loss of vision
- see General Patient teaching and advice for antineoplastic agents (p. 584)

ROMIDEPSIN (Istodax)

Available form

Vial: 10 mg

Action

- histone deacetylase inhibitor

Use

- peripheral T cell lymphoma (in patient with ≥ one prior systemic treatments)

Dose

- 14 mg/m^2 IV over 4 hours on days 1, 8 and 15 of 28-day cycle, repeated every 28 days

Adverse effects

- QT interval prolongation, ECG changes
- see also General Adverse effects of antineoplastic agents (p. 582)

Interactions

- caution if used with warfarin as prothrombin time may be prolonged and INR elevated, therefore INR should be closely monitored especially when starting or stopping therapy
- caution if given with agents known to prolong QT interval or cause electrolyte imbalance (especially hypokalaemia or hypomagnesaemia)
- may reduce effectiveness of oestrogen-containing oral contraceptives
- serum levels may be increased by rifampicin and therefore not recommended together

Nursing points/Cautions

- serum potassium and magnesium should be checked before each infusion
- reconstitute using 2 mL diluent to given concentration of 5 mg/mL, then dilute further with 500 mL sodium chloride 0.9%
- caution if used in those with congenital or acquired prolonged QT interval or electrolyte imbalance
- see also General Nursing points/Cautions for antineoplastic agents (p. 582)

Patient teaching and advice

- advise patient to seek medical advice immediately if irregular or abnormal heartbeat occurs
- see also General Patient teaching and advice for antineoplastic agents (p. 584)

RUXOLITINIB (Jakavi)

Available forms

Tablets: 5 mg, 10 mg, 15 mg, 20 mg

Action

- Janus associated kinases (JAK1, JAK2) inhibitors (JAK1 dysregulation and JAK2 signalling are associated with polycythemia and myelofibrosis)
- two major active metabolites contributing about 20% activity

Use

- disease-related splenomegaly or symptoms of primary myelofibrosis, post-polycythemia vera myelofibrosis or post-essential thrombocythaemia myelofibrosis
- polycythemia (in patients resistant or intolerant to hydroxycarbamide (hydroxyurea))

Dose

- (myelofibrosis, platelet count 50–100 × 10^9/L) 5 mg orally twice daily **OR**
- (myelofibrosis, platelet count 100–200 × 10^9/L) 15 mg orally twice daily **OR**
- (myelofibrosis, platelet count > 200 × 10^9/L) 20 mg orally twice daily **OR**

- (polycythemia vera) initially 10 mg orally daily for 4 weeks, increasing at 5 mg increments at ≥ 2-week intervals based on response (maximum 25 mg twice daily)

Adverse effects
- dizziness, headache
- thrombocytopenia, anaemia, neutropenia
- increased liver enzymes, cholesterol and triglycerides
- herpes zoster (shingles)
- non-melanoma skin cancer
- progressive multifocal leukoencephalopathy (PML)

Interactions
- serum levels may be increased if given with amprenavir, atazanavir, boceprevir, ciprofloxacin, clarithromycin, diltiazem, erythromycin, indinavir, itraconazole, nelfinavir, posaconazole, ritonavir, saquinavir, verapamil, voriconazole, grapefruit and grapefruit juice
- not recommended with fluconazole > 200 mg daily
- decreased serum levels may occur if given with carbamazepine, dexamethasone, phenytoin, phenobarbital (phenobarbitone), rifampicin, rifabutin and St John's wort
- caution if given with aprepitant, budesonide, darifenacin, darunavir, everolimus, lovastatin, midazolam and sirolimus
- may increase serum levels of ciclosporin, dabigatran, digoxin and rosuvastatin

Nursing points/Cautions

- before starting therapy, patient should be assessed for hepatitis B status and active or latent TB because of increased risk of reactivation
- regular skin examinations are recommended during therapy
- liver enzymes, cholesterol and triglycerides should be measured before starting and regularly throughout therapy
- (polycythemia vera) therapy should be stopped after 6 months if there has been no reduction in spleen size or improvement in symptoms
- abrupt discontinuation should be avoided
- see also General Nursing points/Cautions for antineoplastic agents (p. 582)

Patient teaching and advice

- instruct patient to avoid grapefruit and grapefruit juice during therapy
- (myelofibrosis) warn patient against suddenly stopping therapy as symptoms of myelofibrosis may return over about 7 days
- patient should be instructed to seek medical advice if any of the following occur:
    - any new or worsening skin lesions
    - numbness, itching, tingling or burning pain (which may occur days or weeks before rash appears), flu-like symptoms (usually without fever), rash (usually restricted on one side of body) with blisters (blisters may open, ooze and crust over in 5 days) and rash that takes 2–4 weeks to heal. Pain may also occur with rash
    - confusion, trouble thinking, memory loss, blurred vision, loss of vision, balance or walking problems, decreased strength in arms or legs
- see also General Patient teaching and advice for antineoplastic agents (p. 584)

SORAFENIB TOSILATE (SORAFENIB TOSYLATE) (Nexavar)

Available form
Tablets: 200 mg

Action
- tyrosine, serine/threonine kinase inhibitor which stops replication of tumour cells

Use
- advanced renal cell carcinoma
- advanced hepatocellular carcinoma
- locally advanced or metastatic differentiated thyroid cancer (refractory to radioactive iodine)

Dose
- 400 mg orally twice daily

Adverse effects
- hand–foot syndrome (hand/foot numbness, paraesthesia, tingling, erythema, pain, swelling and, at worst, ulceration, blistering or moist desquamation)
- hypertension
- cardiac ischaemia, myocardial infarction, QT prolongation
- (thyroid cancer) hypocalcaemia
- see also General Adverse effects of antineoplastic agents (p. 582)

Interactions
- decreased serum levels may occur if given with rifampicin, phenytoin, carbamazepine, phenobarbital (phenobarbitone), dexamethasone and St John's wort
- caution if given with warfarin; INR should be closely monitored especially when starting or stopping therapy
- caution if used with docetaxel or irinotecan
- decreased availability if given with neomycin
- caution if used with agents known to prolong QT interval or cause electrolyte imbalance (especially hypokalaemia or hypomagnesaemia)
- see also General Interactions of antineoplastic agents (p. 582)

Nursing points/Cautions
- BP should be monitored regularly as hypertension may occur early in therapy
- (differentiated thyroid cancer) calcium levels and TSH should be monitored during therapy. Thyroxine dose should be adjusted if needed
- caution if used in those with recent myocardial infarction or unstable coronary artery ischaemia
- caution if used in those with known congenital or acquired QT prolongation or electrolyte imbalance
- see also General Nursing points/Cautions for antineoplastic agents (p. 582)

Patient teaching and advice
- advise patient that tablet may be taken on an empty stomach or with a moderate fat meal
- symptoms of hand–foot syndrome can be reduced by advising patients to keep hands/feet cool (e.g. not wearing restricting gloves, socks or shoes; soaking hands/feet in cool water) starting 4–7 days after therapy. Other treatment may consist of pyridoxine (50–150 mg daily) and/or corticosteroids. Symptoms usually subside in 7–14 days
- instruct patient to seek medical advice if any of the following occur:
  - abnormal or rapid heart rate
  - chest pain that may spread to shoulder or neck
- see General Patient teaching and advice for antineoplastic agents (p. 584)

SUNITINIB (Sutent)

Available forms
Capsules: 12.5 mg, 25 mg, 37.5 mg, 50 mg

Action
- multiple receptor tyrosine kinase inhibitor which stops replication of tumour cells

Use
- advanced renal cell carcinoma (RCC)

- gastrointestinal stromal tumour (GIST) (after imatinib failure)
- unresectable well-differentiated pancreatic neuroendocrine tumour (NET)

Dose

- (mRCC, GIST) 50 mg orally daily for 4 consecutive weeks, followed by 2-week rest interval (6-week cycle) **OR**
- (pancreatic NET) 37.5 mg orally daily, adjusting in 12.5 mg increments if needed

Adverse effects

- prolongation of QT interval
- skin discolouration, depigmentation of hair, dry skin, rash on palms/soles
- osteonecrosis of the jaw
- thromboembolic events, aneurysm, artery dissection
- proteinuria
- hypoglycaemia
- thyroid dysfunction
- hypertension
- (rare) seizures
- see also General Adverse effects of antineoplastic agents (p. 582)

Interactions

- increased serum levels may occur if given with grapefruit juice, clarithromycin, erythromycin, itraconazole and ritonavir and are not recommended together
- decreased serum levels may occur if given with carbamazepine, dexamethasone, phenobarbital (phenobarbitone), phenytoin, rifampicin and St John's wort, and are not recommended together
- caution if given with other agents known to prolong QT interval (e.g. amiodarone, clarithromycin, disopyramide, methadone, sotalol) or cause electrolyte imbalance (e.g. diuretics)
- increased risk of osteonecrosis of the jaw if given with or after IV bisphosphonates
- see also General Interactions of antineoplastic agents (p. 582)

Nursing points/Cautions

- BP should be monitored regularly as hypertension occurs, especially during the early stages of treatment
- urine should be tested for protein regularly during therapy
- any hypomagnesaemia and hypokalaemia should be corrected before starting therapy
- thyroid function should be measured and any imbalance treated before starting therapy
- in those patients with risk factors (e.g. poor dental hygiene, chronic periodontal disease, head/neck radiotherapy as well as treatment with antineoplastic agents and corticosteroids), a dental examination and any necessary treatment should be carried out before starting therapy with bisphosphonate. Invasive dental procedures should be avoided if possible during therapy to prevent osteonecrosis of the jaw occurring
- caution if given in those with known congenital or acquired prolongation of QT interval or at risk of electrolyte imbalance (especially hypokalaemia and hypomagnesaemia)
- not recommended in those who have had a myocardial infarction, severe or unstable angina, coronary artery bypass graft surgery, stroke, pulmonary embolism or transischaemic attack in last 12 months
- see also General Nursing points/Cautions for antineoplastic agents (p. 582)

Patient teaching and advice

- warn patient to avoid grapefruit and grapefruit juice during therapy
- patient should be advised that hair or skin may change colour

- those with diabetes should be warned to monitor blood glucose levels during therapy as hypoglycaemia may occur
- instruct patient to seek medical advice immediately if any of the following occur:
  - jaw or dental pain, bleeding gums, sores on gums or jaw
  - irregular heart rate
  - cough, shortness of breath, difficulty breathing, swollen calf that is red, warm and tender
- encourage patient to practise good dental hygiene, including brushing teeth and tongue after meals and before bed, daily flossing to remove plaque and using a mirror to check teeth and gums regularly for any sores or bleeding of the gums
- see General Patient teaching and advice for antineoplastic agents (p. 584)

TALIMOGENE LAHERPAREPVEC (Imlygic)

Available forms

Vial: 1 × 10^6 PFU/mL, 1 × 10^8 PFU/mL

Action

- attenuated herpes simplex virus type 1 (HSV-1) oncolytic immunotherapy, which has been modified to replicate inside tumours to produce immune stimulatory proteins (GM CSF), resulting in tumour cell death and release of tumour-derived antigens and GM CSF (which together promote a systemic anti-tumour immune response)

Use

- melanoma (unresectable cutaneous, subcutaneous or nodal lesions after initial surgery)

Dose

- initially 1 × 10^6 (1 million) PFU /mL intralesionally, then 3 weeks later 1 × 10^8 (100 million) PFU, then 2 weeks later 1 × 10^8 (100 million) PFU/mL (maximum 4 mL/session)

Adverse effects

- fever, chills, flu-like symptoms
- fatigue, headache, malaise, dizziness, insomnia, anxiety, depression
- nausea, vomiting, diarrhoea, constipation, decreased appetite, decreased weight
- myalgia, arthralgia, pain in extremity, back or groin pain
- peripheral oedema
- cough, dyspnoea
- herpetic infection (e.g. cold sores, herpes keratitis)
- rash, dermatitis, vitiligo, pruritus
- (injection site) redness, pain, induration, pruritus, swelling, bleeding, inflammation, impaired healing, cellulitis, necrosis, ulceration, plasmacytoma (discrete solitary mass of neoplastic monoclonal plasma cells)
- hypersensitivity

Nursing points/Cautions

- healthcare professionals and close family members should avoid contact with injected lesions and body fluids during and for 30 days after finishing therapy
- patient who is HSV-1 seronegative has a greater risk of fever, chills and flu-like symptoms compared to those who are HSV-1 seropositive (especially in first 12 weeks of therapy)
- (initial intralesional injection) largest lesion(s) should be injected first, then any other lesion prioritised on basis of size until maximum (4 mL) is reached
- (second and subsequent injections) any new lesion(s) that have developed since initial injection, then any other lesion prioritised on basis of size until maximum (4 mL) is reached
- volume injected per lesion is dependent on size of lesion ($>$ 5 cm = up to 4 mL, $>$ 2.5–5 cm = up to 2 mL, $>$ 1.5–2.5 cm = up to 1 mL, $>$ 0.5–1.5 cm = up to 0.5 mL, $\leq$ 0.5 cm = up to 0.1 mL)

- treatment may be restarted if new lesions appear after course of treatment has finished
- vial should be thawed at room temperature (20–25°C) before use for about 30 minutes and gently swirled (not shaken) before use
- lesion may be treated with local anaesthetic (around periphery but not directly into lesion) before administration of talimogene laherparepvec. Multiple injections may be required if radial reach of needle is not sufficient
- new needle should be used each time needle is totally withdrawn from lesion
- pressure should be applied with sterile gauze for 30 seconds to injection site and area then cleaned with alcohol swab before applying absorbent pad and occlusive dressing
- if staff member has accidental contact with material during preparation or administration, area should be washed well for at least 15 minutes
- solution must not be refrozen after being thawed out
- contraindicated in those who are severely immunocompromised due to risk of disseminated herpetic infection

Patient teaching and advice

- instruct patient to:
  - avoid scratching injected lesions as this may transfer talimogene laherparepvec to other sites
  - keep lesion/injection site covered at all times and replace dressing immediately if it falls off
  - place any used dressings and cleaning materials into a sealed plastic bag before disposing of in household waste
  - use latex condom (males) or reliable contraception (females) during therapy
- immunocompromised people, pregnant women and children under 3 months should avoid contact with lesion/injection site during and for 30 days after finishing therapy (i.e. they should not assist with cleaning area or changing dressings)
- seek medical advice immediately if any of the following occur:
  - pain, burning or tingling around mouth, genitals, ear or fingers, followed by blister formation
  - eye pain, red eye, blurry vision, discharge from eye
  - flu-like symptoms
- avoid kissing others if oral cold sore develops, or sexual contact if genital herpes develops
- caregiver assisting patient should be instructed to:
  - wear gloves if changing dressings on injected lesions
  - avoid contact with patient's body fluids
  - wash area well with soap and water or disinfectant if accidental exposure to material occurs
  - seek medical advice if any signs of herpes infection develop (see above)

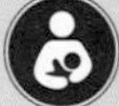
not recommended during pregnancy or breastfeeding

TAMOXIFEN (Genox, Nolvadex-D, Tamosin)

Available forms
Tablets: 10 mg, 20 mg

Action
- anti-oestrogen agent which prevents oestrogen binding to oestrogen receptor (although it has also been shown to have some activity on oestrogen negative tumours, suggesting another mechanism of action)
- active metabolite (which has similar activity to tamoxifen)

Use
- treatment of breast cancer
- risk reduction of breast cancer in those with moderate-to-high risk

Dose
- (treatment) initially 20 mg orally daily, increasing to 40 mg if no response **OR**
- (risk reduction) 20 mg orally daily (for 5 years)

Adverse effects
- hot flushes
- vaginal discharge/bleeding
- endometrial changes (e.g. hyperplasia, polyps, uterine fibroids)
- microvascular flap complications (in delayed breast reconstruction)
- retinopathy, cataract
- thromboembolic events
- paraesthesia, altered taste
- see also General Adverse effects of antineoplastic agents (p. 582)

Interactions
- increased risk of thromboembolic events occurring when given with other cytotoxic agents
- contraindicated with warfarin due to increased anticoagulant effects, therefore INR should be closely monitored, especially when starting or stopping therapy
- decreased efficacy if given with SSRIs
- decreased serum levels may occur if given with rifampicin
- not recommended with oral contraceptives or hormone replacement therapy
- see also General Interactions of antineoplastic agents (p. 582)

Nursing points/Cautions
- regular gynaecological examination is recommended
- in pre-menopausal women, pregnancy should be excluded before starting therapy
- should be stopped during periods of immobility or at least 3 weeks before elective surgery due to increased risk of thromboembolic events
- contraindicated in those with history of pulmonary embolism or deep vein thrombosis
- see also General Nursing points/Cautions for antineoplastic agents (p. 582)

Patient teaching and advice
- patient should be advised to seek medical advice immediately if any of the following occur:
  - vaginal bleeding or any other gynaecological symptoms such as pelvic pain or pressure
  - visual disturbances
- see General Patient teaching and advice for antineoplastic agents (p. 584)

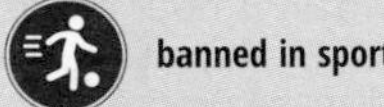

banned in sport

TEMOZOLOMIDE (Temizole, Temodal)

Available forms

Capsules: 5 mg, 20 mg, 100 mg, 140 mg, 180 mg, 250 mg

Action
- imidazotetrazine alkylating agent
- rapidly converted to active compound (monomethyl triazeno imidazole carboxamide)

Use
- newly diagnosed glioblastoma multiforme (with radiotherapy) then as adjunct
- recurrent brain tumours (anaplastic astrocytoma, glioblastoma multiforme) (after standard treatment)
- advanced metastatic malignant melanoma (first-line treatment)

Dose

- (newly diagnosed glioblastoma multiforme) 75 mg/m^2 orally daily 1 hour before food for 42 days (maximum 47 days) with focal radiotherapy (concomitant phase), then after 4-week interval, 150 mg/m^2 orally 1 hour before food for 5 days of 28-day cycle (cycle 1), then increasing to 200 mg/m^2 for next 5 cycles depending on toxicity (adjunctive phase) **OR**
- (recurrent anaplastic astrocytoma or glioblastoma multiforme) 200 mg/m^2 orally 1 hour before food daily (if previously untreated) or 150 mg/m^2 (if previously treated) for 5 days of 28-day cycle, increasing to 200 mg/m^2 from cycle 2 depending on absolute neutrophil count (ANC) or platelet count (for up to 2 years or disease progression) **OR**
- (metastatic malignant melanoma) 200 mg/m^2 orally daily 1 hour before food for 5 days of 28-day cycle (for up to 2 years or disease progression)

Adverse effects

- *Pneumocystis carinii* pneumonia (PCP)
- reactivation of hepatitis B
- see also General Adverse effects of antineoplastic agents (p. 582)

Interactions

- clearance may be decreased if given with sodium valproate
- see also General Interactions of antineoplastic agents (p. 582)

Nursing points/Cautions

- before starting therapy, patient should be assessed for hepatitis B status due to risk of reactivation
- antiemetic premedication is recommended before administration of temozolomide
- prophylactic antibiotics for PCP are recommended for 42-day cycle in those receiving radiotherapy concurrently
- contraindicated in those with hypersensitivity to dacarbazine
- see also General Nursing points/Cautions for antineoplastic agents (p. 582)

Patient teaching and advice

- instruct patient to take 1 hour before food, swallowed whole with water and if vomiting occurs, second dose should not be given
- see also General Patient teaching and advice for antineoplastic agents (p. 584)

TIOGUANINE (THIOGUANINE) (Lanvis)

Available form

Tablets: 40 mg

Action

- purine antimetabolite
- derivative of mercaptopurine; however, detoxification is not dependent on xanthine oxidase

Use

- acute myeloblastic leukaemia (AML)
- less commonly, chronic granulocytic leukaemia (during blast crisis or during busulfan-induced thrombocytopenia)

Dose

- 2–2.5 mg/kg daily orally in 1–2 divided doses (to the closest multiple of 20 mg)

Adverse effects

- phototoxicity
- see also General Adverse effects of antineoplastic agents (p. 582)

Interactions

- increased risk of nodular regenerative hyperplasia, portal hypertension and oesophageal varices if given with busulfan
- caution if given with olsalazine, mesalazine or sulfasalazine

- see also General Interactions of antineoplastic agents (p. 582)

Nursing points/Cautions

- testing for thiopurine methyltransferase deficiency is recommended before starting therapy as low or absent activity may be life threatening
- cross-resistance may exist between tioguanine and mercaptopurine
- if remission has not occurred after 2–3 attempts at induction, therapy should be reconsidered
- not recommended in those lacking hypoxanthine guanine phosphoribosyltransferase (e.g. Lesch-Nyhan syndrome) as conversion to active metabolite will be blocked
- not recommended for maintenance or prolonged therapy due to risk of hepatotoxicity
- see also General Nursing points/Cautions for antineoplastic agents (p. 582)

Patient teaching and advice

- see General Patient teaching and advice for antineoplastic agents (p. 584)

TISAGENLECLEUCEL (Kymriah)

Available form

Suspension bag: 1.2–6.0 $\times$ 10^6 anti-CD19 CAR T-cells in 10–50 mL

Action

- CD19 directed genetically modified autologous T-cell immunotherapy prepared from patient's own T cells, which have been harvested via leukapheresis and then genetically modified by retroviral transduction to express a chimeric antigen receptor (CAR)

Use

- relapsed or refractory diffuse large B-cell lymphoma (DLBCL) (after two or more types of systemic therapy)
- B-cell precursor acute lymphoblastic leukaemia (ALL) (refractory, in relapse post-transplant or in second or later relapse)

Dose

- (B-cell ALL, weight $\leq$ 50 kg) 0.2–5.0 $\times$ 10^6 CAR-positive viable T cells/kg **OR**
- (B-cell ALL, weight $>$ 50 kg) 0.2–2.5 $\times$ 10^8 CAR-positive viable T cells **OR**
- (DLBCL) 0.6–6.0 $\times$ 10^8 CAR-positive viable T cells

Adverse effects

- See Adverse effects for Axicabtagene ciloleucel (Yescarta) (p. 593)

Interactions

- not recommended with or within 6 weeks of live virus vaccines
- may cause false positive result on HIV nucleic acid tests. ELISA or Western blot tests for HIV antibodies are recommended instead

Nursing points/Cautions

- before collecting cells for therapy, patient should be screened for hepatitis B and C and HIV
- after infusion, blood counts, uric acid and immunoglobulin levels should be monitored
- therapy should be delayed if patient has unresolved serious adverse reactions from previous chemotherapy, active uncontrolled infection, active chronic graft versus host disease (GvHD) or significant worsening of leukaemia burden or rapid progression of lymphoma after lymphodepleting chemotherapy (see below)
- lymphodepleting chemotherapy is required unless WBC is $\leq$ 1,000 cells/microL within 1 week of infusion. If there is more than 4 weeks between completing lymphodepleting chemotherapy and infusion, and WBC $>$ 1000 cells/microL, patient should be re-treated with chemotherapy
- infusion is recommended 2–14 days after lymphodepleting chemotherapy is completed

- pretreatment involves lymphodepleting chemotherapy:
  - (B-cell ALL) cyclophosphamide 500 mg/m^2 IV daily for 2 days (starting on same day as fludarabine) and fludarabine 30 mg/m^2 IV daily for 4 days before infusion. If haemorrhagic cystitis occurs with cyclophosphamide or patient is chemorefractory, then cytarabine 500 mg/mg^2 IV daily for 2 days and etoposide 150 mg/m^2 IV for 3 days (starting on first day of cytarabine is recommended)
  - (DLBCL) cyclophosphamide 250 mg/m^2 IV daily for 3 days (starting on same day as fludarabine) and fludarabine 25 mg/m^2 IV daily for 3 days. If haemorrhagic cystitis occurs with cyclophosphamide or patient is chemorefractory, then bendamustine 90 mg/m^2 IV for 2 days is recommended
- premedication (paracetamol and diphenhydramine (or other H1 antihistamine)) is recommended 30–60 minutes before infusion. Corticosteroids are not recommended as part of premedication
- severe or life-threatening cytokine-release syndrome should be treated with tocilizumab (see DMARDs, p. 1003) or tocilizumab and corticosteroids. A minimum of 4 doses of tocilizumab must be readily available in case of cytokine-release syndrome, along with emergency equipment. Treatment and supportive care (e.g. oxygen, fluids, vasopressor and if life threatening, ventilator support, haemodialysis) must be instituted at first signs of cytokine-release syndrome
- if patient has high uric acid levels or high tumour burden, allopurinol (or alternative) is recommended prophylactically before infusion to reduce risk of tumour lysis syndrome
- important to coordinate thaw and infusion timing so that infusion is thawed and available for infusion when the patient is ready
- patient identity must be confirmed (matching patient ID with patient identifiers on infusion cassette). When correctly identified, product bag is removed from cassette and inspected for any breaks or cracks before thawing. Infusion bag should then be placed in second sterile bag and then thawed, either in water bath or by dry thaw method, until there is no visible ice in infusion bag. Bag should be gently mixed to disperse any cellular clumps. If second bag is used, it should not be thawed until all contents of first bag have been infused
- leukodepleting filter should not be used
- only given IV (with central venous line recommended)
- line should be primed with sodium chloride 0.9% before and after infusion
- infused via gravity feed at 10–20 mL/minute
- standard precautions for blood-borne pathogens should be adhered to and handling and disposal should be as per institution biosafety guidelines
- patient should be monitored for at least 7 days post-infusion for any signs of cytokine-release syndrome
- contains dextran and dimethyl sulfoxide which can cause anaphylaxis in sensitive individuals
- not recommended within 4 months of undergoing allogeneic stem cell transplant due to risk of worsening GVHD
- not recommended in those with HIV because of risk of loss of HIV viral suppression
- not recommended in those with relapsed CD19-negative leukaemia

Patient teaching and advice

- see Axicabtagene ciloleucel (Yescarta) Patient teaching and advice (p. 594)

TOPOTECAN HYDROCHLORIDE (Hycamtin)

Available forms

Vial: 4 mg; Vial (solution): 4 mg/4 mL

Action

- topoisomerase1 inhibitor (topoisomerase1 is involved in replication, transcription and DNA damage repair)

Use

- small cell lung cancer (SCLC) (after failure of first-line treatment)
- metastatic ovarian cancer (after failure of first-line or subsequent treatment)
- recurrent or persistent cervical cancer (with cisplatin) (unsuitable for radiation or surgery)

Dose

- (SCLC, ovarian cancer) 1.5 mg/m^2 IV over 30 minutes for 5 days, repeated every 21 days for at least 4 cycles **OR**
- (cervical cancer) 0.75 mg/m^2 IV over 30 minutes for 3 days (with cisplatin), repeated every 21 days for 6 cycles or until disease progression

Adverse effects

- interstitial lung disease
- see also General Adverse effects of antineoplastic agents (p. 582)

Interactions

- see General Interactions of antineoplastic agents (p. 582)

Nursing points/Cautions

- reconstitute powder with 4 mL water for injections and then further dilute with glucose 5% or sodium chloride 0.9% before IV administration
- caution if used in those with interstitial lung disease, pulmonary fibrosis, lung cancer, thoracic irradiation or with use of pneumotoxic agents or colony-stimulating factors, due to increased risk of interstitial lung disease
- see also General Nursing points/Cautions for antineoplastic agents (p. 582)

Patient teaching and advice

- advise patient to seek medical advice if any cough, shortness of breath or difficulty breathing occurs
- see also General Patient teaching and advice for antineoplastic agents (p. 584)

TOREMIFENE (Fareston)

Available form

Tablets: 60 mg

Action

- triphenylethylene derivative
- anti-oestrogen agent that binds to oestrogen receptors in a similar way to tamoxifen and clomifene (clomiphene)

Use

- hormone-dependent metastatic breast cancer (post-menopausal)

Dose

- 60 mg orally daily

Adverse effects

- prolongation of QT interval
- (rare) hypercalcaemia
- see also General Adverse effects of antineoplastic agents (p. 582)

Interactions

- contraindicated with agents that prolong QT interval or cause electrolyte imbalance (especially hypokalaemia and hypomagnesaemia)
- increased risk of hypercalcaemia if given with thiazide diuretics or other agents that decrease calcium excretion
- decreased serum levels may occur if given with phenobarbital (phenobarbitone), phenytoin or carbamazepine

- not recommended with warfarin. If given, INR should be closely monitored
- caution if given with antifungal agents, erythromycin or macrolide antibacterial agents as increased serum levels may occur
- see also General Interactions of antineoplastic agents (p. 582)

Nursing points/Cautions

- gynaecological examination is recommended before starting therapy to exclude any endometrial abnormalities, and then repeated annually
- increased risk of endometrial cancer in those with high BMI (> 30), hypertension, diabetes or history of hormone replacement therapy
- tablets contain lactose and are therefore not recommended in those with rare hereditary problem of galactose intolerance, Lapp lactose deficiency or glucose–galactose malabsorption
- caution if used in those with severe angina or cardiac insufficiency
- not recommended in those with hypersensitivity to other anti-oestrogen agents or with severe thromboembolic disease
- contraindicated in those with severe liver failure, pre-existing endometrial hyperplasia or oestrogen receptor negative tumours
- contraindicated in those with history of congenital or acquired QT interval prolongation or electrolyte disturbance, clinically relevant bradycardia, heart failure with reduced left ventricular ejection fraction or symptomatic arrhythmias
- see also General Nursing points/Cautions for antineoplastic agents (p. 582)

Patient teaching and advice

- advise patient to seek medical advice if any of the following occur:
  - rapid or abnormal heart rate
  - signs of hypercalcaemia including abdominal pain, excessive thirst and urination, muscle pain, weakness, anxiety, depression, confusion, fatigue, loss of concentration
- see also General Patient teaching and advice for antineoplastic agents (p. 584)

banned in sport

TRAMETINIB (Mekinist)

Available forms

Tablets: 0.5 mg, 2 mg

Action

- protein kinase (MEK) inhibitor
- MEK (mitogen activated extracellular signal regulated kinase) proteins are critical in activating mutated BRAF pathways resulting in tumour growth

Use

- BRAF V600 positive unresectable stage III or metastatic stage IV melanoma (with dabrafenib)
- BRAF V600 positive unresectable stage III or metastatic stage IV melanoma (as monotherapy, intolerant to or where BRAF inhibitor can't be used)
- BRAF V600 positive locally advanced or metastatic anaplastic thyroid cancer (with dabrafenib)
- BRAF V600 positive advanced non-small cell lung cancer (with dabrafenib)

Dose

- 2 mg orally daily 1 hour before or 2 hours after food (monotherapy or with dabrafenib)

Adverse effects

- haemorrhage (intracranial, gastric)
- retinal pigment epithelial detachment, retinal vein occlusion, visual impairment
- left ventricular dysfunction
- interstitial lung disease, pneumonitis
- fever
- see also General Adverse effects of antineoplastic agents (p. 582)

Nursing points/Cautions

- BRAF V600 mutation should be confirmed using a valid and reliable test
- left ventricular ejection fraction should be evaluated using echocardiogram before starting, 1 month after starting therapy and then 3-monthly
- urgent (within 24 hours) ophthalmological review should be organised if patient experiences any visual changes
- (melanoma-adjunctive therapy) treatment should be 12 months only
- not recommended for BRAF V600 mutation-positive melanoma that has metastasised to brain
- see also General Nursing points/Cautions for antineoplastic agents (p. 582)

Patient teaching and advice

- instruct patient to seek medical advice immediately if any of the following occur:
  - decreased central vision, blurry vision or loss of vision
  - cough, shortness of breath, difficulty breathing
  - fever > 38.5°C
  - increased heart rate, palpitations, shortness of breath, swelling of ankles, dizziness, light-headedness
  - headache, feeling weak, coughing or vomiting blood, vomiting material that looks like coffee grounds, bloody diarrhoea, black tarry stools
- if patient is taking dabrafenib as well, the two should be taken at same time (morning or evening)
- see also General Patient teaching and advice for antineoplastic agents (p. 584)

TRASTUZUMAB (Herceptin, Herceptin SC, Herzuma, Kanjinti, Ogivri, Ontruzant, Trazimera)

TRASTUZUMAB EMTANSINE (Kadcyla)

Available forms

Vial (powder): 60 mg, 150 mg, 160 mg, 420 mg, 440 mg; Vial (solution): 600 mg/5 mL

Action

- human epidermal growth factor receptor 2 (HER2) recombinant monoclonal antibody
- (Kadcyla) combines HER2 recombinant monoclonal antibody with microtubule inhibitory drug (DM1) and stable thioether linker

Use

- early or locally advanced breast cancer (HER2-positive, after surgery with other chemotherapy and/or radiation therapy)
- metastatic breast cancer (HER2-positive) (monotherapy with other chemotherapy)
- previously untreated HER2-positive stomach or gastric-oesophageal junction cancer (with cisplatin and fluorouracil or capecitabine)

Dose

- (early, locally advanced or metastatic breast cancer – 3-week regimen) 8 mg/kg IV over 90 minutes (loading dose), then 6 mg/kg IV over 30 minutes (if loading dose was well tolerated) at 3-weekly intervals **OR**

- (early or metastatic breast cancer – weekly regimen) 4 mg/kg IV over 90 minutes (loading dose), then 2 mg/kg IV over 30 minutes (if loading dose was well tolerated) at weekly intervals **OR**
- (advanced gastric cancer) 8 mg/kg IV over 90 minutes (loading dose), then 6 mg/kg over 30 minutes (if loading dose was well tolerated) at 3-weekly intervals **OR**
- (early, metastatic or locally advanced breast cancer) 600 mg SC over 2–5 minutes every 3 weeks (Herceptin SC) **OR**
- (early breast cancer) 3.6 mg/kg IV over 90 minutes every 3 weeks, then reducing IV rate to 30 minutes (if first infusion was well tolerated) (21-day cycle) for 14 cycles, unacceptable toxicity or disease progression (Kadcyla)
- (metastatic breast cancer) 3.6 mg/kg IV over 90 minutes every 3 weeks, then reducing IV rate to 30 minutes (if first infusion was well tolerated) until disease progression or unacceptable toxicity (Kadcyla)

Adverse effects

- infusion-related reactions
- congestive cardiac failure, left ventricular dysfunction
- interstitial lung disease
- see also General Adverse effects of antineoplastic agents (p. 582)

Interactions

- decreased clearance if given with paclitaxel
- increased risk of cardiac toxicity if anthracyclines or cyclophosphamide have been previously used
- see also General Interactions of antineoplastic agents (p. 582)

Nursing points/Cautions

- HER2 testing is required before starting therapy
- cardiac assessment (history, physical assessment, ECHO cardiogram and/or MUGA (multigated acquisition) scan) is recommended before starting, 3-monthly during treatment and 6-monthly for 2 years after stopping therapy
- different formulation of trastuzumab (Herceptin and Kadcyla) are not interchangeable. Furthermore, Herceptin IV formulation should not be given SC and Herceptin SC should not be given IV
- loading dose is given over 90 minutes if well tolerated, infusion time can be decreased to 30 minutes if well tolerated
- (early or locally advanced breast cancer) treatment is for 1 year, disease progression or until unacceptable toxicity occurs
- (Herceptin SC) SC sites should be rotated between right and left thigh and at least 2.5 cm from previous injection sites
- (Herceptin SC) no further dilution is required
- chills and/or fever are common during first infusion
- (IV) reconstitute using water for injections (3 mL for 60 mg vial, 7.2 mL for 150 mg, 20 mL for 420–440 mg) and swirl gently to dissolve (do not shake), allowing solution to stand for 15 minutes after reconstitution and further dilute with 250 mL sodium chloride 0.9%
- (Kadcyla) reconstitute using water for injections (5 mL for 100 mg vial, 8 mL for 160 mg vial) and swirl gently to dissolve (do not shake) and then further dilute with 250 mL sodium chloride 0.45% or sodium chloride 0.9%. If sodium chloride 0.45% is used, no inline filter is required. If sodium chloride 0.9% is used, 0.22 micron inline filter is required
- (IV) should not be given as an IV bolus or push
- incompatible with glucose 5%

- (Ogivri) contains sorbitol and is not recommended in those with hereditary fructose intolerance
- caution if used in those with symptomatic intrinsic lung disease or with extensive tumour involvement of the lungs
- caution if used in those with hypertension, congestive cardiac failure, ventricular dysfunction or coronary artery disease due to increased risk of cardiac toxicity
- not recommended in those with dyspnoea at rest due to malignancy complications or co-morbidities
- contraindicated in those with left ventricular ejection fraction less than 45% or symptomatic heart failure or hypersensitivity to Chinese hamster ovary cell proteins
- see also General Nursing points/ Cautions for antineoplastic agents (p. 582)

Patient teaching and advice

- advise patient to seek medical advice if any of the following occur:
  - cough, shortness of breath, difficulty breathing
  - swelling of feet, shortness of breath when lying down or after gentle exercise, such as walking
- see also General Patient teaching and advice for antineoplastic agents (p. 584)

TRETINOIN (Vesanoid)

Available form
Capsules: 10 mg

Action
- retinoid, related to vitamin A, which inhibits proliferation of transformed haemopoietic cells, including human myeloid leukaemic cells

Use
- acute promyelocytic leukaemia (induction of remission)

Dose
- 45 mg/m^2 orally daily in 2 equal doses, continued for 30–120 days unless disease progression occurs (after remission, consolidation therapy should be started)

Adverse effects
- hyperleukocytosis, retinoic acid syndrome (RAS)
- intracranial hypertension/pseudotumour cerebri
- anxiety, mood alteration, depression
- see also General Adverse effects of antineoplastic agents (p. 582)

Interactions
- contraindicated with vitamin A due to risk of hypervitaminosis A
- not recommended with other agents that cause intracranial hypertension/ pseudotumour cerebri such as tetracyclines
- not recommended with ciclosporin, cimetidine, diltiazem, erythromycin, itraconazole and verapamil as increased serum levels may result
- serum levels may be decreased if given with carbamazepine, phenobarbital (phenobarbitone), phenytoin, rifampicin and rifabutin
- caution if used with tranexamic acid, aprotinin and aminocaproic acid due to increased risk of thrombotic complications

Nursing points/Cautions

- pregnancy test (negative) must be performed 2 weeks before starting and then monthly throughout therapy as tretinoin is highly teratogenic
- to be eligible for therapy, female patients of childbearing potential must be suffering from life-threatening malignancy and understand dangers of becoming pregnant (risk of severe fetal malformation) and agree to using effective contraception 4 weeks before, during and 4 weeks after stopping therapy

- caution if used in those with history of depression
- contraindicated in those with hypersensitivity to vitamin A
- see also General Nursing points/ Cautions for antineoplastic agents (p. 582)

Patient teaching and advice

- instruct patient to immediately seek medical advice if any of the following occur:
  - any new or worsening headache
  - fever, difficulty breathing, shortness of breath, sudden weight gain (RAS)
  - anxiety, low mood, depression
- ensure female patient understands the need to use reliable contraception before, during and after therapy, as well as monthly pregnancy testing, due to tretinoin causing severe fetal malformations if taken during pregnancy
- see also General Patient teaching and advice for antineoplastic agents (p. 584)

Note

- contained in ReTrieve Cream and StievaA for management of acne vulgaris

VEMURAFENIB (Zelboraf)

Available form

Tablets: 240 mg

Action

- inhibitor of mutated form of BRAF serine-threonine kinase enzyme (mutated BRAF can cause cell proliferation in the absence of growth factors normally required for proliferation)
- very long half-life (about 57 hours)

Use

- metastatic melanoma (unresectable stage IIIc and IV BRAF V600 positive)

Dose

- 960 mg orally twice daily 1 hour before or 2 hours after food until disease progression or unacceptable toxicity

Adverse effects

- phototoxicity
- skin cancers (melanoma, cutaneous squamous cell, non-cutaneous squamous cell)
- uveitis, blurred vision, iritis, photophobia, retinal vein occlusion
- pancreatitis
- QT prolongation
- Dupuytren's contracture
- see also General Adverse effects of antineoplastic agents (p. 582)

Interactions

- not recommended with agents known to prolong QT interval or cause electrolyte imbalance (such as diuretics)
- not recommended with ipilimumab due to increased risk of liver injury
- may increase serum levels of caffeine, ciclosporin, clozapine, dextromethorphan, methadone, olanzapine, theophylline and TCAs
- may decrease serum levels of midazolam
- may decrease efficacy of oral contraceptives
- caution if given with warfarin; INR should be closely monitored, especially when starting or stopping therapy
- increased serum levels may occur if given with atazanavir, clarithromycin, indinavir, itraconazole, ritonavir, saquinavir and voriconazole
- decreased serum levels may occur if given with carbamazepine, rifabutin, rifampicin, phenytoin, phenobarbital (phenobarbitone) and St John's wort
- may increase serum levels of digoxin increasing risk of toxicity
- may potentiate radiation toxicity (given at same time or sequentially)

- efficacy may be reduced if given with amiodarone, ciclosporin, clarithromycin, itraconazole, ritonavir and verapamil

Nursing points/Cautions

- before starting therapy, BRAF V600 mutation positive tumour status should be confirmed by an accredited laboratory
- ECG and electrolytes should be monitored before starting therapy, after any dose adjustment, monthly for first 3 months, then 3-monthly
- skin examination for any lesions should occur before starting, during and for 6 months after completing therapy
- patient should have ophthalmological examination before starting and regularly during therapy
- not recommended in those with congenital or acquired QT prolongation or electrolyte imbalance (especially hypokalaemia and hypomagnesaemia)
- see General Nursing points/Cautions for antineoplastic agents (p. 582)

Patient teaching and advice

- patient should be instructed to take tablets whole 1 hour before or 2 hours after meals
- warn patient to avoid sun exposure during therapy including wearing sunscreen (SPF 30+), lip balm, long-sleeved clothing and hat when outdoors
- instruct patient to check skin regularly for any new or changing lesions
- advise patient to seek medical advice if any of the following occur:
  - any new or changing skin lesions
  - increased sensitivity to sun, severe sunburn or sunburn occurring more easily
  - changes to vision, eye pain, blurred vision, sensitivity to light
  - irregular heart rate
  - unexplained abdominal pain (especially in first 2 weeks of therapy) sometimes with nausea and vomiting
  - thickening or appearance of visible cords, bands or lumps in palm of one or both hands
- see also General Patient teaching and advice for antineoplastic agents (p. 584)

VINBLASTINE SULFATE (DBL Vinblastine Injection)

Available form

Vial: 10 mg/10 mL

Action

- vinca alkaloid that inhibits cell division and amino acid synthesis
- active metabolite whose activity is greater than parent
- therapeutic effects increased when given with other antineoplastic agents

Use

- advanced (stage III and IV) Hodgkin's disease, lymphocytic lymphoma, advanced testicular cancer, mycosis fungoides, Kaposi's sarcoma, Histiocytosis X, choriocarcinoma (resistant to other agents), breast cancer (unresponsive to hormone therapy or endocrine surgery)

Dose

- 3.7 mg/m^2 IV once every 7 days (dose 1), then 5.5 mg/m^2 (dose 2), 7.4 mg/m^2 (dose 3), 9.25 mg/m^2 (dose 4), 11.1 mg/m^2 (dose 5) (maximum 18.5 mg/m^2)

Adverse effects

- acute shortness of breath, severe bronchospasm
- see also General Adverse effects of antineoplastic agents (p. 582)

Interactions

- phenytoin serum levels may be decreased, increasing the risk of seizures
- increased risk of cardiotoxicity if given with bleomycin and cisplatin
- increased risk of acute pulmonary reaction if given with mitomycin
- see also General Interactions of antineoplastic agents (p. 582)

Nursing points/Cautions

- patient should be observed for any shortness of breath or bronchospasm, especially if vinblastine is given with mitomycin, and should not be readministered if they occur
- jaw and organ pain (in organ containing tumour) is common
- next injection should not be given until WBC is at least 4 × 10^9/L
- not recommended IM, SC or IT (fatal if given intrathecally)
- given as IV injection or into rapidly flowing IV infusion
- should not be diluted in large volumes (100–250 mL) or given by prolonged infusion
- caution if used in those with cachexia or skin ulceration
- contraindicated in those with vinca alkaloid hypersensitivity
- see also General Nursing points/Cautions for antineoplastic agents (p. 582)

Patient teaching and advice

- see General Patient teaching and advice for antineoplastic agents (p. 584)

VINCRISTINE SULFATE (Vincristine Sulfate Injection)

Available forms

Vial: 1 mg/mL, 2 mg/2 mL, 5 mg/5 mL

Action

- vinca alkaloid that inhibits cell division and also has some immunosuppressant activity
- does not readily cross blood–brain barrier

Use

- acute leukaemias
- Ewing's sarcoma, Wilms' tumour, Hodgkin's disease, non-Hodgkin lymphoma, neuroblastoma, sarcomas, breast, uterine, cervical and lung (oat cell) tumours, malignant melanoma, rhabdomyosarcoma (with other agents), mycosis fungoides
- idiopathic thrombocytopenic purpura (resistant to other therapies)

Dose

- 0.4–1.4 mg/m^2 IV weekly

Adverse effects

- acute shortness of breath, severe bronchospasm
- jaw pain
- neurotoxicity
- hyperuricaemia
- see also General Adverse effects of antineoplastic agents (p. 582)

Interactions

- serum levels may be increased if given voriconazole
- increases cellular uptake of methotrexate by malignant cells
- clearance may be decreased by nifedipine
- increased risk of myelosuppression if given with prednisolone and doxorubicin and are therefore not recommended together
- may decrease absorption of digoxin, ciprofloxacin or norfloxacin
- may decrease serum levels of phenytoin increasing risk of seizures
- severe bronchospasm and acute shortness of breath may occur if given with mitomycin

- therapy should be delayed until any radiation therapy is completed
- earlier onset and/or more severe neurotoxicity if given with itraconazole or fluconazole
- see also General Interactions of antineoplastic agents (p. 582)

Nursing points/Cautions

- ensure patient is well hydrated during therapy
- should not be diluted with solutions that raise or lower pH outside the range of 3.5–5.5
- protective clothing should be worn when handling patient urine or faeces for 4–7 days after administration
- may be given IV or into free-flowing IV infusion line
- caution is used in the elderly, those with neuromuscular disease or previous irradiation due to risk of neurotoxicity
- not recommended for CNS leukaemia as vincristine has poor blood–brain penetration
- contraindicated via SC, IM or IT route (fatal if given intrathecally)
- contraindicated in those with demyelinating Charcot-Marie-Tooth disease, hypersensitivity to mannitol or other vinca alkaloid, or who have received previous irradiation through ports that include the liver
- see also General Nursing points/Cautions for antineoplastic agents (p. 582)

Patient teaching and advice

- see General Patient teaching and advice for antineoplastic agents (p. 584)

VINFLUNINE (Javlor)

Available form
Vial: 25 mg/mL

Action
- fluorinated vinca alkaloid
- one active metabolite
- narrow therapeutic threshold

Use
- advanced or metastatic transitional cell urothelial tract cancer (after failure of platinum-based therapy)

Dose
- 320 mg/m^2 IV over 20 minutes every 3 weeks

Adverse effects
- severe constipation
- neuropathy
- QT interval prolongation
- posterior reversible encephalopathy syndrome (PRES)
- severe hyponatraemia, syndrome of inappropriate antidiuretic hormone secretion (SIADH)
- see also General Adverse effects of antineoplastic agents (p. 582)

Interactions
- caution if used with agents that are known to prolong QT interval or cause electrolyte imbalance (especially hypokalaemia and hypomagnesaemia)
- caution if used with opioids due to risk of constipation
- increased serum levels may occur if given with ritonavir, itraconazole and grapefruit juice and not recommended together
- decreased serum levels may occur if given with rifampicin and St John's wort
- increased serum level may occur if used with liposomal (liposomal) doxorubicin while decreasing doxorubicin efficacy

Nursing points/Cautions

- oral hydration, increased fibre intake and laxatives/faecal softeners are recommended during day 1 to 5 or 7

of treatment cycle to prevent constipation occurring
- administration of 100 mL (of 500 mL) sodium chloride 0.9% or glucose 5% to assess vein patency before starting infusion, then continued at 60–120 mL/hour during infusion, followed by remaining 250 mL at 300 mL/hour
- dilute with 100 mL sodium chloride 0.9% or glucose 5%
- not recommended via intrathecal administration or by IV push or bolus
- caution if used in those at risk of constipation including opioid use, prior abdominal surgery, peritoneal cancer or abdominal mass
- caution if used in those with cardiac disease, previous history of myocardial infarction or angina, congenital or acquired prolongation of QT interval or electrolyte imbalance
- contraindicated in those with hypersensitivity to other vinca alkaloids, within 2 weeks of severe infection, baseline absolute neutrophil count (ANC) $< 1.5 \times 10^9$/L (before first administration) or $< 1.0 \times 10^9$/L (subsequent administrations) or platelets $< 100 \times 10^9$/L
- see also General Nursing points/Cautions for antineoplastic agents (p. 582)

Patient teaching and advice

- advise patient to seek medical advice immediately if any of the following occur:
  - confusion, trouble thinking, memory loss, blurred vision, loss of vision, balance or walking problems, decreased strength in arms or legs
  - irregular heart rate
  - confusion, lethargy, altered consciousness
  - persistent constipation with swollen stomach and vomiting
- patient should be warned to avoid grapefruit and grapefruit juices during therapy
- see also General Patient teaching and advice for antineoplastic agents (p. 584)

VINORELBINE (Navelbine, Navelbine Oral)

Available forms

Vial: 10 mg/mL, 50 mg/5 mL; Capsules: 20 mg, 30 mg

Action

- vinca alkaloid that inhibit mitosis at metaphase
- active metabolite with activity greater than parent

Use

- advanced breast cancer (after failure of standard treatment) (as monotherapy or part of combination therapy)
- completely resected, stage 2B or greater non-small cell lung cancer (NSCLC) (with cisplatin)

Dose

- (advanced breast cancer, NSCLC) 60 mg/m^2 orally with food once weekly for 3 weeks, then increasing to 80 mg/m^2 **OR**
- (advanced breast cancer, NSCLC) 25–30 mg/m^2 slow IV bolus over 6–10 minutes or IV infusion over 20–30 minutes weekly (monotherapy) **OR**
- (advanced breast cancer, NSCLC) 25–30 mg/m^2 slow IV bolus over 6–10 minutes or IV infusion over 20–30 minutes on days 1 and 8, or days 1 and 5 every 3 weeks (combination therapy) **OR**
- (resected NSCLC) 25–30 mg/m^2 slow IV bolus over 6–10 minutes or IV infusion over 20–30 minutes weekly for 16 weeks (with cisplatin)

Adverse effects

- acute shortness of breath, severe bronchospasm
- peripheral neuropathy including numbness, paraesthesia
- jaw pain
- (uncommon) inappropriate secretion of antidiuretic hormone, hyponatraemia
- see also General Adverse effects of antineoplastic agents (p. 582)

Interactions

- contraindicated with yellow fever vaccine and not recommended with other live attenuated vaccines
- severe bronchospasm and acute shortness of breath may occur if given with mitomycin
- increased risk of neutropenia if given with lapatinib
- may decrease serum levels of phenytoin increasing risk of seizure activity
- if given with warfarin, INR should be closely monitored especially when starting or stopping therapy
- not recommended with itraconazole due to increased risk of neurotoxicity

Nursing points/Cautions

- premedication with antiemetic (e.g. ondansetron) is recommended before oral administration
- dilute before use (50 mL for bolus, 125 mL for infusion) and give by slow IV bolus over 6–10 minutes or short infusion over 20–30 minutes (Navelbine)
- should not be diluted using alkaline solution as precipitation will occur
- not recommended SC, IM or IT (fatal if given intrathecally)
- contraindicated in those with vinca alkaloid hypersensitivity or requiring long-term oxygen therapy
- see also General Nursing points/Cautions for antineoplastic agents (p. 582)

Patient teaching and advice

- instruct patient that capsules should be swallowed whole with food, not chewed, sucked or opened
- advise patient if capsules are opened, hands should be thoroughly washed with saline or normal saline
- patient should be advised to seek medical advice immediately if any of the following occur:
  - tingling or numbness of extremities
  - ongoing shortness of breath
- see also General Patient teaching and advice for antineoplastic agents (p. 584)

VISMODEGIB (Erivedge)

Available form

Capsules: 150 mg

Action

- Hedgehog pathway inhibitor that blocks genes responsible for cell proliferation, survival and differentiation
- half-life 4 days

Use

- metastatic or locally invasive basal cell carcinoma (where surgery or other treatment was ineffective or inappropriate)

Dose

- 150 mg orally daily until disease progression or unacceptable toxicity

Adverse effects

- severe skin reactions
- see also General Adverse effects of antineoplastic agents (p. 582)

Interactions

- caution if given with statins

Nursing points/Cautions

- pregnancy should be excluded using pregnancy test 7 days before starting

therapy. Pregnancy test should be done monthly during therapy
- see also General Nursing points/Cautions for antineoplastic agents (p. 582)

Patient teaching and advice

- patient should be advised to seek medical advice if any rash or skin blistering occurs
- advise patient to avoid making semen, blood or blood product donation during therapy and for 24 months after last dose
- female patient of childbearing potential should be counselled to use two reliable contraceptive methods during therapy and for 24 months after last dose to avoid pregnancy. Patient should be advised to seek medical advice immediately if pregnancy occurs
- see also General Patient teaching and advice for antineoplastic agents (p. 584)

VORINOSTAT (Zolinza)

Available form

Capsules: 100 mg

Action

- histone deacetylase inhibitor (HDAI) 1, 2, 3 and 6

Use

- cutaneous manifestations of cutaneous T cell lymphoma (progressive, persistent, recurrent disease despite treatment)

Dose

- 400 mg orally daily with food, decreasing dose to 300 mg daily or 300 mg daily for 5 consecutive days if intolerance occurs

Adverse effects

- (rare) hyperglycaemia, thromboembolism
- See General Adverse effects of antineoplastic agents (p. 582)

Interactions

- caution if used with warfarin, therefore INR should be closely monitored, especially when starting or stopping therapy
- not recommended with sodium valproate and related agents due to increased risk of adverse effects

Nursing points/Cautions

- ensure patient is well hydrated and any vomiting or diarrhoea is corrected before starting therapy
- full blood count and electrolytes including electrolytes, glucose and serum creatinine should be measured every 2 weeks for first 8 weeks, then monthly during therapy
- caution if used in those with previous history of thromboembolic events
- contraindicated in those with severe liver impairment

Patient teaching and advice

- instruct patient to drink at least 2 L of fluid per day to prevent dehydration
- if patient has diabetes, blood glucose levels should be monitored closely during therapy
- advise patient to seek medical advice immediately if any of the following occur:
  - swelling of leg/calf, pain/tenderness in calf/leg, redness, warmth
  - excessive diarrhoea or vomiting
- see also General Patient teaching and advice for antineoplastic agents (p. 584)

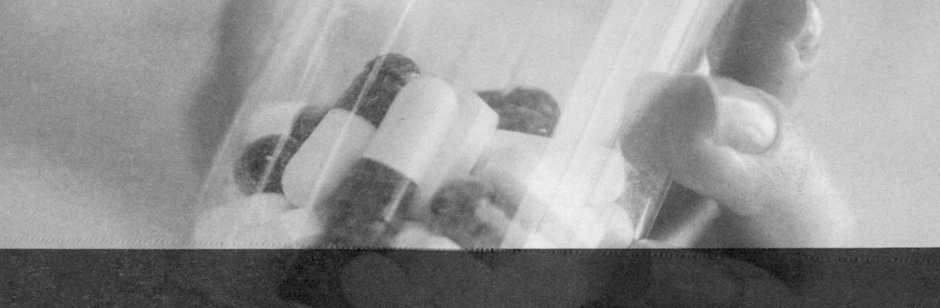

ANTINEOPLASTIC SUPPORT AGENTS

This section contains a heterogenous (diverse) group of agents that are used during or after therapy with antineoplastic agents. Other agents that fulfil a similar supportive role are found in Antiemetic agents (p. 365) and Haemopoietic agents (p. 1118).

AMIFOSTINE (Ethyol)

Available form

Vial: 500 mg

Action

- organic thiophosphate which selectively protects healthy tissues (not tumours) against ionising radiation and alkylating agents
- prodrug, converted to active metabolite
- elimination half-life less than 10 minutes

Use

- decrease neutropenia-related fever and infection induced by alkylating agents
- decrease acute and cumulative nephrotoxicity caused by platinum-based therapy
- protect against acute and late xerostomia associated with radiation therapy for head and neck cancer

Dose

- (before chemotherapy) 740–910 mg/m^2 daily by IV infusion over 15 minutes, 30 minutes before chemotherapy **OR**
- (before radiotherapy) 200 mg/m^2 daily by slow IV push over 3 minutes, 15–30 minutes before radiotherapy

Adverse effects

- hypotension
- dizziness, somnolence
- hiccups, sneezing, cough
- nausea, vomiting, diarrhoea
- rash, pruritus, dermatitis
- diplopia, blurred vision
- flushing, feeling of warmth, chills
- injection site reactions
- (rare) allergic reaction, severe cutaneous reactions, arrhythmias, seizures, hypocalcaemia (usually with multiple doses within 24 hours), transient hypertension

Interactions

- hypotension may be potentiated if given with antihypertensive agents
- caution if given with any agent that can cause seizures

Nursing points/Cautions

- patient should be well hydrated before and during infusion and nursed supine throughout the infusion to decrease risk of hypotension

- before starting therapy, patient should be closely assessed for the appearance of any rash (other than at radiation or injection site) and therapy not commenced if rash exists
- cutaneous reaction can occur for up to 10 days after administration
- BP should be monitored before starting and at 5-minute intervals throughout therapy and therapy stopped if systolic BP decreases significantly (20–50 mmHg, depending on baseline pressure). If patient is asymptomatic and systolic BP returns to normal within 5 minutes, infusion may be restarted
- hypotension can be reversed by postural changes and infusion of fluids (sodium chloride 0.9%)
- if full dose cannot be given because of hypotension, further therapy is at lower dosage
- serum calcium levels should be monitored in patients at risk of hypocalcaemia and calcium supplements given if needed
- antihypertensive agents should be stopped for 24 hours before starting therapy
- when chemotherapy is known to be strongly emetogenic (e.g. cisplatin), dexamethasone 20 mg IV and $5HT_3$ antagonist should be given with amifostine and fluid balance should be closely monitored
- prophylactic antiemetics are also recommended before radiotherapy
- (chemotherapy) risk of adverse effects is greater if infusion is given over more than 15 minutes
- reconstitute using 9.7 mL sodium chloride 0.9% and then dilute further with 100–250 mL for infusion. Further dilution is not required if administered before radiotherapy
- should be administered alone
- caution if used in those with pre-existing cardiovascular or cerebrovascular conditions or kidney insufficiency (especially if other risk factors such as vomiting, dehydration or severe hypotension exist or if patient is over 60 years)
- contraindicated in those with sensitivity to aminothiol preparations, hypotension, dehydration, renal/liver impairment, children, and adults over 70 years

Patient teaching and advice

- patient should be advised to seek medical advice immediately if any rash appears (even up to 10 days after therapy)
- warn patient against driving or operating machinery if blurred or double vision, hypotension or dizziness are ongoing
- see also General Patient teaching and advice (p. xxvii)

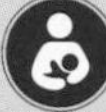

not recommended during pregnancy and breastfeeding

MESNA (Uromitexan)

Available forms

Tablets: 400 mg, 600 mg; Ampoules: 400 mg/mL, 1 g/10 mL

Action

- synthetic sulfhydryl detoxifying agent that is rapidly transported to the kidneys where it detoxifies urotoxic compounds; however, does not protect against renal toxicity

Use

- reduce and prevent haemorrhagic cystitis caused by oxazaphosphorine alkylating agents (ifosfamide, cyclophosphamide)

Dose

- (intermittent alkylating agent therapy) 40% of alkylating agent dose orally 2 hours before alkylating agent therapy and repeated at 2 and 6 hours **OR**

- (intermittent alkylating agent therapy) initially 20% of alkylating agent dose IV with alkylating agent therapy, followed by oral dose (40% of alkylating agent) given at 2 and 6 hours **OR**
- initially 40% of ifosfamide orally at completion of alkylating agent infusion, repeated at 2 and 6 hours **OR**
- initially 20% of alkylating agent IV over 15–30 minutes with alkylating agent therapy, then same dose repeated IV at 4 and 8 hours (total 3 doses)

Adverse effects

- anorexia, nausea, vomiting, diarrhoea, constipation, bad taste in mouth, flatulence, abdominal pain
- headache, fatigue, dizziness, somnolence
- limb pain, arthralgia, back pain
- flushing, fever, rigors, flu-like symptoms
- pharyngitis, cough
- (rare) allergic reaction, severe skin reactions,
- IV site reaction

Interactions

- may cause false positive to ketones, ascorbic acid (vitamin C) or erythrocytes on urinary dipstick

Nursing points/Cautions

- if patient is vomiting or treated with high-dose cyclophosphamide with total body irradiation, oral dose should be replaced with IV dose
- urine output should be maintained at 100 mL/hour
- urine should be checked daily (morning) for protein and blood before starting therapy with ifosfamide or cyclophosphamide. If haematuria develops despite therapy, dose of ifosfamide or cyclophosphamide should be decreased or stopped (depending on severity of haematuria)
- repeated with each administration of alkylating agent
- (IV) incompatible with cisplatin, epirubicin, carboplatin and nitrogen mustard
- can be diluted with glucose 5%, sodium chloride 0.9% or lactated Ringer's solution to give concentration 1.5–3 mg/mL and then administered over 15–30 minutes
- if patient has history of urinary tract lesions, previous cystitis related to ifosfamide or cyclophosphamide or irradiation of small pelvis, an increased dose and/or shorter interval may be required as there is a high risk of haemorrhagic cystitis
- caution if given to those with autoimmune diseases because there is an increased risk of anaphylactic reaction. Medical supervision and readily available resuscitation equipment is recommended
- contraindicated in those with hypersensitivity to thiols (e.g. penicillamine, captopril, amifostine)

Patient teaching and advice

- patient should be advised to avoid driving or operating machinery if dizziness, light-headedness or tiredness are ongoing problems
- see also General Patient teaching and advice (p. xxvii)

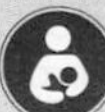

should only be used during pregnancy or breastfeeding if benefits outweigh potential risks

METHOXSALEN (Uvadex)

Available form

Vial: 200 microgram

Action

- on activation by exposure to UVA light, methoxsalen binds to pyrimidine bases of nucleic acids causing a covalent bond between 2 DNA strands; stops proliferation of lymphocytes

- also suppresses photo-treated T cells
- used with Therakos Cellex photopheresis system, which provides UV light to activate methoxsalen

Use

- extracorporeal (ECP) administration with Therakos Cellex photopheresis system for management of:
  - steroid-refractory or steroid-intolerant chronic graft versus host disease (cGvHD) after allogenic stem cell transplant
  - palliative treatment of skin manifestations of cutaneous T-cell lymphoma (CTCL) that is unresponsive to other treatments

Dose

- dose is calculated according to volume of plasma that is collected in photoactivation bag (displayed on side of photopheresis instrument): Treatment volume × 0.017 mL = dose
- (cGvHD) 3 ECP treatments in first week, followed by 2 treatments per week for at least 12 weeks (or as clinically indicated) **OR**
- (CTCL) 2 ECP treatments on 2 successive days each month for 6 months, increasing to 2 treatments on 2 successive days every 2 weeks for 12 weeks if skin scores improve after 8 treatments

Adverse effects

- (cGvHD) diarrhoea, nausea, headache, hypertension, sinus/upper respiratory tract infection, fatigue, fever, cough, dyspnoea, anaemia
- (CTCL) nausea, vomiting, hypotension, infection, transient fever, vascular access complication, headache
- (rare) cataract formation, pulmonary embolism, deep vein thrombosis, allergic reaction

Interactions

- may decrease clearance of caffeine
- decreases activation of paracetamol
- phenytoin may increase metabolism of methoxsalen reducing levels
- caution if given with other medications which may cause sensitivity to light, such as ciprofloxacin, cyclopropamide, doxycycline, haloperidol, isotretinoin, nalidixic acid, and some diuretics

Nursing points/Cautions

- should only be administered by medical practitioners trained and experienced in photopheresis
- patient should be informed of risks before starting procedure, especially risk of ocular damage
- photopheresis collection bag should be visually inspected for any signs of haemolysis
- not injected directly into patient
- photopheresis should only be performed where medical emergency equipment is available, as well as volume replacement fluids or volume expanders
- during therapy, patient's eyes should be protected from UVA light by wearing wrap-around UVA-opaque sunglasses
- photopheresis instrument operating manual should be consulted before starting procedure
- (ECP) process involves patient being attached to photopheresis system via a catheter. RBCs are separated from WBCs and plasma with the RBCs and excess plasma returned to patient. The leukocyte-enriched blood and some plasma is collected in the photoactivation bag on the side of the instrument. This instrument shows the volume collected, which is used to calculate the dose required for each session. Methoxsalen is injected into the photoactivation bag followed by the leucocyte-enriched blood circulating

through the photoactivation unit, exposing it to UVA light. At the end of the photoactivation, the cells are reinfused into the patient over 15–20 minutes with the whole procedure taking up to 3 hours
- should not be diluted
- should be injected into photopheresis system as soon as drawn up into syringe and discarded if not used with 1 hour
- monitoring of albumin, calcium, haematocrit, haemoglobin, potassium and RBC count is recommended during therapy
- (CTCL) an adequate response is a 25% improvement in skin score that is maintained for at least 4 weeks. Skin scores are calculated based on the severity of lesions in each of 29 body sections, percentage surface area to obtain a regional score, followed by adding all regional scores for an overall lesion score
- (CTCL) number of sessions should not exceed 20 in 6 months
- caution if used in those with liver disease, alcoholism, epilepsy or brain injury/disease due to ethanol content (40.55 mg/mL)
- caution if used in those with liver impairment as prolonged photosensitivity may occur
- not recommended in those who have diseases with sensitivity to light such as porphyria, systemic lupus erythematosus or albinism
- contraindicated in those with hypersensitivity to methoxsalen or psoralen compounds or with co-existing melanoma, basal cell or squamous cell carcinoma or aphakia (absence of eye lens)
- photopheresis procedure is contraindicated in those with photosensitive disease, coagulation disorders, previous splenectomy, WBC > 25,000 mm^3, or if unable to tolerate extracorporeal volume loss (e.g. severe anaemia, severe cardiac disease)

Patient teaching and advice

- advise patient not to drive or operate machinery after photopheresis session
- patient should be instructed to:
  - wear sunglasses for 24 hours after therapy (in addition to during therapy)
  - avoid exposure to sun in 24 after therapy to previous burn injury and premature skin aging
- men and women of childbearing potential should be counselled to used adequate contraception during and after completion of therapy
- see General Patient teaching and advice (p. xxvii)

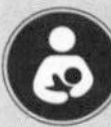

may cause fetal harm if given during therapy and is therefore not recommended

contraindicated during breastfeeding

SAMARIUM (153Sm) (SAMARIUM) LEXIDRONAM (Quadramet)

Available form

Vial: 6 GBq/3 mL

Action

- anti-inflammatory radiopharmaceutical which has an affinity for skeletal tissue concentrating in areas of bone turnover
- accumulates in areas where lesion to normal bone ratio is about 5:1
- rapidly cleared from the blood

Use

- relief of bone pain due to confirmed osteoblastic skeletal metastases

Dose

- 37 MBq/kg as IV bolus over 1 minute

Adverse effects

- myelosuppression (including decreased haemoglobin, WBC and platelet counts), thrombocytopenia

- lymphadenopathy
- haematuria, epistaxis, ecchymosis, purpura
- rash
- arrhythmia, hypertension, chest pain
- flare reactions (worsening of pain)
- dizziness
- cough, bronchitis
- infection, fever, chills
- diarrhoea, nausea, vomiting, abdominal pain, oral thrush
- spinal cord compression

Interactions

- contraindicated with chemotherapy or external beam radiation therapy

Nursing points/Cautions

- bone metastases should be confirmed by bone scan before starting therapy
- blood counts should be monitored 2-weekly after administration for at least 8 weeks until bone marrow function has adequately recovered
- any conditions requiring urgent surgical intervention (e.g. pathological fracture, impending spinal cord compression) should be excluded prior to starting therapy
- treatment should be in a facility where appropriate shielding is available to minimise radiation exposure to other patients and staff
- bone marrow should be allowed to recover before any therapy with chemotherapy or external beam radiation therapy is started or restarted
- repeat administration should be based on patient's previous response to therapy, current symptoms and haematological status
- therapy should not be repeated within 8 weeks of previous administration and only when blood counts (including WBC and platelets) have recovered
- patient should be encouraged to drink at least 500 mL fluid before administration. If patient cannot take fluids orally, IV administration is recommended
- patient should be encouraged to void as often as possible post-administration to reduce bladder exposure to radiation
- if patient is incontinent, bladder catheterisation is recommended post-administration to decrease risk of radiation contamination of patient's environment, including clothing and bed linen
- urinary excretion is usually complete in 6 hours
- product is supplied frozen and should not be used if thawed when received. Vial should be allowed to thaw and administered within 8 hours
- administer alone, as calcium is present in solution which may cause precipitation to occur if mixed with other solutions
- patient dose should be measured using suitable radioactivity calibration system (e.g. radioisotope dose calibrator) immediately before administration. Accurate dose calibration can be done using dose calibrator (available from manufacturer)
- there are currently no Australian standards or guidelines regarding patient discharge from hospital post-administration. United States regulations recommend discharge when external exposure is < 0.05 mSv/hour at a distance of 1 metre (however, generally large doses of about 8 GBq are needed to achieve this exposure)
- storage and disposal of radioactive waste should be carried out in accordance with ARPANSA 'Code of practice for the disposal of radioactive wastes by the user'
- if patient has compromised bone marrow reserve from disease or previous treatment(s), therapy should only be

given if potential benefit is greater than risks, otherwise is not recommended
- contraindicated in those with severe bone marrow depression
- contraindicated in those with hypersensitivity to phosphonates similar to ethylenediamine tetramethylene phosphonic acid (EDTMP)

Patient teaching and advice

- warn patient that bone pain may initially worsen within 3 days of therapy, but this usually passes quickly and is controllable with analgesics
- female patient of childbearing potential should be counselled to use adequate contraception during therapy to avoid pregnancy

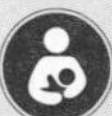

may cause harm to fetus if given during pregnancy, therefore should be avoided

not recommended during breastfeeding

TELOTRISTAT ETHYL (Xermelo)

Available form

Tablets: 250 mg

Action

- telotristat ethyl is a prodrug converted to active metabolite telotristat which inhibits serotonin synthesis
- neuroendocrine tumours can cause too much serotonin to be released into the bloodstream, resulting in symptoms such as diarrhoea, abdominal pain, skin flushing, hypotension, rash and weight loss (referred to as carcinoid syndrome)
- by reducing serotonin production, symptoms of carcinoid syndrome are lessened
- terminal half-life is about 11 hours

Use

- carcinoid syndrome diarrhoea (in combination with somastatin analogues (lanreotide or octreotide))

Dose

- 250 mg orally 3 times daily with food

Adverse effects

- constipation, abdominal pain, decreased appetite, flatulence
- elevated liver enzymes
- fatigue, headache
- fever
- peripheral oedema
- depression, depressed mood

Interactions

- if given with octreotide, octreotide should be given at least 30 minutes before telotristat
- loperamide may decrease formation of active telotristat
- may decrease efficacy of amilodipine, atorvastatin, bupropion, carbamazepine, ciclosporin, diltazem, ethinylestradiol, everolimus, felodipine, midazolam, nifedipine, sertraline, simvastatin, sodium valproate, sunitinib, topiramate, verapamil

Nursing points/Cautions

- liver enzymes should be monitored before starting and during therapy, especially if there is any liver impairment present. If liver injury occurs, therapy should be stopped and not restarted until liver enzymes return to normal
- therapy should be reassessed if clinical response is not achieved within 12 weeks
- caution if used in those with mild-to-moderate kidney impairment
- not recommended in those with severe kidney impairment, end-stage renal failure requiring dialysis or severe liver impairment

Patient teaching and advice

- advise patient not to take double dose if a dose is missed. The subsequent dose should be taken at next scheduled time

- suggest patient take tablet with food, preferably high-fat meal, to improve absorption
- patient should be instructed to drink sufficient water and eat fibre-containing foods to decrease constipation
- warn patient not to drive or operate machinery if fatigue occurs
- patient should be advised to seek medical attention if any of the following occur:
  - nausea, dark urine, yellow skin or eyes, fatigue/tiredness, upper right abdominal pain
  - feelings of sadness or depression
- counsel women of childbearing potential to use effective contraception during therapy to prevent pregnancy occurring
- see General Patient teaching and advice (p. xxvii)

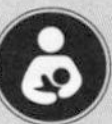

not recommended during pregnancy or breastfeeding

tablet can be crushed and mixed with water or spoonful of yoghurt or apple puree

GRANULOCYTE COLONY STIMULATING FACTOR (G-CSF)

General Actions of G-CSF

- recombinant human granulocyte colony-stimulating factor (G-CSF), which regulates production and release of neutrophils from bone marrow through action on progenitor (stem) cells

General Uses of G-CSF

- decrease incidence and duration of severe neutropenia (and associated infection) after chemotherapy
- reversal of neutropenia and maintenance of neutrophil counts with antiviral and/or myelosuppressive agents in those with HIV
- severe chronic neutropenia
- mobilisation of peripheral blood progenitor cells (PBPC) for autologous or allogenic bone marrow transplantation
- mobilisation of peripheral blood progenitor cells (PBPC) for allogenic peripheral blood stem cell transplantation in normal volunteers
- after autologous or allogenic bone marrow transplant
- decrease incidence of infection after myelosuppressive therapy in non-myeloid malignancy

General Adverse effects of G-CSF

- splenomegaly
- mild-to-moderate medullary bone pain, back pain, myalgia, arthralgia, pain in extremities
- headache, fatigue, malaise, asthenia, dizziness
- fever
- anorexia, diarrhoea, constipation, stomatitis, abdominal pain
- cough, haemoptysis
- alopecia
- rash, exacerbation of pre-existing skin conditions (e.g. psoriasis)
- leucocytosis, thrombocytopenia, anaemia
- injection site reaction
- reversible elevation of levels of uric acid, lactate dehydrogenase and alkaline phosphatase
- (uncommon) haematuria, proteinuria

- (children with chronic severe neutropenia) osteopenia, osteoporosis, decreased bone density
- (rare) adult respiratory distress syndrome (ARDS), rupture of spleen, hypersensitivity, sickle cell crisis, acute febrile dermatosis (Sweet's syndrome), aortitis, pulmonary haemorrhage, pulmonary infiltrates, glomerulonephritis
- (very rare) capillary leak syndrome, cutaneous vasculitis

General Interactions of G-CSF

- caution if used with agents known to lower platelet count
- may affect results of bone imaging scans

General Nursing points/Cautions for G-CSF

- (severe chronic neutropenia) diagnosis should be confirmed before starting therapy and other causes of neutropenia eliminated. Before starting therapy, serial blood count (with differential and platelet count) and bone marrow evaluation (morphology and karyotype) should be performed
- trade name should be recorded in patient history
- not recommended with or within 24 hours of chemotherapy
- allow to come to room temperature before use
- avoid vigorous shaking (shaking should be avoided as it will denature protein)
- contraindicated in those with known hypersensitivity to *Escherichia coli*-derived proteins or G-CSF-related products

General Patient teaching and advice for G-CSF

- warn patient against driving or operating machinery if dizziness is problematic
- patient should be advised to immediately seek medical advice if any of the following occur:
  - pain in shoulder tip or left upper abdominal quadrant
  - unexplained cough, fever, coughing blood or blood-stained sputum, and difficulty breathing (dyspnoea). Chest X-ray is recommended if these symptoms occur
  - fever or painful skin lesions (on arms or legs, sometimes face and neck)
  - blood in urine
- warn patient that mild-to-moderate bone pain commonly occurs at the start of therapy and is controlled with non-opioid analgesics
- see General Patient teaching and advice (p. xxvii)

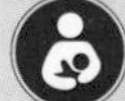

not recommended during pregnancy unless benefits outweigh risks

caution if used during breastfeeding

FILGRASTIM (Neupogen, Nivestim, Zarzio)

Available forms

Vial: 120 microgram/0.2 mL, 300 microgram/mL, 480 microgram/1.6 mL, 480 microgram/0.8 mL; Prefilled syringe: 300 microgram/0.5 mL, 480 microgram/0.5 mL

Action

- see General Actions of G-CSF (p. 722)
- effects reversed within 24 hours of stopping therapy and neutrophils return to normal within 4 days

Use

- see General Uses of G-CSF (p. 722)

Dose

- (cancer patients receiving standard chemotherapy; induction/consolidation chemotherapy for acute myeloid leukaemia) 5 microgram/kg/day SC daily **OR**
- (patients with non-myeloid malignancy after chemotherapy) 5 microgram/kg/day SC or as IV infusion over 15–30 minutes for up to 2 weeks until absolute neutrophil count (ANC) $> 1 \times 10^9$ for 3 consecutive days or 10×10^9/L for 1 day after chemotherapy **OR**
- (patients with non-myeloid malignancy after high-dose toxic chemotherapy with autologous/allogenic bone marrow or peripheral stem cell transplantation) initially 10 microgram/kg/day by SC/IV infusion over 4–24 hours, then increase, decrease or stop infusion depending on ANC **OR**
- (patients with myeloid malignancy after high-dose toxic chemotherapy with autologous/allogenic bone marrow or peripheral progenitor cell transplantation) 5 microgram/kg/day following transplant (24 hours after infusion of bone marrow or progenitor cells or cytotoxic therapy) until neutrophil count recovers (up to 28 days) **OR**
- (autologous progenitor cell collection and therapy) 10 microgram/kg/day daily SC or 24-hour infusion for at least 4 days before first leukapheresis, and continued until last day of leukapheresis. Stem cell collection occurs on day 5 and on consecutive days until sufficient cells have been collected **OR**
- (autologous stem cell collection and therapy after myelosuppressive chemotherapy) 5 microgram/kg/day SC daily starting 24 hours after chemotherapy until neutrophil count has returned to normal range. Leukapheresis can start when ANC $> 5 \times 10^9$/L and occurs on consecutive days until sufficient cells are collected **OR**
- (autologous stem cell collection from normal donor) 10 microgram/kg/day SC for 4–5 consecutive days and leukapheresis starting on day 5 and 6 to collect required amount of cells **OR**
- (congenital severe chronic neutropenia) 12 microgram/kg SC daily or in divided doses **OR**
- (idiopathic/cyclic severe chronic neutropenia) 5 microgram/kg SC daily or in divided doses **OR**
- (HIV infection) initially 1 microgram/kg/day SC daily, increasing gradually to 5 microgram/kg/day until neutrophil count is achieved and maintained (ANC $\geq 2 \times 10^9$/L), then 300 microgram daily SC 3 times per week, adjusting dose if necessary

Adverse effects

- see General Adverse effects of G-CSF (p. 722)

Interactions

- see General Interactions of G-CSF (p. 723)

Nursing points/Cautions

- brands (e.g. Neupogen, Zarzio) should not be substituted without seeking medical advice first
- patient may be taught to self-administer using prefilled syringe
- (patient with HIV infection) absolute neutrophil count (ANC) is recommended during first 2–3 days, then twice weekly for 2 weeks, then weekly
- (peripheral blood progenitor cell (PBPC) collection and therapy) neutrophil count should be monitored 4 days after start of therapy, then regular full blood count (including platelet count) is recommended at

least 3 times weekly after infusion of PBPCs until haemopoietic recovery. If leucocyte count rises above 100 × 109/L, therapy should be stopped

- (stem cell collection) prolonged therapy with some chemotherapy agents (e.g. carboplatin, carmustine and melphalan) may decrease stem cell yield
- (chronic neutropenia) full blood count (with differential) is recommended during initial 4 weeks of therapy and for 2 weeks after any dose adjustment, then monthly for 12 months when patient is clinically stable. If patient has congenital neutropenia, annual bone marrow evaluation is also recommended during therapy
- (cancer patient receiving myelosuppressive therapy) full blood count (with differential, platelet count and haematocrit) is recommended before chemotherapy and then twice weekly during filgrastim therapy
- premature discontinuation of therapy is not recommended
- urinalysis should be conducted regularly during therapy
- for IV or SC infusion, dilute with 25–50 mL glucose 5%. If dilution concentration < 15 microgram/mL, adsorption to plastic may occur. This can be overcome by using albumin (human) to a final concentration of 2 mg/mL
- dilution to < 5 microgram/mL is not recommended
- insertion of CVC line should be avoided
- incompatible with sodium chloride 0.9% as precipitation will occur
- (patients with non-myeloid malignancy after high-dose toxic chemotherapy with autologous/allogenic bone marrow or peripheral stem cell transplantation) if absolute neutrophil count (ANC) > 1 × 10^9/L for 3 consecutive days, dose should be decreased to 5 microgram/kg/day, then discontinue if ANC remains at that level for 3 consecutive days. If ANC < 1 × 10^9/L, infusion can be resumed at 5 microgram/kg/day. If ANC < 1 × 10^9/L during infusion of 5 microgram/kg/day, dose should be increased to 10 microgram/kg/day
- needle shield contains latex, which may cause reaction in latex-sensitive individuals
- caution if used in those with sickle cell disease or trait (as sickle cell crisis may occur) or if used with chemoradiotherapy
- see also Nursing points/Cautions for G-CSF (p. 723)

Patient teaching and advice

- if patient is going to administer SC, education should include:
  - not administering within 24 hours of chemotherapy, radiotherapy, bone marrow transplant or stem cell transplant
  - injection is under the skin (subcutaneous injection)
  - importance of changing injection sites, including thighs and abdomen, but avoiding navel and waistline
  - not injecting into areas that are red or swollen, into muscle or into the same spot
  - not stopping abruptly or without seeking medical advice
- correct technique, such as:
  - wash and dry hands before start of procedure
  - check name and strength of medication and expiry date (and not using if after expiry date)
  - do not use solution if it is cloudy or coloured, or contains lumps or flakes

  - allow prefilled syringe to come to room temperature before use (about 00 minutes) (not in direct sunlight or using any method, such as hot water or microwave, to warm solution)
  - do not shake solution/syringes. If solution is frothy or bubbly, it should be allowed to sit for a few minutes for froth/bubbles to settle
  - do not mix with any other medications or dilute
  - remove needle cover, taking care not to touch exposed needle
  - check the dose prescribed and find the correct volume mark on syringe barrel, and then carefully push plunger until grey upper edge of plunger reaches correct volume (this will get rid of excess fluid and air)
  - clean area with alcoholic swab and allow to dry
  - pinch skin firmly between thumb and finger
  - push prefilled syringe firmly against pinched skin (at 45–90° angle) and inject
  - withdraw needle, press site gently after injection with cotton wool swab to prevent bleeding, but do not rub
  - do not recap needle after use
- correct storage
  - store in fridge, but can remain at room temperature for up to 3 days before use
  - do not freeze
- disposal of used equipment
  - do not reuse needles or syringes
  - do not dispose of syringes and needles in the normal household rubbish
  - use puncture-resistant sharps container to dispose of used needles and syringes
  - container should be disposed of as instructed by doctor, pharmacist or nurse
- see also General Patient teaching and advice for G-CSF (p. 720)

LENOGRASTIM (Granocyte)

Available forms

Vial: 13.4 × 10^6 IU (105 microgram) (Granocyte 13), 33.6 × 10^6 IU (263 microgram) (Granocyte 34)

Action

- see General Actions of G-CSF (p. 722)

Use

- see General Uses of G-CSF (p. 722)

Dose

- (peripheral blood progenitor cell mobilisation after chemotherapy) 5 microgram/kg daily SC starting day after completing chemotherapy until neutrophil count returns to normal, usually 8–14 days **OR**
- (peripheral blood progenitor cell mobilisation alone) 10 microgram (1.28 million IU)/kg daily SC injection for 4–6 days with leukapheresis performed between days 5 and 7 **OR**
- (bone marrow transplantation and post-peripheral blood progenitor cell reinfusion) 5 microgram/kg SC (or IV infusion over 30 minutes post-bone marrow transplantation) daily, starting day after reinfusion of stem cells until neutrophil count returns to normal **OR**
- (peripheral blood progenitor cell mobilisation in healthy donors) 10 microgram/kg daily SC for 5–6 days allowing collection of sufficient stem cells **OR**
- (severe chronic neutropenia) 5 microgram/kg daily SC until neutrophil count recovers **OR**
- (after established chemotherapy) 5 microgram/kg daily SC starting day after completing chemotherapy until neutrophil count returns to normal, usually 8–14 days

Adverse effects
- see General Adverse effects of G-CSF (p. 722)

Nursing points/Cautions
- Granocyte 34 is recommended for patients with body surface area up to 18 m^2, while Granocyte 13 is for those with surface area up to 0.7 m^2
- to reconstitute add 1 mL of water for injections and gently swirl, avoiding vigorous shaking
- no more than 1 mL should be given per SC site
- if given IV, reconstituted solution should be further diluted with glucose 5% or sodium chloride 0.9%
- contraindicated in those with myeloid malignancy
- see also General Nursing points/Cautions for G-CSF (p. 723)

Patient teaching and advice
- see General Patient teaching and advice for G-CSF (p. 723)

LIPEGFILGRASTIM (Lonquex)

Available form
Prefilled syringe: 6 mg/mL

Action
- see General Actions of G-CSF (p. 722)
- sustained form of filgrastim (p. 723)

Use
- decrease incidence and duration of neutropenia in patients treated with chemotherapy

Dose
- 6 mg SC once per chemotherapy cycle

Adverse effects
- hypokalaemia
- see also General Adverse effects of G-CSF (p. 722)

Interactions
- see General Interactions of G-CSF (p. 723)

Nursing points/Cautions
- serum potassium levels should be monitored for hypokalaemia
- contains sorbitol
- see also General Nursing points/Cautions for filgrastim and G-CSF (p. 723)

Patient teaching and advice
- see General Patient teaching and advice for filgrastim and G-CSF (p. 723)

PEGFILGRASTIM (Fulphila, Neulasta Syringe with Automatic Needle Guard, Pelgraz, Ristempa, Tezmota, Ziextenzo)

Available form
Prefilled syringe: 6 mg/0.6 mL

Action
- see General Actions of G-CSF (p. 722)
- long-acting form which has been combined with polyethylene glycol (PEG) molecule reducing renal clearance and prolonging persistence compared to filgrastim (p. 723)

Use
- cancer patients following chemotherapy to decrease duration of severe neutropenia to reduce incidence of infection

Dose
- 6 mg SC once per cycle given 24 hours after chemotherapy

Adverse effects
- see General Adverse effects of G-CSF (p. 722)

Interactions
- see General Interactions of G-CSF (p. 723)

Nursing points/Cautions
- can be given 14 days before chemotherapy

- contraindicated in those with hypersensitivity to filgrastim, polyethylene glycol or *E. coli*-derived proteins
- see also General Nursing points/ Cautions for G-CSF (p. 723)

Patient teaching and advice

- if patient is going to administer SC, education should include points for filgrastim patient teaching and education (p. 725), with the following differences:
  - pull grey needle cap straight out and away from your body
  - pinch skin firmly between thumb and finger
  - insert needle into skin and push plunger slowly until person feels or hears a 'snap' and continue to push all the way down through snap (this is important to ensure full dose)
  - withdraw needle (after releasing plunger, prefilled syringe safety guard will cover injection needle) and press site gently after injection with cotton wool swab to prevent bleeding, but do not rub
  - remove and save label from prefilled syringe
- see also General Patient teaching and advice for G-CSF (p. 723)

ANTI-PARKINSON'S AGENTS

In 1817 James Parkinson described what would become known as Parkinson's disease (PD), and which is now the second most common age-related neurodegenerative disease, behind Alzheimer's disease. Parkinson's disease results from degeneration of the dopaminergic neurons in the substantia nigra, leading to decreased dopamine concentrations in the brain. Other neurons (cholinergic, serotonin, norepinephrine, olfactory) also degenerate, accounting for the non-dopaminergic symptoms. Symptoms of Parkinsonism become evident when more than 80% of the neurons have degenerated. In most cases, the cause of Parkinson's disease is unknown; however, early onset Parkinson's disease is thought to run in families. Secondary Parkinsonism has been associated with some drugs (particularly antipsychotic agents, metoclopramide, chlorpromazine, lithium) and also infection, tumour, trauma, stroke or exposure to neurotoxins (e.g. carbon monoxide, manganese) (Olanow et al 2019).

The four cardinal features of PD are tremor at rest, rigidity/stiffness, bradykinesia (slowing) and gait dysfunction with postural instability. Other motor symptoms include reduced eye blinking, drooling, soft voice, difficulty swallowing, handwriting becoming progressively smaller and cramped, reduced facial expression and freezing (a sudden but temporary inability to move) (Olanow et al 2019). Non-motor features of PD (thought to be due to the degeneration of non-dopaminergic neurons) include loss of smell, sensory disturbance, mood disorders (e.g. depression (which is very common in PD), anxiety, panic attacks), sleep disturbances (e.g. fragmented, sleep apnoea), orthostatic hypotension, GI (e.g. decreased gastric motility, constipation) and genitourinary disturbances, sexual dysfunction and mild cognitive impairment, which may progress to dementia (Olanow et al 2019).

Management of PD may involve:

- *pharmacological treatment* – based on restoring the supply of dopamine to the brain
- *management of non-motor and non-dopaminergic features* – this includes management of anxiety, panic attacks, depression, sweating, sensory issues, freezing and constipation. Other issues can include sleep disturbances, psychosis and dementia
- *non-pharmacological therapy* – involves aids to increase stability and

reduce the risk of falling, such as canes and walkers; exercise to maintain and improve function; access to support groups for both patient and carer

- *surgical treatment* – ablative surgery involves destroying small areas of brain tissue responsible for abnormal activity. This has largely been replaced by deep brain stimulation, which uses electrical stimulation to interfere with abnormal activity. A number of other procedures, including transplantation with stem cells, are still in the experimental stages (Olanow et al 2019).

Pharmacological treatment for PD involves a number of different classes of agents, but none actually stops the progression of the disease. The aim of these pharmacological agents is to reduce the symptoms to a manageable level, and include:

- anticholinergics (e.g. benzatropine, benzhexol)
- catechol-O-methyl transferase (COMT) inhibitors (e.g. entacapone)
- dopaminergic agents
  - levodopa (precursor to dopamine)
  - dopamine agonists (e.g. apomorphine, bromocriptine, cabergoline, pergolide)
  - amantadine (antiviral agent which has dopaminergic activity)
- monoamine oxidase type B enzyme (MAO-B) inhibitors (e.g. selegiline, rasagiline, salfinamide)

ANTICHOLINERGIC ANTI-PARKINSON'S AGENTS

General Actions of anticholinergic anti-Parkinson's agents

- inhibit the action of acetylcholine at the muscarinic receptors of the parasympathetic division of the autonomic nervous system
- reduce production of sweat, saliva, lacrimal, nasal, bronchial, gastric and intestinal secretions
- reduce GI tone and gastric acid production
- increase heart rate by blocking vagal stimulus
- raise intraocular pressure, cause mydriasis and cycloplegia
- inhibit micturition

General Uses of anticholinergic anti-Parkinson's agents

- all types of Parkinsonism (adjunct)
- prevention or treatment of drug-induced extrapyramidal symptoms

General Adverse effects of anticholinergic anti-Parkinson's agents

- nausea, vomiting, dry mouth, constipation
- dizziness, headache, nervousness, euphoria, agitation, delusions, hallucinations, paranoia, impaired memory, confusion, drowsiness, sedation
- dry skin, reduced sweating, heat intolerance, hyperthermia
- rash
- tachycardia or bradycardia, aggravate pre-existing hypertension
- urinary urgency, difficulty and retention
- mydriasis, photophobia, cycloplegia, blurred vision, raised intraocular pressure, dry eyes
- (abrupt dose reduction or discontinuation) neuroleptic malignant syndrome, acute exacerbation of Parkinsonism (e.g. anxiety, bradycardia, hypotension, decreased sleep quality)

- (rare) parotitis, dilation of colon, paralytic ileus, allergic reaction

General Interactions of anticholinergic anti-Parkinson's agents

- may decrease absorption and effects of levodopa
- may increase dopaminergic effects of levodopa
- not recommended with other anticholinergic or antipsychotic agents because of increased risk of tardive dyskinesia
- may decrease effects of metoclopramide
- additive anticholinergic effects (including risk of paralytic ileus) may occur if given with other anticholinergic agents, phenothiazines or MAOIs/TCAs with anticholinergic properties
- increased renal tubular absorption, decreased excretion and increased effects may occur if given with carbonic anhydrase inhibitors (e.g. acetazolamide)
- not recommended with alcohol as serum levels may be decreased
- increased sedation may occur if given with alcohol, hypnotics, sedatives, opioids, barbiturates or cannabinoids
- actions may be antagonised by parasympathomimetic (cholinergic) agents (e.g. acetylcholine)
- caution if used with opioids as there may be additive effects on GI motility and bladder function

General Nursing points/Cautions for anticholinergic anti-Parkinson's agents

- intraocular pressure should be monitored regularly during therapy
- drug abuse potential is present because of stimulating and euphoric effects
- not recommended in those with tardive dyskinesia (unless patient has concurrent Parkinson's disease) or for prevention of drug-induced Parkinsonism
- caution if given to those with a history of seizures
- caution if used in those with arrhythmias, tachycardia, heart failure, coronary/ischaemic heart disease, mitral valve stenosis or hypertension
- caution if used in those with a history of atherosclerosis or idiosyncrasy to other drugs as there is an increased risk of nausea, vomiting, confusion, agitation and disturbed behaviour
- caution if given to those with glaucoma, myasthenia gravis, prostatic hypertrophy, urinary retention or obstructive GI disease because of anticholinergic adverse effects
- caution if given in those with liver or kidney impairment
- caution if used during fever, high environmental temperatures, during physical exercise or by those doing manual work in hot environments because of decreased sweating
- caution if used in those $>$ 60 years due to increased risk of anticholinergic adverse effects
- contraindicated in those with paralytic ileus, megacolon, narrow-angle glaucoma or tardive dyskinesia

General Patient teaching and advice for anticholinergic anti-Parkinson's agents

- if dry mouth is a problem, advise the patient to take medication before

meals or if the patient feels nauseous, it may be taken after or with meals
- advise patient that thirst and/or dry mouth may be relieved by drinking water, chewing gum or mints or sucking hard sweets
- patient should be advised to avoid alcohol
- caution patient to avoid sudden withdrawal of the drug as it may cause an exacerbation of the Parkinsonian symptoms or cause a syndrome similar to neuroleptic malignant syndrome (hyperpyrexia, muscle rigidity, psychological changes, increased serum creatine phosphokinase), which can be life threatening
- patient should be warned to avoid driving or operating heavy machinery if blurred vision, dizziness or drowsiness occur
- patient should be advised to report any blurring of vision and to wear dark glasses if there is continuous dilation of pupils
- patients who wear contact lenses should be instructed to use lubricating drops more frequently during therapy as dry eyes commonly occur
- warn patient to avoid high environmental temperatures, doing physical exercise or manual work in hot environments due to decreased sweating and risk of overheating and heat stroke
- patient should be advised to immediately report any fever, heat intolerance or GI problems (especially if also taking phenothiazines, haloperidol or other anticholinergic agents)
- see also General Patient teaching and advice (p. xxvii)

not recommended during pregnancy and breastfeeding unless benefits outweigh potential risks

BENZATROPINE MESILATE (BENZTROPINE MESYLATE) (Benztrop)

Available forms
Tablets: 2 mg; Ampoules: 2 mg/2 mL

Action/Use
- has both anticholinergic and antihistamine properties
- long duration of action
- main effect is to relieve tremor and rigidity
- onset of action is the same whether given IM or IV
- see General Actions/Uses of anticholinergic anti-Parkinson's agents (p. 730)

Dose
- (arteriosclerotic, post-encephalitic or idiopathic Parkinsonism) initially 0.5–1 mg orally, IV or IM, increasing dose gradually at 0.5 mg increments and 5–6-day intervals (daily maximum 6 mg) **OR**
- (drug-induced Parkinsonism) 1–4 mg orally or IM 1–2 times daily **OR**
- (emergency, acute dystonic reaction) 1–2 mg IM or IV stat, repeated if required

Adverse effects
- (large dose) weakness, inability to move particular muscle groups
- see also General Adverse effects of anticholinergic anti-Parkinson's agents (p. 730)

Interactions
- see General Interactions of anticholinergic anti-Parkinson's agents (p. 731)

Nursing points/Cautions/Patient teaching and advice

- parenteral administration may provide quick results if patient is psychotic with acute dystonic reactions
- other anti-Parkinson's agents should not be stopped suddenly when starting benzatropine
- therapy is cumulative, therefore should be started with low dose, increasing at 5–6-day intervals
- some patients may benefit from taking entire dose at bedtime (i.e. enable them to roll over in bed independently), whereas others prefer divided daily doses
- (drug-induced Parkinsonism) therapy should be stopped after 1–2 weeks to determine if continued use is necessary
- caution if used in those with mental disorders as condition may become intensified or psychosis may be precipitated
- see also General Nursing points/Cautions and Patient teaching and advice for anticholinergic anti-Parkinson's agents (p. 731)

tablet may be dispersed in water or crushed and mixed with spoonful of yoghurt or apple puree

TRIHEXYPHENIDYL (BENZHEXOL) HYDROCHLORIDE (Artane)

Available forms

Tablets: 2 mg, 5 mg

Action/Use

- see General Actions/Uses of anticholinergic anti-Parkinson's agents (p. 730)

Dose

- (Parkinsonism) initially 1 mg orally before or with food, increasing by 2 mg increments at 3–5-day intervals to 6–10 mg daily (in 3 divided doses) according to response. May require 12–15 mg in advanced cases (in 4 divided doses with meals and at bedtime) **OR**
- (drug-induced Parkinsonism) initially 1 mg orally daily, increasing dose gradually to 5–15 mg orally daily in divided doses until extrapyramidal symptoms are controlled

Adverse effects

- see General Adverse effects of anticholinergic anti-Parkinson's agents (p. 730)

Interactions

- increased risk of euphoria if given with large amounts of caffeine
- effects may be decreased if given with citrus and fruit juices
- additive effects may occur if given with cannabis, barbiturates, opioid analgesics or alcohol (increasing risk of abuse)
- decreased blood levels may occur if given with alcohol
- decreased absorption may occur if given with magnesium hydroxide
- increased risk of dry mouth, blurred vision and urine hesitancy if given with memantine
- see General Interactions of anticholinergic anti-Parkinson's agents (p. 731)

Nursing points/Cautions

- patient should be advised against ingesting large amounts of caffeine or fruit/citrus juices
- instruct patient to separate medication by at least 2 hours from magnesium hydroxide (antacid)
- daily doses > 10 mg can be divided into 4 doses (with meals and bedtime)

- (post-encephalitic Parkinsonism) advise patient to take medication before meals due to increased salivation (small amount of atropine may also be required)
- abuse potential exists because of stimulant and euphoric effects
- caution if used in those with liver or kidney impairment
- see also General Nursing points/ Cautions and Patient teaching and advice for anticholinergic anti-Parkinson's agents (p. 731)

Patient teaching and advice

- advise patient to avoid large amounts of coffee, citrus and fruit juice during therapy
- see also General Patient teaching and advice for anticholinergic anti-Parkinson's agents (p. 731)

tablet can be dispersed in water or crushed and mixed with spoonful of yoghurt or apple puree

CATECHOL-O-METHYL TRANSFERASE (COMT) INHIBITORS

ENTACAPONE (Comtan)

Available form

Tablets: 200 mg

Action

- inhibits COMT in peripheral tissues, reducing metabolism of levodopa by COMT, increasing the amount of levodopa and therefore the amount of dopamine
- short half-life (30 minutes)

Use

- Parkinson's disease (adjunct to levodopa to control motor fluctuations)

Dose

- 200 mg orally (with levodopa–carbidopa or levodopa–benserazide) 4–7 times daily (maximum daily dose 2 g)

Adverse effects

- diarrhoea, nausea, vomiting, dry mouth, abdominal pain, constipation, anorexia
- dizziness, drowsiness, fatigue, headache, vertigo, insomnia, daytime somnolence, nightmares, sudden sleep onset
- falls, pain, back pain, leg cramps
- dyskinesia, dystonia, tremor, aggravated Parkinson's, hyper/hypokinesia
- hallucinations, depression, confusion, paranoia
- discoloured urine
- increased sweating
- postural hypotension
- (uncommon) impulse control disorders, including pathological gambling, increased libido, hypersexuality, shopping, eating, repetitive purposeless activity (punding)
- (rare) rhabdomyolysis, neuroleptic malignant syndrome, elevated liver enzymes, decreased haemoglobin, colitis

Interactions

- contraindicated with non-selective or selective MAOIs (except selegiline at doses less than 10 mg)
- not recommended with TCAs, noradrenaline reuptake inhibitors, isoprenaline, adrenaline (epinephrine), noradrenaline (norepinephrine), dopamine, dobutamine, methyldopa sesquihydrate, apomorphine or paroxetine

- may form chelates with dietary iron
- may increase levodopa-induced or antihypertensive-induced hypotension
- may require adjustment of other anti-Parkinson's medication to decrease risk of dyskinesia
- may increase bioavailability of levodopa, increasing the risk of dopaminergic adverse effects (especially if combined with benserazide)
- high doses may decrease bioavailability of carbidopa monohydrate
- may increase serum levels of warfarin, increasing the risk of bleeding, therefore INR should be monitored closely, especially when starting, stopping or altering dose

Nursing points/Cautions

- levodopa dose is usually reduced by 10–30% by either decreasing dose or increasing dosing interval
- if diarrhoea and anorexia is ongoing, weight should be monitored to prevent excessive loss
- drowsiness is a problem at the start of therapy
- levodopa dose will require adjustment
- tablets contain sucrose and therefore are not recommended in those with fructose intolerance, glucose–galactose malabsorption or sucrase–isomaltase insufficiency
- caution if used in those with ischaemic heart disease
- contraindicated in those with liver impairment, phaeochromocytoma, previous history of neuroleptic malignant syndrome or rhabdomyolysis (non-traumatic)

Patient teaching and advice

- instruct patient to take 2–3 hours apart from meals to prevent binding with dietary iron
- advise patient to avoid postural hypotension by moving gradually to a sitting or standing position, especially after sleep
- instruct patient to report any prolonged or persistent diarrhoea
- patient should be advised not to drive or operate machinery if drowsiness, daytime somnolence, sudden sleep onset or dizziness continues
- family/carers should be asked to observe for:
  - any sudden sleep onset, as patients are often unaware that this occurs and it may be dangerous if the person drives or operates machinery, or
  - persistent/recurring gambling, increase in sexual desires or repetitive behaviours with no purpose
- patient should be advised to avoid suddenly stopping therapy as it may cause an exaggeration of the Parkinson's symptoms or may cause overheating, muscle rigidity and psychological changes which can be potentially life threatening
- patient should be warned that urine may appear a harmless reddish-brown colour
- see also General Patient teaching and advice for anticholinergic anti-Parkinson's agents (p. 731)

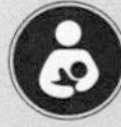

contraindicated during pregnancy or breastfeeding

tablet can be dispersed in 20 mL water or crushed and mixed with spoonful of yoghurt or apple puree

Note

- combined with levodopa, and carbidopa monohydrate in Stalevo preparations, Carlevent preparations and Tridopa preparations

DOPAMINE AGONISTS

General Adverse effects of dopamine agonists

- anorexia, nausea, vomiting, constipation, dyspepsia, indigestion, dry mouth
- dizziness, insomnia, somnolence, sedation, nightmares, drowsiness, light-headedness, ataxia, abnormal dreams, insomnia, headache, asthenia, fatigue, lethargy
- depression, anxiety, agitation, concentration difficulties, nervousness, elevated mood, hallucinations (visual, auditory), confusion, disorientation
- postural hypotension, peripheral oedema
- rash, pruritus, increased sweating
- dyskinesia, hypokinesia
- (rare) somnolence, sudden sleep onset
- (abrupt withdrawal, rare) neuroleptic malignant syndrome, worsening Parkinson's symptoms
- (uncommon, high doses) impulse control disorders, including pathological gambling, increased libido, hypersexuality, binge and compulsive eating, repetitive purposeless activity (punding), compulsive spending and buying

General Interactions of dopamine agonists

- not recommended with agents that antagonise dopamine receptors (e.g. metoclopramide, phenothiazines, butyrophenones, thioxanthenes)
- increased risk of adverse effects (e.g. confusion, hallucinations, nightmares, GI disturbances and other atropine-like effects) if given with anticholinergic agents and therefore not recommended together
- caution if given with alcohol and other CNS-depressing agents as additive CNS effects may occur
- increased risk of dyskinesia, hallucinations and confusion if given with levodopa

General Nursing points/Cautions for dopamine agonists

- before starting therapy, patients should have a cardiovascular assessment (including ECG/echocardiogram), ESR, lung function test, chest X-ray and renal function
- ECG/echocardiogram should be monitored within 3–6 months of starting therapy, then 6–12-monthly
- chest X-ray and ESR are recommended if patient develops any pulmonary symptoms
- drowsiness is a problem at the start of therapy
- dose may require adjusting if given with other anti-Parkinson's agents
- observe patient for suicidal tendencies or depression
- patient should be carefully monitored for any signs of confusion or hallucinations because this may require cessation of therapy
- avoid abrupt withdrawal of therapy to prevent neuroleptic malignant syndrome, worsening of Parkinson's symptoms, catatonia or delirium
- (drug-induced extrapyramidal symptoms) when symptoms have been controlled, dose should be gradually decreased and then ceased
- caution if used in those with epilepsy, confusion, psychosis, hallucinations, underlying psychiatric disorders, gastric ulcers or bleeding, cardiovascular disease, congestive heart failure, postural hypotension, narrow-angle glaucoma, prostatic enlargement,

kidney or liver impairment, Raynaud's syndrome or recurrent eczema

General Patient teaching and advice for dopamine agonists

- advise patient to resume physical activity gradually to avoid injury
- patient should be advised to immediately report:
  - any rash
  - swelling of feet or lower limbs
  - feelings of depression or suicidal thoughts
  - changes to vision, blurred vision
- patient should be advised to avoid suddenly stopping therapy as worsening of Parkinson's symptoms and/or increase in body temperature, sweating, muscle rigidity and psychological changes may occur, which are potentially life threatening
- patients should be warned to avoid alcohol during therapy
- advise patient to avoid postural hypotension by moving gradually to a sitting or standing position, especially after sleep
- patient should be advised not to drive or operate machinery if drowsiness, daytime somnolence, sudden sleep onset or dizziness continues
- family/carers should be asked to observe for any:
  - sudden sleep onset as patients are often unaware that this occurs and it may be dangerous if the person drives or operates machinery
  - persistent/recurring gambling, increase in sexual desires, pathological gambling, increased libido, binge and compulsive eating, repetitive purposeless activity, compulsive spending and buying
  - change in mood, depression or expressions of self-harm or suicide
- see also General Patient teaching and advice (p. xxvii)

AMANTADINE HYDROCHLORIDE (Symmetrel)

Available form

Capsules: 100 mg

Action

- thought to stimulate synthesis and release of dopamine (and other catecholamines) in the brain and also delay reuptake
- may alter D_2 receptors
- some anticholinergic activity
- narrow therapeutic index
- (PD) response usually within 24–48 hours and 7 days
- (influenza) inhibits penetration of the virus (influenza A) into the host cell, preventing viral replication

Use

- Parkinson's disease and other forms of Parkinsonism (not indicated for tardive dyskinesia)
- drug-induced extrapyramidal reactions
- prophylaxis against influenza type A

Dose

- (PD, less than 65 years) initially 100 mg orally daily for 1 week, then increasing to 100 mg orally twice daily **OR**
- (PD, 65 years and over) 100 mg orally daily **OR**
- (drug-induced extrapyramidal effects) initial treatment should be dosage reduction of the drug causing the effects. If this is not practical, then 100 mg orally 2–3 times daily, discontinuing when symptoms have been controlled **OR**
- (influenza prophylaxis) 100 mg orally twice daily after food for 10 days

Adverse effects

- palpitations
- mottling of skin (livedo reticularis)
- blurred vision (transient), slurred speech
- (rare) corneal lesions, seizures
- see General Adverse effects of dopamine agonists (p. 736)

Interactions

- increased serum levels and toxicity may occur if given with hydrochlorothiazide/triamterene fixed-dose combinations
- see also General Interactions of dopamine agonists (p. 736)

Nursing points/Cautions

- adverse effects usually occur within 1–4 days of starting therapy and disappear within 48 hours of stopping
- daily dose should not be exceeded because of narrow therapeutic index
- effectiveness may diminish after several weeks, but may be regained by temporarily stopping therapy gradually
- abrupt withdrawal is not recommended
- see also General Nursing points/Cautions for dopamine agonists (p. 736)

Patient teaching and advice

- female patients of childbearing potential should be counselled to avoid pregnancy by using effective contraception during and for 5 days after stopping therapy
- see also General Patient teaching and advice for dopamine agonists (p. 737)

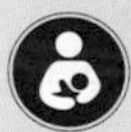

contraindicated during pregnancy and breastfeeding

capsules are difficult to open and contents are oily and waxy

APOMORPHINE HYDROCHLORIDE HEMIHYDRATE (APOMORPHINE HYDROCHLORIDE) (Apomine, Movapo)

Available forms

Ampoules: 20 mg/2 mL, 50 mg/5 mL; Vial: 100 mg/20 mL; Prefilled syringes: 50 mg/10 mL; Multi-dose pen: 30 mg/3 mL

Action

- dopamine agonist acting on pre- and post-synaptic D_2 receptors and antagonising alpha-2-adrenergic receptors
- induces vomiting by stimulating chemoreceptor trigger zone (CTZ) in the medulla
- (SC) onset of action within 5 minutes, half-life is approximately 33 minutes

Use

- reduction in severity and number of motor fluctuations in Parkinson's disease refractory to other conventional treatment ('off' phase of the 'on–off' phenomenon, in which the patient fluctuates between mobility and immobility)

Dose

- threshold dose (considered to be the lowest dose that produces an 'unequivocal' motor response compared with baseline)
- after immobility has been provoked and baseline motor assessment has been completed, initially 1.5 mg SC, then observe the patient for 30 minutes for motor response. If there is no/poor response after 40 minutes, give 3 mg SC and observe patient for another 30 minutes. Give a third dose of 5 mg and a fourth dose of 7 mg at 40-minute intervals, if required, observing the patient for 30 minutes as previously (if still no response, patient is thought to be a 'non-responder'. A 10 mg dose can be given if the patient had a minimal response at 7 mg)
- (restarting anti-Parkinsonian treatment) administer threshold dose (as established above) 2.4–3.6 mg SC at first sign of 'off' phase (maximum daily dose 50 mg; maximum single dose 6 mg) and observe for 1 hour **OR**
- initially 1 mg/hour by continuous SC infusion via portable syringe driver pump, increasing as necessary to achieve motor response during waking hours (maximum daily dose 200 mg)

Adverse effects

- (injection site/continuous SC infusion site) itchy, nodular lesions, local bruising, redness, tenderness, fibrosis and, rarely, necrosis
- nausea, vomiting
- somnolence, drowsiness, sedation
- yawning
- visual hallucinations, confusion
- (uncommon) increasingly severe 'on' phase dyskinesia, transient postural hypotension, rash
- (rare) eosinophilia, haemolytic anaemia, impulse control disorders
- (high dose) QT prolongation

Interactions

- Coombs' positive haemolytic anaemia may occur if used in conjunction with levodopa
- not recommended with metoclopramide as effects of apomorphine may be reduced
- not recommended with ondansetron, dolasetron and granisetron due to risk of toxicity
- increased serum levels may occur if given with entacapone
- not recommended with other agents known to prolong QT interval
- caution if used with clozapine
- may potentiate effects of antihypertensive and cardiac-active medications
- see also General Interactions of dopamine agonists (p. 736)

Nursing points/Cautions

- monitoring FBC and hepatic, renal and cardiovascular function during prolonged therapy is recommended
- patient must be hospitalised during pre-treatment phase
- domperidone (antiemetic) is started 48–72 hours before treatment (10 mg orally 3 times daily or less if renal insufficiency exists), may be reduced by 10 mg daily at weekly intervals until mild nausea reappears and may be stopped after several weeks
- anti-Parkinsonian medications are stopped to provoke the 'off' phase (immobility) after at least 3 days of hospitalisation
- perform baseline motor assessment (unilateral alternate hand-tapping for 30 seconds, time to walk 12 metres, clinical assessment of tremor and dyskinesia (4-point score) and modified Webster disability scale to assess 12 features of Parkinsonism (maximum disability score 36)). Positive motor response consists of 15% increase in hand-tapping, 25% increase in walking time, 2-point increase in tremor score or Webster score increase of 3 or more points
- dose for treatment may be further adjusted to response, if needed
- not recommended IV
- when starting therapy, patient should be closely monitored for adequate therapeutic effects and/or adverse effects
- SC administration sites are usually the thigh and lower abdomen
- prefilled syringe does not require any further dilution. Ampoule is diluted using sodium chloride 0.9% for use in portable syringe-driver pump
- continuous SC infusion via mini pump may be recommended for patients who require 8–10 injections per day, or whose overall control is not satisfactory
- continuous SC infusion is only required during waking hours (unless patient is experiencing night-time problems)
- infusion sites should be rotated every 12 hours
- liver, kidney, blood and heart function should be regularly monitored during therapy
- opioid antagonist (e.g. naloxone) may be used to treat overdosage, respiratory or CNS depression or excessive vomiting

- prefilled syringe should be discarded 24 hours after opening
- caution if used in those with predisposition to nausea/vomiting, at increased risk of respiratory depression (including the elderly) or those with endocrine, pulmonary or cardiovascular disease
- not recommended in those under 18 years
- contraindicated in those with known hypersensitivity to sodium metabisulfite, morphine or related products
- contraindicated in those with dementia or pre-existing neuropsychiatric problems, at risk of QT interval prolongation, liver/kidney impairment, unstable coronary vascular disease, cerebrovascular disease, respiratory or CNS depression or in those with Parkinson's disease in which the 'on' response to levodopa is marred by severe dyskinesia, hypotonia or psychotoxicity

Patient teaching and advice

- patient/carer should be educated regarding injection technique, importance of site rotation, correct storage information and safe disposal of used needles
- patient should be warned that injection site reaction (itchy nodules) is common and disappears within 48 hours; however, care should be taken to prevent nodules ulcerating and becoming infected
- warn patient not to use solution if it has turned green
- see also General Patient teaching and advice for dopamine agonists (p. 737)

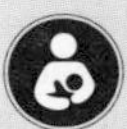

not recommended during pregnancy or breastfeeding

BENSERAZIDE HYDROCHLORIDE

Action

- peripheral inhibitor of dopa decarboxylase, which normally decarboxylates levodopa to dopamine in the tissues, thereby preventing any therapeutic dose from reaching the brain (levodopa but not dopamine can cross the blood–brain barrier). Benserazide prevents this peripheral decarboxylation from occurring, so that the levodopa crosses the blood–brain barrier before conversion to dopamine, allowing substantially lower doses of levodopa to be used (e.g. benserazide and levodopa 200 mg is equal to 1000 mg levodopa alone)
- at therapeutic dose, does not cross the blood–brain barrier

Use

- given with levodopa in the treatment of Parkinson's disease or Parkinsonism

Note

- combined with levodopa in Madopar preparations

BROMOCRIPTINE MESILATE (BROMOCRIPTINE MESYLATE) (Parlodel)

Available forms

Tablets: 2.5 mg

Action

- ergot derivative with no uterotonic and little vasoconstrictor activity
- stimulates dopaminergic receptors
- inhibits release of prolactin
- elimination half-life 2–8 hours

Use

- mild Parkinson's disease (as monotherapy or with other anti-Parkinson's agents)

- preventing onset of lactation, hyperprolactinaemia (where surgery and/or radiotherapy are not indicated or have been ineffective) (see Pregnancy, childbirth and breastfeeding, p. 1419)
- acromegaly (adjunctive therapy)

Dose

- (PD) initially 1.25 mg orally 1–2 times daily with food for 7 days, then increasing by 1.25 mg at weekly intervals until therapeutic response is reached (range 5–40 mg in divided doses 6–8-hourly) **OR**
- (adjunctive therapy in acromegaly) initially 1.25 mg orally at night increasing gradually over 7–14 days to 10 mg in 4 divided doses with food (maximum daily dose 40 mg)

Adverse effects

- nausea, vomiting, constipation
- headache, somnolence, dizziness, syncope
- nasal congestion
- (uncommon) confusion, hypotension, auditory or visual hallucinations
- (very rare, prolonged therapy) reversible pallor of fingers or toes induced by cold
- (PD, rare) pleural/pericardial effusion/fibrosis, cardiac valvulopathy, retroperitoneal fibrosis, diabetic retinopathy, sudden sleep onset, impulse control disorders, gastric ulceration/bleeding
- (PD, high dose) persistent hallucinations (even after stopping therapy)
- (acromegaly, high dose) gastric haemorrhage

Interactions

- increased plasma levels may result if given with erythromycin, clarithromycin or octreotide
- increased risk of adverse effects if given with other ergot alkaloids
- not recommended with alcohol
- hypotensive effects may be enhanced if given with antihypertensive agents or other agents known to decrease BP
- increased risk of hypertension and headache if given with sympathomimetic agents
- may alter serum levels of levodopa, increasing risk of adverse effects
- may have additive effects if given with sumatriptan
- see also General Interactions of dopamine agonists (p. 736)

Nursing points/Cautions

- see General Nursing points/Cautions for dopamine agonists (p. 736)
- dosage increases are made gradually, starting with smallest dose, usually over several days, to reduce adverse effects especially hypotension
- decreasing dose usually stops auditory/visual hallucinations
- (PD) may be given alone or as combination therapy
- (long-term therapy) women should have regular gynaecological examinations (to monitor for any uterine tumour)
- (PD) regular X-ray monitoring is recommended to detect pulmonary fibrosis
- tablets are not recommended in those with galactose intolerance, severe lactase deficiency or glucose–galactose malabsorption
- caution if used in those with suspected/known peptic ulceration, dementia, Raynaud's phenomenon or impaired liver function
- caution if used in those with diabetes due to risk of diabetic retinopathy
- contraindicated in those with hypersensitivity to ergot alkaloids, uncontrolled hypertension, toxaemia, hypertensive disorders associated with pregnancy (including postpartum), coronary artery disease, severe cardiovascular conditions or serious psychiatric disorders

Patient teaching and advice

- patient should be advised to immediately report:
  - any shortness of breath, persistent cough or chest pain (pulmonary fibrosis)
  - loin/flank pain, lower limb swelling or abdominal tenderness (retroperitoneal fibrosis)
  - vomiting blood, bloody diarrhoea, red or black bowel motions, bleeding from rectum
  - any persistent headache or visual problems
  - any visual or auditory hallucinations
- warn patient that alcohol may cause nausea, abdominal pain and bloating if used during bromocriptine therapy
- warn patients with acromegaly to immediately report any GI side-effects
- advise patient to take initial doses at bedtime, to reduce the incidence of hypotension and loss of consciousness
- instruct patient that gastric irritation can be reduced if taken with or immediately after food
- see also General Patient teaching and advice for dopamine antagonists (p. 737)

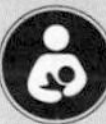

not recommended during breastfeeding as lactation is suppressed/inhibited

tablets can be dispersed in water or crushed and mixed with spoonful of yoghurt or apple puree

CABERGOLINE (Cabaser, Dostinex)

Available forms
Tablets: 500 microgram, 1 mg, 2 mg

Action
- ergot derivative
- stimulates D_2 dopamine receptors, inhibiting prolactin secretion
- long half-life (63–68 hours)

Use
- Parkinson's disease (Cabaser)
- inhibiting physiological lactation, hyperprolactinaemia (Dostinex) (see Pregnancy, childbirth and breastfeeding, p. 1421)

Dose
- (PD monotherapy) initially 0.5 mg orally daily, increasing at 1–2-weekly intervals orally to 2–3 mg daily **OR**
- (PD, with levodopa) initially 1 mg orally daily, increasing at 1–2-weekly intervals orally to 2–3 mg daily

Adverse effects
- palpitations, hypertension
- dyspnoea
- (rare) pleural/pericardial effusion/fibrosis, cardiac valvulopathy, retroperitoneal fibrosis
- see also General Adverse effects of dopamine agonists (p. 736)

Interactions
- not recommended with other ergot alkaloids
- not recommended with macrolide antibacterial agents (e.g. erythromycin)
- hypotensive effects may be enhanced if given with antihypertensive agents or other agents known to decrease BP
- see also General Interactions of dopamine agonists (p. 736)

Nursing points/Cautions
- patient should be screened for any signs of depression or psychiatric history before starting therapy
- doses of levodopa can be gradually decreased while dose of cabergoline is increased
- no data exists to show that 1 and 2 mg tablets are bioequivalent at equal doses
- caution if used in those with severe liver disease
- contraindicated in those with hypersensitivity to any ergot alkaloid
- contraindicated in those with history of pulmonary, pericardial or

retroperitoneal fibrotic disease or anatomical evidence of cardiac valvulopathy
- see also General Nursing points/Cautions for dopamine agonists (p. 736)

Patient teaching and advice

- advise patient that administration with food may lessen GI disturbances
- patient should be advised to immediately report:
  - any shortness of breath, persistent cough or chest pain (pulmonary fibrosis)
  - loin/flank pain, lower limb swelling or abdominal tenderness (retroperitoneal fibrosis)
- female patient of childbearing potential should be counselled that pregnancy should be excluded before starting therapy and at least 1 month should elapse between stopping treatment and becoming pregnant
- see also General Patient teaching and advice for dopamine agonists (p. 737)

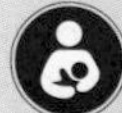

not recommended during pregnancy

lactation will be suppressed/inhibited and therefore not recommended during breastfeeding

tablet can be crushed and mixed with water or spoonful of yoghurt or apple puree

CARBIDOPA MONOHYDRATE (CARBIDOPA)

Action

- inhibits peripheral decarboxylation of levodopa, increasing the amount that enters the brain for conversion to dopamine
- does not cross the blood–brain barrier in therapeutic doses

Use

- given with levodopa to treat Parkinsonism

Note

- combined with levodopa in Duodopa Intestinal Gel, Kinson, Sinadopa, Sinemet and Sinemet CR
- combined with levodopa and entacapone in Stalevo preparations, Carlevent preparations and Tridopa preparations

LEVODOPA

Available forms

Capsules: levodopa 50 mg/benserazide 12.5 mg, levodopa 100 mg/benserazide 25 mg, levodopa 200 mg/benserazide 50 mg; Capsules (sustained-release): levodopa 100 mg/benserazide 25 mg; Tablets: levodopa 100 mg/benserazide 25 mg, levodopa 200 mg/benserazide 50 mg; Tablets (dispersible): levodopa 50 mg/benserazide 12.5 mg, levodopa 100 mg/benserazide 25 mg; Tablets: levodopa 100 mg/carbidopa 25 mg, levodopa 250 mg/carbidopa 25 mg; Tablets (sustained-release): levodopa 50 mg/carbidopa 12.5 mg/entacapone 200 mg, levodopa 200 mg/carbidopa 50 mg, Tablets (film-coated): levodopa 50 mg/carbidopa 12.5 mg/entacapone 200 mg, levodopa 75 mg/carbidopa 18.75 mg/entacapone 200 mg, levodopa 100 mg/carbidopa 25 mg/entacapone 200 mg, levodopa 125 mg/carbidopa 31.25 mg/entacapone 200 mg, levodopa 150 mg/carbidopa 37.5 mg/entacapone 200 mg, levodopa 200 mg/carbidopa 50 mg/entacapone 200 mg; Intestinal cassette gel (plastic): levodopa 20 mg/carbidopa 5 mg/mL

Action

- main therapy for Parkinson's disease since 1960s
- extensively metabolised, mainly to dopamine, but also adrenaline (epinephrine) and noradrenaline

- decarboxylation occurs in peripheral tissues, as well as in the CNS, thereby decreasing the amount of levodopa entering the CNS to be converted to dopamine
- peripheral decarboxylation is inhibited by benserazide or carbidopa monohydrate
- controls akinesia and rigidity more effectively than tremor

Use

- all types of Parkinsonism (except drug-induced Parkinsonian symptoms)

Dose

- rarely used alone

Adverse effects

- muscle cramps, hypotonia
- teeth grinding
- delusions
- depression, suicidal ideation
- dyskinesia, hyperkinesia, involuntary movements, freezing episodes
- dark urine, sweat and saliva, rash, hair loss
- (less frequent) cardiac arrhythmias, palpitations, hypertension and, rarely, chest pain
- (uncommon) haemolytic and non-haemolytic anaemia, transient leucopenia
- (late complications) 'wearing-off effect' (deterioration occurs before next dose is due), 'on–off' phenomenon (abrupt but transient fluctuations in severity of symptoms at frequent intervals)
- (rare) gastrointestinal bleeding and ulceration, melanoma
- (overdose) muscle twitching, blepharospasm, dystonia, dyskinesia
- (intestinal gel) dislocation of tube, occlusion, incision site pain and erythema, abdominal pain
- see also General Adverse effects of dopamine agonists (p. 736)

Interactions

- see General Interactions of dopamine antagonists (p. 736)
- effects enhanced by the peripheral dopa decarboxylase inhibitors, carbidopa monohydrate and benserazide
- not recommended with baclofen as baclofen toxicity and/or worsening of Parkinsonian symptoms may occur
- contraindicated with or within 14 days of MAOIs
- increased risk of hypertension and dyskinesia if given with TCAs
- not recommended with halothane as combination may result in arrhythmia
- bioavailability decreased if given with iron-containing products
- effects may be reduced if given with isoniazid, phenothiazines, metochlopramide, benzodiazepine or phenytoin
- severe hypotension may occur if given with selegiline
- caution if given with antihypertensives or other agents known to reduce BP as symptomatic postural hypotension may occur
- high-protein diet may decrease absorption of levodopa
- increased serum levels may occur if given with penicillamine
- may cause hypotension and/or dyskinesia if given with methyldopa sesquihydrate
- bioavailability may be increased if given with domperidone or COMT inhibitors
- may potentiate effects of epinephrine (adrenaline), norepinephrine (noradrenaline), isoprenaline and dexamphetamine
- may cause false positive for urinary ketone bodies and positive Coombs' test

Nursing points/Cautions

- GI and cardiovascular adverse effects may be decreased when given with peripheral decarboxylase inhibitor
- conduct monthly FBC and monitor liver, kidney and cardiovascular function during prolonged therapy

- sudden fluctuations of effectiveness of levodopa develop after about 2 years of therapy ('on–off' effect)
- appearance of involuntary movements may be a sign of levodopa toxicity
- levodopa therapy is discontinued at least 2–3 days before surgery and restarted as soon as the patient is able to take oral medications
- dispersible tablets are recommended for those with swallowing difficulties or if rapid onset of action is required
- (intestinal gel) gel is administered directly into the duodenum, initially via a temporary nasoduodenal/nasojejunal tube to confirm positive clinical response (maximising functional 'on' time and minimising the disabling 'off' periods) before the insertion of a permanent percutaneous endoscopic gastrostomy (PEG) tube (tube placement should be confirmed before administration). Gel is administered continuously using a portable pump (CADD Legacy Duodopa (CE 0473)). Dosage consists of morning bolus dose (100–200 mg over 10–30 minutes), continuous maintenance dose (20–200 mg/hour) and extra boluses (given if patient becomes hypokinetic during the day, usually between 10 and 40 mg). If extra boluses are given more than 5 times per day, the continuous maintenance dose should be recalculated. The morning bolus dose may also require adjusting (maximum levodopa 300 mg (15 mL)). The gel should only be administered for a total of 16 hours, after which the cassette should be discarded, regardless of whether any gel remains in the cassette or not. If the administration continues overnight, the cassette must still be changed after it has been at room temperature for 16 hours. Continuous administration may result in tolerance and reduction of therapeutic effect. If a sudden deterioration in effect (e.g. bradykinesia) is seen, placement of the tube should be checked as it may become displaced from duodenum into the stomach
- caution if used in those with epilepsy, depression, history of psychosis, severe cardiovascular or pulmonary disease, cardiac arrhythmias or myocardial infarction (therapy should be started as an inpatient), asthma, liver, kidney or endocrine disease or history of peptic ulceration
- not recommended for drug-induced extrapyramidal reactions
- (Madopar) contraindicated in those under 30 years
- contraindicated in those with a history of malignant melanoma or suspicious lesion because therapy may activate a malignant melanoma
- contraindicated in those with any hypersensitivity to sympathomimetic amines or with uncompensated cardiovascular, endocrine, kidney, liver or blood disease, narrow-angle glaucoma, active psychosis or psychoneurosis, pheochromocytoma, hyperthyroidism, Cushing's syndrome, intention tremor or Huntington's chorea

Patient teaching and advice

- patient should be advised to take medication 30–60 minutes before food if possible; however, gastric irritation is reduced by taking with or immediately after food, if needed
- instruct patient to avoid eating a high-protein diet as this may impair absorption of medication
- (sustained-release tablets/capsules) advise patient to swallow whole (not chewed or crushed); however, tablets can be divided without affecting properties. Because the onset of action of sustained-release preparations is long, patient may also need to take an immediate-release preparation for immediate effects

- instruct patient that dispersible tablets should be dissolved in 25–50 mL water (solution is milky white) and drunk within 30 minutes, ensuring that solution is well stirred
- advise patient about the need to continue treatment because it is long-term replacement therapy; maximum improvement may take up to 6 months and is maintained only while therapy continues, so therapy should not be suddenly stopped
- instruct patient to report any loss of movement (a few minutes to a few hours) that may occur when medication has been taken for a long period of time. This may recur and is called 'on–off' effect. It may require an increase in dose or change of medication
- those with diabetes are advised to monitor blood glucose levels closely during therapy
- warn patient that a reddish tinge in the urine is harmless; tears and sweat may also appear brown
- patient/carer should be advised to report any:
  - lowered mood, mental changes or signs of depression or suicidal tendencies
  - appearance of involuntary movements may be a sign of levodopa toxicity and should be reported immediately
  - changes in skin lesions (size, shape, colour)
- (intestinal gel) patient should be advised to avoid swimming or bathing as pump cannot be taken into water. Patient should be warned that disconnecting pump may result in sudden bradykinesia which could result in person drowning if he/she is in water
- see also General Patient teaching and advice for dopamine antagonists (p. 737)

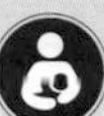
not recommended during pregnancy and breastfeeding

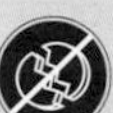
controlled/modified-release tablets/capsules should not be broken or crushed

Plain tablets can be dispersed in water or crushed and mixed with spoonful of apple puree

Note

- combined with benserazide in Madopar preparations, carbidopa monohydrate in Duodopa Intestinal Gel, Kinson, Sinemet, Sinemet CR and Sinadopa, and with carbidopa monohydrate and entacapone in Stalevo

PRAMIPEXOLE DIHYDROCHLORIDE MONOHYDRATE (Sifrol, Sifrol ER, Simipex, Simpral)

Available forms

Tablets: 125 microgram, 250 microgram, 1 mg; Tablets (extended-release): 375 microgram, 750 microgram, 1.5 mg, 2.25 mg, 3 mg, 3.75 mg, 4.5 mg

Action

- dopamine agonist that binds selectively to dopamine D_2 and D_3 receptors
- decreases prolactin levels
- half-life 8–12 hours

Use

- Parkinson's disease (alone or with levodopa)
- restless leg syndrome (RLS)

Dose

- (PD) initially 125 microgram orally 3 times daily, increasing to 250 microgram orally 3 times daily after 5–7 days, then to 500 microgram orally 3 times daily after a further 5–7 days, with further increases at weekly intervals if needed (daily maximum 4.5 mg) (immediate-release tablets) **OR**

- (PD) initially 375 microgram orally daily for 5–7 days, increasing to 750 microgram orally daily for 5–7 days, then 1.5 mg orally daily for 5–7 days, increasing further if needed at 5–7-day intervals (daily maximum 4.5 mg) (extended-release tablets) **OR**
- (RLS) initially 125 microgram orally daily 2–3 hours before bedtime, increasing every 4–7 days to 750 microgram daily if needed (immediate-release tablets)

Adverse effects

- cough, dyspnoea, nasal congestion
- flushing, sweating
- vertigo
- back pain, pain in extremities, arthralgia, muscle cramps, myalgia
- urinary frequency and incontinence
- hallucinations (but more common if given with levodopa)
- (rare) rhabdomyolysis
- (RLS) augmentation (earlier onset of symptoms, increase in severity and spread of symptoms to other body parts)
- see also General Adverse effects of dopamine agonists (p. 736)

Interactions

- serum levels may be increased by cimetidine, diltiazem, ranitidine, triamterene, verapamil, digoxin and trimethoprim
- see also General Interactions of dopamine agonists (p. 736)

Nursing points/Cautions

- if given with levodopa, dose of levodopa should be reduced by 25% to avoid adverse effects
- if discontinuing therapy, dose should be gradually reduced at a rate of 750 microgram/day until 750 microgram daily dose is reached, then reduced by 375 microgram/day
- dose reduction is required in those with mild kidney impairment (creatinine clearance 20–50 mL/min)
- see also General Nursing points/Cautions for dopamine agonists (p. 736)

Patient teaching and advice

- advise patient that extended-release tablets should be swallowed whole, and not chewed, crushed or split
- see General Patient teaching and advice for dopamine agonists (p. 737)

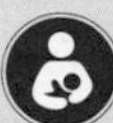

only used during pregnancy if benefits outweigh risks

may inhibit/suppress lactation, therefore not recommended during breastfeeding

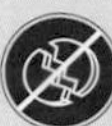

extended-release tablets should not be broken or crushed

plain tablets can be dispersed in water or crushed and mixed with spoonful of yoghurt or apple puree

ROTIGOTINE (Neupro)

Available forms

Transdermal patches: 2 mg/24 hour, 4 mg/24 hour, 6 mg/24 hour, 8 mg/24 hour

Action

- non-ergot dopamine agonist that activates D_1, D_2, D_3, D_4 and D_5 (but particularly D_3) receptors in the brain
- decreases prolactin levels

Use

- Parkinson's disease (alone or with levodopa)
- restless leg syndrome (RLS)

Dose

- (early stage PD) initially 2 mg/24-hour patch applied daily, then increased at weekly intervals of 2 mg/24-hour to an effective dose (maximum 8 mg/24 hours) **OR**
- (advanced stage PD) initially 4 mg/24-hour patch applied daily, then increased at weekly intervals of 2 mg/24-hour to an effective dose (maximum 16 mg/24 hours). For doses above 8 mg/24 hours, combination of patches can be used **OR**

- (RLS) initially 1 mg/24 hours, increasing if needed at weekly intervals (maximum 3 mg/24 hours)

Adverse effects

- (application site) erythema, pruritus, urticaria, rash, irritation, burning, dermatitis, vesicles/papules, exfoliation, swelling, inflammation, discolouration, pain, hypersensitivity
- (RLS) augmentation (earlier onset of symptoms, increase in severity and spread of symptoms to other body parts)
- increase in systolic and/or diastolic blood pressure, increased heart rate, palpitations, atrial fibrillation
- vertigo
- (PD) weight gain, fluid retention
- (uncommon) blurred vision, visual impairment, photopsia (flashes of light), elevated liver enzymes
- (rare) seizures
- see also General Adverse effects of dopamine agonists (p. 736)

Interactions

- see General Interactions of dopamine agonists (p. 736)

Nursing points/Cautions

- regular ophthalmology monitoring is recommended
- patient should be closely monitored for fluid retention and weight gain (especially if pre-existing congestive cardiac failure or kidney insufficiency exists)
- dose reduction is recommended if worsening liver impairment occurs
- (restless leg syndrome) therapy should be evaluated for effectiveness after 6 months
- contains sodium metabisulfite, which can cause allergic reaction in susceptible people
- contraindicated with cardioversion or magnetic resonance imaging (MRI) due to the risk of skin burning because of the aluminium backing layer
- see General Nursing points/Cautions for dopamine agonists (p. 736)

Patient teaching and advice

- patients should be advised to:
  - apply patch at approximately the same time each day and to leave in situ for 24 hours
  - apply patch to clean, dry, intact skin on upper arms, shoulders, hip, flank (side, between rib and hip), thigh or belly, but not in an area that is rubbed by tight clothing
  - avoid any skin that is red, inflamed, irritated or damaged
  - if applying to hairy area, skin should be shaved at least 3 days before applying patch
  - rotate application sites daily and do not use the same site within 14 days
  - leave patch intact when swimming or bathing
  - avoid direct sunlight to any application site rash or irritation until the skin heals
  - avoid external heat (e.g. excessive sunlight, heating pads, sauna, hot bath) to the transdermal patch area
- do not cut transdermal patch into smaller pieces
- if patch falls off, new patch should be applied for the rest of the day
- correctly dispose of used patch (i.e. folded in half without matrix exposed, placed in original sachet and discarded out of the reach of children) as it still contains active substance
- advise patient not to use any skin products (e.g. creams, oils, powders, lotions) on or near the area where the patch is applied
- instruct patient to wash area where patch was applied with water and soap (but not use any alcohol or other dissolving fluids) to remove any residual adhesive
- patients should be advised to report any application site reaction that either

spreads beyond the site or persists for more than 2–3 days or if excessive weight gain/fluid retention occurs
- see also General Patient teaching and advice for dopamine agonists (p. 737)

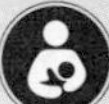

not recommended during pregnancy and breastfeeding. Suppression/inhibition of lactation will occur

MONOAMINE OXIDASE TYPE B ENZYME (MAO-B) INHIBITORS

General Patient teaching and advice for MAO-B inhibitors

- warn patient to avoid driving or operating machinery if dizziness, vertigo, fatigue or hypotension occurs
- advise patient to avoid postural hypotension by moving gradually to a sitting or standing position, especially after sleep
- advise patient to resume physical activity gradually to avoid injury
- patient should be warned not to stop therapy suddenly because it may cause hallucinations and confusion
- patient should be advised to avoid alcohol during therapy
- patient should be advised to avoid excessive amounts of foods with high tyramine content (e.g. aged cheeses, red wine)
- family/carers should be asked to observe for:
  - any signs of depression or altered mood
  - persistent/recurring gambling, increase in sexual desires or repetitive behaviours with no purpose, abnormal buying or selling, meaningless collecting and sorting of objects
- see also General Patient teaching and advice (p. xxvii)

RASAGILINE (Azilect, Rasalect, Rasazil)

Available form

Tablets: 1 mg

Action

- irreversible monoamine oxidase type B (MAO-B) selective inhibitor thought to cause an increase in extracellular dopamine levels

Use

- idiopathic Parkinson's disease (as monotherapy or as adjunct therapy with levodopa/decarboxylase inhibitor)

Dose

- 1 mg orally daily (with or without levodopa/decarboxylase inhibitor therapy)

Adverse effects

- headache, malaise, dizziness, vertigo, daytime drowsiness, somnolence and (if given with dopamine agonists) sudden sleep onset
- depression, hallucinations
- fever, flu-like symptoms
- neck pain, arthralgia, arthritis, joint or tendon disorder
- angina, peripheral vascular disorder, postural hypotension
- dyspepsia, anorexia, vomiting, tooth disorder
- ecchymosis, leucopenia
- decreased libido, impotence, urinary urgency

- pharyngitis, rhinitis, asthma
- alopecia, contact dermatitis, skin carcinoma (including melanoma), rash
- conjunctivitis, otitis media
- albuminaemia
- (adjunct therapy) exacerbate dyskinesia, postural hypotension
- (rare) impulse control disorder, serotonin syndrome (see Glossary), hypertensive crisis, hallucinations

Interactions

- contraindicated with or within 14 days of MAOIs or pethidine
- contraindicated with tramadol, methadone, dextropropoxyphene, dextromethorphan, ciprofloxacin and St John's wort
- not recommended with fluoxetine and fluvoxamine. Fluoxetine should be discontinued for 5 weeks before starting therapy with rasagiline. Rasagiline should be discontinued for at least 2 weeks before starting therapy with fluoxetine or fluvoxamine
- increased risk of serotonin syndrome (see Glossary) if given with SSRIs, SNRIs or TCAs
- not recommended with dextromethorphan or sympathomimetic agents (including nasal and cold preparations)
- clearance may be decreased by entacapone
- increased clearance in smokers
- caution if used with alcohol
- may potentiate dopaminergic adverse effects (including exacerbation of pre-existing dyskinesia) if given with levodopa

Nursing points/Cautions

- before starting therapy, patient should be assessed for any skin lesions
- check supine and standing BP regularly for postural hypotension, especially during first 8 weeks of therapy when it commonly occurs
- recommended dose should not be exceeded due to risk of hypertensive crisis
- not recommended in those under 18 years
- contraindicated in those with liver impairment

Patient teaching and advice

- instruct patient (or carer) to monitor skin for any new or changes to existing skin lesions such as change in colour or size
- if patient is planning to quit smoking while on therapy, he/she should be advised to seek medical advice and not stop suddenly
- advise patient not to take any over-the-counter 'cold and flu' preparations or nasal drops without discussing with doctor or pharmacist first as these may interact with therapy
- see also General Patient teaching and advice for MAO-B inhibitors (p. 749)

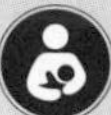

not recommended during pregnancy unless benefits outweigh risks

may inhibit lactation. Caution if used during breastfeeding

tablet can be dispersed in water or crushed and mixed with spoonful of yoghurt or apple puree

SAFINAMIDE (Xadago)

Available forms

Tablets: 50 mg, 100 g

Action

- selectively and reversibly inhibits MAO-B enzyme (breaks down dopamine in the brain), thereby increasing brain levels of dopamine
- elimination half-life 20–30 hours, steady state achieved in about 7 days

Use

- Parkinson's disease (as monotherapy or as adjunct with levodopa in later stage disease)

Dose

- initially 50 mg orally daily, increasing to 100 mg daily after 14 days if needed

Adverse effects
- nausea, dyspepsia, change in appetite, dry mouth, diarrhoea, abdominal pain/distention
- postural hypotension, peripheral oedema
- gait disturbance, falls
- cataract formation and uncommonly, blurred vision, diplopia, photophobia
- dyskinesia, somnolence, dizziness, headache, vertigo
- fatigue, asthenia
- (uncommon) hypertriglyceridaemia, hypercholesterolaemia, hyperglycaemia, urinary tract infection, nocturia, dysuria, erectile dysfunction, cough, dyspnoea, palpitations, tachycardia, bradycardia, arrhythmias, sweating
- (rare) impulse control disorder, serotonin syndrome, suicidal ideation

Interactions
- contraindicated with or within 7 days of MAOIs or pethidine
- not recommended with SSRIs, SNRIs, TCAs, tetracyclic antidepressants, opioids and dexamphetamine due to risk of serotonin syndrome. A washout period of 5 half-lives is recommended when stopping SSRI and starting safinamide
- pre-existing dyskinesia may be exacerbated if given with levodopa and/or dopamine agonists
- caution if used with sympathomimetic agents
- not recommended with dextromethorphan
- may transiently inhibit breast cancer resistance protein (BCRP), therefore a 5-hour interval should be allowed between safinamide and BCRP substrates such as pravastatin, ciprofloxacin, methotrexate, topotecan and diclofenac

Nursing points/Cautions
- if discontinuing therapy, 50 mg daily dose can be stopped without any titration, but 100 mg therapy should be reduced to 50 mg for 7 days before stopping
- tyramine-containing foods do not need to be restricted during therapy
- caution if used in those with moderate liver impairment
- contraindicated in those with severe liver impairment, albinism, retinal degeneration, uveitis, inherited retinopathy or severe progressive diabetic retinopathy

Patient teaching and advice
- see General Patient teaching and advice for MAO-B inhibitors (p. 749)
- female patients of childbearing potential should be advised to use adequate contraception and avoid pregnancy

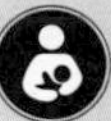
not recommended during pregnancy and breastfeeding

tablets can be crushed and mixed with water or spoonful of yoghurt or apple puree

SELEGILINE HYDROCHLORIDE (Eldepryl)

Available form

Tablets: 5 mg

Action
- selectively and irreversibly inhibits MAO-B enzyme (breaks down dopamine in the brain), thereby increasing brain levels of dopamine
- may also inhibit dopamine reuptake
- three active metabolites with half-lives ranging from 2–20 hours

Use
- Parkinson's disease (as monotherapy in early disease, or as adjunct with levodopa in late stage disease)

Dose
- 5 mg orally twice daily with breakfast and lunch

Adverse effects

- nausea, vomiting, dry mouth
- postural hypotension, syncope
- angina, arrhythmias, bradycardia
- headache, fatigue, dizziness, vertigo, insomnia, sleep disorders
- confusion, hallucinations
- dyskinesia, hypokinesia
- transient increase in liver enzymes (ALT, AST)
- (rare) impulse control disorder

Interactions

- severe hyper/hypotension may result if given with linezolid or other non-selective MAOIs
- increased tyramine sensitivity may result if given with moclobemide. If given together, a low tyramine diet is recommended (see 'cheese reaction' in Glossary for a list of foods to avoid)
- pethidine is contraindicated with or within 14 days of stopping selegiline
- contraindicated with SSRIs. Selegiline should be stopped for 2 weeks before starting SSRIs or SSRIs should be stopped for 5 weeks before starting selegiline
- hypertension may occur if given with dopamine
- increased bioavailability may occur if given with oral contraceptives containing gestodene/ethinylestradiol or levonorgestrel/ethinylestradiol
- increased risk of serotonin syndrome (see Glossary) if given with SSRIs, TCAs, clozapine or ecstasy/MDMA (3, 4-methylenedioxymethamphetamine) or other serotonin potentiating agents
- caution if used with tramadol
- may increase adverse effects of levodopa
- increased risk of CNS toxicity if given with TCAs, therefore these should be stopped 2 weeks before starting selegiline
- not recommended with alcohol
- caution if used with general anaesthetics during surgery due to increased CNS depression

Nursing points/Cautions

- dose of levodopa can be reduced by 10–30% after 2–3 days if levodopa-related adverse effects occur
- check supine and standing BP regularly for postural hypotension
- recommended dose should not be exceeded
- caution if used in those with severe kidney or liver dysfunction

Patient teaching and advice

- see General Patient teaching and advice for MAO-B inhibitors (p. 749)

banned in sport

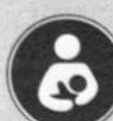

not recommended during pregnancy and breastfeeding unless benefits outweigh the risks

tablets can be dispersed in 10–20 mL water or crushed and mixed with spoonful of yoghurt or apple puree

ANTIPLATELET AGENTS

When a blood vessel is 'damaged', platelets adhere to the site, becoming activated and synthesising factors such as platelet-activating factor, thromboxane A_2, ADP (which binds to $P2Y_{12}$ and $P2Y_1$ receptors) and thrombin, which cause vasoconstriction and platelet aggregation. Platelet aggregation occurs when the platelet receptors (glycoproteins IIb and IIIa) bind with fibrinogen, linking the platelets together. This process is necessary when haemostasis is required, but can sometimes occur when thrombus formation is not required and the thrombus is, in fact, dangerous and may occlude the vessel, leading to conditions such as myocardial infarction, stroke and peripheral arterial thrombosis (Hogg & Weitz 2018).

Antiplatelet agents inhibit this unwanted thrombus formation by decreasing platelet aggregation. As a group, the antiplatelet agents can be subdivided into aspirin (discussed in Analgesics and NSAIDs, p. 11), glycoprotein IIb/IIIa inhibitors and $P2Y_{12}$ inhibitors. They are used in a range of conditions, including the prevention of thromboembolic events (particularly arterial thrombus, which consists mainly of platelets with little fibrin), ischaemic heart disease and prevention of stroke (Hogg & Weitz 2018).

ASPIRIN (Aspro Clear Extra Strength, Aspro preparations, Astrix 100, Astrix Tablets, Cardasa, Cardiprin 100, Cartia, Disprin preparations, Solprin, Spren)

Available forms

Capsules: 100 mg; Tablets: 100 mg, 300 mg, 320 mg, 500 mg; Tablets (enteric coated): 100 mg; Tablets (effervescent): 300 mg, 500 mg

Action

- see General Actions of NSAIDs (p. 12)
- aspirin is converted to salicylic acid mainly in the GI tract
- absorption is dependent on formulation (e.g. soluble formulation increases rate of absorption)
- irreversibly inhibits COX platelet activity (needed for thromboxane synthesis) resulting in prolonged action. It may take 8–12 days (platelet turnover time) after therapy is stopped to fully recover
- half-life of aspirin is about 30 minutes, half-life of salicylate is dose dependent

Use

- analgesic, anti-inflammatory
- antiplatelet therapy (only on medical advice) for prophylaxis against myocardial infarction, unstable angina, transient ischaemic attacks (TIAs) and stroke (see general points for Analgesics and NSAIDs, p. 11)

CLOPIDOGREL (Clovix, Iscover, Piax, Plavicor, Plavix, Plidogrel)

Available forms

Tablets: 75 mg, 300 mg

Action

- inhibits platelet aggregation by irreversibly binding to ADP platelet receptors ($P2Y_{12}$)
- prodrug which is metabolised to active metabolite in a two-step process
- platelet aggregation occurs within 2 hours
- half-life 6–8 hours (active metabolite 30 minutes)
- platelet function returns to normal within 7 days of stopping therapy

Use

- prevention of vascular ischaemia associated with atherothrombotic events (e.g. myocardial infarction, stroke)
- treatment of unstable angina or non-ST-elevation myocardial infarction (NSTEMI) (with aspirin) to prevent early and long-term atherothrombotic events
- treatment of ST elevation myocardial infarction (STEMI) (with aspirin) to prevent atherothrombotic events

Dose

- (unstable angina/NSTEMI) 300 mg orally stat (loading dose), then 75 mg orally once daily (with aspirin 75–325 mg daily) **OR**
- (STEMI) 75 mg orally daily (with or without 300 mg loading dose) with aspirin 75–325 mg daily (with or without fibrinolytic agents) commencing as soon as possible after first symptoms

Adverse effects

- diarrhoea
- rash, pruritus
- bleeding
- (rare) thrombotic thrombocytopenic purpura (TTP), neutropenia, purpura

Interactions

- caution with aspirin or NSAIDs due to increased risk of GI bleeding
- may interfere with metabolism of phenytoin, tamoxifen, warfarin, fluvastatin and some NSAIDs at high doses
- caution if given with heparin, NSAIDs, antiplatelet agents, warfarin or fibrinolytic agents due to increased risk of bleeding
- not recommended with omeprazole, esomeprazole, fluvoxamine, fluoxetine, moclobemide, voriconazole, fluconazole, ciprofloxacin, cimetidine, chloramphenicol, carbamazepine and oxcarbazepine

Nursing points/Cautions

- should be stopped 5 days before any elective surgery (including coronary artery bypass surgery) if antiplatelet effect is not wanted
- blood counts should be closely monitored if any signs of bleeding occur
- in those who have undergone percutaneous coronary intervention (PCI) with stenting, clopidogrel and aspirin should be continued according to type and reasons for stent
- caution if used in those at increased risk of bleeding due to trauma, surgery or other conditions (e.g. recent transient ischaemic attack or stroke, or at risk of recurrent ischaemic events) or with kidney or liver impairment

- extra caution if person is at risk of ophthalmic bleeding due to intraocular lesions
- contraindicated in those with any active gastrointestinal or intracranial bleeding or severe liver impairment

Patient teaching and advice

- warn patient that any bleeding may take longer to stop compared with before therapy
- patient should be advised to tell dentists or doctors of therapy before any invasive procedures (including routine tooth extraction) are undertaken as bleeding may be prolonged
- advise patient not to take over-the-counter NSAIDs as these increase the risk of bleeding
- instruct patient to immediately report any:
    - unusual or prolonged bleeding or bruising (including abnormal blood noses)
    - red/purple skin blotches
    - vomiting blood, black or bloody bowel motions
- tablets are not scored, therefore patient should be advised to use a pill cutter to divide tablet if needed
- see also General Patient teaching and advice (p. xxvii)

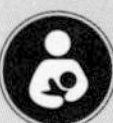

clopidogrel and its metabolites cross the placenta, therefore not recommended during pregnancy

contraindicated during breastfeeding

tablet can be crushed and mixed with 10 mL of water or given with spoonful of yoghurt or apple sauce. 300 mg tablet is very hard to crush

Note

- combined with aspirin in APO-Clopidogrel/Aspirin, Clopidogrel/Aspirin AN, CoPlavix, DuoCover, DuoPlidogrel, and Piax Plus Aspirin

DIPYRIDAMOLE (Persantin Ampoules)

Available form

Ampoules: 10 mg/2 mL

Action

- antiplatelet agent with coronary vasodilator activity
- $P2Y_{12}$ receptor inhibitor
- inhibits adenosine uptake by RBC and platelets, increasing levels of circulating adenosine; inhibits cGMP-phosphodiesterase
- half-life 10–12 hours (oral)

Use

- prevention of ischaemic stroke and transient ischaemic attack (with low-dose aspirin or alone)
- alternative to exercise in cardiac imaging

Dose

- (cardiac perfusion imaging) 0.56 mg/kg infused over 4 minutes (maximum dose 60 mg) **OR**
- (stress echo) 0.56 mg/kg infused over 4 minutes, followed by 4 minutes of no dose, then 0.28 mg/kg over 2 minutes (if no changes were observed on echo monitoring in real time) (total cumulative dose 0.84 mg/kg over 10 minutes)

Adverse effects

- chest pain, angina, ECG changes, arrhythmias, tachycardia
- hypertension, severe hypotension, labile blood pressure
- headache, dizziness, fatigue
- paraesthesia
- nausea, vomiting, diarrhoea, abdominal pain, dyspepsia
- myalgia
- oedema
- dyspnoea
- hot flushes
- rash, urticaria
- pain
- (undiluted IV) vein irritation

- (rare) seizures, non-fatal myocardial infarction, asystole, transient ischaemic attack, AV block, bronchospasm, pulmonary oedema

Interactions

- vasodilating effects decreased by xanthine derivatives (including tea and coffee)
- may counteract anticholinesterase effect of cholinesterase inhibitors (potentially aggravating myasthenia gravis)
- may increase hypotensive effects of antihypertensive agents
- may increase plasma levels and cardiovascular effects of adenosine
- IV dipyridamole is contraindicated in those taking oral dipyridamole

Nursing points/Cautions

- ECG and vital signs should be monitored during and 10–15 minutes after administration
- imaging agents should be given within 5 minutes of IV dipyridamole
- should be diluted to 20–50 mL with glucose 5% or sodium chloride 0.45% before being infused
- administer alone
- slow IV aminophylline (50–100 mg over 30–60 seconds) should be administered if bronchospasm or chest pain occurs. Aminophylline is not recommended if variant angina with ST elevation occurs, as it may be worsened by administration of aminophylline. Glyceryl trinitrate (sublingual or intravenous) may also be given if chest pain continues despite administration of aminophylline
- if severe hypotension occurs, patient should be placed in supine position with head tilted down (if needed)
- caution if used in those with myasthenia gravis as dipyridamole may interact with cholinesterase inhibitors
- caution if used in those with left main coronary stenosis, moderate stenotic valvular disease, electrolyte imbalance, severe arterial hypertension (systolic > 200 mmHg and/or diastolic > 110 mmHg), tachyarrhythmias, bradyarrhythmias, AV block or cardiomyopathy
- not recommended in those with asthma, hypotension (less than systolic BP 90 mmHg), unexplained syncope or transient ischaemic attacks
- contraindicated in those with unstable angina, uncontrolled cardiac arrhythmias, uncontrolled symptomatic heart failure, acute pulmonary embolus or pulmonary infarction, acute myocardial infarction, acute myocarditis or pericarditis, acute aortic dissection and severe aortic stenosis

Patient teaching and advice

- advise patient that side-effects reduce or disappear altogether with continued therapy
- warn patient against driving or operating machinery if severe headache or dizziness occurs
- see also General Patient teaching and advice (p. xxvii)

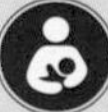

should only be used during pregnancy if benefits outweigh risks

caution if used during breastfeeding as it appears in breastmilk

capsules can be opened and pellets sprinkled onto spoonful of yoghurt or apple puree

Note

- contained with aspirin in Diasp SR

EPTIFIBATIDE (Integrilin)

Available forms

Ampoules: 20 mg/10 mL (for bolus), 75 mg/100 mL (for IV infusion)

Action

- binds to glycoprotein IIb/IIIa receptors inhibiting platelet aggregation by preventing fibrinogen, von Willebrand factor and other ligands binding to the receptor
- platelet inhibition reversed within 6 hours of stopping therapy

Use

- adjunct to non-urgent percutaneous intracoronary (PCI) stenting
- unstable angina
- non-Q wave myocardial infarction

Dose

- (non-urgent PCI stenting with normal renal function) 180 microgram/kg IV bolus immediately before procedure, followed 10 minutes later by second bolus. An infusion of 2.0 microgram/kg/minute should be started with the first bolus and continued until discharge or 18–24 hours after stenting procedure **OR**
- (non-urgent PCI stenting with renal impairment (creatinine clearance < 50 mL/min)) 180 microgram/kg IV bolus immediately before procedure, followed 10 minutes later by second bolus. An infusion of 1.0 microgram/kg/minute should be started with the first bolus and continued until discharge or 18–24 hours after stenting procedure **OR**
- (unstable angina/non-Q-wave myocardial infarction with normal renal function) 180 microgram/kg IV bolus as soon as practicable after diagnosis, followed by an infusion of 2.0 microgram/kg/minute for up to 72 hours, discharge from hospital or coronary artery grafting (whichever comes first). If PCI stenting occurs, infusion should be continued for 20–24 hours post-procedure (maximum therapy duration 96 hours) **OR**
- (unstable angina/non-Q-wave myocardial infarction with renal impairment (creatinine clearance < 50 mL/min)) 180 microgram/kg IV bolus as soon as practicable after diagnosis, followed by an infusion of 1.0 microgram/kg/minute for up to 72 hours, discharge from hospital or coronary artery grafting (whichever comes first). If PCI stenting occurs, infusion should be continued for 20–24 hours post-procedure (maximum therapy duration 96 hours)

Adverse effects

- bleeding (major, minor)
- hypotension
- atrial fibrillation, chest pain, ventricular fibrillation/tachycardia, congestive cardiac failure, AV block, cardiac arrest, shock
- headache
- fever
- nausea, abdominal pain
- (rare) thrombocytopenia, cerebral ischaemia
- (IV site) phlebitis

Interactions

- caution if given with other agents affecting platelet aggregation or haemostasis such as oral anticoagulants, dextran, adenosine, low molecular weight heparins, antiplatelet agents, prostacyclin and NSAIDs
- contraindicated with fibrinolytic agents or other GP IIb/IIIa inhibitors

Nursing points/Cautions

- baseline prothrombin time, APTT, platelet count, serum creatinine, haemoglobin and haematocrit should be

measured within 6 hours of starting therapy and daily thereafter. If platelet count falls to $< 100 \times 10^9$/L therapy should be stopped
- IV infusion should be continued for a minimum of 12 hours
- if patient requires emergency or urgent cardiac surgery during therapy, infusion should be stopped immediately
- if patient requires semi-elective surgery, infusion should be stopped in time to allow platelet function to return to normal
- patient should be closely monitored for any signs of bleeding, especially if there has been an invasive procedure, including catheter insertion sites and intramuscular injection sites (these should be minimised or avoided altogether). If intravenous access is necessary, compressible sites should be used
- use of nasogastric tubes, urinary catheters and nasotracheal intubation should also be minimised
- if arterial sheath is used, it should only be removed after coagulation has returned to normal (APTT < 45 seconds). Site should be observed for at least 4 hours after removal
- women, the elderly and those of low body weight are at greater risk of bleeding and should be carefully monitored
- if serious bleeding occurs (not controlled with pressure), infusion should be stopped. If heparin is being administered at the same time, it should also be stopped
- incompatible with IV furosemide (frusemide)
- administer alone
- usually given with heparin and aspirin (antiplatelet dose) unless contraindicated. Heparin dose is determined by patient's weight and is given as a bolus, followed by IV infusion. APTT should be monitored and heparin adjusted accordingly
- caution if used in those with liver impairment or moderate to severe kidney insufficiency
- contraindicated in patients with abnormal bleeding or within 30 days of active bleeding, abnormal clotting times (INR ≥ 2.0), bleeding disorder or thrombocytopenia ($< 100 \times 10^9$/L), or if patient has had a recent stroke (within 30 days), haemorrhagic stroke or intracranial disease (neoplasm, aneurysm, AV malformation), recent major surgery or trauma (within 6 weeks), hypertension (severe), kidney (including dialysis) or significant liver impairment

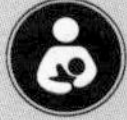

should only be used in pregnancy if benefits outweigh potential risks

not recommended during breastfeeding

PRASUGREL (Prasugrel SCP)

Available forms

Tablets: 5 mg, 10 mg

Action

- irreversible $P2Y_{12}$ receptor inhibitor
- prodrug with active metabolite
- platelet aggregation returned to normal after 7–9 days (single dose) and 5 days (stopping therapy)
- peak concentration within 30 minutes
- half-life of active metabolite is 2–15 hours; however, irreversible binding results in prolonged activity after therapy is stopped

Use

- prevention of atherothrombotic events in patients with unstable angina or non-ST elevation myocardial infarction (NSTEMI) (with aspirin)
- treatment of ST elevation myocardial infarction (STEMI) who will undergo percutaneous coronary intervention

(PCI) (with aspirin) to prevent atherothrombotic events

Dose

- initially 60 mg orally (loading dose), followed by 10 mg orally daily (with aspirin 75–325 mg) **OR**
- (patient weighing < 60 kg) initially 60 mg orally (loading dose), followed by 5 mg orally daily (with aspirin 75–325 mg)

Adverse effects

- bleeding (minor, major)
- hypertension, hypotension, atrial fibrillation, bradycardia, non-cardiac chest pain
- hypercholesterolaemia, hyperlipidaemia
- headache, back pain, pain in extremities
- dyspnoea, cough
- nausea, diarrhoea
- dizziness, fatigue
- leucopenia
- rash
- fever
- peripheral oedema
- (rare) thrombotic thrombocytopenic purpura (TTP), hypersensitivity, angioedema

Interactions

- caution if used with heparin, oral anticoagulants, NSAIDs or fibrinolytic agents because of increased risk of bleeding

Nursing points/Cautions

- for NSTEMI patients, loading dose should be given at time of PCI
- therapy should be discontinued for at least 7 days before elective surgery (if antiplatelet effect is not desired)
- caution in those weighing less than 60 kg or who have had recent surgery or trauma, recent/recurrent gastrointestinal bleeding, active peptic ulcer disease, severe liver or kidney impairment
- contains lactose, therefore not recommended in those with galactose intolerance, Lapp lactase deficiency or glucose–galactose malabsorption
- caution if used in those of Asian origin because of increased risk of bleeding
- not recommended in those over 75 years
- contraindicated in those with active bleeding, history of stroke or transient ischaemic attack or severe liver failure

Patient teaching and advice

- advise patient not to drive or operate machinery if dizziness or fatigue are problems
- instruct patient to take tablets whole and not break in half
- advise patient to report any of the following symptoms immediately:
  - unusual or prolonged bleeding or bruising
  - nosebleeds
  - blue/purple spots under skin or nails
  - vomiting or coughing up blood or dark/black tarry stools
- see also General Patient teaching and advice (p. xxvii)

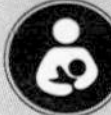

should only be used during pregnancy or breastfeeding if benefits outweigh risks

tablet can be crushed and mixed with water or spoonful of yoghurt or apple puree

TICAGRELOR (Brilinta)

Available form

Tablets/Orodispersible tablets: 90 mg

Action

- selective and reversible $P2Y_{12}$ receptor inhibitor

- active metabolite (half-life 6.5–12.8 hours)
- half-life 4.5–12.8 hours

Use

- prevention of atherothrombotic events in those with unstable angina, non-ST elevation myocardial infarction (NSTEMI), ST elevation myocardial infarction (STEMI) (with aspirin)

Dose

- initially 180 mg orally (loading dose), followed by 90 mg orally twice daily (with aspirin 75–150 mg)

Adverse effects

- epistaxis, bleeding (major, minor)
- dyspnoea, cough
- cardiac failure, atrial fibrillation, bradycardia, chest pain
- hypertension, hypotension
- non-cardiac chest pain, back pain
- increased uric acid, gout, increased creatinine levels
- nausea, vomiting, diarrhoea, constipation, abdominal pain, dyspepsia, gastrointestinal bleeding
- headache, fatigue, dizziness, syncope, vertigo
- fever
- rash
- peripheral oedema
- (rare) hypersensitivity, angioedema

Interactions

- contraindicated with clarithromycin, ritonavir and atazanavir
- not recommended with clopidogrel or prasugrel
- increased dyspnoea (transient) may occur if given with adenosine
- increased risk of bleeding if given with SSRIs
- caution if used with NSAIDs, oral anticoagulants or fibrinolytic agents due to increased risk of bleeding
- caution if used with agents known to induce bradycardia (e.g. digoxin, beta-adrenoceptor blocking agents, verapamil, diltiazem)
- not recommended with ergot alkaloids
- may increase serum levels of ciclosporin and digoxin increasing the risk of toxicity. Serum levels should be closely monitored if given together
- increased serum levels may occur if given with ciclosporin or digoxin
- decreased serum levels may occur if given with rifampicin, dexamethasone, phenytoin, carbamazepine and phenobarbital (phenobarbitone)
- caution if given with simvastatin (doses > 40 mg daily) due to increased risk of myopathy and rhabdomyolysis
- caution if used with angiotensin II receptor blocking agents due to risk of kidney impairment

Nursing points/Cautions

- should be discontinued for 5 days before elective surgery
- renal function should be monitored monthly during therapy; uric acid levels should also be monitored regularly
- if switching from clopidogrel, ticagrelor 90 mg should be given 24 hours after last dose of clopidogrel
- therapy should be continued for at least 12 months
- caution in those with asthma or chronic obstructive pulmonary disorder due to increased risk of dyspnoea
- caution if used in those without a pacemaker and with sick sinus syndrome, second or third degree A-V block or bradycardia-related syncope due to increased risk of bradycardia; in those with hyperuricaemia or gout; in those who have coagulation disorders, history of or recent/active bleeding, recent trauma or surgery, ischaemic stroke, if the patient weighs less than 60 kg or aged 75 years or more

- contraindicated in those with active bleeding, history of intracranial haemorrhage, moderate-to-severe liver impairment

Patient teaching and advice

- warn patient against driving or operating machinery if dizziness or confusion occur
- patient should be advised that shortness of breath is a common side-effect of this medication. However, it is still important to seek medical advice if it occurs or worsens
- if unable to swallow tablets, advise patient to crush tablet to a fine powder using mortar and pestle/crushing device and add 100 mL, stir well and pour into a glass. Another 100 mL of water should be added to mortar and pestle/crushing device, stirred to ensure all fine powder is removed and transferred to glass and drink 200 mL immediately
- advise patient to place dispersible tablet on tongue, allow to dissolve and swallow with or without water
- see also General Patient teaching and advice (p. xxvii)

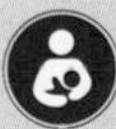
not recommended during pregnancy or breastfeeding

available as an orally dispersible tablet (dissolve on the tongue) or tablet can be crushed and mixed with water

TIROFIBAN HYDROCHLORIDE (Aggrastat, Tirofiban Juno Concentrate)

Available form
Vial: 12.5 mg/50 mL

Action
- glycoprotein IIb/IIIa receptor inhibitor
- half-life 1.4–1.8 hours, prolonged to 1.9–2.2 hours in those with coronary artery disease

Use
- unstable angina or non-Q wave myocardial infarction in the prevention of cardiac ischaemia (with heparin)

Dose
- 0.4 microgram/kg/minute for 30 minutes (with IV bolus of heparin 5000 U), then 0.1 microgram/kg/minute (with heparin infusion 1000 U/hour, titrated to APTT)

Adverse effects
- bleeding (major, minor), thrombocytopenia
- headache
- fever
- nausea
- rash, urticaria

Interactions
- contraindicated with other glycoprotein IIb/IIIa receptor inhibitors
- caution if given with drugs that affect haemostasis such as fibrinolytic agents

Nursing points/Cautions

- take patient history before the procedure to exclude, within the past month, any major surgical procedures or trauma, spinal or epidural anaesthetic, intracranial bleeding, neoplasm or aneurysm, stroke, active internal bleeding, severe uncontrolled hypertension, history or symptoms of aortic dissection or active pericarditis, because these are all contraindications to therapy
- great caution should be taken in patients who have a history of bleeding within the past year
- monitor haemoglobin, haematocrit and platelet count before starting therapy, within 6 hours of loading dose and then daily during therapy
- therapy should be withdrawn if platelet count confirms thrombocytopenia

- APTT should be measured before starting and regularly throughout therapy (it should be twice the normal value) and dose adjusted if needed
- patient should be closely monitored after removal of sheath for any signs of bleeding or haematoma formation. Arterial sheath should only be removed when APTT < 180 seconds or 2–6 hours after stopping heparin therapy
- combination therapy with heparin should be continued for a minimum of 48 hours and may be continued through angiography and for 12–24 hours after if necessary
- monitor urine and faeces for occult blood
- incompatible with IV diazepam
- to dilute, remove 50 mL from 250 mL bag or normal saline 0.9% or glucose 5% and replace with 50 mL of tirofiban to achieve a final concentration of 0.05 mg/mL and administer via infusion pump
- caution if used in those who have had a clinically significant bleed or stroke in the last year, recent epidural procedure, known coagulopathy, platelet disorder or thrombocytopenia, haemorrhagic retinopathy, impaired kidney function (creatinine clearance < 30 mL/minute), chronic haemodialysis or platelet count below 150,000 cells/mm^3
- contraindicated in those with or within 30 days of active internal bleeding, within 30 days of severe trauma, major surgery (including epidural or spinal anaesthesia) or haemorrhagic stroke, with thrombocytopenia following previous exposure to tirofiban, bleeding disorders, severe uncontrolled hypertension, history/symptoms of aortic dissection, acute pericarditis or intracranial haemorrhage, aneurysm, AV malformation or intracranial neoplasm

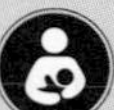

should only be used during pregnancy or breastfeeding if benefits outweigh potential risks

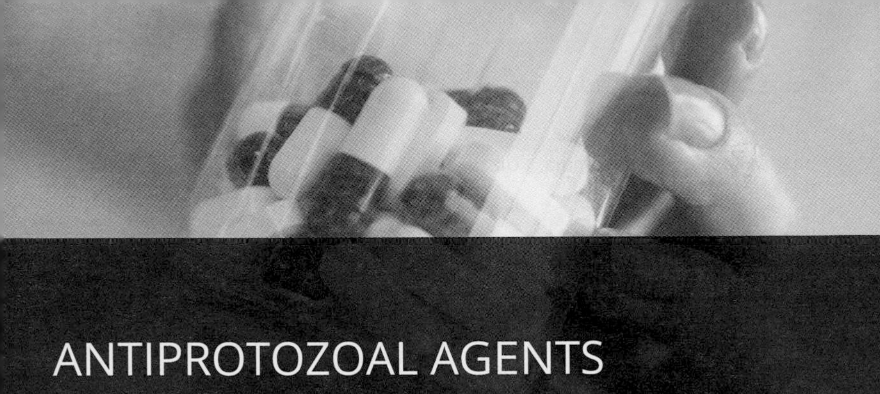

ANTIPROTOZOAL AGENTS

Protozoa are single-celled eukaryotic organisms, some of which are parasitic pathogens that divide within the host, causing a range of diseases. Protozoa are generally classified according to their mode of 'locomotion' and include:

- amoebae, which move using pseudopodia (or false feet), and cause, for example, amoebic dysentery
- flagellates, which move by beating their flagellum (whip) in a whip-like movement, and are responsible for giardiasis, trichomonal vaginitis, leishmaniasis and trypanosomiasis
- ciliates, which move by beating cilia (hair-like appendages)
- sporozoans, the adult forms of which do not appear to have any means of movement (e.g. *Plasmodium* spp., see Antimalarial agents, p. 542) (CDC 2016).

Some human protozoan infections include amoebiasis (second leading cause of death due to parasitic disease), giardiasis, trichomiasis, toxoplasmosis, leishmaniasis (700,000–1 million new cases and 26,000–65,000 deaths annually), cryptosporidiosis and trypanosomiasis (WHO 2019a).

ATOVAQUONE (Wellvone Suspension)

Available form

Suspension: 750 mg/5 mL

Action

- selective and potent inhibitor of nucleic acid and ATP synthesis in some parasitic protozoa, particularly *Pneumocystis carinii*, *Toxoplasma gondii* and *Plasmodium* species
- half-life 2–3 days

Use

- acute treatment of mild-to-moderate *P. carinii* pneumonia (PCP) in adults with AIDS who are intolerant of trimethoprim–sulfamethoxazole (co-trimoxazole) therapy

Dose

- 750 mg orally twice daily with food for 21 days **OR**
- 1500 mg orally once daily with food for 21 days (patients with swallowing difficulties or unable to eat 2 meals per day)

Adverse effects

- nausea, vomiting, diarrhoea, abdominal pain, constipation, dyspepsia, oral monilia (thrush)
- rash, pruritus, sweating
- sinusitis

- headache, fever, insomnia, dizziness, asthenia
- anaemia, neutropenia
- increased liver enzymes
- hyponatraemia, hyperglycaemia
- hypersensitivity

Interactions

- plasma levels decreased when given with rifampicin or metoclopramide
- if given with rifabutin, may decrease plasma levels of both drugs
- may decrease metabolism of zidovudine, therefore use with caution
- caution should be used when given with warfarin
- may decrease serum levels of indinavir

Nursing points/Cautions

- any patient with lung disease should be carefully evaluated before starting therapy for causes of infection and any other therapies (e.g. antiviral, antibacterial, antifungal, antimycotic) which may have been used in the management of the disease
- not recommended prophylactically, in acute cases of PCP or in those who have failed other treatments for PCP

Patient teaching and advice

- advise the patient to shake suspension well before use and not to dilute it with any other fluids
- advise the patient to take suspension with food, particularly high-fat meals, because this significantly increases the availability
- warn patient to avoid driving or operating machinery if dizziness occurs
- any diarrhoea should be immediately reported (because this correlates with therapy failure)
- the patient should be advised to report any sore white mouth or tongue (as this may be due to yeast overgrowth and require treatment)
- see also General Patient teaching and advice (p. xxvii)

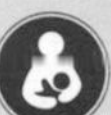

should not be used during pregnancy or breastfeeding unless benefits outweigh potential risks

Note

- contained in antimalarial agent Malarone with proguanil and Promozio 250/100

METRONIDAZOLE (Flagyl, Flagyl S Suspension, Metrogyl, Metronidazole Intravenous Infusion, Metronide, Rozex Cream and Gel, Zidoval Vaginal Gel)

Available forms

IV solution: 500 mg/100 mL; Tablets: 200 mg, 400 mg; Suppositories: 500 mg; Suspension 200 mg/5 mL; Gel: 5 mg/g, 7.5 mg/g; Cream: 7.5 mg/g; Vaginal gel: 0.75%

Action

- effective against a wide range of anaerobic organisms (bactericidal, amoebicidal, trichomonacidal) and protozoa
- disrupts DNA and inhibits synthesis of nucleic acids
- metabolite has some antiprotozoal activity
- widely distributed throughout body tissues and reaches therapeutic levels in abscesses, bile, CSF, synovial and seminal fluid
- inactive against aerobic and facultative anaerobic bacteria
- (IV) half-life 6.3–8.3 hours

Use

- (IV) treatment of severe anaerobic organisms (where oral medication is contraindicated or not possible)
- surgical site prophylaxis where there is potential contamination with anaerobic organisms
- bacterial vaginosis, urogenital trichomoniasis, pelvic abscess/cellulitis, post-delivery sepsis

- amoebiasis (intestinal, extra intestinal)
- anaerobic infections (e.g. septicaemia, osteomyelitis, brain abscess, necrotising pneumonia, giardiasis, acute ulcerative gingivitis, bacteraemia)
- (topical) rosacea (with associated erythema, papules and pustules)
- postoperative wound infection

Dose

- (urogenital trichomoniasis, bacterial vaginosis) 2 g as single oral dose **OR**
- (urogenital trichomoniasis) 200 mg orally 3 times daily for 7 days **OR**
- (bacterial vaginosis) 400 mg orally 3 times daily for 7 days **OR**
- (bacterial vaginosis) 2 g orally daily for 3 days **OR**
- (amoebiasis) 400–800 mg orally 3 times daily for 5–10 days **OR**
- (giardiasis) 2 g orally daily for 3 days **OR**
- (acute ulcerative gingivitis) 200 mg orally 3 times daily for 3 days **OR**
- (anaerobic infection) 400 mg orally 3 times daily for 7 days **OR**
- (surgical prophylaxis) 400 mg orally 1–2 hours before surgery and repeated 8-hourly for 24 hours **OR**
- (surgical prophylaxis) 500 mg IV just prior to surgery and repeated 8-hourly for 24 hours **OR**
- (elective colonic surgery) 2 rectal suppositories (1 g) every 8 hours for 48 hours before and after surgery (with bowel preparation) **OR**
- (anaerobic infection) 2 rectal suppositories (1 g) every 8 hours for 3 days, then 12-hourly if needed **OR**
- (surgical prophylaxis – appendectomy) 2 rectal suppositories (1 g) at diagnosis, then repeated 8-hourly for 48 hours after surgery **OR**
- 500 mg IV every 8 hours, infused over 30 minutes **OR**
- (symptomatic bacterial vaginosis) one applicator full (5 g) intravaginally nightly at bedtime for 5 days **OR**
- (rosacea) apply thin film of cream or gel to affected area and rub in until absorbed twice daily for 3–9 weeks (gel) or 12–16 weeks (cream)

Adverse effects

- metallic taste, anorexia, nausea, vomiting, dyspepsia, dry mouth, abdominal discomfort/cramping, diarrhoea, constipation, oral mucositis
- rash, pruritus
- hypersensitivity (rash, urticaria, nasal congestion, fever, flushing, dry mouth, angioedema)
- superinfection (including glossitis, stomatitis, furry tongue, vaginitis (*Candida* spp.))
- dysuria, cystitis, pruritus of genital area, pelvic pressure, darkening of urine, dryness of vagina or vulva
- headache, dizziness, insomnia
- vertigo, tinnitus, impaired hearing
- syncope
- seizures, confusion, ataxia, lack of coordination, hallucinations, depression, disorientation, dysarthria
- transient joint pain, weakness
- transient leucopenia
- transient blurry or double vision, changes in vision or acuity or colour vision, optic neuritis
- nasal congestion
- flattened T wave, prolonged QT interval
- (prolonged administration) peripheral neuropathy, seizures
- (rare) pancreatitis, abnormal liver function tests, hepatitis, anaphylaxis, aseptic meningitis, encephalopathy with cerebellar toxicity, pseudomembranous colitis, reversible thrombocytopenia, severe skin reactions
- (IV) thrombophlebitis
- (vaginal cream) pelvic discomfort
- (topical) skin irritation, redness, itching, burning, stinging, dryness, aggravated acne/rosacea (transient) eye irritation (if applied too close to eyes)

Interactions

- may result in lithium toxicity in patients on a high dose of lithium
- increased risk of toxicity if used with carmustine or cyclophosphamide
- if taken in combination with alcohol, may produce disulfiram-alcohol reaction (see Glossary)
- may enhance activity of warfarin, therefore prothrombin time should be closely monitored throughout therapy
- may increase serum ciclosporin, busulfan and fluorouracil, increasing risk of toxicity
- serum levels may be increased by cimetidine, prolonging half-life and decreasing clearance
- plasma levels may be reduced by phenobarbital (phenobarbitone) and phenytoin
- may decrease clearance of phenytoin
- increased risk of psychotic reaction (e.g. acute psychoses, confusion) if given with or within 2 weeks of disulfiram
- transient neutropenia may occur if given with fluorouracil or azathioprine
- increased risk of sodium retention and oedema if given with corticosteroids
- may interfere with laboratory tests (AST, ALT, LDH), triglycerides or glucose determination

Nursing points/Cautions

- neurological function (e.g. gait, seizure activity, paraesthesia) and blood counts (e.g. differential leucocyte counts) should be monitored regularly throughout any prolonged therapy (> 10 days) and drug discontinued if leucopenia or neurological symptoms occur
- to reduce the incidence of reinfection, treatment for urogenital trichomoniasis should include sexual partner
- transfer from IV to oral therapy as soon as possible
- oral suspension should not be used to manage acute situations
- suppositories are recommended where oral therapy is contraindicated or not possible
- if re-treatment for urogenital trichomoniasis is required, an interval of 4–6 weeks should be allowed and leucocyte count monitored before starting and during therapy
- (urogenital trichomoniasis) if patient is pregnant and in second or third trimester, 1-day course should not be administered due to increased risk to fetus
- (bacterial vaginosis) gonorrohea should be excluded
- IV daily maximum 4 g
- should be administered IV at a rate of 25 mg/minute
- administer alone
- incompatible with aluminium
- IV solution contains sodium (310 mg/100 mL) and may result in sodium retention in those predisposed to oedema or taking corticosteroids
- caution if used in those with acute or chronic severe peripheral CNS disease or with impaired liver function
- caution if used in those with Cockayne syndrome because of increased risk of hepatotoxicity. If used, liver function should be assessed before starting, during and after completion of therapy and patient alerted to signs of liver impairment
- contraindicated in those with blood dyscrasias, active organic brain disease or hypersensitivity to imidazoles
- (topical, vaginal) contraindicated in those with hypersensitivity to hydroxybenzoates

Patient teaching and advice

- instruct patients that tablets should be taken with meals and swallowed whole (not crushed or chewed); the suspension is taken 1 hour before a meal
- patient should be advised to avoid alcohol while taking metronidazole

and for at least 1 day after stopping therapy

- warn the patient that the urine may become a harmless dark colour during treatment
- patient should be warned against driving or operating machinery if dizziness, vertigo or confusion occur
- advise patient to seek medical advice immediately if any of the following occur:
  - weakness of hands or feet, dizziness, numbness or seizures
  - visual disturbances
  - uncoordinated movements, difficulty speaking, confusion, hallucinations, depression
  - unusual bleeding or bruising
  - frequent infections, fever, chills, sore throat or mouth ulcers, flu-like illness
  - sore, white mouth or tongue (yeast overgrowth)
  - vaginal itching or burning, white discharge (yeast overgrowth in females)
- (vaginal cream) ensure patient understands correct insertion technique
- (suppository) advise patient to empty bowel before insertion of suppository and ensure that he/she has been instructed in correct insertion technique
- (topical) instruct patients in the following:
  - wash hands immediately after applying gel or cream
  - cream or gel should be applied 20 minutes after cleaning affected area
  - avoid contact with eyes
  - avoid use of cosmetic products or medicated soaps that are drying
  - avoid exposure to sunlight or UV radiation during therapy and wear protective clothing and sunscreen with high protective factor (SPF 30+) when exposed to sunlight
  - moisturiser and/or cosmetics can be applied after gel has been allowed to dry
- female patient of childbearing potential should be counselled to use adequate contraception and avoid pregnancy during therapy
- see General Patient teaching and advice (p. xxvii)

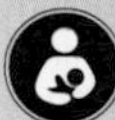

should not be used in the first trimester of pregnancy as it crosses placental barrier and rapidly enters fetal circulation. Use in second or third trimester should be restricted to women with trichomoniasis where palliative treatment has not controlled symptoms

not recommended during breastfeeding

oral suspension is available

PENTAMIDINE ISETIONATE (PENTAMIDINE ISETHIONATE) (DBL Pentamidine Isethionate for Injection)

Available form

Vial: 300 mg

Action

- exact mechanism of action is unknown although thought to interfere with nuclear metabolism
- very low penetration of CNS

Use

- *P. carinii* pneumonia (PCP) (first-line treatment in patients with AIDS, second-line treatment in non-AIDS patients)
- most types of trypanosomiasis (second-line treatment)
- visceral and cutaneous forms of leishmaniasis (second-line treatment)
- *Leishmania aethiopica* (first-line treatment)

Dose

- (PCP) 4 mg/kg daily by IV infusion over 60 minutes for 14 days **OR**

- (visceral leishmaniasis) 3–4 mg/kg by IV infusion over 60 minutes 3 times weekly (alternate days) to a maximum of 10 doses **OR**
- (cutaneous leishmaniasis) 3–4 mg/kg by IV infusion over 60 minutes 1–2 times weekly until condition resolves **OR**
- (trypanosomiasis during haemolymphatic stage) 4 mg/kg daily by IV infusion over 60 minutes or on alternate days to a maximum of 7–10 doses

Adverse effects

- severe hypotension, syncope
- cardiac arrhythmias, cardiac arrest, ventricular tachycardia, tachycardia, bradycardia
- dizziness
- nausea, vomiting, taste disturbance
- acute renal failure
- acute pancreatitis, abnormal liver function
- leucopenia, thrombocytopenia, anaemia
- severe hypoglycaemia, sometimes followed by hyperglycaemia, diabetes mellitus
- fever, rash, flushing
- hypocalcaemia, hyperkalaemia, hyponatraemia
- delirium, Jarisch–Herxheimer reaction (malaise, fever, chills, sore throat, myalgia, headache, tachycardia)
- (local) thrombophlebitis
- (rare) Stevens–Johnson syndrome (see Glossary)

Interactions

- increased risk of nephrotoxicity if given with other nephrotoxic drugs
- caution if given with hepatotoxic agents

Nursing points/Cautions

- following observations are recommended during therapy:
  - daily serum electrolytes, full blood count (including platelet), serum creatinine and blood urea nitrogen (BUN)
  - fasting blood glucose levels before starting, daily during and at regular intervals after completion of therapy
  - daily urinalysis
  - liver function tests before starting, then weekly (if normal) or every 3–5 days if baseline is elevated or if given with hepatotoxic agents
  - weekly serum calcium levels
  - regular ECG
- patient should lie down while receiving pentamidine because of hypotensive risk
- monitor BP before and regularly during IV infusion and hourly after completion of infusion until BP is stable
- not recommended by IV push or bolus
- reconstitute with 3–5 mL of water for injections, then dilute further with 50–250 mL of glucose 5% or sodium chloride 0.9%
- administer infusion over at least 60 minutes
- caution if used in those with malnutrition, hyperglycaemia, hypoglycaemia, liver or kidney dysfunction, hypertension, hypotension or blood disorders

Patient teaching and advice

- warn patient against driving or operating machinery if dizziness or lightheadedness occurs
- patient should be advised to avoid alcohol (or reduce consumption) as it will exacerbate dizziness and lightheadedness
- instruct patient to seek medical advice immediately if any of the following occur:
  - unusual bleeding or bruising
  - flu-like illness, sore throat, fever, chills, mouth ulcers
  - signs of high blood glucose (hyperglycaemia), including increased thirst and urination, tiredness

  - signs of low blood glucose (hypoglycaemia), including trembling/shaking, irritability, light-headedness
  - peeling of skin
  - dizziness or fainting, slow/fast or irregular heart rate
  - fever, chills, headache and muscle pain
  - upper abdominal pain
  - breathlessness or difficulty breathing
- female patients of childbearing potential should be counselled to use adequate contraception to avoid pregnancy occurring during therapy
- see also General Patient teaching and advice (p. xxvii)

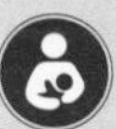

contraindicated during pregnancy or breastfeeding unless benefit outweighs any potential risk

PYRIMETHAMINE (Daraprim)

Available form
Tablets: 25 mg

Action
- antifolate that blocks synthesis of plasmodial nucleic acids by inhibiting dihydrofolate reductase, thereby disrupting protein synthesis and nuclear division
- half-life 90 hours

Use
- toxoplasmosis (usually given with a sulfonamide)

Dose
- initially 50 mg orally, then 25 mg daily for 3–6 weeks (with sulfadiazine 150 mg/kg/day)

Adverse effects
- nausea, vomiting, diarrhoea, colic
- rash
- headache, dizziness
- anaemia, thrombocytopenia, leucopenia (early in treatment)
- (less common) dry mouth and/or throat, dermatitis, depression, abnormal skin pigmentation, fever, malaise
- (rare) convulsions (prolonged therapy or high doses for toxoplasmosis)

Interactions
- increased risk of seizures if given with methotrexate (in children with CNS leukaemia)
- increased risk of bone marrow depression if given with cytostatic agents such as methotrexate, daunorubicin or cytarabine
- may induce hepatotoxicity when given with lorazepam
- may further decrease folate metabolism in those taking folate inhibitors or myelosuppressive agents such as methotrexate, zidovudine, proguanil, trimethoprim or co-trimoxazole
- absorption may be decreased if given with antacids or kaolin
- increased risk of seizures if given with antimalarial agents or methotrexate
- increased risk of megaloblastic anaemia if given in doses > 25 mg/week with trimethoprim/sulfonamide combination
- may increase serum levels if given with agents with low therapeutic index and highly protein bound (e.g. warfarin)

Nursing points/Cautions
- folate supplement (folic acid 5 mg or calcium folinate 6 mg daily) is recommended to decrease risk of bone marrow depression
- monitor blood cell counts weekly during and for 2 weeks after stopping treatment to detect folate deficiency and treat with high-dose calcium folinate if folate deficiency occurs
- treatment for toxoplasmosis should continue for 3–6 weeks. If further

treatment is required, a 2-week rest period is required between treatments
- if given with a sulfonamide, patient should be well hydrated to prevent crystalluria
- tablets contain lactose and are therefore not recommended in those with galactose intolerance, Lapp lactase deficiency or glucose–galactose malabsorption
- caution if used in those with folate deficiency (including megaloblastic anaemia or due to malnutrition) or history of seizures (loading dose should not be given)

Patient teaching and advice

- advise patient to taking antacids within 2 hours of tablets
- see also General Patient teaching and advice (p. xxvii)

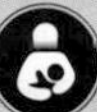

contraindicated during first semester of pregnancy. Folate supplement is recommended if used during pregnancy (second or third trimester) if eye lesions threaten mother's vision or antibody titres against toxoplasma are rising. Toxoplasmosis carries a high risk to the fetus, including malformation and abortion

secreted in breastmilk, therefore not recommended during breastfeeding

tablets can be crushed and mixed with water or spoonful of yoghurt or apple puree

ANTIPSYCHOTIC AND MOOD-STABILISING AGENTS

Antipsychotic (or neuroleptic) agents are used in the management of schizophrenia, psychoses and some agitated states. They are generally classified as typical (first generation) (phenothiazines, butyrophenones and thioxanthenes) or atypical (second generation), which include some of the more recently developed agents, such as clozapine and risperidone. Agents within these groups are not homogenous and the terminology (first or second generation) tends to be associated with the length of time the agents have been available; however, the difference relates to the receptors where they have their main effects. Typical antipsychotic agents inhibit dopamine (D2) receptors, whereas the atypical antipsychotics also act on serotonin (5-hydroxytryptamine, histamine and acetylcholine receptors), resulting in not only therapeutic effects but also adverse effects (Bryant et al 2019; Psychotropic Expert Group 2013).

In general, antipsychotic agents decrease the positive symptoms (e.g. hallucinations, delusions, thought disorders) of schizophrenia, along with some decrease in hostility and excitement, but have limited impact on negative symptoms (e.g. lack of motivation, self-care, blunted affect, reduced speed output and social withdrawal), cognitive impairment (e.g. impaired memory, planning and social cognition) and mood disturbance (including depression and anxiety), so these aspects require added treatment (Psychotropic Expert Group 2013).

Before starting any therapy, a thorough assessment is necessary and medications only used if necessary and then tailored to the patient, starting with the lowest dose and simplest regimen, in combination with non-pharmacological therapies. It is important that the patient understands and agrees to participate in treatment; however, assistance may be required, depending on the level of mental illness experienced by the person (Bryant et al 2019).

Antipsychotics generally need to be taken for several weeks before any clinical improvement is seen. Treatment is often ongoing for many years, and relapses are common when therapy is stopped. Concordance with some of the older antipsychotic agents was poor because of the pronounced side-effects, but this has improved with some of the newer, atypical antipsychotic agents because they have fewer adverse effects. Concordance is complex and can be improved by agreement between patient and doctor on the treatment plan (including discussion of the goals of treatment, advantages and disadvantages of treatment), simplifying treatment regimen (e.g. once-daily compared to more frequent administration), case management and regular contact with healthcare professions (such as community mental health nurses), family/friends/significant others involved in therapy (if the patient agrees), provision of clear, written information (and instructions if appropriate), use of reminders (e.g. for appointments, taking medications), monitoring of concordance (e.g. plasma drug levels, counting tablets) or use of long-acting depot preparations which can be administered 2–4-weekly (Bryant et al 2019; Psychotropic Expert Group 2013).

General Adverse effects of antipsychotics

- neuroleptic malignant syndrome (a rare but potentially fatal reaction to antipsychotic drugs). Symptoms include hyperthermia, muscle rigidity, altered consciousness, tachycardia, labile BP, profuse sweating and arrhythmias. May also include raised creatine phosphokinase, rhabdomyolysis and acute renal failure. Predisposing factors include dehydration, pre-existing organic brain disease and AIDS. Infants and the elderly are particularly susceptible. It is usually managed by discontinuing the antipsychotic drugs and monitoring and treating symptoms
- extrapyramidal reactions or syndrome (may include all or some of the following symptoms and may occur after a single dose, especially in children and young adults):
  - Parkinsonian symptoms: difficulty speaking or swallowing, loss of balance, shuffling gait, rigidity, tremor at rest, mask-like face (occurs commonly in the elderly; usually occurs within 5–30 days of starting therapy; managed with anti-Parkinson's agents, such as benztropine or diphenhydramine)
  - akathisia: motor and mental restlessness (usually occurs within 5–60 days of starting therapy; managed by reducing dose or changing drug or using clonazepam or propranolol)
  - acute dystonia: spasm of muscles (tongue, face, neck and back) resulting in facial grimacing, torticollis, oculogyric crisis (commonly occurs in young or patients not previously treated with antipsychotics; usually occurs within 1–5 days of starting medication; usually managed with anti-Parkinson's agents)
  - tardive dyskinesia: exaggerated and persistent chewing movements, tongue protrusion, lip smacking, uncontrolled movement of legs/arms (elderly patients are at increased risk; occurs months or years into treatment; may be reversible if recognised early and the drug is stopped)
- anticholinergic effects (may include any of the following: dry mouth, thirst, blurred vision, difficulty with accommodation, urinary retention or urgency retention, constipation, flushing and dryness of skin, decreased sweating, tachycardia, palpitations, arrhythmias, mydriasis, photophobia, cycloplegia and (less commonly) raised intraocular pressure)
- disrupted ability to maintain core temperature, increased sweating
- QT interval prolongation and arrhythmias (the risk is increased in

those with bradycardia, hypokalaemia, hypomagnesaemia or a family history of long QT syndrome)

- postural (also referred to as orthostatic) hypotension; may be associated with dizziness, tachycardia and syncope; hypertension sometimes occurs
- raised prolactin levels (and associated symptoms, including galactorrhoea, gynaecomastia, amenorrhoea, menstrual disorders, erectile dysfunction, breast pain, impotence)
- dry mouth, nausea, vomiting, constipation, diarrhoea, dyspepsia, hypersalivation, abdominal pain
- changes in body weight (commonly increased but sometimes, decreased)
- headache, dizziness, sedation, drowsiness, somnolence, insomnia, tremor
- restlessness, nervousness, anxiety, fatigue, lethargy, agitation, impaired judgement, thinking and motor skills
- depression, suicide ideation
- decreased seizure control
- hyperglycaemia and, rarely, ketoacidosis or hyperosmolar coma
- altered liver function, increased serum cholesterol and triglycerides
- sleep apnoea
- dysphagia (decreased motility of oesophagus, increasing risk of aspiration), bronchopneumonia
- leucopenia/neutropenia, agranulocytosis
- (sudden withdrawal effects) vertigo, tachycardia, headache, nausea, vomiting
- (rare) venous thromboembolism, priapism, intraoperative floppy iris syndrome
- (very rare) sudden death

General Interactions of antipsychotics

- contraindicated with agents known to prolong the QT interval (such as amiodarone, arsenic trioxide, chlorpromazine, clarithromycin, disopyramide, droperidol, erythromycin, haloperidol, lithium, methadone, pentamidine, sotalol, ziprasidone), those agents which could cause hypokalaemia (e.g. amphotericin B (amphotericin), diuretics, glucocorticoids, stimulant laxatives, tetracosactides) or induce bradycardia (e.g. beta-adrenergic blocking agents, calcium-channel blockers, clonidine, digoxin)
- may enhance CNS effects of alcohol, anaesthetics, antidepressants, antihistamines, barbiturates, benzodiazepines, hypnotics, MAOIs, opioid analgesics, sedatives and other CNS active agents
- hypotensive effects of antihypertensive agents (especially those with alpha adrenoceptor blocking properties) may be enhanced if given with antipsychotics
- increased risk of neuroleptic malignant syndrome if antipsychotic agents are given together
- antipsychotic agents are generally not recommended together
- anticholinergic effects of antipsychotics may be enhanced if given with anticholinergic agents
- anticholinergic agents may reduce effects of antipsychotic agents
- dopamine antagonism reduces effects of cabergoline, bromocriptine and levodopa, and are therefore contraindicated/not recommended together
- caution if given with other agents that lower seizure threshold as this

may increase the risk of seizure activity
- increased risk of sleep apnoea if given with sedatives

General Nursing points/Cautions for antipsychotics

- initial stabilisation should be done under medical supervision as adverse effects can be unpredictable. Improvement may take days to weeks to achieve and patient should be closely monitored during this time
- before starting therapy, patient should be thoroughly medically assessed (including HR, BP, full blood count, electrolyte levels, fasting glucose levels, liver function, full lipid profile, family history of QT prolongation) to establish any factors which may increase risk of arrhythmias, QT interval prolongation and other adverse effects such as blood dyscrasias
- any hypokalaemia or hypomagnesaemia should be corrected before starting therapy
- liver function, blood counts and serum cholesterol and triglycerides should be monitored regularly throughout therapy
- many antipsychotic agents also have an antiemetic effect, therefore care should be taken as this may mask symptoms of overdosage or obscure diagnosis of other conditions, such as intestinal obstruction or brain tumour
- patient may experience an increase in temperature during the first 4 weeks of therapy and this must be carefully evaluated and distinguished from neuroleptic malignant syndrome, infection or agranulocytosis
- all psychotic illnesses carry an inherent risk of suicide, therefore patients should be closely observed, especially at the start of therapy. Patients should also only have a small supply of antipsychotic agents to lessen the risk of accidental/intentional overdose
- patient should be observed carefully so that a distinction may be made between a return of psychotic behaviour and the onset of extrapyramidal reactions. Rapid mood swings may occur when antipsychotics are used to treat the mania phase of bipolar disorders and should not be used if depression is the major symptom
- therapy should be slowly discontinued over 1–2 weeks before stopping
- caution if used in those with liver impairment as most antipsychotics are metabolised in the liver, and impairment would lead to increased serum levels and therefore increased risk of adverse effects
- caution if used in those with kidney impairment and dose reduction is generally recommended
- caution if used in those with a history of seizures or epilepsy as seizure threshold may be lowered
- caution if used in those with a risk of aspiration pneumonia or chronic respiratory disorders
- caution if used in those with cardiovascular disease (such as myocardial infarction, heart failure), cerebrovascular disease, predisposition to hypotension (including treatment with antihypertensives) or risk factors for venous or arterial thromboembolic events
- caution if used in those with glaucoma, prostatic hypertrophy, paralytic ileus or urinary retention as anticholinergic effects may aggravate these conditions

- caution if used in those with diabetes or risk factors for diabetes including obesity. Blood glucose levels should be carefully monitored during therapy
- caution if used in those with hypothyroidism (susceptible to hypothermia), thyrotoxicosis (higher risk of extrapyramidal adverse effects) or hyperthyroidism (risk of neurotoxicity)
- caution if used in those with pre-existing low WBC, history of drug-induced leucopenia/neutropenia. FBC should be monitored regularly during first months of therapy and therapy should be stopped if severe neutropenia occurs
- caution if used in those with history or risk factors for sleep apnoea
- caution if used in those with history of neuroleptic malignant syndrome. If given, patient should be very closely monitored
- not recommended in elderly patients with dementia-related psychoses (due to increased risk of stroke and/or death) or organic brain syndrome
- contraindicated in those with prolactin-dependent tumours (including breast cancer and pituitary gland prolactinomas), phaeochromocytoma, liver impairment/failure or active liver disease
- contraindicated in those with severe CNS depression (including drug intoxication), coma, Parkinson's disease, circulatory collapse, congenital/acquired long QT interval, known hypokalaemia or hypomagnesaemia, significant bradycardia or arrhythmias (treated with class IA or III antiarrhythmic agents)

General Patient teaching and advice for antipsychotics

- patient/family/carer should be advised that it may take several weeks for there to be improvement in their symptoms and that they should continue to take their medication
- advise patient that initial drowsiness subsides within weeks of starting therapy
- patient should be warned against driving a vehicle or operating machinery if drowsy or dizzy, especially in the first few weeks of therapy
- advise patient to avoid dizziness, light-headedness and/or fainting (due to postural hypotension) by moving gradually to a sitting or standing position, especially after sleep. Warn patient that postural hypotension is made worse by prolonged standing, hot baths or showers, hot weather, physical exertion, large meals and drinking alcohol
- instruct patient to avoid alcohol with therapy because tolerance is reduced
- warn patient against suddenly stopping therapy because this may cause symptoms such as nausea, vomiting and restlessness. Relapse often occurs
- patient should be advised to avoid overheating (including strenuous exercise or work and exposure to extreme temperatures) and dehydration, because antipsychotics disrupt the body's ability to control temperature. Patient should also be aware of risks associated with swimming in cold water, staying cool in hot weather and ensuring a good oral intake in hot weather
- warn patient against taking over-the-counter antihistamine preparations

because of interactions with antipsychotic medications

- advise patient to maintain good mouth hygiene as continued dry mouth may predispose them to tooth decay, gum disease and fungal infection (oral thrush)
- family members/carers should be instructed to monitor the patient closely (especially at the start of therapy or with changes in dose) for any agitation, irritability or change in behaviour or any signs of depression, such as sadness, withdrawal from friends or previously pleasurable activities, or any attempts at self-harm
- patient should be advised to seek medical advice immediately if any of the following occur:
  - increased thirst, increased urination and weakness
  - sore throat, chills, swollen glands, fever or flu-like symptoms (especially 4–10 weeks after starting therapy)
  - fits/seizures
  - hardness or rigidity of muscles, fever, altered mental state, irregular pulse, sweating
  - unwanted muscle movements of mouth, tongue, jaw, cheeks, arms or legs
  - worm-like movements of the tongue
  - prolonged and painful penis erection (not returning to normal flaccid state)
  - sudden fainting for no reason or after exercise/emotional excitement, rapid or erratic heartbeat
  - headache, changes in vision
- patient should be counselled regarding diet as weight gain is a common adverse effect of most antipsychotic agents
- patient with diabetes should be instructed to monitor blood glucose levels closely during therapy
- advise patient that any constipation may necessitate increased fluid intake, added dietary roughage or a laxative
- female patient should be counselled to use adequate contraception during therapy to avoid pregnancy
- see also General Patient teaching and advice (p. xxvii)

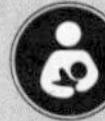

not recommended during pregnancy unless potential benefits are thought to outweigh risks. Infants exposed to antipsychotics during third trimester are at risk of extrapyramidal disturbances and/or withdrawal symptoms after delivery. Newborns should be closely monitored

contraindicated/not recommended during breastfeeding

AMISULPRIDE (Amipride, Amisolan, Solian, Sulprix)

Available forms

Tablets: 100 mg, 200 mg, 400 mg; Suspension: 100 mg/mL

Action

- typical antipsychotic (benzamide) that binds selectively to D_2 and D_3 dopamine receptors (especially presynaptically) with a low affinity for other receptor sites
- has no antiemetic properties
- minimal sedation, hypotensive and anticholinergic effects
- half-life about 12 hours

Use

- acute and chronic schizophrenic disorders (with positive and/or negative symptoms, including those with predominantly negative symptoms)

Dose

- (acute psychotic episodes) 200–400 mg orally twice daily before meals, increasing if needed (daily maximum 1200 mg) **OR**
- (predominantly negative symptoms) 50–300 mg orally daily before meals

Adverse effects

- see General Adverse effects of antipsychotics (not anticholinergic effects) (p. 772)
- blurred vision
- hypotension and uncommonly, hypertension
- pruritus
- (uncommon) bradycardia

Interactions

- caution if given with other renally excreted agents, such as lithium
- serum level may be increased if given with clozapine
- see General Interactions of antipsychotics (p. 773)

Nursing points/Cautions

- see General Nursing points/Cautions for antipsychotics (p. 774)
- doses of 400 mg or less can be given as a single daily dose
- oral solution contains hydroxybenzoates, which may cause hypersensitivity reactions in sensitive individuals
- contraindicated in children up to puberty

Patient teaching and advice

- advise patient that solution should be dispensed using pipette/dosage syringe supplied, which is carefully washed after use
- patient should be instructed that oral solution can be added to water if desired
- see General Patient teaching and advice for antipsychotics (p. 775)

oral solution available. Tablet can be crushed and mixed with water or spoonful of yoghurt or apple puree

ARIPIPRAZOLE (Abilify, Abilify Maintena, Abyraz, Tevaripiprazole)

Available forms

Tablets: 5 mg, 10 mg, 15 mg, 20 mg, 30 mg; Vial: 300 mg, 400 mg

Action

- atypical antipsychotic
- partial agonist (dopamine D_2 and serotonin $5HT_{1A}$ receptors) and serotonin $5HT_{2A}$ antagonist
- no antiemetic properties, minimal sedation, hypotension and anticholinergic actions
- active metabolite has a half-life of 100 hours
- half-life 75 hours

Use

- acute and maintenance treatment of schizophrenia
- prevention of recurrent mania or mixed episodes associated with bipolar I disorder (monotherapy or combination therapy with lithium or sodium valproate)

Dose

- (schizophrenia) initially 10–15 mg orally daily, increasing at 2-week intervals if needed (range 10–30 mg daily) **OR**
- (schizophrenia, prevention of recurrent mania) 400 mg IM monthly **OR**
- (prevention of recurrent mania) initially 15 mg orally daily (alone or with lithium or sodium valproate), increasing to 30 mg (if needed) for at least 9 weeks

Adverse effects

- see General Adverse effects of antipsychotics (p. 772)

- rash
- cough, nasal congestion, pharyngolaryngeal pain, nasopharyngitis
- toothache
- peripheral oedema, hypertension
- blurred vision
- arthralgia, muscle stiffness and/or spasm, musculoskeletal pain, myalgia, pain in extremities, back pain
- (injection site) haematoma, redness, swelling, discomfort/pain, pruritus, induration

Interactions

- see General Interactions of antipsychotics (p. 773)
- increased serum levels may occur if given with amiodarone, ciclosporin, cimetidine, clarithromycin, erythromycin, fluconazole, fluoxetine, indinavir, itraconazole, paroxetine, ritonavir or grapefruit juice
- decreased serum levels may occur if given with carbamazepine, efavirenz, nevirapine, phenobarbital, phenytoin, primidone, rifabutin, rifampicin and St John's wort

Nursing points/Cautions

- see General Nursing points/Cautions for antipsychotics (p. 774)
- in those who have never taken aripiprazole, oral therapy should be initiated to determine tolerability before starting injectable formulation for maintenance therapy
- (IM) oral therapy (with aripiprazole or other antipsychotic agent) should be continued for 14 consecutive days to maintain therapeutic levels
- (IM) dose can be decreased to 300 mg if adverse effects occur
- only given IM (not SC or IV) into gluteal or deltoid muscle
- dose should not be divided
- (oral) if switching from another antipsychotic agent, this may be done by tapering down over 2 weeks while increasing dose of aripiprazole, starting on recommended dose of aripiprazole while tapering down dose of other antipsychotic, or starting aripiprazole and stopping another agent
- if switching from another long-acting injectable antipsychotic, can be replaced at next scheduled injection with 14 days of oral aripiprazole
- reconstitute using 1.9 mL of water for injections (diluent) for 400 mg or 1.5 mL for 300 mg dose
- shake well for at least 30 seconds to dissolve powder. Reconstituted solution is opaque and milky in colour
- use 23-gauge, 1 inch (deltoid) or 22-gauge, 1.5 inch (38 mm) (gluteal) hypodermic needle for non-obese patient or 22-gauge, 1.5 inch (38 mm) (deltoid) or 21-gauge, 2 inch (51 mm) (gluteal) hypodermic needle for obese patient
- solution should be injected slowly and area not massaged after injection
- injection sites should be rotated
- (IM) if second or third monthly dose is missed (> 4 weeks but < 5 weeks), dose should be administered as soon as possible and monthly regimen resumed; if > 5 weeks has elapsed, oral dose should be restarted for 14 consecutive days with IM injection and then monthly regimen resumed
- (IM) if fourth or subsequent monthly dose is missed (> 4 weeks but < 6 weeks), dose should be administered and monthly regimen resumed; if > 6 weeks has elapsed, oral dose should be restarted for 14 consecutive days with IM injection and then monthly regimen resumed
- tablets contain lactose and are therefore not recommended in those with rare hereditary problems of galactose intolerance, Lapp lactase deficiency or glucose–galactose malabsorption
- not recommended in those under 18 years
- not recommended in those with psychosis related to Alzheimer's disease

Patient teaching and advice

- see General Patient teaching and advice for antipsychotics (p. 775)
- patient should be advised to avoid grapefruit juice

ASENAPINE MALEATE (Saphris)

Available forms

Wafer: 5 mg, 10 mg

Action

- atypical antipsychotic
- dibenzoxepino pyrroles
- binds to D_2 and $5HT_{2A}$ receptors
- also binds to other serotonin and alpha-adrenergic receptors
- no antiemetic properties, minimal sedative, hypotensive and anticholinergic actions
- half-life about 24 hours

Use

- treatment of schizophrenia
- treatment and prevention of acute manic or mixed episodes associated with bipolar I disorder (alone or in combination with lithium or sodium valproate)

Dose

- (schizophrenia) initially 5 mg orally twice daily, increasing to 10 mg twice daily if needed **OR**
- (treatment and prevention of manic or mixed episodes in bipolar I disorder: monotherapy) initially 10 mg twice daily, reducing to 5 mg twice daily if needed **OR**
- (treatment and prevention of manic or mixed episodes in bipolar I disorder: combination therapy) initially 5 mg orally twice daily, increasing to 10 mg twice daily if needed (with lithium or sodium valproate)

Adverse effects

- see General Adverse effects of antipsychotics (p. 772)
- oral hyperaesthesia/paraesthesia

Interactions

- caution if given with fluvoxamine
- see also General Interactions of antipsychotics (p. 773)

Nursing points/Cautions

- see General Nursing points/Cautions for antipsychotics (p. 774)

Patient teaching and advice

- see General Patient teaching and advice for antipsychotics (p. 775)
- patient should be given the following instructions regarding administration of wafers
  - wafer should not be removed from blister pack until just before administration
  - hands should be dry
  - wafer should not be pushed through blister pack
  - tab should be pulled back gently
  - wafer should be placed under tongue and allowed to dissolve completely without being chewed, crushed or swallowed
  - if other medications are administered at the same time, wafer should be given last
  - warn patient that mouth may feel numb for up to an hour after using the wafer
  - not to eat or drink for 10 minutes after wafer

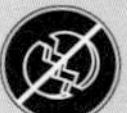

wafer should not be crushed, broken, chewed or swallowed with water

BREXPIPRAZOLE (Rexulti)

Available forms

Tablet: 0.25 mg, 0.5 mg, 1 mg, 2 mg, 3 mg, 4 mg

Action

- atypical antipsychotic

- although action is not completely understood, thought to modulate serotonin–dopamine activity
- terminal half-life about 91 hours

Use
- treatment of schizophrenia

Dose
- initially 1 mg orally daily for 4 days, then increasing to 2 mg for 3 days, then 4 mg depending on clinical response and tolerability, maintenance dose 2–4 mg orally daily (daily maximum 4 mg)

Adverse effects
- toothache
- back pain, pain in extremity, muscle spasms, musculoskeletal pain
- pruritus
- increased blood creatine phosphokinase, increased triglycerides
- see General Adverse effects of antipsychotic agents (p. 772)

Interactions
- serum levels may decrease if given with rifampicin, rifabutin, carbamazepine, phenytoin, phenobarbital (phenobarbitone) and St John's wort
- serum levels may increase if given with amprenavir, atazanavir, boceprevir, darunavir, fosamprenavir, indinavir, itraconazole, nelfinavir, ritonavir, saquinavir, telaprevir
- see also General Interactions for antipsychotic agents (p. 773)

Nursing points/Cautions
- see General Nursing points/Cautions for antipsychotics (p. 774)
- for those with moderate-to-severe liver impairment or moderate, severe or end-stage kidney impairment, daily maximum should not exceed 3 mg
- tablets contain lactose and are not recommended in those with rare hereditary problems of galactose intolerance, Lapp lactase deficiency or glucose–galactose malabsorption

Patient teaching and advice
- see General Patient teaching and advice for antipsychotics (p. 775)

CARBAMAZEPINE (Tegretol)

Available forms
Tablets: 100 mg, 200 mg; Tablets (controlled-release): 200 mg, 400 mg; Suspension: 100 mg/5 mL

Action
- antipsychotic action thought to be related to its effects on dopamine and noradrenaline
- other actions related to its use in epilepsy and neuralgia (see Carbamazepine in Antiepileptics, p. 387)

Use
- mania, bipolar disorder (as monotherapy or as an adjunct to lithium, other antipsychotic agents or antidepressants)
- epilepsy, neuralgia (see Carbamazepine in Antiepileptics, p. 387)

Dose
- (mania: monotherapy) 100–200 mg orally twice daily, increasing by 200 mg daily increments to 800–1000 mg/day (week 1) and if no response in week 2, increasing to 1600 mg daily in divided doses **OR**
- (maintenance) 100–200 mg twice daily, increasing by 100 mg weekly increments until plasma levels are adequate (4–12 microgram/mL; 17–50 micromol/L)

Adverse effects/Interactions/Nursing points/Cautions/Patient teaching and advice
- see general points for antiepileptics (pp. 381–84)
- suspension or tablets (not sustained release) are recommended for establishing dose for treatment of mania

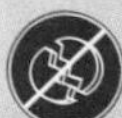

controlled-release tablets should not be crushed, broken or chewed

oral suspension available. Plain tablet can be dispersed in water or crushed and mixed with spoonful of yoghurt or apple puree.

CHLORPROMAZINE HYDROCHLORIDE (Largactil)

Available forms

Tablets: 10 mg, 25 mg, 100 mg; Suspension: 25 mg/5 mL; Ampoules: 50 mg/2 mL

Action

- phenothiazine with typical antipsychotic actions
- alpha adrenergic blocking agent producing hypotension
- dopamine inhibitor
- impairs body temperature regulation
- antiemetic effects, also has sedative and anticholinergic properties, as well as causing hypotension
- stimulates prolactin release

Use

- acute function psychosis (e.g. schizophrenia, mania or psychotic depression)
- schizophrenia (long-term management)
- agitation and/or behavioural disturbance (delirium, dementia) (short term)
- control of nausea and/or vomiting associated with disease, drugs and surgery premedication or terminal illness
- intractable hiccups
- short-term management of agitation, severe depression
- behavioural disturbances (in children with autism or intellectual disability) (with non-pharmacological management program)

Dose

- initially 25 mg orally 3 times daily, increasing gradually if necessary to 25–100 mg orally 3 times daily (maintenance) (daily maximum 600–800 mg)
OR
- 25–50 mg deep IM 6–8-hourly if needed

Adverse effects

- see General Adverse effects of antipsychotics (p. 772)
- nasal stuffiness
- rash, urticaria, contact dermatitis, photosensitivity
- decreased cough reflex, respiratory depression
- pain, irritation (IM site)
- (rare) pigmentation of conjunctivae, discolouration of cornea and sclera, lens/corneal opacities, severe liver toxicity

Interactions

- plasma level may be increased by propranolol, TCAs, SSRIs, oestrogens, antimalarial agents, ciprofloxacin, fluvoxamine and progestogens
- increased risk of neurotoxicity and extrapyramidal side-effects if given with lithium. Antiemetics effects may mask lithium toxicity if given together
- not recommended with citalopram or escitalopram
- increased CNS effects if given with benzodiazepines, anaesthetics, opioids, barbiturates and lithium
- increased risk of toxicity if given with amitriptyline and other TCAs
- effects may be variable if given with phenytoin, therefore patient should be closely monitored for any signs of phenytoin toxicity, loss of psychotic control or increase in seizure frequency
- increased risk of QT interval prolongation if given with other antipsychotics, amiodarone, clonidine, diltiazem, disopyramide, IV amphotericin, IV erythromycin, methadone, pentamidine, sotalol, stimulant laxatives, thiazide diuretics, tetracosactides, verapamil or beta-adrenergic receptor blocking agents

- use with metoclopramide may increase risk of antipsychotic-induced extrapyramidal effects
- absorption may be decreased when given with food, alcohol, antacids or benztropine resulting in decreased serum levels
- decreased serum levels may occur if given with phenobarbital (phenobarbitone) or carbamazepine
- may decrease serum levels of phenobarbital (phenobarbitone)
- anticholinergic effects may be increased (e.g. increased risk of heat stroke, severe constipation, paralytic ileus) if given with anticholinergics or atropine
- increased risk of seizures if given with tramadol
- may antagonise anti-Parkinsonian effect of levodopa, bromocriptine and pergolide
- may increase serum levels of sodium valproate and propranolol
- increased hypotension, sedation and respiratory depression may occur if given with pethidine
- may antagonise effects of antidiabetic agents
- may decrease effects of amphetamines
- may decrease effects of anticoagulants, therefore INR should be monitored regularly, especially when starting or stopping therapy
- increased risk of postural hypotension and extrapyramidal syndrome if given with MAOIs
- may oppose action of adrenaline (epinephrine) and clonidine
- adrenaline (epinephrine) should not be used to treat phenothiazine-induced hypotension or in overdose
- increased risk of transient metabolic encephalopathy if given with desferrioxamine
- may decrease seizure threshold requiring adjustment of antiepileptic dose
- increase risk of postural hypotension if given with thiazide diuretics

Nursing points/Cautions

- see General Nursing points/Cautions for antipsychotics (p. 774)
- regular ophthalmological examination and liver function tests are recommended for patients on long-term therapy
- contact dermatitis may be avoided if injectable preparations are handled using plastic or rubber gloves
- give IM injections slowly and deeply to avoid irritating subcutaneous tissues
- rotate injection sites
- BP and vital signs should be closely monitored after IM administration
- patient to remain recumbent for at least 1 hour after injection to avoid postural hypotension
- syrup is recommended for those with swallowing difficulties or who refuse tablets
- noradrenaline should be available for severe hypotension (adrenaline (epinephrine) is contraindicated) and benztropine for severe extrapyramidal side-effects
- injection and suspension contain sodium metabisulfite and sodium sulfite, which may cause allergic-type reactions in susceptible individuals
- caution if used in those with chronic respiratory disease or at risk of aspiration pneumonia
- caution if used in the elderly, starting dose should be half adult dose
- not recommended in children or adolescents with signs suggestive of Reye's syndrome
- not recommended in those with epilepsy, hypoparathyroidism, myasthenia gravis, Parkinson's disease or prostatic hypertrophy
- contraindicated in those with hypersensitivity to other phenothiazines

(e.g. jaundice, blood dyscrasias), bone marrow depression, severe depression, blood dyscrasias, circulatory collapse, CNS depression (coma or drug intoxication), phaeochromocytoma, liver failure or active liver disease

Patient teaching and advice

- advise patient to seek medical advice immediately if any of the following occur:
  - fever or sore throat, gums or mouth, chills or swollen glands, especially between weeks 4 and 10 of therapy (early signs of bone marrow depression)
  - blurred vision or other visual disturbances, including difficulties with night vision or colour vision defects
- advise patient to avoid extreme sun exposure by wearing a hat, long-sleeved clothing and sunscreen (SPF 30+) to avoid exaggerated reaction to sun causing severe sunburn
- instruct patient that antacids (e.g. aluminium hydroxide or magnesium trisilicate) should be taken either 1 hour before or 2 hours after chlorpromazine
- advise patient that tablets should not be crushed or broken (suspension is available if tablets are difficult to swallow) as skin contact with crushed tablets may lead to dermatitis
- see also General Patient teaching and advice for antipsychotics (p. 775)

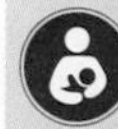
if given during third trimester, increased risk of neonatal respiratory distress, brady- or tachycardia, agitation, hypo- or hypertonia, tremor, somnolence and/or feeding difficulties

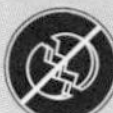
syrup is available. Tablet should not be crushed, broken or chewed

CLOZAPINE (Clopine, Clozaril, Versacloz)

Available forms

Tablets: 25 mg, 50 mg, 100 mg, 200 mg; Oral suspension: 50 mg/mL

Action

- atypical antipsychotic
- tricyclic dibenzodiazepine
- weakly blocks dopamine (D_1 and D_2) receptors
- anticholinergic, antihistamine, antiserotonin with no antiemetic properties
- sedative (inhibits arousal)
- relieves both negative and positive symptoms of schizophrenia
- little or no elevation of prolactin levels
- active metabolite which has weaker action and shorter duration than clozapine
- half-life 14 hours

Use

- treatment-resistant schizophrenia (in those who are unresponsive or intolerant to other antipsychotics)

Dose

- initially 12.5 mg orally 1–2 times daily for day 1, followed by 25 mg orally 1–2 times daily (day 2). If tolerated, then increasing increments of 25–50 mg over 2–3 weeks, up to 300 mg/day. If necessary, further weekly increases of 50–100 mg to a dose of 200–450 mg/day in divided doses, with the larger dose at night (daily maximum 600–900 mg) **OR**
- (maintenance dose) dose decreased to 150–300 mg orally daily in divided doses

Adverse effects

- see General Adverse effects of antipsychotics (p. 772)
- fever
- blurred vision

- tachycardia, ECG changes and less commonly, QT interval prolongation
- (common) leucopenia, neutropenia, eosinophilia, leucocytosis and uncommonly, agranulocytosis
- (rare) myocarditis, cardiomyopathy, myocardial infarction, seizure
- (abrupt discontinuation) cholinergic rebound (profuse sweating, headache, nausea, vomiting, diarrhoea)

Interactions

- see General Interactions of antipsychotics (p. 773)
- use with lithium or other CNS active agents may increase risk of neuroleptic malignant syndrome
- contraindicated with any drugs that may cause bone marrow depression or with long-acting depot antipsychotic agents
- not recommended with carbamazepine due to added bone marrow depression
- caution if given with other agents with anticholinergic, hypotensive or respiratory depression properties as additive effects may occur
- plasma levels may be increased when given with azithromycin, azole antifungal agents, caffeine, cimetidine, ciprofloxacin, citalopram, clarithromycin, erythromycin, fluvoxamine, fluoxetine, paroxetine, protease inhibitors, sertraline, venlafaxine or oral contraceptives
- plasma levels may be decreased when given with phenytoin, carbamazepine, rifampicin, St John's wort, nicotine, pantoprazole or omeprazole, resulting in an exacerbation in symptoms
- increased risk of cardiac and/or respiratory arrest when given with benzodiazepines
- increased risk of seizure and delirium if given with sodium valproate (even in those without epilepsy)
- may antagonise effects of adrenaline (epinephrine) and related products

Nursing points/Cautions

- see General Nursing points/Cautions for antipsychotics (p. 774)
- blood counts (WBC, differential count, absolute neutrophil count (ANC)) should be monitored 10 days before starting, weekly during first 18 weeks and then monthly and for 1 month after stopping therapy. Additional monitoring is recommended if therapy is interrupted after initial 18 weeks of therapy
- if patient has history of bone marrow disorder, he/she should be reviewed by haematologist before starting therapy
- if patient has been on therapy for more than 18 weeks and treatment is stopped for 4–28 days, blood counts (WBC, ANC) should be monitored weekly for 6 weeks; if the interruption is greater than 28 days, monitoring should be weekly for the next 18 weeks
- doses of up to 200 mg may be given as a single dose at night
- 24-hour washout period should be allowed when changing patient from conventional antipsychotic therapy to clozapine, after gradual discontinuation over 7 days
- increased risk of adverse effects if dose $>$ 450 mg/day
- liver function should be regularly monitored in any patient with liver abnormalities
- if therapy is stopped for longer than 2 days, it should be restarted at 12.5 mg 1–2 times daily (day 1) and then titrated upwards more rapidly than the initial titration (within patient tolerance)
- in patients with cardiovascular, respiratory or hepatic disorders or history of seizures, dose should be started at 12.5 mg and increased very slowly, monitoring functions closely
- if family history of cardiac disease exists, cardiac assessment is recommended before starting therapy

- contraindicated in those with a history of bone marrow disorders (including drug-induced agranulocytosis), alcoholic/toxic psychoses, severe renal/cardiac/liver disease, uncontrolled epilepsy, CNS depression, circulatory collapse, paralytic ileus or if patient is unable to undergo regular blood tests

Patient teaching and advice

- see also General Patient teaching and advice for antipsychotics (p. 775)
- advise patient that fever (above 38°C) occurs commonly during first 4 weeks of therapy
- if patient is taking oral suspension, he/she/family member/carer should be instructed in correct use
- warn patient not to suddenly start or stop smoking or drinking coffee/tea/cola drinks without talking to doctor first as this will affect blood levels and effectiveness of medication
- patient should be advised to report immediately any:
  - fever, sore throat, mouth ulcers or other signs of infection or flu-like illness
  - fast or irregular heart rate, shortness of breath, rapid breathing, fatigue, chest pain, fever or flu-like illness (may be signs of cardiomyopathy)

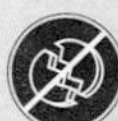

oral solution is available. Tablet can be crushed (but mask and gloves must be worn) and mixed with water or spoonful of yoghurt or apple puree

DROPERIDOL (Droleptan)

Available form
Ampoules: 2.5 mg/mL

Action
- butyrophenone
- antiemetic effect
- onset of action 3–10 minutes (IV, IM), full effect in 30 minutes, duration 2–4 hours
- altered consciousness may last up to 12 hours

Use
- antiemetic, premedication, induction and maintenance of anaesthesia, neuroleptanalgesia
- (psychiatry) management of severe agitation, aggression or hyperactivity in psychotic disorders or disturbed states, including non-psychotic acute excitation states

Dose

Psychiatry
- 5–25 mg IM 4–6-hourly if needed **OR**
- 25–62.5 mg slow IV infusion over 20 minutes, twice daily **OR**
- (psychiatric crisis) ≤ 5 mg IM immediately before transferring patient to hospital

Anaesthesia
- (premedication, diagnostic or minor procedure without anaesthesia) 2.5–10 mg slow IV 30–60 minutes before induction **OR**
- (adjunct to general anaesthetic) 0.25 mg/kg IM or slow IV with an opioid analgesic and/or general anaesthetic agent to provide a smooth induction **OR**
- (maintenance) 1.25–2.5 mg slow IV **OR**
- (adjunct to regional anaesthesia) 2.5–5 mg IM or slow IV when additional sedation is required

Adverse effects
- see General Adverse effects of antipsychotics (p. 772)
- bronchospasm, laryngospasm, increased depth of respiration
- (rare) arrhythmia, prolongation of QT interval

Interactions
- contraindicated with drugs known to prolong QT interval or cause

significant bradycardia, hypokalaemia or hypomagnesaemia
- may potentiate respiratory depression of opioid analgesics and therefore should be given together with caution using ¼ of normal opioid dose
- muscle rigidity may occur if given with opioid analgesic
- adrenaline (epinephrine) may decrease BP when given with droperidol
- may increase effects of barbiturates, general anaesthetics, antipsychotics, benzodiazepines and opioid analgesics
- serum levels may decrease if given with phenytoin, carbamazepine, phenobarbital (phenobarbitone), smoking and alcohol use

Nursing points/Cautions

- see General Nursing points/Cautions for antipsychotics (p. 774)
- any electrolyte imbalance should be corrected before starting therapy
- ECG monitoring before first dose (if possible) is recommended to detect any bradycardia or arrhythmia and up to 7 hours after procedure (if used during surgery). If patient has acute symptoms, ECG should be performed when symptoms have reduced
- vital signs should be monitored during IV therapy
- slow IV infusion will decrease risk of muscle rigidity (especially respiratory muscles) if given with opioids
- (anaesthesia) pulmonary arterial pressure may decrease during therapy and this should be considered if these results require clinical interpretation
- may be given in 250 mL of sodium chloride 0.9% or glucose 5% or Ringer's solution and infused over 20 minutes
- (anaesthesia) caution when repositioning patient due to risk of orthostatic hypotension
- caution if used in those with ventricular arrhythmias, cardiac disease, family history of sudden death, kidney/liver failure, respiratory failure, COPD or electrolyte disturbance (or risk of), including persistent vomiting or diarrhoea
- caution if used in those with a history of epilepsy, epilepsy or risk factors for epilepsy
- not recommended in those with phaeochromocytoma
- contraindicated in those with acute alcohol intoxication (relative contraindication)
- contraindicated in female patients with QT interval > 450 msec or male patients with QT interval > 440 msec, or with acquired or congenital (or family history of) long QT syndrome

Patient teaching and advice

- patient should be warned not to drive or operate machinery for at least 12 hours after administration as consciousness can remain affected
- see General Patient teaching and advice for antipsychotics (p. 775)

FLUPENTIXOL DECANOATE (FLUPENTHIXOL DECANOATE) (Fluanxol)

Available forms

Ampoules: 20 mg/mL, 40 mg/2 mL, 100 mg/mL

Action

- thioxanthene typical antipsychotic
- non-sedating at low to moderate doses
- disinhibiting and mood-elevating properties
- increases prolactin levels
- onset 24–72 hours, symptoms improve for 2–4 weeks
- decanoate allows slow release from oily solution (coconut oil)

Use

- chronic schizophrenia and related chronic psychosis (maintenance therapy)

Dose

- (patients not previously treated with long-acting depot preparations) 20 mg deep IM (after 5–10 days of test dose of 5–20 mg) **OR**
- (previously treated patients) 20–40 mg deep IM, then second dose of 20–40 mg 4–10 days later, then 20–40 mg IM 2–4 weeks later, depending on clinical response and/or side-effects **OR**
- (concentrated depot preparation) for doses greater than 100 mg IM, fortnightly injections are required, concentrated preparation is recommended to reduce volume required

Adverse effects

- see General Adverse effects of antipsychotics (p. 772)
- (IM site) inflammation, abscess
- dysphagia, gingival hypertrophy

Interactions

- see General Interactions of antipsychotics (p. 773)
- may decrease effects of levodopa and adrenergic agents
- increased risk of extrapyramidal adverse effects if given with metoclopramide

Nursing points/Cautions

- see General Nursing points/Cautions for antipsychotics (p. 774)
- blood counts and liver function tests are recommended during first months of therapy
- for those not previously treated with a depot long-acting antipsychotic, a test dose of 5–20 mg is recommended. For patients who are elderly, thin, frail or with a family history of extrapyramidal reactions, 5 mg dose is recommended. For others (long-acting neuroleptic naive), 5–20 mg is recommended
- oral therapy should be continued during test dose period, but at a reduced dose
- patient should be monitored for 5–10 days after test dose for therapeutic response and/or any adverse effects (especially extrapyramidal reactions)
- not given IV
- given by deep IM injection
- if volume required is greater than 2–3 mL of 20 mg/mL solution, then 100 mg/mL solution should be used
- should not be mixed with any other depot preparations containing sesame oil as properties may be altered
- not for short-term treatment (less than 3 months)
- fluphenazine decanoate 25 mg = flupentixol decanoate 40 mg and haloperidol decanoate 50 mg = flupentixol decanoate 40 mg
- concentrated solution (100 mg/mL) is recommended in those requiring large volumes (> 2–3 mL) or high doses
- if patient is having surgery, BP should be closely monitored for any hypotensive phenomena
- not recommended in severely agitated psychotic patients, including confused or agitated elderly as symptoms may be exacerbated
- caution if used in those with liver or kidney damage or insufficiency, severe arteriosclerosis, risk factors for stroke, organic brain syndrome, epilepsy, Parkinsonism, cerebrovascular or cardiovascular disease
- contraindicated in those with hypersensitivity to thioxanthenes and possible cross-sensitivity to phenothiazines, sensitivity to coconut oil, blood dyscrasias, subcortical brain damage, phaeochromocytoma, circulatory collapse, coma or depressed conscious state due to any cause (e.g. alcohol intoxication, barbiturates, opioids)

Patient teaching and advice

- patient should be advised to immediately report any sore mouth, gums or throat, chills, fever or any flu-like symptoms
- instruct patient to maintain good dental hygiene throughout therapy, taking care with use of toothbrush (soft recommended), dental floss or toothpicks, as there is an increased risk of infection, gum bleeding and delayed healing
- see General Patient teaching and advice for antipsychotics (p. 775)

HALOPERIDOL (Serenace)

HALOPERIDOL DECANOATE (Haldol Decanoate)

Available forms

Tablets: 0.5 mg, 1.5 mg, 5 mg; Suspension: 2 mg/mL; Ampoules: 5 mg/mL; Ampoules (depot): 50 mg/mL

Action

- butyrophenone not related to phenothiazines
- some anticholinergic and sedative actions
- inhibits central action of dopamine (D_2) and noradrenaline
- antiemetic
- increase prolactin release
- active metabolite with activity less than haloperidol
- half-life about 24 hours
- decanoate allows slow release from oily solution (sesame oil)

Use

- schizophrenia, psychoses, manic phase of bipolar I disorder
- during alcohol withdrawal (short-term therapy)
- intractable nausea and vomiting related to radiation sickness or cancer (short-term therapy)
- Gilles de la Tourette syndrome
- neuroleptanalgesia

Dose

- (moderate symptoms) 1–5 mg orally daily as single dose or 2 divided doses **OR**
- (severe symptoms) 5–15 mg orally daily as single dose or 2 divided doses, increasing up to 20 mg if necessary to achieve control, then reducing to the lowest dose to maintain control **OR**
- (elderly or debilitated patient) 1–3 mg orally daily as single dose or 2 divided doses **OR**
- (agitation, aggression with acute psychosis, including alcohol withdrawal) initially 0.5–10 mg IM or IV, followed by further dose half-hourly (IV) or hourly (IM) until clinical response is achieved (daily maximum 20 mg) **OR**
- (maintenance) half of IM/IV dose used to achieve control given as 2 divided doses (morning and evening) with first dose administered 4–8 hours after last controlling dose **OR**
- (depot IM injection) initially 10–15 times previous oral daily dose, not exceeding 100 mg at 4-week intervals

Adverse effects

- see General Adverse effects of antipsychotics (p. 772)
- dental caries, periodontal disease, oral thrush
- (depot injection) local reaction

Interactions

- see General Interactions of antipsychotics (p. 773)
- increased risk of hypotension and greater intoxication if given with alcohol
- may inhibit metabolism of TCAs, increasing the risk of toxicity and anticholinergic effects
- may result in acute encephalopathic syndrome if given with lithium
- may interfere with anticoagulant action of warfarin

- may enhance CNS effects (e.g. disorientation, memory loss, aggression, confusion) when given in high doses with methyldopa sesquihydrate
- may antagonise the action of adrenaline (epinephrine) and other sympathomimetic agents
- prolonged carbamazepine, phenobarbital (phenobarbitone), phenytoin, St John's wort or rifampicin therapy may decrease plasma levels
- increased serum levels may occur if given with alprazolam, buspirone, chlorpromazine, duloxetine, fluvoxamine, fluoxetine, itraconazole, paroxetine, ritonavir or venlafaxine
- when given with amphetamines, may decrease stimulant effects of amphetamine and decrease antipsychotic effects of haloperidol
- increased intraocular pressure may occur if given with anticholinergic or anti-Parkinson's agents
- increased risk of hypotension and cardiac arrest if given with propranolol
- anti-Parkinson's agents and haloperidol should not be discontinued simultaneously because of increased risk of extrapyramidal symptoms
- serum levels may be decreased in those who smoke
- may increase serum levels of dextromethorphan including risk of adverse effects
- increased risk of Parkinsonism and neuroleptic malignant syndrome if given with olanzapine
- increased risk of seizures if given with tramadol
- may interfere with actions of levodopa
- decrease effect of both haloperidol and cabergoline if given together and therefore not recommended together
- increased serum prolactin levels may occur if given with bromocriptine

Nursing points/Cautions

- see General Nursing points/Cautions for antipsychotics (p. 774)
- children and elderly patients are more sensitive to medication, therefore starting dose should be low and titration gradual
- should only be used short term for acute mania and discontinued as soon as symptoms are relieved
- parenteral medication should be switched to oral as soon as practicable
- dose titration should be rapid and daily dose reduced to lowest effective dose
- (depot) before starting therapy with depot long-acting haloperidol, patient should be stabilised on oral therapy
- (depot) dose calculated on 10–15 times previous day's oral dose
- (depot) short-acting forms may be used to supplement depot preparation during dose adjustment or psychotic symptom exacerbations
- depot injection given as deep IM injection using 21-gauge needle
- depot must not be given IV
- 3 mL volume should not be exceeded for IM injection
- ECG is recommended during IV therapy. If rapid control of acutely distressed patient is needed or if repeated or large doses are given, ECG monitoring is recommended. Parenteral anti-Parkinson medication and resuscitation equipment should be readily available
- serum levels should be monitored if patient starts or stops smoking
- not recommended in those with bipolar disorder where depression is the predominant feature
- contraindicated in those with known hypersensitivity to sesame products (depot), basal ganglia lesions, CNS depression due to alcohol or

depressant drugs, severe depression, previous spastic disease, prolactin-dependent tumours, patients with pre-existing Parkinsonian symptoms, Parkinson's disease or congenital or acquired long QT syndrome

Patient teaching and advice

- patient should be advised to remain recumbent for at least 1 hour after injection to avoid postural hypotension
- warn patient not to abruptly start or stop smoking as this will impact on blood levels and effectiveness of medication
- caution patient to avoid taking over-the-counter preparations that include dextromethorphan, such as cough mixtures
- instruct patient to maintain good dental hygiene throughout therapy taking care with use of toothbrush (soft recommended), dental floss or toothpicks, as there is an increased risk of infection, gum bleeding and delayed healing
- see also General Patient teaching and advice for antipsychotics (p. 775)

oral liquid is available. Tablet can be dispersed in water or crushed and mixed with spoonful of yoghurt or apple puree

LITHIUM CARBONATE (Lithicarb, Quilonum SR)

Available forms

Tablets: 250 mg; Tablets (slow-release): 450 mg

Action

- lithium ions may compete with sodium ions (which are believed to increase greatly in mania), thereby altering the electrophysiological characteristics of neurons
- thought to inhibit release of dopamine while increasing turnover of noradrenaline and serotonin in the brain, decreasing post-synaptic receptor sensitivity resulting in a correction of overactive catecholamines
- proven efficacy in treatment of mania, but little to no effect in those not experiencing mania
- increased tolerance to lithium when patient is in manic phase
- narrow therapeutic index, with therapeutic serum level from 0.8 to 1.6 mmol/L, above which toxic adverse effects may be expected
- half-life 24 hours (adults), 18 hours (adolescents) and up to 36 hours (elderly)
- pregnancy and alkaline urine increase lithium clearance

Use

- prevention and treatment of mania
- prevention and treatment of mania in manic depressive (bipolar) illness (less effective for depressive swing)
- prevention of recurrent unipolar depressive illness
- chronic schizophrenia, schizoaffective illness

Dose

Prophylaxis

- 0.9–1.2 g orally daily in 2 divided doses (SR preparation) (to maintain serum lithium level 0.6–1.0 mmol/L)

Acute episodes

- initially 0.5–1 g orally daily in divided doses (day 1), 1.25–1.75 g orally in divided doses (day 2), 1.5–2 g orally daily in divided doses (day 3). This should achieve serum levels between 0.8 and 1.6 mmol/L (maximum 2 mmol/L). After 7–14 days, dose should be reduced to maintain therapeutic range (usually 0.5–1 g daily) as a single or divided dose

OR

- 1.8 g orally daily in 2 divided doses (SR preparation) (to maintain serum lithium level 0.8–1.4 mmol/L)

Adverse effects

- (initially, disappear with stabilisation of serum level) nausea, diarrhoea, muscle weakness, dazed feeling, vertigo
- (at therapeutic levels)
  - metallic taste, weight gain, constipation, anorexia, transient nausea, diarrhoea, epigastric discomfort/gastritis, increased salivation
  - thirst, polyuria
  - fine hand tremor
  - headache, fatigue, sedation
  - oedema
  - reversible ECG changes, arrhythmias, hypotension, bradycardia
  - exacerbation of skin conditions (e.g. acne, psoriasis), rash, alopecia, pruritus
  - leucocytosis
  - euthyroid goitre, hypercalcaemia, hyperglycaeamia, hyperparathyroiditis
- (toxic/overdose) increased diarrhoea, persistent nausea and vomiting, slurred speech, blurred vision, marked coarse tremor, ataxia, clonic limb movement, muscle twitching, hyperactive deep tendon reflexes, EEG changes, delirium, seizure, stupor, circulatory collapse, coma
- (rare) nephrogenic diabetes insipidus, hyperthyroidism, hyperparathyroidism

Interactions

- contraindicated with diuretics (loop, thiazide) as excretion of lithium is decreased
- increased risk of toxicity (due to increased serum levels) may result if given with NSAIDs (especially indometacin and piroxicam), metronidazole, methyldopa sesquihydrate, ACE inhibitors, angiotensin II receptor antagonists, calcium-channel blockers, corticosteroids and appetite suppressants
- therapeutic effects of lithium may be reduced by acetazolamide, xanthines (including theophylline and caffeine), urea, mannitol and urinary alkalinalisers (including sodium bicarbonate) because of increased urinary excretion
- may result in neurotoxicity when given with carbamazepine, methyldopa sesquihydrate, SSRIs, TCAs and calcium-channel blockers
- may prolong action of neuromuscular blocking agents
- increased risk of delirium, prolonged seizures and/or confusion if given with ECT therapy
- caution if given with SSRIs or other serotonergic agents as serotonin syndrome may be provoked
- not recommended with other antipsychotic agents due to potentiation of antipsychotic adverse effects as well as risk of encephalopathic syndrome (weakness, lethargy, fever, tremor, confusion, leucocytosis and extrapyramidal symptoms)
- increased risk of QTc interval prolongation if given with ziprasidone
- increased risk of hypothyroidism and QT prolongation if given with amiodarone
- caution if given with antithyroid drugs or iodides
- excretion may be altered if given with corticosteroids or appetite suppressants

Nursing points/Cautions

- see General Nursing points/Cautions for antipsychotics (p. 774)
- therapy should be started in an inpatient setting to closely monitor patient and blood levels
- before starting therapy, patient should have a thorough assessment, including ECG and renal function (e.g. urinalysis, specific gravity, 24-hour urine volume, serum creatinine, creatinine clearance)

- during therapy, regular monitoring of thyroid, cardiac and renal functions is recommended
- narrow margin between therapeutic and toxic serum levels necessitates frequent estimations of lithium level, thereby detecting toxicity early and monitoring adherence
- serum levels monitored twice weekly initially, then weekly for 1 month, then monthly for 1 year, and then 4-monthly with blood samples taken 12 hours after administration of the last dose
- lithium should be stopped for 24 hours before major surgery. Maybe be re-started soon after surgery if electrolytes are normal
- if changing from immediate-release to sustained-release formulation, same total dose should be given and patient should be monitored at 1–2-week intervals for therapeutic effects and/or adverse effects and dose adjusted accordingly
- withdrawal should be gradual over at least 15 days
- overdosage/toxicity treatment includes stopping therapy immediately, maintenance of fluid and electrolyte balance and renal function to prevent hypernatraemia, ECG monitoring and control of hypotension and seizures. Activated charcoal does not absorb lithium
- caution if given to those with vomiting, diarrhoea, fluid restriction, excessive sweating, dehydration, strenuous exercise, low salt diet, fever or infection (which might affect electrolyte balance) or during acute mood swings (as lithium requirements may alter)
- not recommended in those with Brugada syndrome because of increased risk of ventricular arrhythmias
- contraindicated in those with cardiovascular or kidney disease, hypothyroidism, conditions associated with hyponatraemia (e.g. Addison's disease, dehydration, low sodium diet)

Patient teaching and advice

- patient should be warned against driving a vehicle or operating machinery if drowsy or dizzy, especially in the first few weeks of therapy
- patient should be advised to seek medical attention immediately if any of the following occur:
  - vomiting, diarrhoea, dehydration, fever or infection (as this will increase risk of toxicity occurring)
  - excessive thirst or urination
  - signs or symptoms of toxicity including persistent nausea and vomiting, slurred speech, ataxia, muscle twitching and seizures
- patient, relatives and nurses must memorise or retain a written record of serious adverse effects/toxicity requiring immediate cessation of therapy
- instruct patient to take with food to minimise nausea and sustained-release tablets should be taken whole and not broken, crushed, chewed or taken with hot beverages
- ensure patient has been given information regarding the importance of normal diet with adequate salt intake and a fluid intake of up to 3 L/day, especially if exercising strenuously, leading to increased sweating and therefore sodium loss. Salt intake should not suddenly be restricted
- advise patient about the need to continue therapy usually for at least 6–9 months before the full benefits are seen
- abrupt changes to caffeine intake can alter lithium serum levels, especially if normal intake is greater than 4 cups of coffee (or caffeine equivalent) per day. Patient should therefore be warned not to eliminate caffeine from diet without first discussing with doctor

- advise patient against driving or operating machinery if dazed feeling, poor co-ordination, drowsiness or vertigo occur
- patient should be advised to avoid alcohol during therapy as drowsiness may be worsened
- if patient has pre-existing skin condition such as acne or psoriasis, he/she should be warned that it may worsen during therapy
- female patient should be counselled regarding avoiding pregnancy during therapy

crosses the placental barrier and enters fetal circulation, where it may cause thyroid disturbances and/or cardiovascular malformations. If the newborn is showing signs of lithium toxicity (e.g. flaccid appearance), fluid therapy should be started. Serum lithium levels should be carefully monitored during pregnancy, but it is recommended that therapy be stopped before planning pregnancy

not recommended during breastfeeding to avoid infant becoming hypotonic, flaccid and difficult to feed

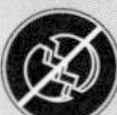

slow-release tablets should not be broken, crushed, chewed or taken with hot liquids

plain tablets can be crushed and mixed with water or spoonful of yoghurt or apple puree

LURASIDONE HYDROCHLORIDE (Latuda)

Available forms
Tablets: 40 mg, 80 mg

Action
- atypical antipsychotic
- benzisothiazol
- antagonises dopamine (D_2) and serotonin ($5HT_{2A}$) receptors

Use
- schizophrenia

Dose
- initially 40 mg orally daily with food, increasing dose if needed (daily maximum 160 mg)

Adverse effects
- blurred vision
- hypertension, tachycardia
- rash, pruritus
- see also General Adverse effects of antipsychotics (p. 772)

Interactions
- contraindicated with clarithromycin, ritonavir, voriconazole, rifampicin, carbamazepine, phenytoin and St John's wort
- serum levels may be increased by grapefruit or grapefruit juice and therefore not recommended together
- caution if given with diltiazem

Nursing points/Cautions
- not recommended in those under 17 years
- not recommended in those with moderate-to-severe liver or kidney impairment. Initial and daily dose reductions are recommended if used
- see also General Nursing points/Cautions for antipsychotics (p. 774)

Patient teaching and advice
- advise patient not to use with grapefruit or grapefruit juice
- see also General Patient teaching and advice for antipsychotics (p. 775)

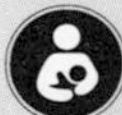

should only be used during pregnancy if benefits outweigh risks

not recommended during breastfeeding

tablet can be crushed and mixed with water or spoonful of yoghurt or apple puree

OLANZAPINE (Olanzacor, Ozin, Pryzex, Pryzex ODT, Zypine, Zypine ODT, Zyprexa, Zyprexa IM, Zyprexa Zydis Wafers)

OLANZAPINE PAMOATE MONOHYDRATE (Zyprexa Relprevv)

Available forms

Tablets: 2.5 mg, 5 mg, 7.5 mg, 10 mg; Wafers (dissolvable/orally disintegrating tablets): 5 mg, 10 mg, 15 mg, 20 mg; Vial: 10 mg; Vial (prolonged-release): 210 mg, 300 mg, 405 mg

Action

- atypical antipsychotic with mood stabilising properties
- dopamine antagonist (affinity for D_1, D_2, D_3, D_4, D_5 receptors)
- also shows affinity for cholinergic, serotonergic, histaminic and alpha-adrenergic receptors
- increases prolactin level
- half-life is about 33 hours. Half-life is prolonged and clearance is reduced in those > 65 years

Use

- schizophrenia, related psychoses
- schizophrenia maintenance in adults stabilised with oral olanzapine (prolonged-release injectable)
- acute mania associated with bipolar I disorder (alone or with lithium or sodium valproate) (short term)
- prevent recurrence of manic/depressive/mixed episodes associated with bipolar I disorder

Dose

- (schizophrenia) initially 5–10 mg orally daily, increasing to 20 mg if necessary **OR**
- (acute mania with bipolar disorder: monotherapy) 10–15 mg orally once daily, increasing dose if needed (daily maximum 20 mg) **OR**
- (acute mania with bipolar disorder with lithium or sodium valproate) 10 mg orally daily, increasing dose if needed (daily maximum 20 mg) **OR**
- (bipolar disorder prevention) initially 10 mg orally daily (or dose achieved in previous point), increasing dose if needed (range 5–20 mg)

Schizophrenia maintenance after stabilisation

- (previous oral dose 10 mg/day) initially 210 mg deep IM every 2 weeks or 405 mg deep IM every 4 weeks for 8 weeks, then 150 mg every 2 weeks or 300 mg every 4 weeks (maintenance) **OR**
- (previous oral dose 15 mg/day) initially 300 mg deep IM every 2 weeks for 8 weeks, then 210 mg every 2 weeks or 405 mg every 4 weeks (maintenance) **OR**
- (previous oral dose 20 mg/day) initially 300 mg deep IM every 2 weeks for 8 weeks, then 300 mg every 2 weeks (maintenance)

Adverse effects

- see General Adverse effects of antipsychotics (p. 772)
- (IM) hypotension, peripheral oedema
- (IM, prolonged-release) post-injection syndrome (including sedation, confusion, agitation, anxiety, dizziness, cognitive impairment, weakness, ataxia)
- (uncommon) secondary amenorrhoea, hypo-oestrogenism, drug reaction eosinophilia and systemic symptoms (DRESS)
- (IM, rare) injection site abscess

Interactions

- see General Interactions of antipsychotics (p. 773)
- increased metabolism may result if taken with carbamazepine or if patient is a smoker
- increased serum levels may occur if given with fluvoxamine or ciprofloxacin

Nursing points/Cautions

- see General Nursing points/Cautions for antipsychotics (p. 774)
- BP should be regularly monitored throughout therapy, especially if patient is aged 65 years or over
- if secondary amenorrhoea occurs (lasting more than 6 months), bone loss can be prevented by using prophylactic treatment with bone and calcium regulating agents
- wafers are bioequivalent to tablets
- parenteral administration is for short-term use only
- only given IM (not SC or IV)
- before starting maintenance therapy with prolonged formulation, patient tolerability should be determined on oral olanzapine
- (IM, maintenance therapy) patient must be observed for 2 hours post-injection (including alertness monitored every 30 minutes) for any signs of post-injection syndrome (sedation and/or delirium related to olanzapine overdose). Observation period should be extended if any signs and symptoms occur. Patient should only be released if alert, oriented and free of any signs and symptoms of overdose
- (IM, maintenance therapy) gloves should be worn when reconstituting solution. If solution makes contact with skin, it should be flushed with water immediately
- dose should be started at 5 mg in those aged 65 years or more
- wafers contain aspartame, therefore caution if used in those with phenylketonuria
- tablets contain lactose and are not recommended in those with rare hereditary problems of galactose intolerance, Lapp lactase deficiency or glucose–galactose malabsorption
- caution if used in those with diabetes, prostatic hypertrophy, glaucoma, paralytic ileus, kidney/liver impairment, elevated liver enzymes, bone marrow depression, history of or predisposition to seizures, myeloproliferative disorders, cardiovascular disease (with syncope, hypotension and/or bradycardia)
- (IM) contraindicated in those with hypersensitivity to polysorbate 80 or mannitol

Patient teaching and advice

- patient should be warned to remain recumbent after injection to avoid postural hypotension
- warn patient that there is a 2-hour observation period required after injection with prolonged formulation to monitor for adverse effects
- (IM for maintenance) patient should be advised not to travel alone post-injection, nor drive or operate heavy machinery
- (IM for maintenance) instruct patient (carer or family member) to immediately seek medical attention if confusion, irritability, excessive sleepiness, dizziness, disorientation, aggression, anxiety, weakness or difficulty talking or walking occurs
- patient should be advised to seek medical attention if any rash, dermatitis, fever, chills, headache or enlarged lymph nodes occur
- instruct patient that wafer should not be handled directly as it is very fragile and should be placed on the tongue directly from the blister pack and allowed to dissolve or can be dissolved in liquids (not cola beverages) if preferred
- female patients (pre-menopausal) should be advised to report any lack of menstruation that occurs for longer than 6 months
- see General Patient teaching and advice for antipsychotics (p. 775)

available as a wafer or oral disintegrating tablets

PALIPERIDONE (Invega, Invega Sustenna, Invega Trinza)

Available forms

Tablets (prolonged-release): 3 mg, 6 mg, 9 mg; Prefilled syringe: 25 mg, 50 mg, 75 mg, 100 mg, 150 mg; 175 mg/0.875 mL, 263 mg/1.315 mL, 350 mg/1.75 mL, 525 mg/2.625 mL

Action

- benzisoxazole that is an active metabolite of risperidone
- binds to D_2 and $5HT_{2A}$ receptors
- also binds to other serotonin, histamine and alpha-adrenergic receptors producing moderately high sedation and antihypertensive properties but no antiemetic actions
- half-life 23 hours

Use

- acute and maintenance treatment of schizophrenia
- acute treatment of schizoaffective disorder (alone or in combination with antidepressants and/or lithium or sodium valproate)

Dose

- (schizophrenia) 6 mg orally daily mane, adjusting dose to 3 or 9 mg after 5 days if needed (maximum daily dose 12 mg) **OR**
- (schizophrenia) initially 150 mg IM (deltoid) (day 1), then 100 mg IM (deltoid) 7 days later (day 8), followed by 25–150 mg IM (deltoid or ventrogluteal) monthly (maintenance) (monthly formulation) **OR**
- (schizophrenia) 3.5 times monthly IM dose (above) (first dose given within 7 days of monthly scheduled IM injection), then 3-monthly (dose range 175–525 mg) **OR**
- (acute exacerbation of schizoaffective disorder) initially 6 mg orally daily mane, increasing at 3 mg daily at 4-day intervals if needed (daily maximum 12 mg)

Adverse effects

- see General Adverse effects of antipsychotics (p. 772)
- (IM) induration, pain, redness or swelling at injection site
- (IM, very rare) hypersensitivity

Interactions

- see also General Interactions of antipsychotics (p. 773)
- not recommended with risperidone (as paliperidone is its active metabolite)
- (oral) absorption may be delayed if given with metoclopramide
- decreased serum levels may occur if given with carbamazepine
- increased risk of extrapyramidal symptoms if given with psychostimulants such as methylphenidate

Nursing points/Cautions

- see General Nursing points/Cautions for antipsychotics (p. 774)
- tolerability should be established before starting IM paliperidone in those who have never previously used paliperidone (orally) or risperidone (orally or parentally)
- (3-monthly IM formulation) monthly IM formulation should be administered for at least 4 months (with last 2 doses being at the same dose) before switching to 3-monthly formulation
- (3-monthly IM formulation) dose response may not be apparent for several months and this should be taken into consideration if adjusting dose
- if switching from monthly to 3-monthly IM dosing, IM dose should be 3.5 times monthly dose and administered when next monthly dose was due, then 3-monthly
- if switching from 3-monthly to monthly IM dosage, IM dose should be divided by 3.5 and administered 3 months after last scheduled dose

- if switching from 3-monthly IM formulation to extended-release tablets, administration should start 3 months from last IM injection with oral dose dependent on IM dose (daily dose range 3–12 mg). Manufacturer's information should be consulted
- if changing from another long-acting injectable antipsychotic agent, therapy can be started at next scheduled injection and continued monthly
- IM doses should not be divided but given as single IM injection
- given by deep IM only (ventrogluteal or deltoid muscles only)
- injections should be alternated between two deltoid or gluteal muscles
- ensure syringe is vigorously shaken (for at least 15 seconds) to mix solution evenly before use within 5 minutes
- (deltoid administration) 23-gauge (1 inch) needle is recommended for patients weighing < 90 kg; if patient weighs > 90 kg, 22-gauge (1½ inch) is recommended
- (gluteal administration) regardless of patient weight, 22-gauge (1½ inch) needle is recommended
- consult manufacturer's information if IM doses are missed for readministration schedule
- increased risk of neuroleptic malignant syndrome if given to those with Parkinson's disease or Lewy body dementia
- caution if used in those with severe liver impairment
- not recommended in those with pre-existing severe gastrointestinal narrowing or motility disorders due to increased risk of obstruction due to non-conformable tablet coating
- not recommended in those with creatinine clearance < 10 mL/min
- contraindicated in those with hypersensitivity to risperidone

Patient teaching and advice

- see General Patient teaching and advice for antipsychotics (p. 775)
- advise patient to take tablets on an empty stomach or with food and always take the same way (with or without food, not alternate between the two)
- instruct patient to take whole (not broken, chewed or crushed) with fluids
- warn patient that outer coating of capsule may appear in stools
- (IM) patient should be advised to seek medical advice immediately if any fever, abnormally high body temperature, light-headedness, dizziness or unusual heart rate (fast, slow, irregular) occurs

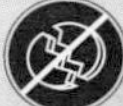

extended-release tablets should not be broken, chewed or crushed

PERICIAZINE (PERICYAZINE) (Neulactil)

Available forms
Tablets: 2.5 mg, 10 mg

Action
- typical antipsychotic with greater sedating action, higher antiemetic and anticholinergic properties than other antipsychotic phenothiazines

Use
- severe anxiety and tension
- psychoses (maintenance)

Dose
- (mild-to-moderate) 15–30 mg orally daily in 2 divided doses with larger dose given in the evening **OR**
- (moderate-to-severe hospitalised patient) 25–75 mg orally daily in 2 divided doses

Adverse effects

- photosensitivity
- see General Adverse effects for antipsychotics (p. 772)

Interactions

- contraindicated with regional or spinal anaesthetics
- caution if given with desferrioxamine due to risk of transient metabolic encephalopathy
- see General Interactions for antipsychotics (p. 773)

Nursing points/Cautions

- see General Nursing points/Cautions for antipsychotics (p. 774)
- (elderly) starting dose should be 10 mg daily in divided doses, increasing if needed to 30 mg daily maximum

Patient teaching and advice

- instruct patient to avoid direct sunlight during therapy as photosensitivity may occur
- see General Patient teaching and advice for antipsychotics (p. 775)

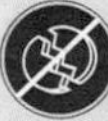

tablets can be dispersed in water or crushed and mixed with spoonful of yoghurt or apple puree. If crushing or dispersing tablets, gloves should be worn as contact may cause contact dermatitis

QUETIAPINE (Delucon, Kaptan, Quetia, Quetia XR, Seroquel, Seroquel XR, Syquet, Tevatiapine XR)

Available forms

Tablets: 25 mg, 100 mg, 200 mg, 300 mg; Tablets (modified-release): 50 mg, 150 mg, 200 mg, 300 mg, 400 mg

Action

- atypical antipsychotic agent with high affinity for serotonin ($5HT_2$) and dopamine (D_1 and D_2) receptors
- affinity also for histamine and alpha-1-adrenergic receptors
- no antiemetic properties, some sedative and hypotensive properties, low anticholinergic actions
- active metabolite (norquetiapine) which has a half-life of 9 hours
- half-life 7 hours

Use

- schizophrenia
- treatment and maintenance of bipolar I disorder (monotherapy or with lithium or sodium valproate)
- treatment of depressive episodes associated with bipolar disorders
- treatment of acute mania associated with bipolar disorders (monotherapy or with lithium or sodium valproate)
- generalised anxiety disorder
- major depressive disorder (in patients intolerant to or who have had inadequate response to other therapies)

Dose

- (schizophrenia) initially 50 mg orally (day 1), increasing to 100 mg daily (day 2), 200 mg daily (day 3) and 300 mg daily (day 4) given in 2 divided doses, and then adjusted according to clinical response (usual effective daily dose 300–450 mg) **OR**
- (schizophrenia) initially 300 mg orally daily (day 1), then 600 mg (day 2) and up to 800 mg (range 400–800 mg daily) (modified-release tablets) **OR**
- (acute mania in bipolar disorder) initially 100 mg orally (day 1), 200 mg (day 2), 300 mg (day 3), 400 mg (day 4), then increasing by increments not greater than 200 mg daily, up to 800 mg by day 6 if needed, given in 2 divided doses (alone or with lithium or sodium valproate) **OR**
- (acute mania in bipolar disorder) initially 300 mg orally daily (day 1), then 600 mg (day 2) and up to 800 mg (alone or with lithium or sodium valproate) (modified-release tablets) **OR**

- (bipolar depression) initially 50 mg orally at bedtime (day 1), then 100 mg (day 2), 200 mg (day 3) and 300 mg (day 4), then increasing at 100 mg daily increments to 600 mg if needed **OR**
- (bipolar disorder maintenance) 300–800 mg orally daily in 2 divided doses (immediate-release tablets) or single daily dose (modified-release tablets) **OR**
- (recurrent major depressive disorder) initially 50 mg orally nocte (day 1 and 2), increasing to 150 mg (day 3 and 4), then adjusting dose to clinical response (range 50–300 mg daily) (modified-release tablets) **OR**
- (generalised anxiety disorder) initially 50 mg orally daily (day 1 and 2), increasing to 150 mg (day 3 and 4), then adjusting dose to clinical response (range 50–150 mg daily) (modified-release tablets)

Adverse effects

- peripheral oedema
- transient decrease in thyroid hormone levels
- (rare) cardiomyopathy, myocarditis, pancreatitis, increased risk of dependence/tolerance
- see General Adverse effects of antipsychotics (p. 772)

Interactions

- decreased serum levels may occur if given with phenytoin, carbamazepine, phenobarbital (phenobarbitone) or rifampicin
- increased serum levels may occur if given with azole antifungal agents, macrolide antibiotics or protease inhibitors
- not recommended with grapefruit juice as increased serum levels may occur increasing risk of toxicity
- may increase serum levels of lorazepam
- not recommended with medications such as atomoxetine, dexamphetamine and methylphenidate used in the management of ADHD
- may cause false positive results for methadone and TCAs in enzyme immunoassays
- see General Interactions of antipsychotics (p. 773)

Nursing points/Cautions

- see General Nursing points/Cautions for antipsychotics (p. 774)
- if switching from immediate-release to modified-release formulation, dose is equivalent but given as a single daily dose (e.g. 300 mg twice daily immediate-release tablets = 600 mg daily dose of modified-release tablets)
- (recurrent major depression disorder) if no clinical response after 6 weeks, therapy should be re-evaluated
- (plain tablets) contain lactose and are not recommended in those with galactose intolerance, Lapp lactase deficiency or glucose–galactose malabsorption
- caution if used in those with history of alcohol or drug abuse due to risk of misuse or abuse

Patient teaching and advice

- instruct patient that modified-release tablets should be taken whole, not crushed, divided or chewed
- advise patient that any somnolence usually resolves within the first few weeks of therapy
- patient should be warned to avoid grapefruit juice during therapy
- see General Patient teaching and advice for antipsychotics (p. 775)

plain tablets can be crushed and mixed with water or spoonful of yoghurt or apple puree

RISPERIDONE (Ozidal, Rispa, Rispernia, Risperdal, Risperdal Consta, Rixadone)

Available forms

Tablets: 0.5 mg, 1 mg, 2 mg, 3 mg, 4 mg; Oral suspension: 1 mg/mL; Vial: 25 mg, 37.5 mg, 50 mg

Action

- benzisoxazole atypical antipsychotic
- antagonises dopamine (D_2) and serotonin ($5HT_2$) receptors
- also weakly binds to alpha-1 and alpha-2 adrenergic and H_1 histamine receptors
- no antiemetic properties and moderate hypotensive action
- increases prolactin level
- active metabolite (paliperidone)

Use

- schizophrenia and related psychoses
- management of acute mania associated with bipolar I disorder (short term)
- treatment of behavioural disturbances (with dementia) (up to 12 weeks) (in those not responding to non-pharmacological management strategies)
- treatment of conduct/disruptive behaviour disorders in those with mental retardation or sub-average intellectual functioning (> 5 years)
- behavioural disorders associated with autism

Dose

- (schizophrenia) initially 1 mg orally twice daily (day 1), increased to 2 mg twice daily (day 2), then increasing gradually if needed (daily dose range 4–6 mg) **OR**
- (bipolar mania) initially 2 mg orally daily, increasing by 1 mg increments at daily intervals if needed (daily dose range 2–6 mg) **OR**
- (behavioural disturbance with dementia) initially 0.25 mg orally twice daily, increasing dose by 0.25 mg increments twice daily every second day if needed **OR**
- (conduct/disruptive behaviour disorders, body weight ≥ 50 kg) initially 0.5 mg orally daily, increasing by 0.5 mg increments every second day if needed (daily maximum 1.5 mg) **OR**
- (conduct/disruptive behaviour disorders, body weight < 50 kg) initially 0.25 mg orally daily, increasing by 0.25 mg increments every second day if needed (daily maximum 0.75 mg) **OR**
- (behaviour disorders associated with autism, body weight ≥ 20 kg) initially 0.5 mg orally daily (days 1–3), increasing to 1 mg (days 4–14). Clinical response should be assessed at day 14 and if needed, may be increased at 0.5 mg increments at 2-week intervals (dose range 1–2.5 mg/day but higher dose will be required if body weight is > 45 kg) **OR**
- (behaviour disorders associated with autism, body weight < 20 kg) initially 0.25 mg orally daily (days 1–3), increasing to 0.5 mg (days 4–14). Clinical response should be assessed at day 14 and if needed, may be increased at 0.25 mg increments at 2-week intervals (dose range 0.5–1.5 mg/day) **OR**
- (schizophrenia) initially 25 mg IM 2-weekly, increasing to 37.5 or 50 mg if necessary (maximum dose 50 mg/2-weekly)

Adverse effects

- see General Adverse effects of antipsychotics (p. 772)
- drooling
- rhinorrhoea, cough, nasal stuffiness, rhinitis, nasopharyngitis, dyspnoea, upper respiratory tract infection, sinusitis
- epistaxis
- rash, dry skin
- secondary amenorrhoea
- (IM) pain and rarely, abscess, cellulitis, ulcer, haematoma or necrosis

Interactions

- see General Interactions of antipsychotics (p. 773)
- carbamazepine and rifampicin may decrease plasma risperidone levels
- plasma levels may be increased if given with phenothiazines, TCAs, protease inhibitors, itraconazole, paroxetine, fluoxetine and some beta-adrenoceptor blocking agents
- not recommended with psychostimulants (e.g. methylphenidate) due to increased risk of extrapyramidal symptoms
- bioavailability may be reduced by topiramate
- increased hypotension may occur if given with antihypertensive agents or TCAs
- caution if given with furosemide (frusemide) (especially in the elderly with dementia) due to increased risk of mortality

Nursing points/Cautions

- see General Nursing points/Cautions for antipsychotics (p. 774)
- in those not previously treated, oral risperidone is recommended before starting parenteral formulation
- during first 3 weeks of therapy with slow-release IM preparation, oral therapy should be continued
- (IM) use diluent (in prefilled syringe) and needles provided for administration (drawing up and administration needle – for deltoid, 1-inch hypodermic needle or for ventrogluteal, 2-inch hypodermic needle is recommended)
- allow components to reach room temperature for 30 minutes before reconstituting
- follow manufacturer's instructions for use of safety device (Needle-Pro)
- shake reconstituted solution well before use to ensure powder is dissolved
- rotate injection sites (alternate ventrogluteals or deltoids, depending on patient's preference). Injection site should be inspected before injection and not used if any signs of inflammation exist
- not given IV
- dose increases should not occur more often than monthly
- if secondary amenorrhoea occurs (lasting more than 6 months), bone loss can be prevented by using prophylactic treatment with bone and calcium regulating agents
- when changing from other antipsychotics to risperidone, there should be a gradual discontinuance. If a depot injection has been previously used, risperidone should not be started until the next injection is due

Patient teaching and advice

- see General Patient teaching and advice for antipsychotics (p. 775)
- patient should be warned that it may take up to 3 weeks for clinical response to increased dose to become apparent
- advise patient that oral suspension may be mixed with mineral water, orange juice, milk or coffee but not tea
- patient should be instructed that oral suspension comes with a calibrated pipette and instructions should be followed regarding its correct use, including rinsing after use before storage
- female patient of menstrual age should be advised to report any lack of menstruation for 6 months or more

oral solution is available. Tablet can be dispersed in 2.5 mL water and then mixed with spoonful of yoghurt or apple puree

SODIUM VALPROATE (Epilim, Epilim IV, Valprease, Valpro)

Available forms
Tablets (sustained-release): 200 mg, 500 mg; Tablets (crushable): 100 mg; Suspension: 200 mg/5 mL; Vial: 400 mg

Action
- anticonvulsant, antipsychotic
- thought to raise brain levels of the inhibitory synaptic transmitter GABA, as well as blocking voltage-dependent sodium channels
- half-life 8–12 hours

Use
- mania (where other agents are ineffective or inappropriate)
- epilepsy (see Sodium valproate in Antiepileptics, p. 409)

Dose
- (mania) initially 600 mg orally daily, increasing by 200 mg/day at 3-day intervals until control is reached (daily maximum 2500 mg)

Adverse effects/Interactions/Nursing points/Cautions/Patient teaching and advice
- see General Adverse effects of antiepileptics (p. 382)

ZIPRASIDONE (Zeldox, Zeldox IM, Ziprox)

Available forms
Capsules: 20 mg, 40 mg, 60 mg, 80 mg; Vial: 20 mg

Action
- indole derivative unrelated to phenothiazine or butyrophenone antipsychotics
- dopamine (D_2) and serotonin ($5HT_2$) antagonist
- also binds to alpha-1 adrenergic and H_1 histamine receptors
- no antiemetic properties, low-to-moderative sedative and hypotensive actions
- half-life 6–10 hours

Use
- schizophrenia and related psychoses
- acute manic or mixed episodes associated with bipolar I disorder (monotherapy, short term)
- (IM) acute management of agitated/disturbed behaviour in schizophrenia and related psychoses where oral therapy is inappropriate (short term)

Dose
- (schizophrenia, bipolar I disorder) initially 40 mg orally twice daily with food, then increasing at 2-day intervals if needed (daily maximum 160 mg) **OR**
- (acute management of agitated/disturbed behaviour) 10 mg IM 2-hourly or 20 mg IM 4-hourly (daily maximum 40 mg) (up to 3 days)

Adverse effects
- see General Adverse effects of antipsychotics (p. 772)
- rash, urticaria and rarely, severe cutaneous reactions
- 'thick tongue' sensation
- (IM) dizziness, tachycardia, postural hypotension

Interactions
- see General Interactions of antipsychotics (p. 773)
- decreased serum levels may occur if given with carbamazepine, rifampicin and St John's wort
- caution if given with lithium due to increased risk of arrhythmias

Nursing points/Cautions
- see General Nursing points/Cautions for antipsychotics (p. 774)
- parenteral therapy should be replaced with oral therapy as soon as possible

- only given IM, not IV
- reconstitute using 1.2 mL water for injections
- contraindicated in those with recent myocardial infarction (MI) or uncompensated heart failure

Patient teaching and advice

- see General Patient teaching and advice for antipsychotics (p. 775)
- advise patient to seek medical advice if any rash develops

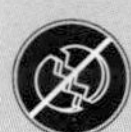

capsules can be opened and contents dispersed in water (gloves should be worn). Pregnant staff should not open capsules

ZUCLOPENTHIXOL (Clopixol) ZUCLOPENTHIXOL ACETATE (Clopixol Acuphase)

ZUCLOPENTHIXOL DECANOATE (Clopixol Depot)

Available forms

Tablets: 10 mg; Vial: 50 mg/mL, 100 mg/2 mL; Vial (depot): 200 mg/mL

Action

- thioxanthene
- dopamine receptor (D_1 and D_2) antagonist
- increases serum prolactin levels
- weak anticholinergic properties, no antiemetic action, some sedative properties
- half-life 20 hours
- decanoate allows slow release from oily solution (coconut oil)

Use

- (tablets) acute and chronic schizophrenia and other psychoses, manic phase of bipolar disorders
- (Acuphase injection) initial treatment of acute psychoses; mania; exacerbation of chronic psychoses
- (depot) maintenance treatment

Dose

- (acute schizophrenia, mania, acute agitation, acute psychoses) initially 10–20 mg orally daily, increasing by 10–20 mg every 2–3 days to 75 mg daily if needed **OR**
- (chronic schizophrenia or psychoses) 20–40 mg orally at bedtime **OR**
- 50–150 mg IM repeated every 2–3 days if necessary (maximum dose 400 mg/course or 4 injections over maximum duration of 2 weeks) **OR**
- (depot preparation) 200–400 mg IM every 2–4 weeks

Adverse effects

- see General Adverse effects of antipsychotics (p. 772)
- injection site reaction

Interactions

- see General Interactions of antipsychotics (p. 773)
- may decrease effects of levodopa and adrenergic drugs
- increased risk of extrapyramidal symptoms if given with metoclopramide

Nursing points/Cautions

- see General Nursing points/Cautions for antipsychotics (p. 774)
- dose stabilisation should occur under close medical supervision
- parenteral treatment should not exceed 2 weeks and is then maintained with either oral or depot medication
- sedation occurs up to 2 hours after injection, lasting about 8 hours and then decreases (parenteral)
- if patient is receiving 100 mg IM, oral treatment is usually started at 40 mg daily as single or divided doses, which can then be increased if necessary
- changing from oral to IM depot formulation, oral daily dose × 8 = depot IM every 2–4 weeks, continuing oral medication at reduced dose for first week after first depot injection

- if changing from parenteral to depot, depot injection (200–400 mg) should be given with last IM parenteral dose
- tablets contain lactose and are therefore not recommended in those with galactose intolerance, Lapp lactase deficiency or glucose–galactose malabsorption
- contraindicated in those with hypersensitivity to coconut oil or thioxanthenes as cross-sensitivity with phenothiazines may exist

Patient teaching and advice

- see General Patient teaching and advice for antipsychotics (p. 775)
- patient should be advised to report any sore throat, chills, fever or flu-like illness

tablet can be crushed and mixed with spoonful of yoghurt or apple puree, but does not disperse readily in water

ANTIULCER AGENTS

The cells of the stomach secrete hydrochloric acid and intrinsic factor (from parietal cells), digestive enzymes (pepsinogen, gastric lipase) (from peptic cells), mucus and bicarbonate (from mucus-secreting cells). Hydrochloric acids performs a number of roles, including killing bacteria, denaturing protein, and converting inactive pepsinogen to active pepsin which further degrade protein. Mucus and bicarbonate form a gel-like protective layer protecting the stomach from acid while also providing lubrication between undigested food and superficial cells. Intrinsic factor (from parietal cells) binds to vitamin B_{12} for absorption in the ileum (Bryant et al 2019).

The parietal cells secrete 1–2 litres of hydrochloric acid daily, so it is vital that the mucosal barrier remains intact in order to prevent ulceration from occurring. Factors that impact on the mucosal barrier include blood flow changes, decreased mucus secretion, bacterial infection and damage by alcohol, aspirin, NSAIDs and other agents (Bryant et al 2019). This breach in the gastric mucosa allows it to be further attacked, resulting in peptic ulcers (Del Valle 2018).

Peptic ulcers can be divided into duodenal or gastric (depending on their location) and share some common features, including epigastric pain (burning or gnawing) and cause (*Helicobacter pylori* (*H. pylori*) and NSAIDs) (Del Valle 2018).

- *duodenal ulcers* occur most commonly in the first part of the duodenum (within 3 cm of the pylorus) and are often silent, only presenting when complications arise. They are rarely malignant. Epigastric pain usually occurs 90 minutes to 3 hours after eating and is frequently relieved by antacids or food. Pain may wake a person from sleep, occurring in about two-thirds of patients
- *gastric ulcers* tend to occur later in life (peak incidence in the sixth decade), are more common in males and less common than duodenal ulcers. Gastric ulcers may be benign or malignant and should therefore be biopsied. Epigastric discomfort may be caused by food with nausea, vomiting and weight loss common symptoms.

Complications of both duodenal and gastric ulcers include bleeding, perforation and gastric outlet obstruction. Furthermore, *H. pylori* infection is associated with an increased risk of gastric cancer (Del Valle 2018; Mitchell & Katelaris 2016).

Antiulcer agents may be used as either treatment or prophylaxis. Eradication of *H. pylori* and prevention of NSAID-induced disease is the mainstay of ulcer treatment. In Australia, recommended eradication treatment of *H. pylori* involves triple therapy (e.g. proton pump inhibitor, clarithromycin and amoxicillin), usually for 7 days, with alternate regimens available if the patient has a proven penicillin allergy. The outcome of the eradication therapy should be assessed not less than 4 weeks after completion, by either gastroscopy or urea breath test (Mitchell & Katelaris 2016).

Some antiulcer agents act by either reducing gastric acid secretion or protecting the mucosa from the effects of acid. Reduction of gastric acid secretion occurs by blocking histamine (H_2) receptors (H_2-receptor antagonists) or by acting directly on the parietal cells (proton pump inhibitors). Some prostaglandins inhibit gastrin and gastric acid secretion, as well as protecting the mucosa (cytoprotective) (Del Valle 2018). Antacids are generally used to relieve symptoms of dyspepsia and are discussed at the end of this section.

HISTAMINE H_2-RECEPTOR ANTAGONISTS

General Actions of H_2-receptor antagonists

- reduce gastric acid secretion by competitively blocking the action of histamine at histamine H_2-receptor sites of parietal cells, thereby reducing hydrochloric acid
- inhibit both daytime and nocturnal basal (non-stimulated) gastric acid secretion
- inhibit stimulated gastric acid secretion by food, histamine, coffee, insulin and pentagastrin
- cross-sensitivity may exist between members of the histamine H_2-receptor antagonists

General Uses of H_2-receptor antagonists

- treatment and maintenance of gastric and duodenal ulcers (short-term therapy)
- maintenance therapy for chronic benign gastric or duodenal ulcers (up to 12 months)
- persistent gastro-oesophageal reflux disease (commonly known as GORD) (up to 12 months)
- short-term management of heartburn and other GORD symptoms (2 weeks)
- gastrinoma (Zollinger–Ellison syndrome)
- scleroderma oesophagitis (short-term therapy)
- erosive and ulcerative oesophagitis

General Nursing points/Cautions for H_2-receptor antagonists

- before starting therapy, any unintentional loss of weight, recurrent vomiting, dysphagia, haematemesis, anaemia, melaena or malignancy should be investigated. It is

also recommended that those with ulceration be re-endoscoped 8–12 weeks after starting therapy to determine if the ulcer is healing
- treatment for GORD and associated reflux symptoms should only be started after conservative measures and antacids are unsuccessful
- may increase the risk of developing community-acquired pneumonia in the elderly, those with diabetes or chronic lung disease, or the immunocompromised
- caution when used in those in intensive care units because agents which suppress acid secretion have been associated with nosocomial lung infections
- caution in those with kidney impairment
- contraindicated in those with hypersensitivity to other H_2-receptor antagonists

General Patient teaching and advice for H_2-receptor antagonists

- patient should be encouraged to continue treatment for 4–6 weeks, after which a maintenance dose may be prescribed
- antacids may be required for symptomatic relief but should be taken 1 hour apart
- patient should be advised against driving or operating machinery if drowsiness or dizziness occur
- patient should be counselled to:
  - stop (or reduce) smoking
  - limit daily caffeine (coffee, tea, cola, chocolate, cocoa) and alcohol intake
  - if possible, reduce aspirin and other NSAIDs intake
  - eat small and frequent meals, ensuring meals are eaten slowly
- see General Patient teaching and advice (p. xxvii)

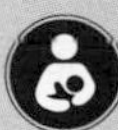

not recommended during pregnancy or breastfeeding unless expected benefit outweighs any potential risk

CIMETIDINE (Magicul)

Available forms

Tablets: 200 mg, 400 mg, 800 mg

Action

- see General Actions of H_2-receptor antagonists (p. 806)
- peak activity 45–90 minutes, half-life 2 hours
- duration of action 4–5 hours (basal), 6–8 hours (nocturnal)

Use

- see General Uses of H_2-receptor antagonists (p. 806)

Dose

- (acute gastric or duodenal ulcer) 200 mg orally 3 times daily with meals and 400 mg at night, increasing to 400 mg 4 times daily if response is inadequate **OR**
- (acute gastric, duodenal ulcer) 400 mg orally with breakfast and 400 mg at bedtime **OR**
- (acute gastric, duodenal ulcer) 800 mg orally at night **OR**
- (recurrent duodenal ulcer) 400 mg orally at night (maintenance) **OR**
- (chronic benign gastric ulceration) 400 mg orally at night (for up to 1 year) (maintenance) **OR**
- (Zollinger–Ellison syndrome) 200 mg orally 3 times daily with meals and 400 mg at night, increasing dose if needed to 1.6–2 g daily **OR**
- (GORD) 800 mg orally at night or in divided doses for 12 weeks **OR**
- (heartburn and symptoms of GORD) 200 mg orally 4 times daily (for up to 2 weeks) **OR**

- (scleroderma oesophagitis) 1.2 g orally daily in divided doses

Adverse effects

- headache, tiredness, dizziness, drowsiness
- diarrhoea, constipation, vomiting, nausea, flatulence
- musculoskeletal pain, myalgia
- rash
- (high dose) (rare) gynaecomastia, impotence
- (rare) reversible confusion, blood dyscrasias, hepatitis

Interactions

- absorption reduced by antacids
- may cause further bone marrow depression when given with drugs known to cause this (e.g. carmustine, epirubicin, fluorouracil), as well as radiation therapy
- may lead to increased serum levels, effects and potential toxicity of alfentanil, aminophylline, calcium-channel blockers, carbamazepine, ciclosporin, diazepam, flecainide, lidocaine (lignocaine), metformin, metoprolol, nifedipine, opioid analgesics, oral sulfonylureas, phenytoin, tacrolimus, theophylline, TCAs and warfarin. Therefore serum levels should be closely monitored, especially when starting and stopping therapy
- prothrombin time should be closely monitored if given with warfarin
- may decrease absorption of posaconazole and itraconazole and therefore should be separated from these agents by 2–3 hours to improve absorption
- may increase absorption of atazanavir which should be separated by a 12-hour interval from cimetidine

Nursing points/Cautions

- see General Nursing points/Cautions for H_2-receptor antagonists (p. 806)

Patient teaching and advice

- instruct patient to swallow tablets whole, not crushed or chewed
- advise patient to immediately seek medical advice if any of the following occur:
  - (men) breast enlargement (gynaecomastia) and impotence
  - yellowing of skin and eyes, loss of appetite, nausea, vomiting, upper abdominal pain, dark urine, pale stools
  - confusion
  - unusual bleeding or bruising
  - looking pale, tiredness, shortness of breath on exercising
- signs of frequent infection such as fever, chills, sore throat, mouth ulcers
- see also General Patient teaching and advice for H_2-receptor antagonists (p. 807)

can be crushed and mixed with water or given with spoonful of yoghurt or apple puree.

FAMOTIDINE (Ausfam)

Available forms

Tablets: 20 mg, 40 mg

Action

- see General Actions of H_2-receptor antagonists (p. 806)
- peak activity 1–3 hours, half-life 2.5–4 hours
- duration of action 10–12 hours

Use

- see General Uses of H_2-receptor antagonists (p. 806)

Dose

- (treatment: duodenal ulcer, benign gastric ulcer) 40 mg orally at night **OR**
- (maintenance: duodenal ulcer) 20 mg orally at night for up to 12 months **OR**

- (Zollinger–Ellison syndrome) initially 20 mg orally 6-hourly, then dose adjusted, and treatment continued, according to clinical need **OR**
- (treatment and maintenance of GORD) 20 mg orally twice daily

Adverse effects
- headache, dizziness
- constipation, diarrhoea

Nursing points/Cautions
- (duodenal and gastric ulcers) treatment is continued for 4–8 weeks, but duration may be shortened if endoscopy reveals that the ulcer has healed
- see General Nursing points/Cautions for H_2-receptor antagonists (p. 806)

Patient teaching and advice
- see General Patient teaching and advice for H_2-receptor antagonists (p. 807)

can be crushed and mixed with water or given with spoonful of yoghurt or apple puree.

NIZATIDINE (Nizac, Tacidine, Tazac)

Available forms
Capsules: 150 mg, 300 mg

Action
- see General Actions of H_2-receptor antagonists (p. 806)
- peak activity 0.5–3 hours, half-life 1–2 hours
- duration of action up to 12 hours

Use
- see General Uses of H_2-receptor antagonists (p. 806)

Dose
- (active duodenal ulcer, benign gastric ulcer, GORD) 150 mg orally twice daily **OR**
- (benign gastric ulcer, active duodenal ulcer) 300 mg orally at night **OR**
- (maintenance: duodenal ulcer) 150 mg orally at night (for up to 12 months)

Adverse effects
- anaemia, hyperuricaemia
- urticaria, sweating, rash, pruritus
- elevated liver enzymes
- (rare) reversible confusion, hepatitis, jaundice, impotence, gynaecomastia, fever, eosinophilia, nausea

Interactions
- may increase serum salicylate levels if given with very high doses of aspirin
- may cause false positive test for urobilinogen using Multistix

Nursing points/Cautions
- not recommended in those with liver failure
- see also General Nursing points/Cautions for H_2-receptor antagonists (p. 806)

Patient teaching and advice
- advise patient to immediately seek medical advice if any of the following occur:
  - (men) breast enlargement and impotence
  - yellowing of skin and eyes, loss of appetite, nausea, vomiting, upper abdominal pain, dark urine, pale stools
  - confusion
- see also General Patient teaching and advice for H_2-receptor antagonists (p. 807)

capsules can be opened and dispersed in 120 mL water (not apple juice) or contents mixed with yoghurt

RANITIDINE HYDROCHLORIDE (Ausran, Rani 2, Zantac preparations, Zantac Concentrate for Injection, Zantac Oral Liquid)

Available forms

Tablets: 150 mg, 300 mg; Effervescent/Dispersible tablets: 150 mg; Syrup: 150 mg/10 mL; Ampoules: 50 mg/2 mL, 50 mg/5 mL

Action

- see General Actions of H_2-receptor antagonists (p. 806)
- less antiandrogenic than cimetidine
- peak activity 1–3 hours, half-life 1–3 hours
- duration of action up to 4 hours (basal), 13 hours (nocturnal)

Use

- see General Uses of H_2-receptor antagonists (p. 806)

Dose

- (acute treatment: duodenal/gastric ulceration) 300 mg orally at night or 150 mg orally twice daily initially for 4–8 weeks **OR**
- (maintenance: duodenal/gastric ulceration) 150 mg orally at night **OR**
- (Zollinger–Ellison syndrome) initially 150 mg orally 3 times daily, increasing as necessary to 600–900 mg/day **OR**
- 50 mg (diluted in 20 mL sodium chloride 0.9%) given IV slowly over at least 5 minutes, may be repeated 6–8-hourly if needed **OR**
- continuous IV infusion at 25 mg/hour for 2 hours, which may be repeated 6–8-hourly **OR**
- (oesophagitis: treatment) 300 mg orally at night or 150 mg orally twice daily **OR**
- (oesophagitis: maintenance) 150 mg orally twice daily (morning and bedtime)

Adverse effects

- headache
- constipation, diarrhoea, nausea, vomiting, abdominal discomfort
- reversible changes in liver function
- rash
- (rare) reversible confusion, impotence, blurred vision, dizziness, porphyria, hepatitis, jaundice
- (IV, rapid) bradycardia
- (prolonged high-dose IV therapy) increase in liver enzymes

Interactions

- antacids and high-dose sucralfate (2 g) significantly reduce absorption of ranitidine
- may increase absorption of triazolam, midazolam and glipizide
- may decrease absorption of atazanavir and gefitinib
- prothrombin time should be closely monitored if given with warfarin

Nursing points/Cautions

- IV administration is only recommended where oral is not appropriate
- (IV) compatible with sodium chloride 0.9%, glucose 5%, sodium bicarbonate or Hartmann's solution
- IV solution should not be rapidly administered because bradycardia, dizziness and peripheral vasodilation may occur
- (effervescent tablets) contain sodium (328 mg) and aspartame and therefore should be used with caution in those on a sodium-restricted diet or with phenylketonuria
- (syrup) contains alcohol (375 mg/5 mL)
- not recommended in those with porphyria
- see General Nursing points/Cautions for H_2-receptor antagonists (p. 806)

Patient teaching and advice

- advise patient to immediately seek medical advice if any of the following occur:
  - (men) breast enlargement (gynecomastia) and impotence
  - yellowing of skin and eyes, loss of appetite, nausea, vomiting, upper abdominal pain, dark urine, pale stools
  - confusion
  - change in heart rate
- instruct patient that syrup should not be diluted
- advise patient that tablets should not be taken with antacids or sucralfate; separate them by at least 2 hours
- instruct patient to dissolve dispersible or effervescent tablets in half a glass of water before swallowing
- see General Patient teaching and advice for H_2-receptor antagonists (p. 807)

PROTON PUMP INHIBITORS

General Actions of proton pump inhibitors

- reduce gastric acid secretion by inhibiting the enzyme $H^+ - K^+$ ATPase (the proton pump) in the parietal cells
- converted to active form by high concentration of acid

General Uses of proton pump inhibitors

- treatment of benign gastric and duodenal ulcers
- symptomatic relief of gastro-oesophageal reflux disease (GORD), including treatment and prevention of erosive reflux oesophagitis
- prevention of re-bleeding of acute, bleeding gastric or duodenal ulcers after IV treatment
- gastrinoma (Zollinger–Ellison syndrome)
- *H. pylori* eradication therapy (in combination with antibiotics)
- prophylaxis or treatment of gastric/duodenal ulcers associated with NSAIDs

General Interactions of proton pump inhibitors

- contraindicated with atazanavir, nelfinavir and cilostazol
- may increase absorption of digoxin
- INR/prothrombin time should be monitored if given with warfarin, especially when starting or stopping therapy or changing dose
- may decrease absorption of iron, ampicillin, erlotinib, posaconazole and itraconazole and should therefore be separated from these agents by 2–3 hours to improve absorption
- may increase serum levels of methotrexate (high dose) increasing risk of adverse effects and toxicity
- caution if used with mycophenolate mofetil in transplant patients
- (prolonged therapy) caution if used with agents (e.g. diuretics) that cause hypomagnesaemia

General Nursing points/Cautions for proton pump inhibitors

- before starting therapy, any unintentional loss of weight, recurrent vomiting, dysphagia, haematemesis, anaemia, melaena or malignancy should be investigated. It is also recommended that those with ulceration be re-endoscoped 8–12 weeks after starting therapy to determine if the ulcer is healing

- IV therapy is only recommended for short-term therapy where oral administration is not appropriate
- serum magnesium levels should be monitored before starting and then regularly if therapy is expected to be prolonged or if given with agents that can reduce magnesium levels (e.g. diuretics)
- use of proton pump inhibitors increases the risk of fundi gland polyps developing, which increase the chance of GI bleeding or intestinal blockage if large or ulcerated
- increased risk of GI infection by Salmonella, *Campylobacter* and *C. difficile* (in hospitalised patient), therefore patients should be closely monitored during therapy
- caution if used in those at risk of osteoporosis and bone fracture
- caution if used in those with impaired liver function as there can be increased availability, decreased plasma clearance and prolonged elimination half-life
- contraindicated in those with hypersensitivity to other proton pump inhibitors

General Patient teaching and advice for proton pump inhibitors

- patient should be encouraged to continue treatment for recommended time (depending on condition), after which a maintenance dose may be prescribed
- advise patient to seek medical advice if symptoms return
- antacids may be required for symptomatic relief, but should be taken 1 hour apart
- patient should be advised against driving or operating machinery if drowsiness or dizziness occur
- instruct patient to immediately seek medical advice if any of the following occur:
  - dizziness, rapid heart rate, confusion, fatigue or tetany (tingling around mouth, hands and feet increasing in intensity, followed by spasm of facial, hand and feet muscles) (signs of hypomagnesaemia)
  - lesions appear on sun-exposed areas of the skin with joint pain
- patient should be counselled to:
  - stop (or reduce) smoking
  - limit daily caffeine (coffee, tea, cola, chocolate, cocoa) intake
  - if possible, reduce aspirin and other NSAIDs intake
  - eat small and frequent meals
  - reduce weight
- see also General Patient teaching and advice (p. xxvii)

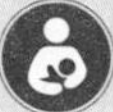

not recommended during pregnancy or breastfeeding

ESOMEPRAZOLE (Esopreze, Guardium Acid Reflux Relief, Mepreze, Nexazole, Nexium, Nexium IV, Nexole, Noxicid, Noxicid Tabs Heartburn Relief)

Available forms

Vial: 42.5 mg (equivalent 40 mg); Tablets: 20 mg, 40 mg; Granules: 10 mg

Action

- see General Actions of proton pump inhibitors (p. 811)
- half-life about 1 hour

Use

- see General Uses of proton pump inhibitors (p. 811)

Dose

- (GORD with oesophagitis) 40 mg orally or IV daily for 4 weeks; may be repeated for a further 4 weeks for patients who have persistent symptoms or if oesophagitis has not healed **OR**
- (healed oesophagitis maintenance) 20 mg orally or IV daily **OR**
- (GORD without oesophagitis) 20 mg orally daily for 4 weeks, then 20 mg orally daily when needed **OR**
- (Zollinger–Ellison syndrome) 40 mg orally twice daily, increasing dose if needed **OR**
- (patients requiring NSAIDs) 20 mg orally daily for up to 4 weeks when starting NSAIDs **OR**
- (healing of gastric ulceration associated with NSAIDs) 20 mg orally daily for up to 8 weeks **OR**
- (prevention of gastric/duodenal ulcers associated with NSAIDs) 20 mg orally daily for up to 6 months **OR**
- (prevention of re-bleeding of gastric/duodenal ulcer) 80 mg IV over 30 minutes, followed by 8 mg/hour by IV infusion for 3 days **OR**
- (prevention of re-bleeding of gastric/duodenal ulcer) 40 mg orally daily **OR**
- (*H. pylori* eradication) 20 mg orally twice daily for 7 days with appropriate antibiotics

Adverse effects

- headache, dizziness
- diarrhoea, flatulence, abdominal pain, nausea, vomiting, constipation, fundic gland polyps
- (uncommon) dermatitis, pruritus, urticaria, rash, elevated liver enzymes, peripheral oedema
- IV site reaction
- (prolonged therapy) vitamin B_{12} deficiency
- (rare) interstitial nephritis, hypomagnesaemia, increased risk of osteoporosis and bone fracture, blood dyscrasias, subacute cutaneous lupus erythematosus

Interactions

- may increase serum levels of phenytoin, citalopram, imipramine, clomipramine, tacrolimus and diazepam
- decreased serum levels may occur if given with St John's wort
- not recommended with clopidogrel
- may interfere with chromogranin A (CgA) estimation for neuroendocrine tumours and should be stopped 5–14 days before measurement
- see General Interactions of proton pump inhibitors (p. 811)

Nursing points/Cautions

- IV therapy is only recommended when oral therapy is inappropriate. Can be continued for up to 10 days, but should be replaced by oral therapy as soon as practicable
- reconstitute with 5 mL sodium chloride 0.9% only and further dilute with 50–100 mL sodium chloride 0.9% for IV infusion administration
- given IV either over 3 minutes or by infusion over 10–30 minutes
- administer alone IV
- see also General Nursing points/Cautions for proton pump inhibitors (p. 811)

Patient teaching and advice

- patient should be advised to swallow tablets or capsules whole (do not crush or chew); however, if patient is unable to swallow, tablets and contents of capsules can be dispersed in water only (non-carbonated) and drunk within 30 minutes
- instruct patient that granules should be used in those with swallowing difficulty or for children. Instructions for using granules should include:
  - disperse granules in non-carbonated water (15 mL for 10 g (1 sachet) or 30 mL for 20 g (2 sachets))
  - contents should be stirred and allowed to thicken

- stir again and drink within 30 minutes
- if anything remains, glass should be rinsed and contents swallowed
- can also be administered via gastric or nasogastric tube after dispersing granules as on previous page. Tube should be flushed well after administration
- advise patient that granules should not be chewed or crushed

- see also General Patient teaching and advice for proton pump inhibitors (p. 812)

tablets and contents of capsules can be dispersed in water only (non-carbonated) and drunk within 30 minutes

Note
- may be used with amoxicillin and clarithromycin (Nexium Hp7, Esomeprazole Sandoz Hp7 Combination) in the treatment of *H. pylori*

LANSOPRAZOLE (Lanzopran, Zopral, Zopral ODT, Zoton FasTabs)

Available forms
Capsules: 15 mg, 30 mg; Tablets (oral disintegrating): 15 mg, 30 mg

Action/Use
- see General Actions and Uses of proton pump inhibitors (p. 811)

Dose
- (reflux oesophagitis) 30 mg orally in the morning before food for 4–8 weeks, then 15–30 mg daily (maintenance) **OR**
- (gastric ulcer) 30 mg orally in the morning before food for 8 weeks **OR**
- (duodenal ulcer) 30 mg orally in the morning before food for 4 weeks, then 15 mg daily (maintenance) **OR**
- (acid-related dyspepsia) 15–30 mg orally in the morning before food for 2–4 weeks **OR**
- (*H. pylori* eradication) 30 mg orally twice daily before food (with appropriate antibiotics)

Adverse effects
- headache, dizziness, fatigue, malaise
- depression, confusion, hallucinations
- diarrhoea, abdominal pain, nausea, vomiting, dyspepsia, constipation, flatulence, dry/sore mouth/throat, fundic gland polyps
- rash, urticaria, pruritus
- altered liver enzymes
- (prolonged therapy) vitamin B_{12} deficiency
- (rare) interstitial nephritis, hypomagnesaemia, increased risk of osteoporosis and bone fracture, subacute cutaneous lupus erythematosus, blood dyscrasias

Interactions
- caution if given with theophylline, phenytoin or carbamazepine
- absorption decreased by antacids and sucralfate and should be separated by at least 1 hour
- serum levels may be increased by fluvoxamine
- serum levels may be decreased by St John's wort
- may increase serum levels of tacrolimus
- may decrease serum levels of posaconazole, levothyroxine and liothyronine
- see General Interactions of proton pump inhibitors (p. 811)

Nursing points/Cautions
- not recommended in those with fructose intolerance, glucose–galactose malabsorption or sucrase–isomaltase insufficiency
- contraindicated in those with severe liver impairment
- see General Nursing points/Cautions for proton pump inhibitors (p. 811)

Patient teaching and advice

- instruct patient that capsules are enteric coated and should not be chewed or crushed. Capsules may be opened and contents sprinkled on a tablespoon of yoghurt, cottage cheese, apple sauce or strained pears or in fluid (e.g. apple, orange or tomato juice) and swallowed immediately. If fluids are used, patient should be advised to rinse glass with a small amount of same fluid and contents swallowed to ensure full dose is taken
- if patient has gastric or nasogastric tube in situ, capsule contents can be sprinkled in 40 mL apple juice (no other fluids) and administered via tube, followed by flush with apple juice to ensure full dose is administered
- advise patient that orally disintegrating tablet should be placed on tongue and gently sucked or swallowed (but not chewed) whole with water
- see General Patient teaching and advice for proton pump inhibitors (p. 812)

OMEPRAZOLE (Acimax, Losec, Maxor, Maxor Heartburn Relief, Omepral, Ozmep, Pemzo, Probitor)

Available forms

Vial: 40 mg; Tablets: 10 mg, 20 mg; Capsules: 20 mg

Action

- see General Actions of proton pump inhibitors (p. 811)
- onset of action within 60 minutes, peak effect 2 hours, duration of action 3–5 days, half-life 30 minutes

Use

- see General Uses of proton pump inhibitors (p. 811)

Dose

- (duodenal/gastric ulcer, ulcerative reflux oesophagitis) 40 mg IV over 20–30 minutes once daily **OR**
- (Zollinger–Ellison syndrome) initially 60 mg IV over 20–30 minutes once daily, increasing as needed. Doses greater than 120 mg IV should be given in divided doses **OR**
- (Zollinger–Ellison syndrome) 60 mg orally once daily, adjusting dose as necessary **OR**
- (GORD) 10–20 mg orally daily for 4 weeks **OR**
- (erosive oesophagitis) 20 mg orally daily for 4–8 weeks, then 10–20 mg daily (maintenance therapy) **OR**
- (erosive oesophagitis refractory to treatment) 40 mg orally daily for 8 weeks **OR**
- (duodenal/gastric ulcer) 20–40 mg orally daily for 4–8 weeks, then 10–20 mg daily as maintenance therapy **OR**
- (NSAID-associated ulceration) 20–40 mg orally daily for 4–8 weeks, then 20 mg orally daily as maintenance **OR**
- (*H. pylori* eradication) 40 mg orally daily or 20 mg orally twice daily (with appropriate antibiotics)

Adverse effects

- nausea, vomiting, diarrhoea, constipation, flatulence, abdominal pain, fundic gland polyps
- headache, drowsiness, somnolence, insomnia
- (prolonged therapy) vitamin B_{12} deficiency
- (rare) interstitial nephritis, hypomagnesaemia, increased risk of osteoporosis and bone fracture, subacute cutaneous lupus erythematosus

Interactions

- may increase serum levels of diazepam, tacrolimus, carbamazepine and phenytoin, increasing the risk of adverse effects including toxicity
- not recommended with St John's wort as serum levels may be decreased
- not recommended with clopidogrel
- caution if given with digoxin

- not recommended with posaconazole or erlotinib
- serum levels increased by fluvoxamine, voriconazole and clarithromycin
- contraindicated as combination therapy for *H. pylori* eradication with clarithromycin in those with liver impairment
- may interfere with chromogranin A (CgA) estimation for neuroendocrine tumours and should be stopped 5–14 days before measurement
- see also General Interactions of proton pump inhibitors (p. 811)

Nursing point/Cautions

- IV therapy is only recommended in severely ill patients and oral therapy resumed as soon as practicable
- if IV therapy is required for > 5 days, daily dose should be reduced
- (Zollinger–Ellison syndrome) if more than 80 mg orally daily, give in divided doses
- reconstitute powder using 100 mL sodium chloride 0.9% or glucose 5%
- see General Nursing points/Cautions for proton pump inhibitors (p. 811)

Patient teaching and advice

- advise patient that tablets and capsules should be swallowed whole with water, not chewed or crushed
- if patient has difficulty swallowing, tablets can be stirred in non-carbonated water or fruit juice until pellets are released and then drunk without chewing or crushing pellets. Glass should be rinsed and drunk to ensure all pellets have been taken
- see General Patient teaching and advice for proton pump inhibitors (p. 812)

PANTOPRAZOLE (Gastenz Heartburn Relief, I-Pantoprazole, Ozpan, Panthron, Panto, Pantofast, Salpraz, Salpraz Heartburn Relief, Somac, Somac Heartburn Relief, Somac Injection, Sozol, Topra, Torzole)

Available forms

Vial: 40 mg; Tablets (enteric-coated): 20 mg, 40 mg; Granules: 40 mg/sachet

Action

- see General Actions of proton pump inhibitors (p. 811)
- half-life about 1 hour

Use

- see General Uses of proton pump inhibitors (p. 811)

Dose

- (duodenal ulcer) 40 mg orally or IV daily for 2–4 weeks **OR**
- (gastric ulcer) 40 mg orally or IV daily for 4–8 weeks **OR**
- (GORD – symptomatic relief) 20 mg orally for 4 weeks **OR**
- (GORD – healed reflux oesophagitis maintenance) 20–40 mg orally daily **OR**
- (GORD – treatment of reflux oesophagitis) 20–40 mg orally daily for 4–8 weeks **OR**
- (lesions refractory to H_2-receptor antagonists) 40 mg orally or IV daily for 4–12 weeks **OR**
- (prophylaxis of gastroduodenal ulceration in patients taking NSAIDs) 20 mg orally daily **OR**
- (Zollinger–Ellison syndrome) 40 mg orally or IV daily **OR**
- (*H. pylori* eradication) 40 mg orally twice daily (with appropriate antibiotics)

Adverse effects

- pruritus, rash
- headache, dizziness, fatigue, asthenia

- sweating
- diarrhoea, constipation, flatulence, dry mouth, metallic taste, upper abdominal pain, nausea, vomiting, fundic gland polyps
- (prolonged therapy) vitamin B_{12} deficiency
- (rare) interstitial nephritis, hypomagnesaemia, increased risk of osteoporosis and bone fracture, subacute cutaneous lupus erythematosus
- (IV) thrombophlebitis

Interactions

- may increase serum levels of tacrolimus increasing risk of toxicity
- may decrease effects of levothyroxine and liothyronine
- caution if given with fluvoxamine
- see General Interactions of proton pump inhibitors (p. 811)

Nursing points/Cautions

- (Zollinger-Ellison) dose should be individually assessed to maintain acid output below 10mmol/L
- IV therapy should be replaced by oral administration as soon as practicable
- reconstitute powder using 10 mL sodium chloride 0.9% and then further dilute to 100 mL using sodium chloride 0.9% or glucose 5% or 10% and then infused over 2–15 minutes
- contraindicated in those with cirrhosis or severe liver disease
- see General Nursing points/Cautions for proton pump inhibitors (p. 811)

Patient teaching and advice

- patient should be advised to swallow tablets whole (not chewed or crushed) with a little water before or during breakfast
- (granules) patient should be instructed to mix granules with 15–30 mL water, apple or orange juice or apple sauce and drink immediately. Glass should be rinsed and contents swallowed to ensure entire dose is taken. If patient has gastric or nasogastric tube, granules should be emptied into catheter-tipped syringe connected to gastric/nasogastric tube, followed by 5 mL of apple or orange (pulp-free) juice or water. Tube should be flushed with water to ensure full dose has been administered
- see General Patient teaching and advice for proton pump inhibitors (p. 812)

RABEPRAZOLE SODIUM (Parbezol, Pariet, Pariet 10, Razit, Zabep)

Available forms

Tablets: 10 mg, 20 mg

Action

- see General Actions of proton pump inhibitors (p. 811)
- acid suppression starts within 1 hour of administration, maximum effect within 2–4 hours

Use

- see General Uses of proton pump inhibitors (p. 811)

Dose

- (active GORD) 20 mg orally daily for 4–8 weeks **OR**
- (prevention of GORD relapse) 10–20 mg orally daily **OR**
- (symptomatic treatment of GORD without oesophagitis) initially 10 mg orally daily, increasing to 20 mg daily for 4 weeks if needed, then decreasing to 10 mg daily when needed **OR**
- (treatment of gastric/duodenal ulcer) 10–20 mg orally daily for 4–12 weeks **OR**
- (*H. pylori* eradication) 20 mg orally twice daily (with appropriate antibiotics)

Adverse effects

- nausea, vomiting, diarrhoea, abdominal pain, flatulence, dry mouth, constipation, metallic taste, fundic gland polyps
- headache, dizziness, fatigue, asthenia, insomnia

- cough, rhinitis, pharyngitis, flu-like symptoms
- myalgia, back pain, pain
- chest pain
- rash
- (prolonged therapy) vitamin B_{12} deficiency
- (rare) interstitial nephritis, hypomagnesaemia, increased risk of osteoporosis and bone fracture, subacute cutaneous lupus erythematosus

Interactions

- see General Interactions of proton pump inhibitors (p. 811)

Nursing points/Cautions/Patient teaching and advice

- instruct patient to swallow tablets whole (not crushed or chewed) with water
- see General Nursing points/Cautions and Patient teaching and advice for proton pump inhibitors (pp. 811–12)

CYTOPROTECTIVE AGENTS

MISOPROSTOL (Cytotec, GyMiso)

Available form

Tablets: 200 microgram

Action

- synthetic prostaglandin E_1 analogue
- acts directly on parietal cells
- reduces gastric acid secretion in basal state, as well as when stimulated by histamine, food and coffee
- decreases nocturnal acid secretion
- mucosal cytoprotective properties
- active metabolite (half-life 1.5 hours)
- peak effect 30 minutes, half-life 20–40 minutes
- inhibits gastric secretion for 3–6 hours

Use

- treatment of acute gastric and duodenal ulcers
- prophylaxis of stress-induced GI bleeding and lesions (postsurgical intensive care (ICU) patients)
- prophylaxis of gastric ulceration (patients taking NSAIDs at high risk of gastric ulceration)
- pregnancy termination (see Pregnancy, childbirth and breastfeeding, p. 1418) (GyMiso)

Dose

- (duodenal/gastric ulcer treatment) 200 microgram orally daily after meals and at night (4 times daily) for 4–8 weeks **OR**
- (prevention of stress-induced bleeding and lesions in ICU) 200 microgram orally 4-hourly after food for up to 14 days **OR**
- (prophylaxis of gastric ulceration in patients taking NSAIDs) 100–200 microgram orally daily with meals and at night (4 times daily), taken with NSAIDs

Adverse effects

- nausea, vomiting, diarrhoea, loose stools, abdominal pain, flatulence, dyspepsia, constipation
- headache
- dizziness
- (uncommon) uterine cramps, menstrual disorders, dysmenorrhoea, menorrhagia, intermenstrual bleeding, spotting, vaginal haemorrhage (including post-menopausal)
- (rare) hypotension

Nursing points/Cautions

- before starting therapy, any unintentional loss of weight, recurrent vomiting, dysphagia, haematemesis, anaemia, melaena or malignancy should be investigated. It is also recommended that those with ulceration be re-endoscoped 8–12 weeks

after starting therapy to determine if the ulcer is healing
- pregnancy must be excluded before commencing therapy
- caution when used in those in intensive care units because agents that suppress acid secretion have been associated with nosocomial lung infections
- caution if used in those with asthma (due to risk of bronchospasm) or those with a predisposition to inflammatory bowel disease, diarrhoea, dehydration, epilepsy or where hypotension may precipitate complications (e.g. cerebrovascular or coronary artery disease)
- not recommended in those under 18 years
- contraindicated in those with known hypersensitivity to prostaglandins

Patient teaching and advice

- patient should be warned against driving or operating machinery if dizziness occurs
- advise patient that diarrhoea is less likely to occur if medication is taken after meals and avoiding magnesium-containing antacids
- women of childbearing potential should receive counselling and written information regarding the importance of adequate contraception before starting therapy
- see General Patient teaching and advice (p. xxvii)

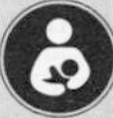

contraindicated during pregnancy. May cause uterine contractions, abortion, fetal death and premature birth, as well as incomplete miscarriage

not recommended during breastfeeding as may cause diarrhoea in newborn

(Cytotec) can be dispersed in water or crushed and given with spoonful of yoghurt or apple puree

Note

- contained in MS-2 Step (for pregnancy termination)

SUCRALFATE (Carafate)

Available form

Tablets: 1 g

Action

- composed of sulfated sucrose and aluminium hydroxide and is non-absorbable
- reacts with acid to produce sticky yellow–white gel which selectively adheres to the ulcer base, protecting it from potential ulcerogenic properties of acid, pepsin and bile
- complexes with pepsin and bile directly and blocks acid diffusion across the ulcer site
- enhances prostaglandin synthesis stimulating mucus and bicarbonate production
- protects mucosa for up to 6 hours

Use

- treatment of acute non-malignant gastric and duodenal ulcers
- prevent recurrence of duodenal ulcers

Dose

- (treatment of gastric/duodenal ulcers) 1 g orally 3 times daily 1 hour before meals and at night for up to 8 weeks **OR**
- (duodenal ulcer maintenance therapy) 1 g orally twice daily 1 hour before meals for up to 12 months

Adverse effects

- nausea, indigestion, constipation, gastric discomfort, diarrhoea, dry mouth
- obstruction of GI tract (bezoars) (especially patients on parenteral feeding with delayed gastric emptying)
- back pain
- urticaria, rash, pruritus
- headache, dizziness, sleepiness, vertigo
- (rare) hypophosphataemia

Interactions

- not recommended with citrate preparation due to risk of increased blood levels of aluminium
- antacids decrease the mucosal binding of sucralfate if taken less than 30 minutes before or after sucralfate
- reduces bioavailability of ciprofloxacin, digoxin, tetracycline, phenytoin, frusemide, proton pump inhibitors, cimetidine and norfloxacin
- may reduce bioavailability of warfarin, therefore INR should be closely monitored, especially when starting or stopping therapy

Nursing points/Cautions

- correct diagnosis is important at start of therapy to exclude any gastric malignancy
- (duodenal ulcers) therapy should continue for up to 8 weeks unless healing has been confirmed
- (gastric ulcers) if no response is seen in 6 weeks, alternative therapy should be considered. However, if ulcer is large, it may require 8 weeks to achieve healing
- caution if used in those with swallowing difficulties including recent and/or prolonged intubation, dysphagia, previous history of aspiration, tracheostomy or other conditions which affect gag/cough reflex or oropharyngeal motility
- caution if used in those with phosphate deficiencies
- not recommended in those under 18 years
- not recommended for patients with severely impaired kidney function (contains 190 mg aluminium) or those with actively bleeding peptic ulcers
- contraindicated as long-term therapy in patients receiving dialysis

Patient teaching and advice

- instruct patient to take antacids at least 30 minutes before or after sucralfate. Other medications should be taken 2–3 hours before sucralfate
- patient should be advised not to drive or operate machinery if dizziness, sleepiness or vertigo occurs
- see General Patient teaching and advice (p. xxvii)

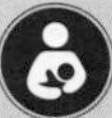

not recommended during pregnancy unless benefits outweigh any potential risks

caution if used during breastfeeding

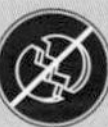

if person is not at risk of aspiration, tablets can be dispersed in water

ANTACIDS

Antacids buffer or neutralise hydrochloric acid in the stomach and in the past, acid neutralisation was seen as the main form of peptic ulcer management. Today, however, antacids are now used mainly as symptom relief for dyspepsia.

The major ingredients of antacids include aluminium hydroxide, calcium carbonate, magnesium salts and sodium bicarbonate, either alone or in combination with the magnesium–aluminium combinations, which are the most commonly used (Bryant et al 2019).

ALUMINIUM HYDROXIDE HYDRATE (ALUMINIUM HYDROXIDE) (Alu-Tab)

Available form

Tablets: 600 mg

Action
- antacid that neutralises gastric hyperacidity
- aluminium hydroxide binds with phosphate ions in the bowel to form insoluble phosphate salts that are excreted by the bowel

Use
- gastric hyperacidity
- relieves symptoms of peptic ulcer (uncomplicated)
- phosphate binding in renal dysfunction

Dose
- 1–2 tablets (600–1200 mg) orally 4 times daily

Adverse effects
- constipation, chalky taste
- (prolonged treatment or high doses) hypophosphataemia (anorexia, malaise, muscle weakness)
- (in chronic renal failure) hyperaluminaemia, dialysis dementia
- intestinal obstruction (in patients who are dehydrated or have reduced bowel motility and develop faecal impaction)

Interactions
- forms a complex with tetracyclines preventing their absorption
- may reduce absorption of many drugs, but particularly digoxin, indometacin, oral iron, naproxen, penicillin, sulfonamides and vitamins

Nursing points/Cautions
- (chronic therapy) serum calcium, aluminium and phosphate levels should be monitored regularly. For those on maintenance haemodialysis, bimonthly monitoring of serum phosphate levels is recommended
- caution if used in those with renal dysfunction due to increased risk of hyperalbuminaemia and associated accumulation in bone, lungs and nerve tissue
- contraindicated in those with hypophosphataemia or chronic renal failure (due to increased risk of aluminium toxicity)

Patient teaching and advice
- advise patient to take aluminium-containing antacids 2 hours before or after other medications
- encourage patient to maintain an adequate fluid intake (within any fluid restriction) during therapy to prevent constipation. If constipation occurs, patient should be advised to seek medical advice
- patient should be advised to seek medical advice if symptoms do not improve within a few days

Note
- contained in De Wit's Antacid Powder, Gastrogel, Mylanta Original, Mylanta Double Strength, Mylanta P

CALCIUM CARBONATE

Action
- antacid that neutralises gastric hyperacidity

Use
- heartburn and indigestion

Adverse effects
- constipation, belching, flatulence, abdominal extension
- (high dose, prolonged use) acid rebound
- (rare) hypercalcaemia, alkalosis, phosphate depletion, renal calculi, milk–acid syndrome

Interactions
- may decrease absorption of tetracyclines, fluoroquinolones, salicylates and iron

Nursing points/Cautions

- contraindicated in those with severe hypercalcaemia or metabolic acidosis, hyperparathyroidism, kidney impairment (because of increased risk of hypercalcaemia)

Patient teaching and advice

- advise patients to take calcium-containing antacids 2–3 hours before or after other medications
- patient should be advised to seek medical advice if symptoms do not improve within a few days

Note

- contained in Gaviscon preparations, Rennie Spearmint Flavour

MAGNESIUM HYDROXIDE, MAGNESIUM TRISILICATE (Magnesium Trisilicate)

Available form

Liquid suspension

Action

- neutralises gastric hyperacidity

Use

- hyperacidity, heartburn

Dose

- 10–20 mL 3 times daily after meals and before bedtime

Adverse effects

- diarrhoea, chalky taste, belching
- (rare) elevated magnesium levels

Interactions

- may form a complex if given with tetracyclines and therefore should be separated by at least 1–2 hours if given together

Nursing points/Cautions

- magnesium trisilicate-containing antacids contain significant amounts of sodium which should be considered if sodium-restricted diet is in place
- caution if used in those with existing diarrhoea as it may be aggravated
- contraindicated in those with kidney impairment due to increased risk of increased magnesium levels

Patient teaching and advice

- advise patients to take magnesium-containing antacids 2–3 hours before or after other medications
- patient should be advised to seek medical advice if symptoms do not improve within a few days

Note

- contained in Gastrogel Antacid Suspension, Magnesium Trisilicate and Belladonna, Mylanta Original and Double Strength Suspension and tablets, Mylanta P Suspension

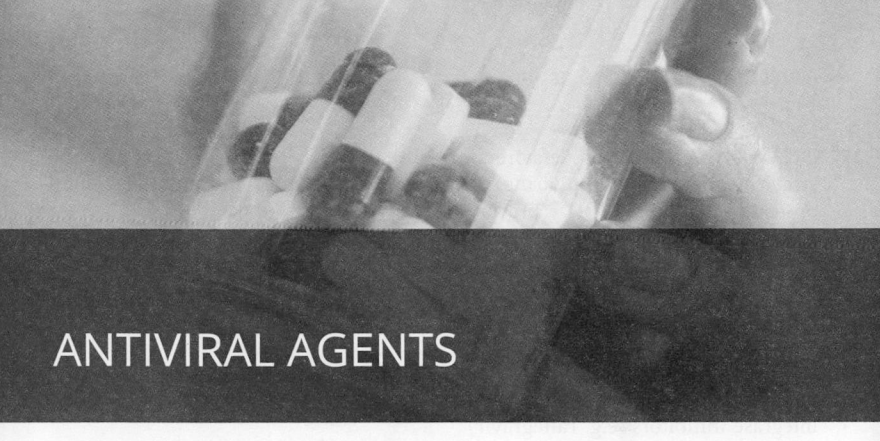

ANTIVIRAL AGENTS

Viruses are true parasites that are unable to replicate independently, requiring a host's metabolic machinery to replicate. Classification of viruses is according to nucleic acid composition (DNA or RNA), double- or single-stranded, and whether a lipoprotein envelope is present or not. Retroviruses are a special class of RNA viruses that have a complex replication mechanism, making them very difficult to treat using standard antiviral agents. Unfortunately, with many viral infections, replication has reached its peak before symptoms are present, making the infection difficult to treat (Bryant et al 2019).

Antiviral agents are a broad group of drugs that inhibit viral replication by selectively inhibiting the reproductive pathway of the virus at different stages (e.g. adsorption of the virion into the cell, penetration, uncoating, assembly or release) or they may inhibit transcription or translation steps that are shared with the host cell (Neal 2015). Antiviral drugs can be divided into *antiretrovirals* (those drugs used to retro) or *non-retroviral* (drugs used to treat non-HIV viral infections) (Bryant et al 2019).

Antiviral (*non-retroviral*) *agents* are subdivided into a number of classes:

- DNA polymerase inhibitors (e.g. aciclovir, cidofovir, famciclovir, foscarnet, ganciclovir, valaciclovir, valganciclovir)
- neuraminidase inhibitors (e.g. oseltamivir, zanamivir)
- NS3/4A protease inhibitors (e.g. grazoprevir, paritprevir, simeprevir)
- NS5A inhibitors (e.g. daclatasvir, elbasvir, ledipasvir, obmitasvir, velpatasvir)
- NS5B RNA-dependent RNA protease inhibitors (e.g. dasabuvir, sofosbuvir)
- other antiviral agents (e.g. adefovir, amantadine, entecavir, ribavirin, telbivudine) (Bryant et al 2019).

Antiretroviral agents are further subdivided depending on their site of action:

- nucleoside reverse transcriptase inhibitors (NRTIs) (prevent viral RNA being converted into viral DNA) (e.g. abacavir, emtricitabine, lamivudine, stavudine, tenofovir, zidovudine)
- non-nucleoside reverse transcriptase inhibitors (NNRTIs) (block RNA-dependent and DNA-dependent

DNA polymerases) (e.g. efavirenz, etravirine, nevirapine, rilpivirine)
- protease inhibitors (PI) (prevent HIV protease from cleaving polypeptide and block maturation of HIV virus) (e.g. atazanavir, darunavir, fosamprenavir, indinavir, lopinavir, ritonavir, saquinavir, tipranavir)
- entry inhibitors (e.g. enfuvirtide, maraviroc)
- integrase inhibitors (e.g. raltegravir) (Bryant et al 2019).

Note
- AIDS: acquired immune deficiency syndrome
- CMV: cytomegalovirus
- HIV: human immunodeficiency virus

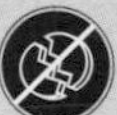

caution if crushing or dispersing antiviral medications as bioavailability may be altered

ANTIVIRAL (NON-RETROVIRAL) AGENTS

DNA POLYMERASE INHIBITORS

ACICLOVIR (Aciclovir Intravenous Infusion, Blistex Antiviral Cold Sore Cream, Nyal Antiviral Cold Sore Cream, Ozvir, Zovirax Cold Sore Cream, Zovirax Ophthalmic Ointment, Zovirax Tablets)

Available forms
Ampoules: 250 mg/10 mL, 500 mg/20 mL; Vial: 250 mg, 500 mg; Tablets: 200 mg, 400 mg, 800 mg; Eye ointment: 30 mg/g; Cream: 50 mg/g

Action
- selectively taken up by herpes virus infected cell where it is converted to an active form that inhibits viral replication by interfering with DNA synthesis
- oral form is poorly absorbed, but still reaches therapeutic levels
- (IV) half-life is about 2.5 hours (increasing to 20 hours in those with kidney impairment)
- resistance to therapy may develop

Use
- prophylaxis and treatment of herpes simplex infections (including types 1 and 2, herpes zoster (shingles) (within 72 hours of rash presentation), herpes simplex keratitis, herpes simplex encephalitis)
- advanced HIV disease

Dose

Genital herpes
- (initial treatment) 200 mg orally 4-hourly (while awake) (total 1 g daily) for 10 days **OR**
- (chronic suppressive therapy for recurrent genital herpes) 200 mg orally 3 times daily for up to 6 months **OR**
- (intermittent therapy for recurrent genital herpes) 200 mg orally 4-hourly (while awake) (total 1 g daily) for 5 days, starting at earliest signs of recurrence

Herpes zoster (shingles)
- 800 mg orally 4-hourly (while awake), starting within 72 hours of rash onset and continuing for 7 days **OR**
- (varicella zoster in immunocompromised patient) 10 mg/kg 8-hourly by slow IV infusion **OR**

- (severe herpes zoster (shingles) infection) 5 mg/kg 8-hourly by slow IV infusion

Herpes simplex infections

- (immunocompetent or immunocompromised) 5 mg/kg 8-hourly by slow IV infusion for 5–7 days **OR**
- apply cream in sufficient amount to cover lesion 5 times daily (approximately 4-hour intervals) to mouth lesion for 5–7 days (approximately 4-hour intervals, omitting night-time application), starting at first signs or symptoms (burning, tingling, itching) **OR**
- (eye infections) 1 cm ointment placed in the lower conjunctival sac 5 times daily (approximately 4-hour intervals) and for 3 days after healing is complete or 14 days (whichever is earlier)

Herpes simplex encephalitis (immunocompetent or immunocompromised)

- 10 mg/kg 8-hourly by slow IV infusion for 10 days

Advanced symptomatic HIV disease

- 800 mg orally 6-hourly (with other antiretrovirals)

Adverse effects

- nausea, vomiting, diarrhoea, abdominal pain, taste alteration, anorexia
- headache, dizziness, lethargy, fatigue, confusion, altered level of consciousness, tremors, somnolence, psychosis, hallucinations, agitation, seizures
- vertigo
- fever
- reversible abnormal liver enzymes and bilirubin
- anaemia, leucopenia, thrombocytopenia
- rash, urticaria, pruritus, photosensitivity, hair loss
- (IV) reversible increased serum urea and creatinine
- (rare) haematuria, jaundice, hepatitis, coma, encephalopathy, hypotension, dyspnoea, anaphylaxis
- (IV bolus) renal damage
- (eye ointment) mild stinging, blepharitis and rarely, sensitivity reactions
- (cold sore cream) (uncommon) mild pain, burning, stinging, skin flaking
- (IV site) inflammation, pain, phlebitis

Interactions

- clearance may be decreased when given with probenecid and cimetidine, increasing risk of crystal precipitation in renal tubules
- serum levels may be increased when given with diuretics (patients aged over 60 years) and mycophenolate mofetil
- caution if used with mycophenolate mofetil, ciclosporin or tacrolimus
- not recommended with nephrotoxic agents
- caution if used with interferon or methotrexate (intrathecally) due to increased risk of encephalopathy
- may cause increase in theophylline serum levels increasing risk of adverse effects

Nursing points/Cautions

- (IV) ensure adequate hydration during therapy (especially in elderly patients) to prevent precipitation of crystals in renal tubules
- (IV) urine output should be closely monitored, especially in the first hours after therapy
- IV bolus doses should not be given
- solution should be added to at least 50–100 mL of IV solution and administered over at least 1 hour at a rate of 25 mg/mL using an infusion pump (to avoid renal damage)
- IV site should be closely monitored to avoid extravasation, which may cause inflammation and/or tissue necrosis
- eye(s) or skin should be thoroughly rinsed with water if contact with IV solutions occurs

- doses need to be adjusted for those with renal impairment
- IV solution should not be refrigerated because it causes precipitation and solution should be discarded if this occurs as crystals will not redissolve at room temperature
- IV solution should not be administered if there are any crystals or it is turbid in appearance
- (herpes labialis) oral aciclovir is recommended (rather than cream) if patient is immunocompromised
- caution if used in those with renal disease or impairment, dehydration, neurological abnormalities, significant hypoxia, serious liver or electrolyte abnormalities or in those who have shown neurological changes when using other cytotoxic agents
- contraindicated in those with hypersensitivity to valaciclovir or aciclovir

Patient teaching and advice

- advise patient that tablets may be swallowed whole or dispersed in 50 mL water
- those with genital herpes should be advised to avoid sexual intercourse during acute episodes and decrease risk of transmission by using a condom at other times because viral shedding occurs even when there are no symptoms
- patient with herpes labialis (cold sores) should be instructed to:
  - apply cream at the first signs of cold sore (e.g. area burning, tingling, itching)
  - use gloves when applying cream to prevent spread to other people or other parts of the body
  - avoid kissing to prevent spread to others
  - not use cream on mucous membranes (mouth, eyes, vagina)
  - avoid cream making contact with eyes
- patient should be instructed in correct use of ophthalmic ointment, including:
  - removal of contact lenses during therapy
  - washing hands before and after using ointment
  - applying 1 cm of ointment inside eye lid of affected eye(s) (without letting the tip of the tube touch the eyelid if possible)
  - closing eye for 30 seconds
  - noting that vision may be blurred for 5–10 minutes after ointment has been applied and transient stinging may occur
  - allowing vision to clear before driving or operating machinery

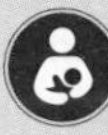

only used during pregnancy and breastfeeding if benefits outweigh risks. If used perinatally for suppression therapy, viral shedding may still occur and risk to fetus or neonate still exists

tablets can be dispersed in 50 mL of water

Note

- contained in Zovirax Duo Cold Sore Cream with hydrocortisone

CIDOFOVIR (Empovir)

Available form

Vial: 375 mg/5 mL

Action

- acyclic nucleoside analogue with activity against CMV
- selectively inhibits viral DNA polymerase preventing DNA synthesis and viral replication
- not metabolised and about 70–85% is excreted unchanged in the urine
- probenecid blocks renal clearance and protects kidneys from nephrotoxicity

Use

- CMV retinitis in patients with AIDS (with probenecid)

Dose

- initially 5 mg/kg by IV infusion over 1 hour weekly for 2 weeks (induction), then every 2 weeks (with probenecid) (maintenance)

Adverse effects

- nausea, vomiting, diarrhoea
- headache, asthenia
- fever, chills
- dyspnoea
- proteinuria, increased serum creatinine, renal failure
- neutropenia
- alopecia, rash
- decreased intraocular pressure, uveitis, iritis, decreased visual acuity
- (rare) acquired Fanconi syndrome (see Glossary)

Interactions

- contraindicated with or within 7 days of other nephrotoxic agents such as aminoglycosides (IV), amphotericin B (amphotericin), foscarnet, pentamidine (IV), NSAIDs and vancomycin
- zidovudine should be temporarily discontinued or dose decreased on days of cidofovir administration, because probenecid decreases zidovudine clearance
- probenecid interferes with metabolism and excretion of a large number of drugs, leading to increased serum levels and risk of adverse effects or toxicity. Drugs affected include paracetamol, aspirin, aciclovir, ACE inhibitors, barbiturates, benzodiazepines, famotidine, furosemide (frusemide), methotrexate, NSAIDs and theophylline

Nursing points/Cautions

- serum creatinine, urine protein and WBC count (with neutrophil differential) should be measured 24–48 hours before each administration
- if urine shows ≥ 2+ protein, IV hydration should be administered (see below) and urine retested. If urine continues to show ≥ 2+ protein, therapy should not be continued
- intravenous pre-hydration and oral probenecid are given with each administration; hydration consists of 1 L sodium chloride 0.9% over 1 hour before the cidofovir infusion, and, if tolerated, a second litre over 1–3 hours either with or immediately after cidofovir infusion
- oral probenecid 2 g is given 3 hours before cidofovir infusion, 1 g 2 hours before, then 1 g 8 hours after completion of IV infusion (total 4 g probenecid)
- should be infused into a large vein to allow rapid dilution
- must be diluted in 100 mL of sodium chloride 0.9% and administered using an infusion pump over 1 hour
- regular ophthalmic examinations (especially intraocular pressure monitoring) are recommended during therapy
- contains 57 mg sodium/vial which may need to be considered if patient is on sodium-restricted diet
- contraindicated as direct intraocular injection
- contraindicated in those with renal impairment, creatinine clearance < 55 mL/minute, proteinuria (> 100 mg/dL, ≥ 2+), clinically significant hypersensitivity to probenecid or other sulfur-containing products

Patient teaching and advice

- ensure patient understands the need for probenecid and hydration before and after therapy to reduce risk of kidney damage
- patient should be advised to immediately report any changes to vision
- advise patient to eat before probenecid to decrease nausea and vomiting

- counsel female patient to use adequate contraception during and for 4 weeks after therapy has stopped to prevent pregnancy occurring
- male patient should be counselled to use barrier method contraception (condom) during and for 12 weeks after stopping therapy

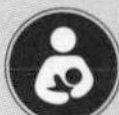

contraindicated during pregnancy

not recommended during breastfeeding

FAMCICLOVIR (Elovax One Dose, Ezovir, Ezovir Cold Sore Relief, Famlo, Famvir, Famvir for Cold Sores, Favic)

Available forms

Tablets: 125 mg, 250 mg, 500 mg

Action

- nucleoside analogue which is an orally active prodrug of penciclovir, which targets virus-infected cells inhibiting viral DNA synthesis and therefore viral replication
- orally well absorbed and converted to active metabolite penciclovir in intestinal wall
- half-life 2–3 hours

Use

- treatment of acute herpes zoster (within 72 hours of rash onset)
- treatment and suppression of herpes simplex
- treatment and suppression of recurrent episodes of genital herpes
- treatment of recurrent episodes of herpes labialis (cold sores)

Dose

Immunocompetent patient

- (herpes zoster) 250 mg orally 3 times daily for 7 days, starting within 48–72 hours of rash onset **OR**
- (recurrent genital herpes) 125 mg orally twice daily for 5 days, starting during prodromal phase or first onset of lesions **OR**
- (recurrent genital herpes) 500 mg orally stat, then 250 mg orally 12-hourly for 3 doses **OR**
- (recurrent genital herpes) 1 g orally twice daily for 1 day **OR**
- (suppression of recurrent genital herpes) 250 mg orally twice daily **OR**
- (recurrent herpes labialis (cold sores)) 1.5 g orally stat at first signs of cold sore (tingling, itching, burning) **OR**
- (recurrent herpes labialis (cold sores)) 750 mg orally twice daily at first signs of cold sore (tingling, itching, burning) for 1 day

Immunocompromised patient

- (herpes zoster) 500 mg orally 3 times daily for 10 days, starting within 48–72 hours of rash onset **OR**
- (recurrent genital herpes) 500 mg orally twice daily for 7 days, starting during prodromal phase or first onset of lesions **OR**
- (suppression of recurrent genital herpes with HIV infection) 500 mg orally twice daily

Adverse effects

- nausea, vomiting, abdominal pain, dry mouth, diarrhoea
- headache, dizziness, anxiety, somnolence, insomnia, fatigue
- nasopharyngitis
- dysmenorrhoea
- back pain
- rash, pruritus
- (rare) confusion in the elderly

Interactions

- serum level of active metabolite may be increased by probenecid
- caution if given with other agents which are nephrotoxic
- efficacy may be decreased if given with raloxifene

Nursing points/Cautions

- (suppression of recurrent genital herpes) therapy should be reviewed after 12 months
- 125 mg and 250 mg tablets contain lactose and are therefore not recommended in those with galactose intolerance, glucose–galactose malabsorption or Lapp lactase deficiency
- caution if used in those with renal impairment
- not recommended for ophthalmic zoster, chicken pox or zoster encephalomyelitis patients

Patient teaching and advice

- advise patient against driving or operating machinery if dizziness occurs or is ongoing
- patients with genital herpes should be advised to avoid sexual intercourse during acute episodes and decrease risk of transmission by using a condom at other times because viral shedding occurs even when patient is asymptomatic
- (recurrent genital herpes) advise patient to start therapy during prodromal period or as soon as possible after onset of lesions
- (recurrent herpes labialis (cold sores)) advise patient to start therapy at first sign/symptom including tingling, burning or itching at site

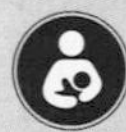

not recommended during pregnancy unless benefits outweigh risks

not recommended during breastfeeding

tablet can be crushed and mixed with water or spoonful of yoghurt or apple puree

FOSCARNET SODIUM (Foscavir)

Available form

Bottle: 6g/250 mL

Action

- virustatic broad-spectrum antiviral agent that inhibits all human herpes viruses, varicella zoster virus, cytomegalovirus (CMV), Epstein Barr virus and some retroviruses, including HIV
- viral replication restarts when drug is discontinued
- chelates bivalent ions such as calcium
- half-life 3.3–6.8 hours

Use

- CMV retinitis in patients with AIDS
- aciclovir-resistant herpes simplex virus infection in patients with HIV

Dose

- (CMV retinitis induction and maintenance therapy) 60 mg/kg by slow IV infusion (over 1 hour) 8-hourly for 2–3 weeks (induction), then 90–120 mg/kg IV infusion over 2 hours daily **OR**
- (herpes simplex virus infections) 40 mg/kg by slow IV infusion (over 1 hour) 8-hourly for 2–3 weeks (or until lesions have healed)

Adverse effects

- anorexia, nausea, vomiting, diarrhoea, dyspepsia, abdominal pain, constipation, GI bleeding, pancreatitis
- paraesthesia, tremor, neuropathy, ataxia, abnormal coordination, hypoaesthesia, involuntary muscle contraction
- aggression, anxiety, confusion, depression, nervousness, agitation
- headache, dizziness, asthenia, fatigue, malaise
- genital ulceration and irritation
- impaired renal function, polyuria, dysuria, decreased creatinine clearance, increased serum creatinine, kidney pain
- abnormal liver function
- hypocalcaemia, hypomagnesaemia, hypokalaemia, hypophosphataemia, hyperphosphataemia, hyponatraemia, hypercalcaemia
- dehydration

- anaemia, leucopenia, thrombocytopenia, granulocytopenia, neutropenia
- chills, fever
- sepsis
- rash, pruritus
- palpitations, tachycardia, hypertension or hypotension, chest pain, ECG abnormalities (including QT interval prolongation)
- seizures (related to impaired electrolyte imbalance)
- (IV site) thrombophlebitis

Interactions

- contraindicated with pentamidine (IV) because it may result in further lowering of calcium levels and both may also cause nephrotoxicity
- caution if given with other drugs known to lower calcium levels
- caution if given with other drugs known to cause QT interval prolongation or cause electrolyte disturbances
- additive renal toxicity may occur when given with other nephrotoxic drugs (e.g. aminoglycosides, amphotericin B (amphotericin), aciclovir, methotrexate, tacrolimus and ciclosporin)
- renal excretion is impaired when given with drugs that inhibit renal tubular secretion
- not recommended with loop diuretics
- increased risk of renal impairment if given with ritonavir and/or saquinavir

Nursing points/Cautions

- hydration will reduce renal toxicity, therefore 0.5–1 L is recommended before first infusion to establish diuresis, then 0.5–1 L added to each infusion
- serum electrolytes (especially calcium, magnesium and creatinine) should be monitored before and during therapy
- serum creatinine should be measured every second day during induction and then weekly during maintenance
- patient should be monitored for any seizure activity
- local irritation and burning sensation may occur if foscarnet contacts eyes or skin, and area should be immediately rinsed with water
- must be given IV only
- if given via peripheral veins, foscarnet should be diluted with glucose 5% or sodium chloride 0.9% to a concentration of 12 mg/mL
- if given via a central vein, solution of 24 mg/mL does not need further dilution
- administration time should not be less than 1 hour
- if patient experiences severe nausea or paraesthesia, infusion rate should be reduced
- an initial induction period of 2–3 weeks is recommended (dependent on clinical response), followed by maintenance therapy as appropriate. Maintenance dose is determined by creatinine clearance
- if expected response is not achieved, resistance should be considered
- incompatible with a range of drugs (especially those containing calcium), therefore it is recommended that foscarnet be infused alone
- each mL contains 5.5 mg sodium which may need to be taken into account in those on sodium-reduced diet
- caution in patients with renal impairment or dehydration
- caution if used in those with pre-existing anaemia, hypomagnesaemia, hypocalcaemia or history of seizures
- caution if used in those with pre-existing or history of QT prolongation, electrolyte imbalance (especially hypokalaemia, hyperkalaemia or hypomagnesaemia), bradycardia or cardiac disease
- contraindicated as long-term treatment in those with reasonable prognosis (e.g. bone marrow transplantation)

Patient teaching and advice

- warn patient not drive or operate machinery if any confusion, dizziness, tremor or abnormal coordination occurs
- patient should be advised to maintain good personal hygiene (washing genital area well after each micturition) to prevent genital irritation and/or ulceration because of high drug level excreted in the urine
- advise patient to seek medical advice immediately if any of the following occur:
  - fast, slow or pounding heart rate
  - tingling or numbness of feet or toes
  - fitting (seizures)
  - feeling abnormally tired, pale, lacking in energy, bruising or bleeding easily
- patients (male and female) should be counselled regarding the importance of avoiding pregnancy during therapy. Male patient should be advised to use condoms during therapy and for at least 6 months after stopping

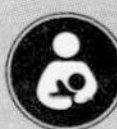

not recommended during pregnancy or breastfeeding

GANCICLOVIR (Cymevene)

Available form

Vial: 500 mg

Action

- nucleoside analogue that inhibits replication of herpes viruses (e.g. CMV, herpes simplex 1 and 2, Epstein-Barr)
- structurally similar to aciclovir
- plasma half-life is 2.5–3.6 hours
- half-life prolonged in those with kidney impairment

Use

- palliative and maintenance treatment of CMV retinitis in AIDS or severely immunosuppressed individuals
- treatment of confirmed CMV pneumonitis in bone marrow transplant patients
- prevention of CMV disease in liver, heart and bone marrow transplant patients

Dose

- (CMV retinitis with normal renal function) initially 5 mg/kg 12-hourly by IV infusion over 1 hour for 14–21 days (induction), followed by either 5 mg/kg daily or 6 mg/kg 5 days a week (maintenance) **OR**
- (prevention of CMV infection in liver transplant patients with normal renal function) initially 5 mg/kg 12-hourly by IV infusion over 1 hour for 7–14 days (induction), followed by either 5 mg/kg for 7 days a week or 6 mg/kg for 5 days a week (for up to 100 days post-transplant) **OR**
- (prevention of CMV in bone marrow transplant patients with normal renal function) initially 5 mg/kg 12-hourly by IV infusion over 1 hour for 7 days (induction), followed by 5 mg/kg daily for up to 100–120 days after transplant (maintenance) **OR**
- (prevention of CMV infection in heart transplant patients with normal renal function) 5 mg/kg 12-hourly IV infused over 1 hour for 14 days (induction), followed by 6 mg/kg daily 5 days per week for up to 100 days after transplant (maintenance) **OR**
- (other transplantation) 5 mg/kg 12-hourly IV infused over 1 hour for 7–14 days (induction), followed by 5 mg/kg for 7 days a week or 6 mg/kg for 5 days a week

Adverse effects

- neutropenia, thrombocytopenia, anaemia, leucopenia, pancytopenia, aplastic anaemia, bone marrow depression

- anorexia, diarrhoea, abdominal pain or distension, dyspepsia, dysphagia, oesophageal candidiasis
- anxiety, headache, confusion
- pruritus
- arthralgia, myalgia
- fever, rigors
- abnormal liver function
- kidney impairment, kidney failure
- infection, sepsis
- lymphadenopathy
- hypertension, hypotension, tachycardia, chest pain
- pleural effusion, cough, dyspnoea, rhinitis
- peripheral neuropathy, hypoaesthesia
- (IV site) phlebitis, pain, inflammation, infection

Interactions

- probenecid may increase plasma half-life, increasing the risk of toxicity
- additive myelosuppression and/or renal impairment may occur when given with some antineoplastic agents (e.g. vinca alkaloids), hydroxycarbamide (hydroxyurea), dapsone, pentamidine, amphotericin B (amphotericin), trimethoprim/sulfonamides, ciclosporin, tacrolimus, mycophenolate mofetil or other nucleoside analogues (e.g. zidovudine)
- zidovudine and ganciclovir should not be given together during ganciclovir induction because severe anaemia and neutropenia may ensue
- not recommended with imipenem–cilastatin due to risk of seizures

Nursing points/Cautions

- CMV retinitis diagnosis should be confirmed by indirect ophthalmoscopy before starting therapy and supported by CMV culture in urine, blood, throat or other sites
- patient should be adequately hydrated before starting IV therapy
- therapy should not be started if neutrophil count is less than 0.5×10^9/L, platelet count is less than 2.5×10^{10}/L or haemoglobin < 80 g/L
- FBC and platelet count should be monitored every second day during first 14 days of therapy, then weekly during maintenance therapy
- serum creatinine or creatinine clearance should be closely monitored if patient has renal impairment
- if disease progresses, can be retreated using induction regime
- avoid contact with skin or mucous membranes, inhalation or ingestion when handling powder or solution. Wash skin with soap and water or eyes with plain water for at least 15 minutes if contact does occur
- safety glasses and latex gloves should be worn when handling. Preparation, handling and disposal should be according to cytotoxic protocol
- administer alone
- patient should be monitored for extraocular CMV when treated for CMV retinitis
- regular ophthalmological examination is recommended for both eyes 4–6-weekly during therapy
- reconstitute using water for injections, and then further dilute with glucose 5%, Ringer's lactated solution or sodium chloride 0.9% to 100 mL for infusion (level not greater than 10 mg/mL)
- should be infused in 100 mL of solution over at least 1 hour (not greater than 10 mg/minute)
- not administered rapidly or by bolus as this increases risk of toxicity
- IM or SC administration will result in severe tissue irritation because of its high pH
- IV site should be closely monitored to avoid phlebitis

- caution if used in those with renal impairment as dose adjustment will be required (based on creatinine clearance and serum creatinine levels)
- caution if given with valaciclovir or aciclovir because cross-hypersensitivity may exist
- caution if used in those with history of cytopenia, previous drug-induced cytopenia or exposure to marrow toxic drugs, chemicals or irradiation
- not recommended for congenital or neonatal CMV disease or for treatment of CMV in immunocompetent patients
- not recommended for CMV prophylaxis in donor negative/receptor negative transplant patients
- not recommended in early post-transplant phase of bone marrow transplantation (about 3 weeks post-transplant) until haemopoietic recovery is evident
- contraindicated in those with hypersensitivity to aciclovir, valaciclovir or valganciclovir or with a neutrophil count less than 0.5×10^9/L, platelet count less than 2.5×10^{10}/L or haemoglobin less than 80 g/L

Patient teaching and advice

- patient should be advised that ganciclovir is not a cure and ophthalmologic examinations are recommended every 4–6 weeks during therapy
- warn patient against driving or operating machinery if any confusion, anxiety or sensory changes occur
- advise patient to seek medical advice if any of the following occur:
  - numbness or tingling or decreased sensation in hands or feet
  - worsening eyesight
  - signs of infection, including fever, chills, sore throat, mouth ulcers, swollen glands
  - unusual tiredness or lack of energy, shortness of breath (especially on exertion), pallor
  - unusual bruising or bleeding, purple spots on skin
- patients (male and female) should be counselled regarding the importance of avoiding pregnancy during therapy. Male patient should be advised to use condoms during therapy and for at least 12 weeks after stopping
- male and female patients should be warned that therapy may inhibit fertility during therapy and this may be permanent or temporary

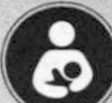

contraindicated during pregnancy because of the embryotoxic and teratogenic potential, therefore use adequate contraception during therapy to avoid pregnancy

contraindicated during breastfeeding

LETERMOVIR (Prevymis)

Available form
Tablets: 240 mg

Action
- inhibits CMV DNA-terminase complex required for viral replication

Use
- prophylaxis of CMV infection or disease in adult CMV-seropositive recipients of allogeneic haemotopoietic stem cell transplant

Dose
- 480 mg orally daily, up to 100 days post-transplant (starting no later than 28 days post-transplant) **OR**
- (with ciclosporin) 240 mg orally daily

Adverse effects
- tachycardia, atrial fibrillation
- nausea, vomiting, diarrhoea, abdominal pain
- peripheral oedema
- headache, fatigue
- cough

Interactions

- combination of letermovir and ciclosporin are contraindicated with simvastatin due to increased risk of myopathy and rhabdomyolysis
- when given with ciclosporin, serum levels of both ciclosporin and letermovir may increase. Ciclosporin levels should be closely monitored during therapy
- may increase serum levels of amiodarone, HMG-CoA reductase inhibitors (statins), sirolimus, tacrolimus, repaglinide, rosiglitazone, alfentanil, fentanyl, midazolam and quinidine, increasing risk of adverse effects
- may decrease serum levels of voriconazole, omeprazole, pantoprazole, phenytoin, warfarin

Nursing points/cautions

- therapy can be started on day of transplant or before or after engraftment but no later than 28 days post-transplant
- if ciclosporin is started after letermovir, next dose of letermovir should be reduced to 240 mg; if ciclosporin is discontinued, letermovir dose should be increased to 480 mg or if ciclosporin is stopped temporarily due to high serum levels, dose of letermovir does not require changing
- not recommended in those with severe liver impairment or in those with moderate liver impairment with concurrent moderate-to-severe renal impairment

Patient teaching and advice

- advise patient that tablets should be swallowed whole, not divided, crushed or broken
- patient should be advised to seek medical advice if any rapid or fluttering heart rate or swelling of feet and ankles occurs

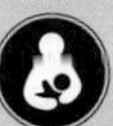

caution if used during pregnancy or breastfeeding

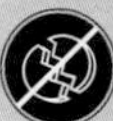

tablet should not be crushed or broken

VALACICLOVIR (Shilova, Valacor, Vaclovir, Valtrex, Zelitrex)

Available form

Tablets: 500 mg

Action

- prodrug that is converted to aciclovir by first pass intestinal and liver metabolism
- inhibits herpes virus DNA synthesis
- half-life 2.5–3.3 hours
- some resistance has developed

Use

- treatment of herpes zoster (shingles) within 72 hours of onset of rash
- treatment and prevention of genital herpes
- treatment of recurrent herpes labialis (cold sores)
- treatment of ophthalmic zoster
- prevention of CMV following solid organ transplantation (in those at risk of CMV infection)

Dose

- (herpes zoster) 1 g orally 3 times daily for 7 days **OR**
- (herpes labialis (cold sores)) 2 g orally 12 hours apart (total 2 doses) (at first signs of cold sores, including tingling, burning or itching) **OR**
- (genital herpes) 500 mg orally twice daily for 5–10 days (first presentation) or 5 days (recurrence) **OR**
- (prevention of genital herpes in immunosuppressed patients) 500 mg orally twice daily **OR**
- (prevention of genital herpes – fewer than 10 episodes/year) 500 mg orally once daily or in divided doses **OR**

- (prevention of genital herpes – more than 10 episodes/year) 1 g orally once daily **OR**
- (reduction of transmission of genital herpes) 500 mg orally daily **OR**
- (prevention of CMV infection and disease) 2 g orally 4 times daily for 90 days, starting as soon as possible after transplantation

Adverse effects

- (transplant patients) hallucinations, confusion
- (prolonged or high dose) thrombotic thrombocytopenic purpura, haemolytic uraemic syndrome
- see Adverse effects of aciclovir (p. 825)

Interactions

- see Interactions of aciclovir (p. 825)

Nursing points/Cautions

- see General Nursing points/Cautions for acyclovir (p. 825)

Patient teaching and advice

- (herpes labialis (cold sore)) advise patient to start therapy at first signs (e.g. tingling, burning, itching) and therapy should not exceed 2 doses taken 12 hours apart
- patient/carer/family member should be advised to immediately seek medical advice if patient displays any confusion or experiences hallucinations
- see Patient teaching and advice for aciclovir (p. 826)

tablet can be crushed and mixed with spoonful of jam, yoghurt or apple puree (has very unpleasant taste)

VALGANCICLOVIR (Valcyte)

Available forms

Tablets: 450 mg; Oral solution: 50 mg/mL

Action

- prodrug that is converted by intestinal and liver enzymes to ganciclovir
- nucleoside analogue

Use

- treatment of CMV retinitis in those with AIDS
- prevention of CMV infection and disease after solid organ transplantation (in those at risk of CMV infection)

Dose

- (treatment of CMV retinitis in AIDS) 900 mg orally twice daily for 21 days with food (induction), followed by 900 mg orally daily (maintenance) **OR**
- (CMV prevention in solid organ transplantation) 900 mg orally daily with food, starting within 10 days of transplant and continuing up to 200 days after kidney transplantation or 100 days after other solid organ transplantation

Adverse effects

- see Adverse effects of ganciclovir (p. 831)

Interactions

- see Interactions for ganciclovir (p. 832)

Nursing points/Cautions

- see also Nursing points/Cautions for ganciclovir (p. 832)

Patient teaching and advice

- advise patient to take tablets with food
- (oral solution) instruct patient to use dispenser provided (25 mg graduations) to measure solution, which should be washed with hot soapy water after use, dried and not used to measure other medications
- patients (male and female) should be counselled regarding the importance of avoiding pregnancy during therapy. Male patients should be advised to use condoms during therapy and for at least 12 weeks after stopping
- male and female patients should be warned that fertility may be inhibited during therapy, and this may be permanent or temporary

- see Patient teaching and advice for ganciclovir (p. 833)

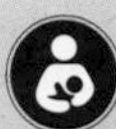

contraindicated during pregnancy because of the embryotoxic and teratogenic potential, therefore use adequate contraception during therapy to avoid pregnancy

contraindicated during breastfeeding

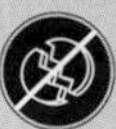

oral solution is available. Tablet should not be crushed, broken or dispersed

NEURAMINIDASE INHIBITORS

OSELTAMIVIR PHOSPHATE (Tamiflu, Taminex)

Available forms
Capsules: 30 mg, 45 mg, 75 mg; Oral suspension: 6 mg/mL

Action
- neuraminidase inhibitor (prodrug) that is converted to active form (oseltamivir carboxylate) in the gastrointestinal tract and liver after absorption
- neuraminidase enzyme is required for replication of both influenza A and B strains as it plays a role in viral release from the cells enabling spread to other cells
- active metabolite half-life 6–10 hours (prolonged in those with kidney impairment)

Use
- treatment of influenza A and B (up to 48 hours after onset of first symptoms)
- influenza prophylaxis (although vaccination is the preferred prophylaxis)

Dose
- (treatment) 75 mg orally twice daily for 5 days, starting within 48 hours of symptom onset **OR**
- (prophylaxis) 75 mg orally daily for 10 days, starting within 48 hours of exposure

Adverse effects
- nausea, vomiting
- headache
- back pain

Nursing points/Cautions
- significantly reduces duration and severity of influenza, as well as reducing risks of secondary infections
- when used prophylactically, protection lasts as long as therapy continues
- only effective against influenza A or B virus
- (oral suspension) not recommended in those with hereditary fructose intolerance because it contains sorbitol
- caution if used in those with kidney impairment or with underlying respiratory or cardiac conditions and complicated influenza (e.g. pneumonia)
- not recommended in those with end-stage kidney disease (creatinine clearance < 10 mL/minute) not undergoing dialysis

Patient teaching and advice
- advise patient to avoid contact with skin or eyes. Rinse area with water if contact occurs
- patient should be advised to take with food to reduce gastrointestinal adverse effects
- (oral solution) instruct patient to shake well before use

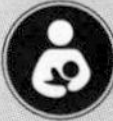

should not be used during pregnancy or breastfeeding unless benefits outweigh risks

oral suspension available. Capsule can be opened and contents mixed with spoonful of yoghurt, apple puree or other sweetened product to mask bitter taste

PERAMIVIR (Rapivab)

Available form
Vial: 20 mg/20 mL

Action
- inhibits influenza virus neuraminidase (enzyme that releases viral particles from infected cells)

Use
- treatment of acute influenza in those who have been symptomatic for up to 2 days

Dose
- 600 mg by IV infusion over 15–30 minutes

Adverse effects
- diarrhoea, constipation
- hypertension
- insomnia
- elevated liver enzymes
- (rare) allergic reactions, serious skin reactions
- (rare, children) delirium, abnormal behaviour, hallucinations

Interactions
- live attenuated vaccines are not recommended with 48 hours of peramivir

Nursing points/Cautions

- should be given within 2 days of developing influenza symptoms
- dilute vial with sodium chloride 0.9% or 0.45%, glucose 5% or Ringer's lactated solution to a volume of 100 mL
- dose reduction is required in those with creatinine clearance < 50 mL/minute
- repeated doses are not recommended as efficacy has not been established
- only suitable for viral illness, bacterial infections may still occur
- not a substitute for vaccination against influenza

Patient teaching and advice

- suggest that patient has yearly influenza vaccination
- advise patient to seek medical advice immediately if any of the following occur
    - rash, itching, hives, swelling of face, tongue or lips
    - severe blistering or peeling of skin, mouth sores, fever, fatigue
    - inflamed, red and raised skin and blisters

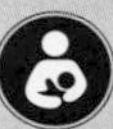

caution if used during pregnancy or breastfeeding if benefits outweigh risks. There may be risks to both mother and fetus if influenza develops during pregnancy

ZANAMIVIR (Relenza)

Available form

Powder for inhalation: 5 mg/dose

Action
- selective viral neuraminidase inhibitor, preventing release of infective particles and thereby reducing propagation of influenza virus
- neuraminidase enzyme is essential for viral replication as it plays a role in releasing the virus from infected cells, enabling spread
- not metabolised and is excreted unchanged in the urine
- half-life 2.5–5.1 hours (inhalation)

Use
- treatment of influenza (A or B) within 48 hours of symptom onset
- prevention of influenza A or B (where strain is not included in annual influenza vaccine)
- reduce transmission among members of infected person's household

Dose
- (treatment) 10 mg (2 inhalations) twice daily for 5 days (starting within 48 hours of symptom onset) (daily total 20 mg) **OR**
- (prevention) 10 mg (2 inhalations) daily for 10 days, which can be increased to 28 days if exposure is > 10 days

Adverse effects

- nausea, vomiting, diarrhoea
- headache
- cough, bronchitis
- (very rare) bronchospasm, dyspnoea, allergic reaction (facial and oropharyngeal oedema), neuropsychiatric events (e.g. delirium, abnormal behaviour), severe skin reaction

Nursing points/Cautions

- maximum benefit if administered within 48 hours of symptom onset
- decreases symptoms and duration of influenza symptoms
- not recommended as routine prevention of influenza
- caution if used in those with asthma or COPD because of the increased risk of bronchospasm
- contraindicated in those with severe milk protein allergy

Patient teaching and advice

- patient should be advised to seek medical advice if any of the following occur:
  - wheezing or shortness of breath
  - abnormal behaviours or mood changes
- if taking with other inhaled medication, instruct patient that they should be administered before zanamivir
- instruct patient that medication can only be administered using Diskhaler device, which is provided, and ensure patient understands technique for correct use

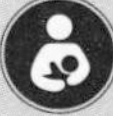

not recommended during pregnancy (especially first trimester) or breastfeeding unless benefits outweigh risks to fetus

NS3/4A PROTEASE INHIBITORS

Medications in this group are only available as a fixed-dose combination

GRAZOPREVIR

Action

- NS3/4A inhibitors disrupt the hepatitis C virus through two mechanisms (blocks viral processing as well as elimination)
- second generation
- fixed-dose combination has good activity against a range of hepatitis C viral genotypes

Use

- management of chronic hepatitis C genotype 1 or 4

Note

- contained in Zepatier with elbasivir (NS5A inhibitor)

NS5A INHIBITORS

A number of the medications included in this group (elbasvir, ledipasvir, velpatasvir) are only available in fixed-dose formulation with other antiviral agents

DACLATASVIR (Daklinza)

Available forms

Tablets: 30 mg, 60 mg

Action

- direct-acting hepatitis C virus (HCV) protein NS5A inhibitor
- NS5A is an essential protein in HCV replication
- inhibits both viral RNA replication and virion assembly
- synergistic activity with interferon alfa, HCV NS3 protease inhibitors, HCV NS5B non-nucleoside inhibitors and HCV NS5B nucleoside analogues
- half-life 12–15 hours

Use

- treatment of chronic hepatitis C (with other agents)

Dose

- (genotype 1 or 3) 60 mg orally daily (with sofosbuvir) for 12 weeks

Adverse effects
- headache, fatigue, dizziness
- fever
- arthralgia, myalgia, back pain
- diarrhoea, nausea
- nasopharyngitis, cough
- pruritus, rash, dry skin, alopecia
- dysglycaemia (in those with diabetes)

Interactions
- contraindicated with phenytoin, carbamazepine, oxcarbazepine, phenobarbital (phenobarbitone), rifampicin, rifabutin, dexamethasone and St John's wort
- may cause severe bradycardia if given in combination with amiodarone and sofosbuvir, therefore patient should be closely monitored especially in first 48 hours of combination therapy
- serum levels may be increased by clarithromycin, erythromycin, dabigatran etexilate, boceprevir, atazanavir/ritonavir, atazanavir/cobicistat, cobicistat/emtricitabine/tenofovir/elvitegravir, itraconazole, posaconazole, voriconazole, diltiazem and verapamil
- serum levels may be decreased by efavirenz, etravirine, nevirapine
- may increase serum levels of digoxin, increasing risk of adverse effects and toxicity
- may increase serum levels of HMG-CoA reductase inhibitors (statins) and should be given with caution
- INR should be closely monitored if given with warfarin

Nursing points/Cautions
- patient should be screened for hepatitis B co-infection before starting therapy as reactivation of hepatitis B may occur
- not recommended as monotherapy
- multidrug regimen is dependent on HCV genotype and prior treatment (e.g. no prior treatment, failed therapy)
- (genotype 3) in patients with cirrhosis, therapy may be extended to 24 weeks
- treatment interruption is not recommended

Patient teaching and advice
- if patient has diabetes, advise close monitoring of blood glucose levels during therapy
- (combination therapy with ribavirin) counsel female patient regarding the importance of not becoming pregnant during therapy and for 6 months after stopping, including the need for two forms of reliable contraception to be used (one by each partner). Patient should be instructed to conduct monthly pregnancy test during therapy
- (combination therapy with ribavirin) male patient should be advised regarding the importance of pregnant female partners avoiding any contact with capsules

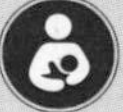

contraindicated with peginterferon alfa and ribavirin during pregnancy

not recommended during breastfeeding

tablet can be crushed and mixed with water or spoonful of yoghurt or apple puree

NS5B RNA-DEPENDENT RNA PROTEASE INHIBITORS

SOFOSBUVIR (Sovaldi)

Available form
Tablets: 400 mg

Action
- NS5B RNA polymerase inhibitor
- nucleotide prodrug that is metabolised to active analogue which is incorporated by HCV NS5B acting as a chain terminator

- half-life 0.4 hours, half-life of active metabolite 27 hours

Use

- chronic hepatitis C (as part of combination antiviral therapy)

Dose

- 400 mg orally daily (with ribavirin or peginterferon alfa and ribavirin)

Adverse effects (combination therapy)

- fatigue, headache, insomnia, asthenia, irritability
- nausea, diarrhoea, loss of appetite
- myalgia
- pruritus, rash
- fever, chills, flu-like illness
- anaemia
- (uncommon) severe depression, suicidal ideation, pancytopenia

Interactions

- symptomatic bradycardia may occur if combination therapy (sofosbuvir, peginterferon alfa and ribavirin) is given with amiodarone and are therefore not recommended together
- not recommended with rifampicin, modafinil, carbamazepine, oxcarbazepine, phenytoin, phenobarbital (phenobarbitone), rifabutin, rifampicin, tipranavir/ritonavir or St John's wort as they decrease plasma levels of sofosbuvir
- INR should be closely monitored if given with warfarin

Nursing points/Cautions

- before starting therapy, patient should be screened for hepatitis B co-infection as reactivation may occur
- not recommended as monotherapy
- if patient is taking amiodarone (with no other alternative), cardiac monitoring as an inpatient is recommended for first 48 hours of therapy, then daily as an outpatient or heart rate monitored at home for first 2 weeks of therapy. If amiodarone is discontinued just before starting therapy, cardiac monitoring as previously described should occur as amiodarone has a long half-life and risk of bradycardia would exist
- (patient with genotype 1, 4, 5 or 6 chronic hepatitis C) given with peginterferon alfa and ribavirin for 12 weeks
- (patient with genotype 2 chronic hepatitis C) given with ribavirin for 12 weeks
- (patient with genotype 3 chronic hepatitis C) given with ribavirin for 16 weeks
- (patient with chronic hepatitis C awaiting liver transplantation) given with ribavirin until liver transplantation occurs
- ribavirin dose is according to weight:
  - $<$ 75 kg: 1000 mg orally in 2 divided doses with food
  - $\geq$ 75 kg: 1200 mg orally in 2 divided doses with food
- (combination therapy with ribavirin) therapy should not be started until a negative pregnancy test has been obtained just before starting therapy
- caution if used in those over 65 years
- caution if used in those with pre-existing history of depression or psychiatric illness
- not recommended in those with genotype 1, 4, 5 and 6 HCV infection, HCV/HCB or HCV/HIV co-infection
- not recommended in patient with severe renal failure or decompensated cirrhosis (if combined with peg interferon alfa, contraindicated in those with liver decompensation)

Patient teaching and advice

- warn patient not to drive or operate machinery if fatigue, asthenia and insomnia occur
- advise patient to seek medical advice immediately if any of the following occur:
  - fainting or near fainting, dizziness, light-headedness, malaise,

weakness, excessive tiredness, shortness of breath, chest pains, confusion, memory problems
  - any signs of depression such as sadness, withdrawal from friends or previously pleasurable activities, or any attempts at self-harm
- female patient should be advised to use high-dose oral contraceptive containing at least 30 microgram of ethinylestradiol combined with norethisterone acetate/norethisterone
- (combination therapy with ribavirin) counsel female patient regarding the importance of not becoming pregnant during therapy and for 6 months after stopping, including the need for two forms of reliable contraception to be used (one by each partner). Patient should be instructed to conduct monthly pregnancy test during therapy
- (combination therapy with ribavirin) male patient should be advised regarding the importance of pregnant female partners avoiding any contact with capsules

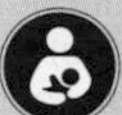

contraindicated in pregnancy if used in combination with ribavirin because of risk of birth defects and fetal death

not recommended during breastfeeding

tablet can be crushed and mixed with water or spoonful of thickened fluid, yoghurt or apple puree

Note
- contained in Harvoni with ledipasvir (NS5A inhibitor), in Epclusa with velpatasir (NS5B RNA inhibitor) and in Vosevi with velpatasir and voxilaprevir (NS3/4A protease inhibitor)

OTHER ANTIVIRAL AGENTS

ADEFOVIR DIPIVOXIL (APO-Adefovir)

Available form
Tablets: 10 mg

Action
- nucleoside analogue with an active metabolite (adefovir diphosphate) which inhibits hepatitis B viral DNA reverse transcriptase
- active metabolite (adefovir diphosphate) has half-life of 12–36 hours

Use
- chronic hepatitis B (with evidence of active viral replication and either elevated serum aminotransferases (ALT, AST) or histologically active disease)

Dose
- 10 mg orally daily

Adverse effects
- abnormal liver function
- kidney failure, abnormal kidney function, nephrotoxicity
- headache, asthenia
- nausea, diarrhoea, flatulence, dyspepsia, abdominal pain
- (rare) lactic acidosis, severe hepatomegaly with steatosis
- post-treatment exacerbation of hepatitis

Interactions
- increased risk of nephrotoxicity if given with other nephrotoxic agents such as ciclosporin, tacrolimus, vancomycin, aminoglycosides and NSAIDs
- contraindicated with tenofovir disoproxil fumarate, tenofovir alafenamide or formulations containing either of them

Nursing points/Cautions

- HIV testing is recommended before starting therapy to identify any HIV co-infection because of the risk of viral resistance developing
- monitoring of liver and renal function (including creatinine clearance) is recommended before starting and regularly during therapy
- dosing interval should be adjusted in those with creatinine clearance < 50 mL/minute
- caution when discontinuing therapy because severe exacerbation of hepatitis can occur. Liver function should be closely monitored for at least 12 weeks when therapy is stopped
- caution if used in women, the obese or those with prolonged exposure to nucleosides because of the increased risk of lactic acidosis and severe hepatomegaly
- caution if used in those with kidney impairment due to risk of nephrotoxicity
- caution if used in those > 65 years

Patient teaching and advice

- warn patient that exacerbation of hepatitis may occur up to 12 weeks after stopping therapy. If symptoms including upper abdominal pain, tiredness, yellowing of eyes and/or skin, dark urine and pale stools (bowel motions) occur, medical advice should be sought immediately

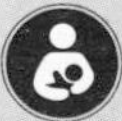

should only be used during pregnancy if benefits outweigh potential risks

not recommended during breastfeeding

tablet can be crushed and mixed with water or spoonful of yoghurt or apple puree (has very bitter taste)

ENTECAVIR MONOHYDRATE (Baraclude, Entac, Enteclude)

Available forms

Tablets: 0.5 mg, 1 mg

Action

- deoxyguanosine nucleoside analogue which is selectively active against hepatitis B virus (HBV) polymerase
- little or no activity against other viruses
- phosphorylated to active form that inhibits HBV DNA replication at three stages
- well absorbed on empty stomach but does not undergo extensive metabolism
- half-life 128–149 hours

Use

- chronic hepatitis B (with evidence of active liver inflammation)

Dose

- 0.5 mg orally daily either 2 hours before or 2 hours after a meal **OR**
- (lamivudine refractory/resistant patient) 1 mg orally daily either 2 hours before or 2 hours after a meal

Adverse effects

- fatigue, headache,
- altered liver enzymes
- (rare) lactic acidosis, severe hepatomegaly with steatosis

Interactions

- caution if used with agents that reduce kidney function or compete for renal tubular secretion
- caution if given with antiretroviral agents due to increased risk of lactic acidosis and severe hepatomegaly with steatosis

Nursing points/Cautions

- liver function should continue to be monitored for several months after stopping therapy

- tablets contain lactose and are not recommended in those with hereditary problems of galactose intolerance, Lapp lactase deficiency or glucose–galactose malabsorption
- caution if used in those > 65 years
- caution if used in those with renal impairment (creatinine clearance < 50 mL/minute)
- caution if used in liver transplant patients receiving immunosuppressants as kidney function may be affected. Kidney function should be closely monitored
- not recommended in those with HIV co-infection, unless being treated with antiretroviral agents

Patient teaching and advice

- advise patient to take tablets on an empty stomach, either 2 hours before or 1 hour after food
- patient should be warned that acute exacerbation of hepatitis may occur after therapy is stopped
- patient should be instructed that therapy does not decrease risk of transmission of hepatitis B virus to others via sexual contact or blood contamination, therefore precautions should be taken (e.g. condoms during sexual contact, not sharing needles)

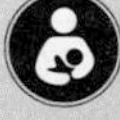

only used during pregnancy if benefits outweigh risks

not recommended during breastfeeding

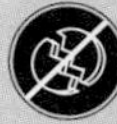

tablet can be dispersed in 10–20 mL of water or crushed and mixed with spoonful of yoghurt or apple puree. Mask and gloves should be worn if dispersing or crushing tablets

RIBAVIRIN (Ibavyr, Virazide)

Available forms

Powder for inhalation: 6 g; Capsules: 200 mg

Action

- antiviral agent (nucleoside analogue) that penetrates virus-infected cells and thought to reduce GTP storage as well as inhibiting RNA and protein synthesis, thereby inhibiting viral replication and spread to other cells (although mechanism is not entirely understood)
- no activity against hepatitis C virus if used alone
- half-life 9.5 hours after inhalation
- very long half-life (274–298 hours) (multiple dosing) (oral)

Use

- treatment of severe lower respiratory tract infection caused by RSV in hospitalised infants and children under 2 years of age (within first 3 days of infection)
- treatment of chronic hepatitis C (in combination therapy with sofosbuvir p. 839)

Dose

RSV infection (paediatric)

- given via aerosol as per manufacturer's directions for 3–7 days for 12–18 hours per day

Hepatitis C (with sofosbuvir)

- (weight < 75 kg) 500 mg orally twice daily with food (with 400 mg sofosbuvir) for 12 weeks (genotype 2), 16 weeks (genotype 3) or until liver transplantation **OR**
- (weight ≥ 75 kg) 600 mg orally twice daily with food (with 400 mg sofosbuvir) for 12 weeks (genotype 2), 16 weeks (genotype 3) or until liver transplantation

Adverse effects

RSV (inhalation)

- apnoea, pneumothorax, worsening respiratory status, cardiac arrest,

- hypotension
- rash, conjunctivitis

Hepatitis C (capsules) (combined with sofosbuvir)

- anorexia, nausea, stomatitis, diarrhoea
- headache, fatigue, asthenia, irritability
- cough, dyspnoea, pharyngitis
- myalgia, arthralgia
- rash, pruritus
- fever, chills, flu-like illness
- anaemia, neutropenia, haemolytic anaemia
- (uncommon) depression, suicidal or homicidal ideation

Interactions

Hepatitis C

- because of very long half-life, interactions with medications may occur up to 2 months after stopping therapy with ribavirin
- not recommended with azathioprine due to increased risk of myelotoxicity

Nursing points/Cautions

RSV

- RSV infection should be confirmed before or within 24 hours of starting therapy and only severe infection treated
- respiratory function and fluid status should be closely monitored throughout therapy
- standard respiratory support and fluid management should be given at same time as ribavirin therapy
- powder for inhalation should be reconstituted with 100 mL water for injections and then further dilute to 300 mL to give final concentration of 20 mg/mL
- administered via infant oxygen hood from SPAG-2 aerosol generator
- any remaining solution should be discarded after 24 hours
- should not be administered with any other aerosol medication or other aerosol devices
- sterilisation of wetted parts of equipment should be done daily
- should not be used for infants requiring assisted ventilation, because the drug may precipitate in respiratory equipment and interfere with safe and effective ventilation

Hepatitis C combination therapy

- not given as monotherapy
- (genotype 3) therapy may be extended to 24 weeks if needed
- complete blood count (with haemoglobin, differential, platelet count, electrolytes, serum creatinine, liver function tests, uric acid, lipid levels), thyroid function and cardiac function are recommended before starting therapy and regularly during combination therapy
- monthly pregnancy testing is required during and for 6 months after stopping therapy for all female patients of childbearing potential or female partners of male patients. Therapy should not be started unless patient and his/her partner are using two reliable forms of contraception during and for 6 months after therapy has stopped
- caution if used in those with history of depression
- caution if used in those with pre-existing severe anaemia (e.g. history of GI bleeding, spherocytosis)
- caution if used in those with pre-existing cardiac disease. If used, ECG monitoring is recommended before starting and regularly during therapy
- not recommended in those with decompensation cirrhosis of the liver, post-liver transplantation or if the patient has co-infection with hepatitis B or HIV

- contraindicated in men whose partners are pregnant
- contraindicated in those with history of pre-existing cardiac disease in previous 6 months, haemoglobinopathies (e.g. thalassaemia, sickle cell anaemia) and renal impairment (creatinine clearance < 50 mL/minute)

Patient teaching and advice

Hepatitis C combination therapy

- warn patient not to drive or operate machinery if fatigue, headache or depression occur or are ongoing
- instruct patient to swallow capsules whole (not opened, broken, crushed or chewed) and taken after food
- advise patient to seek medical advice immediately if any of the following occur:
    - depression, sadness, aggression, mood swings, withdrawal from previously pleasurable activities or friends, thoughts of self-harm or suicide (up to 6 months after therapy has stopped)
    - tiredness, shortness of breath and looking pale
    - unusual bleeding or bruising
- counsel female patient regarding the importance of not becoming pregnant during therapy and for 6 months after stopping, including the need for two forms of reliable contraception to be used (one by each partner). Patient should be instructed to conduct monthly pregnancy test during therapy
- male patient should be advised regarding the importance of female partners not becoming pregnant during therapy or for 6 months after including the need for two forms of reliable contraception to be used (one by each partner). Male patient's female partner should be instructed to conduct monthly pregnancy test during therapy

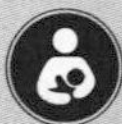
contraindicated during pregnancy and breastfeeding

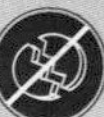
tablet should not be crushed

ANTIRETROVIRAL AGENTS

Retroviruses are RNA viruses that replicate in the host using a reverse transcriptase enzyme producing DNA from an RNA genome, then using the host cell DNA to replicate. Because of this complex replication mechanisms, retroviruses are very difficult to treat (Bryant et al 2019).

General Adverse effects of antiretroviral agents

- headache, dizziness, lethargy, fatigue, asthenia, depression, insomnia, somnolence, dream disturbance, anxiety, concentration level impairment, confusion
- anorexia, nausea, vomiting, diarrhoea, flatulence, abdominal pain, dry mouth, dyspepsia
- fever
- rash
- elevated liver enzymes, elevated cholesterol and triglycerides
- increased risk of opportunistic infections
- (combination therapy) increased risk of myocardial infarction
- (rare) (protease inhibitors) spontaneous bleeding in those with haemophilia
- (rare) lactic acidosis, hepatomegaly

- (rare) osteonecrosis, lipodystrophy syndrome (redistribution/accumulation of body fat), hyperglycaemia, new onset or exacerbation of pre-existing diabetes mellitus
- (rare) immune reconstitution syndrome (is an inflammatory reaction to asymptomatic/opportunistic infections (e.g. cytomegalovirus (CMV) retinitis, mycobacterial infections, *Pneumocystis jiroveci* pneumonia (PCP))
- (nucleoside/nucleotide analogues) mitochondrial dysfunction (in children exposed in utero)

General Interactions of antiretroviral agents

- may increase serum levels and associated risk of myopathy and rhabdomyolysis if given with simvastatin, pravastatin, fluvastatin or atorvastatin
- antacids may decrease absorption
- may decrease serum levels of methadone, increasing the risk of opiate withdrawal syndrome (especially if given with low-dose ritonavir)
- increased risk of hypotension, syncope, visual changes and priapism if given with sildenafil, tadalafil or vardenafil
- if given with warfarin, prothrombin time should be closely monitored, especially when starting, stopping or altering dosage

General Nursing points/Cautions for antiretroviral agents

- HIV testing is recommended before starting therapy to identify any HIV disease because of the increased risk of viral resistance to the drug. This should also include cases of needle stick injury involving a known HIV source
- cardiac risk factors (e.g. hypertension, diabetes mellitus, smoking, hyperlipidaemia) should be assessed and treated before starting therapy to decrease risk of myocardial infarction
- liver function should be tested before starting and during therapy
- in patients with concomitant hepatitis B, recurrent hepatitis may occur when therapy is stopped. Monitoring of liver function and markers of hepatitis B replication is recommended regularly after therapy is stopped
- patient should be examined for any signs of lipodystrophy syndrome (e.g. central obesity, buffalo hump, peripheral wasting, breast enlargement, increase in serum cholesterol and triglycerides and blood glucose), therefore serum triglycerides and cholesterol and blood glucose should be monitored throughout therapy
- if one antiretroviral agent (part of combination therapy) is stopped, all the antiretroviral agents should be restarted together
- combination antiretroviral therapy increases the risk of lipodystrophy syndrome
- combination therapy for treatment of HIV infection is common, as resistance occurs quickly to monotherapy. However, it becomes difficult to establish if adverse effects are caused by a single agent, the combination therapy or progression of the disease itself
- cross-resistance between members of a similar group may exist and should

be taken into consideration when developing treatment regimens

- (protease inhibitors) caution if used in those with haemophilia A and B due to increased risk of bleeding
- (nucleoside analogues) increased risk of lactic acidosis and hepatomegaly in women
- caution if used in those who have hepatitis co-infection. Patients should be closely monitored when therapy is stopped for any evidence of exacerbation of hepatitis
- caution if used in those with mild-to-moderate liver impairment (including active hepatitis B or C)
- contraindicated in those with severe liver failure

General Patient teaching and advice for antiretroviral agents

- therapy with antiretroviral agents does not cure HIV or decrease risk of transmission of the virus and the patient should therefore be encouraged to continue safe sex practices (e.g. use of condoms) and not share needles
- patient should be advised to seek medical advice if any of the following occur:
  - fatigue, loss of appetite, skin or eye yellowing, dark urine and upper abdominal tenderness/pain
  - joint aches and/or pain, stiffness or difficulty moving
  - generalised weakness, tiredness, unusual muscle pain, loss of appetite, unexplained weight loss, nausea, vomiting, unusual stomach discomfort, rapid and/or difficulty breathing, shortness of breath, dizziness, light-headedness
  - signs of infection, such as fever, swollen glands, sore throat
  - very sick with rapid breathing (may be worse in women than men)
  - loss of body fat from arms, legs and face with increased fat on abdomen, breasts and back of neck (buffalo hump)
  - chest pain, which may or may not radiate into neck and/or arm, nausea, sweating, severe anxiety or a sense of impending doom
- patient should be advised to seek medical advice before taking any prescription or non-prescription drugs (including over-the-counter or herbal preparations) as they may interact with antiretroviral agents
- warn patient to avoid driving or operating machinery if dizziness, somnolence, fatigue, asthenia or confusion occur
- if patient has diabetes, advise to monitor blood glucose levels closely during therapy
- patient should be warned that some people (especially those who have been HIV-positive for some time) may develop an inflammatory reaction (e.g. fever, pain, redness, swelling) within weeks of starting therapy, which may be a sign of the body's recovery in its ability to fight infection. The patient should be instructed to discuss any concerns with doctors if this occurs
- some antiretroviral agents decrease the efficacy of oral contraceptives, therefore women of childbearing potential should be advised to use an alternative or additional form of contraception to avoid pregnancy
- see also General Patient teaching and advice (p. xxvii)

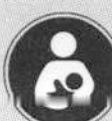

antiretroviral agents are not recommended during pregnancy unless benefits are thought to outweigh potential risks. Mitochondrial damage resulting in anaemia, neutropenia, hyperlactataemia, hyperlipasaemia, hypertonia and convulsion have been demonstrated both in vitro and in vivo

to avoid HIV transmission to a non-infected child, women who are HIV-positive are advised not to breastfeed. Most antiretroviral agents are not recommended during breastfeeding unless benefits are thought to outweigh potential risks

NUCLEOSIDE REVERSE TRANSCRIPTASE INHIBITORS (NRTIS)

ABACAVIR (Ziagen)

Available forms
Tablets: 300 mg; Oral solution: 20 mg/mL

Action
- nucleoside analogue reverse transcriptase inhibitor
- selective against HIV-1 and HIV-2
- half-life about 1.5 hours

Use
- HIV infections (with other antiretroviral agents)

Dose
- 300 mg orally twice daily

Adverse effects
- hypersensitivity (may be life threatening)
- myalgia
- dyspnoea, sore throat, cough
- hyperlactataemia
- see General Adverse effects of antiretroviral agents (p. 845)

Interactions
- caution if given with methadone

Nursing points/Cautions
- testinq for HLA-B*5701 allele is recommended before starting therapy. Those with positive allele are at higher risk of hypersensitivity reactions
- if hypersensitivity is suspected, therapy is immediately stopped and should **never** be restarted
- caution if used in women, those who are obese or who have had prolonged exposure to nucleoside analogues, because these factors increase the risk of lactic acidosis and severe hepatomegaly
- (oral solution) contains sorbitol and is therefore not recommended in those with hereditary fructose intolerance. Sorbitol may also cause diarrhoea and abdominal pain
- see also General Nursing points/Cautions for antiretroviral agents (p. 846)

Patient teaching and advice
- patient should be advised to immediately stop therapy and seek medical advice if any of the following occur:
  - unusual rash, fever, chills, itching, headache, fatigue, muscle pain, nausea, vomiting, diarrhoea, abdominal pain, sore throat, cough or shortness of breath, which may be signs of hypersensitivity (but also adverse effects of the drug) (especially in first 6 weeks of therapy)
- if patient develops hypersensitivity reaction (as described above), he/she should be instructed to **never** take abacavir (or any preparation containing abacavir) again, otherwise a life-threatening reaction can occur within hours
- advise patient to wear or carry some form of identification, such as a MedicAlert or Alert card (contained

in medication packet) with details of hypersensitivity
- (oral solution) instruct patient to use supplied dosing syringe to administer correct dose. Bottle adapter and syringe should be washed after each use
- see also General Patient teaching and advice for antiretroviral agents (p. 847)

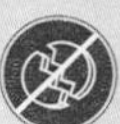

available as oral solution. Tablet may be crushed and mixed with spoonful of yoghurt or apple puree. Staff should wear mask and gloves if crushing. Pregnant staff should not crush tablets

Note
- combined with lamivudine and zidovudine in Trizivir, lamivudine and dolutegravir in Triumeq, and lamivudine in Kivexa

EMTRICITABINE (Emtriva)

Available form
Capsules: 200 mg

Action
- synthetic nucleoside analogue
- analogue of cytosine
- effective against HIV-1, HIV-2 and hepatitis B
- half-life about 10 hours

Use
- treatment of HIV (with other antiretroviral agents)

Dose
- 200 mg orally daily

Adverse effects
- rash, skin discolouration (hyperpigmentation of palms and/or soles)
- neutropenia, anaemia
- arthralgia, myalgia
- neuropathy, peripheral neuritis, paraesthesia
- see General Adverse effects of antiretroviral agents (p. 845)

Interactions
- contraindicated with other preparations containing emtricitabine or lamivudine

Nursing points/Cautions
- not recommended as monotherapy
- increased risk of liver toxicity if given to those with chronic hepatitis B or C treated with combination antiviral therapy
- caution if used in those with kidney impairment as predominantly excreted via kidney. Adjustment to dosing interval is required depending on creatinine clearance
- see General Nursing points/Cautions for antiretroviral agents (p. 846)

Patient teaching and advice
- patient should be advised to seek medical advice immediately if any of the following occur:
  - tingling, numbness or changes to sensation at extremities
  - change in skin colour (palms or soles of feet)

capsule can be opened and contents mixed with water or spoonful of yoghurt or apple puree

Note
- combined with tenofovir disoproxil fumarate in Truvada, tenofovir disoproxil fumarate and efavirenz in Atripla, tenofovir disoproxil fumarate and rilpivirine in Eviplera and Tenofovir EMT, tenofovir disoproxil fumarate, cobicistat and elvitegravir in Stribild, tenofivir alafenamide and bictegravir in Biktarvy, rilpivirine and tenofovir alafenamide in Odefsey, tenofovir alafenamide in Descovy, cobicistat, elvitegravir and tenofovir alafenamide in Genvoya and cobicistat, darumavir and tenofovir alafenamide in Symtuza

LAMIVUDINE (3TC, Zeffix, Zetlam)

Available forms
Tablets: 100 mg, 150 mg, 300 mg; Oral solution: 5 mg/mL, 10 mg/mL

Action
- active against hepatitis B (HBV), as well as HIV-1 and HIV-2
- converted to active metabolite (lamivudine triphosphate) which inhibits HIV reverse transcription by terminating viral DNA chain
- also inhibits RNA and DNA-dependent DNA polymerase functions
- synergism of antiviral activity when given with zidovudine
- active metabolite half-life 10–15 hours

Use
- treatment of HIV infection (with other antiretroviral agents)
- treatment of chronic hepatitis B

Dose
- (HIV-1 treatment) 150 mg orally twice or 300 mg once daily **OR**
- (HBV) 100 mg daily

Adverse effects
- rash, alopecia
- myalgia, muscle cramps
- hyperlactataemia
- neutropenia, anaemia
- pancreatitis (especially in children)
- neuropathy
- see General Adverse effects of antiretroviral agents (p. 845)

Interactions
- increased serum levels may occur if given with trimethoprim as part of trimethoprim/sulfamethoxazole combination
- activity may be decreased by ciprofloxacin, pentamidine and ganciclovir
- not recommended with emtricitabine or formulations that contain emtricitabine
- increased risk of pancreatitis if given with IV pentamidine
- not recommended with other sorbitol-containing medications

Nursing points/Cautions
- not recommended as monotherapy
- (oral solution) contains propylene glycol and hydroxybenzoates, which may cause hypersensitivity reactions in sensitive individuals
- caution if used in those with moderate-to-severe kidney impairment or decompensated liver disease
- caution if used in those with history of pancreatitis or peripheral neuropathy
- see also General Nursing points/Cautions for antiretroviral agents (p. 846)

Patient teaching and advice
- those with diabetes should be advised that oral solution contains sucrose (5 mL = 1 g sucrose), therefore blood glucose levels should be closely monitored during therapy if oral solution is taken
- (HBV) advise patient that there may be an exacerbation/reactivation of hepatitis if therapy is stopped. Liver function should be monitored for at least 16 weeks after stopping therapy (especially in those with advanced liver disease or transplant recipients)
- advise patient that dose for HBV is not appropriate for treatment of HIV
- instruct patient to immediately seek medical advice if any of the following occur:
  - abdominal pain, nausea and vomiting
  - any weakness, pain, numbness or tingling of feet or hands
- see also General Patient teaching and advice for antiretroviral agents (p. 847)

oral solution available. Tablet can be crushed and mixed with water or spoonful of yoghurt or apple puree

Note

- combined with zidovudine in Combivir, abacavir and zidovudine in Trizivir, abacavir in Kivexa, and abacavir and dolutegravir in Dovato and Triumeq

TENOFOVIR ALAFENAMIDE (Vemlidy)

TENOFOVIR DISOPROXIL FUMARATE (Viread)

Available form

Tablets: 300 mg

Action

- nucleoside reverse transcriptase inhibitor
- prodrug that is converted to tenofovir diphosphate in both resting and activated T cells
- competitively inhibits HIV reverse transcriptase
- bioavailability increases if given with food

Use

- treatment of HIV infection (with other antiretroviral agents)
- treatment of chronic hepatitis B

Dose

- 300 mg orally daily with food

Adverse effects

- decrease in bone density
- nephrotoxicity
- peripheral neuropathy
- (post discontinuing treatment) reactivation of hepatitis
- see General Adverse effects of antiretroviral agents (p. 845)

Interactions

- caution if given with other nephrotoxic agents or with agents that increase serum levels (e.g. lopinavir/ritonavir combination)
- contraindicated with other tenofovir disoproxil fumarate-containing agents or tenofovir alafenamide-containing agents or adefovir dipivoxil
- only recommended with atazanavir in combination with ritonavir
- decreased serum levels may occur if given with rifampicin, rifabutin, phenobarbital, phenytoin and St John's wort, therefore not recommended together

Nursing points/Cautions

- testing for HIV–hepatitis B co-infection is recommended before starting therapy
- discontinuing antihepatitis B therapy in those with advanced liver disease or cirrhosis is not recommended because of the increased risk of liver decompensation
- caution if used as part of a triple NRTIs regime as viral resistance may occur. Triple regime therapy should consist of two NRTI agents plus either NNRTI or HIV-1 protease inhibitor
- not recommended in those < 12 years or > 65 years
- see also General Nursing points/Cautions for antiretroviral agents (p. 846)

Patient teaching and advice

- patient should be advised to take with food
- warn patient that acute exacerbation/reactivation of hepatitis may occur when therapy is stopped and therefore regular liver function monitoring is recommended
- advise patient to seek medical advice if any of the following occur:
  - weakness, pain or tingling in hands or feet
  - bone pain

- see also Patient teaching and advice for antiretroviral agents (p. 847)

tablet can be dispersed in 100 mL of water, orange or grape juice or crushed and mixed with spoonful of yoghurt or apple puree

Note

- contained in Descovy, Truvada and Tenofovir EMT with emtricitabine, Atripla with emtricitabine and efavirenz, Odefsey, Eviplera with emtricitabine and rilpivirine and in Genvoya, Stribild with emtricitabine, cobicistat and elvitegravir, Biktarvy with bictegravir and emtricitabine, and Symtuza with cobicistat, metricitabine and darunavir

ZIDOVUDINE (formerly Azidothymidine or AZT) (Retrovir)

Available forms

Capsules: 100 mg, 250 mg; Syrup: 50 mg/5 mL

Action

- thymidine nucleoside analogue
- converted to zidovudine triphosphate which interferes with RNA-dependent DNA polymerase (reverse transcriptase) inhibiting HIV replication

Use

- treatment of HIV infection (as monotherapy or with other antiretroviral agents)

Dose

- 500–600 mg orally daily in 2–5 divided doses

Adverse effects

- anaemia, neutropenia, leucopenia, pancytopenia
- myalgia, paraesthesia
- dyspnoea
- rash, sweating
- see General Adverse effects of antiretroviral agents (p. 845)

Interactions

- probenecid may slow renal excretion of zidovudine
- not recommended with ribavirin or stavudine due to potential exacerbation of anaemia
- increased risk of neutropenia if given with paracetamol
- risk of toxicity increases if given with other nephrotoxic or cytotoxic drugs or those that interfere with white or red blood cell numbers or function such as pyrimethamine, sulfamethoxazole/trimethoprim, doxorubicin, dapsone, pentamidine (IV), amphotericin B (amphotericin), ganciclovir, flucytosine, vincristine, vinblastine, adriamycin and interferon
- metabolism may be altered by paracetamol, aspirin, indometacin, ketoprofen, naproxen, oxazepam, lorazepam, cimetidine, dapsone, codeine, methadone and morphine
- phenytoin levels should be closely monitored if given together as serum levels may vary
- absorption may be decreased if given with clarithromycin
- metabolism may be slowed if given with atovaquone
- increased risk of neurotoxicity if given with aciclovir

Nursing points/Cautions

- regular blood counts every second week for first 3 months of treatment, then monthly are recommended
- therapy should be interrupted if haemoglobin level falls below 7.6 g/dL or neutrophil count falls below 0.75 × 10^9/L (or 750/mm^3)
- if patient develops rash, evaluation for sensitisation is recommended
- caution if used in those with compromised bone marrow or advanced HIV disease
- contraindicated in those with abnormally low neutrophil counts (below

0.75 × 10^9/L) or abnormally low haemoglobin level (< 7.5 g/dL)

- see also General Nursing points/Cautions for antiretroviral agents (p. 846)

Patient teaching and advice

- patient should be advised about the haematological side-effects, which may require treatment by blood transfusion and/or dose modification and the importance of regular blood tests
- warn patient not to take paracetamol while taking zidovudine
- if given with clarithromycin tablets, instruct patient to separate by at least 2 hours
- instruct patient to remain in upright position when taking zidovudine (especially if there are any swallowing difficulties) as oesophageal irritation can occur
- patient should be advised to seek medical advice if any of the following occur:
  - frequent infection such as fever, chills, sore throat, mouth ulcers or flu-like symptoms
  - unusual bleeding or bruising
  - shortness of breath on exertion, tiredness, pale appearance (especially in first 2–4 weeks of therapy)
  - abnormal rash
- see also General Patient teaching and advice for antiretroviral agents (p. 847)

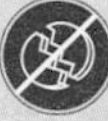

oral solution is available. Capsule can be opened and contents mixed with water or spoonful of yoghurt or apple puree. Staff should wear mask and gloves if opening capsule

Note

- combined with lamivudine in Combivir, and abacavir and lamivudine in Trizivir

NON-NUCLEOSIDE REVERSE TRANSCRIPTASE INHIBITORS (NNRTIS)

EFAVIRENZ (Stocrin)

Available forms

Tablets: 200 mg, 600 mg; Oral solution: 30 mg/mL

Action

- non-nucleoside reverse transcriptase inhibitor of HIV-1 (but not HIV-2)
- blocks RNA-dependent and DNA-dependent DNA polymerases
- viral resistance has occurred when given alone
- onset of action 3–5 hours
- half-life 52–76 hours (single dose) and 40–55 hours (multiple dosing)

Use

- treatment of HIV infections (with other antiretroviral agents)

Dose

- 600 mg orally 1 hour before or 2 hours after food at night (with other antiretroviral agents)

Adverse effects

- rash
- dizziness, abnormal dreams, impaired concentration
- (rare) severe depression, suicidal ideation, aggression, paranoia, delusions, psychoses, pancreatitis, severe rash, seizures, QT prolongation
- see General Adverse effects of antiretroviral agents (p. 845)

Interactions

- contraindicated with triazolam, midazolam, voriconazole, itraconazole and ergot alkaloids
- contraindicated with St John's wort
- contraindicated with elbasvir/grazoprevir combination
- not recommended with sofosbuvir/velpatasvir/voxilaprevir or sofosbuvir/velpatasvir combination

- not recommended with other formulations containing efavirenz
- not recommended with posaconazole, proguanil or atovaquone
- not recommended with alcohol due to risk of added CNS effects
- may decrease serum levels of ciclosporin, tacrolimus and sirolimus reducing efficacy
- caution if given with hepatotoxic agents. If used together, liver function should be closely monitored
- may decrease serum levels of atazanavir, lopinavir/ritonavir, saquinavir, indinavir, simeprevir, rifabutin, diltiazem, sertraline, bupropion, artemether/lumefantrine, maraviroc, pravastatin, simvastatin, carbamazepine and clarithromycin
- if given with ritonavir, increased risk of adverse effects and liver enzymes should be monitored regularly
- may increase serum levels of ethinylestradiol
- decreased serum levels may result if given with rifampicin, phenytoin, phenobarbital (phenobarbitone), carbamazepine or St John's wort
- bioavailability increased if given with food
- caution if given with warfarin because of variable effects. INR should be carefully monitored, especially when starting and stopping therapy
- may decrease plasma levels of methadone leading to opiate withdrawal symptoms
- not recommended with other agents known to prolong QT interval
- may cause false positive urine cannabinoid test

Nursing points/Cautions

- not recommended as monotherapy
- cholesterol and triglyceride monitoring is recommended during therapy
- CNS symptoms usually start in first 2 days of therapy and resolve within 1–4 weeks
- increased risk of psychiatric/nervous system symptoms if given to those with a history of mental illness or substance abuse, therefore should be given with caution
- if patient has (or is suspected of having) hepatitis B or C co-infection or being treated using hepatotoxic agents, liver function monitoring is recommended
- caution if used in those with a history of seizures or moderate-to-severe liver impairment
- contraindicated in those who have previously experienced life-threatening skin reactions
- see General Nursing points/Cautions for antiretroviral agents (p. 846)

Patient teaching and advice

- patient and/or significant others/carers should be advised to immediately report any depression, feelings of self-harm, delusion or hallucinations, aggressive behaviour or psychosis
- advise patient that taking medication at night may alleviate some of the CNS symptoms
- if patient is taking oral solution, instruct to use supplied syringe to measure solution accurately
- warn patient that:
    - rash commonly occurs within 1 to 2 days of starting therapy but resolves with continued therapy. If skin blistering, mouth blisters or fever occur, patient should be advised to seek medical attention immediately
    - symptoms such as dizziness, abnormal dreaming, difficulty sleeping and impaired concentration usually resolve within 2–4 weeks of continued therapy. Patient should be advised not to drive or operate machinery if these occur and/or are ongoing
- patients should be warned to avoid alcohol during therapy

- counsel female patients to use 2 methods of contraception (barrier and oral/hormonal) during and for 12 weeks after stopping therapy to prevent pregnancy
- see General Patient teaching and advice for antiretroviral agents (p. 847)

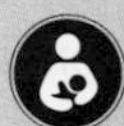

contraindicated during pregnancy

not recommended during breastfeeding

oral solution is available. Tablet can be crushed and mixed with water or no more than 2 spoonfuls of yoghurt (not apple puree as has peppery taste)

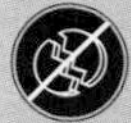

pregnant staff should not disperse or crush tablets. Mask should be worn if crushing tablets

Note
- contained in Atripla with emtricitabine with tenofovir

ETRAVIRINE (Intelence)

Available form
Tablets: 200 mg

Action
- non-nucleoside reverse transcriptase inhibitor of HIV-1
- blocks RNA-dependent and DNA-dependent DNA polymerases
- half-life 30–40 hours

Use
- treatment of HIV-1 infection (in those with evidence of viral replication and resistance to non-nucleoside transcriptase inhibitors and other antiretroviral agents) (as part of combination therapy)

Dose
- 200 mg orally twice daily after food

Adverse effects
- anaemia
- hypercholesterolaemia, hypertriglyceridaemia, hyperlipidaemia, hyperglycaemia
- peripheral neuropathy
- rash
- night sweats
- hypertension
- (rare) severe skin reactions, hypersensitivity reactions, myocardial infarction
- see also General Adverse effects of antiretroviral agents (p. 845)

Interactions
- not recommended with efavirenz, nevirapine, rilpivirine, unboosted atazanavir, ritonavir, other unboosted protease inhibitors (e.g. saquinavir), tipranavir/ritonavir, darunavir/cobicistat
- not recommended with clarithromycin as increased levels of clarithromycin's active metabolite may occur (which does not have the same efficacy against Mycobacterium atrium complex (MAC))
- plasma levels may be decreased by dexamethasone, carbamazepine, phenobarbital (phenobarbitone), phenytoin, rifampicin, maraviroc, dolutegravir, elbasvir/grazoprevir and St John's wort and are therefore not recommended together
- may increase plasma levels of fosamprenavir (unboosted)
- if given with digoxin, digoxin serum levels should be monitored regularly
- if given with warfarin, INR should be monitored regularly, especially when starting or stopping therapy
- may increase plasma levels of diazepam
- may decrease plasma levels of atorvastatin (but increase plasma levels of active metabolite), simvastatin, rosuvastatin and fluvastatin
- caution if used with ciclosporin, tacrolimus or sirolimus
- may decrease activation of clopidogrel to active metabolite and therefore not recommended together
- caution if boosted etravirine is given with rifabutin
- may decrease serum levels of PDE-5 inhibitors such as sildenafil, tadalafil and vardenafil

- may decrease serum levels of daclatasvir
- may decrease serum levels of antiarrhythmic agents such as amiodarone, flecainide, disopyramide and lidocaine (systemic)

Nursing points/Cautions

- see General Nursing points/Cautions for antiretroviral agents (p. 846)

Patient teaching and advice

- warn patient that mild-to-moderate rash occurs commonly during second week of therapy and rarely after week 4
- patient should be advised to seek medical advice immediately if any of the following occur:
    - severe rash
    - rash with fever, malaise, fatigue, muscle and joint aches, blisters, oral lesions, conjunctivitis
    - chest pain, neck/jaw pain, left arm pain, anxiety, sweating, pallor, nausea, vomiting, indigestion, dizziness
- instruct patient to swallow tablet whole with water (if possible). If patient is unable to swallow, advise patient that tablet may be dispersed in water, taking care to stir well and drink immediately. Instruct patient to rinse glass well and swallow to ensure complete dose has been taken
- see also General Patient teaching and advice for antiretroviral agents (p. 847)

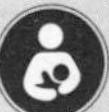

should only be used during pregnancy if benefits outweigh risks

not recommended during breastfeeding

tablet can be dispersed in water

RILPIVIRINE HYDROCHLORIDE (Edurant)

Available form
Tablets: 25 mg

Action
- non-nucleoside reverse transcriptase inhibitor
- blocks RNA-dependent and DNA-dependent DNA polymerases
- effective against HIV-1
- absorption improved if taken with food or high-fat meal
- half-life about 50 hours

Use
- treatment of HIV-1 infection (with other antiretrovirals) in those with viral load ≤ 100,000 copies/mL and treatment naive

Dose
- 25 mg orally daily with food

Adverse effects
- depression
- rash
- (rare) QT interval prolongation
- see General Adverse effects of antiretroviral agents (p. 845)

Interactions
- contraindicated with carbamazepine, oxcarbazepine, phenobarbital (phenobarbitone), phenytoin, rifabutin, rifampicin, proton pump inhibitors, dexamethasone (except as a single treatment) and St John's wort
- caution if used with rifabutin, antacids or H_2-receptor antagonists (famotidine, ranitidine, cimetidine, nizatidine) as decreased serum levels may occur
- increased serum levels may occur if given with darunavir/ritonavir, lopinavir/ritonavir, atazanavir/ritonavir, fosamprenavir/ritonavir, saquinavir/ritonavir, tipranavir/ritonavir, atazanavir, fosamprenavir, indinavir, clarithromycin, erythromycin, itraconazole, fluconazole, voriconazole or posaconazole

- not recommended with efavirenz, etravirine, nevirapine
- caution if given with methadone
- caution if given with agents known to prolong QT interval

Nursing points/Cautions

- not used as monotherapy
- caution if used in those with moderate liver impairment and not recommended in those with severe liver impairment
- see General Nursing points/Cautions for antiretroviral agents (p. 846)

Patient teaching and advice

- instruct patient to take antacids 2 hours before or at least 4 hours after rilpivirine, or for H_2-receptor antagonists (such as ranitidine) 12 hours before or at least 4 hours after rilpivirine
- advise patient to take with a meal to help with absorption
- see also General Patient teaching and advice for antiretroviral agents (p. 847)

tablet can be dispersed in water or crushed and mixed with spoonful of yoghurt or apple puree. Should be administered immediately as rilpivirine is light sensitive

Note

- contained in Eviplera with emtricitabine and tenofovir disoproxil fumarate, Juluca with dolutegravir, and Odefsey with emtricitabine and tenofovir alafenamide

PROTEASE INHIBITORS (PI)

ATAZANAVIR (Reyataz)

Available forms

Capsules: 150 mg, 200 mg, 300 mg

Action

- HIV-1 protease inhibitor
- half-life 6.5–7.9 hours

Use

- treatment of HIV-1 infection (with other antiretroviral agents)

Dose

Therapy-naive patient

- 400 mg orally daily with food **OR**
- 300 mg orally daily (with ritonavir 100 mg daily)

Therapy-experienced patient

- 300 mg orally daily (with ritonavir 100 mg daily)

Adverse effects

- back pain, peripheral neuropathy
- jaundice, scleral icterus, increased bilirubin (asymptomatic)
- prolonged PR interval, and rarely, QT interval prolongation
- rash
- nephrolithiasis, cholelithiasis, haematuria, proteinuria
- see General Adverse effects of antiretroviral agents (p. 845)

Interactions

- contraindicated with midazolam, triazolam, rifampicin, indinavir, alfuzosin, St John's wort, salmeterol, simvastatin, lovastatin, sildenafil (if used for pulmonary arterial hypertension), glecaprevir/pibrentasvir, elbasvir/grazoprevir and ergot alkaloids
- not recommended with efavirenz, nevirapine, voxilaprevir
- atazanavir/ritonavir combination is not recommended with fluticasone or budesonide
- caution if given with other agents which prolong PR interval (e.g. beta-adrenoceptor blocking agents, digoxin)
- may increase serum levels of calcium-channel blockers, further prolonging the PR interval. ECG monitoring is recommended if given together
- decreased serum levels may occur if given with histamine H_2-receptor antagonists (e.g. cimetidine), proton

pump inhibitors, phenytoin, phenobarbital (phenobarbitone), carbamazepine, nevirapine, antacids, boceprevir, tenofovir or efavirenz
- increased serum levels may occur if given with ritonavir, saquinavir, other protease inhibitors, itraconazole or voriconazole
- may decrease efficacy of oral contraceptives or hormone replacement therapy by decreasing serum levels of estradiol
- may increase serum levels of irinotecan, ciclosporin, tacrolimus, sirolimus, clarithromycin, rifabutin, amiodarone, lidocaine (lignocaine), TCAs, colchicine, buprenorphine, saquinavir, sildenafil, tadalafil, vardenafil, midazolam (IV) or atorvastatin increasing risk of adverse effects and toxicity
- may decrease serum levels of phenytoin, lamotrigine and phenobarbital (phenobarbitone)
- caution if given with warfarin as serum levels may be increased. INR should be monitored especially when starting or stopping therapy
- caution if given with other agents known to prolong QT interval or cause electrolyte imbalance
- increased risk of bleeding if given with dabigatran, apixaban or rivaroxaban
- see General Interactions of antiretroviral agents (p. 846)

Nursing points/Cautions

- not recommended as monotherapy. Should be given with ritonavir
- should be given 2 hours apart from histamine H_2-receptor antagonists (e.g. cimetidine)
- dose should be reduced if given with other antiretroviral agents
- tablets contain lactose and therefore not recommended in those with galactose intolerance, glucose–galactose malabsorption or Lapp lactase deficiency
- caution if used in those with pre-existing conduction problems (e.g. AV block), bradycardia, congenital QT syndrome or electrolyte imbalance
- see also General Nursing points/Cautions for antiretroviral agents (p. 846)

Patient teaching and advice

- patient should be advised that rash commonly occurs in first 3 weeks of therapy and then resolves within 2 weeks of stopping medication
- instruct patient to seek medical advice immediately if any of the following occur:
  - yellowing of skin or eyes, loss of appetite, unexplained tiredness, upper abdominal pain, dark urine, pale stools
  - pain in right or middle upper stomach, fever, nausea, vomiting, yellowing of eyes/skin
  - pain in kidney area, pain on urination, blood in urine
  - unusual heart rate
  - any numbness, tingling or changed sensation in extremities
- advise patient to separate by:
  - at least 10 hours if used with H_2-receptor antagonist such as famotidine
  - if taking antacids, they should be separated by 2 hours before or 1 hour after medication
- see General Patient teaching and advice for antiretroviral agents (p. 847)

capsules can be opened and contents mixed with spoonful of yoghurt or apple puree

Note

- combined with cobicistat (pharmacokinetic enhancer) in Evotaz

DARUNAVIR (Prezista)

Available forms
Tablets: 150 mg, 600 mg, 800 mg

Action
- HIV-1 protease inhibitor
- half-life about 15 hours (when combined with ritonavir)

Use
- treatment of HIV-1 infection (in combination with low-dose ritonavir and other antiretroviral agents)

Dose
- 600 mg orally twice daily with food (with ritonavir 100 mg twice daily) **OR**
- 800 mg orally daily with food (with ritonavir 100 mg daily)

Adverse effects
- drug-induced hepatitis
- rash
- (rare) severe skin reaction
- see General Adverse effects of antiretroviral agents (p. 845)

Interactions
- contraindicated with midazolam (oral), triazolam, alfuzosin, lovastatin, simvastatin, St John's wort, ergot derivatives, rifampicin, flecainide, lidocaine (lignocaine), amiodarone, sildenafil (when used for pulmonary arterial hypertension), lurasidone, dapoxetine, apixaban, ivabradine, elbasvir/grazoprevir or colchicine (in those with liver/kidney impairment)
- not recommended with rivaroxaban or dabigatran
- caution if used with other hepatotoxic agents
- caution if given with buprenorphine/naloxone due to increase in active metabolite and risk of opioid toxicity
- caution if given with fentanyl, oxycodone and tramadol as increased serum levels may occur increasing risk of respiratory depression
- increased risk of QT prolongation if given with artemether/lumefantrine
- activity enhanced by ritonavir and is therefore given as combination therapy (low dose ritonavir)
- may decrease serum levels of etravirine, voriconazole, sertraline and paroxetine
- may decrease serum levels of warfarin, therefore INR should be monitored especially when starting or stopping therapy
- may increase serum levels of bosentan, fluticasone, prednisolone, budesonide, betamethasone, fluconazole, clonazepam, digoxin, calcium-channel blockers, itraconazole, posaconazole, rifabutin, clarithromycin, nevirapine, tenofovir, indinavir, efavirenz, rilpivirine, carbamazepine, salmeterol, colchicine, atorvastatin, pravastatin, risperidone, quetiapine, carvedilol, metoprolol, sedatives, hypnotics, maraviroc, dasatinib, nilotinib, vinca alkaloids, irinotecan, sildenafil, vardenafil, tadalafil, TCAs, domperidone, clotrimazole, ticagrelor, ciclosporin, everolimus, tacrolimus or sirolimus increasing risk of adverse effects and toxicity, therefore serum levels should be closely monitored
- may decrease serum levels and efficacy of oral contraceptives and hormone replacement therapy
- serum levels may be decreased if given with oxcarbazepine, modafinil, dexamethasone, efavirenz, phenobarbital (phenobarbitone) or phenytoin
- serum levels may be increased if given with indinavir, rifabutin or posaconazole
- not recommended with boceprevir, simeprevir, elvitegravir, saquinavir or lopinavir/ritonavir combination

Nursing points/Cautions
- not used as monotherapy
- once-a-day dosing is recommended for treatment-naive patients, treatment-experienced patient with no darunavir-resistant mutations and

HIV-1 RNA < 100,000 copies/mL or treatment experienced but HIV protease naive patients where HIV-1 genotype is unavailable
- twice-daily dosing is recommended for treatment-experienced patient with at least one darunavir resistance-associated mutation, HIV protease inhibitor treatment experienced patient where HIV-1 genotype is unavailable or those with plasma HIV-1 RNA ≥ 100,000 copies/mL
- liver function tests should be performed before starting and regularly during therapy
- caution if used in those > 65 years
- caution if used in those with pre-existing liver disease including chronic active hepatitis B or C and not recommended in those with severe liver impairment
- caution if used in those with sulfonamide allergy
- see General Nursing points/Cautions for antiretroviral agents (p. 846)

Patient teaching and advice

- instruct patient to take tablets whole, not divided, crushed or chewed
- patient should be advised to seek medical advice immediately if any of the following occur
    - any rash (with or without fever), tiredness, muscle/joint ache, blisters or conjunctivitis
    - fatigue, loss of appetite, liver tenderness, nausea, dark urine, yellowing of eyes or skin
- see General Patient teaching and advice for antiretroviral agents (p. 847)

Note

- combined with cobicistat in Prescobiv and cobisistat, emtricitabine and tenofovir alafenamide in Symtuza

FOSAMPRENAVIR (Telzir)

Available form

Tablets: 700 mg

Action

- protease inhibitor
- prodrug of amprenavir, hydrolysed in gut epithelium (amprenavir is a potent and selective inhibitor of HIV-1 and HIV-2)
- amprenavir half-life 7.7 hours (prolonged when given with ritonavir)

Use

- treatment of HIV-1 infection (with low-dose ritonavir and other antiretrovirals)

Dose

- (antiretroviral-naive patient) 1.4 g orally daily (with ritonavir 200 mg daily) or 700 mg orally twice daily (with ritonavir 100 mg twice daily) (with other antiretroviral agents) **OR**
- (protease inhibitor experienced patient) 700 mg orally twice daily (with ritonavir 100 mg twice daily) (with other antiretroviral agents)

Adverse effects

- rash
- (rare) severe skin reaction
- see General Adverse effects of antiretroviral agents (p. 845)

Interactions

- metabolism may be inhibited by ritonavir
- fosamprenavir/ritonavir combination is contraindicated with alfuzosin, rifampicin, triazolam, midazolam, flecainide, quetiapine, lurasidone, sildenafil (when used for pulmonary arterial hypertension) and ergot alkaloids
- not recommended with amiodarone, lidocaine (lignocaine), TCAs, rifabutin, St John's wort, boceprevir, PDE5 inhibitors (sildenafil, tadalafil, vardenafil), telaprevir, simeprevir and paritaprevir
- caution if given with warfarin, INR should be closely monitored
- should not given with nevirapine without ritonavir
- caution if used with raltegravir and dolutegravir

- increased risk of adverse effects if given with lopinavir/ritonavir
- increased risk of Cushing's syndrome and adrenal suppression if given with fluticasone or other glucocorticoids
- not recommended with simvastatin and lovastatin due to risk of myopathy and/or rhabdomyolysis and caution if given with atorvastatin
- increased risk of elevated liver enzymes and changes in hormonal levels if fosamprenavir/ritonavir is given with oral contraceptive
- serum levels may be decreased by dexamethasone, phenytoin, carbamazepine, phenobarbital, H_2-receptor antagonists and efavirenz
- fosamprenavir/ritonavir combination may increase serum levels of clarithromycin, erythromycin, TCAs, itraconazole, benzodiazepines, sirolimus, ciclosporin, tacrolimus, everolimus, vinblastine, dasatinib, nilotinib, rifabutin and calcium-channel blockers, thereby increasing the risk of adverse or serious effects
- may decrease serum levels of paroxetine, phenytoin and methadone

Nursing points/Cautions

- once-daily regimen is not recommended in those who have been previously treated with antiviral protease inhibitors
- caution if used in those with hypersensitivity to sulfonamides
- contraindicated in those with hypersensitivity to ritonavir or amprenavir
- see General Nursing points/Cautions for antiretroviral agents (p. 846)

Patient teaching and advice

- advise patient that use of antihistamines may decrease severity and duration of rash
- if vomiting occurs within 30 minutes of administration, advise patient to take dose again
- patient should be warned to seek medical advice immediately if any severe rash, blistering, mouth lesions or fever occur
- see General Patient teaching and advice for antiretroviral agents (p. 847)

tablet can be crushed and mixed with water or spoonful of yoghurt or apple puree

RITONAVIR (Norvir)

Available form

Tablets: 100 mg

Action

- protease inhibitor of both HIV-1 and HIV-2
- HIV protease is needed for viral infectivity and cleaves viral precursor polypeptide into active viral enzymes and structural proteins. Protease inhibitors prevent polypeptide cleaving and block viral maturation
- 5 metabolites but only one (M2) is active
- half-life 3–5 hours

Use

- treatment of HIV-1 infection (in combination with other antiretroviral agents or as monotherapy if combination therapy is not appropriate)

Dose

- 600 mg orally twice daily with food

Adverse effects

- peripheral neuropathy, paraesthesia, myalgia
- throat irritation, pharyngitis
- altered taste
- rash, and rarely, severe skin reactions
- elevated liver enzymes, cholesterol and triglycerides
- pancreatitis
- prolongation of PR interval
- see General Adverse effects of antiretroviral agents (p. 845)

Interactions

- contraindicated with diazepam, midazolam, triazolam, flurazepam and zolpidem because of increased sedation and risk of respiratory depression
- contraindicated with ergot alkaloids because of increased risk of ergot toxicity
- contraindicated with amiodarone, bupropion, clozapine, flecainide, pethidine, piroxicam, colchicine, lurasidone, voriconazole, alfuzosin, St John's wort, sildenafil (when used for pulmonary arterial hypertension), simvastatin, lovastatin, salmeterol, fusidic acid, neratinib, apalutamide, venetoclax and rifabutin
- not recommended with glecaprevir/pibrentasvir
- serum levels may be increased by fusidic acid and efavirenz
- may decrease serum levels of bupropion, theophylline, sulfamethoxazole–trimethoprim, warfarin, voriconazole and zidovudine
- may increase serum levels of amprenavir, bosentan, buspirone, clarithromycin, dasatinib, digoxin, efavirenz, fentanyl, fluticasone, indinavir, maraviroc, nilotinib, quetiapine, simeprevir, saquinavir, vinblastine and vincristine
- increased risk of hepatitis and hepatic decompensation if given with tipranavir (especially in those with hepatitis B or C co-infection)
- increased risk of severe hepatoxicity if given in combination with saquinavir and rifampicin
- increased risk of bleeding if given with rivaroxaban
- not recommended with PDE5 inhibitors (sildenafil, tadalafil, vardenafil)
- doses of clarithromycin $>$ 1 g/day are not recommended with ritonavir
- may produce disulfiram–alcohol-like reaction (see Glossary) if given with disulfiram or metronidazole because the formulation contains alcohol
- may decrease effectiveness of oral contraceptives by decreasing serum levels of estradiol
- increased risk of Cushing's syndrome and adrenal suppression if given with fluticasone, triamcinolone, budesonide or other glucocorticoids (inhaled, injected or intranasally)
- increased risk of cardiac or neurological adverse events if given with disopyramide
- increased risk of serotonin syndrome if given with fluoxetine
- caution if given with verapamil due to increased risk of PR interval prolongation
- caution if used with HMG-CoA reductase inhibitors (statins) atorvastatin and rosuvastatin

Nursing points/Cautions

- caution if used in those with pre-existing prolonged PR interval
- see also General Nursing points/Cautions for antiretroviral agents (p. 846)

Patient teaching and advice

- instruct patient to take with food
- advise patient that tablets should be swallowed whole, not chewed, broken or crushed
- patient should be advised to report any unusual nausea, vomiting and abdominal pain (which may be symptoms of impending pancreatitis)
- counsel female patient to use alternative form of contraception, because oral contraceptives may have reduced effectiveness
- see also General Patient teaching and advice for antiretroviral agents (p. 847)

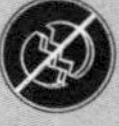

oral solution is available (has unpleasant taste which can be masked with chocolate milk, or something strong tasting such as cheese after dose). Tablet should not be crushed

Note
- contained in Kaletra with lopinavir

SAQUINAVIR (Invirase)

Available form
Tablets: 500 mg

Action
- highly selective protease inhibitor
- HIV protease is needed for viral infectivity and cleaves viral precursor polypeptide into active viral enzymes and structural proteins. Protease inhibitors prevent polypeptide cleaving and block viral maturation

Use
- HIV- or AIDS-related infection (with other antiretroviral agents)

Dose
- (treatment-experienced patient) 1 g orally twice daily within 2 hours of full meal (with ritonavir 100 mg twice daily plus other antiretroviral agents)

OR
- (treatment-naive patient) initially 500 mg orally twice daily within 2 hours of full meal (with ritonavir 100 mg twice daily plus other antiretroviral agents) for 7 days, then increasing to 1 g orally daily

Adverse effects
- anaemia
- altered taste
- prolonged QT and PR interval, cardiac arrhythmias
- rash
- paraesthesia, peripheral neuropathy
- (rare) confusion, ataxia, severe skin reaction, seizures
- see General Adverse effects of antiretroviral agents (p. 845)

Interactions
- food increases bioavailability
- contraindicated with amiodarone, flecainide, disopyramide, quinidine, lidocaine, clarithromycin, erythromycin, dasatinib, sunitinib, tacrolimus, dapsone, alfuzosin, triazolam, midazolam, ergot alkaloids, simvastatin, lovastatin, lurosidone, clozapine, chlorpromazine, quetiapine, rilpivine, atazanavir and rifampicin
- not recommended with nelfinavir, tipranavir, colchicine or salmeterol
- caution if given with fentanyl or alfentanil due to risk of respiratory depression
- caution if given with sotalol, pentamidine, fluconazole, miconazole and itraconazole due to risk of cardiac arrhythmia
- caution if given with PDE5 inhibitors (sildenafil, tadalafil, vardenafil) due to increased risk of hypotension, syncope, visual changes and priapism
- decreased serum levels may result if given with St John's wort, carbamazepine, garlic capsules, dexamethasone, efavirenz, phenobarbital (phenobarbitone), phenytoin, rifabutin or rifampicin
- caution if given with atorvastatin due to risk of myopathy. If required, pravastatin or fluvastatin are preferred
- caution if given with methadone or lopinavir/ritonavir due to increased risk of QT and/or PR interval prolongation
- not recommended with fusidic acid hemihydrate due to risk of mutual toxicity
- increased serum levels may result if given with clarithromycin, fluconazole, indinavir, itraconazole, miconazole or proton pump inhibitors
- serum warfarin levels may be affected, therefore INR should be closely monitored
- may increase serum levels of alprazolam, bosentan, calcium-channel blockers, carbamazepine, clarithromycin, ciclosporin, diazepam, digoxin, flurazepam, maravivoc, midazolam (IV), nifedipine, rifabutin, sirolimus, tacrolimus, TCAs increasing the risk of adverse events and toxicity

- increased risk of Cushing's syndrome and adrenal suppression if given with fluticasone, beclometasone (beclomethasone) and budesonide
- may decrease serum levels and efficacy of oral contraceptives

Nursing points/Cautions

- not used as monotherapy
- once daily dosing is not recommended
- ECG is recommended before starting therapy which should not be commenced if QT interval > 450 msec. ECG should be repeated after 10 days. If QT interval > 480 msec or increased > 20 msec above baseline, therapy should be stopped
- any electrolyte imbalance (especially hypokalaemia) should be corrected before starting therapy
- tablets contain lactose and are therefore not recommended in those with galactose intolerance, glucose–galactose malabsorption or Lapp lactase deficiency
- caution if used in those with prolonged diarrhoea as efficacy may be decreased
- caution if used in those with structural heart disease, pre-existing conduction system abnormalities, cardiomyopathy or ischaemic heart disease due to risk of QT and PR interval prolongation
- contraindicated in those with congenital or acquired QT prolongation or with electrolyte imbalance especially hypokalaemia
- see also General Nursing points/Cautions for antiretroviral agents (p. 846)

Patient teaching and advice

- advise female patient of child-bearing potential to use alternative form of contraception, because oral contraceptives may have reduced effectiveness
- patient should be instructed to take within 2 hours of a meal to increase bioavailability (full meal has greater effect than light meal)
- see also General Patient teaching and advice for antiretroviral agents (p. 847)

tablet can be crushed and mixed with water or spoonful of yoghurt or apple puree. Crushed tablets have an unpleasant taste

TIPRANAVIR (Aptivus)

Available form

Capsules: 250 mg

Action

- non-peptide HIV-1 protease inhibitor
- sulfonamide

Use

- treatment of HIV-1 infection (in those with antiretroviral resistant strains) (with low-dose ritonavir)

Dose

- 500 mg orally twice daily with food (with ritonavir 200 mg twice daily and at least 2 other antiretroviral agents)

Adverse effects

- elevated lipids and cholesterol, hepatitis, hepatic decompensation
- inhibits platelet aggregation
- (uncommon) intracranial haemorrhage (fatal, non-fatal)
- see General Adverse effects of antiretroviral agents (p. 845)

Interactions

- contraindicated with amiodarone, flecainide, simvastatin, lovastatin, rifampicin, St John's wort, vardenafil, sildenafil (when used for pulmonary arterial hypertension), ergot derivatives, quetiapine, alfuzosin, midazolam (oral) and triazolam
- contraindicated with colchicine in those with kidney or liver impairment

- not recommended with boceprevir, etravirine, telaprevir, cobicistat or cobicistat-containing formulations
- not recommended with salmeterol due to risk of QT prolongation, palpitations and tachycardia
- caution if given with warfarin; INR time should be closely monitored especially when starting or stopping therapy
- may decrease serum levels of abacavir, zidovudine, nevirapine, loperamide, pethidine (but increases levels of metabolite), raltegravir, etravirine, bupropion, omeprazole, dolutegravir, amprenavir, lopinavir, saquinavir, atazanavir and theophylline
- may decrease serum level of methadone, increasing risk of opiate withdrawal syndrome
- serum levels may be increased by enfuvirtide and rifabutin
- increased risk of hepatitis and hepatic decompensation if given with ritonavir (especially in those with chronic hepatitis B or hepatitis C infection)
- serum levels may be decreased by rifampicin, carbamazepine, phenobarbital (phenobarbitone), phenytoin and St John's wort
- may increase serum levels of fluoxetine, paroxetine, sertraline, rosuvastatin, atorvastatin, clarithromycin, rifabutin, rilpivirine and desipramine increasing risk of adverse effects and toxicity
- may decrease serum levels and efficacy of oral contraceptives and hormone replacement therapy
- increased liver enzymes may occur if given with valaciclovir
- caution if given with bosentan. Bosentan should be stopped at least 36 hours before starting therapy and then resumed after at least 10 days at an adjusted dose
- may alter serum levels of ciclosporin, sirolimus and tacrolimus, therefore levels should be closely monitored during therapy
- may produce disulfiram–alcohol-like reaction (see Glossary) if given with disulfiram or metronidazole because formulation contains alcohol
- not recommended with fluticasone
- not recommended with fluconazole at doses > 200 mg daily
- caution if given with itraconazole
- may have a variable effect on oral hypoglycaemic agents, therefore blood glucose levels should be closely monitored
- increased risk of non-serious rash if given with oestrogens
- increased risk of hypotension, syncope, visual changes and priapism if given with sildenafil, vardenafil and tadalafil (for erectile dysfunction)
- increased risk of bleeding if given with antiplatelet or anticoagulants with high vitamin E doses

Nursing points/Cautions

- not recommended as monotherapy
- genotyping is recommended before starting therapy in those with HIV-1 strains resistant to more than one protease inhibitor
- liver function (including cholesterol and triglyceride levels) should be measured before starting therapy and regularly throughout
- capsules contain alcohol (7%) which may need to be considered if given to pregnant or breastfeeding women, children, those with liver disease, epilepsy or alcoholism
- contains sorbitol, therefore contraindicated in those with fructose intolerance
- if used in those with chronic hepatitis B or C co-infection, liver function should be closely monitored due to risk of hepatotoxicity
- caution if given to those with advanced HIV/AIDS (increased risk of intracranial haemorrhage), a known hypersensitivity to sulfonamide or at increased risk of bleeding
- see General Nursing points/Cautions for antiretroviral agents (p. 846)

Patient teaching and advice

- advise patient to swallow capsules whole and not chew or open them
- instruct patient to immediately seek medical advice if any of the following occur:
  - rash
  - loss of appetite, tiredness, upper abdominal pain, yellowing of skin or eyes, darkening of urine, light stools
- women taking oral contraceptives should be advised to use an alternative or additional barrier. They should also be warned that they are at increased risk of developing a non-serious rash
- see also General Patient teaching and advice for antiretroviral agents (p. 847)

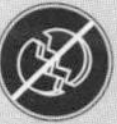

not suitable for those with swallowing difficulties

ENTRY INHIBITORS

ENFUVIRTIDE (Fuzeon)

Available form
Vial: 108 mg

Action
- fusion (HIV entry) inhibitor that specifically binds to virus protein outside the cell, stopping it from penetrating the cell
- half-life about 4 hours

Use
- treatment of HIV-1 infection (with other antiretroviral agents; in patients previously treated with antiretrovirals which were ineffective)

Dose
- 90 mg SC twice daily

Adverse effects
- (injection site reactions) pain, erythema, induration, nodules, cysts, pruritus, ecchymosis
- skin infection, cellulitis, abscess formation, sepsis, acne
- bacterial pneumonia, cough, rhinitis, nasal congestion, sinusitis, flu-like illness
- (occasionally) hypersensitivity
- see General Adverse effects of antiretroviral agents (p. 845)

Nursing points/Cautions
- not recommended as monotherapy
- injection sites should be rotated and not used if injection site reaction has occurred
- first injection should be done under supervision of a healthcare professional
- reconstitute using 1.1 mL water for injections. Vial should be tapped gently for 10 seconds, gently rolled (to avoid foaming) and allowed to stand until completely dissolved (may take up to 45 minutes). Withdraw 1 mL of solution for injection
- caution if used in those with low CD4 counts, high initial viral loads, history of IV drug use, smoking or history of lung disease as there is an increased risk of pneumonia
- see General Nursing points/Cautions for antiretroviral agents (p. 846)

Patient teaching and advice
- patient should be advised to seek medical advice if any of the following occur:
  - pneumonia (chills, fever, cough, shortness of breath, rapid breathing)
  - skin infection (not at injection site), such as red, hot and tender skin (with fever and chills)
- patient should be instructed in self-administration, including:
  - correct reconstitution and injection technique (under skin, not into muscle or veins)
  - choosing injection site that is free of infection, scars, moles or

  irritation and not irritated by clothes that sit on the waistline
  - rotation of sites (upper arm, thigh or abdomen)
  - storage requirements
  - safe disposal of used needles (including not reusing needles and disposing in puncture-resistant container)
- see General Patient teaching and advice for antiretroviral agents (p. 847)

MARAVIROC (Celsentri)

Available forms

Tablets: 150 mg, 300 mg

Action

- chemokine receptor CCR5 antagonist which selectively binds to human cytokine receptor CCR5 blocking interaction between CCR5 and HIV glycoprotein (gp120)
- half-life 13.2 hours

Use

- CCR5 tropic HIV-1 infection (with other retroviral agents)

Dose

- 150, 300 or 600 mg orally twice daily (dose depending on co-administered antiretroviral agent)

Adverse effects

- infection (upper respiratory tract, herpes, oesophageal candidiasis, influenza), fever, cough, rhinitis, sinusitis
- rash, pruritus
- myalgia, muscle spasms, arthralgia
- paraesthesia, dysaesthesia
- postural hypotension, syncope, dizziness
- (uncommon) myocardial infarction, angina
- see General Adverse effects of antiretroviral agents (p. 845)

Interactions

- caution if used with other agents known to lower blood pressure
- serum levels may be decreased if given with efavirenz, etravirine, rifabutin or rifampicin and therefore not recommended together
- serum levels may be increased if given with atazanavir, darunavir, ritonavir (or fixed combinations containing ritonavir), lopinavir, saquinavir, indinavir, clarithromycin, and itraconazole increasing risk of postural hypotension
- not recommended with St John's wort
- may decrease serum levels of fosasmprenavir/ritonavir

Nursing points/Cautions

- liver function (enzymes and bilirubin) monitoring is recommended before starting and regularly during therapy
- only recommended in those with detectable CCR5 tropic HIV-1, therefore tropism and resistance testing is recommended before starting therapy
- caution in those who are at risk of cardiovascular events, history of or risk factors for postural hypotension or pre-existing liver disease
- caution if used in those with severe renal insufficiency due to increased risk of hypotension
- not recommended in those with dual/mixed or CXCR4 tropic HIV-1
- see also General Nursing points/Cautions for antiretroviral agents (p. 846)

Patient teaching and advice

- patient should be advised to report any signs of frequent infection, such as fever, chills, sore throat, mouth ulcers or flu-like symptoms
- instruct patient to immediately seek medical advice if chest pain or angina occurs
- warn patient not to drive or operate machinery if hypotension and dizziness occur

- see also General Patient teaching and advice for antiretroviral agents (p. 847)

tablet can be crushed and mixed with water or spoonful of yoghurt or apple puree

INTEGRASE INHIBITORS

DOLUTEGRAVIR (Tivicay)

Available forms
Tablets: 10 mg, 25 mg, 50 mg

Action
- HIV integrase inhibitor that blocks the strand transfer step of retroviral DNA integration needed for HIV replication
- half-life about 14 hours

Use
- treatment of HIV-1 infection (with other antiretrovirals) in adults and children (over 12 years) weighing more than 40 kg

Dose
- (no resistance to integrase class) 50 mg orally daily **OR**
- (resistance to integrase class) 50 mg orally twice daily

Adverse effects
- rash
- (rare) depression, suicidal ideation
- see General Adverse effects of antiretroviral agents (p. 845)

Interactions
- plasma levels may be decreased by efavirenz, etravirine, nevirapine, tipranavir/ritonavir, fosamprenavir/ritonavir, carbamazepine, phenytoin, phenobarbital (phenobarbitone), St John's wort, oxcarbazepine and rifampicin
- plasma levels may be decreased by antacids containing magnesium or aluminium, calcium or iron supplements
- plasma levels may be increased by atazanavir and atazanavir/ritonavir combination
- may increase serum levels of metformin increasing risk of hypoglycaemia

Nursing points/Cautions
- liver function tests are recommended especially in those with hepatitis B and/or C co-infection
- caution if used in those with pre-existing history of depression or other psychiatric illness
- see General Nursing points/Cautions for antiretroviral agents (p. 846)

Patient teaching and advice
- instruct patient to immediately seek medical advice if any severe rash or rash with fever, malaise, fatigue, muscle or joint pain, blisters, oral lesions, conjunctivitis or facial swelling occurs
- advise patient to take aluminium- or magnesium-containing antacids, calcium or iron supplements either 2 hours before or 6 hours after therapy
- if patient has diabetes treated using metformin, he/she should be warned to closely monitor blood glucose levels as there is an increased risk of hypoglycaemia occurring during therapy
- patient (or carer/family member) should be advised to immediately seek medical advice if any signs of depression such as sadness, withdrawal from friends or previously pleasurable activities, or any attempts at self-harm occur
- see also General Patient teaching and advice for antiretroviral agents (p. 847)

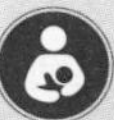

should only be used during pregnancy if benefits outweigh risks

not recommended during breastfeeding

tablet can be crushed and mixed with water or spoonful of yoghurt or apple puree

Note
- contained in Triumeq with abacavir and lamivudine, Jaluca with rilpivine and Dovato with lamivudine

RALTEGRAVIR POTASSIUM (Isentress)

Available forms
Tablets: 400 mg, 600 mg; Chewable tablets: 25 mg, 100 mg

Action
- HIV integrase strand transfer inhibitor (integrase is an HIV encoded enzyme required for viral replication)

Use
- treatment of multi-resistant HIV-1 infection (where current therapy has failed) (with other antiretroviral agents)

Dose
- (treatment-experienced patients) 400 mg orally twice daily (with other antiretroviral agents) **OR**
- (treatment-naive patients) 1200 mg orally once daily (with other antiretroviral agents)

Adverse effects
- elevated creatine kinase levels
- (rare) severe skin reactions
- see also General Adverse effects of antiretroviral agents (p. 845)

Interactions
- serum levels may be decreased by rifampicin, phenytoin, carbamazepine or phenobarbital (phenobarbitone)
- serum levels may be decreased if given with aluminium or magnesium-containing antacids and are therefore not recommended together
- serum levels may be increased if given with omeprazole
- not recommended with atazanavir and tipravir/ritonavit

Nursing points/Cautions
- maximum dose of chewable tablets is 300 mg twice daily
- tablets and chewable tablets are not bioequivalent
- 1200 mg dose should be given as 2 × 600 mg <u>NOT</u> 3 × 400 mg
- chewable tablets contain phenylalanine and are therefore not recommended in those with phenylketonuria
- caution if used in those at risk of myopathy or rhabdomyolysis

Patient teaching and advice
- (400 or 600 mg tablets) advise patient that tablets should be swallowed whole, not chewed, crushed or divided
- (chewable tablets) should be chewed, not swallowed
- instruct patient to separate therapy at least 2 hours from magnesium or aluminium-containing antacids
- patient should be advised to immediately seek medical advice if any rash (especially severe or blistering), fever, malaise or fatigue, joint or muscle ache, facial swelling or mouth ulceration/blistering occurs
- see General Patient teaching and advice for antiretroviral agents (p. 847)

chewable tablets are available

BLADDER FUNCTION DISORDER AGENTS

The bladder, a functional internal sphincter and a striated external sphincter, are responsible for the storage and intermittent evacuation of urine. The bladder and internal sphincter are made up of detrusor muscle. The sphincters control continence and, in the male, the internal sphincter is also responsible for preventing the reflux of semen from the urethra during ejaculation. The sphincters relax, allowing the bladder to push the urine into the urethra; this function involves afferent and efferent nerve fibres in the spinal cord. For a person to urinate, there is relaxation of the perineum (voluntary), increased tension in the abdominal wall, contraction of the detrusor muscle and opening of the internal sphincter, followed by relaxation of the external sphincter (Ropper et al 2019).

Causes of bladder function disorder include:

- destruction of the spinal cord below T12, which causes bladder paralysis, resulting in no awareness that the bladder is full
- diseases of the spinal cord, including the nerves that innervate the bladder
- interruption of afferent fibres from the bladder (e.g. diabetes, tabes dorsalis); urinary retention may also occur
- spinal cord lesions above T12 causing neurogenic bladder (e.g. multiple sclerosis, traumatic myelopathy), resulting in accumulation of urine and distension of the bladder
- stretched bladder wall injury, which may occur because of obstruction of the bladder neck (e.g. prostatic hypertrophy) and repeated overdistension of the bladder, resulting in fibroses of the bladder wall increasing bladder capacity; further, contractions are not sufficient to empty the bladder, resulting in residual urine remaining in the bladder (increasing the risk of infection)
- frontal lobe problems resulting in the person ignoring the urge to void because of a confused mental state; and/**or**
- delay in developing inhibition of micturition, resulting in nocturnal enuresis or urinary incontinence during sleep (Ropper et al 2019).

Agents used in the treatment of bladder function disorders include cholinergic agents that stimulate contraction of the bladder and sympathomimetic agents which relax the urinary sphincter facilitating urination (Ropper et al 2019).

ALFUZOSIN HYDROCHLORIDE (Xatral SR)

Available form

Tablets (prolonged-release): 10 mg

Action

- selective alpha-1 adrenoreceptor antagonist (alpha-1 receptors are found in the trigone of the bladder, urethra and prostate)
- decreases urethral pressure, resulting in decreased resistance to urine flow during micturition
- peak effect 9 hours, half-life 9.1 hours

Use

- symptoms of benign prostatic hyperplasia

Dose

- 10 mg orally daily immediately after food

Adverse effects

- rhinitis, pharyngitis, upper respiratory tract infection
- headache, dizziness, malaise, asthenia, fatigue
- nausea, abdominal pain, gastralgia, vomiting
- arthralgia
- pruritus
- renal calculi
- (rare) intraoperative floppy iris syndrome, priapism

Interactions

- contraindicated with other alpha adrenoceptor blocking agents because of increased risk of postural hypotension
- increased serum levels may occur if given with itraconazole or ritonavir, and are therefore contraindicated together
- caution if used with other antihypertensive agents or agents known to prolong QT interval
- caution if given with nitrates
- not recommended with phenoxybenzamine or labetalol
- increased risk of BP instability if given with general anaesthetics
- caution if taken with grapefruit juice, St John's wort or milk thistle

Nursing points/Cautions

- blood pressure should be measured before starting and regularly during therapy (especially in those taking concurrent antihypertensive agents)
- patient should be thoroughly assessed for prostate cancer (e.g. digital examination, prostate-specific antigen (PSA) blood test) before starting and regularly during therapy
- should be discontinued 24 hours before surgery
- if cataract surgery is planned, surgeon should be notified of therapy because of the risk of intraoperative floppy iris syndrome
- caution in those with known hypersensitivity to other alpha adrenoceptor blocking agents
- caution if used in the elderly or those with cardiac disease and/or concurrent treatment with antihypertensive agents
- caution in those with symptomatic orthostatic hypotension or acquired/congenital prolongation of QT interval
- not recommended in those with Parkinson's disease, multiple sclerosis, unstable angina or severe heart disease
- contraindicated in those with history of liver insufficiency or orthostatic hypotension

Patient teaching and advice

- advise patient to swallow tablet whole (not crushed, chewed or divided)

- warn patient against driving or operating machinery if dizziness occurs
- instruct patient to take care when going from lying or sitting position as light-headedness and dizziness may occur. Further, if any dizziness, fatigue, sweating or feeling faint occurs, patient should be advised to lie down until symptoms totally disappear
- advise patient to avoid grapefruit juice and herbal preparations such as St John's wort during therapy
- patient should be advised to seek medical advice if any of the following occur:
  - irregular heartbeat or palpitations
  - prolonged painful erection
- see also General Patient teaching and advice (p. xxvii)

tablet should not be crushed, broken or chewed or dispersed in water

BETHANECHOL CHLORIDE (Urocarb)

Available form
Tablets: 10 mg

Action
- parasympathomimetic agent that is not inactivated by acetylcholinesterase, so has a prolonged action at receptor sites
- produces rapid but transitory increase in tone and motility of the urinary bladder, stomach and intestine
- effective within 30–90 minutes (oral), duration about 1 hour

Use
- acute postoperative and post-partum urinary retention (non-obstructive)
- neurogenic atony of urinary bladder (with retention)

Dose
- 10–30 mg orally or sublingually 3–4 times daily 1 hour before or 2 hours after food

Adverse effects
- sweating, flushing of skin
- abdominal discomfort, salivation

Nursing points/Cautions
- urinary tract infection should be ruled out before starting therapy
- have atropine (0.6 mg) SC available to reverse undesired effects
- contraindicated in those with asthma, hyperthyroidism, hypotension, bradycardia, coronary insufficiency, peptic ulcer, urinary tract infection, epilepsy or Parkinsonism

Patient teaching and advice
- advise patient to take on an empty stomach to prevent nausea and vomiting
- female patient of childbearing years should be counselled regarding the need to use adequate contraception to avoid pregnancy during therapy
- see also General Patient teaching and advice (p. xxvii)

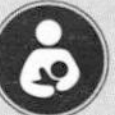

not recommended during pregnancy because of potent excitatory effect on smooth muscle

tablet can be placed under the tongue and allowed to dissolve before swallowing or crushed and mixed with water

DARIFENACIN HYDROBROMIDE (Enablex)

Available forms
Tablets (prolonged-release): 7.5 mg, 15 mg

Action

- selective muscarinic M3 antagonist (M3 receptors appear to control urinary bladder muscle contraction)
- decreases frequency of incontinence, micturition and urgency while increasing functional bladder capacity
- peak effect 6 hours, half-life 12.8–18.7 hours

Use

- treatment of detrusor overactivity (with symptoms of urgency, frequency and/or incontinence)

Dose

- initially 7.5 mg orally daily, increasing to 15 mg daily after 2 weeks if greater symptom relief is required

Adverse effects

- abdominal pain, constipation, dry mouth, dyspepsia, nausea, vomiting, diarrhoea, weight gain
- asthenia, dizziness, headache
- flu-like symptoms
- dry nasal passages, rhinitis, sinusitis, pharyngitis
- arthralgia, back pain
- hypertension
- urinary tract infection, vaginitis
- abnormal vision (including blurred vision), dry eyes
- dry skin
- rash, pruritus
- peripheral oedema

Interactions

- frequency and/or severity of effects increased if given with other anticholinergic agents including anti-Parkinson's agents and TCAs
- caution if given with flecainide or TCAs
- caution if given with agents such as oral bisphosphonates that cause or worsen oesophagitis
- if given with itraconazole, miconazole or ritonavir, dose should be no greater than 7.5 mg
- caution if given with paroxetine, cimetidine or fluoxetine
- may increase serum levels of digoxin, therefore serum levels should be monitored when starting, stopping or adjusting dose

Nursing points/Cautions

- dose should be no greater than 7.5 mg in those with moderate liver impairment
- caution if used in those being treated for narrow-angle glaucoma, decreased gastrointestinal motility, gastro-oesophageal reflux, oesophagitis, autonomic neuropathy, hiatus hernia, significant bladder outflow obstruction, risk of urinary retention, severe constipation (< 2 bowel motions/week), gastrointestinal obstructive disorder or pre-existing cardiac disease
- not recommended in those with severe liver impairment
- contraindicated in those with urinary retention, gastric retention or uncontrolled glaucoma

Patient teaching and advice

- advise patient that prolonged-release tablets should be swallowed whole, not chewed or crushed
- warn patient that dry mouth, nose and/or eyes occur commonly but usually disappear with ongoing therapy
- patient should be advised not to drive or operate machinery if blurred vision, dizziness or drowsiness occurs
- instruct patient to seek medical advice immediately if any of the following occur:
  - painful red eye with associated loss of vision (may be signs of undiagnosed glaucoma) or
  - diarrhoea (which may be the first sign of intestinal obstruction, especially in those with an ileostomy or colostomy)

- see also General Patient teaching and advice (p. xxvii)

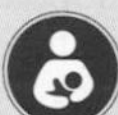

not recommended during pregnancy or breastfeeding unless benefits outweigh potential risks

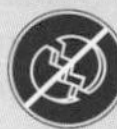

tablets should not be crushed, broken or chewed or dispersed in water

DUTASTERIDE (Avodart)

Available form

Capsules: 500 microgram

Action

- inhibits conversion of testosterone to 5-alpha dihydrotestosterone (DHT) (which is responsible for development and enlargement of prostate gland)
- active metabolite
- very long half-life (3–5 weeks), serum levels remain detectable for 4–6 months after stopping therapy

Use

- symptomatic benign prostatic hyperplasia (monotherapy or with alpha adrenoceptor blocking antagonist)

Dose

- 500 microgram orally daily

Adverse effects

- impotence, decreased libido, ejaculation disorders
- breast enlargement and tenderness
- decrease in prostate-specific antigen (PSA)
- (rare) increased risk of high-grade prostate cancer, alopecia (mainly body hair), breast cancer, testicular pain/swelling

Interactions

- increased serum levels may occur if given with verapamil and diltiazem

Nursing points/Cautions

- patient should be thoroughly assessed for prostate cancer (e.g. digital examination, PSA blood test) before starting and regularly during therapy. It should be noted that dutasteride lowers PSA by almost 50% after 6 months of therapy, even in the presence of prostate cancer. It is recommended that new PSA baseline is established after 6 months of therapy and then monitored regularly thereafter
- total serum PSA returns to baseline within 6 months of stopping therapy
- may take 6 months of therapy before benefits are apparent
- (combination therapy with alpha adrenoceptor blocking antagonist) cardiovascular function should be assessed before starting therapy. Dose titration is required to avoid postural hypotension, dizziness and syncope if given with terazosin and prazosin (but not tamsulosin or alfuzosin)
- caution if used in those with liver disease (because of very long half-life)
- contraindicated in those with known hypersensitivity to other 5-alpha reductase inhibitors, severe liver impairment or in women or children

Patient teaching and advice

- advise patient to swallow capsules whole without breaking or chewing
- patient (and female partner/carer) should be advised that women and children should avoid contact with leaking capsules. If contact occurs, skin should be washed immediately with warm water and soap
- advise patient to seek medical advice immediately if there are any changes in breast tissue, including lumps or discharge from nipples
- instruct patient not to donate blood within 6 months of stopping therapy

- patient should be instructed to wear condom during sex as dutasteride has been detected in semen
- (combination therapy) warn patient against driving or operating machinery if dizziness occurs
- (combination therapy) patient should be advised to take care getting out of bed or standing from sitting position to avoid dizziness or fainting
- see also General Patient teaching and advice (p. xxvii)

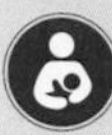

contraindicated in women. Dutasteride is absorbed through the skin and pregnant women should avoid contact with capsules as absorption may result in anomalies to male fetus (i.e. may inhibit the development of male external genitalia)

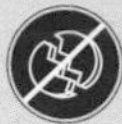

capsules should not be opened, crushed or chewed

Note
- combined with tamsulosin hydrochloride in Duodart and Doubluts

FINASTERIDE (A&M Fintab-1, Finapen, Finasta, Finnacar, Finpro, Propecia, Proscar)

Available forms
Tablets: 1 mg, 5 mg

Action
- inhibits enzyme (type II 5-alpha reductase) that converts testosterone to dihydrotestosterone (DHT), decreasing amounts circulating and in the prostate gland
- hair follicles also contain type II 5-alpha reductase. Finasteride decreases scalp and serum DHT levels, which may reverse balding
- peak effect 2 hours, half-life 6–8 hours

Use
- benign prostatic hyperplasia (with enlarged prostate)
- male pattern baldness (Propecia)

Dose
- (benign prostatic hyperplasia) 5 mg orally daily for 6–12 months **OR**
- (male pattern baldness) 1 mg orally daily (Propecia)

Adverse effects
- impotence, decreased libido, decreased ejaculate, ejaculation disorders, testicular pain
- breast tenderness and enlargement
- rash, pruritus
- depression
- headache
- (rare) increased risk of high-grade prostate cancer, breast cancer, hypersensitivity reaction

Nursing points/Cautions
- patient should be thoroughly assessed for prostate cancer (e.g. digital examination, prostate-specific antigen (PSA) blood test) before starting and regularly during therapy. It should be noted that dutasteride lowers PSA by almost 50% after 6 months of therapy, even in the presence of prostate cancer. It is recommended that new PSA baseline is established after 6 months of therapy and then monitored regularly thereafter
- total serum PSA returns to baseline within 6 months of stopping therapy
- therapy should be reviewed after 6–12 months and continued if appropriate
- (male pattern baldness) effectiveness of treatment (increased hair growth and/or decreased further hair loss) may not be apparent for at least 12 weeks
- (male pattern baldness) efficacy has not been shown in those > 41 years

- tablets contain lactose and are therefore not recommended in those with galactose intolerance, Lapp lactase intolerance or glucose–galactose malabsorption
- caution if used in men with diminished urinary flow and/or large residual volume as obstruction may occur
- contraindicated in women and children

Patient teaching and advice

- patient should be advised that therapy may not decrease symptoms related to prostatic hyperplasia
- advise patient to seek medical advice immediately if there are any changes in breast tissue including lumps or discharge from nipples
- counsel patient that tablets should not be handled by pregnant partner because of risk to male fetus
- see General Patient teaching and advice (p. xxvii)

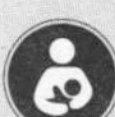

patient should be advised that his sexual partner should avoid exposure to his semen or handling crushed tablets if she is or may become pregnant

tablets can be dispersed in 10–20 mL of water or crushed and mixed with spoonful of yoghurt or apple puree

pregnant women should not crush or disperse tablets

MIRABEGRON (Betmiga)

Available forms

Tablets (prolonged-release): 25 mg, 50 mg

Action

- beta3 adrenergic agonist that relaxes bladder smooth muscle increasing mean voided volume per micturition and decreased frequency of non-voiding contractions with no effect on voiding pressure or residual urine
- may enhance urine storage function by stimulating beta3 adrenoceptors in the bladder
- peak activity 3–4 hours, half-life about 50 hours

Use

- symptomatic treatment of urgency, increased micturition frequency and/or urgency incontinence in those with overactive bladder syndrome

Dose

- 25 mg orally daily, increasing to 50 mg if needed

Adverse effects

- hypertension, tachycardia
- nasopharyngitis
- urinary tract infection, urinary retention
- headache, fatigue
- abdominal pain, diarrhoea, constipation, nausea
- upper respiratory tract infection
- arthralgia
- (infrequently) blurred vision, dizziness, somnolence, angioedema

Interactions

- may increase serum levels of flecainide, metoprolol and desipramine
- may increase serum levels of digoxin, increasing risk of adverse effects, therefore serum levels should be closely monitored
- caution if given with warfarin. INR should be closely monitored, especially when starting or stopping therapy
- caution if given with agents known to prolong QT interval, such as sotalol, amiodarone, haloperidol, erythromycin and clarithromycin

Nursing points/Cautions

- BP should be monitored before starting and regularly during therapy (especially if patient is hypertensive)
- caution if used in those with bladder outlet obstruction or taking antimuscarinic (anticholinergic) agents

- caution if used in those with known prolongation of QT interval or taking medication that prolongs QT interval
- caution if used in those with moderate (grade 2) hypertension (systolic BP 160–190 mmHg or diastolic BP 100–109 mmHg)
- not recommended for those with end-stage kidney disease, requiring haemodialysis or with severe liver impairment
- contraindicated in those with severe uncontrolled hypertension (systolic BP ≥ 180 mmHg and/or diastolic BP ≥ 110 mmHg)

Patient teaching and advice

- advise patient to swallow tablets whole with liquids but tablet should not be chewed, crushed or divided
- patient should be warned not to drive or operate machinery if any dizziness, somnolence or blurred vision occurs
- instruct patient to seek medical advice immediately if any of the following occur:
  - fast or irregular heartbeat
  - any swelling of eyelids, lips, throat or tongue
  - urinary tract infection (burning or pain passing urine, urge to pass urine frequently, cloudy and/or offensive-smelling urine)
- see also General Patient teaching and advice (p. xxvii)

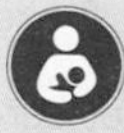

not recommended during pregnancy or breastfeeding

tablets should not be crushed, broken or chewed or dispersed in water

OXYBUTYNIN (Ditropan, Oxytrol Transdermal System)

Available forms

Tablets: 5 mg; Transdermal patch: 3.9 mg/24 hours

Action

- antispasmodic, anticholinergic
- relaxes smooth muscle in bladder, decreasing urgency and frequency during incontinence and voluntary urination
- greater antispasmodic activity than atropine sulfate monohydrate
- active metabolite has activity similar to oxybutynin on detrusor muscle
- (tablets) peak activity 1 hour, half-life 2 hours

Use

- treatment of detrusor over activity (frequency, urgency and/or incontinence)

Dose

- 5 mg orally 2–3 times daily (daily maximum 20 mg) **OR**
- 1 transdermal patch twice weekly

Adverse effects

- dry mouth, constipation, nausea, vomiting, diarrhoea
- headache, confusion, drowsiness, dizziness
- urinary urgency, difficulty and retention
- impotence
- flushing and dryness of skin, decreased sweating
- dry eyes, blurred vision
- suppresses lactation
- (less common) raised intraocular pressure, heat intolerance, hypersensitivity
- (transdermal patch) pruritus, erythema, rash, vesicles, dry mouth, constipation, dysuria, blurred vision, diarrhoea

Interactions

- additive anticholinergic effects with TCAs, phenothiazines, amantadine, digoxin, hyoscine, anti-Parkinson's agents and some antihistamines
- not recommended with alcohol or other sedative agents as drowsiness may be enhanced
- caution if used with agents that exacerbate oesophagitis (e.g. bisphosphonates)

- may alter absorption of other medications given at the same time because of effect on GI motility

Nursing points/Cautions

- patient should be assessed before starting therapy (including cystometry) to determine cause of bladder dysfunction and to treat any infection (if needed). Cystometry is also recommended regularly to assess effectiveness of therapy
- dose should be started at 2.5 mg in the elderly and slowly increased if needed
- caution if used in those with significant bladder outflow obstruction, cognitive disorders, Parkinson's disease, prostatic hypertrophy, tachycardia, hypertension, hyperthyroidism, coronary artery disease, congestive cardiac failure, cardiac arrhythmias and hiatus hernia associated with reflux oesophagitis
- caution if used in those with kidney or liver impairment
- contraindicated in those with urinary or gastric retention, partial or complete gastrointestinal obstruction, paralytic ileus, intestinal atony, uncontrolled glaucoma or increased intraocular pressure associated with shallow anterior chamber, severe ulcerative colitis, megacolon, toxic megacolon, myasthenia gravis, obstructive uropathy or unstable cardiovascular status in acute haemorrhage

Patient teaching and advice

- (transdermal patch) advise patient about correct use of transdermal patch, including:
    - use calendar to record when patch is applied
    - only use one patch at a time
    - apply to clean, dry skin (avoid skin folds or areas that are inflamed, irritated or have rashes)
    - use a different area of skin (stomach area, hips or buttocks) each time and do not reuse same area within 7 days
    - avoid waist area as clothes may rub and cause the patch to roll or be dislodged
    - do not apply to areas that have had oils, lotions or powder applied to them (as these will prevent patch sticking to skin)
    - do not expose patch to sunlight
    - contact with water (e.g. bathing or showering, swimming, exercising) is okay as long as patch is not dislodged during activity
    - if patch partly rolls up or falls off, it should be pressed back into place. However, if it does not stay on, it should be replaced with a new patch
    - remove patch slowly to prevent damaging skin
    - wash area of removed patch with soap and water to remove any adhesive, but do not use alcohol or nail polish remover as these will irritate skin
    - used patches should be folded together and carefully disposed of
- patient should be advised not to drive or operate machinery if blurred vision, dizziness or drowsiness occurs
- warn patient to take care taking medication during high temperatures or physical exercise or if febrile because of increased risk of heat stroke from decreased sweating
- advise patient to avoid alcohol during therapy
- instruct patient to immediately report:
    - painful red eye with associated loss of vision (may be signs of undiagnosed glaucoma) or
    - diarrhoea (which may be the first sign of intestinal obstruction, especially in those with an ileostomy or colostomy)
- see also General Patient and teaching advice (p. xxvii)

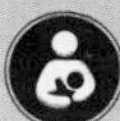
not recommended during pregnancy or breastfeeding unless benefits outweigh potential risks

tablets can be crushed and mixed with water or spoonful of yoghurt or apple puree

PENTOSAN POLYSULFATE SODIUM (Elmiron)

Available form

Capsules: 100 mg

Action

- heparin-like derivative similar to glycosaminoglycans
- inhibits formation of activated factor Xa, resulting in anticoagulant activity which is about 1/15 of heparin
- mobilises tissue plasminogen activator resulting in fibrinolytic activity
- mediates release of lipoprotein lipases
- appears to bind to transitional epithelium in the bladder, coating denuded areas and restoring normal barrier between bladder epithelium and urine

Use

- treatment of interstitial cystitis

Dose

- 100 mg orally 3 times daily 1 hour before meals or 2 hours after

Adverse effects

- headache, dizziness
- peripheral oedema
- nausea, dyspepsia, diarrhoea
- elevated liver function tests
- (rare) mood swings, suicidal ideation

Interactions

- contraindicated with heparin or oral anticoagulants

Nursing points/Cautions

- interstitial cystitis should be confirmed before starting therapy
- complete blood count, PT, APTT, liver and renal function tests and serum calcium levels should be monitored regularly during long-term therapy
- if response is not adequate after 6–8 weeks, symptoms recur or new symptoms arise, cystoscopy is recommended
- symptoms may recur when prolonged therapy is discontinued
- caution if used in those with bleeding disorders or at risk of bleeding (e.g. elderly, alcohol-dependent patient)
- not recommended for undiagnosed urogenital bleeding
- contraindicated in those with haemophilia or active or history of bleeding

Patient teaching and advice

- advise patient it may take 6–8 weeks before a response is seen
- instruct patient to take tablets either 1 hour before or 2 hours after meals
- patient should be warned against driving or operating machinery if dizziness occurs
- instruct patient to seek medical advice immediately if any of the following occur:
  - worsening of bladder symptoms
  - any ongoing sadness, withdrawal from friends or previously pleasurable activities, or any attempts at self-harm
- see also General Patient teaching and advice (p. xxvii)

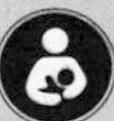
not recommended during pregnancy or breastfeeding

SILODOSIN (Urorec)

Available forms

Capsules: 4 mg, 8 mg

Action

- selective alpha 1A (α_{1A}) adrenoceptor antagonist (mostly located in

prostate, bladder base and neck, prostatic capsule and urethra) causing relaxation of smooth muscle in these tissues, decreasing bladder outlet resistance with any impact on detrusor smooth muscle contraction. This results in improvement of lower urinary tract symptoms associated with benign prostatic hyperplasia, including both storage (irritative) and voiding (obstructive) symptoms
- lower affinity for cardiovascular α_{1B}-adrenoceptors
- active metabolite that reaches plasma concentrations higher than parent compound

Use
- relief of lower urinary tract symptoms associated with benign prostatic hyperplasia in adult men

Dose
- 8 mg orally daily, swallowed whole with food

Adverse effects
- diarrhoea
- dizziness, headache, insomnia
- urinary tract infection, retrograde ejaculation, erectile dysfunction, loss of libido
- influenza, nasal congestion, nasopharyngitis, sinusitis, rhinitis
- hypertension, orthostatic hypotension, tachycardia
- (rare) intraoperative floppy iris syndrome

Interactions
- not recommended with other alpha adrenoceptor blocking agents
- not recommended with itraconazole, ritonavir or ciclosporin
- not recommended with strong P-glycoprotein inhibitors such as clarithromycin, erythromycin and verapamil
- caution if used with sildenafil or tadalafil

Nursing points/Cautions
- patient should be examined before starting therapy to rule out prostatic cancer which may present with similar symptoms
- if cataract surgery is planned, surgeon should be notified of therapy because of the risk of intraoperative floppy iris syndrome
- caution if used in those with moderate kidney impairment. Lower starting dose is recommended and caution if dose is increased to 8 mg
- not recommended in patients with orthostatic hypotension or severe liver impairment
- not recommended in patients who are scheduled for cataract surgery

Patient teaching and advice
- instruct patient to take capsule at same time every day with food. Capsule should be swallowed whole without chewing, crushing or breaking
- instruct patient to take care when going from lying or sitting position as light-headedness and dizziness may occur. Further, if any dizziness, fatigue, sweating or feeling faint occurs, patient should be advised to lie down until symptoms totally disappear
- warn patient not to drive or operate machinery if dizziness occurs
- inform patient that fertility may be temporarily affected during therapy
- see also General Patient teaching and advice (p. xxvii)

capsules can be opened and contents mixed with apple puree and eaten immediately (however, capsule contents should not be chewed)

SOLIFENACIN SUCCINATE (Solicare, Vesicare)

Available forms
Tablets: 5 mg, 10 mg

Action

- muscarinic receptor antagonist (muscarinic receptors are important in urinary bladder smooth muscle contraction as well as stimulating salivary secretion)
- peak activity 3–8 hours, half-life 45–68 hours

Use

- treatment of detrusor overactivity (urgency, frequency and/or incontinence)

Dose

- initially 5 mg orally daily, increasing to 10 mg if needed

Adverse effects

- dry mouth, constipation, dyspepsia, abdominal pain, nausea, vomiting
- fatigue, headache, dizziness, insomnia, depression
- blurred vision, dry eyes
- cough, flu-like symptoms
- hypertension
- peripheral oedema
- urinary retention, dysuria, urinary tract infection
- (rare) QT prolongation, angioedema, anaphylaxis

Interactions

- if given with ritonavir, itraconazole, nelfinavir, ciclosporin or macrolide antibiotics, dose should not exceed 5 mg daily
- caution if given with verapamil, diltiazem, rifampicin, phenytoin or carbamazepine
- caution if given with agents known to prolong QT interval (or cause electrolyte imbalance, especially hypokalaemia) including erythromycin, sotalol, disopyramide, droperidol, chlorpromazine, haloperidol, amiodarone, amitriptyline and fluconazole
- caution if used with medications that increase risk of oesophagitis, such as bisphosphonates

Nursing points/Cautions

- tablets contain lactose and are therefore not recommended in those with galactose intolerance, Lapp lactase intolerance or glucose–galactose malabsorption
- caution in those who have a history or risk of prolonged QT interval, autonomic neuropathy, undergoing treatment for narrow-angle glaucoma, risk of decreased gastrointestinal motility, gastrointestinal obstructive disorders, decreased liver or kidney function, clinically significant bladder overflow obstruction or hiatus hernia associated with reflux oesophagitis
- contraindicated in those with urinary or gastric retention, partial or complete gastrointestinal obstruction, paralytic ileus, intestinal atony, uncontrolled glaucoma or increased intraocular pressure associated with shallow anterior chamber, severe ulcerative colitis, megacolon, toxic megacolon, myasthenia gravis, obstructive uropathy, severe liver impairment or on haemodialysis

Patient teaching and advice

- patients should be advised to take tablets whole (not crushed or broken) with liquid
- warn patient to avoid driving or operating heavy machinery if dizziness or blurred vision occur
- advise patient to immediately seek medical advice if any of the following occur:
  - worsening of bladder symptoms
  - sudden fainting for no reason or after exercise/emotional excitement, rapid or erratic heartbeat
  - any swelling of lips, tongue or eyes
- see also General Patient teaching and advice (p. xxvii)

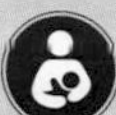

should only be used during pregnancy if potential benefits outweigh risks

not recommended during breastfeeding

tablet can be crushed and mixed with water or spoonful of yoghurt or apple puree

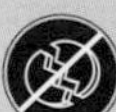

safety glasses should be worn when crushing tablets to avoid any contact with eyes as this can cause eye damage

TAMSULOSIN HYDROCHLORIDE (Flomaxtra, Flosix)

Available form

Tablets (prolonged-release): 400 microgram

Action

- alpha adrenoceptor blocking agent with no effects on beta adrenoceptors (alpha adrenoceptors are found in distal urethral sphincter and bladder neck smooth muscle, as well as hyperplastic prostate gland)
- inhibition reduces bladder outflow resistance, improving urinary flow and frequency of micturition, as well as reducing the volume of residual urine in the bladder
- half-life about 15 hours

Use

- benign prostatic hypertrophy

Dose

- 400 microgram orally daily

Adverse effects

- abnormal ejaculation
- dizziness, insomnia
- blurred vision
- (uncommonly) postural hypotension, palpitations, headache, rash, pruritus, urticaria
- (rare) intraoperative floppy iris syndrome (during cataract surgery), priapism, photosensitivity, severe skin reaction

Interactions

- contraindicated with other alpha adrenoceptor blocking agents
- increased serum levels may occur if given with cimetidine
- caution if used with paroxetine
- decreased serum levels may occur if given with furosemide (frusemide)

Nursing points/Cautions

- prostate cancer and other urological conditions should be ruled out before starting therapy
- if cataract surgery is planned, surgeon should be notified of therapy because of the risk of intraoperative floppy iris syndrome
- caution if used in those with sulfonamide allergy
- not indicated for children or women
- not recommended in those who have experienced angina or myocardial infarction in previous 6 months
- contraindicated in those with a history of orthostatic hypotension, severe kidney or liver impairment

Patient teaching and advice

- patient should be advised to swallow capsule whole (not broken or chewed)
- warn patient against driving or operating machinery if dizziness occurs
- instruct patient to take care when going from lying or sitting position as light-headedness and dizziness may occur. Further, if any dizziness, fatigue, sweating or feeling faint occurs, patient should be advised to lie down until symptoms totally disappear
- advise patient to seek medical advice immediately if any of the following occur:
  - prolonged painful erection
  - severe skin reactions, including blistering
- see also General Patient teaching and advice (p. xxvii)

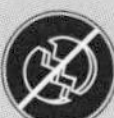

tablet should not be crushed, broken or chewed or dispersed in water

Note

- combined with dutasteride in Duodart

TOLTERODINE TARTRATE (Detrusitol)

Available forms

Tablets: 1 mg, 2 mg

Action

- muscarinic receptor antagonist (anticholinergic) (muscarinic receptors are important in urinary bladder smooth muscle contraction, as well as stimulating salivary secretion)
- active metabolite (same activity as tolterodine)

Use

- treatment of detrusor overactivity (urgency, frequency and/or incontinence)

Dose

- 1–2 mg orally twice daily

Adverse effects

- dry mouth, abdominal pain, constipation, dyspepsia, vomiting, nausea, diarrhoea, ulcerative stomatitis
- palpitations, hypertension, abnormal ECG
- headache, fatigue, malaise, migraine, somnolence, dizziness
- allergy, acne, pruritus, dry skin
- blurred vision, dry eyes
- abnormal liver enzymes
- asthma, bronchitis, cough, rhinitis, sinusitis
- dysuria, urinary tract infection
- leg pain, pain, arthralgia
- (rare) prolongation of QT interval

Interactions

- caution if given with agents known to prolong QT interval (or cause hypokalaemia) including erythromycin, sotalol, disopyramide, droperidol, chlorpromazine, haloperidol, amiodarone, amitriptyline and fluconazole
- not recommended with erythromycin, clarithromycin, itraconazole, miconazole, ritonavir, indinavir
- additive anticholinergic effects with TCAs, phenothiazines, amantadine, digoxin, hyoscine, anti-Parkinson's agents and some antihistamines
- may decrease effects of metoclopramide
- serum levels may be increased by fluoxetine

Nursing points/Cautions

- dose should be limited to 1 mg daily in those with severe kidney or liver impairment
- if there has been no response after 6 months, consideration to an alternative therapy should be given
- caution in those who have a history or risk of prolonged QT interval, autonomic neuropathy, undergoing treatment for narrow-angle glaucoma, risk of decreased gastrointestinal motility, gastrointestinal obstructive disorders, pyloric stenosis, decreased liver or kidney function, clinically significant bladder overflow obstruction or hiatus hernia associated with reflux oesophagitis
- contraindicated in those with urinary or gastric retention, uncontrolled glaucoma, severe ulcerative colitis, megacolon, toxic megacolon, myasthenia gravis

Patient teaching and advice

- warn patient to avoid driving or operating heavy machinery if dizziness or blurred vision occur

- advise patient to immediately seek medical advice if any of the following occur:
  - worsening of bladder symptoms
  - sudden fainting for no reason or after exercise/emotional excitement, rapid or erratic heartbeat
- see also General Patient teaching and advice (p. xxvii)

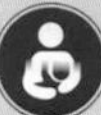

should only be used during pregnancy if potential benefits outweigh risks

not recommended during breastfeeding

tablet can be dispersed in water or crushed and mixed with spoonful of yoghurt or apple puree

BONE AND CALCIUM REGULATING AGENTS

Bone undergoes constant remodelling throughout a person's life and provides the means for mobility (e.g. acts as a lever and site for muscle attachment) and protection (e.g. supporting underlying organs and cavities), as well as acting as a reservoir for many ions necessary for body function (e.g. calcium, phosphorus, magnesium, sodium). Bone is also essential for haematopoiesis where blood cell proliferation and differentiation occur (Bringhurst et al 2019; Bryant et al 2019).

Bone remodelling is achieved by two cell types – osteoblasts and osteoclasts. Osteoclasts are responsible for the resorption of old bone, while new bone is deposited by osteoblasts. Bone mass increases and stabilises until about the age of 20–25 years, after which it is lost slowly during the adult years, with this rate increasing in women after menopause. Bone remodelling is a complex interaction of endocrine factors, vitamin D, parathyroid hormone levels, calcitonin and plasma calcium levels (Bryant et al 2019).

Paget's disease (osteitis deformans) is a disease of disordered bone remodelling (abnormal osteoclasts increase the rate of bone resorption, followed by a compensatory increase in new bone formation by osteoblasts). This results in bone that is expanded, less compact and more vascular, leading to a decrease in bone strength and increasing the likelihood of bowing, deformity and fractures (Favus & Vokes 2019). It is estimated to affect 2–4% of the Australian population, occurring more often in males, and prevalence increases with age, rarely occurring before 55 years (Bryant et al 2019; Favus & Vokes 2019). The bones commonly involved include the pelvis, vertebrae, skull, femur and tibia. Pain is generally the most common presenting symptom and results from increased bone vascularity, expanding lytic lesions, fractures, bowing and other deformities (Favus & Vokes 2019). Femur or tibia bowing causes gait abnormalities with associated mechanical stresses, resulting in secondary osteoarthritis of the hip or knee joints. Other serious complications include bone fractures (commonly long bones) and cardiovascular issues (Favus & Vokes 2019).

Osteoporosis is a disease in which the bones lose their density and structural quality, resulting in bones that are weak, fragile and fracture easily. While males and females have similar rates of osteoporosis up until about 35 years of age, by the time they reach 75 years, 1 in 4 women have osteoporosis compared to 1 in 10 males (AIHW 2019f; ABS 2019). A number of issues contribute to osteoporosis and fractures, including lifestyle factors (e.g. alcohol abuse, smoking, immobility, inadequate physical activity, falling, previous fractures, genetics, hypogonadal states (e.g. anorexia, bulimia, athletic amenorrhoea), endocrine disorders (e.g. thyrotoxicosis, diabetes mellitus types 1 and 2, gastrointestinal disorders (e.g. malabsorption syndromes), medications (e.g. glucocorticoids, lithium, excessive thyroid hormone, parenteral nutrition, ciclosporin, antiepileptic agents, antidepressants) and a number of other diseases (Lindsay & Cosman 2019). For women, other oestrogen-related risk factors include late menarche (time of first menstrual period), episodic amenorrhoea and early menopause. Age-related bone loss and decreasing sex steroid levels result in osteoporosis in older men when compared to women (Bryant et al 2019).

Hypercalcaemia can be associated with a number of conditions, including parathyroid conditions, malignancy related (e.g. breast, lung and kidney cancer, multiple myeloma, lymphoma, leukaemia), vitamin D related, associated with high bone turnover (e.g. hyperthyroidism, immobility), vitamin A intoxication, excessive calcium intake, thiazide or anti-oestrogen treatment) or associated with endocrine disease (Khosla 2019). Before starting treatment, it is essential to ensure diagnosis as a false positive can result from blood collection issues or elevated serum proteins such as albumin. Hypercalcaemia can be asymptomatic or result in fatigue, depression, difficulty concentrating, loss of appetite, nausea, vomiting, constipation, increased urine output, shortened QT interval and in some, cardiac arrhythmias; it can be life threatening (Khosla 2019).

There are a number of agents used to prevent or treat bone disorders, such as bisphosphonates, parathyroid hormone analogues, calcimimetic agents (increase sensitivity of calcium-sensing receptors), calcitonin and vitamin D/analogues.

BISPHOSPHONATES

General Actions of bisphosphonates

- incorporated into bone matrix where they may continue to act for some months, even after therapy has stopped
- inhibit resorption by impairing osteoclast function and decreasing osteoclast numbers
- nitrogen-containing bisphosphonates inhibit bone resorption without inhibiting bone formation (alendronate, ibandronate, pamidronate, risedronate, tiludronate, zoledronic acid)
- low oral availability

General Uses of bisphosphonates

- Paget's disease of the bone
- hypercalcaemia of malignancy (also called tumour-induced hypercalcaemia)

- osteoporosis (prevention and treatment)

General Adverse effects of bisphosphonates

- abdominal pain/distension, nausea, vomiting, diarrhoea, flatulence, dysphagia, constipation, acid regurgitation, dyspepsia, anorexia, gastritis, taste alteration
- oesophagitis, oesophageal ulcer/erosion
- headache, dizziness, fatigue, malaise, asthenia
- asymptomatic hypocalcaemia, symptomatic hypocalcaemia (tetany, paraesthesia), hypophosphataemia, hypokalaemia, hypomagnesaemia, increased serum creatinine
- bone, joint and muscle pain, muscle cramp
- (prolonged therapy) atypical stress fractures
- (rare) conjunctivitis, uveitis, iritis, oesophageal stricture/perforation, renal impairment
- (rare) osteonecrosis of the jaw (generally occurring in those with cancer (especially those with bony metastases or multiple myeloma), existing periodontal disease, oral trauma, poor oral hygiene or being treated with antineoplastic agents, radiotherapy or corticosteroids. Most cases are associated with dental procedures (e.g. tooth extraction) and symptoms include jaw pain, toothache, altered sensation, recurrent infection (including osteomyelitis), non-healing sores of the mouth/jaw and/or exposed bone)
- osteonecrosis of other bones (including hip, knee, femur, humerus, external auditory canal)

General Interactions of bisphosphonates

- calcium supplements, antacids and other oral medications may decrease absorption of bisphosphonates
- caution if used with NSAIDs due to increased risk of gastric irritation/ulceration and kidney dysfunction
- should not be given with other bisphosphonates
- caution if given with aminoglycosides as they may decrease serum calcium
- may interfere with bone scintigraphy examinations

General Nursing points/Cautions for bisphosphonates

- osteoporosis should be confirmed (low bone density mass, two or more standard deviations from normal and/or presence of osteoporotic fracture) before starting therapy
- any hypocalcaemia and dehydration should be corrected before starting therapy
- (IV) serum creatinine should be measured before therapy is administered
- calcium and vitamin D supplements are essential in those with Paget's disease or glucocorticoid-induced osteoporosis
- (tumour-induced hypercalcaemia) rehydration before and after therapy is recommended (especially if patient is older or on concurrent diuretic therapy)
- in those patients with risk factors (e.g. poor dental hygiene, chronic periodontal disease, head/neck radiotherapy, as well as treatment with antineoplastic agents and corticosteroids), a dental examination and any necessary treatment should be

carried out before starting therapy with bisphosphonate. Invasive dental procedures should be avoided if possible during therapy
- caution if used in those with history of nephrolithiasis or hypercalciuria as dietary restriction of calcium may be required during therapy
- not recommended in those with a creatinine clearance of less than 35 mL/minute
- caution if used in those with dysphagia, oesophageal diseases/abnormalities, gastritis, duodenitis or gastric ulceration
- contraindicated in those who are unable to sit/stand upright for 30 minutes after taking medication, have delayed oesophageal emptying (e.g. stricture, achalasia) or hypocalcaemia
- contraindicated in those with hypersensitivity to other bisphosphonates

General Patient teaching and advice for bisphosphonates

- patient should be advised to take tablets with plain water (not mineral water, coffee, tea or fruit juices) at least 30 minutes before first food of the day and remain upright for at least 30 minutes. Tablets should be swallowed whole and not sucked or chewed
- warn patient <u>not</u> to take medication at night or lying down because this increases the risk of oesophageal ulceration
- instruct patient to allow at least 30 minutes before taking any other medications
- advise patient to avoid milk, calcium-rich foods and antacids for at least 2 hours after taking medication
- patient should be advised to immediately report any:
  - difficulty or pain with swallowing
  - new or worsening heartburn or chest pain
  - pain in gums or jaw, swelling or jaw numbness or heavy jaw feeling, loosening of teeth
  - any new or unusual thigh, hip or groin pain
  - visual disturbances (e.g. blurred vision, pain or redness of eyes)
  - ear pain, recurrent or chronic ear infections
- encourage patient to maintain good dental hygiene during therapy, including brushing teeth after meals and before bed, gentle regular flossing to remove plaque and avoiding the use of alcohol-containing mouthwashes. Patient should also be instructed to keep mouth moist and regularly check teeth and gums using a mirror and seek dental advice if there is any tooth or jaw pain or there are loose teeth
- instruct patient to tell dentist of therapy before any invasive dental procedures are performed
- patient taking once-weekly medication should be advised to mark the scheduled day on a calendar as a reminder. If the person forgets to take medication on this day, they should be advised to take it as soon as they remember (in the morning, before food) and then return to the normal scheduled day
- patient should be advised not to drive or operate machinery if dizziness occurs
- advise patient to:
  - exercise regularly to build and maintain bone strength
  - eat a balanced diet, including calcium-rich food

   - decrease smoking and/or excessive drinking on a regular basis
- female patients of childbearing potential should be counselled to avoid pregnancy by using adequate contraception during therapy. Patient should also be advised that effects could continue for months after therapy has stopped because bisphosphonates are slowly released from bone
- see also General Patient teaching and advice (p. xxvii)

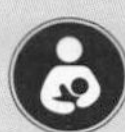
not recommended/contraindicated during pregnancy or breastfeeding

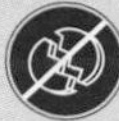
tablets should not be chewed or sucked

ALENDRONIC ACID (ALENDRONATE SODIUM) (Alendro, Alendrobell, Fonat)

Available forms
Tablets: 10 mg, 40 mg, 70 mg

Action
- see General Actions of bisphosphonates (p. 886)
- half-life greater than 10 years

Use
- see General Uses of bisphosphonates (p. 886)

Dose
- (osteoporosis) 10 mg orally daily 30 minutes before food **OR**
- (osteoporosis) 70 mg orally once weekly 30 minutes before food **OR**
- (prevention of osteoporosis in post-menopausal women) 5 mg orally daily 30 minutes before food **OR**
- (Paget's disease) 40 mg orally daily 30 minutes before food for 6 months **OR**
- (treatment of glucocorticoid-induced osteoporosis) 5 mg orally daily 30 minutes before food **OR**
- (glucocorticoid-induced osteoporosis in post-menopausal women not receiving oestrogen) 10 mg orally daily 30 minutes before food

Adverse effects
- see General Adverse effects for bisphosphonates (p. 887)

Interactions
- use with hormone replacement therapy (HRT) may increase bone mass and reduce bone turnover
- see also General Interactions/Nursing points for bisphosphonates (p. 887)

Nursing points/Cautions/Patient teaching and advice
- see General Nursing points/Cautions/Patient teaching and advice for bisphosphonates (pp. 887–88)

Note
- contained in Alendronate Plus D3, FonatPlus, Fosamax Plus Once Weekly and ReddyMax Plus D-Cal

IBANDRONATE SODIUM (Bondronat)

Available forms
Tablets: 50 mg; Injection solution: 6 mg/6 mL

Action
- see General Actions of bisphosphonates (p. 886)
- half-life 10–60 hours

Use
- see General Uses of bisphosphonates (p. 886)

Dose

- (metastatic bone disease) 6 mg by IV infusion over 1–2 hours every 4 weeks **OR**
- (metastatic bone disease) 50 mg orally daily 30 minutes before food **OR**
- (tumour-induced hypercalcaemia) 2–4 mg by IV infusion over 1–2 hours stat

Adverse effects

- peripheral oedema
- flu-like symptoms
- sore throat, tooth disorder
- increased creatinine
- (IV) bone/muscle ache/pain, chills, fever, headache, feeling of warmth, sweating, anaphylaxis
- see also General Adverse effects of bisphosphonates (p. 887)

Interactions

- increased serum levels may occur if given with IV ranitidine
- see also General Interactions of bisphosphonates (p. 887)

Nursing points/Cautions

- renal function and serum calcium, phosphate and magnesium should be monitored throughout therapy
- (IV) resuscitation equipment should be readily available if anaphylaxis occurs
- (metastatic bone disease) if patient has renal impairment, dose adjustment is required
- (tumour-induced hypercalcaemia) dose is dependent on tumour type and severity of hypercalcaemia
- (tumour-induced hypercalcaemia) repeat treatment may be required if hypercalcaemia recurs if therapy does not sufficiently reduce calcium levels
- (IV) should be diluted with 500 mL sodium chloride 0.9% or glucose 5% for infusion
- (IV) should not be mixed with any calcium-containing solutions
- see General Nursing points/Cautions for bisphosphonates (p. 887)

Patient teaching and advice

- see General Patient teaching and advice for bisphosphonates (p. 888)

PAMIDRONATE DISODIUM (DISODIUM PAMIDRONATE) (Pamisol)

Available forms

Solution for injection: 15 mg/5 mL, 30 mg/10 mL, 60 mg/10 mL, 90 mg/10 mL

Action

- see General Actions of bisphosphonates (p. 886)
- biphasic elimination (1.6 hours, 27 hours)

Use

- see General Uses of bisphosphonates (p. 886)

Dose

- (Paget's disease) 60 mg IV as a single infusion (not exceeding 15–30 mg over 2 hours), but may be repeated when necessary **OR**
- (lytic bone metastases – breast cancer and multiple myeloma) 90 mg IV infusion (not exceeding 1 mg/minute) every 4 weeks, or every 3 weeks if receiving chemotherapy every 3 weeks **OR**
- (tumour-induced hypercalcaemia) initially 30–90 mg (depending on serum calcium) IV infusion as a single dose or divided doses on consecutive days, over 2–4 hours; may be repeated if hypercalcaemia recurs or serum calcium concentration does not decrease within 2 days

Adverse effects

- rash
- atrial fibrillation, hypertension
- insomnia, somnolence
- anaemia, thrombocytopenia, lymphocytopenia, leucopenia

- hypertension
- (rare) renal toxicity
- (IV site) redness, swelling, pain, induration, phlebitis
- (tumour-induced hypercalcaemia) (rare) convulsions
- see also General Adverse effects of bisphosphonates (p. 887)

Interactions

- increased risk of renal dysfunction if given with thalidomide when treating those with multiple myeloma
- caution if used with nephrotoxic agents
- added effect if given with calcitonin to lower serum calcium levels in those with hypercalcaemia
- see also General Interactions of bisphosphonates (p. 887)

Nursing points/Cautions

- (Paget's disease) calcium and vitamin D supplements are recommended to prevent hypocalcaemia
- large vein should be used for IV administration to decrease IV site irritation
- not given as IV bolus
- reconstitute using 5–10 mL water for injections and dissolve completely before further diluting using sodium chloride 0.9% or glucose 5%
- for breast cancer, 90 mg is diluted in 250 mL and given over 2 hours; for multiple myeloma 90 mg is diluted in 500 mL and given over 4 hours
- should not be added to IV infusions containing calcium or divalent cations such as Ringer's solution
- serum creatinine should be measured prior to each therapy in those having prolonged therapy, especially if pre-existing (or predisposed to) renal impairment
- serum electrolytes, calcium and phosphate should be monitored regularly after starting therapy
- caution if used in those with liver impairment
- see also General Nursing points/Cautions for bisphosphonates (p. 887)

Patient teaching and advice

- see General Patient teaching and advice for bisphosphonates (p. 888)

RISEDRONATE SODIUM (Actonel, Actonel EC 35 mg Once-a-Week, Actonel 150 mg Once-A-Month)

Available forms

Tablets: 5 mg, 30 mg, 35 mg, 150 mg; Tablets (enteric coated): 35 mg

Action

- see General Actions of bisphosphonates (p. 886)
- biphasic half-life (1.5 hours, 480 hours)

Use

- see General Uses for bisphosphonates (p. 886)

Dose

- (osteoporosis) 5 mg orally mane 30–60 minutes before first food/drink **OR**
- (osteoporosis) 35 mg orally once weekly 30–60 minutes before first food/drink **OR**
- (osteoporosis) 35 mg orally once weekly (enteric-coated tablets) **OR**
- (osteoporosis) 150 mg orally monthly 30–60 minutes before first food/drink **OR**
- (Paget's disease) 30 mg orally daily 30–60 minutes before first food/drink for 8 weeks, repeated if treatment fails

Adverse effects

- hypertension
- pharyngitis, rhinitis, flu-like symptoms
- cataract
- infection
- (uncommon) glossitis, duodenitis
- (rare) abnormal liver function tests
- see also General Adverse effects of bisphosphonates (p. 887)

Interactions

- see General Interactions of bisphosphonates (p. 887)

Nursing points/Cautions/Patient teaching and advice

- (Actonel EC Once-a-Week) advise patient that tablet can be swallowed whole with or without food and should not be chewed, cut or crushed
- see also General Nursing points/Cautions/Patient teaching and advice for bisphosphonates (pp. 887–88)

Notes

- contained in Acris Combi (combination pack) with calcium carbonate
- combined in Actonel Combi-D with calcium carbonate and colecalciferol

SODIUM CLODRONATE (Bonefos)

Available forms

Capsules: 400 mg; Tablets: 800 mg

Action/Use

- see General Actions and Uses for bisphosphonates (p. 886)

Dose

- (hypercalcaemia of malignancy) initially 2.4–3.2 g orally daily in divided doses 1 hour before or 2 hours after meals, then reducing to 1.6 g orally daily **OR**
- (osteolytic bone metastases) initially 1.6 g orally daily in single or divided doses, increasing to 3.2 g daily if necessary

Adverse effects

- see General Adverse effects of bisphosphonates (p. 887)

Interactions

- use with other agents that reduce calcium may potentiate hypocalcaemic effect (depending on tumour type)
- see General Interactions of bisphosphonates (p. 887)

Nursing points/Cautions

- tablets and capsules contain sodium (128 mg in tablets, 64 mg in capsules) so caution if used in those on a sodium-reduced diet or with kidney disease
- see also General Nursing points/Cautions for bisphosphonates (p. 887)

Patient teaching and advice

- if dose is greater than 1600 mg, the patient should be advised to divide it into 2 (1 dose 1600 mg, the second dose is the remainder)
- advise patient that 400 mg tablets should be swallowed whole, but 800 mg tablets may be divided to help with swallowing
- see also General Patient teaching and advice for bisphosphonates (p. 888)

ZOLEDRONIC ACID (Aclasta, Deztron, Osteovan, Zometa)

Available forms

Solution: 4 mg/5 mL, 4 mg/100 mL, 5 mg/100 mL

Action

- see General Actions of bisphosphonates (p. 886)
- triphasic elimination (0.23 hours, 1.75 hours, 167 hours)

Use

- see General Uses of bisphosphonates (p. 886)

Dose

- (bone metastases) 4 mg IV over 15 minutes every 3–4 weeks (4 mg/5 mL solution, 4 mg/100 mL solution) **OR**
- (hypercalcaemia of malignancy) 4 mg IV over 15 minutes (4 mg/5 mL solution, 4 mg/100 mL solution) **OR**

- (osteoporosis, Paget's disease, prevention of fractures) 5 mg by IV infusion over 15 minutes once-yearly (5 mg/100 mL solution)

Adverse effects

- post-dose syndrome (also called acute phase reaction) (flu-like symptoms, fever, rigors, flushing, chills, fatigue, bone pain, myalgia, weakness, arthralgia, headache)
- atrial fibrillation, palpitations, hypertension, hypotension
- sweating
- anaemia
- urinary tract infection, urinary retention
- (uncommon) rash, pruritus, peripheral oedema
- (injection site) redness, swelling, pain
- see also General Adverse effects of bisphosphonates (p. 887)

Interactions

- caution if used with nephrotoxic agents, aminoglycosides or diuretics
- increased risk of renal dysfunction if given with thalidomide when treating patients with multiple myeloma
- see also General Interactions of bisphosphonates (p. 887)

Nursing points/Cautions

- post-dose (acute phase) syndrome symptoms can be reduced by giving paracetamol (not NSAIDs) with IV administration
- (Paget's disease) if re-treatment is required, an interval of at least 12 months should be allowed unless clinical symptoms such as bone pain or compression symptoms worsen
- creatinine clearance should be measured before each treatment (especially in those with kidney impairment)
- concentrated solution (4 mg/5 mL) should be further diluted using 100 mL sodium chloride 0.9% or glucose 5% and infused over 15 minutes
- 4 mg/100 mL does not require further dilution
- infusion should not be mixed with any other calcium-containing solutions (e.g. Ringer's solution)
- administer alone
- see also General Nursing points/Cautions for bisphosphonates (p. 887)

Patient teaching and advice

- patient who experiences post-dose syndrome should be advised that symptoms usually occur within first 3 days of infusion. Paracetamol (not NSAIDs) can be taken to reduce these adverse effects
- advise patient that onset of action is approximately 2–3 months
- see General Patient teaching and advice for bisphosphonates (p. 888)

OTHER BONE AND CALCIUM REGULATING AGENTS

CALCITONIN SALMON (SALCATONIN) (Miacalcic)

Available forms

Ampoules: 50 IU/mL, 100 IU/mL

Action

- synthetic polypeptide hormone structurally identical to salmon calcitonin (called calcitonin salmon (salcatonin)), which is 10–40-fold more potent than human calcitonin in reducing calcium concentrations
- lowers blood calcium concentration by decreasing the rate of bone resorption and increasing urinary calcium, phosphorus and sodium excretion

- thought to also increase osteoclastic activity, thereby promoting bone and collagen formation
- no effect on calcium absorption
- inhibits gastric acid and pancreatic enzyme secretion, stimulates intestinal secretion of water and electrolytes and modifies glucose–insulin relationship
- (Paget's disease) relieves bone pain, lowers skin temperature over affected bones, decreases excessive cardiac output, stabilises hearing and causes regression of bone lesions
- onset of action 15 minutes (IM or SC) or immediately (IV), peak effect 2 hours, duration of action 6–8 hours, half-life 60–90 minutes

Use

- Paget's disease (in those where other treatments are ineffective or unsuitable)
- hypercalcaemia

Dose

- (Paget's disease) 80–100 IU daily or every second day SC or IM, reducing to 50 IU daily when symptoms improve **OR**
- (hypercalcaemia) 5–10 IU/kg daily by slow IV infusion in 500 mL sodium chloride 0.9% over 6 hours **OR**
- (hypercalcaemia) 5–10 IU/kg by slow IV injection or infusion in 2–4 divided doses over 24 hours **OR**
- (hypercalcaemia) 5–10 IU/kg daily IM or SC

Adverse effects

- nausea, vomiting, diarrhoea, abdominal pain, unusual taste
- dizziness, headache, fatigue
- facial flushing, feeling of warmth
- arthralgia
- (injection site) pain, redness, swelling
- (high dose) development of antibodies
- (long-term therapy) escape phenomenon
- (rare) localised or generalised hypersensitivity, visual disturbances, increased risk of malignancy, rash, pruritus

Interactions

- may reduce serum levels of lithium, requiring dose adjustment

Nursing points/Cautions

- any dehydration should be corrected before starting therapy
- skin testing using 1:100 diluted solution intradermally is recommended to determine any sensitivity
- treatment duration should be as short as possible in order to reduce risk of malignancies occurring
- if patient has kidney impairment, dose should be reduced
- IV route is recommended for emergencies or severe cases of hypercalcaemia
- IM is preferable if amount exceeds 2 mL; multiple sites should be used
- nausea and vomiting may be decreased by dividing daily dose or administering antiemetic agent at the same time
- escape phenomenon is due to saturation of the receptor sites, not antibody production. Response is restored by stopping therapy for a short period

Patient teaching and advice

- patient should be advised not to drive or operate machinery if dizziness, fatigue or visual disturbances occur
- patients should be educated in self-administration: injection technique, rotation of sites, safe handling and disposal of needles, storage requirements
- see General Patient teaching and advice (p. xxvii)

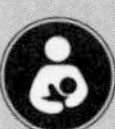
contraindicated during pregnancy or breastfeeding

CALCITRIOL (Calcitrol, Kosteo, Rocaltrol, Sical)

Available form
Capsules: 0.25 microgram

Action
- active form of vitamin D_3 (colecalciferol) normally formed in kidneys by precursor
- regulates bone and calcium homeostasis
- stimulates osteoblastic activity
- active metabolites
- half-life 3–6 hours
- (uraemia) kidney fails to convert precursor to active form

Use
- treatment and prevention of osteoporosis (post-menopausal or corticosteroid-induced)
- hypocalcaemia in patients with uraemic osteodystrophy, hypoparathyroidism, rickets
- vitamin D deficiency

Dose
- (osteoporosis) initially 0.25 microgram orally twice daily, increasing to 0.5 microgram twice daily if needed **OR**
- (corticosteroid-induced osteoporosis) 0.25–0.75 microgram orally daily in divided doses (dose depending on corticosteroid dose) **OR**
- (uraemic osteodystrophy, hypoparathyroidism, rickets) initially 0.25 microgram orally daily, increasing by 0.25 microgram per day at 2–4-week intervals if needed **OR**
- (uraemic osteodystrophy) 0.25 microgram orally second daily (if serum calcium is normal or slightly reduced)

Adverse effects
- hypercalcaemia, pruritus, hyperphosphataemia
- drowsiness, weakness, headache
- nausea, diarrhoea, constipation, abdominal pain, decreased appetite
- rash
- decreased kidney function
- metastatic or ectopic calcification of soft tissue
- (early signs of vitamin D toxicity (acute)) headache, weakness, somnolence, nausea, vomiting, decreased appetite, abdominal pain, dry mouth, metallic taste, constipation, muscle and bone pain
- (late signs of vitamin D toxicity (chronic)) muscle weakness, fever, polyuria, polydipsia, dehydration, nocturia, anorexia, weight loss, pancreatitis, photophobia, sensory disturbance, pruritus, decreased libido, increased urea, cholesterol and albumin levels, elevated liver enzymes, hypertension, cardiac arrhythmias, hyperthermia, rhinorrhoea, growth retardation, apathy, conjunctivitis (calcific) and, rarely, overt psychosis

Interactions
- cardiac arrhythmias may occur if given with digoxin
- actions may be counteracted by corticosteroids
- hypermagnesaemia may occur if given with magnesium-containing antacids
- colestyramine or colestipol may decrease absorption
- metabolism may be increased by phenytoin or phenobarbital (phenobarbitone)
- not recommended with vitamin D or derivatives due to increased risk of hypercalcaemia
- hypercalcaemia may occur if given with thiazide diuretics or calcium supplements

- dose of phosphate-binding agent may require adjusting if given together

Nursing points/Cautions

- serum calcium, phosphorus, magnesium and alkaline phosphatase levels and 24-hour urinary calcium and phosphorus levels should be measured twice weekly initially, then 2–4-weekly, then 2–3-monthly for the remainder of therapy
- if patient becomes immobile, serum calcium levels should be monitored more frequently to avoid hypercalcaemia
- blood samples should be taken without a tourniquet to reduce local calcium effects
- (hypoparathyroidism) malabsorption may be present requiring an increase in dose
- (corticosteroid-induced osteoporosis) calcium intake should not be greater than 1 g/day
- caution if changing from ergocalciferol to calcitriol as it may take months to return to pre-treatment ergocalciferol levels, increasing risk of overdose occurring
- caution if used in those with kidney failure as serum phosphate levels may increase
- contraindicated in those with hypercalcaemia or vitamin D toxicity

Patient teaching and advice

- instruct patient to immediately seek medical advice if any of the following occur:
  - signs of acute vitamin D toxicity, including headache, weakness, nausea, vomiting, dry mouth, metallic taste and bone/muscle pain
  - signs of hypercalcaemia, including fatigue, depression, confusion, anorexia, nausea, vomiting, constipation, increased urine output, unusual heart rate
- patient should be advised to maintain adequate daily fluid intake and avoid becoming dehydrated
- patient should be educated about diet, importance of not exceeding daily calcium intake (800 mg) by suddenly changing calcium intake and the need to avoid magnesium-containing antacids and vitamin D supplements, including multivitamin preparations as these contain both calcium and vitamin D
- warn patient to avoid driving or operating machinery if drowsiness occurs
- see also General Patient teaching and advice (p. xxvii)

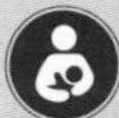
not recommended during pregnancy or breastfeeding unless benefits outweigh risks

CALCIUM CHLORIDE DIHYDRATE (CALCIUM CHLORIDE) (Calcium Chloride Injection, Min-I-Jet Calcium Chloride)

Available forms

Prefilled syringe: 100 mg/mL; Vial: 1 g/10 mL

Action

- calcium is an essential element involved in functioning of the heart, nerves and muscle contraction, blood coagulation, absorption of vitamin B_{12}, storage and release of neurotransmitters and hormones

Use

- hypocalcaemia where rapid increase in calcium is required (e.g. hypocalcaemic tetany or tetany due to parathyroid deficiency)
- severe hyperkalaemia (as an adjunct to antagonise cardiotoxicity)
- magnesium toxicity
- cardiac resuscitation

Dose

- (hypocalcaemia) 0.5–1 g slow IV, at 1–3-day intervals, depending on calcium concentrations **OR**
- (magnesium toxicity) 500 mg slow IV, observing patient for signs of recovery before administering any further doses

Adverse effects

- vein irritation
- (rapid IV) tingling sensation, chalky/calcium taste, hot flushes, sense of oppression (impending doom), decreased BP, bradycardia, cardiac arrhythmias, syncope
- (rare) hypercalcaemia

Interactions

- contraindicated in patient taking digoxin because of risk of arrhythmias
- may reverse effects of non-depolarising neuromuscular blocking agents
- should not be mixed with carbonates, phosphates, magnesium sulfate, tartrates or tetracyclines
- may reduce effects of calcium-blocking agents
- excretion increased by calcitonin, diuretics and growth hormone
- excretion decreased by parathyroid hormone, thiazide diuretic and vitamin D
- use with calcium or magnesium-containing agents is not recommended because of risk of hypercalcaemia or hypermagnesaemia

Nursing points/Cautions

- should not be given IM or SC due to risk of necrosis and tissue sloughing
- administered using a small needle into a large vein at a rate not greater than 0.35–0.7 mmol/minute to reduce risk of adverse effects
- patient should remain recumbent after administration
- only recommended by slow IV administration as rapid injection will cause syncope
- IV site should be monitored for any signs of extravasation
- solution should be warmed to body temperature before administration
- BP should be monitored because vasodilation may occur
- serum and urinary calcium should be closely monitored during therapy
- if patient has hyperkalaemia, constant ECG monitoring is recommended and dose adjusted if needed
- caution if used in those with cardiac disease
- not recommended in those with renal insufficiency-associated hypocalcaemia
- caution if used in those with respiratory failure, respiratory acidosis or cor pulmonale or where there is a risk of hypercalcaemia occurring (e.g. dehydration, electrolyte imbalance, kidney impairment)
- contraindicated in those with hypercalcaemia, hypercalciuria or severe renal disease, including renal calculi, in those with sarcoidosis or if the patient is taking digoxin
- (cardiac resuscitation) contraindicated in those with ventricular fibrillation

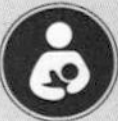

not recommended during pregnancy or breastfeeding

CINACALCET (Sensipar)

Available forms

Tablets: 30 mg, 60 mg, 90 mg

Action

- reduces parathyroid hormone (PTH) levels by increasing sensitivity of calcium receptor to extracellular calcium

- reduces serum calcium–phosphorus product and calcium and phosphorus levels
- biphasic half-life (6 hours, 30–40 minutes)

Use

- secondary hyperparathyroidism (end-stage kidney disease with dialysis) (adjunctive therapy)
- hypercalcaemia (parathyroid cancer)
- primary hyperparathyroidism (where parathyroidectomy is not possible)

Dose

- (end-stage kidney disease) initially 30 mg orally daily with food, increasing dose at 2–4 week intervals to a maximum of 180 mg (to achieve PTH level between 1.5 and 5 times the upper limit of normal) **OR**
- (parathyroid cancer, primary hyperparathyroidism) initially 30 mg orally twice daily with food, increasing dose at 2–4-week intervals to 60 mg twice daily, then 90 mg twice daily, then 90 mg orally 3–4 times daily until calcium level is normal

Adverse effects

- nausea, vomiting, diarrhoea, abdominal pain, dyspepsia, decreased appetite, constipation
- dyspnoea, cough
- headache, dizziness, asthenia, fatigue
- fever
- myalgia, muscle spasm, back pain
- non-cardiac chest pain
- hypertension
- peripheral oedema
- rash
- (uncommon) hypersensitivity
- (rare) hypocalcaemia (paraesthesia, myalgia, cramping, tetany, seizures), adynamic bone disease, hypotension, worsening cardiac failure, seizures, gastrointestinal ulceration/bleeding

Interactions

- may increase serum levels of metoprolol, flecainide, vinblastine and TCAs and therefore should be used with caution
- serum levels may be increased by erythromycin or itraconazole
- serum levels may be decreased by rifampicin, phenytoin and St John's wort
- caution if used with other calcium-lowering agents

Nursing points/Cautions

- serum calcium levels should be monitored before starting, throughout therapy and during any dose titration. Therapy should not be started if serum calcium is below 8.4 mg/dL (2.1 mmol/mL)
- (secondary hyperparathyroidism) serum calcium level should be measured within first week and intact PTH (iPTH) within 1–4 weeks of starting therapy. When maintenance is achieved, serum calcium should be measured monthly and iPTH levels 1–3-monthly
- (parathyroid cancer, primary hyperparathyroidism) serum calcium level should be measured 1 week after starting therapy and dose adjusted accordingly, then 2–3-monthly when maintenance is achieved
- PTH levels should be measured 12 hours after taking cinacalcet. PTH levels should be maintained above 100 picogram/mL to prevent adynamic bone disease
- if hypocalcaemia occurs (between 7.5 and 8.4 mg/dL), calcium-containing phosphate binder and vitamin D sterol should be started to increase calcium levels. However, if low levels persist, therapy with cinacalcet should be stopped or dose reduced
- liver function should be monitored regularly if used in those with any liver impairment
- not recommended for those with chronic kidney disease who are not on dialysis

- caution if used in those with epilepsy as significant decreases in calcium levels may lower seizure threshold
- caution if used in those with hypotension or impaired cardiac function
- caution if used in those with moderate-to-severe liver impairment
- caution if used in those at risk for upper gastrointestinal bleeding (e.g. ulcers, gastritis, severe vomiting)
- contraindicated in those with hypocalcaemia

Patient teaching and advice

- ensure patient understands the need to take tablets with or after food to improve availability. Patient should be advised to swallow tablets whole, not chewed or broken
- warn patient against driving or operating machinery if dizziness occurs
- advise patient to immediately seek medical advice if any of the following occur:
  - any numbness or tingling around the mouth, muscle pain or cramping
  - seizures (fitting)
  - any signs of worsening heart symptoms
  - rash
  - severe vomiting (especially if blood is present), abdominal or stomach pain
- see also General Patient teaching and advice (p. xxvii)

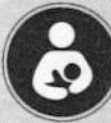

not recommended during pregnancy or breastfeeding unless benefits outweigh risks

tablet can be dispersed in water

DENOSUMAB (Prolia, Xgeva)

Available forms

Prefilled syringe: 60 mg/mL; Vial: 120 mg/1.7 mL

Action

- monoclonal antibody (IgG2) with high affinity and specificity for RANK ligand cytokine (essential for formation, function and survival of osteoclast), inhibiting osteoclast formation, thereby decreasing bone resorption and increasing bone mass and strength
- long half-life 28 days

Uses

- treatment of osteoporosis in postmenopausal women
- osteopenia in men after androgen-deprivation therapy for non-metastatic prostate cancer
- increase bone mass in men and women with osteoporosis at risk of fractures (including due to glucocorticoid therapy)
- prevention of skeletal-related events in patients with multiple myeloma or bone metastases from solid tumours
- treatment of giant cell tumour of the bone (recurrent or unresectable)
- hypercalcaemia of malignancy (not responding to IV bisphosphonates)

Dose

- 60 mg SC 6-monthly (Prolia) **OR**
- 120 mg SC every 4 weeks (Xgeva) **OR**
- (treatment of giant cell tumour, hypercalcaemia of malignancy) initially 120 mg SC day 8 and day 15 (loading dose), then 120 mg SC every 4 weeks

Adverse effects

- arthralgia, back pain, bone pain, musculoskeletal pain, pain in extremity, osteoarthritis
- nasopharyngitis, bronchitis, cough, dyspnoea
- hypertension, angina
- dizziness, headache, insomnia, fatigue, asthenia
- decreased appetite, nausea, vomiting, diarrhoea, constipation, dyspepsia, decreased weight, abdominal pain

- eczema
- fever
- peripheral oedema
- (SC site) pain
- (after discontinuing therapy) hypercalcaemia, multiple vertebral fractures
- (rare) osteonecrosis of the jaw (generally occurring in those with cancer (especially bony metastases or multiple myeloma) also being treated with antineoplastic agents and corticosteroids. Most cases are associated with dental procedures (e.g. tooth extraction), periodontal disease, oral trauma, poor oral hygiene or on chemotherapy, radiation therapy or corticosteroids. Symptoms include jaw pain, toothache, altered sensation, recurrent infection (including osteomyelitis), non-healing sores of the mouth/jaw and/or exposed bone)
- (rare) hypocalcaemia, skin infection (cellulitis), pancreatitis, atypical femoral fractures), hypersensitivity, osteonecrosis of other bones

Interactions

- caution if used with bisphosphonates, glucocorticoids or proton pump inhibitors due to increased risk of atypical femoral fractures
- not recommended with other agents containing denosumab

Nursing points/Cautions

- any hypocalcaemia should be corrected before starting therapy
- regular serum calcium level monitoring is recommended before starting therapy, within 2 weeks of first administration and then regularly throughout therapy especially if hypocalcaemia is suspected or in those at risk of hypocalacaemia (e.g. severe kidney impairment, history of parathyroid or thyroid surgery, malabsorption syndrome)
- calcium and vitamin D supplements are recommended unless hypercalcaemia is present
- in those patients with risk factors (e.g. poor dental hygiene, chronic periodontal disease, head/neck radiotherapy as well as treatment with antineoplastic agents and corticosteroids), a dental examination and any necessary treatment should be carried out before starting therapy. Invasive dental procedures should be avoided if possible during therapy
- (Xgeva) not recommended in those with rare hereditary problem of fructose intolerance
- not recommended in those under 18 years (unless skeletally mature with giant cell tumour of bone)
- not recommended in those with latex allergy as prefilled syringe needle cap contains latex
- caution if used in those with severe kidney impairment (creatinine clearance < 30 mL/minute) or on dialysis due to increased risk of hypocalcaemia
- caution if used in those with vitamin D deficiency, rheumatoid arthritis or hypophosphatasia due to increased risk of atypical femoral fractures
- contraindicated in those with severe untreated hypocalcaemia, unhealed lesions from dental/oral surgery or hypersensitivity to Chinese hamster ovary protein

Patient teaching and advice

- patient should be advised not to stop therapy without medical advice
- instruct patient/carer in correct administration technique, including:
  - give as an injection under the skin (subcutaneous) into upper thigh, belly region (except for 5 cm area around belly button) or upper arm
  - ensure prefilled syringe is intact when taken from packaging (and

hasn't been dropped or damaged in any way), and check the expiry date and solution (should be clear, colourless to slightly yellow)
  - allow it to come to room temperature for 30 minutes before injection to reduce pain (but do not heat by any other means)
  - prefilled syringe should not be shaken
  - wash hands with soap and water
  - clean injection site with alcohol swab and allow it to dry
  - ensure area to be injected is not tender, bruised, red, hard, scarred or stretch marks are present
  - pull grey needle cap straight out and away from body, pinch injection site, insert needle into skin fold and push plunger in slow constant movement until a snap is heard or felt. Continue to push through snap to inject full dose and then release thumb and lift syringe from skin
  - safety guard should automatically cover needle
  - discard used syringe into sharps disposal container
  - used syringe should not be reused
  - store unused syringe in fridge but do not freeze. Once syringe has come to room temperature, it should be used within 30 days
- patient should be advised to use stickers (provided) as a reminder of next injection date
- advise patient to seek medical advice immediately if any of the following occur:
  - signs of skin infection (area that is hot, red, swollen, painful/tender)
  - any new or unusual groin, thigh or hip pain
  - pain in gums or jaw, swelling or jaw numbness or heavy jaw feeling, loosening of teeth or non-healing sores in mouth or jaw
  - numbness or tingling in fingers, toes or around mouth, muscle twitching, spasm or cramps
  - (after therapy is stopped) excessive thirst, frequent urination, stomach pain, bone pain, muscle weakness, fatigue, confusion, lethargy, anxiety, depression
- warn patient against driving or operating machinery if dizziness occurs
- patient should be advised to take calcium (at least 1000 mg) and vitamin D (400 IU) daily
- encourage patient to maintain good dental hygiene during therapy, including brushing teeth after meals and before bed, gentle regular flossing to remove plaque and avoiding the use of alcohol-containing mouthwashes. Patient should also be instructed to keep mouth moist, regularly check teeth and gums using a mirror and seek dental advice if any tooth or jaw pain, unhealed sores in mouth/jaw or loose teeth occur
- women of childbearing potential should be counselled to use adequate contraception to avoid pregnancy occurring
- see also General Patient teaching and advice (p. xxvii)

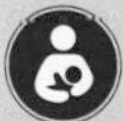
contraindicated during pregnancy or breastfeeding

RALOXIFENE HYDROCHLORIDE (Evifyne, Evista, Fixta 60, Ralovista)

Available form

Tablets: 60 mg

Action

- selective (o)estrogen receptor modulator (SERM) that potentiates the effects of oestrogen on bone and lipid metabolism (decreased oestrogen

levels lead to increased bone resorption, accelerated bone loss and increased fracture risk)
- antagonises negative effects of oestrogen on uterus and breast tissue minimising risk of oestrogen-dependent cancers
- reduces bone absorption and decreases bone turnover caused by oestrogen deficiency
- half-life about 28 hours

Use
- prevention and treatment of osteoporosis (post-menopausal women)
- decrease risk of invasive breast cancer (post-menopausal women at high risk or with osteoporosis)

Dose
- 60 mg orally daily

Adverse effects
- hot flushes, fever, sweating
- headache, depression, insomnia, vertigo
- infection, flu-like symptoms
- conjunctivitis
- rash
- chest pain
- sinusitis, laryngitis, pneumonia, bronchitis, increased cough, pharyngitis
- vaginitis, leucorrhoea, uterine/endometrial disorder, vaginal bleeding
- arthralgia, myalgia, leg cramps, tendon disorder, arthritis
- urinary tract infection, cystitis, urinary tract disorder
- neuralgia
- weight gain, peripheral oedema
- nausea, diarrhoea, vomiting, flatulence, gastric erosion, abdominal pain
- increase serum triglycerides
- deep vein thrombosis, pulmonary embolus, retinal venous thrombosis, stroke, myocardial infarction, acute coronary syndrome

Interactions
- not recommended with colestyramine or colestipol as absorption will be decreased
- serum levels may be reduced by ampicillin
- may decrease prothrombin time if given with warfarin, therefore should be monitored closely, especially when starting, stopping or changing dose
- lowers serum total and LDL cholesterol levels (should be taken into account if given with lipid-lowering agents)
- not recommended with oestrogen or hormone replacement therapy

Nursing point/Cautions
- if patient has a history of oestrogen-induced hypertriglyceridaemia, triglyceride levels should be monitored regularly throughout therapy
- therapy should be stopped if there is prolonged immobilisation. If immobility is due to planned surgery, therapy should be stopped for 3 days before event is planned to occur. Therapy should not be restarted until patient is fully mobile
- calcium supplementation is recommended if patient's diet is inadequate
- caution if used in women with a history of stroke, atrial fibrillation, transient ischaemic attack or oestrogen-induced hypertriglyceridaemia
- not recommended in those with liver impairment
- contraindicated in males or premenopausal women or as treatment for invasive breast cancer
- contraindicated in women with or with a history of deep vein thrombosis, pulmonary embolism, retinal vein thrombosis or liver impairment

Patient teaching and advice
- patient should be advised to report any unexplained vaginal bleeding immediately
- advise patient to ensure they have adequate calcium in their diet
- advise patient to move around regularly during any prolonged travel (especially air travel)

- patient should be instructed to have a breast examination and mammogram before starting therapy, then regularly during therapy as raloxifene does not eliminate risk of breast cancer
- female patient of childbearing potential should be counselled to use adequate contraception to avoid pregnancy during therapy
- see also General Patient teaching and advice (p. xxvii)

banned in sport

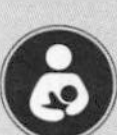

contraindicated during pregnancy or breastfeeding

tablet can be crushed and mixed with water or spoonful of yoghurt or apple puree

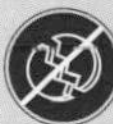

mask and gloves must be worn to crush tablets and a closed tablet crusher used. Pregnant staff must not crush tablets

SODIUM PHOSPHATE (Phosphate Phebra)

Available form

Tablets (effervescent): 500 mg

Action

- high-dose phosphate supplement
- decreases serum calcium concentration in those with hypercalcaemia as serum phosphate levels are inversely proportional to serum calcium levels

Use

- hypercalcaemia (associated with hyperparathyroidism, multiple myeloma and metastatic bone disease)
- hypophosphataemia (associated with vitamin D-resistant rickets)

Dose

- (hypercalcaemia) up to 3 g (6 tablets) orally daily **OR**
- (vitamin D-resistant rickets) 2–3 g (4–6 tablets) orally daily

Adverse effects

- nausea, vomiting, diarrhoea, abdominal pain
- (rare) soft tissue calcification, nephrocalcinosis, acute renal failure

Interactions

- absorption may be decreased by antacids or compounds containing calcium, magnesium, iron or aluminium
- increased risk of ectopic soft tissue calcification if given with calcium supplements
- increase risk of hyperphosphataemia due to increased absorption if given with vitamin D supplements

Nursing points/Cautions

- dose should be adjusted according to individual requirements
- tablets contain 469 mg sodium (20.4 mmol) and 123 mg potassium (3.1 mmol); therefore caution if used in those with congestive heart failure, hypertension, pre-eclamptic toxaemia, impaired kidney function or electrolyte imbalance

Patient teaching and advice

- advise patient that effervescent tablets should be dissolved in 1/2 glass of water and swallowed when fizzing stops. Warn patient that tablets should not be swallowed whole
- patient should be warned to avoid calcium and vitamin D supplements (or multivitamin preparations)
- see also General Patient teaching and advice (p. xxvii)

TERIPARATIDE (Forteo)

Available form

Prefilled pen: 250 microgram/mL

Action

- recombinant human parathyroid hormone (PTH) fragment that activates

osteoblasts via specific PTH cell receptors, stimulating formation of new bone
- action is the same as parathyroid hormone (regulates bone metabolism, renal tubular reabsorption of calcium and phosphate, and absorption of intestinal calcium)
- half-life about 1 hour (SC)

Use
- osteoporosis (post-menopausal women)
- primary osteoporosis (men at risk of fractures where other agents are unsuitable)
- osteoporosis (associated with glucocorticoid therapy)

Dose
- 20 microgram daily SC

Adverse effects
- nausea, vomiting, dyspepsia, tooth disorder, constipation, diarrhoea
- leg cramps, arthralgia
- asthenia, dizziness, depression, insomnia, vertigo, headache
- angina, hypertension, syncope, transient hypotension
- increased cough, dyspnoea, pneumonia, pharyngitis, rhinitis
- rash, sweating
- neck pain, muscle spasm
- (uncommon) hyperuricaemia
- (rare) antibody development, increased risk of osteosarcoma, exacerbation of hypercalcaemia
- (injection site) pain, swelling, erythema, pruritus, localised bruising

Interactions
- caution if used with digoxin as hypercalcaemia may predispose to digoxin toxicity

Nursing points/Cautions
- patient should be observed and BP monitored during the first 4 hours of treatment and advised to go slowly from sitting to standing because orthostatic hypotension may occur
- treatment is for 24 months only, after which patient may commence other therapy for osteoporosis
- if patient becomes immobile, serum calcium must be closely monitored until fully mobile
- (males) any primary or secondary hypogonadism should be excluded (and treated) before starting therapy
- calcium and vitamin D supplementation is recommended in those whose diet is inadequate
- should not be used in children or young adults with open epiphyses
- caution if used in those with or with recent urolithiasis because condition may be exacerbated
- not recommended in those with kidney impairment, hyperparathyroidism, hypercalcaemia or those who have an increased risk of developing osteosarcoma (including those with unexplained alkaline phosphatase levels, open epiphyses or prior skeletal radiation therapy) or who have bone metastases or skeletal malignancies
- contraindicated in those with Paget's disease

Patient teaching and advice
- patient needs to be fully informed of length of treatment (24 months only) and the implications of the development of osteosarcoma during animal experiments. Patient should be asked to sign an informed consent form
- advise patient to go slowly from sitting to standing because dizziness and fainting may occur
- warn patient that transient low blood pressure may occur during first few treatments and happens within 4 hours of administration and usually resolves spontaneously. However,

patient is advised to lie down during this time
- instruct patient to maintain adequate amounts of calcium and vitamin D in the diet and add supplements if necessary
- patient should be instructed that each pen can be used for up to 28 days and then discarded
- educate patient in self-administration including correct SC technique, rotation of sites, storage requirements and correct disposal
- patients are advised not to drive or operate machinery if dizziness, insomnia or vertigo occur

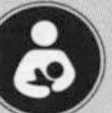
not recommended during pregnancy or breastfeeding

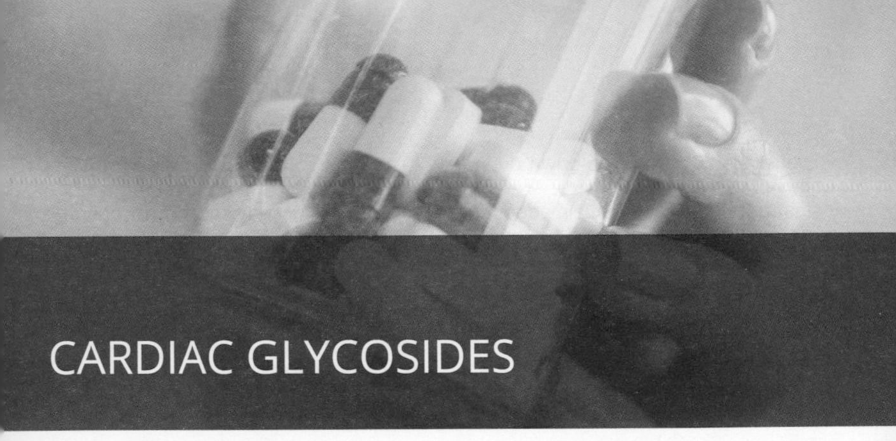

CARDIAC GLYCOSIDES

Cardiac glycosides increase the force of contraction of the myocardium. While the term 'digitalis' is used to describe the entire group of cardiac glycosides being obtained from the *Digitalis* (or foxglove) plant, digoxin is the only cardiac glycoside used clinically. In the past, digoxin was considered to be the basis of management for heart failure, but it is largely being replaced by more effective medications, such as ACE inhibitors, loop and thiazide diuretics, angiotensin II receptor antagonists and beta-adrenoceptor blocking agents (beta blockers). Digoxin remains valuable in the management of chronic heart failure in those who have concurrent atrial fibrillation (Bryant et al 2019). While milrinone lactate is not a cardiac glycoside, it has a positive inotropic effect by increasing myocardial contraction, and therefore has been included in this section.

DIGOXIN (Lanoxin, Sigmaxin)

Available forms

Tablets: 62.5 microgram; 250 microgram; Elixir (paediatric): 50 microgram/mL; IV solution: 500 microgram/2 mL; IV solution (paediatric): 50 microgram/2 mL

Action

- cardiac glycoside
- increases the force of myocardial contraction in the failing heart (positive inotropic action) by inhibiting sodium–potassium pump exchange in cardiac myocytes
- slows and reduces conduction rate particularly through the AV node (negative chronotropic action) by increasing vagal activity, resulting in prolonged refractory rate and decreasing ventricular rate
- in those with heart failure, increased vascular resistance and venous tone occurs
- decreases plasma renin activity and serum aldosterone
- improved kidney function as a result of increased kidney perfusion leading to diuresis
- (IV) onset of action is 5–30 minutes, peak activity 1–5 hours (undigitalised patient)
- (oral) onset of action is approximately 30 minutes to 2 hours and has maximal effect in 2–6 hours (undigitalised patient)
- half-life 36–48 hours, increased to $\geq$ 4.5 days in those with kidney failure
- steady state is achieved in approximately 5–7 days

- action may persist for 3–4 days after drug withdrawal (digitalised patient)
- narrow therapeutic index
- adult therapeutic range: 0.5–2 nanogram/L

Use

- congestive heart failure
- atrial fibrillation
- paroxysmal atrial tachycardia

Dose

Digitalising loading dose

If no cardiac glycoside has been given in last 2 weeks:

- 0.75–1.5 mg (10–20 microgram/kg) orally as a single dose or 3–4 divided doses 4–6-hourly **OR**
- (elderly) 500–750 microgram orally as a single dose or 3–4 divided doses 4–6 hourly **OR**
- (adults, children >10 years) 0.5–1 mg slowly IV over at least 5 minutes as a single dose or in divided doses of 0.25–0.5 mg 4–6-hourly **OR**
- (elderly) 250–500 microgram slowly IV over at least 5 minutes as a single dose or in divided doses of 125–250 microgram 4–6-hourly

Maintenance dose

- (normal renal function) 250 microgram orally once or twice daily **OR**
- (elderly or impaired renal function) 125 microgram orally daily or in 2 divided doses

Adverse effects

- anorexia, nausea, vomiting, diarrhoea, abdominal pain
- rash, urticaria
- blurred vision, visual disturbances (including yellow/green/white vision or coloured haloes)
- dizziness, headache, drowsiness, CNS disturbances
- arrhythmias, bradycardia, bigeminy (coupled beats), trigeminy, PR-prolongation, conduction disturbances
- (uncommon) depression
- (rare) intestinal ischaemia, thrombocytopenia, allergic reaction (rash, eosinophilia), gynaecomastia (long-term therapy)
- (digoxin toxicity) dysrhythmias, decreased appetite, nausea, vomiting, fatigue, malaise, muscle weakness, blurred vision or visual disturbances (such as yellow or green haloes), headache, drowsiness, dizziness, confusion, disorientation, seizures and, rarely, hallucinations and psychosis

Interactions

- risk of digoxin toxicity is increased by hypokalaemia, which may result from the associated administration of alcohol, amphotericin B (amphotericin), beta-2 adrenergic bronchodilators, corticosteroids, corticotrophin, diuretics, edetate disodium, insulin, laxatives, lithium salts, potassium-losing diuretics, sodium polystyrene sulfonate hydrogen or sodium bicarbonate, therefore potassium levels should be closely monitored if given together
- effects of digoxin are enhanced by hypokalaemia, hypomagnesaemia and hypoxia, increasing the risk of digoxin toxicity
- increased risk of digoxin-induced arrhythmias if given to those with hypercalcaemia or hyperkalaemia. Hyperkalaemia may result from administration of medication that increases serum potassium levels, such as ACE inhibitors, amiloride, ciclosporin, indometacin, potassium supplements, spironolactone, suxamethonium, tacrolimus and high doses of potassium-containing penicillins, therefore potassium levels should be closely monitored if given together
- ineffective if given when patient is hypocalcaemic, therefore calcium levels should be rectified before therapy is started
- risk of toxicity is increased with agents that lower extracellular potassium,

such as glucagon, large doses of dextrose and dextrose–insulin infusions, therefore potassium levels should be closely monitored if given together
- serum digoxin levels may be increased by ACE inhibitors, alprazolam, amiodarone, atorvastatin, IV calcium salts, captopril, ciclosporin, diazepam, diltiazem, diphenoxylate with atropine, erythromycin, felodipine, flecainide, gentamicin, indometacin, itraconazole, nifedipine, prazosin, propantheline, quinine, spironolactone, tetracyclines, trimethoprim and verapamil
- serum digoxin levels are reduced by acarbose, adrenaline (epinephrine), metoclopramide, penicillamine, phenytoin, rifampicin, salbutamol, St John's wort and some bulk-forming laxatives
- absorption of digoxin is reduced by some antacids, colestyramine, kaolin–pectin, neomycin, rifampicin and sulfasalazine
- beta-adrenoceptor blocking agents may potentiate bradycardia and heart block. ECG and serum digoxin levels should be carefully monitored during therapy
- may increase risk of arrhythmias when given with adrenaline (epinephrine), calcium salts (IV), ephedrine, pancuronium, pseudoephedrine and suxamethonium. ECG monitoring is recommended if given together
- risk of toxicity increases with hypoxia
- excessive bradycardia may occur if given with verapamil or diltiazem, therefore ECG is recommended if combination is given
- extreme caution if given with IV magnesium salts as heart block may occur

Nursing points/Cautions

- dosage is highly individualised and toxicity can occur at or close to therapeutic range in some people
- consideration should be given to whether a digitalising loading dose is required or not. If there is no emergency or urgency, the maintenance dose may be started as the initial dose, but optimal effect will take 5–7 days to occur
- distribution into body fat is poor, so the dose should be based on ideal lean body weight rather than total body weight
- therapeutic serum digoxin level is close to the toxic concentration, leaving only a narrow margin of safety, so serum levels should be monitored in premature infants, the elderly and in patients with impaired kidney or thyroid function or electrolyte imbalance
- symptoms of toxicity commonly occur at serum levels > 2 nanogram/mL
- blood sample for establishing serum digoxin levels should be taken 6–8 hours after the last dose or immediately before next dose is due
- serum electrolytes and kidney function (serum creatinine) should be monitored regularly during therapy
- predisposing factors to toxicity include hypercalcaemia, hypokalaemia, hypomagnesaemia and/or co-existing conditions such as renal factors; therefore, these conditions should be treated before starting therapy with digoxin if possible. Caution if used in those with hypercalcaemia or hyperkalaemia as there is an increased risk of primary heart block and/or digitalis-induced arrhythmias
- hypokalaemia sensitises the heart to digoxin and so may induce toxicity. Hypokalaemia can be caused by malnutrition, diarrhoea, dialysis, long-standing heart failure, increased age, prolonged vomiting and some drugs (e.g. corticosteroids, diuretics such as frusemide (furosemide) and thiazides). Patient should be closely monitored if any of these occur

- severe vitamin B_1 deficiency (beriberi) should be corrected before starting therapy
- note any improvement, such as return of heart rate to within normal limits, reduced cyanosis, easier breathing, reduced oedema, reduced pulse deficit and increased urinary output
- select the correct preparation, noting especially when the weaker formulations of digoxin are prescribed: Lanoxin PG (paediatric–geriatric), Lanoxin Paediatric Elixir (50 microgram/mL) or Lanoxin Paediatric Injection (50 microgram/2 mL)
- for a dose of 0.125 mg, give 2 tablets of 62.5 microgram, not half a 0.25 mg tablet
- not recommended IM or SC as digoxin absorption may be unpredictable and cause prolonged intense pain and muscle necrosis
- may be added to sodium chloride 0.9%, glucose 5% or glucose 4% plus sodium chloride 0.18% and given slowly IV over at least 5 minutes, avoiding extravasation
- rapid IV administration should be avoided because it may cause vasoconstriction and hypertension and/or reduced coronary flow
- not given by continuous IV infusion
- anorexia, nausea and vomiting may occur in the absence of digoxin toxicity because of gastric irritation and stimulation of the vomiting centre by the drug itself or because of the congestive heart failure
- patients receiving both digoxin and diuretics should have electrolytes measured regularly
- digoxin should be withdrawn 1–2 days before cardiac surgery or cardioversion. In emergency situations, such as cardiac arrest, the lowest possible energy should be applied
- patients with digoxin toxicity are at greater risk of arrhythmias when cardioverted
- digoxin-specific immune antigen binding fragment – f(Ab) – is used for overdosage (see Antidotes, antagonists and chelating agents, p. 332). It may be several days before a reduction in digoxin dose is reflected in a new serum concentration; however, neurological and visual symptoms may continue after other signs of toxicity have resolved
- digoxin is tissue bound, therefore not removed by peritoneal or haemodialysis
- have facilities available for cardiac monitoring, defibrillation and resuscitation
- patients with malabsorption syndrome or GI reconstruction may require higher dose to achieve clinical effect
- caution if used in those with kidney impairment or failure
- caution if used in those with thyroid disease as hyperthyroidism will make the person less sensitive and hypothyroidism will make the person more sensitive to the effects of digoxin. Half-life is prolonged in hypothyroidism and decreased in hyperthyroidism
- caution if used in those with carotid sinus hypersensitivity, acute glomerulonephritis with cardiac failure, idiopathic hypertrophic subaortic stenosis, hypoxia or sick sinus syndrome
- caution if used in those with ischaemic heart disease, acute phase of post-myocardial infarction, myxoedema or severe pulmonary/respiratory disease due to increased risk of digitalis-induced arrhythmias
- not recommended in those with constrictive pericarditis, heart failure associated with cardiac amyloidosis or myocarditis
- contraindicated in those with intermittent complete heart block, second-degree AV block (especially if Stokes–Adams attacks have previously

occurred), ventricular tachycardia, ventricular fibrillation, arrhythmias due to digoxin toxicity, supraventricular arrhythmia with accessory AV pathway (e.g. Wolff-Parkinson-White syndrome), hypertrophic obstructive cardiomyopathy or hypersensitivity to other digitalis glycosides

Patient teaching and advice

- advise patient to seek medical advice immediately if any of the following occur:
  - o loss of appetite, nausea, vomiting or diarrhoea
  - o slow heart rate
  - o unusual tiredness or extreme weakness
  - o blurred vision or coloured haloes around objects
- discuss with patient the importance of not taking vitamin or potassium supplements, or taking any medications (including herbal preparations or OTC preparations) without first discussing these with doctor or pharmacist
- warn patient against driving or operating machinery if dizziness or blurred vision occurs
- if elixir is used, calibrated dropper should be used to administer dose
- if patient is female and of childbearing capacity, counsel regarding the importance of not becoming pregnant or immediately seeking medical advice if she becomes pregnant
- see also General Patient teaching and advice (p. xxvii)

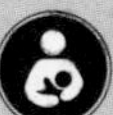

dose adjustment may be necessary during pregnancy to avoid toxicity because digoxin may cause adverse fetal effects

tablets do not disperse easily in water. Tablet can be crushed and given with spoonful of yoghurt or apple sauce

Note

- 1000 microgram = 1 milligram

MILRINONE LACTATE (Milrinone Concentrate for Infusion, Primacor Injection)

Available form

IV solution: 1 mg/mL

Action

- phosphodiesterase 3 (PDE_3) inhibitor which increases cAMP levels increasing intracellular calcium and force of contraction (positive inotrope) and improving diastolic function
- not related to digoxin or catecholamines
- vasodilator
- half-life 2.3 hours, duration of action 3–6 hours

Use

- congestive heart failure (short-term (48 hours) management, not responding to other therapy)
- low output states after cardiac surgery (including weaning from bypass pump)

Dose

- 50 microgram/kg by slow IV over 10 minutes (loading dose), then 0.375–0.75 microgram/kg/minute by continuous IV infusion (maintenance)

Adverse effects

- ventricular and supraventricular arrhythmias
- hypotension, chest pain
- headache
- infusion site reaction
- (rare) rash, abnormal liver enzymes
- (very rare) torsades de pointes (see Glossary)

Nursing points/Cautions

- any hypokalaemia or hypotension should be corrected before therapy starts

- use should be restricted to ICU or cardiac units
- heart rate, blood pressure, ECG, renal function, fluid and electrolyte status should be monitored throughout therapy
- infusion rate should be adjusted according to haemodynamic and clinical response
- dose should not exceed 1.13 mg/kg/day
- if severe hypotension occurs, infusion should be stopped until resolved and restarted at a lower rate if needed
- IV site should be closely monitored to avoid extravasation
- solution should be further diluted using diluents before use
- incompatible with frusemide (furosemide) or bumetanide because of precipitation in the infusion line
- should not be diluted with sodium bicarbonate
- infusion should be discarded after 24 hours
- caution If used in those with arrhythmias, including atrial flutter/fibrillation not controlled with digoxin, hypotension, severe renal impairment or previous vigorous treatment with diuretics
- not recommended in those in the acute phase of post-myocardial infarction
- contraindicated in those with severe obstructive aortic or pulmonary valve disease, hypertrophic subaortic stenosis or hypersensitivity to bipyridine

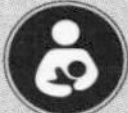

should only be used in pregnancy or if breastfeeding if benefits outweigh risks

CHOLINERGIC AND ANTICHOLINERGIC AGENTS

The nervous system (NS) is divided into the central nervous system (CNS) and the peripheral nervous system (PNS), which is further split into the somatic and autonomic NS. The autonomic nervous system has two subdivisions – the sympathetic and the parasympathetic NS (Bryant et al 2019).

CHOLINERGIC (PARASYMPATHOMIMETIC) AGENTS

The major transmitter substance for the parasympathetic NS is acetylcholine. After it has been released and activates receptors at the postsynaptic membrane, acetylcholine is broken down into acetate and choline by the enzyme acetylcholinesterase, with the choline actively transported back into the presynaptic axon terminals for reuse (Bryant et al 2019). Two classes of agents acting on the parasympathetic nervous system are:

- cholinergic agents (also called cholinergic agonists, cholinomimetics or parasympathomimetics), which mimic the action of acetylcholine at the postsynaptic receptor sites
- anticholinesterase agents, which inhibit cholinesterase, thereby allowing the amount of acetylcholine to increase and be available at the receptor sites.

Other cholinergic (parasympathomimetic) agents may be found in the chapters on Eye, ear, nose and throat agents (p. 1064) and Anti-Alzheimer's agents (p. 53).

General Actions of cholinergic agents

- miosis
- decreased heart rate
- bronchoconstriction
- increased gastric and pancreas secretions
- increase in stomach and intestinal motility
- increases skeletal muscle tone
- contracts bladder wall and relaxes trigone and urinary sphincter

General Adverse effects of cholinergic agents

- nausea, vomiting, diarrhoea, abdominal cramps, flatulence, increased peristalsis, increased salivation

- miosis, nystagmus, increased lacrimation
- headache, agitation, fear, slurred speech, drowsiness, dizziness, decreased consciousness
- increased desire to urinate or defecate, involuntary urination or defecation
- muscle cramps and fasciculation, weakness, ataxia
- bradycardia, hypotension, syncope
- rash, urticaria, increased sweating
- dyspnoea, bronchospasm, tight chest, wheezing, increased secretions (bronchial, pharyngeal, oral)
- (rare) cardiac arrest, coma, convulsions, paralysis, respiratory depression, allergic reaction

NEOSTIGMINE METHYLSULFATE (Neostigmine Injection BP)

Available forms

Ampoules: 0.5 mg/mL, 2.5 mg/mL

Action

- reversible cholinesterase inhibitor
- see General Actions of cholinergic agents (p. 912)
- at moderate doses, does not cross the blood–brain barrier
- half-life 47–60 minutes (IV) or 50–91 minutes (IM)

Use

- reverses effects of non-depolarising neuromuscular blocking agents
- treatment of myasthenia gravis (acute exacerbation)
- prevention and treatment of postoperative intestinal atony and urinary retention

Dose

- (reversal of non-depolarising muscle relaxants) 0.5–2.5 mg IV (with 0.6–1.2 mg atropine, in separate syringes) slowly IV over 1 minute (maximum dose 5 mg) **OR**
- (myasthenia gravis) 1–2.5 mg SC or IM daily in several daily doses when greatest strength is required, up to 20 mg daily **OR**
- (prophylaxis of intestinal atony and urinary retention) 0.25 mg IM or SC before or immediately after operation, repeated 4–6-hourly for 2–3 days **OR**
- (treatment of urinary retention) 0.5 mg IM or SC and apply heat to lower abdomen. After patient has voided, 0.5 mg IM or SC 3-hourly for at least 5 injections

Adverse effects

- see General Adverse effects of cholinergic agents (p. 912)

Interactions

- may antagonise neuromuscular blockade of aminoglycosides
- prolonged respiratory depression and apnoea may occur if given with suxamethonium
- effects may be decreased if given with corticosteroids
- when concurrent corticosteroids are stopped, increased effect may be seen
- effects may be reversed by atropine
- effects may be decreased if given with quinine, hydroxychloroquine, beta-adrenoreceptor antagonists or lithium

Nursing points/Cautions

- may be given IV, IM or SC
- 0.5 mg IV = 1–1.5 mg IM or SC
- (myasthenia gravis) record muscle strength variations because severity can vary and increased risk of overdosage
- (myasthenia gravis) duration of action is 2–4 hours
- (non-depolarising neuromuscular blockage reversal) should not be attempted until spontaneous recovery from paralysis is obvious, and it is recommended that patient is well

ventilated with patent airway until normal respiration is achieved
- complete reversal of non-depolarising neuromuscular blocking agents occurs within 5–15 minutes
- have atropine sulfate available to reverse the effects if necessary
- administer alone
- (bladder dysfunction) if patient has not voided within 1 hour of first dose, catheterisation is recommended
- caution if used in those who have had recent intestinal or bladder surgery, or have asthma, cardiac disease, arrhythmias, bradycardia, recent myocardial infarction or coronary occlusion, hypotension, epilepsy, peptic ulcer, Parkinsonism, vagotonia, kidney impairment, hyperthyroidism or Addison's disease
- contraindicated in those with peritonitis or mechanical obstruction of intestinal or urinary tract

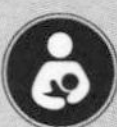

anticholinesterase agents may irritate the uterus and induce premature labour when given IV near term, therefore should only be used in pregnancy if benefits outweigh risks

Note
- is contained in Novistig with glycopyrronium bromide

PYRIDOSTIGMINE BROMIDE (Mestinon, Mestinon Timespan)

Available forms
Tablets: 10 mg, 60 mg; Tablets (controlled-release): 180 mg

Action
- cholinesterase inhibitor
- direct effect on skeletal muscle
- onset of action 30–45 minutes, duration 3–6 hours, half-life 1.5–4.25 hours
- see General Actions of cholinergic agents (p. 912)

Use
- myasthenia gravis

Dose
- 60–180 mg orally 2–4 times daily **OR**
- 180–540 mg orally 1–2 times daily (Timespan tablets)

Adverse effects
- see General Adverse effects of cholinergic agents (p. 912)

Interactions
- may prolong phase I block of depolarising muscle relaxants (e.g. suxamethonium)
- atropine antagonises action of pyridostigmine
- may antagonise neuromuscular blockade of aminoglycosides
- caution if given with aminoglycosides, local and some general anaesthetics, antiarrhythmic agents and other agents known to interfere with neuromuscular transmission in patients with myasthenia gravis
- additive effects may occur if given with dexpanthenol (vitamin B_5)

Nursing points/Cautions
- dose and frequency of administration is dependent on severity of disease plus level of physical and/or emotional stress and may vary from day to day
- dose interval should not be less than 6 hours
- lung function (especially vital capacity) should be regularly monitored and dose adjusted to maintain good respiratory function. Facilities for cardiopulmonary resuscitation, cardiac monitoring, endotracheal intubation and assisted respiration should be readily available during dose adjustment
- patient may become resistant to therapy with prolonged treatment, which may be restored by temporarily discontinuing therapy for several days (under medical supervision)

- lower incidence of adverse effects when compared to other anticholinesterases
- if patient shows little clinical improvement, it may be the result of under- or overdosage. Overdosage may result in cholinergic crisis, whereas underdosage may result in myasthenia crisis
- caution if atropine is used to counteract adverse effects as it may mask signs of cholinergic or myasthenic crisis
- caution if given to those with epilepsy, asthma, bradycardia, recent coronary occlusion, vagotonia, hyperthyroidism, arrhythmias, peptic ulcers or impaired kidney function
- large doses are not recommended in those with megacolon or decreased GI motility
- contraindicated in those with hypersensitivity to anticholinesterases or bromides, or in those with intestinal or urinary tract obstruction (mechanical)

Patient teaching and advice

- ensure patient understands that drug does not restore muscle strength to normal and therefore patient is not to increase dose in order to improve response
- instruct patient that dose should be taken when he/she experiences greatest fatigue and has the greatest need (e.g. given 30–45 minutes before meals if person has problems when eating)
- patient should be advised that different muscle groups respond differently to therapy, sometimes resulting in weakness of one muscle group and strength in another. Neck muscles and those involved in chewing and swallowing are usually the first to show signs of overdosage, followed by the muscles of the upper extremities and shoulder girdle, with the pelvic girdle, leg muscles and the extraocular muscles being the last to be affected
- see also General Patient teaching and advice (p. xxvii)

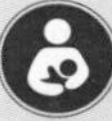

only given during pregnancy if benefits outweigh risks and in the case of myasthenia gravis, maternal requirements are often absolute. Transient muscle weakness may occur in newborn

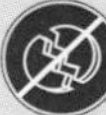

controlled-release tablets should not be crushed. Plain tablet can be crushed and mixed with water or spoonful of yoghurt or apple puree

ANTICHOLINERGIC AGENTS

These drugs are also known as antimuscarinic agents because they act by inhibiting the action of acetylcholine at the muscarinic receptors of the parasympathetic division of the autonomic nervous system (Bryant et al 2019). Muscarinic receptors are found in:

- the CNS, peripheral neurons and gastric parietal cells (neuroparietal or M1 receptors)
- the heart and peripheral neurons (neurocardiac or M2 receptors)
- smooth muscle and glands (smooth muscle–glandular or M3 receptors)
- the eye (ocular or M4 receptors).

Other anticholinergic agents may be found in the chapters on Antiasthma agents, bronchodilators and respiratory agents (p. 108), Eye, ear, nose and throat agents (p. 1064) and Anti-Parkinson's agents (p. 730).

General Actions of anticholinergic agents

- reduce production of sweat, saliva, lacrimal, nasal, bronchial, gastric and intestinal secretions
- reduce stomach and intestinal motility
- reduces gastric acid production
- increase heart rate (by blocking vagal stimulus)
- bronchodilation
- inhibit micturition
- mydriasis, cycloplegia, raises intraocular pressure

General Adverse effects of anticholinergics

- dry mouth, dysphagia, thirst, constipation, nausea, vomiting, taste alteration, bloating
- headache, nervousness, insomnia, confusion, drowsiness, dizziness
- urinary urgency, difficulty and retention
- impotence
- flushing and dryness of skin, decreased sweating
- tachycardia, palpitations, arrhythmias, bradycardia (at high doses)
- mydriasis, photophobia, cycloplegia, blurred vision
- suppresses lactation
- (less common) raised intraocular pressure, angina, heat intolerance, hypersensitivity, hyperpyrexia
- injection site reaction

General Interactions of anticholinergics

- may delay absorption of other oral agents given at same time
- increased intraocular pressure may occur if given with corticosteroids
- additive anticholinergic effects with disopyramide, TCAs, MAOIs, phenothiazines, amantadine, antispasmodics, anti-Parkinson's agents, other anticholinergics (e.g. ipratropium) and some antihistamines
- may cause an increase in intraocular pressure if given with corticosteroids
- may antagonise GI effects of metoclopramide
- urinary excretion may be delayed by urinary alkalisers
- increased risk of severe constipation, urinary retention and paralytic ileus if given with opioid analgesics
- may interfere with antipsychotic effectiveness of haloperidol if given to those with schizophrenia
- should not be administered 24 hours before gastric acid secretion test
- mydriasis and cycloplegia caused by anticholinergic may interfere with neuroradiological tests for intracranial neoplasm, subdural haematoma or aneurysm

General Nursing points/Cautions for anticholinergics

- caution if used in the elderly or brain damaged as there is an increased risk of mental confusion
- caution if used in children or those with Down syndrome as they have greater sensitivity to effects, whereas those with albinism have reduced sensitivity
- caution if used in those who are febrile as decreased sweating may lead to hyperpyrexia by inhibiting heat loss
- caution if used in debilitated patients because decreased bronchial secretions

may lead to formation of bronchial plug

- caution if used in those with ileostomy or colostomy as diarrhoea may be sign of incomplete intestinal obstruction
- caution if used in those with diarrhoea, gastric ulcer, GI infection (known or suspected), porphyria, hyperthyroidism, liver, kidney or metabolic impairment, hypertension, cardiac arrhythmias, tachycardia, severe heart disease, ulcerative colitis, paralytic ileus, chronic lung disease, autonomic neuropathy, prostatic hypertrophy, oesophageal reflux or hiatus hernia
- contraindicated in those with hypersensitivity to other anticholinergic agents, severe ulcerative colitis, toxic megacolon, GI obstructive disease, intestinal atony (in elderly or debilitated patients), closed-angle glaucoma, myasthenia gravis, bladder neck obstruction, tachycardia (because of thyrotoxicosis or cardiac insufficiency), acute haemorrhage (in which cardiovascular status is unstable), prostatic enlargement or fever

General Patient teaching and advice for anticholinergics

- patient should be advised not to drive or operate machinery if blurred vision, confusion, dizziness or drowsiness occur
- warn patient to take care taking medication during high temperatures or physical exercise or if febrile because of increased risk of heat stroke from decreased sweating
- caution patient to keep medications out of reach of infants and young children because they are especially susceptible to toxicity, even from the absorption of eye preparations, so note irritability, dry mouth, tachycardia, mydriasis, fever and rash
- instruct patient to seek medical advice immediately if any of the following occur:
  - painful red eye with associated loss of vision (may be signs of undiagnosed glaucoma)
  - diarrhoea (which may be the first sign of intestinal obstruction, especially in those with an ileostomy or colostomy)
- see General Patient teaching and advice (p. xxvii)

ATROPINE SULFATE MONOHYDRATE (ATROPINE SULFATE) (Atropine Injection BP, Atropt, Min-I-Jet Atropine Sulfate Solution for Injection, Minims Atropine Eye Drops)

Available forms

Ampoules: 600 microgram/mL, 1.2 mg/mL; Prefilled syringe: 100 microgram/mL; Eye drops: 10 mg/mL

Action

- see General Actions of anticholinergic agents (p. 916)
- more accurately described as antimuscarinic
- well absorbed IM, peak 30 minutes, duration 4–6 hours with longer ocular effects
- salivation inhibited within 30 minutes, peak 1–2 hours, duration 4 hours

Use

- premedication before induction of general anaesthesia to reduce salivary and bronchial secretions
- given with anticholinesterase, which reverses the effects of non-depolarising muscle relaxants

- acute myocardial infarction and sinus bradycardia (with associated hypotension and increased ventricular irritability)
- to prevent cholinergic cardiac effects such as bradycardia, hypotension and arrhythmias
- treatment of poisoning by organophosphate insecticides (with anticholinesterase reactivator e.g. pralidoxime)
- mydriatic and cycloplegic drops (see Eye, ear, nose and throat agents, p. 1064)

Dose
- (premedication) 0.3–0.6 mg SC or IM, usually with opioid, 30–60 minutes before anaesthesia **OR**
- (premedication) 0.3–0.6 mg IV immediately before induction of anaesthesia **OR**
- (reversal of effects of non-depolarising muscle relaxants) 0.6–1.2 mg slowly IV for each 0.5–2.5 mg neostigmine **OR**
- (cardiopulmonary resuscitation) 0.4–1 mg IV, repeated at 5-minute intervals until desired heart rate is achieved (total dose maximum 2 mg) **OR**
- (organophosphate poisoning) initially 1–2 mg IV, then 2 mg IM or IV every 5–60 minutes until symptoms have subsided (and repeated if they reappear) (total dose of 50 mg in first 24 hours) with a cholinesterase reactivator **OR**
- (severe organophosphate poisoning) initially 2–6 mg IV, then 2–6 mg IM or IV every 5–60 minutes if necessary (total dose of 50 mg in first 24 hours) with a cholinesterase reactivator

Adverse effects
- see General Adverse effects of anticholinergics (p. 916)

Interactions
- antagonises actions of bethanechol, carbachol, anticholinesterase agents (e.g. neostigmine) and cholinomimetic agents (e.g. pilocarpine)
- may interfere with anti-Alzheimer's agents (e.g. donepezil, rivastigmine)
- see also General Interactions of anticholinergics (p. 916)

Nursing points/Cautions
- (organophosphate poisoning) doses are repeated until signs and symptoms of poisoning disappear and repeated if symptoms reappear
- administer alone
- (organophosphate poisoning) should be withdrawn slowly when treating severe cases to avoid recurrence of symptoms such as pulmonary oedema
- incompatible with adrenaline (epinephrine), ampicillin, chloramphenicol, heparin, metaraminol, nitrofurantoin, sodium bicarbonate, sulfadiazine, thiopentone, vitamin B complex with ascorbic acid, and warfarin (may cause precipitation)
- see General Nursing points/Cautions for anticholinergics (p. 916)

Patient teaching and advice
- see General Patient teaching and advice for anticholinergics (p. 917)

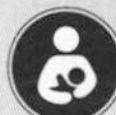

caution if used during pregnancy as it may cause tachycardia in the fetus

inhibits lactation and therefore not recommended during breastfeeding

Note
- contained in Donnatab, Lofenoxal, Lomotil

GLYCOPYRRONIUM (GLYCOPYRROLATE) BROMIDE (Robinul)

Available form
Vial: 0.2 mg/mL

Action
- see General Actions of anticholinergic agents (p. 916)
- does not cross the blood–brain barrier, therefore there are far fewer CNS-related side-effects than for atropine sulfate monohydrate or hyoscine hydrobromide
- onset of action within 1 minute (IV), action peaks 30–45 minutes (IM), duration of vagal effects 2–3 hours

Use
- preoperative or intraoperative use to prevent bradycardia
- preoperative to reduce secretions
- reversal of neuromuscular block

Dose
- (preoperatively) 0.2–0.4 mg IV or IM before induction of anaesthesia **OR**
- (intraoperatively) 0.2–0.4 mg IV as a single dose (may be repeated) **OR**
- (reversal of neuromuscular block) 0.2 mg IV per 1 mg neostigmine or equivalent dose of pyridostigmine

Adverse effects
- see General Adverse effects of anticholinergics (p. 916)

Interactions
- see General Interactions of anticholinergics (p. 916)

Nursing points/Cautions
- any tachycardia should be investigated before surgery
- (neuromuscular blockade) may be administered in same syringe as anticholinesterase
- stability may be compromised if mixed with dexamethasone, sodium phosphate or a buffered lactated Ringer's solution as this alters pH
- incompatible with thiopentone, chloramphenicol, diazepam, dimenhydrinate or sodium bicarbonate
- caution if used in those with latex sensitivity (closure system contains dry natural rubber)
- see General Nursing points/Cautions for anticholinergics (p. 916)

Patient teaching and advice
- see General Patient teaching and advice for anticholinergics (p. 917)

not recommended during pregnancy or breastfeeding unless benefits outweigh potential risks

Note
- contained in Novistig with neostigmine methylsulfate

HYOSCINE BUTYLBROMIDE (Buscopan, Gastro-Sooth, Hyoscine Butylbromide SXP for Injection, Trust Stomach Ease)

HYOSCINE HYDROBROMIDE (DBL Hyoscine Injection BP, Kwells, Travacalm HO)

Available forms
Ampoules: 400 microgram/mL, 20 mg/mL; Tablets: 300 microgram, 10 mg, 20 mg

Action
- see General Actions of anticholinergics (p. 916)
- belladonna alkaloid that has more potent effects than atropine on the iris, ciliary body and some secretory glands, but less potent effects on heart, intestine and bronchial muscle
- produces CNS depression at therapeutic doses with CNS stimulation at higher doses or in the presence of pain
- does not increase respiratory rate or blood pressure
- (IM) onset of action 30 minutes, duration 4 hours
- known as scopolamine in USA

Use
- premedication (for sedation, amnesia and decreased secretions)
- prevention and treatment of motion sickness

- spasm of GI tract, biliary spasm, renal spasm, diagnostic aid in radiology

Dose

- (premedication) 0.3–0.6 mg SC, IV or IM 30–60 minutes before induction of anaesthesia **OR**
- (travel sickness) up to 1 mg IM, SC or IV **OR**
- (travel sickness) 300–600 microgram orally taken 30–60 minutes before travelling and repeated 4–6-hourly if needed (daily maximum 1.2 mg) (300 microgram tablet) **OR**
- (antispasmodic) 20 mg orally 4 times daily **OR**
- (antispasmodic) 20–40 mg IM or slow IV injection (maximum daily dose 100 mg)

Adverse effects

- (parenteral) anaphylaxis, including shock
- see also General Adverse effects of anticholinergics (p. 916)

Interactions

- may have additive antivagal effects on AV node conduction if given with procainamide
- see also General Interactions of anticholinergics (p. 916)

Nursing points/Cautions

- (Buscopan) should not be taken for prolonged length of time without investigating cause of abdominal pain
- (Buscopan) tablets contain sucrose, which is not recommended in those with rare hereditary fructose intolerance
- (Buscopan Forte) tablets contain lactose, which is not recommended in those with rare hereditary galactose intolerance, Lapp lactase intolerance or glucose–galactose malabsorption
- (parenteral) may be given IV, IM or SC
- (parenteral) if given IV, should be diluted with water for injections and administered slowly
- (parenteral) patient should be closely monitored for any signs of shock or anaphylaxis and emergency equipment readily available
- (parenteral) incompatible with alkalis
- contraindicated IM in those concurrently taking anticoagulant therapy due to risk of intramuscular haematoma
- contraindicated in those with porphyria
- see also General Nursing points/Cautions for anticholinergics (p. 916)

Patient teaching and advice

- patient should be advised to seek medical advice immediately if any of the following occur:
  - abdominal pain or cramps persists or worsens
  - fever, nausea, vomiting, change in bowel movements, blood in stools or fainting
- (antispasmodic) advise patient not to take tablets for more than 2–3 days. If symptoms persist, patient should seek medical advice
- (motion sickness) tablets may be chewed, sucked or swallowed whole
- see General Patient teaching and advice for anticholinergics (p. 917)

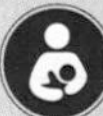

if given before onset of labour, may result in CNS depression in newborn and may add to risk of newborn haemorrhage due to decreased vitamin K dependent clotting factors

not recommended during breastfeeding unless benefits outweigh potential risks

tablet can be crushed and mixed with water or spoonful of yoghurt or apple puree

Note

- contained in Donnatab and Travacalm Original

PROPANTHELINE BROMIDE (Pro-Banthine)

Available form
Tablets: 15 mg

Action
- see General Actions of anticholinergic agents (p. 916)
- does not cross the blood–brain barrier, therefore does not have central effects
- half-life 9 hours

Use
- gastric and duodenal ulcers (adjunctive therapy)
- neurogenic bladder, urinary incontinence, hyperhidrosis

Dose
- (gastric/duodenal ulcer) 15 mg orally 3 times daily 30 minutes before meals and 30 mg at night (maximum daily dose 120 mg) **OR**
- (other indications) 15–30 mg orally 4 times daily

Adverse effects
- see General Adverse effects of anticholinergics (p. 916)

Interactions
- may increase severity of potassium chloride-induced GI lesions if given with potassium chloride (especially wax matrix preparations)
- absorption may be decreased if given with antacids or absorbent antidiarrhoeals
- may decrease absorption of levodopa
- intestinal motility may be further reduced if given with pyridostigmine
- may increase serum levels of digoxin increasing risk of toxicity
- see also Interactions of anticholinergics (p. 916)

Nursing points/Cautions
- see General Nursing points/Cautions for anticholinergics (p. 916)

Patient teaching and advice
- patient should be advised to take 2–3 hours apart from antacids or antidiarrhoeals
- see General Patient teaching and advice for anticholinergics (p. 917)

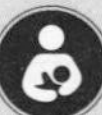

should only be used during pregnancy or breastfeeding if potential benefits outweigh risks

tablet can be crushed and mixed with water or spoonful of yoghurt or apple puree (tablet has very bitter taste)

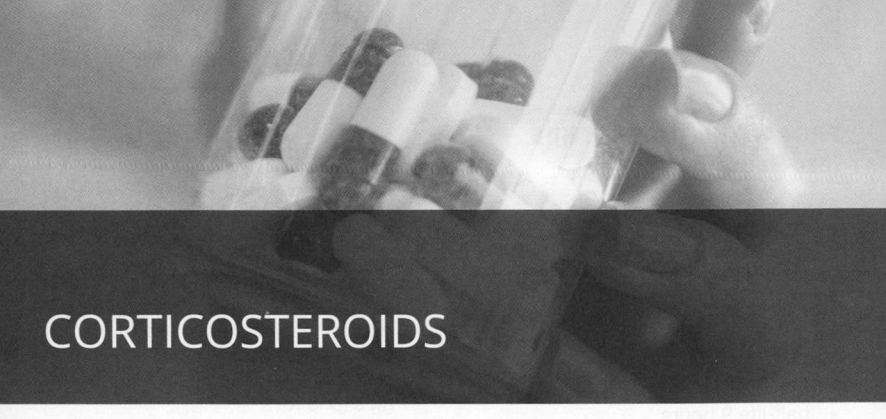

CORTICOSTEROIDS

The adrenal cortex produces three groups of hormones with a steroid structure known as corticosteroids (or adrenocorticosteroids):

- *mineralocorticoids* (e.g. aldosterone), which have electrolyte and fluid balance effects, including sodium and fluid-retaining properties
- *glucocorticoids* (e.g. cortisol), which affect metabolism, as well as having immunosuppressive and anti-inflammatory properties
- *androgens* (i.e. precursors of sex hormones), which regulate reproduction and development of sex organs (see Sex hormones, p. 1448) (Bryant et al 2019).

The corticosteroids are synthesised from cholesterol when needed, rather than being stored. This synthesis and release is controlled by a negative feedback system involving the hypothalamus, the anterior pituitary and the adrenal glands. When the body is stressed, injured or infected, the hypothalamus releases corticotrophin-releasing factor (CRF), which in turn acts on the anterior pituitary gland to release adrenocorticotropic hormone (ACTH). ACTH reaches the adrenal glands via the bloodstream, signalling the synthesis and release of cortisol. The cortisol level exerts a negative feedback effect, 'turning off' the release of CRF and ACTH. This is referred to as hypothalamic-pituitary-adrenal (HPA) axis suppression (Bryant et al 2019).

General Actions of corticosteroids

- increase gluconeogenesis and decrease peripheral glucose utilisation, maintaining blood glucose levels and glycogen content in muscle and liver
- increase protein breakdown from muscle and extra-hepatic tissue, increasing plasma amino acid levels
- inhibit protein synthesis, delaying wound healing
- promote mobilisation of fatty acid from adipose tissue to plasma; however, also increases fat deposition in face, shoulders and abdomen
- decreases calcium absorption from gut while increasing urinary calcium excretion, inducing increased osteoclastic activity in order to increase blood calcium levels (leading to osteoporosis with prolonged therapy)
- suppresses inflammatory response, including inhibiting inflammatory

mediators such as prostaglandins, thromboxanes, prostacyclin and leukotrienes
- causes atrophy of thymus gland, as well as blocking synthesis and release of cytokines and other immune mediators, and affecting T and B lymphocytes, macrocytes and monocytes, resulting in suppression of immune and allergic responses
- inhibits extraneuronal uptake of noradrenaline (norepinephrine) and other catecholamines, potentiating vasoconstriction
- affects mood and behaviour and possibly neuronal/brain excitability, leading to euphoria, depression, insomnia, anxiety and increased motor activity
- (high levels) suppress the hypothalamic-pituitary-adrenal (HPA) axis decreasing glucocorticoid secretion and long-term adrenal cortex atrophy
- glucocorticoids are well absorbed after oral, topical or local administration

General Uses of corticosteroids

- replacement therapy for primary or secondary adrenocortical insufficiency
- suppress undesirable inflammatory or immune responses in conditions such as:
  - cerebral oedema
  - neonatal respiratory distress syndrome (antenatal prophylaxis)
  - chronic inflammatory conditions of skin, gut, joints, liver
  - allergic conditions (e.g. allergic rhinitis), anaphylaxis, urticaria, drug reaction
  - rheumatic disorders, collagen and dermatological diseases
  - gastrointestinal (e.g. ulcerative colitis, Crohn's disease) and respiratory diseases (e.g. asthma)
  - haematological and neoplastic diseases
  - autoimmune disorders (e.g. SLE, rheumatoid arthritis)
  - prevention of organ or tissue transplantation
  - ophthalmic conditions (e.g. blepharitis and blepharoconjunctivitis (non-infected, allergic conjunctivitis, inflammatory ocular conditions)

General Adverse effects of corticosteroids

- sodium and fluid retention, potassium and calcium depletion, hypokalaemia, negative nitrogen balance
- hypertension, congestive cardiac failure (in susceptible patients), arrhythmias (associated with hypokalaemia)
- muscle wasting, weakness, steroid myopathy, osteoporosis, bone pain, pathological fractures of long bones, vertebral compression fractures, tendon rupture, avascular necrosis
- abdominal distension, indigestion, ulcerative oesophagitis, gastric irritation and ulceration, pancreatitis, diarrhoea, constipation
- headache, dizziness, depression, psychosis, mood swings, personality changes, euphoria, nervousness, anxiety, insomnia, restlessness, aggravation of pre-existing psychiatric conditions
- delayed wound healing, easy bruising, red/purple striae on thighs/buttocks/shoulders; hirsutism; acne-type eruption on face, chest and back; facial erythema; skin thinning;

petechiae; ecchymosis; purpura; increased sweating
- raised intracranial pressure, vertigo, seizures
- menstrual irregularities
- altered number, mobility and motility of sperm
- decreased carbohydrate tolerance, decreased insulin sensitivity, hyperglycaemia, glycosuria, activation of latent diabetes mellitus, hypertriglyceridaemia
- cataract, glaucoma, raised intraocular pressure, increased risk of eye infection, blurred vision
- increased frequency and severity of infection, may mask signs of infection (fever, inflammation)
- development of latent infections, including tuberculosis
- (Cushingoid state) increased appetite, weight gain, obesity, fat redistribution (e.g. moon face, buffalo hump), osteoporosis, hyperglycaemia, negative nitrogen balance, muscle wasting, poor wound healing
- growth restriction in children on prolonged therapy
- increased WBC count
- acute adrenal insufficiency may be precipitated by sudden withdrawal or reduction in dosage or an increase in corticosteroid requirements associated with stress caused by injury, surgery or infection
- (withdrawal effects) muscle weakness, hypotension, hypoglycaemia, headache, nausea, vomiting, restlessness, muscle and joint pain
- steroid resistance (decreased responsiveness to therapy)
- (IM) pain, sterile abscess formation, hypopigmentation, hyperpigmentation
- (severe, life threatening) suppression of hypothalamic-pituitary-adrenal axis
- (rare) anaphylactoid or anaphylactic reaction, pseudotumour cerebri/ benign intracranial hypertension, blindness (associated with intradermal administration around face and head)

General Interactions of corticosteroids

- clearance may be increased by rifampicin, phenytoin, carbamazepine, ephedrine, phenobarbital (phenobarbitone) and other barbiturates decreasing serum levels
- clearance may be decreased by aprepitant, ciclosporin, clarithromycin, diltiazem, erythromycin, indinavir, isoniazid, itraconazole, ritonavir and grapefruit juice, increasing serum levels and risk of adverse effects
- response to anticoagulants (heparin and oral) may be altered when given with corticosteroids, therefore prothrombin time should be closely monitored, especially when starting or stopping therapy
- excessive potassium loss and hypokalaemia may occur if used with potassium-depleting diuretics
- may decrease effects of potassium-sparing agents including diuretics, amphotericin B (amphotericin), xanthines and beta2 agonists
- may enhance potassium depletion caused by amphotericin B (amphotericin) leading to severe hypokalaemia
- may increase risk of gastric ulceration and bleeding if given with alcohol, aspirin or NSAIDs
- may decrease plasma levels of salicylates by increasing clearance

- may increase efficacy and risk of toxicity if given with sympathomimetic agents
- CNS adverse effects may be potentiated by CNS active agents such as antianxiety agents and antipsychotics
- hyperglycaemic effect of corticosteroids may counteract hypoglycaemic agents requiring dose adjustments
- excessive effects may occur if given with oestrogen or oestrogen-containing contraceptives
- increased risk of hypoprothrombinaemia if given with aspirin
- increased risk of arrhythmia or digoxin toxicity associated with hypokalaemia if given with digoxin
- may decrease effects of somatotropin
- may antagonise effects of anticholinesterase (precipitating myasthenic crisis in those with myasthenia gravis)
- increased risk of acute myopathy if high-dose corticosteroids are given with anticholinergics, including neuromuscular blocking agents
- increased serum levels may occur if given with HIV protease inhibitors
- may decrease serum levels of HIV protease inhibitors by increasing metabolism
- may decrease or enhance actions of neuromuscular blocking agents
- may decrease serum levels of isoniazid by increasing metabolism
- may decrease metabolism of ciclosporin, increasing serum levels and risk of toxicity including convulsions
- metabolism may be decreased by ciclosporin, increasing serum levels of corticosteroid
- not recommended with live attenuated virus vaccination (unless replacement therapy is being used)
- decreased absorption may occur if given with antacids, colestyramine and colestipol and should be separated by 2 hours
- caution if used in those treated with antithyroid agents
- may suppress reaction to skin tests
- may cause false negative reactions using nitroblue tetrazolium test for systemic bacterial infections
- may decrease I^{131} uptake and protein-bound iodine concentration, making it difficult to monitor response to therapy for thyroiditis

General Nursing points/Cautions for corticosteroids

- patient should be monitored for any changes in mood, psychosis or emotional lability
- salt-restricted diet (< 1 g/day) and potassium supplements may be necessary
- serum electrolytes (especially potassium) should be monitored regularly (especially in those also taking potassium-depleting agents such as thiazide diuretics or prolonged laxative use)
- check urine for glycosuria; blood glucose monitoring may also be necessary (especially for those with pre-existing diabetes mellitus)
- fluid balance chart (if hospitalised) and daily weight should be monitored to detect fluid retention
- monitor BP, haematological and adrenal function regularly during therapy
- IM route is recommended for allergic, dermatological, rheumatic or other conditions such as bursitis that respond to systemic corticosteroids; intra-lesion injections are recommended for dermatological conditions;

intra/periarticular injections are recommended for treatment of osteoarthritis and rheumatoid arthritis; injection into soft tissue is recommended for bursitis, fibrositis and myositis
- alternate day oral therapy may be suitable for some patients receiving long-term therapy to minimise adverse effects such as protein catabolism and adrenal suppression and growth suppression in children
- during trauma, surgery or severe illness, patient will require extra doses of corticosteroids to prevent drug-induced adrenal insufficiency
- select correct corticosteroid preparation and strength
- rapid IV administration should be avoided as it may cause cardiovascular collapse
- IM preparation given deep into large muscle mass (e.g. buttock) rather than the deltoid muscle to avoid subcutaneous atrophy
- small-bore needle (23 or 25 gauge) should be used for intralesional injections
- care should be taken when injecting into lesions not to produce blanching because this can cause sloughing
- (osteoarthritis) joint destruction may occur with repeated injections
- may cause tendon rupture if injected directly into tendon rather than tendon sheath
- suitable intra-articular joints for corticosteroid injections are knee, ankle, wrist, hip, shoulder, elbow and phalangeal joints
- intra-articular corticosteroids are often given with local anaesthetics (e.g. lidocaine (lignocaine), procaine)
- corticosteroids should not be injected into unstable joints, infected or previously infected areas or intravertebral spaces. Joints should be inspected for any signs of intra-articular infection before injection
- infants' and children's growth requires close monitoring during long-term corticosteroid therapy. They should also be closely observed and monitored for any obesity, osteoporosis and/or adrenal suppression
- live attenuated vaccines should not be administered while the patient is undergoing corticosteroid therapy
- long-term follow-up and monitoring is recommended for up to 12 months after discontinuing corticosteroid therapy
- ensure that all relevant medical and nursing personnel are aware that the patient is undergoing corticosteroid therapy, especially if undergoing surgery as wound healing may be delayed depending on dose, route and duration of therapy (e.g. inhaled corticosteroids have less impact on healing than chronic systemic therapy)
- dose adjustment may be required with disease remission or exacerbation and patient response to emotional or physical stress (e.g. surgery, serious infection, injury)
- (long-term therapy) transfer from parenteral to oral administration should be considered after weighing risks versus benefits carefully
- not recommended via epidural administration
- soft tissue, intralesional, intra-articular and topical corticosteroids (applied to large areas, when skin is broken or under occlusive dressings) may produce systemic effects
- caution if used in those with ocular herpes simplex infection because

of the increased risk of corneal perforation

- caution if used in post-menopausal women or others at risk of osteoporosis
- caution if used in those with thyroid disease because metabolic clearance of corticosteroid is increased in hypothyroidism and decreased in hyperthyroidism, requiring a dose adjustment of corticosteroid
- caution if used in those with epilepsy, uraemia or diminished cardiac reserve or congestive cardiac failure
- caution if used in those with active or latent tuberculosis (TB) as TB may be reactivated
- caution if used in those with impaired liver function or cirrhosis, the elderly, those with non-specific ulcerative colitis with a possibility of perforation, abscess or infection
- great caution if used in those with *Strongyloides* (threadworm) infestation as corticosteroid-induced immunosuppression can lead to hyperinfection and widespread larval migration, resulting in severe enterocolitis and potentially fatal Gram-negative septicaemia
- caution if used in those with renal insufficiency
- not recommended in the management of traumatic brain injury
- corticosteroid therapy is contraindicated (unless a life-threatening situation exists) in those with osteoporosis, marked emotional instability, psychosis/psychoneurosis or peptic ulceration, systemic fungal infections, active or quiescent tuberculosis, acute or chronic infection (including HIV infection or AIDS, measles, chicken pox), ocular herpes simplex, glaucoma (or family of), diverticulitis, recent intestinal anastomosis, thromboembolic tendency, diabetes mellitus (or family history of diabetes mellitus), myasthenia gravis, pheochromocytoma, hypertension or management of hyaline membrane disease after birth
- contraindicated in those with hypersensitivity to other corticosteroid agents
- should only be used during pregnancy after cautious consideration of benefit versus potential risks. Adrenocortical hormones may cause transient postnatal hypoadrenalism in infants and have caused malformations in animal studies
- women should be monitored for adrenal insufficiency during and after labour if treated with corticosteroids during pregnancy

Topical

- topical corticosteroids provide a way of delivering large doses locally without serious systemic effects
- corticosteroid creams and ointments are applied thinly and not rubbed in, preferably after showering or bathing
- lotions are recommended for use on hairy areas such as the scalp
- occlusive dressings are generally not recommended with corticosteroid cream (and especially not if a primary skin infection is present) unless ordered by a doctor as this increases risk of absorption and systemic effects. If an occlusive dressing is used, miliaria, folliculitis or pyodermas may occur
- generally not recommended for longer than 7 days
- should be applied with an applicator, gauze or gloved hand to protect against cutaneous absorption

- should be used alone or in combination with one or more other preparations, such as soothing, cleansing or antibacterial agents or cell growth stimulants, allowing sufficient time between application of individual preparations
- lower strength/potency preparations should be used on the face, with more potent preparations applied to palms, soles and any lichenified areas
- ointments are generally more potent than creams due to better absorption
- caution if applied to eyelids as skin is very thin in this area
- caution if applying creams, lotions and ointments to children as there is an increased risk of systemic absorption and effects due to higher skin permeability properties and larger surface area to body mass ratio
- not recommended in those with impaired circulation as skin ulceration may occur
- not recommended on skin that is inflamed, broken or ulcerated (or near chronic ulcerated areas) as systemic absorption may occur
- caution if used in those with psoriasis as exacerbation of psoriasis or pustular psoriasis may occur during or on withdrawal of therapy
- caution if used in those receiving immunosuppressant therapy or who have impaired T cell function
- contraindicated in those with hypersensitivity to corticosteroids, peri-oral dermatitis, skin reaction post-vaccination, viral skin infections (e.g. shingles, chicken pox), acne vulgaris, rosacea or TB or syphilis of the skin or untreated skin infection

Ophthalmic

- corticosteroid eye drops should not be used without a doctor's prescription as healing is impaired and herpes simplex virus is potentiated, resulting in a dendritic ulcer, cataract may start to form in the lens and intraocular pressure may be increased in some patients
- ocular corticosteroids should not be prescribed for > 2 weeks without supervision from ophthalmologist, unless facilities for monitoring corneal epithelium and intraocular pressure are readily available
- ocular infections can be masked, enhanced or activated by corticosteroids
- prolonged use may suppress ocular tissue immune response, leading to the possibility of secondary ocular infection (including fungal)
- take care with any conditions that may cause thinning of the cornea, because perforation may occur
- heavy or prolonged use (> 1 year) of corticosteroids may lead to posterior subcapsular opacities
- may cause increased intraocular pressure in susceptible individuals and pressure should be measured 2–3 weeks after starting corticosteroid therapy and then as determined by other factors such as the presence of diabetes mellitus
- fungal infections of the cornea may occur with long-term therapy
- pre-existing cataracts and glaucoma may be exacerbated
- caution if used in those with diabetes mellitus, because the therapy may predispose patients to increased intraocular pressure and/or cataract formation

- contraindicated in those with acute superficial herpes simplex keratitis, mycobacterial or viral diseases of the cornea or conjunctiva, tuberculosis of the eye, fungal diseases of ocular structures, acute purulent untreated infections or those with known hypersensitivity to corticosteroid preparations

Withdrawal

- corticosteroid withdrawal should always be gradual to prevent adrenal insufficiency syndrome. The rate of withdrawal is dependent on several factors, including the disease being treated, dose, duration of therapy and patient's response to therapy (e.g. less likely to occur if dose is lower than 7.5 mg prednisolone (or equivalent) or if therapy is less than 21 days)
- symptoms of adrenal insufficiency precipitated by sudden withdrawal and/or decrease in dose include headache, malaise, mental changes, restlessness, fever, muscle weakness, muscle and joint pain, dyspnoea, anorexia, nausea, vomiting, hypoglycaemia, hypotension and dehydration (muscle weakness and joint pains may last for 3–6 months after stopping corticosteroids)
- gradual withdrawal allows normal adrenal function to deal with daily needs, but a longer time is required before it can deal with infection, surgery or trauma

General Patient teaching and advice for corticosteroids

- patient should be advised to:
  - wear a MedicAlert bracelet or pendant that contains information such as dose and emergency instructions
  - avoid alcohol, NSAIDs (except paracetamol) and aspirin during therapy
  - avoid grapefruit juice
  - reduce sodium intake to less than 1 g/day
  - have an adequate protein intake to counteract any weight loss or muscle wasting
  - have regular medical check-ups during therapy
  - not overuse joint(s) that have been injected
  - not suddenly stop therapy as adverse effects will occur
  - report infection, inflammation, persistent backache, chest pain and changes in body shape
  - avoid contact with chicken pox and measles (especially children) and seek medical advice promptly if exposure occurs as follow-up will be required
  - take antacids or prescribed antiulcer agent between meals (but at least 2 hours apart from corticosteroid) to help prevent peptic ulcer development
- warn patient that corticosteroid therapy may mask signs of infection (fever and inflammation)
- instruct patient that long-term therapy is ceased gradually over several days, weeks or months to allow return of adequate adrenocortical function, but it may be 1 or 2 years before normal function returns. If patient becomes stressed (e.g. trauma, illness) during tapering process, dose may need to be reintroduced or increased. Patient should also be warned that

muscle weakness and joint stiffness may persist for 3–6 months after stopping therapy
- patient on reduction regimen should be advised to immediately report any vomiting, weakness or faintness
- patient needs to be aware that monitoring for up to 12 months after stopping long-term or high-dose corticosteroid therapy is required
- relatives or other household members should also be aware of implications and precautions during corticosteroid therapy, including the need to monitor for any signs of mood changes or depression
- patients with diabetes mellitus should be instructed regarding the need to carefully monitor blood glucose levels during therapy

Topical (cream, ointment, lotion)
- instruct the patient to only use topical preparation as prescribed (amount and frequency) as there is no benefit to more frequent administration or excess amount and it may result in adverse effects
- warn patient to avoid contact with eyes and wash well with copious amounts of water if contact occurs
- advise patient that topical corticosteroids should not be used on infected, broken or inflamed areas
- patient should be instructed to smooth preparation on skin (and not to rub in)
- patient should be instructed to shake lotion well before application
- instruct patient to wash hands well after using topical agent
- advise patient to allow corticosteroid preparation sufficient time to be absorbed before applying second skin preparation such as a moisturiser

Nasal spray instillation
- if using a nasal spray, instruct the patient in correct use (see Anti-asthma agents, bronchodilators and respiratory agents, p. 112)

Eye drop instillation
- instruct patient in correct technique for instilling eye drops (see Eye, ear, nose and throat agents, p. 1062)
- advise patient to seek medical advice immediately if any ocular trauma, infection or surgery occurs, or if patient develops conjunctivitis or lid reaction while using corticosteroid eye preparation
- see also General Patient teaching and advice (p. xxvii)

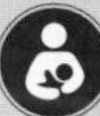

topical preparations are only recommended during pregnancy in minimal quantities for minimal duration

systemic preparations should be avoided during pregnancy unless benefits outweigh risks. Not recommended in pregnant women with pre-eclampsia, eclampsia or signs of placental damage when used for prophylaxis of hyaline membrane disease in premature infants

not recommended during breastfeeding because growth retardation or hypoadrenalism may occur in the infant

BETAMETHASONE ACETATE, BETAMETHASONE SODIUM PHOSPHATE (Celestone Chronodose)

BETAMETHASONE DIPROPIONATE (Diprosone, Diprosone OV, Eleuphrat)

BETAMETHASONE VALERATE (Antroquoril, Betnovate preparations, Celestone M Cream and Ointment, Cortival)

Available forms

Ampoules: 5.7 mg/mL; Cream: 0.2 mg/g, 0.5 mg/g, 1 mg/g; Ointment: 0.2 mg/g, 0.5 mg/g, 1 mg/g; Lotion: 0.5 mg/mL, 1 mg/mL

Action

- glucocorticoid with much higher potency than hydrocortisone
- combines rapid and depot forms to provide both rapid and steady effect (Celestone Chronodose)
- OV refers to optimised vehicle which increases penetration and enhances local effects (Diprosone OV)
- see also General Actions of corticosteroids (p. 922)

Use

- see General Uses of corticosteroids (p. 923)

Dose

Parenteral (1 mL = 5.7 mg beclomethasone)

- (allergic states, collagen diseases) initially 1–2 mL IM, followed by 1 mL weekly **OR**
- (prevention of respiratory distress syndrome in premature infants) 2 mL IM 24 hours before expected delivery, followed by 2 mL 24 hours later if delivery has not occurred **OR**
- (bursitis, fibrositis, myositis) initially 1 mL, repeated at 1–2-week intervals injected into bursae, tendon sheath **OR**
- 0.25–2 mL into joint capsules (amount dependent on size of the joint) (intra-articular) **OR**
- (joint capsule ganglions) 0.5 mL injected directly into ganglion cysts **OR**
- (intralesional treatment) 0.2 mL/cm^2 intradermally (not exceeding 1 mL/week total)

Topical

- small amount of cream/ointment applied to affected area 1–3 times daily, may be covered by a dry dressing if necessary **OR**
- (psoriasis) (pulse dose regimen) up to 3.5 g applied to lesions previously treated for 3 consecutive applications 12 hours apart (e.g. morning, evening, morning) each week (Diprosone OV) **OR**
- (seborrhoea, scalp psoriasis) part hair with comb and apply lotion directly to scalp twice daily for 4 weeks

Adverse effects

- see General Adverse effects of corticosteroids (p. 923)
- (intra-articular) post-injection flare, pain, irritation/discomfort at injection site, sterile abscess formation, hypopigmentation, hyperpigmentation, degeneration of joint with loss of sensation, joint instability (repeated injections), Charcot-type arthropathy (see Glossary)
- (intradermal/intralesional) local discomfort, sterile abscess formation, hypopigmentation, hyperpigmentation, subcutaneous/cutaneous atrophy
- (topical) burning, itching, irritation, dryness, erythema
- (topical) (prolonged/excessive therapy) telangiectasis, skin atrophy, striae
- (topical) (rare) folliculitis, pustules, hypertrichosis, hypopigmentation, contact or perioral dermatitis, skin maceration, secondary infection, miliaria, acne-form eruptions, visual disturbances

Interactions

- see General Interactions of corticosteroids (p. 924)

Nursing points/Cautions/Withdrawal

- not given IV or SC
- lotion is recommended for areas where hair may impede access to skin conditions

- (pulse dosing regimen) recommended for patients who have shown at least 80% improvement in lesion/s. If relapse occurs, therapy should return to 1–2 times daily application
- (Celestone M) recommended for maintenance therapy
- (Celestone Chronodose) caution if given IM to those with idiopathic thrombocytopenic purpura
- see also General Nursing points/Cautions/Withdrawal for corticosteroids (p. 925–29)

Patient teaching and advice

- (Celestone M preparations) instruct patient that these may be used 2–3 times daily and some conditions (e.g. chronic lichen simplex, hypertrophic lichen planus, atopic dermatitis, chronic eczematous and lichenified hand eruptions, recalcitrant pustular eruptions of palms/soles) are more responsive if occlusive dressing (light gauze covered by transparent film dressing, edges sealed with adhesive tape) is used
- (osteoarthritis, rheumatoid arthritis) advise patient that joint pain, soreness and/or stiffness is usually relieved 2–4 hours after injections and relief should last for 1–4 weeks
- see General Patient teaching and advice for corticosteroids (p. 929)

banned in sport for oral, rectal or systemic use. Permitted in sport for intra-articular, local injection and use via anal, respiratory, oromucosal, ocular, nasal, cutaneous/topical and auricular routes

Note

- contained in Calcipotriol/Betamethasone Sandoz 50/500 ointment, Daivobet 50/500 Ointment and Gel and Enstilar Foam spray with calcipotriol

BUDESONIDE (Budamax, Budenofalk, Budenofalk Foam Enema, Cortiment, Entocort, Jorveza, Pulmicort, Rhinocort, Rhinocort Hayfever & Allergy)

Available forms

Nebulising solution (respules): 0.5 mg/2 mL, 1 mg/2 mL; Turbuhaler: 100 microgram/inhalation, 200 microgram/inhalation, 400 microgram/inhalation; Nasal spray: 32 microgram/dose, 64 microgram/dose; Capsules: 3 mg; Orally disintegrating tablets: 1 mg; Enema: 2 mg; Tablets (prolonged release): 9 mg

Action

- glucocorticoid related to hydroxyprednisolone, with fewer systemic effects than beclometasone, although twice as potent

Uses

- (asthma) symptom preventer and induction of remission in those with mild-to-moderate Crohn's disease (see Antiasthma agents, bronchodilators and respiratory agents, p. 126)

CLOBETASOL PROPIONATE (Clobex)

Available form

Shampoo: 500 microgram/mL

Action

- see General Actions of corticosteroids (p. 922)

Use

- moderate-to-severe scalp psoriasis

Dose

- apply 7.5 mL to dry scalp, massage well into lesions and leave uncovered for 15 minutes. Rinse hair thoroughly, then wash with normal shampoo and dry as usual

Adverse effects
- skin burning sensation, acne, folliculitis
- (uncommon) irritation, pruritus, urticaria, skin atrophy, telangiectasis, headache, visual disturbances
- (prolonged or extensive use, use on broken skin) systemic adverse effects (see General Adverse effects for corticosteroids, p. 923)

Nursing points/Cautions/ Withdrawal
- for use on scalp only
- recommended for 4 weeks maximum
- if no improvement is seen in 4 weeks, reassessment should be conducted
- not recommended for acne, rosacea or perioral dermatitis
- contraindicated in children < 2 years
- see also General Nursing points/ Cautions/Withdrawal for corticosteroids (p. 925–29)

Patient teaching and advice
- ensure patient understands instructions for correct use (massage well into lesions on scalp, leave uncovered for 15 minutes and then rinse well, followed by normal washing with shampoo. Hair can be dried normally)
- advise patient that shampoo should not be applied to other parts of the body
- instruct patient that when improvement is seen, frequency of administration can be decreased or changed to other products
- warn patient to avoid contact with eyes and wash with copious amounts of water if contact occurs
- see General Patient teaching and advice for corticosteroids (p. 929)

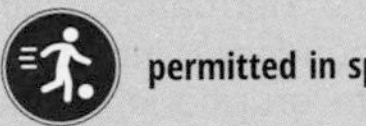
permitted in sport

should be avoided in pregnancy or breast-feeding unless benefits outweigh risks

CLOBETASONE BUTYRATE (Eumovate, Kloxema)

Available form
Cream: 0.5 mg/g (0.05%)

Action
- see General Actions of corticosteroids (p. 922)

Use
- short-term management of mild eczema, dermatitis and other inflammatory skin conditions

Dose
- apply a thin layer to affected area twice daily for up to 7 days

Adverse effects
- (topical) burning, itching, irritation, dryness, erythema
- (topical) (prolonged/excessive therapy) telangiectasis, skin atrophy, striae
- (topical) (rare) folliculitis, pustules, hypertrichosis, hypopigmentation, contact or perioral dermatitis, skin maceration, secondary infection, miliaria, acne-form eruptions, visual disturbances
- (prolonged or extensive use, use on broken skin) systemic adverse effects (see General Adverse effects of corticosteroids, p. 923)

Interactions
- not recommended with other topical or systemic corticosteroids

Nursing points/Cautions/ Withdrawal
- not recommended in those with rosacea, acne, pruritus, perioral dermatitis, untreated bacterial, viral or fungal infections or in those with impaired circulation

- see General Nursing points/Cautions/Withdrawal for corticosteroids (p. 925–29)

Patient teaching and advice

- advise patient to seek medical advice if condition has not improved in 7 days
- instruct patient that cream should not be applied to face, groin, genitals or between toes
- see General Patient teaching and advice for corticosteroids (p. 929)

permitted in sport

CORTISONE ACETATE (Cortate)

Available forms
Tablets: 5 mg, 25 mg

Action
- mineralocorticoid and glucocorticoid activity that is converted to active form (hydrocortisone) in the liver, which has:
  - half-life of about 100 minutes
  - half-life prolonged in those with cirrhosis and shortened in those with thyrotoxicosis
- see also General Actions of corticosteroids (p. 922)

Use
- Addison's disease, allergic disorders, status asthmaticus, angioneurotic oedema, serum sickness, drug sensitisation, giant cell arteritis, periarteritis nodosa, disseminated lupus erythematosus

Dose
- (initially 25 mg orally 6-hourly (until remission is achieved), then reduced by 10–20 mg every few days until optimal maintenance dose is reached (dose is individualised)

Adverse effects/Interactions/Nursing points/Cautions/Withdrawal/Patient teaching and advice
- larger doses may be required in those with acute and severe sensitivity or anaphylaxis
- see general points for corticosteroids (p. 922–30)

banned in sport

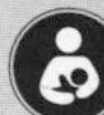
only used in pregnancy if benefits outweigh risks

tablets can be dispersed in water or crushed and mixed with spoonful of yoghurt or apple puree

DESONIDE (Desowen)

Available form
Lotion: 0.5 mg/g

Action
- see General Actions of corticosteroids (p. 922)

Use
- relief of inflammatory and pruritic signs of dermatoses

Dose
- apply a thin layer to affected area 2–3 times daily for a maximum of 8 weeks

Adverse effects
- (topical) burning, itching, irritation, dryness, erythema
- (topical) (prolonged/excessive therapy) telangiectasis, skin atrophy, striae
- (topical) (rare) folliculitis, pustules, hypertrichosis, hypopigmentation, contact or perioral dermatitis, skin maceration, secondary infection, miliaria, acne-form eruptions, visual disturbances

Nursing points/Cautions/Withdrawal/Patient teaching and advice

- occlusive dressing may be used for psoriasis or recalcitrant conditions management
- advise patient to shake lotion well before use
- see General Nursing points/Cautions/Withdrawal/Patient teaching and advice for corticosteroids (pp. 925–29)

permitted in sport

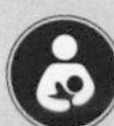
avoid use to breast area if breastfeeding

DEXAMETHASONE (Dexmethsone, Maxidex (Eye Drops), Ozurdex)

DEXAMETHASONE PHOSPHATE (DBL Dexamethasone Sodium Phosphate Injection, Dexamethasone Mylan Injection)

Available forms

Tablets: 0.5 mg, 4 mg; Ampoules: 4 mg/mL; Vial: 8 mg/2 mL; Eye drops: 0.1%; Intravitreal implant: 700 microgram

Action

- glucocorticoid that is 25–30 times more potent than hydrocortisone with little mineralocorticoid activity (few sodium and water-retaining properties)
- see also General Actions of corticosteroids (p. 922)

Use

- diabetic macular oedema (DME), oedema due to retinal vein occlusion (BRVO), central vein occlusion (CRVO) or non-infectious uveitis of posterior eye segment (intravitreal implant)
- see also General Uses of corticosteroids (p. 923)

Dose

- initially 0.5–10 mg orally daily with food in 3 or 4 divided doses, then reducing 0.5–1 mg daily as maintenance **OR**
- (cerebral oedema) initially 10 mg IV, then 4 mg IM 6-hourly until symptoms disappear (usually 12 to 24 hours), reducing dose after 2–4 days and stopping over 5–7 days **OR**
- (acute life-threatening cerebral oedema) initially 50 mg IV, then 8 mg IV 2-hourly for 3 days, 4 mg IV 2-hourly for 1 day, 4 mg IV 4-hourly for the next 3 days, then reducing by 4 mg daily **OR**
- (cerebral oedema associated with cerebral malignancy) initially 10 mg IV, then 2 mg IM or IV 2–3 times daily (as maintenance) **OR**
- (severe shock associated with haemorrhage, trauma or surgery) 2–6 mg/kg IV stat, repeated in 2–6 hours if shock persists and usually no longer than 48–72 hours **OR**
- (severe shock) initially 20 mg IV, followed by 3 mg/kg/day by IV infusion **OR**
- (intrasynovial, soft tissue injections) 0.4–6 mg into joint or site (depending on size of joint), may be repeated in 3–5 days (bursae) or 2–3-weekly (joints) **OR**
- 700 microgram intravitreal implant, repeated at 5–7-month intervals if needed (DME), or at least 6-month intervals based on visual acuity and/or anatomical parameters (uveitis, RVO) **OR**
- 1–2 drops instilled into the conjunctival sac(s) hourly (severe inflammation) or 4–6 times daily (mild inflammation)

Adverse effects

- see also General Adverse effects of corticosteroids (p. 923)
- (intra-articular) post-injection flare, pain, irritation/discomfort at injection site, sterile abscess formation, hypopigmentation, hyperpigmentation, degeneration of joint with loss of sensation, joint instability (repeated injections), Charcot-type arthropathy (see Glossary)
- (ophthalmic) transient stinging and burning, irritation, tearing, discharge, itching, eye oedema, eye pain, conjunctival and ocular hyperaemia
- (ophthalmic, rare) increased intraocular pressure, optic nerve damage, glaucoma, secondary ocular infections, cataract formation, decreased visual acuity, visual disturbances, blurred vision
- (ophthalmic, long-term therapy) corneal and scleral thinning, corneal perforation
- (vitreous implant) vitreous floaters/detachment/opacities, anterior chamber inflammation, ocular hypertension, increased intraocular pressure, cataract, lens opacities, conjunctival oedema, decreased visual acuity

Interactions

- see General Interactions of corticosteroids (p. 924)
- (ophthalmic) may increase intraocular pressure, decreasing efficiency of antiglaucoma agents
- (ophthalmic) increased risk of intraocular hypertension if given with anticholinergic agents (in those predisposed to acute angle closure)
- (intravitreal) increased risk of vitreous haemorrhage if inserted into those taking anticoagulants or antiplatelet agents
- increased serum levels may occur if given with aprepitant. However, prolonged use of dexamethasone may induce aprepitant metabolism resulting in lowered serum levels
- false negative results for dexamethasone suppression tests may occur if patient is also treated with indometacin or high doses of benzodiazepines or cyproheptadine

Nursing points/Cautions/Withdrawal

- IM/IV route should only be used for life-threatening situations or acute illness and replaced with oral therapy as soon as possible
- for IV infusion, may be diluted with glucose 5% or sodium chloride 0.9% (as long as sodium restriction is not present)
- (eye drops) if used for > 10 days, intraocular pressure should be monitored
- (intravitreal implant) (uveitis, RV) if vision improves and is maintained, retreatment is not required
- (intravitreal implant) for DME, retreatment with > 7 implants is not recommended; for RVO, up to 2 implants are recommended; for uveitis, repeat administration is not recommended
- (intravitreal implant) after insertion, patient monitoring is recommended, including checking optic nerve perfusion, tonometry (within 30 minutes of procedure) and biomicroscopy 2–7 days after injection
- (intravitreal implant) administration to both eyes concurrently is not recommended
- (eye drops) not recommended for Sjögren's keratoconjunctivitis
- (intravitreal implant) caution if used in those who have had cataract surgery or iridectomy due to increased risk of implant migration into anterior chamber
- (8 mg/2 mL) contraindicated in those with sulfite hypersensitivity
- (intravitreal implant) contraindicated in those with advanced glaucoma, aphakic eyes with rupture of posterior lens capsule, eyes with anterior

intraocular lens, iris or translateral fixated intraocular lens and rupture of posterior lens capsule or active/suspected ocular or periocular infection
- see also General Nursing points/Cautions/Withdrawal for corticosteroids (p. 925–29)

Patient teaching and advice

- (intravitreal implant) patient should be advised to seek medical advice if any of the following occur:
  - pain, redness, lid swelling
  - blurred vision, loss of visual acuity, discharge from the eye, photophobia
  - headache
  - inflammation in and around the eye
- (intravitreal implant) patient should be instructed not to drive or operate machinery until visual blurring has cleared after procedure
- see also General Patient teaching and advice for corticosteroids (including instillation of eye drops, p. 929)

eye drops and intravitreal implants are permitted in sport

other preparations are banned in sport via rectal, parenteral or oral use

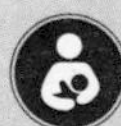

not recommended during pregnancy unless benefits outweigh risks

tablets can be crushed and mixed with water or spoonful of yoghurt or apple puree

Note

- contained in Otodex and Sofradex ear drops

FLUDROCORTISONE ACETATE (Florinef)

Available form

Tablets: 0.1 mg

Action

- mineralocorticoid with strong glucocorticoid effects similar to hydrocortisone, but with greater effects on electrolyte balance
- duration of action 24–48 hours
- see also General Actions of corticosteroids (p. 922)

Use

- Addison's disease
- salt-losing adrenogenital syndrome

Dose

- (Addison's disease) 0.1 mg orally daily (usually given with cortisone or hydrocortisone) **OR**
- (salt-losing adrenogenital syndrome) 0.1–0.2 mg orally daily

Adverse effects/Interactions/Nursing points/Cautions/Withdrawal

- (Addison's disease) dose can vary from 0.1 mg 3 times weekly to 0.2 mg daily
- (Addison's disease) dose may be reduced by 0.05 mg daily if transient hypertension occurs
- heart failure may be exacerbated if there is fluid and electrolyte imbalance
- not recommended in those with heart disease, hypertension or impaired kidney function
- see General Adverse effects/Interactions/Nursing points/Cautions/Withdrawal for corticosteroids (pp. 923–29)

Patient teaching and advice

- advise patient to seek medical advice if any severe or persistent headache, joint pain, dizziness, weakness or swelling of feet or legs occurs
- see General Patient teaching and advice for corticosteroids (p. 929)

banned in sport

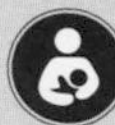
should not be used in pregnancy unless benefits outweigh risks

tablets can be dispersed in water or crushed and mixed with spoonful of yoghurt or apple puree

FLUOROMETHOLONE (Flucon, FML)

FLUOROMETHOLONE ACETATE (Flarex)

Available form
Eye drops: 1 mg/mL (0.1%)

Action
- glucocorticoid that inhibits ocular inflammatory response

Use
- palpebral and bulbar conjunctival inflammation, inflammation of the cornea and anterior segment of the globe

Dose
- 1–2 drops instilled into the conjunctival sac(s) 2–4 times daily. If needed, initial treatment can be 2 drops 1–2-hourly for first 24–48 hours

Adverse effects
- taste disturbance
- transient irritation, tearing, eye pain, ocular hyperaemia, foreign body sensation
- increased intraocular pressure, optic nerve damage, glaucoma
- secondary ocular infections, cataract formation, decreased visual acuity, blurred vision

Interactions
- decreased corneal healing may occur if used with topical NSAIDs
- (ophthalmic) increased risk of raised intraocular pressure if given with anticholinergics in those at risk of acute angle closure
- (ophthalmic) chronic/prolonged use may increase intraocular pressure and decrease efficacy of anti-glaucoma agents

Nursing points/Cautions/Patient teaching and advice
- fluorometholone acetate is more potent than fluorometholone and the two formulations are therefore not interchangeable
- see general points for corticosteroids (p. 922–30)

permitted in sport

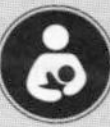
only used during pregnancy if clearly needed

HYDROCORTISONE (DermAid 1% Spray and Solution, DermAid Cream, DermAid Soft Cream, Hysone)

HYDROCORTISONE ACETATE (Colifoam Rectal Foam, CorticDS, Hysoderm, Sigmacort, Siguent Hycor Eye Ointment)

HYDROCORTISONE SODIUM SUCCINATE (SoluCortef)

Available forms
Tablets: 4 mg, 20 mg; Vial: 100 mg; Act-O-Vials: 100 mg/2 mL, 250 mg/2 mL, 500 mg/4 mL; Topical spray: 10 mg/mL; Topical cream/ointment: 0.5 mg/g (0.5%), 1 mg/g (1%); Solution: 10 mg/g (1%); Eye ointment: 1 mg/mL (1%); Rectal foam: 100 mg/g (10%)

Action

- glucocorticoid with some mineralocorticoid properties
- peak concentration achieved in about 1 hour, duration of action 8–12 hours, half-life 1.5–2 hours
- topical products are considered mild potency
- see General Actions of corticosteroids (p. 922)

Use

- see General Uses of corticosteroids (p. 923)
- (rectal foam) ulcerative colitis, proctosigmoiditis, granular proctitis
- (topical) facial and flexure dermatitis, psoriasis, nappy dermatitis, minor skin irritation

Dose

- 100–500 mg IV injection or continuous infusion, repeated at 2-, 4- or 6-hourly intervals, depending on severity of the condition and the patient's response **OR**
- (Addison's disease, chronic adrenocortical insufficiency secondary to hypopituitarism) 30 mg orally daily in divided doses with food, increasing to 75–150 mg daily during illness or surgery **OR**
- (cream, ointment) apply a small amount to affected area 2–4 times daily **OR**
- (solution) apply few drops to affected area 2–3 times daily and massage gently **OR**
- (topical spray) 1–2 sprays to affected area 2–3 times daily and massage gently **OR**
- (eye ointment) apply ointment to affected eye(s) 2–4 times daily **OR**
- (rectal foam) one applicator full (90–100 mg) 1–2 times daily for 2–3 weeks, then reducing to every second day

Adverse effects

- see General Adverse effects of corticosteroids (p. 923)
- (topical) slight stinging, burning, itching, irritation, dryness, erythema
- (topical) (prolonged/excessive therapy) telangiectasis, skin atrophy, striae
- (topical) (rare) folliculitis, pustules, hypertrichosis, hypopigmentation, contact or perioral dermatitis, skin maceration, secondary infection, miliaria, acne-form eruptions
- (ophthalmic) transient blurred vision
- (ophthalmic, uncommon/rare) burning, stinging, redness, tearing, glaucoma, corneal thinning, eye pain, secondary ocular infection, decreased visual acuity
- (rectal) redness, irritation, burning, dryness, anorectal discomfort, proctalgia

Interactions

- (ophthalmic) increased risk of raised intraocular pressure if given with anticholinergics in those at risk of acute angle closure
- (ophthalmic) chronic/prolonged use may increase intraocular pressure and decrease efficacy of antiglaucoma agents
- see General Interactions of corticosteroids (p. 924)

Nursing points/Cautions/ Withdrawal

- (IV) increased risk of hypernatraemia if high-dose therapy is continued beyond 48–72 hours and should be replaced with agent such as methylprednisolone with little or no salt retention properties
- (oral) divided doses should be ⅔ dose in the morning (20 mg) and ⅓ at about 4 pm (10 mg)
- (IV) reconstitute using water for injections and then dilute with glucose 5% or sodium chloride 0.9% depending on patient's sodium restriction
- administration rate is dependent on dose (e.g. 100 mg over 30 seconds, 500 mg or more over 10 minutes)

- ensure manufacturer's instructions are consulted before using Act-O-Vial system
- frequency of administration can be reduced once condition has improved
- (Solu-Cortef) contraindicated by local, intrathecal or epidural injection
- (rectal foam) contraindicated if anal infection or warts are present, or any obstruction, abscess, perforation, peritonitis, extensive fistulae, fresh intestinal anastomoses, or if patient has hypersensitivity to components (including hydroxybenzoates, propane, propylene glycol, emulsifying wax)
- see also General Nursing points/Cautions/Withdrawal for corticosteroids (p. 925–29)

Patient teaching and advice

- (oral) patient should be advised to take tablets with food or milk to reduce gastric acidity
- (topical spray) hold spray 10 cm from area to be sprayed
- (topical) advise patient to decrease frequency of administration when inflammation subsides
- instruct patient in correct eye ointment insertion (see Eye, ear, nose and throat agents, p. 1063), including:
  - allow 10 minutes between ointment and any other topical ophthalmic agent
- ensure patient understands instructions for rectal foam use (see Gastrointestinal agents (miscellaneous) p. 1100)
- see General Patient teaching and advice for corticosteroids (p. 929)

eye ointment and topical preparations are permitted in sport

other preparations are banned in sport via rectal, parenteral or oral use

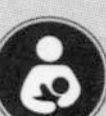

not recommended during pregnancy unless benefits outweigh risks

tablets can be dispersed in water or crushed and mixed with spoonful of yoghurt or apple puree

Note

- contained in Candacort Cream, Canesten Extra Clotrimazole and Hydrocortisone Cream, Canesten Plus Clotrimazole Plus Hydrocortisone Cream, Ciproxin HC Ear Drops, Hydrozole, Proctosedyl Ointment and Suppositories, Resolve Plus 1.0, Resolve Plus 0.5, SOOV IT, Xyloproct and Zovirax Due Cold Sore Cream

METHYLPREDNISOLONE ACEPONATE (Advantan)

METHYLPREDNISOLONE ACETATE (Depo-Medrol, Depo-Nisolone)

METHYLPREDNISOLONE SODIUM SUCCINATE (Solu-Medrol)

Available forms

Vial: 40 mg/mL, 125 mg, 500 mg, 1 g; Act-O-Vials: 40 mg/mL, 125 mg/2 mL; Cream: 1 mg/g; Ointment: 1 mg/g; Lotion: 1 mg/g

Action/Use

- potent glucocorticoid
- see General Actions and Uses of corticosteroids (pp. 922–23)

Dose

- (high dose > 250 mg) 30 mg/kg IV over at least 30 minutes, repeated 4–6-hourly if needed, for up to 48 hours **OR**
- 10–500 mg IV daily (with larger doses being for short-term treatment of acute conditions) **OR**

- (rheumatoid arthritis, osteoarthritis) 4–80 mg intra-articularly, dose depending on severity of disease and size of joint, repeated every 1–5 weeks **OR**
- (bursitis, ganglion, tendinitis, epicondylitis) 4–30 mg into site, repeated as needed in chronic or recurrent conditions **OR**
- (adrenogenital syndrome) 40 mg IM every 2 weeks **OR**
- (rheumatoid arthritis maintenance) 40–120 mg IM weekly **OR**
- (seborrhoeic dermatitis) 80 mg IM weekly **OR**
- (multiple sclerosis, acute exacerbation) 160 mg IM daily for 1 week, then 64 mg every second day for 1 month **OR**
- (*Pneumocystis jiroveci* pneumonia (PCP)) 40 mg IV 6-hourly for 5–7 days, then converting to oral tapering regimen (for up to 21 days or the end of antipneumocystis therapy) **OR**
- (skin lesions) 40–120 mg IM weekly for 1–4 weeks or every 5–10 days (contact dermatitis) **OR**
- (dermatological conditions) 20–60 mg intradermally into lesions, repeated 1–4 times (interval depends on type of lesions) **OR**
- (allergic rhinitis) 80–120 mg IM stat (may provide relief in 6 hours, lasting for up to 3 weeks) **OR**
- (asthma) 80–120 mg IM stat (may provide relief in 6–48 hours, lasting up to 2 weeks) **OR**
- (cream/ointment) apply thinly to affected area once daily (twice daily for psoriasis) for up to 12 weeks **OR**
- (lotion) apply sparingly to affected area (including scalp) and massage until lotion disappears for up to 12 weeks

Adverse effects

- see General Adverse effects of corticosteroids (p. 923)
- (intra-articular) post-injection flare, pain, irritation/discomfort at injection site, sterile abscess formation, hypopigmentation, hyperpigmentation, degeneration of joint with loss of sensation, joint instability (repeated injections), Charcot-type arthropathy (see Glossary)
- (intradermal/intralesional) local discomfort, sterile abscess formation, hypopigmentation, hyperpigmentation, subcutaneous/cutaneous atrophy
- (IV, large doses) bradycardia
- (IV, rapid administration) cardiac arrhythmias, circulatory collapse, cardiac arrest
- (topical) burning, itching, irritation, dryness, erythema, rash
- (topical) (prolonged/excessive therapy) telangiectasis, skin atrophy, striae
- (topical) (rare) folliculitis, pustules, secondary infection, miliaria, acneform eruptions

Interactions

- increased serum levels may occur if given with aprepitant
- increased risk of convulsions if given with ciclosporin
- may alter serum levels of tacrolimus, therefore levels should be monitored especially when stopping methylprednisolone
- see General Interactions of corticosteroids (p. 924)

Nursing points/Cautions/Withdrawal

- Achilles tendon should not be injected
- (AIDS-related PCP) diagnosis of PCP should be confirmed because of potential to mask other untreated lung infection. If person shows positive response to skin test for TB, antimycobacterial therapy should be started with antipneumocystis therapy

- (AIDS-related PCP) adjunctive corticosteroid therapy should be commenced at maximum dose within 72 hours of starting antipneumocystis therapy
- IM injections (250 mg or less) should only be injected into large muscles
- doses of up to 250 mg IV should be given over at least 5 minutes; doses greater than 250 mg should be given over 30 minutes
- high doses (> 250 mg) should only be continued for 48–72 hours until patient's condition has stabilised
- follow manufacturer's instructions for reconstitution of powder as amount of diluent is dependent on product strength and recommended concentration
- reconstituted solution should be diluted with glucose 5% or sodium chloride 0.9% for IV infusion
- administer alone
- ensure manufacturer's instructions are consulted before using Act-O-Vial system
- (topical) if skin shows excessive drying, a change of formulation with a higher fat content (e.g. Advantan Fatty Ointment) is recommended
- (ointment) suitable for non-weeping, dry, fissured, scaly or hyperkeratinised skin
- (lotion) suitable for hirsute areas
- see General Nursing points/ Cautions/Withdrawal for corticosteroids (p. 925–29)

Patient teaching and advice

- (lotion) patient should be instructed that lotion should not be used on axilla, groin or skin folds
- see General Patient teaching and advice for corticosteroids (p. 929)

topical preparations are permitted in sport

other preparations are banned in sport via rectal, parenteral or oral use

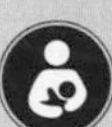

should only be used during pregnancy if benefits outweigh risks

MOMETASONE FUROATE (Azonaire Hayfever & Allergy Prevention Nasal Spray, Elocon, Momasone, Nasonex Aqueous Nasal Spray, Novasone, Sensease Nasal Allergy Relief Nasal Spray, Zatamil)

Available forms

Lotion: 1 mg/g; Cream: 1 mg/g; Ointment: 1 mg/g; Hydrogel: 1 mg/mL; Nasal spray: 50 microgram/dose

Action

- potent topical glucocorticoid
- (nasal) decreases capillary permeability and mucus production as well as causing vasoconstriction in the nasal mucosa
- see General Actions of corticosteroids (p. 922)

Use

- psoriasis, dermatitis
- treatment of allergic and perennial rhinitis, prevention of seasonal allergic rhinitis
- prevention and treatment of seasonal or perennial allergic rhinitis
- nasal polyps
- acute rhinosinusitis (without signs/ symptoms of severe bacterial infection)

Dose

- (psoriasis, dermatitis) thin film of cream/ointment/hydrogel applied to affected area once daily **OR**
- (psoriasis, dermatitis) apply few drops of lotion to affected area, including scalp, massage gently until solution disappears **OR**
- (allergic rhinitis) initially 2 sprays per nostril (50 microgram per spray) daily until symptoms are controlled, then reduced to 1 spray per nostril (maximum daily dose 200 microgram) **OR**
- (nasal polyps) 2 sprays per nostril (50 microgram per spray) daily, increasing to twice daily if symptoms are not controlled, then reducing dose (maximum daily dose 400 microgram) **OR**
- (acute rhinosinusitis) 2 sprays per nostril (50 microgram per spray) twice daily for 15 days. If no improvement, therapy should be stopped (maximum daily dose 400 microgram)

Adverse effects

- (topical) burning, stinging, itching, irritation, dryness, erythema
- (topical) (prolonged/excessive therapy) telangiectasis, skin atrophy, striae
- (topical) (rare) folliculitis, pustules, hypertrichosis, hypopigmentation, contact or perioral dermatitis, skin maceration, secondary infection, miliaria, acne-form eruptions
- (nasal spray) nasal stinging, itching, irritation, epistaxis, sneezing, sore throat, dry mouth, cough, headache, pharyngitis, visual disturbances
- (nasal spray) (rare) nasal septum perforation, increased intraocular pressure, glaucoma, hypersensitivity, taste/smell disturbances

Nursing points/Cautions/Withdrawal

- (cream) suitable for lesions
- (ointment) suitable for dry, scaling skin with fissures
- (lotion) recommended for scalp psoriasis and seborrhoeic dermatitis
- (nasal spray) not recommended after recent nasal surgery or trauma as healing may be delayed
- (nasal spray) contraindicated if severe nasal infection is present, bleeding disorders or if there is a history of nose bleeding
- (topical) contraindicated in those with rosacea, perioral dermatitis, viral or fungal skin infection or ulcerative conditions
- see General Nursing points/Cautions/Withdrawal for corticosteroids (p. 925–29)

Patient teaching and advice

- (prevention of seasonal allergic rhinitis) patient should be advised to start therapy 2–4 weeks before start of pollen season
- advise patient to seek medical advice if any of the following occur:
  - symptoms persist after 7 days of continuous use
  - fever, persistent/severe one-sided face or tooth pain, swelling around eyes
  - worsening of symptoms after an initial improvement
- see General Patient teaching and advice for corticosteroids (p. 929)

permitted in sport

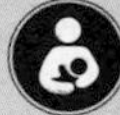

should only be used during pregnancy or breastfeeding if benefits outweigh risks

PREDNISOLONE SODIUM PHOSPHATE (Minims Prednisolone Eyedrops)

PREDNISOLONE (Panafcortelone, Predsolone, Predmix Oral Solution, Predsol Retention Enema and Suppositories, Redipred Solone)

Available forms

Tablets: 1 mg, 5 mg, 25 mg; Eye drops: 5 mg/mL; Oral liquid: 5 mg/mL; Retention enema: 20 mg/100 mL; Suppositories: 5 mg

Action

- glucocorticoid with greater activity than hydrocortisone but less mineralocorticoid effects (less sodium retention, oedema and electrolyte imbalance)
- peak concentration after 1–2 hours orally, half-life 2–4 hours
- see also General Actions of corticosteroids (p. 922)

Use

- see General Uses of corticosteroids (p. 923)
- proctitis (haemorrhagic, granular or post-radiation), rectal complications of Crohn's disease

Dose

- initially 20–80 mg orally daily in 2–4 divided doses, as a single dose or on alternate days, reducing gradually to 5–20 mg daily (maintenance) **OR**
- (ulcerative colitis, Crohn's disease) contents of 1 disposable enema unit nightly for 2–4 weeks as a retention enema until progressive improvement occurs **OR**
- (proctitis) suppository inserted twice daily (at bedtime and after morning defecation) with treatment continuing until tissue appears normal **OR**
- 1 drop instilled into the conjunctival sac(s) hourly (for intensive treatment) or 2–4 times daily

Adverse effects

- (ophthalmic) transient blurred vision or discomfort
- (ophthalmic, uncommon/rare, prolonged use) glaucoma, secondary ocular infection, visual acuity defect, optic nerve damage, ocular hypertension, ptosis, mydriasis
- (rectal) mucosal atrophy, itching, burning
- see also General Adverse effects of corticosteroids (p. 923)

Interactions

- see General Interactions of corticosteroids (p. 924)
- topical corticosteroids are not recommended concurrently with oral or IV corticosteroids

Nursing points/Cautions/Withdrawal

- doses > 40 mg are not recommended for prolonged therapy to minimise adverse effects
- alternate day therapy is recommended for long-term/maintenance treatment providing symptom relief while minimising adrenal suppression and other adverse effects
- (enema) therapy should not be continued if there is no improvement in condition
- caution if used in those with systemic sclerosis due to risk of scleroderma renal crisis with hypertension and decreased urinary output if daily dose greater than 15 mg is given. BP and renal function should be closely monitored
- (oral solution) contraindicated in those with hypersensitivity to hydroxybenzoates
- (rectal) caution if diverticulitis is present or there is any possibility of impending perforation, abscess or other infection

- (rectal) contraindicated if there is any impaired circulation (as rectal ulceration may occur) or any trauma or infection in anorectal region
- (eye drops) contraindicated in those with glaucoma or if any eye infection is present
- see also General Nursing points/Cautions/Withdrawal for corticosteroids (p. 925–29)

Patient teaching and advice

- advise patient that 1 mg tablets should not be broken even though they are scored
- (oral solution) instruct patient that oral solution should be refrigerated after opening (not frozen) and discarded after 28 days
- (oral solution) solution can be taken alone or with milk, cordial, soft drink or soft food if needed
- (rectal) patient should be advised to stop therapy if irritation, rash or rectal bleeding occurs and seek medical advice
- patient should be instructed in correct technique for eye drop instillation (see Eye, ear, nose and throat agents, p. 1062)
- instruct patient in correct technique for suppository insertion (see Gastrointestinal agents (miscellaneous) p. 1100)
- ensure patient understands correct enema instillation technique (see Gastrointestinal agents (miscellaneous) p. 1099)
- see General Patient teaching and advice for corticosteroids (p. 929)

banned in sport via rectal, parenteral or oral route

permitted in sport for intra-articular injection use, local injection, and use via anal, respiratory, oral mucosal, ocular, nasal, cutaneous and auricular routes

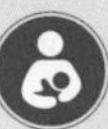

should only be used during pregnancy if benefits outweigh risks

available as oral solution. Tablet can be crushed and mixed with yoghurt or apple puree

Note

- contained in Prednefrin Forte and Scheriproct

PREDNISONE (Panafcort, Predsone, Sone)

Available forms

Tablets: 1 mg, 5 mg, 25 mg

Action

- synthetic glucocorticoid that is converted in the liver to its active metabolite, prednisolone, within 60 minutes
- duration of action 12–36 hours
- see also General Actions of corticosteroids (p. 922)

Use

- see General Uses of corticosteroids (p. 923)

Dose

- initially 20–80 mg daily in 2–4 divided doses, as a single dose or on alternate days after meals, then 5–20 mg daily (maintenance)

Adverse effects/Interactions/Nursing points/Cautions/Withdrawal/Patient teaching and advice

- advise patient that 1 mg tablets should not be broken even though they are scored
- doses > 40 mg are not recommended for prolonged therapy to minimise adverse effects
- alternate day therapy is recommended for long-term/maintenance

treatment providing symptom relief while minimising adrenal suppression and other adverse effects
- see general points for corticosteroids (p. 922–30)

banned in sport

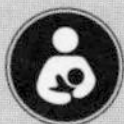

only used during pregnancy if benefits outweigh risks

tablets can be dispersed in water (has strong bitter taste) or crushed and mixed with spoonful of yoghurt or apple puree

TRIAMCINOLONE ACETONIDE (Aristocort, Kenacort-A 10, Kenacort-A 40, Kenalog in Orabase, Tricortone)

Available forms

Ampoules: 10 mg/mL, 40 mg/mL; Cream: 0.2 mg/g; Ointment: 0.2 mg/g; Oral paste: 1 mg/g;

Action

- moderately potent glucocorticoid with activity similar to prednisolone (4 mg triamcinolone = 5 mg prednisolone)
- see also General Actions of corticosteroids (p. 922)

Use

- see General Uses of corticosteroids (p. 923)

Dose

- initially 60 mg deep IM into buttock, then dose adjusted according to response (range 20–80 mg) (solution strength 40 mg/mL) **OR**
- (hay fever, pollen asthma unresponsive to other treatment) 40–100 mg IM stat (solution strength 40 mg/mL) **OR**
- 2.5–15 mg depending on size of joint and disease (intra-articular, intrabursal, injection into ganglia or tendon sheath) (solution strength 10 mg/mL) **OR**
- 10–40 mg depending on size of joint and disease (intra-articular, intrabursal, injection into ganglia or tendon sheath) (solution strength 40 mg/mL) **OR**
- (intradermally) initial dose dependent on specific disease but limited to 1 mg (0.1 mL) per site, repeated weekly or less frequently as needed **OR**
- (inflamed skin lesions) apply cream or ointment 3–4 times daily to affected area **OR**
- (mouth ulcers) cover lesion with sufficient paste (about 1 cm) to form a thin film each night, increasing to 2–3 times daily after meals if lesions are severe

Adverse effects

- (topical) burning, itching, irritation, dryness, erythema
- (topical) (prolonged/excessive therapy) telangiectasis, skin atrophy, striae
- (topical) (rare) folliculitis, pustules, hypertrichosis, hypopigmentation, contact or perioral dermatitis, skin maceration, secondary infection, miliaria, acne-form eruptions
- (intra-articular) post-injection flare, pain, irritation/discomfort at injection site, sterile abscess formation, hypopigmentation, hyperpigmentation, degeneration of joint with loss of sensation, joint instability (repeated injections), Charcot-type arthropathy (see Glossary)
- (intradermal/intralesional) local discomfort, sterile abscess formation, hypopigmentation, hyperpigmentation, subcutaneous/cutaneous atrophy
- see also General Adverse effects of corticosteroids (p. 923)

Interactions

- see General Interactions of corticosteroids (p. 924)

Nursing points/Cautions/Withdrawal

- (intradermal) if multiple sites are to be injected intradermally, there should be at least 1 cm between sites
- (ampoules) shake well before use
- (intra-articular) not recommended for unstable joints
- (oral paste) contraindicated if bacterial or fungal infection is present in mouth or throat, or in those with viral herpetic oral or intra-oral lesions
- (ampoules) contain benzyl alcohol and are therefore contraindicated in newborn or premature infants
- see also General Nursing points/Cautions/Withdrawal for corticosteroids (p. 925–29)

Patient teaching and advice

- (oral paste) advise patient not to rub paste in as it will crumble
- (cream, ointment) patient should be advised if treating eczematised psoriasis, occlusive non-permeable dressing may be applied over cream or ointment to improve effectiveness
- (intra-articular) advise patient to seek medical advice if local swelling, restricted joint movement, fever or malaise occurs
- see General Patient teaching and advice for corticosteroids (p. 929) and correct instillation of nasal spray (see Antiasthma agents, bronchodilators and respiratory agents, p. 112)

banned in sport via rectal, parenteral or oral route

permitted in sport for intra-articular injection use, local injection, and use via anal, respiratory, oral mucosal, ocular, nasal, cutaneous and auricular routes

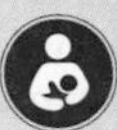

only used in pregnancy if benefits outweigh risks

Note

- contained in Kenacomb, Kenacomb Otic, Otocomb Otic

COUGH SUPPRESSANTS AND EXPECTORANTS

Under normal circumstances, coughing is a protective mechanism that clears the airways of secretions and any foreign materials. Combinations of cough suppressants, expectorants, sympathomimetics or analgesics are widely used in various cough and cold preparations that are commonly available as over-the-counter (OTC) preparations. It is important that the patient is aware of the constituents of these preparations because they often have adverse interactions with other medications.

Cough suppressants (antitussives) have a central and/or peripheral action on the cough reflex and are used to suppress irritating unproductive coughs (e.g. dextromethorphan, codeine phosphate hemihydrate, dihydrocodeine and pholcodine).

Although their exact action is unknown, expectorants are thought to increase the volume of secretions in the respiratory tract and therefore facilitate their removal by ciliary action and coughing. Some are thought to have an irritant effect on the gastric mucosa (e.g. ammonium chloride, guaifenesin, ipecacuanha, senega and ammonia).

Decongestants are cough preparations that contain an antihistamine (decreasing capillary permeability) and a sympathomimetic agent (causing vasoconstriction) with the combination resulting in less congested mucous membranes.

AMMONIUM CHLORIDE (Nyal Bronchitis Cough Medicine)

Available form

Syrup: 110 mg/10 mL

Action

- increases quantity and decreases viscosity of respiratory tract secretions, allowing easier removal by ciliary action and coughing

Use

- expectorant, relief from cough associated with common cold

Dose

- 110 mg (10 mL) orally 4-hourly if needed

Nursing points/Cautions

- not recommended in children under 6 years

Patient teaching and advice

- instruct patient to shake bottle well before use

- patient should be advised to seek medical advice if symptoms persist after 7 days or if fever and increased bronchial secretions occur

Note

- contained in Benadryl Oral Liquid with diphenhydramine hydrochloride

BROMHEXINE HYDROCHLORIDE (Bisolvon Chesty Forte Oral Liquid, Bisolvon Chesty Oral Liquid, Bisolvon Chesty Forte Tablets, DuroTuss Chesty Cough Liquid Bromhexine (1.6 mg/mL), DuroTuss Chesty Cough Liquid Regular)

Available forms

Elixir: 4 mg/5 mL, 8 mg/5 mL; Tablets: 8 mg; Sachets: 8 mg/5 mL

Action

- mucolytic that reduces the viscosity of mucus and promotes flow of thin bronchial secretions, gradually reducing the volume of mucus
- facilitates expectoration, eases cough
- half-life 6.6–31.4 hours (single dose) or 1 hour (multiple dosing)

Use

- breakdown of viscid mucus in those with common cold, influenza or other bronchial conditions causing excessive mucus production

Dose

- (tablets) initially 8–16 mg orally 3 times daily for 7 days, then 8 mg 3 times daily if needed **OR**
- (elixir/sachets) 8–16 mg (10–20 mL) orally 3 times daily

Adverse effects

- (occasionally, mild) nausea, vomiting, diarrhoea, indigestion, upper abdominal pain
- headache, dizziness, sweating
- (rare) hypersensitivity reaction, severe skin reactions

Interaction

- may increase concentration of amoxicillin or erythromycin in bronchial secretions if taken concurrently

Nursing points/Cautions

- soluble tablets are not recommended in children under 12 years
- soluble tablets contain fructose and are therefore not recommended in those with fructose intolerance
- (oral liquid, tablets, sachets) contain lactose and are therefore not recommended in those with Lapp lactase intolerance or glucose–galactose malabsorption
- contains sorbitol, which may cause diarrhoea
- caution if used in those with gastric ulceration or severe kidney/liver disease

Patient teaching and advice

- patient should be advised to seek medical attention if any new skin or mucosal lesions occur
- warn patient to expect an initial increase in the flow of secretions
- instruct patient to dissolve soluble tablets in either hot or cold water and drink immediately
- patient should be advised to seek medical advice if symptoms persist after 7 days or if fever and increased bronchial secretions occur

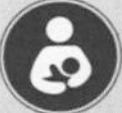

not recommended during first trimester of pregnancy

not recommended during breastfeeding

available as solution and soluble tablets. Tablet can be crushed and mixed with spoonful of yoghurt or apple puree

Note

- contained in Benadryl Chesty Forte (New formulation) Oral liquid, Demazin Chesty Cough Relief, Duro-Tuss Chesty Cough Liquid Forte, Du-roTuss Chesty Cough Liquid Oral, DuroTuss Chesty Cough Liquid plus Nasal Decongestant, DuroTuss Chesty Cough Lozenges, DuroTuss Cough Liquid Expectorant, DuroTuss PE Chesty Cough Plus Nasal Decongestant, Robitussin Chesty Cough Forte, Robitussin Mucus Relief Double Action Oral Liquid

DEXTROMETHORPHAN HYDROBROMIDE MONOHYDRATE (DEXTROMETHORPHAN HYDROBROMIDE) (Bisolvon Dry (Oral Liquid), Bisolvon Dry Pastilles, Robitussin Dry Cough Forte)

Available forms

Syrup: 10 mg/5 mL, 15 mg/5 mL, 30 mg/10 mL; Pastilles: 10 mg

Action

- non-opioid antitussive which is centrally acting (medulla)
- metabolised to weak codeine analogue
- no analgesic, sedative or respiratory depressant effects at antitussive dose
- weak serotonergic properties
- onset of action within 60 minutes, duration 3–6 hours
- half-life 1.2–3.9 hours (extended in poor metabolisers)

Use

- relief of dry, irritating, unproductive cough
- (pastilles) also soothe throat

Dose

- 10–30 mg orally 4–6-hourly (10 mg/5 mL) (daily maximum 4 doses, maximum duration 5 days) **OR**
- 30 mg (10 mL) 6–8-hourly (30 mg/10 mL) (maximum duration 5 days) **OR**
- suck 1–3 (10–30 mg) pastilles every 4–6 hours as needed (maximum daily dose 12 pastilles (120 mg))

Adverse effects

- nausea, vomiting, diarrhoea, abdominal pain, constipation
- dizziness, drowsiness, fatigue, confusion, somnolence
- abuse, dependency
- tolerance (with prolonged use)
- (overdose) confusion, excitation, psychosis, nervousness, restlessness, severe nausea and vomiting, respiratory depression, serotonin syndrome (see Glossary)

Interactions

- contraindicated with or within 14 days of MAOIs
- caution if used with other serotonergic agents, including SSRIs and TCAs
- may increase CNS effects if given with alcohol or CNS depressants
- serum levels may increase if given with amiodarone, bupropion, fluoxetine, haloperidol, cimetidine, ritonavir, flecainide and paroxetine increasing risk of adverse effects

Nursing points/Cautions

- has addictive potential and tolerance may develop with prolonged use
- caution if used in those with tendency towards abuse or dependence (e.g. history of alcohol/drug abuse or psychiatric disorders). Should only be used for short period of time under medical supervision
- (Bisolvon Dry) contains fructose and is therefore not recommended in those with fructose intolerance
- caution if used in those with liver or kidney impairment or impaired cough reflex (e.g. Parkinson's disease, dementia) or at risk of developing respiratory failure

- not recommended in those with mastocytosis
- not recommended for productive cough with mucus production (e.g. cystic fibrosis, bronchiectasis)
- contraindicated in those with asthma, chronic obstructive pulmonary disease, pneumonia, respiratory failure or depression

Patient teaching and advice

- advise patient to sip undiluted linctus slowly; will be more effective if not followed immediately by liquid (e.g. milk or water)
- some oral formulations contain sorbitol, which may cause diarrhoea
- patient should be advised not to drive or operate machinery if drowsiness or dizziness occurs
- warn patient to avoid alcohol while taking this medication
- patient should be advised to seek medical advice if symptoms have not been relieved or fever with increasing bronchial secretions occurs

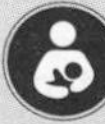

not recommended during first trimester of pregnancy and only if benefits outweigh risks in second or third trimester. Medical supervision is recommended if used during pregnancy

contraindicated during breastfeeding

Note

- contained in Benadryl PE Dry Cough and Nasal Congestion Oral Liquid, Codral Original Cold & Flu + Cough Day & Night Capsules, Demazin Cough and Cold Relief, Dimetapp preparations, Panadol Cold & Flu Relief + Cough, Robitussin Cough & Cold Congestion

DIHYDROCODEINE TARTRATE (Rikodeine Oral Liquid)

Available form

Syrup: 19 mg/10 mL

Action

- semi-synthetic opioid with cough suppressant properties

Use

- unproductive or intractable (dry) cough

Dose

- 9.5–19 mg (5–10 mL) orally 4–6-hourly

Adverse effects

- drowsiness, diarrhoea

Interactions

- may increase effects of alcohol and CNS depressants

Nursing points/Cautions

- contains sorbitol which may cause diarrhoea

Patient teaching and advice

- patient should be advised not to drive or operate heavy machinery if drowsiness occurs
- patient should be advised to seek medical advice if symptoms persist after 7 days or if fever and increased bronchial secretions occur
- warn patient to avoid alcohol with this medication

GUAIFENESIN (Robitussin Chesty Cough Oral Liquid, Vicks Cough Syrup for Chest Coughs)

Available forms

Syrup: 20 mg/mL, 200 mg/15 mL

Action

- increases the volume and reduces the viscosity of bronchial and tracheal secretions
- half-life 60 minutes

Use
- expectorant for productive cough providing symptomatic relief from congested chest and cough

Dose
- 200–400 mg orally 4-hourly (daily maximum 6 doses)

Adverse effects
- nausea, vomiting, abdominal pain, diarrhoea
- dizziness, headache, drowsiness
- rash
- (rare) hypersensitivity

Nursing points/Cautions
- caution if used in those with porphyria
- not recommended in those with chronic/persistent cough associated with asthma, bronchitis, emphysema, smoker's cough, chronic obstructive pulmonary disease (COPD) or cough associated with excessive secretions
- contraindicated in those under 6 years

Patient teaching and advice
- patient should be advised to seek medical advice if symptoms persist after 7 days or if fever and increased bronchial secretions occur

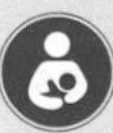
not recommended during breastfeeding unless benefits outweigh potential risks

Note
- contained in Benadryl Chesty Forte, Benadryl PE Chesty Cough and Nasal Congestion, DuroTuss Chesty Cough Liquid Forte, DuroTuss Chesty Cough Forte Tablets, Lemsip Multi-Relief Cold and Flu, Nyal Chesty Cough Medicine, Robitussin preparations

PHOLCODINE (Benadryl Dry Tickly Cough, Benadryl Dry Tickly Cough Forte, DuroTuss Dry Cough Liquid Forte, DuroTuss Dry Cough Liquid Regular, Gold Cross Pholcodine Linctus APF)

Available forms

Elixir: 1 mg/mL, 3 mg/mL, 4 mg/mL

Action
- opioid related to morphine, with no analgesic properties
- depresses cough centre in the medulla, without affecting the respiratory centre
- mild sedative effect
- has no euphoric properties, therefore dependence is unlikely to be a problem

Use
- relief of unproductive (dry) cough

Dose
- 10–15 mg (10–15 mL) orally up to 4 times daily (1 mg/mL solution) **OR**
- 15 mg (5 mL) orally up to 4 times daily (3 mg/mL solution) **OR**
- 15 mg (3.75 mL) orally 3–4 times daily (4 mg/mL solution)

Adverse effects
- diarrhoea
- drowsiness

Interactions
- not recommended with alcohol
- caution if used with other cough and cold preparations

Nursing points/Cautions
- preparations contain benzoates which can cause hypersensitivity reaction in sensitive individuals
- (Benadryl) contraindicated in children under 12 years
- (DuroTuss) not recommended in children under 6 years

Patient teaching and advice

- instruct patient to shake bottle before use
- advise patient not to drive a vehicle or operate machinery if drowsy
- patient should be advised to seek medical advice if symptoms persist after 7 days or if fever and increased bronchial secretions occur

Note

- contained in Difflam plus Sore Throat and Cough Lozenges, DuroTuss preparations

DERMATOLOGICAL AGENTS

The skin is the largest organ of the body and is subject to a range of disorders, including viral, bacterial and fungal infections, parasitic infestations, cancers, ulcers, allergic reactions, as well as skin-specific conditions, such as disorders of the hair follicles and sebaceous glands, and those of unknown aetiology, such as psoriasis, pityriasis rosea and lichen planus.

Absorption of dermatological agents is influenced by a number of factors, such as age (e.g. skin is thin at the extremes of age), condition and site (e.g. palms and soles of feet have thick layers that are not easily penetrated), metabolism and circulation (i.e. poor circulation impedes healing) and formulation of the agent (e.g. water-soluble drugs are poorly absorbed through the skin; alcohol-containing agents have a drying effect).

Goals of therapy for dermatological agents include:

- treating the cause (e.g. infection)
- relieving symptoms (e.g. redness, pruritus, inflammation), and/or
- restoring and maintaining normal skin function (if possible).

It should be noted that while dermatological agents are used for their local effects, they may also have systemic effects, especially if applied to large areas, broken skin or under occlusive dressings.

TOPICAL ECTOPARASITICAL AGENTS

Ectoparasites are multicellular organisms that live or feed off human skin, and include ticks, fleas and mites. Pediculicides are agents which are used to treat lice, while scabicides or acaricides are used to treat mite infestation (Bryant et al 2019).

PEDICULOSIS (LICE INFESTATION)

There are three types of lice which cause infestation of the body (body louse), hair (head louse) or pubic area (pubic or crab louse). Lice are small, wingless, blood-sucking organisms that can only crawl (not fly or jump), therefore spread is by close contact. For example, outbreaks of head lice frequently occur in schools, childcare centres and families where children have close contact with each other.

General Patient teaching and advice for pediculicides

- lice do not distinguish between clean and dirty hair
- hair should be checked regularly for head lice (use hair conditioner on dry hair and comb using fine-toothed comb, looking for lice or eggs (nits))
- children may return to school after treatment for head lice has started
- none of the treatments kill all eggs, therefore treatment must be repeated 7–10 days apart
- all members of the family should be checked for head lice and only treated if head lice/nits are present
- children should be instructed not to share hats, scarves, hair ribbons/bands or combs/brushes
- fine-toothed combs (used for removal of lice/nits) should be washed in hot water and allowed to air dry
- apply lotion/cream/mousse to dry hair and massage into hair to completely cover and wet hair/scalp
- leave in situ for 10 minutes
- comb out dead lice and nits, starting at the top of the head and lifting a 2 cm section of hair. Comb should be touching scalp and, using a firm motion, comb away from the scalp towards the end of the hair. Nits/lice should be wiped on tissue before moving to next section of hair
- wash hair with usual shampoo
- avoid contact with eyes and mucous membranes. If contact occurs, area should be flushed with water
- gloves should be worn, or wash hands thoroughly after applying lotion
- ensure patient/parent/carer understands that lotion should not be swallowed

BENZYL ALCOHOL (NeutraLice Advance)

Available form

Lotion: 5% w/w

Action

- suffocates lice by blocking respiratory system

Use

- head lice

Dose

- apply generous amount of lotion to dry hair, rubbing vigorously into hair and scalp, concentrating on areas behind ears and back of neck. Leave lotion on hair for at least 10 minutes, using plastic comb provided to remove lice and nits. Wash with water and towel dry

Adverse effects

- skin irritation

Nursing points/Cautions

- not recommended in children under 6 months

Patient teaching and advice

- see General Patient teaching and advice for pediculicides (above)

SCABIES

Scabies is a highly contagious skin infestation with female mites burrowing under the skin after mating to lay their eggs for 4 to 6 weeks. Mites and eggs are contained in lesions (small, wavy, threadlike, slightly elevated, greyish-white burrows) ranging in length from 1 to 10 mm with a terminal end capped with a small blister. Lesions are commonly found between the toes and fingers, anterior surfaces of wrists and elbows, axillae, lower abdomen, under female breasts and genitalia of both sexes, with face and neck unaffected (Gunning et al 2012).

The main symptom is intense itching, which is usually worse after a hot bath or at night, and scratching may lead to secondary infection. Outbreaks of scabies occur in childcare centres, kindergartens, nursing homes and institutions. Transmission of scabies involves either skin contact with the infected person or infected towels, bedclothes or undergarments (contaminated within past 4–5 days). The incubation period is usually 2–6 weeks (not previously infected) or 1–4 days (re-infection). Diagnosis is via skin scraping (Gunning et al 2012).

General Patient teaching and advice for scabicides

- ensure patient understands that cream/lotion should be applied to skin only and not taken orally
- avoid contact with face, neck and eyes. If contact occurs, area should be washed thoroughly with water
- solution should be diluted for use in children
- personal garments, towels and bedclothes should be washed in hot water
- blankets should be dry-cleaned or placed in tumble dryer for 30 minutes on hot setting
- all members of the household or sexual contacts should be treated at the same time
- a hot bath and gentle scrubbing before application of lotion/cream is recommended to open up burrows; dry thoroughly
- lotion/cream is applied to whole body from neck to toes, especially in areas known for infestation, but avoiding the face and head. Care should be taken to work cream or lotion into skin folds (especially between fingers and toes, wrists, armpits and genital areas)
- if area is washed (e.g. hands) during contact time, lotion/cream should be reapplied
- lotion/cream is allowed to dry and remain in situ for 8–24 hours (depending on brand) and then washed off using soap and water
- re-treatment is recommended after 5–7 days if mites are still present
- patient is non-infectious within 24 hours of treatment
- itch may persist for up to 4 weeks after treatment (which may be due to reaction to dead mites under the skin rather than treatment failure)

BENZYL BENZOATE (Ascabiol, McGloin's Benzemul)

Available form
Lotion: 250 mg/mL

Action
- ectoparasiticidal

Use
- pediculosis (body lice)
- scabies

Dose
- (pediculosis) apply lotion thinly to affected area, leave for 24 hours, then remove with soap and water **OR**
- (scabies) apply lotion thinly to whole body from neck, allow to dry and leave for 24 hours before washing off

Adverse effects
- skin irritation and burning sensation

Nursing points/Cautions
- skin testing 10 minutes before general application is recommended to detect any severe skin reaction. If stinging occurs, solution should be diluted with equal quantity of water and skin re-tested

- if used in children under 12 years, lotion should be diluted in equal parts with water, and with 3 parts water if used on babies
- (pediculosis) treatment may be repeated after 7 days if lice are still present. May be repeated multiple times
- (scabies) re-treatment may be necessary after 5 days if live mites are still present

Patient teaching and advice

- see General Patient teaching and advice for scabicides (p. 956)

Note

- contained in Anusol with zinc oxide

CROTAMITON (Eurax)

Available forms

Cream: 10%; Lotion: 10%

Action

- antipruritic and acaricide with some antiseptic effect, which prevents secondary infection
- duration of effect 6–10 hours

Use

- pruritus (due to insect bites and stings, nettle rash, allergies, prickly heat (miliaria)) or senile, anal and genital pruritus
- itching due to head or pubic lice (lotion)
- scabies

Dose

- (pruritus) rub gently into affected areas 2–3 times daily **OR**
- (scabies infestation) apply thinly and evenly over whole body (avoiding face and scalp) at bedtime, then repeated daily for 3–5 days depending on response

Adverse effects

- (uncommon) pruritus
- (rare) contact dermatitis, rash, eczema, erythema, irritation, angioedema

Nursing points/Cautions

- lotion is preferred for use on hairy areas of the body
- contains propylene glycol, which can cause skin irritation, and sorbic acid, cetostearyl alcohol and wool fat, which can cause contact dermatitis in sensitive individuals
- (children) not recommended for application to whole body

Patient teaching and advice

- (pruritus) if itch is not relieved in 5 days, patient should be advised to seek medical attention
- advise patient to not reapply more than once daily if washing of area with soap and water has occurred
- see General Patient teaching and advice for scabicides (p. 956)

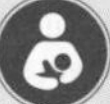

contraindicated during pregnancy

not recommended during breastfeeding

PERMETHRIN (Lyclear)

Available form

Cream: 50 mg/g (5%)

Action

- scabicide that alters conductivity of cells leading to paralysis

Use

- scabies

Dose

- (adults, children > 12 years) apply to whole body below neck and wash off 8–12 hours later

Adverse effects

- burning, stinging, erythema, oedema, eczema, rash, pruritus

Nursing points/Cautions

- nursing staff who apply permethrin routinely should wear gloves to avoid hand irritation

- not recommended in the elderly or children under 2 years without medical advice
- contraindicated in those with known hypersensitivity to permethrin, synthetic pyrethroids or pyrethrins

Patient teaching and advice

- patients should be advised to reapply to hands if handwashing with soap and water has occurred within 8 hours of application
- see General Patient teaching and advice for scabicides (p. 956)

OTHER DERMATOLOGICAL PREPARATIONS

AMINOLEVULINIC ACID HYDROCHLORIDE (Alacare)

Available form

Dermal patch: 8 mg

Action

- sensitiser for photodynamic therapy (PDT)
- after application of aminolaevulinic acid hydrochloride, protoporphyrin IX (PPIX) accumulates intracellularly in actinic keratosis lesion. PPIX is a photoactive compound and when activated in presence of oxygen, damage is caused to the targeted cells' mitochondria

Use

- treatment of mild-to-moderate actinic keratosis lesion on face and scalp (hairless areas)

Dose

- apply patch to lesion ensuring it is completely covered. Up to 8 lesions can be treated in one session of PDT. Patch(es) left in situ for 4 hours, then removed and lesion(s) exposed to red light

Adverse effects

- (application site) redness, exfoliation, irritation, pain, pruritus, scab, bleeding, scaling, discharge, discomfort, erosion, hyper/hypopigmentation, swelling, vesicle/pustule formation
- headache

Interactions

- hypericin can increase phototoxic reactions caused by PDT and should therefore be discontinued 2 weeks before therapy. Hypericin-containing products include St John's wort
- phototoxicity may be potentiated if given with etretinate, griseofulvin, iron chelators, methotrexate, phenothiazines, quinolones, St John's wort, sulfonamides, sulfonylureas, tetracyclines, thiazide diuretics and vitamin D analogues
- efficacy may be decreased by tryptophan, glutathione, acetylcysteine, melatonin and methionine
- not recommended with other topical medications

Nursing points/Cautions

- any UV therapy should be stopped before starting treatment
- avoid contact with eyes
- should only be used by health professionals experienced in using photodynamic therapies
- if patch does not stick to lesion, it can be fixed with adhesive strip
- lamp should have filters and mirrors to minimise exposure to heat, blue light and UV radiation
- light dose is determined by size of light field, distance between lamp and skin surface and illumination time
- patient and operator should wear appropriate protective goggles during illumination period

- untreated skin surrounding lesions does not require protection
- treated lesions should be assessed after 12 weeks
- not recommended for use on very thick, red, scaly, indurated actinic keratosis lesions or in those with moderate brown to black skin
- contraindicated in those with porphyria or who have been previously unresponsive to PDT with aminolaevulinic acid preparations, with known photodermatoses or varying pathology (e.g. aminoaciduria, polymorphic light reaction) or diseases/conditions precipitated or aggravated by light exposure (e.g. lupus erythematosus)

Patient teaching and advice

- advise patient to avoid sun exposure to treated lesion site and surrounding area for at least 48 hours post-treatment
- warn patient about common skin reactions post-treatment. Cooling area may decrease skin reactions
- see General Patient teaching and advice (p. xxvii)

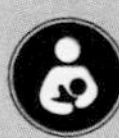

not recommended during pregnancy unless benefits outweigh risks

breastfeeding should be discontinued for 48 hours post-treatment

BRIMONIDINE (Mirvaso)

Available form

Gel: 3.3 mg/g

Action

- highly selective alpha-2-adrenergic agonist which reduces erythema by direct cutaneous vasoconstriction

Use

- facial erythema of rosacea

Dose

- 5 small pea-sized amounts of cream applied daily to forehead, chin, nose, each cheek

Adverse effects

- erythema, pruritus, flushing, skin-burning sensation, skin warmth, skin irritation, acne, pain
- contact dermatitis, dermatitis, rosacea
- paraesthesia, headache
- blurred vision
- nasal congestion, nasopharyngitis, upper respiratory tract infection
- increased intraocular pressure

Interactions

- contraindicated with MAOIs and tricyclic or tetracyclic antidepressants
- caution if used with CNS depressants (e.g. alcohol, barbiturates, opioids, sedatives or anaesthetics) as additive effects may occur
- caution if used with agents that affect metabolism and uptake of circulating amines (e.g. chlorpromazine, methylphenidate)
- caution if used with antihypertensives and digoxin as additive cardiac effects may occur
- caution if used with isoprenaline and prazosin as they may interfere with alpha adrenergic receptor agonists

Nursing points/Cautions

- medical diagnosis of rosacea should be made before starting therapy
- before starting therapy, response and tolerance can be determined by applying a small amount of gel daily for at least 7 days
- if therapy is stopped because of adverse effects, it should be recommenced by using a small amount for at least 1 full day before full face application
- contains methylparahydroxybenzoate, which may cause allergic

reactions and propylene glycol which may cause skin irritation

- not recommended for irritated skin or open wounds
- caution if used in those with severe, unstable or uncontrolled cardiovascular disease, depression, cerebral or coronary insufficiency, Raynaud's phenomenon, orthostatic hypotension, thromboangitis obliterans, scleroderma or Sjögren's syndrome
- contraindicated in those under 18 years

Patient teaching and advice

- instruct patient not to exceed maximum dose or frequency of application
- patient should be advised that cooling the treatment area and use of NSAIDs and/or antihistamines may alleviate symptoms of redness and flushing
- advise patient to wash and dry skin and then smoothly apply cream over all areas of face, avoiding missing areas
- warn patient to avoid applying cream to eyes, eyelids, lips, mouth and inner nose membrane. If contact occurs, area should be washed with copious amount of water
- patient should be instructed that other creams and lotions (e.g. cosmetics, sunscreen) can be applied after cream has dried
- advise patient to avoid excess sunlight or sunlamps and wear protective clothing and sunscreen with high protective factor (SPF 30+) when going outdoors

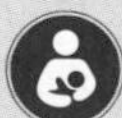

should only be used during pregnancy if benefits outweigh risks

not recommended during breastfeeding

CALCIPOTRIOL

Available form

Cream: 50 microgram/g

Action

- derived from vitamin D and suppresses proliferation, reversing abnormal keratinocytic changes associated with psoriasis

Use

- chronic stable plaque psoriasis

Adverse effects

- skin and/or scalp irritation, peeling, bullous eruption
- initial exacerbation of psoriasis
- photosensitivity, skin discolouration
- (uncommon) contact dermatitis, allergic reaction
- (rare) hypercalcaemia

Interactions

- not recommended with calcium or vitamin D supplements or other agents which increase availability of calcium

Nursing points/Cautions

- serum calcium and renal function should be monitored 3-monthly during therapy. If serum calcium becomes elevated, therapy should be stopped and serum calcium measured weekly until it returns to normal
- dose should not exceed total of 100 g per week
- not recommended for severe extensive psoriasis, generalised pustular psoriasis, guttate psoriasis or erythrodermic exfoliative psoriasis
- not recommended for use on the face
- contraindicated in those with calcium metabolism disorders

Patient teaching and advice

- instruct patient to wash hands immediately after use to avoid transfer to face or other unaffected areas. If contact occurs, area should be rinsed with water
- patient should be advised to avoid calcium or vitamin D supplements during therapy
- warn patient that psoriasis may be exacerbated initially but this will subside
- patient should be warned to use cream with caution in skin folds as this may increase risk of irritation occurring
- advise patient to avoid excess sunlight or sunlamps and wear protective clothing and sunscreen with high protective factor (SPF 30+) when going outdoors
- warn patient that occlusive dressings should not be used
- advise patient that cream is not recommended for use on the face
- instruct patient that refrigeration of cream is not recommended as it becomes more difficult to spread

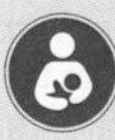

should only be used during pregnancy and breastfeeding if benefits are thought to outweigh risks. If breastfeeding, cream should not be applied in breast area

Note

- contained in Daivobet 50/500 with betamethasone, Enstilar Foam Spray and Calcipotriol/Betamethasone 50/500

CRISABOROLE (Staquis)

Available form

Ointment: 20 mg/g (2%w/w)

Action

- phosphodiesterase-4 (PDE-4) inhibitor that suppresses inflammation and secretion of some cytokines

Use

- mild-to-moderate atopic dermatitis in patient over 2 years old

Dose

- apply thin layer to affected areas twice daily

Adverse reaction

- application site pain, infection
- eczema, contact dermatitis
- fever
- headache
- cough, nasopharyngitis, upper respiratory tract infection, oropharyngeal pain, sinusitis, asthma, pharyngitis
- vomiting

Nursing points/Cautions

- contraindicated in those with hypersensitivity to paraffin, propylene glycol or sodium calcium edetate

Patient teaching and advice

- instruct patient (or whoever is applying ointment) to wash hands after application (unless hands are being treated)

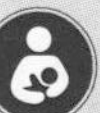

only recommended during pregnancy if benefits outweigh risks

should not be applied to breast if woman is breastfeeding

DEOXYCHOLIC ACID (Belkyra)

Available form

Solution for injection: 10 mg/mL

Action

- causes lysis of adipocyte cell membranes, resulting in macrophages being attracted to the area to remove cellular debris and lipids by natural processes

Use

- non-surgical fat removal under chin (submental convexity fullness) for contoured neck profile and jawline

Dose

- 2 mg/cm^2 SC (consisting of up to 50 injections of 0.2 mL spaced 1 cm apart)

Adverse effects

- (injection site) pain, swelling, haematoma, induration, erythema, pruritus, numbness, bleeding, warmth, bruising, discomfort, discolouration to area, nerve injury
- hypertension
- headache
- nausea
- swallowing difficulties
- (uncommon) taste alteration, hoarseness
- (uncommon) alopecia of area (male), urticaria, ulcer formation, hypersensitivity
- (rare) skin ulceration and necrosis (due to superficial dermal injection)

Nursing points/Cautions

- before starting therapy, patient should be screened for other potential causes for submental (chin) convexity fullness, such as thyromegaly or cervical lymphadenopathy
- should only be administered by medical practitioner who has good knowledge of submental anatomy, neuromuscular structures and any alterations to anatomy in that particular patient (e.g. due to previous surgery). Needle placement with respect to mandible is important in reducing potential injury to marginal mandibular nerve (which could result in paralysis of lip depressor muscle)
- number of injections and number of treatments is dependent on patient's fat distribution and treatment goals. Up to 6 single treatments may be given at intervals of at least 4 weeks apart
- patient comfort can be increased by use of topical or injectable local anaesthetic or ice/cold packs
- only administer SC
- vial should be inverted gently several times before use
- solution should not be diluted before administration
- pressure may be applied to injection sites to minimise bleeding
- contains 4.23 mg (184 mmol) sodium per mL, which may need to be considered if patient is on sodium-restricted diet
- caution if used in those over 65 years and not recommended in those under 18 years
- caution if there is any inflammation or induration in area to be injected
- caution if used in patients who have had other procedures to the area, such as surgery, liposuction or other injections, such as Botox
- caution if used in those who have excessive skin laxity, prominent platysmal bands or other conditions that may result in suboptimal results
- caution if used in those with bleeding abnormalities or taking antiplatelet or anticoagulant medication due to risk of excessive bleeding and bruising
- not recommended in patients with previous or current history of dysphagia as condition may be exacerbated
- not recommended in patients with mild or extreme submental (chin) fat
- contraindicated if there is infection at treatment site

Patient teaching and advice

- patient should be advised to seek medical attention if any of the following occur:
  - troubling swallowing or taste disturbance
  - uneven smile
  - discolouration or ulceration at injection site
  - tingling or reduced sensation around mouth
  - (male) unusual hair loss around injection site

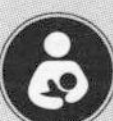

not recommended during pregnancy or breastfeeding

HEPARINOIDS (HEPARINOID) (Hirudoid)

Available form
Cream: 0.3%

Action
- topical anticoagulant and thrombolytic agent

Use
- accidental/surgical injury, including bruises, contusions, sprains and haematomas
- to speed up the resolution of traumatic oedema and exudates (including haematomata associated with vein stripping)
- treatment of superficial thrombophlebitis (e.g. superficial phlebitis associated with IV infusion or phlebitis associated with varicose veins)
- loosen scar tissue

Dose
- apply 3–5 cm to affected area 1–2 times daily, massaging gently until cream is absorbed **OR**
- (scars) massage into scar firmly

Adverse effects
- erythema

Interactions
- may increase effects of IV heparin

Patient teaching and advice
- advise patient that cream should not be applied to bleeding or infected areas
- instruct patient to avoid contact with eyes

IMIQUIMOD (Aldara, Aldiq)

Available form
Cream: 50 mg/g (5%)

Action
- topical immune response modifier with no direct antiviral activity

Use
- superficial basal cell carcinoma (where surgery is inappropriate)
- solar (actinic) keratosis (face/scalp)
- external genital and perianal warts (condyloma acuminate)

Dose
- (external genital and perianal warts) apply thin layer of cream 3 times weekly at bedtime until warts disappear or up to 16 weeks maximum

Adverse effects
(for use in external genital and anal warts)
- (application site) erythema, oedema, erosion, scabbing, itching, burning or stinging sensation, tenderness, rash, irritation, excoriation/flaking, induration, pain
- headache, flu-like symptoms, myalgia, fatigue
- (uncommon) infection, hypopigmentation

Interactions
- caution if used with other immunosuppressing agents

Nursing points/Cautions
- repeat courses are not recommended if patient is immunocompromised
- efficacy may be reduced in those with HIV (although the reason for this is unclear)
- not recommended on broken skin, therefore area should be allowed to heal before starting therapy
- not recommended for urethral, intravaginal, cervical, rectal or intra-anal warts

Patient teaching and advice

- advise patient that it usually takes 8–10 weeks for warts to disappear, but may clear sooner
- patient should be advised to seek medical attention if warts recur
- instruct patient that sexual (genital, anal, oral) contact should be avoided while cream is on skin
- if skin reaction is severe, advise patient to wash area with mild soap and water and stop therapy for several days until irritation has settled and then restart (there is no need to make up missed doses)
- cream may weaken condoms and vaginal diaphragms, therefore alternate forms of contraception are recommended during therapy
- advise patient to select 3 days for therapy (e.g. Monday, Wednesday and Friday or Tuesday, Thursday and Saturday) as this will improve adherence with therapy regimen
- instruct patient to avoid application of excessive cream as this will only increase risk of irritation
- if severe irritation occurs, advise patient that area can be covered with non-occlusive dressing (such as cotton gauze or cotton underwear), but occlusive dressing should not be used
- female patient should be advised to avoid applying cream near vaginal opening as skin reactions on mucosal membrane may occur resulting in pain and/or swelling, which may further result in difficulty passing urine
- uncircumcised male patient with wart(s) under foreskin should be instructed to retract foreskin and clean area daily to prevent foreskin tightness and stricture, which may occur with cream use. Patient should be advised to immediately report any local skin reactions (induration, swelling, erosion, ulceration) or difficulty retracting foreskin
- instruct patient as follows:
  1. cream is available in single-use sachets or pump
  2. after removing protective cap, pump should be primed until cream appears in nozzle
  3. 4 pump actuations = 250 mg sachet (and is sufficient to cover an area of 20 cm^2)
  4. hands should be washed thoroughly before and after cream application
  5. wash application area with mild soap, rinse and dry
  6. apply cream and rub in until not visible
  7. leave cream on wart(s) for 6–10 hours (overnight) and then wash off with mild soap and water
  8. patient should not bathe or shower while cream is on skin
  9. replace protective cap on pump
  10. pump should be discarded 4 weeks after opening
- see General Patient teaching and advice (p. xxvii)

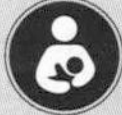

not recommended during pregnancy or breastfeeding

INGENOL MEBUTATE (Picato Gel)

Available forms

Gel: 150 microgram/g (0.015%), 500 microgram/g (0.05%)

Action

- action not fully understood, but thought to induce local lesion cell death and promote inflammatory response characterised by pro-inflammatory cytokine and chemokines production and infiltration of immunocompetent cells

Use

- treatment of solar (actinic) keratosis on face, scalp and body

Dose

- (solar (actinic) keratosis of face and scalp) 0.015% gel applied to affected area of face and/or scalp once daily for 3 consecutive days **OR**
- (solar (actinic) keratosis of body) 0.05% gel applied to affected area on body once daily for 2 consecutive days

Adverse effects

- (application site) pain, pruritus, irritation, erythema, flaking, crusting, scaling, swelling, ulceration, vesiculation
- periorbital oedema, eyelid oedema
- infection
- application site paraesthesia
- headache
- (rare) dermal necrosis, hypersensitivity

Nursing points/Cautions

- patient should be reassessed after 8 weeks for response to treatment
- not recommended until skin has healed from any previous open wounds or medical or surgical treatment

Patient teaching and advice

- warn patient that local skin reactions (redness, flaking/scaling, crusting, swelling, ulceration) commonly occur and usually within 1 day of treatment, peak after about 1 week and resolve within 2 weeks (face, scalp) or 4 weeks (body and extremities) of completing treatment
- ensure patient understands that gel is available in two strengths and they should only be used for the specified area (e.g. 0.015% gel is for face and scalp only). Each tube is single use only
- patient should be advised to avoid gel contact with eyes or mouth. If contact occurs, area should be washed immediately with copious amounts of water
- advise patient to avoid excess sunlight or sunlamps and wear protective clothing and sunscreen with high protective factor (SPF 30+) when going outdoors
- patient should be instructed to squeeze gel from tube onto fingertip and spread over affected area evenly and allow area to dry for 15 minutes without touching it
- advise patient to avoid applying gel immediately before or after showering or less than 2 hours before bedtime
- instruct patient to wash hands with soap and water immediately after applying gel
- if hands are also being treated, advise patient that only fingertip applying gel should be washed after application
- warn patient not to touch and wash treated area for 6 hours after applying gel. After this time the area may be cleansed with mild soap and water
- patient should be instructed not to cover treated area(s) with occlusive bandages
- instruct patient to store gel in refrigerator

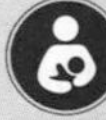

not recommended during pregnancy

if mother is breastfeeding, she should be advised that baby should not make contact with treated area for 6 hours after gel application

MINOXIDIL (Hair A-Gain, Loniten, Men's Regaine Extra Strength, Women Regaine)

Available forms

Liquid: 20 mg/mL (2%), 50 mg/mL (5%); Foam: 50 mg/mL (5%); Tablets: 10 mg

Action

- (topical) stimulates hair growth, although exact mechanism of action is unknown
- (other actions) see Antihypertensive agents (Loniten) (p. 538)

Use

- alopecia androgenetica (hereditary/common baldness) (in healthy males and females)

Dose

- (solution) 1 mL (2% solution for females, 5% solution for males) applied and massaged gently into scalp twice daily (maximum daily dose 2 mL) **OR**
- (foam – male) up to ½ capful (depending on size of hair loss) applied and massaged gently into scalp twice daily **OR**
- (foam – female) up to ½ capful (depending on size of hair loss) applied and massaged gently into scalp once daily

Adverse effects

- (topical) dermatitis, rash, acne, redness, scaling, burning, itching, dry skin/scalp, transient hair shedding
- headache, peripheral oedema, dyspnoea, pruritus, rash
- (rare) (women) hypertrichosis (including facial hair growth)
- (rare) allergic reactions

Interactions

- not recommended with topical retinoids, topical corticosteroids or other skin preparations
- caution if given with other vasodilators
- not recommended with other topical scalp preparations

Nursing points/Cautions

- scalp should be examined before starting therapy for any signs of infection or inflammation and, if they exist, therapy should not be started until conditions have resolved
- therapy should be discontinued after 6 months if no regrowth has occurred
- not recommended for any areas of the body other than the scalp
- not recommended in those with heart disease
- contraindicated in those with hypersensitivity to other formulations of minoxidil or propylene glycol or ethanol
- contraindicated in those with non-familial baldness, unexplained hair loss, scalp inflammation or if any pain, infection or irritation of scalp exists
- contraindicated in those over 65 years or under 18 years

Patient teaching and advice

- ensure patient understands that foam/lotion should be applied to scalp only (no other parts of the body)
- warn patient that there may be some transient hair loss at the start of therapy (first 2–6 weeks)
- patient should be advised to immediately report any fluid retention or unexplained weight gain, swollen feet or hands, chest pain, rapid heartbeat, faintness or dizziness
- warn patient not to drive or operate machinery if dizziness occurs
- instruct patient that hair and scalp should be dry before applying lotion/foam
- advise patient not to use hair drier to speed up the drying process, because heat may decrease effectiveness
- instruct patient to wash hands thoroughly after applying lotion/foam
- (lotion) patient should be instructed to use dropper applicator and apply to centre of affected area first (not exceeding 2 mL daily dose) regardless of size of bald spot, massaged

gently into scalp and then left for at least 2 hours (up to 4 hours)
- (foam) instruct patient to hold can upside down and press nozzle down to dispense up to 1/2 capful into palm, massaged gently into scalp and then left for at least 2 hours (up to 4 hours)
- (foam) warn patient that hands should be cold when using foam otherwise it will melt on contact with warm hands. Rinse hands under cold water and ensure they are dry before using foam
- warn patient that hair regrowth usually takes at least 4 months of twice-daily application for males (once per day for females) to become noticeable and when therapy is discontinued, hair growth will stop and pre-treatment appearance will be restored in 3–4 months
- patient should be advised to allow 1 hour before applying protective headgear (e.g. bicycle or motorbike helmet)
- warn patient to avoid contact with eyes, mucous membranes or abraded skin. If contact occurs, area should be washed with copious quantities of cold water

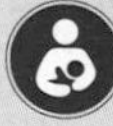
contraindicated during pregnancy and breastfeeding

PIMECROLIMUS (Elidel)

Available form
Cream: 10 mg/g (1%)

Action
- ascomycin macrolactam derivative calcineurin inhibitor

Use
- atopic dermatitis (eczema) (short-term management of signs and symptoms, or intermediate long-term management of emerging or resolving lesions where corticosteroids are not yet warranted, no longer needed or not recommended) in those over 3 months of age

Dose
- apply a thin layer to affected area and rub in completely twice daily for up to 6 weeks

Adverse effects
- transient skin burning/warmth sensation
- irritation, pruritus, erythema, folliculitis
- lymphadenopathy
- (rare) skin cancer, lymphoma, hypersensitivity, allergic reactions

Nursing points/Cautions
- any bacterial or fungal infection should be treated during therapy. If infection continues, pimecrolimus should be ceased until infection is controlled
- not recommended if acute viral skin infection (e.g. cold sore) is present, on skin post-vaccination
- not recommended with phototherapy
- not recommended for skin areas where skin cancer has been removed, affected by premalignant changes (e.g. actinic keratoses) or in those with Netherton syndrome or generalised erythroderma (severely inflamed, damaged skin) or if immunocompromised
- contraindicated in those with hypersensitivity to macrolactams

Patient teaching and advice
- instruct patient that cream should be completely rubbed in
- patient should be warned that feeling of warmth and/or burning sensation is common on application and is transient

- advise patient/carer to avoid excess sunlight or sunlamps and wear protective clothing and sunscreen with high protective factor (SPF 30+) when going outdoors
- patient should be instructed to only apply cream to areas that are eczematous
- instruct patient to avoid using excessive amounts of cream. In an adult, a fingertip of cream is sufficient to cover an area equivalent to two hands
- patient/carer should be instructed to wash hands after application
- warn patient to avoid contact with eyes, nose or mouth, areas of viral infection (such as cold sores), areas post-vaccination or breasts (if breastfeeding)
- advise patient that treatment should be restarted at the first sign of recurrence (e.g. itching, scratching, persistent redness, thickening of skin)
- if using a moisturiser, patient should be instructed to use it after pimecrolimus cream. If having a shower or bath, use moisturiser first, then apply pimecrolimus cream
- ensure patient/carer understands that occlusive dressings over cream are not recommended
- advise patient to seek medical advice if any of the following occur:
  - condition worsens
  - condition shows no improvement after 6 weeks
  - any skin infection occurs

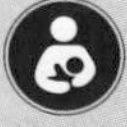

not recommended during pregnancy

caution if used during breastfeeding

PODOPHYLLOTOXIN (Condyline Paint)

Available form

Paint: 5 mg/mL

Action

- antimitotic agent that causes necrosis of wart tissue

Use

- anogenital warts (condylomata acuminate) in males and females

Dose

- sufficient paint using provided applicator to cover wart is applied twice daily for 3 consecutive days with 4 drug-free days, repeated initially for 4 weeks; if wart is not removed, seek medical advice

Adverse effects

- tenderness, pain, itching, smarting, burning, erythema, superficial epithelial ulceration, skin discolouration
- (males) inflammation of glans and foreskin (balanoposthitis)

Interactions

- contraindicated with any other preparations containing podophyllotoxin

Nursing points/Cautions

- medical supervision is recommended for lesions in females or if $> 4\ cm^2$ in males
- increased risk of systemic adverse effects with prolonged use, involvement of an extensive area of skin, if the skin is friable or bleeding, or if applied to recently biopsied skin. This risk is also increased if applied to mucous membrane or healthy skin
- treatment can be repeated for a total of 5 weeks if needed
- contraindicated in those with open surgical wounds, inflamed or bleeding lesions or in children

Patient teaching and advice

- instruct patient to wash hands before and after applying paint
- patient should be advised to wash area thoroughly with soap and water and dry before application of paint. Allow paint to dry after applications

- warn patient to avoid contact with eyes and mucous membranes; rinse with water immediately if contact occurs
- instruct patient to apply using applicator supplied
- patient should be advised that local irritation may increase on day 2 or 3 of therapy as the wart starts to respond (i.e. become necrotic), but it will decrease with ongoing treatment
- warn patient to apply paint to wart only and avoid healthy surrounding tissue, because prolonged exposure may harm healthy skin or increase risk of systemic absorption
- instruct patient to discard paint solution 6 weeks after opening

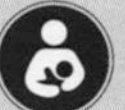

contraindicated during pregnancy and breastfeeding

DISEASE-MODIFYING ANTIRHEUMATIC DRUGS (DMARDs)

Arthritis is a term used to describe diseases of the joints, with common forms including rheumatoid arthritis (RA), osteoarthritis, juvenile idiopathic arthritis and spondyloarthropathies (e.g. ankylosing spondylitis). An estimated 7 million (or one in seven) Australians suffer from some form of arthritis, with rheumatoid arthritis accounting for nearly 2% (or 458,000) of that total (AIHW 2019g).

RA is a chronic autoimmune disease characterised by inflammation and thickening of the synovial membrane (synovitis). This unrelenting inflammation leads to destruction of tissue, cartilage erosion and, at times, rupturing of tendon fibres. However, it can affect the entire body, including organs (heart, respiratory system, nerves and eyes) (AIHW 2019g). Symptoms include pain, swelling, stiffness and loss of joint function. Most commonly, the small joints of the hands and feet are involved. RA is a rapidly progressing disease which often takes an erratic and unpredictable course (AIHW 2019g). Even with treatment, RA sometimes still progresses, with destruction of the affected joints, deformity, disability and possible reduction in life expectancy (RACGP 2009). Early diagnosis and treatment with DMARDs is essential in slowing disease progression and achieving remission. There is some evidence to suggest that early use of DMARDs is associated with an improvement in quality of life and long-term functional outcomes, compared to now-superseded treatments using NSAIDs as first-line management (Bryant et al 2019).

The DMARDs are a diverse group of drugs, many of which have unknown actions resulting in their anti-rheumatic properties. Although mainly used to treat RA, they are also used to treat other autoimmune diseases such as Crohn's disease, psoriatic arthritis and systemic lupus erythematosus (SLE). DMARDs can be divided into the 'conventional' DMARDs (e.g. methotrexate, gold, sulfasalazine), the immunosuppressants (e.g. ciclosporin, azathioprine, leflunomide), the cytokine modulators (e.g. abatacept, anakinra, rituximab) and the tumour necrosis factor alpha (TNF-α) antagonists (e.g. adalimumab, infliximab). Onset of action of the DMARDs is often slow, taking weeks to months before clinical improvement is apparent. They are used alone, or in combination with other DMARDs, NSAIDs and/or corticosteroids (Bryant et al 2019).

Adjunctive treatment for RA should also include physiotherapy, occupational therapy, exercises and, most importantly, patient education and access to support services (e.g. Arthritis Australia).

CONVENTIONAL DMARDs

AURANOFIN (Ridaura)

Available forms

Tablets: 3 mg; Capsules 3 mg

Action

- synthetic gold complex that decreases inflammation, levels of rheumatoid factor and elevated immunoglobulin levels
- may slow progression of joint erosion
- anti-inflammatory action
- clinical improvement seen in 3–4 months after initiation of therapy (although some people may take longer)
- half-life increased from about 17 days to 26 days after 6 months of therapy

Use

- rheumatoid arthritis (unresponsive or intolerant to NSAIDs)

Dose

- initially 6 mg orally daily with food, increasing to 9 mg in 3 divided doses if needed after 4–6 months

Adverse effects

- diarrhoea or loose stools, constipation, flatulence
- anorexia, nausea, vomiting, abdominal pain/cramps, dyspepsia, distorted taste, stomatitis, glossitis
- conjunctivitis
- rash, pruritus, phototoxicity
- hair loss
- leucopenia, granulocytopenia, anaemia, thrombocytopenia
- haematuria, proteinuria, increased blood urea and serum creatinine, nephrotoxicity
- increased liver enzymes
- (rare) ulcerative enterocolitis

Interactions

- contraindicated with other agents causing blood dyscrasias or bone marrow depression
- contraindicated with leflunomide
- contraindicated with clozapine, antimalarial agents, penicillamine or immunosuppressants
- caution if used with warfarin, clonidine or dextropropoxyphene
- may increase effects of radiotherapy
- caution if given with ACE inhibitors due to risk of vasomotor reaction (see Glossary)
- increased risk of nephrotoxicity and/or haemotoxicity if given with alcohol, aminoglycosides, amphotericin B, penicillins, phenytoin, sulfonamides, NSAIDs and aciclovir
- may increase serum levels of phenytoin, increasing risk of adverse effects, including skin reactions, therefore phenytoin levels should be closely monitored
- delayed hypersensitivity may occur if given with aspirin, penicillins or quinidine
- absorption may be decreased if given with prokinetic agents (e.g. loperamide) or laxatives
- caution if given with theophylline

Nursing points/Cautions

- diabetes, heart failure or hypertension should be controlled or corrected before starting therapy
- renal and liver function tests, blood count (with differential white cell

count), haemoglobin and complete urinalysis (with urinary protein levels) should be performed before starting therapy
- monthly blood counts (with differential white cell count), platelet count and urinary protein levels are recommended
- ophthalmological examination is recommended periodically throughout therapy
- annual chest X-ray is recommended
- GI symptoms are dose-related and those with low body weight are at greatest risk
- auranofin-induced diarrhoea can be controlled by decreasing dose
- daily dose > 9 mg is not recommended
- overlap or washout period not required if transferring from injectable gold preparations
- tablets contain lactose and are therefore not recommended in those with galactose intolerance, Lapp lactase deficiency or glucose–galactose malabsorption
- caution if used in those with inflammatory bowel disease, history of bone marrow depression or atopy, or liver/kidney dysfunction
- not recommended in those with porphyria, systemic sclerosis or Sjögren's syndrome
- not recommended in those who have undergone recent radiotherapy
- contraindicated in those with previous toxicity or sensitivity to gold or heavy metals, severe liver/kidney disease, severe chronic dermatitis, bone marrow depression, bone marrow aplasia, haematological disorders or gold-induced pulmonary fibrosis, necrotising enterocolitis or systemic lupus erythematosus (SLE)

Patient teaching and advice

- patient should be warned that diarrhoea is a common adverse effect, especially in those of low body weight
- advise patient to avoid alcohol during therapy
- instruct patient to avoid exposure to strong direct sunlight and if outdoors, patient should wear protective clothing and SPF 30+ sunscreen
- patient should be advised to seek medical advice immediately if any of the following occur:
  - diarrhoea with rectal bleeding or rectal bleeding alone
  - any metallic taste, sore throat or tongue, mouth ulceration, easy bruising, bleeding gums, blood nose, heavy menstrual bleeding, bleeding under the skin resembling purple rash (sign of impending toxicity)
  - itching (pruritus), rash (early sign of intolerance)
- counsel women of childbearing age to use adequate contraception during and for at least 6 months after stopping therapy because gold is slowly excreted from the body, which may have negative effects on a developing fetus
- see also General Patient teaching and advice (p. xxvii)

not recommended during pregnancy or breastfeeding. Gold is slowly excreted from the body after stopping therapy; this should be taken into account if a woman wants to breastfeed

tablet can be dispersed in water or crushed and mixed with spoonful of yoghurt or apple puree

CICLOSPORIN (CYCLOSPORIN) (Neoral, Sandimmun)

Available forms

Capsules: 10 mg, 25 mg, 50 mg, 100 mg; Oral solution: 100 mg/mL; Ampoules: 50 mg/mL

Action

- potent immunosuppressive agent (calcineurin inhibitor)
- thought to act by blocking both lymphocytes and antigen-triggered lymphokine release by activated T cells
- half-life 6.3 hours, increasing to 20.4 hours in those with severe liver disease

Use

- prevent or delay organ rejection after transplantation
- prevention of graft versus host disease in organ transplantation
- induction and/or maintenance of remission in nephrotic syndrome (when other therapies have been ineffective or inappropriate and renal function is still intact)
- severe, active rheumatoid arthritis (when other therapies have been ineffective or inappropriate)
- severe psoriasis (when other therapies have been ineffective or inappropriate)
- severe atopic dermatitis (when other therapies have been ineffective or inappropriate)

Dose

- (rheumatoid arthritis) 3 mg/kg daily orally in 2 divided doses for first 6 weeks of therapy (which may be continued to 12 weeks for full effectiveness). If no clinical response in 4–8 weeks, dose may be increased by 0.5–1.0 mg/kg/day at 1–2-month intervals to 5 mg/kg/day maximum. If the patient has been stable for at least 3 months, the dose may be decreased by 0.5 mg/kg/day at 1–2-month intervals to achieve the lowest effective dose **OR**
- (psoriasis) 2.5 mg/kg orally daily in 2 divided doses, increasing to 5 mg/kg if there is no clinical response in 4 weeks (daily maximum 5 mg/kg) **OR**
- (nephrotic syndrome) 2.5–5 mg/kg/day, decreasing to lowest effective dose (maintenance) **OR**
- (atopic dermatitis) initially 2.5–5 mg/kg orally daily in 2 divided doses, reducing dose gradually when satisfactory response has been achieved **OR**
- (organ transplantation) initially 10–15 mg/kg orally 4–12 hours pre-transplant, continued for 1–2 weeks postoperatively, then gradually reduced to 2–6 mg/kg/day as single or 2 divided doses (maintenance) **OR**
- (organ transplantation) 3–5 mg/kg/day by IV infusion over 2–6 hours, started 4–12 hours pre-transplant, then starting oral dosing as soon as possible post-transplant

Adverse effects

- hypertension
- fluid retention and oedema, weight increase
- hyperkalaemia, hyperuricaemia, hypomagnesaemia, hyperlipidaemia
- fever, flushing
- tremor, fatigue, burning sensation in hands and feet (initially)
- muscle cramps, myalgia
- headache/migraine, paraesthesia, convulsions
- hirsutism, rash, acne
- dysmenorrhoea/amenorrhoea (reversible)
- gingival hypertrophy
- anorexia, nausea, vomiting, diarrhoea, abdominal pain, peptic ulceration
- anaemia, leucopenia
- increased susceptibility to or aggravation of infection (local or general)
- impaired renal function, hepatic dysfunction, acute pancreatitis
- increased risk of malignancy
- (IV) anaphylactoid reactions

Interactions

- increased risk of nephrotoxicity when low-dose ciclosporin is given with NSAIDs, requiring regular monitoring of kidney function

- may increase serum levels of sirolimus, everolimus and anthracyclines (e.g. doxorubicin) increasing risk of toxicity
- may lead to increase in blood pressure if given with recombinant human erythropoietin
- increased risk of nephrotoxicity if given with tacrolimus
- increase in BP may result if given with recombinant human erythropoietin
- caution if given with lercanidipine as serum level of both agents may be increased
- increased risk of hyperkalaemia if given with potassium-containing or potassium-sparing medications, including potassium-sparing diuretics, ACE inhibitors and angiotensin II receptor antagonists
- not recommended with UVB irradiation or PUVA photochemotherapy because of increased risk of skin cancer development
- reversible renal impairment may occur if given with fenofibrate or other fibric acid derivatives
- not recommended with other known nephrotoxic drugs such as aminoglycosides, amphotericin B (amphotericin), ciprofloxacin, colchicine, histamine H_2 antagonists, melphalan, methotrexate, NSAIDs, trimethoprim and vancomycin. If used together, serum creatinine and renal function should be closely monitored
- serum levels may be increased if given with allopurinol, amiodarone, azole antifungal agents, cholic acid, colchicine, danazol, diltiazem, doxycycline, grapefruit juice, imatinib, macrolide antibiotics, metoclopramide, methylprednisolone (high dose), oral contraceptives, protease inhibitors, verapamil and voriconazole, increasing risk of toxicity
- not recommended with atorvastatin or simvastatin due to increased risk of muscle toxicity (muscle pain, weakness, myositis, rhabdomyolysis) because of decreased clearance. Caution if used with pravastatin, fluvastatin or rosuvastatin
- may increase serum levels of repaglinide, increasing risk of hypoglycaemia occurring
- serum levels may be decreased if given with barbiturates, bosentan, carbamazepine, ciprofloxacin, isoniazid, octreotide, orlistat, oxcarbazepine, phenytoin, rifampicin, St John's wort, sulfamethoxazole/trimethoprim (IV)
- not recommended with thiazide or loop diuretics because of increased risk of hyperuricaemia and gout. Serum uric acid levels should be monitored if any signs of gout occur
- not recommended with live or live attenuated vaccines
- caution if used with alcohol
- increased risk of gingival hyperplasia if given with nifedipine or amlodipine
- may decrease clearance (and therefore increase blood levels) of ambrisentan, bosentan, colchicine, dabigatran, digoxin, etoposide, prednisolone and statins, and increasing risk of toxicity

Nursing points/Cautions

- capsules and oral solution are bioequivalent; however, changing between brands should be done carefully. Ciclosporin serum level, serum creatinine level and blood pressure should be measured at 2, 4 and 8 weeks (or within 4–7 days if used for transplant) after changeover. If blood pressure or creatinine levels are greater than the pre-changeover levels, decreasing the dose is recommended
- any infections should be identified and treated before starting therapy
- adverse effects are more common when ciclosporin is used for

transplant patients than when used for other conditions because the dose is higher

- routine serum ciclosporin levels should be monitored in transplant patients, but not required in non-transplant patients unless indicated by risk of adverse reactions or potential drug interaction
- blood taken to measure routine serum levels should be taken immediately before next dose is due and collection time recorded
- blood pressure should be monitored regularly throughout therapy and hypertension treated with appropriate antihypertensive medication if it occurs. However, diuretic therapy should be avoided. If hypertension cannot be controlled, ciclosporin therapy should be stopped
- blood lipids should be measured before starting therapy and after 4 weeks of therapy. If lipids increase, dose should be decreased and a fat-reduced diet commenced
- creatinine levels should be measured twice before and every 2 weeks during the first 3 months of therapy, then monthly. Doses should then be adjusted accordingly. Therapy should stop if reducing the dose does not reduce creatinine levels within 1 month. Creatinine levels should be measured more frequently when the dose of ciclosporin is increased or if the patient is taking NSAIDs concurrently
- serum bilirubin and urea should be measured before starting and regularly throughout therapy
- serum potassium levels should be monitored regularly, as should serum uric acid levels in high-risk patients (e.g. gout) and serum magnesium (as hypomagnesaemia increases risk of neurotoxicity)
- (nephrotic syndrome) dose is dependent on renal function. If improvement is not seen in 12 weeks, therapy should be stopped
- (nephrotic syndrome) renal biopsy is recommended if therapy continues for 12 months
- (psoriasis) any unusual lesions should be biopsied before starting therapy to decrease risk of cancer occurring
- (psoriasis) if there is no improvement within 6 weeks of therapy at 5 mg/kg/day, therapy should be stopped
- (atopic dermatitis) active herpes infection and skin infections should be treated before starting therapy
- (atopic dermatitis) lymphadenopathy should be monitored during therapy. If lymphadenopathy is present after skin improves with therapy, a biopsy is recommended to rule out lymphoma
- (atopic dermatitis) course can be continued for up to 12 months if tolerated
- (atopic dermatitis) not recommended with PUVA photochemotherapy
- (rheumatoid arthritis) patients appear to be at greater risk of nephrotoxicity
- (rheumatoid arthritis) discontinue therapy if there is no improvement in 6 months where maximum tolerable dose has been achieved for 3 months
- (organ transplant) if given as part of triple or quadruple drug therapy with other immunosuppressants (including corticosteroids) decreased dose may be used (e.g. renal transplant patients may require dose less than 5 mg/kg/day if given with corticosteroid)
- IV should only be used if patient is unable to tolerate oral formulation
- (IV) glass container should be used if available
- care should be taken during IV administration because solution is highly irritant and can cause tissue damage if extravasation occurs

- IV concentrate should be diluted using sodium chloride 0.9% or glucose 5% to 1:20–1:100 concentration and infused over 2–6 hours
- any unused diluted solution should be discarded after 48 hours
- (oral solution) 0.1 mL solution = 10 mg ciclosporin
- solution and capsules contain up to 12–13% v/v alcohol while IV concentrate contains 34% v/v, which may need to be considered in patients with epilepsy, alcohol abuse problems or if pregnant or breastfeeding
- (oral) caution if used in those with malabsorption problems as reaching therapeutic level may be difficult
- not recommended in those with severe heart, lung or peripheral vessel complications
- (non-transplant use) contraindicated in those with uncontrolled hypertension or infection, primary or secondary immunodeficiency, impaired baseline renal function with serum creatinine greater than 200 micromol/L (nephrotic syndrome use), any renal impairment (other uses), or any existing malignant or premalignant conditions
- (IV) contraindicated in those with hypersensitivity to polyoxyethylated castor oil

Patient teaching and advice

- advise patients to avoid heavy alcohol use while taking ciclosporin, especially red wine
- instruct patients to take doses 12 hours apart at the same time each day
- caution patients to swallow capsules whole, with or without food
- advise patients that oral solution comes with two syringes (1 mL and 4 mL). The 1 mL syringe should be used for doses less than or equal to 1 mL, while the 4 mL syringe is used for doses between 1 mL and 4 mL
- instruct patients to dilute oral solution of ciclosporin with apple or orange juice (not grapefruit) or soft drink and stir well before drinking immediately. Glass should be rinsed with more juice or soft drink to ensure whole dose is taken
- warn patient to avoid grapefruit juice during therapy
- instruct patient that the dose-dispensing syringe should not come into contact with juice or soft drink when diluting solution and should be wiped clean, not rinsed with water or other fluids
- patient should be advised to avoid foods high in potassium (e.g. sweet potatoes, potatoes, bananas, milk, spinach), potassium-containing or potassium-sparing medications to avoid an increase in potassium levels
- counsel patient to avoid excessive unprotected sun exposure due to increased risk of skin cancer and wear a hat, use SPF 30+ sunscreen and protective clothing if sun exposure cannot be avoided
- educate patient regarding care of teeth and gums during therapy
- instruct patient to discard oral solution 2 months after opening
- advise patient that oral solution should be stored in a cool dark place (20–25°C), but not refrigerated. Oily components of ciclosporin may solidify below 20°C and a jelly-like substance may also result. This is reversible at warmer temperatures and does not affect the safety or efficacy

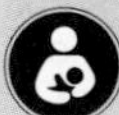

not recommended during pregnancy or breastfeeding as it can cause immunosuppression of newborn

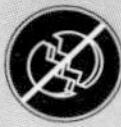

oral solution available. Capsule should not be opened or crushed

HYDROXYCHLOROQUINE SULFATE (Hequinel, Plaquenil, Rusquen)

Available form

Tablets: 200 mg

Action

- aminoquinoline antimalarial that has unknown therapeutic actions in rheumatoid arthritis and systemic and discoid lupus erythematosus
- active against erythrocytic forms of *Plasmodium vivax* and *Plasmodium malariae* and most strains of *Plasmodium falciparum* (not gametocytes of *P. falciparum*)
- does not prevent relapses because it is not active against exo-erythrocytic phases
- stops acute attacks and lengthens the time between treatment and relapses (*P. vivax*, *P. malariae*). With *P. falciparum*, complete cure may be possible if organism is not resistant to hydroxychloroquine
- not effective against chloroquine-resistant strains of *P. falciparum*
- onset of action: may take 2–6 months before benefits are apparent

Use

- rheumatoid arthritis
- systemic and discoid lupus erythematosus (mild)
- treatment and suppression of malaria

Dose

- (lupus erythematosus) initially 400–800 mg orally daily for several weeks, reducing to maintenance dose of 200–400 mg daily **OR**
- (rheumatoid arthritis) initially 400–600 mg orally daily with food, increasing dose slowly after 5–10 days until optimal dose is achieved without adverse effects for 4–12 weeks, reducing to a maintenance dose of 200–400 mg daily when clinical improvement is established (daily maximum 6 mg/kg) **OR**
- (acute malaria treatment) initially 800 mg orally, then 400 mg 6–8 hours later, followed by 400 mg daily for 2 consecutive days or 800 mg as a single oral dose (total dose 2 g) **OR**
- (malaria suppression/prophylaxis) 400 mg orally as a single weekly dose starting 2 weeks before exposure and continuing for 8 weeks after leaving a malarial area (if unable to start 2 weeks before exposure, 2 doses of 400 mg are taken 6 hours apart)

Adverse effects

- nausea, abdominal pain, diarrhoea, vomiting, anorexia
- blurred vision
- rash, pruritus, skin dryness, increased skin pigmentation
- alopecia
- headache
- hypoglycaemia
- (uncommon) vertigo, tinnitus, corneal or retinal changes, photophobia, halos, dizziness, nerve deafness, bleaching of hair
- (rare) bone marrow depression, muscle weakness, decreased/absent deep tendon reflexes, exacerbate or precipitate porphyria, cardiomyopathy, seizures
- (very rare) suicidal behaviours, extrapyramidal disorder

Interactions

- incompatible with MAOIs
- use with digoxin may increase plasma digoxin levels, leading to toxicity, therefore digoxin levels should be closely monitored during therapy
- may enhance hypoglycaemic action of insulin or oral hypoglycaemic agents
- may lower convulsive threshold, increasing risk of seizures. This is enhanced if given with other antimalarial agents

- may impair antiepileptic effect, so should be used with caution
- caution if given with antiarrhythmic agents due to risk of inducing ventricular arrhythmias
- may increase serum levels of ciclosporin

Nursing points/Cautions

- because the effect of hydroxychloroquine accumulates, maximum clinical effects may take several months to be achieved; however, side-effects may appear much earlier
- ophthalmological examination (colour vision, fundoscopy, visual fields) should be done before starting therapy and continued every 6 months during treatment or more often in those at high risk (e.g. dose > 6 mg/kg, elderly, kidney/liver impairment, visual problems in previous 8 years, low body weight). Visual disturbances/retinal changes can continue to occur after therapy has stopped
- patients on long-term therapy should have regular full blood counts, blood glucose levels and testing of knee and ankle reflexes to monitor muscle strength. If any weakness occurs, medication should be stopped
- if rash appears, the drug should be withdrawn and recommenced at a lower dose
- (rheumatoid arthritis) any corticosteroid and/or salicylate dose may be decreased once hydroxychloroquine has been used for several weeks. Gradual reduction in corticosteroid dosage is recommended
- (rheumatoid arthritis) therapy should be stopped if there is no clinical improvement (e.g. improved mobility, decreased joint swelling) in 6 months
- patients should be monitored for any signs of cardiomyopathy
- caution if used in those with diabetes, kidney or liver impairment, quinine sensitivity or G6PD deficiency
- not recommended in those with porphyria or psoriasis as symptoms may become exacerbated, or in those with severe GI, neurological or blood disorders
- contraindicated in those with pre-existing maculopathy, hypersensitivity to 4-aminoquinolone compounds or as long-term therapy in children under 6 years

Patient teaching and advice

- patient should be advised to seek medical advice if any of the following occur:
  - visual disturbances (e.g. blurred vision, changes to night vision, light flashes or streaks)
  - rash, itchiness, dry skin or changes to pigmentation
- advise patient that visual disturbance may occur or progress after therapy has ceased
- warn patients about dangers of driving or operating machinery if blurred vision occurs
- patient should be advised to wear sunglasses in strong sunlight
- inform patients that clinical effect may take months to be noticeable; however, adverse effects may occur sooner
- if patient has diabetes, he/she should be instructed to monitor blood glucose levels closely as etanercept may cause hypoglycaemia. Dose of antidiabetic medications may need to be adjusted accordingly
- (malaria prophylaxis) patient should be advised to take dose on same day of each week to increase likelihood of adherence to regime
- see General Patient teaching and advice (p. xxvii)

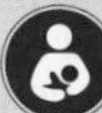

not recommended during pregnancy unless benefits outweigh the risks. May cause CNS damage, ototoxicity, retinal haemorrhage and abnormal retinal pigmentation in newborn (Note: this is the recommendation for use as an antimalarial)

use with great caution during breastfeeding

tablet can be crushed (has a bitter taste) and mixed with water or spoonful of yoghurt or apple puree

LEFLUNOMIDE (Arabloc, Arava, Ataris, Lunava)

Available forms
Tablets: 10 mg, 20 mg, 100 mg

Action
- immunomodulating and immunosuppressant actions
- weak anti-inflammatory properties
- converted to active metabolite by first-pass metabolism in the gut wall and liver
- active metabolite has a long half-life of approximately 1–4 weeks
- clinical improvement may occur in 4 weeks, and usually occurs in 4–6 months

Use
- active rheumatoid arthritis
- active psoriatic arthritis

Dose
- initially 100 mg orally daily for 3 days (loading dose), then 10–20 mg daily (maintenance)

Adverse effects
- rash, hair loss (reversible), pruritus, dry skin, hair and skin discolouration
- allergic reaction
- diarrhoea, abdominal pain, dyspepsia, nausea, anorexia, vomiting, mouth ulceration, stomatitis, weight loss, dry mouth, altered taste
- sleep disorder
- anxiety
- reversible elevation of liver enzymes (ALT, AST)
- urinary tract infection
- flu-like symptoms
- hypertension, chest pain, angina, tachycardia
- respiratory infection, bronchitis, cough, pharyngitis, sinusitis, rhinitis, pneumonia
- dizziness, headache, migraine
- paraesthesia, asthenia
- blurred vision
- hypokalaemia
- arthralgia, leg cramps, synovitis, tenosynovitis, back pain, neck pain, tendon rupture
- (rare) haematological disorder, hepatitis, jaundice, severe infection
- (very rare) severe skin reaction, interstitial lung disease, peripheral neuropathy

Interactions
- colestyramine and activated charcoal rapidly decrease plasma levels
- may increase plasma levels of rifampicin and phenytoin
- excessive alcohol intake should be avoided
- vaccination with live or live attenuated vaccines should be avoided during and for at least 6 months after finishing therapy
- not recommended with other agents that are hepatotoxic or haemotoxic/myelotoxic (e.g. methotrexate). If used together, increased monitoring of adverse effects is recommended
- caution if given with NSAIDs (including COX-2 inhibitors) because of increased risk of hepatotoxicity
- increased risk of peripheral neuropathy if used with other neurotoxic agents
- if given with warfarin, INR should be closely monitored

- may alter efficacy of combined oral contraceptives (ethinylestradiol, levonorgestrel)
- may increase serum levels of repaglinide, pioglitazone, paclitaxel and rosiglitazone
- may decrease efficacy of theophylline and duloxetine
- caution if used with benzylpenicillin, cefaclor, cimetidine, ciprofloxacin, indometacin (indomethacin), furosemide (frusemide), ketoprofen and zidovudine
- may increase serum levels of rifampicin, doxorubicin, methotrexate, sulfasalazine, daunorubicin, topotecan and HMG-CoA reductase inhibitors (e.g. rosuvastatin, simvastatin), increasing risk of toxicity or adverse effects

Nursing points/Cautions

- before starting, every 4 weeks for 6 months and then 6–8-weekly during therapy patients should have a full blood count (including differential white cell count), platelet count and liver function tests
- patient should be carefully evaluated for any active or latent tuberculosis and closely monitored for any reactivation
- BP should be monitored before starting and throughout therapy
- treatment should be immediately ceased if ulcerative stomatitis is evident
- because of the long half-life (1–4 weeks) of the active metabolite, recovery from any adverse effects may take some time after ceasing therapy
- risk of adverse effects when given with methotrexate may be lessened by avoiding giving the loading dose
- (washout procedure) leflunomide is stopped, then colestyramine 8 g orally 3 times daily or 50 g orally activated charcoal 4 times daily for 11 days total. Colestyramine and activated charcoal may both interfere with oral contraceptives, and therefore barrier forms of contraception should also be used. Plasma levels should be measured twice, 2 weeks apart after washout
- caution if used in those over 60 years or with diabetes mellitus due to the increased risk of peripheral neuropathy
- caution if used in those with kidney impairment
- contraindicated in those with severe immunodeficiency states, impaired bone marrow function, blood dyscrasias, significant anaemia, severe uncontrolled infection, liver impairment, severe hypoproteinaemia or those who have (or had) severe skin reactions (e.g. Stevens–Johnson syndrome, toxic epidermal necrolysis or erythema multiforme)

Patient teaching and advice

- patients should be advised to swallow the tablet whole with water, at the same time every day
- warn patients to avoid excessive alcohol intake
- instruct patient to seek medical advice immediately if any of the following occur:
  - sore throat, rash, excessive tiredness or flu-like symptoms
  - persistent cough, coughing up blood, fatigue or weight loss
  - fever, cough, breathing difficulties
  - pins, needles or numbness or weakness in arms or legs
  - recurring or persistent painful mouth ulcers
  - skin reaction
- caution patients against driving or operating machinery if dizziness or blurred vision occur

- patient should be warned that clinical improvement may take 4 weeks; however, it may take longer
- before starting treatment, pregnancy must be excluded
- if female patient is undergoing washout procedure prior to conception (see above), advise her to use a barrier method of contraception in addition to oral contraceptive, as failure may occur due to the colestyramine or activated charcoal
- counsel women of childbearing potential to use reliable contraception during therapy and the importance of telling their doctor if menstruation is delayed
- men and women are advised that levels of active metabolite should be below 0.02 mg/L on two separate tests taken 14 days apart before considering pregnancy after washout procedure (see p. 980)
- see General Patient teaching and advice (p. xxvii)

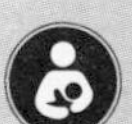

contraindicated during pregnancy and breastfeeding. Very high risk of causing permanent damage to the fetus

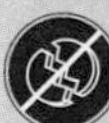

tablet should not be crushed or broken. Can be dispersed in 10–20 mL water (2–7 minutes dispersion time). Person handling tablet should wear disposable gloves

METHOTREXATE (Methoblastin, Methotrexate Injection and Tablets, Trexject)

Available forms

Tablets: 2.5 mg, 10 mg; Vial: 5 mg/2 mL, 50 mg/2 mL, 500 mg/5 mL, 500 mg/20 mL, 1000 mg/10 mL, 5000 mg/50 mL; Prefilled syringe: 7.5 mg/0.15 mL, 7.5 mg/0.3 mL, 10 mg/0.2 mL, 10 mg/0.4 mL, 15 mg/0.3 mL, 15 mg/0.6 mL, 20 mg/0.4 mL, 20 mg/0.8 mL, 25 mg/0.5 mL, 25 mg/mL

Action

- antimetabolite antineoplastic agent
- inhibits metabolism of folic acid, thereby interfering with cell replication (especially in rapidly dividing cells such as dermal epithelial cells, buccal, urinary bladder and intestinal cells)
- (rheumatoid arthritis) decreases swelling, pain and stiffness in rheumatoid arthritis, but does not induce remission or affect bone erosion
- (psoriasis) rate of epithelial cell production in skin is increased; therefore, methotrexate's action is due to its interference with this process
- may accumulate in third-space compartments (e.g. pleural effusions, ascites), resulting in prolonged half-life and toxicity
- onset of action may take 3–6 weeks, peak activity 1–4 hours (oral), 0.25–1 hour (IM) and 0.25–1.5 hours (SC)

Use

- antineoplastic chemotherapy (see Antineoplastic agents, p. 664)
- severe psoriasis that is unresponsive to other treatments
- severe rheumatoid arthritis that is unresponsive to other treatments

Dose

Rheumatoid arthritis

- 7.5 mg orally once weekly. May be increased by 15 mg/week after 6 weeks if no response (weekly maximum 20 mg). Once a response is established, dose should be decreased to the lowest that produces a clinical effect **OR**
- 2.5 mg orally for 3 doses at 12-hourly intervals weekly. May be increased by 15 mg/week after 6 weeks if no response (weekly maximum 20 mg). Once a response is established, dose should be decreased to the lowest that produces a clinical effect **OR**

- initially 7.5 mg SC weekly, increasing by 2.5 mg weekly (maximum 20–25 mg/weekly), then reduce to lowest effective dose as maintenance

Psoriasis

- (patient weight ≥ 70 kg) 10–25 mg IM or IV once weekly, gradually increasing to achieve optimal response, but not exceeding 50 mg/week. Once a response is established, dose should be decreased to the lowest that produces a clinical effect **OR**
- initially 7.5 mg SC weekly, then increasing gradually to 20–25 mg/weekly, then reducing to lowest effective dose as maintenance **OR**
- 10–25 mg orally once weekly, increasing gradually until adequate response is achieved (weekly maximum 50 mg) **OR**
- 2.5 mg orally for 3 doses at 12-hourly intervals weekly, gradually increasing to achieve optimal response, but not exceeding 30 mg/week. Once a response is established, dose should be decreased to the lowest that produces a clinical effect **OR**
- 2.5 mg orally for 4 doses at 8-hourly intervals weekly, gradually increasing to achieve optimal response, but not exceeding 30 mg/week. Once a response is established, dose should be decreased to the lowest that produces a clinical effect **OR**
- 2.5 mg orally daily for 5 days, followed by 2-day rest period, gradually increasing to achieve optimal response, but not exceeding 6.25 mg/day. Once a response is established, dose should be decreased to the lowest that produces a clinical effect

Adverse effects

- nausea, abdominal pain, diarrhoea, anorexia, vomiting, haematemesis, melaena, GI ulceration
- ulcerative stomatitis, mucositis (gingivitis, pharyngitis, glossitis)
- decreased serum albumin, altered liver function
- rash, pruritus, urticaria, acne, dermatitis, photosensitivity, hyperpigmentation/depigmentation
- nail changes
- hair loss (reversible)
- cystitis, haematuria, dysuria, proteinuria, urogenital dysfunction, renal failure
- dry non-productive cough, dyspnoea, pneumonia, interstitial pneumonitis, pulmonary fibrosis
- menstrual dysfunction, infertility, transient oligospermia, azotaemia
- abortion, fetal defects, fetal death
- osteoporosis, arthralgia, myalgia
- bone marrow depression, neutropenia, leucopenia, pancytopenia
- hypotension, pericarditis, pericardial effusion, thromboembolic events
- malaise, fatigue, chills and fever, headache, dizziness, drowsiness, paraesthesia
- tinnitus
- blurred vision, eye discomfort
- decreased resistance to infection
- increased risk of secondary tumour formation, increased risk of infection
- (high and prolonged therapy) hepatotoxicity, haemorrhagic enteritis, liver fibrosis and cirrhosis
- (psoriasis) burning, erythema (1–2 days after treatment), skin ulceration and rarely, anaphylactoid reactions
- (rare) tumour lysis syndrome (if rapidly growing tumour is present), severe skin reactions

Interactions

- (intrathecal) contraindicated with CNS radiotherapy
- contraindicated with acitretin or other retinoids
- contraindicated with alcohol and other hepatotoxic agents (e.g. retinoids, azathioprine, leflunomide, sulfasalazine)

- contraindicated with live or live attenuated vaccines
- not recommended with other DMARDs
- serum levels (and associated risk of toxicity) may be increased by salicylates, sulfonamides, sulfonylureas, phenytoin, penicillins, ciprofloxacin, tetracyclines, chloramphenicol, probenecid, proton pump inhibitors (e.g. omeprazole, pantoprazole) and aminobenzoic acid and therefore not recommended together
- (high dose) not recommended with NSAIDs due to increased risk of myelosuppression and GI toxicity because half-life of methotrexate is prolonged. Caution should also be used with lower doses of methotrexate
- toxicity may be increased by folate deficiency
- serum levels may be decreased by colestyramine
- risk of toxicity increased if given with other antineoplastic agents
- (antineoplastic agent) not recommended with vitamin supplements containing folic or folinic acid
- (rheumatoid arthritis) folic acid or folinic acid may decrease adverse effects but also decrease the efficacy of methotrexate and should not be administered on the same day
- if used with nitrous oxide, may potentiate methotrexate's effects on folate metabolism
- increased risk of bone marrow depression if given with allopurinol, trimethoprim, trimethoprim/sulfamethoxazole and pyrimethamine
- (use in psoriasis) increased risk of skin ulceration if given with amiodarone
- may decrease clearance of theophylline, thereby increasing risk of toxicity. Theophylline levels should be closely monitored during concurrent therapy
- may impair absorption of phenytoin, increasing risk of seizures
- may be antagonised by asparaginase
- (IV infusion) increased risk of toxicity if given with transfusion of packed red blood cells
- absorption and metabolism may be decreased by chloramphenicol, tetracycline and non-absorbable broad-spectrum antibiotics
- may increase plasma levels of mercaptopurine
- increased risk of pancytopenia and hepatotoxicity if given with leflunomide
- increased risk of soft tissue necrosis and osteonecrosis if given with radiotherapy
- half-life may be increased if given with probenecid or phenylbutazone
- increased risk of skin cancer if given with PUVA therapy
- may interfere with folic acid detection assay

Nursing points/Cautions

- pregnancy should be excluded before starting therapy
- adverse effects are generally dose related
- SC administration is for psoriasis and rheumatoid arthritis therapy only
- if switching from oral to parenteral administration, a dose reduction may be required because of variable methotrexate bioavailability after oral administration. No dose adjustment is required if switching from IM to SC route or vice versa
- (SC, rheumatoid arthritis) therapeutic response occurs after 4–8 weeks
- (SC, psoriasis) therapeutic response occurs after 2–6 weeks
- (SC) first self-administration should be under medical supervision
- (IM or IV, psoriasis) single 5–10 mg IV or IM dose may be given as a test

dose before starting therapy to identify any patient idiosyncrasies. Complete blood counts with platelets should be evaluated 7–10 days later

- full blood count (with differential and platelet count), haematocrit, renal function test, liver function test (including serum albumin and prothrombin time), urinalysis (urine should be alkaline), hepatitis B or C infection testing and chest X-ray should all be completed before, during (4–8-weekly) and after therapy. Liver biopsy may be recommended if patient has history of excessive alcohol use, chronic hepatitis B or C infection or persistently abnormal liver function test. Testing should be more frequent if changing dosage or if dehydration occurs increasing risk of elevated levels
- patient should be closely monitored for any lung symptoms. Lung function tests are recommended if methotrexate-induced lung disease is suspected
- (psoriasis) liver biopsy is recommended before, during (2–4-monthly), after a cumulative dose of 1.5 g and then after each additional 1–1.5 g
- liver biopsy and/or bone marrow aspiration is recommended for those receiving high-dose or long-term therapy
- (rheumatoid arthritis) hepatotoxicity is related to age of first dose and duration of therapy
- urine should be kept alkaline during therapy
- pregnant staff should be cautioned not to handle methotrexate
- tablets contain lactose and are therefore not recommended in those with galactose intolerance, Lapp lactase deficiency or glucose–galactose malabsorption
- (IV) incompatible with cytarabine, fluorouracil and prednisolone
- caution if used in those with inactive chronic infections (e.g. TB, herpes zoster, hepatitis B or C) as these may be reactivated
- caution if used in those who are debilitated or at extremes of age (young, elderly)
- contraindicated in those with poor nutrition, bone marrow depression, blood dyscrasias, severe liver or kidney impairment, alcoholic or alcoholic liver disease, immunodeficiency syndromes, blood dyscrasias, peptic ulcer disease, ulcerative colitis or severe acute or chronic infection

Patient teaching and advice

- it is important to ensure the patient has a good understanding of the dosing regimen as accidental daily dosing (instead of weekly) may be fatal
- caution patients not to crush or chew tablets, and to swallow tablets with a full glass of water
- hands should be washed immediately after handling tablets
- advise patient to avoid alcohol during therapy
- (SC, psoriasis, rheumatoid arthritis) patient can be taught to self-administer:
    - See p. 990 in General teaching and advice for TNF-α antagonists for self-administration teaching and advice. The following should also be included:
        - if patient weight $>$ 100 kg, administration site should be upper thigh only
        - if patient has psoriasis, advice should include avoiding injections into psoriatic lesion
        - if carer is administering injection, disposable gloves should be worn and hands washed before and after administration

  - if any spills occur, area should be cleaned with paper towels, which are disposed of in 'sharps container' and area
  - if any solution makes contact with eyes or skin, it should be washed with copious amounts of water and medical attention sought
- (psoriasis) warn patients that burning and redness is common in psoriatic area for 1–2 days post-therapy
- (rheumatoid arthritis) patient should be advised that improvement may be seen in 3–6 weeks after starting therapy, and improvement seen for a further 12 weeks or more
- (rheumatoid arthritis) warn patient that symptoms may worsen within 3–6 weeks of stopping therapy
- advise patient to maintain good hydration throughout therapy and seek medical advice if any vomiting, diarrhoea or stomatitis (sore inflamed gums, inside of lips, cheeks or tongue) occurs that might lead to dehydration
- instruct patient to immediately seek medical advice if any of the following occur:
  - dry persistent non-productive cough, fever, chest pain, shortness of breath (lung disorder)
  - fever, sore throat, chills (signs of infection)
  - vomiting, diarrhoea, inflamed gums or mouth ulcers
  - headache, shortness of breath, dizziness, looking pale (signs of anaemia)
  - blood in urine or bowel motions, black tarry bowel motions, black vomit, pinpoint red spots on skin (bleeding disorders or internal bleeding)
  - pain or difficulty urinating, lower back or side pain (possible kidney disorder)
- patient should be advised to avoid people with infections if possible
- instruct patient to avoid excessive sun exposure or sunlamps, as photosensitivity reaction may occur, or to wear a hat and long-sleeved shirt/garment and SPF 30+ sunscreen to protect skin if sun exposure cannot be avoided
- caution patients not to drive or operate machinery if dizziness, drowsiness, blurred vision or fatigue occur
- advise pregnant women that they should not handle tablets
- before treatment begins, all patients (male and female) should be counselled regarding potential benefits and risks of therapy, including effects on reproduction, and the importance of using effective contraception throughout therapy and for a minimum of 3 months after therapy has stopped. Female patients should be instructed to seek medical advice immediately if menstruation does not occur and pregnancy is suspected
- see also General Patient teaching and advice (p. xxvii)

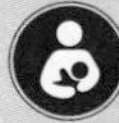

contraindicated during pregnancy and breastfeeding. Has been proven to cause fetal death and/or congenital abnormalities, as well as severe and/or toxic adverse effects

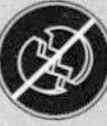

tablet should not be broken or crushed. Tablet can be dispersed in 10–20 mL of water. Disposable gloves should be worn by staff dispersing tablet. Pregnant staff should not disperse tablet

PENICILLAMINE (D Penamine)

Available forms

Tablets: 125 mg, 250 mg

Action

- degradation product of penicillin
- forms a stable complex (chelate) with heavy metals such as copper, lead, gold and mercury

- reduces urinary levels of cystine by combining with cystine to form a more soluble, readily excretable complex, so reducing formation of cystine calculi
- effect in rheumatoid arthritis is due to unknown action
- half-life about 90 hours

Use

- severe active rheumatoid arthritis
- Wilson's disease (deficiency of copper-binding protein)
- treatment of heavy metal poisoning
- treatment of cystinuria (where high fluid regimens are not adequate or as an adjunct to them)

Dose

- (rheumatoid arthritis) up to 250 mg orally daily in divided doses 1 hour before or 2 hours after food for 1 month, then increasing by the same amount monthly to a maximum of 1500 mg daily. The dose is then lowered to achieve the lowest effective dose (maintenance dose) **OR**
- (Wilson's disease) 1500–2000 mg orally daily 1 hour before or 2 hours after meals **OR**
- (heavy metal poisoning) 250–1000 mg orally in divided doses 1 hour before or 2 hours after meals **OR**
- (cystinuria) 750–1000 mg orally in divided doses 1 hour before or 2 hours after meals (maximum daily dose 2 g) **OR**
- (cystinuria) 500 mg orally before retiring, followed by free fluids during the day

Adverse effects

- erythematous or maculopapular rash, fever, joint pains, urticaria, lymphadenopathy
- impaired taste (reversible), anorexia, nausea, vomiting, diarrhoea, cheilosis, glossitis
- drug fever (in second or third week of therapy)
- tinnitus
- hair loss
- hepatic dysfunction, pancreatitis
- proteinuria, nephrotic syndrome
- iron-deficiency anaemia (prolonged use), agranulocytosis, thrombocytosis, eosinophilia, leukocytosis, leucopenia, thrombocytopenia
- impaired wound healing, increased skin friability (at pressure points), purpuric skin lesions
- increased excretion of other heavy metals
- (rarely) pyridoxine deficiency, reversible optic neuritis, breast enlargement (male and female), glomerulonephritis (Goodpasture's syndrome) (see Glossary)

Interactions

- enhances urinary excretion of copper, lead, zinc, gold, mercury and other heavy metals
- may potentiate isoniazid
- contraindicated in those taking antimalarial agents or receiving gold therapy for arthritis

Nursing points/Cautions

- neurological examination is recommended before starting therapy
- blood count (including WBC count, differential cell count and direct platelet count) should be measured weekly for the first 4 weeks, then every second week for 5 months, then monthly. Urinalysis should occur at the same time. Skin and mucous membranes should also be assessed for any allergic reaction. Therapy should be stopped if fever or reaction in urine, blood or skin appears or if blood count declines over three successive tests
- if albumin > 2 g/day, therapy should be stopped
- liver function should be monitored 6-monthly for 18 months

- annual ophthalmological examination is recommended
- (rheumatoid arthritis) if no response occurs in 6 months at full maintenance dose, therapy should be discontinued
- should be discontinued at least 6 weeks before any surgery as penicillamine may interfere with collagen cross-links and therefore interrupt the healing process
- (cystinuria) annual chest X-ray is recommended
- may require daily prophylactic pyridoxine (25 mg) if central and/or peripheral nervous system symptoms occur
- (Wilson's disease, lead poisoning) if patient is vomiting or unable to swallow, parenteral EDTA is recommended
- (Wilson's disease) some clinical deterioration may occur at start of therapy before improvement
- iron supplementation may be required if iron deficiency occurs
- caution if used in penicillin-hypersensitive patients because cross-allergy may occur

Patient teaching and advice

- instruct patient to check temperature, skin and urine each day before taking medication and any fever, chills, bruising, bleeding, rash, sore throat, proteinuria or haematuria should be reported immediately to the doctor because it indicates the need to stop the drug
- (rheumatoid arthritis) warn patient that it may take 6–8 weeks for a response to be seen
- warn patient that drug fever (with or without skin reactions) commonly occurs in first 2–3 weeks of therapy
- advise patient against abrupt withdrawal of therapy
- instruct patient to take medication on an empty stomach (1 hour before or 2 hours after food, and at least 1 hour apart from other medication, milk or snacks)
- patient should be advised to immediately seek medical advice if any of the following occur:
  - visual disturbances
  - become pale and tired, short of breath
  - develop muscle weakness, double vision, drooping eyelids
- female patients should be counselled regarding the need to avoid becoming pregnant while taking medication
- see also General Patient teaching and advice (p. xxvii)

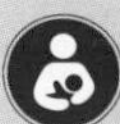

not recommended during pregnancy because cutis laxa (a connective tissue disorder) has occurred in the fetus

tablet can be crushed and mixed with water or spoonful of apple puree (NOT yoghurt)

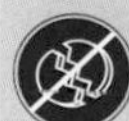

pregnant staff should not crush or disperse tablet

SULFASALAZINE (Pyralin EN, Salazopyrin, Salazopyrin EN-Tabs)

Available forms

Tablets: 500 mg; Tablets (enteric-coated): 500 mg

Action

- broken down in the colon by bacteria to 5-aminosalicylic acid and sulfapyridine

producing an anti-inflammatory effect by its action on prostaglandin synthesis, leukotrienes and arachidonic acid metabolites
- onset of action may take 6–12 weeks

Use
- ulcerative colitis and Crohn's disease (see Gastrointestinal agents (miscellaneous) p. 1093)
- rheumatoid arthritis (unresponsive to other drug therapy)

Dose
- (rheumatoid arthritis) initially 500 mg orally at night for 1 week, 500 mg twice daily for 1 week, 500 mg in the morning and 1 g at night for 1 week, then 1 g twice daily for 1 week (to daily maximum of 3 g)

OR
- (ulcerative colitis, Crohn's disease) initially 1–2 g orally 4 times daily after meals, then 500 mg 4 times daily

TUMOUR NECROSIS FACTOR ALPHA (TNF-α) ANTAGONISTS

General Actions of TNF-α antagonists
- recombinant monoclonal antibody (IgG1) that neutralises activity of tumour necrosis factor (TNF). (TNF is a naturally occurring cytokine that is involved in inflammatory and immune responses. It is found in high levels in the synovial fluid of those with RA. It is thought to be involved in both joint inflammation and erosion. Raised TNF levels are also found in those with psoriatic arthritis, psoriatic plaques and ankylosing spondylitis)

General Adverse effects of TNF-α antagonists
- (infusion site reaction) erythema, pain, itching, swelling
- headache, fatigue, fever, dizziness, vertigo, asthenia
- flushing
- nausea, vomiting, abdominal pain, diarrhoea, dyspepsia
- upper and lower respiratory tract infections, pneumonia, dyspnoea, sinusitis, pharyngitis, nasopharyngitis, cough
- viral infection
- other infections (urinary tract, soft tissue, joints, reproductive tract, ear, oral, fungal)
- chest pain, hypertension
- rash, pruritus, urticaria, dry skin, increased sweating
- autoantibody development
- (long-term) development of malignancy and blood dyscrasias
- (rare) reactivation of tuberculosis, demyelinating diseases, peripheral neuropathy, transverse myelitis, seizure disorders, new or worsening psoriasis, aplastic anaemia, pancytopenia, worsening heart failure, lupus-like syndrome, hypersensitivity

General Interactions of TNF-α antagonists
- contraindicated with anakinra, abatacept, other cytokine modulators and other TNF-α antagonists due to increased risk of infection
- not recommended with live or live attenuated vaccines

General Nursing points/Cautions for TNF-α antagonists

- before starting therapy, all patients should be:
  - screened for any signs of infection. This should include screening for hepatitis B and C, and tuberculosis (TB) (clinical history, chest X-ray, skin tuberculin test) as these can become reactivated. If latent TB is diagnosed, it should be treated with appropriate antimycobacterial agents before starting therapy. If active TB is found, therapy should not be started
  - asked about any travel to areas at high risk of TB or endemic mycoses (e.g. histoplasmosis)
  - examined for skin cancer
  - checked to ensure their immunisations are up to date before starting therapy
- any infection should be identified, treated and controlled before starting therapy
- before starting therapy, full blood count, creatinine and liver function tests are recommended and repeated if signs of infection or blood dyscrasias occur
- trade name and batch number should be recorded in patient history
- infusion-related reactions occur more frequently in those who develop autoantibodies
- do not mix with other agents in the syringe
- patient may be taught to self-administer medication SC. They should be educated about rotation of sites, injection technique, storage requirements and safe disposal of used needles
- rotate injection sites (thigh or abdomen) avoiding skin that is reddened, bruised, tender or hard or within 3 cm of previous injection sites
- if undergoing surgery, patient should be closely monitored for any signs of infection
- needle covers of prefilled syringes contain latex and should not be handled by or administered to anyone with a latex sensitivity
- therapy should be stopped if new, serious infection develops
- if switching from one biological agent to another, patient should be carefully monitored for any signs of infection
- development of autoantibodies may worsen or induce lupus-like syndrome
- cardiac status should be closely monitored in those with mild congestive cardiac failure and stopped if there is any worsening
- caution if used in those who live or travel to areas where mycoses are endemic. Fungal infection should be suspected if the person develops a serious systemic infection
- caution if used in those aged 65 years or more as they are at increased risk of infection and malignancy
- caution if used in those who have recently been diagnosed with CNS or peripheral demyelinating disease, on concurrent immunosuppressive therapy (as there is an increased risk of infection) or mild heart failure (as it may be worsened)
- caution if used in those with chronic or recurring infection or conditions that may predispose them to infection, including asthma or poorly controlled diabetes

- caution if used in heavy smokers or those with chronic obstructive pulmonary disease (COPD) as there is an increased risk of lung, neck and head cancer
- contraindicated in those with serious or untreated infections (including active tuberculosis), sepsis, moderate-to-severe heart failure, lupus-like syndrome or history of blood dyscrasias

General Patient teaching and advice for TNF-α antagonists

- patients should be counselled to immediately seek medical advice if they develop any:
  - persistent cough, coughing up blood, loss of weight or low-grade fever (signs of TB)
  - persistent fever, bruising, bleeding, pallor
  - numbness or tingling in arms or legs
  - any changes to skin lesions (new ones appearing or existing ones changing in size or appearance)
- advise patient to have regular skin examinations (self-examination and by qualified health professional)
- warn patient that needle covers of prefilled syringes and pens contain latex
- patients may be taught to self-administer medication SC. Information should include:
  - if not confident about the techniques, do not attempt to self-inject
  - do not inject through clothing
  - wash hands before self-injecting
  - collect prefilled syringe/autoinjector and alcohol pad
  - check expiry date before using and do not use if after month/year shown
  - solution should be checked to ensure that colour has not changed and that there are no particles present. If cloudy, discoloured or if flakes are present, syringe should not be used
  - allow syringe to come to room temperature before administration (15–30 minutes) (this will reduce pain). Should not be warmed in any other way, such as water bath or microwave
  - choose injection site (thigh or stomach) 3 cm away from previous injection site or navel (do not choose an area that is red, tender, hard, bruised, scarred or has broken skin)
  - it is important to rotate or change injection sites so that area does not become too painful. Areas should be rotated between thigh and stomach
  - clean injection site using alcohol wipe, wiping the area in a circular motion
  - don't touch this area again before injecting
  - gently invert, but do not shake, syringe before administration. If solution looks frothy, it should be allowed to rest until it clears before using
  - remove cap from needle (being careful not to touch the needle or let it touch any surface)
  - grasp cleaned skin area with one hand, gently but firmly
  - with the other hand, hold syringe at 45–90° angle with the grooved side up

  - using a quick, short motion, push needle completely into skin
  - release the skin and push plunger to completely inject solution (may take 2–5 seconds)
  - when syringe is empty, remove needle from skin
  - using thumb and piece of gauze or cottonwool ball (not the alcohol swab), apply pressure (but do not rub) over injection site for 10 seconds
  - can apply a plaster (e.g. Band-Aid) if required
  - syringe should not be recapped; dispose of according to instructions (e.g. patient may have been supplied with sharps container for safe disposal)
  - protect prefilled syringes from light before use and store them at 2–8°C, but not frozen
  - if travelling, ensure syringes are kept at the correct temperature
  - if injection site reactions occur, applying cold pack to site will relieve any pain, swelling or itching
- see also General Patient teaching and advice (p. xxvii)

ADALIMUMAB (Amgevita, Hadlima, Humira, Hyrimoz, Idacio)

Available forms

Prefilled syringe: 20 mg/0.4 mL, 40 mg/0.8 mL; Prefilled pen: 40 mg/0.8 mL

Action

- see General Actions of TNF-α antagonists (p. 988)
- long half-life 10–20 days

Use

- moderate-to-severe rheumatoid arthritis (alone or with methotrexate)
- moderate-to-severe psoriatic arthritis (unresponsive to other DMARDs)
- active ankylosing spondylitis
- moderate-to-severe polyarticular juvenile idiopathic arthritis (over 2 years of age) (unresponsive to other DMARDs) (alone or with methotrexate)
- moderate-to-severe plaque psoriasis
- moderate-to-severe Crohn's disease (inadequate response to conventional therapies or intolerant/unresponsive to infliximab)
- moderate-to-severe ulcerative colitis (inadequate response to conventional therapies)
- moderate-to-severe non-infectious intermediate posterior uveitis (inadequate response to corticosteroids)
- moderate-to-severe Hidradenitis Suppurativa (HS) (acne inversa) (inadequate response to conventional therapies)

Dose

- (rheumatoid arthritis) 40 mg SC fortnightly (or weekly if not given concurrently with methotrexate) **OR**
- (psoriatic arthritis, ankylosing spondylitis) 40 mg SC fortnightly **OR**
- (psoriasis) initially 80 mg SC, then 1 week later 40 mg SC, repeated fortnightly **OR**
- (polyarticular juvenile idiopathic arthritis) 20 mg SC fortnightly (weight 10 kg to < 30 kg) or 40 mg SC fortnightly (weight 30 kg or more) **OR**
- (Crohn's disease, ulcerative colitis, HS) initially 160 mg SC as 4 injections (day 0) or 80 mg SC as 2 injections (day 0) and repeated on day 1, followed by 80 mg as 2 injections on day 14 (induction), then 40 mg SC on day 28 and continuing fortnightly (maintenance) **OR**
- (uveitis) initially 80 mg SC, then 40 mg SC fortnightly starting 1 week after initial dose

Adverse effects

- see General Adverse effects of TNF-α antagonists (p. 988)

- visual impairment, conjunctivitis, eye swelling
- impaired healing
- nail disorder
- cough, asthma
- migraine
- musculoskeletal pain, muscle spasm
- paraesthesia
- tachycardia, oedema
- depression, anxiety, insomnia
- elevated liver enzymes
- gastrointestinal haemorrhage, gastroesophageal reflux disease (GORD)
- haematuria, renal impairment
- leucopenia, thrombocytopenia, anaemia, neutropenia
- hyperlipidaemia, hypokalaemia, hypocalcaemia, hypophosphataemia, hyperglycaemia, increased uric acid, abnormal serum sodium
- prolonged activated PTT

Interactions

- see General Interactions of TNF-α antagonists (p. 988)

Nursing points/Cautions

- see General Nursing points/Cautions for TNF-α antagonists (p. 989)
- (uveitis) because of association between uveitis and central demyelinating disorders, neurological assessment is recommended before starting therapy
- (ulcerative colitis) if patient has previous history or is at risk of dysplasia or colon cancer (e.g. long-standing ulcerative colitis or primary sclerosing cholangitis), screening for dysplasia (e.g. colonoscopy, biopsy) is recommended before starting and regularly during therapy
- (psoriasis) not recommended with phototherapy or other systemic agents
- (uveitis) can be given with corticosteroids and/or non-biological immunotherapy. Corticosteroid dose may be tapered 2 weeks after starting therapy
- (HS) antibiotic therapy may be continued if necessary
- (HS) therapy should be stopped after 12 weeks if there is no clinical response
- (Crohn's) aminosalicylates, corticosteroids and/or azathioprine or mercaptopurine can be continued during therapy
- (ankylosing spondylitis, psoriatic arthritis) glucocorticoids, salicylates, NSAIDs or DMARDs can be continued during therapy

Patient teaching and advice

- see General Patient teaching and advice for TNF-α antagonists (p. 990)
- patients can be instructed to self-administer using prefilled syringe or pen. For patient teaching and advice for prefilled syringe see pp. 990–91. For prefilled pen, instructions are as follows:
  - leave at room temperature for 15–30 minutes before administration, but do not use any other method to warm (e.g. microwave, water bath)
  - check expiry date and do not use if it has passed
  - hold pen with grey cap pointing up (viewing solution through window)
  - ensure solution is clear, colourless and contains no particles
  - do not remove grey or plum-coloured caps until ready to inject
  - follow instructions on pp. 990–91 for choosing and rotating sites, cleaning skin and handwashing
  - remove grey cap and discard, exposing white needle sleeve
  - remove plum cap and discard, revealing activation button
  - it is important not to put pen down as this might activate and release the solution

- with free hand, pinch clean skin at injection site and hold firmly
- place white end of pen at 90 degrees (right angle) to the skin, pressing down slightly and observing window
- when ready to inject press plum-coloured button. A click will be heard as the needle is released and a small prick felt. Keep pressing, holding pen steady for about 10 seconds to complete injection. A yellow indicator will move into the window during the injection and will stop moving when injection is complete
- lift pen away from injection site and discard into a sharps-disposal container
- if there is a drop of blood at injection site, press site with gauze or cotton wool ball but do not rub the injection site
- store pen at 2–8°C but do not freeze. Pen can be stored at room temperature (< 25°C) for up to 14 days (write down date of removal from fridge) and protected from the light. If not used in this time, pen should be discarded and not refrigerated again. This is important if the patient is travelling

- women of childbearing age should be counselled to use adequate contraception during and for 5 months after stopping therapy
- if newborn has been exposed to adalimumab during pregnancy, live vaccines should not be administered for at least 5 months after last administration

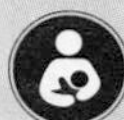

not recommended during pregnancy and breastfeeding or for at least 5 months after stopping therapy

CERTOLIZUMAB PEGOL (Cimzia)

Available forms

Prefilled syringe: 200 mg/mL; Prefilled pen: 200 mg/mL

Action

- immunomodifier
- recombinant humanised antibody fragment (Fab)
- expressed in *E. coli* and conjugated (pegylated) to polyethylene glycol (PEG) increasing half-life
- high affinity for human TNF-α which is a pro-inflammatory cytokine that plays a central role in the inflammatory process
- long half-life (14 days)

Use

- moderate-to-severe rheumatoid arthritis (RA) (alone or with methotrexate)
- active ankylosing spondylitis (unresponsive or intolerant to at least one NSAID)
- active psoriatic arthritis (unresponsive to other DMARDs)
- moderate-to-severe plaque psoriasis

Dose

- (all uses) initially 400 mg (2 injections of 200 mg) SC at weeks 0, 2 and 4, then either 200 mg SC second weekly or 400 mg SC monthly (maintenance) (alone or with methotrexate)

Adverse effects

- see General Adverse effects of TNF-α antagonists (p. 988)
- prolonged aPTT
- anaemia, eosinophilia
- conjunctivitis
- gastritis
- abnormal liver function
- back ache, muscle spasm, pain in extremities
- oropharyngeal pain

Interactions

- see General Interactions of TNF-α antagonists (p. 988)
- may interfere with some coagulation assays resulting in falsely elevated aPTT

Nursing points/Cautions

- see General Nursing points/Cautions for TNF-α antagonists (p. 989)
- (RA) if no response within 12 weeks, use should be re-evaluated
- (psoriasis) if no response within 16 weeks, use should be re-evaluated

Patient teaching and advice

- see General Patient teaching and advice for TNF-α antagonists (p. 990)
- patients can be instructed to self-administer using prefilled syringe or pen. For patient teaching and advice for prefilled syringe see p. 990. For prefilled pen, instructions are similar to those for adalimumab (p. 992) with the following differences:
    - hold pen firmly by black handle and remove clear cap
    - injection should occur within 5 minutes of cap removal
    - holding pen firmly by black handle, press down firmly on skin at 90 degrees. Click will be heard starting the injection and a second click is heard (this may take up to 15 seconds). The window on the side of the pen should be orange indicating the injection is complete.
- counsel female patients about the importance of using adequate contraception to avoid pregnancy during and for at least 5 months after stopping therapy

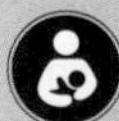

women should be advised to use adequate contraception during and for 5 months after stopping therapy to prevent pregnancy occurring

women should breastfeed only if benefits outweigh risks

ETANERCEPT (Brenzys, Enbrel)

Available forms

Vial: 25 mg; Prefilled syringe: 50 mg/mL; Autoinjector: 50 mg/mL

Action

- see General Actions of TNF-α antagonists (p. 988)
- reaches maximum concentration in 24–96 hours after SC administration
- long half-life (about 80 hours)

Use

- rheumatoid arthritis (unresponsive to other DMARDs) (alone or with methotrexate)
- active polyarticular course juvenile chronic arthritis (unresponsive to other DMARDs)
- psoriatic arthritis (unresponsive to other DMARDs)
- active ankylosing spondylitis
- moderate-to-severe chronic plaque psoriasis
- non-radiographic axial spondyloarthritis (inadequate response to NSAIDs)

Dose

- (rheumatoid arthritis, polyarticular juvenile chronic arthritis, psoriatic arthritis, ankylosing spondylitis, axial spondyloarthritis) 50 mg SC weekly or 25 mg SC twice weekly 3–4 days apart **OR**
- (plaque psoriasis) 50 mg SC weekly or 25 mg SC twice weekly 3–4 days apart. Dose may be increased to 50 mg SC twice weekly for up to 12 weeks if necessary, then reduced

Adverse effects

- see General Adverse effects of TNF-α antagonists (p. 988)
- (rare) uveitis, inflammatory bowel disease, autoimmune hepatitis
- (very rare) fatal pancytopenia, aplastic anaemia

Interactions

- see General Interactions of TNF-α antagonists (p. 988)
- caution if given with sulfasalazine as a decrease in WBC may occur
- not recommended with cyclophosphamide

Nursing points/Cautions

- see General Nursing points/Cautions for TNF-α antagonists (p. 989)
- (vial) reconstitute powder by gently injecting water for injections into vial using vial adapter attached to syringe and swirl gently, avoiding vigorous agitation or shaking
- (vial) clear and colourless solution should result within 10 minutes of reconstitution
- (vial) solution should not be filtered, nor used if discoloured, cloudy or containing particulate matter
- (vial) use within 6 hours of reconstitution
- caution if used in those with diabetes as there is an increased risk of hypoglycaemia, necessitating a decreased dose in hypoglycaemic medication
- caution in those with moderate-to-severe alcoholic hepatitis

Patient teaching and advice

- see General Patient teaching and advice for TNF-α antagonists (p. 990)
- inform patient that injection site reaction reduces after initial 4 weeks
- if patient has diabetes, he/she should be instructed to monitor blood glucose levels closely as etanercept may cause hypoglycaemia. Dose of hypoglycaemic medications may need to be adjusted accordingly
- advise patient to seek medical advice immediately if they are exposed to chickenpox or shingles during therapy
- prefilled syringe/autoinjector can be stored at up to 25°C for 4 weeks; however, it should be discarded if not used in that time or if exposed to high temperature

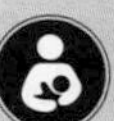

use during pregnancy only if benefits clearly outweigh potential risks to fetus

live vaccine should not be given to infant within 16 weeks of last dose

not recommended during breastfeeding

GOLIMUMAB (Simponi)

Available forms

Prefilled syringe/injector pen: 50 mg/0.5 mL, 100 mg/mL

Action

- see General Actions of TNF-α antagonists (p. 988)
- half-life 9–15 days

Use

- moderate-to-severe active rheumatoid arthritis (with methotrexate)
- active, progressive psoriatic arthritis (alone or with methotrexate)
- active ankylosing spondylitis
- moderate-to-severe ulcerative colitis (unresponsive to other treatments)
- non-radiographic axial spondyloarthritis (inadequate response to NSAIDs)

Dose

- (rheumatoid arthritis, psoriatic arthritis, ankylosing spondylitis, axial spondyloarthritis) 50 mg SC monthly **OR**
- (ulcerative colitis) initially 200 mg SC, 100 mg SC after 2 weeks, then 100 mg SC monthly

Adverse effects

- see General Adverse effects of TNF-α antagonists (p. 988)
- constipation
- elevated liver enzymes
- bone fractures

Interactions

- see General Interactions of TNF-α antagonists (p. 080)

Nursing points/Cautions

- see General Nursing points/Cautions for TNF-α antagonists (p. 989)
- long half-life should be taken into consideration if patient is undergoing surgery
- (post-surgery) patients should be closely monitored during and after therapy for any signs of infection
- (ulcerative colitis) because of increased risk of bowel cancer and dysplasia, colonoscopy and biopsy are recommended before starting therapy and at regular intervals in those with long-standing ulcerative colitis, primary sclerosing cholangitis or previous history of colon dysplasia or cancer
- (ulcerative colitis) corticosteroid dose may be tapered during maintenance therapy according to clinical practice guidelines
- patients with active rheumatoid arthritis (especially if treated previously with immunosuppressant agents) are at increased risk of leukaemia and lymphoma and should be carefully monitored during and after therapy

Patient teaching and advice

- see General Patient teaching and advice for TNF-α antagonists (p. 990)
- if multiple injections are required, different sites should be used
- women of childbearing potential should be counselled to use reliable contraception during therapy and for 6 months post-therapy, and also the importance of telling their doctor if menstruation is delayed

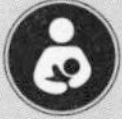

not recommended during pregnancy

live vaccines should not be administered to infants within 6 months of stopping therapy

not recommended during breastfeeding and should not be commenced within 6 months of stopping therapy

INFLIXIMAB (Iflectra, Remicade, Remsima, Renflexis)

Available form

Vial: 100 mg

Action

- see General Actions of TNF-α antagonists (p. 988)
- half-life 8–9.5 days

Use

- moderate-to-severe Crohn's disease (in patients over 6 years) to induce and maintain remission (unresponsive to conventional treatment)
- moderately severe to severe active ulcerative colitis (unresponsive to conventional treatment)
- treatment of refractory fistulising Crohn's disease
- rheumatoid arthritis (with methotrexate)
- ankylosing spondylitis
- psoriatic arthritis (unresponsive to other DMARDs) (alone or with methotrexate)
- severe plaque psoriasis (unresponsive to other conventional treatment)

Dose

- (rheumatoid arthritis) initially 3 mg/kg IV over 2 hours, then 3 mg/kg IV given at 2 and 6 weeks after the first infusion, then 3 mg/kg IV 8-weekly (with methotrexate). Dose may be increased by 1.5 mg/kg incrementally to a maximum of 7.5 mg/kg for optimal response **OR**
- (ankylosing spondylitis) initially 5 mg/kg IV over 2 hours, then 5 mg/kg IV given at 2 and 6 weeks after the first infusion, followed by 5 mg/kg IV 6-weekly **OR**

- (psoriatic arthritis, plaque psoriasis) 5 mg/kg IV over 2 hours, then 5 mg/kg at 2 and 6 weeks after initial dose, then 8-weekly (maintenance) **OR**
- (moderate-to-severe Crohn's disease, refractory fistulating Crohn's disease, ulcerative colitis) initially 5 mg/kg by IV infusion over 2 hours, then 2 and 6 weeks after initial infusion (induction), followed by 5 mg/kg by IV infusion 8-weekly (maintenance)

Adverse effects

- see General Adverse effects of TNF-α antagonists (p. 988)

Interactions

- see General Interactions of TNF-α antagonists (p. 988)

Nursing points/Cautions

- see General Nursing points/Cautions for TNF-α antagonists (p. 989)
- for doses > 6 mg/kg, infusion should be > 2 hours
- gently add 10 mL water for injections down the inside of the vial, swirl gently and avoid shaking to dissolve. Foaming may occur
- allow solution to stand for 5 minutes before administering
- solution may be colourless to light yellow and clear
- should be diluted to 250 mL with sodium chloride 0.9%, gently mixed and then given as an IV infusion (rate not greater than 2 mL/min) over at least 2 hours
- a filter (micron size 1.2 or less) should be added to the infusion set
- administer alone
- patient should be carefully observed for at least 2 hours post-infusion (especially after the first and second dose), because infusion reactions are most likely to occur during this time
- if infusion reaction occurs, infusion should be slowed or stopped until symptoms subside, then started at a lower rate
- paracetamol, antihistamines, corticosteroids, adrenaline (epinephrine) and artificial airway should be readily available for infusion reaction
- premedication with paracetamol, hydrocortisone and/or antihistamine may prevent mild and transient effects of infusion reaction
- in adult patients who have tolerated three 2-hour infusions and are receiving maintenance therapy, consideration may be given to decreasing infusion time (no less than 1 hour). If infusion reaction occurs, subsequent infusions should be at a slower rate
- readministration after a 16-week drug-free interval is not recommended because of increased risk of hypersensitivity reaction
- (refractory fistulating Crohn's disease, ulcerative colitis) if no response after initial 3 doses, therapy should be stopped
- (Crohn's disease – maintenance) dose can be increased to 10 mg/kg if response is inadequate
- (rheumatoid arthritis) clinical response is usually seen within 12 weeks. Dose may be increased if response is inadequate or lost
- contraindicated in those with hypersensitivity to other murine proteins

Patient teaching and advice

- women of childbearing age should be counselled to use adequate contraception during and for 6 months after stopping therapy
- see General Patient teaching and advice for TNF-α antagonists (p. 990)

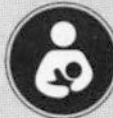

not recommended during pregnancy

not recommended during breastfeeding, which should also be avoided within 6 months of therapy

CYTOKINE MODULATORS

General Adverse effects of cytokine modulators

- headache, dizziness, fatigue, asthenia, paraesthesia, insomnia
- nausea, abdominal pain, diarrhoea, dyspepsia, mouth ulceration, stomatitis
- infection (lower respiratory, urinary tract, upper respiratory), rhinitis, herpes simplex, herpes zoster
- limb pain, back pain, myalgia, arthralgia
- hypertension, chest pain
- development of antibodies
- (uncommon) hypersensitivity, anaphylaxis, reactivation of hepatitis B, non-melanoma skin cancers, malignancies
- (rare) chronic inflammatory, demyelinating polyneuropathy, multiple sclerosis

General Interactions of cytokine modulators

- not recommended with tumour necrosis factor (TNF) inhibitors, rituximab or anakinra
- not recommended with or within 3 months of live or live attenuated vaccine

General Nursing points/Cautions for cytokine modulators

- patient should be screened for any signs of infection before starting therapy. This should include screening for hepatitis B and tuberculosis (clinical history, chest X-ray, skin tuberculin test). If latent tuberculosis is diagnosed, it should be treated with appropriate antimycobacterial agents before starting therapy
- patients with previous tuberculosis should be closely monitored for any reactivation
- regular skin examinations are recommended
- if changing from TNF blocking agent, patient should be closely monitored for any sign of infection
- vaccinations should be up to date before starting therapy
- needle covers of prefilled syringes contain latex and should not be handled by or administered to anyone with a latex sensitivity
- caution if used in those $\geq$ 65 years, as they are at greater risk of infections and malignancy
- caution if used in those with moderate-to-severe kidney impairment
- caution if used in those with previous history or at increased risk of skin cancers
- caution if used in those with chronic obstructive pulmonary disease (COPD) as respiratory symptoms (cough, dyspnoea, rhonchi) may be exacerbated
- not recommended in those with active (including chronic or localised) infection and caution if used in those with chronic or recurrent infection, those who have been exposed to TB, history of serious or opportunistic infection, lived or travelled in areas of endemic TB or endemic mycoses

General Patient teaching and advice for cytokine modulators

- patient should be counselled to immediately seek medical advice if they develop:
  - persistent cough, coughing up blood, unexplained weight loss, loss of energy or low-grade fever (signs of TB)
  - any new skin spots, including spots that have changed, become larger, bleed or don't heal
  - stomach ache or pain that does not go away, change in bowel habits
  - symptoms of infection such as fever, sweating or chills, muscle aches
  - tiredness, headache, shortness of breath when exercising, looking pale
- if patient has pre-existing COPD, he/she should be advised to immediately report to doctor any worsening symptoms, trouble breathing, cough or development of pneumonia
- advise patient to have regular screening for any skin cancers, avoid sunburn and wear sunscreen (SPF 30+), long-sleeved clothing and a hat when outdoors
- warn patient not to drive or operate machinery if dizziness, fatigue or insomnia occur
- women of childbearing age should be advised to use adequate contraception during therapy
- see General Patient teaching and advice (p. xxvii)

ABATACEPT (Orencia)

Available forms

Vial: 250 mg; Prefilled syringe: 125 mg/mL; Autoinjector: 125 mg/mL

Action

- modulates key co-stimulatory signal required for full activation of T-lymphocytes which are found in the synovium of those with rheumatoid arthritis
- (RA) half-life about 14 days (IV, SC)

Use

- moderate-to-severe rheumatoid arthritis (with methotrexate) (intolerant or unresponsive to other DMARDs or never previously treated with methotrexate)
- moderate-to-severe active polyarticular juvenile idiopathic arthritis (unresponsive to other DMARDs) (alone or with methotrexate)
- active psoriatic arthritis (inadequate response to DMARDs) (alone or with non-biologic DMARD)

Dose

- (rheumatoid arthritis, psoriatic arthritis) (patient weight < 60 kg) 500 mg, (60–100 kg) 750 mg or (> 100 kg) 1 g IV over 30 minutes given 2 and 4 weeks after initial infusion, then monthly **OR**
- (rheumatoid arthritis) initially 500 mg, 750 mg or 1 g IV (loading dose) (according to body weight, as above) then 125 mg SC within 24 hours of loading dose, then weekly **OR**
- (rheumatoid arthritis, psoriatic arthritis) 125 mg SC weekly **OR**
- (polyarticular juvenile idiopathic arthritis) (patient weight < 75 kg) 10 mg/kg IV over 30 minutes given 2 and 4 weeks after initial infusion, then monthly (if patient weight is > 75 kg, regimen for rheumatoid arthritis is followed (maximum 1 g))

Adverse effects

- (IV infusion-related reaction – within 1 hour) dizziness, hypotension, nausea, headache, flushing
- (IV peri-infusion reaction – up to 24 hours of infusion) dizziness, nausea, vomiting, flushing, rash

- (SC) local injection site reaction including redness, pruritus, haematoma
- cough
- rash, alopecia
- elevated liver enzymes
- increased BP
- (uncommon) leucopenia, thrombocytopenia
- see also General Adverse effects of cytokine modulators (p. 998)

Interactions

- see General Interactions of cytokine modulators (p. 998)
- may cause a falsely elevated blood glucose reading on the day of IV infusion (not SC injection) (if test strips contain glucose dehydrogenase pyrroloquinoline-quinone as this reacts with maltose in the solution)

Nursing points/Cautions

- see General Nursing points/Cautions for cytokine modulators (p. 998)
- if switching from IV to SC therapy, first SC dose should be given when monthly IV dose is due
- patients should be monitored during and after infusion for any signs of infusion-related events
- patient may be taught to self-administer medication SC. They should be educated about rotation of sites, injection technique, storage requirements and safe disposal of used needles. First self-administration should be done under supervision
- rotate injection sites (thigh or abdomen) avoiding skin that is reddened, bruised, tender or hard or within 3 cm of previous injection sites
- (polyarticular juvenile idiopathic arthritis) vaccinations should be up to date before starting therapy
- IV dosage dependent on body weight
- (IV) reconstitute by gently injecting 10 mL water for injections into vial, swirl gently, avoiding vigorous agitation or shaking to prevent foaming. After reconstitution, vial should be vented with a needle to dispel any foam formed. Reconstituted solution should be clear and colourless to pale yellow. This should be added to a 100 mL bag of 0.9% sodium chloride, first removing the equivalent amount of sodium chloride (e.g. if 4 vials have been reconstituted totalling 40 mL, then 40 mL of sodium chloride should be removed before adding the reconstituted solution). Bag should be gently inverted, not shaken
- (IV) administer alone
- (IV) contains 8.6 mg sodium per vial, which may need to be considered for those on a sodium-controlled diet

Patient teaching and advice

- see General Patient teaching and advice for cytokine modulators (p. 999)
- warn patient that hair loss may occur
- for SC self-administration instructions, see General Patient teaching and advice for TNF-α antagonists (p. 990)
- if newborn has been exposed to abatacept during pregnancy, live vaccines should not be administered for at least 5 months after last administration

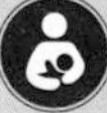

not recommended during pregnancy or breastfeeding

ANAKINRA (RBE) (Kineret)

Available form

Prefilled syringe: 100 mg/0.67 mL

Action

- recombinant, non-glycosylated human interleukin-1 receptor antagonist

(interleukin-1 is thought to play a part in both inflammatory and immunological responses, including the degradation of cartilage and stimulation of bone resorption)
- half-life 4–6 hours

Use
- active rheumatoid arthritis (with methotrexate) (unresponsive to other DMARDs)

Dose
- 100 mg daily SC (same time every day)

Adverse effects
- see General Adverse effects of cytokine modulators (p. 998)
- mild injection site reaction (erythema, ecchymosis, inflammation, pain)
- elevated total cholesterol levels
- depression
- rash, pruritus
- (uncommon) transient elevation of liver enzymes
- (rare) neutropenia, thrombocytopenia, bone fractures

Interactions
- see General Interactions of cytokine modulators (p. 998)
- caution if given with agents that have narrow therapeutic index (e.g. warfarin). Serum levels should be closely monitored, especially when starting or stopping therapy

Nursing points/Cautions
- see General Nursing points/Cautions for cytokine modulators (p. 998)
- baseline blood counts (WBC, platelets, absolute neutrophil count) should be measured before starting, monthly for 6 months and then every 4 months throughout therapy
- patient may be taught to self-administer medication SC. They should be educated about rotation of sites, injection technique, storage requirements and safe disposal of used needles. First self-administration should be done under supervision
- not recommended in those with severe renal impairment
- contraindicated in those with known hypersensitivity to *E. coli*-derived products or if patient is neutropenic (ANC $< 1.5 \times 10^9$/L)

Patient teaching and advice
- see General Patient teaching and advice for cytokine modulators (p. 999)
- for SC self-administration instructions, see General Patient teaching and advice for TNF-α antagonists (p. 990)
- if patient is experiencing discomfort at the administration site, advice can include rotation of sites, cooling site after administration with cold cloth, ensuring solution is at room temperature before administration and, if prescribed, use of topical corticosteroids or antihistamines

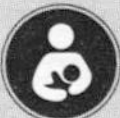

should only be used during pregnancy if benefits outweigh potential risks

caution if used during breastfeeding

RITUXIMAB (Mabthera, Mabthera SC, Riximyo, Truxima)

Available forms

Vial: 100 mg/10 mL, 1400 mg/11.7 mL

Action
- murine/human anti CD 20 monoclonal antibody that depletes B lymphocytes
- action in rheumatoid arthritis may be due to suppression of inflammation by

reducing B lymphocyte-induced T cell activation and cytokine production

Use

- relapsed or refractory CD 20 positive diffuse large B-cell non-Hodgkin lymphoma, chronic lymphocytic leukaemia, severe granulomatosis with polyangiitis (Wegener's), microscopic polyangiitis
- severe rheumatoid arthritis (unresponsive or intolerant to TNF-α antagonists) (with methotrexate)

Dose

- (rheumatoid arthritis) 1 g by IV infusion, then 1 g by IV infusion 2 weeks later (with methotrexate) (see General Nursing points/Cautions p. 998 regarding rate of administration)

Adverse effects

- see General Adverse effects of cytokine modulators (p. 998)
- acute infusion reactions (hypo/hypertension, nausea, rash, pruritus, urticaria, chills, fever, rhinitis, throat irritation, flushing)
- hypercholesterolemia
- transient hypophosphataemia, hyperuricaemia
- transient neutropenia
- (rare) progressive multifocal leukoencephalopathy (PML), severe bronchospasm, hypoxia, dyspnoea, acute respiratory failure

Interactions

- see General Interactions of cytokine modulators (p. 998)

Nursing points/Cautions

- see General Nursing points/Cautions for cytokine modulators (p. 998)
- premedication with paracetamol/salicylate/NSAID, antihistamine and glucocorticoid (e.g. methylprednisolone 100 mg IV) is recommended 30–60 minutes before infusion to reduce severity and frequency of infusion-related reaction
- patient should be monitored during and at least 2 hours after first infusion for any signs of cytokine release syndrome (dyspnoea, bronchospasm, hypoxia, chills, fever, rigors, urticaria and angioedema).
- if severe cytokine release syndrome occurs, infusion should be stopped
- ensure emergency treatment for anaphylaxis (adrenaline (epinephrine), antihistamine, corticosteroid) is readily available
- for first infusion, rate should be started at 50 mg/hour and patient carefully monitored. If no hypersensitivity or infusion-related event occurs, rate may be increased by 50 mg/hour at 30-minute intervals to maximum of 400 mg/hour. If hypersensitivity reaction occurs, infusion rate should be halved. If no hypersensitivity occurs, subsequent infusions can be started at 100 mg/mL and increased at 100 mg increments at 30-minute intervals to 400 mg/hr maximum
- if no serious infusion reaction has occurred, a more rapid infusion may be given for second and subsequent infusions using 4 mg/mL in 250 mL volume. Rate can be started at 250 mg/hr for first 30 minutes, then 600 mg/hr for next 90 minutes. Infusion will be completed in 2 hours using this rate
- (RA) response is usually seen in about 16 weeks
- (RA) further courses may be given. Repeat courses should not be given at intervals less than 16 weeks
- antibody development has been associated with worsening infusion or allergic reactions after second infusion

- any concurrent antihypertensive agent may need to be withheld for 12 hours before and during infusion because of added risk of severe hypotension occurring
- reconstitute with 4 mL water for injections, then dilute further with 50–250 mL sodium chloride 0.9% or glucose 5% and gently invert to mix, but prevent foaming
- administer alone
- not given as SC, IV push or bolus
- patient should be carefully monitored for any signs or symptoms that might suggest progressive multifocal leukoencephalopathy (PML) (e.g. cognitive, neurological or psychiatric symptoms). If signs occur, therapy should be stopped and further evaluation including MRI, CSF testing and repeat neurological assessments completed
- contains sodium chloride (100 mg vial = 52.6 mg sodium; 500 mg vial = 263.2 mg sodium) which may need to be considered if patient is on sodium-reduced intake
- patient with cardiovascular disease (including arrhythmias) or previous serious reaction to other biologic therapy or rituximab, should not be given rapid (2-hour) IV infusion and closely monitored during infusion
- not recommended in patients with severely immunocompromised (CD4 or CD8 are very low)
- contraindicated in those with murine protein hypersensitivity

Patient teaching and advice

- see General Patient teaching and advice for cytokine modulators (p. 999)
- warn patient that reactions (e.g. fever, chills, shivering) may occur after infusion (especially within the first 2 hours of the first infusion) and are transient. They occur less frequently after first infusion
- patient/carer/family members should be advised to seek medical advice immediately if any confusion, disorientation, memory loss, changes in moving, talking and/or walking, decreased strength, increased weakness or blurred or loss of vision occurs
- women of childbearing potential should be counselled to use adequate contraception during and for 12 months after stopping therapy

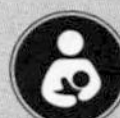

not recommended during pregnancy or breastfeeding unless benefits outweigh risks

Note

- Mabthera SC and Riximyo are used as an antineoplastic agent (see p. 691), not as a DMARD

TOCILIZUMAB (Actemra)

Available forms

Vial: 80 mg/4 mL, 200 mg/10 mL, 400 mg/20 mL; Prefilled syringe: 162 mg/0.9 mL; Prefilled pen: 162 mg/0.9 mL

Action

- recombinant humanised monoclonal antibody of IgG1 that bind to interleukin 6 receptors which are thought to be involved in pathogenesis of inflammatory disease including rheumatoid arthritis and juvenile idiopathic arthritis
- produced by recombinant DNA technology using mammalian Chinese hamster ovary cell culture
- (IV) long half-life (11–13 days) and even longer in younger patients with juvenile arthritis (up to 23 days)

Use

- moderate-to-severe rheumatoid arthritis (RA) (either alone or in combination with methotrexate or other non-biologic DMARDs)

- active systemic juvenile idiopathic arthritis (sJIA) (> 2 years) (alone or with methotrexate)
- moderate-to-severe polyarticular juvenile idiopathic arthritis (pJIA) (> 2 years) (alone or with methotrexate)
- giant cell arteritis (GCA)
- cytokine release syndrome (CRS)

Dose

- (RA) 8 mg/kg by IV infusion over 1 hour every 4 weeks (maximum 800 mg) (alone or with methotrexate and/or other non-biologic DMARD) **OR**
- (RA) 162 mg SC weekly (alone or with methotrexate and/or non-biologic DMARD) **OR**
- (sJIA < 30 kg) 12 mg/kg by IV infusion over 1 hour every 2 weeks (alone or with methotrexate) **OR**
- (sJIA ≥ 30 kg) 8 mg/kg by IV infusion over 1 hour every 2 weeks (alone or with methotrexate) **OR**
- (pJIA < 30 kg) 10 mg/kg by IV infusion over 1 hour monthly (alone or with methotrexate) **OR**
- (pJIA ≥ 30 kg) 8 mg/kg by IV infusion over 1 hour monthly (alone or with methotrexate) **OR**
- (pJIA < 30 kg) 162 mg SC every 3 weeks (alone or with methotrexate) **OR**
- (pJIA ≥ 30 kg) 162 mg SC every 2 weeks (alone or with methotrexate) **OR**
- (GCA) 162 mg SC weekly or every 2 weeks (with tapering corticosteroids or alone after corticosteroids have been discontinued) **OR**
- (CRS) 8 mg/kg (if patient weight ≥ 30 kg) or 12 mg/kg (if patient weight < 30 kg) by IV infusion over 1 hour (alone or with corticosteroids) (800 mg maximum per infusion)

Adverse effects

- see General Adverse effects of cytokine modulators (p. 998)
- IV infusion reaction (hypo/hypertension, nausea, headache, dizziness, rash, urticaria)
- SC site reaction (erythema, pruritus, pain, haematoma)
- cough, dyspnoea
- weight increase
- rash, pruritus, urticaria
- leucopenia, neutropenia
- hypercholesterolaemia, hypertriglyceridaemia
- hypofibrinogenemia
- (sJIA) (rare) macrophage activation syndrome
- (CRS) elevated liver enzymes, cytopenias
- (rare) GI perforation, hepatotoxicity

Interactions

- see General Interactions of cytokine modulators (p. 998)
- may decrease serum levels of simvastatin
- caution if given with atorvastatin, calcium-channel blockers, theophylline, warfarin, phenytoin, ciclosporin or benzodiazepines, especially when starting or stopping therapy as serum levels may be altered
- caution if used with other hepatotoxic agents

Nursing points/Cautions

- see General Nursing points/Cautions for cytokine modulators (p. 998)
- ensure correct formulation is selected for administration as IV and SC formulations are not interchangeable
- if absolute neutrophil count (ANC) $< 0.5 \times 10^9$/L, therapy should not be started

- IV dose adjusted according to liver enzymes, ANC and platelet count
- patient should be monitored during and for 30 minutes post-infusion for any signs of infusion reaction, which can occur up to 24 hours after completion
- serum lipids (LDL, HDL, total cholesterol) should be measured 4–8 weeks after starting therapy, then regularly or (pIA) 12-weekly
- ensure emergency treatment (adrenaline (epinephrine), antihistamine, corticosteroid) and resuscitation equipment are readily available
- (RA) increased risk of cardiovascular disorders and therefore should be thoroughly assessed for any risk factors (e.g. hypertension, hyperlipidaemia) before starting therapy. Serum lipids should be monitored 4–8-weekly during first 6 months of therapy
- (RA, GCA) liver enzymes (ALT, AST), neutrophil and platelet count should be measured 4–8-weekly during first 6 months of therapy, then 12-weekly or (sJIA, pJIA) at time of second infusion, then 4–8-weekly (pJIA) or (sJIA) 2–4-weekly
- it is recommended that all patients (and especially those with sJIAv) are up to date with vaccinations; these should be completed before starting therapy
- (GCA) if condition relapses, corticosteroid therapy may be restarted or dose increased according to clinical need
- (CRS) if no improvement after first dose, up to 3 further doses may be given at intervals not less than 8-hourly
- (RA, sJIA, pJIA ≥ 30 kg) dilute to a total volume of 100 mL with sodium chloride 0.9% and administer over 1 hour or (sJIA, pJIA < 30 kg) to a total volume of 50 mL. Equivalent amount of sodium chloride should be removed from infusion bag first before adding tocilizumab
- instruct patient on SC administration technique. First SC injection should be under medical supervision
- contains 26.55 mg (1.17 mmol) of sodium per maximum dose of 1200 mg, which may need to be taken into consideration if patient is on sodium-restricted diet
- caution if used in those with history of diverticulitis or intestinal ulceration due to risk of GI perforation
- caution if used in those with liver impairment or active liver disease
- caution if used in those with low neutrophil (ANC $< 2 \times 10^9$/L) or platelet count ($< 100 \times 10^9$/L)
- contraindicated in those with hypersensitivity to other recombinant human or humanised antibodies or Chinese hamster ovary cell products or if active severe infection is present

Patient teaching and advice

- warn patient/carer that infusion-related reaction (headache, rash, hives, diarrhoea, arthralgia, stomach pains) may occur up to 24 hours after infusion
- for SC self-administration instructions for prefilled syringe, see General Patient teaching and advice for TNF-α antagonists (p. 990), with the following difference:
  - allow syringe to stand at room temperature for 25–30 minutes and injection should be completed within 5 minutes
- for SC self-administration instruction for prefilled pen, instructions are similar to those for adalimumab

(see Patient teaching and advice for adalimumab, p. 992) (read those instructions first) with the following differences:

- allow pen to come to room temperature for at least 45 minutes (not in direct sunlight, nor using any other means such as microwave or water bath)
- hold pen with green cap pointing down and view solution through window on side (should be clear and colourless to pale yellow)
- remove green cap and discard
- pinch skin to make fold, hold needle guard against skin at 90 degrees
- unlock green activation button by pressing pen firmly against skin until needle shield is pushed in
- press green activation button until a click is heard. Continue pressing green button until purple indicator in window has stopped moving (second click may be heard) – the injection may take up to 10 seconds. When purple indicator has stopped, remove pen from skin (at 90 degrees). Needle shield should move into place and cover the needle
- do not rub injection site. If there is any blood, press gauze or cotton ball on the site to stop the bleeding. A small dressing such as a Band-Aid can be used if needed
- injection should be completed within 3 minutes of removing green cap

- see General Patient teaching and advice for cytokine modulators (p. 999)

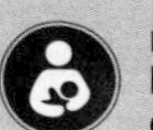
not recommended during pregnancy and breastfeeding unless benefits clearly outweigh risks

TOFACITINIB (Xeljanz)

Available form
Tablets: 5 mg

Action
- Janus kinase (JAK1-3) inhibitor (these cytokines are thought to have a role in immune function modulation)
- peak activity in 0.5–1 hour, rapid half-life about 3 hours

Use
- treatment of moderate-to-severe active rheumatoid arthritis (RA) (with or without non-biological DMARDs) in patients who have intolerance or inadequate response to methotrexate
- active psoriatic arthritis (PA) (with conventional DMARDs) in patients who have had inadequate response to DMARDs
- moderate-to-severe ulcerative colitis (UC) in patients where response has been lost or who are intolerant to other therapies

Dose
- (RA, PA) 5 mg orally twice daily **OR**
- (UC) initially 10 mg orally twice daily for 8 weeks (induction), then 5 mg orally twice daily (maintenance)

Adverse effects
- see General Adverse effects of cytokine modulators (p. 998)
- anaemia, neutropenia, lymphocytosis,
- hypercholesterolaemia, hyperlipidaemia
- altered liver enzymes
- increased heart rate
- fever
- cough
- peripheral oedema
- acne
- (uncommon) prolongation of PR interval

- (rare) interstitial lung disease, gastrointestinal perforation

Interactions
- see General Interactions of cytokine modulators (p. 998)
- not recommended with other agents that decrease heart rate or prolong PR interval such as antiarrhythmics, beta-adrenoceptor blocking agents, alpha-2 agonists, cholinesterase inhibitors, some calcium-channel blockers, some HIV protease inhibitors and digoxin
- serum levels may be increased by fluconazole
- serum levels may be decreased by rifampicin
- contraindicated with ciclosporin
- not recommended with tacrolimus

Nursing points/Cautions
- see General Nursing points/Cautions for cytokine modulators (p. 998)
- before starting, a full blood count (including differential white cell count), platelet count and liver function tests are recommended, then monitoring:
  - lymphocytes, neutrophils and haemoglobin after 4–8 weeks, then 3-monthly
  - lipids after 4–8 weeks
  - liver function routinely
- therapy should not be started if ALC $< 0.75 \times 10^9$/L, ANC $< 1 \times 10^9$/L or Hb $<$ 90g/L
- (UC) if adequate clinical response is not achieved by week 8, induction dose (10 mg twice daily) can be used for an extra 8 weeks (16 weeks total). If there is no clinical response after this time, therapy should be stopped. If clinical benefit is not maintained on 5 mg twice daily maintenance dose, this can be increased to 10 mg twice daily
- caution if used in those with low heart rate ($<$ 60 beats/minute), history of arrhythmias or syncope, sick sinus syndrome, SA or AV block, ischaemic heart disease or congestive cardiac failure
- caution if used in those with or at risk of interstitial lung disease, especially Asian patients who are at greater risk of interstitial lung disease, herpes zoster, elevated liver enzymes, opportunistic infections and decreased white blood counts
- caution if used in those at risk of gastrointestinal perforation (e.g. history of diverticulitis)
- caution if used in those with kidney impairment. Dose adjustment is required if GFR $\leq$ 50 mL/min
- contraindicated in those with severe liver impairment

Patient teaching and advice
- see General Patient teaching and advice for cytokine modulators (p. 999)
- if patient is Asian, warn of increased risk of infection and lung problems
- advise patient to seek medical advice if any of the following occur:
  - change in heart rate
  - stomach pain/ache that does not go away, change in bowel habits
  - dry persistent cough, shortness of breath, fatigue
- women of childbearing potential should be counselled to use adequate contraception during therapy

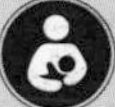

should not be used during pregnancy or by women attempting to become pregnant

not recommended during breastfeeding

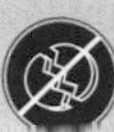
tablet should not be crushed or broken

UPADACITINIB (Rinvoq)

Available form
Tablets: 15 mg

Action
- Janus kinase (JAK1-3) inhibitor (these cytokines are thought to have a role in immune function modulation)
- half-life 9–14 hours

Use
- treatment of moderate-to-severe rheumatoid arthritis (RA) in patients who are intolerant to or have had inadequate response to one or more DMARDs

Dose
- 15 mg orally daily (as monotherapy or with methotrexate or other conventional DMARDs)

Adverse effects
- serious infections (e.g. pneumonia, cellulitis, bacterial meningitis), reactivation of tuberculosis and herpes zoster, oral/oesophageal candidiasis, cryptococcosis, pneumocytosis, bronchitis, nasopharyngitis, sinusitis, urinary tract infection
- neutropenia, lymphopaemia, anaemia
- elevated lipids (total cholesterol, low-density lipoprotein (LDL) cholesterol, high-density lipoprotein (HDL) cholesterol
- increased liver enzymes, elevated creatine phosphokinase (CPK)
- headache, dizziness
- hypertension
- cough
- fever
- diarrhoea, nausea, vomiting
- (rare) thrombosis (deep vein thrombosis, pulmonary embolism, arterial thrombosis), non-melanoma skin cancer, increased risk of malignancy

Interactions
- contraindicated with biologic DMARDs
- not recommended with other JAK inhibitors or potent immunosuppressants (e.g. azathioprine, ciclosporin, tacrolimus) because of the added immunosuppression
- caution if used with itraconazole, posaconazole, voriconazole and clarithromycin
- therapeutic effect may be decreased if given with rifampicin and phenytoin

Nursing points/Cautions
- patient should be screened for any signs of infection before starting therapy. This should include screening for hepatitis B and tuberculosis (clinical history, chest X-ray, skin tuberculin test). If latent tuberculosis is diagnosed, it should be treated with appropriate antimycobacterial agents before starting therapy
- before starting therapy neutrophil, lymphocyte and haemoglobin levels should be monitored and not started if absolute lymphocyte count (ALC) < 500 cells/mm^3, absolute neutrophil count (ANC) < 1000 cells/mm^3 or haemoglobin < 8 g/dL. Therapy should be interrupted if neutrophil, lymphocyte and haemoglobin levels fall below these levels and restarted once they return to normal
- lipids and liver enzymes should be monitored before starting and regularly throughout therapy
- patients with previous tuberculosis should be closely monitored for any reactivation
- therapy should be interrupted if patient develops a serious or opportunistic infection and restarted once the infection has been treated and controlled

- regular skin examinations are recommended
- vaccinations should be up to date before starting therapy
- caution if used in those with severe kidney impairment
- not recommended in those with severe liver impairment
- not recommended in those with active (including chronic or localised) infection and caution if used in those with chronic or recurrent infection, those who have been exposed to TB, history of serious or opportunistic infection, lived or travelled in areas of endemic TB or endemic mycoses

Patient teaching and advice

- patient should be counselled to immediately seek medical advice if they develop:
  - persistent cough, coughing up blood, unexplained weight loss, loss of energy or low-grade fever (signs of TB)
  - any new skin spots, including spots that have changed, become larger, bleed or don't heal
  - symptoms of infection such as fever, sweating or chills, muscle aches
  - tiredness, headache, shortness of breath when exercising, looking pale
  - swelling, pain, redness, warmth in the calf area
  - shortness of breath, rapid breathing, sudden sharp chest pain made worse on coughing or deep breathing, rapid heart rate, coughing up pink frothy sputum, sweating
  - cold pulseless limb, muscle pain or spasm in affected area, numbness or tingling in area
- advise patient to have regular screening for any skin cancers, avoid sunburn and wear sunscreen (SPF 30+), long-sleeved clothing and a hat when outdoors
- warn patient not to drive or operate machinery if dizziness occurs
- women of childbearing age should be advised to use adequate contraception during therapy
- see General Patient teaching and advice (p. xxvii)

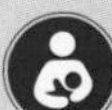

not recommended during pregnancy or breastfeeding

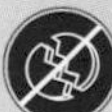

modified-release tablets should not be crushed, broken, divided or chewed

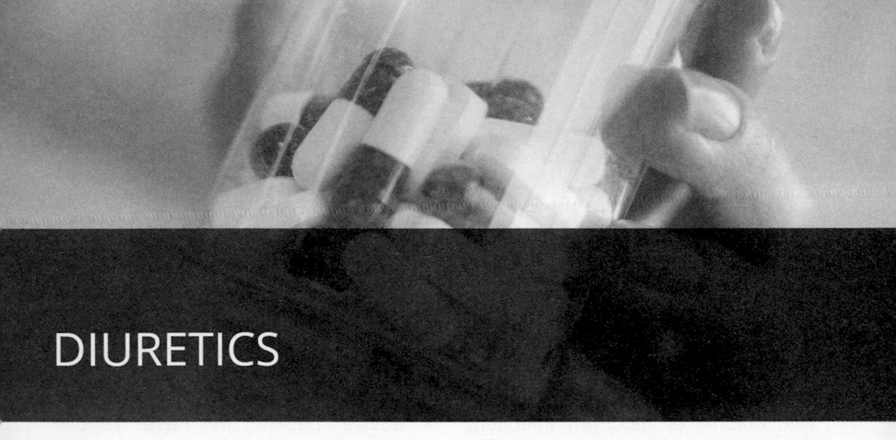

DIURETICS

Diuretics increase the rate of urine formation by reducing the reabsorption of sodium, chloride and water by the renal tubules, either by interfering with active transport mechanisms or by altering tubular permeability. Uses for diuretics include treatment of hypertension, oedema (e.g. acute and chronic congestive cardiac failure), chronic renal failure, nephrotic syndrome and cirrhosis (Bryant et al 2019).

Classes of diuretics include:

- *carbonic anhydrase inhibitors* block the enzyme carbonic anhydrase (which normally promotes reabsorption of bicarbonate in the proximal tubule), thereby increasing the excretion of bicarbonate, sodium and water; however, carbonic anhydrase inhibitors are weak diuretic agents and today are rarely used alone for the diuretic action
- *loop diuretics* limit the amount of sodium reabsorbed in the peritubular capillaries surrounding the loop of Henle, with reabsorption of calcium and magnesium also blocked
- *thiazide diuretics* interfere with sodium chloride reabsorption in the distal tubules, leading to increased excretion of sodium, chloride and water
- *potassium-sparing diuretics* are aldosterone antagonists that reduce sodium reabsorption and potassium excretion at the end of the distal tubule and at the collecting duct
- *osmotic diuretics* affect the proximal tubule and descending loop of Henle, and the strong osmotic pressure in the nephron prevents water reabsorption into the peritubular capillaries increasing urine volume.

General Nursing points/Cautions for diuretics

- excessive dose or diuresis may result in electrolyte imbalance
- monitor fluid intake and output and patient's weight
- observe patient for dehydration, especially in hot weather
- note increase or reduction in oedema
- check supine and standing BP regularly for postural hypotension
- observe for features of electrolyte imbalance (e.g. anorexia, nausea, vomiting, dry mouth, thirst, excessive diuresis, oliguria, weakness, lethargy,

drowsiness, restlessness, muscle pain/cramp/fatigue, hypotension, tachycardia and arrhythmias)
- observe for features of hyponatraemia (lethargy, weakness, anorexia, nausea, slowing of cerebration)
- observe for features of hypokalaemia (drowsiness, muscle weakness and cramps, paraesthesia, cardiac arrhythmias or corresponding ECG changes), especially in patients also on digitalis therapy, because this may cause digitalis toxicity
- if hypovolaemia or dehydration occurs, diuretic should be stopped and any fluid, electrolyte and/or acid–base balance corrected
- caution if used in those with diabetes mellitus as glucose tolerance may become impaired

General Patient teaching and advice for diuretics

- advise patient of expected diuresis and take medication early in the day to avoid getting up at night to urinate (nocturia). If taken twice daily, the second dose should be at approximately midday (and definitely before 6 pm)
- instruct patient to take with or following meals to minimise nausea or other gastrointestinal side-effects
- ensure patient understands importance of drinking sufficiently (especially after exercise or being in hot water) to prevent dehydration occurring. However, patient should understand any fluid restriction that may be present
- warn patient to sit or lie down if faintness occurs (postural hypotension). This can be avoided by moving gradually to a sitting or standing position, especially after sleep, and can be aggravated by prolonged standing, hot baths or showers, hot weather, physical exertion, large meals and drinking alcohol
- patient should be advised to avoid driving or handling heavy machinery if dizziness, drowsiness, lethargy, faintness or confusion occur
- if patient is taking high doses of non-potassium-sparing diuretics for prolonged periods, encourage high-potassium foods (such as apricots, avocados, bananas, rockmelon, dates, grapefruit, oranges, potatoes, prunes, raisins, spinach, strawberries, watermelon and orange, grapefruit, prune and pineapple juice)
- advise patient to seek medical advice immediately if any of the following occur:
  - weak and rapid pulse, clammy skin, rapid breathing, dry mouth, nose and other mucous membranes, reduced urinary output (hypovolaemia)
  - nausea, vomiting, headache, confusion, loss of energy, fatigue, restlessness, irritability, muscle weakness, spasm or cramps, seizures (fitting), coma (hyponatraemia)
  - weakness, cramps or spasms, heart palpitations (hypokalaemia)
  - numbness and/or tingling of hands/feet or lips, muscle cramps or spasms, seizures (fitting), facial twitching, muscle weakness, light-headedness, slow heart rate (hypocalcaemia)
- see also General Patient teaching and advice (p. xxvii)

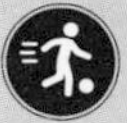

diuretics are banned in sport

CARBONIC ANHYDRASE INHIBITORS

ACETAZOLAMIDE (Diamox, Glaumox Powder for Injection)

Available forms
Tablets: 250 mg; Vial: 500 mg

Action
- non-bacterial sulfonamide derivative that inhibits the action of carbonic anhydrase
- inhibits secretion of aqueous humour, reducing intraocular pressure
- thought to retard abnormal, paroxysmal excessive discharge from CNS neurons
- increases bicarbonate excretion in the renal tubules and consequently sodium, potassium and water excretion, resulting in an alkaline diuresis

Use
- adjunctive treatment in chronic simple (open-angle) glaucoma, secondary glaucoma and preoperatively in acute closed-angle glaucoma (see Antiglaucoma agents, p. 455)
- some types of epilepsy (see Antiepileptics, p. 385)
- cardiac- and drug-induced oedema (adjunct)

Dose
- (cardiac failure induced oedema) initially 250–375 mg (5 mg/kg) orally or IV each morning. If response is not sustained, then therapy should be continued on alternate days or for 2 days, followed by a rest day if there is not a continued weight loss **OR**
- (drug-induced oedema) 250–375 mg orally or IV for 1–2 days, alternating with a rest day

Adverse effects
- paraesthesia with tingling feeling in extremities and face
- fatigue, headache, dizziness, flushing, drowsiness, malaise
- anorexia, nausea, vomiting, diarrhoea
- polyuria, polydipsia, thirst
- fever
- depression, excitement, confusion, ataxia
- abnormal liver function
- crystalluria, renal colic, renal calculi
- transient myopia
- (uncommon) convulsions
- (rare) allergic skin reactions, photosensitivity, tinnitus, hearing disturbances
- (rare, but occasionally fatal) blood dyscrasias, anaphylaxis, anaphylactoid reaction
- (prolonged therapy) electrolyte imbalance (hypokalaemia, metabolic acidosis, hyponatraemia, osteomalacia, hypoglycaemia, hyperglycaemia)
- (injection site) pain

Interactions
- may potentiate effects of oral anticoagulants and folic acid antagonists
- increased risk of osteomalacia if given with chronic phenytoin therapy
- risk of cardiac glycoside toxicity may be increased by acetazolamide-induced hypokalaemia
- use with salicylates may result in severe metabolic acidosis
- may decrease serum levels of lithium or primidone
- increased risk of renal calculi if given with sodium bicarbonate
- may prevent urinary antiseptic effect of methenamine hippurate
- not recommended with other carbonic anhydrase inhibitors
- may increase effects and duration of amphetamines by decreasing excretion
- may increase or decrease blood glucose levels, therefore treatment with hypoglycaemic agents may be affected

- may increase serum levels of ciclosporin or phenytoin, increasing risk of adverse effects and toxicity
- caution if used with antihypertensive agents
- increased risk of anorexia, tachypnoea, lethargy and coma if given with high-dose aspirin
- may interfere with HPLC assay method for theophylline
- may give false negative or decreased result for urinary protein, serum non-protein and serum uric acid

Nursing points/Cautions

- FBC, platelet count and serum electrolytes should be monitored before starting and regularly throughout therapy
- effectiveness as a diuretic diminishes with continuous use
- hypokalaemic acidosis corrected by administering bicarbonate and/or potassium
- increasing dose does not increase diuresis (or may decrease diuresis), and may increase risk of dizziness, drowsiness and/or paraesthesia
- therapy should be stopped if any skin reactions occur
- IV route is only recommended when oral route cannot be used
- reconstitute vial using 5 mL water for injections
- caution if used in those with diabetes mellitus or impaired glucose tolerance
- caution if used in those with a predisposition to electrolyte and acid–base imbalance, such as those with renal impairment
- contraindicated in those with pre-existing depression of serum sodium and/or potassium levels, glomerular filtration rate < 10 mL/min, kidney/liver dysfunction, suprarenal gland failure or hyperchloraemic acidosis; long-term administration contraindicated in those with chronic, non-congestive angle-closure glaucoma
- contraindicated in those with hypersensitivity to sulfonamide or related products
- see also General Nursing points/Cautions for diuretics (p. 1010)

Patient teaching and advice

- advise patient against taking high doses of aspirin during therapy
- those with diabetes should be advised to closely monitor blood glucose levels during therapy
- see also General Patient teaching and advice for diuretics (p. 1011)

banned in sport

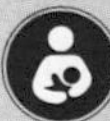
teratogenic in animal studies at high doses, therefore should not be used during pregnancy, especially in the first trimester

use with caution during breastfeeding

tablet can be crushed and mixed with water or spoonful of yoghurt or apple puree

LOOP DIURETICS

General Actions of loop diuretics

- also known as high-ceiling diuretics
- potent diuretics that inhibit sodium, potassium and chloride reabsorption in the proximal and distal renal convoluted tubules, but mainly in the ascending limb of the loop of Henle, resulting in increased water excretion
- some direct vascular effect, which may be due to reduced response to angiotensin II and noradrenaline (both vasoconstrictors)
- rapid onset of action

General Uses of loop diuretics

- oedema associated with heart failure, cirrhosis, nephrotic syndrome and renal impairment
- acute pulmonary oedema (where other diuretics have been ineffective)
- hypertension (alone or with antihypertensive agent)

General Adverse effects of loop diuretics

- electrolyte imbalance (hyperglycaemia, hypokalaemia, hypomagnesaemia, hyponatraemia, metabolic acidosis, increased creatinine and blood urea nitrogen (BUN))
- hypovolaemia, dehydration (thirst, dizziness, headache, dry mouth, visual disturbances)
- urinary retention
- deafness, tinnitus, vertigo, sense of fullness in the ears
- anorexia, nausea, vomiting, dysphagia, abdominal pain/discomfort, diarrhoea
- malaise, fatigue, confusion, apprehension, headache
- hypotension, dizziness, syncope
- muscle cramps, weakness, musculoskeletal pain, arthralgia
- blurred vision
- hyperuricaemia, precipitation of gout
- rash, pruritus, urticaria
- fever, chills
- (rare) blood dyscrasias

General Interactions of loop diuretics

- not recommended with lithium because lithium serum levels and toxicity are increased
- effects of antihypertensive agents may be enhanced
- loop diuretic-induced hypokalaemia may increase risk of toxicity and arrhythmias of digoxin
- increased risk of ototoxicity and nephrotoxicity if given with aminoglycosides
- effects may be inhibited by probenecid
- caution if used with angiotensin receptor antagonists or ACE inhibitors because of increased risk of first dose hypotension (severe)
- effects reduced by NSAIDs and may predispose patient to kidney failure, especially in the presence of preexisting hypovolaemia
- increased risk of nephrotoxicity if given with cisplatin
- increased risk of hypokalaemia if given with potassium-lowering agents (e.g. thiazide diuretics)
- profound diuresis and electrolyte imbalance may occur if given with thiazide diuretics
- may reduce glucose tolerance in patients with diabetes mellitus, necessitating dose adjustment of insulin and/or oral hypoglycaemics

General Nursing points/Cautions for loop diuretics

- any induced electrolyte imbalance should be corrected before therapy starts
- serum electrolytes and blood urea nitrogen (BUN) should be monitored regularly (especially potassium) and potassium supplements (or patient encouraged to eat potassium-rich food) added if needed (especially if patient is on long-term therapy)
- encourage salt in the diet to prevent hyponatraemia and hypochloraemia (if allowed)

- should be discontinued if patient with renal disease develops oliguria or if there is an increase in blood urea nitrogen or creatinine
- if excessive diuresis or electrolyte loss occurs, therapy should be stopped temporarily
- patients with diabetes should be encouraged to monitor blood glucose levels more frequently
- caution if excessive doses or frequent administration occurs as patient could become severely dehydrated and experience electrolyte disturbance (especially the elderly)
- caution if used in those with advanced liver cirrhosis (as sudden electrolyte imbalance can precipitate encephalopathy and coma), severe myocardial disease treated with digoxin (increased risk of arrhythmias associated with hypokalaemia), renal impairment or severely decompensated liver cirrhosis with ascites (with or without encephalopathy)
- caution if given to those with prostatic hypertrophy and impaired micturition (due to risk of urinary retention), gout, predisposition to hypotension, hepatorenal syndrome, hypoproteinaemia, diabetes mellitus or SLE (which may be precipitated or exacerbated)
- contraindicated in those with hypersensitivity to sulfonamides or loop diuretics (as cross-sensitivity may occur) or those with anuria, complete renal shutdown, hepatic coma or pre-coma or conditions causing electrolyte depletion
- contraindicated in those with severe electrolyte imbalance until corrected
- see also General Nursing points/Cautions for diuretics (p. 1010)

General Patient teaching and advice for loop diuretics

- patient should be advised to immediately seek medical advice if any hearing loss or ringing in ears occurs
- instruct patient with diabetes to closely monitor blood glucose levels as impaired glucose tolerance may occur
- see also General Patient teaching and advice for diuretics (p. 1011)

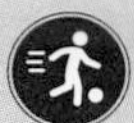

banned in sport

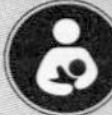

only used during pregnancy and breastfeeding if potential benefits outweigh risks and then at lowest possible dose to achieve desired results. Loop diuretics enter fetal circulation and/or may cause fetal electrolyte disturbances and neonatal thrombocytopenia

BUMETANIDE (Burinex)

Available form
Tablets: 1 mg

Action
- effect on distal tubule is small
- decreases uric acid excretion, thereby increasing uric acid level
- onset of action 30 minutes (oral), peak effect in 1–2 hours, duration approximately 4–6 hours, half-life 60–90 minutes
- diuretic effect: 1 mg bumetanide = 40 mg furosemide (frusemide) (oral)
- diuretic effect is dose related and increasing dose produces diuresis
- see also General Actions of loop diuretics (p. 1013)

Use
- see General Uses of loop diuretics (p. 1014)

Dose

- 1 mg orally daily (morning or early evening) (daily maximum 10 mg) **OR**
- 1 mg orally 4–5-hourly to achieve diuresis in refractory patients (daily maximum 10 mg) **OR**
- 1 mg orally daily (morning or evening) on alternate days (daily maximum 10 mg) **OR**
- 1 mg orally daily for 3–4 days, followed by 1–2 drug-free days (daily maximum 10 mg)

Adverse effects

- see General Adverse effects of loop diuretics (p. 1014)
- dyspnoea, cough
- peripheral oedema
- (high-dose, prolonged therapy) increased creatinine, hyperuricaemia, azotaemia

Interactions

- increased risk of electrolyte imbalance and cardiotoxicity if given with class III antiarrhythmic agents (e.g. amiodarone)
- increased sensitivity to neuromuscular blocking agents may occur if hypokalaemia results
- caution if used with proton pump inhibitors due to increased risk of hypomagnesaemia
- also see General Interactions of loop diuretics (p. 1014)

Nursing points/Cautions

- tablets contain lactose and are not recommended in those with hereditary problems of galactose intolerance, Lapp lactase deficiency or glucose–galactose malabsorption
- contraindicated in those with hypersensitivity to furosemide (frusemide) as cross-sensitivity may exist
- see also General Nursing points/Cautions for diuretics (p. 1010) and loop diuretics (p. 1014)

Patient teaching and advice

- see General Patient teaching and advice for diuretics (p. 1011) and loop diuretics (p. 1015)

tablet can be crushed and mixed with water or spoonful of yoghurt or apple puree

ETACRYNIC (ETHACRYNIC) ACID (Edecrin)

Available form

Tablets: 25 mg

Action

- see General Actions of loop diuretics (p. 1013)
- onset of action 30 minutes, peak effect 2 hours, half-life 0.2–2.6 hours
- (diuretic effect) 50 mg etacrynic acid = 40 mg furosemide (frusemide) (oral)

Use

- see General Uses of loop diuretics (p. 1014)

Dose

- initially 50 mg orally daily after breakfast, increasing by 25–50 mg daily if needed, to 50–150 mg (maintenance) (daily maximum 400 mg)

Adverse effects

- (rare) nausea, vomiting, profuse diarrhoea, gastric bleeding, acute pancreatitis, haematuria
- see also General Adverse effects of loop diuretics (p. 1014)

Interactions

- may enhance effects of warfarin, therefore prothrombin time should be closely monitored
- increased risk of gastric haemorrhage if given with corticosteroids
- also see General Interactions of loop diuretics (p. 1014)

Nursing points/Cautions

- dosage may be given on alternate days or for 2–3 days with 2–3 drug-free days
- effective dose is that which produces gradual weight decrease of 0.5–1 kg
- daily doses of more than 50 mg should be given in 2 divided doses
- see also Nursing points/Cautions for diuretics (p. 1010) and for loop diuretics (p. 1014)

Patient teaching and advice

- advise patient that tablets should not be divided
- instruct patient to stop drug immediately if profuse watery diarrhoea occurs and seek medical advice
- see also Patient teaching/advice for diuretics (p. 1011) and for loop diuretics (p. 1015)

FUROSEMIDE (FRUSEMIDE) (Frusemix, Frusemix-M, Lasix, Lasix High Dose, Uremide, Urex, Urex-M, Urex Forte)

Available forms

Ampoules: 20 mg/2 mL, 40 mg/4 mL, 250 mg/25 mL; Tablets: 20 mg, 40 mg, 500 mg; Oral solution: 10 mg/mL

Action

- sulfonamide
- diuresis onset within 1 hour (oral), peak 1–2 hours, duration 6–8 hours
- diuresis onset within 10–15 minutes (IM), 5 minutes (IV), peak 30 minutes, duration 2 hours (IM, IV)
- biphasic half-life is about 100 minutes (prolonged in those with kidney or liver impairment or in newborns)
- oral bioavailability is about 50% of IV (e.g. 20 mg IV = 40 mg oral)
- oral bioavailability may be reduced in those with severe heart failure or renal impairment
- see also General Actions of loop diuretics (p. 1013)

Use

- see General Uses of loop diuretics (p. 1014)
- treatment of severe hypercalcaemia (with adequate rehydration)
- oliguria or oedema in patients with severely impaired renal function (high-dose formulations)

Dose

- (oedema) initially 20–80 mg orally daily, increasing by 20–40 mg at 6–8-hourly intervals until required diuresis is seen (maximum daily dose 400 mg) **OR**
- (hypertension) initially 40 mg orally twice daily, then add antihypertensive agent if response is unsatisfactory **OR**
- (oedema) 20–40 mg IM or IV slowly; may be repeated in 2 hours if necessary **OR**
- (acute pulmonary oedema) initially 40 mg IV slowly, increasing to 80 mg if there is no response within 1 hour **OR**
- (cerebral oedema) 20–40 mg IV 3 times daily **OR**
- (oedema in patients with severely impaired renal function) 250 mg diluted with 250 mL sodium chloride 0.9%, glucose 5% or lactated Ringer's solution and infused over 60 minutes at a rate not greater than 4 mg/minute. A second infusion of 500 mg diluted as above may be given 1 hour after completion of first infusion if diuresis of 40–50 mL/hour has not occurred (maximum daily dose 1000 mg) (high-dose IV formulation) **OR**
- (oedema in patients with severely impaired renal function) (after no response to conventional therapy) initially 250 mg orally daily, increasing by 250 mg every 4–6 hours until required diuresis of at least 2.5 L/day occurs (maximum daily dose 1000 mg) (high-dose oral formulation)

Adverse effects

- increased serum cholesterol and triglyceride levels
- decreased serum calcium, and rarely, tetany
- (uncommon) impaired glucose tolerance
- transient increase in blood urea, creatinine and uric acid, gout
- (rapid administration) ototoxicity
- (rare) exacerbation/activation of SLE, vasculitis, acute pancreatitis, cholestasis, jaundice
- (very rare, IV) anaphylaxis
- see also General Adverse effects of loop diuretics (p. 1014)

Interactions

- increased risk of hypotension and/or decreased renal function may occur if given with ACE inhibitors. Furosemide (frusemide) should be stopped or dose decreased for 3 days before starting therapy with ACE inhibitors or angiotensin II receptor antagonists
- (IV) not recommended within 24 hours of chloral hydrate as sweating, flushing, nausea, tachycardia and increased BP may occur
- (IV) may increase serum levels of theophylline
- not recommended with etacrynic acid or cisplatin (increased risk of ototoxicity)
- increased risk of nephrotoxicity if given with cisplatin (unless furosemide (frusemide) is given in low doses and fluid balance is positive)
- increased risk of ototoxicity and nephrotoxicity if given with some cephalosporins (especially in high doses)
- (oral) absorption may be decreased by sucralfate
- increases risk of salicylate toxicity if given with high-dose salicylate therapy
- may result in excessive loss of potassium if given with corticosteroids or amphotericin B (amphotericin)
- effect may be antagonised by indometacin, aspirin and other NSAIDs, as well as increased risk of renal failure if hypovolaemia also exists
- may potentiate or antagonise neuromuscular blocking agents, depending on dosage of both agents
- response may be decreased if given with antiepileptic agents
- effects may be reduced if given with phenytoin, methotrexate or probenecid
- may decrease elimination of phenytoin, methotrexate and probenecid, resulting in elevated serum levels
- caution if used with risperidone as toxicity may result (especially in the elderly)
- furosemide (frusemide)-induced hypokalaemia or hypomagnesaemia may increase toxicity to agents that prolong the QT interval
- corticosteroids, laxatives (prolonged use) and liquorice (large amounts) predispose the patient to hypokalaemia and excessive potassium loss may occur if given with furosemide (frusemide)
- increased risk of gouty arthritis if given with ciclosporin
- may reduce effects of epinephrine (adrenaline) and norepinephrine (noradrenaline)
- (high dose) caution if given with levothyroxine. If given together, thyroid hormone levels should be monitored regularly
- may increase deterioration of renal function if given to those with radiocontrast nephropathy
- see also General Interactions of loop diuretics (p. 1014)

Nursing points/Cautions

- any fluid, electrolyte or acid–base imbalance should be corrected before starting therapy with parenteral furosemide (frusemide)

- IM route is generally not recommended unless both oral and parenteral routes are not available
- (250 mg/25 mL) should not be given as IV bolus
- (high-dose formulations, IV or oral) test dose of 40–80 mg IV over 2–5 minutes may be given to test diuretic response before administration
- not mixed with other drugs for injection or infusion
- should not be added to tubing of already running IV infusion
- may precipitate if added to solutions of pH less than 5.5
- add only to sodium chloride 0.9%, glucose 5% or compound sodium lactate for infusion and use within 24 hours (high-dose formulation)
- for hypervolaemic patients, high-dose formulation may be administered undiluted or in a small volume (50 mL) using a volumetric pump to ensure 4 mg/minute limit is not exceeded (to prevent ototoxicity)
- parenteral therapy should be replaced with oral (high-dose) therapy as soon as practicable
- maximum injection and infusion rate 4 mg/minute (or 2.5 mg/minute if renally impaired) to avoid hearing impairment/ototoxicity
- monitor vital signs and fluid balance (input and output) if given parenterally
- oral salt restriction is not recommended
- if starting therapy with ACE inhibitor, furosemide (frusemide) should be stopped or dose decreased for 3 days prior
- recommended to discontinue furosemide (frusemide) 7 days before elective surgery
- (IV) if stored at low temperatures, crystals may form in solution. These can be dissolved by warming solution to 40°C
- (oral solution) available in two formulations, so manufacturer's instructions should be followed regarding correct storage conditions
- (oral solution) contains sorbitol, which may cause diarrhoea
- (oral solution – not requiring refrigeration) contains alcohol (0.5 g/5 mL), which may be harmful in those with alcoholism, children or those with epilepsy or liver disease
- (high-dose formulations) recommended for use in those with greatly reduced glomerular filtration rate (< 20 mL/minute but > 5 mL/minute)
- (high-dose formulation) contraindicated in those with impaired renal function, severe dehydration or electrolyte imbalance, hypotension
- (high-dose formulation) contraindicated in those with normal renal function because of increased risk of severe fluid and electrolyte loss, or hepatitis, cirrhosis, existing or impending hepatic coma or nephrotoxic agent induced renal failure
- see also General Nursing points/Cautions for loop diuretics (p. 1014) and diuretics (p. 1010)

Patient teaching and advice

- advise patient to take tablets or oral solution on empty stomach
- patient should be advised to separate furosemide (frusemide) by at least 2 hours from sucralfate
- see General Patient teaching and advice for loop diuretics (p. 1015) and diuretics (p. 1011)

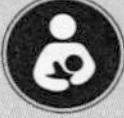

contraindicated during pregnancy and breastfeeding

available as oral solution. Tablet can be dispersed in water or crushed and mixed with water or spoonful of yoghurt or apple puree

THIAZIDE DIURETICS

General Actions of thiazide diuretics

- chemically related to sulfonamides
- increase excretion of sodium and chloride ions and water, principally in the proximal segment (diluting) of the distal tubule
- increase excretion of potassium, magnesium and bicarbonate ions
- reduce calcium excretion
- ineffective if creatinine clearance is less than 30 mL/minute
- will not lower blood pressure in normotensive patients
- some vasodilator activity

General Uses of thiazide diuretics

- oedema, including cirrhosis with ascites
- hypertension (as primary therapy in those with creatinine clearance > 30 mL/min or combined with antihypertensive agents)
- mild-to-moderate stable, chronic heart failure (creatinine clearance > 30 mL/min)

General Adverse effects of thiazide diuretics

- electrolyte disturbances (hyperglycaemia, hypochloraemia, hypokalaemia, hyponatraemia, hypomagnesaemia, impaired glucose tolerance, hyperuricaemia, alkalosis)
- hypovolaemia, dehydration
- dizziness, vertigo, headache, asthenia, fatigue
- blurred vision
- reversible tinnitus and hearing loss (rarely permanent)
- weakness, muscle cramps
- polyuria
- hypotension
- rash, urticaria, photosensitivity
- male impotence
- increased serum total cholesterol, LDL cholesterol and triglyceride levels, decreased HDL cholesterol
- anorexia, mild GI disturbances, dry mouth
- (rare) blood dyscrasias
- (rare) hypersensitivity reactions, attack of gout, hypercalcaemia, glycosuria, activation or exacerbation of systemic lupus erythematosus

General Interactions of thiazide diuretics

- thiazide diuretic-induced hypokalaemia or hypomagnesaemia may increase sensitivity of heart to digoxin, increasing risk of cardiac arrhythmias
- not recommended with lithium because it may increase serum levels and toxicity of lithium
- orthostatic hypotension may be enhanced when given with alcohol, barbiturates, opioid analgesics, sedatives or imipramine-related antidepressants
- may impair glucose tolerance and hypoglycaemic control in those with diabetes, therefore adjustment to insulin and/or oral hypoglycaemic agent may be required
- decreased antihypertensive effect may occur if given with corticosteroids
- increased risk of renal impairment if given with ACE inhibitor and

NSAID (including COX-2 inhibitor and high-dose aspirin)
- may potentiate the hypotensive effect of antihypertensive agents (especially ACE inhibitors)
- absorption may be reduced by colestyramine
  - increased effects may occur if given with anticholinergic agents (due to decreased GI motility and gastric emptying rate)
- increased hyperglycaemic effect if given with diazoxide
- increased risk of adverse effects if given with amantadine
- decreased diuretic and antihypertensive effects may occur if given with indometacin and some other NSAIDs
- increased risk of hypersensitivity reaction if given with allopurinol
- increase in hypokalaemia may occur if given with corticosteroids, ACTH, beta-2 agonists, amphotericin B (amphotericin)
- caution if used with potassium-sparing diuretics due to alterations to serum potassium levels
- may increase serum calcium level if given with vitamin D or calcium salts
- increased risk of hyperuricaemia and gout-like complications if given with ciclosporin
- caution if given with tacrolimus or ciclosporin due to risk of increased plasma creatinine
- not recommended with metformin if plasma creatinine is $>$ 15 mg/L (men) or 12 mg/L (women) due to risk of lactic acidosis
- may interfere with parathyroid function tests, therefore should be discontinued before test

General Nursing points/Cautions for thiazide diuretics

- any induced electrolyte imbalance should be corrected before therapy starts
- serum electrolytes and blood urea nitrogen (BUN) should be monitored regularly (especially potassium) and potassium supplements (or patient encouraged to eat potassium-rich food) added if needed (especially if patient is on long-term therapy)
- should be stopped for 2–3 days before starting antihypertensive therapy with ACE inhibitors or angiotensin II inhibitors
- discontinue before parathyroid function tests
- sulfonamide derivatives may activate or exacerbate SLE in susceptible patients, therefore should be given with caution
- caution if used in the elderly as they are more susceptible to electrolyte imbalance and orthostatic hypotension
- caution if used in those with diabetes mellitus or if receiving treatment (diet/combination) for hypercholesterolaemia with renal or liver impairment
- contraindicated in those with anuria, severe oliguria, severe kidney or liver failure (including hepatic pre-coma and coma, cirrhosis), untreated Addison's disease, refractory hypokalaemia, hyponatraemia or hypercalcaemia, history of gout or uric acid calculi, pregnancy-related hypertension, creatinine clearance less than 30 mL/minute and conditions involving potassium loss or heart failure with significant oedema

- contraindicated in those with thiazide or sulfonamide sensitivity
- see also General Nursing points/ Cautions for diuretics (p. 1010)

General Patient teaching and advice for thiazide diuretics

- advise patient to avoid vitamin D and calcium-containing supplements during therapy
- warn patient to avoid alcohol during therapy
- patient should be instructed to protect skin from sun (e.g. protective long-sleeved clothing, hat, SPF 30+ sunscreen) and artificial UV light and seek medical attention immediately if severe sunburn develops
- see also General Patient teaching and advice for diuretics (p. 1011)

banned in sport

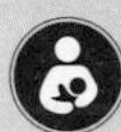

only used during pregnancy if potential benefits outweigh risks and then at lowest possible dose to achieve desired results. Thiazide and related diuretics enter fetal circulation and may cause fetal electrolyte disturbances and/or neonatal thrombocytopenia. May also decrease uteroplacental perfusion because of reduced maternal blood volume

not recommended during breastfeeding

CHLORTALIDONE (CHLORTHALIDONE) (Hygroton)

Available form
Tablets: 25 mg

Action
- see General Actions of thiazide diuretics (p. 1020)
- onset of diuresis 2–3 hours, peak effect in 4–24 hours, duration 48–72 hours, half-life 24–55 hours

Use
- see General Uses of thiazide diuretics (p. 1020)

Dose
- (oedema) up to 50 mg orally daily or on alternative days **OR**
- (chronic stable congestive heart failure) initially 25–50 mg orally daily or 100 mg every second day, then either 12.5–50 mg daily or 25–50 mg every second day (maintenance) **OR**
- (hypertension) initially 12.5–25 mg orally daily; if ineffective after 3–4 weeks, may be combined with antihypertensive agent

Adverse effects
- see General Adverse effects of thiazide diuretics (p. 1020)

Interactions
- see General Interactions of thiazide diuretics (p. 1020)

Nursing points/Cautions

- not recommended as first-line treatment in those with diabetes mellitus or hypercholesterolaemia
- see also General Nursing points/ Cautions for thiazide diuretics (p. 1021) and diuretics (p. 1010)

Patient teaching and advice

- see General Patient teaching and advice for thiazide diuretics (p. 1022) and diuretics (p. 1011)

tablets can be dispersed in water or crushed and mixed with spoonful of yoghurt or apple puree

HYDROCHLOROTHIAZIDE (Dithiazide)

Available form
Tablets: 25 mg

Action
- see General Actions of thiazide diuretics (p. 1020)

- onset of action within 2 hours, peak action in 4 hours, duration 6–12 hours, half-life 2.5 hours

Use
- see General Uses of thiazide diuretics (p. 1020)
- premenstrual tension (PMT) with oedema

Dose
- (oedema) 25–100 mg orally 1–2 times daily, or on alternate days or 3–5 times/week (maximum daily dose 200 mg) **OR**
- (hypertension) 25–50 mg orally as single or divided dose (or 12.5 mg if given with antihypertensive agent) (maximum daily dose 100 mg) **OR**
- (PMT with oedema) 25–50 mg orally 1–2 times daily from onset of symptoms until start of menses

Adverse effects
- acute transient myopia, acute secondary angle-closure glaucoma, increased risk of non-melanoma skin cancers
- see also General Adverse effects of thiazide diuretics (p. 1020)

Interactions
- see General Interactions of thiazide diuretics (p. 1020)

Nursing points/Cautions
- caution if used in those with penicillin allergy due to increased risk of acute secondary angle-closure glaucoma
- caution if used in patients with history of non-melanoma skin cancers
- see also General Nursing points/Cautions for thiazide diuretics (p. 1021) and diuretics (p. 1010)

Patient teaching and advice
- advise patient to seek medical advice immediately if any eye pain, blurred or changes to vision occur (especially at the start of therapy)
- instruct patient to check skin regularly for any new or changing skin lesions and seek medical advice immediately if any occur. Patient should also be advised to avoid exposure to sunlight or UV light and ensure protection with sunscreen (SPF 30+), hat and long-sleeved garments
- if used for PMT, counsel patient to start therapy when symptoms start up to the start of period
- see General Patient teaching and advice for thiazide diuretics (p. 1021) and diuretics (p. 1010)

Note
- contained in Accuretic with quinapril, Adeson HCT, Candesartan HCT, Candesartan HCTZ, Atacand Plus, Candesartan Plus with candesartan cilexetil, Moduretic with amiloride, Arbisart HCT, Avsartan HCT, Irbesartan HCT, Avapro HCT, Karvezide with irbesartan, Enalapril/HCT and Renitec Plus 60/6 with enalapril, Exforge HCT and Valsartan/Amlodipine/HCT with valsartan and amlodipine, Fosinopril HCTZ, Fositec 20/125, Olmertan Combi, Olmesartan HCT, Olmetsartan HCT-MXL, Olmetec Plus or Sevikar HCT with olmesartan, Telmisartan HCT, Teltartan HCT, Micardis Plus and Mizart HCT with telmisartan, Teveten Plus with eprosartan, Co-Diovan with valsartan and Sevikar HCT 20/5/12.5 with amlodipine and olmesartan

plain tablets can be dispersed in water or crushed and mixed with spoonful of yoghurt or apple puree

INDAPAMIDE HEMIHYDRATE (DapaTabs, Insig, Natrilix, Natrilix SR, Odaplix SR, Tenaxil SR)

Available forms

Tablets: 2.5 mg; Tablets (sustained-release): 1.5 mg

Action

- non-thiazide indole derivative of chlorosulfonamide
- onset of action 30 mins–2 hours, peak effect 1–3 hours, biphasic half-life 14 and 25 hours
- antihypertensive effect may be due to decreased vascular reactivity to pressor amines
- see also General Actions of thiazide diuretics (p. 1020)

Use

- see General Uses of thiazide diuretics (p. 1020)

Dose

- (hypertension) 2.5 mg orally each morning **OR**
- (hypertension) 1.5 mg orally each morning (SR formulation)

Adverse effects

- (rare) severe skin reaction
- see General Adverse effects of thiazide diuretics (p. 1020)

Interactions

- see also General Interactions of thiazide diuretics (p. 1020)
- increased risk of antihypertensive effects if given with baclofen
- not recommended with disopyramide, amiodarone, sotalol, some antipsychotic agents, erythromycin (IV), pentamidine and moxifloxacin due to risk of QT prolongation and cardiac arrhythmias
- if given with iodinated contrast media, patient should be well hydrated to prevent acute renal failure

Nursing points/Cautions

- optimum hypotensive effect is seen in approximately 4–6 weeks
- hypotensive effect may continue for up to 1–2 weeks after stopping therapy
- tablets contain lactose and are therefore not recommended in those with rare hereditary problems of galactose intolerance, Lapp lactase deficiency or glucose–galactose malabsorption
- see also General Nursing points/Cautions for thiazide diuretics (p. 1021) and diuretics (p. 1010)

Patient teaching and advice

- advise patient that SR preparations should not be chewed or broken, but swallowed whole
- instruct patient to seek medical advice immediately if any of the following occur:
    - rapid or irregular heartbeat
    - skin rash with purple spots and some blistering, mainly on legs, arms, neck and around ears
- see also General Patient teaching and advice for thiazide diuretics (p. 1022) and diuretics (p. 1011)

Note

- contained in Coversyl Plus, Idraprex Combi 4/1.25, Indopril Combi 4/1.25, Indosyl Combi 4/1.25, Perindopril and Indapamide CH 4/1.25, Perindo Combi 4/1.25 and Prexum Combi 5/125 with perindopril

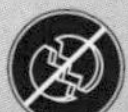

sustained-release tablets should not be crushed or broken.

plain tablets (2.5 mg) can be crushed and mixed with water or spoonful of yoghurt or apple puree

POTASSIUM-SPARING DIURETICS

AMILORIDE HYDROCHLORIDE DIHYDRATE (Kaluril)

Available form
Tablets: 5 mg

Action
- potassium-sparing diuretic that increases excretion of sodium in the distal convoluted tubule but conserves potassium
- does not antagonise aldosterone, therefore does not require aldosterone to be present to be effective
- mild diuretic and antihypertensive effect when used alone
- onset of action about 2 hours, peak action 6–10 hours, duration 24 hours, half-life 17–26 hours

Use
- oedema due to heart failure, hepatic cirrhosis or nephrotic syndrome
- hypertension
- adjunct to thiazide or loop diuretic

Dose
- (hypertension) 5–10 mg orally daily, increasing dose if needed (maximum daily dose 20 mg) (with another diuretic) **OR**
- (oedema – hepatic cirrhosis) initially 5 mg daily, increasing dose if necessary to achieve result, then decreasing dose when patient's weight is stable (daily maximum 20 mg) **OR**
- (oedema – cardiac) 5–10 mg orally daily, then reducing dose if possible (with another diuretic) **OR**
- 5 mg twice daily, increasing dose as necessary to achieve diuresis, then reducing dose in 5 mg increments (daily maximum 20 mg)

Adverse effects
- fluid and electrolyte imbalance (hyponatraemia, hypochloraemia, increased blood urea nitrogen (BUN))
- hyperkalaemia (muscle weakness, fatigue, paraesthesia, flaccid paralysis, bradycardia, ECG abnormalities)
- dizziness, weakness, paraesthesia, headache, fatigue
- anorexia, nausea, vomiting, abdominal pain, flatulence, dry mouth, thirst, diarrhoea
- mild rash, pruritus, alopecia
- impotence, decreased libido
- polyuria, dysuria, bladder spasm, increased micturition
- hypotension, palpitations, arrhythmias
- cough, dyspnoea
- joint pain, back pain, pain in extremities
- (rare) jaundice

Interactions
- increased risk of hyperkalaemia if given with ciclosporin, tacrolimus, angiotensin II receptor antagonists or ACE inhibitors
- increased risk of hyperkalaemia and renal failure if given with NSAIDs
- contraindicated with other potassium-sparing diuretics (triamterene or spironolactone) or potassium supplements
- not recommended with lithium because of risk of toxicity due to increased serum levels

Nursing points/Cautions
- renal function and electrolyte levels should be checked before starting and regularly throughout therapy (especially if patient is taking NSAID concurrently)
- observe for features of hyponatraemia and hyperkalaemia
- discontinue for 3 days prior to patients with diabetes having a glucose tolerance test
- caution if used in those with known or suspected diabetes mellitus

(especially if uncontrolled) because of increased risk of hyperkalaemia
- caution if potassium serum levels > 3.5 mmol/L
- caution if used in those with respiratory or metabolic acidosis or liver cirrhosis
- contraindicated in those with hyperkalaemia (> 5.5 mmol/L), anuria, acute renal failure, severe progressive renal failure or diabetic nephropathy
- see also General Nursing points/Cautions for diuretics (p. 1010)

Patient teaching and advice

- advise patient to avoid foods high in potassium (such as apricots, avocados, bananas, rockmelon, dates, grapefruit, oranges, potatoes, prunes, raisins, spinach, strawberries, watermelon and orange, grapefruit, prune and pineapple juice) or potassium supplements
- patient should be advised to seek medical attention immediately if he/she experiences any muscle weakness, tiredness, nausea, slow heart rate or weak pulse, numbness or tingling in hands or feet (signs of hyperkalaemia)
- see also General Patient teaching and advice for diuretics (p. 1011)

banned in sport

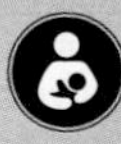

not recommended during pregnancy or breastfeeding unless the expected benefit outweighs any potential risk. Maternal use may result in electrolyte disturbance in the fetus

tablet can be dispersed in water or crushed and mixed with spoonful of yoghurt or apple puree

Note

- combined with hydrochlorothiazide in Moduretic

EPLERENONE (Espler, Inpler, Inspra)

Available forms

Tablets: 25 mg, 50 mg

Action

- selective mineralocorticoid receptor antagonist that competitively inhibits aldosterone
- peak concentration within 1.5 hours, half-life 3–5 hours

Use

- to decrease risk of cardiovascular death in patients with heart failure/left ventricle impairment (within 3–14 days of myocardial infarction) (adjunct)
- to decrease risk of mortality and morbidity in those with chronic heart failure and left ventricular systolic dysfunction (adjunct)

Dose

- initially 25 mg orally daily, increasing to 50 mg within 4 weeks of starting therapy according to serum potassium levels

Adverse effects

- hypotension, syncope
- myocardial infarction, angina, non-cardiac chest pain
- dehydration
- dizziness
- nausea, vomiting, diarrhoea, constipation, flatulence
- hyperkalaemia, increased blood urea
- abnormal kidney function, increased creatinine
- muscle spasm, musculoskeletal pain
- cough
- pruritus
- infection

Interactions

- contraindicated with fluconazole, itraconazole, erythromycin, clarithromycin, verapamil, ritonavir and saquinavir
- contraindicated with other potassium-sparing diuretics

- not recommended with ciclosporin or tacrolimus due to risk of hyperkalaemia and renal impairment
- increased risk of hyperkalaemia if given with trimethoprim
- increased risk of hypotension if given with prazosin, alfuzosin, TCAs, amifostine and baclofen
- not recommended with lithium
- caution if given with NSAIDs due to risk of reduced antihypertensive effect, hyperkalaemia and renal impairment
- caution if given with ACE inhibitors or angiotensin II receptor antagonists due to risk of hyperkalaemia
- serum levels may be decreased if given with St John's wort, rifampicin, carbamazepine, phenytoin and phenobarbital (phenobarbitone) and therefore not recommended together

Nursing points/Cautions

- serum potassium should be measured before starting therapy, after first week and first month, then regularly and dose adjusted accordingly
- if serum potassium level is ≥ 6 mmol/L, therapy should be stopped and restarted at 25 mg second daily when serum potassium level has fallen to below 5.5 mmol/L
- chronic heart failure should be reassessed after 12 months to determine effectiveness of therapy
- caution if used in those with diabetes mellitus (with cardiac failure post-myocardial infarction)
- contraindicated in those with hyperkalaemia (> 5.5 mmol/L when starting therapy), moderate-to-severe kidney impairment (glomerular filtration rate < 30 mL/minute) or severe liver impairment

Patient teaching and advice

- advise patient to avoid foods high in potassium (such as apricots, avocados, bananas, rockmelon, dates, grapefruit, oranges, potatoes, prunes, raisins, spinach, strawberries, watermelon and orange, grapefruit, prune and pineapple juice) and potassium supplements
- patient should be advised to seek medical advice immediately if he/she experiences any muscle weakness, tiredness, nausea, slow heart rate or weak pulse, numbness or tingling in hands or feet (signs of hyperkalaemia)
- also see General Patient teaching and advice for diuretics (p. 1011)

banned in sport

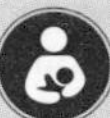

only used during pregnancy or breastfeeding if benefits are thought to outweigh risks

if crushing tablets, mask, gloves and safety glasses must be worn. May cause eye and skin irritation

SPIRONOLACTONE (Aldactone, Spiractin)

Available forms

Tablets: 25 mg, 100 mg

Action

- competitive inhibitor of aldosterone in the distal convoluted tubule that increases sodium and water excretion but decreases potassium excretion
- effect is directly related to plasma concentration of circulating aldosterone
- does not interfere with renal tubule transport of sodium and chloride
- does not inhibit carbonic anhydrase
- has both diuretic and antihypertensive effects

- moderate antiandrogen effects
- active metabolite (canrenone) (half-life 18–20 hours)
- onset of action 24–48 hours, peak response in 48–72 hours, effects last 3 days after discontinuation, half-life 1.5 hours

Use

- oedema associated with congestive heart failure and hepatic cirrhosis and ascites
- diagnosis and treatment of primary hyperaldosteronism
- adjunctive therapy in malignant hypertension (excessive aldosterone secretion, hypokalaemia and metabolic acidosis)
- female hirsutism
- essential hypertension
- prevention and treatment of diuretic-induced hypokalaemia (when other measures are ineffective or inappropriate)
- nephrotic syndrome

Dose

- (essential hypertension) 50–100 mg orally daily as single or divided dose **OR**
- (oedema – congestive heart failure) initially 100 mg orally daily as single or divided dose, increasing to 200 mg if needed, then reducing to 25–200 mg daily (maintenance) **OR**
- (cirrhosis – sodium:potassium ratio > 1) 100 mg orally daily **OR**
- (cirrhosis – sodium:potassium ratio < 1) 200–400 mg orally daily **OR**
- (hypokalaemia) up to 100 mg orally daily **OR**
- (female hirsutism) 50–200 mg orally daily in divided doses for 12 months as either continuous therapy or 3 weeks of therapy followed by 1 drug-free week **OR**
- (malignant hypertension) initially 100 mg orally daily, increasing at 2-weekly intervals to 400 mg daily (with other antihypertensive agents) **OR**
- (nephrotic syndrome) 100–200 mg orally daily **OR**
- (primary hyperaldosteronism diagnosis – long test) 400 mg orally daily for 3–4 weeks **OR**
- (primary hyperaldosteronism diagnosis – short test) 400 mg orally daily for 4 days

Adverse effects

- headache, drowsiness, confusion, ataxia, lethargy, drug fever, malaise, dizziness
- rash, urticaria, pruritus
- nausea, vomiting, gastritis, gastric bleeding, gastric ulceration, abdominal cramp, diarrhoea, constipation
- alopecia, hypertrichosis
- electrolyte disturbance: hyponatraemia (tachycardia, hypotension, oliguria), hyperchloraemia, hyperkalaemia (paraesthesia, muscle weakness, fatigue, flaccid paralysis, bradycardia, serum potassium > 5.5 mmol/L, ECG changes)
- (prolonged or high-dose therapy) (females) menstrual disturbances, post-menopausal bleeding, breast pain, changes to libido, benign breast neoplasm
- (prolonged or high-dose therapy) (males) gynaecomastia, impotence, decreased libido
- abnormal liver function
- (female hirsutism, cyclical dosing) menstrual irregularities (in women with previously regular cycles)
- (rare) agranulocytosis, thrombocytopenia, severe skin reactions

Interactions

- contraindicated with eplerenone
- increased risk of hyperkalaemia if given with indometacin or ACE inhibitors
- diuretic effect may be weakened by NSAIDs, in particular, aspirin, indometacin or mefenamic acid
- may increase half-life of digoxin increasing serum levels and risk of toxicity

- not recommended with other potassium-sparing diuretics or potassium supplements, angiotensin II inhibitors, aldosterone blockers, potassium-rich diet, NSAIDs, heparin, low molecular weight heparins or ACE inhibitors due to risk of hyperkalaemia
- may potentiate action of other diuretics and antihypertensive agents, therefore doses should be reduced
- caution if used with noradrenaline (norepinephrine) as vascular response is reduced
- hyperkalaemic metabolic acidosis may occur if given with colestyramine or ammonium chloride
- may interfere with assay for digoxin plasma levels

Nursing points/Cautions

- (primary hyperaldosteronism diagnosis) correction of hypokalaemia and hypertension is evidence for diagnosis of hyperaldosteronism (long test)
- (primary hyperaldosteronism diagnosis) if serum potassium increases during therapy and then decreases when stopped, this is suggestive evidence for hyperaldosteronism (short test)
- monitor fluid intake, output and body weight and note increase or decrease in oedema
- check BP at start, then regularly during therapy
- maximum effect for essential hypertension may not be seen for up to 2 weeks
- serum electrolytes should be monitored regularly and therapy stopped if serum potassium > 5 mEq/L or serum creatinine > 4 mg/dL
- (heart failure) potassium and creatinine levels should be measured 1 week after starting therapy, then monthly for 3 months, then 4 times for 1 year, and 6-monthly when increasing dose
- observe for features of hyponatraemia and hyperkalaemia
- (hirsutism) cyclical dosing of 3 weeks with 1 week drug-free may decrease menstrual irregularities in women with previously regular cycle
- (hirsutism) clinical improvement may be seen in 3–6 months, but should be continued for at least 12 months initially
- (essential hypertension only) dose of diuretic or antihypertensive agent should be decreased by 50% when aldosterone is added and then doses adjusted according to response
- caution if used in those with kidney or liver impairment
- caution if used in the elderly as they are at greater risk of electrolyte imbalance and hypotension
- not recommended in those with severe heart failure
- contraindicated in those with anuria, acute renal failure, significant renal impairment, Addison's disease or pre-existing hyperkalaemia (> 5 mmol/L)

Patient teaching and advice

- instruct patient to take with food or immediately after to increase absorption
- advise patient to avoid foods high in potassium (such as apricots, avocados, bananas, rockmelon, dates, grapefruit, oranges, potatoes, prunes, raisins, spinach, strawberries, watermelon and orange, grapefruit, prune and pineapple juice) and potassium supplements
- patient should be advised to seek medical attention immediately if any of the following occur:
  - muscle weakness, tiredness, nausea, slow heart rate or weak pulse, numbness or tingling in hands or feet (signs of hyperkalaemia)
  - (male) breast enlargement or inability to get or maintain erection
  - (female) menstrual changes
  - changes in sex drive

  - breast pain, breast lump
  - excessive hair growth
  - hair loss or thinning
  - yellowing of skin or eyes
- (female hirsutism, cyclical dosing) warn female patients that menstrual cycle may become irregular during therapy
- female patients of childbearing potential should be counselled to use adequate contraceptive measures throughout therapy and advise doctor immediately if pregnancy occurs
- also see General Patient teaching and advice for diuretics (p. 1011)

banned in sport

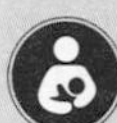
contraindicated during pregnancy because it may cause demasculinisation of male fetus

not recommended during breastfeeding as active metabolite appears in breastmilk

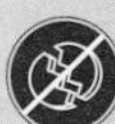
mask and gloves must be worn if crushing tablets, which should then be mixed with water or spoonful of yoghurt or apple puree

OSMOTIC DIURETICS

GLUCOSE (Glucose 50%)

Available form
Vial: 25 g/50 mL (50%)

Action
- monosaccharide
- strongly hypertonic solution that promotes diuresis by increasing osmotic pressure of glomerular filtrate
- metabolised to carbon dioxide and water releasing energy
- cerebrospinal fluid (CSF) pressure reduced for 2–4 hours after injection

Use
- severe hypoglycaemia (from insulin excess)
- reduce CSF pressure and/or oedema caused by acute alcohol intoxication or delirium tremens

Dose
- (acute hypoglycaemia) 12.5–25 g (25–50 mL) by slow IV injection at 3 mL/minute, then evaluate response

Adverse effects
- fever
- venous thrombosis, phlebitis, extravasation, thrombophlebitis
- generalised flush, local pain, vein irritation (if given too rapidly)
- precipitate vitamin B deficiency, oedema, hypokalaemia, hypophosphataemia, hypomagnesaemia
- exacerbation of diabetes mellitus
- (overdosage) hyperglycaemia, glycosuria
- (rare) anaphylaxis

Nursing points/Cautions
- patient should be closely monitored for:
  - signs of dehydration, including observation of skin (decreased skin turgor) and tongue (dry), and haematocrit measurement
  - signs of fluid overload or electrolyte imbalance including hyperglycaemia
- prolonged administration may affect insulin production
- (acute hypoglycaemia) after desired response has been achieved, patient should be commenced on oral feeding to prevent relapse
- hypertonic solution is for IV use only
- injection should be given slowly to avoid thrombosis

- should be given using small-bore needle to avoid venous trauma
- tourniquet should be removed as soon as venipuncture is completed
- warming patient's arm and the IV solution may decrease risk of thrombosis
- flushing may occur due to rapid administration and should subside in about 10 minutes
- should not be administered with blood or blood products, because agglutination may occur
- caution if used in those with carbohydrate intolerance, thiamine deficiency (e.g. chronic alcohol abuse), diabetes mellitus, severe malnutrition, thiamine deficiency, hypokalaemia, hypophosphataemia, hypomagnesaemia, haemodilution, sepsis or trauma
- contraindicated in those with diabetic coma (while blood glucose is excessively high), anuria, at risk of or after ischaemic stroke, intracranial or intraspinal haemorrhage, delirium tremens with dehydration, or with hypersensitivity to corn or corn products
- contraindicated in those with glucose–galactose malabsorption syndrome

banned in some sports and not others

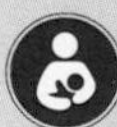

not used during pregnancy or breastfeeding unless expected benefit outweighs any potential risk

MANNITOL (Osmitrol Intravenous Infusion)

Available forms

Solution: 10% w/v, 20% w/v

Action

- pharmacologically inert
- produces osmotic diuresis by inhibiting tubular reabsorption of water and enhancing sodium and chloride excretion by increasing osmolarity of glomerular filtrate
- alters plasma osmotic pressure, lowering intraocular and cerebrospinal fluid pressures

Use

- promoting diuresis (prevention and/or treatment of acute renal failure before it becomes irreversible)
- reducing intracranial pressure (ICP) and oedema
- reducing raised intraocular pressure (where other treatments are ineffective)
- promoting urinary excretion of toxic substances by forced diuresis

Dose

- 50–100 g/24 hours by IV infusion to maintain urine output of at least 30–50 mL/hour **OR**
- (reduce intraocular pressure) 1.5–2 g/kg body weight infused over 30 minutes using 20% solution (may be given 1–1.5 hours preoperatively) **OR**
- (ICP reduction) 0.25 g/kg body weight by IV infusion 6–8-hourly **OR**
- (prevention of acute renal failure – oliguria) 50–100 g as a 10% or 20% solution by IV infusion (during surgery) **OR**
- (oliguria treatment) 100 g as 20% solution by IV infusion **OR**
- (adjunct treatment to intoxication) 10–20% solution, depending on fluid requirements and urinary output

Adverse effects

- fluid and electrolyte imbalance, hyponatraemia, hypernatraemia, acidosis
- dehydration (oedema, cramps, thirst, dry mouth), hypovolaemia, haemoconcentration
- hypotension, hypertension, tachycardia, chest pain, arrhythmia, pulmonary oedema, congestive cardiac failure
- excessive diuresis, urinary retention, acute renal failure, osmotic nephrosis

- nausea, vomiting
- headache, dizziness, raised intracranial pressure
- chills, fever
- blurred vision
- urticaria
- hypersensitivity reaction (rhinitis, angioedema, allergic reaction, anaphylaxis)
- CNS toxicity (confusion, lethargy, coma)
- (injection site) pain, necrosis, inflammation, rash, thrombophlebitis

Interactions

- increased risk of renal failure if given with nephrotoxic agents
- effects may be potentiated by diuretics
- may increase excretion of lithium and methotrexate
- increased risk of nephrotoxicity if given with ciclosporin
- caution if given with aminoglycosides due to risk of ototoxicity
- may enhance effects of neuromuscular blocking agents
- may decrease effects of oral anticoagulants
- increased risk of digoxin toxicity if mannitol-induced hypokalaemia occurs
- may cause false positive for blood ethylene glycol concentrations

Nursing points/Cautions

- cardiovascular evaluation is recommended before starting therapy
- rapid infusion of hypertonic solutions is not recommended
- administration should be via large peripheral veins or central line to decrease venous irritation
- IV site should be closely monitored to avoid extravasation
- infusion rate should be regulated to maintain a urine output of 30–50 mL/hour or as directed
- monitor vital signs during infusion, noting changes in heart and respiratory rate and BP
- monitor fluid intake and output carefully, noting signs of circulatory overload, excessive diuresis or urinary retention
- monitor serum electrolytes (especially sodium and potassium), acid–base balance, renal function and osmolarity levels closely during mannitol administration
- patient should be monitored for any signs of hypersensitivity reaction and infusion stopped immediately if any signs occur
- test dose should be given before therapy if the patient has marked oliguria or inadequate renal function (may require 1 or 2 test doses of 0.2 g/kg over 3–5 minutes to produce urine flow of 30–50 mL/hour). No more than 2 test doses should be given
- no more than 50 g of mannitol should be administered at any one time
- (ICP reduction) rebound increase in ICP may occur 12 hours after mannitol administration
- should not be administered with blood or blood products, because agglutination may occur
- incompatible with cefepime, cilastatin and imipenem
- should not be administered with solutions containing potassium or sodium chloride
- any crystals formed at low temperature can be redissolved by warming solution to approximately 70°C, then allowing it to cool to room temperature before administration via an IV administration set containing a filter. Solution should not be microwaved
- caution if used in the elderly, children, women and those with psychogenic polydipsia due to increased risk of developing hyponatraemia (which may lead to acute symptomatic hyponatraemic encephalopathy)
- not recommended in children < 12 years

- not recommended in acute traumatic brain injury or acute shock
- not recommended for those in shock and/or kidney dysfunction until fluid and electrolyte balance has been restored
- contraindicated in those with established anuria (due to severe kidney disease), pre-existing plasma hyperosmolarity, blood–brain barrier disturbance, severe heart failure, severe pulmonary congestion or frank pulmonary oedema, active intracranial bleeding (except during craniotomy), severe dehydration or if there was no response to test dose(s) or hypersensitivity to mannitol
- contraindicated in those with progressive renal damage/dysfunction, progressive heart failure or pulmonary congestion after mannitol therapy has been started

banned in sport

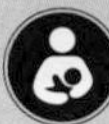

not used during pregnancy or breastfeeding unless expected benefit outweighs any potential risk

Note

- also available as Bronchitol Powder for Inhalation and Aridol Diagnostic kit

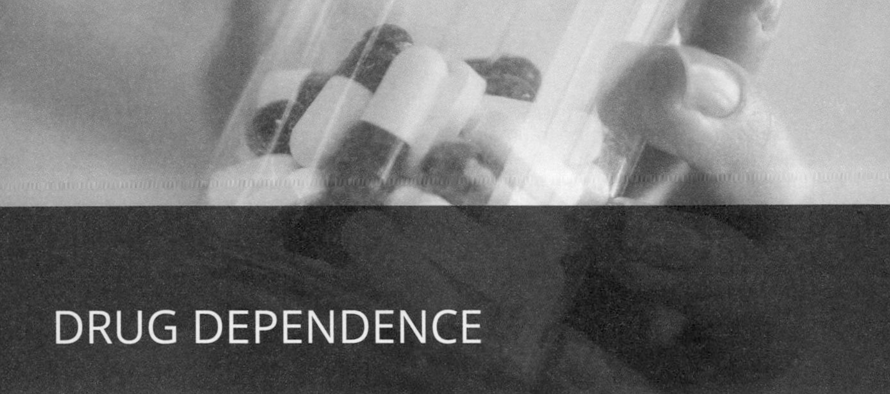

DRUG DEPENDENCE

Any drug (prescribed, over-the-counter (OTC) or recreational) has the capacity to be abused or misused. *Drug abuse* is defined as 'self-administration of a drug in chronically excessive quantities in a manner that deviates from approved medical or social patterns in a given culture resulting in physical or psychological harm', while *drug misuse* is considered to be 'inappropriate or indiscriminate use of drugs' (Bryant et al 2019, p. 426). Factors leading to drug abuse and dependence include sociocultural (e.g. drug availability, peer-group pressure), personality (e.g. rebelliousness, tolerance of deviance, school performance, genetic predisposition to dependence, antisocial tendencies, depression) and pharmacological factors (e.g. drug's CNS effects provide relief from problems and/or achieve pleasure) (Bryant et al 2019).

Physical dependence occurs when the body progressively adapts to a drug, producing tolerance whereby the same dose produces a smaller effect. Many drugs given at therapeutic doses can result in physical dependence and also withdrawal symptoms if the drug is suddenly stopped. Physical dependence, tolerance and withdrawal symptoms are natural biological phenomena and not suggestive of addiction, which is compulsive drug-taking (Bryant et al 2019). The distinction between addiction and dependence is an important one for health professionals to understand as it is the underlying reason for many patients with pain being under-medicated, especially with opioid analgesics.

ACAMPROSATE CALCIUM (Campral)

Available form

Tablets (enteric coated): 333 mg

Action

- structurally similar to neuromediators gamma amino butyric acid (GABA) and taurine
- decreases voluntary intake of alcohol without affecting food and fluid intake
- appears to reduce elevation of brain concentration of glutamate during withdrawal from ethanol, although mechanism of action is not completely understood
- half-life 13–28 hours

Use

- maintenance of abstinence in alcohol-dependent patients (combined with counselling)

Dose
- (weight ≥ 60 kg) 666 mg (2 tablets) orally 3 times daily **OR**
- (weight < 60 kg) 666 mg (2 tablets) orally each morning, 333 mg (1 tablet) orally at midday and at night

Adverse effects
- nausea, vomiting, abdominal pain, diarrhoea
- pruritus, rash
- decreased libido, frigidity, impotence

Interactions
- bioavailability decreased by food

Nursing points/Cautions
- tablets should be swallowed whole
- treatment should be started after alcohol withdrawal period, maintained even if relapse occurs and continued for up to 1 year
- should be used in combination with counselling
- patients should be monitored for any signs of depression or suicidal ideation
- tablets contain 33.3 mg of calcium, therefore caution should be observed in those who may need to limit calcium intake
- not recommended in those over 65 years
- contraindicated in those with severe kidney or liver failure

Patient teaching and advice
- advise patient to swallow tablets whole, not crush or break them
- patient (or partner/family member) should be advised to report any thoughts/talk about self-harm, harm to others, suicide or death or recent attempts at self-harm or change in mood including signs of depression
- see also General Patient teaching and advice (p. xxvii)

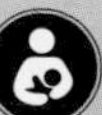
contraindicated during pregnancy or breastfeeding

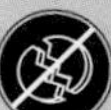
tablet should not be crushed, chewed or broken

BUPRENORPHINE (Bupredermal Transdermal, Buvidal Monthly, Buvidal Weekly, Norspan Transdermal Patch, Sublocade, Subutex, Temgesic)

Available forms
Sublingual tablets: 200 microgram, 400 microgram, 2 mg, 8 mg; Transdermal patches: 5 mg, 10 mg, 15 mg, 20 mg, 25 mg, 30 mg, 40 mg; Ampoules: 300 microgram/mL; Modified-release solution (prefilled syringe): 8 mg/0.16 mL, 16 mg/0.32 mL, 24 mg/0.48 mL, 32 mg/0.64 mL, 64 mg/0.18 mL, 96 mg/0.27 mL, 100 mg/0.5 mL, 128 mg/0.36 mL, 300 mg/1.5 mL

Action
- synthetic opioid that has both opioid agonist and antagonist properties
- more potent than morphine and longer acting (6–8 hours IM, IV or sublingual, 7 days of transdermal patches)
- active metabolite (norbuprenorphine)
- half-life about 35 hours (sublingual)

Use
- moderate-to-severe pain (short-term management), opioid dependence (detoxification or maintenance) (see Opioid analgesics, p. 1369)

BUPROPION HYDROCHLORIDE (Zyban SR)

Available form
Tablets (sustained-release): 150 mg

Action

- selectively inhibits noradrenaline and dopamine reuptake
- originally developed as antidepressant
- unknown mechanism increases ability to refrain from smoking
- has equivalent efficacy to nicotine replacement therapy but not as efficacious as varenicline, therefore considered second-line management
- use with nicotine replacement therapy does not improve efficacy
- half-life is about 20 hours
- three active metabolites (half-life range from 20 to 37 hours)

Use

- nicotine dependence (short-term adjunct with counselling)

Dose

- initially 150 mg orally daily (days 1–3), then 150 mg orally twice daily for 7–9 weeks (daily maximum 300 mg)

Adverse effects

- headache, dizziness, insomnia, abnormal dreams, agitation, anxiety, asthenia, impaired concentration, tremor, nervousness
- anorexia, nausea, vomiting, dry mouth, constipation, altered taste sensation, abdominal pain, mouth ulcers
- urticaria, rash, pruritus, sweating, flushing
- neck pain, myalgia, arthralgia
- rhinitis, pharyngitis, sinusitis, epistaxis
- visual disturbances, increased intraocular pressure, glaucoma, mydriasis
- fever
- (uncommon) hypertension, tachycardia, tinnitus
- (rare) seizures, depression, psychosis, mania, suicidal ideation

Interactions

- contraindicated with or within 14 days of MAOIs
- increased risk of hypertension if used with nicotine replacement therapy
- may decrease efficacy of tamoxifen
- caution if given with ifosfamide, cyclophosphamide, ticlopidine, clopidogrel or orphenadrine
- may reduce tolerance to alcohol and increase risk of neuropsychiatric adverse effects
- caution if given with St John's wort
- decreased serum levels may occur if given with phenytoin, phenobarbital (phenobarbitone), carbamazepine, efavirenz or ritonavir
- may increase serum levels of sodium valproate increasing risk of adverse effects
- lowers seizure threshold, therefore not recommended in those taking antidepressants, antipsychotic agents, antihistamines (sedating), corticosteroids (systemic), theophylline, tramadol, antimalarials, sedatives, stimulants, anorectic agents or those with high alcohol intake
- caution if used with TCAs, SSRIs, antipsychotic agents, some beta-adrenoceptor blocking agents or antiarrhythmic agents
- smoking cessation itself may alter pharmacokinetics of some medications taken concurrently
- may decrease serum levels of digoxin
- increased risk of neuropsychiatric adverse effects if given with amantadine or levodopa, therefore should be given together with caution
- may result in false positive results in some rapid urine drug screening tests

Nursing points/Cautions

- before starting therapy, patient should be assessed for any factors that might lower seizure threshold, such as medications known to lower threshold, head trauma, diabetes, use of stimulants or anorectic agents or excessive use of alcohol or sedatives

- patient should start therapy while they are still smoking to allow sufficient time for therapy to have its therapeutic effect. If they are still smoking after 7 weeks, it is unlikely that therapy will be of benefit
- may be combined with nicotine replacement program (although this does increase risk of hypertension occurring) and if used together, blood pressure should be monitored weekly
- should be part of a multifaceted program that includes counselling
- caution if used in those with psychiatric disorders (e.g. bipolar disorder) because neuropsychiatric symptoms may be precipitated or exacerbated
- caution if used in those with renal impairment, raised intracranial pressure, at risk of glaucoma, history of head trauma, epilepsy, diabetes, high alcohol or sedative intake, recent myocardial infarction or unstable heart disease
- caution if used in those with liver impairment (especially liver cirrhosis). Dose should not be greater than 150 mg every second day
- contraindicated in those with history of seizures, CNS tumour, abrupt withdrawal from alcohol or benzodiazepines, current or history of eating disorder

Patient teaching and advice

- patient should be warned not to drive or operate heavy machinery if dizziness, visual disturbances or impaired concentration occur
- instruct patient that insomnia can be reduced by not taking second dose close to bedtime (but at least 8 hours after last dose)
- advise patients to take tablets whole, not broken or crushed
- patient should be advised not to exceed the recommended dose
- counsel patient to avoid alcohol during therapy as this may increase the risk of having a seizure
- advise patient to report any insomnia, dry mouth or seizures (as these signs may indicate high drug or metabolite levels)
- patient (or partner/family member) should be advised to report any thoughts/talk about self-harm, harm to others, suicide or death or recent attempts at self-harm or change in mood including signs of depression
- counsel patient to identify other strategies to help quit including other activities (e.g. eating healthy snacks, exercise, drinking water slowly, chewing sugar-free gum) that take his/her mind off smoking, as well as identifying other situations (such as socialising with other friends that smoke, drinking alcohol, reducing coffee intake) where smoking is a 'normal' activity for that person
- see also General Patient teaching and advice (p. xxvii)

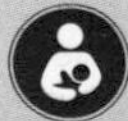

not recommended during pregnancy and breastfeeding unless benefits outweigh potential risks

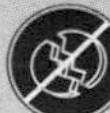

tablets should not be crushed, broken or chewed

Note

- combined with naltrexone in Contrave

DISULFIRAM (Antabuse)

Available form

Tablets (effervescent): 200 mg

Action

- interferes with alcohol metabolism by inhibition of aldehyde dehydrogenase, causing an accumulation of

acetaldehyde, resulting in the 'aldehyde' or 'disulfiram–alcohol' reaction (intense flushing starting at face, throbbing headache, nausea, vomiting, sweating, palpitation, difficulty breathing)
- prodrug
- inert in small doses
- half-life about 10 hours
- effect may persist for 7–14 days

Use
- deterrent to alcohol consumption in the management of chronic alcoholism (as part of a multidiscipline, holistic management strategy)

Dose
- initially 100 mg orally daily on waking (at night if sedation is a problem) for 1–2 weeks, increasing dose to a maximum of 300 mg daily if needed, then decreased to 200 mg daily for 6 weeks to 6 months as necessary

Adverse effects
- drowsiness, lassitude
- peripheral neuropathy, polyneuritis (numbness, tingling, pain or weakness in feet/hands)
- optic neuritis (eye pain, tenderness, visual changes)
- (during first 1–2 weeks) metallic or garlic aftertaste, fatigue, headache, acne rash, stomach upset, seizures
- (rare) mood and psychotic changes, altered liver function tests, jaundice, hepatitis

Interactions
- contraindicated with paraldehyde and metronidazole
- contraindicated with alcohol and alcohol-containing preparations (e.g. cough syrup, vinegar)
- use with phenytoin may result in increased levels of phenytoin and associated risk of toxicity
- use with isoniazid may result in ataxia and changes in mood
- effects of diazepam may be prolonged
- may prolong prothrombin time, requiring dose adjustments of oral anticoagulants (e.g. warfarin)
- may increase toxicity of morphine, pethidine, amphetamines and barbiturates

Nursing points/Cautions
- should be part of a multifaceted program that includes counselling
- therapy commences only after abstinence from alcohol for 24 hours
- intensity of reaction is proportional to the amount of alcohol ingested
- duration of reaction is dependent on ethanol concentration in the blood, but the disulfiram reaction can occur within 5–10 minutes of alcohol ingestion and last for 2–4 hours or longer (in severe cases, until there is no alcohol in blood)
- disulfiram reaction is treated using IV ascorbic acid (1 g) and chlorpromazine (5–100 mg IM). Patient should be closely monitored and any hypotension, hypoxia, fluid or electrolyte imbalance treated using supportive measures, including elevation of foot of bed 20–25 cm
- if therapy is prolonged, liver function monitoring and FBC are recommended regularly
- caution if used in those with diabetes, epilepsy, hypothyroidism, impaired liver or kidney function, heart disease, asthma or allergic contact dermatitis
- contraindicated in those with known hypersensitivity to thiuram products (e.g. pesticides, rubber products), severe myocardial heart disease, ischaemic heart disease, known psychosis or severe kidney or liver impairment or if intoxicated

Patient teaching and advice

- patient and relatives or responsible household member must be counselled and understand the basis of treatment and be educated about the disulfiram–alcohol reaction (e.g. intense flushing, sensation of heat, sweating, palpitations, tachycardia, pounding headache, hyperventilation, dyspnoea) and its consequences before starting therapy
- patient should be strongly cautioned against taking alcohol or alcohol-containing preparations, including some cough syrups, sauces, vinegar and food prepared in wine. Alcohol-based backrubs and aftershave lotions should also be avoided
- warn patient to avoid alcohol during therapy and for at least a week after stopping as disulfiram–alcohol reaction can occur for up to 3 weeks post-therapy
- advise patient that effervescent tablets should be dissolved in water
- patient should be advised not to drive or operate machinery if drowsiness, visual changes or numbness/tingling in feet occur
- warn patient that during first 1–2 weeks of therapy a number of side-effects (e.g. metallic or garlic aftertaste, fatigue, headache, acne, rash, stomach upset, seizures, impotence) may occur, but these subside after this time
- instruct patient to seek medical advice immediately if any of the following occur:
  - weakness, tiredness, loss of appetite, nausea, vomiting, dark urine, abdominal pain or yellowing of skin or eyes
  - numbness, tingling, pain or weakness in hands or feet
  - eye pain or tenderness or changes in vision
  - mood changes or abnormal thoughts
- see General Patient teaching and advice (p. xxvii)

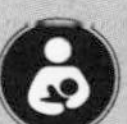

contraindicated during pregnancy

caution if used during breastfeeding

tablet can be dissolved in water or crushed and mixed with spoonful of yoghurt or apple puree

METHADONE HYDROCHLORIDE (Aspen Methadone Syrup, Biodone Forte, Physeptone)

Available forms

Oral liquid: 5 mg/mL; Tablets: 10 mg; Ampoules: 10 mg/mL

Action

- synthetic opioid with properties similar to morphine but less hypnotic
- duration of action 4–24 hours (oral, IM or IV)
- long half-life of 15 hours in non-tolerant (opioid-naive) people, increasing to 22 hours with chronic use (with variation of 15–60 hours being reported)

Use

- severe pain (especially visceral), substitution therapy in the treatment of opioid dependence (Biodone Forte) (see Opioid analgesics, p. 1378)

NALTREXONE HYDROCHLORIDE (Naltrexone GH)

Available form

Tablets: 50 mg

Action

- opioid antagonist related to naloxone which blocks physical dependence to opioids
- produces some pupillary constriction by unknown mechanism

- does not cause disulfiram-like reaction when used as part of an alcohol dependence program
- elimination half-life 4 hours
- active metabolite (half-life about 13 hours)

Use

- part of alcohol dependence program
- adjunctive treatment in maintenance of abstinence from opioids

Dose

- (alcohol dependence) 50 mg orally daily for up to 12 weeks **OR**
- (opioid dependence) initially 25 mg orally daily, increasing to 50 mg if no signs of withdrawal occur

Adverse effects

- nausea, vomiting, decreased appetite, diarrhoea, constipation, increased thirst, abdominal pain/cramps
- headache, dizziness, nervousness, fatigue, anxiety, lethargy, irritability, low mood
- insomnia, somnolence
- joint and muscle pain
- rash
- chills
- (large doses) hepatotoxicity
- (rare) depression, suicidal ideation

Interactions

- not recommended with other hepatotoxic agents
- not recommended with neuroleptic agents, barbiturates, benzodiazepines, antianxiety agents, hypnotics, sedatives, centrally acting antihypertensives, sedating antidepressants, sedating antihistamines, baclofen and thalidomide
- may counteract effects of any opioid-containing preparations (including cough/cold preparations, antidiarrhoeals or combination analgesics)
- may increase rate and extent of absorption of acamprosate

Nursing points/Cautions

- naloxone (Narcan) challenge test should not be performed if patient's urine is positive for opioids or there are any clinical signs of opioid withdrawal
- if there is any concern that the patient is still using opioids or has used in the last 7–10 days, urine should first be tested for the presence of opioids. Naloxone (Narcan) challenge test should then be performed: 0.2 mg naloxone (Narcan) IV and observe patient for signs of withdrawal for 30 seconds, then further 0.6 mg IV and observe for 20 minutes. Alternatively, 0.8 mg SC and observe for 20 minutes for signs of withdrawal. Signs and symptoms of withdrawal include nausea, vomiting, abdominal cramps, yawning, sweating, weeping eyes, stuffy nose, rhinorrhoea, opioid craving, dysphoria, disrupted sleep, sweating, fidgeting, pupil dilation, inability to concentrate or focus, piloerection (goose bumps), anxiety, feeling of skin crawling, fasciculations, change in BP, pulse or temperature, muscle aches or cramps. If test is positive, therapy should not begin. Re-test 24 hours later and if test is still positive, therapy should not begin. If negative, therapy may begin
- risk of hepatoxicity is increased if dose > 50 mg, especially if therapy is prolonged
- treatment should be ceased if there are any signs of hepatitis
- patient should be closely monitored throughout therapy because risk of suicide is increased in those with a substance abuse problem
- if patient requires opioid analgesic in an emergency situation, a larger than usual dose may be needed to obtain the required analgesic

effect, greatly increasing the risk of deeper and more prolonged respiratory depression. Respiratory status should be closely monitored during this time
- motivation and social supports as part of a treatment plan are required for successful withdrawal and ongoing abstinence
- tablets contain lactose and are therefore not recommended in those with rare hereditary galactose intolerance, Lapp lactase or glucose malabsorption
- caution if used in those with liver or kidney impairment
- contraindicated in those who are currently receiving or have a dependence on opioids, experiencing opioid withdrawal, failed the naloxone (Narcan) challenge test, have a positive urine test for opioids or have acute hepatitis or hepatic failure

Patient teaching and advice

- caution patient against driving or operating machinery if dizziness or somnolence occur
- patient should be advised to seek medical advice immediately if loss of appetite, lethargy or tiredness, abdominal pain, dark urine, pale bowel motions or yellowing of eyes or skin occur
- counsel patient regarding the risk of opioid sensitivity and therefore increased risk of overdose and death if he/she stops therapy and resumes heroin (opioid) habit at previous level
- see also General Patient teaching and advice (p. xxvii)

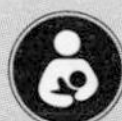

use with great caution during pregnancy or breastfeeding

tablet can be dispersed in water or crushed and mixed with spoonful of yoghurt or apple puree

Note
- combined with bupropion in Contrave (modified-release tablet which should not be crushed, chewed or broken)

NICOTINE (Herron Nicaway Lozenges, Nicabate preparations, Nicorette preparations, Nicotinell preparations, QuitX preparations)

Available forms

Transdermal patches: 7 mg/day, 14 mg/day, 21 mg/day, 10 mg/16 hours, 15 mg/16 hours, 25 mg/16 hours; Lozenges: 1.5 mg, 2 mg, 4 mg; Chewing gum: 2 mg, 4 mg; Inhalator: 15 mg; Oral spray: 1 mg/spray

Action
- main alkaloid found in tobacco which is rapidly absorbed through skin and respiratory tract
- acts on nicotinic receptors in the peripheral and central nervous systems
- cardiovascular effects include vasoconstriction, tachycardia and increased BP
- stimulates cerebral cortex resulting in alertness and increased cognitive performance and produces 'stimulating' and 'reward/pleasure' effects in different parts of the brain. In low doses, produces stimulant effects. At high doses, reward effects are produced
- all formulations are equally efficacious
- evidence suggests combination nicotine replacement therapy is more effective than monotherapy

Use
- treatment of nicotine dependence, as an aid to the cessation of smoking

Dose

- (transdermal patch e.g. Nicabate, QuitX) initially patch of 30 cm^2 (21 mg/day) applied daily for 4–6 weeks, then 20 cm^2 (14 mg/day) for 2–4 weeks and finally 7 cm^2 (7 mg/day) for last 2–4 weeks **OR**
- ($<$ 10 cigarettes/day, weighing less than 45 kg or having cardiovascular disease) (transdermal patch e.g. Nicabate, QuitX) initially patch of 20 cm^2 (14 mg/day) applied daily for 4–6 weeks, decreasing gradually to 7 cm^2 (7 mg/day) for last 2–8 weeks **OR**
- (transdermal patch (e.g. Nicorette), $>$ 15 cigarettes per day) initially patch 22.5 cm^2 (25 mg/16 hours) applied in the morning and removed each night for 8 weeks, then reducing to 13.5 cm^2 (15 mg/16 hours) for 2 weeks and finally 20 cm^2 (10 mg/16 hours) for 2 weeks **OR**
- (transdermal patch (e.g. Nicorette), $<$ 15 cigarettes per day) initially 13.5 cm^2 (15 mg/16 hours) applied in the morning and removed each night for 8 weeks, then reducing to 20 cm^2 (10 mg/16 hours) for 4 weeks **OR**
- (chewing gum) one piece of gum when the person feels the urge to smoke, normally 8–12 pieces of 2 mg strength gum or 8–10 pieces of 4 mg strength gum per day, for 12 weeks, then reducing amount over next 4 weeks (daily maximum 40 mg) **OR**
- (inhalator) 3–6 cartridges daily taking puffs that mimic normal cigarette smoking for 12 weeks, then reducing dose over 6–8 weeks (daily maximum 6 cartridges) **OR**
- (lozenge) 1 lozenge orally 1–2-hourly for 6 weeks, then 1 lozenge orally 2–4-hourly for 3 weeks, then 1 lozenge 4–8-hourly for 3 weeks, then 1 lozenge when strongly tempted to smoke for next 12 weeks (daily maximum 15–20 lozenges depending on cigarette habit) **OR**
- (oral spray) 1–2 sprays when person feels urge to smoke (up to 64 sprays per 24 hours) for 6 weeks, then decreasing number of sprays over next 3 weeks (to about half previous number), then further reducing number of sprays to no more than 4 per day for 3 weeks

Adverse effects

- headache, dizziness, nervousness, tremor, sleep disturbances, including insomnia and abnormal dreams
- nausea, vomiting, dyspepsia, flatulence, abdominal pain, diarrhoea, dry mouth, constipation
- palpitations
- increased sweating
- cough, dyspnoea, pharyngitis
- arthralgia, myalgia
- nicotine withdrawal syndrome (craving, irritability, anxiety, impaired concentration, dizziness, nausea, vomiting, abdominal pain, sweating, flushing, confusion)
- (chewing gum) hiccups, jaw muscle ache, sore mouth/throat, diarrhoea
- (transdermal patch) erythema, urticaria, itching, rash, swelling, pain, burning, tingling, numbness, heavy sensation at application site or surrounding limb and uncommonly, hypersensitivity
- (inhaler) mouth/throat irritation, cough, nasal congestion, hiccups
- (lozenge) hiccups, mouth/throat irritation and ulceration, burning sensation, dry mouth, bloating, belching, dysphagia, heartburn, indigestion
- (oral spray) mouth/throat irritation, hiccups, cough, mouth ulcers, gum bleeding, nasopharyngitis

Interactions

- cessation of smoking may alter response to concurrently used medications, with or without nicotine substitutes
- smoking increases metabolism (and decreases blood levels) of caffeine,

theophylline, insulin, fluvoxamine, olanzapine, clomipramine, clozapine, paracetamol, oestrogens, prazosin, labetalol, lidocaine (lignocaine), warfarin and imipramine, and therefore ceasing smoking will lead to increased blood levels. Other agents that require close monitoring include antiepileptics, furosemide, propranolol, H_2-antagonists, isoprenaline, phenylephrine and nifedipine
- may enhance effects of adenosine

Nursing points/Cautions

- if person relapses on monotherapy, combination (e.g. transdermal patch plus gum/lozenge/oral spray/inhaler) may be used. However, only 2 mg strength lozenge/gum should be used as combination therapy (not 4 mg strength)
- (transdermal patches) available in a variety of strengths, so ensure the correct strength is selected (e.g. a patch labelled 21 mg/day means that a total of 21 mg of nicotine is absorbed over 24 hours). Dimensional measures (cm^2) refer to the drug releasing area, not patch size
- (oral spray) therapy should be stopped when patient is only using 2–4 sprays per day. Regular use for longer than 6 months is not recommended
- (chewing gum) contains sorbitol, which is not recommended in those with hereditary fructose intolerance and may have laxative effect in others
- (chewing gum) caution if used by those with dentures (as chewing may be difficult) or if oral inflammation is present
- (inhalator) offers an alternative to patches and gum that addresses behavioural dependence ('hand-to-mouth' action) as well as physical dependence
- (inhaler/inhalator) caution if used in those with asthma or chronic throat conditions
- (lozenge) contains 15 mg sodium per lozenge which may need to be considered in a low-sodium diet
- (lozenge) contains aspartame and is therefore contraindicated in those with phenylketonuria
- (lozenge) caution if used in those with any oral inflammation
- (transdermal patches) caution if used in those with history of dermatitis
- caution if used in those with diabetes when nicotine replacement therapy is started, as carbohydrate metabolism may be affected and therefore impact on blood glucose levels. Vasoconstriction may also reduce insulin absorption
- combination therapy (using more than one nicotine preparation at the same time) is not recommended in those with known cardiovascular disease
- (oral) caution if used in those with active gastric/duodenal ulcers or oesophagitis as symptoms may become exacerbated
- caution if used in those with moderate-to-severe liver or kidney impairment, uncontrolled hypertension, vasospasm, heart failure, stable angina, cerebrovascular disease or occlusive peripheral arterial disease
- caution if used in those with hyperthyroidism or pheochromocytoma
- caution if used in those with susceptibility to angioedema and/or urticarial
- (Nicabate P) contraindicated in those who smoke < 10 cigarettes/day or weigh < 45 kg
- (transdermal patches) contraindicated in those with chronic dermatological conditions such as urticaria and psoriasis

- (all nicotine products) contraindicated in those who are non-tobacco users, within 3 months of myocardial infarction, in those who have unstable angina, variant (Prinzmetal) angina, severe cardiac arrhythmias or acute phase of stroke

Patient teaching and advice

- advise patient of counselling facilities that may assist, such as Quitline (Australia: 13 78 48; New Zealand: 0800 778778)
- instruct patient to keep nicotine-containing products out of reach of children and ensure used products are safely disposed of, because poisoning in children can be fatal
- patient with diabetes should be advised to monitor blood glucose levels during therapy, as well as after quitting smoking altogether
- warn patient that if they continue to smoke while using nicotine-containing products (or using multiple products concurrently), the risk of adverse effects (especially cardiovascular) is greatly increased
- patient should be cautioned against abrupt withdrawal from nicotine products to avoid withdrawal syndrome (dysphoria, depression, insomnia, irritability, anger, frustration, anxiety, impaired concentration, impatience, restlessness, decreased heart rate, increased appetite and weight gain)
- nicotine is dangerous in small children and can be fatal. Patients should be warned to keep nicotine replacement therapy products out of reach of children

Transdermal patches

- advise patient to:
  - rotate sites daily (using upper thigh, upper body and upper outer arm)
  - apply to clean, non-hairy skin
  - avoid areas that are red, irritated or broken skin or creases
  - same application site should not be reused within 7 days to avoid adverse skin reaction
  - bathing, swimming and showering are permissible as long as patch is correctly applied
  - wash hands thoroughly after application or removal of patch
  - avoid contact with eyes or sensitive skin
  - remove transdermal patch if undergoing MRI procedure
  - discard used patches safely (folded in half with sticky side innermost)
- Nicorette patches should be applied in the morning and removed at night (16-hour use), whereas QuitX and Nicabate are left on the skin for 24 hours. However, if the person is experiencing sleep disturbance, the patch may be removed at bedtime
- withdrawal from patches should be gradual, beginning at about 12 weeks and being completed by approximately week 16. Withdrawal consists of reducing patch strength over a number of weeks (e.g. for a person starting on a 30 cm^2 patch, reduce to a 20 cm^2 patch for 2 weeks, followed by a 10 cm^2 patch for 2 weeks before final withdrawal). Soft gum or lozenges may be used with the patches during this withdrawal period
- patient should be advised that if they continue to smoke or chew nicotine-containing gum while using transdermal patches, they are at risk of greater adverse effects because of the added amount of nicotine
- instruct patient to stop using patches and seek medical advice if they experience persistent (4 days) or severe local skin reactions at application site or generalised skin reactions, including rash, hives or urticaria

Chewing gum

- gum is available in different strengths, so ensure that correct strength is selected with 4 mg gum recommended for those who smoke > 20 cigarettes/day
- patient should be instructed in the correct use of the gum before starting therapy, including:
  - only use 1 piece of chewing gum at a time and no more than 20 pieces/day (2 mg) or 10 pieces/day (4 mg)
  - use 1 piece of chewing gum per hour only
  - chew gum slowly until strong taste or slight tingling is felt
  - when this occurs, gum should be placed under the tongue or between the cheek and gums until the taste or tingling has disappeared
  - chewing may then be slowly resumed and the procedure repeated until the effects are no longer felt (about 30 minutes)
  - avoid rapid chewing as this may result in hiccups, nausea or irritation to the mouth/throat
  - any nicotine swallowed is destroyed by the liver
- if indigestion or heartburn occurs with 4 mg gum, changing to 2 mg gum, chewing slowly and increasing frequency of use (if needed) may reduce symptoms
- instruct patient to avoid acidic drinks (e.g. coffee, soft drinks) for 15 minutes before using gum, because the acid interferes with nicotine absorption
- patient should be warned that overdose may occur if multiple pieces of gum are chewed together or in rapid succession
- after 3 months, patient should be advised to reduce the number of pieces chewed daily gradually to 1–2 pieces/day and then stop completely
- if therapy extends beyond 9 months, patient should be advised to seek medical advice as alternate strategies may be required for successful quitting to occur
- warn patient that because of mannitol and sorbitol content in gum, excessive use may result in diarrhoea
- advise patient that gum (2 mg) may be used with transdermal patches

Inhaler/Inhalator

- instruct patient on correct use including:
  - sealed cartridge is put into mouthpiece, which is then reassembled and seals both ends of the broken cartridge. Nicotine is vaporised and absorbed as air is inhaled through the cartridge
  - technique depends on person's preference and smoking habit (e.g. can be used intensely or using a slower technique)
  - each cartridge equals 7 cigarettes (about 80 puffs)
  - if craving is not relieved, number of puffs, size of puffs or how often used should be increased (however, not greater than 6 cartridges over 24 hours)
  - opened cartridge should only be used for 24 hours and then discarded
- patient should be instructed not to eat or drink during inhaler therapy
- instruct patient to avoid acidic drinks (e.g. coffee, soft drinks) for 15 minutes before using inhaler, because the acid interferes with nicotine absorption

Lozenge

- those who have first cigarette of day more than 30 minutes after waking should be advised to use 2 mg strength lozenge; however, if person has first cigarette of day less than 30 minutes after waking, 4 mg strength lozenge should be used

- advise patient that lozenge should not be chewed or swallowed whole. The lozenge should be placed in mouth and allowed to dissolve over 20–30 minutes, moving lozenge from one side of the mouth to the other
- patient should be advised to only use one lozenge at a time
- patient should be instructed to refrain from eating or drinking until lozenge is totally dissolved
- instruct patient to avoid acidic drinks (e.g. coffee, soft drinks) for 15 minutes before using lozenge, because the acid interferes with nicotine absorption
- after 12 weeks of therapy, patient should be counselled to take 1 lozenge if smoking urge is strong

Oral spray

- ensure patient understands how to use oral spray, including:
  - prime device before first use, or if unused for 2 days, by pointing nozzle away from self or anyone else and pressing several times until a fine spray occurs
  - pointing spray nozzle towards open mouth (as close as possible) and pressing to release one spray (avoiding lips)
  - not inhaling while spraying to prevent spray in throat
  - not swallowing for a few seconds after spraying
  - if second spray is required, repeat steps
  - avoiding contact with eyes. If this occurs, eye should be rinsed thoroughly with water
  - ensuring device is safely closed after each use
- advise patient to not use more than 2 sprays per episode and no more than 64 sprays in 24 hours (4 sprays per hour over 16 hours)
- may be combined with transdermal patches (no more than 2 sprays per hour, or 32 sprays per day)
- instruct patient to avoid acidic drinks (e.g. coffee, soft drinks) for 15 minutes before using oral spray, because the acid interferes with nicotine absorption

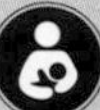

nicotine is harmful to the fetus, but risk from nicotine replacement therapy appears to be lower than from smoking. Nicotine affects fetal breathing and has a dose-dependent impact on placental/fetal circulation. Lozenges and gum are preferred as daily dose is lower than for patches

nicotine is found in breastmilk. Patches are not recommended during breastfeeding. Gum or lozenges should be used just before breastfeeding to allow maximum time between therapy and breastfeeding

VARENICLINE TARTRATE (Champix)

Available forms

Tablets: 0.5 mg, 1 mg

Action

- has both agonist (alleviating craving and withdrawal symptoms) and antagonist (blocking reward and reinforcing effects of smoking) activity
- highly selective, binding to alpha-4 beta-2 receptor, thereby blocking nicotine from binding to the same site
- as efficacious as combination nicotine replacement therapy (NRT) but greater efficacy than monotherapy NRT
- considered first-line treatment
- half-life 10–58 hours

Use

- aid to smoking cessation

Dose

- 0.5 mg orally daily (days 1–3), then 0.5 mg orally twice daily (days 4–7), then 1 mg orally twice daily (day 8 and remainder of therapy)

Adverse effects

- nausea, vomiting, dyspepsia, dry mouth, diarrhoea, constipation, flatulence, abdominal pain/distention, altered taste, increased or decreased appetite, weight gain
- headache, fatigue, dizziness, somnolence, insomnia, abnormal dreams, nightmares, agitation, irritability, disturbed attention
- nasopharyngitis, sinusitis, cough, dyspnoea
- rash, pruritus
- back pain, arthralgia, myalgia
- (uncommon) altered mood, abnormal thinking, restlessness, decreased libido
- (uncommon) hypertension, chest pain
- (rare) seizures, angioedema, severe skin reactions, sleepwalking

Interactions

- smoking impacts on pharmacokinetics of many agents and this should be considered when ceasing smoking as dose adjustments may be necessary
- not recommended with cimetidine in those with severe kidney impairment
- increased risk of adverse effects if taken with nicotine replacement therapy
- caution if used with alcohol as it may increase risk of neuropsychiatric adverse effects as well as increasing alcohol's effects

Nursing points/Cautions

- before starting therapy, patient should set a target date to stop smoking and therapy started 1–2 weeks before the target date. Alternatively, patient can start therapy and stop smoking between days 8 and 35
- therapy should go for 12 weeks: for those who successfully stop smoking in this time, 1 mg twice daily is recommended for a further 12 weeks to reinforce abstinence; for those not successful in 12 weeks (or who relapse), factors contributing to failure should be identified and dealt with before recommencing therapy
- stopping smoking may be associated with exacerbation of underlying psychiatric diseases and these should be identified before starting therapy
- caution if used in those with history of seizures or cardiovascular disease

Patient teaching and advice

- instruct patient to take tablets whole (not divided or chewed) with glass of water
- patient should be advised not to drive or operate machinery if fatigue, dizziness and sleep problems are ongoing problems
- warn patient that when therapy is stopped, increased irritability, urge to smoke, depression and/or insomnia commonly occur
- counsel patient to identify other strategies to help quit including other activities (e.g. eating healthy snacks, exercise, drinking water slowly, chewing sugar-free gum) that take his/her mind off smoking, as well as identifying other situations (such as socialising with other friends who smoke, drinking alcohol, reducing coffee intake) where smoking is a 'normal' activity for that person
- patient (or partner/family member) should be advised to report any thoughts/talk about self-harm, harm to others, suicide or death or recent attempts at self-harm or change in mood including signs of depression, agitation and/or anxiety
- advise patient to seek medical advice immediately if any of the following occur:
    - rash or sudden severe itching
    - severe painful red blisters, chills, fever, feeling unwell
    - swelling of face, lips, eyes, throat
    - fitting (seizures)

  - sleepwalking
  - any new or worsening heart symptoms including chest pain
- warn patient that intoxicating effects of alcohol may be increased, as well as increasing risk of neuropsychiatric adverse effects such as altered mood or abnormal thinking
- see also General Patient teaching and advice (p. xxvii)

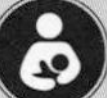

not recommended during pregnancy or breastfeeding

ERECTILE DYSFUNCTION AGENTS

Sensory or mental stimulation begins penile erection, as impulses from the brain and local nerves cause relaxation of the corpora cavernosa muscles, allowing blood to flow in. This causes an increase in pressure, resulting in expansion of the penis. The erection is maintained because the tunica albuginea traps the blood. When the penile muscles contract, the inflow of blood is stopped and the outflow channels open, thereby reversing the erection.

Erectile dysfunction commonly (10–25%) occurs in middle-aged or elderly men, but is not considered a normal part of ageing (McVary 2019). Erectile dysfunction usually occurs for one of three reasons (although these can occur together or separately):

- failure to initiate (psychogenic, endocrinologic or neurogenic)
- failure to fill (arteriogenic), and/or
- failure to store adequate blood volume within lacunar network (veno-occlusive dysfunction) (McVary 2019).

Commonly implicated conditions in erectile dysfunction include penile problems (e.g. injury to the penis); problems with the muscles, fibrous tissues, veins or arteries (arteriogenic) in or near the corpora cavernosa; diabetes mellitus; obesity; heart disease; hypertension; general systemic inflammatory diseases (e.g. rheumatoid arthritis); chronic alcoholism; neurological diseases (e.g. multiple sclerosis) or spinal cord injury. Surgery or radiation therapy (e.g. prostate or bladder surgery for cancer), commonly prescribed medications (e.g. antihypertensive agents, diuretics, SSRIs, TCAs, lithium, phenothiazines and cimetidine) and recreational agents (e.g. alcohol, cocaine, marijuana) can also produce erectile dysfunction as an adverse effect (McVary 2019). Furthermore, smoking, hormonal abnormalities and psychological (psychogenic) factors (e.g. stress, anxiety, guilt, depression, anger) are also implicated.

It is important that underlying causes are investigated and treated (if possible) before starting therapy with erectile dysfunction agents. Other management strategies include androgen therapy, vacuum constriction devices, surgery and sex therapy (McVary 2019).

INTRACAVERNOSAL ADMINISTRATION

General Adverse effects of intracavernosal administration

- pain (including burning sensation and tension) in penis during erection, penile fibrosis, prolonged erection (lasting 4–6 hours), priapism (erection lasting > 6 hours)
- (injection site) bleeding, haematoma, oedema, inflammation, itching, swelling

General Interactions of intracavernosal administration

- increased risk of bleeding if given with anticoagulants
- not recommended with other erectile dysfunction agents

General Nursing points/Cautions for intracavernosal administration

- medical causes of erectile dysfunction should be examined before use of erectile dysfunction agents and penile fibrosis should be excluded
- first injection should be administered by medical personnel and the patient educated in self-administration techniques
- dose should be sufficient for erection lasting no longer than 1 hour for satisfactory sexual intercourse
- contraindicated in women or children
- contraindicated in men who are predisposed to priapism (e.g. leukaemia, sickle cell anaemia), have a deformed penis, penile fibrosis or penile implant or if sexual activity is not advisable or contraindicated

General Patient teaching and advice for intracavernosal administration

- patient should be advised to visit specialist regularly to establish efficacy and dose, as well as for examination for penile fibrosis
- instruct and assess patient (or partner) in:
  - correct self-injection technique
  - reconstitution of powder or dialling of dose
  - not injecting more than once daily or 3 times per week
  - cleaning area with alcohol swab before injection
  - rotating injection sites, not using midline or underside of penis for injection, and taking care to avoid veins
  - not using bent needles or attempting to straighten bent needles, because this increases the risk of needle breakage during administration. If needle breakage occurs, patient should attend emergency department immediately
  - performing injection while upright, standing or slightly reclining
  - massaging after injection to help solution distribute through penis
  - applying pressure to injection site for 5 minutes or until bleeding stops
  - using equipment once only
  - safe disposal of injection equipment
- in titrating dose, patient should be advised to halve dose if erection lasts for more than 1 hour
- small amounts of blood may be present at the injection site and patient

should be advised about the possibility of blood-borne diseases and their spread
- counsel patient regarding the need to use barrier methods (e.g. condom) to protect against sexually transmitted or blood-borne diseases
- instruct patient to seek medical attention immediately if:
  - erection lasts for longer than 4 hours. Patient should be advised to empty bladder, try walking around, take a shower and avoid sexual contact before seeking medical attention
  - any new or increased penile pain, penile bending or nodule formation in shaft occurs
- see also General Patient teaching and advice (p. xxvii)

ALPROSTADIL (prostaglandin E1) (Caverject Impulse, Prostin VR)

Available forms
Disposable syringe device (powder and diluent): 10 microgram, 20 microgram; Ampoules: 500 microgram/mL (for treatment of ductus arteriosus)

Action
- vasodilator, prevents platelet aggregation
- relaxes trabecular smooth muscle and dilates cavernosal arteries, inducing erection in men with erectile dysfunction, with erection starting 5–20 minutes after administration and duration being dose dependent

Use
- erectile dysfunction in adult men (treatment and diagnosis)
- to maintain patency of the ductus arteriosus in neonates with congenital heart failure until surgery is possible (see Vasodilators, p. 1569)

Dose
- (erectile dysfunction treatment) initially 2.5–5 microgram intracavernosally, increasing by 2.5–5.0 microgram increments until satisfactory response is achieved (usually 10–20 microgram) (no more than once daily or 3 times per week) **OR**
- (erectile dysfunction diagnosis) initially 2.5 microgram intracavernosally, increasing by 2.5 microgram increments

Adverse effects/interaction
- see General Adverse effects and Interactions of intracavernosal administration (p. 1050)

Nursing points/Cautions
- starting dose is dependent on cause of erectile dysfunction. If cause is unknown or due to neurogenic/psychogenic causes, starting dose is 2.5 microgram, increasing in 2.5 microgram increments. If cause is arteriogenic (or other cause), starting dose is 5 microgram with increments of 5 microgram
- see General Nursing points/Cautions for intracavernosal administration (p. 1050)

Patient teaching and advice
- instruct patient that reconstituted solution can be refrigerated for up to 24 hours if not used
- patient (and partner) should be advised not to inhale particles or expose skin to alprostadil
- see General Patient teaching and Advice for intracavernosal administration (p. 1050)

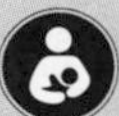

semen may contain small amounts of alprostadil, which stimulates uterine smooth muscle. Use of condoms is therefore recommended if partner is pregnant

Note
- Prostin VR is not used for erectile dysfunction

PAPAVERINE HYDROCHLORIDE (DBL Papaverine Hydrochloride Injection)

Available forms
Ampoules: 30 mg/mL, 120 mg/10 mL

Action
- relaxes arteriolar smooth muscle, leading to penile erection
- spasmolytic effect is pronounced in coronary, cerebral, pulmonary and peripheral vessels
- relaxes smooth muscles of bronchial, GI, biliary and urinary tracts
- direct inotropic effect, increasing myocardial oxygen consumption, decreasing myocardial excitability, prolonging refractory period and depressing myocardial conductivity
- erection within 10 minutes of injection, duration > 1 hour, short half-life 1–2 hours

Use
- erectile dysfunction

Dose
- initially 15 mg intracavernosally, increasing or decreasing dose to achieve required result (up to 60 mg) **OR**
- (erectile dysfunction caused by spinal cord injury) initially 5 mg intracavernosally, then titrating dose to required response

Adverse effects
- liver function abnormalities
- headache, flushing, heat sensation in pelvis, dizziness
- retinal irritation (seeing sparks or flashes)
- tachycardia, hypotension
- syncope, vasovagal reaction
- allergic reaction, urticaria
- tolerance (with long-term use)
- impaired ejaculation, loss of penile sensation, thrombophlebitis
- (high dose) cardiac arrhythmias, apnoea
- see also General Adverse effects of intracavernosal administration (p. 1050)

Interactions
- may be potentiated by CNS depressants
- may result in synergistic action if given with morphine
- may interfere with levodopa, therefore not recommended for use together
- not recommended with alprostadil due to risk of dizziness and syncope
- see General Interactions of intracavernosal administration (p. 1050)

Nursing points/Cautions
- see General Nursing points/Cautions for intracavernosal administration (p. 1050)
- ECG is recommended in the elderly before starting therapy to rule out any cardiac conduction disorders
- if patient does not respond to 60 mg dose, other therapies should be considered
- if erection lasts longer than 4 hours, dose should be reduced
- if tolerance occurs with long-term use, an increase in dose may be required
- baseline and 6-monthly liver function tests are recommended in those males who have liver disease or a history of alcohol abuse
- patients with psychogenic erectile dysfunction are more likely to respond to lower doses while higher doses may be required in those with vasculogenic erectile dysfunction
- incompatible with lactated Ringer's solution as precipitate will form

- caution in those males who have liver impairment, cardiac conduction disorders or who have unstable cardiovascular disease
- contraindicated in men with complete AV block

Patient teaching and advice

- advise patient to take care rising from lying or sitting position or when climbing stairs due to risk of postural hypotension
- patient should be instructed to seek medical advice immediately if any of the following occur:
  - rapid or unusual heart rate, fainting
  - yellowing of eyes or skin, dark urine, upper abdominal pain, lethargy, nausea, loss of appetite, light bowel motions
- see also General Patient teaching and advice for intracavernosal administration (p. 1050)

PHOSPHODIESTERASE TYPE 5 (PDE5) INHIBITORS

General Actions of PDE5 inhibitors

- sexual stimulation leads to an increase in nitrous oxide levels that leads to an increase in cyclic guanosine monophosphate (cGMP) which relaxes smooth muscle
- inhibits specific phosphodiesterase type 5 (main phosphodiesterase in human corpora cavernosa) (commonly known as a PDE5 inhibitor) that breaks down cGMP, resulting in relaxation of smooth muscle and flow of blood into penile tissue producing erection
- effective in a broad range of reasons for erectile dysfunction, including psychogenic, diabetic, vasculogenic, post-radical prostatectomy (nerve-sparing procedures) and spinal cord injury
- may also inhibit phosphodiesterase type 6 involved in phototransduction cascade in the retina

General Adverse effects of PDE5 inhibitors

- headache, flushing, dizziness
- dyspepsia, diarrhoea
- nasal and sinus congestion, rhinitis
- urinary tract infection
- abnormal vision (including increased sensitivity to light, blurred vision, colour tinge in vision)
- rash
- (uncommon) angina, tachycardia, palpitations, transient hypotension, dyspnoea, hearing impairment, tinnitus
- (rare) myocardial ischaemia, arrhythmias, non-arteritic anterior ischaemic optic neuropathy (NAION), prolonged erection, priapism, allergic reaction

General Interactions of PDE5 inhibitors

- contraindicated with nitrates (via any route), including glyceryl trinitrate, isosorbide salts, sodium nitroprusside, amyl nitrite and nicorandil
- serum levels may be increased if given with cimetidine, clarithromycin, erythromycin, indinavir, itraconazole, saquinavir, ritonavir, telithromycin or voriconazole, and are therefore contraindicated together

- serum levels may be decreased if given with rifampicin, phenobarbital (phenobarbitone), phenytoin or carbamazepine
- caution if given with alpha adrenoceptor blocking agents (e.g. prazosin) as hypotension may occur. Patient should be haemodynamically stable for introduction of PDE5 inhibitor therapy, which should be started at a low dose
- increased risk of hypotension if given with riociguat
- not recommended with alcohol

General Nursing points/Cautions for PDE5 inhibitors

- patient should have a thorough medical and physical examination (especially cardiovascular assessment) before starting therapy. Reasons for erectile dysfunction should be investigated before starting therapy
- erectile dysfunction agents are not indicated for use in women
- caution if used in men with severe kidney impairment, cardiovascular disease with left ventricular outflow obstruction (e.g. aortic stenosis), predisposition to priapism (e.g. sickle cell anaemia, leukaemia, multiple myeloma), deformity of the penis, diabetic retinopathy, bleeding disorders, conditions that are sensitive to hypotension or multiple system atrophy (with impaired blood pressure control)
- contraindicated in those men for whom sexual activity is not recommended due to heart failure, unstable angina or uncontrolled arrhythmias, recent stroke (within 6 months) or myocardial infarction (90 days), hypertension (BP > 170/110), hypotension (BP < 90/50), severe liver impairment, known hereditary degenerative retinal disorders (e.g. retinitis pigmentosa), if they have had vision loss due to NAION or hypersensitivity to PDE5 inhibitors

General Patient teaching and advice for PDE5 inhibitors

- warn patient not to exceed daily dose and only use once per day
- patient should be advised not to combine therapies for erectile dysfunction
- instruct patient to take medication about 1 hour before intending to have sex
- advise patient against driving or operating machinery if dizziness or visual disturbances occur
- patient should be advised to stop therapy and immediately seek medical advice if any of the following occur:
  - loss of vision to one or both eyes occurs (non-arteritic anterior ischaemic optic neuropathy (NAION))
  - changes to vision (blurring, sensitivity to light, blue tinge)
  - decrease or loss of hearing or ringing/buzzing in the ears
  - persistent headache
  - unusual heart rate or chest pain
  - prolonged erection lasting longer than 4 hours (as damage to penile tissue may occur)
- ensure patient understands that alcohol may impair the ability to obtain an erection
- see also General Patient teaching and advice (p. xxvii)

AVANAFIL (Spedra)

Available forms
Tablets: 50 mg, 100 mg, 200 mg

Action
- see General Actions of PDE5 inhibitors (p. 1053)
- active metabolites
- half-life 6–17 hours

Use
- erectile dysfunction in adult males

Dose
- 100 mg orally once daily 15–30 minutes before sexual activity (maximum daily dose 200 mg)

Adverse effects
- see General Adverse effects and Interactions of PDE5 inhibitors (p. 1053)
- backache, arthralgia
- nasopharyngitis, sinusitis, bronchitis, influenza
- hypertension

Interactions
- see General Interactions of PDE5 inhibitors (p. 1053)
- contraindicated with nitrates (via any route), including glyceryl trinitrate, isosorbide salts, sodium nitroprusside, amyl nitrite and nicorandil. If nitrates are medically needed because of a life-threatening situation, a minimum of a 12-hour interval should be allowed between avanafil and nitrate
- caution if used with vasodilators or antihypertensive agents due to risk of symptomatic hypotension
- not recommended with bosentan or grapefruit juice
- increased serum levels may occur if given with erythromycin, amprenavir, aprepitant, diltiazem, fluconazole, fosamprenavir or verapamil. If used together, avanafil dose should be restricted to 100 mg every 48 hours

Nursing points/Cautions
- dose can be decreased to 50 mg or increased to 200 mg once daily if needed
- contraindicated in those with severe liver impairment (Child-Pugh C) or severe kidney impairment (creatinine clearance < 30 mL/minute), chronic kidney disease stage 4 or end-stage kidney failure
- see also General Nursing points/Cautions for PDE5 inhibitors (p. 1054)

Patient teaching and advice
- see General Patient teaching and advice for PDE5 inhibitors (p. 1054)
- advise patient to avoid grapefruit juice for at least 24 hours before taking avanafil
- warn patient that onset of activity may be delayed if taken with food

SILDENAFIL (Noumed, Revatio, Silcap, Sildatio PHT, Vasafil, Vedafil, Viagra, Wafesil)

Available forms
Tablets: 20 mg, 25 mg, 50 mg, 100 mg; Wafers: 25 mg, 50 mg; Vial: 10 mg/12.5 mL

Action
- see General Actions of PDE5 inhibitors (p. 1053)
- PDE5 is also found in pulmonary vascular smooth muscle, therefore in those with pulmonary hypertension it can lead to selective vasodilation of pulmonary vascular bed and some vasodilation of systemic circulation
- active metabolite (half-life 4 hours)
- half-life 3–5 hours

Use
- erectile dysfunction in adult males (Noumed, Silaran, Silcap, Sildatio, Vasafil, Vedafil, Viagra, Wafesil)

- pulmonary arterial hypertension (PAH) (WHO functional classes II and III) to improve exercise capacity or secondary to connective/collagen tissue disease (Revatio)

Dose

- (erectile dysfunction) 25–100 mg orally once daily 1 hour before sexual activity (maximum daily dose 100 mg) **OR**
- (erectile dysfunction) initially 50 mg sublingually once daily 1 hour before sexual activity (maximum daily dose 100 mg) (wafers) **OR**
- (PAH) 20 mg orally 3 times daily **OR**
- (PAH) 10 mg by IV bolus 3 times daily

Adverse effects

- (PAH) myalgia, cough, fever, epistaxis, vertigo
- fluid retention, weight increase, paraesthesia
- (IV) flushing, flatulence
- see also General Adverse effects of PDE5 inhibitors (p. 1053)

Interactions

- (PAH) serum levels may be decreased by bosentan
- (PAH) may increase serum levels of bosentan
- (PAH) not recommended with other PDE5 inhibitors
- (PAH) increased risk of epistaxis if given with vitamin K antagonist such as warfarin
- (PAH) contraindicated with ritonavir
- serum levels may increase if given with grapefruit juice
- see also General Interactions of PDE5 inhibitors (p. 1053)

Nursing points/Cautions

- (PAH) IV administration is recommended in those who are temporarily unable to take oral therapy but are haemodynamically stable
- (PAH) blood pressure should be carefully monitored during IV administration
- (PAH) therapy should be stopped gradually and patient carefully monitored during this period
- (PAH) caution if used in those with bleeding disorders or active peptic ulceration or over 65 years
- (IV) not recommended if patient is clinically or haemodynamically unstable, under 18 years or with pulmonary veno-occlusive disease
- (PAH) not recommended in those with severe pulmonary hypertension (functional class IV) or with pulmonary arterial hypertension with previous episode of non-arteritic anterior ischaemic optic neuropathy (NAION)
- (PAH) contraindicated in those with severe liver impairment
- see also General Nursing points/Cautions for PDE5 inhibitors (p. 1054)

Patient teaching and advice

- patient should be warned that absorption will be decreased if taken with a high-fat meal and therefore take longer to work
- advise patient not to take with grapefruit juice
- (wafers) instruct patient on the following:
    - do not remove wafer from foil until just before administration
    - do not push wafer through foil packet
    - handle wafer with dry hands
    - rinse mouth with water before administration
    - do not chew, suck, swallow, eat or drink until wafer has totally dissolved
    - (one wafer dose) place wafer under tongue and allow to dissolve
    - (two wafer dose) place wafers under tongue on opposite sides and allow to dissolve
- see also General Patient teaching and advice for PDE5 inhibitors (p. 1054)

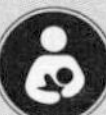

caution if used during pregnancy as no adequate or controlled studies have been conducted in pregnant women

not recommended during breastfeeding

available as sublingual wafer which will dissolve in mouth. Tablet can be dispersed in water and mixed with strong-flavoured drink to disguise taste or crushed and mixed with spoonful of yoghurt, apple puree, honey or jam

TADALAFIL (Adcirca, Cialis, Ciavor, Cidala, Tadacip, Tadalaccord, Tadalca, Tadalis)

Available forms

Tablets: 5 mg, 10 mg, 20 mg

Action

- see General Actions of PDE5 inhibitors (p. 1053)
- PDE5 is also found in pulmonary vascular smooth muscle, therefore in those with pulmonary hypertension, can lead to selective vasodilation of pulmonary vascular bed and some vasodilation of systemic circulation
- half-life 17.5 hours (prolonged to 22 hours in those over 65 years)

Use

- erectile dysfunction in adult males (Cialis)
- moderate-to-severe lower urinary tract symptoms associated with benign prostatic hyperplasia (Cialis)
- pulmonary arterial hypertension (PAH) (WHO functional classes II and III) to improve exercise capacity, idiopathic PAH or PAH secondary to connective/collagen tissue disease (Adcirca)

Dose

- (erectile dysfunction, on demand dosing) 10–20 mg orally 30–60 minutes prior to sexual activity once daily only (daily maximum 20 mg) **OR**
- (erectile dysfunction) 2.5–5 mg orally once daily **OR**
- (benign prostatic hyperplasia) 5 mg orally daily **OR**
- (PAH) 40 mg orally daily

Adverse effects

- myalgia, back pain, pain in extremities
- epistaxis
- (PAH) abnormal or excessive menstrual bleeding
- see also General Adverse effects of PDE5 inhibitors (p. 1053)

Interactions

- (PAH) not recommended with other PDE5 inhibitors
- serum levels may be decreased by bosentan
- see also General Interactions of PDE5 inhibitors (p. 1053)

Nursing points/Cautions

- (benign prostatic hyperplasia) prostate cancer and other causes for lower urinary tract symptoms should be excluded before starting therapy
- tablets contain lactose, therefore not recommended in those with rare hereditary problems of galactose intolerance, Lapp lactase deficiency or glucose–galactose malabsorption
- (PAH) caution if used in those who could be affected by vasodilation such as those with severe left ventricular outflow obstruction, fluid depletion, autonomic hypotension or resting hypotension
- (PAH) not recommended in those with pulmonary veno-occlusive disease
- caution if used in those with creatinine clearance ≤ 50 mL/minute
- see also General Nursing points/Cautions for PDE5 inhibitors (p. 1054)

Patient teaching and advice

- (daily dosing) advise patient to take dose at the same time every day
- see General Patient teaching and advice for PDE5 inhibitors (p. 1054)

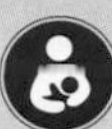

(PAH) should only be used during pregnancy if benefits are thought to outweigh risks

caution if used during breastfeeding

tablet can be crushed and mixed with water or spoonful of yoghurt or apple puree

VARDENAFIL (Levitra)

Available forms
Tablets: 5 mg, 10 mg, 20 mg

Action
- see General Actions of PDE5 inhibitors (p. 1053)
- active metabolite
- half-life 4–5 hours

Use
- erectile dysfunction in adult males

Dose
- initially 10 mg orally once daily 25–60 minutes before sexual intercourse, increasing or decreasing dose if needed (daily maximum dose 20 mg)

Adverse effects
- see General Adverse effects of PDE5 inhibitors (p. 1053)

Interactions
- see General Interactions of PDE5 inhibitors (p. 1053)
- not recommended with agents that prolong QT interval

Nursing points/Cautions
- not recommended in those with history of QT prolongation
- contraindicated in those with end-stage kidney disease requiring dialysis
- see also General Nursing points/Cautions for PDE5 inhibitors (p. 1054)

Patient teaching and advice
- see General Patient teaching and advice for PDE5 inhibitors (p. 1054)

tablet can be crushed and mixed with spoonful of yoghurt or apple puree

OTHER AGENTS

DAPOXETINE (Priligy)

Available form
Tablets: 30 mg

Action
- selective serotonin reuptake inhibitor (SSRI)
- ejaculation is mediated by sympathetic nervous system and action is thought to be due to inhibition of serotonin uptake and potentiation at pre- and post-synaptic receptors
- equipotent active metabolite
- half-life 19 hours (with similar half-life for active metabolite)

Use
- treatment of premature ejaculation in men (18–64 years) who have intravaginal ejaculatory latency time < 2 minutes; persistent or recurrent ejaculation with minimal sexual stimulation before, on or shortly after penetration and before patient wishes; marked personal distress; interpersonal difficulty as a consequence of premature ejaculation and poor control over ejaculation

Dose
- 30 mg orally 1–3 hours before sexual activity (daily maximum 30 mg)

Adverse effects

- syncope (with or without prodromal symptoms)
- orthostatic/postural hypotension
- headache, dizziness, somnolence, insomnia, disturbed dreams, irritability, anxiety, fatigue, restlessness, disturbed attention, tremor
- paraesthesia
- back pain
- blurred vision
- tinnitus
- flushing, sweating
- nausea, diarrhoea, dry mouth, vomiting, constipation, abdominal pain, flatulence, dyspepsia
- nasopharyngitis, influenza, sinusitis, yawning
- cough
- erectile dysfunction, decreased libido
- (uncommon) depression, loss of libido, tachycardia, visual disturbances, eye pain, mydriasis, bleeding

Interactions

- contraindicated with or within 14 days of stopping MAOIs because of increased risk of serotonin syndrome. MAOIs should not be administered within 7 days of stopping dapoxetine
- contraindicated with or within 14 days of stopping SSRIs, SNRIs, TCAs or serotonergic agents such as linezolid, sumatriptan, tramadol, tryptophan, fentanyl, lithium, St John's wort. These agents should not be administered within 7 days of stopping dapoxetine
- contraindicated with azole antifungal agents (e.g. itraconazole) and HIV retroviral agents (e.g. ritonavir, saquinavir, atazanavir)
- increased serum levels may occur if given with erythromycin, clarithromycin, aprepitant, verapamil, diltiazem, amprenavir and fluconazole
- use with alcohol should be avoided
- not recommended within 24 hours of grapefruit juice
- caution if given with agents that lower seizure threshold
- caution if given with other centrally acting agents
- caution if used with other vasodilating agents such as alpha adrenergic receptor antagonists, nitrates and PDE5 inhibitors due to increased risk of postural hypotension
- caution if used with agents known to affect platelet function (e.g. atypical antipsychotics, phenothiazines, TCAs, aspirin, antiplatelet agents, NSAIDs, anticoagulants)

Nursing points/Cautions

- patient should be evaluated for any depressive or psychiatric disorder before starting therapy
- before starting therapy, an orthostatic test should be performed to assess patient for orthostatic hypotension
- risk versus benefit of therapy should be evaluated after 12 weeks or 6 doses (whichever comes first)
- syncope (with or without prodromal symptoms) can occur at any time, but commonly occurs within 3 hours of taking dapoxetine, after first dose or after procedures such as blood taking
- not recommended in those under 18 years
- not recommended in those with history of mania/hypomania, bipolar disorder, depressive disorder, schizophrenia or unstable epilepsy
- caution if used in those with a history of bleeding disorders, with epilepsy or history of seizures, mild liver impairment, raised intraocular pressure or narrow-angle glaucoma or mild-to-moderate kidney impairment

- caution if used in men with other forms of sexual dysfunction as condition might worsen
- not recommended in those with underlying structural cardiovascular disease (e.g. carotid stenosis, coronary artery disease, valvular heart disease), history of orthostatic reaction, or severe kidney impairment
- contraindicated in those with significant cardiac disease (e.g. heart failure, second or third degree AV block, sick sinus syndrome) not treated with pacemaker, significant ischaemic heart disease or valvular disease or moderate-to-severe liver impairment

Patient teaching and advice

- advise patient to take tablet with at least 1 full glass of water
- warn patient not to exceed 1 tablet per day as this increases risk of side-effects such as fainting
- counsel patient against using recreational drugs (e.g. ecstasy, LSD, ketamine, narcotics, benzodiazepines) with dapoxetine due to combined side-effects
- patient should be advised not to drink alcohol due to increased risk of fainting and accidental injury
- advise patient to avoid grapefruit juice within 24 hours of dapoxetine
- warn patient to take care not to stand up quickly after prolonged lying or sitting as light-headedness, dizziness and fainting may occur
- warn patient about syncope (loss of consciousness) which may occur with or without warning signs (including nausea, dizziness, light-headedness, sweating). If symptoms occur, patient should lie down (so head is lower than body) or put head between knees until symptoms have passed
- instruct patient to avoid driving, operating machinery or other situations where injury could occur if syncope or other side-effects (e.g. dizziness, blurred vision, somnolence, disturbance in attention) occur

tablet can be dispersed in 5–20 mL water or crushed and mixed with spoonful of yoghurt or apple puree

LIDOCAINE (LIGNOCAINE) (Stud 100 Desensitising Spray For Men)

Available form
Metered dose spray: 9.6%

Action
- local anaesthetic

Use
- local surface penile desensitiser to delay ejaculation

Dose
- 3–8 sprays applied to head and shaft of penis 5–15 minutes before intercourse (maximum daily dose 24 sprays)

Adverse effects
- rash, irritation

Nursing points/Cautions

- caution if used in those with liver or kidney disorders
- contraindicated if partner is pregnant, if either partner is allergic to local anaesthetics or if skin is broken or inflamed

Patient teaching and advice

- instruct patient that number of sprays and timing before intercourse will depend on individual needs
- warn patient not to apply spray to any broken or inflamed skin
- patient should be advised to wash spray off after intercourse

- warn patient that therapy should be stopped if either partner develops rash or irritation
- instruct patient that therapy should only be used for 12 weeks without medical supervision
- instruct patient to avoid spray contact with eyes or nostrils. If contact occurs, area should be thoroughly washed with water
- also see General Patient teaching and advice (p. xxvii)

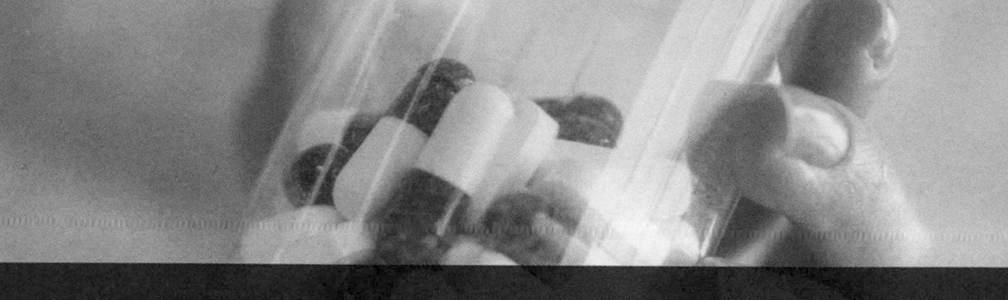

EYE, EAR, NOSE AND THROAT AGENTS

THE EYE

There are a number of eye conditions that require treatment with medications most commonly applied topically. These conditions include glaucoma (which results in raised intraocular pressure, damage to the optic nerve and changes to visual fields) (see Antiglaucoma agents, p. 452), macular degeneration, infection, inflammation and irritation. Furthermore, ocular agents are used to diagnose damaged tissue by staining (e.g. fluorescein, Bengal rose), mydriatic and cycloplegic agents (used for diagnostic procedures) and ocular decongestants (to reduce redness and tearing) (Bryant et al 2019).

It should also be noted that there are a number of systemic medications that have ocular adverse effects, such as blurred or impaired vision, dry eyes, nystagmus, raised intraocular pressure, diplopia, optic neuritis and cataract formation. Conversely, ocular agents can have systemic effects after nasolacrimal absorption and include bradycardia, hypo/hypertension, palpitations, nausea, sweating and tremors (Bryant et al 2019).

General Nursing points/Cautions for eye preparations

Instillation of eye drops

- patient should be sitting or lying comfortably
- select correct drug preparation including strength, and check which eye is to be treated
- check expiry date before use
- wash hands before instilling
- ensure contact lenses are removed, if worn
- shake drops before use
- evert lower lid and ask patient to look up
- instil correct number of drops into the lower conjunctival sac, midway between the inner and outer canthus, avoiding contact between the container and the skin or lashes
- ask patient to close the eye gently and not squeeze the lids or rub eyes
- systemic absorption may be reduced by compressing the lacrimal sac (tear duct) for 2 minutes after instilling the drops

- when separate solutions of a miotic and adrenaline (epinephrine) are to be instilled, adrenaline (epinephrine) is instilled 2–10 minutes after the miotic
- allow 5–10 minutes between preparations if instilling one or more antiglaucoma agents.

Insertion of eye ointment

- crust or exudate should be cleaned from lid margins, first using cooled boiled water or sterile saline solution, if available
- patient should be sitting or lying comfortably
- advise patient that the ointment may cause blurred vision
- select correct drug preparation and check which eye is to be treated
- wash hands before insertion
- ensure contact lenses are removed, if worn
- the first centimetre of ointment from the tube should be discarded onto a sterile swab to prevent contamination of the eye
- evert lower lid and ask the patient to look up
- starting at the inner canthus, squeeze the tube and insert the ointment along the lower fornix, ending at the outer canthus, avoiding contact of the container with the skin or lashes
- ask patient to close the eye gently to spread ointment over the eye

General Patient teaching and advice for eye preparations

- advise patient that eye drops should not be instilled if soft or gas-permeable contact lenses are in situ. Lenses should be removed before instillation and reinserted after at least a 15-minute interval
- patient should be instructed to thoroughly wash their hands before handling contact lenses and ensure that the correct solution is used with the particular lens type (i.e. either hard lens, soft lens or gas permeable)
- warn patient that many eye preparations contain benzalkonium chloride (preservative), which can cause irritation and also discolours soft contact lenses
- advise patient to report if the eye drops cause burning or visual disturbances
- the presence of pus and other exudates can decrease the effectiveness of anti-infective agents, therefore advise patient to cleanse the eye with saline or cooled boiled water
- patient should be escorted to and from an ophthalmological examination in which cycloplegic mydriatic drops are used for retinoscopy, because accommodation is paralysed for several hours. They should be advised not to drive or operate machinery during this time
- instruct patient to write the expiry date on eye preparations and discard accordingly (usually 28 days)
- advise patients that eye preparations are for one patient only
- patients should be warned not to stop treatment suddenly
- patients should be instructed to seek medical advice if eye infection does not show some improvement within 24–48 hours of starting eye drops or completely clear after 7 days
- instruct patient in correct technique for instilling eye drops, including:
  - do not allow tip of dispensing container to touch the eye as it may cause injury and/or contaminate the eye drops

- if the container is new, remove the protective seal, otherwise it is important to check the expiry date
- wash hands thoroughly with soap and water
- remove lid/cap and hold container upside down in one hand between thumb and forefinger or index finger
- using other hand, gently pull down on lower eyelid to form a pouch/pocket and tilt head back, looking up
- place tip of container close to lower eyelid (taking care not to make contact between tip and eye). Squeezing bottle gently, release one drop into pouch/pocket formed between eye and eyelid, taking care not to allow tip to touch eye
- gently close eye, but do not blink or rub eye
- while eye is closed, place index finger against inside corner of eye and press against nose for about 2 minutes (this stops medicine from draining through tear duct into nose and throat)
- blot any excess solution from around the eye with a tissue
- replace lid/cap tightly
- wash hands again to remove any residue

- instruct patient in correct eye ointment application, including:
  - check expiry date
  - wash hands thoroughly before applying eye ointment
  - tilt head back gently and gently pull lower eyelid down
  - squeeze 1.5 cm of eye ointment inside lower eyelid (however, do not allow tip of tube to touch eye, eyelid or lashes)
  - release eyelid slowly and close eyes gently for 1–2 minutes or blink a few times to help spread the ointment over the eye
  - blot any excessive ointment from around the eye with a tissue
  - wash hands thoroughly after finishing applying eye ointment
- see also General Patient teaching and advice (p. xxvii)

CYCLOPLEGIC AND MYDRIATIC DROPS

General Actions of cycloplegic and mydriatic drops

- acetylcholine normally causes miosis and allows accommodation (focusing for near vision), but antimuscarinic (anticholinergic) drugs block the actions of acetylcholine, causing mydriasis (dilation of pupil) and block ciliary muscles of the lens, resulting in paralysis of accommodation (cycloplegia)

General Adverse effects of cycloplegic and mydriatic drops

- dilation of the pupil (resulting in photophobia and loss of accommodation)
- blurred vision, irritation, redness, follicular conjunctivitis, vascular congestion, oedema, contact dermatitis, transient stinging, photophobia
- increased intraocular pressure

- (uncommon) CNS disturbance (ataxia, incoherent speech, hallucinations, hyperactivity, disorientation, seizures) (children are particularly susceptible)
- (rare, systemic absorption) dry mouth, thirst, flushing, dry skin, blurred vision, rapid and irregular pulse, fever, lack of coordination, atrial fibrillation, drowsiness, confusion, decreased bladder tone, increased risk of urinary retention (especially in older men), decreased GI motility which may lead to constipation

General Interactions of cycloplegic and mydriatic drops

- increased risk of convulsions and extrapyramidal symptoms if systemic absorption occurs and if given with phenothiazines, antiemetics or barbiturates
- if systemic absorption occurs, may potentiate actions of other anticholinergic agents
- may interfere with antiglaucoma actions of carbachol or pilocarpine

General Nursing points/Cautions for cycloplegic and mydriatic drops

- intraocular pressure and estimation of anterior chamber depth should be measured before starting therapy
- atropine is never put into an eye without a doctor's prescription, because its effects cannot be reversed quickly and it will cause an increase in intraocular pressure in susceptible patients
- systemic absorption of atropine or atropine-like drugs can result in toxicity, including increased pulse and respiratory rate, hypotension, restlessness, confusion, delirium, coma
- atropine-like agents can increase intraocular pressure in patients predisposed to glaucoma
- caution if used in the elderly as they are more sensitive to effects and also more prone to adverse effects
- caution if used in those who have had severe reactions to systemic atropine in the past
- caution if atropine or atropine-like agents are used in high ambient temperatures due to risk of hyperpyrexia (especially in children)
- caution if used in those with Down syndrome or predisposed to narrow-angle (angle-closure) glaucoma or anatomically narrow angles
- contraindicated in those with or suspected narrow-angle (angle-closure) glaucoma
- see general points for eye preparations (p. 1062)

General Patient teaching and advice for cycloplegic and mydriatic drops

- warn patient not to drive while pupils are dilated
- patient should be warned that eyes may be sensitive to light and that sunglasses should be worn outside
- see General Patient teaching and advice for eye preparations, which includes instructions on eye drop instillation (p. 1063)

ATROPINE SULFATE MONOHYDRATE (ATROPINE SULFATE) (Atropt, Minims Atropine Eye Drops)

Available form

Eye drops: 10 mg/mL (1%)

Action
- belladonna alkaloid that blocks acetylcholine
- dilates pupil (mydriasis), paralyses accommodation (cycloplegia)
- maximum mydriatic effects in 30–40 minutes, duration 7–12 days
- maximum cycloplegic effects in 3–6 hours, duration 7–14 days
- see also General Actions of cycloplegics and mydriatics (p. 1064)
- for other actions of atropine sulfate monohydrate, see Anticholinergic section of Cholinergic and anticholinergic agents (p. 915)

Use
- diagnostic procedures requiring mydriasis and cycloplegia

Dose
- 1 drop into eye(s) as required

Interactions
- may antagonise antiglaucoma action of ecothiopate
- if systemic absorption occurs, may decrease gastric motility increasing risk of adverse effects and/or toxicity if given with potassium supplements, potassium citrate or anti-myasthenics (e.g. neostigmine, pyridostigmine)
- see General Interactions of cycloplegic and mydriatic drops (p. 1065)

Adverse effects/Nursing points/Cautions/Patient teaching and advice
- infants and young children are especially susceptible to atropine toxicity, even from the absorption of eye preparations, so note irritability, dry mouth, tachycardia, mydriasis, fever and rash
- onset and duration of action is prolonged in patients with heavily pigmented eyes
- not recommended in infants under 3 months
- not recommended in those with keratoconus or synechiae between iris and lens
- see also General Adverse effects/Nursing points/Cautions/Patient teaching and advice for cycloplegic and mydriatic drops (pp. 1064–65)

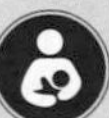

breastfed infants may show rapid pulse, fever and dry skin if mother is using atropine-containing eye preparations

CYCLOPENTOLATE HYDROCHLORIDE (Cyclogyl, Minims Cyclopentolate Eye Drops)

Available forms
Eye drops: 5 mg/mL (0.5%), 10 mg/mL (1%)

Action
- anticholinergic with rapid action but shorter duration than atropine sulfate monohydrate (p. 1065)
- maximum mydriatic effect 30–60 minutes, duration 24 hours
- maximum cycloplegic effect 25–75 minutes, duration 6–24 hours

Use
- diagnostic procedures requiring mydriasis and cycloplegia
- treatment of uveitis

Dose
- (refraction, examination of back of eye) 1 drop (0.5% but 1% in heavily pigmented eyes) to affected eye(s), followed 5 minutes later by 1 drop **OR**
- (anterior/posterior uveitis, breakdown of posterior synechiae (adhesion)) 1–2 drops (0.5%) to affected eye(s) 6–8-hourly

Adverse effects
- (children) psychotic reactions and behavioural disturbances (more common than other anticholinergic agent)

- (rare) seizures, acute psychosis
- see General Adverse effects of cycloplegic and mydriatic drops (p. 1064)

Interactions

- see General Interactions of cycloplegic and mydriatic drops (p. 1065)

Nursing points/Cautions

- infants should be observed for at least 30 minutes after instillation for any behavioural or psychotic reactions
- caution if used in children with epilepsy
- (1% solution) not recommended in young children
- see General Nursing points/Cautions for cycloplegic and mydriatic drops (p. 1065)

Patient teaching and advice

- patient should be advised that full recovery will take approximately 24 hours
- see General Patient teaching and advice for cycloplegic and mydriatic drops (p. 1065)

PHENYLEPHRINE HYDROCHLORIDE (Minims Phenylephrine Eye Drops)

Available forms

Eye drops: 25 mg/mL (2.5%), 100 mg/mL (10%)

Action

- sympathomimetic agent that causes mydriasis by direct stimulation of alpha-adrenoceptors (alpha-1 and alpha-2)
- no cycloplegic action or effect on intraocular pressure
- mydriasis occurs in 10–90 minutes, recovery 5–7 hours

Use

- mydriasis for diagnostic or therapeutic purposes

Dose

- (diagnostic) (2.5%, 10%) 1 drop to each eye, repeated once only after 1 hour

Adverse effects

- (rare) significant increase in BP, aneurysm, arrhythmias
- see General Adverse effects of cycloplegic and mydriatic drops (p. 1064)

Interactions

- may reverse action of antihypertensive agents
- absorption is increased if ocular hyperaemia is present
- increased risk of arrhythmias if given with or within several days of stopping TCAs
- increased risk of arrhythmias if given with digoxin
- not recommended with or within 3 weeks of MAOIs

Nursing points/Cautions

- local anaesthetic eye drops may be used before phenylephrine to reduce stinging
- caution if used in those with hyperthyroidism, asthma, arteriosclerosis, hypertension, cardiovascular problems, aneurysms, tachycardia and long-standing insulin-dependent diabetes mellitus
- caution if used in those with closed-angle glaucoma (unless treated with iridectomy) or narrow-angle glaucoma sensitive to mydriatic-provoked glaucoma
- not recommended if corneal epithelium is damaged due to risk of increased absorption
- contraindicated in those with hypersensitivity to sodium metabisulfite
- (10% solution) contraindicated in children and elderly
- see also General Nursing points/Cautions for cycloplegic and mydriatic drops (p. 1065)

Patient teaching and advice

- patients should be warned that they may experience transient floaters for 30–45 minutes after administrations
- see General Patient teaching and advice for cycloplegic and mydriatic drops (p. 1065)

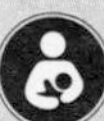

only used during pregnancy and breast-feeding if thought to be necessary

Note

- contained in Prednefrin Forte (Eye Drops) with prednisolone

TROPICAMIDE (Minims Tropicamide, Mydriacyl)

Available forms

Eye drops: 5 mg/mL (0.5%), 10 mg/mL (1%)

Action

- anticholinergic with action and adverse effects similar to those of atropine sulfate monohydrate but with more rapid onset and shorter duration
- mydriasis occurs in 20–40 minutes, duration 6 hours
- maximum cycloplegia occurs within 30–40 minutes, recovery in 2–6 hours

Use

- diagnostic purposes

Dose

- (examination of fundus) 1–2 drops 0.5% solution 15–20 minutes before examination of the fundus **OR**
- (refraction examination) 1–2 drops 1% solution, repeated after 5 minutes; may be repeated after 20–30 minutes if necessary

Interactions

- effects may be enhanced if given with other agents with anticholinergic effects
- may interfere with hypotensive effects of carbachol, pilocarpine or ophthalmic cholinesterase inhibitors

Adverse effects

- (children) CNS disturbances
- see General Adverse effects of cycloplegic and mydriatic drops (p. 1064)

Nursing points/Cautions

- those with heavily pigmented irises may require more doses or higher strength solution
- contains benzalkonium chloride which may cause eye irritation
- caution if eye is inflamed as increased absorption may occur
- (1% solution) not recommended in infants
- see General Nursing points/Cautions for cycloplegic and mydriatic drops (p. 1065)

Patient teaching and advice

- see General Patient teaching and advice for cycloplegic and mydriatic drops (p. 1065)

MIOTICS AND OCULAR DECONGESTANTS

ACETYLCHOLINE CHLORIDE (Miochol-E)

Available form

Vial: 20 mg/2 mL

Action

- parasympathomimetic
- very short-acting chemical transmitter that acts directly on cholinergic synapses and neuroeffector junctions

- activates neuromuscular junctions of parasympathetic fibres in the iris sphincter, resulting in very rapid miosis
- rapidly inactivated by acetylcholinesterase to choline and acetic acid

Use
- rapid miosis during ocular surgery (e.g. placement of intraocular lens after cataract surgery), penetrating keratoplasty, iridectomy

Dose
- 0.5–2 mL by gentle intraocular irrigation (instilled into anterior chamber with or after sutures are secured)

Adverse effects
- (uncommon) corneal clouding or oedema (infrequent)
- (systemic, rare) bradycardia, hypotension, flushing, sweating, breathing difficulties

Nursing points/Cautions/Patient teaching and advice
- reconstitute using diluent provided
- if used after cataract surgery, should only be used after placement of intraocular lens
- solution is prepared immediately before use and the remainder discarded after use as it becomes rapidly unstable
- see general points for eye preparations (p. 1062)

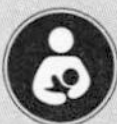
only used during pregnancy if needed

caution if used during breastfeeding

CARBACHOL (Miostat)

Available form
Vial: 150 microgram/1.5 mL (0.01%)

Action
- parasympathomimetic agent that stimulates the parasympathetic nervous system, but is not inactivated by acetylcholinesterase
- causes contraction of ciliary muscle, resulting in accommodation for near vision
- miosis occurs in 2–5 minutes
- decreases intraocular pressure

Use
- miosis during surgery

Dose
- (miosis during surgery) 50 microgram (0.5 mL of 0.01% solution) gently instilled into anterior chamber before or after securing sutures

Adverse effects
- blurred vision, redness, eye pain
- (uncommon) headache, increased intraocular pressure
- (rare) retinal detachment, corneal clouding, persistent bullous keratopathy and postoperative iritis (after cataract extraction)

Nursing points/Cautions
- patient should be carefully monitored as therapy may increase surgically induced intraocular inflammation
- vial stopper contains latex, which may cause allergic reaction in sensitive individuals
- caution if used in those with acute heart failure, asthma, active peptic ulceration, hyperthyroidism, GI spasm, urinary tract obstruction or Parkinson's disease

Patient teaching and advice
- patient should be advised to wait until vision has cleared before driving or operating machinery

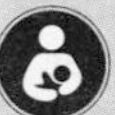
only use in pregnancy or breastfeeding if benefits outweigh risks

LODOXAMIDE TROMETAMOL (Lomide Eye Drops 0.1%)

Available form
Eye drops: 1 mg/mL (0.1%)

Action
- mast cell stabiliser that inhibits IgE mediated (immediate) hypersensitivity reaction
- inhibits increase in cutaneous vascular permeability, but has no vasoconstricting, antihistamine or anti-inflammatory activity

Use
- seasonal allergic conjunctivitis (prophylaxis and treatment)
- vernal keratoconjunctivitis

Dose
- 1 drop in each eye 4 times daily at regular intervals

Adverse effects
- transient burning/stinging/discomfort, ocular pruritus, blurred vision, lid margin crusting, dry eye, tearing, hyperaemia
- (uncommon) warm sensation, headache, nausea, dizziness, dry nose, sneezing, rash

Nursing points/Cautions
- (vernal keratoconjunctivitis) contact lenses should not be worn
- eye drops contain benzalkonium chloride which can cause eye irritation and also discolours soft contact lenses
- not recommended in children under 4 years

Patient teaching and advice
- (prophylaxis of seasonal allergic conjunctivitis) advise patient to begin therapy about a week before start of allergy season and continue for duration of season
- emphasise need to use drops as directed to be effective. Improvement in symptoms may be seen in a few days but some patients may require longer (4 weeks)
- warn patient that some transient stinging or burning may occur when drops are first instilled; however, if this continues, advise patient to seek medical advice
- if patient normally wears soft contact lenses, instruct patient to remove before instilling eye drops and not reinsert for at least 15 minutes
- advise patient to wait at least 10 minutes after instilling medication before instilling any other eye drops
- see also General Patient teaching and advice for eye preparations (p. 1063)

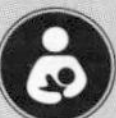

should only be used during pregnancy or breastfeeding if clearly needed

NAPHAZOLINE HYDROCHLORIDE (Albalon, Murine Clear Eyes, Naphcon Forte, Optrex Eye Drops, Systane Red Eyes)

Available forms
Eye drops: 0.12 mg/mL (0.012%), 0.1 mg/mL (0.01%), 1 mg/mL (0.1%)

Action
- sympathomimetic agent

Use
- minor irritation (redness and dryness)

Dose
- 1–2 drops to affected eye(s) 3–4-hourly (Albalon, Systane Red Eyes) or up to 4 times daily (Murine, Naphcon Forte, Optrex Eye Drops)

Adverse effects
- raised intraocular pressure with pupil dilation
- transient stinging, blurred vision, hyperaemia, eye irritation, oedema, eye pain

- (systemic, rare) drowsiness, hypersensitivity

Interactions

- contraindicated with MAOIs
- caution if used with methyldopa sesquihydrate or TCAs

Nursing points/Cautions

- caution if used in men with prostatic enlargement
- caution if used in those with hypertension, hyperthyroidism, diabetes mellitus or cardiac disease
- caution if used on inflamed eyes as hyperaemia increases systemic absorption
- contraindicated in those with narrow-angle glaucoma or anatomically narrow angle
- see also General Nursing points/ Cautions for eye preparations (p. 1062)

Patient teaching and advice

- instruct patient that eye drops should not be used for more than 2 weeks
- if condition does not improve in 48 hours or symptoms recur, patient should be advised to seek medical advice
- see also General Patient teaching and advice for eye preparations (p. 1063)

Note

- contained in Albalon-A, Naphcon-A Eye Drops, Visine Allergy

TETRYZOLINE (TETRAHYDROZOLINE) HYDROCHLORIDE (Murine Sore Eyes, Visine Advanced, Visine Clear)

Available form

Eye drops: 0.5 mg/mL (0.05%)

Action

- sympathomimetic with marked alpha adrenergic activity
- conjunctival decongestant

Use

- minor eye irritation

Dose

- 1–2 drops to affected eye(s) up to 4 times daily

Adverse effects

- eye pain, blurred vision, hyperaemia

Nursing points/Cautions

- contraindicated in those with narrow-angle glaucoma, anatomically narrow angle, or if serious eye infection is present
- contraindicated in children under 6 years
- see also General Nursing points/ Cautions for eye preparations (p. 1062)

Patient teaching and advice

- advise patient to seek medical advice if symptoms persist for more than 72 hours
- see also General Patient teaching and advice for eye preparations (p. 1063)

AGENTS USED FOR MACULAR DEGENERATION

General Adverse effects for macular degeneration treatment agents

- (very common) conjunctival or retinal haemorrhage, eye pain, vitreous floaters, vitreous detachment, intraocular inflammation, eye irritation, foreign body sensation, increased lacrimation, blepharitis, ocular hyperaemia, dry eye, ocular pruritus, subretinal fibrosis, vitritis
- (common) retinal degeneration or detachment, retinal tear, decreased

visual acuity, vitreous haemorrhage, blurred vision, eyelid pain or oedema, conjunctival hyperaemia, corneal abrasion, eye discharge, photophobia, iritis, uveitis, iridocyclitis, subcapsular cataract, conjunctivitis
- transient increased intraocular pressure
- (rare) arterial thromboembolic events, endophthalmitis, retinal detachment, hypersensitivity

General Nursing points/Cautions for macular degeneration treatment agents

- should only be administered by qualified ophthalmologist who is experienced in intravitreal injection
- intraocular pressure and optic nerve head perfusion should be measured immediately after intravitreal injection
- bilateral treatment at the same time may increase risk of systemic exposure and is generally not recommended
- dose interval should not be less than 1 month
- treatment should be withheld if intraocular surgery is planned or performed within the previous or next 28 days
- treatment should be withheld if rhegmatogenous retinal detachment or stage 3 or 4 macular holes occur
- if a retinal break occurs, dose should be withheld and not restarted until break has been repaired
- treatment should be withheld (and not resumed until next scheduled interval) if there is a decrease in visual acuity (decrease of ≥ 30 letters compared to last assessment), subretinal haemorrhage involving fovea centre occurs or if haemorrhage is ≥ 50% of total lesion area
- caution if used in those with poorly controlled glaucoma
- caution if used in those with a history of stroke or transient ischaemic attack (TIA) due to increased risk of thromboembolic events
- caution if used in those with risk factors for retinal pigment epithelial tears
- contraindicated in those with ocular or periocular infection or active severe intraocular inflammation

General Patient teaching and advice for macular degeneration treatment agents

- patient should be advised not to drive or operate machinery until visual function has recovered post-injection and any associated eye examinations
- advise patient to immediately seek medical advice if any of the following occur:
  - severe eye pain, redness, blurred vision or increased sensitivity to light
  - sudden decrease in vision or swelling of eyelid in the injected eye
  - perception of or increase in having something floating in the eye (floaters) or visual disturbances such as blurred vision or dark spots
  - increased tear production
  - weakness or numbness in limbs or face, difficulty swallowing or speaking (signs of stroke)
  - chest pain and pain that spreads to shoulders and neck (signs of heart attack)

AFLIBERCEPT (Eylea)

Available form
Vial: 4 mg/0.1 mL

Action
- anti-vascular endothelial growth factor (VEGF), placental growth factor monoclonal antibody fragment
- antineovascularisation action

Use
- neovascular (wet) age-related macular degeneration (AMD)
- visual impairment due to diabetic macular oedema (DME)
- visual impairment secondary to central retinal vein occlusion (CRVO), branch retinal vein occlusion (BRVO) or myopic choroidal neovascularisation (myopic CNV)

Dose
- (wet AMD) 2 mg by intravitreal injection monthly for 3 consecutive months, followed by 1 injection every 2 months, then treatment interval adjusted based on visual and/or anatomic outcomes **OR**
- (DME) 2 mg by intravitreal injection monthly for 5 consecutive months, followed by 1 injection every 2 months for 12 months, then treatment interval adjusted based on visual and/or anatomic outcomes **OR**
- (BRVO, CRVO) 2 mg by intravitreal injection monthly for 3 consecutive months, then treatment interval adjusted based on visual and/or anatomic outcomes **OR**
- (myopic CNV) 2 mg by intravitreal injection, dose repeated if disease persists

Adverse effects
- (injection site) irritation, pain, haemorrhage
- see also General Adverse effects for macular degeneration treatment agents (p. 1071)

Nursing points/Cautions
- see General Nursing points/Cautions for macular degeneration treatment agents (p. 1072)
- (wet AMD) dosing interval can be extended from every 2 to every 3 months once visual acuity is optimised and there is no active disease present
- not recommended in those with clinical signs of irreversible ischaemic visual function loss

Patient teaching and advice
- see General Patient teaching and advice for macular degeneration agents (p. 1072)

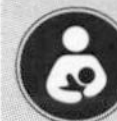

not recommended during pregnancy or breastfeeding unless benefits outweigh risks

BROLUCIZUMAB (Beovu)

Available form
Prefilled syringe: 6 mg/0.05 mL

Action
- anti-vascular endothelial growth factor (VEGF) that suppresses endothelial cell proliferation reducing neovascularisation and decreasing vascular permeability
- monoclonal antibody fragment

Use
- treatment of neovascular (wet) age-related macular degeneration

Dose
- 6 mg by intravitreal injection every 4 weeks for 3 doses, then according to disease activity (for active disease, every 8 weeks; for no disease activity, every 12 weeks)

Adverse effects
- hypersensitivity reaction
- see also General Adverse effects for macular degeneration treatment agents (p. 1071)

Interactions

- not recommended with other VEGF agents (ocular or systemic)

Nursing points/Cautions

- see General Nursing points/Cautions for macular degeneration treatment agents (p. 1072)
- patient should be assessed 16 weeks after starting therapy

Patient teaching and advice

- see General Patient teaching and advice for macular degeneration treatment agents (p. 1072)
- women of childbearing potential should be counselled to use effective contraception during and for at least 4 weeks after stopping therapy
- see General Patient teaching and advice (p. 1072)

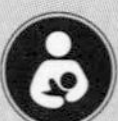

not recommended during pregnancy unless benefits outweigh risks

breastfeeding is not recommended during therapy or for at least 4 weeks after stopping therapy

RANIBIZUMAB (Lucentis)

Available forms

Vial: 2.3 mg/0.23 mL; Prefilled syringe: 1.65 mg/0.165 mL

Action

- recombinant monoclonal antibody fragment that targets vascular endothelial growth factor A

Use

- neovascular (wet) age-related macular degeneration (AMD)
- visual impairment due to diabetic macular oedema (DME)
- treatment of proliferative diabetic retinopathy (PDR)
- visual impairment secondary to retinal vein occlusion (RVO)
- visual impairment due to choroidal neovascularisation (CNV) secondary to pathologic myopia
- visual impairment due to macular oedema secondary to retinal vein occlusion (RVO)

Dose

- initially 0.5 mg by intravitreal injection monthly until visual acuity has optimised or there are no signs of active disease. For AMD, DME, PDR and RVO, 3 or more monthly injections are usually required

Adverse effects

- nasopharyngitis, cough, flu-like syndrome
- anaemia
- nausea
- rash, urticaria, pruritus, erythema
- arthralgia
- headache, anxiety, stroke
- urinary tract infection
- (injection site) haemorrhage, pain
- see also General Adverse effects for macular degeneration treatment agents (p. 1071)

Nursing points/Cautions

- (vial) 5 micrometre filter (supplied) should be used when drawing up solution
- (prefilled syringe) attach 30-gauge 1/2 inch needle for intravitreal injection
- administer alone
- intraocular pressure should be monitored pre- and post-injection (60 minutes)
- patient should be reviewed 1 week post-injection to allow early treatment of infection if it occurs
- treatment may be fixed (monthly) or variable (patient is seen regularly and treated when disease is active)
- (CNV) patient may only require 1–2 injections per year; however, some patients require more

- (macular oedema due to RVO) if no improvement to visual acuity is seen after 3–4 injections, therapy may be stopped
- if given with laser photocoagulation therapy, a 30-minute interval should be allowed between the two therapies with injection administered first
- caution if used in those with type 1 diabetes mellitus, especially those with HbA1c > 12% or uncontrolled hypertension
- not recommended in patients with RVO with clinical signs of irreversible ischaemic visual function loss
- see also General Nursing points/ Cautions for macular degeneration treatment agents (p. 1072)

Patient teaching and advice

- see General Patient teaching and advice for macular degeneration treatment agents (p. 1072)
- counsel female patient of childbearing potential to use adequate contraception during and for 12 months after stopping therapy
- see General Patient teaching and advice (p. xxvii)

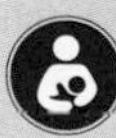

not recommended during pregnancy and breastfeeding

VERTEPORFIN (Visudyne)

Available form

Vial: 15 mg

Action

- antineovascularisation agent
- therapy is a two-step process involving verteporfin and non-thermal red light
- laser light activates drug to generate oxygen radicals, which damage vascular endothelium, leading to occlusion of abnormal vessels
- half-life 5–6 hours

Use

- subfoveal choroidal neovascularisation due to age-related macular degeneration or other macular diseases

Dose

- 6 mg/m^2 given by IV infusion over 10 minutes; 15 minutes after start of infusion, a non-thermal laser light (600 mW/cm^2) is shone into the affected eye for 83 seconds

Adverse effects

- blurry, hazy or fuzzy vision, flashes of light, decreased vision, scotoma, black spots, grey or black haloes, visual field defects, cataract formation, blepharitis
- nausea, constipation
- back pain, chest pain
- asthenia
- flu-like symptoms, cough
- pruritus
- hypercholesterolaemia
- leucopenia
- (injection site) pain, oedema, inflammation, localised skin necrosis
- photosensitivity reaction (e.g. sunburn within 24 hours of therapy)
- (extravasation) severe pain, inflammation, swelling, discolouration, blistering
- (rare) vasovagal reaction, hypersensitivity (headache, malaise, fainting, sweating, dizziness, rash, urticaria, flushing, dyspnoea, changes in BP and heart rate)

Interactions

- increased uptake in vascular endothelium may occur if given with calcium-channel blockers or radiation therapy
- increased risk of photosensitivity reactions if given with tetracyclines, sulfonamides, phenothiazines, sulfonylurea antidiabetic agents, thiazide diuretics and griseofulvin
- decreased activity may occur if given with mannitol, beta carotene (vitamin A), ethanol, dimethyl sulfoxide or

formate as these agents reduce free oxygen radicals
- decreased activity may occur if given with agents that decrease clotting, vasoconstriction or platelet aggregation such as thromboxane A_2 inhibitors

Nursing points/Cautions

- patient should be closely monitored throughout infusion as fainting, sweating, dizziness, rash, dyspnoea, flushing and changes to BP and heart rate commonly occur
- reconstitute using 7 mL water for injections and then dilute using glucose 5% to a final volume of 30 mL
- sodium chloride 0.9% is not recommended
- reconstituted solution is opaque green; it should be protected from light and used within 4 hours
- administer alone
- should be given via large blood vessel to decrease risk of extravasation
- if extravasation occurs, infusion should be stopped immediately, cold compress applied and area protected from sunlight until swelling and discolouration have disappeared
- if patient requires emergency surgery in first 48 hours after procedure, as much internal tissue as possible should be shielded from light
- if vision decreases (decrease of 4 or more lines on reading chart) within 1 week of the procedure, retreatment is not recommended until vision has completely returned to pre-procedural level
- patient should be re-examined after 3 months
- treatment may be repeated 3-monthly if vessels continue to leak or bleed
- staff are advised to wear gloves and eye protection during administration and avoid contact with eyes or skin. If contact occurs, area should be thoroughly rinsed with water. If spill occurs, should be contained and wiped up with damp cloth
- incompatible lasers should not be used
- caution if used in those with biliary tract obstruction, unstable heart disease, uncontrolled hypertension or moderate liver impairment
- contraindicated in those with severe liver impairment or porphyria

Patient teaching and advice

- warn patient not to drive or operate machinery until visual disturbances have stopped
- patient should be instructed to wear wristband to remind him/her to avoid direct sunlight or bright indoor light (normal household indoor lighting is acceptable) for first 48 hours following procedure. If patient does go outside during daylight hours during first 48 hours, protective clothing and dark sunglasses should be worn. UV sunscreens are NOT effective
- see General Patient teaching and advice (p. xxvii)

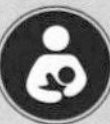

only recommended during pregnancy if benefits are thought to outweigh risks

not recommended during breastfeeding

OTHER OPHTHALMIC AGENTS

LIFITEGRAST (Xiidra)

Available form

Eye drops: 50 mg/mL (5%)

Action

- targets interaction between lymphocyte function-associated antigen-1 (LFA-1) (protein found on leukocytes that mediates immune and inflammatory responses) and intercellular adhesion molecule-1 (ICAM-1). ICAM-1 is normally found in low levels in leukocytes but thought to increase when inflammatory cytokines are present, including dry eye conditions

Use

- moderate-to-severe dry eye disease where artificial tear use has not been sufficient

Dose

- one drop to affected eye(s) twice daily

Adverse effects

- eye irritation, eye pain, eye pruritus, increased lacrimation, blurred vision
- altered taste
- headache
- (rare) allergic reactions

Nursing points/Cautions

- comprehensive examination is recommended before starting therapy to determine reason for symptoms that may be reversible and treatable
- see also General Nursing points/Cautions for eye preparations (p. 1062)

Patient teaching and advice

- see General Patient teaching and advice for eye preparations (p. 1063)

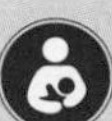

caution if used during breastfeeding

OCRIPLASMIN (Jetrea)

Available form

Vial: 0.5 mg/0.2 mL

Action

- ocular proteolytic enzyme developed by recombinant DNA technology
- acts against vitreous body and vitreoretinal interface proteins (e.g. laminin, fibronectin, collagen) dissolving protein matrix responsible for abnormal vitreomacular adhesion. Tight protein binding leads to vitreomacular traction, visual impairment and/or macular holes
- half-life several hours

Use

- treatment of vitreomacular traction, including when associated with macular hole diameter ≤ 400 micron

Dose

- 0.125 mg (0.1 mL of diluted solution) injected into mid-vitreous of affected eye

Adverse effects

- blurred vision, vitreous floaters, eye pain, photopsia (perceived flashes of light), conjunctival haemorrhage, decreased visual acuity, visual impairment, macular oedema, photophobia, ocular discomfort, iritis, vitreous detachment, dry eye, eye pruritus/irritation, foreign body sensation, increased lacrimation
- intraocular inflammation/infection, intraocular haemorrhage, increased intraocular pressure
- dyschromatopsia (yellowish vision)
- (uncommon) long-term loss of visual acuity
- lens subluxation, phacodonesis (lens tremulous)
- new or enlarged macular holes

Interactions

- remains in the eye for several days after intravitroal injection, therefore administration of other agents to treated eye is not recommended as activity of both agents may be affected

Nursing points/Cautions

- before treatment, complete clinical picture (patient history, clinical examination and investigations including optical coherence tomography) should be obtained
- patient monitoring after injection (between 2 and 7 days) is recommended to detect any inflammation, infection or increase in intraocular pressure
- patient should be monitored for any loss of visual acuity, especially in first week after treatment
- for intravitreal use only
- both eyes should not be treated concurrently or within 7 days of initial injection
- repeat administration to same eye is not recommended
- allow to thaw at room temperature before use (about 2 minutes), then dilute with 0.2 mL sodium chloride 0.9%, gently swirl and use within 15 minutes of reconstitution
- caution if used in those with non-proliferative diabetic retinopathy, history of uveitis or significant eye trauma
- not recommended in those with large diameter macular holes (> 400 micron), high myopia (> 8 dioptre spherical correction or axial length > 28 mm), aphakia, history of rhegmatogenous retinal detachment, lens zonule instability, recent ocular surgery or intraocular injection (including laser therapy), proliferative diabetic retinopathy, ischaemic retinopathies, retinal vein occlusion, exudative age-related macular degeneration or vitreous haemorrhage
- not recommended in those with panretinal disease associated with electroretinography (ERG) findings (e.g. retinitis pigmentosa, chorioderaemia)
- contraindicated in those with active or suspected ocular or periocular infection

Patient teaching and advice

- patient should be advised of risk of transient loss of visual acuity during first week after treatment
- instruct patient not to drive or operate machinery if any visual disturbances occur (and these are most likely in first 7 days after treatment)

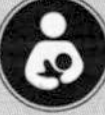

should only be used during pregnancy or breastfeeding if benefits outweigh risks

THE EAR

Common ear conditions include infections (bacterial and fungal), ear wax accumulation, painful, inflammatory and allergic conditions, deafness and balance issues. Medications/agents used to treat ear conditions include anti-inflammatories (analgesics, topical anaesthetics, corticosteroids), antibacterial or antifungal agents, analgesic and decongestants (Bryant et al 2019). Most of these agents are discussed in other sections, including corticosteroids, antibacterial agents, antifungal agents and non-steroidal anti-inflammatory agents (NSAIDs). It should also be noted that there are a number of medications that can cause ear disturbances, including tinnitus and ototoxicity, such as aminoglycosides, salicylates and loop diuretics (Bryant et al 2019).

General Nursing points/Cautions for ear preparations

- some systemic absorption may occur
- contraindicated if there is inflammation or perforation of the tympanic membrane

Instillation of ear drops

- patient should sit or lie comfortably
- select the correct preparation and strength, and check which ear is to be treated
- cleanse ear canal before instilling ear drops
- ensure that drops are at room temperature before instillation as cold solution may provoke dizziness
- with the affected ear uppermost, pull the auricle upwards and backwards to straighten the external auditory canal (for children, pull the auricle downwards)
- instil required number of drops into the canal without touching the ear with the dropper and return dropper to bottle without washing
- press the tragus over the meatus
- position maintained for 2–3 minutes so that drops reach the ear drum
- saturated wick may be used for the first 24–48 hours

General Patient teaching and advice for ear preparations

- warn patient not to drive or operate machinery if dizziness or lightheadedness occurs
- advise patient to stop use if any pain or inflammation is experienced
- patient should be advised to seek medical advice if pain or irritation occurs or condition continues
- instruct patient in correct instillation technique for ear drops, including:
  - check expiry date
  - if the ear drops are new, break safety cap and open
  - wash hands thoroughly with soap and water
  - hold bottle upside down in one hand (between thumb and middle finger)
  - tilt head to one side with affected ear facing up (it may be easier in sitting or lying position)
  - place dropper tip close to (but not touching) ear and gently tap or press base of container to release drops
  - continue holding head in same position for 1 minute to allow drops to reach deeper into the ear
  - repeat for other ear if needed
  - replace cap on bottle and close tightly
  - wash hands to remove any residue
- warn patient that feeling of drops flowing deeper into ear may be unpleasant
- advise patient that a bad taste in the mouth may occur after using ear drops
- patient should be advised to note opening date and discard after that date (e.g. 28 days)
- see General Patient teaching and advice (p. xxvii)

WAX SOFTENERS

CARBAMIDE PEROXIDE (Ear Clear for Ear Wax Removal)

Available form
Ear drops: 65 mg/mL

Action
- loosens wax by effervescent action

Use
- wax removal

Dose
- tilt head to one side and instil 5–10 drops in affected ear(s) twice daily for up to 4 days

Nursing points/Cautions/Patient teaching and advice
- see general points for ear preparations, including instillation advice (p. 1078–79)
- not recommended for children under 12 years
- not recommended for swimmer's ear, inflamed tissue or itching in ear canal
- not recommended if there is any dizziness, ear perforation or ear pain or within 6 weeks of ear surgery

DOCUSATE SODIUM (Waxsol)

Available form
Ear drops: 0.5%

Action
- penetrates ceruminous mass, reducing solid mass to semi-solid, allowing it to be removed normally by physiological process or syringing process

Use
- softening or loosening of ear wax to help in removal

Dose
- fill affected ear(s) for 2 nights preceding syringe procedure

Nursing points/Cautions/Patient teaching and advice
- contraindicated if there is any perforation or inflammation of tympanic membrane present
- see also general points for ear preparations, including instillation advice (p. 1078–79)

THE NOSE

Olfaction (sense of smell) receptors are found on the top of the nasal cavity, synapse to the olfactory bulb, forming the olfactory tract passing through the temporal lobe of the cortex and to the limbic system and hypothalamus. Decreased lack of smell (hyposmia) resulting from colds, rhinitis and nasal passage obstruction is common and may result in food becoming tasteless (because it can't be smelt) (Bryant et al 2019). A number of medications can decrease or impair smell, including calcium-channel blockers (nifedipine, diltiazem), some diuretics (e.g. acetazolamide, spironolactone), some antimicrobial agents (e.g. ciprofloxacin, metronidazole), corticosteroids (e.g. prednisolone) and antiepileptics (e.g. carbamazepine, phenytoin) (Bryant et al 2019). Agents are introduced into the nose to treat infection, sinusitis, various types of rhinitis and relieve nasal congestion.

General Nursing points/Cautions for nasal preparations

Instillation of nasal drops

- ask patient to blow nose
- have the patient recumbent, but with a pillow under the shoulders so that the neck is hyperextended (if possible) to prevent entry of drops into the throat
- select correct preparation and strength
- ask patient to breathe through the mouth
- instil the prescribed volume of drops into each nostril, turning the head to the same side as the nostril being dealt with
- maintain the position for several seconds to enable wide coverage of the nasal mucosa
- excessive use of topical sympathomimetic nasal decongestants can lead to drug-induced rhinitis and rebound nasal congestion

General Patient teaching and advice for nasal preparations

- if using a nasal spray, instruct the patient to:
  - ensure nasal spray is primed for use if new, dust cover has been left off or device has been unused for some time (priming instructions vary from nasal spray to nasal spray, but essentially involve vigorously shaking container (with cap on) for 10 seconds and then priming by releasing 6–7 sprays until spray is uniform)
  - blow nose
  - insert spray adapter/nozzle into nostril while closing other nostril
  - tilt head slightly forwards keeping nasal spray container upright
  - avoid tilting head back as this will result in bitter smell/taste
  - depress pump while breathing gently and slowly through the nostril
  - repeat procedure in same nostril if second spray per nostril is required
  - remove adapter/nozzle from nostril and repeat in other nostril
  - after prescribed amount has been delivered, remove adapter/nozzle from nostril and wipe with tissue
  - wash spray adapter/nozzle regularly with warm water
  - re-prime with 2 sprays after cleaning
  - if nozzle/adapter becomes blocked, pins or other sharp devices should not be used to unblock device as it may become damaged and not deliver required amount of nasal spray
  - nasal spray should be vigorously shaken for at least 10 seconds before each use
  - replace dust cap after each use
- see General Patient teaching and advice (p. xxvii)

SYMPATHOMIMETIC NASAL DECONGESTANTS

General Actions of sympathomimetic nasal decongestants

- sympathomimetic agent that stimulates alpha-adrenergic receptors
- vasoconstricting agents that act on small arterioles of the nasal passage

General Uses of sympathomimetic nasal decongestants

- temporary relief of nasal congestion (colds, influenza, allergy, sinusitis)

General Adverse effects of sympathomimetic nasal decongestants

- burning/stinging in nose or throat
- sneezing
- nose/mouth/throat dryness or irritation
- increase in nasal discharge, epistaxis
- nausea, taste disturbance
- headache, insomnia, tiredness, dizziness, light-headedness
- nervousness, tremors
- hypertension, palpitations, reflex bradycardia
- rebound congestion
- (rare) allergy

General Interactions of sympathomimetic nasal decongestants

- not recommended with or within 2 weeks of MAOIs or TCAs
- not recommended with other cold or cough medications

General Nursing points/Cautions for sympathomimetic nasal decongestants

- see General Nursing points/Cautions for nasal preparations (p. 1081)
- caution if used in those with heart disease (including angina), diabetes mellitus, hypertension, prostatic enlargement, congenital porphyria or thyroid disease
- not recommended in children under 6 and only used in those 6–11 years with medical advice
- contraindicated in those with hypersensitivity to other nasal decongestants or with narrow-angle glaucoma
- contraindicated in those with recent transsphenoidal hypophysectomy, transnasal or transoral surgical procedures where dura mater has been exposed

General Patient teaching and advice for sympathomimetic nasal decongestants

- advise patient to avoid contact with eyes
- patient should be advised not to share preparations to prevent spreading infection
- instruct patient that nasal decongestant should not be used for more than 3–5 days because rebound nasal congestion may occur
- advise patient not to exceed recommended dose
- see General Patient teaching and advice for nasal preparations, including instillation advice (p. 1081)

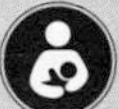

not recommended during pregnancy or breastfeeding

OXYMETAZOLINE HYDROCHLORIDE (Demazin 12 Hour Relief, Dimetapp 12 Hour Nasal Spray, Drixine Decongestant Nasal Spray, Drixine No Drip Formula, Logicin Rapid Relief Nasal Spray, Vicks Sinex Nasal Spray)

Available forms

Metered-dose nasal spray: 500 microgram/mL; Squeeze spray: 500 microgram/mL

Action

- see General Actions and Uses of sympathomimetic nasal decongestants (p. 1081)
- action in 5–10 minutes, duration 5–6 hours, gradual decline over next 6 hours

Dose

- 1–3 sprays in each nostril twice daily 10–12-hourly (not exceeding twice in 24 hours) (Dimetapp) **OR**
- 1–2 sprays to each nostril 2–3 times daily (Logicin, Vicks Sinex) **OR**
- 2–3 sprays in each nostril twice daily (Demazin, Drixine)

Uses/Adverse effects/Interactions/ Nursing points/Cautions/Patient teaching and advice

- see general points for sympathomimetic nasal decongestants (p. 1081–82)

TRAMAZOLINE HYDROCHLORIDE (Spray Tish, Spray Tish Menthol)

Available form

Metered-dose nasal spray: 82 microgram/ dose

Action

- see General Actions and Uses of sympathomimetic nasal decongestants (p. 1081)
- action within 5 minutes, duration up to 8 hours

Dose

- 1–2 sprays in each nostril up to 4 times daily

Uses/Adverse effects/Interactions/ Nursing points/Cautions

- see general points for sympathomimetic nasal decongestants (p. 1081–82)
- contraindicated in those with rhinitis sicca (dry disease of nasal mucosa forming crusts and scabs) or with hypersensitivity to benzalkonium chloride (preservative)

Patient teaching and advice

- should not be used for more than 7 days
- instruct patient that pump should be re-primed if not used for 2 weeks
- see General Patient teaching and advice for sympathomimetic nasal decongestants (p. 1082)

XYLOMETAZOLINE HYDROCHLORIDE (Flo Rapid Relief, Otrivin Menthol Spray, Otrivin Nasal Drops Adult, Otrivin Nasal Drops Junior, Otrivin Nasal Spray Adult, Otrivin Nasal Spray Junior, Sudafed Xylo Nasal Decongestant Nasal Spray)

Available forms

Metered-dose nasal spray (adult): 1 mg/mL; Nasal drops (adult): 1 mg/ mL; Metered-dose nasal spray (junior): 0.5 mg/mL; Nasal drops (junior): 0.5 mg/mL

Action

- see General Actions and Uses of sympathomimetic nasal decongestants (p. 1081)
- action within few minutes, duration up to 10–12 hours

Dose

- (nasal spray, adult) 1 spray to each nostril 2–3 times daily **OR**
- (nasal drops, adult) 2–3 drops to each nostril 2–3 times daily (8–10-hourly)

Uses/Adverse effects/Interactions/ Nursing points/Cautions/Patient teaching and advice

- see general points for sympathomimetic nasal decongestants (p. 1081–82)
- should not be used for more than 3 days
- (Flo Rapid Relief) can be used for up to 12 weeks after opening

Note

- contained in Otrivin Plus Nasal Spray with ipratropium bromide

THE OROPHARYNX

The mouth contains the four main taste receptors (sour, sweet, bitter and salty) where the information is received and relayed via the taste pathways through the pons and medulla to the thalamus and on to the cerebral cortex where taste is perceived (Bryant et al 2019). A number of medications can alter, decrease or impair the sense of taste and include ACE inhibitors (e.g. captopril, enalapril), antineoplastic agents (e.g. fluorouracil, methotrexate, bleomycin, doxorubicin), nicotine, some antidepressants, antiepileptics and anti-Parkinson's agents, NSAIDs and antimicrobial agents (Bryant et al 2019).

Agents are introduced into the mouth and throat to treat mouth ulcers, infections and inflammation.

General Nursing points/Cautions for mouth and throat preparations

- ensure that analgesic or anaesthetic agents are given to patients with painful mouth ulcers a few minutes before eating
- do not give anything to drink if the patient has had the pharynx anaesthetised until at least 1 hour after application to prevent aspiration of fluid
- mouth washes are beneficial before as well as after meals

General Patient teaching and advice for mouth and throat preparations

- patient should be advised not to eat or drink within 15 minutes of applying mouth gel
- instruct patient that lozenges should not be chewed, but allowed to dissolve slowly
- advise patient to remove dentures when necessary to allow access to ulcers
- instruct patient that rinsing/gargling solution should not be swallowed, but spat out after gargling and that rinsing/gargling solution is generally used undiluted, but if stinging/burning occurs, may be diluted with water
- see General Patient teaching and advice (p. xxvii)

ANTI-INFECTIVE AGENTS

CETYLPYRIDINIUM CHLORIDE (Cepacol)

Available form
Solution: 500 microgram/mL

Action
- antibacterial

Use
- sore, irritated, inflamed or infected throat or mouth
- after dental treatments

Dose
- gargle or rinse 10–15 mL for 10–15 seconds and expel every 2–3 hours **OR**
- (dental treatments/plaque reduction) rinse for 10–15 seconds after brushing teeth and meals

Nursing points/Cautions/Patient teaching and advice

- patient should be advised not to swallow solution

- instruct patient to seek medical advice if symptoms persist, recur or worsen or if other symptoms (fever, headache, vomiting, nausea) develop
- see general points for mouth and throat preparations (p. 1084)

Note
- contained in Cepacaine, Difflam preparations, Duro-Tuss Chesty Cough Lozenges, Duro-Tuss Dry Cough Lozenges and Sodium Bicarbonate Mouthwash 1% w/v solution

CHLORHEXIDINE GLUCONATE (Rivacol Chlorhexidine 0.2% Mouthwash, Savacol Mouth & Throat Rinse)

Available form
Solution: 2 mg/mL (0.2%)

Action
- antiseptic

Use
- mouth ulcer, minor throat infection
- plaque reduction and prevention of gingivitis

Dose
- (mouth ulcer, throat infection) rinse or gargle 10 mL for 1–2 minutes 3 times daily after meals **OR**
- (dental hygiene) rinse or gargle 10 mL for 1–2 minutes daily

Adverse effects
- teeth staining, taste alteration

Nursing points/Cautions/Patient teaching and advice
- patient should be advised not to swallow solution after rinsing or gargling
- instruct patient to seek medical advice if symptoms persist, recur or worsen or if other symptoms (fever, headache, vomiting, nausea) develop
- (children under 10 years) dilute solution (5 mL in 5 mL warm water)
- see general points for mouth and throat preparations (p. 1084)

Note
- contained in Difflam C Inflammatory Antiseptic Solution and Savacol Freshmint Antiseptic Mouth and Throat Rinse

POVIDONE–IODINE (Betadine Sore Throat Gargle, Betadine Sore Throat Gargle – Ready To Use, Difflam Sore Throat Gargle with Iodine Concentrate, Riodine Concentrated Gargle Solution)

Available forms
Solution (diluted): 10 mg/mL; Solution (undiluted): 75 mg/mL (7.5%)

Action
- topical microbicidal antiseptic

Use
- sore throat

Dose
- (undiluted preparations) dilute according to directions (1 mL solution to 20 mL water) and gargle for up to 30 seconds 3–4-hourly daily **OR**
- (diluted preparation) 15 mL gargled for 30 seconds 3–4-hourly

Adverse effects
- allergy

Interactions
- not recommended with hydrogen peroxide mouthwash

Nursing points/Cautions/Patient teaching and advice
- patient should be advised not to swallow solution

- if condition does not improve in 2 days, patient should be advised to seek medical advice
- contraindicated in those with hypersensitivity to iodine, thyroid disease or within 4 weeks of thyroid cancer treatment
- see also general points for mouth and throat preparations (p. 1084)

not recommended during pregnancy or breastfeeding

Note

- povidone–iodine is also used as a skin antiseptic and in wound dressing products

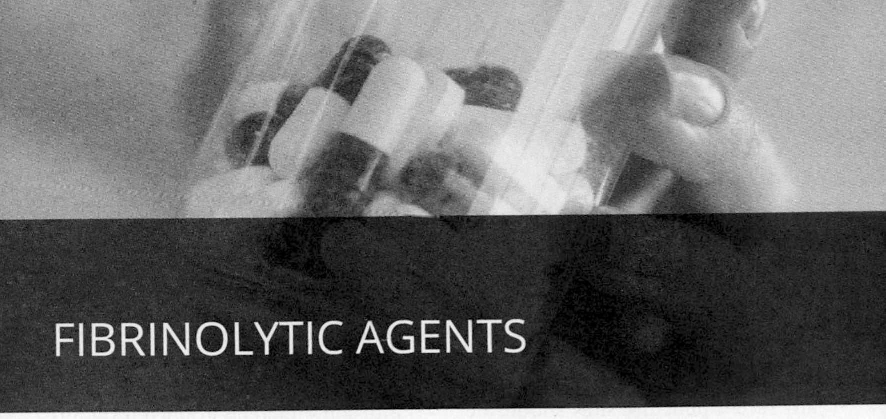

FIBRINOLYTIC AGENTS

Thrombosis is formation of a clot that may occlude either the arterial circulation (and may lead to myocardial infarction or peripheral ischaemia) or the venous circulation (and may lead to pulmonary embolism or deep vein thrombosis). Blood stasis is often a cause of venous thrombi because it allows platelets and fibrin to build up, which also makes these thrombi amenable to treatment with fibrinolytic agents. Because arterial thrombi consist mainly of platelets, fibrinolytic agents are not as effective (Hogg & Weitz 2018).

Fibrinolytic agents (also known as thrombolytic agents) activate plasminogen to form the proteolytic enzyme plasmin, which breaks down fibrin and therefore dissolves the clot wherever it can be reached by the plasmin. Fibrinolytic agents have a greater impact on haemostasis compared to anticoagulants, resulting in bleeding that is more severe and difficult to control (in part, because the clots may be located in areas that are not amenable to compression) (Bryant et al 2019). Some agents, such as alteplase, are fibrin-specific and have little or no effect on circulating unbound plasminogen, whereas the fibrin non-specific agents affect circulating unbound plasminogen as well as fibrin-bound plasminogen. Potency is generally expressed in units that are not comparable between agents in this class.

General Adverse effects of fibrinolytic agents

- minor or major bleeding (intracranial, internal or superficial)
- (IV site) haemorrhage
- arrhythmias (associated with reperfusion), tachycardia or bradycardia
- hypotension
- (rare) anaphylactoid reaction (rash, urticaria, bronchospasm, laryngeal oedema, periorbital oedema, angioedema), cholesterol embolus, seizures

General Interactions of fibrinolytic agents

- increased risk of bleeding if given before, during or within 24 hours of anticoagulants (INR > 1.3), antiplatelet agents or other fibrinolytic agents, and these agents are therefore not recommended/contraindicated together

General Nursing points/Cautions for fibrinolytic agents

- treatment should be started as soon as possible after onset of symptoms
- should only be used in hospital setting by experienced doctors with facilities that allow monitoring and have readily available resuscitation equipment
- any recent puncture sites should be carefully observed for bleeding
- IM injections, arterial punctures, venipuncture and undue patient handling should be avoided during therapy; however, if arterial puncture is necessary, choose a site that can be manually compressed and apply pressure for 30 minutes; pressure dressing should be applied and site frequently observed
- patient should be closely monitored for:
  - any signs of cholesterol embolism, including 'purple toe' syndrome, gangrenous digits, livedo reticularis (see Glossary), hypertension, myocardial infarction, bowel infarction and rhabdomyolysis
  - any signs of bradycardia or ventricular irritability as this can become life threatening. Antiarrhythmic agents should be readily available
  - any signs of angioedema (during infusion and for 24 hours after)
- patient should be advised to report any visual disturbances that might be indicative of ophthalmic bleeding
- should not be mixed with any other drugs
- diluent should be added gently to vial to reconstitute it and solution should not be shaken or vial inverted. If reconstituted solution is further diluted, infusion bag should not be agitated, but should be gently inverted to ensure even mixing of solution
- do not administer if any discolouration or particulate matter is present
- discard any unused solution
- should be administered via a dedicated line/lumen and infusions given via infusion pump
- infusion should be stopped if significant bleeding occurs
- fibrinolytic agents are generally not recommended within 10 days of surgery or trauma unless exceptional circumstances exist (e.g. pulmonary embolus) where risk versus benefit must be carefully weighed
- (acute myocardial infarction) generally not recommended in those with only ST depression on ECG, except in those with true posterior infarct (tall R waves with marked ST depression in leads V1 to V3)
- caution if used in those with left heart thrombus (e.g. mitral stenosis, atrial fibrillation) as there is an increased risk of thromboembolism
- consider analysis of benefits versus risks in patients with the following conditions, who have increased risk of adverse effects: within 6 months of transient ischaemic attacks or ischaemic stroke, over 75 years of age, over 70 years of age with hypertension, mitral stenosis with atrial fibrillation, diabetic haemorrhagic retinopathy, recent head or cranial trauma, pregnancy, septic thrombophlebitis, occluded arteriovenous cannula at seriously infected site, recent minor traumas within 10 days (e.g. biopsy, IM injections), systolic BP $>$ 160 mmHg, indwelling urethral

catheter in situ, open tuberculosis or low body weight (< 60 kg)

- contraindicated in those with bleeding disorders (or within last 6 months), coagulation problems, intracranial bleed, neoplasm (likely to bleed), intracranial or spinal surgery, recent head trauma, aneurysm, severe uncontrolled hypertension (systolic BP > 180 mmHg, diastolic > 110 mmHg), within 10 days of obstetric delivery (or abortion), prolonged or traumatic cardiopulmonary resuscitation (> 2 minutes) within 10 days, organ biopsy or puncture of subclavian or jugular vein, within 12 weeks of major surgery, significant trauma or ulcerative GI disease, oesophageal varices, acute pancreatitis, arterial aneurysm, arterial/venous malformation, subacute bacterial endocarditis, pericarditis, severe liver or kidney disease/dysfunction (especially if associated with coagulation problems), recent history of stroke (< 6 months), diabetic haemorrhagic retinopathy or other haemorrhagic ophthalmic conditions

ALTEPLASE (Actilyse)

Available forms

Vial: 10 mg, 50 mg

Action

- recombinant tissue plasminogen activator (r-tPA) which acts on fibrin in thrombus with little or no effect on circulation unbound plasminogen
- minimal systemic effects
- duration of fibrinolytic effect 4 hours
- (acute myocardial infarction) reperfuses occluded vessels in approximately 90 minutes in most patients

Use

- acute myocardial infarction (within 12 hours of onset of symptoms)
- pulmonary embolism
- acute ischaemic stroke within 4.5 hours of onset of symptoms (and exclusion of intracranial bleed)

Dose

- (pulmonary embolus) 100 mg IV given as a 10 mg IV bolus over 1–2 minutes, then remaining 90 mg over 2 hours (not exceeding 1.5 mg/kg if weight is < 65 kg) **OR**
- (myocardial infarction) 10 mg IV bolus over 1–2 minutes, 50 mg by IV infusion over 60 minutes, then 40 mg over the next 2 hours (not exceeding 1.5 mg/kg if weight is ≤ 65 kg) **OR**
- (myocardial infarction, weight > 65 kg) 100 mg IV given as a 15 mg IV bolus over 1–2 minutes, 50 mg by IV infusion over 30 minutes, then 35 mg over the next 60 minutes **OR**
- (myocardial infarction, weight < 65 kg) 100 mg IV given as a 15 mg IV bolus over 1–2 minutes, then 0.75 mg/kg by IV infusion over 30 minutes, then 0.5 mg/kg over the next 60 minutes **OR**
- (acute ischaemic stroke) 0.9 mg/kg (maximum 90 mg) by IV infusion over 60 minutes, with 10% of total dose as initial IV bolus

Adverse effects

- nausea, vomiting
- fever
- see General Adverse effects of fibrinolytic agents (p. 1087)

Interactions

- increased risk of anaphylactoid reaction if given with ACE inhibitors
- (acute ischaemic stroke) increased risk of bleeding if patient has been pretreated with aspirin
- see General Interactions of fibrinolytic agents (p. 1087)

Nursing points/Cautions

- (pulmonary embolus) diagnosis should be confirmed before starting therapy. Any underlying deep vein thrombosis should also be treated, taking into consideration that lysis of any deep vein thrombi may cause re-embolisation and therefore patient should be closely monitored
- (acute ischaemic stroke) intracranial haemorrhage should be excluded (e.g. CT scan) before starting therapy
- (acute ischaemic stroke) BP monitoring is recommended during therapy and 24 hours post-infusion
- trade name and batch number should be recorded in patient medical notes
- reconstitute using water for injections (without preservatives). Dissolve powder by swirling vial gently to prevent excessive foaming. Allow to stand for several minutes to allow any foaming to settle and clear, then dilute with sodium chloride 0.9% only
- when reconstituting 50 mg vial, use transfer cannula (provided) to inject water for injections into vial
- solutions containing preservatives or carbohydrates (e.g. glucose) should be avoided for reconstitution or dilution as this increases turbidity of fluid
- administer alone
- (acute myocardial infarction, pulmonary embolism) usually given with IV heparin to reduce risk of re-occlusion. An IV bolus of 5000 units is given before the start of fibrinolytic therapy or within the first hour, followed by infusion of 1000 units/hour for 24–48 hours, adjusted according to aPTT (1.5–2.5 of normal limits, 50–70 seconds)
- aspirin 160 mg should be started immediately and continued (160–325 mg daily) for the first few months after myocardial infarction
- heparin and alteplase infusions should be stopped immediately if uncontrolled bleeding occurs
- readministration should be undertaken with great caution because there is a possibility of antibody formation and hypersensitivity reaction
- stopper contains latex, which may cause hypersensitivity reaction in sensitive individuals
- increased risk of intracranial bleeding if total dose > 100 mg (myocardial infarction, pulmonary embolus) or > 90 mg (acute ischaemic stroke)
- (acute ischaemic stroke) caution if used in those who have received previous aspirin therapy, have uncontrolled diabetes, who have had a prior stroke, late presentation, have small asymptomatic cerebral aneurysms or over 80 years
- (acute ischaemic stroke) contraindicated if > 4.5 hours have elapsed since onset of symptoms or if onset time is unknown, in those showing minor neurological deficit showing improvement or in those with severe stroke, if seizure occurred with stroke, within 48 hours of heparin therapy or elevated APTT, combination of prior stroke and diabetes, within 12 weeks of previous stroke or head trauma, if platelet count is < 100,000/mm^3, systolic BP > 185 mmHg or diastolic BP > 110 mmHg, blood glucose < 50 mg/dL (2.8 mmol/L) or > 400 mg/dL (22.2 mmol/L), or if the patient is aged less than 18 or greater than 80 years or with an intracranial bleed (including symptomatic subarachnoid bleed with normal CT)
- (myocardial infarction, pulmonary embolus) contraindicated in those with haemorrhagic stroke, stroke of unknown origin or within 6 months of ischaemic stroke or transient ischaemic attack

- contraindicated in those with hypersensitivity to gentamicin (traces may remain from the manufacturing process)
- see General Nursing points/Cautions for fibrinolytic agents (p. 1088)

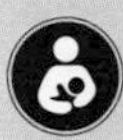

should only be used in pregnancy or breastfeeding when benefits outweigh the risks. Animal studies have shown placental haemorrhage resulting in prematurity and fetal loss

RETEPLASE (Rapilysin)

Available form
Vial: 10 U

Action
- recombinant plasminogen activating factor (r-tPA), similar to alteplase
- reduction in plasma fibrinogen levels is dose dependent
- peak effect 2 hours
- fibrinogen levels return to normal in approximately 2 days

Use
- thrombolysis for acute myocardial infarction within 6 hours of symptom onset

Dose
- initially 10 U as slow IV bolus (over not more than 2 minutes), followed by a second 10 U bolus 30 minutes after the first

Adverse effects
- (injection site) burning sensation
- see General Adverse effects of fibrinolytic agents (p. 1087)

Interactions
- not recommended with abciximab
- see General Interactions of fibrinolytic agents (p. 1087)

Nursing points/Cautions
- reconstitute using reconstitution spike and 10 mL solvent (both provided), swirling gently to dissolve powder
- reconstituted solution is clear and colourless
- incompatible with heparin and should be administered via a dedicated line
- if dedicated IV line is not available, line should be well flushed with sodium chloride 0.9% or glucose 5% before and after bolus administration
- 5000 IU bolus of heparin is given before first bolus, followed by 1000 IU/hour infusion after second bolus and continued for at least 24–72 hours to maintain APTT at 1.5–2 normal limits (50–75 seconds)
- aspirin therapy (250–350 mg orally should be started as soon as possible after onset of symptoms, then 75–150 mg/daily until discharge) is usually started at the same time to prevent re-thrombosis
- readministration is not recommended
- contraindicated in those with hypersensitivity of reteplase or polysorbate 80
- see General Nursing points/Cautions for fibrinolytic agents (p. 1088)

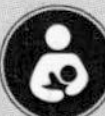

contraindicated during pregnancy unless situation is life threatening

breastmilk should be discarded for 24 hours after therapy

TENECTEPLASE (Metalyse)

Available forms
Vial: 40 mg (8000 IU), 50 mg (10,000 IU)

Action
- genetically engineered tissue plasminogen activator (tPA), similar to alteplase, although structural differences make it fibrin specific
- biphasic elimination with initial half-life about 18.5–29.5 minutes and terminal half-life 42–206 minutes

- improves blood flow within 90 minutes of injection
- no antibody formation has been observed

Use

- thrombolysis for acute myocardial infarction within 12 hours of onset of symptoms

Dose

- 30–50 mg (6000–10,000 IU) as a single IV bolus (dose is weight dependent)

Adverse effects

- nausea, vomiting
- fever
- see General Adverse effects of fibrinolytic agents (p. 1087)

Interactions

- see General Interactions of fibrinolytic agents (p. 1087)

Nursing points/Cautions

- reconstitute using water for injections (provided in prefilled syringe), swirling gently to dissolve powder, avoiding excessive foaming
- given as a single bolus injection over 10 seconds
- should only be injected into IV lines containing sodium chloride 0.9%
- incompatible with glucose solutions
- administer alone
- heparin is usually started with a 4000–5000 IU bolus, then continued at 800–1000 IU/hour IV infusion for at least 48–72 hours to maintain APTT at 50–75 seconds
- aspirin (150–325 mg) is usually started as soon as possible after onset of symptoms and continued daily until discharge
- caution if used in those ≥ 75 years
- contraindicated in those with gentamicin or polysorbate 20 hypersensitivity
- see General Nursing points/Cautions for fibrinolytic agents (p. 1088)

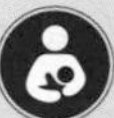

should only be used in pregnancy or breastfeeding when the benefits outweigh the risks

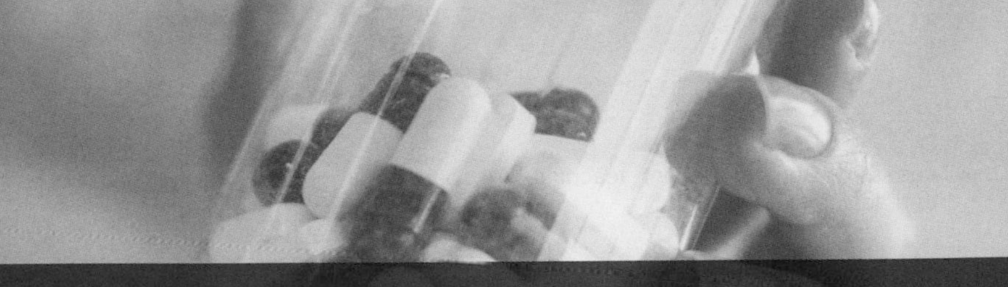

GASTROINTESTINAL AGENTS (MISCELLANEOUS)

Numerous agents exert their effects on the GI tract, including agents from the following drug classes covered in other sections of this book:

- antidiarrhoeal agents
- antiemetics
- antiulcer agents (including antacids)
- laxatives
- topical rectal medication.

Gastrointestinal agents that do not fall into these categories are included in this section.

MEBEVERINE HYDROCHLORIDE (Colese, Colofac)

Available form
Tablets: 135 mg

Action
- antispasmodic
- non-specifically relaxes vascular, cardiac and other smooth muscle

Use
- management of irritable bowel syndrome (IBS) symptoms

Dose
- 135 mg orally 3 times daily before or with food until desired effect is achieved, then gradually decrease dose

Adverse effects
- dizziness, headache, insomnia, general malaise
- indigestion, heartburn, anorexia, constipation
- decreased pulse rate
- (rare) hypersensitivity, angioedema

Nursing points/Cautions
- liver function tests are recommended if patient develops gastrointestinal symptoms or jaundice
- contains lactose (Colese: 100 mg/tablet; Colofac: 80 mg/tablet) and should not be given to patients with lactose intolerance
- caution if used in those with cardiac arrhythmias, AV heart block, angina or ischaemic heart disease or advanced liver or kidney dysfunction
- not recommended in those with galactose intolerance, Lapp lactase deficiency or glucose–galactose malabsorption

Patient teaching and advice
- warn patient that it may take several weeks before desired effects are achieved
- patient should be advised not to drive or operate machinery if dizziness occurs

- see also General Patient teaching and advice (p. xxvii)

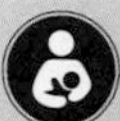

not used during pregnancy or breastfeeding unless expected benefit outweighs any potential risk

TEDUGLUTIDE (Revestive)

Available form
Vial: 5 mg

Action
- analogue of GLP-2 (peptide secreted by L-cells of distal intestine) (GLP-2 increases intestinal and portal blood flow, decreases intestinal motility and inhibits gastric acid secretion)
- binds to GLP-2 receptors releasing mediators such as insulin-like growth factors (IGF-1), nitric oxide and keratinocyte growth factor (KGF)
- preserves mucosal integrity by promoting repair and normal intestine growth, increasing villus height and crypt depth
- half-life is 1.1 hours (in patient with short bowel syndrome)

Use
- treatment of patients with short bowel syndrome (who are dependent on parental support)

Dose
- 0.05 mg/kg SC daily

Adverse effects
- abdominal pain and distention, nausea, vomiting, flatulence, diarrhoea, loss of appetite
- colonic polyps, pancreatitis, small intestinal stenosis, intestinal obstruction
- cholecystitis
- fatigue, headache, insomnia
- fever
- arthralgia
- nasopharyngitis, flu-like illness
- cough, dyspnoea
- peripheral oedema, congestive cardiac failure
- (injection site) haematoma, erythema
- (uncommon) increase in blood amylase and lipase, pancreatic duct stenosis, pancreas infection, fluid overload, antibody development

Interactions
- caution if used with benzodiazepines, opioid analgesics, digoxin and antihypertensive agents

Nursing points/Cautions
- patient should be stable for 4 or more weeks on parental nutrition before starting therapy
- therapy should be started under medical supervision
- bilirubin and alkaline phosphatase should be measured before starting and regularly during therapy
- colonoscopy of whole colon with removal of any polyps is recommended before starting therapy (up to 6 months) and then within 1–2 years after starting therapy and then every 5 years (or more often for patients at high risk of colorectal polyps). If polyps are found, removed and found to be colorectal cancer, therapy should be stopped
- patient should be closely monitored for any signs of small bowel and hepatobiliary malignancy
- patient should be monitored for any fluid overload, especially at the start of therapy. Parenteral nutrition needs should be assessed and re-evaluated during the first months of therapy to minimise risk of fluid overload
- therapy should be continued in those patients who have weaned off parenteral nutrition
- when therapy is stopped, fluid and electrolyte levels should be carefully monitored as discontinuation may result in fluid and electrolyte imbalance and potential dehydration

- should only be administered SC, rotating sites (thigh, upper arm or abdomen)
- not for IM or IV administration
- reconstitute using 0.5 mL water for injections giving a concentration of 10 mg/mL
- when reconstituting, vial should not be shaken but can be rolled between palms and turned gently upside down once and used within 3 hours of reconstitution
- reconstituted solution should not be shaken or frozen or used if cloudy or containing particles
- in patients with active non-gastrointestinal malignancy or at risk of malignancy, decision to start therapy should be based on risk versus benefit
- caution if used in those with a history of cardiovascular disease (e.g. cardiac insufficiency, hypertension)
- contraindicated in those with active gastrointestinal (gastrointestinal tract, hepatobiliary, pancreatic) malignancy or with a history of gastrointestinal malignancy within last 5 years

Patient teaching and advice

- patient should be instructed to seek medical advice immediately if any of the following occur:
  - sudden weight gain, swollen ankles, difficulty breathing (fluid overload)
  - upper abdominal pain which spreads to right shoulder or back, abdominal tenderness, nausea, vomiting, fever (cholecystitis)
  - upper abdominal pain radiating to back, abdominal pain that is worse after eating, abdominal tenderness, nausea, vomiting, rapid pulse (pancreatitis)
  - intermittent crampy abdominal pain, loss of appetite, vomiting, abdominal swelling, inability to pass gas or have bowel movements (intestinal obstruction)

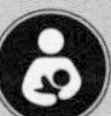

should only be used during pregnancy and breastfeeding if benefits outweigh risks

URSODEOXYCHOLIC ACID (Ursodox GH, Ursofalk, Ursosan)

Available forms

Capsules: 250 mg; Tablets: 500 mg; Suspension: 50 mg/mL

Action

- alters bile salt composition, decreasing the concentration of more toxic bile salts and increasing bile acid output and bile flow
- half-life 3.5–5.8 days

Use

- chronic cholestatic liver disease (including associated with primary sclerosing cholangitis (PSC), primary biliary cholangitis (PBC) and cystic fibrosis (CF) related cholestasis)

Dose

- (PSC) 10–15 mg/kg/day orally in 2–3 divided doses, increasing to 20 mg/kg/day if needed **OR**
- (CF-related cholestasis) up to 20 mg/kg/day orally in 2–3 divided doses **OR**
- (PBC, non-CF chronic cholestasis) 12–16 mg/kg/day orally in 2–3 divided doses until liver function improves, then decreasing to a single nightly dose

Adverse effects

- diarrhoea, nausea, vomiting, right upper abdominal pain
- increased pruritus
- sleep disturbance
- increased cholestasis
- (rare) allergic reaction, calcification of gallstones, hepatitis, cirrhosis, urticaria

Interactions

- absorption may be inhibited by colestyramine, colestipol, charcoal and

antacids containing aluminium hydroxide or aluminium oxide
- may increase absorption of ciclosporin, therefore ciclosporin serum levels should be closely monitored
- may decrease the absorption of ciprofloxacin

Nursing points/Cautions

- liver enzymes (AST, ALT and glutamyl transferase) should be measured monthly for the first 3 months, then 3-monthly
- if patient weighs less than 34 kg or is unable to swallow, suspension is recommended
- (PBC) if pruritus increases initially, dose should be decreased to 250 mg daily, then slowly increased at weekly intervals
- 5 mL suspension contains 11.39 mg sodium, which may need to be considered if patient is on sodium-restricted diet
- not recommended in those with acute gallbladder or bile duct inflammation or obstruction of common bile duct or cystic duct

Patient teaching and advice

- advise patient to swallow capsules and tablets whole
- patient should be advised to separate by 2 hours from colestyramine, colestipol, charcoal and some antacids
- instruct patient to shake suspension well before use and discard 4 months after opening
- warn patient to seek medical advice immediately if right-sided upper abdominal pains occurs or if itching (pruritus) gets worse
- see also General Patient teaching and advice (p. xxvii)

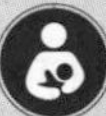

not recommended in first month of pregnancy or during breastfeeding

suspension is available for those with swallowing difficulties

AGENTS USED IN INFLAMMATORY BOWEL DISEASE

Australia has one of the highest incidence rates of inflammatory bowel disease (IBD) in the developed countries (29.3 per 100,000). While this incidence has plateaued in most developed countries, the figure is now increasing in developing countries (Wright et al 2018). IBD is made up of Crohn's disease and ulcerative colitis. *Crohn's disease* may affect the entire intestine and causes inflammation of both the mucosal and the submucosal layers, while *ulcerative colitis* affects the colon and rectum and, in severe cases, abscesses may erode the colon wall, leading to perforation (Wright et al 2018). Early diagnosis and management is vital in inducing and maintaining remission rather than just symptom control as subclinical inflammation may lead to intestinal damage (Wright et al 2018).

Aminosalicylic acid-based agents (e.g. sulfasalazine, mesalazine) are used to induce remission and prevent relapse in mild-to-moderate ulcerative colitis; however, these are less efficacious in Crohn's disease. For moderate-to-severe disease, corticosteroids such as prednisolone are used for remission of active disease (see Corticosteroids p. 943). Immunomodifying agents (such as azathioprine) are recommended for maintenance of remission in moderate-to-severe Crohn's disease or ulcerative colitis not responding to other treatment. More recently, anti-tumour necrosis-α factor (e.g. adalimumab, infliximab) (see DMARDs pp. 991 and 996) and monoclonal antibodies (e.g. vedolizumab, ustekinumab) have been used for induction and maintenance of remission. Faecal microbiota transplantation has shown good results in induction of remission in patients with ulcerative colitis; however, this therapy is still in its infancy and requires further research (Wright et al 2018).

BALSALAZIDE SODIUM (Colazide)

Available form

Capsules: 750 mg

Action

- aminosalicylate
- prodrug, active metabolite is mesalazine which is an intestinal anti-inflammatory agent action on colonic mucosa
- onset of action 1–2 hours

Use

- treatment of mild-to-moderate ulcerative colitis, and maintenance of remission in those intolerant to sulfasalazine

Dose

- initially 2.25 g (3 capsules) 3 times daily until remission or 12 weeks, then 1.5 g (2 capsules) twice daily (maintenance)

Adverse effects

- abdominal pain, diarrhoea, nausea, vomiting, dyspepsia, anorexia, constipation, dry mouth
- headache, fatigue, dizziness
- arthralgia, back pain, myalgia
- flu-like illness, dyspnoea
- rectal bleeding
- aggravated ulcerative colitis
- pruritus
- (rare) blood dyscrasias

Interactions

- caution if used with digoxin, therefore plasma levels should be closely monitored during therapy, especially when starting or stopping therapy
- caution if used with agents with a narrow therapeutic range if secreted in the renal tubules
- caution if given with warfarin
- may impair absorption of folic acid
- may increase risk of myelosuppression if given with mercaptopurine and azathioprine
- caution if given with oral antibacterial agents

Nursing points/Cautions

- blood counts, blood urea nitrogen (BUN), creatinine and urine analysis is recommended during therapy
- rectal or oral corticosteroids can be used at the same time if needed
- caution if used in those with asthma, history of kidney disease or mild kidney impairment, or mild-to-moderate liver impairment
- not recommended in those under 18 years
- contraindicated in those with hypersensitivity to mesalazine or salicylates, severe liver impairment, moderate-to-severe kidney impairment, those with bleeding tendency or active peptic ulceration

Patient teaching and advice

- advise patient to seek medical advice if any unexplained bruising, bleeding, sore throat, fever or tiredness occurs
- see General Patient teaching and advice (p. xxvii)

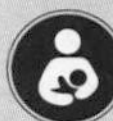

not recommended during the first stages of pregnancy unless expected benefit outweighs any potential risk; and contraindicated in the last weeks of pregnancy

not recommended during breastfeeding

MESALAZINE (Asacol, Mesasal, Mezavant, Pentasa preparation, Salofalk preparations)

Available forms

Tablets (modified release): 250 mg, 500 mg, 800 mg, 1.2 g; Granules (modified release): 500 mg/sachet, 1 g/sachet, 1.5 g/sachet, 2 g/sachet, 3 g/sachet, 4 g/sachet; Suppositories: 1 g; Enema: 1 g/100 mL, 2 g/60 mL, 4 g/60 mL; Enema (foam): 80 g

Action

- active component of sulfasalazine (5-aminosalicylic acid)
- anti-inflammatory action by inhibiting prostaglandin synthesis, chemotactic leukotriene synthesis and leucocytic motility

Use

- acute inflammatory large bowel disease
- maintenance of remission of ulcerative colitis and Crohn's disease in patients intolerant to sulfasalazine
- ulcerative proctitis, ulcerative proctosigmoiditis

Dose

- (ulcerative colitis) 1.5–3 g orally daily in 1–3 divided doses 30–60 minutes before food (treatment), then 250 mg orally 3 times daily (maintenance of remission) **OR**
- (Crohn's disease) 2.4–4.8 g orally once daily (induction of remission), then 2.4 g daily (maintenance) (prolonged-release tablets) **OR**
- (Crohn's disease – maintenance) 250 mg orally 3 times daily **OR**
- (ulcerative colitis) 2.4–4.8 g orally daily in single or divided doses (induction of remission), then 1.6–2.4 g orally daily (maintenance of remission) (modified-release tablets) **OR**
- (ulcerative colitis) up to 4 g once daily or in divided doses (induction of remission), then 1.5–2 g daily in divided doses (maintenance) (Pentasa – prolonged-release tablets, granules) **OR**
- (Crohn's disease) up to 4 g daily in divided doses (treatment), then 4 g daily (maintenance) (Pentasa – prolonged-release tablets, granules) **OR**
- (ulcerative colitis) 2–4 g enema/foam enema nightly per rectum (acute treatment and maintenance) **OR**
- (ulcerative proctosigmoiditis, left-sided ulcerative colitis) 1 g enema nightly per rectum (Pentasa) **OR**
- (ulcerative proctitis) 1 g rectally at bedtime (suppository)

Adverse effects

- nausea, vomiting, diarrhoea, abdominal pain, flatulence, dyspepsia, exacerbation of ulcerative colitis
- headache, neuropathy, fatigue, asthenia
- fever
- hypertension
- rash, alopecia, pruritus, urticaria
- arthralgia, myalgia, back pain
- decreased sperm count, impaired sperm motility
- haematuria, ketouria
- chest pain
- (transient) changes in liver function tests
- (rare) interstitial nephritis, reversible pancreatitis, colitis, blood dyscrasias, myocarditis, pericarditis, hypersensitivity, kidney failure, photosensitivity

Interactions

- not recommended with anticoagulants as effects may be potentiated, therefore prothrombin time should be closely monitored
- may potentiate effects of sulfonylureas, increasing risk of hypoglycaemia, therefore blood glucose levels should be closely monitored
- may delay excretion of methotrexate, increasing risk of toxicity
- may antagonise probenecid and sulfinpyrazone

- may decrease effects of rifampicin, furosemide and spironolactone
- not recommended with lactulose or similar drugs that lower gastric or stool pH and prevent the release of mesalazine
- increased risk of nephrotoxicity if given with nephrotoxic agents including NSAIDs and azathioprine
- increased risk of myelosuppression if given with azathioprine, thioguanine or mercaptopurine
- increased risk of gastric adverse effects if given with glucocorticoids

Nursing points/Cautions

- kidney (including urinalysis) and liver function and differential blood counts should be monitored before starting, monthly for 3 months, then 3-monthly
- if patient weighs less than 40 kg, half-dose should be given
- (acute ulcerative colitis) remission usually occurs in about 8 weeks
- (foam enema) contains sodium metasulfite and therefore should be used with caution in those with allergies or asthma
- (Salofalk granules) contain aspartame and therefore not recommended in those with phenylketonuria
- (Pentasa enema) contains sodium metabisulfite and therefore should be used with caution in those with allergies or asthma
- (Asacol) not recommended in those with galactose intolerance, Lapp lactase deficiency or glucose–galactose malabsorption
- caution if used in patients with preexisting skin conditions (e.g. eczema, dermatitis) due to increased risk of photosensitivity reaction
- caution if given to patients with renal impairment or renal failure (with proteinuria and elevated blood urea nitrogen (BUN)), hypersensitivity to sulfasalazine, liver impairment or predisposed to myocarditis or pericarditis
- caution in those with organic/functional obstruction of upper GI tract as this may delay onset of action of tablets or granules
- contraindicated in those with hypersensitivity to salicylates or sulfasalazine, severe kidney impairment, active peptic ulcer or bleeding tendency

Patient teaching and advice

- advise patient that tablets should not be crushed or chewed, but swallowed with plenty of water
- warn patient that empty tablet shells may appear in faeces. If intact tablet is present, medical advice should be sought
- instruct patient to place granules on the tongue, not crushed or chewed, and then wash them down with water or juice. They may also be dispersed in 50 mL of cold water
- (enema) warn patient that enema may cause staining to clothing and fabrics
- (enema) ensure patient understands correct instillation technique, including:
    - bowel should be emptied before instillation
    - wash hands with soap and water
    - cut along dotted line of enema pack, taking care not to damage bottle
    - shake bottle for 30 seconds
    - remove applicator cap
    - lie on left side with left leg outstretched and right leg bent
    - guide applicator into rectum and squeeze bottle gently until empty
    - remove and remain lying down for at least 30 minutes
    - wash hands and try not to open bowels until next morning if possible

- (foam enema) ensure patient understands the following:
  - 2 g = 2 applications
  - empty bowel before application
  - use foam enema at room temperature (20–25°C)
  - wash hands thoroughly with soap and water
  - shake for 15 seconds after fitting applicator to canister
  - remove safety tab under pump dome, twist dome until semicircular gap is underneath in line with nozzle
  - insert applicator into rectum (while standing with one foot on floor and other on chair/stool)
  - push pump dome and hold for 5 seconds and then release to administer one application (1 g) and wait 15 seconds
  - after second administration, applicator should be left in rectum for 30 seconds before withdrawal
  - remove applicator from canister and dispose of appropriately
  - wash hands
  - instruct patient to store canister away from direct sunlight, flames or sparks. Canister should not be frozen or refrigerated or punctured when empty
- (suppository) instruct adult patient in correct technique for suppository insertion, including:
  - the need to empty bowel if possible before suppository insertion
  - wash hands with soap and water
  - if suppository feels soft, place it (unwrapped) in the fridge or hold it under cold water to firm it up
  - put on disposable glove, if wanted
  - remove wrapper from suppository and moisten slightly by dipping in cool water
  - lie on side with knees raised to chest
  - push suppository (blunt end first) gently into rectum, taking care not to break suppository
  - remain lying down for a few minutes to allow suppository to dissolve
  - wash hands thoroughly after insertion
- advise patient to seek medical advice if any of the following occur:
  - unusual bleeding or bruising, fever, chills, sore throat, mouth ulcers
  - severe stomach ache and/or cramps, fever, rash, severe headache
  - skin rash, hives, itching
  - yellowing of eyes or skin, itching, upper abdominal pain, lethargy, loss of appetite, nausea, dark urine, pale stools
- male patient should be counselled regarding the possibility of transient reduction in sperm and sperm mobility during therapy
- female patients should be counselled to use contraception and avoid pregnancy occurring during therapy
- see General Patient teaching and advice (p. xxvii)

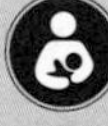

not recommended during the first stages of pregnancy unless expected benefit outweighs any potential risk. Contraindicated in the last weeks of pregnancy and during breastfeeding

granules are recommended for those with swallowing difficulties

OLSALAZINE SODIUM (Dipentum)

Available forms

Capsules: 250 mg; Tablets: 500 mg

Action

- poorly absorbed by the GI tract
- consists of 2 molecules of 5-aminosalicylic acid
- cleaved by bacteria in the colon to the clinically active form

Use

- ulcerative colitis (in those intolerant to sulfasalazine)

Dose

- (treatment of acute ulcerative colitis) initially 250 mg orally daily after meals (day 1), then increasing by 250 mg per day to 2 g orally daily in divided doses after meals (capsules) **OR**
- (treatment of acute ulcerative colitis) initially 500 mg orally daily after meals (day 1), then increasing by 500 mg per day to 2 g orally daily in divided doses (tablets) **OR**
- (maintenance of remission) 500 mg orally twice daily after meals

Adverse effects

- nausea, diarrhoea, abdominal pain, upset stomach, dry mouth
- headache, dizziness, insomnia, mood swings, irritability
- blurred vision, dry eyes, watery eyes
- fever, chills
- rash, urticaria, photosensitivity, alopecia
- dysuria, haematuria, proteinuria, impotence, menorrhagia
- arthralgia, myalgia, joint pain
- (rare) blood dyscrasias, hepatitis, pancreatitis, peripheral neuropathy, angioedema, rectal bleeding/discomfort, interstitial lung disease, nephritis

Interactions

- not recommended with salicylates or low molecular weight heparins due to increased risk of bleeding
- prothrombin time should be closely monitored if given with warfarin; however, not recommended together
- increased risk of myelosuppression if given with mercaptopurine or tioguanine
- increased risk of Reye's syndrome if given within 6 weeks of varicella vaccine

Nursing points/Cautions

- bioequivalence of capsules and tablets has not been established
- single dose should not be greater than 1 g
- daily dose can be increased to 3 g if needed
- kidney function (serum creatinine) should be measured before starting therapy, 3-monthly for first year, 6-monthly for next 4 years, then yearly for life
- caution if used in those with known allergies, asthma or impaired kidney or liver function
- contraindicated in those with hypersensitivity to salicylates, bleeding tendency/blood dyscarsias, peptic ulcer or erosive gastritis

Patient teaching and advice

- warn patient that diarrhoea occurs commonly during therapy
- advise patient that tablets should not be divided
- patient should be advised not to drive or operate machinery if dizziness occurs
- instruct patient to seek medical advice if any of the following occur:
  - diarrhoea (as watery diarrhoea requires dose reduction)
  - fever, chills, sore throat, mouth ulcers, unusual bleeding or bruising
- see also General Patient teaching and advice (p. xxvii)

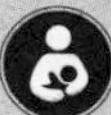

not used during pregnancy or breastfeeding unless expected benefits outweigh any potential risks

SULFASALAZINE (Pyralin EN, Salazopyrin, Salazopyrin EN-Tabs)

Available forms
Tablets: 500 mg; Tablets (enteric-coated): 500 mg

Action
- broken down in the colon by bacteria to 5-aminosalicylic acid and sulfapyridine producing an anti-inflammatory effect by its action on prostaglandin synthesis, leukotrienes and arachidonic acid metabolites
- onset of action may take 6–12 weeks

Use
- ulcerative colitis
- treatment of active Crohn's disease with colonic involvement
- rheumatoid arthritis (unresponsive to NSAIDs)

Dose
- (ulcerative colitis, Crohn's disease) initially 1–2 g orally 4 times daily after meals, then 500 mg 4 times daily as maintenance **OR**
- (rheumatoid arthritis) initially 500 mg orally at night for 1 week, 500 mg twice daily for 1 week, 500 mg in the morning and 1 g at night for 1 week, then 1 g twice daily for 1 week (to daily maximum of 3 g) then 2–3 g orally daily in 2–3 divided doses (maintenance)

Adverse effects
- anorexia, nausea, vomiting, diarrhoea
- fever, headache, pallor
- erythema, pruritus, rash
- reversible oligospermia, proteinuria, haematuria, crystallurian
- (rare) hypersensitivity reaction (including drug rash with eosinophilia and systemic symptoms (DRESS)), agranulocytosis, aplastic anaemia, microcytosis, pancytopenia, folate deficiency

Interactions
- may potentiate oral anticoagulants, methotrexate and sulfonylureas, increasing risk of adverse effects
- reduces absorption and metabolism of folic acid, resulting in folic acid deficiency, macrocytosis and pancytopenia
- reduces absorption of digoxin, therefore serum levels should be monitored
- increased blood levels may occur in patients taking oral anticoagulants, indometacin, sulfinpyrazone, urinary acidifiers or salicylates
- decreased absorption may occur if given with antacids or ferrous sulfate heptahydrate
- increased risk of bone marrow depression and leucopenia if given with azathioprine or mercaptopurine
- activity may be decreased if given with para-aminobenzoic acid-type local anaesthetics
- increased GI disturbances (especially nausea) may occur if given with methotrexate

Nursing points/Cautions
- therapy should be discontinued if serious infection develops
- enteric-coated tablets are available if GI intolerance is experienced
- monitor blood counts (including differential white cell count), liver function tests and renal function analysis (including urinalysis) before starting therapy, second-weekly for 3 months and then every 3 months
- adverse effects are mainly dose dependent
- encourage adequate fluid intake to reduce risk of crystalluria and stone formation
- serious skin reactions are most likely to occur in first 4 weeks of therapy
- caution if given to those with G6PD deficiency (as risk of haemolytic anaemia is increased) or severe

allergy, bronchial asthma, atopic disease or recurring or chronic infection
- not recommended in those with blood dyscrasias or impaired liver or kidney function
- contraindicated in those with any allergy/hypersensitivity to sulfonamide or salicylate derivatives, intestinal/urinary obstruction, porphyria or blood dyscrasias

Patient teaching and advice

- instruct patients that enteric-coated tablets should not be crushed or broken but swallowed whole with plenty of water
- advise patient to allow a 2-hour interval if taking antacids
- (inflammatory bowel disease) patient should be advised that no more than 8 hours should elapse between overnight doses
- warn patient that urine may become orange-yellow colour if alkaline
- instruct patient to immediately report any:
  - sore throat, fever, pallor
  - swollen glands
  - skin rash
  - pinpoint bleeding on the skin (purpura)
  - yellow-orange discolouration of skin, urine and other body fluids
- instruct patient to drink plenty of water during therapy
- counsel male patients about reversible male infertility (effects reversed within 8–12 weeks of stopping therapy) and female patients regarding potential harm to developing fetus
- see also General Patient teaching and advice (p. xxvii)

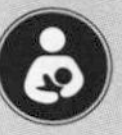

may inhibit absorption and metabolism of folic acid leading to folic acid deficiency, potentially resulting in blood disorders or harm to developing fetus, therefore should only be used if benefits outweigh risks

not recommended during breastfeeding unless the expected benefits outweigh any potential risk

VEDOLIZUMAB (rch) (Entyvio)

Available form

Vial: 300 mg

Action

- humanised IgG1 monoclonal antibody that binds to alpha4beta7 ($\alpha4\beta7$) integrin (integrin $\alpha4\beta7$ is expressed on leucocytes including T-lymphocytes that migrate into GI tract causing inflammation)
- selectively inhibits $\alpha4\beta7$ integrin preventing inflammation

Use

- moderate-to-severe ulcerative colitis or Crohn's disease in those with inadequate response or intolerant to conventional therapy or tumour necrosis factor alpha (TNFα) antagonist

Dose

- 300 mg by IV infusion over 30 minutes, repeated after 2 and 6 weeks, then every 8 weeks

Adverse effects

- infusion-related reaction (including flushing, hypertension, increased heart rate, rash, urticaria, bronchospasm, dyspnoea)
- nausea
- nasopharyngitis, upper respiratory tract infection, cough, bronchitis, influenza
- arthralgia, back pain, pain in extremities
- rash, pruritus
- fever
- fatigue, headache, dizziness
- oropharyngeal pain
- (rare) progressive multifocal leukoencephalopathy, increased liver enzymes, hypersensitivity reaction, development of anti-vedolizumab antibodies, malignancy

Interactions

- not recommended with live or attenuated live vaccines or within 3 months of stopping vedolizumab
- caution if used with or within 12 weeks of natalizumab
- not recommended concurrently with biologic immunosuppressants

Nursing points/Cautions

- all patients should be carefully screened for history or symptoms of tuberculosis (TB), including detailed medical history and possible previous exposure to TB. Chest X-ray and tuberculin skin test (Mantoux) may also be performed (however, there is a risk of false negative skin test occurring in patients who are severely ill or immunocompromised)
- any patient with latent TB should be treated with antimycobacterials before starting therapy
- any other active infections should be treated before starting therapy
- patient should be up to date with current immunisation guidelines before starting therapy
- patient should be reviewed for signs of clinical response within 12–14 weeks of starting therapy. If no response is seen within 14 weeks, therapy should not be continued
- patient should be closely monitored during and after infusion for any signs of infusion reaction which can occur up to several hours post-infusion. If infusion reaction occurs, infusion should be slowed or stopped until symptoms subside, then started at a lower rate. Infusion reactions have occurred after 2 hours and more than 2 days after infusion
- paracetamol, antihistamines, corticosteroids, adrenaline (epinephrine) and artificial airway should be readily available for infusion reaction
- premedication with paracetamol, hydrocortisone and/or antihistamine may prevent mild and transient effects of infusion reaction
- patient should be carefully monitored for any signs of symptoms that might suggest progressive multifocal leukoencephalopathy (e.g. cognitive, neurological or psychiatric symptoms). If signs (progressive one-sided weakness, clumsiness, visual disturbances, changes to thinking, memory or orientation, confusion, personality changes) occur, therapy should be stopped and further evaluation including MRI, CSF testing and repeat neurological assessments completed
- not given via IV bolus or push
- reconstitute using 4.8 mL of water for injections, vial swirled gently for at least 15 seconds to dissolve powder. Reconstituted solution should be allowed to sit for 20 minutes to allow any foam to settle. Vial can be swirled further if needed. If not fully dissolved, wait another 10 minutes. Invert reconstituted solution 3 times before withdrawing 5 mL and adding to 250 mL sodium chloride 0.9% and then gently mixing infusion bag before administration
- administer alone
- trade name and batch number should be recorded in patient's medical records
- caution if used in those with controlled severe infection or history of severe infection
- not recommended in those under 18 years
- contraindicated in those with active severe infections (including active tuberculosis), sepsis and serious abscesses

Patient teaching and advice

- instruct patient to carry a Patient Alert Card at all times
- patients should be advised to seek medical advice immediately if any of the following occur:

- recurrent or persistent infection
- persistent fever, pallor, unexplained bleeding or bruising (blood dyscrasia)
- persistent cough, weight loss and low-grade fever (possible TB)
- progressive one-sided arm or leg weakness, clumsiness or loss of balance, blurred or double vision, disorientation, confusion, personality changes, difficulty speaking, persistent numbness, decreased or loss of sensation

- women of childbearing age should be counselled to use adequate contraception during and for 18 weeks after stopping therapy to avoid pregnancy
- see General Patient teaching and advice (p. xxvii)

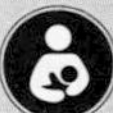

not recommended during pregnancy or breastfeeding unless benefits are thought to outweigh risks

ENZYME REPLACEMENT

Pancreatic enzyme replacement is used when the pancreas is unable to produce sufficient amounts of the enzymes necessary for the digestion of fats, carbohydrates and proteins. Conditions requiring enzyme replacement therapy include cystic fibrosis, chronic pancreatitis or after pancreatectomy (Sharkey & Wallace 2018).The goal of pancreatic enzyme replacement therapy for those with cystic fibrosis is to improve nutritional status and growth while controlling maldigestion symptoms (such as steatorrhoea). Currently marketed pancreatic enzyme replacement preparations differ in their composition, enzymatic activities, formulation, stability and bioavailability.

PANCRELIPASE (Creon Capsules, Creon Micro, Panzytrat 25000)

Available forms

Capsules: contain lipase, protease and amylase; Enteric-coated granules

Action

- mimics the enzymes that assist in the digestion of fats to fatty acids and glycerol, proteins to amino acids and carbohydrates to dextrins and sugars

Use

- malabsorption caused by pancreatic insufficiency, including cystic fibrosis, chronic pancreatitis and after some types of abdominal surgery (e.g. post-pancreatectomy, gastric bypass surgery)

Dose

- usually 1 capsule orally with meals and 1 capsule with snacks (6 capsules daily) **OR**
- (cystic fibrosis ≥ 4 years) 500 lipase units/kg of body weight with meal (titrating the dose to the disease severity, control of steatorrhoea and maintenance of good nutritional status) **OR**
- (patients with pancreatic insufficiency due to other causes) 25,000–40,000 BP units of lipase (5–8 scoops of granules) with meals and half-dose with snacks, adjusting dose if necessary

Adverse effects

- skin reaction (rash, pruritus, urticaria)
- diarrhoea, constipation, abdominal pain or distention, nausea, flatulence
- (high dose) fibrosing colonopathy

Interactions

- not recommended with antacids

Nursing points/Cautions

- patients with a history of gastrointestinal complications should be closely assessed for risk of fibrosing colonopathy
- 1 measuring scoop = 100 g of granules = 5000 units of lipase
- dose should be adjusted according to food and disease severity; however, a rapid increase in dose is not recommended due to risk of constipation
- dose should not exceed 10,000 lipase units/kg/day or 4000 lipase units/g fat intake
- of porcine origin, and therefore should not be given to patients who have cultural or religious objections, such as those of the Muslim or Jewish faith
- contraindicated in those with hypersensitivity to porcine protein, in early stages of acute pancreatitis or acute attack of chronic pancreatitis

Patient teaching and advice

- advise patient that capsules should not be crushed or chewed, although if swallowing is problematic capsules may be opened and contents sprinkled on food and eaten immediately
- instruct patient that capsule content should not be sprinkled on food with a pH greater than 5.5 (e.g. milk, ice-cream) because the protective coating may dissolve
- if antacids are necessary, patient should be advised to allow at least 1 hour between antacids and pancrelipase
- instruct patient to use measuring scoop provided for administration of granules (1 measuring scoop = 100 g of granules = 5000 units of lipase)
- advise patient that granules may be sprinkled on small amount of acidic soft food (pH < 5.5) such as apple sauce or mashed banana and eaten immediately (not stored) without chewing or crushing granules, followed by water or juice to ensure entire dose has been swallowed
- patient should be instructed to ensure he/she drinks sufficiently to prevent dehydration and constipation from occurring
- advise patient (especially if he/she has cystic fibrosis) to immediately seek medical advice if severe or prolonged abdominal pain occurs
- see General Patient teaching and advice (p. xxvii)

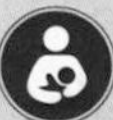

not used during the first trimester of pregnancy

not used during breastfeeding unless the expected benefit outweighs any potential risks

capsules can be opened and granules sprinkled on food and eaten immediately without chewing or crushing granules

GENERAL ANAESTHETICS

General anaesthetic agents cause a loss of sensation associated with a reversible loss of consciousness and absence of pain (Bryant et al 2019). There is no one anaesthetic agent that can produce muscle relaxation, abolition of reflexes, unconsciousness and analgesia, so several agents are used together during a procedure. The anaesthetic procedure is made up of the following:

- *Premedication* – given to reduce anxiety, apprehension, pain and decrease secretions, and sometimes to produce sedation and amnesia. Premedication agents also assist with induction of anaesthesia and are usually given 30–60 minutes (IM or SC) or IV just before induction. Agents given as premedications include opioid analgesics (e.g. morphine, fentanyl), benzodiazepines (e.g. midazolam, flunitrazepam), phenothiazines (e.g. prochlorperazine, promethazine), H_2-receptor antagonists (e.g. cimetidine, ranitidine) and anticholinergics (e.g. atropine, glycopyrronium (glycopyrrolate) bromide, hyoscine).
- *Induction* – render the patient unconscious and unreactive to stimuli, usually by means of a short-acting barbiturate or benzodiazepine given IV, often with a short-acting muscle relaxant to allow intubation.
- *Maintenance* – unconsciousness is maintained, usually with an inhalation anaesthetic, and supplemented with IV analgesics and muscle relaxants.
- *Reversal* – anticholinesterases (e.g. neostigmine) are used to reverse the effects of the non-polarising muscle relaxants.
- *Recovery* – recovery period lasts until the patient is fully conscious, has stable cardiovascular status, is able to maintain airway unaided and is comfortable.

There are two groups of general anaesthetics:

- *inhalation anaesthetics* (including gases (e.g. nitrous oxide) and volatile liquids (e.g. desflurane)
  - mixed with oxygen, allowing administration by inhalation where they rapidly reach a concentration in the blood and brain to depress CNS causing anaesthesia
  - lung function is critical for effectiveness
  - abolish both superficial and deep reflexes

    - good anaesthetic agents, but not very useful as analgesics, requiring combination with other agents such as opioid analgesics
    - rapid recovery when administration is stopped
    - allergic reactions uncommon (Bryant et al 2019).
- *intravenous anaesthetics* (e.g. thiopental and propofol)
    - can be used for induction and maintenance of general anaesthesia, conscious sedation, induce amnesia and as an adjunct to inhalation anaesthetics
    - induce unconsciousness and suppress reflexes rapidly, allowing external control of airway
    - reduce amount of inhalation agent required
    - allow prompt recovery
    - minimal analgesic properties (except ketamine) or muscle relaxation actions
    - have amnesic properties (especially midazolam)
    - commonly cause hypersensitivity reactions
    - may cause hypotension, laryngospasm and respiratory failure after overdosage or prolonged administration (Bryant et al 2019).

Dose

- doses have not been stated because anaesthetic agents are generally given by anaesthetists and are calculated for individual patients using body weight or mass and can also be based on the procedure required, patient's physical condition and patient's response

General Adverse effects of general anaesthetics

- cardiovascular and respiratory depression
- (during induction) coughing, breath holding, apnoea, laryngospasm, bronchospasm, increased salivary secretions, hiccups
- involuntary muscle movements, shivering
- (halogenated anaesthetic) dose-dependent hypotension
- decreased reflexes
- postoperative nausea and vomiting, headache, convulsions
- kidney and liver toxicity
- (halogenated anaesthetic) intraoperative hyperkalaemia and/or hyperglycaemia
- increased intracranial pressure (in those with space-occupying lesions)
- (rare) hypersensitivity, malignant hyperthermia/hyperpyrexia (see Glossary)
- (rare) hepatitis, jaundice

General Interactions of general anaesthetics

- additive CNS depressant effects if given with opioid analgesic, resulting in lower general anaesthetic dose being required
- alcohol, antihistamines, antianxiety agents, opioid analgesics, sedatives and hypnotics intensify cardiovascular, respiratory and CNS depressant effects
- cardiovascular suppression may be enhanced if given with calcium-channel blockers, beta-adrenergic blocking agents or ACE inhibitors

General Nursing points/Cautions for general anaesthetics

- some long-term therapy (e.g. aspirin, oral anticoagulants) may require change of dose or cessation before surgery
- dose adjustments may be necessary for patients with chronic conditions, such as diabetes and hypertension
- (halogenated anaesthetic) repeated administration within short period of time is not recommended and if undertaken, great caution is needed
- potassium levels should be closely monitored in those with latent or overt neuromuscular disorders to avoid development of cardiac arrhythmias
- hyperventilation before or during anaesthesia prevents increase in intracranial pressure
- repeat administration within short period of time should be undertaken with great caution
- if patient is a heavy or regular alcohol user, close monitoring is recommended as alcohol withdrawal syndrome may occur. Anaesthetic requirements may also be increased
- caution if used in those with mitochondrial disorders
- caution if used in those with myasthenia gravis as these people are very sensitive to agents that depress respiration
- caution if used in those with latent or overt neuromuscular disorders as cardiac arrhythmias may occur
- caution if used in those with space occupying brain lesions as intracranial pressure or CSF may be increased or those at risk of raised intracranial pressure
- caution if used in those with hypovolaemia, hypotension, haemodynamically unstable, kidney/liver impairment, cardiac or respiratory diseases/impairment (where bronchoconstriction may occur), hypertension or in those who are debilitated
- contraindicated in those with history/risk of malignant hyperthermia/hyperpyrexia
- contraindicated in those who developed jaundice, liver dysfunction, unexplained fever, leucocytosis after exposure to halogenated anaesthetics
- contraindicated as sole agent for general anaesthesia induction

General Patient teaching and advice for general anaesthetics

- patient should be advised to avoid alcohol in the immediate postoperative period
- instruct patient to have an adult to escort them home
- warn patient that their intellectual functioning may decrease or be clouded for 2–3 days after a general anaesthetic and therefore it is recommended that they do not drive, operate machinery, make important decisions or sign legal documents during this time
- alert patient that he/she may experience mood changes for up to 6 days after an anaesthetic
- see General Patient teaching and advice (p. xxvii)

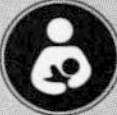

all general anaesthetics cross the placenta and may potentially depress the CNS and respiratory system of the newborn. Caution should be taken if fetus is known to be compromised and anaesthetic agent selected carefully, if used at all. Many

general anaesthetics are uterine relaxants and decrease placental blood flow

breastfeeding is not recommended for 12 hours after an anaesthetic agent and any milk produced during this time should be discarded

DESFLURANE (Suprane)

Available form
Liquid for inhalation (240 mL)

Properties and actions
- non-flammable volatile liquid agent given by inhalation (halogenated anaesthetic)
- similar to isoflurane
- fast washout from the body allowing rapid recovery
- excreted mainly via lungs

Use
- maintenance of surgical anaesthesia

Adverse effects
- pharyngitis
- (rare) QT prolongation
- see also General Adverse effects of general anaesthetics (p. 1108)

Interactions
- may potentiate actions of non-depolarising muscle relaxants
- recovery from neuromuscular blockade is longer for desflurane than isoflurane
- anaesthesia is more pronounced when given with nitrous oxide
- interacts with dry carbon dioxide absorbents to form carbon monoxide and carboxyhaemoglobin in some patients
- see also General Interactions of general anaesthetics (p. 1108)

Nursing points/Cautions
- see General Nursing points/Cautions for general anaesthetics (p. 1109)
- caution if used in those with coronary artery disease or where increase in heart rate or blood pressure is undesirable, in order to avoid myocardial ischaemia
- caution if used in those with history of QT prolongation
- not recommended in pregnancy termination
- not recommended for mask induction due to respiratory adverse effects
- contraindicated in those with hypersensitivity to halogenated anaesthetics or as inhalational induction agent in children

Patient teaching and advice
- see General Patient teaching and advice for general anaesthetics (p. 1109)

ISOFLURANE (Aerrane, Forthane)

Available forms
Liquid for inhalation (100 mL, 250 mL)

Properties and actions
- non-flammable volatile liquid agent given by inhalation (halogenated anaesthetic)
- slightly irritating to mucous membranes
- ether smell
- rapid induction and recovery
- excreted via lungs
- analgesic and muscle relaxant properties, as well as profound respiratory depressant
- peripheral vasodilation
- stimulates secretions weakly

Use
- induction and maintenance of surgical anaesthesia (usually with nitrous oxide and oxygen)

Adverse effects
- shivering, sweating, chills
- delirium, asthenia, fatigue
- (during induction) agitation, retching

- hypotension, cardiac arrhythmias
- myalgia
- increased WBC count
- increased liver enzymes and bilirubin, liver dysfunction, hepatitis
- rash
- (uncommon) nightmares, mood changes
- (rare) QT prolongation
- see also General Adverse effects of general anaesthetics (p. 1108)

Interactions

- contraindicated with or within 15 days of MAOIs
- not recommended with isoprenaline, adrenaline (epinephrine) or noradrenaline (norepinephrine) due to risk of ventricular arrhythmia. Adrenaline (epinephrine) used for haemostatic action (SC, gingival) should also be limited
- increased respiratory depression may occur if given with opioid analgesic (including as premedication) or other respiratory depressants
- caution if used with beta-adrenergic receptor blockers due to increased hypotension and negative inotropic effects
- decreases requirements for neuromuscular blocking agents
- caution if used with calcium-channel blockers as marked hypotension may occur
- may potentiate actions of non-depolarising muscle relaxants
- anaesthesia is more pronounced when given with nitrous oxide
- increased risk of hepatotoxicity if given with isoniazid. Should be stopped 7 days before and restarted 15 days after administration of isoflurane
- increased risk of hypersensitivity if given with dexamphetamine and related agents, appetite suppressants or ephedrine and related products. Should be stopped several days before isoflurane administration
- interacts with dry carbon dioxide absorbents to form carbon monoxide
- increased risk of severe hypotension and delayed emergence if used in those treated long term with St John's wort
- see also General Interactions of general anaesthetics (p. 1108)

Nursing points/Cautions

- see General Nursing points/Cautions for general anaesthetics (p. 1109)
- caution if used in those with history of QT prolongation
- caution if used in those with coronary artery disease (especially those with subendocardial ischaemia)
- contraindicated in those undergoing obstetric procedures

Patient teaching and advice

- see General Patient teaching and advice for general anaesthetics (p. 1109)

KETAMINE HYDROCHLORIDE (Ketalar, Ketamine Solution for Injection)

Available form

Vial: 200 mg/2 mL

Action

- non-barbiturate short-acting general anaesthetic agent (dissociative anaesthetic that causes amnesia and dissociation from surroundings/event)
- non-competitive antagonist at NMDA receptors increasing extracellular glutamate in prefrontal cortex
- pharyngeal and laryngeal reflexes remain intact
- marked analgesic properties, but transient minimal respiratory depression
- active metabolite
- induction of anaesthesia in 30 seconds (IV) and lasts 5–10 minutes

- induction of anaesthesia in 3–4 minutes (IM) and lasts 12–25 minutes

Use
- induction of anaesthesia
- diagnostic or short painful surgical operations not requiring skeletal muscle relaxation
- to supplement low potency agents such as nitrous oxide
- chronic and postoperative pain

Adverse effects
- involuntary muscle movement (may resemble seizures)
- hypotension, hypertension, bradycardia, tachycardia, cardiac arrhythmias
- emergence reactions (pleasant or unpleasant, including vivid dreams, nightmares, hallucinations, irrational behaviour, confusion, delirium)
- postoperative nausea, vomiting, anorexia, hypersalivation, laryngospasm
- (rapid IV, high dose) respiratory depression, apnoea
- diplopia, nystagmus, slight increased intraocular pressure
- abuse/dependence potential
- (misuse) severe urinary tract symptoms
- (rare) anaphylaxis
- (injection site) pain, erythema, rash

Interactions
- prolonged recovery time may occur if given with barbiturates and/or opioid analgesics
- increased half-life may occur if given with halogenated anaesthetics or benzodiazepines, resulting in prolonged recovery
- increased risk of bradycardia, hypotension and/or decreased cardiac output if given with high-dose halogenated anaesthetics (especially if given rapidly or in high doses)
- may antagonise hypnotic effect of thiopental
- increased risk of hypertension and tachycardia may result if given with thyroxine
- increased risk of hypotension if given with antihypertensive agents. Cardiac function should be monitored if given together
- seizure threshold may be decreased if given with theophylline
- increased risk of CNS and respiratory depression may occur if given with alcohol, phenothiazines, muscle relaxants or some antihistamines
- decreased dose may be required if given with antianxiety agents, sedatives or hypnotics
- may potentiate neuromuscular blocking effect and respiratory depression if given with atracurium

Nursing points/Cautions
- see General Nursing points/Cautions for general anaesthetics (p. 1109)
- given IV or IM
- emergence reaction usually lasts for a few hours, but in some patients has lasted up to 24 hours postoperatively
- great care should be taken not to disturb or overstimulate the patient during recovery to avoid emergence reaction
- risk of emergence reaction is decreased if given IM
- severe emergence reaction can be treated with low dose of short-acting or ultra short-acting barbiturate
- cardiac monitoring is recommended in those with hypertension or cardiac decompensation
- should not be mixed in the same syringe as barbiturates as precipitation will occur
- respiratory depression may occur if given by rapid IV injection, therefore should be given over at least 1 minute
- caution if used in those with alcohol abuse problems or who are intoxicated or have known raised intracranial pressure, glaucoma, schizophrenia, acute psychosis, porphyria, epilepsy, hyperthyroidism or receiving

thyroid hormone replacement, lung or upper respiratory tract infection, hydrocephalus, head injury or intracranial mass
- caution if used in those with hypovolaemia, dehydration or who have cardiac disease, moderate hypertension or arrhythmias
- not recommended as sole agent for surgery or diagnostic procedures of pharynx, larynx or bronchial tree as pharyngeal and laryngeal reflexes are active
- contraindicated in those with severe/poorly controlled hypertension, severe cardiovascular disease, heart failure, recent myocardial infarction, history of stroke, kidney or liver impairment, cerebral trauma or haemorrhage or intracerebral mass

Patient teaching and advice

- see General Patient teaching and advice for general anaesthetics (p. 1109)

METHOXYFLURANE (Penthrox)

Available forms
Liquid for inhalation (1.5 mL, 3 mL)

Properties and actions
- non-flammable volatile anaesthetic with mildly pungent odour
- powerful inhalation analgesic. Onset of analgesia occurs after a few breaths; intermittent use provides analgesia for 20–30 minutes
- slower metabolism and longer half-life than other halogenated anaesthetics
- renal toxicity limits use as anaesthetic

Use
- self-administration to haemodynamically stable, conscious patients (under supervision of trained staff) in trauma situations
- in monitored, conscious patients requiring analgesia for short surgical procedures (e.g. dressing changes)

Adverse effects
- cough, oropharyngeal pain
- dry mouth, nausea, vomiting
- retrograde amnesia, drowsiness, dizziness, euphoria, somnolence, anxiety, depression
- sensory neuropathy
- feeling drunk, increased risk of falls and accident
- fever, headache or migraine
- back pain
- sweating
- elevated liver enzymes
- hypotension, hypertension
- rash
- (rare) hepatic damage, nephrotoxicity, malignant hyperthermia/hyperpyrexia

Interactions
- use with tetracyclines may result in fatal renal toxicity
- may enhance renal toxicity of gentamicin, colistin and amphotericin B (amphotericin)
- increased metabolism may occur if given with barbiturates, alcohol, isoniazid, phenobarbital or rifampicin
- caution if given with adrenaline (epinephrine) or noradrenaline (norepinephrine)
- increased risk of hypotension if given with beta-adrenergic blocking agents
- caution if used with CNS depressants as added depression may occur

Nursing points/Cautions

Penthrox inhaler
- patient using inhaler should be supervised by trained personnel at all times
- activated carbon (AC) chamber should be inserted on top of inhaler
- loosen lid of methoxyflurane bottle (bottom of inhaler can be used for this) and contents poured into inhaler, which is tipped at 45° while rotating
- place wrist loop over patient's wrist
- instruct patient to inhale through mouthpiece with first few breaths

being gentle, then breathing normally (exhaled breath goes through AO chamber which absorbs exhaled methoxyflurane)
- if stronger analgesia is required, patient can cover dilutor hole with finger during inhalation

General
- see General Nursing points/Cautions for general anaesthetics (p. 1109)
- health workers regularly exposed to methoxyflurane should be aware of occupational health and safety guidelines for inhalational agents
- cumulative doses should be less than 6 mL/day or 15 mL/week to avoid nephrotoxicity, therefore not recommended on consecutive days
- caution if used in those with decreased renal blood flow, urine output or glomerular filtration rate
- caution if used in those with diabetes (especially in those who are obese, poorly controlled, have polyuria or kidney impairment) due to increased risk of nephropathy
- not recommended for use in toxaemia of pregnancy due to possibility of existing kidney impairment
- not recommended as an anaesthetic agent due to risk of nephrotoxicity
- not recommended in those with methoxyflurane or halothane-induced liver damage
- contraindicated in those with renal failure/impairment, sensitivity to fluorinated anaesthetics, respiratory depression, cardiovascular instability, head injury, loss of consciousness or history/family history of adverse reactions following anaesthetics including malignant hyperthermia/hyperpyrexia

Patient teaching and advice
- patient should be instructed in use of inhaler before starting (take gentle breaths initially, then normal inhalation and exhalation) and the expected effects (relief of pain/discomfort within 6–10 breaths; however, pain may not be totally eliminated)
- instruct patient to use inhaler intermittently rather than continuously
- advise patient of fruity smell of agent
- patient should be warned to take care as a pedestrian and not drive or operate machinery until doctor advises that normal activities can be resumed

NITROUS OXIDE

Properties and actions
- colourless gas given by inhalation
- although non-flammable, supports combustion
- strong analgesic properties (thought to be mediated through opioid receptors); however, has weak anaesthetic and muscle relaxant properties
- inhaled and absorbed by lungs and has low solubility in blood and tissue
- excreted unchanged through the lungs
- often combined with other (volatile) anaesthetics to enhance effects
- rapid onset of action and recovery time

Use
- used with other agents in induction and maintenance of surgical anaesthesia
- used with oxygen in dentistry
- used with oxygen in obstetrics by self-administration

Adverse effects
- hypoxia (unless adequate oxygen administered)

- mild cardiac depression
- nausea, vomiting
- delirium
- (prolonged (> 6 hours) administration) bone marrow depression, neurological effects

Nursing points/Cautions

- supplied in a blue metal gas cylinder
- increased risk of hypoxia if inadequate oxygen is given
- supplementary oxygen is usually given for 3–5 minutes to clear nitrous oxide from lungs at end of anaesthesia

PROPOFOL (Diprivan, Fresofol 1% Injection, Fresofol 1% MCT/LCT, Propofol-Lipuro 1% and 2%, Provive 1%, Provive MCT/LCT 1%)

Available forms

Prefilled syringe: 500 mg/50 mL; Ampoule: 10 mg/mL; Vial: 10 mg/mL

Action

- non-barbiturate hypnotic
- short-acting IV agent with onset of action approximately 30 seconds with no analgesic properties
- no analgesic effects
- effects thought to be mediated through GABA receptors
- onset of action within 30 seconds, duration 3–5 minutes, recovery usually within 5–10 minutes
- elimination half-life 3–8 hours

Use

- induction and maintenance of general anaesthesia in adults
- sedation of mechanically ventilated adult patients in intensive care setting
- monitored conscious sedation for surgical/diagnostic procedures

Adverse effects

- involuntary muscle movement, shivering, twitching, tremors, hiccups
- cough
- hypotension, bradycardia (sometimes profound), hypertension
- postoperative nausea, vomiting
- respiratory depression, transient apnoea
- increased intracranial pressure
- headache, euphoria
- flushing, rash
- raised serum triglycerides
- (injection site) pain, burning, stinging, tingling, phlebitis
- (rare) (prolonged therapy > 48 hours, high dose > 5 mg/hour) (intensive care) propofol infusion syndrome (cardiac failure, arrhythmias, metabolic acidosis, rhabdomyolysis, kidney failure), urine discolouration, hyperkalaemia, potential for abuse

Interactions

- increased sedation and respiratory depression may occur if given with other CNS depressants, including fentanyl
- decreased dose may be required if given after premedication with opioid analgesics and/or benzodiazepines, barbiturates, chloral hydrate or droperidol
- decreased dose may be used when adjunct to regional anaesthesia
- lower dose may be required when used as an adjunct to regional anaesthetic techniques

Nursing points/Cautions

- see General Nursing points/Cautions for general anaesthetics (p. 1109)
- emulsion is formulated for IV injection or infusion
- not recommended as rapid bolus injection
- calorific value is similar to Intralipid 10% (1.0 mL = 1.1 kcal)
- urine may become discoloured with prolonged use
- incompatible with atracurium and mivacurium

- prefilled syringe should be administered using syringe driver
- compatible with glucose 5% if dilution is required
- administer alone
- do not use if emulsion is separated or discoloured
- shake well before use
- caution if used in those with epilepsy as there is an increased risk of seizures during recovery period
- caution if used in those with hyperlipidaemia or a disorder of fat metabolism
- not recommended for obstetric anaesthesia
- contraindicated in those with known hypersensitivity to egg lecithin, peanut, glycerol, soya oil or sodium hydroxide, sodium oleate or sodium edetate
- contraindicated in children under 16 years in intensive care or for monitored conscious sedation for surgery or diagnostic procedures

Patient teaching and advice

- see General Patient teaching and advice for general anaesthetics (p. 1109)
- warn patient that urine may become discoloured if administration has been prolonged

SEVOFLURANE (Sevorane)

Available form

Liquid for inhalation (250 mL)

Properties and actions

- inhalation anaesthetic
- volatile, non-flammable liquid
- faster induction and emergence than isoflurane, but slightly slower than desflurane
- excreted mainly via lungs
- pleasant smell
- half-life 15–23 hours

Use

- induction and maintenance of general anaesthesia

Adverse effects

- fever, hypothermia
- hypotension, bradycardia, tachycardia
- agitation, headache, somnolence, dizziness
- (rare) cardiac arrhythmias, QT prolongation
- see also General Adverse effects of general anaesthetics (p. 1108)

Interactions

- may potentiate actions of non-depolarising muscle relaxants
- anaesthesia is more pronounced when given with nitrous oxide
- increased risk of respiratory depression if given with opioid analgesics or other respiratory depressing agents
- caution if used with isoprenaline, adrenaline (epinephrine) and noradrenaline (norepinephrine) due to risk of ventricular arrhythmias
- not recommended with or within 14 days of MAOIs
- caution if given with calcium-channel blockers due to risk of additive negative inotropic effects and marked hypotension
- decreased dose may be required if given with benzodiazepines or opioid analgesics
- increased metabolism may occur if given with alcohol or isoniazid
- increased risk of hypotension and chills if given with alfentanil

Nursing points/Cautions

- see General Nursing points/Cautions for general anaesthetics (p. 1109)
- caution if used in those with cardiac arrhythmias or history of QT prolongation
- contraindicated in those with hypersensitivity to other halogenated anaesthetics or with rebreathing apparatus containing Baralyme

Patient teaching and advice

- see General Patient teaching and advice for general anaesthetics (p. 1109)

THIOPENTAL SODIUM (Pentothal)

Available form
Ampoules: 500 mg

Action
- very short-acting IV barbiturate with poor analgesic and muscle-relaxing properties
- depresses the myocardium and respiration
- decreases intracranial pressure, laryngeal reflexes and lower oesophageal sphincter tone
- accumulates in fatty tissue if repeated doses are given
- recovery usually occurs within 10–30 minutes
- half-life 3–8 hours (single dose)

Use
- induction of anaesthesia before other anaesthetic agents
- anaesthesia of short duration
- control convulsions (short term)
- supplement to regional anaesthesia or nitrous oxide

Adverse effects
- hiccups, sneezing
- prolonged somnolence
- tachycardia, cardiac arrhythmias
- (rare) anaphylactic reaction
- see also General Adverse effects of general anaesthetics (p. 1108)

Interactions
- increased risk of hypotension if given with diazoxide, diuretics, antihypertensives, ketamine (high dose, rapid IV administration) or phenothiazines
- may be antagonised by aminophylline
- alcohol and CNS depressants may increase depressant and hypotensive effects
- increased risk of respiratory depression and hypotension when given with ketamine
- action may be prolonged by probenecid
- increased CNS depressant effect may occur if given with IV magnesium sulfate heptahydrate
- increased effects if given with benzodiazepines
- decreased analgesic effect if given with opioid analgesics
- may decrease uptake of sodium iodide by thyroid

Nursing points/Cautions
- see General Nursing points/Cautions for general anaesthetics (p. 1109)
- small test dose (25–75 mg) is usually given to test tolerance and sensitivity with patient observed for 1 minute post-administration
- extravasation and intra-arterial injection should be avoided
- may form a precipitate with acidic solutions (e.g. suxamethonium)
- caution if used in those who are debilitated or with severe cardiovascular disease, hypotension, shock, excessive premedication, Addison's disease, liver or kidney dysfunction, myxoedema, myasthenia gravis, severe anaemia, severe uraemia, increased intracranial pressure, asthma, endocrine insufficiency, muscular dystrophies or myotonias
- contraindicated in those with hypersensitivity to barbiturates, status asthmaticus, inadequate airway maintenance perioperatively, porphyria, constrictive pericarditis, respiratory depression/impairment, mouth, jaw and/or neck inflammation
- contraindicated if suitable veins are not available

Patient teaching and advice
- patient should be advised that they may experience the taste sensation of garlic after thiopentone is given and before onset of anaesthesia
- see also General Patient teaching and advice for general anaesthetics (p. 1109)

HAEMOPOIETIC AGENTS

Erythropoiesis is the process of producing new red blood cells and occurs in the bone marrow in adults (and liver and spleen in the fetus). There are a number of steps required for a haematopoietic stem cell to become a mature erythrocyte requiring adequate nutrients, including iron, vitamin B_{12} and folate. These steps are controlled by the hormone erythropoietin (also known as EPO or epoetin) which is produced in the kidneys (Hendrick 2017).

Haemopoietic agents are termed erythropoietin-stimulating agents (ESA) and are similar to the human erythropoietin, but are produced by recombinant DNA technology. They are used to increase the production of erythrocytes, primarily in anaemia, due to causes such as chronic renal failure, and during chemotherapy with agents that cause bone marrow depression. Unfortunately, ESAs are also used illegally in some sports to improve aerobic performance and have led to the deaths of athletes (Bryant et al 2019). EPO and ESA are banned in all sports, both in and out of competition (WADA 2021).

General Actions of haemopoietic agents

- glycoproteins produced by recombinant technology
- erythropoiesis stimulating agent (ESA) that stimulates production and differentiation of erythroid stem cells and stimulates proliferation and maturation of red blood cells causing increased haemoglobin formation
- haemoglobin levels may take 2–10 weeks to rise
- endogenous erythropoietin production is impaired in chronic renal failure, resulting in anaemia

General Adverse effects of haemopoietic agents

- flu-like symptoms, fever, chills
- headache, dizziness, asthenia, fatigue
- insomnia, depression, anxiety
- hypertension (including increase in BP in normotensive patient or aggravation of existing hypertension), hypotension
- non-cardiac chest pain
- peripheral oedema, fluid overload
- dyspnoea, cough, bronchitis, upper respiratory tract infection
- arthralgia, myalgia, limb or back pain
- mild rash, urticaria, pruritus, alopecia
- anorexia, nausea, diarrhoea, vomiting, abdominal pain, constipation
- (dialysis patients) haemodialysis graft occlusion/shunt thrombosis

- increased liver enzymes, decreased serum ferritin and transferrin
- (injection site) pain
- pure red cell aplasia, anaemia, neutralising antibody development
- (rare) myocardial ischaemia/infarction, cerebrovascular haemorrhage/infarction, transient ischaemic attacks, deep vein thrombosis, pulmonary emboli, retinal thrombosis, hypertensive encephalopathy, seizures, hyperkalaemia, tumour growth
- (rare) anaphylactoid reactions, angioedema, severe skin reactions

General Nursing points/Cautions for haemopoietic agents

- ESAs are not equivalent and should not be substituted without authorisation from treating doctor
- any hypertension should be controlled before starting therapy
- potentially correctable anaemia should be investigated and treated before considering use of ESA
- folic acid and vitamin B_{12} deficiencies should be excluded before starting therapy as effectiveness may be reduced
- monitor haemoglobin, serum iron, ferritin and total iron-binding capacity before starting, then monthly for first 3 months, then 3-monthly
- blood pressure, platelet count and serum potassium and phosphate levels should be monitored throughout regular therapy. Any elevated potassium levels should be treated
- if blood pressure cannot be controlled during therapy (with standard measures), therapy should be withheld until haemoglobin level falls, to decrease risk of hypertensive encephalopathy and seizures
- lowest dose possible should be used and haemoglobin level should not be allowed to rise above 120 g/L and increase rate not more than 10 g/L over 2 weeks to reduce the risk of cardiovascular/thrombotic events
- (chronic renal failure) 200–300 mg oral iron daily is recommended if serum ferritin < 100 nanogram/mL or serum transferrin $< 20\%$
- (non-myeloid malignancies) 200–300 mg oral iron daily is recommended if transferrin saturation $< 20\%$
- (autologous pre-donation) 200 mg oral iron daily is recommended for several weeks before donation
- for dialysis patients, IV is the preferred route
- first SC injection should be done by health professional/under supervision and then patient may be taught to self-administer
- for non-dialysis patients, SC route is recommended to avoid peripheral vein puncture
- rotate SC sites
- volumes greater than 1 mL should be given in different SC sites
- IV route should only be used by health professionals
- administer alone
- do not dilute
- guidelines for autologous pre-donation cover principles for blood donation, including that haemoglobin should be $\geq$ 110 g/L and volume of blood withdrawn should not be greater than 12% of person's estimated blood volume
- any vigorous shaking should be avoided as it will denature the protein
- pure red cell aplasia is associated with neutralising antibodies (to native erythropoietin) and results in

loss of response, therefore any loss of response should be investigated and therapy ceased if neutralising antibodies are found

- (non-myeloid malignancies) only recommended to treat anaemia in cancer patients when anaemia is due to chemotherapy. ESAs have been associated with increased mortality and should only be used if blood transfusion is considered inappropriate
- (chronic renal failure) caution in those who are hyporesponsive as there is an increased risk of cardiovascular events and mortality
- (chronic renal failure, dialysis) caution if used in those with hypotension or if arteriovenous fistulae shows any signs of complications as there is an increased risk of shunt thrombosis
- caution if used in those with pre-existing hypertension, ischaemic vascular disease, refractory anaemia, epilepsy or history or seizures, CNS infections, brain tumours/metastases, chronic liver failure, thrombocytosis, porphyria or gout
- not recommended in those with active malignant disease not receiving chemotherapy or radiation therapy
- contraindicated in those with known sensitivity to mammalian cell derived products (e.g. Chinese hamster ovary protein used in DNA recombinant technology)
- contraindicated in those with uncontrolled hypertension or severe cardiovascular disease, or who have developed pure red cell aplasia after treatment with erythropoietin, or those scheduled for elective surgery who have severe coronary, peripheral, arterial, carotid or cerebrovascular disease, recent (within 4 weeks) myocardial infarction or cerebrovascular accident, or if scheduled for surgery and cannot receive antithrombotic therapy

General Patient teaching and advice for haemopoietic agents

- advise patient to seek medical advice immediately if any of the following occur:
  - rapid pulse, difficulty breathing, feeling faint, sweating
  - swelling of face, lips, mouth, tongue or throat
  - shortness of breath
  - rash or hives
- patient should be advised of the importance of maintaining dietary restrictions and continue to take antihypertensive medication throughout therapy
- warn patient not to drive or operate machinery if dizziness or changes to blood pressure occur
- patient should be instructed to immediately seek medical advice if stabbing severe migraine/headache occurs
- patient should be advised that ESAs are not necessarily equivalent and should not be switched or dose changed without consulting doctor
- if patient is going to self-administer SC, education should include:
  - injection is under the skin (SC)
  - importance of rotating injection sites, including thighs and abdomen, but avoiding navel and waistline
  - do not inject into areas that are red or swollen, into muscle or into the same spot as previous injection

- correct technique, such as:
  - wash and dry hands before start of procedure
  - check name and strength of medication and expiry date (and do not use if after expiry date)
  - allow prefilled syringe/pen to come to room temperature before use (about 30 minutes) (not in direct sunlight or using any method such as hot water or microwave to warm solution)
  - do not shake solution/syringes
  - do not mix with any other medications or dilute
  - clean area with alcoholic swab and allow to dry
  - pinch skin firmly between thumb and finger
  - push prefilled syringe/pen firmly against pinched skin and inject
  - press site gently after injection with cotton wool swab to prevent bleeding, but do not rub
- correct storage
  - store in fridge, but can remain at room temperature for up to 3 days before use
- disposal of used equipment
  - do not recap needles
  - do not reuse needles, pens or syringes
  - syringes, pens and needles should not be disposed of in normal household rubbish
  - use puncture-resistant sharps container to dispose of used needles and syringes
  - container should be disposed of as instructed by doctor, pharmacist or nurse

- (chronic renal failure) female patient of childbearing potential should be counselled that menses may restart with therapy and therefore adequate contraception may be needed to prevent unwanted pregnancy occurring
- see also General Patient teaching and advice (p. xxvii)

banned in sport at all times (in and out of competition). Misuse by healthy people may lead to an excessive increase in packed cell volume, increasing the risk of cardiovascular and thrombotic events

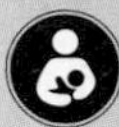

should only be used during pregnancy if benefits outweigh potential risks

caution if used during breastfeeding

DARBEPOETIN ALFA (Aranesp)

Available forms

Prefilled syringe: 10 microgram/0.4 mL, 20 microgram/0.5 mL, 30 microgram/0.3 mL, 40 microgram/0.4 mL, 50 microgram/0.5 mL, 60 microgram/0.3 mL, 80 microgram/0.4 mL, 100 microgram/0.5 mL, 150 microgram/0.3 mL; Prefilled pen: 20 microgram/0.5 mL, 40 microgram/0.4 mL, 60 microgram/0.3 mL, 80 microgram/0.4 mL, 100 microgram/0.5 mL, 150 microgram/0.3 mL

Action

- see General Actions of haemopoietic agents (p. 1118)
- terminal half-life is 3 times longer than erythropoietin
- half-life 12–40 hours (IV) or 35–39 hours (SC, chronic renal failure) or 124–144 hours (SC, non-myeloid malignancy)

Use

- anaemia associated with chronic renal failure
- prevention and treatment of anaemia in those with non-myeloid malignancies

receiving chemotherapy where blood transfusion is not appropriate

Dose

- (chronic renal failure: on dialysis) initially 0.45 microgram/kg SC or IV weekly, increasing dose by 25% at monthly intervals if response is inadequate (i.e. if haemoglobin increase < 10 g/L in 4 weeks) and iron stores are adequate. For maintenance, dose should be given weekly or every 2 weeks to maintain target haemoglobin **OR**
- (chronic renal failure: no dialysis) initially either 0.45 microgram/kg SC weekly, 0.75 microgram/kg SC every 2 weeks or 1.5 microgram/kg SC monthly, increasing dose by 25% at monthly intervals if response is inadequate (i.e. if haemoglobin increase < 10 g/L in 4 weeks) and iron stores are adequate. For maintenance, dose should be given weekly, every 2 weeks or monthly to maintain target haemoglobin **OR**
- (non-myeloid malignancies) 500 microgram (or 6.75 microgram/kg) every 3 weeks SC or 2.25 microgram/kg SC weekly, increasing to 4.5 microgram/kg weekly if haemoglobin response is less than 10 g/L after 1 month, continuing for 4 weeks after the end of chemotherapy or until haemoglobin concentration normalises. If no/poor response after 9 weeks, further treatment is unlikely to be beneficial

Adverse effects

- see General Adverse effects of Haemopoietic agents (p. 1118)

Nursing points/Cautions

- needle cover of prefilled syringe contains latex and is not recommended in those with known latex allergy
- (chronic renal failure) if changing from 2–3 times weekly r-HuEPO, once-weekly darbepoetin is recommended. If changing from once-weekly r-HuEPO, 2-weekly darbepoetin is recommended. Dose of darbepoetin should be based on r-HuEPO dose and administered via same route
- (chronic renal failure) haemoglobin should be measured every 1–2 weeks
- (chronic renal failure) if no response or response is not maintained, other causes of anaemia should be investigated
- (chronic renal failure) dose changes during maintenance period should not occur more often than every 1–2 weeks
- (chronic renal failure) as haemoglobin (Hb) approaches 120 g/L, dose should be decreased by 25%. If Hb continues to increase, therapy should be stopped until Hb level has decreased and then restarted at 25% lower than previous dose
- (non-myeloid malignancy) therapy should not be started until Hb < 100–110 g/L
- (non-myeloid malignancy) as haemoglobin (Hb) approaches 120 g/L, dose should be decreased by 25–50%. If Hb > 120 g/L, therapy should be stopped until Hb decreases to 110 g/L and then restarted at 25–50% lower than previous dose
- (non-myeloid malignancy) therapy should be continued for 4 weeks post-chemotherapy or until Hb approaches 120 g/L
- if changing route of administration, same dose should be used and Hb monitored, with subsequent dose adjustment if needed
- see also General Nursing points/Cautions for haemopoietic agents (p. 1119)

Patient teaching and advice

- if patient is going to self-administer, ensure that each prefilled syringe

type is demonstrated so patient is confident in administration technique
- see also General Patient teaching and advice for haemopoietic agents (p. 1120)

EPOETIN ALFA (Eprex)

Available forms
Prefilled syringe: 1000 IU/0.5 mL, 2000 IU/0.5 mL, 3000 IU/0.3 mL, 4000 IU/0.4 mL, 5000 IU/0.5 mL, 6000 IU/0.6 mL, 8000 IU/0.8 mL, 10,000 IU/mL, 20,000 IU/0.5 mL, 30,000 IU/0.75 mL, 40,000 IU/mL

Action
- see General Actions of haemopoietic agents (p. 1118)
- also known as EPO
- half-life 4–6 hours (increasing to 6–9 hours in those with renal failure)

Use
- anaemia associated with chronic renal failure
- prevention and treatment of anaemia in those with non-myeloid malignancies receiving chemotherapy where blood transfusion is not appropriate
- elective surgery (expecting moderate blood loss (900–1800 mL)) in those with mild-to-moderate anaemia (haemoglobin 100–130 g/L)
- augment autologous blood collection

Dose
- (chronic renal failure, anaemia: correction phase) initially 50 IU/kg IV over 1–2 minutes 3 times weekly, increasing to 75 IU/kg if haemoglobin has not increased by 10 g/L after 1 month, increasing by 25 IU/kg 3 times weekly at monthly intervals to achieve a haemoglobin concentration of not greater than 120 g/L (maximum dose 3 × 200 IU/kg/week) **OR**
- (chronic renal failure, anaemia: maintenance phase) maintenance phase is individually tailored, usually 75–300 IU/kg IV or SC weekly to maintain target haemoglobin (maximum dose is less than the maintenance maximum dose) **OR**
- (elective surgery) 600 IU/kg SC weekly for 3 weeks before surgery and on day of surgery **OR**
- (elective surgery where lead time is less than 3 weeks) 300 IU/kg SC daily for 10 consecutive days before surgery, on the day of surgery and for 4 days after surgery, stopping when haemoglobin reaches 150 g/L regardless of the number of doses given **OR**
- (autologous pre-donation program) 300–600 IU/kg IV twice weekly for 3 weeks (with 200 mg oral iron) **OR**
- (non-myeloid malignancies) initially 150 IU/kg SC 3 times weekly for 1 month, then adjusting the dose according to haemoglobin and reticulocyte count

Adverse effects
- see General Adverse effects of haemopoietic agents (p. 1118)

Interactions
- may increase heparin required during dialysis to prevent clotting in dialyser
- serum level of ciclosporin should be closely monitored and dose adjusted if necessary if given together
- caution if used with agents that decrease erythropoiesis as effectiveness will be reduced

Nursing points/Cautions
- (elective surgery) antithrombic therapy is recommended
- (chronic renal failure) administer after completion of haemodialysis
- (chronic renal failure) IV route is recommended for patients who undergo dialysis, SC is suggested for non-dialysis patients

- if converting from SC to IV route, same dose should be given and haemoglobin monitored and dose adjusted if needed
- (chronic renal failure) if haemoglobin (Hb) approaches 120 g/L, dose should be decreased by 25%. If Hb continues to increase, therapy should be stopped until Hb level has decreased and then restarted at 25% lower than previous dose. If Hb increases by > 10 g/L in any 2-week period, dose should be decreased or dosing interval increased or both
- slow injection may prevent flu-like symptoms
- (elective surgery) therapy should not be started if haemoglobin > 130 g/L because of increased risk of postoperative thrombotic vascular events
- (non-myeloid malignancies) therapy should not be started unless haemoglobin < 100–110 g/L
- caution if used in patients with chronic liver failure
- see also General Nursing points/Cautions for haemopoietic agents (p. 1119)

Patient teaching and advice

- see General Patient teaching and advice for haemopoietic agents (p. 1120)

EPOETIN BETA (NeoRecormon)

Available forms

Prefilled syringe: 2000 IU/0.3 mL, 3000 IU/0.3 mL, 4000 IU/0.3 mL, 5000 IU/0.3 mL, 6000 IU/0.3 mL, 10,000 IU/0.6 mL

Action

- see General Actions of haemopoietic agents (p. 1118)
- half-life is 4–12 hours (IV) or 13–28 hours (SC)

Use

- anaemia associated with chronic renal failure
- prevention and treatment of anaemia in those with non-myeloid malignancies receiving chemotherapy where blood transfusion is not appropriate
- increase yield of autologous blood (pre-donation) to avoid use of homologous blood
- prevention of anaemia in premature infants (less than 34 weeks gestation and weight 750–1500 g)

Dose

- (chronic renal failure: correction) 60 IU/kg/week SC either as single weekly dose or 7 divided doses given daily, increasing at monthly intervals by 60 IU/kg/week if haemoglobin increase is not adequate (< 1.5 g/L/week) **OR**
- (chronic renal failure: correction) 120 IU/kg/week IV over 2 minutes in 3 divided doses, increasing to 240 IU/kg/week after 1 month (if haemoglobin increase is not adequate (< 1.5 g/L/week). If response still remains inadequate, further increases by 60 IU/kg/week at monthly intervals may be needed **OR**
- (chronic renal failure: maintenance) dose is initially halved and then adjusted to maintain haemoglobin between 100 and 120 g/L, given as either single weekly dose or up to 7 divided doses (weekly maximum 720 IU/kg) **OR**
- (autologous pre-donation program) 400–1600 IU/kg/week IV over 2 minutes or 300–1200 IU/kg/week SC given in 2 divided doses for a maximum of 4 weeks **OR**
- (anaemia in non-myeloid malignancy) 450 IU/kg/week SC as single weekly dose or in 3–7 divided doses. If response is inadequate after 4 weeks, dose should be increased to 900 IU/kg/week **OR**
- (prevention of anaemia in premature infants) 750 IU/kg/week SC in 3 divided doses (starting by day 3 of life) for 6 weeks

Adverse effects

- see General Adverse effects of haemopoietic agents (p. 1118)
- overhydration
- menstrual disorders
- leucopenia, thrombocytopenia
- lower respiratory tract infection, infection

Nursing points/Cautions

- see General Nursing points/Cautions for haemopoietic agents (p. 1119)
- (non-myeloid malignancy) therapy should be continued for up to 4 weeks after end of chemotherapy. If haemoglobin falls by more than 10 g/L during next cycle of chemotherapy in spite of therapy with epoetin beta, further treatment is not warranted
- (prevention of anaemia in premature infants) less effective if premature infant has had blood transfusion
- (prevention of anaemia in premature infants) oral iron (2 mg/day) should be started as soon as possible (by day 14 at the latest). If serum ferritin < 100 nanogram/mL or there are other signs of iron deficiency, oral iron dose should be increased to 5–10 mg/day
- increase in heparin may be required in dialysis patients to prevent occlusion of dialysis system/shunt thrombosis
- dose adjustments should be no more frequent than monthly and dependent on Hb (maintaining Hb < 120 g/L)
- (non-myeloid malignancy) not recommended if haemoglobin is > 110 g/L
- caution if used in those with refractory anaemia (with blasts in transformation), thrombocytosis or chronic liver failure
- contains phenylalanine and is therefore not recommended in those with severe phenylketonuria
- contraindicated in those with angina pectoris or history of thromboembolic disease (autologous blood collection) or who have suffered myocardial infarction or stroke in preceding 4 weeks

Patient teaching and advice

- see General Patient teaching and advice for haemopoietic agents (p. 1120)

EPOETIN LAMBDA (Novicrit)

Available forms

Prefilled syringe: 1000 IU/0.5 mL, 2000 IU/mL, 3000 IU/0.3 mL, 4000 IU/0.4 mL, 5000 IU/0.5 mL, 6000 IU/0.6 mL, 8000 IU/0.8 mL, 10,000 IU/mL

Action

- see General Actions of haemopoietic agents (p. 1118)
- similar to epoetin alfa
- half-life 2.5–6.7 hours (IV) or 24 hours (SC)

Use

- anaemia associated with chronic renal failure
- prevention and treatment of anaemia in those with non-myeloid malignancies receiving chemotherapy where blood transfusion is not appropriate
- patients with anaemia (Hb > 100 – ≤ 130 g/L) scheduled for elective surgery where moderate blood loss (900–1800 mL) is expected to reduce exposure to allogeneic blood transfusion
- augment autologous blood collection in patients scheduled for major elective surgery

Dose

- (elective surgery scheduled) 600 IU/kg SC over 1–2 minutes weekly for 3 weeks before surgery and on day of surgery (total 4 doses) (with 200 mg oral elemental iron daily) **OR**
- (elective surgery, shortened lead-in time) 300 IU/kg SC over 1–2 minutes daily for 10 consecutive days before

surgery, day of surgery and 4 days post-surgery (total 15 doses) **OR**

- (autologous pre donation program) 300–600 IU/kg IV over 1–2 minutes twice weekly for 3 weeks (with 200 mg oral elemental iron daily) **OR**
- (chronic renal failure) initially 50 IU/kg IV over 1–2 minutes 3 times weekly. If haemoglobin (Hb) does not increase by 10 g/L after 4 weeks, dose may be increased to 75 IU/kg IV over 1–2 minutes 3 times weekly to achieve Hb not greater than 120 g/L (correction) (maximum weekly dose 3 × 200 IU/kg), then 75–300 IU/kg weekly IV over 1–2 minutes (maintenance) to maintain Hb in target range **OR**
- (non-myeloid malignancies) initially 150 IU/kg SC over 1–2 minutes 3 times weekly. If Hb has increased by 10 g/L or reticulocyte count ≥ 40,000 cells/microlitre above baseline after 4 weeks, dose continues at 150 IU/kg. If Hb increases < 10 g/L and reticulocyte count < 40,000 cells/microlitre above baseline, dose is increased to 300 IU/kg. After a further 4 weeks at 300 IU/kg, if there is no improvement in Hb or reticulocyte count, therapy should be discontinued as response is unlikely

Adverse effects

- see General Adverse effects of haemopoietic agents (p. 1118)
- seizures

Interactions

- effects may be decreased if given with agents that decrease erythropoiesis
- may increase serum levels of ciclosporin, therefore blood levels should be closely monitored during therapy

Nursing points/Cautions

- blood pressure and prodromal neurological symptoms of seizures should be closely monitored during therapy (especially in first 3 months)
- if patient is on dialysis, administration should be after completion
- if patient experiences flu-like symptoms administration can be slowed to 5 minutes
- (non-myeloid malignancy) therapy should not start until Hb < 100–110 g/L
- (elective surgery) therapy should be stopped if Hb is 150 g/L regardless of the number of doses given
- see General Nursing points/Cautions for haemopoietic agents (p. 1119)

Patient teaching and advice

- patient should be advised against driving or operating machinery during the first 3 months of therapy because of the increased risk of seizures
- see General Patient teaching and advice for haemopoietic agents (p. 1120)

METHOXY POLYETHYLENE GLYCOL EPOETIN BETA (Mircera)

Available forms

Prefilled syringes (with colour-coded plunger): 30 microgram/0.3 mL (aqua), 50 microgram/0.3 mL (yellow), 75 microgram/0.3 mL (red), 100 microgram/0.3 mL (turquoise), 120 microgram/0.3 mL (calcium oxide), 200 microgram/0.3 mL (purple), 360 microgram/0.6 mL (salmon)

Action

- see General Actions of haemopoietic agents (p. 1118)
- chemically synthesised ESA with longer half-life (15–20 times) than erythropoietin
- longer half-life allows monthly administration
- increase in haemoglobin is usually seen 7–15 days after administration

Use

- anaemia associated with chronic kidney disease

Dose

- (chronic kidney disease, not currently receiving ESA, not on dialysis) initially 1.2 microgram/kg SC monthly **OR**
- (chronic kidney disease, not currently receiving ESA, no dialysis) initially 0.6 microgram/kg IV or SC every second week **OR**
- (chronic kidney disease, not currently receiving ESA, dialysis) initially 0.6 microgram/kg IV or SC every second week **OR**
- (chronic kidney disease, receiving ESA) initial dose is dependent on previous weekly dose:
  - o darbepoetin alfa < 40 microgram/week or epoetin < 8000 IU/week, starting dose 120 microgram/month
  - o darbepoetin alfa 40–80 microgram/week or epoetin 8000–16,000 IU/week, starting dose 200 microgram/month
  - o darbepoetin alfa > 80 microgram/week or epoetin > 16,000 IU/week, starting dose 360 microgram/month

Adverse effects

- see General Adverse effects of haemopoietic agents (p. 1118)

Nursing points/Cautions

- if changing route of administration, Hb should be closely monitored to ensure it remains in target range
- haemoglobin should be monitored second weekly until stable and then regularly to maintain target (100–120 g/L). If haemoglobin (Hb) increase is < 10 g/L over 4 weeks, dose should be increased by 25–50%. Further increases of 25–50% may be required at monthly intervals to achieve target Hb
- if haemoglobin (Hb) approaches 120 g/L, dose should be decreased by 25%. If Hb continues to increase, therapy should be stopped until Hb level has decreased and then restarted at 25% lower than previous dose. If Hb increases by > 10 g/L in any 2-week period, dose should be decreased or dosing interval increased or both
- dose adjustments should be no more frequent than monthly
- when converting from epoetin or darbepoetin alfa, administration can be monthly or every 2 weeks
- see General Nursing points/Cautions for haemopoietic agents (p. 1119)

Patient teaching and advice

- see General Patient teaching and advice for haemopoietic agents (p. 1120)

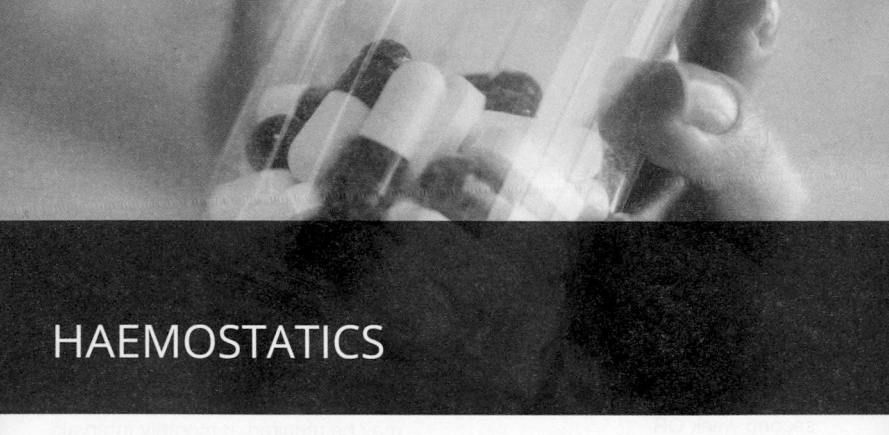

HAEMOSTATICS

Haemostasis is the process of stopping bleeding from a damaged blood vessel and occurs in three steps: (1) constriction of the blood vessel, (2) platelet plug formation, and (3) clot (mainly fibrin) formation. Once vessel repair has started, the fibrin clot is broken down by the action of plasmin on the fibrin (fibrinolysis). For clot formation to occur, a series of steps (the clotting cascade) involving an intrinsic or extrinsic pathway (which converge to a common pathway) must occur (Arruda & High 2018). Deficiency in coagulation factors results in inadequate clot formation occurring and continued bleeding.

Examples of coagulation factor deficiencies include:

- haemophilia A (also called 'classic' haemophilia), a genetically transmitted deficiency of factor VIII affecting males (although transmitted by females), which occurs in mild, moderate or severe forms (Arruda & High 2018)
- haemophilia B (also called 'Christmas disease'), a deficiency of factor IX, occurring less commonly than haemophilia A and also occurring in mild, moderate or severe forms (Arruda & High 2018)
- von Willebrand disease (VWD), the most common inherited bleeding disorder and a deficiency of von Willebrand's factor, which circulates in the blood attached to factor VIII, binding platelets to minor ruptures in blood vessels. There are three types of VWD with type 2 having four sub-types (Konkie 2018).

Bleeding associated with coagulation factor deficiencies is sometimes spontaneous, as a result of mild trauma or associated with surgical or dental procedures. Bleeding into joints (haemarthrosis) can become chronic, leading to joint damage (e.g. synovial thickening and synovitis) and deformity (Arruda & High 2018). Management using haemostatic agents may be prophylactic (to prevent spontaneous bleeding or bleeding associated with a surgical or dental procedure) or it may be to treat the bleeding when it occurs.

Some haemostatic agents act by inhibiting the breakdown of the fibrin clot, whereas others replace the missing coagulation factors, with the aim of both types of agents being to reduce blood loss.

ELTROMBOPAG OLAMINE (Revolade)

Available forms
Tablets: 25 mg, 50 mg

Action
- thrombopoietin (TPO) receptor agonist, resulting in proliferation of megakaryocytes from bone marrow stem cells
- pharmacokinetics influenced by race and gender, with those from East Asia having increased plasma levels when compared to Caucasians. Plasma levels in females > males
- half-life 21–32 hours, prolonged in those with idiopathic thrombocytopenic purpura (ITP)

Use
- treatment of idiopathic thrombocytopenic purpura (in those patients who are intolerant or had ineffective response to corticosteroids and immunoglobulins)
- chronic hepatitis C-associated thrombocytopenia that prevents initiation of interferon-based therapy
- severe aplastic anaemia (SAA) (with standard immunosuppressive therapy)
- refractory SAA (where response to immunosuppressive therapy was ineffective)

Dose
- (chronic ITP) initially 50 mg orally daily, then adjusting dose in 25 mg daily increments at intervals of at least 2 weeks to maintain platelet count ≥ 50 × 10^9/L for at least 4 weeks (daily maximum 75 mg) **OR**
- (hepatitis C-associated thrombocytopenia) initially 25 mg orally daily, adjusting dose in 25 mg intervals at 2-week intervals to achieve target platelet count to start interferon therapy (daily maximum 100 mg) **OR**
- (SAA) 150 mg orally daily for 6 months with dose adjustment according to platelet count (with immunosuppressive therapy) **OR**
- (refractory SAA) 50 mg orally daily with dose adjustment of 50 mg increments every 2 weeks according to platelet count (daily maximum 150 mg)

Adverse effects
- diarrhoea, nausea, vomiting
- pharyngolaryngeal pain, pharyngitis
- myalgia, back pain, musculoskeletal chest pain, musculoskeletal pain, muscle spasms, bone pain
- alopecia, rash, phototoxicity
- elevated liver enzymes, elevated bilirubin
- paraesthesia
- menorrhagia
- thromboembolic/thrombotic events, bone marrow reticulin formation, bone marrow fibrosis, cytogenic abnormalities
- dry eye, cataract formation

Interactions
- serum levels may be decreased by lopinavir/ritonavir combination or with dietary calcium (e.g. dairy products)
- may increase serum levels of rosuvastatin increasing risk of toxicity
- chelates polyvalent cations, including aluminium, calcium, iron, magnesium, selenium and zinc

Nursing points/Cautions
- (ITP, East Asian patients) dose should be started at 25 mg daily
- (East Asian patients) dose should be started at 75 mg daily (SAA) or 25 mg (refractory SAA)
- platelet count usually increases within 1–2 weeks of starting therapy
- any loss in response should be investigated
- (ITP, refractory SAA, hepatitis-associated thrombocytopenia) liver function should be measured before starting therapy, then 2-weekly during dose adjustment and then monthly once

maintenance has been established. If abnormal liver enzymes occur, testing should be carried out within 3–5 days and therapy discontinued if levels are elevated ($\geq$ 3 times upper limit of normal (ULN) or baseline), progressive or persist for $\geq$ 4 weeks, or if clinical symptoms or an increase in direct bilirubin also exist

- (SAA) liver function should be measured before starting and regularly throughout therapy. If liver enzymes (ALT) are $> 6 \times$ ULN, therapy should be discontinued and restarted at same dose when ALT $< 5 \times$ ULN. If ALT again increases to $> 6 \times$ ULN with reason (e.g. sepsis, azole therapy), therapy should be again stopped and ALT measured every 3–4 days, and restarted at a reduced dose (25 mg less than previous dose) when ALT $< 5 \times$ ULN. If ALT remains $> 6 \times$ ULN, therapy should be stopped. If ALT $< 5 \times$ ULN, therapy should be restarted at reduced dose. If ALT again increases to $> 6 \times$ ULN, dose should be reduced by 25 mg daily until ALT $< 5 \times$ ULN
- peripheral blood smears and full blood count (with white blood cell count differential) should be assessed before starting and weekly during therapy until platelet count is stable for at least 4 weeks, and then monitored monthly
- blood smears should be checked for any red blood cell abnormalities or cytopenia and therapy should be stopped if abnormalities are found
- platelet count returns to baseline within 14 days of discontinuing therapy, increasing risk of bleeding. Platelet count should be monitored for 4 weeks after stopping therapy
- (ITP) if platelet count does not increase to expected level with 4 weeks of therapy at maximum dose, stopping therapy is recommended
- (hepatitis C-associated thrombocytopenia) if there is no response after 12 weeks, therapy should be stopped
- (refractory SAA) therapy should be stopped if no response is evident in 16 weeks, if new cytogenic abnormality appears, if there is an excessive platelet response or if liver abnormalities occur
- (refractory SAA) if platelet count $> 50 \times 10^9$/L, Hb $>$ 100g/L and absolute neutrophil (ANC) $> 1 \times 10^9$/L for more than 8 weeks dose should be reduced by 50%. If counts remain stable after 8 weeks at reduced dose, therapy can be stopped and blood counts monitored regularly
- (ITP, liver impairment) dose adjustment intervals should be 3 weeks
- baseline ocular examinations should be performed before starting therapy, then regularly throughout monitoring for signs and symptoms of cataracts
- (hepatitis C-associated thrombocytopenia) therapy should only be started in patients with chronic hepatitis C where thrombocytopenia prevents interferon therapy from being initiated or limits ability to maintain optimal interferon therapy
- (hepatitis C-associated thrombocytopenia) platelet count should be monitored weekly before starting and during interferon therapy until platelet count is stable, then monthly (and should include full blood count, platelet count and peripheral blood smears)
- (hepatitis C-associated thrombocytopenia) therapy should be stopped when interferon therapy is ceased
- caution if used in those with liver or kidney impairment, advanced age or at risk of thromboembolism (e.g. prolonged periods of immobilisation, malignancies, surgery, trauma,

obesity, smoking, factor V Leidan, ATIII deficiency or antiphospholipid syndrome)

Patient teaching and advice

- advise patient that dairy products, antacids and mineral supplements should be taken at least 4 hours apart from medication. Tablets can be taken with food with little or no calcium
- instruct patient to avoid unnecessary UV exposure, including direct sunlight or artificial sources (such as tanning beds). Sunscreen, hat and protective clothing are recommended to avoid sunburn
- patient should be advised to seek medical advice immediately if any of the following occur:
  - yellowing of eyes or skin, dark urine, tiredness, loss of appetite, right upper stomach pain
  - swelling or pain/tenderness in legs
- see General Patient teaching and advice (p. xxvii)

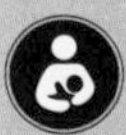

not recommended during pregnancy or breastfeeding unless benefits are thought to outweigh risks

FIBRINOGEN (RiaSTAP)

Available form

Vial: 1 g

Action

- coagulation factor I derived from human plasma
- converted to haemostatic clot in the presence of thrombin, activated coagulation factor XIII and calcium ions

Use

- acute bleeding episodes in patients with congenital fibrinogen deficiency (e.g. afibrinogenaemia, hypofibrinogenaemia)

Dose

- (fibrinogen level not known) initially 70 mg/kg IV, dose then adjusted according to target level (e.g. 1 g/L for minor event such as epistaxis, intramuscular bleeding or menorrhagia or 1.5 g/L for major event such as head trauma or intracranial haemorrhage. Target levels should be maintained for at least 3 days after minor bleeding or for 7 days after major bleeding

OR

- calculated according to following equation:

$$\text{Dose of fibrinogen (mg/kg body weight)} = \frac{[\text{target level (g/L)} - \text{measured level (g/L)}]}{0.017\ (\text{g/L per mg/kg body weight})}$$

Adverse effects

- fever
- thromboembolic events
- (uncommon) allergic/anaphylactic reactions

Nursing points/Cautions

- fibrinogen level should be measured before starting therapy and during dose adjustment
- dose is dependent on severity of disorder, location and extent of bleeding, and clinical condition of patient
- normal fibrinogen level 2.0–4.5 g/L, with bleeding occurring at levels of 1.0 g/L and below
- patient should be closely monitored during infusion for any signs of allergy or thrombosis
- product is made from human plasma, which may contain infectious agents such as viruses. Current manufacturing processes are effective against HIV, hepatitis B, hepatitis C and hepatitis A
- contains 164 mg (7.1 mmol) sodium per vial, which may need to be

considered in those with sodium-restricted diet
- vial and water for injections should be at room temperature before reconstitution. Reconstitute by adding 50 mL water for injections to vial and swirling gently (avoid shaking vial) until solution is clear and colourless
- administer alone
- rate should not exceed 5 mL/minute
- name and batch number of product should be recorded in patient notes
- caution if used in those with coronary heart disease, myocardial infarction, liver impairment, peri- or postoperative patients, at risk of thromboembolic events or DIC
- caution if used in those with congenital dysfibrinogenaemia because of increased risk of thrombosis

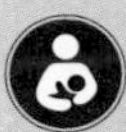

only used during pregnancy and breastfeeding if benefits are thought to outweigh risks

Note
- contained in Tisseel VH S/D solution with aprotinin, factor XIII and thrombin, TachoSil and Evisel Topical with thrombin, and Artiss with aprotinin and factor XIII

ORNIPRESSIN (Por-8 Ferring)

Available form
Ampoule: 5 IU/mL

Action
- vasoconstrictor similar in action to vasopressin, but weaker antidiuretic activity
- local ischaemia occurs within 10 minutes of administration, lasting 1–2 hours

Use
- local administration to induce ischaemia and haemostasis (plastic surgery, obstetrics, gynaecology, ENT surgery, other types of surgery)

Dose
- maximum dose 5 IU (diluted) by regional infiltration

Adverse effects
- facial/general pallor, sweating
- increased bowel motility
- rise/fall in BP, arrhythmias, angina pain
- (systemic absorption) increased heart rate, cardiac fibrillation
- (rare) allergy

Interactions
- contraindicated as adjunct to local anaesthetics in regions of terminal arteries such as fingers
- caution if used with other vasoconstricting agents

Nursing points/Cautions
- should be diluted with sodium chloride 0.9% before use (50–60 mL for gynaecological surgery, laparotomy; 20 mL for ENT surgery)
- caution if used in those where a rise in blood pressure would be unwanted, or in those with ischaemic heart disease
- contraindicated in those with coronary heart disease, severe hypertension, advanced arteriosclerosis, toxaemia of pregnancy, epilepsy or as spinal anaesthetic

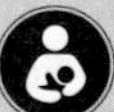

contraindicated during pregnancy (animal studies have shown it to be teratogenic)

ROMIPLOSTIM (Nplate)

Available forms
Vial: 375 microgram (extractable dose 250 microgram/0.5 mL), 625 microgram (extractable dose 500 microgram/mL)

Action

- thrombopoietin (TPO) mimetic class agent
- increases platelet production by binding to and activating thrombopoietin receptor similar to action of endogenous thrombopoietin

Use

- thrombocytopenia (in those with chronic idiopathic thrombocytopenia (ITP), who have been splenectomised with inadequate response or have not been splenectomised with inadequate response or where immunoglobulins and corticosteroids are inappropriate)

Dose

- initially 1 microgram/kg SC weekly, then adjusting dose at weekly intervals and increments of 1 microgram/kg (to maintain platelet count $\geq 50 \times 10^9$/L but $\leq 200 \times 10^9$/L) (maximum weekly dose 10 microgram/kg)

Adverse effects

- anaemia, thrombocytopenia, idiopathic thrombocytopenic purpura
- haematoma, petichiae, ecchymosis
- nosebleed
- hypertension
- diarrhoea, nausea, vomiting, abdominal pain, bleeding gums or mouth, constipation
- headache, dizziness, paresthesia, fatigue, asthenia, anxiety, insomnia, confusion
- peripheral oedema
- fever
- rash, pruritus
- arthralgia, myalgia, back/leg pain, muscle spasm, musculoskeletal pain, chest pain, pain
- toothache
- hypokalaemia
- upper respiratory tract infection, cough, dyspnoea, nasopharyngitis, sinusitis, bronchitis, nasal congestion, rhinorrhoea
- urinary tract infection
- development of neutralising antibodies (inhibitors)
- (rare) increase in bone marrow reticulum, thrombotic/thromboembolic events, progression of existing myelodysplastic syndromes, hypersensitivity

Nursing points/Cautions

- before starting and during therapy, peripheral blood smears and blood count should be monitored for any red blood cell abnormalities or cytopenia. Therapy should be stopped if abnormalities are found. Blood counts should be monitored for at least 4 weeks after stopping therapy
- platelet count should be measured weekly until count is stable at $\geq 50 \times 10^9$/L for at least 4 weeks without any dose adjustment
- if maximum weekly dose of 10 microgram/kg is reached for 4 weeks without platelet improvement, therapy should be stopped
- if, after initial response, there is a failure to maintain or there is a loss of the platelet response, causative factors may be the development of neutralising antibodies or increased bone marrow reticulin
- thrombocytopenia may recur when therapy is stopped
- patient may be taught to self-administer once platelet count has been stable for 4 weeks. After 4 weeks of self-administration, patient technique for reconstitution and administration should be checked
- should be administered using syringe with 0.01 graduations
- reconstitute using sterile water for injections (0.72 mL for 375 mg vial and 1.2 mL for 625 mg vial), swirl gently and invert vial until solution is clear and colourless; however, do not shake vial

- caution if used in those with severe liver or kidney impairment, or with known or acquired factors for thromboembolism including factor V Leidan, antiphospholipid syndrome, advanced age, prolonged immobilisation, malignancy, surgery, trauma, smoking and obesity
- contraindicated in those with hypersensitivity to *Escherichia coli* (*E. coli*) products

Patient teaching and advice

- warn patient against driving or operating machinery if dizziness, numbness or fatigue occurs
- if patient is going to self-administer SC, education should include:
  - injection is under the skin (SC)
  - importance of rotating injection sites, including thighs and abdomen, but avoiding navel and waistline
  - not injecting into areas that are red or swollen, into muscle or into the same spot as previous injection
  - correct technique, such as:
    - wash and dry hands before start of procedure
    - checking name and strength of medication and expiry date (and not using if after expiry date)
    - reconstituting powder using water for injections as demonstrated by nurse or physician
    - swirling vial gently to dissolve powder (but not shaking) until solution is clear and colourless
    - cleaning area with alcoholic swab and allowing to dry
    - pinching skin firmly between thumb and finger
    - pushing syringe against pinched skin and injecting solution
    - pressing site gently after injection with cotton wool swab to prevent bleeding but do not rub
  - correct storage
    - powder should be stored in fridge but not frozen
    - after reconstituting powder, solution can be kept in fridge for up to 24 hours if not given immediately
    - any unused solution should be discarded
  - disposal of used equipment
    - not recapping needles
    - using puncture-resistant sharps container to dispose of used syringes
    - container should be disposed of as instructed by doctor, pharmacist or nurse
- see General Patient teaching and advice (p. xxvii)

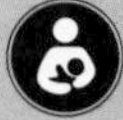

should only be used during pregnancy or breastfeeding if benefits outweigh potential risks

TRANEXAMIC ACID (Cyklokapron, Tranexamic Acid Solution for Injection, Zamic)

Available forms

Tablets: 500 mg; Ampoule: 500 mg/5 mL, 1 g/10 mL, 2 g/20 mL

Action

- competitive inhibitor of plasminogen activation
- inhibits fibrinolysis by reducing the conversion of plasminogen to plasmin (high doses)
- more potent than aminocaproic acid
- half-life about 2 hours

Use

- hereditary angioneurotic oedema
- hyphaema (short term)
- in patients with established coagulopathies having minor procedures

- menorrhagia
- (IV) reduce blood loss peri- and post-surgery (cardiac surgery, total knee arthroplasty, total hip arthroplasty)

Dose

- (traumatic hyphaema) 1–1.5 g orally 8-hourly for 6–7 days **OR**
- (known coagulopathy: cervical conisation) 1–1.5 g orally 8–12-hourly for 12 days postoperatively **OR**
- (known coagulopathy: prostatectomy) 1 g orally 6 hours preoperatively, followed by 1 g 3–4 times daily until macroscopic haematuria disappears **OR**
- (known coagulopathy: dental procedures) 25 mg/kg orally 2 hours before the procedure (with factor VIII and IX), followed by 25 mg/kg 3–4 times daily for 6–8 days **OR**
- (hereditary angioneurotic oedema) 1–1.5 g orally 2–3 times daily (continuously or until symptoms subside) **OR**
- (menorrhagia) 1 g orally 4 times daily, increasing to 1.5 g 4 times daily if necessary for a total of 4 days, starting with onset of visible bleeding **OR**
- (cardiac surgery, after anaesthetic induction, before skin incision) 15 mg/kg IV bolus (loading dose), then 4.5 mg/kg/hour IV infusion for duration of surgery (0.6 mg/kg of infusion dose may be given as part of priming volume of heart–lung machine) **OR**
- (total knee arthroplasty) 15 mg/kg IV bolus (before release of tourniquet), then 15 mg/kg IV bolus 8-hourly for 2 doses (last bolus given 16 hours after initial dose) **OR**
- (total hip arthroplasty) 15 mg/kg IV bolus (before skin incision), then 15 mg/kg IV bolus 8-hourly for 2 doses (last bolus given 16 hours after initial dose)

Adverse effects

- nausea, vomiting, diarrhoea
- dermatitis
- (rapid IV) dizziness, hypotension
- (IV) cardiogenic shock, renal failure, respiratory failure, stroke, myocardial infarction, arrhythmias
- (rarely) colour vision impairment, altered vision, giddiness, thromboembolic events, seizures, death

Interactions

- not recommended with factor IX complex concentrates or anti-inhibitor coagulant concentrates due to increased risk of thrombosis

Nursing points/Cautions

- IV bolus should not exceed 50 mg/minute to avoid dizziness and/or hypotension
- should be discontinued if the patient develops a colour vision or other vision defect as these may be indicative of retinotoxicity
- (menorrhagia) patient should be reassessed after 3 months of therapy
- (prostatectomy) treatment > 14 days is not recommended
- if treatment is to be prolonged (> 7 days), a baseline ophthalmological examination (visual acuity, colour vision, eyeground and visual fields) is recommended before starting and regularly throughout therapy
- (IV) should not be mixed with blood or penicillin
- use with caution if blood exists in body cavities (pleural space, joint spaces, urinary tract), because undissolvable clots may occur, or in those with disseminated intravascular coagulation (DIC) or impaired kidney function
- should only be used in those at high risk of thrombosis if benefits outweigh risks and under close medical supervision
- (menorrhagia) not recommended in females with irregular menstrual bleeding due to unknown cause

- not recommended for haematuria caused by renal parenchymal disease
- contraindicated in those with history/risk of thrombosis (unless treated with anticoagulants), active thromboembolic disease, subarachnoid haemorrhage or acquired disturbance of colour vision

Patient teaching and advice

- patient should be advised to immediately seek medical advice if any of the following occur:
  - visual disturbances, including colour vision
  - dizziness, light-headedness, rapid heart rate, weakness, sweating, cold, clammy skin, restlessness
- see General Patient teaching and advice (p. xxvii)

should only be used during pregnancy if benefits outweigh potential risks

caution if used during breastfeeding

tablet can be dispersed in water (2–5 minutes) or can be crushed and mixed with a spoonful of yoghurt or apple puree

COAGULATION FACTORS

Coagulation factors treat coagulation factor deficiencies and may be produced by recombinant technology or extracted from human plasma. Recombinant technology consists of taking the human coagulation factor and expressing in non-human cells (e.g. hamster kidney cells). The coagulation factors produced are expressed as international units (IU), but each coagulation factor has its own discrete units and they are therefore not interchangeable.

FACTOR VII

Activated factor VII (factor VIIa) triggers factor X into factor Xa, which then starts the conversion of prothrombin to thrombin and fibrinogen to fibrin. For factor VII to be active, it needs to form a complex with the tissue factor exposed when the vessel wall is injured.

EPTACOG ALFA (NovoSeven RT)

Available forms

Vial: 1 mg (50,000 IU), 2 mg (100,000 IU), 5 mg (250,000 IU); Prefilled syringe: 1 mg (50,000 IU), 2 mg (100,000 IU), 5 mg (250,000 IU), 8 mg (400,000 IU)

Action

- recombinant coagulation factor VIIa

Use

- treatment and prophylaxis of bleeding in patients with inhibitors to coagulation factors VIII or IX
- treatment and prophylaxis of bleeding in patients with congenital deficiency of factor VII
- Glanzmann's thrombasthenia (with GPIIb-IIIa and/or HLA antibodies, refractory to platelet transfusion)

Dose

Inhibitors to clotting factors VIII or IX

- (bleeding control) 35–120 microgram/kg by IV bolus over 2–5 minutes

2-3-hourly until bleeding is controlled, then 3-12-hourly if treatment is still needed **OR**
- (mild-to-moderate bleeding episodes) 90 microgram/kg by IV bolus over 2–5 minutes at 3-hourly intervals for 2–3 doses **OR**
- (mild-to-moderate bleeding episodes) 270 microgram/kg by IV bolus over 2–5 minutes stat **OR**
- (surgical prophylaxis) 35–120 microgram/kg by IV bolus over 2–5 minutes 2–3-hourly for 1–2 days, then 2–6-hourly if treatment is still needed **OR**
- (prophylaxis to decrease frequency of bleeding episodes) 90 microgram/kg daily by IV bolus over 2–5 minutes for up to 12 weeks

Congenital factor VII deficiency
- 15–30 microgram/kg 4–6-hourly until haemostasis is achieved

Glanzmann's thrombasthenia
- 80–120 microgram/kg for at least 3 doses 2.5 hours apart

Adverse effects
- fever, headache
- nausea
- pruritus, urticaria, rash
- (rare) (injection site) reaction, pain
- (rare) anaphylaxis, neutralising antibody production (inhibitors), thromboembolic events, DIC

Interactions
- not recommended with prothrombin complex concentrate or recombinant coagulation factor XIII
- may shorten prothrombin time if given at 15–30 microgram/kg 4–6-hourly

Nursing points/Cautions
- prothrombin time and factor VII coagulant activity should be measured before starting and regularly throughout therapy. If expected level is not reached or uncontrolled bleeding continues, this may be due to development of neutralising antibodies and should be investigated
- patient should be closely monitored for any sign of thrombosis or unwanted activation of the coagulation system (e.g. inducing DIC)
- if bleeding is severe, administration of coagulation factor VIII or IX inhibitors is recommended
- reconstitute using provided solvent/diluent (1.1 mL for 1 mg vial, 2.1 mL for 2 mg and 5.2 mL for 5 mg), swirling gently to dissolve until solution is clear
- administer alone
- not recommended in those with fructose intolerance, glucose malabsorption or sucrase–isomaltase insufficiency
- caution if used in those with advanced atherosclerotic disease, crush injury, septicaemia, disseminated intravascular coagulopathy (DIC), coronary heart disease, liver disease or after major surgery due to increased risk of thromboembolic event
- caution if used in those with platelet and/or blood product sensitivity
- contraindicated in those with a known hypersensitivity to mouse, hamster or bovine proteins or factor VIIa complexes

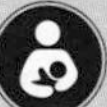
should only be used during pregnancy or breastfeeding if benefits outweigh potential risks

FACTOR VIII

Factor VIIIa acts as a cofactor for factor IXa, accelerating the conversion of factor X to factor Xa, which then converts prothrombin to thrombin, which in turn converts fibrinogen to fibrin and the clot is formed.

EFMOROCTOCOG ALFA (Eloctate)

MOROCTOCOG ALFA (Xyntha)

OCTOCOG ALFA (Advate, Kogenate FS)

RURIOCTOCOG ALFA PEGOL (Adynovate)

Available forms
Vial: 250 IU, 500 IU, 750 IU, 1000 IU, 1500 IU, 2000 IU, 3000 IU, 4000 IU

Action
- recombinant coagulation factor VIII
- (rurioctocog alfa pegol) octocog alfa has been conjugated with PEG reagent to extend plasma half-life
- (efmoroctocog alfa) recombinant fusion protein of factor VIII bonded to IgG1 prolonging half-life

Use
- treatment and prophylaxis of bleeding in patients with haemophilia A

Dose
- dose is calculated to determine amount required for a given response or the response expected from a given amount. Formula used is:

  Required IU = weight (kg) × desired factor VIII rise (as % of normal) × 0.5

- (mild muscle or oral bleeding, early haemarthrosis) 10–20 IU/kg IV repeated 12–24-hourly for 1–3 days until bleeding and pain resolves **OR**
- (mild-to-moderate bleeding) 20–30 IU/kg IV repeated 24–48-hourly until bleeding and pain resolves (Eloctate) **OR**
- (moderate muscle bleeding, bleeding into oral cavity, known trauma, definite haemarthrosis) 15–30 IU/kg IV, repeated 12–24-hourly for 3 or more days, until bleeding resolves **OR**
- (major/significant bleed, fractures, head trauma) initially 30–50 IU/kg IV, repeated 8–24-hourly until bleeding resolves **OR**
- (major bleed) 40–50 IU/kg IV every 12–24 hours until bleeding resolves (Eloctate) **OR**
- (perioperative, minor surgery) 30–50 IU IV bolus within 1 hour of surgery, with additional dosing 12–24-hourly if needed **OR**
- (perioperative, minor surgery including tooth extraction) 25–40 IU/kg IV, repeated every 24 hours if needed (Eloctate) **OR**
- (perioperative, major surgery) preoperatively 40–60 IU IV bolus (verifying 100% activity has been achieved before surgery), then 40–60 IU 8–24-hourly (depending on desired level of factor VIII and state of healing) **OR**
- (long-term prophylaxis) 10–50 IU/kg IV 3 to 5 times weekly **OR**
- (long-term prophylaxis) 65 IU/kg IV weekly (Eloctate)

Adverse effects
- (injection site) inflammation, pain
- headache, chills, flushing, sweating, fever
- dizziness, tremor
- nausea, vomiting, altered taste, abdominal pain
- rash, urticaria, pruritus
- dyspnoea
- palpitations
- fatigue, malaise
- development of neutralising antibodies (inhibitors)
- (uncommon/rare) allergy, hypersensitivity

Nursing points/Cautions
- 1 IU is equal to the concentration of factor VIII in 1 mL of fresh human plasma (pooled) (WHO standard)
- dose, frequency and duration of therapy is dependent on patient's

weight, site and extent of bleeding, severity of disorder, titre of inhibitors and desired concentration of factor VIII. For example, the minimum plasma factor VIII activity required will be different for minor surgical procedures than for major surgical procedures or life-threatening haemorrhage
- risk of developing neutralising antibodies is highest in first 20 days of exposure (but can occur after 100 days) and therefore patient should be closely monitored (clinical observation and laboratory values), which may result in bleeding not being controlled
- blood levels for factor VIII should be measured 3–6 hours after start of IV infusion and then daily using one-stage clotting assay
- if switching between factor VIII products, therapeutic response should be closely monitored
- if bolus administration results in increase in pulse rate, rate should be decreased or temporarily stopped
- (Advate) can be given as bolus injection at a rate not greater than 10 mL/minute or by continuous infusion for 500 IU, 1000 IU or 1500 IU doses (by syringe driver at a rate of 0.4 mL/hour or greater)
- (Advate) initial reconstitution should be with 5 mL of diluent until no hypersensitivity is established. If no hypersensitivity occurs, diluent volume can be reduced to 2 mL
- reconstitution should occur at room temperature and according to the manufacturer's specific instructions (different products are not interchangeable in terms of use or reconstitution instructions)
- add diluent provided (amount according to manufacturer's instructions) to powder and swirl gently to dissolve
- solution should be used within 3 hours of reconstitution
- (Adynovate) contains 10 mg sodium per vial, which may need to be taken into consideration in those who have a low-sodium diet
- not recommended in those with von Willebrand disease
- contraindicated in those with a known hypersensitivity to mouse, hamster or bovine proteins

Patient teaching and advice

- patient should be advised to immediately report any skin reaction (such as hives), chest pain/tightness, wheezing, flushing, feeling faint or difficulty breathing
- ensure patient/carer understands and is able to demonstrate correct administration technique, including reconstitution of powder, use of connection device (provided), attaching infusion needle, administration rate, safe disposal of used needles and cleaning requirements if any blood is spilled
- if patient is planning travel, ensure they understand the importance of having adequate supply for length of trip
- see General Patient teaching and advice (p. xxvii)

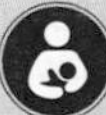

should only be used during pregnancy if benefits outweigh potential risks

not recommended during breastfeeding

FACTOR VIII (Biostate)

Available forms

Vial (contains 1 : 2.4 ratio of factor VIII to von Willebrand factor): 250/600 IU, 500/1200 IU, 1000/2400 IU

Action

- human purified coagulation factor VIII plus von Willebrand factor complex (promotes platelet aggregation and adhesion on damaged endothelium and carrier protein for precoagulant protein factor VIII)

Use

- treatment and prophylaxis in those with factor VIII deficiency caused by haemophilia A
- treatment of bleeding associated with von Willebrand disease (where desmopressin is ineffective or contraindicated)

Dose

Haemophilia A

- (minor haemorrhage) 10–15 IU/kg IV 12–24-hourly for 1–2 days **OR**
- (moderate-to-severe haemorrhage) 15–40 IU/kg IV 8–24-hourly for 1–4 days **OR**
- (life-threatening haemorrhage) initially 50–60 IU/kg IV, then 20–25 IU/kg 8–12 hourly (days 2–10) **OR**
- (minor surgery) 20–30 IU/kg IV stat (loading dose preoperatively), followed by 20–25 IU/kg twice daily (days 1–3), then 20–30 IU daily **OR**
- (major surgery) 40–50 IU/kg IV stat (loading dose preoperatively), followed by 20–25 IU/kg 8–12-hourly (days 1–3), 15–20 IU/kg 8–12-hourly (days 4–6), then 10–20 IU/kg twice daily **OR**
- (dentistry) 35–40 IU/kg IV stat (loading dose preoperatively), followed by 25–30 IU/kg twice daily for 1–3 days (maintenance) **OR**
- (prophylaxis) 25–40 IU/kg IV 3 times weekly

von Willebrand disease

- (spontaneous bleeding) initially 10–20/25–50 IU/kg IV, then 10–20 IU/kg IV 12–24-hourly until bleeding stops (usually 2–4 days) **OR**
- (minor surgery) 25/60 IU/kg IV daily until healing is complete (usually 2–4 days) **OR**
- (major surgery) initially 25–35/60–80 IU/kg IV, then 15 25/[illegible] IU/kg IV 12–24-hourly, usually 5–10 days until healing is complete **OR**
- (prophylaxis) 10–15/25–40 IU/kg IV 1–3 times per week

Adverse effects

- hypersensitivity (tachycardia, chest pain/discomfort, back pain)
- altered taste
- fever, headache
- abnormal liver enzymes
- development of neutralising antibodies (inhibitors)
- (rare) allergy, anaphylactic reaction, thromboembolic events, thrombophlebitis

Nursing points/Cautions

- for surgical indications, loading dose is given day before procedure
- risk of developing neutralising antibodies is greatest in first 20 days (although in some it will develop after 100 days of exposure) or in those who are switching from one factor VIII product to another who have previously had $>$ 100 exposure days with a previous development of neutralising antibodies. If bleeding is not controlled or target levels not reached, investigation for neutralising antibodies is recommended
- immunisation with hepatitis A and hepatitis B vaccines is recommended for those with no antibodies to these viruses before administration of factor VIII
- product is made from human plasma, which may contain infectious agents such as viruses. Current manufacturing processes are effective against HIV, hepatitis B, hepatitis C and hepatitis A
- vial should be allowed to reach room temperature before reconstitution. The appropriate amount of water for injections should be drawn into the syringe and attached to preparation

device. A plastic cannula of preparation device is then inserted into the stopper using a push and twist action and water Is drawn into the vial using vacuum. Contents are gently swirled to dissolve without excessive frothing (2–5 minutes to produce clear solution)
- name and batch number should be recorded for each treatment
- reconstituted solution should not be refrigerated
- if clots or gel form, it should not be used (return to Australian Red Cross Lifeblood)
- administer over at least 5 minutes (or as tolerated). Infusion rate should not exceed 6 mL/min
- administer alone
- do not mix with whole bleed
- any spills should be cleaned with sodium hypochlorite 1% for 15 minutes
- patient and/or family member can be instructed in preparation and administration
- caution if used in those with allergy to factor VIII and/or von Willebrand factor concentrates or human albumin
- contraindicated in those with history of anaphylaxis or severe systemic response to factor VIII or von Willebrand factor preparations

Patient teaching and advice

- patient should be advised to immediately report any skin reaction (such as hives), chest pain/tightness, wheezing, flushing, feeling faint or difficulty breathing
- ensure patient/carer understands and is able to demonstrate correct administration technique, including reconstitution of powder, use of connection device (provided), attaching infusion needle, administration rate, safe disposal of used needles and cleaning requirements if any blood is spilled
- if patient is planning travel, ensure they understand the importance of having adequate supply for length of trip
- see General Patient teaching and advice (p. xxvii)

FACTOR VIII INHIBITOR BYPASSING FRACTION (Feiba-NF)

Available forms

Vial: 500 IU, 1000 IU, 2500 IU

Action

- blood coagulation factor complex
- contains factors II, IX and X (mainly non-activated), factor VII (activated) and 1–6 units of factor VIII coagulation antigen
- those with haemophilia A and B can acquire inhibitors to factor VIII or IX during factor VIII or IX replacement therapy. This prevents the formation of the complex that catalyses Xa production
- generates Xa and thrombin without needing factor VIIIa–IXa complex, bypassing inhibitory action of factor VIII or IX inhibitors

Use

- routine prophylaxis, control of spontaneous bleeding or in surgery in those with haemophilia A or B with neutralising antibodies (inhibitors)

Dose

- (joint, muscle and soft tissue haemorrhage – minor-to-moderate bleed) 50–75 IU/kg IV 12-hourly until bleeding resolves (pain decreases, reduction in swelling or joint mobilisation) (daily maximum 200 IU/kg) **OR**
- (joint, muscle and soft tissue haemorrhage – major bleed) 100 IU/kg IV 12-hourly until bleeding resolves (pain decreases, reduction in swelling or joint mobilisation) (daily maximum 200 IU/kg) **OR**

- (mucous membrane haemorrhage) 50 IU/kg IV 6-hourly, increasing to 100 IU/kg if bleeding does not stop (daily maximum 200 IU/kg) **OR**
- (other severe haemorrhage) 100 IU/kg IV 12-hourly, reducing to 6-hourly if needed (daily maximum 200 IU/kg) **OR**
- (surgery) 50–100 IU/kg IV up to 6-hourly (daily maximum 200 IU/kg) **OR**
- (routine prophylaxis) 70–100 IU/kg IV 3–4 times weekly, adjusting dose on clinical response (daily maximum 200 IU/kg)

Adverse effects

- hypersensitivity reaction
- dizziness, headache
- hypotension
- rash
- hepatitis B surface antibody positive
- (rare) thrombotic and thromboembolic events, allergic and anaphylactoid reactions

Interactions

- not recommended with antifibrinolytic agents due to risk of thrombotic event. If required, they should be administered 12 hours apart
- may decrease active immunity from live attenuated vaccine if given together
- may interfere with Coomb's test (antiglobulin test)

Nursing points/Cautions

- increased risk of thromboembolic events if high doses are given, therefore dose should not exceed 100 IU/kg (as a single dose) or 200 IU/kg (daily maximum)
- dose is independent of patient's inhibitor titres
- patient should be monitored carefully for any signs including changes in BP, pulse rate, respiratory distress, chest pain and cough. If these occur, infusion should be stopped and diagnostic tests conducted to determine if DIC is present (decreased fibrinogen, decreased platelet count and/or presence of fibrin-fibrinogen degradation product, significantly prolonged thrombin time, prothrombin time or partial thromboplastin time)
- infusion rate should not exceed 2 IU/kg/minute
- vial should be allowed to reach room temperature before reconstitution. Appropriate amount of water for injections should be drawn into syringe and attached to preparation device. A plastic cannula of the preparation device is then inserted into the stopper using a push and twist action and water drawn into the vial using vacuum. The contents are gently swirled to dissolve without excessive frothing
- solution should not be refrigerated and should be used within 3 hours of reconstitution
- product is made from human plasma, which may contain infectious agents such as viruses. Current manufacturing processes are effective against HIV, hepatitis B, hepatitis C and hepatitis A
- appropriate vaccination (hepatitis A and B) should be considered if the patient is receiving regular or repeated therapy
- contains sodium (80–200 mg/vial), which may need to be taken into consideration in those who have a low-sodium diet
- caution if used in those with liver impairment
- caution if used in those with disseminated intravascular coagulation (DIC), advanced arterial disease, crush injury, septicaemia, arterial or venous thrombosis or if receiving concurrent therapy with recombinant factor VIIa

- contraindicated in those with normal coagulation, DIC, fibrinolysis, coronary heart disease, acute thrombosis and/or embolism
- contraindicated during cardiac surgery involving cardiopulmonary bypass and procedures involving extracorporeal membrane oxygenation (ECMO) due to high risk of thrombotic adverse events

Patient teaching and advice

- patient should be advised to immediately report any skin reaction (such as hives), chest pain/tightness, wheezing, flushing, feeling faint or difficulty breathing
- see General Patient teaching and advice (p. xxvii)

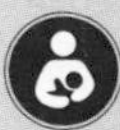

should only be used during pregnancy if benefits outweigh risks

caution if used during breastfeeding

EMICIZUMAB (Hemlibra)

Available form

Vial: 30 mg/mL, 60 mg/0.4 mL, 105 mg/0.7 mL, 150 mg/mL

Action

- humanised monoclonal antibody IgG4 whose structure bridges activated factor IX and factor X to restore function of missing activated factor VIII
- does not induce or enhance development of neutralising antibodies (inhibitors)
- produced by recombinant DNA technology in Chinese hamster ovary cells
- long half-life resulting in effects on coagulation assays persisting for up to 6 months after therapy has been stopped

Use

- prophylaxis to prevent bleeding in those with haemophilia A

Dose

- 3 mg/kg SC once weekly for 4 weeks, then either 1.5 mg/kg SC weekly, 3 mg/kg SC every 2 weeks or 6 mg/kg SC monthly

Adverse effects

- (injection site) redness, pain, pruritus
- fever
- headache
- diarrhoea
- arthralgia, myalgia
- (uncommon) thrombotic microangiopathy, thrombosis, skin necrosis, thrombophlebitis

Interactions

- increases risk of microangiopathy and thrombotic events if given with activated prothrombin complex concentrate (cumulative dose > 100 IU/kg/24 hours) for 24 hours or more. If given together, patient should be monitored closely for any signs of thrombotic microangiopathy or thromboembolism
- caution if given with activated factor VII or factor VIII as lower doses may be required
- may interfere with intrinsic pathway clotting-based tests

Nursing points/Cautions

- any bypassing agents (e.g. Feiba-NF) should be discontinued 24 hours before starting therapy. If required during prophylaxis with emicizumab, doctor should discuss dose with patient as this may be lower than used without emicizumab prophylaxis. However, it should be avoided unless there are no other treatment options or alternatives available. Initial dose should not exceed 50 IU/kg and total dose not greater than 100 IU/kg in first 24 hours
- factor VIII prophylaxis therapy can be continued for first 7 days of therapy

- trade name and batch number of product should be recorded in patient medical notes
- SC injection sites should be rotated avoiding any areas that are hard, tender, red, bruised, scarred or there are moles present
- injection of other SC agents should be at different anatomical sites
- patient may be taught to self-administer
- if patient develops thrombotic microangiopathy, supportive care with or without plasmapheresis and haemodialysis is recommended. Improvement in patient condition should be seen within a week
- contraindicated in those with known hypersensitivity to hamster-derived proteins

Patient teaching and advice

- self-administration instruction should include rotation of injection sites, preparation of skin and solution, injection technique, correct storage and disposal advice
- ensure patient understands the importance of following doctor's instruction regarding use of bypassing agent (e.g. Feiba NF) as serious adverse effects may occur if instructions are not followed
- patient should be advised to immediately seek medical advice if any of the following occur:
    - confusion, weakness, arm or leg swelling, yellowing of skin and eyes, abdominal or back pain, nausea, vomiting or urinating less (may be signs of thrombotic microangiopathy)
    - swelling, warmth, redness or pain (may be signs of blood clot in veins near skin surface)
    - headache, face numbness, eye pain or swelling, vision impairment (may be signs of blood clot in eye blood vessel)
    - blackening of skin
- see also General Patient teaching and advice (p. xxvii)

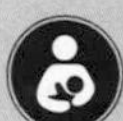
should only be used during pregnancy and breastfeeding if benefits outweigh risks

FACTOR IX

Factor IX is synthesised by the liver and is involved in the intrinsic pathway for blood coagulation. Factor XIa activates factor IX, which then activates factor X (in the presence of factor VIIIa). This leads to the conversion of prothrombin to thrombin and the formation of a fibrin clot.

FACTOR IX (MonoFIX-VF)

Available forms

Vial: 500 IU, 1000 IU

Action

- human purified coagulation factor IX
- contains heparin sodium
- half-life is about 24 hours

Use

- treatment and prophylaxis of bleeding in patients with haemophilia B (Christmas disease)

Dose

- (minor haemorrhage) 20–30 IU/kg IV daily for 1–2 days **OR**
- (moderate-to-severe haemorrhage) 30–50 IU/kg IV 1–2 times daily for 1–5 days **OR**
- (minor surgery, including dental extraction) 40–60 IU/kg IV stat (loading dose), then 15–40 IU/kg 1–2 times daily for 7–10 days **OR**
- (major surgery) 70–100 IU/kg IV stat (loading dose), then 20–90 IU/kg 1–2 times daily for 10–12 days **OR**
- (prophylaxis) 25–40 IU/kg IV twice weekly

Adverse effects

- injection site reaction
- nausea, altered taste
- dizziness
- clammy skin
- thrombocytopenia (because of the heparin component)
- development of neutralising antibodies (inhibitors)
- (rare) allergy, anaphylactic reaction, fever, thrombosis, DIC

Nursing points/Cautions

- any coagulation test results should be carefully interpreted in view of the heparin content
- made from human plasma, therefore carries a potential risk of transmission of infectious agents (despite the manufacturing process which removes and inactivates a number of known viruses, including HIV, hepatitis B and C viruses)
- hepatitis A and hepatitis B vaccination is recommended for patients who have no antibody titre to hepatitis A or B
- plasma factor IX levels should be monitored in those with severe haemorrhage or undergoing surgery
- if expected activity is not achieved or bleeding is not controlled, blood assay for factor IX neutralising antibodies (inhibitors) should be performed
- vial contains 50–140 IU heparin per reconstituted 500 IU vial or 100–280 IU per reconstituted 1000 IU vial
- vial should be allowed to reach room temperature before reconstitution. Appropriate amount of water for injections should be drawn into syringe and attached to preparation device. A plastic cannula of the preparation device is then inserted into the stopper using a push and twist action and water drawn into the vial using vacuum. Contents are gently swirled to dissolve without excessive frothing (2–5 minutes to produce clear solution)
- should not be refrigerated once reconstituted
- if clots or gel form or vacuum is not present in vial, should not be used (return to Australian Red Cross Lifeblood)
- administer alone at a rate not greater than 3 mL/minute
- spillage should be cleaned using sodium hypochlorite 1% for 15 minutes
- not indicated for treatment of factor II, VII or X deficiency or in those with haemophilia A with factor VIII neutralising antibodies (inhibitors)
- caution if used in those with previous severe reaction to factor IX concentrates or in those with fibrinolysis, myocardial infarction, DIC or liver disease

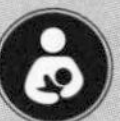

contains heparin, therefore may cause maternal haemorrhage if given during pregnancy

Note

- contained in Prothrombinex-VF

NONACOG ALFA (BeneFIX)

Available forms

Vial: 250 IU, 500 IU, 1000 IU, 2000 IU, 3000 IU

Action

- recombinant coagulation factor IX

Use

- treatment and prophylaxis of bleeding in patients with haemophilia B (Christmas disease)

Dose

- (patients aged ≥ 15 years) dose calculated using the following formula:

Number of factor IX IU required (IU) = weight (kg) × desired factor IX increase (% or IU/dL) × 1.2 IU/kg per IU/dL

Adverse effects

- reaction at IV site
- (uncommon) headache, dizziness, tremor
- (uncommon) nausea, altered taste
- (uncommon) cough, dyspnoea
- (rare) allergy, anaphylaxis, thrombosis, fever, burning sensation in jaw/skull, chest tightness, GI upset
- development of neutralising antibodies (inhibitors)

Nursing points/Cautions

- initial 10–20 doses should be given under medical supervision because of the risk of allergic reaction
- patient changing from plasma-derived factor IX products to nonacog (alfa) should be instructed that recovery may be slower and higher doses may be required
- length of therapy is dependent on reason for administration:
  - (minor bleeding) given 12–24-hourly for 1 to 2 days
  - (moderate bleeding) given 12–24-hourly for 2–7 days (until bleeding stops, healing occurs)
  - (major bleeding) given 12–24-hourly for 7–10 days
- (prophylaxis) may be given as a regular schedule (2–3 times weekly)
- reconstitute by injecting diluent provided (in prefilled syringe) into vial, swirling gently until dissolved and then drawing clear solution back into syringe using vial adapter. Administer using provided infusion kit
- during administration, blood should not be allowed to enter syringe containing reconstituted solution. If this occurs, syringe, tubing and solution should be discarded
- should be administered at a rate of 1–2 mL/minute IV
- administer alone
- reconstituted solution should be used as soon as possible to decrease time spent in plastic syringe as solution absorbs PVC from syringe surface
- caution if used in those with liver disease, post-surgically or with signs/risk of fibrinolysis, DIC or thromboembolic events
- contraindicated in those with known allergy to hamster protein

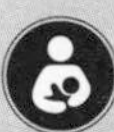

only used during pregnancy or breastfeeding if benefits outweigh risks

NONACOG GAMMA (Rixubis)

Available forms

Vial: 250 IU, 500 IU, 1000 IU, 2000 IU, 3000 IU

Action

- recombinant coagulation factor IX
- specific activity is ≥ 200 IU factor IX/mg

Use

- treatment and prophylaxis of bleeding in patients with haemophilia B (Christmas disease)

Dose

- (≥ 12 years of age) calculated using the following formula:

  Number of factor IX IU required (IU)
  = weight (kg) ×
  desired factor IX increase
  (% or IU/dL) × 1.1 dL/kg **OR**

- (< 12 years of age) calculated using the following formula:

  Number of factor IX IU required (IU)
  = weight (kg) ×
  desired factor IX increase
  (% or IU/dL) × 1.4 dL/kg **OR**

- (routine prophylaxis in those with moderate-to-severe haemophilia B, ≥ 12 years and previously treated) 40–60 IU by IV bolus infusion twice weekly **OR**

- (routine prophylaxis in those with moderate-to-severe haemophilia B, <12 years and previously treated) 40 80 IU by IV bolus infusion twice weekly

Adverse effects

- altered taste
- pain in extremity
- rash, urticaria
- (rare) hypersensitivity, allergy, anaphylaxis, thromboembolism, disseminated intravascular coagulation (DIC)
- development of neutralising antibodies (inhibitors), nephrotic syndrome

Nursing points/Cautions

- factor IX activity levels should be monitored using a one-stage clotting assay to confirm adequate factor IX levels have been achieved and maintained
- risk of hypersensitivity is highest in those previously untreated and with high-risk gene mutations
- length of therapy is dependent on reason for administration:
    - (minor bleeding) given daily until bleeding resolves
    - (moderate bleeding) given daily for 3–4 days or until bleeding stops and healing occurs
    - (life-threatening bleeding) given 8–12-hourly until threat has resolved
    - (minor surgery, including tooth extraction) repeated daily after bolus, continued until healing occurs
    - (major surgery) repeated 8–24-hourly after bolus until adequate healing occurs, then for at least another 7 days (to maintain factor IX activity of 30–60% IU/dL)
- neutralising antibodies (inhibitors) may develop and should be suspected if plasma factor IX activity levels are not achieved or bleeding is not controlled with expected dose. If this occurs, factor IX inhibitor concentration levels should be measured
- those with high levels (titres) of factor IX inhibitors are at increased risk of severe hypersensitivity or anaphylaxis if re-exposed to factor IX
- only plastic syringes should be used
- allow vial and diluent (water for injections) to come to room temperature before reconstitution
- reconstitute by using diluent provided (water for injections) and following manufacturer's instructions
- should be administered by IV bolus at a rate that is comfortable for the patient (up to 10 mL/minute)
- should not be given by continuous IV infusion
- administer alone
- solution should be used within 3 hours of reconstitution
- patient/carer may be taught administration technique
- caution if used in those with liver disease, post-surgically or with signs/risk of fibrinolysis, DIC or thromboembolic events
- contraindicated in those with known allergy to hamster protein

Patient teaching and advice

- advise patient to immediately seek medical advice if any rash/hives, itching, throat tightness, chest pain/tightness, difficulty breathing, lightheadedness, dizziness, nausea or fainting occurs (especially if early in therapy)
- ensure patient/carer understands and is able to demonstrate correct administration technique including reconstitution of powder, use of connection device (provided), attaching infusion needle, administration rate, safe disposal of used needles and

cleaning requirements if any blood is spilled
- if patient is planning travel, ensure they understand the importance of having adequate supply for length of trip
- see General Patient teaching and advice (p. xxvii)

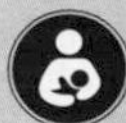

only used during pregnancy or breastfeeding if benefits outweigh risks

EFTRENONACOG ALFA (Alprolix)

Available forms

Vial: 250 IU, 500 IU, 1000 IU, 2000 IU, 3000 IU

Action

- long-acting fusion protein made up of factor IX and IgG1, resulting in a longer plasma half-life

Use

- prophylaxis and treatment of bleeding in patients with haemophilia B

Dose

- (minor-to-moderate bleed) 30–60 IU/kg IV, repeated every 48 hours until bleeding has resolved **OR**
- (surgical prophylaxis – minor surgery including uncomplicated dental extraction) 50–80 IU/kg IV, repeated after 24–48 hours if needed **OR**
- (major bleed; surgical prophylaxis – major surgery) initially 100 IU/kg IV, then 80 IU/kg after 6–10 hours, then daily for 3 days, may be extended to every 48 hours after day 3 if needed **OR**
- (prophylaxis) 50 IU/kg IV weekly or 100 IU/kg IV every 10 days

Adverse effects

- headache, dizziness
- oral paresthesia
- obstructive uropathy
- (uncommon) haematuria, renal colic
- (uncommon) decreased appetite, breath odour, altered taste
- development of neutralising antibodies (inhibitors), nephrotic syndrome
- (rare) allergic reaction, anaphylaxis, thromboembolic events

Nursing points/Cautions

- factor IX activity levels should be monitored using a one-stage clotting assay to confirm adequate factor IX levels have been achieved and maintained
- neutralising antibodies (inhibitors) may develop and should be suspected if plasma factor IX activity levels are not achieved or bleeding is not controlled with expected dose. If this occurs, factor IX inhibitor levels should be measured
- patient may be taught to self-administer
- allow vial and diluent (water for injections) to come to room temperature before reconstitution
- reconstitute by using diluent provided (water for injections) and following manufacturer's instructions
- swirl vial gently to dissolve but do not shake

Patient teaching and advice

- advise patient to immediately seek medical advice if any rash/hives, itching, throat tightness, chest pain/tightness, difficulty breathing, light-headedness, dizziness, nausea or fainting occurs (especially if early in therapy)
- ensure patient/carer understands and is able to demonstrate correct administration technique, including reconstitution of powder, use of connection device (provided), attaching infusion needle, administration rate, safe disposal of used needles and cleaning requirements if any blood is spilled

- if patient is planning travel, ensure they understand the importance of having adequate supply for length of trip
- see also General Patient teaching and advice (p. xxvii)

FACTOR XIII

Factor XIII is the last enzyme in the blood coagulation cascade. When vessel wall damage occurs, factor XIII is activated by thrombin at the site and is responsible for haemostasis maintenance through cross-linking of fibrin and other proteins at the fibrin clot. In the plasma, it circulates as two A-subunits and two B-subunits, which are held together by non-covalent bonds.

CATRIDECACOG (NovoThirteen)

Available form

Vial: 2500 IU

Action

- recombinant coagulation factor XIII A-subunit produced in yeast cells

Use

- prophylaxis of bleeding in patients with congenital factor XIII A-subunit deficiency

Dose

- 35 IU/kg IV monthly with any dose adjustment based on factor XIII activity level

Adverse effects

- nausea, diarrhoea, gastroenteritis
- fever
- headache
- rash
- nasopharyngitis, sinusitis, upper respiratory tract infection, nasal congestion, oropharyngeal pain
- cough
- confusion
- arthralgia, back pain, musculoskeletal pain, myalgia, extremity pain, limb pain
- leucopenia, aggravated neutropenia
- injection site pain
- neutralising antibody development (inhibitors)
- allergic reaction, anaphylaxis

Interactions

- not recommended with factor VII-containing products

Nursing points/Cautions

- not recommended for bleeding prophylaxis in those with congenital factor XIII B-subunit deficiency, therefore it is important that the subunit deficiency is identified before starting therapy
- monitoring factor XIII activity using standard factor XIII assay technique is recommended
- neutralising antibodies (inhibitors) may develop and should be suspected if plasma factor XIII activity levels are not achieved or bleeding is not controlled with expected dose. If this occurs, factor XIII inhibitor levels should be measured
- reconstitute using provided vial adapter and diluent (water for injections) using manufacturer's instructions
- swirl solution gently to dissolve but do not shake as this causes foaming
- solution should be clear and colourless and used within 3 hours of reconstitution
- if dilution of reconstituted solution is needed (e.g. for children under 24 kg), 6 mL of sodium chloride 0.9% is recommended
- caution if used in those with predisposition to thrombosis as fibrin stabilisation effect may lead to increased risk of vessel occlusion
- caution if used in those with severe liver impairment. Factor XIII activity

levels should be closely monitored if used
- may contain traces of yeast, therefore not recommended in those with known yeast hypersensitivity
- not recommended in those with known neutralising antibodies to factor XIII without close monitoring

Patient teaching and advice

- advise patient to immediately seek medical advice if any rash/hives, itching, throat tightness, chest pain/tightness, difficulty breathing, lightheadedness, dizziness, nausea or fainting occurs (especially if early in therapy)
- see also General Patient teaching and advice (p. xxvii)

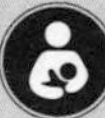

only used during pregnancy or breastfeeding if benefits outweigh risks

HYPOTHALAMIC AND PITUITARY HORMONES

The hypothalamus and pituitary gland are located inferior to the midbrain and work in unison to regulate the synthesis and release of hormones throughout the body. The pituitary gland (also called the hypophysis) is linked to the hypothalamus via a stalk (the infundibulum) (Tortora & Derrickson 2018).

The hypothalamus secretes a range of hormones and releasing factors, including thyrotropin-releasing hormone (TRH), gonadotropin-releasing hormone (GnRH), somatostatin (also called growth hormone release-inhibiting hormone (GHRIH)), growth hormone-releasing hormone (GHRH), corticotropin-releasing hormone (CRH), substance P and prolactin release-inhibiting factor (PRIH). The secretion of hormones and releasing factors is controlled or regulated by a series of complex feedback mechanisms. In turn, all of these hormones and releasing factors regulate the synthesis and secretion of hormones from the anterior pituitary (Tortura & Derrickson 2018).

The pituitary gland itself is divided into two distinct lobes – the anterior pituitary (adenohypophysis) and the posterior pituitary (neurohypophysis). The anterior pituitary secretes a number of hormones that have their effects on various target organs throughout the body, producing other hormones, which are part of the feedback loop to the hypothalamus and/or pituitary, regulating further synthesis and release. Hormones secreted from the anterior pituitary include:

- human growth hormone (GH) (somatotropin) (stimulates growth and regulates metabolism), secretion stimulated by GHRH
- thyroid-stimulating hormone (TSH, or thyrotropin) (stimulates secretion of hormones from the thyroid gland), secretion stimulated by TRH
- adrenocorticotropic hormone (ACTH) (stimulates secretion of glucocorticoids, mineralocorticoids and, to a lesser extent, sex hormones from the adrenal cortex), secretion stimulated by CRH
- gonadotrophins, such as follicle-stimulating hormone (FSH) (stimulates maturation of ovarian follicles and oestrogen production in females and sperm production in males) and luteinising hormone (LH) (stimulates ovulation and oestrogen production in females and testosterone production in males), secretion stimulated by GnRH
- prolactin (promotes lactation), secretion stimulated by prolactin-releasing hormone (PRH)

- melanocyte-stimulating hormone (stimulates production of the melatonin that darkens the skin), secretion stimulated by CRH (Tortura et al 2018).

The posterior pituitary is responsible for only two hormones and their release is mediated by the sympathetic and parasympathetic nervous systems:

- oxytocin (stimulates uterine smooth muscle contraction, as well as stimulating milk ejection from mammary glands. Role in non-pregnant female is unknown) and
- antidiuretic hormone (ADH, or vasopressin) (regulates reabsorption of water in the renal tubules, decreasing urine production) (Tortura & Derrickson 2018).

A number of hypothalamic and pituitary hormone-related agents are discussed in the Pregnancy, childbirth and breastfeeding section (p. 1389).

GONADOTROPHIN-RELEASING HORMONE

GOSERELIN ACETATE (Zoladex 3.6 mg Implant, Zoladex 10.8 mg Implant)

Available forms
Subcutaneous implant: 3.6 mg, 10.8 mg

Action

- GnRH agonist, which causes the release of LH from the pituitary gland (also called luteinising hormone-releasing hormone (LHRH))
- (chronic administration) inhibits gonadotrophin (LH) production resulting in gonadal suppression and regression of sex organs
- (males) testosterone concentration decreases to within castrate range, resulting in prostate tumour regression and symptom improvement
- (females) serum estradiol (oestradiol) levels decrease to post-menopausal levels
- implant releases consistent doses over at least 28 days

Use

- advanced prostate cancer (palliative management of stages C or D (metastatic or locally advanced), suitable for hormonal manipulation or as adjunctive treatment with radiotherapy)
- advanced breast cancer in pre-menopausal women
- early breast cancer (as adjunct therapy in pre-menopausal or peri-menopausal women)
- assisted reproduction (in preparation for controlled ovarian super-stimulation)
- endometrial thinning (prior to endometrial ablation)
- endometriosis (visually proven) (to reduce size and number of lesions, as well as relieving pain)
- uterine fibroids (to reduce size and symptoms, including pain)

Dose

- (prostate cancer) 3.6 mg SC implant into anterior abdominal wall every 28 days **OR**
- (prostate cancer) 10.8 mg SC implant into anterior abdominal wall 3-monthly **OR**
- (early breast cancer, alternative to combination chemotherapy) 3.6 mg SC implant into anterior abdominal wall every 28 days for 2 years **OR**
- (early breast cancer, as adjunct post-combination chemotherapy) 3.6 mg SC implant into anterior abdominal wall every 28 days for 5 years **OR**

- (advanced breast cancer) 3.6 mg SC implant into anterior abdominal wall every 28 days **OR**
- (endometrial thinning) 3.6 mg SC implant into anterior abdominal wall followed by surgery 28 days later, or course of 2 implants 28 days apart with surgery within 14–28 days of second implant **OR**
- (benign gynaecological disorders) 3.6 mg SC implant into anterior abdominal wall every 28 days for 6 months **OR**
- (uterine fibroids) 3.6 mg SC implant into anterior abdominal wall every 28 days for 3–6 months

Adverse effects

- (injection site) pain, haematoma, bleeding and, rarely, vascular injury
- decrease in bone density
- (males) flushing, sweating, gynaecomastia, breast tenderness, decreased libido, erectile dysfunction, decreased glucose tolerance, change in BP, cardiac failure, myocardial infarction, paraesthesia, spinal cord compression, rash, bone pain, arthralgia, weight increase
- (males – after radiotherapy) incontinence, urinary frequency
- (females) headache, flushing, sweating, decreased libido, mood changes, depression, breast enlargement, vaginal dryness, change in BP, arthralgia, paraesthesia, alopecia, rash, acne, weight increase
- (temporary) increase in bone pain (in patients with bony metastases), increase in signs and symptoms of breast cancer (in patients with breast cancer)
- (rare) hypersensitivity reactions, ovarian hyperstimulation syndrome (OHSS) (if given with gonadotrophins), QT prolongation
- (endometrial thinning) increased risk of cervical tearing during procedures

Interactions

- increased risk of QT prolongation if given with agents known to prolong QT interval (e.g. Class IA and Class III antiarrhythmic agents (e.g. amiodarone, sotalol)) or cause electrolyte imbalance (especially hypokalaemia and hypomagnesaemia) (e.g. diuretics)
- increased risk of bleeding when implant is inserted if patient is taking anticoagulants

Nursing points/Cautions

- any electrolyte imbalance should be corrected before starting therapy
- any osteoporosis risk should be assessed before starting therapy and bone density measured if any significant risk factor exists. Risk factors include family history, slight build, heavy smoker, low dietary calcium intake, chronic immobility, chronic anovulatory menstrual disturbances, or taking glucocorticoids
- blood glucose levels and/or glycosylated haemoglobin (HbA1c) should be monitored regularly during therapy (especially in those with existing diabetes mellitus)
- (benign gynaecological conditions) therapy should not exceed 6 months, nor should it be repeated
- implant should be visible in applicator window
- plunger should not be withdrawn when needle is in position
- plunger should be fully depressed to ensure implant enters SC site
- SC sites should be rotated
- injections should not be omitted or delayed, because serum testosterone concentration will rise
- 10.8 mg implant is not for use in females
- (endometriosis) patient should be assessed after 6 months for any risk of osteoporosis and a 2-year interval

should be allowed between repeat course

- caution if used in those with cancer who are at risk of spinal cord compression or ureteric obstruction. These patients should be closely monitored for the first 4 weeks of therapy
- caution if used in those with polycystic ovarian syndrome due to increased risk of ovarian hyperstimulation syndrome (OHSS)
- caution if used in those with congenital long QT syndrome, congestive heart failure, frequent electrolyte imbalance or taking agents that prolong QT interval as androgen deprivation may also prolong QT interval
- contraindicated in those with known hypersensitivity to LH agonist analogues

Patient teaching and advice

- male patients with pre-existing diabetes mellitus should be warned that there may be a loss of glycaemic control and blood glucose levels should be monitored frequently, especially at the start of therapy
- patients with advanced cancer and/or bony metastases should be warned that they may experience an increase in bone pain or other symptoms for up to 2 weeks at the start of therapy
- patient should be instructed to immediately seek medical advice if any of the following occur:
  - any bone pain
  - numbness, tingling or weakness of legs or arms

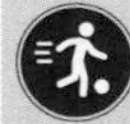

permitted in sport for females only

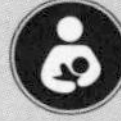

contraindicated during pregnancy or breastfeeding

Note

- contained in ZolaCos CP with bicalutamide

LEUPRORELIN ACETATE (Eligard, Lucrin, Lucrin Depot)

Available forms

Dual-chamber syringe: 7.5 mg, 22.5 mg, 30 mg, 45 mg; Multi-dose vial: 5 mg/mL

Action

- analogue of GnRH that inhibits growth of some hormone-dependent tumours
- (central precocious puberty) suppresses pituitary gonadotropins and peripheral sex steroids and stops progression of secondary sex characteristics

Use

- advanced prostatic cancer (stages C or D, palliative treatment)
- central precocious puberty (CPP) in children

Dose

- (advanced prostatic cancer) 1 mg SC daily **OR**
- (advanced prostatic cancer) 7.5 mg IM monthly (depot) **OR**
- (advanced prostatic cancer) 22.5 mg IM 3-monthly (depot) **OR**
- (advanced prostatic cancer) 30 mg IM 4-monthly (depot) **OR**
- (advanced prostatic cancer) 45 mg IM 6-monthly (depot) **OR**
- (CPP) 30 mg IM 3-monthly (depot)

Adverse effects

- hot flushes, sweating, clamminess, night sweats
- dizziness, headache, asthenia, fatigue, malaise, vertigo, insomnia, depression
- (children) emotional lability, tearfulness
- paraesthesia, neuromuscular disorders

- decreased testicular size, testicular pain, gynaecomastia/breast tenderness, decreased libido, erectile dysfunction
- urinary frequency, urgency and retention, nocturia, haematuria, incontinence
- rash, pruritus, alopecia, acne
- general pain, arthralgia, bone pain, myalgia, joint disorders
- peripheral oedema, oedema
- nausea, vomiting, GI disorders, gastroenteritis/colitis, weight gain
- hyperglycaemia
- decreased bone density
- flare phenomenon (increased bone pain, ureteric obstruction and spinal cord compression)
- (rare) spinal cord compression, ureteric obstruction, myocardial infarction, stroke, convulsions
- (very rare) pituitary apoplexy (rare condition in those with pituitary adenoma caused by infarction of the pituitary gland, which can occur within hours or weeks of the first dose; symptoms include sudden headache, vomiting, visual disturbances, altered mental state and, sometimes, cardiovascular collapse)
- (injection site) pain, burning, stinging, redness, mild bruising

Interactions

- increased risk of QT prolongation if given with agents known to prolong QT interval (e.g. Class IA and Class III antiarrhythmic agents (e.g. amiodarone, sotalol))

Nursing points/Cautions

- flare phenomenon/reaction can be reduced by use of non-steroidal antiandrogen agent
- blood glucose levels and glycosylated haemoglobin (HbA1c) should be monitored regularly during therapy
- serum testosterone and prostate-specific antigen levels should be measured regularly during therapy
- (CPP) must be diagnosed and therapy supervised by paediatric endocrinologist
- rotate injection sites
- depot preparations have different release properties and are not interchangeable, nor should part doses be used
- manufacturer's instructions should be followed for preparation and administration of depot preparations
- (Eligard) product should be allowed to come to room temperature before reconstitution (to reduce pain) and then used within 30 minutes
- caution if used in men with urinary tract obstruction or metastatic vertebral lesions, epilepsy, history of seizures, CNS disorders or tumours
- caution if used in those with or at risk of QT prolongation, electrolyte abnormalities or congestive cardiac failure

Patient teaching and advice

- patient should receive adequate education in correct use of equipment, correct SC injection technique, importance of rotating sites, storage information and safe disposal of used equipment before self-administration can begin
- patients with pre-existing diabetes mellitus should be warned that there may be a loss of glycaemic control and blood glucose levels should be monitored frequently, especially at start of therapy
- warn patient that symptoms (especially bone pain) may initially worsen in first 1 to 2 weeks of therapy (especially if bony metastases are present)
- advise patient to seek medical advice immediately if any of the following occur:
    - any sudden headache, visual disturbance, vomiting or altered mental state

- weakness, tingling or numbness of arms or legs
- blood in the urine or difficulty passing urine
- chest pain or irregular heart rate

- warn patient against driving or operating machinery if dizziness, vertigo, fatigue or paraesthesia occur

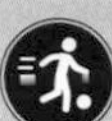

permitted in sport for females only

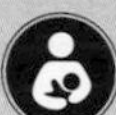

contraindicated during pregnancy and breastfeeding

GROWTH HORMONE RELEASE-INHIBITING FACTOR

General Adverse effects of growth hormone release-inhibiting factor

- (injection site, transient) redness, swelling, stinging, pain, burning, irritation, rash
- anorexia, nausea, vomiting, abdominal pain, bloating, flatulence, dyspepsia, loose stools, diarrhoea, constipation, discolouration of stools, steatorrhoea, decreased weight
- impaired glucose tolerance, hyperglycaemia, hypoglycaemia
- thyroid dysfunction, hypothyroidism
- headache, dizziness, weakness, fatigue, asthenia
- pruritus, rash, transient alopecia
- bradycardia
- reduced gallbladder motility, cholelithiasis, elevated liver enzymes, decreased pancreatic enzymes

General Interactions for growth hormone release-inhibiting factor

- may decrease or delay absorption of ciclosporin
- dose of insulin/oral hypoglycaemic agents may need adjustment when therapy is commenced
- increased risk of bradycardia if given with beta-adrenoceptor blocking agents or other agents that decrease heart rate
- caution if given with agents that have a low therapeutic index

General Patient teaching and advice for growth hormone release-inhibiting factor

- patient should receive adequate education in correct use of equipment, correct SC injection technique, the importance of rotating sites, storage information and safe disposal of used equipment before self-administration can begin
- patient with diabetes mellitus should be advised to closely monitor blood glucose levels during therapy as there is an increased risk of hypo- or hyperglycaemia
- warn patient to avoid driving or operating machinery if dizziness or weakness occur
- instruct patient to seek medical advice immediately if any of the following occur:
  - feeling more thirsty or tired than usual, dry mouth
  - feeling hungry, shaky or sweating more than usual, confusion
  - severe or sudden abdominal pain, high fever, yellowing of skin or eyes, loss of appetite, itchy skin
  - slow heart rate

- any sudden headache, visual disturbance, vomiting or altered mental state

LANREOTIDE ACETATE (Somatuline Autogel)

Available forms

Prefilled syringe (prolonged-release solution): 60 mg/0.5 mL, 90 mg/0.5 mL, 120 mg/0.5 mL

Action

- somatostatin analogue with a long duration of action
- inhibits secretion of GH, serotonin and gastroenteropancreatic (GEP) peptides (gastrin, insulin, glucagon, secretin, motilin, pancreatic polypeptide and vasoactive intestinal peptide)
- inhibits secretion of insulin and glucagon

Use

- acromegaly (after surgery and/or radiotherapy where GH and IGF-1 levels remain high or unresponsive to dopamine agonist treatment)
- carcinoid tumour
- management of symptoms of GEP neuroendocrine tumours (unresectable, locally advanced or metastatic disease)

Dose

Acromegaly

- (not previously treated) initially 60 mg SC every 28 days, then dose increased or decreased according to GH/IGF-1 levels **OR**
- (previously treated with Somatuline LA every 14 days) initially 60 mg SC every 28 days, then dose increased or decreased according to GH/IGF-1 levels **OR**
- (previously treated with Somatuline LA every 10 days) initially 90 mg SC every 28 days, then dose increased or decreased according to GH/IGF-1 levels **OR**
- (previously treated with Somatuline LA every 7 days) initially 120 mg SC every 28 days, then dose Increased or decreased according to GH/IGF-1 levels

Carcinoid tumour

- 60–120 mg SC every 28 days, with dose adjusted according to response

GEP neuroendocrine tumours

- 120 mg SC every 28 days

Adverse effects

- see General Adverse effects for growth hormone release-inhibiting factor (p. 1156)
- myalgia, musculoskeletal pain

Interactions

- see General Interactions for growth hormone release-inhibiting factor (p. 1156)

Nursing points/Cautions

- gallbladder ultrasound is recommended when starting therapy and then 6-monthly
- thyroid function tests are recommended if there are any signs of decreasing thyroid function during therapy
- (carcinoid tumour) obstructive intestinal tumour should be excluded before starting therapy
- should be given deep SC into upper outer quadrant of buttocks, or if self-administered, upper outer thigh
- blood glucose levels should be monitored when starting therapy or adjusting dose (especially in those with pre-existing diabetes)
- kidney and liver function monitoring is recommended in those with renal/hepatic dysfunction
- heart rate monitoring is recommended in those with underlying cardiac disease
- caution if used in those with bradycardia

Patient teaching and advice

- see General Patient teaching and advice for growth hormone release-inhibiting factor (p. 1156)

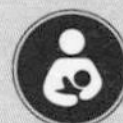

caution if used during pregnancy

contraindicated during breastfeeding

OCTREOTIDE (DBL Octreotide Solution for Injection, Octreotide GH, Octreotide MaxRx, Octreotide Sun, Sandostatin, Sandostatin LAR)

Available forms

Vial/Prefilled syringes (modified-release solution): 10 mg, 20 mg, 30 mg; Vial: 0.05 mg/mL, 0.1 mg/mL, 0.5 mg/mL

Action

- synthetic analogue of somatostatin (GH inhibitor) with prolonged duration of action
- inhibits secretion of GH, serotonin and gastroenteropancreatic (GEP) peptides (gastrin, insulin, glucagon, secretin, motilin, pancreatic polypeptide and vasoactive intestinal peptide)

Use

- treatment of acromegaly (inadequately controlled by surgery, radiotherapy or dopamine agonists, unfit or unwilling to undergo surgery, or until radiotherapy becomes fully effective)
- management of symptoms of GEP endocrine tumours (e.g. carcinoid tumours and vasoactive intestinal peptide-secreting tumours)
- reduction of complications post-pancreatic surgery
- treatment of advanced neuroendocrine tumours of midgut

Dose

Acromegaly

- initially 0.05–0.1 mg SC 8–12-hourly, then dose adjusted monthly depending on clinical symptoms, tolerance and GH and/or insulin-like growth factors (IGF) (maximum daily dose 1.5 mg) **OR**
- (patients controlled with octreotide SC) 20 mg IM monthly for 3 months, starting the day after octreotide SC, then reducing to 10 mg monthly (if symptoms are controlled) or increasing to 30 mg monthly (if symptoms are only partially controlled) (modified-release preparation)

GEP endocrine tumour

- initially 0.05 mg SC 1–2 times daily, increasing gradually to 0.2 mg 3 times daily (depending on tolerance and clinical response) **OR**
- (patients controlled with octreotide SC) 20 mg IM monthly for 3 months with previous SC dose for first 2 weeks of therapy with modified-release preparation, then reduced to 10 mg monthly (if symptoms controlled) or increased to 30 mg monthly (if symptoms only partially controlled) (modified-release preparation) **OR**
- (patients not previously treated with octreotide) 0.1 mg SC 3 times daily for 2 weeks, then assess suitability for modified-release preparation

Complications after pancreatic surgery

- 0.1 mg SC 3 times daily for 7 consecutive days starting 1 hour before surgery

Advanced neuroendocrine tumour of midgut

- 30 mg IM monthly (modified-release preparation)

Adverse effects

- see General Adverse effects for growth hormone release-inhibiting factor (p. 1156)

- dyspnoea
- (prolonged use) biliary sludge, hyperbilirubinaemia, decreased vitamin B_{12} levels, thrombocytopenia
- (rare) hypersensitivity, acute pancreatitis, liver/biliary dysfunction, QT prolongation, arrhythmias, ECG changes, increase in size of pre-existing GH-secreting pituitary tumour

Interactions

- may decrease/delay absorption of cimetidine
- may increase bioavailability of bromocriptine
- caution if given with agents that prolong QT interval (e.g. disopyramide, amiodarone, sotalol, some antipsychotic agents, some antibacterial agents (e.g. IV erythromycin, pentamidine, clarithromycin), antifungal agents or some antihistamines) or cause hypokalaemia or hypomagnesaemia (e.g. diuretics)
- see also General Interactions for growth hormone release-inhibiting factors (p. 1156)

Nursing points/Cautions

- gallbladder ultrasound is recommended before starting therapy and at 6–12-month intervals and any symptomatic gallstones treated
- (acromegaly) those not previously treated with octreotide should be commenced on SC preparation to assess response, then switched to IM preparation
- (acromegaly) monthly assessment of GH and/or IGF-1 levels, clinical symptoms and biochemical markers should occur. If no change after 3 months, therapy should be stopped
- (GEP endocrine tumours) SC doses may be required in addition to IM modified preparation for first 8 weeks of therapy until therapeutic levels are reached and symptoms are controlled
- (Sandostatin LAR) allow provided diluent and vial to come to room temperature, then diluent should be injected slowly down side of vial (but not directly onto powder), allow 2–5 minutes undisturbed (or longer if needed) for powder to become wet, then swirl very gently to form an even, milky suspension. Withdraw the required amount without inverting vial. Change needle before IM administration
- rotate injection sites
- IM injection into deltoid muscle is not recommended because of pain and discomfort
- (long-term therapy) thyroid function, blood glucose levels and vitamin B_{12} levels should be monitored regularly in those with a history of or at risk of vitamin B_{12} deficiency
- patient should be monitored regularly for any signs or symptoms of the growth hormone-secreting tumour increasing in size (e.g. visual field defects)
- caution if used in those with cardiovascular disease, history of gallstones or vitamin B_{12} deficiency or those with concurrent bleeding gastro-oesophageal varices
- caution if used in those with liver cirrhosis as half-life may be increased

Patient teaching and advice

- see General Patient teaching and advice for growth hormone release-inhibiting factor (p. 1156)
- if patient is experiencing gastrointestinal adverse effects, suggest injecting between meals and at bedtime to reduce them
- female patients treated for acromegaly should be advised that fertility may be restored during therapy and contraception should be used to avoid pregnancy if not wanted

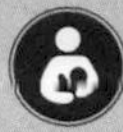

not recommended during pregnancy or breastfeeding unless clearly necessary

PASIREOTIDE (Signifor, Signifor LAR)

Available forms

Ampoule (for SC injection): 300 microgram/mL, 600 microgram/mL, 900 microgram/mL; Vial (for IM injection): 20 mg, 40 mg, 60 mg

Action

- somatostatin analogue
- has a high binding affinity for four of the five human somatostatin receptor subtypes, which are expressed in many tissues, especially neuroendocrine tumours (secreting hormones such as adrenocorticotropic hormone (ACTH) in Cushing's syndrome)

Use

- treatment of adults with Cushing's syndrome where surgery has failed or is unsuitable
- treatment of adults with acromegaly where surgery is not an option or has not been curative or inadequately controlled with other somatostatin analogues

Dose

- (Cushing's syndrome) initially 600 microgram or 900 microgram SC twice daily, then dose titrated to 300–900 microgram SC twice daily **OR**
- (acromegaly) initially 40 mg IM every 4 weeks, increasing to 60 mg if GH and/or IGF-1 levels are not controlled after 12 weeks or decreased by 20 mg increments if adverse reactions or over-response to treatment (IGF-1 < lower normal limit) occur (modified-release preparation)

Adverse effects

- myalgia, arthralgia, back pain, muscle spasm
- fever
- nasopharyngitis, bronchitis, influenza, upper respiratory tract infection, cough, oropharyngeal pain
- hypokalaemia
- prolonged QT interval
- hypocortisolism
- see also General Adverse effects of growth hormone release-inhibiting factors (p. 1156)

Interactions

- see General Interactions of growth hormone release-inhibiting factors (p. 1156)
- may increase availability of bromocriptine
- increased serum levels may occur if given with ciclosporin, verapamil and clarithromycin
- caution if given with agents that prolong QT interval (e.g. disopyramide, amiodarone, sotalol, some antipsychotic agents, some antibacterial agents (e.g. IV erythromycin, pentamidine, clarithromycin), antifungal agents or some antihistamines) or cause hypokalaemia or hypomagnesaemia (e.g. diuretics)

Nursing points/Cautions

- any hypokalaemia or hypomagnesaemia should be corrected before starting therapy
- baseline ECG is recommended before starting and then after 21 days of therapy
- blood glucose levels (BGL) (HbA1c and/or fasting plasma glucose levels) should be measured before starting therapy, then weekly for 8–12 weeks, then regularly afterwards
- cortisol levels should be closely monitored during therapy, especially in the first 8 weeks as temporary glucocorticoid therapy or interruption of

pasireotide therapy may be required if hypocortisolism occurs

- electrolyte levels (especially potassium and magnesium) and pituitary function (e.g. TSH, free T4, GH, IGF-1) should be measured before starting and then regularly during therapy
- liver function should be monitored before starting, then after first 2–3 weeks, monthly for 3 months and then regularly during therapy. If transaminases are elevated (after second test to confirm results), more frequent monitoring is recommended until pre-treatment levels are reached. If jaundice or other signs of liver impairment develop, therapy should be stopped
- heart rate should be monitored (especially at the start of therapy and if patient is taking other agents that cause bradycardia)
- (Cushing's syndrome) response to therapy (decrease in urinary free cortisol and/or improvement in signs and symptoms) should be determined after 8 weeks
- if patient has uncontrolled diabetes mellitus, intense antidiabetic therapy is recommended before starting pasireotide therapy. Additional BGL monitoring is also suggested
- if hyperglycaemia develops during therapy, antidiabetic therapy should be started or adjusted to control BGL. If hyperglycaemia persists, pasireotide dose should be reduced or therapy stopped
- (Cushing's syndrome) dose should be started at 300 microgram twice daily for those with moderate liver impairment to a maximum of 600 microgram twice daily
- (Cushing's syndrome) a starting dose of 600 mg twice daily should be considered for those with diabetes mellitus
- (Cushing's syndrome) patient can be instructed to self-inject
- (acromegaly) IM injection sites should be alternated between left and right gluteal muscles
- (acromegaly) injection kit (powder, prefilled syringe containing diluent, vial adapter and injection needle) should be allowed to come to room temperature for at least 30 minutes before administration
- (acromegaly) manufacturer's instructions should be followed to reconstitute solution, including shaking vial in horizontal position for at least 30 seconds after addition of diluent
- (acromegaly) to avoid sedimentation occurring, syringe may be shaken gently to maintain a uniform suspension
- caution if patient has poor glycaemic control (HbA1c $>$ 8%) as there is an increased risk of severe hyperglycaemia and ketoacidosis
- caution and monitoring is recommended if patient has cardiac disease and/or risk factors for bradycardia (e.g. history of clinically significant bradycardia or acute myocardial infarction, high-grade heart block, congestive cardiac failure, unstable angina, ventricular tachycardia/fibrillation)
- caution if used in those at risk of QT prolongation including congenital long QT syndrome, uncontrolled or significant cardiac disease
- not recommended for treatment of paediatric Cushing's syndrome or in those under 18 years
- contraindicated in those with severe liver impairment

Patient teaching and advice

- see General Patient teaching and advice for growth hormone release-inhibiting factor (p. 1156)
- advise patient to seek medical advice immediately if any of the following occur:
  - weakness, fatigue, loss of appetite, nausea, vomiting, hypotension

(light-headedness, dizziness or fainting), hyponatraemia (nausea, vomiting, headache, confusion, loss of energy and fatigue, irritability, restlessness, muscle weakness/cramps/spasms or fitting), hypoglycaemia (cool pale skin, fatigue, drowsiness, unusual tiredness, sweating, shaking, anxiety, crying, vomiting, headache, excessive hunger, visual changes, palpitations, confusion)

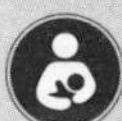

should only be used during pregnancy if benefits outweigh risks

not recommended during breastfeeding

PEGVISOMANT (Somavert)

Available forms
Vial: 10 mg, 15 mg, 20 mg

Action
- growth hormone (GH) analogue that has been structurally altered to produce GH receptor antagonist which binds to GH receptor sites blocking endogenous GH from binding, resulting in decreased levels of insulin-like growth factor-I (IGF-I)
- protein is bonded to propylene glycol

Use
- acromegaly (in patient with inadequate response to surgery, radiation or medical therapy or where these therapies are inappropriate)

Dose
- initially 80 mg SC (loading dose), then 10 mg SC daily, with dose adjustments of 5 mg daily according to serum IGF-I (daily maximum 30 mg)

Adverse effects
- injection site reaction
- chest pain, peripheral oedema
- pain, back pain
- dizziness, paraesthesia
- hypertension
- diarrhoea, nausea
- influenza, sinusitis, respiratory infections
- abnormal liver function
- rash, erythema, pruritus, urticaria
- (rare) increase in size of pre-existing GH-secreting pituitary tumour

Interactions
- caution if used with opioids as higher doses of pegvisomant may be required in order to achieve appropriate IGF-I suppression
- dose of insulin or oral hypoglycaemic agent may require adjustment especially at the start of therapy

Nursing points/Cautions
- before starting therapy, patient should have liver function tests and not start if any signs of liver disease are present. Liver function tests are recommended at least every 6 months after IGF-I levels have become normal
- serum IGF-I level should be measured before starting therapy, then every 4–6 weeks
- because pegvisomant is structurally similar to GH and may cross-react in commercially available assays, serum GH levels should not be used to monitor treatment. Dose adjustments should only be based on serum IGF-I levels
- reconstitute using 1 mL water for injections (provided)
- SC injection sites should be rotated daily to prevent lipohypertrophy
- caution if used in the elderly or those with diabetes mellitus

Patient teaching and advice
- see General Patient teaching and advice for growth hormone release-inhibiting factor (p. 1156)

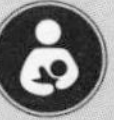

not recommended during pregnancy

caution if used during breastfeeding

ANTERIOR PITUITARY HORMONES

GROWTH HORMONE (SOMATOTROPIC HORMONES)

SOMATROPIN (SOMATOTROPHIN/ SOMATOTROPIN) (Genotropin, Genotropin GoQuick, Genotropin MiniQuick, Humatrope, Norditropin, NutropinAQ, Omnitrope, Saizen, SciTropin A)

Available forms

Prefilled pen: 5 mg/1.5 mL, 6 mg/1.03 mL, 10 mg/1.5 mL, 12 mg/1.5 mL, 15 mg/ 1.5 mL, 20 mg/2.5 mL; Cartridge solution: 5 mg/1.5 mL, 10 mg/1.5 mL, 15 mg/ 1.5 mL; 10 mg/2 mL; Cartridge (with syringe of diluting solution): 6 mg, 12 mg, 24 mg; Two-compartment cartridge (with preservative): 5 mg, 12 mg; Two-compartment cartridge (without preservative): 0.4 mg, 0.6 mg, 0.8 mg, 1 mg, 1.2 mg, 1.4 mg, 1.6 mg, 1.8 mg, 2 mg; Vial: 3 mg, 4 mg, 8 mg, 10 mg

Action

- human growth hormone (GH) is normally secreted at night during sleep, promoting growth through action of insulin-like growth factors (IGF)
- synthetic human GH produced by recombinant DNA technology with therapeutic equivalence to human GH
- normalises insulin-like growth factor 1 (IGF-1)
- promotes skeletal and cell (increasing number and size of muscle cells) growth
- stimulates protein, carbohydrate, mineral and lipid metabolism
- increases retention of sodium, potassium and phosphorus
- gender differences, with adult females requiring higher doses than males for GH deficiency
- choose the appropriate patient, dose and management, and only to be undertaken by those specialised in this field
- special approval is required for the prescribing of this medication
- 1 mg = 3 IU

Use

- decreased or failed secretion of pituitary GH, resulting in short stature
- growth disturbance associated with gonadal dysgenesis (Turner's syndrome)
- adults with severe deficiency of GH
- paediatric patients with Prader-Willi syndrome (to treat short stature and improve body composition)
- growth disturbance in children with chronic renal insufficiency (height or growth velocity ≤ 25th percentile)

Dose

- (children, GH deficiency) initially 0.175–0.255 mg/kg/week SC divided into either 7 daily doses, 6 doses or 3 doses given on alternate days, then gradually titrated to desired response (maximum weekly dose 0.26 mg/kg) **OR**
- (adults, GH deficiency) initially 0.04 mg/kg/week SC divided into 7 daily doses, then increased gradually to maximum dose 0.08 mg/kg/ week **OR**
- (Turner's syndrome) 0.3–0.35 mg/kg/ week SC divided into 6–7 daily doses, preferably in the evening (with concurrent sex steroid therapy) **OR**
- (Turner's syndrome) 0.045–0.05 mg/ kg/day SC, increasing dose in following year if response is not satisfactory **OR**

- (Prader-Willi syndrome) 0.035–0.05 mg/kg SC daily **OR**
- (chronic renal insufficiency) 0.045–0.05 mg/kg SC daily (up to the time of renal transplant)

Adverse effects

- (injection site) pain, redness, swelling
- (adults, common) paraesthesia/abnormal sensation, muscle stiffness, peripheral oedema, facial oedema, arthralgia, myalgia, localised muscle pain, hyperglycaemia (mild), dyspnoea, sleep apnoea, hypertension, carpal tunnel syndrome, insomnia, gynaecomastia
- (adults, uncommon) headache, muscle weakness, glycosuria
- (children) scoliosis, slipped epiphysis of hip, mild transient urticaria at the injection site, mild and transient oedema
- (children, uncommon) muscle stiffness, arthralgia, myalgia, peripheral oedema
- (Turner's syndrome) otitis media, ear disorders, hypothyroidism, peripheral oedema
- antibody formation
- rash, pruritus, urticaria
- (rare) lipoatrophy (SC), antibody formation
- (rare) myositis, benign intracranial hypertension, diabetes mellitus
- (very rare, children) leukaemia, pancreatitis, gynaecomastia

Interactions

- large doses of glucocorticoids may inhibit growth promotion effects
- dose adjustment of insulin or oral hypoglycaemic agents may be necessary
- caution if used with thyroid hormones as GH preparations may alter T3 and T4 concentrations
- larger dose may be required in adult women on oral oestrogen therapy
- may decrease plasma levels of ciclosporin, some antiepileptic agents and sex steroids

Nursing points/Cautions

- before starting therapy, pituitary function (including provocation tests) should be investigated thoroughly
- fasting insulin and IGF-1 levels should be measured before starting therapy and then twice yearly
- urine testing and/or blood glucose levels should be monitored regularly in all patients (as insulin resistance can occur with GH therapy). If the patient is at risk of developing diabetes, oral glucose tolerance testing is also recommended
- regular growth monitoring and measuring of biochemical markers are recommended throughout therapy
- any other pituitary hormone deficiencies or pituitary tumours should be treated before starting therapy (especially in adults)
- any anti-tumour therapy should be completed before starting therapy with somatotropin
- thyroid function test is recommended after start of therapy, along with any dose adjustment (especially in those receiving treatment with thyroid hormones) as hypothyroidism can develop with therapy
- if GH deficiency is due to malignant disease treatment, patient should be closely monitored for any malignancy relapse
- (childhood GH deficiency) GH level should be retested before starting treatment as an adult
- may also be given IM, although SC is preferred route
- (Prader-Willi syndrome) diagnosis should be confirmed by genetic testing before starting therapy
- (Prader-Willi syndrome) evaluation of any upper respiratory obstruction and sleep apnoea should occur before starting therapy. Therapy should be interrupted if any signs of airway

obstruction, including onset or worsening of snoring

- (Prader-Willi syndrome) any respiratory infection should be diagnosed as soon as symptoms appear and treated aggressively
- (Prader-Willi syndrome) a calorie-controlled diet is also recommended with GH therapy
- (Turner's syndrome) girls should have regular ear examinations, including hearing tests as they have an increased risk of ear or hearing disorders
- (chronic renal insufficiency) conservative treatment for renal insufficiency should be established and maintained before starting therapy
- (chronic renal insufficiency) growth retardation should be established for at least 1 year before starting therapy
- (chronic renal insufficiency) treatment should be stopped if renal transplantation is to occur
- reconstitution should be with provided diluents and according to manufacturer's instructions
- some solutions are stable for 14–28 days after reconstitution if refrigerated at 2–8°C. However, some need to be used within 24 hours of reconstitution. It is important to read and follow manufacturer's instructions with regard to storage requirements
- do not shake vial vigorously as protein will be denatured
- (Zomacton) may be administered using Zomajet device
- (Zomacton) contraindicated in adults
- (Genotropin) bioequivalence between formulations has not been demonstrated
- (Humatrope) not indicated for use in those with Prader-Willi syndrome
- caution if used in those who have had renal allograft (who have experienced two or more episodes of rejection) as there is an increased risk of kidney rejection
- caution if used in those with diabetes mellitus due to decreased insulin sensitivity and glucose intolerance. Any existing antidiabetic therapy may require adjustment
- (Humatrope, Zomacton, Genotropin) contraindicated in those with known sensitivity to metacresol or glycerol
- contraindicated in those with evidence of active tumours, children with closed epiphyses, acute respiratory failure, active proliferative or severe non-proliferative diabetic retinopathy, acute critical illness (following trauma, burns or surgery), or those with Prader-Willi syndrome (with severe obesity or severe respiratory impairment, including sleep apnoea)

Patient teaching and advice

- patient should receive adequate education in correct use of equipment (differs from brand to brand), correct injection technique, importance of rotating sites, storage information and safe disposal of used equipment before self-administration can begin
- parent/carer should be advised to observe children for any limping (which may indicate slipped epiphyses of the hip)
- instruct patient to seek medical advice if any of the following occur:
    - any muscle pain or severe pain at the injection site (disproportional to injection) (as this may require changing to a metacresol-free preparation)
    - any nausea/vomiting, severe or recurrent headaches or visual problems (signs of intracranial hypertension)
    - weakness or numbness of legs or arms
- female patients taking oral oestrogen therapy should be advised not to stop oestrogen therapy suddenly without seeking medical advice

banned in sport

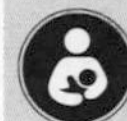
only used during pregnancy if clearly needed

TETRACOSACTIDE (TETRACOSACTRIN) (Synacthen, Synacthen Depot)

Available forms

Ampoules: 250 microgram/mL; Ampoules (depot): 1 mg/mL

Action

- synthetic long chain polypeptide with properties similar to those of endogenous ACTH stimulating the synthesis of glucocorticoids, mineralocorticoids and, to a lesser extent, androgens
- 1 mg tetracosactrin = 100 IU ACTH
- (depot) inorganic zinc complex is added to solution to prolong release

Use

- diagnostic investigation of adrenocortical insufficiency
- exacerbation of multiple sclerosis (MS) (depot)
- hypsarrhythmia and/or infantile spasm (depot)

Dose

- (diagnostic) 250 microgram as single dose deep IM **OR**
- (exacerbation of MS) initially 1 mg daily deep IM, or 1 mg 12-hourly until symptoms abate, then reducing to 0.5–1 mg every 2–3 days or 1 mg weekly (depot)

Adverse effects

- (rare) hypersensitivity reactions (e.g. nausea, vomiting, dizziness, urticaria, flushing, malaise, dyspnoea, angioedema, injection site reaction)
- (long-term or repeated administration) corticosteroid like adverse effects, including:
  - osteoporosis, muscle weakness and loss of mass, bone fractures, steroid myopathy, tendon rupture,
  - peptic ulcer/perforation/haemorrhage, abdominal distension/discomfort
  - hyperpigmentation, thin fragile skin, increased sweating, impaired wound healing, hirsutism
  - decreased resistance to infection
  - decreased carbohydrate metabolism, hyperglycaemia
  - headache, vertigo, seizures, increased intracranial pressure
  - fluid retention, electrolyte disturbance, hypertension
  - Cushing's syndrome
  - euphoria, insomnia, mood swings, personality changes, depression, psychosis, aggravation of existing emotional instability or psychosis
- (prolonged therapy) glaucoma, cataracts
- (depot) salt and water retention
- injection site reaction
- (rare) antibody formation
- (very rare) adrenal haemorrhage

Interactions

- tetracosactrin depot may necessitate adjustment to doses of insulin and/or antihypertensive agents
- spironolactone may cause false positive on fluorometric analysis, therefore should be withheld on morning of test
- not recommended with sodium valproate due to risk of jaundice
- caution if used with phenytoin, clonazepam, nitrazepam, phenobarbital (phenobarbitone) or primidone due to risk of liver damage
- not recommended with live attenuated viruses because of decreased antibody response

- (diagnostic) endogenous and synthetic oestrogens can cause an increase in total cortisol levels (alternative methods (e.g. salivary cortisol, free cortisol index, plasma-free cortisol) are recommended for interpretation of results

Nursing points/Cautions

- before therapy, patient should be assessed for any allergic conditions, especially asthma, and risk versus benefit analysis conducted due to increased risk of hypersensitivity reaction occurring
- treatment should be kept at the lowest possible dose and gradually withdrawn to prevent adrenocorticoid insufficiency
- patient should be observed for first 30 minutes after administration, because this is when hypersensitivity reaction is most likely to occur. If this occurs, IM/IV adrenaline (epinephrine) and IV hydrocortisone should be given
- (depot) shake suspension well before use until it is uniformly cloudy
- depot preparation should never be given IV
- diagnostic test for adrenocortical insufficiency should be done between 6 am and 9 am
- if diagnosis is by the 30-minute test, blood sample should be taken immediately before administration, tetracosactide (tetracosactrin) given IM and a second blood sample taken exactly 30 minutes later. If plasma cortisol increases to at least 200 nanomol/L (70 microgram/L) above baseline, or if post-administration level $>$ 500 nanomol/L (180 microgram/L) (regardless of baseline levels), adrenocortical function is considered normal
- cortisone and hydrocortisone should be withheld on day of diagnostic testing
- if patient is to have surgery or sustains an injury within 12 months of stopping therapy, it may be recommenced or continued at an increased dose or with rapidly acting corticosteroids
- (depot) caution if used in those with emotional instability or psychotic tendencies as these may become aggravated by therapy
- (depot) caution if used in those with hypothyroidism or cirrhosis because effect may be increased
- (depot) caution if used in those with myasthenia gravis, osteoporosis, predisposition to thromboembolism, hypertension, renal insufficiency, recent intestinal anastomosis, diverticulitis or ulcerative colitis
- (depot) caution if used in those with latent TB or amoebiasis, because disease may become reactivated
- (depot) caution if used in those with ocular herpes simplex, because there is an increased risk of corneal perforation
- caution if used in those with asthma or known allergies, because of increased risk of anaphylactic reaction
- (depot) contraindicated in neonates, because of benzyl alcohol content
- contraindicated in those with a current viral disease, recent vaccination with live attenuated virus, acute psychoses, untreated infection, peptic ulcer, Cushing's syndrome, refractory heart failure, diabetes mellitus, moderate/severe hypertension, treatment of adrenocortical insufficiency or adrenogenital syndrome or known hypersensitivity to ACTH

Patient teaching and advice

- patient should be advised to avoid contact with anyone with an infectious disease as he/she is more susceptible to infection

- patient should be advised to have regular ophthalmic examination with prolonged therapy
- low-salt diet should be recommended to prevent water and salt retention problems. Potassium substitutes may be required if therapy is prolonged
- instruct patient to seek medical advice if any of the following occur:
  - severe pain/tenderness in stomach, with nausea and/or vomiting
  - vomiting blood (or material that looks like coffee grounds)
  - fitting (seizures)
  - eye pain or difficulty seeing
  - sudden severe headache, loss of coordination, slurred speech, arm/leg numbness, pain in calves, thighs or chest
  - shortness of breath and leg/ankle swelling (due to fluid build-up)
  - unusual hair growth on body
  - rapid mood swings (e.g. from being very happy to very sad)

banned in sport

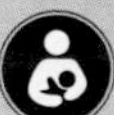
not recommended during pregnancy or breastfeeding

PROLACTIN SUPPRESSION

QUINAGOLIDE HYDROCHLORIDE (Norprolac)

Available forms
Tablets: 25 microgram, 50 microgram, 75 microgram

Action
- selective dopamine D_2 receptor agonist that only inhibits prolactin (not other pituitary hormones)
- prolonged duration of action, allowing once-daily administration
- action within 2 hours, maximum effect within 4–6 hours, duration up to 24 hours

Use
- hyperprolactinaemia (idiopathic, prolactin-secreting pituitary microadenoma or macroadenoma induced)

Dose
- initially 25 microgram orally at night with food for 3 days, then 50 microgram for 3 days, then 75 microgram daily. Dose may be further increased at weekly intervals if needed

Adverse effects
- nausea, vomiting, anorexia, abdominal pain, diarrhoea, constipation
- headache, dizziness, fatigue, insomnia
- hypotension
- muscle weakness
- nasal congestion
- (rare) acute psychosis, somnolence, impulse control disorders (including pathological gambling, increased libido, hypersexuality, compulsive buying or spending, binge eating, repetitive purposeless activity (punding))

Interactions
- effects may be reduced by agents with strong dopaminergic properties (e.g. neuroleptic agents)
- tolerability may be reduced by alcohol

Nursing points/Cautions
- standing and lying BP should be monitored in first days of therapy and when dose is adjusted
- maintenance dose is usually 75–150 microgram/day, but some patients may require doses of up to 300 microgram/day

- contains galactose, therefore not recommended in those with galactose intolerance, Lapp lactase deficiency or glucose–galactose malabsorption
- caution if used in those with history of psychiatric disorders
- contraindicated in those with liver or kidney impairment

Patient teaching and advice

- instruct patient to take tablets with food
- warn patient that adverse effects generally occur in first days of therapy and then decrease
- patient should be advised to avoid alcohol during therapy
- advise patient not to drive or operate machinery if dizziness, fatigue, somnolence or hypotension occurs (especially in first few days of therapy)
- patient/family/carers should be asked to observe and report any:
  - sudden sleep onset as patients are often unaware that this occurs and it may be dangerous if the person drives or operates machinery
  - persistent/recurring gambling, increase in sexual desires (increased libido or hypersexuality), compulsive spending or buying, binge eating or repetitive behaviours with no purpose
- women of childbearing years who do not wish to become pregnant should be advised to use a reliable form of contraception as quinagolide may restore fertility

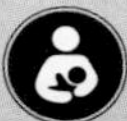

not recommended during pregnancy

suppresses lactation

tablets can be dispersed in water or crushed and mixed with spoonful of yoghurt or apple puree

POSTERIOR PITUITARY HORMONES

ANTIDIURETIC HORMONE (ADH)

ARGIPRESSIN (Pitressin)

Available form

Ampoule: 20 U (pressor units)/mL

Action

- direct antidiuretic action on the distal renal tubule by increasing permeability to water reabsorption
- causes contraction of smooth muscle of GI tract and vascular bed (especially capillaries, small arterioles and venules)

Use

- symptomatic control of diabetes insipidus
- prevention and control of abdominal distension
- dispelling gas shadows in abdominal X-rays

Dose

- (abdominal distension) initially 0.25 mL (5 units) IM or SC, increasing to 0.5 mL (10 units) if needed, given 3–4-hourly **OR**
- (abdominal radiography) 0.5 mL (10 units) IM or SC given twice, once at 2 hours, then 30 minutes before films are exposed **OR**
- (diabetes insipidus) 0.25–0.5 mL (5–10 units) IM or SC 2–3 times daily

Adverse effects

- pallor
- nausea, vomiting, abdominal cramping, flatulence

- tremor, sweating, pounding in head, vertigo
- urticaria, bronchial constriction
- arrhythmias, angina, peripheral vasoconstriction
- (rare) water intoxication, anaphylaxis (shortly after injection), gangrene

Interactions

- antidiuretic effect may be potentiated by carbamazepine, urea, fludrocortisone and TCAs
- antidiuretic effect may be reduced by noradrenaline, lithium, heparin and alcohol
- caution if given with H_2 antagonists as bradycardia and heart block may occur

Nursing points/Cautions

- patient should be closely monitored for any signs of anaphylaxis after administration
- should not be given by IV administration
- SC or IM doses should not exceed 0.75 mL
- (radiology) enema before first dose may be recommended by radiologist
- caution if given to those with epilepsy, migraine, asthma, toxaemia associated with pregnancy, nephritis (with arterial hypertension), goitre (with cardiac complications), coronary thrombosis, angina or arteriosclerosis
- not recommended in those with vascular disease, especially coronary artery disease as angina or myocardial infarction may be precipitated (depending on dose)
- contraindicated in those with chronic nephritis (with nitrogen retention)

Patient teaching and advice

- patient should be advised to immediately report any drowsiness, listlessness or headache (signs of water intoxication)
- warn patient to avoid driving or operating machinery if vertigo, pounding in head or tremor occur

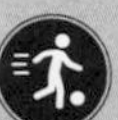

banned in sport

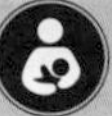

not recommended during pregnancy unless benefits outweigh risks

DESMOPRESSIN (Minirin Melt, Minirin Tablets, Nocdurna)

DESMOPRESSIN ACETATE (Minirin Injection, Minirin Nasal Spray or Drops, Octostim Injection)

Available forms

Metered-dose nasal spray: 10 microgram/dose; Nasal drops: 100 microgram/mL; Tablets: 200 microgram; Ampoules: 4 microgram/mL, 15 microgram/mL; Sublingual wafers: 25 microgram, 50 microgram, 60 microgram, 120 microgram, 240 microgram

Action

- synthetic analogue of vasopressin, but with greater antidiuretic activity, more prolonged action and less pressor activity
- acts on renal collecting tubules, increasing permeability to water reabsorption
- high doses increase factor VIII coagulant activity and von Willebrand factor activity and also release of plasminogen activator
- reduces skin bleeding time by unknown mechanisms
- slight oxytocic effect
- vasodilatory effect reducing BP

Use

- diabetes insipidus

- nocturia due to nocturnal polyuria (in adults who wake ≥ 2 times per night, unresponsive to lifestyle measures)
- diagnostically to determine renal concentrating capacity
- before dental or minor surgery in mild and moderate haemophilia A and von Willebrand disease to increase factor VIII levels
- bleeding in patients with platelet dysfunction (e.g. congenital or drug-induced dysfunction)
- primary nocturnal enuresis (in those aged 6 or more who are refractory to enuresis alarm)

Dose

- (diabetes insipidus) 10–40 microgram intranasally daily or in 2 divided doses **OR**
- (diabetes insipidus) 1–4 microgram IM or IV daily or in 2 divided doses (Minirin) **OR**
- (diabetes insipidus) initially 100 microgram orally 3 times daily, increasing dose according to response, then 100–200 microgram 3 times daily (maintenance) **OR**
- (diabetes insipidus) initially 60 microgram sublingually 3 times daily, then 60–120 microgram 3 times daily (maintenance) **OR**
- (diagnostic) 40 microgram intranasally as a single dose **OR**
- (diagnostic) 4 microgram IM as a single dose (Minirin) **OR**
- (nocturnal enuresis) initially 20 microgram intranasally at night, then adjusting dose as needed to 10–40 microgram (maintenance) **OR**
- (nocturnal enuresis) initially 120 microgram sublingually at night, increasing to 240 microgram if needed **OR**
- (nocturnal enuresis) initially 200 microgram orally at bedtime, increasing to 400 microgram if needed **OR**
- (adult nocturia) 25 microgram (women) or 50 microgram (men) sublingually daily 1 hour before bed (Nocdurna) **OR**
- (mild-to-moderate bleeding – haemophilia A or von Willebrand disease) 0.4 microgram/kg IV, diluted to 10–100 mL with sodium chloride 0.9% and infused over 15–20 minutes 30 minutes before procedure (with tranexamic acid). This may be repeated 12-hourly if cover is needed and response is adequate **OR**
- (non-surgical bleeding in patients with platelet dysfunction) 0.3 microgram/kg IV, diluted to 50 mL with sodium chloride 0.9% and infused over 30 minutes (RBC transfusion may also be given to improve haemostasis in uraemic patients). This may be repeated 12-hourly if cover is needed and response is adequate **OR**
- (before general surgery (except cardiac surgery) in patients with platelet dysfunction) 0.3 microgram/kg IV, diluted to 50 mL with sodium chloride 0.9% and infused over 30 minutes, given 30 minutes before surgery **OR**
- (before cardiac surgery in patients with platelet dysfunction) 0.3 microgram/kg IV, diluted to 50 mL with sodium chloride 0.9% and infused over 30 minutes when cardiopulmonary bypass is complete and protamine has been given

Adverse effects

- (diabetes insipidus) headache, cold, increased weight, dizziness, sore throat, depression
- (nocturnal enuresis) headache, respiratory disorders, coughing, sore throat, nasal congestion, asthma, vomiting, abdominal pain and cramping, nausea, diarrhoea, fever, flu-like symptoms, allergy, earache, ear infection
- (nasal preparations) headache, nausea, abdominal pain, nasal congestion, rhinitis, flushing, nosebleed, upper

respiratory infection, insomnia, nightmares, aggression, nervousness, labile mood
- (rare) water intoxication, hyponatraemia, oedema

Interactions

- additive antidiuretic effects may result if given with TCAs, SSRIs, chlorpromazine, carbamazepine or sulfonylurea antidiabetic agents, increasing the risk of water retention and hyponatraemia
- NSAIDs may induce water retention and hyponatraemia, therefore increased effect may be expected if given together
- increased plasma levels may occur if given with loperamide
- magnitude (not duration) of response may be increased if given with indometacin

Nursing points/Cautions

- fluid balance should be restored before starting therapy and therapy not started if patient is dehydrated or overhydrated
- (haemophilia) fluid restriction is required and patient should be weighed daily. If weight increases gradually or there is a decrease in serum sodium (< 130 mmol/L) or plasma osmolality (< 270 mOsm/kg), further fluid restriction will be required and therapy interrupted
- bladder dysfunction and outlet obstruction should be investigated and ruled out as cause of primary nocturnal enuresis before starting therapy
- if patient becomes acutely unwell during therapy (e.g. systemic infection, fever, gastroenteritis) leading to electrolyte and/or fluid imbalance, therapy should be stopped
- (diabetes insipidus) dose is determined by adequate sleep and adequate, but not excessive, water turnover
- (diagnostic purpose) fluid should be restricted to 500 mL for 1 hour before and 8 hours after administration
- (diabetes insipidus) serum and urinary sodium and osmolality should be closely monitored during therapy
- (diabetes insipidus) if patient develops headache, nausea/vomiting, weight gain (and convulsions in severe cases), therapy should be stopped, dose adjusted and fluids restricted (signs and symptoms of water intoxication and hyponatraemia)
- (diabetes insipidus) usually given as 2 divided doses, but single dose may be administered if patient tolerates it and diabetes insipidus is controlled adequately
- (platelet dysfunction) skin bleeding time should be monitored before surgery and during therapy. Prolonged bleeding may indicate risk of increased blood loss
- (nocturnal enuresis) serum electrolytes should be monitored if therapy continues for more than 7 days
- (nocturnal enuresis, nasal preparations) therapy should be interrupted if patient has nasal infection and/or rhinorrhoea as therapy may be ineffective or unreliable
- (nocturnal enuresis) therapy should be continued for 4–12 weeks and then stopped for 1 week to establish effectiveness of treatment
- baseline blood tests (VIII:C or VIIIR:Ag assays) should be carried out before and repeated 20 minutes after infusion for haemophilia A or von Willebrand disease
- IV/IM dose is 1/10th of intranasal dose
- 15 microgram/mL solution is recommended for IV use only
- caution should be taken to prevent hyponatraemia from occurring, especially in those at high risk (e.g.

those with cystic fibrosis or cardiac failure, those at risk of intracranial pressure, the elderly or those taking medications that may affect fluid balance or induce syndrome of inappropriate secretion of antidiuretic hormone)

- caution is used in those with other causes of urinary frequency (e.g. multiple sclerosis, urge incontinence) or in those with diabetes mellitus or kidney impairment (creatinine clearance < 50 mL/min)
- not recommended in patients who are dehydrated or overhydrated
- (Minims tablets) contain lactose and are therefore not recommended in those with Lapp lactase deficiency, rare hereditary problems of galactose intolerance or glucose–galactose malabsorption
- contraindicated to treat bleeding in patients with type IIB von Willebrand disease
- contraindicated in those with psychogenic/habitual polydipsia (resulting in urine output > 40 mL/kg/24 hours), hyponatraemia, moderate/severe kidney insufficiency (creatinine clearance < 50 mL/min), syndrome of inappropriate secretion of antidiuretic hormone (SIADH) or cardiac insufficiency or other conditions requiring diuretic therapy

Patient teaching and advice

- advise patient to immediately report any sudden or severe headache, lethargy, malaise, dizziness, confusion, blackouts, fitting, nausea/vomiting or sudden weight gain (signs of water retention)
- (nasal spray) patients with nasal infections or rhinorrhoea (runny nose) should be instructed to stop therapy until condition resolves as intranasal absorption will be ineffective/unreliable
- instruct patient in intranasal pump spray use, including:
    - priming pump by pressing at least 4 times before first use (or until even spray is achieved)
    - priming pump by pressing several times if not used in past 2 days to achieve even spray
    - intranasal pump spray delivers 10 microgram per dose. If smaller dose is needed, rhinyle delivery system should be used. Doses greater than 10 microgram should be administered into each nostril (i.e. 20 microgram dose = 10 microgram per nostril)
- patient using nasal drops for the first time should have adequate instruction in the correct technique (one end of the plastic rhinyle (catheter, supplied) is placed in mouth, the other end in the nostril, and the dose is delivered by blowing into the nasal cavity (blowing prevents inhaling))
- (nocturnal enuresis) advise patient/parent/carer that fluid intake should be limited 1 hour before and at least 8 hours after administration to prevent water retention/hyponatraemia from occurring
- (oral wafers) patient should be advised to place wafer under the tongue and allow it to dissolve

banned in sport

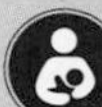

should only be used during pregnancy if benefits outweigh risks

not recommended during breastfeeding

available as dissolvable wafers. Tablets can be dispersed in 10–20 mL water or crushed and mixed with spoonful of yoghurt or apple puree

TERLIPRESSIN (Glypressin Solution, Lucassin, Terlipressin Solution for Injection)

Available forms

Ampoule: 0.85 mg/8.5 mL; Vial: 0.85 mg

Action

- synthetic vasopressin analogue
- prodrug that is converted to active lysine vasopressin
- dose-dependent reduction of portal venous pressure and marked vasoconstriction
- increases mean arterial pressure with reflexic decrease in heart rate
- minimal effects on fibrinolytic system in those with cirrhosis

Use

- treatment of bleeding oesophageal varices
- treatment of hepatorenal syndrome type 1 (reduced renal perfusion and glomerular filtration with preserved tubular function) in patients considered for renal transplant

Dose

- (bleeding oesophageal varices) initially 1.7 mg by slow IV 4-hourly until bleeding is controlled, then adjusting dose to 0.85 mg IV 4-hourly if patient weight < 50 kg or adverse effects occur **OR**
- (treatment of hepatorenal syndrome type 1) 0.85 mg by slow IV injection 6-hourly, increasing dose to 1.7 mg after 3 days if serum creatinine has not decreased from baseline levels by at least 30% for 7–14 days (with albumin 20%)

Adverse effects

- headache, anxiety
- facial pallor
- bradycardia, hypotension, peripheral vasoconstriction, peripheral ischaemia, hypertension, arrhythmias, chest pain
- fluid overload, pulmonary oedema
- fever
- pain in extremities
- abdominal pain, diarrhoea, vomiting, flatulence
- wheezing, bronchospasm, dyspnoea, respiratory failure, pneumonia
- (rare) prolonged QT interval, torsade de pointes, cardiac failure
- (IV site) necrosis

Interactions

- caution if used with agents that can prolong QT interval (e.g. Class IA or III antiarrhythmic agents, erythromycin, some antihistamines and TCAs) or cause hypokalaemia or hypomagnesaemia (e.g. diuretics) as cardiac arrhythmias may be induced
- may increase hypotensive effect of non-selective beta adrenoceptive blocking agents
- caution if used with other agents known to cause bradycardia (e.g. propofol) as heart rate and cardiac output may be lowered

Nursing points/Cautions

- fluid balance and electrolytes (especially serum creatinine) should be monitored daily during therapy
- IV site should be closely monitored to prevent necrosis
- (bleeding oesophageal varices) therapy should not continue for more than 48 hours
- therapy should be continued until hepatorenal syndrome has been resolved for at least 2 days, patient undergoes dialysis or liver transplant, or if serum creatinine remains at or above baseline for 7 days
- dose should not be increased in those with significant ongoing adverse effects (such as pulmonary oedema) or pre-existing cardiovascular disease

- (Lucassin) reconstitute powder using 5 mL of sodium chloride 0.9%
- incompatible with glucose solutions
- administer by slow IV bolus ensuring line is flushed with sodium chloride 0.9% before and after terlipressin
- caution if used in those with kidney insufficiency
- caution if used in those with uncontrolled hypertension, cardiac arrhythmias, coronary artery disease, previous myocardial infarction or cerebral/peripheral vascular disease
- caution if used in those with a history of QT interval prolongation or electrolyte abnormalities (hypokalaemia, hypomagnesaemia)
- caution if used in those who are morbidly obese or have peripheral venous hypertension as they are at increased risk of infusion site necrosis
- caution if used in those with severe asthma or chronic obstructive pulmonary disease (COPD) as smooth muscle constriction may occur
- not recommended in those with unstable angina or recent acute myocardial infarction

banned in sport

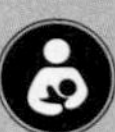
contraindicated during pregnancy

not recommended during breastfeeding

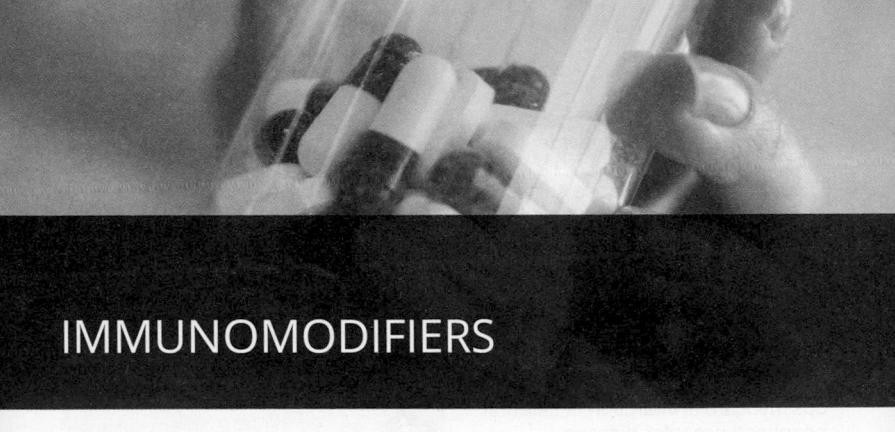

IMMUNOMODIFIERS

As the name suggests, immunomodifiers are drugs that modify the immune system in some way. They are used in a range of conditions, the prime ones being the prevention and treatment of organ rejection after transplantation, and the treatment of autoimmune diseases, such as rheumatoid arthritis, psoriasis and multiple sclerosis.

The success of allograft transplantation can, in part, be directly attributed to the use of immunomodifiers such as ciclosporin and, more recently, the interferons and monoclonal antibodies, which have decreased the risk of graft rejection.

Unfortunately, suppression of the immune system carries with it the increased risk of bacterial, viral and fungal infection, and may also increase the risk of developing neoplasms.

General Adverse effects of immunomodifiers

- increased risk of developing malignancies (especially skin)
- increased risk of infections (viral, bacterial and/or fungal)
- reactivation of chronic infection (e.g. tuberculosis (TB), hepatitis)
- hypersensitivity reaction (e.g. headache, dizziness, malaise, fever, rigors, myalgia, arthralgia, nausea, vomiting, diarrhoea)

General Interactions of immunomodifiers

- use of live attenuated vaccines should be avoided and only be given 6 months after stopping immunosuppressive therapy. Close contacts should not be vaccinated with live poliomyelitis vaccine. If patient is exposed to chicken pox or measles, immunoglobulin should be given immediately
- lower doses are usually required if given with corticosteroids or other immunomodifiers
- decreases efficacy of other vaccinations (especially if given with corticosteroids)

General Nursing points/Cautions for immunomodifiers

- all patients should be carefully screened for history or symptoms of TB or hepatitis, including detailed medical history, possible previous exposure to TB

- chest X-ray and tuberculin skin test (Mantoux) may also be performed (however, there is a risk of false negative skin test occurring in patients who are severely ill or immunocompromised)
- any patient with latent TB should be treated with antimycobacterials before starting therapy with immunomodifier(s)
- patient's immunity to varicella zoster virus (chicken pox, herpes zoster (shingles)) should be assessed (including serological testing) before starting therapy because the response to the virus may be severe if exposed and unprotected
- any other active infections should be treated before starting therapy with immunomodifier
- caution if used in those with history of hepatitis B infection or positive for hepatitis B surface antigen for > 6 months due to risk of reactivation

General Patient teaching and advice for immunomodifiers

- instruct patient to seek medical advice if any of the following occur:
  - recurrent or persistent infection
  - persistent fever, pallor, unexplained bleeding or bruising, shortness of breath on exertion (blood dyscrasia)
  - persistent cough, weight loss and low-grade fever (possible TB)
  - contact with anyone suffering from chicken pox or shingles
- warn patient to limit exposure to direct sunlight and UV light, wear protective clothing (including hat and sunglasses) and use sunscreen with high protective factor (SPF 30+) to decrease risk of skin cancers
- advise patient to immediately report any new or changes to existing moles, cysts, polyps or unusual lumps
- see also General Patient teaching and advice (p. xxvii)

ANTITHYMOCYTE GLOBULIN (EQUINE) (Atgam)

ANTITHYMOCYTE GLOBULIN (RABBIT) (Thymoglobuline)

Available forms

Ampoules: 250 mg/5 mL; Vial: 25 mg

Action

- purified, concentrated gamma globulin (IgG) derived from horse or rabbit plasma
- lymphocyte selective immunosuppressant that reduces circulating thymus-dependent T-lymphocytes, as well as in the spleen and lymph nodes

Use

- renal transplant (to delay onset of allograft rejection)
- treatment of steroid-resistant moderate-to-severe renal transplant rejection
- treatment of refractory or relapsing aplastic anaemia

Dose

- (delaying rejection of renal transplant) 15 mg/kg daily by IV infusion for 14 days, then every second day for 14 days, starting within 24 hours of transplant (total 21 doses) (Atgam) **OR**
- (treatment of rejection of renal transplant) 10–15 mg/kg daily by IV infusion for 14 days, starting when rejection has been diagnosed. Additional doses on alternate days can be given (total 21 doses) (Atgam) **OR**
- (prevention of renal transplant graft rejection) 1–1.5 mg/kg IV daily for

3–9 days after transplantation (cumulative dose 3–13.5 mg/kg) **OR**
- (treatment of steroid-resistant moderate-to-severe renal transplant graft rejection) 1.5 mg/kg IV daily for 7–14 days post-transplant (cumulative dose 10.5–21 mg/kg) **OR**
- (refractory or relapsing aplastic anaemia) 2.5–3.75 mg/kg IV daily for 5 consecutive days (cumulative dose 12.5–18.75 mg/kg)

Adverse effects
- fever, chills, shivering, night sweats
- leucopenia, thrombocytopenia
- rash, pruritus, urticaria, weal, flare
- arthralgia, chest/back/flank pain
- peripheral oedema
- hyperkalaemia
- nausea, vomiting, diarrhoea, stomatitis, dysphagia
- dyspnoea
- headache, malaise, dizziness, asthenia
- hypotension, hypertension, tachycardia
- abnormal renal function tests
- pain at infusion site, clotted arteriovenous fistula, peripheral thrombophlebitis
- (uncommon) anaphylactoid reaction, anaphylaxis, serum sickness, antibody development
- (rare) cytokine-release syndrome, lymphoma, lymphoproliferative disorders
- see also General Adverse effects of immunomodifiers (p. 1176)

Interactions
- see General Interactions of immunomodifiers (p. 1176)

Nursing points/Cautions
- usually given with azathioprine and corticosteroids
- white blood cell and platelet counts should be monitored during and after therapy
- premedication with corticosteroids, antipyretic and/or antihistamine 1 hour before infusion is recommended to decrease likelihood and/or severity of infusion-related reaction
- name and batch number of product should be recorded in patient's medical history
- (Atgam) skin testing is recommended using undiluted solution pricked into skin initially. If there is no reaction (weal) after 10 minutes, 0.02 mL of diluted solution (1 : 1000 with sodium chloride 0.9%) given intradermally and area read after 10 minutes. A sodium chloride control should also be injected. A positive reaction is a weal 3 mm or larger (compared to sodium chloride control) and this indicates an increased risk of allergic reaction. However, allergic reactions can occur with negative skin test, and it does not predict delayed serum sickness reaction
- patient should be observed throughout infusion
- adrenaline (epinephrine), antihistamines, corticosteroids and resuscitation equipment must be readily available in the event of an allergic reaction
- administer alone
- (Atgam) should be diluted before use. Suitable IV solution container should be inverted and antithymocyte globulin solution injected directly into solution (not allowing it to make contact with air) and container gently inverted to mix solution. Solution (diluted or undiluted) should not be shaken as it will become denatured
- (Atgam) suitable IV solutions include sodium chloride 0.9%, glucose 5% with sodium chloride 0.45% and glucose 5% with sodium chloride 0.225%

- (Atgam) not recommended for dilution using glucose-only solutions (as precipitation may occur) or highly acidic solution (become unstable)
- (Thymoglobuline) if patient is obese, dose should be calculated on ideal weight, not actual weight
- (Thymoglobuline) vial should be allowed to come to room temperature for 30 minutes before reconstituting
- (Thymoglobuline) reconstitute powder with 5 mL water for injections, injecting diluent gently down side of vial and gently tilting or rolling to dissolve powder. Vial should not be inverted, shaken or swirled as the protein will be denatured
- (Thymoglobuline) dilute reconstituted solution with 50–500 mL (50 mL/vial) of either sodium chloride 0.9% or glucose 5% and gently invert infusion bag to ensure even distribution
- (Thymoglobuline) precipitation will occur if added to glucose 5% containing heparin and hydrocortisone
- may be administered via high-flow central vein, existing vascular shunt or arterial-venous fistula using inline filter (0.2–1 micron)
- (Thymoglobuline) first dose should be administered over 6 hours, and subsequent doses over 4 hours
- (Atgam) infusion should be over at least 4 hours
- (Atgam) solution may be clear, colourless to light brown in colour and may develop flaky deposit when stored
- repeat courses should be given with great caution due to increased risk of hypersensitivity reaction
- contraindicated in those with hypersensitivity to equine gamma globulin (immunoglobulin) (Atgam) or rabbit protein hypersensitivity (Thymoglobuline) or if person has acute or chronic infection

Patient teaching and advice

- patient should be advised that the possibility of transmitting infectious diseases (e.g. HIV, viral hepatitis), while remote, does exist
- warn patient not to drive or operate machinery if dizziness, malaise or hypotension occur
- see also General Patient teaching and advice for immunomodifiers (p. 1177)

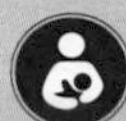

only used during pregnancy if benefits outweigh risks

APREMILAST (Otezla)

Available forms

Tablets: 10 mg, 20 mg, 30 mg

Action

- phosphodiesterase 4 inhibitor (phosphodiesterase 4 is thought to be involved in the inflammatory process), resulting in a decrease in pro-inflammatory cytokines (e.g. interleukin-23) and increase in anti-inflammatory cytokines (e.g. interleukin-10)
- elimination half-life 9 hours

Use

- active psoriatic arthritis
- moderate-to-severe plaque psoriasis in those who are candidates for phototherapy or systemic therapy

Dose

- initially 10 mg orally daily (day 1), then 10 mg twice daily (day 2), 10 mg (morning) and 20 mg (night) (day 3), 20 mg orally twice daily (day 4), 20 mg (morning) and 30 mg (night) (day 5), then 30 mg twice daily

Adverse effects

- decreased appetite, diarrhoea, nausea, vomiting, weight loss, frequent bowel motions, abdominal pain,

gastroesophageal reflux disease (GORD), dyspepsia, gastroenteritis
- headache, migraine, tension headache, fatigue, insomnia
- depression, lowered mood
- upper respiratory tract infection, bronchitis, nasopharyngitis, sinusitis
- cough
- back pain, arthralgia
- hypertension
- urinary tract infection
- hypersensitivity

Interactions
- serum levels decreased by phenytoin, rifampicin, carbamazepine, phenobarbital (phenobarbitone) and St John's wort

Nursing points/Cautions
- renal function should be assessed before starting therapy
- weight should be monitored during therapy and if there is clinically significant weight loss, interruption to therapy should be considered
- caution if used in those with history of depression and/or suicidal ideation
- caution if used in those with severe kidney impairment; dose should be reduced to 30 mg daily
- caution if used in those aged > 65 years or those at risk of volume depletion or hypotension as they should be closely monitored for diarrhoea, nausea and vomiting
- tablets contain lactose and are therefore not recommended in those with rare hereditary problems of galactose intolerance, Lapp lactase deficiency or glucose–galactose malabsorption

Patient teaching and advice
- advise patient to swallow tablets whole, not chewed, broken or divided
- warn patient (and carer/family member) to immediately seek medical advice if there is any change in mood, sadness or thoughts of self-harm

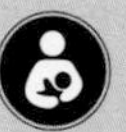
contraindicated during pregnancy and breastfeeding

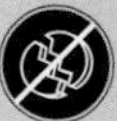
tablets should not be crushed or broken

AZATHIOPRINE (Azapin, Imazan, Imuran, Thioprine)

Available forms
Tablets: 25 mg, 50 mg; Vial: 50 mg

Action
- imidazole, with immune response suppression
- derivative of mercaptopurine (see Antineoplastic agents, p. 663)
- therapeutic effects may only become apparent after weeks to months of therapy when used for other conditions
- half-life about 5 hours

Use
- organ transplantation (with corticosteroids and/or other immunosuppressive agents)
- chronic autoimmune diseases (e.g. severe rheumatoid arthritis, SLE) (with or without corticosteroids and/or other immunosuppressive agents)

Dose
- (transplantation) initially 5 mg/kg IV or orally 1 hour before or 3 hours after food daily, then reducing to 1–4 mg/kg IV or orally daily as maintenance **OR**
- (other conditions) initially 1 mg/kg IV or orally 1 hour before or 3 hours after food daily, then increasing by 0.5 mg/kg/day over several weeks (maximum daily dose 2.5 mg/kg), then dose reduced as appropriate

Adverse effects

- skin rash
- anaemia, leucopenia, thrombocytopenia
- nausea, vomiting, sores on mouth and lips, diarrhoea, GI discomfort, altered taste or smell
- pancreatitis
- (renal transplantation with corticosteroids) reversible alopecia
- (uncommon) decreased liver function, hepatotoxicity, formication (sensation of ants on skin), meningitis
- (rare) reversible pneumonitis, progressive multifocal leucoencephalopathy (PML) (if given with other immunosuppressants), exacerbation of myasthenia gravis, macrophage activation syndrome
- see also General Adverse effects of immunomodifiers (p. 1176)

Interactions

- dose reduction (to one-quarter) may be required if given with allopurinol or related substances
- may increase neuromuscular blockade of suxamethonium
- may decrease neuromuscular blockade of non-depolarising neuromuscular blocking agents such as pancuronium or vecuronium
- may inhibit anticoagulant activity of warfarin, requiring increase in dosage, therefore INR should be closely monitored, especially when starting or stopping therapy or with any dose adjustment
- caution if given with ACE inhibitors and captopril due to increased susceptibility to leucopenia
- myelosuppressive effects may be enhanced if given with cimetidine, indometacin, penicillamine or other bone marrow depressing agents and therefore not recommended together
- caution if given with olsalazine, mesalazine or sulfasalazine
- metabolism may be impaired by furosemide (frusemide) or febuxostat
- clearance may be altered by phenytoin, phenobarbital (phenobarbitone), rifampicin or erythromycin
- not recommended with ribavirin
- dose adjustment may be required if given with high-dose methotrexate
- caution if given with infliximab
- see also General Interactions of immunomodifiers (p. 1176)

Nursing points/Cautions

- see also General Nursing points/Cautions for immunomodifiers (p. 1176)
- testing for thiopurine methyltransferase deficiency is recommended before starting therapy
- IV should only be used when oral route is impractical or unavailable. Oral therapy should replace IV as soon as possible
- any dental work should be completed before start of therapy or postponed until therapy is completed and/or blood counts have returned to normal
- blood counts (including platelet count) should be monitored weekly for first 8 weeks (or more frequently if dose is high or renal/liver disorder is present), then monthly
- should be handled as per cytotoxic protocol
- reconstitute powder using 5–15 mL water for injections and then dilute with 20–200 mL sodium chloride 0.9%, sodium chloride 0.45% or sodium chloride (0.18%) and glucose (4%) solution
- reconstituted solution may be given over at least 1 minute, followed by at least 50 mL of suitable dilution fluid (see previous point) if patient is unable to tolerate large volumes of fluid
- administer alone
- avoid extravasation

- withdrawal should be gradual and under supervision
- caution if used in those with myasthenia gravis as condition may become exacerbated
- caution if used in those with thiopurine methyltransferase deficiency as they are sensitive to myelosuppressive effects
- not recommended in those with hypersplenism or Lesch-Nyhan syndrome (hypoxanthine-guanine-phosphoribosyl transferase deficiency) or with liver dysfunction (regular blood counts and liver function tests are recommended)
- contraindicated in those with known hypersensitivity to mercaptopurine or with rheumatoid arthritis treated previously with alkylating agents (e.g. cyclophosphamide, melphalan) (due to increased risk of neoplasm development)

Patient teaching and advice

- patient should be advised to report immediately any infection, unexpected bruising or bleeding, black tarry stools or blood in urine or stools
- (renal transplantation with corticosteroids) warn patient that alopecia (hair loss) occurs commonly but in most cases is reversible even with continuation of therapy
- advise patient that tablets should be swallowed whole, not crushed or chewed
- counsel patient to use adequate contraception during therapy to avoid pregnancy occurring
- see General Patient teaching and advice for immunomodifiers (p. 1177)

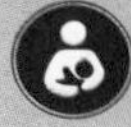

contraindicated during pregnancy or breastfeeding. Pregnancy should be excluded before starting therapy and adequate contraception used if either partner is receiving therapy

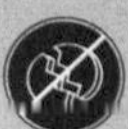

tablets are cytotoxic and should not be crushed or broken

BARICITINIB (Olumiant)

Available forms
Tablets: 2 mg, 4 mg

Action
- selective and reversible inhibitor of Janus kinases (JAK1 and JAK2) (Janus kinases are enzymes that relay signals from cell surface receptors to a number of cytokines and growth factors involved in haematopoiesis, inflammation and immune function)

Use
- treatment of moderate-to-severe rheumatoid arthritis in those who are intolerant to or have had an inadequate response to one or more DMARDs (as monotherapy or with cDMARDs)

Dose
- 2–4 mg orally daily

Adverse effects
- thrombocytosis
- nausea, vomiting, upper abdominal pain, increased weight
- fatigue, headache, depression
- oropharyngeal pain
- upper respiratory tract infection, urinary tract infection, pharyngitis, vulvovaginal candidiasis, influenza
- elevated creatine phosphokinase (CPK), hypercholesterolaemia
- deep venous thrombosis, pulmonary embolism
- see also General Adverse effects for immunomodifiers (p. 1176)

Interactions
- not recommended with other JAK inhibitors or biological DMARDs
- see also General Interactions for immunomodifiers (p. 1176)

Nursing points/Cautions

- see General Nursing points/Cautions for immunomodifiers (p. 1176)
- before starting therapy, lipids, absolute neutrophil count (ANC), absolute lymphocyte count (ALC) haemoglobin and liver function should be measured, and then regularly during treatment. Treatment should be interrupted if ANC, ALC, haemoglobin or liver transaminases become abnormal. Any hyperlipidaemia should be treated if it develops
- caution if used in those with risk factors for deep vein thrombosis or pulmonary embolism (e.g. older age, obesity, history of either, undergoing surgery, immobilisation)
- caution if used in those with moderate renal impairment; 2 mg dose is recommended
- caution if used in the elderly and those with diabetes due to the increased risk of infection
- not recommended in patient with severe and end-stage renal impairment

Patient teaching and advice

- advise patient to seek medical advice immediately if any of the following occur:
  - any shortness of breath or sudden chest pain, cough, light-headedness, dizziness, rapid heart rate
  - sudden painful or tender leg swelling, increased limb warmth, skin discolouration
- female patients of childbearing potential should be counselled to avoid pregnancy by using effective contraception during and for at least 1 week after stopping therapy

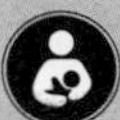

not recommended during pregnancy unless benefits outweigh risks

not recommended during breastfeeding

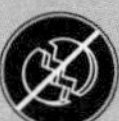

tablets should not be crushed or broken

BASILIXIMAB (Simulect)

Available form

Vial: 20 mg

Action

- recombinant IgG1-kappa that binds to the CD25 antigen on activated T-lymphocyte surface preventing interleukin 2 binding and production of T cells
- does not cause cytokine release or myelosuppression
- half-life 4–10.4 days

Use

- prophylaxis of acute organ rejection (renal transplantation)

Dose

- 20 mg as IV bolus or infusion over 20–30 minutes 2 hours before transplantation, then 20 mg IV 4 days after transplantation

Adverse effects

- pain
- fever
- headache, insomnia
- peripheral oedema, general oedema
- nausea, vomiting, diarrhoea, constipation, abdominal pain
- anaemia
- hyperkalaemia
- hypertension
- antibody development
- see also General Adverse effects of immunomodifiers (p. 1176)

Interactions

- see General Interactions of immunomodifiers (p. 1176)

Nursing points/Cautions

- first dose should only be given when it is certain that transplantation will

occur (with immunosuppressive therapy)
- second dose should not be given if there is severe hypersensitivity or if patient experiences postoperative complication(s)
- reconstitute using 5.0 mL water for injections and then dilute with at least 50 mL sodium chloride 0.9% or glucose 5% for IV infusion
- not recommended for other organ transplantation except kidney
- contraindicated in those with hypersensitivity to murine antibody preparations
- see also General Nursing points/Cautions for immunomodifiers (p. 1176)

Patient teaching and advice

- ensure female patients receive adequate counselling regarding the importance of using adequate contraception during and for 16 weeks after stopping therapy to avoid pregnancy occurring. She should also be advised to seek immediate medical advice if she thinks she may be pregnant
- see also General Patient teaching and advice for immunomodifiers (p. 1177)

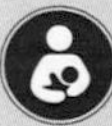

women should be advised to use adequate contraception during and for 16 weeks after stopping therapy to prevent pregnancy occurring

not recommended during breastfeeding; women should also not breastfeed for 16 weeks after stopping therapy

BELIMUMAB (Benlysta)

Available forms

Vial: 120 mg, 400 mg

Action

- human B lymphocyte stimulator neutralising antibody
- B lymphocyte stimulator is a member of the tumour necrosis factor (TNF) family that inhibits B cell apoptosis and stimulates differentiation of B cells into immunoglobulin producing plasma cells and is overexpressed in those with systemic lupus erythematosus (SLE)
- belimumab is a human IgG1γ monoclonal antibody that inhibits survival of B cells reducing differentiation

Use

- add-on therapy in those with active autoantibody positive SLE with a high degree of disease activity (ANA titre ≥ 1:80 or anti-dsDNA titre ≥ 30 IU/mL) despite standard treatment

Dose

- 10 mg/kg by IV infusion over 60 minutes on days 0, 14 and 28, then monthly

Adverse effects

- infusion-related reaction (fatigue, fever, dizziness, headache, shortness of breath, hypertension)
- fever
- headache, migraine, fatigue, insomnia
- nausea, diarrhoea
- arthralgia
- nasopharyngitis, bronchitis, pharyngitis
- leucopenia
- depression and less commonly, suicidal ideation and behaviour
- hypersensitivity, anaphylaxis, angioedema
- (rare) progressive multifocal leucoencephalopathy (PML)
- see also General Adverse effects of immunomodifiers (p. 1176)

Interactions

- see General Interactions of immunomodifiers (p. 1176)

Nursing points/Cautions

- premedication with oral antihistamines with or without antipyretic may be given

- patient should be closely monitored during and after administration for any signs of hypersensitivity
- risk of hypersensitivity is highest during first 2 days of therapy, decreasing with duration. However, delayed sensitivity has occurred
- if patient presents with signs of neurological deterioration, referral to neurologist is recommended as it may be a sign of PML
- therapy should be re-evaluated if there has been no improvement in 6 months
- allow to come to room temperature for 10–15 minutes before administration
- reconstitute 120 mg vial with 1.5 mL of water for injections and 400 mg vial with 4.8 mL to give a concentration of 80 mg/mL
- water for injections should be added to side of vial to avoid frothing. Gently swirl (not shake) for 60 seconds every 5 minutes to dissolve powder. This usually takes 10–15 minutes, but may take up to 30 minutes
- reconstituted solution should be further diluted to 250 mL with sodium chloride 0.9% (withdraw and discard volume equal to the amount to be added). Gently invert infusion bag to ensure solution is adequately mixed
- not compatible with glucose 5%
- not given as IV push or bolus
- administer alone
- caution if used in patient with chronic infection and therapy should not be started if patient is currently receiving therapy for chronic infection
- caution if used in those with a history of malignancy or depression
- caution if used in those with a history of multiple drug allergies or significant hypersensitivity as there is an increased risk of hypersensitivity or infusion-related reaction
- see also General Nursing points/Cautions for immunomodifiers (p. 1176)

Patient teaching and advice

- advise patient to seek medical advice immediately if any of the following occur:
  - rash, nausea, fatigue, muscle pain, headache, facial swelling (which may occur up to 5 days after administration)
  - changes in mood, sadness or signs/talk of self-harm
- women of childbearing potential should be counselled to use adequate contraception during and for at least 4 months after stopping therapy
- see General Patient teaching and advice for immunomodifiers (p. 1177)

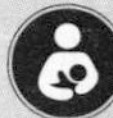

not recommended during pregnancy or breastfeeding

BEZLOTOXUMAB (Zinplava)

Available form

Vial: 1 g/40 mL

Action

- *Clostridium difficile* colonises and infects large intestine expressing two exotoxins, toxin A and toxin B. These toxins target host colonic epithelial cells leading to tissue injury which disrupts normal gut barrier function, as well as causing the release of pro-inflammatory mediators which recruit neutrophils and other immune cells to infection site, contributing to tissue damage persisting
- monoclonal antibody (IgG1) that binds to *C. difficile* toxin B with high affinity, neutralising its activity and preventing it from binding to host cells
- does not bind to *C. difficile* toxin A

Use

- prevention of recurrence of *C. difficile* infection in those at high risk of recurrence and who are receiving treatment

Dose
- 10 mg/kg at single IV infusion over 60 minutes

Adverse effects
- nausea, diarrhoea
- fever
- headache
- heart failure
- (infusion-related reaction) fatigue, fever, dizziness, headache, shortness of breath, hypertension

Nursing points/Cautions
- should be administered as part of course of antibacterial treatment for *C. difficile* infection
- vial should not be shaken
- required amount (according to body weight) should be withdrawn from vial and transferred to IV bag containing either sodium chloride 0.9% or glucose 5% to give concentration of 1–10 mg/mL
- bag should be gently inverted to mix contents
- should be administered alone using low-protein binding 0.2–0.5 micron inline or add-on filter
- should not be given as IV push or bolus
- not indicated for treatment of *C. difficile* infection
- not recommended in those with history of congestive heart failure unless benefits outweigh risks

Patient teaching and advice
- advise patient to seek medical advice immediately if any of the following occur:
  - shortness of breath, swollen legs, tiredness, rapid heart beat (signs of heart failure)

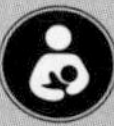
not recommended during pregnancy or breastfeeding

DUPILUMAB (Dupixent)

Available forms
Prefilled syringe: 200 mg, 300 mg

Action
- recombinant IgG4 monoclonal antibody that inhibits interleukin-4 and interleukin-13 (that are known to be cytokines involved in atopic disease)

Use
- treatment of moderate-to-severe atopic dermatitis in those who are candidates for chronic systemic therapy
- as add-on maintenance therapy in those with moderate-to-severe asthma with type 2 inflammation (elevated eosinophils of FeNO (fractional exhaled nitrous oxide))

Dose
- (atopic dermatitis) initially 600 mg SC, followed by 300 mg every second week **OR**
- (asthma) initially 400 mg SC, followed by 200 mg every second week **OR**
- (oral corticosteroid-dependent asthma or with co-morbid moderate-to-severe atopic dermatitis) initially 600 mg SC, followed by 300 mg every second week

Adverse effects
- conjunctivitis (allergic, bacterial), keratitis, eye pruritus, blepharitis, dry eye
- herpes simplex
- oropharyngeal pain
- (asthma) eosinophilic conditions (e.g. eosinophilic pneumonia, vasculitis)
- injection site reactions (redness, oedema, pruritus)
- (rare) hypersensitivity

Interactions
- see General Interactions for immunomodifiers (p. 1176)

Nursing points/Cautions
- any helminth infestation should be treated before starting therapy

- 600 mg or 400 mg doses should be given as two injections consecutively into different injection sites
- trade name and batch number should be recorded in patient's medical history or dispensing record
- patient can be taught to self-administer. First dose should be given under medical supervision
- (atopic dermatitis) not recommended for episodic use
- see also General Nursing points/ Cautions for immunomodifiers (p. 1176)

Patient teaching and advice

- (asthma) ensure patient understands that dupilumab is not for management of acute asthma, acute asthma exacerbations, acute bronchospasm or status asthmaticus
- (asthma) warn patient not to stop corticosteroid therapy when starting therapy with dupilumab
- see Patient teaching and advice for icatibant (p. 1195) for self-administration instructions
- advise patient that if dose is forgotten it can be administered within 7 days from missed dose and then resume previous dosing schedule. If missed dose is not given within 7 days, advise patient to wait until next dose is due
- patient should be instructed to seek medical advice if any of the following occur:
    - new or worsening eye symptoms
    - (asthma) rash, worsening lung symptoms, flu-like symptoms, pins and needles or numbness to arms or legs

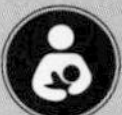

should only be used during pregnancy or breastfeeding if benefits are thought to outweigh risks

ECULIZUMAB (Soliris)

Available form

Vial: 300 mg/30 mL

Action

- genetic mutation in those with paroxysmal nocturnal haemoglobinuria leads to abnormal blood cells that are deficient in terminal complement inhibitors, causing these blood cells to be sensitive to terminal complement-mediated destruction with ensuing anaemia, fatigue, difficulty in function, pain, dark urine, kidney disease, shortness of breath and blood clots
- in atypical haemolytic uraemic syndrome, complement activity regulation impairment leads to uncontrolled terminal complement activation, resulting in platelet activation, endothelial cell damage and thrombotic microangiopathy
- monoclonal antibody hybrid (IgG2-IgG4 $_{kappa}$) specifically binds to complement protein C5 inhibiting its cleavage to C5a and C5b, preventing generation of terminal complement complex C5b-p
- half-life about 12.4 days

Use

- treatment of atypical haemolytic uraemic syndrome (aHUS)
- haemolysis reduction in paroxysmal nocturnal haemoglobinuria (PNH)
- neuromyelitis optica spectrum disorder (NMOSD) (in those who are anti-aquaporin-4 antibody positive) (as adjunct therapy)

Dose

- (PNH) initially 600 mg IV over 25–45 minutes weekly for 4 weeks, followed by 900 mg IV (week 5), then 900 mg IV every 12–16 days (depending on monitoring results) **OR**
- (aHUS, NMOSD) initially 900 mg IV over 25–45 minutes weekly for 4 weeks, followed by 1200 mg

(week 5), then 1200 mg IV every 12–16 days (depending on monitoring results)

Adverse effects

- headache, fatigue, dizziness, insomnia, paraesthesia, asthenia and less commonly, depression, mood swings
- fever
- hypertension
- cough, oropharyngeal pain
- nasopharyngitis, sinusitis, bronchitis, pneumonia, pharyngitis, upper respiratory tract infection
- back pain, myalgia, arthralgia, muscle spasm, pain in extremities
- nausea, diarrhoea, vomiting, abdominal pain, dyspepsia, altered taste, decreased appetite
- alopecia, rash, pruritus, dry skin
- conjunctivitis
- dysuria, cystitis, urinary tract infection
- herpes simplex infection, flu-like illness
- anaemia, leucopenia, thrombocytopenia
- meningococcal infection
- infusion reaction
- antibody development
- anaphylaxis

Nursing points/Cautions

- all patients must be vaccinated against meningococcal disease at least 2 weeks before starting therapy. If the patient is less than 2 years of age or if vaccination has occurred less than 2 weeks before starting therapy, prophylactic antibiotics are required until 2 weeks after vaccination
- if patient is under 18 years, they must also be vaccinated against *Haemophilus influenzae* and pneumococcal infections
- all patients should be monitored for at least 1 hour post-infusion
- (PNH) patient should be monitored for signs and symptoms of intravascular haemolysis, including serum lactate dehydrogenase (LDH) levels, which may result in dose adjustment during maintenance
- (aHUS) patient should be monitored for thrombotic microangiopathy by measuring platelet count, serum LDH levels and serum creatinine, which may result in dose adjustment during maintenance
- (NMOSD) given as an adjunct to existing immunotherapy
- should not be given by IV bolus or push
- administer alone
- requires further dilution to achieve concentration of 5 mg/mL; 600 mg dose should be added to 120 mL of suitable dilution fluid or 180 mL for 900 mg dose
- infusion bag should be gently inverted to mix solution
- may be infused using gravity feed, syringe pump or infusion pump over 25–45 minutes
- (PNH) patient should be monitored for at least 8 weeks after stopping therapy to detect any haemolysis or other reactions. If serious haemolysis occurs, treatment may include blood transfusion, exchange transfusion, anticoagulation, corticosteroids or restarting therapy
- (aHUS) patient should be monitored for at least 12 weeks after stopping therapy to detect any severe thrombotic microangiopathy complications. If these complications occur, treatment may include restarting therapy, anticoagulation, respiratory support with mechanical ventilation or renal support with dialysis
- contains 5 mmol sodium/30 mL, which may need to be taken into consideration if patient is on a sodium-restricted diet

- caution if used in those with active systemic infections
- contraindicated in those with hypersensitivity to murine proteins or with unresolved *Neisseria meningitidis* infection, if not currently vaccinated against *N. meningitides* or those who have not received prophylactic treatment with appropriate antibiotics until 2 weeks after vaccination

Patient teaching and advice

- (PNH, aHUS) patient should be instructed to seek medical advice immediately if any of the following occur (as they may be signs of meningococcal disease):
  - fever > 39°C
  - headache with nausea or vomiting
  - headache with fever and/or stiff neck/back
  - rash
  - confusion
  - severe muscle aches with flu-like symptoms
  - sensitivity to light
- (PNH, aHUS) patient must be given a 'Patient Safety Card' and instructed to carry the card at all times, which is to be given to any health professional if any treatment is required
- (PNH) patient should be advised to seek medical advice if any of the following occur:
  - tiredness, headaches, shortness of breath when exercising, dizziness, looking pale
  - confusion or change in alertness
  - chest pain or angina
  - dark urine
  - blood clots
- (aHUS) patient should be advised to seek medical advice if any of the following occur:
  - bruising or bleeding more than normal
  - tiredness, headaches, shortness of breath on exercising, dizziness, looking pale
  - confusion or change in alertness
  - fitting (seizures)
  - chest pain or angina
  - kidney problems
  - shortness of breath
  - blood clots
- (PNH, aHUS) warn patient not to drive or operate machinery if they experience dizziness or vertigo
- (PNH, aHUS) female patient of child-bearing capacity should be counselled to use adequate contraception during and for up to 5 months after stopping therapy to avoid pregnancy occurring
- see also General Patient teaching and advice for immunomodifiers (p. 1177)

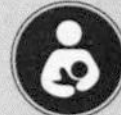

should only be used during pregnancy or breastfeeding if benefits outweigh risks

EVEROLIMUS (Afinitor, Certican, Everocan)

Available forms

Tablets: 0.25 mg, 0.5 mg, 0.75 mg, 1 mg, 5 mg, 10 mg; Dispersible tablets: 2 mg, 3 mg, 5 mg

Action

- protein kinasemTOR inhibitor
- inhibits proliferation of activated T cells by binding to T cell growth factor receptor sites, thereby blocking G_1 stage of cell cycle
- narrow therapeutic index

Use

- prevention of organ rejection in those at risk after receiving allogeneic renal or heart transplant (with ciclosporin and corticosteroids) or liver transplant (with tacrolimus with corticosteroids) (Certican)
- treatment of advanced HER2-negative hormone receptor-positive breast cancer in post-menopausal women (after letrozole or anastrozole failure), advanced renal cancer (after

sorafenib or sunitinib failure), well or moderately differentiated progressive unresectable or metastatic neuroendocrine tumours (of pancreatic origin), tuberous sclerosis complex (TSC) associated with subependymal giant cell astrocytoma (SEGA) (requiring therapeutic intervention but not suitable for curative surgery), TSC with renal angiomyolipoma (not requiring immediate surgery, TSC with refractory seizures (as adjunct) (Afinitor))

Dose

- (renal or heart transplant) initially 0.75 mg orally twice daily starting as soon as possible after transplantation (Certican) **OR**
- (liver transplant) 1 mg orally twice daily starting 4 weeks post-transplant (Certican) **OR**
- (breast cancer, renal cancer, neuroendocrine tumours, TSC with renal angiomyolipoma) 10 mg orally daily (Afinitor) **OR**
- (TSC with SEGA) 4.5 mg/m^2 orally daily (rounded to nearest strength of tablet) (Afinitor) **OR**
- (TSC with refractory seizures, aged $\geq$ 6 years) 5 mg/m^2 orally daily (rounded to nearest strength of tablet) (Afinitor Dispersible)

Adverse effects

- leucopenia, neutropenia, thrombocytopenia, anaemia, pancytopenia, thrombotic microangiopathies
- epistaxis
- hypertension
- decreased appetite, nausea, vomiting, abdominal pain, diarrhoea, stomatitis, constipation, oropharyngeal pain, mouth ulcers, oral mucositis, decreased weight, altered taste, dry mouth, dyspepsia, dysphagia, gastritis, flatulence
- hypokalaemia
- dehydration
- fever
- headache, insomnia, anxiety, fatigue, asthenia, irritability, aggression
- abnormal liver enzymes
- peripheral oedema, lymphoedema
- pain, myalgia, arthralgia
- hypercholesterolaemia, hyperlipidaemia, hypertriglyceridaemia
- cough, dyspnoea, pleural effusion, pneumonitis
- nasopharyngitis
- hypophosphataemia
- acne, rash, pruritus, dry skin, nail disorder
- impaired wound healing, lymphocele
- proteinuria, renal failure
- decreased testosterone, erectile dysfunction
- menstruation irregularities, amenorrhoea, menorrhagia, ovarian cyst, vaginal bleeding
- hyperglycaemia, new onset diabetes mellitus
- angioedema
- renal graft thrombosis
- (rare) interstitial lung disease/non-infectious pneumonitis
- see also General Adverse effects of immunomodifiers (p. 1176)

Interactions

- not recommended with itraconazole, voriconazole, clarithromycin, ritonavir, rifampicin or rifabutin
- may increase renal toxicity of ciclosporin
- serum levels may be increased by ciclosporin, fluconazole, itraconazole, posaconazole, erythromycin, clarithromycin, verapamil, diltiazem, indinavir, amprenavir, metoclopramide, bromocriptine, cimetidine, danazol, fosamprenavir, aprepitant
- not recommended with grapefruit, grapefruit juice, star fruit or Seville oranges
- serum levels may be decreased by St John's wort, carbamazepine, phenobarbital (phenobarbitone), rifampicin, phenytoin, rifabutin,

dexamethasone, prednisolone, prednisone, efavirenz and nevirapine
- caution if used with other agents which affect renal function
- increased risk of angioedema if given with ACE inhibitors
- may increase bioavailability of midazolam
- increased risk of thrombotic microangiopathy, thrombotic thrombocytopenic purpura and/or haemolytic uraemic syndrome if given with calcineurin inhibitors (e.g. ciclosporin, tacrolimus)
- increased risk of acute rejection if not given with either ciclosporin or tacrolimus
- increased risk of serious infection if everolimus/corticosteroid/ciclosporin combination is given with antithymocyte globulin (rabbit) in heart transplant patients
- see also General Interactions of immunomodifiers (p. 1176)

Nursing points/Cautions

- renal function (including urine protein, serum creatinine, blood urea nitrogen (BUN)), serum lipids, full blood count and blood glucose levels should be monitored regularly during therapy
- therapeutic serum levels should be monitored regularly during therapy (especially in those with liver impairment)
- (TSC with SEGA, TSC with seizures) therapeutic levels should be measured 1–2 weeks after starting therapy or altering dose
- if patient is treated for pneumonia with antibiotics and does not show improvement, interstitial lung disease/non-infectious pneumonitis should be considered
- increased risk of hypertension, pneumonitis and/or hyperglycaemia if used in Asian patients
- Afinitor and Afinitor Dispersible tablets are not interchangeable, nor should they be mixed together to achieve the dosage
- (Afinitor) if switching between formulations, dose should be estimated to closest mg and serum levels measured 2 weeks later
- (TSC with SEGA) SEGA volume should be measured 12 weeks after starting therapy and dose adjusted accordingly
- (TSC with SEGA, TSC with refractory seizures) once dosage has stabilised, trough concentration should be measured every 3–6 months if patients have changing surface area (e.g. growth) or 6–12-monthly if surface area is stable
- (Afinitor) dose interruption, reduction or stopping is recommended if patient develops adverse effects (e.g. non-infectious pneumonitis, stomatitis, thrombocytopenia)
- caution if used in those with severe refractory hyperlipidaemia, impaired kidney or liver function
- caution if used in peri-surgical period as delayed wound healing may occur
- tablets contain lactose and are not recommended in those with galactose intolerance, Lapp lactase deficiency or glucose–galactose malabsorption
- (Afinitor) not recommended in children with cancer, TSC with renal angiomyolipoma, TSC with SEGA (if under 1 year) or TSC with refractory seizures (if under 2 years)
- (Afinitor) not recommended in those under 18 years with liver impairment and TSC with SEGA or TSC with refractory seizures
- (Afinitor) not recommended in those with severe liver impairment. Dose reduction is recommended with mild-to-moderate liver impairment

- contraindicated in those with hypersensitivity to sirolimus
- see also General Nursing points/Cautions for immunomodifiers (p. 1176)

Patient teaching and advice

- instruct patient to take tablets whole, not chewed or broken and to consistently take either with or without food (but not switch between the two) and at the same time
- (dispersible tablets) advise patient that dispersible tablets should not be swallowed whole, chewed or crushed
- (dispersible tablets) patient should be given the following instructions regarding dispersion of tablets:
  - (using syringe) place dose (up to 10 mg) in 10 mL syringe and add 5 mL water and 4 mL air. If dose is greater than 10 mg, second syringe should be used. Allow syringe to stand (tip up) in a container for 3 minutes until tablet has dispersed into suspension. Syringe should then be inverted 5 times to mix suspension and then drunk. A further 5 mL water and 4 mL of air should be added to syringe and swirled to suspend any remaining particles and drunk
  - (using glass) place tablet (up to 10 mg) in 25 mL water and allow to disperse for 3 minutes, stir gently with a spoon and drink. A further 25 mL water should be added to glass, stirred with same spoon to resuspend any remaining particles and drunk
- if mouth ulcers or oral mucositis occur, patient should be advised not to use alcohol, hydrogen peroxide, iodine or thyme-containing mouthwashes as they may make the condition worse. Antifungal preparations should only be used if fungal infection exists
- patient should be instructed to avoid grapefruit, grapefruit juice, star fruit or Seville oranges during therapy
- advise patient to seek medical advice if any persistent or worsening cough, wheezing, difficulty breathing or shortness of breath occurs
- counsel patient regarding the importance of avoiding pregnancy during therapy, including the need to use adequate contraception before starting, during and for 8 weeks after therapy is stopped
- see also General Patient teaching and advice for immunomodifiers (p. 1177)

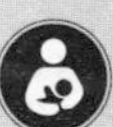

not recommended during pregnancy or during breastfeeding or for 2 weeks after last dose

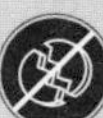

tablets should not be crushed or broken. Mask and gloves should be worn when dispersing tablets

GUSELKUMAB (Tremfya)

Available form
Prefilled syringe/pen: 100mg/mL

Action
- human IgG1 monoclonal antibody that selectively binds to interleukin-23 (known to be elevated in skin of those with plaque psoriasis)

Use
- treatment of moderate-to-severe plaque psoriasis in those who are candidates for systemic therapy or phototherapy

Dose
- 100 mg SC at weeks 0, 4 and then every 8 weeks afterwards

Adverse effects
- diarrhoea, gastroenteritis
- upper respiratory tract infection, herpes simplex infections, tinea
- arthralgia

- headache, migraine
- injection site reactions
- (uncommon) hypersensitivity, rash, urticaria

Interactions
- see General Interactions for immunomodifiers (p. 1176)

Nursing points/Cautions
- see General Nursing points/Cautions for immunomodifiers (p. 1176)
- trade name and batch number should be recorded in patient medical history
- patient may be taught to self-administer. First injection should be under medical supervision

Patient teaching and advice
- see Patient teaching and advice for icatibant (p. 1195) for self-administration instructions
- see General Patient teaching and advice for immunomodifiers (p. 1177)

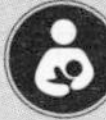
should only be used during pregnancy or breastfeeding if benefits are thought to outweigh risks

HUMAN C1 ESTERASE INHIBITOR (Berinert, Cinryze)

Available forms
Vial: 500 IU, 2000IU, 3000IU

Action
- belongs to serine protease inhibitor group (that includes antithrombin III) and inhibits activated serine proteinases (C1r and C1s), kallikrein and coagulation factors XIIa and XIa
- inhibits complement system, contact system, fibrinolytic system and coagulation cascade
- produced from human plasma
- long elimination half-life (> 60 hours)

Use
- treatment of acute attacks in those with hereditary angioedema
- pre-procedure prevention in those with C1 esterase deficiency
- prevention of angioedema in those experiencing frequent attacks who are intolerant to or inadequately protected by oral therapy

Dose
- (acute attack treatment) 20 IU/kg as slow IV injection at 4 mL/minute (Berinert IV) **OR**
- (treatment of acute attack) 1000 IU IV at 1 mL/minute at first sign of attack, with second dose given if no response after 60 minutes (Cinryze) **OR**
- (routine prophylaxis) 1000 IU IV at 1 mL/minute every 3–4 days, adjusting interval according to response (Cinryze) **OR**
- (routine prophylaxis) 60 IU/kg SC twice weekly (every 3–4 days) (Berinert SC) **OR**
- (pre-procedure prevention) 1000 IU IV at 1 mL/minute within 24 hours of medical, dental or surgical procedure (Cinryze)

Adverse effects
- nausea, vomiting, altered taste, abdominal pain
- headache, dizziness
- rash, erythema, pruritus
- nasopharyngitis
- flushing
- muscle spasms, pain
- peripheral oedema
- fever
- hypersensitivity
- (injection site) redness, pain, bruising, irritation, haematoma and uncommonly, burning sensation, thrombosis, phlebitis
- (uncommon) thrombotic events
- (rare) allergic reaction, anaphylaxis

Nursing points/Cautions

- if patient has a known allergy tendency (e.g. asthma), antihistamines and corticosteroids should be given prophylactically
- (Cinryze, acute attack) second dose is more likely to be required if patient has severe attack, laryngeal attack or if treatment has been delayed
- contains 486 mg of sodium/100 mL (Berinert) or 11.5 mg (Cinryze), which may need to be considered as part of salt-restricted diet
- patient can be taught to self-administer with first injection under medical supervision
- because it is derived from human plasma, there is a theoretical risk, although remote, of transmission of infectious material such as viruses
- reconstituted using diluent provided (water for injections) and manufacturer's instructions
- (IV) administer alone
- do not shake solution as this will denature protein
- name and batch number of product should be recorded in patient history
- caution if used in those at risk of thrombotic events (including presence of indwelling catheter)
- not recommended for treatment of capillary leak syndrome (Berinert IV)

Patient teaching and advice

- caution patient against driving or operating machinery if dizziness persists
- instruct patient in correct self-administration technique, including reconstitution of solution, administration and correct disposal of used needles. It is important to ensure the patient understands the importance of seeking medical attention immediately if any laryngeal swelling or airway obstruction occurs
- counsel patient regarding medication being a human plasma derivative and the theoretical risk of transmission of infectious material

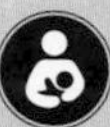

only recommended during pregnancy and breastfeeding if clearly needed

ICATIBANT (Firazyr)

Available form

Prefilled syringe: 30 mg/3 mL

Action

- selective antagonist at bradykinin type 2 receptors
- hereditary angioedema attacks are accompanied by bradykinin release which is responsible for many of the clinical symptoms (subcutaneous and/or submucosal oedema of upper respiratory tract, skin and GI tract)

Use

- symptomatic treatment of hereditary angioedema attack (in adults with C1 esterase inhibitor deficiency)

Dose

- 30 mg SC slowly. If symptoms recur or are not relieved, a further 30 mg SC can be given after 6 hours, and repeated again if necessary (daily maximum 90 mg at 6-hour intervals)

Adverse effects

- (injection site) irritation, erythema, swelling, burning sensation, itching, pain
- prolonged prothrombin time, increase in blood creatine phosphokinase (CPK) and transaminases, and uncommonly abnormal liver function tests, hyperglycaemia, hyperuricaemia
- dizziness, headache and uncommonly fatigue, asthenia

- fever
- rash, pruritus, erythema and uncommonly urticaria
- nausea and uncommonly, vomiting, weight increase
- (uncommon) hot flush
- (uncommon) cough, asthma, nasal congestion, pharyngitis
- (uncommon) herpes zoster
- (uncommon) muscle spasm

Interactions

- may antagonise actions of ACE inhibitors (which are not recommended for those with hereditary angioedema due to risk of inducing attack)

Nursing points/Cautions

- patient may be taught to self-administer. First injection should be under medical supervision
- caution if used in those with acute ischaemic heart disease, unstable angina pectoris or within weeks of having a stroke

Patient teaching and advice

- patient should be advised to seek medical attention immediately if attack involves face, lips, throat or voice box area or patient has difficulty breathing (regardless of response to self-injection)
- advise patient to seek medical advice if there is no resolution in attack within 2 hours of self-injection
- instruct patient in correct SC self-administration technique, including:
    - patient has demonstrated SC administration and is comfortable with technique
    - remove syringe from fridge 30–45 minutes before injection and allow solution to come to room temperature but do not warm in any way
    - check prefilled syringe for any signs of particles or cloudiness (and do not use if these are present)
    - check expiry date and do not use if date has passed
    - do not shake syringe
    - rotate injections sites (abdomen (at least 5 cm from navel), thighs (front, avoiding area 5 cm above knees and below groin) and upper arms (fleshy area at back)
    - do not inject into skin that is red and inflamed, has stretch marks, scarred, tender, bruised or has psoriasis
    - wash hands with soap and water
    - clean injection site with alcohol site and allow to dry for at least 10 seconds (and do not touch site again)
    - remove needle cover and hold syringe in dominant hand (similar to holding a pencil)
    - pinch skin between thumb and index finger (about 5 cm fold) and insert needle at 45–90 degree angle
    - release skin and push plunger down to inject entire content of syringe
    - release plunger and remove syringe
    - if there is blood present, press with cotton ball or gauze but do not rub injection site
    - safely dispose of syringe (e.g. sharps container, puncture-proof hard plastic or glass container with lid) and store container out of reach of children. When full, see advice from pharmacist or doctor regarding disposal
    - prefilled syringes should only be used once
    - store unused syringes in fridge but do not freeze
    - if vial of powder and diluent (water for injections) requires mixing, this must be done carefully and according to directions, taking care not to shake solution in order to mix it

- nothing else should be mixed in same syringe
- instruct patient to inject slowly
- warn patient against driving or operating machinery if dizziness, asthenia or fatigue occur

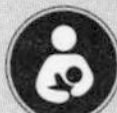

not recommended during pregnancy unless benefits outweigh risks

breastfeeding is not recommended within 12 hours of therapy

IXEKIZUMAB (RCH) (Taltz)

Available form

Autoinjector/Prefilled syringe: 80 mg/mL

Action

- IgG4 monoclonal antibody with high affinity for proinflammatory cytokine IL-17A (IL-17A plays a major role in excess keratinocyte proliferation and activation in psoriasis)
- half-life 13 days (plaque psoriasis), clearance increases as body weight increases

Use

- moderate-to-severe plaque psoriasis
- active psoriatic arthritis (in patients who have not responded to or are intolerant to other DMARDs)

Dose

- (plaque psoriasis) initially 160 mg SC (week 0), then 80 mg SC every 2 weeks for 12 weeks (weeks 2, 4, 6, 8, 10, 12), then 80 mg SC monthly

OR

- (psoriatic arthritis) initially 160 mg SC, then 80 mg SC monthly

Adverse effects

- upper respiratory tract infection, nasopharyngitis, rhinitis, influenza
- nausea
- oropharyngeal pain
- tinea
- conjunctivitis
- oral candidiasis
- transient neutropenia
- (injection site) pain, redness
- (rare) anaphylaxis, angioedema, urticaria, development of antibodies

Interactions

- not recommended with live vaccines

Nursing points/Cautions

- if patient has psoriatic arthritis and moderate-to-severe plaque psoriasis, dosage for plaque psoriasis should be used
- patient should be assessed for TB before starting therapy. Anti-TB therapy should be considered for patients with latent or active TB if adequate treatment cannot be confirmed. Patients must be closely monitored for any signs of TB
- patient can be taught to self-administer
- caution if used in those with Crohn's disease or ulcerative colitis as exacerbation of the condition may occur
- caution if used in those with clinically important chronic or active infection

Patient teaching and advice

- advise patient to seek medical advice if any of the following occur:
  - fever, flu-like symptoms, night sweats, cough that lasts for weeks, shortness of breath, fatigue, unintentional weight loss, coughing up blood
- instruct patient in correct SC self-administration technique (see Patient teaching and advice for icatibant, p. 1195). Warn patient not to shake autoinjector/prefilled syringe
- warn patient not to use solution if it has been frozen
- autoinjector/prefilled syringe should be stored at 2–8°C and protected from light. If not refrigerated and

unused for 5 days, autoinjector/prefilled syringe should be discarded

> not recommended during pregnancy or breastfeeding unless benefits outweigh risks

LENALIDOMIDE (Revlimid)

Available forms

Capsules: 5 mg, 10 mg, 15 mg, 25 mg

Action

- immunomodulator with antiangiogenic, antineoplastic and pro-erythropoietic properties
- inhibits growth of some haemopoietic tumour cells (including multiple myeloma plasma tumour cells), increases T cell and natural killer cell mediated immunity, increases number of natural killer T cells, inhibits monocyte production of pro-inflammatory cytokines and inhibits formation of micro vessels
- structurally related to thalidomide and carries the same risk of teratogenic effects

Use

- treatment of multiple myeloma (MM) (with dexamethasone) in patients where disease has progressed despite one treatment
- treatment of newly diagnosed multiple myeloma (with dexamethasone and bortezomib) in patients ineligible for autologous stem cell transplantation or as induction before stem cell transplantation in those who are eligible
- treatment of relapsed or refractory mantle cell lymphoma
- treatment of transfusion-dependent anaemia due to low or intermediate-1 risk myelodysplastic syndromes (MDS) (associated with deletion 5q cytogenetic abnormality, with or without other cytogenetic abnormalities)

Dose

- (previously treated MM) initially 25 mg orally daily (1 hour before or 2 hours after food) on days 1–21 of a 28-day cycle (with dexamethasone 40 mg orally daily on days 1–4, 9–12 and 17–20 for 4 cycles, then decreasing dexamethasone to 40 mg orally daily on days 1–4 only of 28-day cycle) (with dose adjustment dependent on platelet and absolute neutrophil count (ANC)) and continued until disease progression or unacceptable toxicity occurs **OR**
- (newly diagnosed MM, not eligible for stem cell transplant) initially 25 mg orally daily on days 1–14 of 21-day cycle (with dexamethasone 20 mg orally daily on days 2, 4, 5, 8, 9, 11 and 12 of 21-day cycle and bortezomib IV or SC 1.3 mg/m^2 on days 1, 4, 8 and 11 of 21-day cycle), then 25 mg orally daily on days 1–21 of 28-day cycle (with dexamethasone 40 mg orally daily on days 1, 8, 15 and 22 of 28-day cycle) **OR**
- (newly diagnosed MM, not eligible for stem cell transplant, $\leq$ 75 years, no renal impairment) initially 25 mg orally daily on days 1–21 of 28-day cycle (with dexamethasone 40 mg orally daily on days 1, 8, 15 and 22 of 28-day cycle) **OR**
- (newly diagnosed MM, eligible for stem cell transplant) 25 mg orally daily on days 1–14 of 21-day cycle (with dexamethasone 20 mg orally daily on days 2, 4, 5, 8, 9, 11 and 12 of 21-day cycle and bortezomib IV or SC 1.3 mg/m^2 on days 1, 4, 8 and 11 of 21-day cycle) **OR**
- (newly diagnosed MM, eligible for stem cell transplant) 25 mg orally daily on days 1–21 of 28-day cycle (with dexamethasone 20 mg orally

daily on days 1–4 and 9–12 of 28-day cycle and bortezomib IV or SC 1.3 mg/m² on days 1, 4, 8 and 11 of 28-day cycle) **OR**
- (newly diagnosed MM, post-stem cell transplant) 10 mg orally daily for days 1–28 of 28-day cycle for repeated cycles. If tolerated, dose may be increased to 15 mg orally daily after 12 weeks **OR**
- (MDS) initially 10 mg orally daily on days 1–21 of 28-day cycle (with dose adjustment dependent on platelet and ANC) **OR**
- (relapsed or refractory mantle cell lymphoma) 25 mg orally daily on days 1–21 of 28-day cycle, continued until disease progression or unacceptable toxicity occurs

Adverse effects
- neutropenia, thrombocytopenia, anaemia, leucopenia, febrile neutropenia, pancytopenia
- atrial fibrillation, tachycardia, hypotension, hypertension, chest pain, cardiac failure, myocardial infarction
- peripheral oedema
- dyspnoea, cough, oropharyngeal pain, dysphonia
- anorexia, nausea, vomiting, diarrhoea, abdominal pain, constipation, dyspepsia, altered taste, dry mouth, weight decrease, toothache
- headache, fatigue, asthenia, insomnia, depression, dizziness, tremor
- vertigo
- syncope
- fever
- muscle weakness, muscle spasm, myalgia, arthralgia, bone pain, musculoskeletal pain, back pain, pain in extremities
- hyperglycaemia, hypocalcaemia, hypokalaemia, hypomagnesaemia, iron overload
- transient altered liver enzymes, hyperbilirubinaemia, liver damage
- hypothyroidism, and less commonly, hyperthyroidism
- thromboembolism (deep vein thrombosis (DVT), pulmonary embolus (PE))
- kidney failure
- rash, pruritus, dry skin, increased sweating
- peripheral neuropathy, paraesthesia, neuralgia
- (rare) angioedema, severe dermatological reactions, tumour lysis syndrome, tumour flare reaction, progressive multifocal leukoencephalopathy (with dexamethasone)
- see also General Adverse effects of immunomodifiers (p. 1176)

Interactions
- caution if given with other agents that increase risk of thrombosis
- (MM) increased risk of thromboembolism when given with dexamethasone
- caution if used with agents that impair liver function
- not recommended with combined oral contraceptives or hormone replacement therapy due to increased risk of thromboembolism
- caution if given with other myelosuppressive agents
- caution if given with warfarin, therefore INR should be closely monitored especially when starting or stopping therapy
- may increase serum levels of digoxin increasing risk of toxicity, therefore serum levels should be monitored during therapy

Nursing points/Cautions
- only doctors and pharmacists who are registered with restricted distribution program can prescribe and dispense lenalidomide to patients who meet all requirements and are registered with this program. Patients must be fully aware of the consequences if pregnancy occurs and be willing to abide by the conditions

(e.g. pregnancy testing, contraception) before, during and after treatment is completed

- to be eligible for therapy, a female patient (or female partner of male patient) is considered to no longer be of childbearing potential if she:
  - is over 50 years and has been naturally amenorrhoeic for 1 year (however, amenorrhoea post-chemotherapy does not rule out childbearing potential)
  - has premature ovarian failure (confirmed by specialist gynaecologist)
  - has had a hysterectomy or bilateral salpingo-oophorectomy
  - has uterine agenesis, Turner syndrome or XY genotype
- it is recommended that women of childbearing potential should have a pregnancy test before starting therapy, weekly during first month and then monthly (if menstrual cycles are regular) or 2-weekly (if menstrual cycles are irregular)
- (MM, MDS) complete blood count (including white blood cell count with differential, platelet count, haemoglobin and haematocrit) should be performed before starting therapy, then weekly for 8 weeks, and then monthly
- (newly diagnosed MM, transplant ineligible) complete blood count (including white blood cell count with differential, platelet count, haemoglobin and haematocrit) should be performed before starting therapy, then weekly for first 2 cycles of treatment, then day 1 and 15 of cycle 3 and monthly thereafter
- (newly diagnosed MM, with dexamethasone and bortezomib) complete blood count (including white blood cell count with differential, platelet count, haemoglobin and haematocrit) should be performed before starting therapy, then weekly for first cycle of treatment, then before start of each subsequent cycle, and then monthly afterwards
- (mantle cell lymphoma) complete blood count (including white blood cell count with differential, platelet count, haemoglobin and haematocrit) should be performed before starting therapy, then weekly for first cycle of treatment, every 2 weeks (for cycles 2–4), then before start of each subsequent cycle
- absolute neutrophil count (ANC) and platelet count should be measured before starting therapy
- (MM) if ANC $< 1.0 \times 10^9$/L and/or platelet count $< 75 \times 10^9$/L (or $< 30 \times 10^9$/L depending on bone marrow infiltration by plasma cells), therapy should not be started
- (newly diagnosed MM) if ANC $< 1.5 \times 10^9$/L and/or platelet count $< 50 \times 10^9$/L therapy should not be started
- (MDS) if ANC $< 0.5 \times 10^9$/L and/or platelet count $< 50 \times 10^9$/L therapy should not be started
- thyroid and renal function monitoring is recommended before starting and regularly during therapy
- (MM, eligible for stem cell transplant) up to 8 cycles of 21 days or 6 cycles of 28-day treatment are recommended. Autologous stem cell transplant should occur within 4 cycles
- tablets contain lactose and are not recommended in those with galactose intolerance, lactase deficiency or glucose–galactose malabsorption
- caution if used in those with hypertension, congestive cardiac failure, electrolyte imbalance or infection as they are at increased risk of atrial fibrillation
- caution if used in those with hypertension, hyperlipidaemia or if a smoker, due to increased risk of myocardial infarction
- caution if used in those with high tumour burden (e.g. previously

treated mantle cell lymphoma) due to increased risk of tumour lysis syndrome or tumour flare syndrome
- caution if used in those with liver or renal impairment (dose reduction is recommended in those with renal impairment)
- caution if used in those who have undergone solid organ transplantation due to increased risk of organ rejection
- increased risk of venous and arterial thromboembolism (when given with dexamethasone), therefore caution if used in those with history of thrombosis or with risk factors such as smoking, hypertension or hyperlipidaemia
- not recommended in those who have experienced thalidomide-induced rash
- not recommended for management of chronic lymphocytic leukaemia due to increased mortality
- contraindicated if ANC $< 1.0 \times 10^9$/L or platelet count $< 75 \times 10^9$/L (or $< 30 \times 10^9$/L depending on bone marrow infiltration by plasma cells) (MM), ANC $< 1.0 \times 10^9$/L or platelet count $< 50 \times 10^9$/L (newly diagnosed MM) or if ANC $< 0.5 \times 10^9$/L (MDS)
- contraindicated in women of childbearing potential unless all conditions have been met

Patient teaching and advice

- patient should be advised to take capsules at same time every day and swallow whole (not opened, chewed or divided) with water 1 hour before or 2 hours after food
- patient should be advised if dose is missed by more than 12 hours, it should not be taken. Next dose should be taken at the normal time the next day
- patient must receive counselling to ensure good understanding of the potential therapy risks and outcomes (i.e. risks to unborn child), and contraceptive requirements associated with lenalidomide before giving a full and written consent prior to starting therapy. Patient's sexual partner should also receive counselling and information
- important patient advice should include:
  - do not drive or operate machinery if fatigue, dizziness, blurred vision and/or somnolence occurs
  - seek medical advice if any of the following occur:
    - any shortness of breath, chest pain or arm/leg swelling (symptoms of DVT and PE)
    - febrile illness (neutropenia)
    - bleeding and nosebleeds
    - rash, especially if accompanied with fever and/or swollen glands
    - any numbness, tingling or pain in hands or feet
  - do not donate blood during therapy or within 1 week of stopping therapy
  - male patient must not donate semen during or within 1 week of stopping therapy
  - male patients should be advised that lenalidomide is present in semen and therefore adequate contraceptive methods (latex or polyurethane condoms) must be used during sexual activity with women of childbearing potential (or who have not been menopausal for at least 2 years); condom use must continue for at least 4 weeks after stopping therapy
  - explain the importance of having a medically supervised pregnancy test at the time of consultation (or within 3 days prior to visit) to exclude pregnancy before the start of therapy, with a medically supervised pregnancy

test repeated every 4 weeks, including when therapy is stopped
- women of childbearing potential (who have not had a hysterectomy, salpingo-oophorectomy or are not > 50 years and postmenopausal for more than 1 year) must use one reliable contraceptive measure (e.g. intrauterine device, hormone implant or depot contraception, tubal ligation, partner vasectomy (with 2 negative semen analyses), oral progesterone-only contraceptive pill) for 1 month before, during and 1 month after stopping therapy
- copper-releasing intrauterine devices (IUD) are not recommended due to risk of infection (at time of insertion) and menstrual blood loss, which can compromise female patients with neutropenia or thrombocytopenia
- combined oral contraceptive pill is not recommended because of increased risk of venous thrombotic event
- any woman (either taking lenalidomide or whose partner is taking lenalidomide) who is of childbearing potential and who experiences menstrual irregularities or suspects she is pregnant must seek medical advice immediately

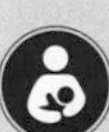

under NO circumstances should lenalidomide be used during pregnancy because of its relationship to thalidomide. Thalidomide is a known human teratogen causing mortality at or just after birth and birth defects, which include absence or shortness of limbs, external ear abnormalities, eye abnormalities, facial palsy, congenital heart defects and malformation of the alimentary tract, urinary tract and/or genital tract

contraindicated during breastfeeding

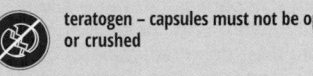

teratogen – capsules must not be opened or crushed

MYCOPHENOLATE MOFETIL (CellCept, Cellplant, Ceptolate, MycoCept)

MYCOPHENOLATE SODIUM (Myfortic)

Available forms

Capsules: 250 mg; Tablets: 500 mg; Tablets (enteric coated): 180 mg, 360 mg; Oral solution: 1 g/5 mL; Vial: 500 mg

Action

- immunosuppressant
- selectively inhibits inosine monophosphate dehydrogenase thereby inhibiting proliferation of T and B cells, decreasing monocyte and lymphocyte recruitment to chronic inflammatory sites
- narrow therapeutic index
- metabolised to active form (mycophenolic acid)

Use

- prevention of solid allogeneic organ rejection
- lupus nephritis (WHO class III, IV or V) (induction and maintenance)

Dose

- (renal transplant) 1 g orally or IV over 2 hours twice daily **OR**
- (cardiac transplant) 1.5 g orally or IV over 2 hours twice daily **OR**
- (liver transplant) initially 1 g IV over 2 hours twice daily, then 1.5 g orally twice daily **OR**
- (other transplant) 1–1.5 g orally or IV over 2 hours twice daily **OR**
- (renal transplant) 720 mg orally twice daily, starting within 48 hours of transplantation (enteric-coated capsules) **OR**

- (lupus nephritis) 720 mg orally twice daily (with corticosteroids) (induction) then dose reduction once clinical response has been achieved (Myfortic)

Adverse effects

- anorexia, diarrhoea, loose stools, constipation, dyspepsia, nausea, vomiting, oral thrush, gastritis, flatulence, GI thrush, abdominal pain/tenderness/distention, oesophagitis and uncommonly, GI ulceration and haemorrhage, and rarely, perforation
- headache, dizziness, fatigue, anxiety, asthenia, insomnia, tremor
- arthralgia, myalgia
- hypertension, hypotension
- cough, dyspnoea, dyspnoea on exertion
- hyperlipidaemia, abnormal liver function tests, hepatitis
- elevated blood creatinine
- peripheral oedema
- hypocalcaemia, hypokalaemia, hyperuricaemia, hyperkalaemia, hypomagnesaemia
- fever
- leucopenia, thrombocytopenia, anaemia, neutropenia
- (IV site) phlebitis, thrombosis
- (rare) progressive multifocal leukoencephalopathy, pure red cell aplasia
- see also General Adverse effects of immunomodifiers (p. 1176)

Interactions

- not recommended with azathioprine due to increased risk of bone marrow depression
- caution if given with aciclovir or valaciclovir as combination may lead to increased serum levels of both agents
- absorption may be decreased if given with aluminium/magnesium hydroxide, phosphate binders or colestyramine
- caution if used with proton pump inhibitors
- dose reduction may be required if given with ganciclovir in those with renal impairment
- not recommended with live attenuated virus vaccines
- caution if given with tacrolimus or sirolimus
- availability may be reduced if given with iron or iron supplements
- serum levels may be decreased by rifampicin and telmisartan
- may decrease efficacy of combined oral contraceptives
- caution if given with ciprofloxacin or amoxicillin with clavulanic acid and metronidazole as serum levels may decrease

Nursing points/Cautions

- see also General Nursing points/Cautions for immunomodifiers (p. 1176)
- therapy should be started within 24 hours of transplantation
- therapy should be changed from IV to oral as soon as possible
- blood counts should be measured weekly for first month, twice monthly for 2 months, then monthly for first year. Therapy should be interrupted and/or dose decreased if absolute neutrophil count (ANC) $< 1.5 \times 10^9$/L
- pregnancy should be excluded before starting therapy in female patients using 2 urine or serum pregnancy tests. The second test should be performed 8–10 days after first test and just before the start of therapy. Pregnancy tests should be repeated if there is any gap in contraception
- therapeutic serum levels should be monitored regularly during therapy
- (IV) reconstitute using glucose 5% only and dilute according to manufacturer's instructions to a concentration of 6 g/mL and administered by IV infusion over 2 hours

- (IV) not recommended by rapid or bolus IV
- (IV) administer alone
- (IV) incompatible with sodium chloride 0.9%, Ringer's or lactated Ringer's solutions
- (IV) reconstituting should be gentle, avoiding foaming
- if oral solution is given via nasogastric tube, tube should have diameter of not less than 1.7 mm
- preparations are not equivalent nor interchangeable (2 g mycophenolate mofetil = 1.44 g mycophenolate sodium)
- (oral suspension) caution if used in those with phenylketonuria as suspension contains aspartame
- caution if used in those with chronic renal impairment (dose should not be greater than 1 g twice daily in those with severe renal impairment), GI disease or Lesch-Nyhan syndrome (hypoxanthine-guanine-phosphoribosyl transferase deficiency)
- caution if used in those over 65 years due to increased risk of adverse effects
- contraindicated in those with hypersensitivity to mycophenolate or mycophenolic acid or polysorbate 80 (if given IV)

Patient teaching and advice

- see also General Patient teaching and advice for immunomodifiers (p. 1177)
- instruct patient to take iron supplements 3 hours after mycophenolate preparations
- patient should be advised to take antacids 2 hours apart from mycophenolate preparations
- advise patient to swallow enteric-coated capsules whole, without chewing or breaking them
- ensure patient understands the importance of consistently taking medication in relation to food (i.e. always before food or always after, not mixing the two) to ensure consistent absorption
- advise patient and carer to seek medical advice if any confusion, apathy, one-sided paralysis, difficulty walking or cognitive impairment occurs
- all patients should be advised not to donate blood during or for 6 weeks after stopping therapy
- (male patient) instruct patient not to donate semen during or for 90 days after stopping therapy
- warn patient not to drive or operate machinery if dizziness, fatigue or anxiety occur
- (male patient) counsel patient regarding the need to wear a condom during and for 13 weeks after stopping therapy (regardless of whether he has had a vasectomy or not as there is a risk of transmission in seminal fluid). Female partner of male patient should also be counselled regarding the need to use highly effective contraception during and for 13 weeks after their partner has ceased therapy
- ensure female patient of childbearing potential understands the importance of using two forms of highly effective contraception before, during and 6 weeks after therapy to avoid pregnancy and to seek medical advice immediately if pregnancy occurs. Patient should be warned that combined oral contraceptives may not be effective during therapy

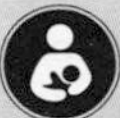

contraindicated during pregnancy as fetal loss and/or congenital abnormalities may occur

contraindicated during breastfeeding

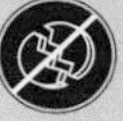

oral solution is available. Capsule should not be opened or tablets broken or crushed

PALIVIZUMAB (Synagis)

Available form
Vial: 100 mg/mL

Action
- IgG_1 monoclonal antibody that has inhibitory activity against respiratory syncytial virus (RSV)

Use
- prevention of serious respiratory tract disease caused by RSV in high-risk children (e.g. bronchopulmonary dysplasia, prematurity (< 35 weeks gestation), significant congenital heart disease)

Dose
- 15 mg/kg IM monthly, starting at the beginning of the RSV season

Adverse effects
- upper respiratory infection, rhinitis, cough, wheeze, bronchiolitis, pneumonia, dyspnoea, pharyngitis, flu-like symptoms, apnoea, croup
- otitis media
- fever
- rash, eczema, fungal dermatitis
- diarrhoea, vomiting, oral thrush, gastroenteritis, constipation, flatulence, feeding abnormalities
- conjunctivitis
- pain
- viral, bacterial and fungal infections
- nervousness, somnolence
- coagulation disorder, haemorrhage, thrombocytopenia, anaemia
- hypokalaemia
- elevated liver enzymes
- failure to thrive
- hypotonia
- (rare) anaphylaxis, allergic reaction
- injection site reaction

Interactions
- may interfere with immune-based RSV diagnostic test and viral culture assays

Nursing points/Cautions
- first dose should be given before start of RSV season
- use may be delayed if the child has severe acute infection or acute febrile illness, unless RSV risk is high
- if child develops RSV, monthly injections are still recommended to prevent reinfection
- adrenaline (epinephrine) (1:1000), corticosteroid, antihistamines, oxygen and resuscitation equipment should be readily available in the event of anaphylaxis
- volume greater than 1 mL should be given as divided IM doses
- gluteal muscle is not routinely used for IM injection in children
- solution should not be diluted for IM administration
- not recommended for use in adults
- caution if given IM to those with thrombocytopenia or coagulation disorder
- contraindicated in those with known hypersensitivity to other recombinant monoclonal antibodies

PIRFENIDONE (Esbriet)

Available forms
Capsule: 267 mg; Tablets: 267 mg, 801 mg

Action
- antifibrotic, anti-inflammatory immunomodifier

Use
- treatment of idiopathic pulmonary fibrosis

Dose
- 267 mg orally 3 times daily with food (days 1–7), then 534 mg 3 times daily (days 8–14), then 801 mg 3 times daily (day 15 onwards)

Adverse effects
- nausea, vomiting, diarrhoea, anorexia, dyspepsia, abdominal pain, gastroesophageal reflux disease (GORD)
- weight loss
- upper respiratory tract infection, sinusitis
- photosensitivity, rash
- angioedema, anaphylaxis
- dizziness, fatigue, headache, insomnia
- arthralgia

Interactions
- contraindicated with fluvoxamine
- not recommended with other agents known to cause photosensitivity
- decreased serum levels in smokers
- caution if given with ciprofloxacin as increased serum levels may occur
- decreased serum levels may occur if given with omeprazole and rifampicin

Nursing points/Cautions
- liver function (ALT, AST and bilirubin) should be measured before starting therapy, then monthly for 6 months and 3-monthly for remainder of treatment
- patient weight should be monitored during therapy and dietary advice recommended if weight loss of clinical significance occurs
- if therapy is interrupted for 14 or more consecutive days, it should be restarted by undergoing the initial 2 weeks of titration up to the recommended daily dose. If therapy is interrupted for less than 14 days, dose can be resumed at previous recommended dose without titration
- caution if used in those with mild, moderate or severe kidney impairment or mild-to-moderate liver impairment
- contraindicated in those with history of pirfenidone-induced angioedema, severe liver impairment, end-stage liver disease, severe kidney impairment (creatinine clearance < 30 mL/minute) or end-stage kidney disease requiring dialysis

Patient teaching and advice
- instruct patient not to drive or operate machinery if dizziness or fatigue occur
- remind patient to take capsules or tablets with food to reduce gastrointestinal adverse effects
- patient should be advised to avoid or minimise exposure to direct sunlight and sunlamps during therapy. If sun exposure cannot be avoided, instruct patient to wear protective clothing and sunscreen (SPF 30+)
- encourage patient to stop smoking before and during therapy and discuss any changes to smoking habit with doctor
- advise patient to seek medical advice immediately if any of the following occur:
  - swelling of face, lips and/or tongue
  - rash or photosensitivity (exaggerated sunburn)
  - dizziness
  - weight loss
  - fatigue, loss of appetite, right upper quadrant abdominal pain, dark urine, yellowing of skin and/or whites of the eyes

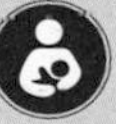
not recommended during pregnancy or breastfeeding

capsule can be opened or tablet crushed and mixed with water or spoonful of yoghurt or apple puree

PLERIXAFOR (Mozobil)

Available form
Vial: 24 mg/1.2 mL

Action
- CXCR4 chemokine receptor antagonist

- stem cells secrete CXCR4 and migrate to bone marrow through a chemo-attractant effect of stromal cell-derived factor-1α (SDF-1α) produced by bone marrow stromal cells. CXCR4 is thought to assist in binding the stem cells in the marrow
- by using a CXCR4 receptor antagonist, leukocytosis is induced and mature and stem cells appear in the circulation

Use
- mobilise stem cells to peripheral blood for collection and subsequent autologous transplantation in those with lymphoma and multiple myeloma (with granulocyte-colony stimulating factor (G-CSF))

Dose
- therapy is initiated after granulocyte-colony stimulating factor (G-CSF) (10 microgram/kg) has been given daily for 4 days, then 0.24 mg/kg SC 6–11 hours before apheresis for 2–4 consecutive days (but up to 7 days)

Adverse effects
- (post-injection reaction) urticaria, periorbital swelling, dyspnoea, hypoxia
- nausea, vomiting, diarrhoea, abdominal pain, flatulence
- headache, dizziness, insomnia, abnormal dreams, fatigue
- arthralgia
- (uncommon) vasovagal reaction (orthostatic hypotension and/or syncope)
- (injection site) pain, redness
- (rare) myocardial infarction, splenic enlargement

Nursing points/Cautions
- WBC and platelet count should be monitored during therapy and apheresis
- patient should be closely monitored for 60 minutes for any post-injection reactions or hypotension and/or syncope
- injection-related reaction can be treated using antihistamines, corticosteroids, hydration and oxygen
- abdomen is preferred SC injection site
- caution if used in those with moderate-to-severe kidney impairment (dose should be reduced to 0.16 mg/kg)
- caution if used in those with neutrophil count $> 50 \times 10^9$ cells/L
- not recommended in those with leukaemia
- not recommended for haemopoietic stem cell mobilisation and harvest in those with leukaemia

Patient teaching and advice
- advise patient to immediately report any left upper abdominal pain and/or shoulder pain (may be sign of spleen problem)
- warn patient that vasovagal reaction may occur up to 1 hour after injection
- patient should be advised not to drive or operate machinery if dizziness, fatigue or vasovagal reaction occurs
- female patient of childbearing capacity should be counselled to use adequate contraception during therapy to prevent pregnancy from occurring

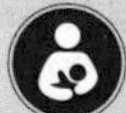

not recommended during pregnancy or breastfeeding unless benefits outweigh risks

POMALIDOMIDE (Pomalyst)

Available forms
Capsules: 1 mg, 2 mg, 3 mg

Action
- thalidomide analogue with direct antimyeloma tumouricidal activity, immunomodulatory activities and

inhibits stromal cells support for multiple myeloma tumour cell growth
- inhibits proliferation and induces apoptosis of haematopoietic tumour cells
- inhibits proliferation of lenalidomide-resistant multiple myeloma cell lines and synergises with dexamethasone in both lenalidomide-sensitive and lenalidomide-resistant cell lines to induce apoptosis
- enhances T cell and natural killer cell-mediated immunity, inhibiting production of pro-inflammatory cytokines by monocytes
- half-life about 9.5 hours

Use
- relapsed refractory multiple myeloma (with dexamethasone) in patients who have received two or more prior treatments (including lenalidomide) with disease progression
- relapsed or refractory multiple myeloma (with dexamethasone and bortezomib) who have received one prior treatment

Dose
- 4 mg orally daily on days 1–21 (of 28-day cycle) with dexamethasone 40 mg orally on days 1, 8, 15 and 22 (of 28-day cycle) **OR**
- 4 mg orally daily on days 1–14 (of 21-day cycle) with dexamethasone 20 mg on days 1, 2, 4, 5, 8, 9, 11 and 12, and bortezomib 1.3 mg/m^2 IV or SC on days 1, 4, 8 and 11 (for cycles 1 to 8), then dexamethasone 20 mg orally daily on days 1, 2, 8 and 9, and bortezomib 1.3 mg/mg^2 IV or SC on days 1 and 8 (for cycle 9 and onwards)

Adverse effects
- dizziness, fatigue, tremor, insomnia, depression
- peripheral neuropathy, paraesthesia
- syncope
- constipation, diarrhoea, nausea, vomiting, decreased weight, altered taste, abdominal pain, stomatitis, dry mouth, abdominal distension
- fever
- peripheral oedema
- anaemia, neutropenia, febrile neutropenia, thrombocytopenia, leucopenia
- pneumonia, upper and lower respiratory tract infection, bronchitis, nasopharyngitis
- dyspnoea, cough, pulmonary embolism
- rash
- atrial fibrillation, hypotension, hypertension
- cataract
- non-cardiac chest pain
- bone pain, back pain, muscle spasm, muscular weakness
- hyperkalaemia, hypokalaemia, hyperglycaemia, hypermagnesaemia, hypophosphataemia, hypocalcaemia
- elevated liver enzymes and bilirubin
- urinary retention, renal failure
- deep vein thrombosis
- (rare) angioedema, severe dermatological reactions, malignancies, tumour lysis syndrome, interstitial lung disease, pneumonitis

Interactions
- caution if used with warfarin. INR should be monitored during therapy, especially when starting, stopping or altering dose
- effectiveness reduced by smoking

Nursing points/Cautions

- only doctors and pharmacists who are registered with restricted distribution (i-access) program can prescribe and dispense pomalidomide to patients who meet all requirements and are registered with this program
- unless other contraindicated, anticoagulation therapy (e.g. aspirin, warfarin, heparin, clopidogrel) is recommended to decrease risk of thromboembolic events

- blood counts should be monitored weekly for first 8 weeks, then monthly during therapy
- liver function should be monitored regularly during therapy
- therapy should only be started when platelet count $\geq 50 \times 10^9$/L and neutrophil count $\geq 1.0 \times 10^9$/L. Dose modification or interruption to therapy is required for haematological issues such as a fall in platelets or a fall in absolute neutrophil count (ANC)
- to be eligible for therapy, a female patient (or female partner of male patient) is considered to no longer be of childbearing potential if she:
  - is over 50 years and has been naturally amenorrhoeic for $\geq$ 1 year (however, amenorrhoea post-chemotherapy does not rule out childbearing potential)
  - has premature ovarian failure (confirmed by specialist gynaecologist)
  - has had a hysterectomy or bilateral salpingo-oophorectomy
  - has uterine agenesis, Turner syndrome or XY genotype
- it is recommended that women of childbearing potential should have a pregnancy test before starting therapy, weekly during first month and then monthly (if menstrual cycles are regular) or 2-weekly (if menstrual cycles are irregular)
- if patient > 75 years, dexamethasone dose should be decreased to 20 mg
- if pregnancy occurs in a female treated with pomalidomide or she has a male partner taking pomalidomide, therapy should be stopped and the woman referred to a physician specialising/experienced in teratology for evaluation and advice
- caution if used in those with peripheral neuropathy
- caution if used in those with renal impairment or high tumour burden due to increased risk of tumour lysis syndrome
- contraindicated in females of child-bearing potential and male patients unless all of the conditions of the i-access program have been met
- contraindicated in those who have had previous allergic reactions to thalidomide or lenalidomide

Patient teaching and advice

- instruct patient to take capsules at same time every day and swallow whole (not chewed, broken, opened or divided). If powder from capsules makes contact with skin, the skin should be immediately washed with soap and water. If powder makes contact with mucous membranes, the area should be flushed well with water
- patient should be advised that if a dose is missed by more than 12 hours it should not be taken. The next dose should be taken at the normal time on the next day
- advise patient to stop smoking before starting therapy. However, any changes to smoking habit during therapy should be discussed with doctor as smoking alters effectiveness of pomalidomide
- patient must receive counselling to ensure good understanding of the potential therapy risks and outcomes (i.e. risks to unborn child), and contraceptive requirements associated with pomalidomide before giving a full and written consent prior to starting therapy. The patient's sexual partner should also receive counselling and information
- important patient advice should include:
  - do not drive or operate machinery if fatigue, dizziness, blurred vision and/or somnolence occurs

- seek medical advice immediately if any of the following occur:
  - any shortness of breath, sudden chest pain, cough or arm/leg swelling/tenderness, discolouration or warmth of limb (symptoms of DVT and PE)
  - febrile illness (neutropenia)
  - unusual bruising or bleeding, nosebleeds
  - numbness, tingling or pain in hands or feet
  - fever, chills, muscle/joint pain, headache, cough, shortness of breath, fatigue, loss of appetite
- do not donate blood during therapy or within 1 week of stopping therapy (all patients with multiple myelomas are permanently excluded from donating blood in Australia)
- male patient must not donate semen during or within 1 week of stopping therapy
- male patients should be advised that pomalidomide is present in semen and therefore adequate contraceptive methods (latex or polyurethane condoms) must be used during sexual activity with women of childbearing potential (or who have not been menopausal for at least 2 years); condom use must continue for at least 4 weeks after stopping therapy
- emphasise the importance of having a medically supervised pregnancy test at the time of consultation (or within 3 days prior to visit) to exclude pregnancy before the start of therapy, with a medically supervised pregnancy test repeated every 4 weeks, including when therapy is stopped
- women of childbearing potential (who have not had a hysterectomy, salpingo-oophorectomy or are not ≥ 50 years and post-menopausal for more than 1 year) must use one reliable contraceptive measure (e.g. intrauterine device, contraceptive hormonal implant, tubal ligation, partner vasectomy (with 2 negative semen analyses), progesterone-only pills, medroxyprogesterone acetate depot) for 1 month before, during and 1 month after stopping therapy
- copper-releasing intrauterine devices (IUD) are not recommended due to risk of infection (at time of insertion) and menstrual blood loss, which can compromise female patients with neutropenia or thrombocytopenia
- combined oral contraceptive pills are not recommended due to the increased risk of venous thromboembolism
- any woman (either taking pomalidomide or whose partner is taking pomalidomide) who is of childbearing potential and who experiences menstrual irregularities or suspects she is pregnant must seek medical advice immediately
- emphasise the importance of not sharing this medication with anyone and returning any unused capsules to the pharmacist at the end of therapy

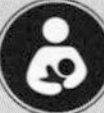

under NO circumstances should pomalidomide be used during pregnancy because of its relationship to thalidomide. Thalidomide is a known human teratogen that causes life-threatening human birth defects. If taken during pregnancy it may cause death to unborn baby or birth defects, which include absence or shortness of limbs, external ear abnormalities, eye abnormalities, facial palsy, congenital heart defects and malformation of the alimentary tract, urinary tract and/or genital tract

contraindicated during breastfeeding

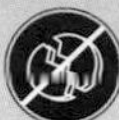

teratogen – capsules must not be opened or crushed

RISANKIZUMAB (Skyrizi)

Available form
Prefilled syringe: 75 mg/0.83 mL

Action
- humanised IgG1 monoclonal antibody that selectively binds to interleukin-23 (subunit p19) (known to be involved in inflammation and immune response)

Use
- treatment of moderate-to-severe plaque psoriasis in those who are candidates for systemic or phototherapy

Dose
- 150 mg SC at week 0, week 4 and every 12 weeks afterwards

Adverse effects
- upper respiratory tract infection, tinea infection, folliculitis
- headache, fatigue
- injection site reaction
- (rare) hypersensitivity

Interactions
- see General Interactions for immunomodifiers (p. 1176)

Nursing points/Cautions
- see General Nursing points/Cautions for immunomodifiers (p. 1176)
- patient may be taught to self-administer. First injection should be under medical supervision

Patient teaching and advice
- see Patient teaching and advice for icatibant (p. 1195) for self-administration instructions
- see also General Patient teaching and advice for immunomodifiers (p. 1177)

should only be used during pregnancy or breastfeeding if benefits are thought to outweigh risks

SECUKINUMAB (Cosentyx)

Available form
Prefilled pen: 150 mg/mL

Action
- monoclonal antibody IgG_{1kappa} that inhibits interleukin 17A, which is a pro-inflammatory cytokine that is involved in normal inflammatory and immune responses
- half-life 14–41 days (in those with plaque psoriasis)

Use
- treatment of moderate-to-severe plaque psoriasis in those who are candidates for systemic or phototherapy
- psoriatic arthritis (where previous response to DMARD was inadequate)
- ankylosing spondylitis

Dose
- (plaque psoriasis) initially 300 mg SC at weeks 0, 1, 2, 3 and 4, followed by 300 mg monthly (as maintenance) **OR**
- (psoriatic arthritis, ankylosing spondylitis) initially 150 mg SC at weeks 0, 1, 2, 3 and 4, followed by 150 mg monthly (as maintenance)

Adverse effects
- nasopharyngitis, rhinitis, pharyngitis, upper respiratory tract infections, rhinorrhoea
- oral herpes
- diarrhoea
- urticaria
- elevated liver enzymes, cholesterol and triglycerides
- (uncommon) conjunctivitis, neutropenia, sinusitis, otitis externa
- (rare) antibody development

- see also General Adverse effects of immunomodifiers (p. 1176)

Interactions

- see General Interactions of immunomodifiers (p. 1176)

Nursing points/Cautions

- 300 mg dose is given as 2 SC injections of 150 mg
- prefilled pen cap contains a latex derivative which may cause a reaction in latex-sensitive individuals
- patient may be taught to self-administer. First administration should be under medical supervision
- caution if used in those with active Crohn's disease as it may be exacerbated by therapy
- caution if used in those with chronic infection or history of recurrent infection
- contraindicated in those with active infection such as tuberculosis. Infection should be treated before starting therapy
- see also General Nursing points/Cautions for immunomodifiers (p. 1176)

Patient teaching and advice

- instruct patient in SC self-administration technique (see Patient teaching and advice for icatibant, p. 1195), including avoiding injecting into areas not affected by psoriasis
- see also General Patient teaching and advice for immunomodifiers (p. 1177)

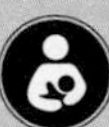

should only be used during pregnancy if benefits outweigh risks. If used during pregnancy, infants should not be vaccinated with live vaccines for at least 16 weeks after mother's last dose

caution if used during breastfeeding

SIPONIMOD (Mayzent)

Available forms

Tablets: 0.25 mg, 2 mg

Action

- sphingosine 1-phosphate receptor modulator that is metabolised to active metabolite fingolimod phosphate
- binds to specific receptors on lymphocytes leading to a redistribution rather than depletion of lymphocytes, reducing the infiltration into the CNS (and associated nerve inflammation and tissue damage)
- readily crosses blood–brain barrier

Use

- treatment of secondary progressive MS

Dose

- 0.25 mg orally daily (days 1 and 2), then 0.5 mg (day 3), 0.75 mg (day 4), 1.25 mg (day 5), then 2 mg (day 6 and maintenance)

Adverse effects

- headache, dizziness, asthenia, tremor
- seizures
- diarrhoea, nausea
- change in lung function
- infection (herpes zoster)
- eye pain, blurred vision, decreased visual acuity, macular oedema
- pain in extremity
- bradycardia, hypertension, AV block
- peripheral oedema
- lymphopenia
- abnormal liver tests, increased liver enzymes
- (rare) posterior reversible encephalopathy syndrome (PRES), progressive multifocal leukoencephalopathy (PML), lymphomas, skin cancers

Interactions

- not recommended with Class Ia or Class III (amiodarone, sotalol) antiarrhythmic agents

- not recommended with digoxin, ivabradine, calcium-channel blockers (that lower heart rate) or beta adrenoreceptor blocking agents due to risk of increased bradycardia
- caution if given with antineoplastic or immunosuppressive therapy (including corticosteroids) due to additive effects on immune system
- not recommended with or within 1 month of live or live attenuated vaccines
- not recommended after therapy with alemtuzumab (unless benefits clearly outweigh risks)

Nursing points/Cautions

- before starting therapy, patient's CYP2C9 genotype should be determined
- patient's immunity to varicella zoster virus (chicken pox, herpes zoster (shingles)) should be assessed (including serological testing) before starting therapy because the response to the virus may be severe if exposed and unprotected
- any infection should be excluded or treated before starting therapy
- complete blood count, liver function test and ophthalmologic examination (including visual acuity and fundus examination) should be performed before starting therapy. Ophthalmologic examination should be repeated after 3–4 months of therapy (especially in those with diabetes mellitus or history of uveitis)
- an ECG is recommended before starting therapy (especially in those with pre-existing slow or irregular heartbeat, cardiac risk factors or taking medications with antiarrhythmic actions)
- (first dose procedure for those with sinus bradycardia, AV block or history of myocardial infarction or heart failure) monitoring heart rate and BP hourly for 6 hours after initial dose is recommended, along with an ECG at the completion of the monitoring time
- if one dose is missed during titration period (days 1 to 6) or if therapy is interrupted for 4 or more days, titration regimen needs to be restarted
- if switching from other immunomodifying agents, half-life and mode of action should be considered before starting therapy to avoid additive immunosuppression. Remains in blood for up to 10 days
- if therapy is discontinued, patient should be closely monitored as severe exacerbation of disease may occur
- caution if used in those with history of uveitis or diabetes mellitus due to increased risk of macular oedema
- caution if used in those with history of recurrent syncope or symptomatic bradycardia
- caution if used in those with asthma
- not recommended in those with risk factors for QT prolongation such as hypokalaemia, hypomagnesaemia or congenital QT prolongation
- not recommended in patient with history of myocardial infarction or cardiac arrest, congestive heart failure, uncontrolled hypertension, cerebrovascular disease or untreated sleep apnoea
- not recommended in those with SA block, second degree AV block or higher, sick sinus syndrome (unless patient has pacemaker) or with QTc interval prolongation (≥ 500 msec)
- contraindicated in those with CYP2C9*3*3 genotype

Patient teaching and advice

- patient should be advised that after first dose procedure involves hourly heart rate and blood pressure monitoring for 6 hours with ECG at the end
- warn patient that heart rate may slow down during therapy

- patient should be advised not to drive or operate machinery if dizziness or visual disturbances occur
- advise patient to seek medical advice immediately if any of the following occur:
  - changes to vision (e.g. centre of vision is blurry or has shadows, blindspot, difficulty seeing colour or fine details), especially in first 4 months of therapy
  - nausea, vomiting, abdominal pain, fatigue, loss of appetite, yellowing of skin or eyes, dark urine
  - sudden severe headache, nausea, vomiting, visual disturbances, fitting or altered mental state
  - any signs of infections including flu-like symptoms, fever, chills, sore throat, joint or aching muscles, cough (up to 8 weeks after stopping therapy)
  - any new or changed skin lesions
- patient and carer/partner should be advised to immediately report any unusual, worse or prolonged neurological symptoms, including difficulty performing mental tasks, unusual behaviour, confusion or personality changes (may be signs of PML or progression of MS)
- female patients of childbearing potential should be counselled to use effective contraception during and for at least 10 days after stopping therapy. If pregnancy occurs patient should be advised to immediately seek medical advice
- see General Patient teaching and advice (p. xxvii)

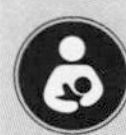
not recommended during pregnancy or breastfeeding

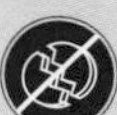
tablet should not be crushed or broken

SIROLIMUS (Rapamune)

Available forms

Oral solution: 1 mg/mL; Tablets: 0.5 mg, 1 mg, 2 mg

Action

- selective immunosuppressant agent that inhibits T cell activation
- blocks calcium-dependent and calcium-independent intracellular signals that cause T cell activation suppressing immune-mediated reactions (e.g. allograft rejection)
- long half-life (48–78 hours)

Use

- prevention of organ rejection in those at mild-to-moderate risk after receiving a renal transplant (with ciclosporin and corticosteroids)

Dose

- initially 6 mg orally (as soon as possible after transplantation) (loading dose), followed by 2 mg orally daily (with ciclosporin and corticosteroids). After 2–4 months, ciclosporin is gradually withdrawn over 4–8 weeks; sirolimus dose should be adjusted to maintain blood concentration of 12–20 nanogram/mL (daily maximum 40 mg)

Adverse effects

- peripheral oedema, oedema and rarely, lymphoedema
- delayed wound healing, wound dehiscence, lymphocele
- fever
- tachycardia, thromboembolism (DVT, PE), hypertension, pericardial effusion
- nausea, abdominal pain, diarrhoea, stomatitis, constipation, ascites, pancreatitis
- anaemia, thrombocytopenia, leucopenia, neutropenia, haemolytic uraemic syndrome, and uncommonly, thrombotic thrombocytopaenic purpura
- abnormal liver function tests, elevated liver enzymes and creatinine

- hypertriglycidaemia, hyperlipidaemia, hypophosphataemia, hypokalaemia, hyperglycaemia
- arthralgia, bone necrosis
- epistaxis
- pleural effusion, pneumonia, pneumonitis
- acne, rash
- pyelonephritis, proteinuria
- headache
- pain
- amenorrhoea, menorrhagia, ovarian cyst
- (rare) interstitial lung disease, pneumonitis, angioedema
- see also General Adverse effects of immunomodifiers (p. 1176)

Interactions

- not recommended with grapefruit juice
- long-term therapy with ciclosporin is not recommended
- increased risk of angioedema if given with ACE inhibitors
- serum levels may increase if given with voriconazole, fluconazole, itraconazole, clarithromycin, erythromycin, ciclosporin, metoclopramide, bromocriptine, cimetidine, danazol, diltiazem, verapamil and protease inhibitors (e.g. ritonavir, indinavir), therefore not recommended together
- serum levels may be decreased if given with rifampicin, rifabutin, phenytoin, phenobarbital (phenobarbitone), carbamazepine and St John's wort, therefore not recommended together
- caution if given with other agents that impair kidney function
- increased risk of rhabdomyolysis if given with HMG-CoA reductase inhibitors or ciclosporin
- see General Interactions of immunomodifiers (p. 1176)

Nursing points/Cautions

- renal function, serum cholesterol and triglyceride levels should be monitored throughout therapy (especially during concurrent ciclosporin therapy)
- urine should be monitored for traces of protein
- combined therapy with ciclosporin should not exceed 3 months post-transplantation
- when measuring blood levels, same dose should be maintained for 3 days (with loading dose) or 7–14 days (without loading dose) to achieve steady-state before adjusting dosage
- blood levels should be measured 7–14 days after switching between different tablet strengths (e.g. 2 mg to 5 mg tablets)
- 2 mg of oral solution = 2 × 1 mg tablets and are therefore interchangeable
- new loading dose may be required if a large dose increase is necessary; calculated according to the following: loading dose = 3 × (new maintenance dose – current maintenance dose)
- if the calculated dose is greater than 40 mg daily maximum dose, dose should be split into two loading doses given over 2 days. Trough level should be measured 3–4 days after new loading dose
- antimicrobial prophylaxis should be given for 12 months to prevent *Pneumocystis carinii* pneumonia (PCP) and for 3 months to prevent cytomegalovirus (CMV) infection
- increased risk of delayed wound healing if used in those with BMI > 30 kg/m^2
- caution if used in those with severe liver impairment as clearance will be decreased and lower maintenance dose required
- not recommended for liver or lung transplantation
- see also General Nursing points/Cautions for immunomodifiers (p. 1176)

Patient teaching and advice

- advise patient to take tablets or oral solution consistently either with or after food, but not switch between the two
- instruct patient to swallow tablets whole, not broken or chewed
- patient should be advised to withdraw dose from bottle using syringe, then add to glass or plastic cup and mix thoroughly with at least 60 mL of water or orange juice (no other liquids should be used) and drink immediately. Glass should be refilled with at least 120 mL of water or orange juice, stirred thoroughly again and drunk
- instruct patient to discard any oral solution 4 weeks after opening
- patient should be advised that it is common for solution to appear white to off-white when mixed with water or orange juice
- patient should be warned to avoid grapefruit juice during therapy
- instruct patient to take 4 hours after ciclosporin and at the same time every day consistently with or without food
- warn patient that refrigerating solution may result in harmless haze, which disappears when solution is allowed to stand at room temperature
- if solution comes into contact with skin or mucous membranes (e.g. eyes), skin should be washed with soap and water or eyes rinsed with water
- advise patient to seek medical advice immediately if any of the following occur:
  - any shortness of breath, sudden chest pain, cough or arm/leg swelling/tenderness, discolouration or warmth of limb (symptoms of DVT and PE)
  - febrile illness (neutropenia)
  - unusual bruising or bleeding, nosebleeds
  - fever, chills, muscle/joint pain, headache, cough, shortness of breath, fatigue, loss of appetite
- counsel female patient of childbearing potential regarding the importance of using reliable contraception during and for 12 weeks after stopping therapy to avoid pregnancy and seeking medical advice if pregnancy occurs
- see General Patient teaching and advice for immunomodifiers (p. 1177)

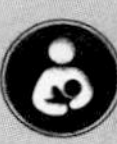
should only be used during pregnancy or breastfeeding if benefits outweigh potential risks

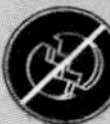
oral solution is available. Tablet should not be divided, broken or crushed

TACROLIMUS (Advagraf XL, Pacrolim, Prograf, Tacrograf)

Available forms
Capsules: 0.5 mg, 1 mg, 5 mg; Capsules (extended release): 0.5 mg, 1 mg, 5 mg; Ampoule: 5 mg/mL

Action
- macrolide lactone that inhibits lymphocyte formation thought to be responsible for graft rejection
- suppresses T cell activation, T helper cell dependent B cell proliferation and lymphokine formation
- half-life about 43 hours

Use
- adjunct to lung, heart, liver or kidney allograft transplantation

Dose
- (liver transplantation) 0.10–0.20 mg/kg orally daily 1 hour before food in 2 divided doses (Prograf, Pacrolim, Tacrograf) or single dose (Advagraf XL),

starting 6 hours after liver transplantation **OR**

- (liver transplantation) 0.01–0.05 mg/kg by IV infusion over 24 hours (if oral administration is not possible) **OR**
- (kidney transplantation) 0.15–0.30 mg/kg orally daily 1 hour before food in 2 divided doses (Prograf, Pacrolim, Tacrograf) or single dose (Advagraf XL), starting within 24 hours of kidney transplantation **OR**
- (kidney transplantation) 0.04–0.06 mg/kg by IV infusion over 24 hours (if oral administration is not possible) **OR**
- (lung transplantation) 0.10–0.30 mg/kg orally daily 1 hour before food in 2 divided doses (Prograf, Pacrolim, Tacrograf) or single dose (Advagraf XL), starting 24 hours after lung transplantation **OR**
- (lung transplantation) 0.01–0.05 mg/kg by IV infusion over 24 hours (if oral administration is not possible) **OR**
- (heart transplantation) 0.075 mg/kg orally daily 1 hour before food in 2 divided doses (Prograf, Pacrolim, Tacrograf) or single dose (Advagraf XL), starting 24 hours after lung transplantation **OR**
- (heart transplantation) 0.01–0.02 mg/kg by IV infusion over 24 hours (if oral administration is not possible)

Adverse effects

- tremor, headache, abnormal dreams, insomnia, depression, anxiety, confusion, dizziness, disorientation, seizures, asthenia, mood disorder, depression, hallucination
- paraesthesia, peripheral neuropathy
- anorexia, diarrhoea, nausea, vomiting, dyspepsia, flatulence, abdominal pain/distention, constipation, stomatitis, bloating, gastrointestinal ulceration and perforation
- fever
- hypertension, tachycardia, fluid overload, ventricular/septal hypertrophy (cardiomyopathy), heart failure, arrhythmias, QT interval prolongation
- thromboembolic and ischaemic events, peripheral vascular disease
- renal dysfunction, renal failure, oliguria, bladder/urethral symptoms
- abnormal liver function tests, cholestasis, jaundice, hepatitis, ascites
- hyperkalaemia, hypomagnesaemia, hyperphosphataemia, hyperuricaemia, hypokalaemia, hypocalcaemia, hyponatraemia, hyperglycaemia, diabetes mellitus, post-transplant diabetes mellitus
- hypercholesterolaemia, hyperlipidaemia, hypertriglyceridaemia
- anaemia, leucopenia, thrombocytopenia, leukocytosis, pure red cell aplasia
- pruritus, rash, acne, sweating, alopecia
- blurred vision, photophobia, eye disorder
- tinnitus
- arthralgia, myalgia, muscle cramps, limb and back pain
- dyspnoea, pleural effusion, cough, nasal congestion, pharyngitis
- neurotoxicity (e.g. tremor, headache, insomnia, seizures, motor function changes, mental status changes), posterior reversible encephalopathy syndrome (PRES) (e.g. headache, visual disturbances, altered mental state)
- primary graft dysfunction
- anaphylaxis, allergic reaction
- see also General Adverse effects of immunomodifiers (p. 1176)

Interactions

- contraindicated with ciclosporin, because of additive nephrotoxicity and increase in ciclosporin half-life. An interval of 24 hours should be allowed between stopping one therapy and starting the other and

ciclosporin blood levels should be closely monitored
- contraindicated with potassium-sparing diuretics
- caution if used with other nephrotoxic agents such as aminoglycosides, amphotericin B (amphotericin), cotrimoxazole, vancomycin, NSAIDs, acyclovir, ganciclovir and ibuprofen
- increased risk of hyperkalaemia if potassium supplements or potassium-sparing diuretics are given
- caution if given with other agents known to prolong QT interval
- serum levels may increase if given with grapefruit juice
- caution if given with mycophenolate products. Mycophenolate serum levels should be monitored during therapy
- increased serum level may occur if given with amiodarone, amphotericin B (amphotericin), bromocriptine, cimetidine, clarithromycin, clotrimazole, cortisone, danazol, dapsone, diltiazem, erythromycin, ethinylestradiol, fluconazole, gestodene, itraconazole, lidocaine (lignocaine), methylprednisolone (high dose) midazolam, nelfinavir, nifedipine, omeprazole, prednisolone (high dose), ritonavir, saquinavir, tamoxifen, telaprevir, verapamil and voriconazole
- may increase serum levels of phenytoin, increasing the risk of toxicity
- decreased serum level may occur if given with dexamethasone, rifampicin, sodium bicarbonate, aluminium hydroxide, magnesium oxide, phenobarbital (phenobarbitone), carbamazepine, phenytoin, isoniazid and St John's wort
- absorption may be increased by metoclopramide. Serum levels of tacrolimus should be closely monitored
- see also General Interactions of immunomodifiers (p. 1176)

Nursing points/Cautions

- oral administration should start as soon as possible. First oral dose should be given 8–12 hours after stopping IV infusion
- for first few months after transplantation, BP, ECG, visual status, blood glucose, creatinine, urea and electrolyte concentrations (especially potassium), urinary output, haematology, coagulation, liver and renal function tests should be monitored frequently
- if switching from ciclosporin, therapy should be started 12–24 hours after stopping ciclosporin. If ciclosporin serum levels are high, therapy should not be started and ciclosporin levels closely monitored
- patient should not be switched between different formulations of tacrolimus once effective dosage has been established
- trough serum levels should be measured 12 hours after immediate-release preparations or 24 hours after extended-release capsules
- care should be taken when selecting dose/formulations of tacrolimus as medication errors have resulted in the past
- refrigerating IV solution may result in harmless haze, which disappears when solution is allowed to stand at room temperature
- if IV solution comes into contact with skin or mucous membranes (e.g. eyes), skin should be washed with soap and water or eyes rinsed with water
- not recommended as IV bolus
- IV concentrate should be diluted using glucose 5% or sodium chloride 0.9%
- IV solution is incompatible with PVC plastic
- caution if used in those with neurological or CNS disorders (because they can be exacerbated), diabetes mellitus, pre-existing heart disease,

liver or kidney impairment, renal/liver dysfunction, fluid overload or hypertension
- caution if given to those who have previously received polyoxyethylene hydrogenated castor oil or have allergic predisposition, because they have increased risk of anaphylaxis
- caution if used in those with congenital or acquired QT prolongation
- contraindicated in those with known hypersensitivity to other macrolides or polyoxyethylene hydrogenated castor oil (found in Prograf Concentrated Injection)
- see also General Nursing points/Cautions for immunomodifiers (p. 1176)

Patient teaching and advice

- instruct patient to take tablets on an empty stomach either 1 hour before or 2 hours after food
- advise patient to avoid grapefruit juice during therapy
- patient should be advised to avoid high-potassium diet during therapy
- warn patient against driving or operating machinery if visual disturbances, dizziness or hallucinations occur
- patient should be advised to seek medical advice immediately if any of the following occur:
  - numbness or tingling in hands or feet (signs of peripheral neuropathy)
  - tremor
  - headache, insomnia, changes in motor function, sensory function, mental status or fitting (signs of neurotoxicity)
  - headache, altered mental state, visual disturbances or fitting (signs of PRES)
  - yellowing of eyes/skin, tiredness, loss of appetite, nausea, vomiting, dark urine, upper abdominal pain (jaundice, hepatitis)
  - palpitation, abnormal heart rate
  - severe abdominal pain, nausea, vomiting, fever, chills (GI perforation signs)
- see also General Patient teaching and advice for immunomodifiers (p. 1177)

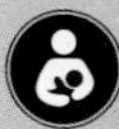

should only be used during pregnancy if benefits outweigh risks as therapy has been linked to neonatal hyperkalaemia and kidney dysfunction. If used during pregnancy, maternal BP and blood glucose levels should be closely monitored

not recommended during breastfeeding

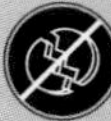

immediate-release capsules only – capsules can be opened and contents dispersed in water. Mask and gloves must be worn

TEMSIROLIMUS (Torisel)

Available form

- Vial: 25 mg

Action

- metabolised to sirolimus (metabolite is equally potent)
- selective immunosuppressant agent that inhibits T cell activation
- blocks calcium-dependent and calcium-independent intracellular signals that cause T cell activation

Use

- advanced renal cell carcinoma
- relapsed and/or refractory mantle cell lymphoma

Dose

- (renal cell carcinoma) 25 mg by IV infusion over 30–60 minutes weekly
OR
- (mantle cell lymphoma) 175 mg by IV infusion over 30–60 minutes weekly for 3 weeks, then reducing to 75 mg IV weekly

Adverse effects

- hypersensitivity/infusion reaction (flushing, chest pain, dyspnoea, hypotension, apnoea, unconsciousness, anaphylaxis)
- rash, pruritus, dry skin, nail disorder, acne
- asthenia, headache, anxiety, dizziness, insomnia, somnolence, fatigue, depression, seizures
- paraesthesia
- back pain, pain, arthralgia, myalgia, muscle cramps
- fever, chills
- oedema (generalised, facial, peripheral, genital)
- hypertension, chest pain, venous thromboembolism (including DVT, PE), pericardial effusion
- mucositis, nausea, vomiting, anorexia, diarrhoea, abdominal pain/distention, constipation, anorexia, dysphagia, altered taste, stomatitis, gastrointestinal haemorrhage, bowel perforation, decreased weight, gingivitis, gastritis, mouth pain
- dehydration
- cataract formation, conjunctivitis, eye haemorrhage
- hyperglycaemia, glucose intolerance, diabetes mellitus
- hyperlipidaemia, hypertriglyceridaemia, hypophosphataemia, hypokalaemia
- delayed wound healing
- thrombocytopenia, neutropenia, anaemia, lymphopenia, leucopenia
- elevated liver enzymes, liver impairment
- elevated creatinine, renal failure
- dyspnoea, cough, epistaxis, pleural effusion, rhinitis, sinusitis, pharyngitis
- (IV) thrombophlebitis
- (rare) interstitial lung disease
- see General Adverse effects of immunomodifiers (p. 1176)

Interactions

- caution if used with anticoagulants as there is an increased risk of intracerebral bleeding
- increased risk of angioedema if given with ACE inhibitors or calcium-channel blockers
- not recommended with carbamazepine, phenytoin, barbiturates, rifabutin, rifampicin or St John's wort as serum levels may be decreased
- not recommended with atazanavir, indinavir, ritonavir, saquinavir, itraconazole, clarithromycin and SSRIs as serum levels may be increased
- caution if given with sunitinib due to risk of increased toxicity
- see General Interactions of immunomodifiers (p. 1176)

Nursing points/Cautions

- liver function, serum bilirubin and serum lipids should be measured before starting and regularly during therapy
- hypersensitivity reaction usually occurs early during first infusion (but can occur in following infusions) and patients should be closely monitored during this time
- premedication with antihistamine IV 30 minutes before infusion is recommended to decrease the likelihood of hypersensitivity reaction
- if hypersensitivity occurs despite the use of antihistamine, infusion should be stopped and patient monitored for 30–60 minutes. Depending on the severity of the reaction, the doctor may order the infusion restarted at a slower rate with an H_1-receptor antagonist (if not previously given) and/or H_2-antagonist (e.g. ranitidine) (given 30 minutes before restarting infusion)
- add 1.8 mL of provided diluent to vial and invert. When bubbles subside, solution should be colourless to light yellow and free from particles
- withdraw 2.5 mL of reconstituted fluid and add to 250 mL sodium chloride 0.9% and invert gently to mix. Solution should be infused over 30–60 minutes

- avoid shaking as this may cause foaming
- PVC tubing or infusion sets/bags made of soft plastic (e.g. ethylene vinyl acetate) should not be used
- inline filter (less than 5 microns) and infusion pump are recommended for IV administration
- administer alone
- reconstituted solution should be protected from excessive room or sun light
- caution if used in those with hypersensitivity to sirolimus, mild liver impairment, CNS tumours or metastases (as there is an increased risk of intracerebral bleeding) or renal insufficiency
- caution if used in peri-surgical period due to risk of delayed wound healing
- contraindicated in those with bilirubin > 1.5 times upper limits of normal levels
- see also General Nursing points/Cautions for immunomodifiers (p. 1176)

Patient teaching and advice

- see also General Patient teaching and advice for immunomodifiers (p. 1177)
- warn patient not to drive or operate machinery if dizziness, anxiety or visual disturbances occur
- patients should be advised to report any:
  - excessive thirst or increase in the frequency or amount of urination (may indicate glucose intolerance)
  - cough, fever, shortness of breath or difficulty breathing (interstitial lung disease)
- counsel female patient regarding the importance of using reliable contraception before starting, during and for 12 weeks after stopping therapy to avoid pregnancy and immediately seek medical advice if pregnancy occurs
- male patient should be counselled regarding the unknown effects on sperm or fetus and therefore the importance of using adequate contraception during and for 12 weeks after stopping therapy

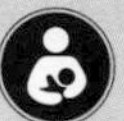

not recommended during pregnancy or breastfeeding

TILDRAKIZUMAB (Ilumya)

Available form
Prefilled syringe: 100 mg/mL

Action
- IgG1/kappa monoclonal antibody that binds specifically to interleukin 23 (subunit p19) (which is involved in inflammatory and immune responses)

Use
- moderate-to-severe plaque psoriasis (in those eligible for systemic therapy)

Dose
- 100 mg SC at week 0, 4 and every 12 weeks afterwards

Adverse effects
- headache, fatigue
- nausea, diarrhoea
- nasopharyngitis, sinusitis
- arthralgia, back pain, pain in extremity
- (injection site) pain
- see also General Adverse effects of immunomodifiers (p. 1176)

Interactions
- see General Interactions of immunomodifiers (p. 1176)

Nursing points/Cautions

- see General Nursing points/Cautions for immunomodifiers (p. 1176)
- patient may be taught to self-administer. First injection should be under medical supervision

- caution if used in those with chronic infection or history of recurrent infection

Patient teaching and advice

- see Patient teaching and advice for icatibant (p. 1195) for self-administration instructions
- female patient of childbearing potential should be counselled to use effective contraception during and for at least 17 weeks post therapy
- see also General Patient teaching and advice for immunomodifiers (p. 1177)

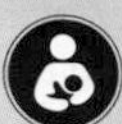

not recommended during pregnancy or breastfeeding unless benefits outweigh risks

USTEKINUMAB (Stelara)

Available forms

Vial: 45 mg/0.5 mL (SC); Vial: 130 mg/26 mL (IV)

Action

- IgG1 kappa monoclonal antibody that binds to interleukin (IL) 12 and 23 interrupting signalling and cytokines involved in psoriasis

Use

- treatment of moderate-to-severe plaque psoriasis in those who are candidates for phototherapy or systemic therapy and over 18 years
- active psoriatic arthritis (with methotrexate) (in those with inadequate response to non-biologic DMARDs)
- moderate-to-severe active Crohn's disease or ulcerative colitis (in those with inadequate or lost response)

Dose

- (plaque psoriasis, psoriatic arthritis) 45 mg SC at weeks 0 and 4 and then 3-monthly **OR**
- (plaque psoriasis, psoriatic arthritis, patient weight > 100 kg) 90 mg SC at weeks 0 and 4 and then 3-monthly **OR**
- (Crohn's disease, ulcerative colitis) initially 260 mg (weight ≤ 55 kg), 390 mg IV (weight > 55 kg but ≤ 85 kg) or 520 mg (weight > 85 kg) by IV infusion over 1 hour, then 90 mg SC after 8 weeks, then 90 mg SC every 12 weeks

Adverse effects

- upper respiratory tract infection, nasopharyngitis, sinusitis
- dizziness, headache, fatigue and less commonly, depression
- pruritis
- oropharyngeal pain
- nausea, vomiting, diarrhoea
- back pain, myalgia, arthralgia
- (injection site) redness, pain
- antibody development
- (rare) reversible posterior leukoencephalopathy syndrome
- see General Adverse effects of immunomodifiers (p. 1176)

Interactions

- see General Interactions of immunomodifiers (p. 1176)
- caution if given with medications with narrow therapeutic index. Serum levels should be closely monitored if used together

Nursing points/Cautions

- (plaque psoriasis) if response is inadequate, therapy may be increased to every 8 weeks
- (psoriatic arthritis) if no response after 28 weeks, therapy should be re-evaluated
- (Crohn's disease) if therapy is interrupted, it may be resumed with SC administration every 8 weeks
- (Crohn's disease, ulcerative colitis) if response is inadequate during maintenance period, frequency can be reduced to every 8 weeks
- patient may be instructed to self-inject SC. First self-administration should be under medical supervision

- (IV) calculate number of vials required (and therefore volume). Withdraw and discard volume to be added from 250 mL sodium chloride 0.9% infusion bag (e.g. if 3 vials are required (390 mg), 78 mL should be discarded). Add required volume, gently invert infusion bag (do not shake) and infuse over 1 hour
- caution if used in those receiving or have undergone allergy treatment especially for anaphylaxis
- caution if used in those > 60 years, with prolonged use of immunosuppressants or history of PUVA therapy due to increased risk of non-melanoma skin cancer
- not recommended in those with past history of malignancy
- contraindicated if active clinically important infection is present (e.g. tuberculosis)
- see also General Nursing points/ Cautions for immunomodifiers (p. 1176)

Patient teaching and advice

- warn patient against driving or operating machinery if dizziness occurs
- advise patient to seek medical advice if any headache, seizures, confusion or visual disturbances occur
- see instructions for SC self-administration (see Patient teaching and advice for icatibant, p. 1195)
- counsel female patients of child-bearing potential of the importance of using effective contraception during and for 15 weeks after stopping therapy
- see also General Patient teaching and advice for immunomodifiers (p. 1177)

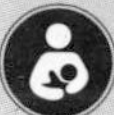

should only be used during pregnancy if benefits outweigh risks

not recommended during breastfeeding or for 15 weeks after stopping therapy

INTERFERONS

General Actions of interferons

- naturally occurring, small protein molecules produced and secreted by cells in response to viral infections or to various synthetic and biological inducers
- bind to specific cell surface receptors that are linked to inner cell networks that control enzyme activity, cell proliferation and immune activity enhancement (e.g. inhibit viral replication in virus-infected cells; enhance activity of macrophages and lymphocytes)
- produced by recombinant DNA technology

General Adverse effects of interferons

- flu-like symptoms (including fever, malaise, chills, sweating, fatigue, myalgia, arthralgia, loss of appetite, headache)
- drowsiness, somnolence, insomnia, dizziness, depression, anxiety, confusion, impaired concentration, nervousness
- vertigo
- nausea, vomiting, anorexia, diarrhoea, abdominal pain, weight loss, taste alteration, dry mouth
- anaemia, leucopenia, thrombocytopenia

- elevated liver enzymes, hypertriglyceridaemia
- reversible alopecia, pruritus, dry skin
- arthralgia, myalgia
- visual disturbances, retinopathy, retinal haemorrhage, cotton wool spots, retinal artery or vein thrombosis, optic neuropathy
- palpitations, transient hypotension or hypertension, chest pain, arrhythmias, oedema, cyanosis
- (alfa interferons, uncommon) cough, dyspnoea, pneumonia, pneumonitis, pulmonary infiltrates
- (alfa interferons) graft rejection
- (uncommon) altered liver function tests, elevated liver enzymes
- thyroid dysfunction
- (rare) hypersensitivity reaction (including bronchospasm, urticaria, anaphylaxis, angioedema), suicidal ideation, hyperglycaemia, diabetes mellitus, jaundice, hepatitis, seizures, development of anti-interferon antibodies, injection site reaction, exacerbation of psoriasis
- see also General Adverse effects of immunomodifiers (p. 1176)

General Nursing points/Cautions for interferons

- patient should be well hydrated before and during therapy (especially during initial stages of treatment) to prevent fluid depletion and hypotension
- monitor blood cell counts (with WBC differential, platelet count), electrolytes, serum creatinine, serum protein, serum lipids, thyroid and liver function before therapy, then at monthly or appropriate intervals during treatment. Ophthalmological examination is also recommended. Furthermore, ECG is recommended in those with pre-existing cardiac disease or advanced cancer
- (hepatitis B or C) liver biopsy should be performed before starting treatment to exclude other causes of hepatitis and determine extent of disease
- paracetamol 0.5–1 g can be taken orally 30 minutes before administration of interferon to alleviate symptoms of fever and headache, then up to 1 g 4 times daily
- chest X-ray is recommended if patient develops cough, dyspnoea or other respiratory symptoms
- any persistent fever should be investigated thoroughly
- all patients should be monitored for any signs of depression or suicidal ideation
- at the discretion of the doctor, patient may be educated to self-administer medication. First self-administered injection should be done under medical supervision
- ensure administered product name and batch number is documented in patient medical history
- when reconstituting solution, care should be taken to avoid foaming or shaking the solution when dissolving
- administer alone
- patients with chronic hepatitis not caused by hepatitis B or C should not be treated with interferon therapy
- (alfa interferons) caution if used in those with liver or other organ transplant due to increased risk of graft rejections
- caution if used in those with diabetes mellitus, because antidiabetic

therapy may need adjusting to control blood glucose levels, as well as increased risk of retinopathy and ketoacidosis occurring
- caution if used in those with psoriasis as disease may be exacerbated
- caution if used in those with severe bone marrow suppression due to increased risk of infection and/or bleeding
- caution if used in those with pre-existing cardiac disease; lung disease; severe kidney, liver or myeloid dysfunction; thyroid disease; history of seizures; compromised CNS function or neuropsychiatric disorders, including depression
- contraindicated in those with hypersensitivity to interferons (natural or recombinant), autoimmune disease, autoimmune hepatitis, chronic hepatitis with advanced decompensated liver disease or cirrhosis, chronic hepatitis recently treated with immunosuppressive therapy
- contraindicated in neonates and children under 3 years due to benzyl alcohol content
- see also General Nursing points/Cautions for immunomodifiers (p. 1176)

General Patient teaching and advice for interferons

- advise patient not to change brands without doctor's supervision
- warn patient about alopecia which sometimes continues for weeks after stopping therapy
- patients should be advised not to drive or operate machinery if adverse effects such as dizziness, confusion, somnolence, visual disturbance or fatigue occur
- instruct patient/family member/carer in correct administration (see Patient teaching and advice for icatibant, p. 1195)
- patient should be advised to seek medical advice immediately if any of the following occur:
  - loss or decrease in vision
  - increase in thirst and urination
  - persistent fever
  - fever, cough and difficulty breathing
  - depression, sadness, loss of appetite, withdrawal from friends or previously pleasurable activities, ideas of or attempts at self-harm or thoughts of suicide

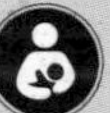

not recommended during pregnancy or breastfeeding unless benefits outweigh risks

INTERFERON ALFA 2A (Roferon-A)

Available forms

Prefilled syringe: 3 million IU/0.5 mL, 9 million IU/0.5 mL

Action

- see General Actions of interferons (p. 1222)

Use

- hairy cell leukaemia
- AIDS-related Kaposi's sarcoma
- chronic active hepatitis B (with no cirrhosis but elevated serum ALT)
- chronic hepatitis C (with ribavirin) (in previously untreated or relapsed patients)
- chronic hepatitis due to hepatitis C (with elevated serum ALT for at least 6 months without liver decompensation)
- low-grade non-Hodgkin lymphoma (with chemotherapy)

- cutaneous T cell lymphoma (mycosis fungoides, Sézary syndrome)
- chronic myelogenous leukaemia (CML)
- thrombocytosis associated with CML and other myeloproliferative disorders
- advanced and/or renal cell carcinoma

Dose

- (hairy cell leukaemia) initially 3 million IU SC daily for 16–24 weeks, then 3 million IU reduced to 3 times weekly (maintenance) for at least 6 months **OR**
- (Kaposi's sarcoma) initially 36 million IU SC daily for 4 weeks, but up to 12 weeks if tolerated, then frequency reduced to 3 times weekly **OR**
- (chronic active hepatitis B) 4.5 million IU SC 3 times weekly for 6 months, dose may be increased to a maximum of 18 million IU 3 times weekly if serum hepatitis B antigen does not decrease within 4 weeks **OR**
- (chronic hepatitis C – monotherapy) 3 million IU SC 3 times weekly for 12 months **OR**
- (chronic hepatitis C with ribavirin) 4.5 million IU SC 3 times weekly for 24 weeks (ribavirin dose 1–1.2 g daily depending on patient weight) **OR**
- (low-grade non-Hodgkin lymphoma) 3 million IU SC 3 times weekly for up to 12 months (as maintenance after treatment with chemotherapy with or without radiotherapy or as part of a chemotherapy regimen) **OR**
- (cutaneous T cell lymphoma) initially 3 million IU daily SC for 3 days, then 9 million IU daily for 3 days, then 18 million IU daily for 3 days, then frequency reduced to 3 times weekly for 8–12 weeks to establish responsiveness **OR**
- (CML) initially 3 million IU SC daily for 3 days, then increasing to 6 million IU for the next 3 days, then increasing to 9 million IU daily for 3–18 months **OR**
- (thrombocytosis associated with CML and other myeloproliferative disorders) 3 million IU SC daily for 3 days, then 6 million IU for 27 days, then frequency reduced to 1–3 million IU 2–3 times weekly (to maintain platelets in normal range) **OR**
- (advanced and/or metastatic renal cell carcinoma–monotherapy) 3 million IU SC 3 times weekly for 1 week, 9 million IU 3 times weekly for 1 week, then 18 million IU 3 times weekly, reducing to 9 million IU if higher dose is not tolerated, for 3–12 months **OR**
- (advanced and/or metastatic renal cell carcinoma – combined therapy with bevacizumab) initially 3–6 million IU 3 times weekly, increasing to 9 million IU 3 times weekly within 2 weeks for up to 12 months or disease progression. May be reduced to 3 million IU 3 times weekly if not tolerated

Adverse effects

- see General Adverse effects of interferons (p. 1222)

Interactions

- caution if given with other neurotoxic, haematotoxic or cardiotoxic agents
- not recommended with Chinese herbal medicine Xiao-Chai-Hu (also known as sho-saiko-to) because it may increase the risk of pulmonary symptoms
- clearance of theophylline may be reduced

Nursing points/Cautions

- when used with ribavirin or bevacizumab, see Adverse effects, Interactions and other points in Antiviral agents (ribavirin, p. 843), or Antineoplastic agents (bevacizumab, p. 599)
- (AIDS-related Kaposi's sarcoma) lesions should be measured and counted before starting therapy and then monthly throughout therapy

- (hairy cell leukaemia) quantification of peripheral hairy cells and bone marrow hairy cells should occur before starting therapy
- (hairy cell leukaemia) treatment should be continued for at least 6 months to determine clinical response
- (CML) treatment should continue for 8–12 weeks before deciding responsiveness
- (CML) not recommended in those who have a planned (or possible) allogeneic bone marrow transplantation
- (chronic hepatitis C, monotherapy) if serum ALT has not normalised in first 12 weeks, therapy should be re-evaluated
- if patient has pre-existing cardiac abnormalities or has an advanced stage of cancer, an ECG is recommended before starting and regularly during therapy
- caution when used in those with severe myelosuppression, because there is a further increased risk of infection or haemorrhage
- see also General Nursing points/Cautions for interferons (p. 1223)

Patient teaching and advice

- instruct patient in correct SC administration technique (see Patient teaching and advice for icatibant, p. 1195)
- see also General Patient teaching and advice for interferons (p. 1224)

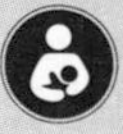

contraindicated during pregnancy as combination therapy with ribavirin, but not alone (see Antiviral agents, p. 843)

INTERFERON GAMMA 1B (Imukin)

Available form

Vial: 2 million IU (100 microgram)/0.5 mL

Action

- see General Actions of interferons (p. 1222)

Use

- chronic granulomatous disease (as adjunct therapy) to decrease frequency of serious infections

Dose

- (patient surface area $\leq$ 0.5 m^2) 30,000 IU (1.5 microgram)/kg SC 3 times weekly **OR**
- (patient surface area $>$ 0.5 m^2) 1 million IU (50 microgram)/m^2 SC 3 times weekly

Adverse effects

- see General Adverse effects of interferons (p. 1222)

Interactions

- caution if given with other hepatotoxic, myelosuppressive and/or nephrotoxic agents
- not recommended with vaccines or other heterologous serum protein preparations due to unexpected effects on immune system

Nursing points/Cautions

- see General Nursing points/Cautions for interferons (p. 1223)
- patient or carer can be taught administration technique. First injection should be under medical supervision
- vial stopper contains rubber which causes allergic reaction in those with latex allergy
- caution if used in those with compromised CNS function as increased risk of gait disturbance, dizziness or decreased mental function (especially if high doses are administered)

Patient teaching and advice

- instruct patient in correct SC administration technique (see Patient teaching and advice for icatibant, p. 1195)

- advise patient/carer to seek medical advice if any dizziness, gait disturbance or change in mental function occurs
- see also General Patient teaching and advice for interferons (p. 1224)

PEGINTERFERON ALFA 2A (Pegasys)

Available forms

Prefilled syringe: 135 microgram/0.5 mL, 180 microgram/0.5 mL

Action

- see General Actions of interferons (p. 1222)
- combination (termed pegylated) of recombinant interferon alfa 2a and monomethoxy polyethylene glycol (PEG reagent) prolonging half-life

Use

- chronic hepatitis B (with evidence of viral replication, liver inflammation and compensated liver disease)
- chronic hepatitis C (in those not receiving previous interferon therapy or have failed interferon alfa therapy (alone or with ribavirin) and with compensated liver disease)

Dose

- (chronic hepatitis B) 180 microgram SC weekly for 48 weeks **OR**
- (chronic hepatitis C – treatment naive) 180 microgram SC weekly for 24–48 weeks (depending on viral genotype) (with ribavirin 0.8–1.2 g orally daily depending on patient weight) **OR**
- (chronic hepatitis C – non-responder or relapsed) 180 microgram SC weekly for 48–72 weeks (depending on viral genotype) (with ribavirin 1–1.2 g orally daily depending on patient weight) **OR**
- (HIV–hepatitis C co-infection) 180 microgram SC weekly for 48 weeks (alone or with ribavirin 800 mg orally daily)

Adverse effects

- (hepatitis C, combined with ribavirin, children 5–17 years) inhibited growth, decreased weight
- see General Adverse effects of interferons (p. 1222)

Interactions

- not recommended with Chinese herbal medicine Xiao-Chai-Hu (also known as sho-saiko-to) because it may increase the risk of pulmonary symptoms
- may decrease metabolism of theophylline leading to increased serum levels and risk of toxicity
- may increase serum levels of methadone
- increased risk of peripheral neuropathy if given with telbivudine
- increased risk of severe anaemia and neutropenia if given with zidovudine
- increased risk of myelotoxicity if given with azathioprine

Nursing points/Cautions

- (hepatitis C, combined with ribavirin, children 5–17 years) growth and weight of children should be monitored regularly during therapy
- dose may be decreased if moderate-to-severe adverse effects occur
- therapy may be discontinued if there has been no response after 12 weeks
- (HIV-hepatitis C co-infection) patient should be closely monitored during therapy for any signs of liver decompensation (e.g. ascites, variceal bleeding, encephalopathy) and therapy should be stopped if this occurs
- (hepatitis B) disease exacerbation (transient increase in serum ALT) occurs commonly during therapy which may require dose reduction or interruption to therapy
- contraindicated in those with hypersensitivity to *E. coli*-derived products, polyethylene glycol or HIV–hepatitis C co-infection with cirrhosis

(unless due to medication-related indirect hyperbilirubinaemia), autoimmune hepatitis, decompensated cirrhosis, thalassaemia or sickle cell anaemia
- see also General Nursing points/ Cautions for interferons (p. 1223)

Patient teaching and advice

- instruct patient in correct SC administration technique (see Patient teaching and advice for icatibant, p. 1195)
- see also General Patient teaching and advice for interferons (p. 1224)

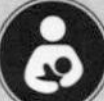

contraindicated during pregnancy as combination therapy with ribavirin (see Antiviral agents, p. 843)

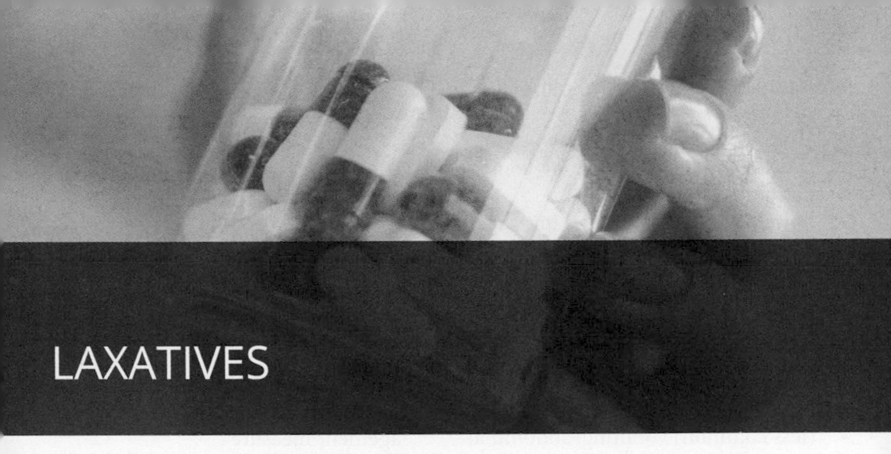

LAXATIVES

Constipation is difficult to define because normal bowel habits vary considerably from person to person. The diagnosis of constipation may include low stool frequency and/or excessive straining, hard stools, lower abdominal fullness or a sense of incomplete evacuation (Camilleri & Murray 2018). Chronic constipation results from inadequate dietary fibre or fluid intake or from disordered colonic transit or anorectal function (resulting from advanced age, medications (e.g. calcium-channel blockers, some antidepressants), colonic obstruction (e.g. diverticular disease, tumour), anal fissure, painful haemorrhoids, pelvic floor dysfunction, neurologic disease (e.g. multiple sclerosis, Parkinson's disease), psychiatric disorders (e.g. depression) and endocrine-related diseases (e.g. hypothyroidism, hypercalcaemia)) (Camilleri & Murray 2018).

Laxatives, also known as aperients, purgatives, cathartics or evacuants, promote defecation. Given orally, by suppository or evacuant enema, laxatives are also used to reduce straining, reduce pain in anorectal disorders and before surgery, radiological or endoscopic procedures (Sharkey & Wallace 2018).

Most laxatives act by increasing retention of fluid in the colon and/or altering motility. Bulk-forming laxatives are hydrophilic, causing an increase in faecal mass, resulting in stimulation of peristalsis. *Stimulant* (irritant) *laxatives* stimulate accumulation of water and electrolytes, which increases intestinal motility. *Osmotic* (non-absorbable inorganic salts or sugars) *laxatives* are poorly absorbed, concentrated solutions that increase intracolonic osmotic pressure, causing decreased absorption of fluid in the bowel, resulting in a fairly rapid, semi-fluid evacuation. *Emollient laxatives* (faecal softeners) soften faeces by decreasing surface tension and increasing penetration of intestinal fluids into the faecal mass, while *prokinetic agents* act primarily on motility (Sharkey & Wallace 2018).

General Uses of laxatives

- prophylactically to prevent straining during defecation (e.g. haemorrhoids, anal fissures)

- short-term management of constipation
- bowel evacuation before investigational procedures (proctoscopy, sigmoidoscopy, colonoscopy, radiology) or surgery

General Adverse effects of laxatives

- (common) nausea, abdominal bloating/discomfort, flatulence
- (less common) vomiting, abdominal cramps, rectal irritation, proctitis
- (prolonged use or overdose) diarrhoea, excessive loss of water and electrolytes, especially potassium
- (rare) intestinal impaction

General Nursing points/Cautions for laxatives

- sufficient lubrication will be produced by warming the suppository in the hand before removing it from the foil wrapper
- entire suppository does not need to dissolve to be effective
- suppositories are effective within 20–60 minutes of insertion
- micro-enema usually effective within 5–15 minutes
- (enemas/suppositories) not recommended in those with anal fissures, ulcerative proctitis with mucosal damage or ulcerated haemorrhoids
- (all laxatives) contraindicated in those with intestinal obstruction, faecal impaction, bowel perforation (frank or suspected), gastric retention, paralytic ileus, undiagnosed abdominal pain and/or nausea/vomiting (including suspected appendicitis), acute surgical abdomen, undiagnosed rectal bleeding, toxic megacolon, toxic colitis, colonic atony

General Patient teaching and advice for laxatives

- warn patient not to drive or operate machinery if any dizziness or fatigue occurs
- advise patient that laxatives should only be used as a short-term management measure
- the patient should be advised to seek medical advice before taking laxatives if bowel habits have changed suddenly over 2 weeks. Medical advice should also be sought if constipation continues for 7 days or more despite treatment or if rectal bleeding occurs
- warn patient to avoid the 'laxative habit' and encourage normal bowel function by increasing fibre and fluid intake, and regular exercise
- patient should be warned not to take laxative in powdered form, because oesophageal obstruction may occur
- instruct patient that it may take 24–48 hours for normal bowel habits to return
- the patient should be instructed in the correct technique for insertion of enema, including:
  - lying on the left side with knees drawn up
  - lubricating the tip of the enema and gently inserting into the rectum, discontinuing the procedure if there is any resistance
  - maintaining position until the urge to evacuate the bowel is strong
  - not retaining enema for prolonged length of time

- instructions for insertion of suppository, including:
  - washing hands thoroughly before insertion
  - removing foil wrapper
  - lying on left side with knees drawn up towards chest
  - gently inserting suppository (pointed end first) into rectum

BULK-FORMING LAXATIVES

General Actions of bulk-forming laxatives

- increase the volume, bulk and moisture of faeces by absorbing water, distending the bowel, so stimulating peristalsis
- generally consist of natural plant gums that are not broken down by normal digestive processes
- do not interfere with absorption of food, but do require adequate fluids for maximal effect
- effective in 12–24 hours, although the full effect may take 2–3 days
- also improve stool consistency for those with diarrhoea or colonoscopy/ileostomy patients

ISPAGHULA (Fybogel)

Available form

Powder: 3.5 g/sachet

Dose

- 1 sachet (3.5 g) orally twice daily morning and evening after meals

Use/Adverse effects

- see General Uses and Adverse effects for laxatives (pp.1229–30)

Interactions

- advise patient to take oral medication 2 hours before or after oral laxative therapy

Nursing points/Cautions

- contains aspartame, therefore caution should be used if given to those with phenylketonuria
- caution if used in those with dysphagia
- see also General Nursing points/Cautions for laxatives (p. 1230)

Patient teaching and advice

- instruct patient that sachet should be stirred into 250 mL glass of water or fruit juice and drunk immediately
- see also General Patient teaching and advice for laxatives (p. 1230)

powder can also be mixed with half cup of yoghurt or apple puree

PSYLLIUM (Fibre Health Natural Granular, Metamucil)

Available forms

Powder: 3.4 g/7 g, 3.4 g/5.9 g, 3.4 g/11 g

Use

- constipation
- lower cholesterol

Dose

- (constipation) 2 level medicinal teaspoons (5 mL spoon) 1–3 times daily in 250 mL of cool water, followed by an additional glass of water **OR**

- (cholesterol) 2 level medicinal teaspoons (5 mL spoon) orally 3 times daily

Adverse effects
- see General Adverse effects for laxatives (p. 1230)

Interactions
- advise patient to take oral medication 2 hours before or after oral laxative therapy

Nursing points/Cautions
- contains aspartame, therefore not recommended in those with phenylketonuria (Metamucil Smooth Texture)
- caution if used in those with dysphagia
- see also General Nursing points/Cautions for laxatives (p. 1230)

Patient teaching and advice
- advise patient to drink generous amounts of water to prevent laxative swelling and blocking throat or oesophagus
- see also General Patient teaching and advice for laxatives (p. 1230)

Note
- contained in GIT 1, H-Bio-Juven Vascurem 2, Herb-a-lax, Lax-Active

STERCULIA (Normafibe)

Available form
Granules

Action
- see General Actions of bulk-forming laxatives (p. 1231)
- vegetable gum that absorbs up to 60 times its own volume in water

Dose
- 1–2 heaped medicinal teaspoons (5 mL spoon) of granules 1–2 times daily

Use/Adverse effects/Nursing points/Cautions
- see General Use/Adverse effects/Nursing points/Cautions for laxatives (pp. 1229–30)

Interactions
- advise patient to take oral medication 2 hours before or after oral laxative therapy

Patient teaching and advice
- patients should be advised not to take laxative immediately before sleep
- advise patients that granules (small amount) can be placed dry on the tongue and swallowed whole with plenty of water or given mixed with jam, honey or ice-cream
- instruct patient to drink generous amounts of water to prevent laxative swelling and blocking throat or oesophagus
- see also General Patient teaching and advice for laxatives (p. 1230)

Note
- contained in Normacol Plus with frangula

OSMOTIC LAXATIVES

General Actions of osmotic laxatives
- not absorbed, but action is via osmotic effect which causes an increase in fluid volume in the lumen, which accelerates transfer to gut contents, thereby increasing defecation

COLON ELECTROLYTE LAVAGE (ColonLYTELY, Glycoprep, Glycoprep-C, Lax-Sachets, Macrovic Powder, Molaxole, Movicol preparations, Moviprep, Pico Prep, Plenvu)

Available forms

Powder: 15.546 g/sachet, 68.58 g/sachet, 70 g/sachet, 200 g/sachet, 210 g/sachet, 123 g/2 sachets (A & B); Oral solution: 25 mL/sachet

Action

- see General Actions of osmotic laxatives (p. 1232)
- polyethylene glycol-electrolyte solution that cleanses bowel by inducing diarrhoea, while causing little change in water and electrolyte balance
- polyethylene glycol (macrogel) acts as an osmotic agent
- electrolyte combinations vary between preparations
- action usually within 1–4 hours of administration

Use

- short-term management of constipation (under supervision)
- bowel preparation before investigational procedures (proctoscopy, sigmoidoscopy, colonoscopy, radiology) or surgery

Dose

- (evening before morning investigation or surgery or morning before afternoon investigation) dissolve sachet in water (according to instructions), then 250 mL orally every 10 minutes until 3–4 L have been consumed or rectal effluent is clear **OR**
- (before radiological procedure) dissolve 15.546 g sachet in 250 mL water at 3 pm (day before procedure), followed by clear fluids (minimum 250 mL/hour), then further 15.546 g sachet at 9 pm while continuing clear fluids (PicoPrep) **OR**
- (constipation) 2 L over 2 hours (may be dissolved in cordial or fruit juice) **OR**
- (constipation) initially 1 sachet daily dissolved in 125 mL water, increasing to 2–3 sachets if needed **OR**
- (constipation – ready to use solution) 1 sachet daily, increasing to 2–3 sachets, if needed **OR**
- (nasogastric) 20–30 mL per hour **OR**
- (before barium enema) 2 L orally (with 10 mg bisacodyl) night before procedure **OR**
- (faecal impaction) 8 sachets over 6 hours for up to 3 days (if patient has cardiac impairment, dose should be reduced to 2 sachets per hour) (daily maximum 8 sachets) (Movicol)

Adverse effects

- rhinorrhoea, skin reactions
- see also General Adverse effects of laxatives (p. 1230)

Interactions

- any oral medications taken within 1 hour may not be absorbed
- may reduce effect of benzylpenicillin
- caution if used with calcium-channel blockers, diuretics or other agents that may affect electrolyte levels
- may interfere with oral contraceptive

Nursing points/Cautions

- any dehydration should be corrected before starting therapy
- patient to fast for 3–4 hours before administration
- (endoscopy/colonoscopy) no solid food should be taken on day prior to procedure. Only clear, sugar-free liquids are allowed
- reconstitute powder using 250 mL water for 15.546 sachet, 1 L water for 68–70 g sachet or 3 L for 200–210 g sachet (other clear fluids may be allowed by doctor)

- (Moviprep) to reconstitute, mix sachet A and sachet B together with 1 L water and then drink over 1–2 hours; repeat with second litre
- (nasogastric) rate should be decreased if patient experiences nausea and/or bloating
- (nasogastric) observe patient closely if there is impaired gag reflex or unconscious
- (ColonLYTELY) no additional flavouring should be added unless instructed by doctor
- contain aspartame and are therefore not recommended in those with phenylketonuria
- first bowel action occurs about 1 hour after starting solution
- preparation is considered to be complete when the patient is passing clear fluid from the bowel
- caution if used in those with severe ulcerative colitis, diabetes, impaired kidney function (creatinine clearance < 30 mL/min), pre-existing electrolyte imbalance or dehydration, congestive cardiac failure, at risk of arrhythmias, thyroid disease, impaired gag reflex, unconscious or semiconscious, prone to aspiration/regurgitation or the elderly
- contraindicated in those with stoma or weight < 20 kg
- see also general points for laxatives (p. 1229–30)

Patient teaching and advice

- advise patient that mixture may be more palatable if refrigerated and can be kept for up to 72 hours
- patient should be advised to slow drinking rate if nausea and bloating become severe
- if patients are ordered to take clear fluids only as part of bowel preparation, these may include water, tea or coffee (without milk or non-dairy creamer), soft drink (non-carbonated) or cordial (but no red or purple colouring as these may interfere with investigations), strained fruit juice (no pulp) or strained soup or clear broth
- advise patient to seek medical advice immediately if any swelling, shortness of breath or fatigue occur
- for constipation, instruct patient that Movicol powder requires dilution in 125 mL water but Movicol Ready-to-Take solution can be taken directly from sachet without dilution
- patient should be advised to take fluids orally before and after bowel preparation to prevent dehydration
- female patients should be counselled regarding possible oral contraceptive failure during therapy and should be advised to use an alternative form of contraception during this time to avoid unwanted pregnancy occurring

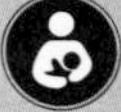

only used during pregnancy if clearly needed

LACTULOSE (Actilax, Dulose)

Available form

Syrup: 3.34 g/5 mL

Action

- administered orally as 50% w/w syrup, which is poorly absorbed from gastrointestinal tract
- metabolised in the colon by bacteria to acetic and lactic acids
- reduces colon pH to 5.0, causing ammonia to be trapped as ammonium, so that less ammonia is absorbed into the blood and is instead excreted in the faeces (this is thought to be mechanism of action in portal systemic encephalopathy (PSE))

- change in osmotic pressure and colon acidification increases water content of stools, promoting peristalsis and evacuation
- also thought to promote growth of healthy promoting bacteria (probiotic action) while potentially suppressing pathogenic bacteria (e.g. *E. coli*, *Clostridium*)

Use
- chronic constipation
- treatment and prevention of portal systemic encephalopathy (including hepatic pre-coma and coma)

Dose
Chronic constipation
- initially 15–45 mL orally daily after breakfast for 3 days, decreasing to 15–30 mL daily (maintenance)

Portal systemic encephalopathy (PSE)
- initially 30–45 mL orally 3–4 times daily, adjusting dose every 1–2 days to produce 2–3 soft stools daily **OR**
- 30–45 mL orally hourly for 24–48 hours for more rapid response, then 30–45 mL 3–4 times daily **OR**
- (acute) 50 mL orally 1–2-hourly until 2 soft stools are produced, then decreasing to 30–45 mL orally 3–4 times daily **OR**
- 300 mL diluted with 700 mL water/ sodium chloride 0.9% and given as retention enema, repeated 4–6-hourly until patient is able to take orally

Interactions
- avoid other laxatives during lactulose therapy because loose stools resulting from their use may be mistaken for adequate lactulose dosage
- caution if given with neomycin (conflicting information about interaction)

Adverse effects
- see General Adverse effects of laxatives (p. 1230)

Nursing points/Cautions
- (PSE) overall management should include dietary protein restriction, correction of any fluid and/or electrolyte imbalance, bowel cleansing and sterilisation, provision of nutritional/ caloric needs and treatment of underlying liver disease
- use cautiously in those with diabetes, especially if therapy is prolonged
- caution if used in those with lactose intolerance
- caution if used in those undergoing electrocautery procedures during colonoscopy or proctoscopy. Bowel should be thoroughly cleansed with non-fermentable solution before procedure
- not recommended in those with rare hereditary problems of galactose intolerance, Lapp lactase deficiency or glucose–galactose malabsorption
- contraindicated in those with galactosaemia
- see General Nursing points/Cautions for laxatives (p. 1230)

Patient teaching and advice
- advise patient that solution may be taken undiluted or diluted with water, milk or fruit juice
- patient should be advised that it may take 24–48 hours before a result is seen
- instruct patient to seek medical advice if painful abdominal symptoms occur
- see General Patient teaching and advice for laxatives (p. 1230)

SODIUM PHOSPHATE (DiaCol, Fleet Ready-to-Use-Enema, Phospho-Soda)

Available forms
Tablets: 1.5 g; Oral solution: 23.1 g/45 mL; Enema: 26 g/133 mL

Action

- see General Actions of osmotic laxatives (p. 1232)

Use

- constipation (under supervision)
- bowel preparation for colon X-ray or colonoscopy
- postoperatively, or relief of faecal/barium impaction

Dose

- contents of 1 disposable enema unit (133 mL) **OR**
- 15 mL mixed with 250 mL of clear fluids and drunk, repeated twice more in next 20 minutes (first dose), followed by at least 3 glasses (250 mL) of clear fluids. Second dose is repeated as per first dose 10–12 hours later (timing is dependent on whether procedure is morning or afternoon) **OR**
- 4 tablets orally with at least 250 mL water or clear fluids every 15 minutes for 75 minutes (or 5 doses) (20 tablets) evening before procedure, then 4 tablets orally with 250 mL water or clear fluids every 15 minutes for 45 minutes (12 tablets) 3–5 hours before procedure (total 32 tablets)

Adverse effects

- (rare) nephrocalcinosis associated with renal insufficiency or renal failure, seizures, QT prolongation
- see also General Adverse effects of laxatives (p. 1230)

Interactions

- caution if given with diuretics, NSAIDs, calcium-channel blockers, ACE inhibitors, angiotensin receptor blockers, lithium or other agents that may affect electrolyte balance and increase risk of QT prolongation
- not recommended with colon electrolyte lavage solutions containing polyethylene glycol (macrogol)

Nursing points/Cautions

- any electrolyte imbalance should be corrected before starting therapy, especially in those with pre-existing electrolyte abnormalities
- calcium and phosphate levels should be closely monitored
- patient should be monitored for any signs of dehydration as life-threatening dehydration and/or electrolyte imbalance can occur
- enema should be warmed to body temperature
- repeat administration of bowel preparation is not recommended within 7 days
- (enema) contains 4.4 g sodium
- (oral solution) caution if used in those on salt restriction as oral solution contains 4.82 mEq sodium and 12.45 mEq/mL phosphate
- caution if used in those with pre-existing dehydration (including taking diuretics), at risk of hyponatraemia (e.g. SIADH, inadequate treatment of hypothyroidism, electrolyte imbalance), diabetes, heart disease or renal impairment
- caution if used in those at risk of hyponatraemia as risk of seizures is increased
- caution if used within 3 months of cardiac surgery or acute myocardial infarction
- caution if used in those with inflammatory bowel disease as an acute exacerbation of the condition may occur
- (Phospho-soda) not recommended in children under 12 years
- not recommended in patients with a colostomy, because of the increased risk of hypocalcaemia, hyperphosphataemia, hypernatraemia and acidosis
- contraindicated in those with imperforate anus, faecal impaction, kidney impairment, fluid/electrolyte disturbance (or at risk of), congestive cardiac

failure, ascites, unstable angina, gastric retention, paralytic ileus, bowel obstruction, severe chronic constipation, bowel perforation, acute colitis, active inflammatory disease, congenital or toxic megacolon or hypomotility syndrome
- contraindicated in those with hypersensitivity to sodium phosphate salt
- see General Nursing points/Cautions for laxatives (p. 1230)

Patient teaching and advice

- advise patient to drink clear fluids only for 12 hours before first dose
- patient should be instructed to avoid laxative use (with any type of laxative) for 7 days after procedure
- instruct patient to seek medical advice if there is no return of liquid after enema administration or no bowel motion within 6 hours of taking oral solution
- if patients are ordered to take clear fluids only as part of bowel preparation, these may include water, tea or coffee (without milk or non-dairy creamer), soft drink (carbonated or non-carbonated) or cordial (but no red or purple colouring as these may interfere with investigations), strained fruit juice (no pulp) or strained soup or clear broth
- if patient has diabetes, frequent monitoring of blood glucose levels is recommended. Adjustment to insulin and/or oral hypoglycaemic agents may be required
- (Phospho-soda) ensure patient understands that solution must be diluted before use
- see General Patient teaching and advice for laxatives (p. 1230)

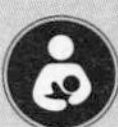

only used during pregnancy and breast-feeding if benefits clearly outweigh risks

SORBITOL (Sorbilax, Sorbisol)

Available form

Syrup: 70% sorbitol solution (14 g/20 mL)

Action

- osmotic laxative, similar to lactulose
- see General Actions of osmotic laxatives (p. 1232)

Use

- relief of constipation

Dose

- initially 20 mL daily, increasing to 20 mL 3 times daily if needed either 1 hour before or 3 hours after food; dose may then be reduced

Adverse effects

- see General Adverse effects of laxatives (p. 1230)

Interactions

- effectiveness may be reduced by antacids and opioid analgesics
- if used with stimulant laxatives, diarrhoea may occur

Nursing points/Cautions

- (chronic use) electrolytes should be monitored regularly with prolonged use
- caution if used in those with insulin-dependent diabetes. If the patient has adequate insulin reserves and is stabilised on insulin there should be an impact on blood glucose levels. However, an increase in blood glucose levels may occur if the patient has insulin-depleted reserves
- contraindicated in those with fructose intolerance
- see General Nursing points/Cautions for laxatives (p. 1230)

Patient teaching and advice

- advise patient to avoid refrigeration of syrup as crystals may form. Warm to room temperature and shake bottle if this occurs

- warn patient that eating fructose-containing foods (e.g. apples, pears) at the same time may cause diarrhoea
- see General Patient teaching and advice for laxatives (p. 1230)

Note
- contained in Microlax enema and Micolette micro-enema
- contained in Carbosorb XS with charcoal

STIMULANT LAXATIVES

General Actions of stimulant laxatives
- promote accumulation of water and electrolytes in lumen and stimulate sensory nerve endings in mucosa, resulting in increased peristalsis of colon
- primary effect is on small and large intestines, hence the tendency to cause cramping
- often used as preparation for bowel procedures and surgery

BISACODYL (Bisalax, Dulcolax, Lax-Tab, Petrus Bisacodyl Suppositories)

Available forms
Suppositories: 10 mg; Tablets: 5 mg; Micro-enema: 2 mg/mL

Action
- see General Actions of stimulant laxatives above
- action in 6–8 hours (empty stomach), increasing to 10–12 hours (with food)

Use
- constipation

Dose
- 10 mg orally at night, or 30 minutes before breakfast (for effect 6–8 hours later) **OR**
- 1 enema rectally after breakfast (on days where defecation is desired) **OR**
- 10 mg (1 suppository) rectally

Adverse effects
- see General Adverse effects of laxatives (p. 1230)

Interactions
- not recommended within 1 hour of antacids or milk

Nursing points/Cautions
- sufficient lubrication will be produced by warming the suppository in the hand before removing it from the foil wrapper
- suppositories are effective within 20–60 minutes of insertion; enema usually effective within 5–15 minutes; tablets effective within 6–8 hours
- enema should be warmed to body temperature
- (Dulcolax) tablets contain lactose and are therefore not recommended in those with hereditary conditions of galactose intolerance, Lapp lactase deficiency or glucose–galactose malabsorption
- (tablets) not recommended in children under 6 years
- see General Nursing points/Cautions for laxatives (p. 1230)

Patient teaching and advice
- instruct patient that tablets should be swallowed whole, not chewed or broken
- patient should have no antacids or milk within 60 minutes of taking tablets

Note
- contained in Go Kit and Glycoprep-C combination pack as complete bowel preparation before abdominal radiographic examination

GLYCEROL (Glycerol Suppositories BP)

Available forms

Suppository: 2.8 g (adult), 1.4 g (child), 700 mg (infant)

Dose

- insert 1 suppository high into rectum against the rectal wall and allow it to remain for 15–30 minutes

Use/Adverse effects/Nursing points/Cautions/Patient teaching and advice

- entire suppository does not have to dissolve to be effective
- also has an osmotic effect
- see general points for laxatives (pp. 1229–30)

SENNOSIDES A AND B (formerly known as Senna) (Bekunis Senna Tablets, Laxettes with Senna, Laxettes with Sennosides, Senna-Gen, Senokot)

Available forms

Tablets: 7.5 mg, 20 mg; Chocolate squares: 12 mg

Dose

- (Senokot) 2–4 tablets orally at night **OR**
- (Laxettes with Senna) initially 1–2 tablets daily with water at bedtime, increasing to 3 tablets if needed **OR**
- (Laxettes with Sennosides) 1–3 squares orally daily at bedtime **OR**
- (Bekunis Senna Tablets) 1–2 tablets daily before bedtime

Use/Adverse effects/Nursing points/Cautions/Patient teaching and advice

- acts within 8–12 hours
- advise patient that tablets should be swallowed whole
- see general points for laxatives (pp. 1229–30)

Note

- contained in Colaxsen, Coloxyl with Senna, Co-Senna, Sennesoft

tablet can be crushed and mixed with spoonful of yoghurt or apple puree

FAECAL SOFTENERS

General Actions of faecal softeners

- soften faeces by decreasing surface tension
- onset of action 1–3 days

General Uses of faecal softeners

- constipation

DOCUSATE SODIUM (Coloxyl Tablets)

Available forms

Tablets: 50 mg, 120 mg

Dose

- 240 mg orally daily after evening meal (120 mg tablets) **OR**
- 100–150 mg orally twice daily (50 mg tablets)

Use/Adverse effects/Nursing points/Cautions/Patient teaching and advice

- see general points for laxatives (pp. 1229–30)

Note

- combined with sennoside b in Colaxsen, Coloxyl with Senna, Co-Senna, Sennesoft and Trust ColoxEase

- combined with sorbitol in Klyx enema
- can also be used to soften ear wax (Waxsol)

PARAFFIN, LIQUID (Agarol, Parachoc)

Available forms
Suspension: 2.5 mL/5 mL, 4.83 mL/15 mL

Dose
- 15–40 mL orally at bedtime, increasing or decreasing dose by 5 mL to produce soft stool without oily leakage

Use/Adverse effects/Nursing points/Cautions/Patient teaching and advice
- see general points for laxatives (pp. 1229–30)

POLOXAMER (formerly known as poloxalkol) (Coloxyl Drops)

Available form
Drops: 10%

Action
- increases penetration of fluid into faeces, softening stool

Use
- faecal softener for children and infants

Paediatric dose
- (< 6 months) 10 drops (0.3 mL) orally 3 times daily **OR**
- (6–18 months) 15 drops (0.5 mL) orally 3 times daily **OR**
- (18 months–3 years) 25 drops (0.8 mL) orally 3 times daily

Adverse effects
- see General Adverse effects for laxatives (p. 1230)

Interactions
- not recommended with other laxatives

Nursing points/Cautions
- effective within 2–3 days
- chronic use should be avoided as this may increase potassium loss from intestine leading to electrolyte imbalance
- contraindicated if appendicitis or intestinal obstruction is suspected, or if undiagnosed rectal bleeding or abdominal pain is present
- see General Nursing points/Cautions for laxatives (p. 1230)

Patient teaching and advice
- advise parent/carer to give the dose orally 3 times daily in a feeding bottle or in fruit juice
- instruct parent/carer to use syringe (provided) to measure dose accurately and then rinse with warm water after use

SODIUM PICOSULFATE (Dulcolax SP Drops, Picolax)

Available forms
Drops: 7.5 mg/mL; Powder: 20 g sachet

Action
- hydrolysed by bacteria in the colon to form the active ingredient, which stimulates the colon and increases motility, decreasing transit time and softening stool

Use
- bowel preparation before gastrointestinal examination
- constipation

Dose
- (bowel preparation) prepare sachet (see Patient teaching and advice, p. 1241) and then take 250 mL at 3 pm and 9 pm (2-sachet schedule) or 1 pm, 5 pm and 9 pm (3-sachet schedule) (Picolax) **OR**
- initially 10 drops (5 mg) orally at night, increasing to 20 drops (10 mg) if needed (Durolax SP Drops)

Adverse effects
- dizziness, syncope
- (rare) skin reactions
- see General Adverse effects of laxatives (p. 1230)

Interactions
- increased risk of electrolyte imbalance if given with diuretics or corticosteroids
- decreased action may occur if given with broad-spectrum antibiotics
- if electrolyte imbalance occurs, it may result in increased sensitivity to digoxin
- efficacy decreased if given with bulk-forming laxatives
- may increase bowel transit time, which will impact on orally administered medications
- caution if used with NSAIDs, TCAs, SSRIs, carbamazepine and antipsychotic agents, as these may increase water retention and/or electrolyte imbalance

Nursing points/Cautions

- caution if used in the elderly or those with kidney impairment, diabetes, mild-to-moderate dehydration, at risk of hypokalaemia or hyponatraemia, inflammatory bowel disease, recent gastrointestinal surgery or impaired gag reflex
- not recommended in those with severe kidney impairment as magnesium accumulation in the plasma may occur
- (Dulcolax SP Drops) contraindicated in those with fructose intolerance
- contraindicated in those with rhabdomyolysis or triarylmethane substance hypersensitivity
- see General Nursing points/Cautions for laxatives (p. 1230)

Patient teaching and advice

- advise patient to ensure that other medications are taken 2 hours before or at least 6 hours after sodium picosulfate
- (drops) patient should be advised not to shake bottle and use dropper provided for correct dosage. Water can be added
- (bowel preparation) instruct patient to prepare sachet by adding 250 mL of cold water and stirring until effervescence stops and then drinking
- (bowel preparation) instruct patient that low-residue diet should be started 2 days before procedure, then no solid foods, milk, milk products or alcohol taken on day of procedure. Clear fluids are allowed up to 6 hours before examination

Note
- contained in Picosalax, Picoprep and Prep Kit C

OTHER AGENTS

METHYLNALTREXONE BROMIDE (Relistor)

Available form
Vial: 12 mg/0.6 mL

Action
- opioid antagonist with selectivity for mu opioid receptors (> kappa receptors) and no significant interaction with delta receptors
- peripherally acting as is not able to cross blood–brain barrier, therefore has no effect on opioid-mediated analgesic effect
- terminal half-life about 8 hours

Use
- opioid-induced constipation in those with advanced illness where response to laxative therapy has been inadequate

Dose
- (weight 38 to < 62 kg) 8 mg SC every second day **OR**
- (weight 62–114 kg) 12 mg SC every second day **OR**
- (< 38 kg or > 114 kg) 0.15 mg/kg SC every second day

Adverse effects
- abdominal pain, flatulence, nausea, diarrhoea
- dizziness
- sweating
- (rare) gastrointestinal perforation (stomach, duodenum, colon)

Interactions
- caution if given with NSAIDs, corticosteroids or bevacizumab as there may be an increased risk of gastrointestinal perforation

Nursing points/Cautions
- no known risk of abuse and/or dependence
- dosing interval can be increased if needed
- only given SC
- administer alone
- rotate administration; sites and areas that are scarred, tender, inflamed or bruised should not be used
- caution if used in those with advanced illness/disease (e.g. cancer, peptic ulcer, pseudo obstruction) which may impact on integrity of GI wall as there may be increased risk of bowel perforation
- caution if used in those with GI tract lesions, active diverticular disease, faecal impaction, colostomy or peritoneal catheter
- not recommended in those with severe liver impairment or end-stage kidney disease requiring dialysis
- not recommended in those with post-operative ileus or those who have undergone gastrointestinal resection
- contraindicated in those with known or suspected mechanical GI obstruction or acute surgical abdomen

Patient teaching and advice
- instruct patient to seek medical advice if severe, persistent diarrhoea or severe or persistent abdominal pain occurs
- advise patient that action usually occurs within 30 minutes and therefore they should remain near toilet facilities
- warn patient to avoid driving or operating machinery if dizziness occurs
- see General Patient teaching and advice (p. xxvii)

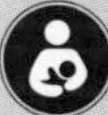

not recommended during pregnancy unless clearly needed

caution if used during breastfeeding

PRUCALOPRIDE (Resotrans)

Available forms
Tablets: 1 mg, 2 mg

Action
- $5HT_4$ agonist
- decreases small bowel transit time, increasing gastric emptying with no impact on colon transit time

Use
- chronic functional constipation that has not been relieved after therapy with laxatives from two or more different classes at highest tolerated dose for ≥ 6 months

Dose
- 2 mg orally daily **OR**
- (adults > 65 years) initially 1 mg orally daily, increasing to 2 mg if needed **OR**
- (adults with kidney or liver impairment) 1 mg orally daily

Adverse effects

- headache, dizziness, fatigue
- decreased appetite, nausea, diarrhoea, abdominal pain, abdominal distension, vomiting, dyspepsia, rectal bleeding, flatulence, unusual bowel sounds
- polyuria
- (uncommon) palpitations, rectal bleeding, tremor, migraine
- (rare) suicidal ideation

Interactions

- if diarrhoea results after use, failure of oral contraceptives may occur
- decreased effectiveness if given with atropine-like agents
- caution if used with agents that prolong QT interval

Nursing points/Cautions

- thorough assessment should be conducted before starting therapy to exclude any secondary causes of constipation
- if therapy is not effective after 4 weeks, patient should be reassessed
- patient should be reassessed after 12 weeks of therapy
- tablets contain lactose and are not recommended in those with galactose intolerance, Lapp lactase deficiency or glucose–galactose malabsorption
- caution if used in those with arrhythmias, ischaemic cardiovascular disease, severe liver or kidney impairment
- not recommended in those with constipation due to secondary causes such as endocrine, neurological or metabolic disorders or related to opioid use
- contraindicated in those with renal impairment requiring dialysis, intestinal perforation or obstruction, paralytic ileus, acute inflammatory intestinal conditions (e.g. Crohn's disease), ulcerative colitis, toxic megacolon or recent bowel surgery

Patient teaching and advice

- warn patient to avoid driving or operating machinery if dizziness or fatigue occurs
- advise patient to seek medical advice if any tremor, rectal bleeding or pounding heart sensation occurs
- patient should be warned that abdominal pain, nausea and/or diarrhoea commonly occur at the start of therapy, but these symptoms abate with continued therapy
- family members or carers should be advised to monitor patient closely and seek medical advice immediately if any lowered mood, talk of self-harm or self-harm behaviours occur
- females of childbearing years should be counselled to use adequate contraception to avoid pregnancy during therapy

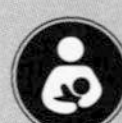

not recommended during pregnancy or breastfeeding

tablet can be dispersed in water or crushed and mixed with spoonful of yoghurt or apple puree

LIPID REGULATING AGENTS

Atherosclerosis describes the process by which plaque is deposited in moderate- to large-sized arteries, resulting in narrowing of the lumen over a period of years to decades. Plaque is comprised of cholesterol, lipid, collagen and modified monocytes. Atherosclerosis may predispose a person to coronary artery disease (e.g. myocardial infarction, angina pectoris), cerebrovascular disease (e.g. stroke, transient cerebral ischaemia), peripheral vascular disease (e.g. intermittent claudication, gangrene) and/or renal artery insufficiency, depending on the location and severity of the plaque deposition (Bryant et al 2019).

Cholesterol is essential in the production of steroid hormones (adrenocorticosteroids) and is produced from carbohydrates, proteins and lipids from the diet. Chylomicrons are responsible for transporting cholesterol and fatty acids from the GI tract to the liver. Oversupply of cholesterol from the diet in the form of saturated fat and/or a hereditary factor causing the overproduction of cholesterol leads to high serum levels of cholesterol known as hypercholesterolaemia (Bryant et al 2019).

Lipids (e.g. triglycerides, cholesterol) are transported from the liver in the blood, in complexes called lipoproteins. The liver synthesises approximately two-thirds of the total plasma lipoproteins. Low-density lipoproteins (LDLs) are responsible for transporting cholesterol to the arteries, where it is deposited, whereas high-density lipoproteins (HDLs) transport cholesterol from peripheral cells to the liver, where it is processed into bile salts. The liver contains LDL receptors which remove LDLs from the plasma – the main mechanism for controlling LDL levels. The number of LDL receptors can be modulated. High levels of HDL are considered to be beneficial (preventing accumulation of cholesterol in artery walls), whereas high levels of LDLs are harmful and predispose a person to the development of atherosclerosis (Bryant et al 2019).

Large amounts of triglycerides (and small amounts of cholesterol) are transported via very-low-density lipoproteins (VLDL). Lipoprotein lipase (an enzyme found in the endothelium of adipose and muscle tissue capillaries) releases the triglycerides from the VLDL, resulting in a short-lived intermediate-density lipoprotein (IDL), which is then either returned to the liver or converted to LDL (Bryant et al 2019).

Apolipoproteins are proteins found on the surface of the lipoproteins and appear to confer properties on the lipoprotein. These apolipoproteins are classified using a letter and Roman numeral (e.g. A-I, A-II). Apolipoprotein A-I appears to confer the beneficial effects of HDL, whereas apolipoprotein C-II deficiency in VLDL results in impaired triglyceride metabolism and hypertriglyceridaemia (Bryant et al 2019).

Dyslipidaemias (hyperlipidaemias) are disorders in which there are elevated levels of triglycerides (hypertriglyceridaemia), cholesterol (hypercholesterolaemia) or both (mixed lipidaemia). Primary hyperlipidaemia is subdivided into six subgroups (I, IIa, IIb, III, IV and V), with the different types carrying differing risks of atherosclerosis and being amenable to treatment by different classes of lipid regulating agents. For example, IIa (familial hypercholesterolaemia) has elevated LDL and cholesterol levels and may be managed using a statin, bile acid binding resin or a combination of both. Secondary causes of dyslipidaemia include disease (e.g. diabetes mellitus, obesity, hypothyroidism, nephrotic syndrome), excess alcohol consumption and some medications (e.g. thiazide diuretics, corticosteroids) (Bryant et al 2019).

Management should include appropriate dietary modification (low in cholesterol, saturated and total fats), correction of any underlying disease (diabetes mellitus, hypothyroidism, alcoholism), avoidance of precipitating factors (smoking, obesity, hypertension) and lifestyle changes (e.g. increasing physical activity) before instituting drug therapy.

Lipid regulating agents can be divided into several classes:

- hydroxymethylglutaryl co-enzyme A (HMG-CoA) reductase inhibitors (statins) (e.g. pravastatin, simvastatin), which are used to treat hypercholesterolaemia or mixed hyperlipidaemia
- fibrates (e.g. gemfibrozil), which are used to treat hypertriglyceridaemia or mixed hyperlipidaemia
- bile acid binding agents (e.g. colestyramine), which are used to treat hypercholesterolaemia or combined hyperlipidaemia
- PCSK9 inhibitors (e.g. alirocumab, evolocumab)
- other agents (e.g. nicotinic acid, ezetimibe, omega-3 fatty acids)

HMG-CoA REDUCTASE INHIBITORS (STATINS)

General Actions of statins

- HMG-CoA reductase is the rate-limiting enzyme that converts 3-hydroxy-3-methylglutaryl co-enzyme A to mevalonate (precursor of sterols, including cholesterol). Statins reversibly inhibit HMG-CoA reductase, reducing cholesterol synthesis and increasing the number of liver LDL receptors, thereby reducing LDL concentration
- also thought to have an effect on endothelial function, modify inflammatory response, decrease platelet

aggregation, modify thrombus formation, stabilise atherosclerotic plaque, decrease smooth muscle cell migration and proliferation, increase fibrolytic action and decrease C-reactive protein
- effect on LDL cholesterol is dependent on specific statin and dose
- reach peak concentration within 5 hours

General Uses of statins
- hypercholesterolaemia (types IIa, IIb) (adjunct to diet)
- mixed hyperlipidaemia
- prevention of cardiovascular disease in those with two or more risk factors

General Adverse effects of statins
- constipation, flatulence, dyspepsia, abdominal pain, nausea, diarrhoea
- headache, dizziness, asthenia, fatigue
- insomnia, nightmares
- rash, pruritus
- back pain, myalgia, arthralgia
- hyperglycaemia
- elevated liver enzymes and creatine kinase (CK) levels, hyperglycaemia
- (high dose) increase risk of type 2 diabetes
- (rare) myopathy (muscle aching or weakness with increase in CPK), rhabdomyolysis, hypersensitivity, interstitial lung disease (long-term therapy), haemorrhagic stroke
- (very rare) immune-mediated necrotising myopathy

General Interactions of statins
- contraindicated with sodium fusidate because of increased risk of rhabdomyolysis. Statin should be stopped for at least 7 days longer than sodium fusidate therapy
- increased serum levels may occur if used with ciclosporin, erythromycin, clarithromycin, antifungal (azole) agents, diltiazem, increasing risk of myalgia and/or rhabdomyolysis
- caution if used with fibrates or nicotinic acid
- caution if used with cimetidine or spironolactone as these may decrease levels or activity of naturally occurring steroid hormones
- if given within 4 hours of colestyramine, decreased serum levels may result

General Nursing points/Cautions for statins

- any secondary causes of hypercholesterolaemia (e.g. poorly controlled diabetes mellitus, hypothyroidism, obstructive liver disease, alcoholism, nephrotic syndrome, dysproteinaemia, drug therapy) should be identified and treated before starting therapy, as well as weight reduction and diet modification
- serum lipid levels should be monitored regularly throughout therapy, 4 weeks after starting therapy and dose adjusted if necessary
- liver function test should be performed before starting therapy and at 6 and 12 weeks, then twice-yearly
- ophthalmological testing is recommended after 5 years of therapy
- CK levels should be measured before starting therapy in those with renal impairment, hypothyroidism, history of hereditary muscular disorders, previous history of muscle toxicity caused by statin or fibrate, alcohol abuse or if aged over 70 years, because there is an increased risk of myopathy and rhabdomyolysis.

CK concentration should not be measured after strenuous exercise

- therapeutic response is expected in 2 weeks, with maximal response in 4 weeks
- statins with short half-life (fluvastatin, pravastatin, simvastatin) should be taken in the evening to maximise efficiency as cholesterol synthesis in the liver is at its maximum between midnight and 2 am
- should be withheld if any condition occurs that predisposes patient to rhabdomyolysis, such as trauma, severe infection, hypotension, major surgery, uncontrolled epilepsy or metabolic, endocrine or electrolyte imbalances
- less effective in homozygous familial hypercholesterolaemia, possibly because there are fewer functioning LDL receptors
- caution if used in those with history of liver disease, impaired liver function or who consume substantial quantities of alcohol
- caution if used in those > 65 years, female or those with uncontrolled hypothyroidism due to increased risk of myopathy
- caution if used in those with renal impairment due to increased risk of myopathy and rhabdomyolysis. Renal function and CK levels should be monitored regularly
- caution if used in those at risk of developing diabetes (e.g. metabolic syndrome, BMI > 30 kg/m^2, elevated glycated haemoglobin A1c (HbA1c), impaired fasting glucose). Blood glucose levels should be closely monitored during therapy
- contraindicated in those with active liver disease or unexplained elevation in serum transaminases (ALT, AST) or who have a history of myopathy related to other lipid-lowering agents

General Patient teaching and advice for statins

- advise patient to seek medical advice immediately if any of the following occur:
  - muscle pain, cramps, tenderness or weakness (not related to exercise), malaise, dark urine or fever
  - non-productive cough, difficulty breathing, fatigue, weight loss or fever
  - itching, yellowing of skin or eyes, loss of appetite, tiredness, dark urine
- advise patient to take medication at least 1 hour before or 4 hours after colestyramine
- patient should be warned against drinking large amounts of alcohol because of increased risk of liver damage
- women of childbearing potential should be counselled to use adequate contraception during therapy
- see also General Patient teaching and advice (p. xxvii)

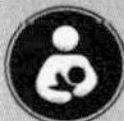

contraindicated during pregnancy or breastfeeding

ATORVASTATIN (Atorvachol, Lipitor, Lorstat, Torvastat, Trovas)

Available forms

Tablets: 10 mg, 20 mg, 40 mg, 80 mg

Action

- see General Actions of statins (p. 1245)
- second generation synthetic statin

- active metabolites
- elimination half-life 15–30 hours

Use

- see General Uses of statins, p. 1246

Dose

- initially 10 mg orally daily, titrating dose at 4-week intervals (range 10–80 mg)

Adverse effects

- nasopharyngitis
- muscle spasm, joint swelling
- (rare) haemorrhagic stroke
- see also General Adverse effects of statins (p. 1246)

Interactions

- serum level may be increased by HIV protease inhibitors, clarithromycin, itraconazole, diltiazem, boceprevir and grapefruit juice (especially excessive amounts > 1.2 L/day)
- caution if given with colchicine due to increased risk of myopathy
- may affect efficacy of oral contraceptives containing norethisterone and ethinylestradiol
- serum levels may be decreased by antacids (magnesium or aluminium hydroxide)
- caution if given with phenytoin, rifampicin or efavirenz as effect may be variable
- if given 1 hour after rifampicin, decreased serum levels may occur. However, if given simultaneously no effect on serum levels
- not recommended with St John's wort
- caution if given with digoxin. If given together, serum digoxin levels should be closely monitored
- see also General Interactions of statins (p. 1246)

Nursing points/Cautions

- patient should be assessed for history of stroke or transischaemic attacks (TIAs) within last 6 months before starting therapy because of increased risk of haemorrhagic stroke
- see General Nursing points/Cautions for statins (p. 1246)

Patient teaching and advice

- see General Patient teaching and advice for statins (p. 1247)
- patient should be advised to avoid grapefruit during therapy
- instruct patient to take 2 hours apart from antacids

tablet can be dispersed in water (5–6 minutes) or crushed and mixed with spoonful of yoghurt or apple puree

Note

- contained in Cadivast and Caduet with amlodipine, and Atozet and Ezetast with ezetimibe

FLUVASTATIN (Lescol XL)

Available forms

Tablets (prolonged-release): 80 mg

Action/Use

- see General Actions/Uses of statins (pp. 1245–46)
- elimination half-life 0.5–2.3 hours

Dose

- (lipid lowering) 80 mg orally nocte **OR**
- (post-coronary transcatheter therapy) 80 mg orally nocte

Adverse effects

- see General Adverse effects of statins (p. 1246)

Interactions

- bioavailability may be increased if given with cimetidine, ranitidine or omeprazole
- bioavailability may be decreased if given with rifampicin

- if given with warfarin, INR should be monitored, especially when starting, stopping or altering dose
- may increase plasma levels of phenytoin, increasing the risk of toxicity
- increased plasma levels may occur if given with phenytoin
- increased risk of myalgia and/or rhabdomyolysis if given with colchicine
- see also General Interactions of statins (p. 1246)

Nursing points/Cautions

- see General Nursing points/Cautions for statins (p. 1246)

Patient teaching and advice

- patients should be advised that prolonged-release tablets should be swallowed whole, not broken, crushed or chewed
- see General Patient teaching and advice for statins (p. 1247)

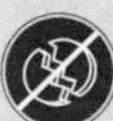

tablet should not be broken or chewed

PRAVASTATIN SODIUM (Cholstat, Cholvastin, Lipostat, Pravachol)

Available forms

Tablets: 10 mg, 20 mg, 40 mg, 80 mg

Action

- see General Actions of statins (p. 1245)
- half-life 1.3–2.8 hours

Use

- see General Uses of statins (p. 1246)
- previous myocardial infarction with normal cholesterol levels, unstable angina
- (adolescents) heterozygous familial hypercholesterolaemia

Dose

- (lipid lowering) initially 10–20 mg orally nocte, increasing at 4-week intervals to 80 mg daily if necessary **OR**
- (coronary heart disease, prevention of myocardial infarction) 40 mg orally nocte **OR**
- (heterozygous familial hypercholesterolaemia, 8–13 years) 20 mg orally nocte **OR**
- (heterozygous familial hypercholesterolaemia, 14–18 years) 40 mg orally nocte

Adverse effects

- dyspnoea
- visual disturbances, including blurred vision
- see also General Adverse effects of statins (p. 1246)

Interactions

- see General Interactions of statins (p. 1246)

Nursing points/Cautions

- not recommended for hypertriglyceridaemia
- not recommended for homozygous familial hypercholesterolaemia
- see also General Nursing points/Cautions for statins (p. 1246)

Patient teaching and advice

- advise patient to take pravastatin on an empty stomach
- patient should be instructed to take tablets whole
- warn patient against driving or operating machinery if blurred vision occurs
- see also General Patient teaching and advice for statins (p. 1247)

tablet can be crushed and mixed with water (but does not disperse readily) or spoonful of yoghurt or apple puree

ROSUVASTATIN (Cavstat, Crestor, Crosuva, Noumed, Rostor)

Available forms
Tablets: 5 mg, 10 mg, 20 mg, 40 mg

Action
- see General Actions of statins (p. 1245)
- metabolite has some activity
- elimination half-life 14–26 hours

Use
- see General Uses of statins (p. 1246)

Dose
- (lipid lowering) initially 5–10 mg orally daily, increasing at 4-week intervals if needed (daily maximum 20 mg) **OR**
- (lipid lowering, Asian patients) initially 5 mg orally daily, increasing at 4-week intervals if needed (daily maximum 20 mg) **OR**
- (prevention of cardiovascular disease) 20 mg orally daily

Adverse effects
- see General Adverse effects of statins (p. 1246)

Interactions
- may decrease serum levels if given with antacids
- caution if used with HIV protease inhibitors
- (Asian patients) contraindicated with fibrates
- see also General Interactions of statins (p. 1246)

Nursing points/Cautions
- tablets contain lactose and are therefore not recommended in those with rare hereditary problems of galactose intolerance, Lapp lactase deficiency or glucose–galactose malabsorption
- 40 mg tablets are contraindicated in those with predisposition to myopathy or rhabdomyolysis
- see also General Nursing points/Cautions for statins (p. 1246)

Patient teaching and advice
- see General Patient teaching and advice for statins (p. 1247)
- instruct patients to take rosuvastatin 2 hours apart from antacids

tablet can be dispersed in water or crushed and mixed with spoonful of yoghurt or apple puree

Note
- contained in Ezalo or Rosuzet Composite Pack with ezetimibe

SIMVASTATIN (Lipex, Simvacor, Simvar, Zimstat, Zocor)

Available forms
Tablets: 5 mg, 10 mg, 20 mg, 40 mg, 80 mg

Action
- see General Actions of statins (p. 1245)
- prodrug requires activation in the liver
- active metabolites
- decreases cholesterol levels by 30–50%
- half-life 2–3 hours

Use
- see General Uses of statins (p. 1246)
- heterozygous familial hypercholesterolaemia (adolescents, 10–17 years)

Dose
- (lipid lowering) initially 10–20 mg orally nocte, increasing at 4-week intervals if needed (daily maximum 80 mg) **OR**
- (heterozygous familial hypercholesterolaemia, adolescents, 10–17 years) initially 10 mg orally nocte, increasing to maximum of 40 mg if needed **OR**

- (coronary heart disease) 40–80 mg orally nocte

Adverse effects
- transient hypotension
- (uncommon) peripheral neuropathy, paraesthesia
- see also General Adverse effects of statins (p. 1246)

Interactions
- contraindicated with gemfibrozil, ciclosporin, danazol, clarithromycin, erythromycin, HIV protease inhibitors and azole antifungals
- caution if used with warfarin; INR should be closely monitored, especially when starting or stopping therapy
- not recommended with grapefruit juice
- caution if given with digoxin. If given together serum digoxin levels should be closely monitored
- increased risk of rhabdomyolysis if given with amiodarone, verapamil, diltiazem, amlodipine or niacin (≥ 1g/day)
- caution if given with colchicine in those with renal insufficiency
- (Asian patients) not recommended with niacin (≥ 1 g/day)
- see also General Interactions of statins (p. 1246)

Nursing points/Cautions
- risk of myopathy increases with dose; 80 mg dose should only be used in patients with high risk of cardiovascular complications who have not achieved treatment goals and where benefits outweigh risks
- see General Nursing points/Cautions for statins (p. 1246)

Patient teaching and advice
- see General Patient teaching and advice for statins (p. 1247)
- instruct patient to avoid grapefruit juice during therapy
- advise patient to report any numbness or tingling in hands or feet

tablet can be crushed and mixed with water or spoonful of yoghurt or apple puree

Note
- contained in Ezetorin, EzSimva, Vytorin and Zelden with ezetimibe

BILE ACID BINDING AGENTS

General Actions of bile acid binding agents
- cholesterol is the major precursor of bile salts. Bile acid binding agents bind cholesterol-containing bile acids in the intestine, preventing them from being reabsorbed. This increases hepatic LDL receptor activity, promoting hepatic uptake and subsequent breakdown of plasma LDL cholesterol for conversion to replacement bile acids, thus lowering the plasma cholesterol concentration

General Uses of bile acid binding agents
- hypercholesterolaemia (adjunctive therapy)
- mixed hyperlipidaemia

- diarrhoea (ileal resection or disease)
- relief of pruritus associated with biliary obstruction and primary biliary cirrhosis

General Adverse effects of bile acid binding agents

- constipation, faecal impaction, haemorrhoids or aggravation of pre-existing haemorrhoids
- (less common) nausea, vomiting, anorexia, abdominal pain and distension, heartburn, indigestion, flatulence, diarrhoea, steatorrhoea
- (less common) headache, migraine, sinus headache, dizziness, fatigue
- (less common) reduced absorption of fat-soluble vitamins, increased risk of bleeding (hypoprothrombinaemia, vitamin K), night blindness (vitamin A) and osteoporosis (vitamin D)
- (less common) rash, irritation of skin, tongue and perianal area
- (prolonged use) hyperchloraemic acidosis

General Interactions of bile acid binding agents

- may reduce or delay absorption of thyroid hormones, warfarin, digoxin, phenobarbital (phenobarbitone), tetracycline, propranolol, benzylpenicillin, gemfibrozil, frusemide, mycophenolate mofetil, mycophenolate sodium, inorganic iron and oral phosphate supplements

General Nursing points/Cautions for bile acid binding agents

- any secondary causes of hypercholesterolaemia (e.g. poorly controlled diabetes mellitus, hypothyroidism, obstructive liver disease, alcoholism, nephrotic syndrome, dysproteinaemia, drug therapy) should be identified and treated before starting therapy, as well as weight reduction and diet modification
- baseline cholesterol and triglyceride levels should be established, then monitored during therapy
- GI function should be evaluated before starting therapy to identify any risks for severe constipation and/or faecal impaction
- if therapy is prolonged, supplementary fat-soluble vitamins A and D may be required and, if there is a bleeding tendency, vitamin K
- therapy should be discontinued if cholesterol level does not fall or triglyceride levels increase
- caution in those with pre-existing constipation (reduced dose required) or if > 60 years
- contraindicated in those with complete biliary obstruction

General Patient teaching and advice for bile acid binding agents

- advise patient that powder/granules must not be taken in dry form
- patient should be instructed to place prescribed amount of sachet contents on the surface of 100–150 mL (for 4 g sachet) or 200–300 mL (for 8 g sachet) of water, milk, carbonated beverage (taking care with excess foaming/frothing), tomato or fruit juice, thin soups, cereals, apple sauce or puree, pears, peaches, fruit cocktail or crushed pineapple in a large glass. Stir vigorously or shake in Questran Lite shaker (for colestyramine only) until the mixture is evenly suspended.

Rinse glass after use and drink contents to ensure total dose is taken
- advise patient that for better absorption take other oral drugs either 1 hour before or 4–6 hours after
- addition of cereal bran and good fluid intake is recommended to minimise constipation
- patient should be advised to seek medical advice if constipation occurs
- see also General Patient teaching and advice (p. xxvii)

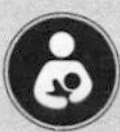

not recommended during pregnancy, because interference with fat-soluble vitamins may be detrimental to the developing fetus

only use during breastfeeding if benefits outweigh risks

COLESTYRAMINE (CHOLESTYRAMINE) (Questran Lite)

Available form
Powder: 4 g

Action
- see General Actions of bile acid binding agents (p. 1251)
- insoluble in water
- not absorbed by GI tract and not affected by digestive enzymes
- decreases cholesterol levels by about 20–40%

Use
- see General Uses of bile acid binding agents (p. 1251)

Dose
- (lipid lowering) initially 4 g (1 sachet) orally daily, increasing over next 2–4 weeks to the required dose
OR
- (other uses) 12–16 g orally daily

Adverse effects
- (uncommon) osteoporosis
- see General Adverse effects of bile acid binding agents (p. 1251)

Interactions
- caution if given with aldosterone antagonists (e.g. spironolactone) because of increased risk of hyperchloraemic acidosis
- may interfere with oestrogen metabolism
- see General Interactions of bile acid binding agents (p. 1252)

Nursing points/Cautions
- (diarrhoea use) response should be seen within 3 days
- large doses (24 g per day) may interfere with fat absorption and result in steatorrhoea
- those with phenylketonuria should be advised that colestyramine contains phenylalanine (16.8 mg/4 g colestyramine)
- see General Nursing points/Cautions for bile acid binding agents (p. 1252)

Patient teaching and advice
- advise patient to avoid holding in mouth for prolonged length of time to avoid tooth decay or discolouration
- see General Patient teaching and advice for bile acid binding agents (p. 1252)

FIBRATES

General Actions of fibrates

- stimulates lipoprotein lipase, reducing the amount of triglyceride in VLDL and chylomicrons
- stimulates liver to increase LDL uptake and therefore LDL clearance
- reduces plasma levels of triglycerides
- increases plasma level of HDL by a moderate amount, variate effect on LDL

General Uses of fibrates

- types II, III, IV and V dyslipidaemia
- mixed hyperlipidaemia
- dyslipidaemia associated with type 2 diabetes
- hypercholesterolaemia (second line)

General Adverse effects of fibrates

- nausea, vomiting, diarrhoea, constipation, dyspepsia, abdominal pain, flatulence
- rash
- elevated liver enzymes and CPK
- gall stone formation
- (uncommon) myopathy, myalgia, myositis
- (uncommon) photosensitivity reaction
- (rare) rhabdomyolysis, hepatitis, pancreatitis, hypersensitivity
- (rare) anaemia, leucopenia, thrombocytopenia

General Interactions of fibrates

- contraindicated with other fibrates
- not recommended with statins because of increased risk of myopathy and rhabdomyolysis
- may enhance effects of oral anticoagulants, therefore INR should be carefully monitored, especially when starting, stopping or altering doses
- caution if used with ciclosporin
- increased risk of myotoxicity if given with colchicine

General Nursing points/Cautions for fibrates

- any secondary causes of hypercholesterolaemia (e.g. poorly controlled diabetes mellitus, hypothyroidism, obstructive liver disease, alcoholism, nephrotic syndrome, dysproteinaemia, drug therapy) should be identified and treated before starting therapy, as well as weight reduction and diet modification
- ineffective in patients with raised cholesterol but normal triglyceride levels
- baseline liver function tests (including liver enzymes, serum lipids, lipoproteins and ratios) should be performed before starting, 3-monthly for first 12 months and then regularly throughout treatment
- if HDL-C levels become severely depressed, therapy should be stopped and restarted when the levels return to baseline
- full blood count should be measured before starting and regularly during first 12 months of therapy
- if not effective in 12 weeks at maximum dose, different or adjunct therapy should be considered
- caution if used in those with hepatobiliary disease
- increased risk of myopathy and/or rhabdomyolysis if given to those over 70 years, history of hereditary muscular disorders, kidney impairment, hypoalbuminaemia, hypothyroidism or high alcohol intake

- contraindicated in those with photoallergy/phototoxic reaction to other fibrates or ketoprofen
- contraindicated in those with liver/renal dysfunction, primary biliary cirrhosis, liver function abnormalities, existing gallbladder disease or chronic/acute pancreatitis (except due to hypertriglyceridaemia)

General Patient teaching and advice for fibrates

- warn patient against drinking large quantities of alcohol
- patient should be advised against driving or operating machinery if dizziness/vertigo occurs
- warn patient to avoid direct exposure to UV and when outdoors, wear protective garment and hat, sunscreen (SPF 30+) and sunglasses
- advise patient to seek medical advice immediately if any of the following occur:
  - muscle pain, cramps, tenderness or weakness, dark urine, malaise or fever
  - yellowing of skin or eyes, tiredness, loss of appetite, abdominal pain, dark urine
  - sudden intense pain in upper right abdomen, sudden rapidly intensifying pain just below breastbone, pain between shoulder blades or right shoulder tip or vomiting

FENOFIBRATE (Fenocopia, Fenocol, Lipidil)

Available forms

Tablets: 48 mg, 145 mg

Action

- see General Actions of fibrates (p. 1254)
- active metabolite (fenofibric acid) which has half-life of about 20 hours
- significantly reduces triglyceride levels by 20–50%
- some uricosuric effect decreasing uric acid levels by about 25%

Use

- see General Uses of fibrates (p. 1254)
- decrease progression of diabetic retinopathy in those with type 2 diabetes and existing diabetic retinopathy

Dose

- (dyslipidaemia, diabetic neuropathy) 145 mg orally daily with food

Adverse effects

- increase in serum creatinine
- (uncommon) headaches
- (rare) urticaria, rash, pulmonary embolism, deep vein thrombosis
- see General Adverse effects of fibrates (p. 1254)

Interactions

- reversible renal impairment may occur if given with ciclosporin. Renal function should be monitored carefully
- caution if used with pioglitazone
- caution if used with agents that have a narrow therapeutic index
- see General Interactions of fibrates (p. 1254)

Nursing points/Cautions

- 48 mg capsules should only be used for reduced doses in kidney impairment
- creatinine clearance should be measured during first 12 weeks of therapy and then regularly (especially in the elderly or those with diabetes)
- caution if used in those with renal impairment (creatinine clearance < 60 mL/minute) as dose may need to be reduced
- not recommended in those with lecithin hypersensitivity or hereditary problems of fructose/galactose

intolerance, Lapp lactase deficiency, glucose–galactose malabsorption or sucrase–isomaltase insufficiency
- contraindicated in those with photoallergy/phototoxic reaction to ketoprofen
- contraindicated in children
- contraindicated in those with allergy to peanuts, arachis oil, soya lecithin or related products
- see also General Nursing points/ Cautions for fibrates (p. 1254)

Patient teaching and advice

- patient should be advised to swallow capsule/tablets whole
- see General Patient teaching and advice for fibrates (p. 1255)

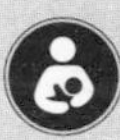
not recommended during pregnancy or breastfeeding

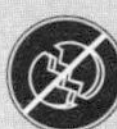
tablet does not disperse readily in water and is hard to crush

GEMFIBROZIL (Ausgem, Lipigem)

Available form
Tablets: 600 mg

Action
- see General Actions of fibrates (p. 1254)
- decreases triglycerides
- slight decrease in cholesterol, increase in HDL
- onset of action 2–5 days, peak effect 4 weeks
- half-life about 1.5 hours

Use
- see General Uses of fibrates (p. 1254)

Dose
- 600 mg orally twice daily 30 minutes before the morning and evening meal

Adverse effects
- acute appendicitis, altered taste
- atrial fibrillation
- fatigue, vertigo, headache, dizziness
- eczema
- (rare) subcapsular bilateral cataracts, urticaria, pruritus
- see also General Adverse effects of fibrates (p. 1254)

Interactions
- see General Interactions of fibrates (p. 1254)
- caution if used with rosiglitazone maleate
- caution if given with hypoglycaemic agents as hypoglycaemia may occur

Nursing points/Cautions
- contraindicated in those with type I hyperlipoproteinaemia
- see General Nursing points/Cautions for fibrates (p. 1254)

Patient teaching and advice
- patient should be advised to swallow tablets whole before meals. However, if this is not tolerated, it can be taken with food
- advise patient not to drive or operate machinery if dizziness or vertigo occur
- instruct those with diabetes to carefully monitor blood glucose levels during therapy as hypoglycaemia may occur
- women of childbearing potential should be counselled to use adequate contraception during therapy to avoid pregnancy
- see General Patient teaching and advice for fibrates, p. 1255

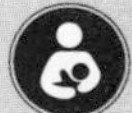
contraindicated during pregnancy and breastfeeding

PCSK9 INHIBITORS

General Actions of PCSK9 inhibitors

- monoclonal antibody (IgG2) that has high affinity for proprotein convertase subtilisin/kexin type 9 (PCSK9)
- inhibits circulation PCSK9 from binding to low-density lipoprotein receptor (LDLR) on liver cell surface preventing PCSK9-mediated LDLR degradation, increasing liver levels of LDLR, resulting in an associated decrease in serum low-density lipoprotein cholesterol (LDL-C)
- maximum inhibition occurs 4–8 hours after administration, peak concentration 3–4 days

General Adverse effects for PCSK9 inhibitors

- nasopharyngitis, influenza, upper respiratory tract infection, cough, sinusitis, bronchitis, flu-like illness
- back pain, arthralgia, myalgia, muscle spasms, pain in extremity
- headache, fatigue, dizziness, insomnia
- nausea, diarrhoea, constipation, gastroenteritis, upper abdominal pain
- hypertension, angina
- rash, urticaria, pruritus
- diabetes mellitus, gout
- antibody development
- (rare) hypersensitivity
- (injection site) redness, pain, bruising

General Interactions of PCSK9 inhibitors

- clearance may be increased by statins

General Nursing points/Cautions for PCSK9 inhibitors

- patient may be instructed to self-administer
- caution if used in those with severe liver impairment or severe/very severe kidney impairment
- contraindicated in those with hypersensitivity to hamster ovary protein or polysorbate

General Patient teaching and advice for PCSK9 inhibitors

- advise patient to seek medical advice immediately if there are any skin reactions, including swelling, itching or hives
- instructions for SC administration should include the following:
  - SC injections are given under the skin
  - injection sites include upper arm, thigh and abdomen, and sites should be rotated
  - injections should not be given into skin that is tender, red, sunburnt, bruised, hard, broken or inflamed
  - prefilled pen/syringe should be allowed to come to room temperature for at least 30–40 minutes before administration; however, it should not be warmed in other ways
  - prefilled pen/syringe should not be shaken
  - no other injections should be given into the same site
  - if prefilled pen/syringe is removed from refrigerator, it should be used within 30 days
  - store in refrigerator but do not freeze

  - used pen/syringe should be disposed of into puncture-resistant container
- see also General Patient teaching and advice (p. xxvii)

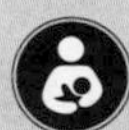

not recommended during pregnancy or breastfeeding unless benefits outweigh risks

ALIROCUMAB (Praluent)

Available forms

Prefilled syringe: 75 mg/mL, 150 mg/mL

Action

- see General Actions for PCSK9 inhibitors (p. 1257)
- half-life 17–20 days (or 12 days if given with a statin)

Use

- primary hypercholesterolaemia (as adjunct to diet and exercise in adults with heterozygous familial or non-familial hypercholesterolaemia at moderate to very high cardiovascular risk)
- as monotherapy or in combination with statin or other lipid-lowering agents in patients with primary hypercholesterolaemia unable to reach LDL-C goals with maximum dose of statin, if intolerant to statin or statin is contraindicated
- reduce risk of cardiovascular events (e.g. myocardial infarction, stroke, unstable angina requiring hospitalisation) in those with established cardiovascular disease in combination with statin or other lipid-lowering agent

Dose

- initially 75 mg SC every 2 weeks, increasing to 150 mg SC every 2 weeks if further LDL-C reduction is required **OR**
- 300 mg SC monthly

Adverse effects

- see General Adverse effects of PCSK9 inhibitors (p. 1257)
- oropharyngeal pain
- peripheral oedema
- musculoskeletal pain
- palpitations
- epistaxis
- haematuria
- increase in liver enzymes

Interactions

- see General Interactions of PCSK9 inhibitors (p. 1257)

Nursing points/Cautions

- LDL-C levels should be measured before starting therapy, after 4–8 weeks and during dose titration
- see also General Nursing points/Cautions for PCSK9 inhibitors (p. 1257)

Patient teaching and advice

- see General Patient teaching and advice for PCSK9 inhibitors (p. 1257)
- if dose is missed, advise patient to administer within 7 days of missed dose and then resume previous administration schedule
- if dosing schedule is every 2 weeks and dose is missed and not administered within 7 days, advise patient that administration should be delayed until next scheduled injection. If dosing schedule is monthly and dose is not administered within 7 days, advise patient to administer dose and then start a new schedule based on this date
- for 300 mg dose, instruct patient to administer two 150 mg injections into 2 different injection sites

EVOLOCUMAB (Repatha)

Available forms

Prefilled pen: 140 mg/mL; Prefilled cartridge with injection device: 420 mg/3.5 mL

Action
- see General Actions for PCSK9 inhibitors (p. 1257)
- half-life 11–17 days

Use
- primary hypercholesterolaemia (heterozygous familial or non-familial hypercholesterolaemia (HeFH) (adjunct to diet, exercise and/or statin and other lipid-lowering therapies)
- homozygous familial hypercholesterolemia (with other lipid-lowering therapies)
- prevention of cardiovascular events in those with established cardiovascular disease with statin or other lipid-lowering agents

Dose
- (primary hypercholesterolaemia or prevention of cardiovascular disease) 140 mg SC every 2 weeks or 420 mg SC once monthly **OR**
- (homozygous familial hypercholesterolemia) initially 420 mg SC monthly, increasing dose to 420 mg SC every 2 weeks if no response after 12 weeks

Adverse effects
- see General Adverse effects of PCSK9 inhibitors (p. 1257)
- nausea, gastroenteritis

Interactions
- see General Interactions of PCSK9 inhibitors (p. 1257)

Nursing points/Cautions
- (homozygous familial hypercholesterolemia) if patient is having apheresis, dose can be started at 420 mg SC every 2 weeks to correspond with apheresis schedule
- see General Nursing points/Cautions for PCSK9 inhibitors (p. 1257)

Patient teaching and advice
- see General Patient teaching and advice for PCSK9 inhibitors (p. 1257)
- if 420 mg dose is required, dose should be given as three (3) SC injections, which should be consecutively within 30 minutes
- see also General Patient teaching and advice (p. xxvii)

OTHER LIPID-LOWERING AGENTS

EICOSAPENTEANOIC ACID ETHYL ESTER/DOCOSAHEXAENOIC ACID ETHYL ESTER (Omacor)

Available form
Capsules: 1 g

Action
- omega-3 fatty acids
- docosahexaenoic acid is an omega-3 fatty acid and a natural component of fish oil found in oily fish such as mackerel, salmon and tuna
- omega-3 fatty acids are thought to reduce formation of VLDL and accelerate metabolism of VLDL to LDL, thereby reducing triglyceride levels, but may also potentially increase LDL levels
- also thought to upregulate metabolism of fatty acids in the liver

Use
- hypertriglyceridaemia (type IV and V as monotherapy; type IIb (with statin))

Dose
- (hypertriglyceridaemia) 4 g orally daily with glass of water

Adverse effects
- abdominal pain, dyspepsia, gastroesophageal reflux disease (GORD), belching, nausea, vomiting, abdominal distention, flatulence, diarrhoea, constipation, taste disturbance
- headache
- mildly elevated ALT

- (uncommon) headache, dizziness, hypotension, angina, rash

Interactions

- increased bleeding time may occur if given with aspirin or warfarin, therefore INR should be monitored carefully, especially when starting or stopping therapy

Nursing points/Cautions

- lipids should be closely monitored during therapy, especially LDL in those with type IV or V dyslipidaemia
- caution if used in those with sensitivity or allergy to fish
- caution if used in those with liver impairment. Liver function should be monitored during therapy especially if daily dose > 4 g
- not recommended for exogenous hypertriglyceridaemia (type 1 hyperchylomicronaemia)
- contraindicated in those with hypersensitivity to soya, including soya milk, soya beans or peanuts

Patient teaching and advice

- advise patient to swallow capsules whole with water; however, they can take the capsules with food if GI disturbances occur
- see General Patient teaching and advice (p. xxvii)

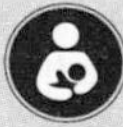

not recommended during pregnancy or breastfeeding unless benefits outweigh risks

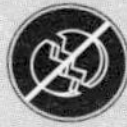

capsules should not be opened or crushed

EZETIMIBE (Ezetrol, Ezemichol, Zient)

Available form

Tablets: 10 mg

Action

- inhibits absorption of cholesterol in the small intestine, decreasing the amount of intestinal cholesterol reaching the liver, resulting in reduced liver cholesterol stores and increasing clearance in the blood
- does not increase bile acid excretion (as with bile acid binding agents)
- does not inhibit liver cholesterol synthesis (as with statins)
- conjugated to active compound in liver
- does not inhibit absorption of fat-soluble vitamins or nutrients
- reduce LDL by about 18% with little impact on triglyceride or HDL levels
- half-life of both parent and conjugated compound is about 22 hours

Use

- (adult) primary hypercholesterolaemia (alone or with statin)
- (adult) homozygous familial hypercholesterolaemia (with statin)
- (adolescent, 10–17 years) heterozygous familial hypercholesterolaemia (with simvastatin) (adjunctive therapy)
- (adolescent, 10–17 years) homozygous familial hypercholesterolaemia (with simvastatin) (adjunctive therapy)
- prevention of cardiovascular disease in patients with coronary heart disease and history of acute coronary syndrome (with statin)

Dose

- 10 mg orally daily (with or without statin)

Adverse effects

- elevated liver enzymes
- headache, fatigue
- abdominal pain, diarrhoea, flatulence and uncommonly, dyspepsia, gastrointestinal reflex disease, decreased appetite
- (uncommon) cough, muscle spasm, neck pain
- (with statin) myalgia
- (with fenofibrate) abdominal pain

Interactions

- not recommended with fibrates (other than fenofibrate)
- caution if used with ciclosporin, therefore ciclosporin levels should be closely monitored during therapy
- decreased plasma level may occur if given within 4 hours of colestyramine
- contraindicated with fenofibrate in those with gallbladder disease
- increased risk of myopathy and/or rhabdomyolysis if given with statin
- if given with warfarin, INR should be closely monitored especially when starting and stopping therapy

Nursing points/Cautions

- any secondary causes of hypercholesterolaemia (e.g. poorly controlled diabetes mellitus, hypothyroidism, obstructive liver disease, alcoholism, nephrotic syndrome, dysproteinaemia, drug therapy) should be identified and treated before starting therapy, as well as weight reduction and diet modification
- liver function tests should be performed at start and regularly throughout therapy if given with a statin
- not recommended in those with impaired liver function
- not recommended in children under 10 years or in premenarchal girls or prepubertal boys
- contraindicated with fenofibrate in those with gallbladder disease
- contraindicated with statin in those with active liver disease or unexplained raised serum transaminases

Patient teaching and advice

- advise patient to report any muscle pain, cramps, tenderness or weakness (not caused by exercise), malaise or fever. If this occurs, CPK concentration should be measured
- if taken with statin, can be taken at the same time
- if taken with bile acid sequestering agent such as cholestyramine, take 2 hours before or 4 hours later
- see also General Patient teaching and advice (p. xxvii)

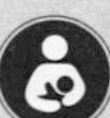

contraindicated with statins during pregnancy or breastfeeding

tablet can be crushed and mixed with water or spoonful of yoghurt or apple puree

Note

- combined with simvastatin in Ezotorin, EziSimva GH, Vytorin and Zeklen, atorvastatin in Alozet, Ezetast and Ezalo, and rosuvastatin in Rosuzet Composite Pack

NICOTINIC ACID (Nicotinic Acid)

Available form

Tablets: 250 mg

Action

- inhibits synthesis of lipoproteins (VLDL) in the liver, thereby decreasing LDL and cholesterol. Cholesterol level decreases by 10–20%, while triglycerides decrease by 40–80%
- promotes lipoprotein lipase activity
- decreases mobilisation of free fatty acids from adipose tissue, increasing sterol in the faeces
- vasodilator at therapeutic levels (not nutritional dose)
- essential dietary element (water soluble B complex vitamin (vitamin B_3, niacin)) (see Vitamins, minerals and electrolytes, p. 1575)
- elimination half-life 45 minutes

Use

- hypercholesterolaemia and hypertriglyceridaemia
- hyperlipoproteinaemia types II, IIB, III, IV and V (adjunctive therapy)
- pellagra

Dose

- (lipid lowering/hypertriglyceridaemia) initially 250 mg orally 3 times daily after meals, increasing by 250 mg every fourth day to a daily maximum of 3–4.5 g **OR**
- (pellagra) 250 mg orally twice daily after meals

Adverse effects

- flushing, headache, pounding head, heat sensation
- atrial fibrillation, cardiac arrhythmias (if coronary heart disease), hypotension
- dry skin, urticaria, rash, pruritus, hyperpigmentation (brown), hyperkeratosis
- nausea, vomiting, diarrhoea, flatulence, heartburn
- activation of peptic ulcer
- jaundice, impaired liver function, ascites, hepatomegaly
- decrease in glucose tolerance, hyperglycaemia
- hyperuricaemia
- hypothyroidism
- toxic amblyopia
- nervousness

Interactions

- vasodilation and hypotensive effects may be enhanced by antihypertensive drugs, including adrenergic blocking agents
- may require increased insulin or oral hypoglycaemic requirement in patients with diabetes
- caution if used with alcohol as delirium and/or lactic acidosis may occur
- may have increased and prolonged effect if given with aspirin, increasing risk of toxicity
- flushing and warm sensation may be reduced by aspirin or clonidine
- increased risk of myopathy, rhabdomyolysis and acute renal failure if given with statins
- increased flushing and dizziness may occur if used with transdermal nicotine
- may cause false positive result for blood bilirubin or urinary glucose (Benedict's agent) or falsely elevated urinary catecholamines

Nursing points/Cautions

- plasma cholesterol and triglyceride levels should be monitored regularly and dose adjusted accordingly
- liver function monitoring is recommended at 4–6-week intervals during the first 3 months of therapy or after any increase in dose, then 3-monthly for 1 year and annually thereafter
- glucose tolerance should be monitored regularly and diet adjusted and/or oral hypoglycaemic dose also adjusted if needed
- serum uric acid levels should be monitored regularly during long-term therapy
- caution if used in those with history of peptic ulceration or GI irritation
- contraindicated in patients with recent myocardial infarction and should be stopped immediately if the patient has a myocardial infarction during therapy
- contraindicated in those with liver dysfunction, peptic ulcers, diabetes mellitus, gout or hyperuricaemia, or in large doses in those with heart or gallbladder disease, glaucoma, arterial bleeding or a sudden fall in peripheral vascular resistance

Patient teaching and advice

- patient should be warned that vasodilation occurs approximately 20 minutes after administration and may persist for 20–60 minutes
- advise patient to seek medical advice immediately if there is fever, malaise, yellowing of skin and eyes, dark urine or abdominal pain

- counsel patient about use of alcohol, hot drinks and aspirin during therapy. Alcohol and hot drinks increase flushing and itching
- if patient is concurrently using nicotine replacement therapy (e.g. nicotine patches), he/she should be advised of the increased risk of flushing and/or dizziness, especially when driving or operating machinery
- patients with diabetes should be warned to closely monitor blood glucose levels as insulin and/or oral hypoglycaemic dose may be altered
- women of childbearing potential should be counselled to use adequate contraception during therapy to avoid pregnancy
- see General Patient teaching and advice (p. xxvii)

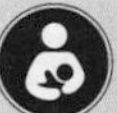

contraindicated during pregnancy or breastfeeding

tablet can be dispersed in water or crushed and mixed with yoghurt or apple puree

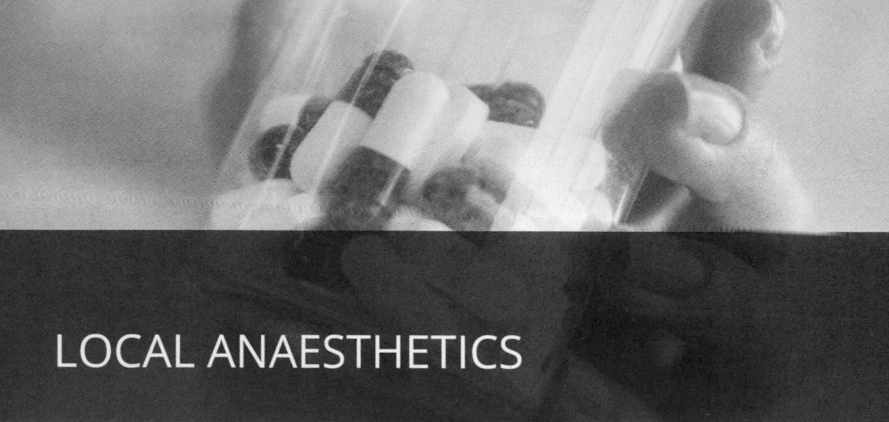

LOCAL ANAESTHETICS

Local anaesthetics are a group of chemically related agents that produce a reversible loss of sensation (without a loss of consciousness), as well as producing a local analgesic action without loss of control. They are administered either topically (e.g. lotions, creams, lozenges, sprays) or parenterally, but not orally (Bryant et al 2019).

General Actions of local anaesthetics

- amide type or ester type
- block or diminish nerve conduction reversibly by inhibiting depolarisation and ion (sodium) exchange (membrane stabiliser)
- do not produce loss of consciousness
- ester-like local anaesthetics are rapidly metabolised by plasma enzyme to p-aminobenzoic acid (PABA) metabolites, which may cause allergic reaction in some people
- amide-like local anaesthetics are not metabolised to PABA metabolites and are less likely to cause allergic reactions
- onset and duration of action is dependent on the agent's lipid solubility, volume and concentration, local blood flow and speed on injection, as well as the patient's liver, kidney and cardiovascular function. Short-acting local anaesthetics (e.g. benzocaine, cocaine) have a duration of 30–60 minutes, intermediate-acting local anaesthetics (e.g. prilocaine, lidocaine (lignocaine)) have a duration of 30 minutes to 4 hours, while long-acting local anaesthetics (e.g. bupivacaine, tetracaine) have a duration of action 3–10 hours
- most local anaesthetics produce vasodilation, therefore the addition of vasoconstrictors (usually adrenaline (epinephrine) or felypressin) decreases blood flow in the area and prolongs the anaesthesia by reducing absorption
- half-life is generally short (1–2 hours)

Surface or topical anaesthesia

- blocks sensory nerve endings in the skin, mucous membranes and the eye

Infiltration anaesthesia

- solution is injected into and around site causing nerve endings (but not motor nerves) to become anaesthetised

Intravenous regional anaesthesia (Bier's block)

- specialised technique for anaesthesia of the upper limbs

Nerve block anaesthesia

- sensory nerve pathways are blocked by injecting into or around nerve trunks or ganglia supplying the affected area
- single nerves or nerve trunks emerging from spinal cord (paravertebral) may be blocked
- epidural and spinal blocks are specialised central nerve blocks. Analgesia can be enhanced if co-administered with an opioid
- dermatome assessment is used to monitor levels and extent of analgesia

Spinal anaesthesia

- regional anaesthesia blocking transmission in spinal nerves in contact with the anaesthetic agent
- agent is injected intrathecally after lumbar puncture procedure
- the somatic level of anaesthesia depends on the specific gravity of the anaesthetic solution and the position of the patient

General Uses of local anaesthetics

- procedures where patient's cooperation and consciousness are needed or wanted
- minor procedures where general anaesthetic is not warranted or hazardous
- sympathetic blockade
- postoperative analgesia

General Doses for local anaesthetics

- dose is dependent on site, vascularity of area, number of neuronal segments to be blocked, individual tolerance and technique, as well as other factors, including age, weight, and kidney and liver function

General Adverse effects of local anaesthetics

- hypotension, bradycardia
- headache, dizziness, drowsiness, nervousness
- tremor, twitching, shaking
- blurred or double vision
- tinnitus
- nausea, vomiting
- increased temperature, chills/rigors
- slurred speech, numbness of tongue
- (uncommon) muscle rigidity and/or muscle twitching
- (injection site) inflammation, haematoma, nerve injury, abscess formation, necrosis
- (spinal or epidural anaesthesia) hypotension, headache, backache, paraesthesia, neuropathy, infection, autonomic dysfunction
- (epidural or intrathecal blockade) hypotension, bradycardia
- (epidural or spinal anaesthesia) epidural/spinal haematoma
- (uncommon) convulsions, unconsciousness, severe hypotension, cardiovascular collapse, bradycardia and possible cardiac arrest
- (rare, spinal anaesthetic) high or total blockade (resulting in respiratory or cardiovascular depression/arrest)
- (rare, intrathecal) paraesthesia, anaesthesia, motor weakness, paralysis, loss of bladder control
- (rare) allergic dermatitis, anaphylaxis (more common with ester-type local anaesthetics), bronchospasm

General Interactions of local anaesthetics

- amide-type local anaesthetics should be used with caution with antiarrhythmic agents, because the cardiac effect may be potentiated

- caution if used with other amide local anaesthetics or chemically related agents as adverse effects are additive
- not recommended with agents that prolong QT interval or cause dysrhythmias
- (epidural/spinal) increased hypotension can occur if given with antihypertensive agents
- (spinal/epidural anaesthesia) increased risk of epidural/spinal haematoma if given to patients on anticoagulant therapy with low-molecular-weight heparins/heparinoids or if taking other agents that affect haemostasis (e.g. NSAIDs, antiplatelet agents, other anticoagulant agents)

General Nursing points/Cautions for local anaesthetics

- before receiving local anaesthetic agent, patient should have any hypoxia, hypotension, fluid or acid–base imbalance corrected to decrease risk of toxic reactions
- monitor heart rate, respiratory rate, oxygen saturation, level of consciousness and BP of patients during and for at least 4 hours after spinal anaesthesia
- (spinal/epidural anaesthesia) patients should be closely monitored for any neurological impairment
- test doses are sometimes given if large dose or epidural anaesthesia is to be administered
- nurse patient in a recumbent position
- have equipment (including oxygen) available for assisted ventilation and mucus extraction in the event of emergency resuscitation. Diazepam and/or thiopentone should be readily available for convulsions and/or vasopressors for bradycardia and hypotension
- local anaesthetics react with some metals and may cause local irritation if injected after being in contact with them; therefore the local anaesthetics should not have prolonged contact with metal bowls, cannulae or syringes with metal parts
- adrenaline (epinephrine) must not be used when producing a nerve block in an appendage such as the digits, ears, nose or penis, because these are supplied by end arteries and therefore subject to gangrene
- spinal cord may be damaged if spinal anaesthetic contains adrenaline (epinephrine)
- caution if used in the head and neck area as systemic adverse effects may occur and respiratory and cardiovascular function should be closely monitored
- all local anaesthetics should be used with caution in those with known drug allergy or sensitivity
- not recommended in those with porphyria unless no safer alternative is available
- caution if epidural anaesthetics are used in those with impaired cardiovascular function
- caution if local anaesthetics are used in those with predisposition to malignant hyperthermia or pre-existing neurological condition
- caution if used in those with renal or liver impairment, epilepsy, partial or complete heart block or conduction disorders, severe bradycardia,

shock, hyperthyroidism or digoxin intoxication
- (spinal/epidural) contraindicated in those with CNS or spinal disease, including meningitis, spinal fluid block, syphilis, poliomyelitis, TB or metastatic lesions of the spinal cord, uncorrected hypotension or cranial/spinal haemorrhage
- contraindicated in those with myasthenia gravis, Stokes–Adams syndrome or Wolff-Parkinson-White syndrome, impaired cardiac conduction, severe shock, known deficiency in plasma cholinesterase activity, serious disease or infection of CNS, or uncorrected hypotension
- contraindicated for extensive surgery requiring large doses that could be toxic
- contraindicated for IV regional anaesthesia (Bier's block) or obstetric paracervical block (due to increased risk of fetal bradycardia and acidosis)
- contraindicated if there is infection or inflammation at the site of the proposed injection or if the patient has septicaemia

General Patient teaching and advice for local anaesthetics

- patient should be advised to avoid driving or operating machinery until any possible impaired coordination, dizziness, drowsiness or other adverse effects have resolved
- warn patient about temporary loss of sensation and muscle function after infiltration and nerve block injection and should not drive after procedure
- see also General Patient teaching and advice (p. xxvii)

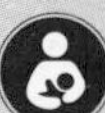

should only be used during pregnancy (not obstetric use) if benefits outweigh risks as local anaesthetics cross placenta rapidly

breastfeeding is not recommended within 48 hours of local anaesthetic

ARTICAINE HYDROCHLORIDE

Action

- amide type, similar to prilocaine and lidocaine (lignocaine)
- see General Actions of local anaesthetics (p. 1264)
- onset of action 1–6 minutes, duration about 68 minutes, half-life about 1.5 hours
- adrenaline (epinephrine) added as vasoconstrictor to reduce bleeding and prolong tissue concentration

Use

- local or regional anaesthesia, for simple and complex dental procedures

Adverse effects

- gingivitis
- tachypnoea, followed by bradypnoea and apnoea
- decreased heart rate and blood pressure
- facial oedema
- see also General Adverse effects of local anaesthetics (p. 1265)

Interactions

- contraindicated with or within 2 weeks of MAOIs, with TCAs or phenothiazines due to risk of prolonged hypotension or hypertension
- caution if used with sympathomimetic agents which may be antagonised by adrenaline (epinephrine)
- see also General Interactions of sympathomimetic agents (p. 1499)

Nursing points/Cautions

- contains sodium metasulfite and is therefore contraindicated in those with hypersensitivity to sulfites

- contraindicated IV
- contraindicated in children under 4 years
- not recommended (because of adrenaline (epinephrine)) in those with diabetes or untreated thyrotoxicosis and with caution in those with hypertension, cardiac disease, cardiac conduction abnormalities or epilepsy
- contraindicated in those with hypersensitivity to amide-type local anaesthetics
- see General Nursing points/Cautions for local anaesthetics (p. 1266)

Patient teaching and advice

- see General Patient teaching and advice for local anaesthetics (p. 1267)

Note

- contained in Articadent Dental, Deltazine, Septanest, Ubistesin and Ubistesin Forte with adrenaline (epinephrine)

BUPIVACAINE HYDROCHLORIDE MONOHYDRATE (BUPIVACAINE HYDROCHLORIDE) (Bupivacaine Injection BP, Bupivacaine Spinal Heavy BNM, Marcain, Marcain Epidural, Marcain Spinal 0.5%, Marcain Spinal 0.5% Heavy)

Available forms

Vial: 50 mg/20 mL, 100 mg/20 mL; Ampoules: 50 mg/10 mL, 20 mg/4 mL; Infusion bag: 125 mg/100 mL, 250 mg/200 mL, 250 mg/100 mL

Action

- long-acting amide with duration up to 12 hours (peripheral nerve block) and 2–5 hours (single epidural injection)
- four-fold potency and toxicity of lidocaine (lignocaine)
- onset of action 10–15 minutes (topical and/or infiltration), 15–30 minutes (nerve block)
- duration of action 3–4 hours (infiltration), 2–6 hours (minor nerve block), 7–14 hours (major nerve block), 3–4 hours (epidural)
- half-life 2–5.5 hours
- accumulation may occur with repeated doses

Use

- surgical anaesthesia (epidural block, infiltration, caudal and regional nerve block)
- analgesia (epidural)

Adverse effects/Interactions/ Patient teaching and advice

- see General Adverse effects, Interactions, Nursing points/Cautions/ Patient teaching and advice for local anaesthetics (pp. 1265–67)

Nursing points/Cautions

- contraindicated IV
- contraindicated in those with pernicious anaemia combined with subacute degeneration of the spinal cord
- contraindicated in those with hypersensitivity to amide-type local anaesthetics
- see General Nursing points/Cautions for local anaesthetics (p. 1266)

Note

- may be combined with fentanyl (Marcain with Fentanyl) or adrenaline (epinephrine) (Bupivadren with Adrenaline, Bupivacaine with Adrenaline, Marcain with Adrenaline (epinephrine))

LEVOBUPIVACAINE HYDROCHLORIDE (Chirocaine)

Available forms

Ampoule: 25 mg/10 mL, 50 mg/10 mL, 75 mg/10 mL; Infusion bags: 250 mg/200 mL

Action

- amide, which is equipotent to bupivacaine
- onset of action 10–15 minutes (infiltration), 15–30 minutes (nerve block)
- duration of action 3–4 hours (infiltration), 2–6 hours (minor nerve block), 7–14 hours (major nerve block), 3–4 hours (epidural)
- half-life 2–3 hours

Use

- surgical anaesthesia (epidural, intrathecal, peripheral nerve block, local infiltration, peribulbar block in ophthalmic surgery)
- pain management (epidural)

Adverse effects

- anaemia
- pruritus
- fetal distress, delayed delivery
- see also General Adverse effects of local anaesthetics (p. 1265)

Interactions

- increased serum levels and risk of toxicity may occur if given with rifampicin, phenytoin, phenobarbital (phenobarbitone), clarithromycin, erythromycin, ritonavir, omeprazole, azole antifungal agents and verapamil
- see also General Interactions of local anaesthetics (p. 1265)

Nursing points/Cautions

- (epidural) test dose (3–5 mL) is recommended, followed by patient monitoring (HR, BP, verbal contact) 5 minutes after dose. If accidental IV administration has occurred, HR will increase immediately, or if given intrathecally, patient will show signs of spinal block
- not given as rapid IV bolus
- not recommended if fast onset of action is required
- (epidural analgesia) not recommended for > 24 hours
- (7.5 mg/mL solution) contraindicated for obstetric use due to increased risk of cardiotoxicity
- contraindicated in those with hypersensitivity to amide-type local anaesthetics
- see also General Nursing points/Cautions for local anaesthetics (p. 1266)

Patient teaching and advice

- see General Patient teaching and advice for local anaesthetics (p. 1267)

LIDOCAINE (LIGNOCAINE) (Lignocaine Gel 2%, Lignocaine Injection, LMX4, Min-I-Jet Lignocaine Hydrochloride Injection, Mucosoothe, Nervoderm, Seda Lotion, Stud 100 Desensitising Spray for Men, Versatis, Xogel Dental Gel, Xylocard, Xylocaine preparations, Ziagel)

Available forms

Ampoules: 10 mg/mL, 20 mg/mL, 500 mg/5 mL; Aerosol pump: 10 mg/actuation; Ointment (dental): 100 mg/g; Dental gel: 5 g/100 g; Gel (sterile or preserved): 20 mg/g (2%); Prefilled syringe: 20 mg/mL (2%); Oral solution: 5 mg/mL (2.5%), 220 mg/mL (2%); Topical ointment: 50 mg/g; Transdermal patch: 50 mg/g (5%); Cream: 40 mg/g (4%)

Action

- amide-type local anaesthetic with Class I antiarrhythmic action
- onset of action 5–10 minutes (infiltration or topical), 5–15 minutes (nerve block, other administration methods), 3–5 minutes (oral)
- duration of action (dependent on concentration and increases when used with a vasoconstrictor) 0.5–1 hour (topical), 1–2.5 hours (infiltration),

1–2 hours (minor nerve block), 3–4 hours (major nerve block), 1–3 hours (epidural)

- half-life 90–120 minutes (doubled in those with liver dysfunction)
- active metabolites
- (transdermal patch) hydrogel protects hypersensitive area with lidocaine (lignocaine) diffusing into skin providing analgesia

Use

- local and regional anaesthesia by infiltration, regional anaesthesia, nerve block, epidural and caudal anaesthesia
- surface anaesthesia of mucous membranes (e.g. endoscopy, cystoscopy, urethral catheterisation, ear, nose and throat procedures)
- ventricular arrhythmias (see Antiarrhythmic agents, p. 84)
- erectile dysfunction (see Erectile dysfunction agents, p. 1060)
- relief of pain or discomfort of mucous membranes of mouth, pharynx and upper gastrointestinal tract (e.g. post-tonsillectomy, mouth ulcers, dental scaling procedures, fitting new dentures)
- relief of neuropathic pain (postherpetic neuralgia) (transdermal patch)
- cutaneous anaesthesia (before venipuncture or IV catheter insertion) or temporary pain relief (e.g. associated with minor burns, non-blistered sunburn, insect bites, sore nipples)

Dose

- (transdermal patch) apply patch to affected area once daily, leaving in situ for 12 hours (maximum of 3 patches) **OR**
- (oral solution) 15 mL of undiluted solution either swished (mouth) or gargled (pharynx) for 30 seconds every 3 hours if needed (daily maximum 120 mL) (2% oral solution) **OR**
- (cutaneous) 1–2.5 g cream applied to skin for 30 minutes before procedure **OR**
- (cutaneous) apply thin layer to unbroken skin 3–4 times daily as needed **OR**
- (dental ointment) apply thin layer to oral mucosa and wait 3–5 minutes before procedure **OR**
- (topical – lotion) apply to affected area (mouth ulcer, sore gum) 2-hourly

Adverse effects

- (transdermal patch) burning, redness, pain and pruritus at application site, headache, nausea, rash, nasopharyngitis
- (cream) redness, itching, irritation, rash
- (aerosol spray) sore throat, hoarseness, loss of voice
- (dental ointment) numb tongue
- See also General Adverse effects of local anaesthetics (p. 1265)

Interactions

- metabolism of IV lidocaine (lignocaine) may be decreased by propranolol and metoprolol, increasing the risk of toxicity
- increased cardiac depressant effects may occur if given with phenytoin
- metabolism of lidocaine (lignocaine) may be increased by antiepileptic agents
- may prolong duration of suxamethonium
- caution if given with antiarrhythmic agents due to added cardiac effects
- decreased clearance and therefore increased serum levels if given IV with amiodarone or cimetidine
- half-life may be prolonged if given with acute severe alcohol intoxication
- decreases minimum effective concentration of inhalation anaesthetics such as nitrous oxide
- caution if given with other amide local anaesthetics
- if given IM, may cause a risk in creatine kinase (CK) for 48 hours which may interfere with myocardial infarction diagnosis

- may cause elevated creatinine levels when enzymatic estimation is used
- see General Interactions of local anaesthetics (p. 1265)

Nursing points/Cautions

- excessive doses and/or short interval between doses can result in elevated serum levels and increase risk of adverse effects
- avoid contact with eyes. Area should be washed well with copious amount of water if contact occurs
- (cream) 1 g cream = 5 cm squeezed from 5 g tube or 3.5 cm from 30 g tube
- (cream) cream may be covered with occlusive dressing if needed and left undisturbed for 30 minutes. Cream can then be removed using gauze and area prepared as per usual protocol for venipuncture or IV cannulation
- (transdermal patch) no more than 3 patches should be used at one time and there should be a 12-hour drug-free interval between applications
- (Xylocaine 4% topical solution) should not be used as a gargle or as an injection
- (gel) ineffective if applied to intact skin
- (gel/oral solution) caution if applied topically to traumatised mucosa or if infection is present at application site
- (aerosol pump) prime pump spray before use
- prolonged use or application to large body area is not advised
- (oral solution) not recommended in infants and children for teething pain
- not recommended in those with porphyria
- (Mucosoothe oral gel) contraindicated in those with hypersensitivity to hydroxybenzoate
- see also General Nursing points/Cautions for local anaesthetics (p. 1266)

Patient teaching and advice

- patient should be warned not to exceed recommended dose or shorten intervals between doses
- see also General Patient teaching and advice for local anaesthetics (p. 1267)

Oral solution/spray

- instruct patient to shake bottle well before use
- advise patient to swish (if mouth is painful) or gargle (if pharynx is painful) 15 mL solution undiluted for 30 seconds. If pharynx is involved, solution may be swallowed after gargling
- patient should be instructed not to eat or drink within 60 minutes of oral solutions due to increased risk of biting and damaging numbed mucous membranes or burning if hot food or liquid is ingested

Cream

- instruct patient that cream should not be applied to wounds, mucous membranes, irritated or broken skin or areas of atopic dermatitis

Ointment

- if used for sore nipples, patient should be instructed to wash area well before breastfeeding
- (dental ointment) advise patient not to exceed daily maximum (8.5–10 g) or single dose (2.5 g = 7.5 cm length of ointment)
- (dental ointment) if inserting new dentures, patient should be instructed to apply ointment to denture surface that will make contact with gum and not eat or drink for at least 1 hour afterwards

Transdermal patch

- ensure patient understands that transdermal patches should be

applied for 12 hours only when pain is greatest (e.g. if pain is worse at night, patch should be applied for night coverage)
- instruct patient in the following:
  - separate protective liner and apply to hairless skin (trim hair with scissors if needed but do not shave area)
  - skin folds, scars, inflamed or irritated areas should not be used. Herpetic lesions should be completely healed if patch is applied in that area
  - do not apply to mucous membranes
  - avoid contact with eyes
  - patch can be cut into smaller pieces (before removing liner) to better fit painful area; however, no more than 3 patches total can be used at one time
  - press patch to skin for about 10 seconds to ensure patch adheres well
  - wash hands thoroughly before and after applying patch
  - if possible, avoid bathing or showering with patch in place and allow skin to cool down before applying patch if bathing or showering first
  - avoid area with patch making contact with external heat source such as electric blanket or heating pads
  - used patches should be disposed of appropriately as they still contain lidocaine (lignocaine)
  - used and unused patches should be kept out of the reach of children at all times
  - store patches in cool place to avoid extremes of temperature and humidity but do not refrigerate or freeze

Note
- contained in CoPhenylcaine Forte, Difflam Plus Sore Throat Lozenges and Anaesthetic Lozenges, EMLA, Lidocaine (lignocaine) 2% Gel with Chlorhexidine 0.05%, Hemocane, Juvederm preparations, Lignospan Special, Minims Lidocaine (lignocaine) with Fluorescein, Medijel Gel, Numit, Oraqix (Peridontal Gel), Paxyl Sunburn Relief Spray, SM-33, SM-33 Adult Formula, SOOV preparations, Strepsils Numbing, Virasolve, Xylocaine Dental with Adrenaline (epinephrine), Xylocaine with Adrenaline (epinephrine), Xyloproct

MEPIVACAINE HYDROCHLORIDE (Scandonest 3%)

Available form
Cartridge: 66 mg/2.2 mL

Action
- amide-type local anaesthetic with anaesthetic properties greater than procaine
- onset is more rapid than procaine and slightly more rapid than lidocaine (lignocaine)
- onset of action 5–10 minutes (infiltration), 5–15 minutes (nerve blockade)
- duration of action 1–2.5 hours (infiltration), 1–2 hours (minor nerve block)
- equipotent to lidocaine (lignocaine) but less toxic

Use
- infiltration or nerve block (dental procedures)

Adverse effects
- see General Adverse effects of local anaesthetics (p. 1265)

Interactions
- contraindicated with or within 2 weeks of MAOIs or with TCAs
- lower dose required if given with sedatives or anti-anxiety agents

- increased risk of toxicity if given with beta-adrenoreceptor blocking agents
- increased serum levels may occur if given with cimetidine
- increased risk of seizures, bradycardia and long sinoatrial arrest if given with amiodarone
- additive cardiac depression may occur if given with phenytoin
- see General Interactions of local anaesthetics (p. 1265)

Nursing points/Cautions

- contraindicated IV
- contraindicated in those with hypersensitivity to amide-type local anaesthetics
- contraindicated if there is a possibility that a general anaesthetic may be required to complete procedure
- see General Nursing points/Cautions/ Patient teaching and advice for local anaesthetics (pp. 1266–67)

Patient teaching and advice

- see General Patient teaching and advice for local anaesthetics (p. 1267)

Note

- contained in Scandonest 2% Special (with Adrenaline (epinephrine))

PRILOCAINE HYDROCHLORIDE (Citanest)

Available forms

Ampoules: 5 mg/mL (0.5%)

Action

- amide local anaesthetic with similar onset and potency as lidocaine (lignocaine), but less vasodilator activity and CNS toxicity
- active metabolite, which may be responsible for methaemoglobinaemia if prilocaine is given in large doses
- onset of action 5–10 minutes (infiltration), 5–15 minutes (nerve blockade)
- duration of action 1–2.5 hours (infiltration), 1–2 hours (minor nerve block), 3–4 hours (major nerve block), 1–3 hours (epidural)
- half-life about 2 hours

Use

- local or regional anaesthesia (infiltration, intravenous regional anaesthesia, nerve block, major plexus block, epidural and subarachnoid block)

Adverse effects

- (high dose) methaemoglobinaemia, cyanosis
- see also General Adverse effects of local anaesthetics (p. 1265)

Interactions

- risk of methaemoglobin formation may be increased if given with sulfonamides, antimalarial agents or some nitric compounds
- see also General Interactions of local anaesthetics (p. 1265)

Nursing points/Cautions

- see General Nursing points/Cautions for local anaesthetics (p. 1266)
- skin testing for suspected hypersensitivity is of limited value
- patient should be observed closely for any cyanosis of lips and/or nails (sign of methaemoglobinaemia)
- (epidural) test dose (3–5 mL) is recommended (preferably with 15 microgram adrenaline (epinephrine)), followed by patient monitoring (HR, BP, verbal contact) 5 minutes after dose. If accidental IV administration has occurred, HR will increase immediately, or if given intrathecally, patient will show signs of spinal block
- increased risk of methaemoglobinaemia if given in high doses to those with hypoxia (e.g. due to severe anaemia, cardiac insufficiency)
- caution if using pulse oximetry as methaemoglobinaemia (even at low levels) may interfere with readings

- may precipitate in alkaline solutions
- not recommended as obstetric paracervical or pudendal block due to risk of methaemoglobinaemia in neonate
- not recommended in infants < 6 months due to increased risk of methaemoglobinaemia
- contraindicated in those with congenital or idiopathic methaemoglobinaemia or with hypoxaemia
- contraindicated in those with hypersensitivity to amide-type local anaesthetics

Note

- contained in 3% Citanest Dental with Octapressin (with felypressin)
- contained in EMLA (Cream and Patches), Numit 5% and Oraqix with lidocaine (lignocaine)

ROPIVACAINE HYDROCHLORIDE (Naropin, Ropibam)

Available forms

Ampoules: 2 mg/mL, 7.5 mg/mL, 10 mg/mL

Action

- amide with both anaesthetic and analgesic properties
- vasoconstriction at lower concentrations and vasodilation at higher concentrations
- duration and intensity is not improved by adrenaline (epinephrine)
- similar analgesic potency to bupivacaine, but less potent for motor block
- onset of action 10–15 minutes (infiltration), 15–30 minutes (nerve block)
- duration of action 3–4 hours (infiltration), 2–6 hours (minor nerve block), 7–14 hours (major nerve block), 3–4 hours (epidural)
- two-phase half-life (14 minutes, 4 hours) due to biphasic absorption

Use

- epidural block, minor nerve block and infiltration, major nerve block, intrathecal anaesthesia
- postoperative pain management

Adverse effects

- urinary retention, oliguria
- back pain, pain, chest pain
- dyspnoea
- (rare) cardiac arrest/arrhythmia, spinal/epidural haematoma
- see also General Adverse effects of local anaesthetics (p. 1265)

Interactions

- clearance may be decreased if given with fluvoxamine and ciprofloxacin leading to increased serum level, duration and risk of toxicity and are therefore not recommended together
- ECG monitoring is recommended if given with Class III antiarrhythmic agents such as amiodarone
- see also General Interactions of local anaesthetics (p. 1265)

Nursing points/Cautions

- (epidural) test dose (3–5 mL) is recommended (preferably with 15 microgram/mL adrenaline (epinephrine)) followed by patient monitoring (HR, BP, verbal contact) 5 minutes after dose. If accidental IV administration has occurred, HR will increase immediately, or if given intrathecally, patient will show signs of spinal block
- skin testing is thought to be of limited value
- administered slowly (25–50 mg/minute)
- if given by two or more routes, total dose should be calculated to avoid toxicity
- precipitation may occur if added to alkaline solution
- increased risk of spinal/epidural haematoma if procedure is traumatic or repeated or if an indwelling epidural catheter is used
- not recommended as paracervical block during pregnancy
- caution if used in those with acute porphyria (if given at all) or severe liver impairment

- contraindicated IV
- contraindicated in those with hypersensitivity to amide-type local anaesthetics
- see General Nursing points/Cautions for local anaesthetics (p. 1266)

Patient teaching and advice

- see General Patient teaching and advice for local anaesthetics (p. 1267)

Note

- contained in Naropin with Fentanyl

LOCAL ANAESTHETIC EYE DROPS

General Actions of local anaesthetic eye drops

- reversibly blocks propagation and conduction of nerve impulses, stabilising membrane and preventing generation of action potential

General Adverse effects of local anaesthetic eye drops

- transient stinging or burning sensation, tearing, blurred vision
- conjunctival redness
- corneal damage (prolonged administration)
- allergic conjunctivitis
- (uncommon) severe keratitis
- (rare) hypersensitivity, allergic reactions

General Interactions of local anaesthetic eye drops

- ester-type local anaesthetics may be blocked by anticholinesterases, prolonging activity
- ester-type local anaesthetics may enhance neuromuscular blockade of suxamethonium chloride

General Nursing points/Cautions for local anaesthetic eye drops

- local anaesthetics should never be put into an eye without a doctor's prescription, because healing is impaired and secondary bacterial infection is possible
- should only be administered by clinician
- systemic absorption can be reduced by compressing lacrimal sac at medial canthus for 60 seconds during and after instillation
- if more than one ophthalmic agent is to be used, a 5-minute interval should be allowed between instillations with eye ointment applied last
- prolonged use will slow wound healing
- any remaining solution should be discarded (single patient use only) to prevent transmission of infection
- for topical ophthalmic application only and should not be injected
- caution if used in the elderly or children
- not recommended after corneal staining
- repeated instillation is contraindicated due to risk of corneal damage
- caution if used in those with known allergies, epilepsy, cardiac disease, hyperthyroidism, myasthenia gravis or respiratory disease
- contraindicated in those with known allergy or hypersensitivity to ester-type local anaesthetics or in premature babies

General Patient teaching and advice for local anaesthetic eye drops

- warn patient that burning/stinging may occur for up to 30 seconds after instillation

- instruct patient that eye should be protected from dust and bacterial contamination while anaesthetised (e.g. eye may be covered with patch until blink reflex returns)
- warn patient not to drive or operate machinery until normal sensation returns to eye(s)
- patient should be advised not to touch or rub eye(s) until anaesthetic effect has worn off

OXYBUPROCAINE HYDROCHLORIDE (Minims Oxybuprocaine)

Available form

Eye drops: 4 mg/mL (0.4%)

Action

- ester-type local anaesthetic
- onset of action 1 minute, peak response 1–15 minutes, duration 20–30 minutes, full sensation returns in 40 or more minutes
- see also General Actions of local anaesthetic eye drops (p. 1275)

Use

- anaesthesia for short ophthalmological procedures

Dose

- (tonometry) 1 drop to affected eye(s) 1 minute before procedure **OR**
- (fitting contact lens) 1 drop, followed 90 seconds later by 1 drop **OR**
- (removal of foreign body, minor surgery) 3–6 drops to affected eye(s) **OR**
- (pterygium surgery) 1 drop per minute to affected eye(s) for 10 minutes **OR**
- (deeper anaesthesia) 1 drop at intervals of greater than 90 seconds

Adverse effects

- see General Adverse effects of local anaesthetic eye drops (p. 1275)
- (rare) nausea, vomiting, dysphagia

Interactions

- see General Interactions of local anaesthetic eye drops (p. 1275)

Nursing points/Cautions

- contraindicated if eye infection is present
- see also General Nursing points/Cautions for local anaesthetic eye drops (p. 1275)

Patient teaching and advice

- see General Patient teaching and advice for local anaesthetic eye drops (p. 1275)

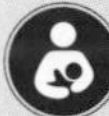

only used during pregnancy or breastfeeding if benefits outweigh risks

PROXYMETACAINE HYDROCHLORIDE (Alcaine Eye Drops 0.5%)

Available form

Eye drops: 5 mg/mL (0.5%)

Action

- ester-type local anaesthetic
- onset of action within 30 seconds, duration of action 15 minutes or more
- see also General Actions of local anaesthetic eye drops (p. 1275)

Use

- short ophthalmic procedures requiring short anaesthesia (e.g. minor surgery, tonometry, removal of foreign body, conjunctival scraping for diagnostic procedures)

Dose

- (tonometry) 1–2 drops just before evaluation **OR**
- (minor surgical procedure (e.g. foreign body or suture removal)) 1–2 drops every 5–10 minutes for 1–3 doses **OR**

- (prolonged anaesthesia (e.g. cataract extraction) 1–2 drops every 5–10 minutes for 3–5 doses

Adverse effects
- see General Adverse effects of local anaesthetic eye drops (p. 1275)

Interactions
- see General Interactions of local anaesthetic eye drops (p. 1275)

Nursing points/Cautions
- avoid contact with skin as contact dermatitis may occur
- contains preservative benzalkonium chloride which may cause eye irritation as well as discolouring and depositing on soft contact lenses
- see also General Nursing points/Cautions for local anaesthetic eye drops (p. 1275)

Patient teaching and advice
- advise patient to avoid wearing contact lenses until local anaesthesia has worn off
- see also General Patient teaching and advice for local anaesthetic eye drops (p. 1275)

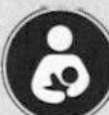
only used during pregnancy if clearly needed

TETRACAINE (AMETHOCAINE) HYDROCHLORIDE (Minims Amethocaine Eye Drops)

Available forms
Eye drops: 5 mg/mL (0.5%), 10 mg/mL (1%)

Action
- ester-type local anaesthetic
- onset of action 10–20 seconds, duration 10–20 minutes, but 1% solution can have a duration up to 1 hour
- see also General Actions of local anaesthetic eye drops (p. 1275)

Dose
- 1 drop to affected eye(s), may be repeated as necessary

Adverse effects
- see General Adverse effects of local anaesthetic eye drops (p. 1275)

Interactions
- contraindicated with sulfonamides
- see also General Interactions of local anaesthetic eye drops (p. 1275)

Nursing points/Cautions
- see General Nursing points/Cautions for local anaesthetic eye drops (p. 1275)

Patient teaching and advice
- see General Patient teaching and advice for local anaesthetic eye drops (p. 1275)

METABOLIC DISORDERS AGENTS

Inborn errors of metabolism are disorders in which a single gene defect causes a significant block in the metabolic pathway, generally with an accumulation of macromolecules in tissues and cells, with associated morbidity and mortality. In the past, these were considered rare but with better detection (such as genetic sequencing), these disorders are now thought to affect as many as 1 in 1500 children in the United States (Thomas et al 2020). These inborn error of metabolism disorders can be due to a large number of causes, including disorders of amino acid, purine and carbohydrate metabolism and lysosomal storage diseases. For example, there have been about 50 different lysosomal storage diseases identified, including Tay-Sachs disease, Fabry disease, Gaucher disease and Niemann-Pick disease (Hopkins & Grabowski 2019).

Treatments include enzyme replacement therapy, dietary restrictions of precursor, enzyme inhibition of precursor or removal of accumulated substrate using either pharmacological agents or dialysis (Thomas et al 2020).

AGALSIDASE ALFA (GHU) (Replagal)

Available form

Vial: 3.5 mg/3.5 mL

Action

- alpha-galactosidase A enzyme that hydrolyses glycosphingolipids (e.g. globotriaosylceramide (GL-3, also called Gb3)) to ceramide and galactose
- in Fabry disease, there is a deficiency in alpha-galactosidase which leads to an accumulation of glycosphingolipids (especially GL-3 (Gb3)) in tissues and fluids, ultimately resulting in narrowing and thrombosis of arteries and arterioles, peripheral neuritis, renal failure, myocardial and cerebral infarction
- enzyme replacement produced by recombinant DNA technology

Use

- long-term enzyme replacement therapy in those with alpha-galactosidase A deficiency (Fabry disease)

Dose

- 0.2 mg/kg by IV infusion over 40 minutes every 2 weeks

Adverse effects

- infusion-related reaction (commonly, rigors/chills, headache, nausea, fever, flushing, fatigue and uncommonly (more serious) fever, rigors, tachycardia, urticaria, nausea, vomiting, angioedema, throat tightness, stridor, swollen tongue)
- peripheral oedema, tachycardia, palpitation, hypertension
- flushing, acne, erythema, pruritus, rash
- cough, throat tightness, hoarseness dyspnoea, rhinorrhoea, pharyngitis, nasopharyngitis, flu-like symptoms
- headache, dizziness, tremor, fatigue, malaise, asthenia
- paraesthesia, hypoaesthesia
- increased lacrimation
- tinnitus, aggravation of pre-existing tinnitus
- neuropathic pain
- myalgia, back and limb pain, arthralgia, joint swelling
- taste alteration, nausea, vomiting, diarrhoea, abdominal pain/discomfort
- antibody development
- (rare) hypersensitivity, anaphylaxis

Interactions

- not recommended with amiodarone or gentamicin

Nursing points/Cautions

- infusion-related reactions usually occur in first 2–4 months of therapy
- infusion can be interrupted for 5–10 minutes until infusion-related reaction subsides and then restarted
- if infused-related reaction occurs, pre-treatment with antihistamine and/corticosteroid 1–24 hours before next infusion is recommended
- administer alone
- standard 0.2 micron filter is recommended
- dilute with 100 mL sodium chloride 0.9% before IV administration
- do not shake solution as protein will be denatured
- not recommended in children under 6.5 years

Patient teaching and advice

- warn patient/carer that infusion-related reactions commonly occur within first 2–4 months of therapy
- advise patient to avoid driving or operating machinery if dizziness occurs
- see General Patient teaching and advice (p. xxvii)

only used during pregnancy if benefits outweigh risks

caution if used during breastfeeding

AGALSIDASE BETA (RCH) (Fabrazyme)

Available forms

Vial: 5 mg, 35 mg

Action

- alpha-galactosidase A enzyme that hydrolyses glycosphingolipids (e.g. globotriaosylceramide (GL-3) also called Gb3) to ceramide and galactose
- in Fabry disease, there is a deficiency in alpha-galactosidase which leads to an accumulation of glycosphingolipids (especially GL-3 (Gb3)) in tissues and fluids, ultimately resulting in narrowing and thrombosis of arteries and arterioles, peripheral neuritis, renal failure, myocardial and cerebral infarction
- enzyme replacement produced by recombinant DNA technology

Use

- long-term enzyme replacement therapy in those with alpha-galactosidase deficiency (Fabry disease)

Dose

- 1 mg/kg by IV infusion every 2 weeks

Adverse effects

- infusion-related reaction (pallor, tachycardia, chest discomfort/pain, chills, fever, feeling hot or cold, headache, dizziness, somnolence, pruritus, urticaria)
- injection site reaction
- nausea, vomiting, abdominal pain
- palpitations, tachycardia, peripheral oedema, hypertension
- flushing
- oral or facial oedema
- asthenia, malaise, paraesthesia, lethargy, fatigue
- dyspnoea, nasal stuffiness, throat tightness, cough, wheezing
- rash, erythema, pruritus, urticaria
- pain in extremities, myalgia, back pain or spasm, arthralgia, muscle tightness, musculoskeletal stiffness
- increased lacrimation
- development of anti-drug antibodies

Interactions

- not recommended with amiodarone or gentamicin

Nursing points/Cautions

- resuscitation equipment should be readily available in the event of infusion-related reaction or anaphylaxis
- initial infusion rate should be no greater than 15 mg/hour to decrease risk of infusion-related reactions. If rate is tolerated and no reactions occur, rate may be gradually increased over subsequent infusions
- pre-treatment with antipyretics (e.g. paracetamol, ibuprofen) and/or antihistamines (e.g. diphenhydramine) is recommended 60 minutes before infusion in those who have experienced a single mild-to-moderate infusion-related reaction. Infusion rate should be 10 mg/hour
- if patient has experienced previous infusion-related reaction (single severe event or recurrent moderate-to-severe events), corticosteroids are recommended 13 hours, 7 hours and 1 hour before infusion (in addition to pre-treatment as described in previous point)
- slowing IV rate or temporarily stopping infusion will improve infusion-related reactions
- reconstitute vial(s) using water for injections for a final concentration of 5 mg/mL (see manufacturer's recommendations), then further dilute using sodium chloride 0.9% and administer by IV infusion
- administer alone
- inline low protein binding 0.2 micron filter can be used
- IgG antibody testing is recommended before starting therapy, 3-monthly for 18 months, then 6-monthly
- caution if given to patient who has experienced infusion-related reaction or in those with liver impairment
- not recommended in children under 8 years

Patient teaching and advice

- warn patient to avoid driving or operating machinery if dizziness or somnolence occurs
- see also General Patient teaching and advice (p. xxvii)

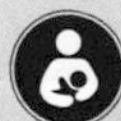

caution if used during pregnancy

not recommended during breastfeeding

ALGLUCOSIDASE ALFA (RHU) (Myozyme)

Available form

Vial: 50 mg

Action

- lysosomal enzyme replacement for Pompe disease
- Pompe disease is a glycogen storage disease (type II) caused by deficiency of lysosomal acid alfa-glucosidase

which breaks down lysosomal glycogen resulting in an accumulation of glycogen in various tissues, including cardiac and skeletal muscle

Use

- long-term treatment of patients with Pompe disease (acid alfa-glucosidase deficiency)

Dose

- 20 mg/kg by IV infusion every 2 weeks

Adverse effects

- infusion-related reaction (hypo/hypertension cyanosis, tachycardia, bradycardia, pallor, flushing, peripheral coldness, tachypnoea, wheezing, throat tightness, hypoxia, dyspnoea, cough, respiratory tract irritation, decreased oxygen saturation, angioedema, urticaria, rash, erythema, periorbital oedema, pruritus, sweating)
- fever
- rhinorrhoea, respiratory distress/failure, rhinitis, cough, tachypnoea
- tachycardia, bradycardia
- pneumonia, otitis media, upper respiratory tract infection, ear infection, pharyngitis, gastroenteritis, oral candidiasis, bronchiolitis, nasopharyngitis
- rash, urticaria
- diarrhoea, vomiting, constipation, upper abdominal pain, gastro-oesophageal reflux disease
- anaemia
- antibody development
- (rare) hypersensitivity, anaphylaxis, severe cutaneous reaction, nephrotic syndrome

Nursing points/Cautions

- resuscitation equipment should be readily available in the event of infusion-related reaction or anaphylaxis
- antibody levels (IgG) should be measured 3-monthly during therapy
- initial infusion rate should not exceed 1 mg/kg/hour, which may then be increased by 2 mg/kg/hour every 30 minutes if patient tolerates it and no infusion-related reactions occur. Maximum rate of 7 mg/kg/hour should not be exceeded
- infusion rate should be slowed or stopped if infusion-related reactions occur
- if patient has experienced infusion-related reaction, decreasing the rate and/or pre-treatment with antihistamines and/or corticosteroids is recommended for next infusion
- do not shake reconstituted or diluted solution as protein will be denatured
- vial(s) should be allowed to reach room temperature for 30 minutes before reconstitution. Reconstitute using 10.3 mL water for injections, slowly injecting it down the inside wall of the vial to prevent foaming, giving a concentration of 5 mg/mL. Reconstituted solution may contain thin white strands or translucent fibres which are removed by inline filter without losing any strength or affecting the purity of the solution
- reconstituted solution should be protected from light
- airspace should be removed from infusion bag to minimise particle formation as solution is sensitive to air–liquid interface, then dilute reconstituted solution in sodium chloride 0.9% to give a final concentration of 0.5–4 mg/mL taking care to avoid foaming in the infusion bag. Invert gently to mix thoroughly
- standard inline 0.2 micron filter is recommended
- administer alone
- infusion solution should be protected from light during administration
- increased risk of hypersensitivity reactions in those with infantile or late-onset Pompe disease, therefore should be given with great caution

Patient teaching and advice

- warn patient/carer that recurrent reaction including flu-like symptoms or combination of chills, fever, muscle or bone pain and fatigue may occur after the infusion has finished and last for a few days in some patients
- advise patient/carer to immediately seek medical advice if any skin reactions occur
- see General Patient teaching and advice (p. xxvii)

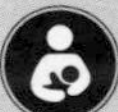

should only be given during pregnancy or breastfeeding if benefits outweigh risks

ALPHA-1-PROTEINASE INHIBITOR (Prolastin C Liquid, Prolastin C Powder for Injection)

Available forms

Vial (solution): 1 g/20 mL; Vial (powder) 1 g

Action

- increases serum alpha-1-proteinase inhibitor levels in those with congenital alpha-1-antitrypsin deficiency and with clinically significant emphysema (FEV1 < 80%)
- congenital alpha-1-antitrypsin deficiency is a hereditary disorder characterised by low serum and lung levels of alpha-1-P1-proteinase inhibitor. Those with levels < 11 micrometre are at increased risk of developing emphysema with levels of 9–23 micrometre considered to be at moderate risk
- smoking increases the risk of developing emphysema in those with the deficiency

Use

- congenital alpha-1-antitrypsin deficiency

Dose

- 60 mg/kg IV weekly at a rate of 0.08 mL/kg/m

Adverse effects

- rash, pruritus, urticaria
- diarrhoea, nausea
- fatigue, headache, dizziness
- fever, chills, flu-like illness
- nasopharyngitis, exacerbation of chronic obstructive pulmonary disease (COPD), dyspnoea
- arthralgia
- urinary tract infection
- tachycardia
- hypersensitivity reaction

Nursing points/Cautions

- treatment should be started and monitored by respiratory doctor in conjunction with other appropriate therapies
- for therapy to commence, patient must be diagnosed with alpha-1-antitrypsin deficiency based on genotype, clinical symptoms of emphysema and alpha-1-antitrypsin level < 11 micrometre
- for IV administration alone
- should be administered alone, within 3 hours of preparation
- recommended dose of 60 mg/kg should take about 15 minutes to administer
- (solution) vial should be allowed to come to room temperature and carefully inspected. Vial should contain few protein particles and be clear to slightly opalescent, colourless or pale yellow/green/brown and not discoloured or cloudy
- (powder) allow vials with powder and diluent to come to room temperature. Insert short end of transfer needle into diluent vial, then remove cover from other end. Invert diluent vial and insert transfer needle into powder vial at 45° to allow diluent to

run down wall of vial to prevent foaming. Vacuum will draw diluent into vial. Swirl for 10–15 seconds to wet powder and then continue until powder is fully dissolved
- may contain trace amounts of IgA, which will increase risk of hypersensitivity reaction in those with selective or severe IgA deficiency
- derived from pooled human plasma collected from donors and carries the risk of transmissible infectious agents. Risk versus benefit should be discussed with patient before prescription or administration of solution
- contraindicated in those with IgA deficiency and antibodies against IgA or those with history of anaphylaxis or other systemic reactions to alpha-1-proteinase inhibitor

Patient teaching and advice

- patient should be counselled to avoid smoking with this condition to decrease risk of developing emphysema
- see also General Patient teaching and advice (p. xxvii)

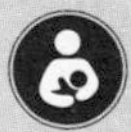

should only be given during pregnancy if benefits outweigh risks

caution if used during breastfeeding

ASFOTASE ALFA (Strensiq)

Available forms

Vial: 18 mg/0.45 mL, 28 mg/0.7 mL, 40 mg/mL, 80 mg/0.8 mL

Action

- recombinant human tissue nonspecific alkaline phosphatase (ALP)
- produced by recombinant DNA technology using mammalian Chinese hamster ovary cell culture
- promotes skeletal mineralisation in patients with hypophosphatasia
- hypophosphatasia is a rare, serious and potentially fatal genetic disorder caused by loss of function mutation in gene encoding TNSALP. Deficiency in TNSALP enzymatic activity leads to increased concentrations of TNSALP substrates, including inorganic pyrophosphate (PPi). Elevated extracellular PPi levels block hydroxyapatite crystal growth inhibiting bone mineralisation and causing accumulation of unmineralised bone matrix (rickets and bone deformations in children) and osteomalacia (bone softening) when growth plates have closed, along with muscle weakness
- half-life 1.06–3.62 days

Use

- enzyme replacement in paediatric-onset hypophosphatasia

Dose

- 2 mg/kg 3 times per week or 1 mg/kg 6 times per week SC

Adverse effects

- craniosynostosis, increased intracranial pressure
- ectopic calcifications (conjunctival and corneal calcification, nephrocalcinosis)
- weight gain
- headache
- tooth loss, dental caries
- vomiting, diarrhoea, constipation, gastro-oesophageal reflux disease
- respiratory tract infection, nasopharyngitis, pneumonia, otitis media, rhinitis, influenza
- cough, oropharyngeal pain
- conjunctivitis
- anaemia
- pain in extremity, arthralgia, back pain
- injection site reaction (redness, rash, pruritus, pain, papule, nodule, atrophy, cellulitis)
- localised lipodystrophy including lipoatrophy and lipohypertrophy

- development of anti-drug antibodies
- hypersensitivity

Interaction

- may interfere with routine measurement of serum alkaline phosphatase

Nursing points/Cautions

- regular monitoring for increased intracranial pressure (including fundoscopy for signs of papilloedema) is recommended for patients < 5 years
- before starting therapy ophthalmology examination and renal ultrasound are recommended, then regularly throughout treatment
- serum parathyroid hormone and calcium levels should be monitored regularly and calcium and vitamin D supplements given if needed
- dietary advice is recommended to avoid disproportionate weight gain
- not given IM or IV
- maximum 1 mL per SC injection site
- SC sites should be rotated and monitored regularly for any signs of potential reactions
- response should be regularly reviewed especially when progressing to adolescence or adulthood
- patient can be taught to self-administer after supervision
- caution if readministered to patient who has previously experienced hypersensitivity reaction. If administered, it should be under medical supervision with emergency equipment readily available
- contraindicated in those with hypersensitivity to Chinese hamster ovary protein

Patient teaching and advice

- patient should be advised to seek medical attention immediately if any hypersensitivity reaction occurs, including difficulty breathing, choking sensation, swelling around eyes and dizziness, which can occur within minutes of administration
- ensure patient has been instructed in SC administration, including:
  - injection technique
  - importance of rotating injection sites including abdomen, thigh, buttock and upper arm
  - correct disposal of sharps, including not reusing needles
  - correct storage (refrigerated but removed an hour before administration)
- female patients of childbearing potential should be counselled to use reliable contraception during therapy and if pregnancy occurs, doctor should be informed immediately
- see also General Patient teaching and advice (p. xxvii)

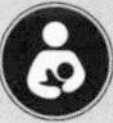

not recommended during pregnancy or breastfeeding

BETAINE (Cystadane)

Available form

Dissolvable powder: 1 g/g

Action

- anti-homocysteine agent (elevated homocysteine blood levels may cause cardiovascular thrombosis, osteoporosis, skeletal abnormalities and optic lens dislocation)
- reduces homocysteine levels by 20–30% of pre-treatment levels
- betaine occurs naturally in the body and some foods, such as seafood, spinach, beets and cereals

Use

- adjunct in management of homocystinuria
- decrease raised homocysteine levels in patients with cystathionine beta-synthase (CBS) deficiency type of homocystinuria

- increase methionine and S-adenosylmethionine levels in patients with methylenetetrahydrofolate reductase (MTHFR) deficiency and cobalamin co-factor metabolism type of homocysteine

Dose

- initially 3 g orally twice daily, increasing gradually until plasma homocysteine is undetectable

Adverse effects

- nausea, diarrhoea, gastrointestinal distress
- (CBS deficiency) cerebral oedema

Nursing points/Cautions

- plasma homocysteine levels should be monitored throughout therapy
- response usually seen within a week of starting therapy
- can be given with folate, vitamin B_6 and vitamin B_{12}
- (CBS deficiency) plasma methionine levels should be monitored during therapy and kept below 1000 micromol/L. Dietary modification and reduced betaine dose may be required

Patient teaching and advice

- instruct patient to use provided scoop (1 g) to measure required amount and dissolve in 120–180 mL water, then drink immediately
- see also General Patient teaching and advice (p. xxvii)

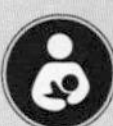

should only be used during pregnancy and breastfeeding with caution

CARGLUMIC ACID (Carbaglu)

Available form

Tablets (for oral solution): 200 mg

Action

- N-acetylglutamate (NAG) analogue
- NAG is naturally occurring activator of carbamoyl phosphate synthetase 1 (CPS 1) (first enzyme in urea cycle), therefore if deficiency occurs, urea cycle is not triggered resulting in elevated levels of ammonia
- half-life up to 28 hours

Use

- treatment of hyperammonaemia due to NAG synthase primary deficiency or organic acidaemias (e.g. due to isovaleric acidaemia, methylmalonic acidaemia or propionic acidaemia)

Dose

- (acute hyperammonaemia) initially 100–250 mg/kg orally or via nasogastric tube daily in 2–4 divided doses (rounded to closest 100 mg), titrating to plasma ammonia levels and clinical symptoms

Adverse effects

- anaemia
- ear infection, infection, influenza, pneumonia, nasopharyngitis, tonsillitis
- abdominal pain, diarrhoea, vomiting, taste perversion, decreased weight, anorexia
- asthenia, headache, somnolence
- rash
- fever, sweating
- cardiac murmur, decreased oxygen saturation
- hyperglycaemia

Nursing points/Cautions

- therapy can be started as early as first day of life as acute symptomatic hyperammonaemia can be life threatening
- regular neurological and cardiac status assessment, laboratory tests (kidney, liver and blood) and clinical response to treatment should be monitored regularly during therapy to maintain plasma levels of ammonia and amino acids within normal levels

- individual responsiveness should be tested before starting long-term therapy (e.g. in a comatose child, 100–250 mg/kg daily is given and ammonia plasma levels measured before each administration. Should normalise within a few hours of starting therapy)
- protein restriction during acute phase and protein supplementation during maintenance phase may be required and, if needed, dietetic advice is recommended
- if administration is via nasogastric tube, 200 mg tablet should be dissolved in 5–10 mL water and then administered via nasogastric tube, followed by water to flush tube

Patient teaching and advice

- advise patient/parent/carer that tablets should not be swallowed whole or crushed. Each 200 mg tablet should be dissolved in 5–10 mL water and given before meals or feed. If undissolved particles remain, container should be rinsed with 5–10 mL water and swallowed immediately (tablets do not completely dissolve)
- warn patient/parent/carer that suspension has a slightly acidic taste
- see also General Patient teaching and advice (p. xxvii)

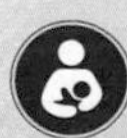

contraindicated during breastfeeding

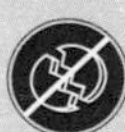

tablets should not be swallowed but should be dissolved in water

CERLIPONASE ALFA (Brineura)

Available form

Vial: 150 mg/5 mL

Action

- recombinant form of human tripeptidyl peptidase 1 (TPP1)
- inactive proenzyme (zymogen) form of a protease that is activated in the lysosome
- inadequate levels of TPPI cause CLN2 disease resulting in neurodegeneration, loss of neurological function (e.g. decline of motor and language functions) and death during childhood.

Use

- treatment of neuronal ceroid lipofuscinosis type 2 (CLN2) disease (also known as tripeptidyl peptidase 1 (TPP1) deficiency)

Dose

- (2 years and older) 300 mg by intracerebroventricular infusion every second week at a rate of 2.5 mL/hour

Adverse effects

- device-related infection (including meningitis)
- hypersensitivity, anaphylactic reactions
- fever
- low CSF protein
- ECG abnormalities, bradycardia
- vomiting, constipation, diarrhoea, dysphagia, abdominal pain, tongue or oral mucosa blistering
- upper respiratory tract infection, nasopharyngitis, rhinitis, viral infection, pharyngitis, tonsillitis, cough
- seizures
- tremor, headache, insomnia, irritability
- rash, urticaria
- development of anti-drug antibodies

Nursing points/Cautions

- first dose should be given at least 5 to 7 days after intracerebroventricular access device (surgically implanted reservoir and catheter) implantation
- medical support and equipment should be readily available in the event of anaphylaxis occurring
- pre-treatment with antihistamines +/− antipyretic 30–60 minutes before the infusion is recommended

- if patient is unable to tolerate the infusion, dose may be reduced by 50% and/or infusion rate decreased
- if the infusion is stopped because of hypersensitivity reaction, it should be restarted at 50% initial infusion rate at which the reaction occurred
- child should be closely monitored for any increase in intracranial pressure (headache, nausea, vomiting, decreased mental state) during infusion and infusion stopped or rate slowed if these occur
- vital signs should be monitored before start of infusion, during infusion and post infusion. Longer monitoring is recommended in children under 3 years
- ECG is recommended during infusion if the child has any history of conduction disorders of the heart (including bradycardia and structural heart disease). If child has no cardiac history, 12-lead ECG is recommended every 6 months
- strict aseptic techniques must be adhered to during administration to prevent device-related infection occurring
- cerliponase alfa and flushing solution should be thawed at room temperature for about 60 minutes before administration (should not be thawed or warmed in any other way)
- vials should not be shaken
- when thawed cerliponase alfa should be clear to slightly opalescent and colourless to pale yellow (thin translucent fibres or opaque fibres may be present but these are removed by inline filter). Flushing solution should be clear and colourless
- cerliponase alfa and flushing solution should not be refrozen if not used
- a programmable syringe pump and 0.2 micron inline filter must be used for administration
- after infusion of cerliponase alfa, a calculated amount of flushing solution must be used to ensure full dose has been administered and maintain patency of the device
- to administer:
  - one unused sterile syringe should be labelled 'Brineura' and using aseptic technique, the required volume should be removed from vial
  - solution should not be diluted or mixed with any other agents
  - amount of flushing solution should be determined to ensure complete dose is administered (flush volume should be calculated by adding priming volume of all infusion components including access device)
  - one unused sterile syringe should be labelled 'flushing solution' and calculated dose removed from vial using aseptic technique
  - infusion line should be primed with cerliponase alfa solution
  - scalp should be closely inspected for signs of potential infection or access device leakage or failure (e.g. swelling, scalp erythema, extravasation of fluid, scalp bulging around or above access device site) (and not administered if any occur)
  - scalp should be prepared according to workplace policy and port needle inserted into access device
  - empty sterile syringe (no larger than 3 mL) should be attached to port needle and 0.5 to 1 mL of CSF should be withdrawn to check patency of access device. CSF sample should be sent for infection monitoring
  - infusion set should be connected to port needle and secured
  - syringe with 'Brineura' should be placed in syringe drive pump and program set to deliver infusion rate of 2.5 mL/hour and infusion commenced

  - when complete, syringe containing flushing solution should be placed in syringe drive pump and set at same rate
  - when infusion is complete, port needle should be removed and gentle pressure and dressing applied to infusion site
- contains 17.42 mg sodium per vial (including flushing solution) which may need to be considered if patient requires sodium-controlled diet
- contraindicated in CLN2 patients with ventriculo-peritoneal shunts, if there is any sign of infection or evidence of access device leakage or failure, or if patient has sensitivity to Chinese hamster ovary cells

Patient teaching and advice

- parents should be instructed to seek medical advice immediately if child develops fever, nausea, vomiting, headache, neck stiffness, becomes sensitive to light and/or has changes in mental status (e.g. becomes sleepy, confused or irritable)

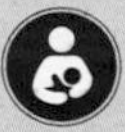

Not recommended during pregnancy or breastfeeding

ELIGLUSTAT (Cerdelga)

Available form
Capsules: 84 mg

Action
- Gaucher disease is a lysosomal storage disease in which there is a deficiency of acid β-glucosidase resulting in accumulation of glucosylceramide (GL-1), especially in the liver, spleen and bone marrow
- potent and specific inhibitor of glycosylceramide synthase in order to reduce the rate of synthesis to match impaired rate of catabolism, preventing accumulation and the associated clinical manifestations

Use
- long-term management of patients with Gaucher disease (type I)

Dose
- (CYP2D6 intermediate and extensive metabolisers) 84 mg orally twice daily **OR**
- (CYP2D6 poor metabolisers) 84 mg orally once daily

Adverse effects
- headache, dizziness
- palpitations
- dyspepsia, upper abdominal pain, diarrhoea, nausea, constipation, gastro-oesophageal reflux, abdominal distension, gastritis
- arthralgia
- fatigue

Interactions
- contraindicated in CYP2D6 immediate or extensive metabolisers who are taking paroxetine, fluoxetine, quinidine, bupropion, duloxetine, moclobemide, tipranavir/ritonavir, dronedarone, cinacalcet with itraconazole, posaconazole, voriconazole, clarithromycin, boceprevir, cobicistat, indinavir, lopinavir, saquinavir, tipranavir/ritonavir, teaprevir, grapefruit juice, saquinavir, fluconazole, ciprofloxacin, erythromycin, ciclosporin, cimetidine, diltiazem, verapamil, imatinib, amprenavir, atazanavir/ritonavir, darunavir, darunavir/ritonavir and apreritant (dose dependent)
- contraindicated in CYP2D6 poor metabolisers who are taking itraconazole, posaconazole, voriconazole, clarithromycin, boceprevir, cobicistat, indinavir, lopinavir, saquinavir, tipranavir/ritonavir, grapefruit juice, saquinavir
- not recommended with grapefruit or grapefruit juice
- not recommended with class IA (e.g. quinidine) or class III (e.g. amiodarone, sotalol) antiarrhythmic agents

- decreased serum levels may occur if given with rifampicin, carbamazepine, phenobarbital (phenobarbitone), phenytoin, rifabutin and St John's wort and are not recommended in CYP2D6 immediate, extensive or poor metabolisers
- may increase serum levels of digoxin, colchicine, dabigatran, phenytoin, pravastatin, metoprolol, amitriptyline, imipramine, clomipramine, desipramine, dextromethorphan, atomoxetine, flecainide and phenothiazines

Nursing points/Cautions

- before starting therapy, patients should be genotyped to determine metabolic status for CYP2D6
- in patients switching from enzyme replacement therapy to eliglustat, disease progression should be monitored at 6-monthly intervals. If there is a suboptimal response, reinstitution of enzyme replacement therapy or an alternate treatment should be considered
- contains lactose, therefore are not recommended in those with rare hereditary problems of galactose intolerance, Lapp lactase deficiency or glucose–galactose malabsorption
- not recommended in those with congestive cardiac failure, recent acute myocardial infarction, bradycardia, heart block, ventricular arrhythmias or structural heart disease associated with arrhythmias, long QT syndrome
- not recommended in those who are CYP2D6 ultra-rapid metabolisers or whose status is indeterminate
- not recommended in those with moderate-to-severe kidney impairment or end-stage renal disease
- contraindicated in those with liver impairment who are intermediate or poor CYP2D6 metabolisers

Patient teaching and advice

- instruct patient to avoid grapefruit and grapefruit juice during therapy
- advise patient to swallow capsules whole with glass of water
- warn patient not to drive or operate machinery if dizziness is an ongoing problem

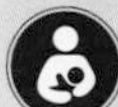

should only be used during pregnancy and breastfeeding if benefits outweigh risks

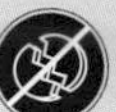

capsules should not be crushed, dispersed in water or opened

ELOSULFASE ALFA (RCH) (Vimizim)

Available form

Vial: 1 mg/mL

Action

- purified human enzyme produced by recombinant DNA technology in Chinese hamster ovary
- mucopolysaccharidosis type IVA is characterised by absence or reduction in N-acetylgalactosamine-6-sulfatase activity leading to accumulation of glycosaminoglycans (GAGs) resulting in cellular, tissue and organ dysfunction

Use

- treatment of mucopolysaccharidosis type IVA (MPS IVA – Morquio A syndrome)

Dose

- 2 mg/kg IV over 4 hours once per week

Adverse effects

- infusion reactions
- headache
- nausea, vomiting, diarrhoea, abdominal pain
- fever, chills

- otitis media, ear infection
- chest discomfort
- oropharyngeal pain, dyspnoea, throat irritation
- headache, dizziness, paraesthesia, somnolence, agitation
- neck pain, myalgia
- urticaria, flushing
- corneal opacity
- development of neutralising antibodies
- (infusion site) pain
- (rare) spinal/cervical cord compression, anaphylaxis, hypersensitivity

Nursing points/Cautions

- patient should be assessed for any acute febrile or respiratory illness before infusion because of increased risk of severe hypersensitivity reaction. Therapy should be postponed if illness is present
- evaluation of airway patency is recommended before starting therapy as sleep apnoea is common in MPS IVA patients. If patient is using supplemental oxygen or continuous positive airway pressure (CPAP) to manage sleep apnoea, these should be immediately available in the event of an emergency
- infusion-related reactions occur more frequently in first 12 weeks of therapy and incidence decreases with time
- pre-treatment with antihistamine with or without antipyretic is recommended before infusion to decrease risk of infusion-related reaction
- patient should be monitored for any signs of hypersensitivity or anaphylaxis. Hypersensitivity reaction occurs within 30 minutes of starting or up to 6 days after completing infusion while anaphylaxis commonly occurs within 30 minutes of starting and up to 3 hours after completion
- if infusion-related reaction occurs, infusion should be slowed or stopped and/or additional antihistamines, antipyretics and/or corticosteroids administered
- calculate total amount required and round up to whole next vial
- vials should be removed from refrigerator but not warmed artificially or shaken
- withdraw and discard volume of sodium chloride 0.9% from infusion bag (equal to volume to be added). Add required volume of elosulfase alfa slowly to infusion bag, taking care not to agitate bag. Infusion bag should be gently rotated (not shaken) to evenly distribute solution
- dilute with sodium chloride 0.9% to final volume of 100 mL (if weight < 25 kg) or 250 mL (if weight ≥ 25 kg)
- if final volume is 100 mL, initial infusion rate should be 3 mL/hour, increasing to 6 mL/hour after 15 minutes, then increasing further by 6 mL/hour at 15-minute intervals until a maximum rate of 36 mL/hour is reached if tolerated by patient
- if final volume is 250 mL, initial infusion rate should be 6 mL/hour, increasing to 12 mL/hour after 15 minutes, then increasing further by 12 mL/hour at 15-minute intervals until a maximum rate of 72 mL/hour is reached if tolerated by patient
- should be administered using low protein binding infusion set with low protein binding 0.2 micron inline filter
- administer alone
- each vial contains 8 mg sodium (plus sodium in infusion solution) which may need to be taken into account if patient is on sodium-controlled diet
- contains sorbitol and is not recommended in those with rare hereditary problems of fructose intolerance
- not recommended in those under 5 or over 65 years
- contraindicated in those with hypersensitivity to Chinese hamster ovary protein

Patient teaching and advice

- patient should be advised not to drive or operate machinery if dizziness occurs
- advise patient to immediately seek medical advice if any of the following occur:
  - back pain, numbness or paralysis, urinary or faecal incontinence
  - cough, redness, throat tightness, hives, flushing, rash, difficulty breat-hing, light-headedness or fainting, chest discomfort with nausea, abdominal pain, retching and vomiting

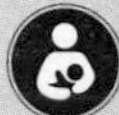

not recommended during pregnancy or breastfeeding unless benefits outweigh risks

GALSULFASE (Naglazyme)

Available form

Vial: 5 mg/5 mL

Action

- Mucopolysaccharidosis VI is characterised by a lack of N-acetylgalactosamine 4-sulfatase, resulting in an accumulation of GAG substrate (dermatan sulfate) throughout the body, leading to widespread cellular, tissue and organ dysfunction
- provides an exogenous enzyme to be taken up into lysosomes and increasing catabolism of GAG
- half-life about 9 hours (first week) increasing to 26 hours by week 24 of therapy

Use

- long-term enzyme replacement therapy in patients with Mucopolysaccharidosis VI (also called Maroteaux-Lamy syndrome or N-acetylgalactosamine 4-sulfatase deficiency)

Dose

- 1 mg/kg body weight IV once weekly over 4 hours

Adverse effects

- apnoea, respiratory distress, dyspnoea, laryngeal oedema, pharyngitis, nasal congestions
- conjunctivitis
- chest pain
- fever, chills, rigors
- malaise
- abdominal pain
- rash
- anaphylaxis, allergic reactions
- immune-mediated reaction (e.g. membranous glomerulonephritis)
- infusion-related reaction (serious or severe)
- onset or worsening of cervical cord compression
- development of anti-drug antibodies

Nursing points/Cautions

- medical staff and resuscitation equipment should be readily available
- airway patency should be assessed before starting therapy
- pre-treatment with antihistamines +/− antipyretics is recommended before infusion to decrease risk of infusion-related reactions. Patients who use supplemental oxygen or continuous positive airway pressure (CPAP) should have them readily available during infusion in the event of infusion reaction or extreme sleepiness/drowsiness related to antihistamine
- if infusion-related reactions occur, infusion rate should be stopped or slowed and additional administration of antihistamine, antipyretic and possibly corticosteroid is recommended
- infusion rate should be set to run infusion over at least 4 hours using infusion pump. Initially rate should be set at 6 mL/hour for first hour and then if well tolerated, rate can be

increased to 80 mL/ hour for last 3 hours. If infusion reaction occurs, rate can be extended
- when calculating the number of vials required according to patient weight, amount should be rounded to next whole vial
- vials should be allowed to come to room temperature before administration (but should not be heated)
- dilute with sodium chloride to a final volume of 250 mL by withdrawing and discarding volume of sodium chloride equal to the volume of the vials to be added. Infusion bag should be gently rotated to mix but not shaken or agitated
- vials should not be shaken as this will denature protein
- 0.2 micron inline filter should be used
- contains 18.5 mg sodium per vial (and is given in sodium chloride 9 mg/mL) which may need to be taken into consideration if patient is on a sodium-restricted diet
- caution if used in patients who have experienced anaphylaxis or allergic reactions previously to galsulfase. During re-challenge, trained personnel and emergency equipment must be readily available
- caution if used in patients susceptible to fluid volume overload (e.g. weighing less than 20 kg, compromised cardiac and/or respiratory system, acute underlying respiratory illness) due to risk of acute cardiorespiratory failure

Patient teaching and advice

- patient/carer should be advised that anaphylaxis and allergic reactions can occur during and up to 24 hours after infusion
- advise patient/carer to seek medical attention immediately if any back pain, limb paralysis, urinary or faecal incontinence occurs

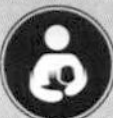

should only be used during pregnancy if benefits outweigh risks

caution if used during breastfeeding

IDURSULFASE (Elaprase)

Available form
Vial: 6 mg/3 mL

Action
- iduronate-2-sulfatase replacement therapy for Hunter syndrome
- Hunter syndrome is caused by insufficient levels of iduronate-2-sulfatase (lysosomal enzyme). Iduronate-2-sulfatase breaks down glycosaminoglycan dermatan sulfate and heparin sulfate, therefore insufficient enzyme levels result in glycosaminoglycan build-up in lysosomes at cell, tissue and organ level and, subsequently, organ dysfunction and tissue destruction

Use
- long-term treatment of Hunter syndrome (mucopolysaccharidosis II)

Dose
- 0.5 mg/kg by IV infusion weekly

Adverse effects
- (IV site) reaction, swelling
- infusion-related reactions (rash, urticaria, pruritus, fever, headache, nausea, vomiting, wheezing, hypertension and flushing)
- headache
- fever
- cyanosis, arrhythmias, tachycardia, hypotension, hypertension, chest pain
- wheezing, dyspnoea, tachypnoea, bronchospasm, hypoxia
- nausea, abdominal pain, dyspepsia, swollen tongue
- erythema, rash, pruritus, urticaria
- facial oedema, peripheral oedema
- antibody development

- (rare) hypersensitivity, late emergent (biphasic) anaphylactoid/anaphylactic reactions

Nursing points/Cautions

- patient should be assessed for any signs of acute febrile respiratory illness before infusion and therapy delayed if signs exist
- some patients may experience late emergent or biphasic anaphylactic reaction where the person has a second reaction about 24 hours after the first, therefore prolonged observation is recommended
- resuscitation equipment should be readily available in the event of infusion-related reaction or anaphylaxis
- if infusion-related reactions occur, infusion rate should be slowed or stopped, or administration of antihistamines, antipyretic, low-dose corticosteroid or beta-agonist nebulisation
- should be diluted in 100 mL of sodium chloride 0.9%
- inline low protein binding filter (0.2 micron) can be used
- diluted solution should be administered within 3 hours. Initial infusion rate should be 8 mL/hour for first 15 minutes, then increasing by 8 mL/hour at 15-minute intervals if tolerated by patient. Infusion rate should not exceed 100 mL/hour
- if 3-hour infusion is well tolerated, infusion time can be gradually decreased for subsequent infusions. Minimum time for infusion should not be less than 1 hour. Infusion time can be increased if patient experiences infusion-related reactions; however, this should not be greater than 8 hours
- infusion time of less than 3 hours is not recommended in children under 5 years
- infusion in the home environment by health professional may be considered if patient is tolerating infusions well, has received at least 6 months of treatment and has been infusion-related reaction-free for that period of time, as well as having stable airway disease. The health professional must be adequately trained in cardiopulmonary resuscitative measures, have ready access to emergency services and be trained to recognise and manage serious infusion-related reactions, hypersensitivity reactions and medical emergencies
- caution if used in those with acute respiratory disease or compromised respiratory function as respiratory compromise may occur as a result of infusion reaction
- caution if used in those who are at risk of fluid overload, acute respiratory disease or compromised cardiac/respiratory function. Fluid restriction and prolonged observation is recommended if used in these patients
- caution if used in children with severe form of Hunter syndrome because of increased risk of developing neutralising antibodies and infusion-related reactions, as well as showing a reduced response to therapy
- not recommended in those over 65 years

Patient teaching and advice

- warn patient/carer that second infusion-related reactions may occur within 24 hours of the first and it is important to seek medical advice immediately
- see also General Patient teaching and advice (p. xxvii)

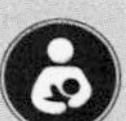

only recommended during pregnancy if benefits outweigh risks

not recommended during breastfeeding

IMIGLUCERASE (RCH) (Cerezyme)

Available form
Vial: 400 U

Action
- recombinant macrophage (variant of human beta-glucocerebrosidase) that catalyses hydrolysis of glucocerebroside (derived from haemopoietic cell turnover) to glucose and ceramide
- a deficiency of glucocerebrosidase results in an accumulation of glucocerebroside in tissue macrophages which become swollen (Gaucher cells)
- Gaucher cells are commonly found in the liver, spleen and bone marrow, as well as the lung, kidney and intestine
- consequences include anaemia, thrombocytopenia, hepatosplenomegaly and debilitating skeletal complications such as osteonecrosis, osteopenia with secondary pathological fractures, remodelling failure, osteosclerosis and bone crisis

Use
- long-term enzyme replacement for those with non neuronopathic (type 1) Gaucher disease or chronic neuronopathic (type 3) (with anaemia, thrombocytopenia, bone disease, hepatomegaly or splenomegaly)

Dose
- 2.5 U/kg 3 times weekly – 60 U/kg every 2 weeks by IV infusion over 1–2 hours

Adverse effects
- (IV site) discomfort, pruritus, burning, swelling, sterile abscess
- infusion-related reactions (pruritus, flushing, urticaria, angioedema, chest discomfort, dyspnoea, coughing, cyanosis, hypotension)
- nausea, abdominal pain, vomiting, diarrhoea
- rash
- chills, fever
- backache
- tachycardia
- fatigue, headache, dizziness
- transient peripheral oedema
- development of IgG antibodies
- (rare) anaphylactoid reactions, hypersensitivity, pulmonary hypertension

Nursing points/Cautions
- dose and frequency of administration is dependent on severity of disease
- regular monitoring for the development of IgG antibodies is recommended during first 12 months of therapy. Development of antibodies increases risk of hypersensitivity reactions
- if patient has experienced infusion-related reaction, decreasing the rate and/or pre-treatment with antihistamines and/or corticosteroids is recommended for next infusion
- if patient develops respiratory symptoms, evaluation for pulmonary hypertension is recommended
- reconstitute with water for injections, mixing gently and avoiding frothing, then dilute further with sodium chloride 0.9% (100–200 mL), rotating infusion bag gently to ensure even distribution before administration
- inline low protein binding filter (0.2 micron) can be used
- diluted solution should be administered within 3 hours
- not recommended in the management of type 2 or type 3 Gaucher disease or acute bone crises associated with Gaucher disease
- caution if given to those with IgG antibodies or previous hypersensitivity reactions to imiglucerase
- not recommended in those with hypersensitivity to Chinese hamster ovary cells

Patient teaching and advice

- warn patient to avoid driving or operating machinery if dizziness occurs
- see also General Patient teaching and advice (p. xxvii)

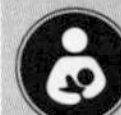

only recommended during pregnancy if benefits outweigh risks

caution if used during breastfeeding

LARONIDASE (RCH) (Aldurazyme)

Available form
Vial: 500 U/5 mL

Action
- lysosomal enzyme alpha L-iduronidase required for glycosaminoglycan catabolism deficiency results in mucopolysaccharide (lysosomal) storage disorder. Deficiency in this enzyme results in accumulation of glycosaminoglycan and associated cell, tissue and organ dysfunction
- enzyme replacement produced by recombinant DNA technology

Use
- long-term enzyme replacement therapy for those with mucopolysaccharidosis (alpha-L-iduronidase deficiency) for treatment of non-neurological manifestations

Dose
- 100 U/kg weekly by IV infusion

Adverse effects
- infusion-related reaction (commonly fever, headache, flushing and rash and, less commonly, cough, bronchospasm, dyspnoea, urticaria, angioedema, pruritus)
- injection site reaction and pain, abscess formation
- upper respiratory tract infection
- corneal opacities
- thrombocytopenia
- bilirubinaemia
- hyperreflexia, paraesthesia
- rash
- hypotension, oedema, chest pain
- cough, oxygen desaturation/hypoxia, dyspnoea, tachypnoea, cyanosis, angioedema, facial/laryngeal oedema
- erythema
- feeling cold
- development of IgG antibodies
- anaphylaxis, allergic reaction

Interaction
- not recommended with procaine

Nursing points/Cautions/Patient teaching and advice

- patient should be assessed before administration as acute illness may increase risk of infusion-related reactions
- resuscitation equipment should be readily available in the event of infusion-related reaction or anaphylaxis
- pre-treatment with antipyretics (e.g. paracetamol, ibuprofen) and/or antihistamines (e.g. diphenhydramine) is recommended 60 minutes before infusion to decrease infusion-related reactions
- slowing IV rate or temporarily stopping infusion will lessen infusion-related reactions
- volume of infusion is dependent on weight ($\leq$ 20 kg total of 100 mL, $>$ 20 kg total of 250 mL)
- initial infusion rate 2 U/kg/hour, rate doubling every 15 minutes for first hour (if tolerated), to maximum of 43 U/kg/hour and maximum rate maintained for remainder of infusion (2–3 hours)
- do not shake solution as protein will be denatured
- allow vial(s) to come to room temperature while calculating amount required. Withdraw and discard this amount of sodium chloride 0.9%

from infusion bag. Gently withdraw required amount from vial(s) and slowly add to sodium chloride infusion bag, taking care not to agitate the solution. Gently rotate infusion bag to ensure distribution and administer IV

- infusion set should contain an inline low protein 0.2 micron filter
- administer alone
- not recommended in children under 5 years or those over 65 years
- caution if used in those with compromised lung function or acute respiratory disorders as infusion-related reactions may compromise respiration and require extra monitoring and/or support

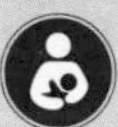

not recommended during pregnancy unless benefits outweigh risks

caution if used during breastfeeding

MERCAPTAMINE (CYSTEAMINE) BITARTRATE (Cystagon)

Available forms

Capsules: 50 mg, 150 mg

Action

- cystinosis causes abnormal transport of cystine out of lysosomes, which may result in accumulation of cystine in organs, especially the kidneys. The cystine crystals damage the kidneys, retina, muscles and CNS, resulting in photophobia, failure to grow, rickets and kidney failure
- cysteamine converts cystine into cysteine and cysteine–cysteamine compound, which can be removed
- half-life 1.5 hours

Use

- management of nephropathic cystinosis

Dose

- (patients > 12 years and > 50 kg) initially 0.2–0.3 g/m^2 orally daily in 4 divided doses, increasing over 4–6 weeks to 2 g daily in 4 divided doses (maintenance) **OR**
- (patients < 12 years) initially 0.2–0.3 g/m^2 orally daily in 4 divided doses, increasing over 4–6 weeks to 1.3 g/m^2 g daily in 4 divided doses (maintenance)

Adverse effects

- fever
- lethargy
- diarrhoea, nausea, vomiting, anorexia, bad breath, constipation, dyspepsia, abdominal pain, GI bleeding/ulceration
- rash, urticaria
- hair colour changes
- (uncommon) abnormal liver function, reversible leucopenia, anaemia, kidney failure, seizures, dehydration, somnolence, depression, lethargy, encephalopathy, headache, confusion, dizziness, nervousness
- (rare) benign intracranial hypertension (pseudotumour cerebri), papilloedema, serious skin reactions

Nursing points/Cautions

- leucocyte cysteine levels should be monitored 5–6 hours after administration and levels should be kept at less than 1 nanomol of half cystine/mg protein. Levels should be repeated 3-monthly
- therapy should be stopped if rash develops and restarted at a lower dose after rash has cleared and slowly titrated to therapeutic dose if possible
- blood counts and liver function tests should be monitored regularly throughout therapy
- eyes should be examined regularly during therapy

- contraindicated in those with hypersensitivity to mercaptamine (cysteamine) or penicillamine

Patient/carer teaching and advice

- patient/carer should be warned that GI symptoms are common at the start of therapy
- if patient is an adult, he/she should be advised not to drive or use machinery if drowsiness or decreased alertness occur
- if patient is a child, he/she should be advised to be careful when partaking in activities such as bike-riding and climbing trees if dizziness or decreased alertness occur
- if patient is child under 6 years, parent/carer should be instructed to sprinkle contents of capsules over food to decrease risk of aspiration by trying to swallow capsule whole
- advise patients/carers to seek medical advice if any of the following occur:
    - nausea, vomiting, loss of appetite, stomach pain or vomiting blood
    - rash
    - skin lesions (resembling stretch marks), leg pain, bone fractures or deformities or joint problems
    - fitting, depression, excessive sleepiness
    - headache, ringing or whooshing in ears (tinnitus), dizziness, nausea, double or blurry vision, loss of vision, pain behind eye or on eye movement
- see also General Patient teaching and advice (p. xxvii)

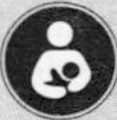

should only be used during pregnancy if benefits outweigh risks

capsules can be opened and contents mixed with water or spoonful of smooth food such as yoghurt

MIGALASTAT (Galafold)

Available form

Capsules: 123 mg

Action

- Fabry disease is a progressive X-linked lysosomal storage disorder that causes a deficiency of lysosomal enzyme α-galactosidase A (α-Gal A) that is needed for glycosphingolipid substrate metabolism. Deficiency in the enzyme results in accumulation of substrate in organs and tissues leading to morbidity and mortality
- selectively and reversibly binds with some mutant forms of α-Gal A stabilising these in the endoplasmic reticulum leading to restoration of α-Gal A
- elimination half-life 3–5 hours

Use

- long-term treatment of Fabry disease in adults and adolescents over 16 years who have amenable mutations of α-Gal A

Dose

- 123 mg orally every second day at same time of day at least 2 hours apart from food

Adverse effects

- palpitations
- vertigo
- nausea, diarrhoea, abdominal pain, constipation, dry mouth, urge to defecate, dyspepsia, weight increase
- fatigue, headache, dizziness
- muscle spasm, myalgia, torticollis, extremity pain
- paraesthesia, hypoaesthesia
- depression
- proteinuria
- dyspnoea, epistaxis
- rash, pruritus

Interactions

- not recommended at the same time as enzyme replacement therapy

Nursing points/Cautions

- kidney function, ECG and biochemical markers should be monitored at least 6-monthly
- not recommended for patients with non-amenable mutations
- not recommended in patients with severe kidney insufficiency
- not recommended in women of childbearing potential who are not using contraception

Patient teaching and advice

- advise patient that capsules should be taken at least 2 hours after food and food should not be eaten within 2 hours of taking medication
- instruct patient that capsules should not be taken on 2 consecutive days
- patient should be advised not to drive or operate machinery if dizziness is an ongoing problem
- women of childbearing potential should be advised to use adequate contraception during therapy

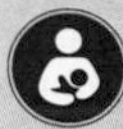

not recommended during pregnancy

should only be used during breastfeeding if benefits outweigh risks

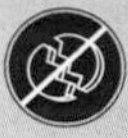

capsules should not be opened or crushed

MIGLUSTAT (Zavesca)

Available form

Capsules: 100 mg

Action

- glucosylceramide synthase inhibitor
- beta-glucocerebrosidase catalyses hydrolysis of glucocerebroside (derived from haemopoietic cell turnover) to glucose and ceramide
- deficiency of glucocerebrosidase results in an accumulation of glucocerebroside in tissue macrophages, which become swollen (Gaucher cells) and are commonly found in the liver, spleen and bone marrow, as well as the lung, kidney and intestine
- consequences of Gaucher disease include anaemia, thrombocytopenia, hepatosplenomegaly and debilitating skeletal complications such as osteonecrosis, osteopenia with secondary pathological fractures, remodelling failure, osteosclerosis and bone crisis
- neurological characteristics of Niemann-Pick type C disease are thought to be due to accumulation of glycosphingolipids in neurons and glial cells
- half-life 6–7 hours

Use

- mild-to-moderate type 1 Gaucher disease (where enzyme replacement is not an option)
- treatment of progressive neuropathy in Niemann-Pick type C disease

Dose

- (type 1 Gaucher disease) 100 mg orally 3 times daily **OR**
- (Niemann-Pick type C disease) 200 mg orally 3 times daily

Adverse effects

- thrombocytopenia
- weight loss, anorexia, diarrhoea, flatulence, abdominal pain, nausea, constipation, vomiting, dyspepsia, abdominal distension/discomfort
- muscle spasm
- tremor, insomnia, decreased libido, peripheral neuropathy, headache, dizziness, paraesthesia, hypoaesthesia, ataxia, fatigue, asthenia
- abnormal nerve conduction tests
- decreased fertility, increased number of abnormal sperm

Nursing points/Cautions

- regular monitoring of vitamin B_{12} is recommended during therapy as deficiency occurs commonly in those with Gaucher disease
- neurological examination should be conducted before starting therapy then at 6-monthly intervals
- regular blood counts are recommended
- dose reduction may be required because of diarrhoea
- enzyme replacement therapy is standard management of type 1 Gaucher disease
- any pre-existing tremor should be assessed before starting therapy
- (Niemann-Pick type C disease) 6-monthly patient assessment is recommended to evaluate neurological manifestations and benefits of treatment
- (Niemann-Pick type C disease) weight and growth should be monitored in children
- not recommended in those with severe kidney impairment (creatinine clearance < 30 mL/min)
- not recommended in those with severe type 1 Gaucher disease (Hb < 90 g/L, platelet $< 50 \times 10^9$/L, active bone disease)

Patient teaching and advice

- warn patient to avoid driving or operating machinery if dizziness or tremor occurs
- patient/carer should be warned that tremor commonly occurs in first month of therapy and usually resolves within 4–12 weeks (although dose reduction is sometimes required)
- patient/carer should be advised to decrease lactose or sucrose-containing foods or take tablets on empty stomach to reduce GI side-effects, especially diarrhoea
- advise patient/carer to report any:
  - numbness or tingling in hands or feet
  - tremor
- counsel male patient to use reliable contraception during and for 12 weeks after stopping therapy due to increased incidence of abnormal sperm production and decreased fertility
- female patient should be advised to use effective contraception to avoid pregnancy occurring during therapy
- see General Patient teaching and advice (p. xxvii)

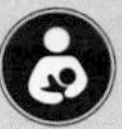
not recommended during pregnancy or breastfeeding

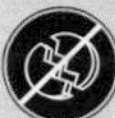
if capsules are opened, mask and safety glasses should be worn and pregnant staff must not handle

content of capsules can be mixed with water or sprinkled on spoonful of yoghurt or apple puree

NITISINONE (Nityr, Orfadin)

Available forms

Capsules: 2 mg, 5 mg, 10 mg, 20 mg; Oral suspension: 4 mg/mL

Action

- competitive 4-hydroxyphenylpyruvate dioxygenase inhibitor which prevents accumulation of toxic intermediates (succinylacetone, succinylacetoacetate) from tyrosine metabolism (which further inhibit porphyrin synthesis pathway and accumulation of 5-aminolevulinate)

Use

- treatment of hereditary tyrosinaemia type 1 (with dietary restriction of tyrosine and phenylalanine)

Dose

- (patients weighing > 20 kg) initially 1 mg/kg/day divided orally after food in 2 divided doses, decreasing to once daily if urine succinylacetone is undetectable after 4 weeks of therapy. Dose may need to be increased to 1.5 mg/kg/day in 2 divided doses if urine succinylacetone is detectable after 4 weeks of therapy (maximum 2 mg/kg/day)

Adverse effects

- thrombocytopenia, leucopenia, granulocytosis
- conjunctivitis, corneal ulcers and opacity, keratitis, photophobia, eye pain
- increased liver enzymes, hepatomegaly, liver failure
- (uncommon) rash, pruritus, dermatitis

Interactions

- may increase serum levels of warfarin and phenytoin increasing risk of adverse effects. If given together, serum levels should be closely monitored

Nursing points/Cautions

- ophthalmological examination (slit lamp examination) is recommended before starting therapy
- liver function tests (including serum alpha-fetoprotein levels) and liver imaging studies are recommended regularly during therapy. If liver nodules appear or serum alpha-fetoprotein levels increase, patient should be immediately assessed for liver malignancy
- WBC and platelet count should be monitored 6-monthly during therapy
- dose adjustment is dependent on urine succinylacetone levels, liver function tests and serum alpha-fetoprotein levels, as well as any changes to body weight
- for patient weighing < 20 kg, dose should be administered as 2 divided doses
- if diet is not restricted in tyrosine and phenylalanine, plasma tyrosine levels increase leading to toxic effects in the eyes, skin and nervous system. Plasma tyrosine levels should be measured regularly
- (suspension) contains sodium benzoate, which can cause bilirubin displacement from albumin potentially causing jaundice (especially in neonates). Bilirubin levels should be measured before starting and regularly throughout therapy. If bilirubin level is elevated in premature infants (with risk of acidosis and low albumin levels), treatment with capsule/tablet (rather than oral suspension) is recommended
- (suspension) contains 0.7 mg sodium per mL suspension. Therapy with capsules should be considered if sodium content is problematic
- (suspension) contains 500 mg glycerol per mL suspension, which can cause headache, stomach upset and diarrhoea if 20 mL or more of suspension is administered. If patient does not tolerate suspension (develops these adverse effects), therapy with capsules/tablets should be considered

Patient teaching and advice

- advise patient/carer to administer with food
- patient/carer should be instructed to maintain dietary restriction of tyrosine and phenylalanine (to maintain plasma tyrosine levels below 500 micromol/L)
- advise patient/carer to immediately report any eye pain, changes to vision, inflammation in cornea/eye/eyelid or sensitivity to light
- patient/carer should be instructed in correct administration of oral suspension, including:
    - suspension should be administered directly into mouth using syringe provided without any dilution

- oral suspension is supplied with 3 oral syringes (1 mL, 3 mL, 5 mL)
  - 1 mL syringe should be used for doses less than 1 mL. Syringe is marked from 0.1 to 1 mL, with graduations of 0.01 mL
  - 3 mL syringe should be used for doses from 1 to 3 mL and has 0.1 mL graduations
  - 5 mL syringe should be used for doses > 3 mL and has 0.2 mL graduations
- New bottle:
  - new bottle should be stored upright in refrigerator in its box
  - remove bottle from refrigerator, label with the date the bottle was removed and opened
  - shake vigorously for at least 20 seconds to ensure suspension is uniformly dispersed and mixed
  - remove cap, place bottle upright on table and insert plastic adapter firmly into bottle neck (as far as it goes)
  - cap can then be replaced
- Administering dose:
  - shake bottle for at least 5 seconds
  - open cap and syringe plunger into the top of the adapter and carefully turn bottle upside down (with syringe in place)
  - pull plunger slowly down until top edge of black ring is exactly level with dose marking
  - if air bubbles are present in syringe, push plunger back up until air bubble is expelled and slowly pull plunger down to dose level required
  - turn bottle upright and remove syringe by gently twisting
  - administer directly into mouth slowly (rapid administration may cause choking)
  - replace cap and store bottle in refrigerator or below 25°C
  - discard 2 months after opening
- syringe should be cleaned immediately with water, separating barrel and plunger and rinsing both. Allow to air dry

- see General Patient teaching and advice (p. xxvii)

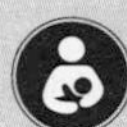

not recommended during pregnancy unless benefits are thought to outweigh risks

contraindicated during breastfeeding

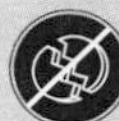

available as oral suspension. Tablet can be crushed or capsule opened and contents mixed with formula or spoonful of yoghurt or oral suspension

SAPROPTERIN DIHYDROCHLORIDE (Kuvan)

Available forms

Tablets (soluble): 100 mg; Powder for oral solution (sachet): 100 mg, 500 mg

Action

- synthetic form of naturally occurring 6R-tetrahydrobiopterin (co-factor for hydroxylases for phenylalanine, tyrosine and tryptophan)
- enhances activity of defective phenylalanine hydroxylase enzyme, increasing/restoring phenylalanine metabolism, preventing (or decreasing) accumulation in the blood
- sustained phenylalanine levels in those with phenylketonuria or tetrahydrobiopterin deficiency can result in neurological damage including severe mental retardation, microcephaly, delayed speech, seizures and behavioural abnormalities
- half-life is 6–7 hours

Use

- treatment of hyperphenylalaninaemia in those with phenylketonuria (PKU) or 6R-tetrahydrobiopterin (BH_4) deficiency

Dose

- (phenylketonuria) initially 10 mg/kg orally once daily with food, adjusting dose according to blood levels (recommended range 5–20 mg/kg/day)

OR

- (BH_4 deficiency) initially 2–5 mg/kg orally daily with food in 2–3 divided doses, adjusting dose according to blood levels (recommended range 2–20 mg/kg/day in 2–3 divided doses)

Adverse effects

- headache
- fever
- rash
- rhinorrhoea, pharyngolaryngeal pain, cough, nasal stuffiness, upper respiratory tract infection
- diarrhoea, vomiting, abdominal pain
- hypophenylalaninaemia
- (rare) seizures, hypersensitivity reaction, gastritis, oesophagitis

Interaction

- caution if used with levodopa due to risk of increased excitability and irritability
- caution if used with glyceryl trinitrate, isosorbide dinitrate, sodium nitroprusside, minoxidil and PDE-5 inhibitors (e.g. sildenafil) that are nitric oxide donors
- caution if used with methotrexate, trimethoprim or other dihydrofolate reductase inhibitors

Nursing points/Cautions

- therapy should be initiated as early as possible to prevent non-reversible neurological disorders in children and cognitive deficits and psychiatric disorders in adults
- phenylalanine blood levels should be measured before and then 1 week after starting therapy. If blood level is not sufficiently reduced, dose can be increased to 20 mg/kg/day maximum and blood levels monitored weekly for 4 weeks with dietary restrictions being maintained. A reduction of 30% or more in blood phenylalanine level is considered satisfactory. If this is not achieved after 4 weeks of therapy, patient is considered non-responder and therapy should be stopped
- (PKU) blood levels of phenylalanine should reduce within 24 hours of single dose, although about 4 weeks is needed for maximum effect to occur
- phenylalanine blood levels should also be measured 1–2 weeks after any dose adjustment, especially in children
- blood phenylalanine levels may increase above pre-treatment levels if therapy is suddenly stopped
- not recommended in children under 4 years
- caution if used in those with history of seizures, kidney or liver impairment, or over 50 years

Patient teaching and advice

- patient/carer should be instructed to maintain strict phenylalanine diet and have regular clinical assessment including serum phenylalanine and tyrosine levels, nutrient intake and psychomotor development
- advise patient/carer to take with food (preferably high-fat, high-calorie meal) at the same time each day for maximum effect
- patient/carer should be warned not to stop therapy suddenly
- instruct patient/carer to seek medical advice if illness occurs as this may cause phenylalanine levels to rise

- adult patient should be instructed to dissolve tablets or sachets in 120–240 mL of water or apple juice and drink within 15–20 minutes. For children, doses above 100 mg should be dissolved in 120 mL or less of water. For doses less than 100 mg, 1 tablet (100 mg) should be dissolved in 100 mL of water and the required amount given
- advise patient/carer that tablets will dissolve faster if they are crushed
- female patients should be counselled that strict control of maternal serum phenylalanine levels is recommended before and during pregnancy due to potential risks to mother and fetus (e.g. high incidence of neurological, cardiac, facial dysmorphism and growth abnormalities). Therapy is recommended only if strict dietary management is inadequate to control serum phenylalanine levels
- patient/carer should be advised to seek medical advice if any of the following occur:
  - abdominal pain, belching, heartburn, nausea, vomiting, loss of appetite, indigestion (symptoms of gastritis)
  - difficulty swallowing, pain on swallowing, sore throat, hoarse voice, heartburn, acid reflux, nausea, chest pain which is worse on swallowing (symptoms of oesophagitis)
- see General Patient teaching and advice (p. xxvii)

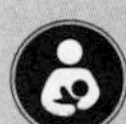

caution if used during pregnancy

not recommended during breastfeeding

tablets are soluble but can also be crushed and mixed with small amount of yoghurt or mashed banana

SEBELIPASE ALFA (Kanuma)

Available form
Vial: 20 mg/20 mL

Action
- lysosomal acid lipase deficiency is a rare autosomal recessive lysosomal storage disorder characterised by a decrease or loss of lysosomal acid lipase activity, resulting in accumulation of cholesteryl esters and triglycerides in liver, spleen, intestine and blood vessel walls. This can result in hepatomegaly, progressive liver disease, cirrhosis and end-stage liver disease; splenomegaly, anaemia and thrombocytopenia; malabsorption in the intestine and growth retardation; dyslipidaemia and increased risk of cardiovascular disease and atherosclerosis

Use
- long-term enzyme replacement therapy in patients with lysosomal acid lipase deficiency

Dose
- (infants < 6 months) initially 1 mg/kg by IV infusion once weekly, increasing dose to 3 mg/kg weekly if required **OR**
- (children and adults) 1 mg/kg by IV infusion every second week

Adverse effects
- diarrhoea, vomiting, nausea, constipation
- headache, asthenia
- fever
- rhinitis, cough, nasopharyngitis, oropharyngeal pain
- anaemia
- urticaria
- transient hyperlipidaemia (occurring within first 2–4 weeks and improving by week 8)
- development of anti-drug antibodies
- anaphylaxis, hypersensitivity reactions

Nursing points/Cautions

- patient should be closely monitored for any anaphylaxis (e.g. fever, chills, abdominal pain, rash, nausea, vomiting, diarrhoea, laryngeal oedema) which can occur during or within 4 hours of infusion. Anaphylaxis can occur within 6 infusions or as late as 1 year after starting therapy
- medical personnel and emergency equipment should be readily available during administration and post infusion
- if reaction occurs, infusion may be stopped or rate reduced and antihistamines, antipyretic and corticosteroid administered depending on severity of reaction
- allow vial to come to room temperature before administration
- do not shake vial
- dilute with sodium chloride 0.9% (10–250 mL depending on weight) and mix gently
- administer using a low-protein binding infusion set with inline 0.2 micron filter
- contraindicated in those with life-threatening hypersensitivity to egg

Patient teaching and advice

- patient should be instructed that anaphylaxis can occur within 4 hours of infusion completion and to seek medical advice immediately if any signs or symptoms occur

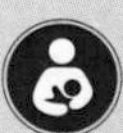

not recommended during pregnancy

should only be used during breastfeeding if benefits outweigh risks

SODIUM PHENYLBUTYRATE (Pheburane)

Available form

Granules: 483 mg/174 g

Action

- nitrogen scavenger
- prodrug, converted to phenylacetate
- reduces raised plasma ammonia and glutamine levels in patients with urea cycle disorders
- phenylbutyrate peak concentration in 1 hour, elimination half-life 0.8 hours
- phenylacetate peak concentration 3.55 hours, elimination half-life 1.3 hours

Use

- hyperammonaemia management associated with urea cycle disorders (with dietary protein restriction +/− dietary supplements)

Dose

- (infants and children < 20 kg) up to 600 mg/kg per day orally in divided doses with meals **OR**
- (children > 20 kg, adolescents, adults) up to 13 g/m^2 per day orally in divided doses with meals

Adverse effects

- anaemia, thrombocytopenia, leucopenia, leucocytosis, thrombocytosis
- metabolic acidosis, alkalosis
- decreased appetite, abdominal pain, vomiting, nausea, constipation, change in taste, increased weight
- rash, abnormal skin odour
- depression, irritability, headache
- syncope
- oedema
- renal tubular acidosis, increased liver enzymes, bilirubin, uric acid, chloride and sodium, decreased potassium, albumin, total protein and phosphate
- amenorrhoea, irregular menstruation
- neurotoxicity (somnolence, fatigue, light-headedness, headache, disorientation, impaired memory, lack or change in taste, partial loss of hearing)

Interactions

- excretion may be inhibited by probenecid

- corticosteroids may cause breakdown of protein increasing plasma ammonia levels
- increased risk of hepatotoxicity if used with rifampicin
- increased risk of hyperammonaemia if given with haloperidol, sodium valproate, carbamazepine, phenobarbital or topiramate

Nursing points/Cautions

- therapy should be started and managed by a practitioner with expertise in urea cycle disorder management
- urinalysis and plasma levels of ammonia, arginine, essential amino acids (especially branched chain amino acids), carnitine and serum proteins should be monitored during therapy. If needed, levels of phenylbutyrate (and metabolites) should be measured. Dose should be adjusted according to levels
- serum potassium should be monitored during therapy as there may be increased potassium excretion
- calibrated dosing spoon dispenses up to 3 g in 250 mg increments
- may be given via nasogastric or gastrostomy tube if needed
- contains 124 mg sodium/g sodium phenylbutyrate and therefore should be used with great caution (if at all) in those with congestive heart failure or severe kidney insufficiency or with care in those on a sodium-controlled diet or where there is sodium retention with oedema
- contains sucrose (768 mg/g) and therefore is not recommended in those with rare hereditary problems of fructose intolerance, glucose–galactose malabsorption or sucrase–isomaltase insufficiency and should be taken into consideration by those with diabetes mellitus
- caution if used in those with liver or kidney impairment
- not recommended for management of acute hyperammonaemia which is life threatening and requires rapid response

Patient teaching and advice

- patient/carer should be instructed to use dosing spoon provided to measure dose only (no other measuring spoons should be used). Instructions include:
  - lines on the spoon indicate the amount in grams
  - pour granules into spoon
  - tap spoon on table to give horizontal level and add more if needed
  - if more than 3 g is needed (maximum amount held by spoon), instructions should be repeated to give total dose
- advise patient/carer that granules can be taken directly with a drink (water, fruit juice, protein-free infant formula) or sprinkled on spoonful of solid food (mashed potato or apple puree/sauce), but should be eaten or drunk straight away
- patient/carer should be aware of need for dietary protein restriction and, if needed, essential amino acid and carnitine supplementation
- if dose is missed, patient/carer should be instructed to take dose as soon as possible with next meal but there should be at least 3 hours between doses
- those with diabetes mellitus should be warned of the sucrose content and need to monitor blood glucose levels
- instruct patient/carer to discard bottle after 45 days of opening
- patient should be advised to seek medical attention if any of the following occur:
  - nausea, vomiting, somnolence, fatigue, light-headedness, headache, disorientation, impaired

memory, lack or change in taste, partial loss of hearing
- women of childbearing potential should be counselled to use effective contraception during therapy to avoid pregnancy occurring

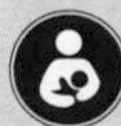

contraindicated during pregnancy and breastfeeding

TALIGLUCERASE ALFA (RPC) (Elelyso)

Available form
Vial: 200 U

Action
- recombinant form of human beta-glucocerebrosidase
- a deficiency of glucocerebrosidase results in an accumulation of glucocerebroside in tissue macrophages which become swollen (Gaucher cells)
- Gaucher cells are commonly found in the liver, spleen and bone marrow, as well as the lung, kidney and intestine
- consequences include anaemia, thrombocytopenia, hepatosplenomegaly and debilitating skeletal complications such as osteonecrosis, osteopenia with secondary pathological fractures, remodelling failure, osteosclerosis and bone crisis

Use
- type 1 Gaucher disease associated with splenomegaly, hepatomegaly, anaemia or thrombocytopenia

Dose
- 30–60 U/kg once every 2 weeks via IV infusion over 60–120 minutes (maximum dose 67 U/kg)

Adverse effects
- infusion-related reactions
- headache, dizziness, fatigue
- flushing, pruritus, rash, erythema
- eye swelling and pruritus, increased lacrimation
- sneezing, runny nose, throat irritation
- vomiting, abdominal pain, nausea, weight increase
- arthralgia, pain in extremity, bone pain, back pain
- peripheral oedema
- hypersensitivity
- infusion site pain
- (rare) development of antibodies, pulmonary hypertension

Nursing points/Cautions
- any pulmonary hypertension should be evaluated regularly during therapy
- infusion-related reactions usually occur within 24 hours of infusion
- if infusion-related reactions occur, rate should be slowed or stopped, then resumed at a reduced rate
- pre-treatment with antihistamines and/or corticosteroids may be used to prevent subsequent reactions
- hypersensitivity reactions commonly occur in first 12 weeks of therapy
- can be switched from imiglucerase using same dose
- reconstitute using 5.1 mL water for injections and mix vial gently (do not shake)
- withdraw 5 mL of reconstituted solution and dilute with 100–200 mL sodium chloride 0.9% and administer by IV infusion
- inline low protein binding 0.2 micron filter is recommended
- contains sodium and is administered in sodium chloride, which may need to be considered if patient has sodium restriction
- caution if used in those with allergy to carrots (as agent has been developed in carrot plant)
- not recommended in those with type 2 Gaucher disease

- contraindicated in those with known allergy to similar glucocerebrosidase enzymes

Patient teaching and advice

- warn patient to avoid driving or operating machinery if dizziness occurs
- see also General Patient teaching and advice (p. xxvii)

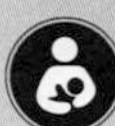

should only be used during pregnancy or breastfeeding if benefits outweigh risks

VELAGLUCERASE ALFA (GHU) (VPRIV)

Available form

Vial: 400 U

Action

- glycoprotein produced by gene activation technology
- recombinant macrophage (variant of human beta-glucocerebrosidase) that catalyses hydrolysis of glucocerebroside (derived from haemopoietic cell turnover) to glucose and ceramide
- a deficiency of glucocerebrosidase results in an accumulation of glucocerebroside in tissue macrophages which become swollen (Gaucher cells)
- Gaucher cells are commonly found in the liver, spleen and bone marrow, as well as the lung, kidney and intestine
- consequences include anaemia, thrombocytopenia, hepatosplenomegaly and debilitating skeletal complications such as osteonecrosis, osteopenia with secondary pathological fractures, remodelling failure, osteosclerosis and bone crisis

Use

- long-term enzyme replacement for those with type 1 Gaucher disease (with anaemia, thrombocytopenia or hepato-splenomegaly)

Dose

- 60 U/kg every 2 weeks by IV infusion over 60 minutes

Adverse effects

- (IV site) discomfort, pruritus, burning, swelling, sterile abscess
- infusion-related reactions (headache, dizziness, hypotension, hypertension, nausea, fatigue, asthenia, fever)
- nasopharyngitis, rhinitis, bronchitis, dyspnoea
- cystitis, urinary tract infection
- headache, dizziness
- paraesthesia
- cough, epistaxis
- abdominal pain, diarrhoea, vomiting, nausea
- urticaria, pruritus, rash, flushing
- chest discomfort, hypertension, hypotension, tachycardia
- arthralgia, bone/back pain, muscle spasm, myalgia, neck pain
- fever, flu-like illness
- peripheral oedema
- development of IgG antibodies, prolonged APPT
- (rare) hypersensitivity, anaphylactoid reaction, allergic dermatitis

Nursing points/Cautions

- infusion-related reactions occur most commonly in the first 6 months of therapy for patients previously untreated with enzyme replacement therapy
- if patient experiences infusion-related reaction, decreasing the rate and/or pre-treatment with antihistamines and/or corticosteroids is recommended for next infusion
- if patient has severe infusion-related reaction or lack/loss of response, antibody testing is recommended
- reconstitute using 4.3 mL water for injections

- do not shake as this will denature protein
- dilute further with 100 mL sodium chloride 0.9%, rotating gently to ensure even distribution before administration
- inline low protein binding filter (0.2 micron) should be used
- diluted solution should be administered over 60 minutes
- infusion in the home environment by health professional may be considered if patient has received at least 3 infusions in the hospital environment and has tolerated them well (infusion-related reaction-free). The health professional must be adequately trained in cardiopulmonary resuscitative measures, have ready access to emergency services and be trained to recognise and manage serious infusion-related reactions, hypersensitivity reactions and medical emergencies
- not recommended in the management of type 2 or type 3 Gaucher disease
- caution if used in those with kidney or liver impairment
- caution if used in those with previous hypersensitivity reactions to other enzyme replacement therapies

Patient teaching and advice

- warn patient to avoid driving or operating machinery if dizziness occurs
- see also General Patient teaching and advice (p. xxvii)

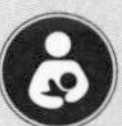

only recommended during pregnancy if benefits outweigh risks

caution if used during breastfeeding

MOVEMENT DISORDER AGENTS

Movement disorders in this section include multiple sclerosis and motor neurone disease (also known as amyotrophic lateral sclerosis in other parts of the world).

MULTIPLE SCLEROSIS

Multiple sclerosis (MS) is an autoimmune disease of the CNS characterised by chronic inflammation, demyelination, plaques or scarring and neuronal loss, with brain lesions developing at different times in different parts of the brain. While MS occurs more commonly in women, with risk factors including vitamin D deficiency, exposure to Epstein-Barr virus after early childhood and smoking, the exact cause is unknown (Cree & Hauser 2019). MS is thought to affect about 2.3 million people worldwide, with over 25,600 of those people being Australian. Interestingly, the further away from the equator that people live, the higher the prevalence of MS, with the highest prevalence being in islands off Scotland. In Australia, Tasmania has twice the prevalence of Queensland (Cree & Hauser 2019; MS Australia 2019).

Onset may be abrupt or insidious, with symptoms that can be trivial or severe. Common symptoms include pain, sensory loss (e.g. reduced sensation, numbness, 'dead' feeling), optic neuritis, limb weakness (e.g. loss of strength, speed or dexterity, fatigue, disturbed gait), diplopia, paraesthesia (e.g. tingling or prickling sensation, 'pins and needles'), ataxia and vertigo (Cree & Hauser 2019). Types of MS include:

- *relapsing/remitting MS*, which accounts for about 85% of cases and is characterised by attacks that evolve over days to weeks, followed by recovery, with patients neurologically stable between attacks. However, as attacks continue, recovery may be less evident
- *secondary progressive MS*, which begins as relapsing/remitting MS, but the patient then experiences a steady deterioration in function not connected to acute attacks
- *primary progressive MS*, which accounts for about 10% of cases with

patients experiencing a steady functional decline from the onset (but no acute attacks) (Cree & Hauser 2019).

Management includes treatment of acute attacks (usually with corticosteroids to control the initial attacks or acute exacerbations), therapies for relapsing forms of MS (pharmacological agents discussed in this section) and symptomatic therapy (e.g. management of ataxia, tremor, spasticity, spasms, weakness, pain, bladder dysfunction and depression), as well as encouraging a healthy lifestyle, including a healthy diet and regular exercise as tolerated (Cree & Hauser 2019).

ALEMTUZUMAB (Lemtrada, MabCampath)

Available forms

Vial: 12 mg/mL (Lemtrada), 30 mg/mL (MabCampath)

Action

- anti-CD52 antibody (CD52 is a surface antigen on T and B lymphocytes, killer cells, monocytes and macrophages)
- MS activity is thought to be related to alteration in number, proportion and properties of some lymphocytes post-treatment

Use

- relapsing/remitting MS (in those with active disease) (Lemtrada)
- B-cell chronic lymphocytic leukaemia (MabCampath) (see Antineoplastic agents, p. 587)

Dose

- initially 12 mg daily by IV infusion over 4 hours for 5 consecutive days (60 mg total), followed by second course 12 mg daily by IV infusion over 4 hours for 3 consecutive days (36 mg total) after 12 months. Third and fourth courses (same as second course) can be given at 12-month intervals if needed

Adverse effects

- infusion-related reaction (headache, rash, fever, nausea, urticaria, pruritus, insomnia, chills, flushing, fatigue, dyspnoea, taste alteration, chest discomfort, tachycardia, dyspepsia, dizziness, pain)
- flushing, fever, chills, fatigue
- rash, urticaria, pruritus, erythema
- peripheral oedema, tachycardia
- back pain, pain in extremities, arthralgia, muscle weakness, myalgia, muscle spasm
- nausea, diarrhoea, vomiting, abdominal pain, dyspepsia, altered taste
- depression (new or worsened), anxiety, confusion, insomnia
- cough, dyspnoea, oropharyngeal pain, flu-like illness, pneumonitis
- paraesthesia, dizziness, hypoaesthesia, headache
- neutropenia, haemolytic anaemia, pancytopenia, leucopenia
- elevated serum creatinine, haematuria, proteinuria
- infection (nasopharyngitis, urinary tract infection, upper respiratory tract infection, sinusitis, oral herpes, influenza, bronchitis, *Listeria monocytogenes*, cervical infection)
- elevated liver enzymes, liver dysfunction, acute liver failure
- stroke, cervicocephalic arterial dissection
- superficial fungal infections (oral and vaginal candidiasis)
- hyper/hypothyroidism
- autobody development
- immune thrombocytopenic purpura (ITP)
- malignancy (thyroid cancer, breast cancer, basal cell carcinoma)
- (rare) Graves' disease, reactivation of tuberculosis, haemophagocytic lymphohistiocytosis, acute acalculous cholecystitis

Interactions

- not recommended with live or live attenuated vaccines
- 28-day interval should be allowed between stopping interferons or glatiramer acetate and starting therapy

Nursing points/Cautions

- all patients should be carefully screened for history of tuberculosis (TB), hepatitis B and C or active infection and therapy delayed if treatment is required
- FBC (with differential), thyroid function tests, serum creatinine and urinalysis (with cell count) is recommended before starting therapy and then at monthly intervals (thyroid function tests 3-monthly) during therapy and continuing for 4 years after last infusion
- premedication with corticosteroid (1 g methylprednisolone), antihistamine and/or antipyretic is recommended just before infusion on first 3 days of any course
- patient should be observed during and for 2 hours after infusion
- prophylactic oral anti-herpes agent (e.g. 200 mg aciclovir twice daily) should be started on first day of therapy and continued for at least 4 weeks after each course
- immunisation should be up to date and completed at least 6 weeks before starting therapy
- patient's immunity to varicella zoster virus (chicken pox, herpes zoster (shingles)) should be assessed (including serological testing) before starting therapy because the response to the virus may be severe if exposed and unprotected
- female patients should be screened for human papilloma virus (HPV) on a yearly basis
- administer alone
- dilute with 100 mL sodium chloride 0.9% or glucose 5% and administer IV over 4 hours
- caution if used in those with cardiac history as infusion-related reactions can include cardiac symptoms
- caution if used in those who are hepatitis B or C carriers because of increased risk of liver damage due to reactivation of virus
- caution if used in those with pre-existing or ongoing malignancy
- not recommended in those with stable or inactive MS
- contraindicated in those with murine protein hypersensitivity or HIV

Patient teaching and advice

- patient should be advised to carry Patient Wallet Guide during and for 4 years post-therapy in case the person develops a severe infection or autoimmune condition that requires medical treatment
- advise patient not to drive or operate machinery if dizziness occurs
- ensure that patient understands the importance of the blood and urine tests taken before starting and monthly for up to 4 years after stopping treatment
- warn patient that infusion-related reactions commonly occur within 24 hours and that he/she will need to be monitored during and for 2 hours after the infusion. Patient will be given medication before the infusion to try and minimise any reactions
- patient should be instructed regarding avoidance of foods that may increase the risk of *L. monocytogenes* infections (e.g. salads from salad bars, soft and semi-soft cheeses, soft serve ice cream, unpasteurised dairy products, ready-to-eat meals, raw shell fish and seafood)

- advise patient to seek medical advice immediately if any of the following occur:
  - bruising or bleeding that is hard to stop or if skin develops any small, scattered, red, pink or purple spots
  - signs of infection, including fever, chills, aching muscles or joints, swollen glands
  - shortness of breath, cough, wheezing, chest pain or tightness, cough, blood-stained sputum
  - abdominal pain and tenderness, fever, nausea and vomiting
  - nausea, vomiting, abdominal pain, fatigue, anorexia, dark urine, yellow skin or whites of the eyes
  - sudden numbness or weakness of face, arm or leg (especially one side of the body), confusion, difficulty speaking or slurring, loss of balance or coordination, dizziness
  - headache, neck pain
- women of childbearing potential should be advised to use effective contraception during and for 16 weeks after stopping therapy
- see General Patient teaching and advice (p. xxvii)

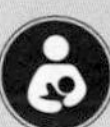

should only be used during pregnancy if benefits outweigh risks

breastfeeding is not recommended during or for 16 weeks after stopping therapy

CLADRIBINE (Leustatin, Litak, Mavenclad)

Available forms

Vial: 10 mg/5 mL, 10 mg/10 mL (Leustatin, Litak); Tablets: 10 mg (Mavenclad)

Action

- antimetabolite (purine nucleoside analogue)
- prodrug

Use

- hairy cell leukaemia, Waldenstrom's macroglobulinaemia (after failure of alkylating agents), B-cell chronic lymphocytic leukaemia (CLL) (after failure of alkylating agents) (Leustatin, Litak) (see Antineoplastic agents p. 617)
- treatment of relapsing remitting multiple sclerosis (MS) to decrease frequency of clinical relapses and delay physical disability progression (Mavenclad)

Dose

- (relapsing remitting MS) 20–30 mg orally daily for 4–5 days (week 1, month 1, year 1), repeated at the start of month 2. Regimen is repeated for year 2 (recommended cumulative dose 3.5 mg/kg over 2 years)

Adverse effects

- infections (nasopharyngitis, upper respiratory tract infection, urinary tract infection, influenza, oral herpes, herpes zoster)
- nausea, diarrhoea
- rash, alopecia
- headache
- lymphopenia, leucopenia
- back pain, arthralgia, pain in extremities
- fatigue, flu-like symptoms
- pharyngolaryngeal pain
- depression, insomnia
- vertigo
- (rare) progressive multifocal leukoencephalopathy (PML), increased risk of malignancies

Interactions

- contraindicated with immunosuppressive or myelosuppressive agents (excepts corticosteroids)
- may increase lymphocyte count reduction if given with beta-interferon
- not recommended within 3 hours of other oral medications
- not recommended with or within 6 weeks of live or live attenuated vaccines

- not recommended with any other multiple sclerosis (MS) modifying treatment
- not recommended with dipyridamole, nifedipine, nimodipine, cilostazol, sulindac or eltrombopag during 4–5 days of cladribine therapy
- caution if given with carbamazepine or NSAIDs due to additive haematological adverse effects
- decreased serum levels may occur if given with corticosteroids, rifampicin or St John's wort

Nursing points/Cautions

- patient should not receive any more than 2 treatment courses over 2 consecutive years
- before starting therapy, patient should be screened for any active tuberculosis, HIV and/or hepatitis B and C and any infection treated
- any active infection should be treated before starting therapy
- patient's immunity to varicella zoster virus (chicken pox, herpes zoster (shingles)) should be assessed (including serological testing) before starting therapy because the response to the virus may be severe if exposed and unprotected. If patient is antibody negative, vaccination is recommended 4–6 weeks before starting therapy
- lymphocyte count should be measured before each course and at 2 and 6 months after each course of treatment. Second course should not be started unless count is at least 800 cells/mm^3. If lymphocyte count does not recover within 6 months, second course of therapy should not be given. Additionally, red blood cell, neutrophil and platelet counts, haemoglobin and haematocrit should also be measured
- if patient is switching from another MS medication that has a risk of progressive multifocal leukoencephalopathy (PML), a baseline magnetic resonance imaging (MRI) is recommended
- pregnancy must be excluded before starting therapy in year 1 and year 2
- if patient requires a blood transfusion, irradiation of cellular blood components is recommended to decrease risk of transfusion-related graft versus host disease
- tablets contain 64 mg sorbitol/tablet and are not recommended in those with fructose intolerance
- not recommended in those over 65 years or under 18 years
- not recommended in patients with active malignancy
- contraindicated in those with HIV infection, active chronic infections (tuberculosis, hepatitis) or who are immunosuppressed (including taking immunosuppressive agents) or with moderate-to-severe kidney impairment

Patient teaching and advice

- instruct patient to swallow tablets whole without chewing. They should be taken at the same time every day and can be taken with or without food
- advise patient to handle tablets with dry hands and wash hands thoroughly after administration
- patient should be instructed to separate cladribine administration from any other oral medications by at least 3 hours
- patient should be advised to conduct regular self-examinations for any new or changing skin lesions, have an annual examination by a dermatologist, seek medical advice if any new or changing skin lesions occur, avoid direct sun exposure and use skin protection (including clothing and sunscreen)

- female patients of childbearing potential should be counselled to use adequate and reliable contraception to prevent pregnancy occurring during and for 6 months after last dose of therapy. If using hormonal contraceptive, an additional barrier method is recommended
- male patients should be counselled to take precautions to avoid pregnancy of their partner occurring during therapy and for at least 6 months after last dose

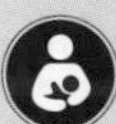
contraindicated during pregnancy or breastfeeding

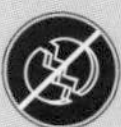
tablets are cytotoxic and must not be broken or crushed

DIMETHYL FUMARATE (Tecfidera)

Available forms
Capsules (enteric-coated): 120 mg, 240 mg

Action
- activates nuclear factor (erythroid-derived 2)-like 2 transcriptional pathway
- anti-inflammatory and immunomodulatory properties reduce release of pro-inflammatory cytokines
- active metabolite (monomethyl fumarate) whose half-life is about 1 hour

Use
- relapsing/remitting MS (to reduce frequency of relapses and delay disease progress)

Dose
- initially 120 mg orally twice daily for 7 days, then increasing to 240 mg orally twice daily

Adverse effects
- flushing, burning sensation, feeling hot
- diarrhoea, nausea, abdominal pain, vomiting, dyspepsia, gastritis
- rash, pruritus, erythema
- gastroenteritis
- lymphopenia, leucopenia
- proteinuria, microalbuminuria, urine albumin present, elevated liver enzymes
- (rare) prolonged lymphopenia, progressive multifocal leukoencephalopathy (PML), anaphylaxis, herpes zoster infections (including disseminated, ophthalmicus, meningoencephalitis, meningomyelitis)

Interactions
- not recommended with live or live attenuated vaccines
- caution if used with nephrotoxic agents such as aminoglycosides, diuretics, NSAIDs and lithium
- not recommended with other topical or systemic fumaric acid derivatives

Nursing points/Cautions
- complete blood count (including lymphocytes) and urinalysis are recommended before starting therapy (within 6 months) and then every 6–12 months
- if lymphocyte count falls below 0.5×10^9/L for more than 6 months, interrupting therapy is recommended
- therapy should be interrupted if severe infection occurs
- dose can be decreased to 120 mg twice daily temporarily if flushing and gastrointestinal adverse effects are severe
- caution if used in those under 18 and over 65 years or if patient has pre-existing low lymphocyte count

Patient teaching and advice
- warn patient that flushing and gastrointestinal adverse effects (nausea, vomiting, diarrhoea, abdominal pain, dyspepsia) are common in first month

and decrease with use. Taking capsules with food may decrease adverse effects

- advise patient that taking 325 mg aspirin before therapy may decrease flushing
- instruct patient to swallow capsules whole and not to crush, divide or dissolve them
- ensure patient understands the importance of completing the urine test before starting therapy and then once per year
- patient should be advised to wear a MedicAlert bracelet outlining the risks of PML
- patient and carer/partner should be advised to immediately report any unusual, worse or prolonged neurological symptoms, including difficulty performing mental tasks, unusual behaviour, confusion or personality changes (may be signs of PML or progression of MS)
- advise patient to seek medical advice immediately if any of the following occur:
    - any signs of infection including fever, chills, swollen glands, feeling unwell
    - skin rash, itching, hives, swelling of lips/throat/tongue, wheezing, difficulty breathing, dizziness, nausea, vomiting, feeling of dread (signs of anaphylaxis)
    - any signs of herpes zoster infection which can vary depending on location but could include headache, one-sided stabbing pain, fever, chills, headache, tingling/burning/itching or stinging sensation before rash appears
- see General Patient teaching and advice (p. xxvii)

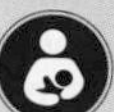

only recommended during pregnancy or breastfeeding if benefits outweigh risks

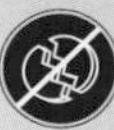

capsules should not be crushed, divided or dissolved

FAMPRIDINE (Fampyra)

Available form

Tablets (modified-release): 10 mg

Action

- non-selective potassium channel blocker that blocks potassium channels in demyelinated nerves, reducing current leakage from axons and restoring neuronal conduction and action potential formation
- readily crosses blood–brain barrier
- elimination half-life about 6 hours

Use

- symptomatic improvement of walking ability in adults with MS

Dose

- 10 mg orally twice daily (12 hours apart)

Adverse effects

- insomnia, anxiety, dizziness, headache, tremor, paraesthesia, asthenia
- pharyngolaryngeal pain
- nausea, vomiting, constipation, dyspepsia
- dyspnoea
- back pain
- balance disorder
- urinary tract infection
- nasopharyngitis
- seizures
- exacerbation of pre-existing trigeminal neuralgia

Interactions

- contraindicated with any form of fampridine/4-aminopyridine
- caution if given with agents which lower seizure threshold
- caution if given with agents which are renally excreted

Nursing points/Cautions

- before starting therapy, patient should be assessed for any history or predisposing factors for seizures or which may lower seizure threshold
- therapy should be re-evaluated after 8 weeks and only continued if walk test shows positive response
- caution if used in those with mild kidney impairment (creatinine clearance 50–80 mL/min) (monitoring renal function regularly is recommended)
- contraindicated in those with moderate-to-severe kidney impairment (creatinine clearance < 50 mL/minute) or history of seizures

Patient teaching and advice

- instruct patient that tablets should be swallowed whole (not broken, crushed or divided)
- advise patient that walking will be assessed after 8 weeks and therapy stopped if no improvement has occurred
- warn patient against driving or operating machinery if dizziness, balance problems or tremor occur
- patient should be advised to immediately report any seizures (fitting)
- see General Patient teaching and advice (p. xxvii)

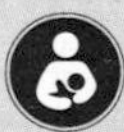

only used during pregnancy if benefits are thought to outweigh risks

not recommended during breastfeeding

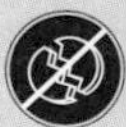

tablets should not be crushed, divided, broken, chewed or dispersed in water

FINGOLIMOD (Gilenya)

Available forms

Capsules: 0.25 mg, 0.5 mg

Action

- sphingosine 1-phosphate receptor modulator that is metabolised to active metabolite fingolimod phosphate
- binds to specific receptors on lymphocytes leading to a redistribution rather than depletion of lymphocytes, reducing the infiltration into the CNS (and associated nerve inflammation and tissue damage)
- readily crosses blood–brain barrier

Use

- relapsing/remitting and secondary progressive MS (to delay disability and/or reduce number of relapses)

Dose

- 0.5 mg orally daily

Adverse effects

- headache, dizziness, migraine, paraesthesia, asthenia
- eczema, alopecia, pruritus, decreased weight
- diarrhoea
- cough, dyspnoea
- infection (influenza, sinusitis, bronchitis, herpes zoster, tinea)
- depression
- eye pain, blurred vision, decreased visual acuity, macular oedema
- back pain
- bradycardia, hypertension
- leucopenia, lymphopenia
- abnormal liver tests, increased liver enzymes, increased triglycerides
- (rare) posterior reversible encephalopathy syndrome (PRES), progressive multifocal leukoencephalopathy (PML), lymphomas, skin cancers, seizures

Interactions

- contraindicated with Class Ia or Class III (amiodarone, sotalol) antiarrhythmic agents
- not recommended with digoxin, ivabradine, calcium-channel blockers (that lower heart rate) or beta-adrenoreceptor blocking agents due to risk of increased bradycardia

- caution if given with antineoplastic or immunosuppressive therapy (including corticosteroids) due to additive effects on immune system
- decreased serum levels may occur if given with carbamazepine
- not recommended with or within 2 months of live or live attenuated vaccines
- not recommended with citalopram, chlorpromazine, haloperidol, methadone or erythromycin due to increased risk of QT prolongation and torsades de pointes
- not recommended with phototherapy with UV-B radiation or PUVA photochemotherapy

Nursing points/Cautions

- patient's immunity to varicella zoster virus (chicken pox, herpes zoster (shingles)) should be assessed (including serological testing) before starting therapy because the response to the virus may be severe if exposed and unprotected
- vaccination against human papilloma virus (HPV) is recommended before starting therapy
- any infection should be excluded or treated before starting therapy
- complete blood count and ophthalmologic examination (including visual acuity and fundus examination) should be performed before starting therapy. Ophthalmologic examination should be repeated after 3–4 months of therapy (especially in those with diabetes mellitus or history of uveitis)
- an ECG is recommended before starting therapy (especially in those with pre-existing slow or irregular heartbeat, cardiac risk factors or taking medications with antiarrhythmic actions)
- (first dose procedure) monitoring heart rate and BP hourly for 6 hours after initial dose is recommended, along with an ECG at the completion of the monitoring time. If post-procedure ECG shows QTc interval prolongation (> 470 msec in female patients, > 450 msec in male patients), patient should be monitored overnight in hospital setting
- after 6 hours, extra observation is required if patient's heart rate < 45 beats/minutes or if ECG shows any new onset second degree or higher AV block
- first dose procedure (as above) will need to be repeated if therapy is discontinued or interrupted for:
  - more than 2 weeks after first 4 weeks, or
  - 1 day or more in first 2 weeks, or
  - 7 days during weeks 3 and 4
- because of very long half-life, patient should be monitored for adverse effects (such as infection) for up to 8 weeks after stopping therapy
- if switching from other immunomodifying agents, half-life and mode of action should be considered before starting therapy to avoid additive immunosuppression
- can be started immediately after interferons, glatiramer acetate or dimethyl fumerate are stopped
- not recommended after alemtuzumab
- allow interval of 2–3 months after natalizumab
- accelerated elimination of teriflunomide is recommended (see p. 1323)
- if therapy is discontinued, patient should be closely monitored as severe exacerbation of disease may occur within 12 weeks of stopping
- caution if used in those > 65 years or < 10 years
- caution if used in those with history of uveitis or diabetes mellitus due to increased risk of macular oedema
- caution if used in those with history of recurrent syncope or symptomatic bradycardia or QT prolongation (QTc > 470 msec (females), > 450 msec

(males)) (cardiology advice is recommended before starting therapy)
- caution if used in those with severe liver disease
- not recommended in those with risk factors for QT prolongation, such as hypokalaemia, hypomagnesaemia or congenital QT prolongation
- not recommended in patient with ischaemic heart disease, history of myocardial infarction or cardiac arrest, congestive heart failure, uncontrolled hypertension, cerebrovascular disease or untreated sleep apnoea
- contraindicated in those with SA block, second degree AV block or higher, sick sinus syndrome (unless patient has pacemaker) or with QTc interval prolongation (≥ 500 msec)
- contraindicated in those who, in the last 6 months, have experienced myocardial infarction, unstable angina, stroke, transient ischaemic attacks (TIAs), decompensated heart failure or Class III/IV heart failure requiring hospitalisation

Patient teaching and advice

- patient should be advised after first dose procedure involving hourly heart rate and blood pressure monitoring for 6 hours with ECG at the end. This will need to be repeated if there is a break in therapy for any length of time
- warn patient that heart rate may slow down during therapy
- patient should be advised not to drive or operate machinery if dizziness or visual disturbances occur
- caution patient to avoid exposure to sunlight without protection and have regular skin examinations during therapy
- advise patient to seek medical advice immediately if any of the following occur:
  - changes to vision (e.g. centre of vision is blurry or has shadows, blindspot, difficulty seeing colour or fine details), especially in first 4 months of therapy
  - nausea, vomiting, abdominal pain, fatigue, loss of appetite, yellowing of skin or eyes, dark urine
  - sudden severe headache, nausea, vomiting, visual disturbances, fitting or altered mental state
  - any signs of infections including flu-like symptoms, fever, chills, sore throat, joint or aching muscles, cough (up to 8 weeks after stopping therapy)
  - any new or changed skin lesions
- patient and carer/partner should be advised to immediately report any unusual, worse or prolonged neurological symptoms, including difficulty performing mental tasks, unusual behaviour, confusion or personality changes (may be signs of PML or progression of MS)
- female patients of childbearing potential should be counselled to use effective contraception during and for at least 8 weeks after stopping therapy. If pregnancy occurs patient should be advised to immediately seek medical advice. If patient plans to become pregnant, therapy should be stopped for at least 8 weeks before conception
- see General Patient teaching and advice (p. xxvii)

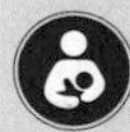

not recommended during pregnancy or breastfeeding

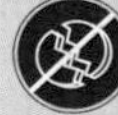

teratogenic, therefore should not be opened by pregnant staff. If no option exists, capsule can be opened and dispersed in water, but gloves and mask must be worn

GLATIRAMER ACETATE (Copaxone Prefilled Syringe)

Available forms

Prefilled syringe: 20 mg/mL, 40 mg/mL

Action

- immunomodulator thought to modify the immune process responsible for pathogenesis of MS

Use

- relapsing/remitting MS (to reduce frequency of relapses and delay progression)
- treatment of patients with single clinical event and at least 2 silent brain lesions (confirmed on MRI) suggestive of MS

Dose

- 20 mg SC daily **OR**
- 40 mg SC 3 times weekly

Adverse effects

- mild injection site reactions (erythema, pain, inflammation, pruritus, oedema, mass)
- (post-injection reaction) flushing, chest pain, palpitations, anxiety, dyspnoea, throat constriction, urticaria
- vasodilation
- tachycardia, palpitations, transient chest pain, hypertension
- visual field defects, diplopia
- infection (influenza, rhinitis, bronchitis, gastroenteritis, vaginal or oral candidiasis, herpes zoster)
- back pain
- syncope
- nausea, vomiting, dysphagia, increase in weight, enlarged salivary glands, tooth caries, bowel urgency, ulcerative stomatitis
- anxiety, tremor, asthenia, nervousness, migraine, abnormal dreams, emotional lability, stupor
- dyspnoea, cough, hyperventilation
- fever, chills
- pruritus, urticaria, rash, sweating, eczema
- lymphadenopathy
- peripheral oedema, facial oedema
- urinary urgency, impotence
- menorrhagia, amenorrhoea, haematuria, vaginal haemorrhage
- autobody development
- skin neoplasm (benign)
- (rare) hypersensitivity, seizures, allergic reactions
- (injection site, rare) lipoatrophy, necrosis

Nursing points/Cautions

- should not be given IV or IM
- should only be discontinued under medical supervision
- caution if used in those with a history of asthma, previous anaphylactoid reaction or kidney impairment
- contraindicated in those with known hypersensitivity to mannitol

Patient teaching and advice

- instruct patient/family member/carer in correct administration, including:
  - remove prefilled syringe from refrigerator 20 minutes before injection and allow to come to room temperature before use (this reduces pain)
  - wash hands before administration
  - check prefilled syringe for any signs of particles or cloudiness (and do not use if these are present) and expiry date
  - the importance of rotating administration sites (abdomen (avoiding area 5 cm around navel), thighs (front, avoiding area 5 cm above knees and below groin), arms (fleshy area at back) and upper hips (below waist area)), and do not use the same site more than once per week
  - injection technique into fatty layer under skin (not into muscle); hold syringe in dominant hand, similar to holding a pencil; pinch skin between thumb and index finger (about 5 cm fold); insert needle and release skin fold; inject medication by pushing plunger down until none remains; pull syringe straight out; using a cotton wad, press down on injection site but do not massage

  - (40 mg/mL) given 3 times per week with at least 48 hours between injections
  - dispose of used syringe in appropriate container, such as a hard-walled detergent container that has a lid and can be stored out of reach of children; when full, seek advice from doctor or pharmacist regarding correct disposal
  - prefilled syringes should only be used once
  - unused syringes should be stored in fridge, but not frozen
- advise patient that post-injection reaction (reddening of face and/or neck, chest tightness, rapid heartbeat, anxiety and/or difficulty breathing) is transient, will pass quickly, generally does not require treatment and usually occurs several months after start of therapy
- see General Patient teaching and advice (p. xxvii)

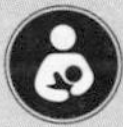

should only be used during pregnancy or breastfeeding if benefits outweigh potential risks

NATALIZUMAB (Tysabri)

Available form
Ampoules: 300 mg/15 mL

Action
- IgG4 humanised monoclonal antibody that binds to alpha-4 integrin found on leucocyte (except neutrophil) cell surface, preventing migration of leucocytes into inflamed parenchymal tissue

Use
- relapsing/remitting MS (to reduce frequency of relapses and delay progression)

Dose
- 300 mg by IV infusion over 1 hour every 4 weeks

Adverse effects
- headache, fatigue, depression, somnolence, vertigo, dizziness
- arthralgia, muscle cramp, joint swelling, pain in extremities
- rigors, fever
- diarrhoea, abdominal pain/discomfort, nausea, vomiting, weight increase or decrease
- rash, dermatitis, pruritus, night sweating, urticaria
- irregular menstruation, dysmenorrhoea, amenorrhoea, ovarian cyst
- chest discomfort
- infection (urinary tract infection, lower respiratory tract infection, tonsillitis, gastroenteritis, vaginitis, tooth infection, herpes encephalitis, herpes meningitis, acute retinal necrosis)
- development of antibodies (transient or persistent)
- increased liver enzymes, elevated bilirubin, liver injury
- nasopharyngitis
- infusion-related reaction (headache, dizziness, fatigue, rigors, localised or generalised hypersensitivity reaction)
- progressive multifocal leucoencephalopathy (PML) (an opportunistic viral brain infection which may lead to death or disability), immune reconstitution inflammatory syndrome (IRIS) if therapy is stopped due to PML, John Cunningham virus (JCV) granule cell neuronopathy

Interactions
- contraindicated with beta interferons, glatiramer acetate or other antineoplastic or immunosuppressive agents because of the increased risk of opportunistic infection and progressive multifocal leukoencephalopathy (PML)

Nursing points/Cautions

- therapy should be started in centre with MRI facilities and under the supervision of neurologist
- antibody testing for JCV (John Cunningham virus) is recommended before starting therapy (using JCV antibody assay) and repeated 6-monthly in negative patients or in positive patients with lower index values
- a recent (within 3 months) MRI scan is required before starting therapy, and then repeated yearly. The scan would assist in differentiating between PML symptoms and MS. More frequent MRI is recommended in those at higher risk of PML (i.e. having all 3 risk factors; having anti-JVC antibody index > 1.5 without prior immunosuppression and > 2 years on therapy)
- therapy should be interrupted if PML is suspected. A new MRI scan may be necessary to compare pre- and post-therapy. Other tests include neurological assessment and testing the CSF for JC viral DNA
- therapy must not be resumed if patient has PML or develops an opportunistic infection
- FBC and liver function tests are recommended in those with active or history of liver disease
- natalizumab remains in the blood for up to 12 weeks after last dose
- patient should be re-evaluated by neurologist 3 months after first infusion, 6 months after first infusion and then at 6-month intervals
- testing for persistent antibodies is recommended if patient has had a long interruption (12 weeks or more) to therapy and has had antibodies detected twice, 6 weeks apart. Persistent antibodies are related to a decrease in treatment effectiveness
- if plasma exchange procedure is performed, an interval of 14 days should be allowed before serum anti-JVC antibody testing
- patient should be monitored during and for 1 hour post-infusion for any signs of infusion-related reaction
- dilute in 100 mL sodium chloride 0.9%, invert gently (do not shake) and infuse over 1 hour
- not recommended by IV bolus or IV push
- administer alone
- risk of hypersensitivity is increased early in therapy and if patient is re-exposed to therapy after being stopped (short course e.g. 3 infusions) and long period (over 12 weeks) without treatment
- caution if used in those with liver disease. If used, liver function should be closely monitored during therapy
- contraindicated in those with or who have had PML, with a murine hypersensitivity or at high risk of opportunistic infection, HIV, organ transplant, active malignancy or who are immunocompromised

Patient teaching and advice

- before starting therapy, patients should be advised of the importance of continuing therapy uninterrupted, especially at the start. The neurologist is required to obtain individual, written, fully informed consent from the patient or legal guardian to the use of natalizumab and the possible adverse effects (PML, opportunistic infection)
- warn patient not to drive or operate machinery if dizziness or vertigo occur
- patient should be advised to wear a MedicAlert bracelet and carry a Patient Alert Card outlining the risks of PML
- patient and carer/partner should be advised to seek medical advice immediately if any of the following occur:

  - unusual, worse or prolonged neurological symptoms, including difficulty performing mental tasks, unusual behaviour, confusion, personality changes
  - severe or prolonged symptoms of infection, including prolonged dizziness, unexplained fever, severe diarrhoea, headache, stiff neck, weight loss, listlessness
  - decreased visual acuity, eye redness, painful eye
- see General Patient teaching and advice (p. xxvii)

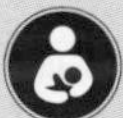

only recommended during pregnancy if benefits outweigh potential risks

caution if used during breastfeeding

OCRELIZUMAB (Ocrevus)

Available form
Vial: 300 mg/10 mL

Action
- recombinant humanised monoclonal antibody
- selectively targets CD-20 expressing B cells reducing their number and function
- terminal half-life 26 days

Use
- treatment of patients with relapsing MS to delay progression of physical disability and reduce frequency of relapses
- treatment of primary progressive MS to delay progression of physical disability

Dose
- 600 mg IV every 6 months, given as:
  - (initial dose) initially, 300 mg IV given at 30 mL/hour, then 2 weeks later, 300 mg IV starting at 30 mL/hour and increasing rate every 30 minutes by 30 mL/hour to a maximum of 180 mL/hour, then
  - (subsequent doses) 600 mg IV starting at 40 mL/hour, then increasing every 30 minutes by 40 mL/hour to a maximum of 200 mL/hour

Adverse effects
- infusion-related reactions
- infections (upper respiratory tract infection, nasopharyngitis, sinusitis, bronchitis, influenza, gastroenteritis, oral herpes, viral infection, herpes zoster, conjunctivitis, cellulitis)
- cough, increased sputum
- neutropenia
- (rare) increased risk of malignancy, progressive multifocal leukoencephalopathy (PML)

Interactions
- not recommended with immunosuppressive agents (except corticosteroids) due to increased risk of serious infections
- not recommended with other disease-modifying multiple sclerosis therapies
- not recommended with live or live attenuated vaccines

Nursing points/Cautions
- any active infection should be treated before starting therapy
- patient should be screened for hepatitis B virus (HBV) as reactivation can occur during therapy. If patient has active HBV, therapy should not be started. If patient has positive serology (negative for hepatitis B surface antigen, positive for HB core antibody and carriers of HBV) patient should consult liver disease expert before starting therapy and monitored closely if therapy occurs
- immunisation should be complete and up to date 6 weeks before starting therapy
- because hypotension can occur as part of infusion-related reactions,

consideration should be given to withholding any antihypertension medication 12 hours before each infusion
- patient should be premedicated with 100 mg IV methylprednisolone (or equivalent) about 30 minutes before infusion, along with antihistamine (given 30–60 minutes before infusion). Antipyretic may also be administered with antihistamine
- not given as IV push or bolus
- initial infusions given over about 2.5 hours, subsequent infusions administered over 3.5 hours
- initial infusions (300 mg) diluted in 250 mL sodium chloride 0.9% and subsequent infusions (600 mg) diluted in 500 mL sodium chloride 0.9%
- observe patient for at least 1 hour after infusion is completed for any symptoms of infusion-related reactions (which can occur within 24 hours of infusion but more commonly during first infusion):
    - if life-threatening (e.g. bronchospasm, asthma exacerbation) reaction occurs, infusion should be stopped and patient treated using supportive therapies. Therapy should be discontinued permanently
    - if serious reaction (e.g. flushing, fever, throat pain) occurs, infusion should be stopped and patient receive symptomatic treatment. Infusion can be restarted when symptoms have totally resolved at a rate half the infusion rate when the reaction occurred
    - if mild-to-moderate reaction (e.g. headache) occurs, infusion rate should be reduced to half that at onset of symptom and this rate maintained for at least 30 minutes. If tolerated, infusion rate can be increased according to patient's original infusion schedule

Patient teaching and advice

- patient should be warned that infusion-related reactions (e.g. rash, pruritus, flushing, throat irritation, oropharyngeal pain, shortness of breath, flushing, fever, fatigue, dizziness, headache) can occur within 24 hours of infusion and patient should seek medical attention immediately if any reaction occurs
- patient and carer/partner should be advised to seek medical advice immediately if any of the following occur:
    - unusual, worse or prolonged neurological symptoms, including difficulty performing mental tasks, unusual behaviour, confusion, personality changes (signs of PML or worsening MS)
    - any signs of infection including fever, chills, swollen glands, fatigue
- women of childbearing potential should be counselled to use effective contraception during therapy and for 6 months after last infusion

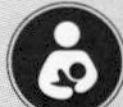

not recommended during pregnancy unless benefits outweigh risks

breastfeeding should be discontinued during therapy

TERIFLUNOMIDE (Aubagio, Teriflagio, Terimide)

Available form

Tablets: 14 mg

Action

- immunomodulator that selectively and reversibly inhibits dihydroorotate dehydrogenase needed for pyrimidine synthesis, thereby blocking the activation and proliferation of stimulated lymphocytes. This is thought to reduce the number of activated

lymphocytes which can migrate into the CNS
- long terminal half-life (about 19 days)

Use
- relapsing/remitting MS (to reduce frequency of relapses and delay progression)

Dose
- 14 mg orally daily

Adverse effects
- nausea, vomiting, diarrhoea, upper abdominal pain, toothache
- paraesthesia
- palpitations, hypertension
- alopecia, rash
- musculoskeletal pain, myalgia, arthralgia
- menorrhagia
- elevated liver enzymes, elevated creatine phosphokinase
- neutropenia
- influenza, sinusitis
- (rare) severe liver injury, thrombocytopenia, interstitial lung disease, peripheral neuropathy, pancreatitis, severe skin reactions, hypersensitivity

Interactions
- caution if switching from one immunomodifying agent to another as added haemotoxicity may occur
- not recommended with or within 6 months of live or live attenuated vaccines
- serum levels may be reduced if given with carbamazepine, phenobarbital (phenobarbitone), rifampicin, phenytoin and St John's wort and should therefore be given with caution
- may increase serum levels of paclitaxel, pioglitazone, repaglinide, rosiglitazone, rosuvastatin, methotrexate, topotecan, sulfasalazine, daunorubicin, doxorubicin, atorvastatin, simvastatin, pravastatin, rifampicin
- caution if used with cefaclor, penicillin G, ciprofloxacin, indomethacin, ketoprofen, furosemide (frusemide), cimetidine, methotrexate and zidovudine
- may decrease serum levels of caffeine, duloxetine, ondansetron, theophylline and agomelatine
- may decrease INR if given with warfarin, therefore careful monitoring is recommended
- caution if given with NSAIDs due to added hepatotoxicity

Nursing points/Cautions

- FBC (including differential WBC count and platelets) and liver function tests (ALT, AST and bilirubin) should be measured before starting therapy, then monthly for 6 months, then 6–8-weekly if stable
- if liver enzyme levels are more than 3 times normal, therapy should be stopped and colestyramine or activated charcoal administered to reduce levels rapidly. If levels are mildly or moderately elevated 2–4-weekly monitoring is recommended
- blood pressure should be measured before starting therapy and then regularly during therapy
- all patients should be carefully screened for history or symptoms of acute or chronic infection (including pneumonia, urinary tract infection), tuberculosis (TB) or hepatitis, including detailed medical history, possible previous exposure to TB. Before starting therapy, any infection should be treated
- if switching from another MS medication to teriflunomide, the following are recommended:
  - interferon beta or glatiramer acetate: no waiting period is required
  - fingolimod: 6-week interval should be allowed between discontinuing fingolimod for clearance and 4–8 weeks for lymphocyte recovery before starting teriflunomide
  - natalizumab: caution if switching as natalizumab has a very long half-life and will cause added

effects on the immune system for 2–3 months if natalizumab is discontinued and teriflunomide started immediately

- pregnancy must be excluded before starting therapy. Therapy should only be started if effective contraception is being used in females of child-bearing potential
- (accelerated elimination procedure) if rapid elimination is required, an 11-day program of either colestyramine (4 g 3 times a day or 8 g 3 times a day) or activated charcoal (50 g twice daily) is recommended, with colestyramine being faster to reduce levels. Choice between the three procedures is dependent on patient tolerability. The 11 days do not need to be consecutive unless rapid elimination is needed. Plasma levels should be measured and verified on two separate tests 14 days apart and be ≤ 0.02 mg/L to reduce risk
- caution if used in those with history of interstitial lung disease or kidney impairment
- not recommended in those under 18 or over 65 years
- contraindicated in those with hypersensitivity to leflunomide
- contraindicated in those with severe immunodeficiency (e.g. AIDS), significant bone marrow impairment, significant anaemia, leucopenia or thrombocytopenia, severe uncontrolled infections, severe hypoproteinaemia or severe liver function impairment
- contraindicated in those who have (or have had) Stevens–Johnson syndrome, toxic epidermal necrolysis or erythema multiforme

Patient teaching and advice

- patient should be advised to seek medical advice immediately if any of the following occur:
  - unexplained nausea and vomiting, abdominal pain, fatigue, loss of appetite, yellowing of eyes or skin, dark urine
  - any signs of infection including unexplained fever, chills, aching muscles or joints, cough
  - any skin or mucosal reactions
  - bilateral numbness or tingling of hands or feet
  - cough, shortness of breath, with/without fever
- warn patient that if accelerated elimination procedure is used, disease activity may potentially return
- women of childbearing potential should be counselled to use effective contraception during therapy and notify doctor immediately if pregnancy is suspected. If pregnancy occurs, accelerated elimination procedure should be performed to lower plasma levels to ≤ 0.02 mg/L

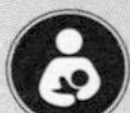
contraindicated during pregnancy or those attempting to become pregnant and breastfeeding

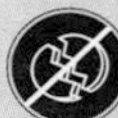
tablets should not be crushed by pregnant staff. If crushing tablet, gloves and eye protection must be worn and closed pill crusher used

INTERFERONS

General Actions of interferons

- naturally occurring, small protein molecules produced and secreted by cells in response to viral infections or to various synthetic and biological inducers

- bind to specific cell surface receptors that are linked to inner cell networks that control enzyme activity, cell proliferation and immune activity enhancement (e.g. inhibit viral replication in virus-infected cells; enhance activity of macrophages and lymphocytes)
- three main forms: interferons alpha and beta (type I) and interferon gamma (type II)
- produced by recombinant DNA technology

General Adverse effects of interferons

- flu-like symptoms (including fever, malaise, chills, sweating, fatigue, myalgia, loss of appetite, headache)
- malaise, fatigue, asthenia, insomnia, dizziness, depression, confusion, vertigo
- fever, chills
- headache, migraine
- nausea, vomiting, anorexia, diarrhoea, abdominal pain, constipation, weight change
- sinusitis, dyspnoea, rhinitis, cough, upper respiratory tract infection, bronchitis, nasopharyngitis
- anaemia, leucopenia, thrombocytopenia, neutropenia
- elevated liver enzymes, hypertriglyceridaemia
- transient mild skin rash, reversible alopecia, sweating/flushing
- arthralgia, myalgia, back pain, musculoskeletal weakness, pain and/or stiffness, pain in extremities, muscle spasm
- palpitations, chest pain, oedema
- menorrhagia, metrorrhagia
- cystitis, urinary frequency, urinary tract infection
- (uncommon) serum neutralising antibodies
- (rare) hypersensitivity reaction (including bronchospasm, urticaria, anaphylaxis, angioedema), suicidal ideation, liver injury, seizures, thyroid dysfunction, nephrotic syndrome, thrombotic microangiopathy (thrombotic thrombocytopenia purpura, haemolytic anaemia)
- (injection site) pain, swelling, redness, pruritus, haematoma
- (rare) injection site necrosis

General Interactions of interferons

- caution if given with agents with narrow therapeutic index
- caution if given with other myelosuppressive agent
- caution if used with other agents that are hepatotoxic including alcohol
- not recommended with other immunomodifying agents

General Nursing points/Cautions for interferons

- treatment should be started and supervised by neurologist experienced in management of MS
- monitor blood cell counts (with WBC differential, platelet count), thyroid and liver function before starting therapy, then at monthly or appropriate intervals during treatment
- paracetamol 0.5–1 g can be taken orally 30 minutes before administration of interferon to alleviate symptoms of fever and headache, then up to 1 g 4 times daily
- chest X-ray is recommended if patient develops cough, dyspnoea or other respiratory symptoms
- any persistent fever should be investigated thoroughly

- all patients should be monitored for any signs of depression or suicidal ideation
- patient should be monitored for any signs of nephrotic syndrome, including proteinuria, oedema and changes in kidney function
- if patient develops seizures, therapy should be stopped and aetiology of seizures established
- at the discretion of the doctor, patient may be educated to self-administer medication
- first self-administered injection should be done under supervision
- when reconstituting solution, care should be taken to avoid foaming or shaking the solution when dissolving
- administer alone
- caution if used in those with severe bone marrow suppression due to increased risk of infection and/or bleeding
- caution if used in those with history of seizures (especially if not well controlled), history of liver disease or active liver disease
- caution if used in those with kidney impairment (kidney function should be monitored regularly)
- caution if used in those with cardiac disorders such as angina, congestive cardiac failure or arrhythmias (cardiac function should be closely monitored)
- contraindicated in those with severe depression and/or suicidal ideation
- contraindicated in those with hypersensitivity to interferons (natural or recombinant), autoimmune disease

General Patient teaching and advice for interferons

- patients should be advised not to drive or operate machinery if adverse effects such as dizziness, confusion, somnolence, visual disturbance or fatigue occur
- advise patient that flu-like syndrome usually occur within hours to days of injection
- patient should be advised to report any skin breaks, swelling, pain, fluid drainage or multiple sores at the injection sites as this may require a temporary stopping of therapy until the skin heals. Therapy may continue if single sore exists and skin cell death (necrosis) is small
- instruct patient/family member/carer in correct administration, including:
  - self-administration instructions including importance of aseptic technique
  - ensure patient/family member/carer is clear about the route (SC or IM)
  - importance of rotation of SC injection sites (abdomen, thigh, upper outer arm) and not using areas that show any signs of redness, scarring
  - if vial of powder and diluent (water for injections) are required to be mixed, this must be done carefully and according to instructions, especially not shaking the solution to mix it
  - not mixing anything else in the same syringe with the interferon
- advise patient to seek medical advice immediately if any of the following occur:
  - nausea, vomiting, abdominal pain, itchiness, yellowing of eyes or skin, dark urine
  - feelings of sadness, anxiety, nervousness or hopelessness, getting

upset easily, or having thoughts of hurting yourself or suicide
- skin reactions, including any swelling or drainage at injection site
- swelling of feet or legs, shortness of breath, irregular heartbeat
- signs of frequent infections such as fever, sore throat, unusual bleeding or bruising

- women of childbearing potential should be counselled to use adequate and effective contraception to avoid pregnancy during therapy
- see General Patient teaching and advice (p. xxvii)

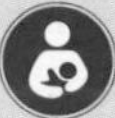

contraindicated during pregnancy

not recommended during breastfeeding

INTERFERON BETA 1A (Avonex, Rebif)

Available forms

Prefilled syringe: 44 microgram (12 million IU)/0.5 mL; 30 microgram (6 million IU)/0.5 mL; Prefilled syringe with autoinjector: 44 microgram (12 million IU)/0.5 mL Multi-dose cartridge: 132 microgram (36 million IU)/1.5 mL

Action

- interferon beta-1A
- see General Actions of interferons (p. 1325)

Use

- relapsing/remitting MS
- single demyelinating event at risk of progression to clinical MS (based on MRI)
- secondary progressive MS with continuous relapse or relapse in last 12 months

Dose

- (relapsing/remitting MS, single demyelinating event) initially 1.5 million (7.5 microgram) IU IM weekly (week 1), then 3.0 million (15 microgram) IU IM (week 2), 4.5 million (22.5 microgram) IU IM (week 3), then 6 million (30 microgram) IU IM (week 4) and thereafter (Avonex) **OR**
- (secondary progressive MS with recent or continuing relapse) 12 million (60 microgram) IU IM weekly (Avonex) **OR**
- (relapsing/remitting MS, single demyelinating event) 12 million IU (44 microgram) SC 3 times weekly (dose may be reduced to 6 million IU (22 microgram) if patient does not tolerate higher dose) (Rebif)

Adverse effects/Interactions

- see General Adverse effects and Interactions of interferons (p. 1326)

Nursing points/Cautions

- see General Nursing points/Cautions for interferons (p. 1326)
- (secondary progressive MS) not recommended unless relapse is continuous or has occurred in last 12 months
- (Rebif) dose should be started at 20% of final dose for weeks 1–2, 50% for weeks 3–4 and full dose from week 5 to avoid anaphylaxis
- (Avonex) not recommended SC
- not recommended in those under 12 or over 65 years
- contraindicated in those with hypersensitivity to any interferon beta (natural or recombinant) or albumin

Patient teaching and advice

- see General Patient teaching and advice for interferons (p. 1327), along with some extra information regarding the specific injection devices:
- allow pen/syringes to come to room temperature for at least 30 minutes before administration to reduce pain
- Rebif available as prefilled syringe or RebiDose (a single-use pre-assembled autoinjector)

- Rebif multi-dose cartridge (RebiSmart) is used with a reusable autoinjecting device and should be discarded after 3 weeks, even if solution remains
- Avonex is available either as a prefilled syringe with needle that needs to be attached before administration IM (either thigh or arm)

INTERFERON BETA 1B (Betaferon)

Available form

Vial: 8 million IU (0.3 mg)

Action

- interferon beta 1b
- see General Actions of interferons (p. 1325)

Use

- treatment of single event suggestive of MS (with 2 lesions proven on magnetic resonance imaging (MRI))
- relapsing/remitting MS (2 attacks in 2 years with recovery intervals)
- reduction in frequency and severity of relapses in those with secondary progressive MS

Dose

- (single event suggestive of MS) initially 2 million IU SC every second day for 3 doses (days 1, 3, 5), 4 million IU SC for 3 doses (days 7, 9, 11), 6 million IU SC for 3 doses (days 13, 15, 17) then 8 million IU every second day **OR**
- (relapsing MS, secondary progressive MS) 8 million IU SC every second day

Adverse effects

- see General Adverse effects of interferons (p. 1326)
- hypertension
- dysmenorrhoea, intermenstrual bleeding
- conjunctivitis, abnormal vision
- (rare) systemic capillary leak syndrome (with shock-like symptoms and fatal outcomes), pancreatitis

Interactions

- see General Interactions of interferons (p. 1326)

Nursing points/Cautions

- see General Nursing points/Cautions for interferons (p. 1326)
- to reconstitute, connect vial adapter to vial with attached needle, then connect prefilled syringe containing diluent and inject 1.2 mL into vial and dissolve powder gently without shaking. Resultant solution should be clear to light yellow. Withdraw 1 mL of reconstituted solution
- contains human plasma, therefore theoretical risk exists for transmission of Creutzfeldt-Jakob disease (CJD) and viral diseases
- caution if used in those with preexisting monoclonal gammopathy due to the increased risk of systemic capillary leak syndrome
- not recommended in those under 18 years
- contraindicated in those with hypersensitivity to any interferon (natural or recombinant), mannitol or albumin

Patient teaching and advice

- see General Patient teaching and advice for interferons (p. 1327) with modification to syringe preparation for SC administration

PEGINTERFERON BETA-1a (Plegridy)

Available form

Prefilled pen: 63 microgram/0.5 mL, 94 microgram/0.5 mL, 125 microgram/0.5 mL

Action

- combination (termed pegylated) of recombinant interferon beta-1a and mono methoxy polyethylene glycol (PEG reagent)
- prolonged half-life compared to nonpegylated interferon beta-1a

Use

- treatment of remitting/relapsing MS

Dose

- initially 63 microgram SC, then 94 microgram SC 2 weeks later, followed by 125 microgram SC after a further 2 weeks, then continued at 125 microgram SC every 2 weeks

Adverse effects/Interactions

- see General Adverse effects and Interactions of interferons (p. 1326)

Nursing points/Cautions

- see General Nursing points/Cautions for interferons (p. 1326)
- contraindicated in those with hypersensitivity to natural or recombinant interferon beta or peginterferon

Patient teaching and advice

- see General Patient teaching and advice for interferons (p. 1327)

MOTOR NEURONE DISEASE (MND)

Motor neurone disease is known as amyotrophic lateral sclerosis in some parts of the world and Lou Gehrig disease in the United States. In Australia, it is estimated that there are currently about 2174 people living with MND (MND Australia n.d.).

Although the onset of MND may only involve loss of upper or lower motor neurone function, it eventually progresses to involve both. Clinical manifestations include asymmetric weakness (usually distal in one limb), cramping (especially in early hours of the morning while stretching in bed), weakness with progressive muscle wasting and atrophy and twitching/fasciculation. If facial muscles are involved, problems chewing and swallowing are experienced, along with movement issues of the tongue and face (Brown 2019). No one muscle group is known to be the first one to show signs; however, with time, as the disease progresses, more muscle groups become involved until there is a symmetrical distribution with both upper and lower motor neurone involvement. Unfortunately, the disease is relentlessly progressive ending in death due to respiratory paralysis with a 3–5-year median survival time from diagnosis (Brown 2019). The cause of MND is unknown with a small number of cases being inherited. Currently, there is no treatment for MND that prevents the disease's progress with only one drug available that lengthens survival time (Brown 2019).

RILUZOLE (Rilutek, Teglutik)

Available forms

Tablets: 50 mg; Oral suspension: 5mg/mL

Action

- glutamate antagonist (hypothesis suggests that vulnerable motor neurones are injured by glutamate)
- inactivates voltage-dependent sodium channels and impairs glutamatergic neurotransmission
- crosses blood–brain barrier
- decreases cerebral glucose metabolism
- neuroprotective
- myorelaxant, sedative and antiepileptic properties at high doses
- elimination half-life is approximately 9–15 hours

Use
- MND (amyotrophic lateral sclerosis)

Dose
- 50 mg orally twice daily

Adverse effects
- anorexia, nausea, abdominal pain, vomiting, flatulence, constipation, diarrhoea, dysphagia, dry mouth, dyspepsia, weight loss
- asthenia, pain, back pain, stiffness, arthralgia, myalgia
- increased or abnormal liver enzymes (ALT, AST)
- headache, dizziness, somnolence, insomnia, paraesthesia, nervousness, anxiety
- decreased lung function, apnoea, rhinitis, increased sputum, aspiration pneumonia, cough, dyspnoea
- tachycardia, peripheral oedema, hypertension
- infection (bronchitis, pneumonia, pharyngitis)
- eczema, pruritus, sweating
- urinary frequency
- (rare) neutropenia, interstitial lung disease

Interactions
- absorption decreased by fat-containing meals
- increased serum levels may occur if given with quinolone antibacterial agents, diazepam, diclofenac, caffeine, clomipramine, imipramine, fluvoxamine, theophylline and amitryptyline
- decreased serum levels may occur if given with rifampicin, omeprazole, and cigarette smoking

Nursing points/Cautions

- serum transaminases should be measured before starting therapy, monthly for 3 months, then 3-monthly for the first year and regularly thereafter
- chest X-ray is recommended if patient develops dry cough and/or dyspnoea
- (oral suspension) contains sorbitol which may have laxative effect or cause diarrhoea in some people and is not recommended in those with rare hereditary problems of fructose intolerance
- caution if given to those with kidney dysfunction, abnormal liver function or neutropenia
- contraindicated in those with liver disease/impairment (transaminase level three times greater than normal)

Patient teaching and advice

- instruct patient to swallow tablet whole
- patient should be advised not to take medication with meals containing fat, because this will reduce absorption
- patient should be instructed in correct administration of oral suspension, including:
  - shake bottle gently for at least 30 seconds before use
  - after opening bottle, insert syringe into bottle neck adapter and turn bottle upside down
  - pull plunger down slightly to allow suspension to enter syringe, then push plunger upward again to remove any air bubbles
  - pull plunger down to the graduation mark that corresponds with prescribed dose
  - turn bottle upright and remove syringe
  - administer suspension direction into mouth (no dilution is needed)
  - recap bottle
  - take syringe apart and wash barrel and plunger separately with water and allow to air dry
  - discard oral suspension 15 days after opening (bottle should be dated on opening)
  - store in cool place below 25°C

- advise patient to seek medical advice immediately if any of the following occur:
  - frequent infections, including fever, chills, mouth ulcers and sore throat
  - dry cough, shortness of breath, difficulty breathing
  - irregular or rapid heart rate
  - swelling of feet, legs or hands
  - itchy or yellow skin, yellow whites of the eyes, severe abdominal pain, nausea and vomiting, fatigue
- warn patient against driving or operating machinery if dizziness, vertigo or somnolence occurs
- female patients of childbearing potential should be counselled to use adequate contraception during therapy to avoid pregnancy occurring
- see General Patient teaching and advice (p. xxvii)

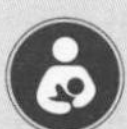

contraindicated during pregnancy and breastfeeding

oral suspension is available. Tablet can be crushed and mixed with spoonful of yoghurt or apple puree

CANNABIDIOL, TETRAHYDROCANNABINOL, NABIXIMOLS (Sativex)

Available form

Oromucosal spray

Action

- there are at least two types of cannabinoid (CB) receptors in the brain, with CB1 found mainly in nerve terminals in the CNS where it modulates neurotransmitter release. CB2 are found mainly in cells within the immune system
- tetrahydrocannabinol (THC) is the main psychotropic constituent of cannabis and acts as a partial agonist at both CB1 and CB2 receptors
- in animal models of multiple sclerosis (MS), CB receptor agonists have been shown to improve both limb stiffness and motor function
- cannabidiol (CBD) has little activity at CB receptors but has neuroprotective properties thought to be due to an ability to modulate intracellular calcium, as well as inhibiting microglial activity and T-cell proliferation

Use

- symptom improvement in patients with moderate-to-severe spasticity due to multiple sclerosis (MS) who have not responded adequately to other anti-spasticity medication and who have shown clinical improvement in spasticity-related symptoms during initial trial

Dose

- (titration period) initially 1 spray in the evening (days 1 and 2), then 2 sprays in the evening (days 3 and 4), then 1 spray in the morning and 2 sprays in the evening (day 5), then 1 spray in the morning and 3 sprays in the evening (day 6), then 1 spray in the morning and 4 sprays in the evening (day 7), then 2 sprays in the morning and 4 sprays in the evening (day 8), then 2 sprays in the morning and 5 sprays in the evening (day 9), then 3 sprays in the morning and 5 sprays in the evening (day 10), then 3 sprays in the morning and 6 sprays in the evening (day 11), then 4 sprays in the morning and 6 sprays in the evening (day 12), then 4 sprays in the morning and 7 sprays in the evening (day 13) and then 5 sprays in the morning and 7 sprays in the evening (day 14)

Adverse effects

- mild-to-moderate dizziness, disorientation, euphoric mood, dissociation, insomnia
- tachycardia, hypertension
- vertigo, dizziness, somnolence, headache, disturbed attention, lethargy, memory impairment, amnesia, tremor, paraesthesia
- blurred vision
- nausea, dry mouth, diarrhoea, vomiting, constipation, dyspepsia, abdominal pain, altered taste, anorexia or increased appetite
- fatigue, asthenia, feeling drunk or abnormal, pain, malaise
- infections (urinary tract, nasopharyngitis, pharyngitis, viral, respiratory tract)
- muscle spasm, back pain, pain in extremities, muscle weakness, arthralgia, balance disorder
- cough, pharyngolaryngeal pain
- (application site) stinging, pain, discomfort, altered taste, mouth ulceration, glossodynia
- (high doses) psychosis, hallucinations, delusions, homicidal and suicidal ideation

Interactions

- may reduce effectiveness of hormonal contraceptive
- may increase metabolism of warfarin, statins, beta-adrenergic blocking agents, and corticosteroids
- caution if itraconazole, ritonavir or clarithromycin is started or stopped with therapy
- decreased serum levels may occur if given with rifampicin, carbamazepine, phenytoin, phenobarbital or St John's wort
- caution if used with hypnotics, sedatives or other agents with sedating properties as increased sedation may occur
- caution if used with alcohol as coordination, concentration and reflexes may all be affected

Nursing points/Cautions

- patient should be assessed by neurologist or rehabilitation physician for suitability. Patient should then be reassessed after 4 weeks of therapy for clinical improvement (defined as 20% improvement in spasticity-related symptoms on a 0–10 patient reported numeric rating scale). If there is no significant clinical improvement, therapy should be discontinued
- therapy should be given in addition to patient's current anti-spasticity medication
- if adverse effects occur, depending on their seriousness or intensity, dose may be continued, dose may be reduced or interrupted temporarily
- a titration period is required to achieve the optimal dose (number and timing of sprays will vary between patients). Caution during titration as there may be alterations in pulse rate or blood pressure
- afternoon/evening dose can be given any time between 4 pm and bedtime. Morning dose can be taken any time between rising and midday
- there should be at least 15 minutes between sprays
- maximum number of consecutive sprays should not exceed 7 within a 3-hour period
- once optimum dose is achieved, patient can spread doses out during the day according to response and tolerance
- dose may require re-titration upwards or downwards if there are any changes in severity of patient's condition
- doses should not exceed 12 sprays in any 24-hour period
- contains 50% v/v ethanol with each spray containing 0.04 g ethanol, therefore caution if used in patients with severe alcohol use disorder

- caution if used in those with moderate-to-severe liver impairment
- caution if used in those with history of epilepsy or recurrent seizures
- caution if used in those with history of depression. If used, patient should be closely monitored and therapy stopped if there is significant worsening of depression
- caution if used in those with history of substance abuse as there is an increased risk of abuse
- caution if used in those > 65 years as there is increased risk of CNS adverse effects
- not recommended in those under 18 years
- not recommended in those with serious cardiovascular disease
- contraindicated in those with hypersensitivity to cannabinoids, known or suspected history or family history of schizophrenia or other psychotic illness, history of severe personality disorder or other significant psychiatric disorder (other than depression associated with MS)

Patient teaching and advice

- advise patient that it might take 2 weeks to find optimal dose
- warn patient that side-effects can occur during this time, especially dizziness, but these are usually mild and resolve within a few days
- patient should be warned not to exceed maximum dose
- advise patient to avoid alcohol during therapy
- caution patient that there is an increased risk of falls when spasticity is reduced if patient has insufficient muscle strength to maintain posture or gait
- advise patient not to drive, operate machinery or participate in activities that are potentially dangerous (e.g. cooking, handling hot foods or liquids) if adverse effects such as dizziness, vertigo, blurred vision or disorientation occur
- patient should be instructed in use of spray, including:
  - prime container before first use and if not used for 21 days shake container gently, removing cap and pressing actuator 2–3 times into a tissue until a fine spray appears
  - (after first use) shake container gently before use and direct spray at different sites on oromucosal surface changing site each time product is used
  - spray should not be applied to areas that are sore or inflamed
  - mouth should be inspected regularly
  - if mouth lesions occur or persist, therapy should be interrupted until area resolves
  - unopened container can be stored upright in refrigerator
  - open container does not need to be refrigerated, but should be stored below 25°C and discarded 42 days after opening
- female patients of childbearing potential should be counselled to use effective contraception during and for 12 weeks after discontinuing therapy. Barrier method should be used in addition to hormonal contraception

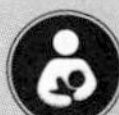

not recommended during pregnancy unless benefits outweigh risks

contraindicated during breastfeeding as high levels of cannabinoids are concentrated in breastmilk

TETRABENAZINE (Tetrabenazine)

Available form

Tablets: 25 mg

Action

- depletes amines (such as dopamine) in CNS
- inhibits monoamine transportation into presynaptic neuronal vesicles
- active metabolite thought to be responsible for therapeutic effects

Use

- management of movement disorders such as chorea, tardive and buccolingual dyskinesia and some dystonic syndromes

Dose

- initially 25 mg orally twice daily, increasing by 25 mg every 3–4 days (to a maximum of 200 mg daily or until therapeutic control is achieved)

Adverse effects

- drowsiness, Parkinsonism (at higher doses)
- postural hypotension, small prolongation of QT interval
- dysphagia, choking attacks
- agitation, insomnia, confusion, depression, anxiety
- (rare) neuroleptic malignant syndrome, suicidal ideation, bronchopneumonia (resulting from dysphagia and choking)

Interactions

- contraindicated with or within 14 days of MAOIs
- blocks action of levodopa, therefore therapies should be separated by at least 1 day and are contraindicated together
- extreme caution if given with other agents known to prolong QT interval
- increased dopamine depletion may occur if given with haloperidol, chlorpromazine or metoclopramide resulting in Parkinsonism and, rarely, neuroleptic malignant syndrome
- sedative effects may be additive if given with alcohol or other CNS depressants
- may potentiate hypotensive action of antihypertensive agents
- increased serum levels may occur if given with fluoxetine, paroxetine, duloxetine, sertraline or amiodarone

Nursing points/Cautions

- check supine and standing BP regularly for postural hypotension
- if no improvement in symptoms is seen after 7–10 days of therapy at maximum dose, therapy should be re-evaluated
- dose reduction may be required in those with kidney or liver impairment or the elderly
- caution if used in those with history of depression or previous suicidal ideation or attempts
- caution if used in those with congenital QT prolongation or history of cardiac arrhythmias
- contains lactose, therefore not recommended in those with galactose intolerance, Lapp lactase deficiency or glucose–galactose malabsorption
- contraindicated in those with depression or Parkinsonism as conditions may be worsened

Patient teaching and advice

- advise patient to avoid postural hypotension by moving gradually to a sitting or standing position, especially after sleep
- warn patient to avoid alcohol during therapy
- patient should be warned not to drive or operate machinery if drowsiness occurs
- patient should be carefully observed during meals if dysphagia and choking attacks are problems, especially early in therapy
- advise patient to seek medical attention if any of the following occur:
  - sweating, uncontrolled movements of legs, arms, hands or

    - head or stiffness/tightness in arms or legs
    - feeling of depression, sadness or thoughts of self-harm or suicide
    - difficulty swallowing or choking attacks
- see also General Patient teaching and advice (p. xxvii)

not recommended during pregnancy

contraindicated during breastfeeding

tablets can be crushed and mixed with spoonful of yoghurt or apple puree

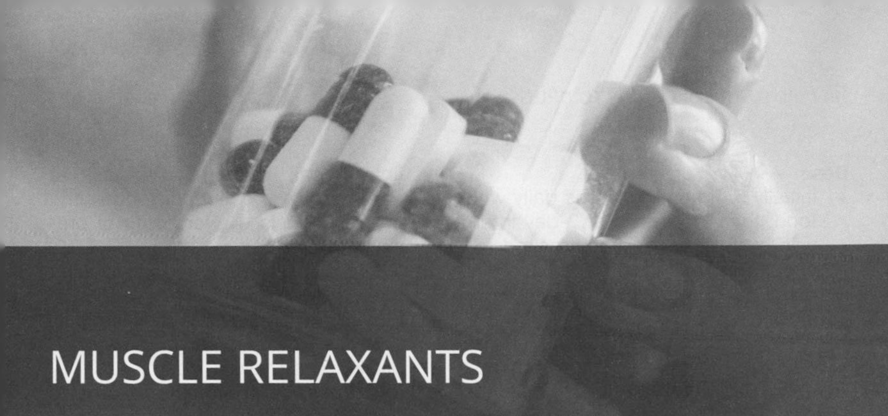

MUSCLE RELAXANTS

Several neurological disorders (such as cerebral palsy, spinal injury, multiple sclerosis and stroke) may cause spasticity, requiring the combined use of muscle relaxants (also called spasmolytic drugs) and physiotherapy to achieve the best outcome for the patient. Spasticity may be intermittent or sustained and is an involuntary contraction of skeletal muscle, leading to stiffness which may interfere with a person's mobility and/or speech (Kruidering-Hall & Campbell 2018).

Muscle relaxants act by modifying the stretch or directly interfering with the skeletal muscle. Although currently available agents relieve the painful spasm, they are generally not effective in improving function such as mobility (Kruidering-Hall & Campbell 2018).

BACLOFEN (Bacthecal, Clofen, Lioresal, Lioresal Intrathecal, Sintetica Baclofen Intrathecal, Stelax)

Available forms

Tablets: 10 mg, 25 mg; Ampoules: 0.05 mg/mL (for screening), 10 mg/20 mL, 10 mg/5 mL

Action

- derivative of gamma aminobutyric acid (GABA)
- selective agonist at pre-synaptic $GABA_B$ receptors
- inhibits adenylyl cyclase blocking calcium channels and release of transmitter
- antispasticity activity via spinal cord inhibiting motor neurone activation
- thought to reduce pain threshold associated with spasticity by inhibiting substance P in the spinal cord
- does not affect neuromuscular transmission
- does not reduce overall muscle strength as much as dantrolene
- stimulates gastric acid secretion
- (intrathecal bolus) onset of action 30–60 minutes, peak response about 4 hours, duration of action 4–8 hours, half-life 1–5 hours
- (intrathecal – continuous) response seen in 6–8 hours, maximum efficacy 24–48 hours
- (oral) onset of action is variable (hours to weeks), half-life 2.5–6 hours

Use

- (oral) skeletal muscle spasm in multiple sclerosis and spinal cord injuries
- (intrathecal) used when there is no response to oral therapy and/or adverse effects are unacceptable

Dose

- initially 5 mg orally 3 times daily with food, then increasing at 3-day intervals by 5 mg/dose until desired response is achieved (optimal daily range 30–75 mg) **OR**
- initially 25–50 microgram intrathecally (via spinal catheter or lumbar puncture), increasing by 25 microgram daily until response lasts for 4–8 hours (screening dose). Screening dose is then doubled and given over 24 hours via intrathecal pump. Dose may be further adjusted to maintain muscle tone as normal as possible and reduce frequency and severity of muscle spasm without intolerable adverse effects

Adverse effects

- decreased appetite, nausea, retching, vomiting, diarrhoea, dry mouth, constipation, increased salivation
- muscle weakness/hypotonia, ataxia, myalgia, disturbed gait, paraesthesia
- headache, insomnia, somnolence, nightmares, drowsiness, dizziness, sedation, tremor, fatigue, asthenia
- confusion, hallucination, depression, disorientation, abnormal thinking, agitation, anxiety, concentration difficulty
- seizures
- tinnitus, vertigo
- double or blurred visual disturbance, nystagmus
- slurred speech
- rash, pruritus, urticaria, hyperhidrosis
- dysuria, enuresis, urinary retention, daytime urinary frequency, urinary incontinence
- sexual dysfunction
- pain, fever, chills
- facial and peripheral oedema
- respiratory depression, dyspnoea, chest tightness, pneumonia
- hypotension, decreased cardiac output, hypertension
- tolerance (may occur after several months)
- (intrathecal) inflammatory mass at catheter tip, infection, dislodgement
- (rare) scoliosis or worsening of pre-existing scoliosis
- (withdrawal syndrome) initially high fever, altered mental state, aggravation of spasticity, muscle rigidity, seizures, coagulopathy, rhabdomyolysis, organ failure, death
- (overdose symptoms) excessive muscular hypotonia, drowsiness, light-headedness, dizziness, somnolence, seizures, loss of consciousness, hypothermia, increased salivation, nausea and vomiting, respiratory depression, bradycardia, apnoea, coma

Interactions

- increased sedation and respiratory depression may occur if given with CNS depressants and alcohol
- may lower seizure threshold
- may increase confusion, hallucinations, agitation, nausea and headaches in patients with Parkinson's disease if given with levodopa–carbidopa
- may be potentiated by TCAs, resulting in pronounced muscular hypotonia
- may potentiate hypotensive effect of antihypertensive agents
- caution if given with MAOIs as increased CNS effects and hypotension may occur
- (oral) may aggravate hyperkinesia if given with lithium and therefore should be given with caution
- may increase blood glucose, requiring a dose adjustment of insulin and/or oral hypoglycaemic agents
- increased risk of sedation and respiratory depression if given with opioid analgesics
- (intrathecal) increased risk of seizures and cardiac disturbances if given with propofol or fentanyl
- caution if used with other agents that impact on kidney function. If used

together, kidney function should be closely monitored

Nursing points/Cautions

- initiation of therapy should be done in a hospital setting for close patient monitoring to reduce spasticity to an acceptable level where muscle tone is sufficient for independence and adverse effects are minimal
- (spasticity due to head injury) symptoms of spasticity should be stable and at least 1 year post-injury before intrathecal therapy is started
- (post-traumatic spasticity) myelography of subarachnoid space is recommended before starting therapy and not commenced if any signs of arachnoiditis is evident (see Glossary)
- intrathecal route is only recommended when patient has been unresponsive to other treatment, including oral baclofen
- patient should be gradually withdrawn from oral antispasmodic agent (including baclofen) to decrease the risk of adverse effects (rebound spasticity and CNS disturbances)
- clinical effect is usually noticeable in 6–8 weeks
- liver enzymes should be monitored in those with liver impairment or diabetes mellitus
- resuscitation equipment should be readily available during initial intrathecal administration
- (intrathecal) no dose increase should occur in first 24 hours of therapy
- (intrathecal) incompatible with glucose 5%
- intrathecal bolus test dose of 100 microgram should not be exceeded
- intrathecal pump should not be implanted until patient response to test dose (intrathecal bolus) and dose titration has been adequately evaluated and it is advisable that patient is free of infection before pump insertion as systemic infection can complicate dose adjustments
- monitor respiratory and cardiovascular function closely (especially in those with cardiopulmonary disease or respiratory muscle weakness)
- patient with intrathecal implant should be very carefully monitored whenever dosage is increased
- (intrathecal) patient should be carefully monitored for any signs that intrathecal catheter tip may be occluded by a mass which may include any decrease in response when previously well controlled, withdrawal symptoms, poor response to increasing doses, pain or neurological dysfunction
- only experienced staff should fill intrathecal pump reservoir and refill schedule should be calculated in a manner to prevent sudden stopping of therapy, which may induce withdrawal syndrome
- for programmable pump, dose increase should be limited to once per 24 hours. If using non-programmable pump (76 cm catheter delivering 1 mL/24 hours), dose increase should be once every 48 hours to evaluate response. Pump function and catheter patency should be checked if there is no clinical effect after substantial dose increase
- once patient is stabilised on therapy, the regimen may be tailored to individual circumstances, such as the patient who experiences increased spasm at night. In this case the infusion rate may be increased overnight, but this should only be done under medical advice. Altered flow rate should be programmed to occur 2 hours before time of desired clinical effect
- for patient with spasticity of spinal origin, dose increments should be

limited to 10–30%. For patients with spasticity of cerebral origin, dose increments should be no greater than 5–15% to decrease risk of overdose

- if withdrawal syndrome occurs, therapy should be restarted and withdrawn over a longer timeframe. Those receiving intrathecal therapy are at increased risk of withdrawal syndrome
- with chronic therapy, there is usually an increased dose requirement with time and some patients develop tolerance. In some cases tolerance can be overcome by stopping therapy gradually and restarting after a 2–3-day break at the initial continuous infusion dose, followed by titration as previously
- if overdose occurs, solution should be removed as soon as possible from the pump and emergency medical advice sought. Patient should be intubated and ventilated in the event of respiratory depression occurring and IV diazepam administered for seizures. Cardiovascular function should be closely monitored and supported until patient recovers
- adverse effects are more common and severe in the elderly and those with psychiatric illness, stroke or cortical/organic brain disorders
- (intrathecal) caution if used in those with abnormal CSF flow as response may be suboptimal
- caution if patient uses spasticity to maintain upright position or balance when moving as use of baclofen may decrease independence
- caution if used in those with pre-existing bladder sphincter hypertonia as urine retention may occur
- caution if used in those with schizophrenia, confusion, psychosis, depression or mania (as these may be exacerbated), or those with epilepsy, significant EEG abnormalities, brain damage, peptic ulcers, cerebrovascular disease, respiratory, liver or kidney failure/impairment, hypertension, porphyria, alcoholism or diabetes mellitus
- extreme caution if used in children under 6 years
- not recommended in those with Parkinson's disease or if spasticity is caused by cerebral palsy, stroke or rheumatoid disorders
- (intrathecal) contraindicated IV, IM, SC or via epidural, or in those with epilepsy that is refractory to therapy

Patient teaching and advice

- instruct patient to take tablets with food to decrease the gastrointestinal side-effects
- advise patients with diabetes mellitus to monitor blood glucose levels more frequently
- warn patient against driving a vehicle or operating machinery if drowsy, dizzy or experiencing double or blurred vision
- instruct patient not to stop therapy abruptly. Withdrawal should be gradual and over 1–2 weeks
- warn patient to avoid alcohol during therapy because of increased sedation
- (intrathecal) everyone caring for patient should receive adequate instruction in caring for the insertion site and pump, as well as being aware of signs and symptoms of overdose and knowledge of what to do if this occurs as this is an emergency situation. It is also important that everyone understands withdrawal symptoms may occur if the pump is allowed to run out of medication, catheter becomes blocked or dislodged, battery on pump runs out or pump malfunctions. This is an emergency situation which could be potentially fatal

- overdose symptoms include unusual muscle weakness, sleepiness, dizziness, light-headedness, nausea and vomiting, excessive saliva, breathing problems, fainting, fitting
- withdrawal symptoms include uncontrolled spasms, difficulty with muscle movement, dizziness, light-headedness, severe itching, numbness/tingling of hands/feet, anxiety, high fever, agitation, confusion, hallucinations, abnormal thinking
- see also General Patient teaching and advice (p. xxvii)

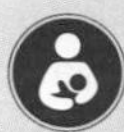

not recommended during pregnancy or breastfeeding unless benefits outweigh potential risks

tablet can be dispersed in water or crushed and mixed with spoonful of yoghurt or apple puree

BOTULINUM TOXIN TYPE A (Botox, Dysport)

Available forms
Vial: 100 U, 200 U; Ipsen units: 125, 300, 500

Action
- purified neurotoxin from *Clostridium botulinum* (toxin type A) that blocks neuromuscular conduction by binding to motor nerve terminals
- enters nerve terminals and inhibits release of acetylcholine
- when given IM, causes localised chemical denervation, flaccid muscle paralysis, including decreased muscle tone and contractility, leading to muscle atrophy
- when given intradermally, causes localised chemical denervation of sweat gland, decreasing sweating in that local area

Use
- blepharospasm associated with dystonia including hemi-facial spasm associated with nerve VII disorder and benign blepharospasm (in those over 12 years)
- strabismus (children and adults)
- spasmodic dysphonia
- cervical dystonia (spasmodic torticollis)
- focal spasticity of upper and lower limbs including dynamic equinus foot deformity due to juvenile cerebral palsy (over 2 years)
- focal spasticity (adults)
- severe primary hyperhidrosis of axillae
- chronic migraine (where person has headaches at least 15 days per month, 8 of which are migraine)
- overactive bladder (with symptoms of incontinence, frequency and urgency where adult patient is intolerant or response has been inadequate to anticholinergics)
- neurogenic detrusor overactivity (due to multiple sclerosis or spinal cord injury, not controlled by anticholinergics)
- (cosmetic use) glabellar lines, crow's feet, forehead lines

Dose
- dependent on site (see manufacturer's instructions)

Adverse effects

General
- generalised weakness, headache, fatigue, flu-like symptoms
- (injection site) pain, inflammation, erythema, oedema/swelling, bleeding, bruising, tenderness, paraesthesia, hypoaesthesia, localised infection
- development of antibodies that reduce the effectiveness of subsequent injections requiring an increase in dosage
- (rare) allergic reaction, spread of toxin effect (adverse effects away from injection site)

As well as general adverse effects (listed above), specific adverse effects for conditions include:

Blepharospasm

- diplopia, ptosis, dry eyes, photophobia, inability to close eyelids completely, entropion, ectropion
- facial muscle weakness

Strabismus

- partial ptosis, vertical deviation, diplopia
- (infrequent) cycloplegia, ocular vertigo, corneal irritation
- (rare) retrobulbar haemorrhage, sclera perforation, spatial disorientation, past pointing

Spasmodic dysphonia

- breathy dysphonia (paralytic dysphonia), dysphagia, aspiration, persistent cough

Cervical dystonia (spasmodic torticollis)

- dysphagia (lasting up to 3 weeks), dry mouth, nausea
- neck pain, asthenia, dizziness, general muscle weakness or stiffness, myalgia, facial paresis, hypertonia, hyperaesthesia
- upper respiratory tract infection, flu-like illness, rhinitis
- malaise, somnolence
- dysphonia

Nerve VII disorder (hemifacial spasm)

- blurred vision, facial droop, dizziness, tiredness (plus adverse effects for strabismus)

Focal spasticity (adult, upper and lower limb, post-stroke)

- (upper limb) arm pain, hypertonia, muscle weakness, arthralgia, musculoskeletal pain, pain in extremities
- (lower limb) falls, injury, lack of coordination, paraesthesia, hypertonia, asthenia, headache, hyperkinesia, peripheral oedema, arthralgia
- fever, flu-like illness
- ecchymosis

Focal spasticity (children)

- local and general weakness, clumsiness, falling, hypokinesia, paraesthesia, muscle spasm, leg/knee/ankle pain, leg cramps, myalgia, abnormal gait, joint dislocation, trigger finger
- vomiting
- lethargy, somnolence
- fever
- nasopharyngitis, flu-like illness, pneumonia, viral infection, ear infection
- rash
- increased micturition, urinary incontinence
- seizures

Hyperhidrosis

- increased non-axillary sweating, pain, hot flushes, transient arm weakness
- headache, asthenia, paraesthesia
- nausea
- pruritus

Chronic migraine

- worsening migraine/headache
- facial paresis, eyelid ptosis
- neck pain, myalgia, muscle spasm/tightness/weakness/stiffness
- pruritus, rash
- (uncommon) dysphagia, jaw pain, skin pain

Overactive bladder/Neurogenic detrusor overactivity

- urinary tract infection, bacteriuria, dysuria, urinary retention, increase in residual urine volume, frequent urination
- fatigue, insomnia

Glabellar lines

- headache, blepharoptosis, eyelid oedema, face pain, local muscle weakness, skin tightness, nausea, paraesthesia, ecchymosis

Crow's feet

- headache, flu-like symptoms, temporary lower lid droop

Forehead lines

- headache, eyebrow ptosis, eyelid swelling, aching/itching forehead, nausea, tension, flu-like symptoms

Interactions

- effects may be potentiated if given with aminoglycosides, colistimethate (polymyxin), tetracyclines, lincomycin, penicillamine, muscle relaxants or other agents that interfere with neuromuscular transmission and acetylcholine release, and should therefore be given with caution

Nursing points/Cautions

- administration should only be performed by suitable qualified and experienced clinician (e.g. intradetrusor administration for bladder dysfunction should only be done by urologist or urogynaecologist)
- dosage is kept as low as possible
- increasing frequency of treatment may result in tolerance developing. More than one ineffective treatment course should occur before patient is classified as non-responder
- neutralising antibodies are more likely to develop if dose is high, there is a short interval (< 3 months) between treatments and/or booster injections are given within 4 weeks of treatment
- denatured by violent agitation, therefore instil diluent and swirl gently to dissolve powder
- reconstitute using sodium chloride 0.9% (1–10 mL) for concentration of 1.25–40 U/0.1 mL (Botox) or sodium chloride 0.9% (0.6–2.5 mL) for concentration of 20–50 units/0.1 mL (Dysport). Manufacturer's instructions should be followed for dilution
- use within 24 hours of reconstitution if refrigerated
- avoid contact with eyes and skin and wash area thoroughly with water if contact occurs
- wear gloves and eye protection when reconstituting solution
- given IM generally; however, can be injected SC (blepharospasm) or intradermally (hyperhidrosis)
- preparations from different manufacturers may not be equipotent, therefore do not substitute brands
- (bladder dysfunction) urinary tract infection should not be present at time of administration
- (bladder dysfunction) any antiplatelet therapy should be discontinued 3 days before injection
- (bladder dysfunction) prophylactic antibiotics (not aminoglycosides) are recommended for 1–3 days before and 1–3 days post-injection
- (overactive bladder) clinical improvement may be seen within 2 weeks, duration about 24 weeks. Further injection not within 3 months
- (overactive bladder) patient should be observed for at least 30 minutes post-injection or until a spontaneous void has occurred
- (overactive bladder) clinical trials showed response to therapy was far greater in females when compared to male patients who, in many cases, had either no response or the condition was worsened
- (overactive bladder) urinary tract infection (as an adverse effect) occurs more commonly in patient with diabetes mellitus than those without
- (neurogenic detrusor overactivity) clinical improvement may be seen within 2 weeks. Fixed interval retreatment is not recommended and reinjection should occur when there is a reduced clinical effect, but no sooner than 3 months
- (bladder dysfunction) post-void residual urine volume should be measured 2 weeks post-treatment and regularly for 12 weeks
- (primary hyperhidrosis of the axillae) before starting therapy, any underlying causes for the hyperhidrosis (e.g. hyperthyroidism, pheochromocytoma) should be investigated first

- (primary hyperhidrosis of the axillae) repeat injections at less than 16-week intervals are not recommended
- (spasmodic dysphonia) diagnosis using a laryngoscope (preferably a nasendoscope) should be made to rule out any other structural disorder of the larynx
- (chronic migraine) retreatment schedule is every 12 weeks; however, if no response is seen after 2 treatment cycles, therapy should be discontinued
- (blepharospasm) ecchymosis of soft eyelid tissue can be decreased by applying light pressure to site immediately after injection
- (blepharospasm) after first injection, effect seen within 3 days, peaking at 1–2 weeks and lasting about 12 weeks. Dose may be increased if subsequent injections do not last longer than 8 weeks. Cumulative dose in 8 weeks should be greater than 200 U
- (strabismus) several drops of anaesthetic eye drops and an ocular decongestant should be applied prior to the injection
- (strabismus) paralysis occurs within 1–2 days, increasing in intensity during first week, lasting 2–6 weeks and gradually resolving over 2–6 weeks
- (nerve VII disorders/hemifacial spasm) cumulative dose over 2 months should not exceed 200 U
- (cervical dystonia) clinical improvement is usually seen in 1–2 weeks, peak effect about 6 weeks, duration 12–16 weeks. Retreatment in less than 8 weeks is not recommended. Total dose of 360 U every 8 weeks should not be exceeded
- (focal spasticity, children) clinical improvement is usually seen in 1–2 weeks, therapy repeated when clinical effects diminish but not more frequently than every 12 weeks
- (focal spasticity, adults) maximum treatment dose of 360 U (upper limbs) or 400 U (lower limbs) divided between muscles. Clinical improvement occurs within 2 weeks, peaking 4–6 weeks after treatment
- (glabellar lines) improvement seen in 1 week, lasting up to 16 weeks
- any leftover solution should be inactivated using dilute hypochlorite (0.5–1%) solution for 5 minutes and then disposed of as medical waste
- (blepharospasm) caution if used in those at risk of acute angle closure glaucoma
- contains albumin, therefore there is a theoretical risk for transmission of viral or prion diseases
- caution if used in those predisposed to seizures
- caution if given to those with prolonged bleeding time because of increased risk of bleeding and bruising at injection site(s)
- caution if used in those with pre-existing swallowing or breathing problems, or any defective neuromuscular transmission
- caution if administered in lung region (especially lung apex) due to risk of pneumothorax
- (spasmodic dysphonia) not recommended in those due to have elective surgery with general anaesthetic because of increased risk of aspiration due to relaxed vocal cords
- not recommended in those with motor neurone disease or motor neuropathy
- (overactive bladder) not recommended in men with overactive bladder and signs of urinary obstruction
- (focal spasticity, adults) not recommended for treatment of lower limb spasticity in adult post-stroke patients if reduced muscle tone is not expected to improve function (e.g. gait) or symptoms (e.g. pain) or to facilitate care

- contraindicated in those with myasthenia gravis or Eaton-Lambert syndrome or if any infection is present at injection site
- (bladder dysfunction) contraindicated in those with acute urinary tract infection or acute retention who do not routinely or are not willing to self-catheterise post-treatment (if required)

Patient teaching and advice

- warn patient to resume activity gradually to prevent falls and accidental injury if previously sedentary
- all patients should be advised that headache, flu-like symptoms and injection site reactions occur commonly post-injection
- instruct patient to seek medical advice if any drooping of upper eyelid, double or blurred vision, difficulty speaking or swallowing, generalised or local muscle weakness or numbness occurs
- (cervical dystonia) patient should be warned of the possibility of difficulty swallowing and breathing. A soft diet may be recommended until swallowing returns to normal. However, if swallowing, speaking or breathing difficulties occur after administration, patient should seek medical advice immediately
- (chronic migraine) warn patient that there may be initial worsening of headache/migraine in the first month after injection
- (bladder dysfunction) patient should be warned that there may be some blood in the urine after injection
- (bladder dysfunction) ensure that patient is aware that he/she will need to see doctor again about 2 weeks after injection to measure the amount of urine that is left in the bladder using ultrasound. This test needs to be done a number of times in the following 12 weeks
- (bladder dysfunction) instruct patient to seek medical advice immediately if he/she experiences difficulties passing urine as catheterisation (passing a small plastic tube into the bladder) may be required
- (bladder dysfunction) patient should be alerted to the signs of urinary tract infection (increase in frequency, difficulty passing urine, stinging/burning sensation) and the need to seek medical advice if they occur
- (bladder dysfunction) female patients should be advised to pass urine after sexual intercourse in order to avoid urinary tract infection
- (strabismus) if patient experiences any spatial disorientation, double vision or past point after therapy, covering the affected eye with a patch may alleviate these symptoms
- see also General Patient teaching and advice (p. xxvii)

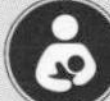

not recommended during pregnancy or breastfeeding unless benefits outweigh risks

DANTROLENE SODIUM HEMIHEPTAHYDRATE (DANTROLENE SODIUM) (Dantrium Capsules, Dantrium Powder for Injection)

Available forms

Capsules: 25 mg, 50 mg; Vial: 20 mg

Action

- hydantoin derivative (related to phenytoin) that interferes with release of calcium ions from skeletal muscle sarcoplasmic reticulum, thus producing muscle relaxation. However, cardiac and smooth muscle are minimally depressed

- no effect on neuromuscular transmission
- half-life 5 hours (IV) or about 8.7 hours (oral)

Use

- relieves long-standing spasticity associated with multiple sclerosis, stroke and spinal cord injury
- malignant hyperthermia (with supportive measures) (IV)

Dose

- (muscle relaxation) initially 25 mg orally daily, increasing to 25 mg 2, 3 or 4 times daily, then by increments of 25 mg up to 50 mg orally 2, 3 or 4 times daily (daily maximum 200 mg)
  OR
- (malignant hyperthermia) initially 1 mg/kg by IV push, up to a total dose of 10 mg/kg or until symptoms subside; may be repeated

Adverse effects

- drowsiness, dizziness, arm/leg weakness, fatigue, malaise
- loss of appetite, diarrhoea, nausea, vomiting, abdominal cramps, altered taste, swallowing difficulties, constipation
- disturbed speech
- chills, fever
- depression, confusion, nervousness
- increased liver enzymes, hepatitis, hepatotoxicity
- photosensitivity, abnormal hair growth, acne-like rash, pruritus, urticaria, sweating
- headache, insomnia
- visual disturbance, diplopia, excessive tearing
- pleural effusion, pericarditis
- seizures
- myalgia, backache
- tachycardia, erratic blood pressure
- haematuria, increased urinary frequency, crystalluria, nocturia, urinary retention, difficult urination
- difficult erection
- (IV) thrombophlebitis, erythema, urticaria, anaphylaxis, loss of grip strength, leg weakness, drowsiness, dizziness
- (IV, rare) malignant hyperthermia crisis

Interactions

- (IV) not recommended with calcium-channel blockers
- caution if given with oestrogen therapy (especially in women over 35 years) because of increased risk of hepatotoxicity
- may potentiate neuromuscular blockade of non-depolarising muscle relaxants such as vecuronium
- effects may be potentiated by alcohol and CNS depressants

Nursing points/Cautions

- baseline liver function tests are recommended before starting and then regularly during therapy (especially in females and those over 35) because of risk of hepatotoxicity
- patient should be observed during meals, because swallowing difficulties may lead to choking
- (oral) dose should not exceed 400 mg
- (oral) when establishing dose by titration, each dose level should be maintained for up to 7 days to determine response
- usually not continued for more than 45 days if there is no response
- (capsules) should not be used for management of neuroleptic malignant syndrome
- (IV) prevent extravasation as solution has a high pH and will cause tissue necrosis
- reconstitute vial for IV use with 60 mL water for injections, shaking the solution until clear
- (malignant hyperthermia) dose is dependent on patient's susceptibility, amount and time of exposure to triggering agent and time between symptoms occurring and treatment

- (malignant hyperthermia) supportive measures include oxygen, managing metabolic acidosis and electrolyte imbalance, cooling patient (if needed) and ensuring adequate urinary output
- caution if used in those with pre-existing liver disease/dysfunction, pulmonary, kidney or cardiac impairment
- not recommended for spasticity related to electroconvulsive treatment (ECT) or rheumatic disorders
- contraindicated in those with active hepatitis, active cirrhosis or those where spasticity to maintain upright position or balance when moving as use with baclofen may decrease independence

Patient teaching and advice

- warn patient against driving a vehicle or operating machinery if drowsy, dizzy or fatigued or within 48 hours of IV treatment
- patient (and family members/carers) should be instructed that muscle strength may diminish, resulting in a risk of swallowing difficulties and choking at mealtime and therefore patient should be closely observed
- patient should be advised to avoid prolonged exposure to sunlight and to wear protective clothing, hat, sunglasses and sunscreen (SPF 30+ or greater) if going outdoors
- instruct patient to immediately seek medical advice if any of the following occur:
  - yellowing of eyes or skin, dark urine, nausea, vomiting or loss of appetite, fever, itching or general feeling of being unwell (signs of liver impairment)
  - severe diarrhoea
  - fitting
  - crystal or blood in urine, difficulty passing urine
- counsel patient to avoid alcohol or any medications that reduce anxiety during therapy to avoid enhancement of dizziness and drowsiness
- see also General Patient teaching and advice (p. xxvii)

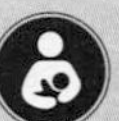

should only be used during pregnancy if benefits outweigh risks

not recommended during breastfeeding

capsule can be opened and mixed with water or orange juice until the suspension is even and then drink. Contents can be mixed with spoonful of yoghurt or apple puree

INCOBOTULINUMTOXINA (Xeomin)

Available forms
Vial: 50 LD50 U, 100 LD50 U

Action
- purified neurotoxin synthesised from *Clostridium botulinum* type A which has had complexing proteins removed making it low molecular weight
- blocks acetylcholine transmission at the neuromuscular junction

Use
- cervical dystonia (adults)
- blepharospasm (adults)
- spasticity of upper limb (adults)
- upper facial lines (glabellar frown lines, horizontal forehead lines, crow's feet) (adults)

Dose
- (cervical dystonia) 0.1–0.5 mL/injection site, not exceeding 200 U/treatment session or 50 U/injection site during first course of treatment, repeated no more frequently than 6-weekly. For second and subsequent treatment, 300 U/treatment session **OR**

- (blepharospasm) 1.25–2.5 U (0.05–0.1 mL)/ injection site, not exceeding 25 U per eye. Total dose should not exceed 100 U/treatment session, repeated no more frequently than 6-weekly **OR**
- (post-stroke spasticity) initially 10–80 U/ injection site, then 5–200 U/injection site (1–4 injection sites per muscle). Maximum dose 400 U/treatment session, repeated no more frequently than 3-monthly. No more than 250 U in shoulder muscles **OR**
- (glabellar frown lines) 4 U (0.1 mL) into each of 5 injection sites (2 into each corrugator muscle, 1 into procerus muscle). Standard dose is 20 U, increasing to 30 U if needed. Injection interval ≥ 3 months **OR**
- (crow's feet) 4 U bilaterally into 3 injection sites (1 injection 1 cm lateral from bony orbital rim, 2 injections approximately 1 cm above and 1 cm below first injection site). Total dose 24 units (12 per side) **OR**
- (crow's feet) 3 U bilaterally into 4 injection sites (first 2 injections 0.5 cm above and below point that is 1 cm lateral from bony orbital rim; second 2 injections 1 cm above and below this point). Total dose 24 units (12 per side) **OR**
- (horizontal forehead lines) 10–20 U into frontalis muscles at 5 injection sites at least 2 cm above bony orbital rim

Adverse effects

General

- general or local weakness
- (injection site) pain, burning, stinging, erythema, oedema/swelling, ecchymosis, bruising, rash, paraesthesia
- development of antibodies that reduce the effectiveness of subsequent injections requiring an increase in dosage
- (rare) hypersensitivity, flu-like symptoms
- (very rare) toxin spread (resulting in adverse effects spreading to sites away from injection site), exaggerated muscle weakness, dysphagia, dysphonia, aspiration pneumonia, breathing difficulties

As well as general adverse effects (listed above), specific adverse effects for conditions include:

Blepharospasm

- dry eye, ptosis, blurred vision, visual disturbance, increased tearing
- dry mouth, diarrhoea, dysphagia, lip disorder, gastroenteritis,
- nasopharyngitis, respiratory tract infection
- urinary tract infection
- asthenia, headache
- dyspnoea
- muscle strain
- hypertension
- tooth infection

Cervical dystonia (spasmodic torticollis)

- neck pain, muscle spasm/pain/ stiffness/weakness
- dysphagia, nausea
- headache, dizziness, light-headedness
- sinusitis, asthma, upper respiratory tract infection
- oropharyngeal pain
- sweating

Spasticity (upper limb, post-stroke)

- headache
- diarrhoea, dry mouth
- seizures (new onset or recurrent)

Glabellar lines

- headache
- bronchitis, sinusitis, nasopharyngitis, flu-like illness
- eye disorders
- gastrointestinal disorders
- outer end of eyebrow located above inner end (Mephisto sign)

Crow's feet

- viral infection
- eyelid oedema, dry eye

Horizontal forehead lines

- eyelid ptosis, dry eye, brow ptosis, outer end of eyebrow located above inner end (Mephisto sign)
- headache
- hypoaesthesia

Interactions

- caution if given with aminoglycosides, colistimethate, tetracyclines, lincomycin, penicillamine, tubocurarine-like muscle relaxants or other agents that interfere with neuromuscular transmission

Nursing points/Cautions

- recommended doses and frequency of administration should be adhered to in order to decrease the risk of adverse effects occurring away from the site of the injection due to spread of the toxin
- optimal dose and frequency should be individualised for each patient by physician
- if areas to be injected are marked with pen, these areas should not be injected through as permanent tattooing may result
- (post-stroke spasticity) initial and maintenance dose is dependent on the muscle group being treated (e.g. biceps muscle (flexed elbow) requires 80 U initially, followed by 75–200 U spread over 1–4 injection sites/muscle)
- (cervical dystonia) onset of effect within 7 days of injection, lasting 3–4 months
- (blepharospasm) onset of effect within 4 days of injection, lasting 3–4 months
- (blepharospasm) immediate gentle pressure at injection site will limit ecchymosis
- (blepharospasm) corneal sensation testing is recommended
- (post-stroke spasticity) onset of effect within 4 days of injection, maximum improvement within 4 weeks, lasting 12 weeks
- (glabellar frown lines) onset of effect within 2–3 days of injection, maximum effect on day 30, lasting up to 4 months
- (crow's feet) duration up to 12 weeks
- (crow's feet) injection close to zygomaticus major muscle should be avoided to prevent lip ptosis
- (horizontal forehead lines) duration up to 16 weeks
- (horizontal forehead lines) avoid injecting near orbit rim to decrease risk of brow ptosis
- increasing frequency of treatment may result in tolerance developing
- neutralising antibodies are more likely to develop if dose is high or there is a short interval between injections
- botulinum toxin products are not interchangeable
- denatured by violent agitation, therefore instil diluent and swirl gently to dissolve powder
- avoid contact with eyes and skin and wash area thoroughly with water if contact occurs
- wear gloves and eye protection when reconstituting solution
- reconstitute using sodium chloride 0.9% according to manufacturer's recommendations. If vacuum does not pull diluent into vial, it should be discarded
- reconstituted solution should be clear and colourless and free of particles
- any leftover solution should be inactivated using diluted sodium hypochlorite (at least 1%) solution, diluted sodium hydroxide solution, 70% ethanol or 50% isopropanol for 5 minutes and then disposed of as medical waste

- any reconstituted solution spill should be wiped up using dry absorbent material or absorbent material impregnated with one of the solutions listed in above point if powder is spilt
- contains albumin, therefore there is a theoretical risk for transmission of viral or prion diseases
- caution if used in those with bleeding disorders or taking anticoagulants
- caution if used in those with motor neurone disease, peripheral neuromuscular dysfunction or if targeted muscles show pronounced weakness or atrophy
- extreme caution if used for neurological indications in those with history of dysphagia or aspiration because of increased risk of excessive muscle weakness
- (cervical dystonia) caution if used in those with respiratory disorders who are dependent on accessory muscles. Caution in those with smaller neck muscles or require bilateral injections into sternocleidomastoid muscles because of increased risk of dysphagia
- (blepharospasm) caution if used in those who at risk of developing narrow-angle glaucoma
- (glabellar frown lines, crow's feet, horizontal forehead lines) not recommended in those with history of dysphagia or aspiration
- contraindicated in those with myasthenia gravis, Lambert-Eaton syndrome or other muscle activity disorders, if there is inflammation or infection at the injection site or if the person has a sensitivity to botulinum toxin or albumin

Patient teaching and advice

- (cervical dystonia) patient should be warned of the possibility of difficulty swallowing (dysphagia) and difficulty breathing (dyspnoea). A soft diet may be recommended until swallowing returns to normal. However, if swallowing, speaking or breathing difficulties occur after administration, patient should seek medical advice immediately
- instruct patient to seek medical advice immediately if any of the following occur:
  - drooping of upper eyelid, double or blurred vision,
  - difficulty breathing, speaking or swallowing,
  - generalised or local muscle weakness (can occur within hours to weeks of injection)
- patient should be warned to avoid driving, operating machinery or engaging in hazardous activities if muscle weakness, blurred vision, tiredness, dizziness or drooping eyelids occur
- see also General Patient teaching and advice (p. xxvii)

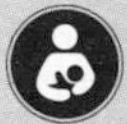

not recommended during pregnancy or breastfeeding

ORPHENADRINE CITRATE (Norflex)

Available form
Tablets: 100 mg

Action
- skeletal muscle relaxant

Use
- painful muscle spasm associated with strains, sprains, fibrositis, whiplash injuries, torticollis or prolapsed intervertebral disc
- tension headache, persistent hiccups

Dose
- 100 mg orally twice daily (may be increased to 300 mg/24 hours in severe cases)

Adverse effects
- nausea, dry mouth
- blurred or double vision
- (rare) rash, drowsiness

Interaction
- caution if used with other agents with anticholinergic action

Nursing points/Cautions
- adverse effects related to anticholinergic activity
- if used long term, monitoring of liver function, blood counts and urine testing are recommended
- caution if used in those with tachycardia, arrhythmias, coronary insufficiency or coronary decompensation
- contraindicated in patients with glaucoma, myasthenia gravis, urinary retention or obstruction of bladder neck, or prostatic hypertrophy because of anticholinergic properties

Patient teaching and advice
- patient should be advised against driving or operating machinery if blurred vision or drowsiness occurs
- if dry mouth is an ongoing problem, instruct patient to suck sweets, sugarless gum or ice, or use saliva substitute. However, if this continues for more than 2 weeks a dentist should be consulted because the patient is at risk of tooth decay, gum disease and fungal infection
- see also General Patient teaching and advice (p. xxvii)

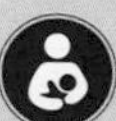
caution if used during pregnancy

tablet can be crushed and mixed with water or spoonful of yoghurt or apple puree

Note
- contained in Norgesic with paracetamol

ROPINIROLE HYDROCHLORIDE (Appese, Repreve)

Available forms
Tablets: 0.25 mg, 0.5 mg, 2 mg

Action
- non-ergot dopamine receptor (D2/D3) agonist
- half-life 6 hours

Use
- primary restless leg syndrome

Dose
- initially 0.25 mg orally daily at bedtime for 2 days, increased to 0.5 mg daily if tolerated for remainder of week 1, then increasing to 1 mg daily (week 2), 1.5 mg daily (week 3), 2 mg daily (week 4), 2.5 mg daily (week 5), 3 mg daily (week 6) and 4 mg daily (week 7) until optimal therapeutic response is reached

Adverse effects
- nausea, vomiting, abdominal pain, diarrhoea, dry mouth
- headache, migraine, dizziness, drowsiness, somnolence, fatigue, vertigo, syncope, sudden sleep onset, paradoxical worsening of restless leg syndrome (earlier onset, increased intensity, spread of symptoms to other limbs, symptoms recurring in early morning)
- nervousness
- arthralgia, myalgia
- paraesthesia
- increased sweating
- coughing, rhinitis, sinusitis, upper respiratory tract infection
- (rare) impulse control disorder, aggression, hypersensitivity, fibrotic complications (e.g. retroperitoneal fibrosis, pericarditis, cardiac valvulopathy)

Interactions

- not recommended with antipsychotic (neuroleptic) agents or centrally active dopamine antagonists (e.g. metoclopramide) because effects of ropinirole may be decreased
- increased serum levels may occur if given with ciprofloxacin or fluvoxamine
- not recommended with alcohol
- increased drug clearance may occur in those who smoke cigarettes. Dose adjustment may be necessary if patient starts or stops smoking cigarettes during therapy with ropinirole
- caution if used with CNS depressants, such as benzodiazepines, antipsychotics and antidepressants due to added sedative actions
- dose adjustment may be required if hormone replacement therapy (HRT) is stopped or started during therapy

Nursing points/Cautions

- before starting therapy, patient should be assessed for the presence of any sleep disorders or use of sedating medications
- if therapy is interrupted for more than a few days, it should be restarted using titration method described in dose section until optimal effects are seen
- caution if used in those with severe cardiovascular diseases, Parkinson's disease or major psychotic disorders
- not recommended in those under 18 years
- not recommended for treatment of neuroleptic-induced akathisia (muscular quivering, urge to constantly move and inability to sit still) or in those with liver impairment or kidney impairment (creatinine clearance < 30 mL/min)

Patient teaching and advice

- patient should be warned that sudden onset of sleep may occur without prior warning of daytime sleepiness. If significant daytime sleepiness or episodes of falling asleep occur, patient should be advised to avoid operating heavy machinery, driving or performing any other hazardous task(s)
- instruct patient that bedtime dose can be taken up to 2 hours before retiring
- patient should be advised to avoid alcohol during therapy
- patient should be warned to advise doctor if smoking cigarettes is started or stopped, because dose adjustment may be needed
- patient (and family member/carer) should be advised to seek medical advice immediately if:
  - symptoms worsen (e.g. start earlier, are more intense, move to other limbs, recur early in the morning) or
  - if patient suddenly develops compulsive behaviours such as urge to gamble or increased sexual urges or behaviours
- female patients of childbearing years should be counselled to use adequate contraception to avoid pregnancy occurring
- see also General Patient teaching and advice (p. xxvii)

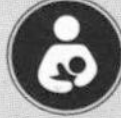

contraindicated during pregnancy or breastfeeding

tablet can be dispersed in 10–20 mL of water or crushed and mixed with water or spoonful of yoghurt or apple puree

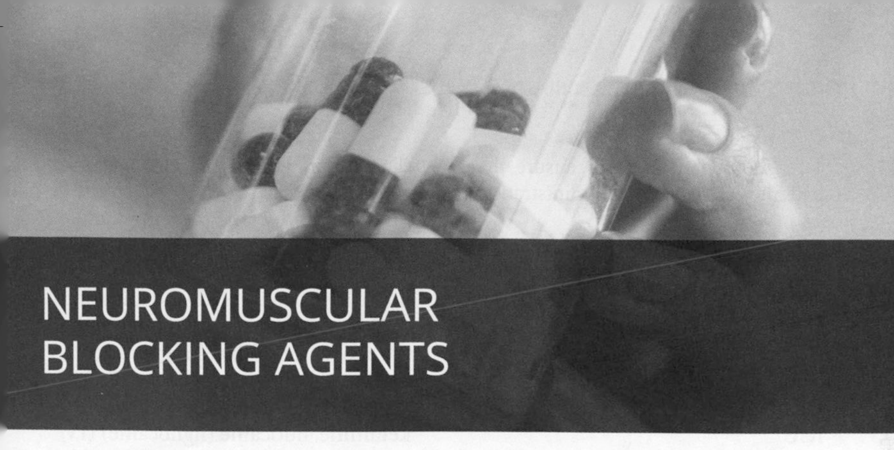

NEUROMUSCULAR BLOCKING AGENTS

The neuromuscular junction is a narrow gap between the motor neurone and muscle cell. The nerve's action potential depolarises its terminal causing an influx of calcium ions into nerve cytoplasm cause storage vesicles to release their contents (acetylcholine). The acetylcholine molecules diffuse across the gap (synaptic cleft) and bind to receptors (nicotinic cholinergic receptors) on the post-synaptic muscle cell membrane. For muscle contraction to occur, it requires activation of these receptors. The acetylcholine is rapidly hydrolysed to acetate and choline by the enzyme acetylcholinesterase. This allows the muscle end-plate to repolarise and the muscle cell relaxes (Butterworth et al 2018).

Neuromuscular blocking agents are drugs that act on the neuromuscular junction. There are two classes of agents:

- *non-depolarising agents* compete at the receptor site with acetylcholine, thereby reducing the response at the postsynaptic receptor site (or end-plate)
- *depolarising agents* act at the motor end-plate and maintain depolarisation, resulting in the receptor sites being unable to respond to any other stimulation, causing paralysis.

NON-DEPOLARISING BLOCKING AGENTS

General Actions of non-depolarising blocking agents

- antagonises acetylcholine by competing at the cholinergic receptor sites at motor end-plate, producing a rapid blockade, causing motor weakness that progresses to total flaccid paralysis
- small muscles are the first to be affected (e.g. eyelids), followed by limbs, neck and trunk, then diaphragm and intercostal muscles. Recovery is the opposite, with the respiratory muscles recovering first
- action blocked by anticholinesterase agents (e.g. neostigmine), increasing amount of acetylcholine available to compete at the receptor site
- no effect on consciousness, pain threshold or cerebration and therefore

care should be taken to ensure the patient is asleep before administration

General Uses of non-depolarising blocking agents

- as an adjunct to general anaesthesia
- facilitate endotracheal intubation
- relax skeletal muscles during surgery or mechanical ventilation
- facilitate mechanical ventilation in ICU

General Adverse effects of non-depolarising blocking agents

- mild transient hypotension, hypertension
- tachycardia, bradycardia
- erythema, pruritus, rash, urticaria, localised skin reaction
- skin flushing on the neck and upper chest
- bronchospasm, wheezing, increase in bronchial secretions, hypoxia, dyspnoea, laryngospasm
- pain and reaction at injection site, phlebitis
- (rare) malignant hyperthermia (signs include muscle rigidity, tachycardia, tachypnoea, increased oxygen requirements, increased carbon dioxide production, increased temperature and metabolic acidosis), anaphylactoid reaction, anaphylactic reaction, muscle weakness, myopathy

General Interactions of non-depolarising blocking agents

- inhalation anaesthetics (e.g. isoflurane) increase the blockade and duration of non-depolarising neuromuscular blocking agents
- potentiated by some antibiotics, including some of the aminoglycosides, tetracyclines, polymyxin (colistimethate), clindamycin, lincomycin, metronidazole and vancomycin
- potentiated by magnesium sulfate heptahydrate
- effects reversed by calcium salts
- intensity is increased and duration prolonged by acetazolamide, alpha adrenoceptor blocking agents, calcium-channel blockers, furosemide (frusemide), glucocorticoids, ketamine, lidocaine (lignocaine) (IV, high dose), lithium salts, possibly mannitol, MAOIs, oral contraceptives, organophosphates, phenytoin, propranolol, protamine, quinine, SSRIs and thiazide diuretics
- onset of action may be lengthened and duration of blockade shortened by chronic use of antiepileptic agents (e.g. phenytoin)
- effects are variable if given with muscle relaxants
- prior administration of suxamethonium hastens onset and increases depth of blockade if given as part of same procedure
- evidence of spontaneous recovery from suxamethonium should be evident before administration of non-depolarising neuromuscular blocking agents
- suxamethonium should not be used to extend the blockade of non-depolarising blocking agents because the prolonged blockade may be difficult to reverse
- activity is decreased (duration shortened) by corticosteroid (high dose), phenytoin, adrenaline (epinephrine), carbamazepine, azathioprine, theophylline (high dose), potassium chloride, sodium chloride or calcium chloride dihydrate and anticholinesterases (e.g. donepezil)

- hypokalaemia can potentiate neuromuscular blockade, therefore agents that cause hypokalaemia (e.g. amphotericin B (amphotericin), cisplatin, thiazide or loop diuretics, corticosteroids) should be given with caution
- (ICU) increased risk of myopathy if given long term with corticosteroids
- some agents (some antibiotics, propranolol, procainamide, chloroquine, D-penicillamine) may aggravate or unmask latent myasthenia gravis, increasing the person's sensitivity to non-depolarising neuromuscular blocking agents

General Nursing points/Cautions for non-depolarising blocking agents

- a small number of people have an atypical cholinesterase gene, which results in the person being very sensitive to neuromuscular blocking agents
- generally administered in the operating theatre or ICU by an anaesthetist or experienced doctor with resuscitation equipment and anticholinesterase reversal agents readily available
- any dehydration, altered blood pH and electrolyte imbalance should be corrected before administering a non-depolarising blocking agent, otherwise the neuromuscular blocking effect will be increased
- appropriate neuromuscular monitoring technique should be used to monitor blockage and recovery
- if given as IV infusion, degree of blockade should be monitored continually
- non-depolarising neuromuscular blocking agents may cause some histamine release locally and systemically, leading to adverse effects including hypersensitivity or anaphylactic reaction. Resuscitation equipment should be readily available
- each agent should be adequately flushed through the IV cannula using sodium chloride 0.9% before the introduction of the next drug
- reversed by neostigmine or pyridostigmine with anticholinergic (e.g. atropine)
- treatment for malignant hyperthermia includes stopping the anaesthetic agent and neuromuscular agent, administration of oxygen, lowering temperature, restoring fluid and electrolyte balance, maintaining urine output, reversing any acidosis and administration of IV dantrolene
- (ICU) prolonged (> 48 hours) administration with corticosteroids should be avoided
- should not be mixed with alkaline solutions (e.g. barbiturates) because a precipitate may occur
- caution if used in severely obese patients (weight > 30% ideal body weight) as dose estimation should be based on lean body weight, not actual weight, to prevent overdosage and prolonged blockade
- caution if used in those with conditions which may lead to electrolyte imbalance, such as adrenal insufficiency
- caution if used in those with pulmonary disease, asthma, cardiovascular diseases, history of anaphylactic reaction or family history of malignant hyperthermia
- caution if used in those with known hypersensitivity to a non-depolarising

blocking agent as cross-sensitivity between agents may exist
- caution if used in those with neuromuscular disease/disorders (e.g. polio, Eaton-Lambert syndrome and myasthenia gravis) as effects may be potentiated when given normal doses of neuromuscular blocking agents
- patients with burns may have a resistance to non-depolarising blocking agents and the dose will be dependent on the extent of the burns and the time elapsed since the burns occurred
- prolonged use over several days for maintenance of intubation and muscle paralysis is contraindicated
- contraindicated in patients known to be homozygous for atypical plasma cholinesterase gene because of increased sensitivity blocking effects

General Patient teaching and advice for non-depolarising blocking agents

- patient should be advised not to drive or operate machinery within 12–24 hours of treatment with a non-depolarising blocking agent
- see also General Patient teaching and advice (p. xxvii)

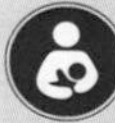

should not be used during pregnancy unless benefits outweigh potential risks. Respiratory depression may occur in the newborn if used during delivery via caesarean section. If patient has received magnesium sulfate heptahydrate for toxaemia during pregnancy, the dose of non-depolarising neuromuscular blocking agent should be reduced

caution if used during breastfeeding

ATRACURIUM BESYLATE (DBL Atracurium Besylate Injection, Tracrium Injectable)

Available forms
Vial: 25 mg/2.5 mL, 50 mg/5 mL

Action
- see General Actions of non-depolarising blocking agents (p. 1353)
- onset within 2–6 minutes, duration 30–60 minutes, half-life about 20 minutes
- recovery time is 25–45 minutes (depending on the type of anaesthesia used)
- causes histamine release from mast cells at higher clinical doses

Dose
- initially 0.4–0.5 mg/kg by IV bolus, then 0.08–0.10 mg/kg (maintenance) 20–45 minutes later, then at 15–25-minute intervals if needed

Adverse effects
- flushing, rash, hypotension, bronchospasm
- (rare) seizures
- see also Adverse effects of non-depolarising blocking agents (p. 1354)

Use/Interactions
- see General Uses/Adverse effects and Interactions of non-depolarising blocking agents (p. 1354)

Nursing points/Cautions/Patient teaching and advice
- should not be given IM
- should not be administered in same IV line as blood transfusion
- if body temperature is reduced, the dose also needs to be reduced
- if patient has hypovolaemia, administration should be over 60 seconds
- causes histamine release, therefore should be used with caution in those who have increased sensitivity to histamine release (e.g. previous

severe anaphylactoid reaction) or those with significant respiratory or cardiovascular disease
- contraindicated on a long-term basis (continuous over a period of days) due to accumulation of laudanosine (metabolite) which has CNS activating properties
- contraindicated in those with hypersensitivity to cisatracurium or benzenesulfonic acid
- see General Nursing points/Cautions/Patient teaching and advice for non-depolarising blocking agents (pp. 1355–56)

CISATRACURIUM (DBL Cisatracurium Injection Concentrate, Nimbex)

Available forms
Vial: 5 mg/mL, 5 mg/2.5 mL, 10 mg/5 mL, 150 mg/30 mL

Action
- stereoisomer of atracurium but more potent
- onset within 2–7 minutes, duration 10–35 minutes, half-life 22–29 minutes
- less likely to cause histamine release than atracurium (therefore less flushing, hypotension and/or bronchospasm)
- see also General Actions of non-depolarising blocking agents (p. 1353)

Dose
- initially 0.15 mg/kg by IV bolus, then 0.03 mg/kg (maintenance) at 20-minute intervals (if needed) **OR**
- initially 0.18 mg/kg/hour by IV infusion, then reduced to 0.06–0.12 mg/kg/hour (maintenance)

Use/Adverse effects/Interactions
- see General Uses/Adverse effects and Interactions of non-depolarising blocking agents (p. 1354)

Nursing points/Cautions/Patient teaching and advice
- incompatible with Ringer's solution, propofol, ketorolac
- should not be given with alkaline solutions (e.g. thiopentone)
- should not be administered in same IV line as blood transfusions
- solution is pale yellow or greenish in colour
- contraindicated in those with hypersensitivity to atracurium or benzenesulfonic acid
- see General Nursing points/Cautions/Patient teaching and advice for non-depolarising blocking agents (pp. 1355–56)

MIVACURIUM CHLORIDE (Mivacron)

Available form
Ampoules: 20 mg/10 mL

Action
- effective within 1–4 minutes, duration of 15–30 minutes, half-life 1.5–3 minutes
- causes histamine release from mast cells
- see also General Actions of non-depolarising blocking agents (p. 1353)

Dose
- (tracheal intubation) 0.2 mg/kg by IV bolus over 30 seconds **OR**
- 0.5–0.6 mg/kg/hour by IV infusion following bolus dose (above)

Use/Adverse effects/Interactions/Nursing points/Cautions/Patient teaching and advice
- IV infusion rate should be maintained for 3 minutes before altering rate
- solution is pale yellow in colour
- caution if used in those with TB, severe or chronic infection, malnutrition, chronic anaemia, malignancy, myxoedema, collagen disease, peptic

ulcer, end-stage liver failure, acute/chronic/end-stage kidney failure
- see general points for non-depolarising blocking agents (pp. 1353–56)

PANCURONIUM BROMIDE (Pancuronium Bromide Injection)

Available form
Ampoules: 2 mg/mL

Action
- effective within 4–6 minutes, duration 60–120 minutes, half-life is triphasic and about 2 hours
- half-life prolonged in those with kidney impairment
- see also General Actions of non-depolarising blocking agents (p. 1353)

Dose
- initially 0.04–0.15 mg/kg IV (depending on procedure), then 0.01 mg/kg at 25–60-minute intervals (maintenance)

Adverse effects
- slight-to-moderate increase in BP and HR
- increased salivation
- significant fall in intraocular pressure, miosis
- (ICU, prolonged use) prolonged paralysis, disuse atrophy, areflexia
- see General Adverse effects of non-depolarising blocking agents (p. 1354)

Interactions
- hydrocortisone and prednisone may decrease effects
- blockade may be prolonged when piperacillin is given preoperatively
- effects of botulism toxin A or B may be potentiated
- increased risk of arrhythmias if given with cardiac glycosides
- intensity of blockade decreased by hypothermia and increased by hyperthermia
- effect may be potentiated if given with large infusion of citrate-anticoagulated blood
- see General Interactions of non-depolarising blocking agents (p. 1354)

Use/Nursing points/Cautions/Patient teaching and advice
- those with bronchial cancer may show increased sensitivity to pancuronium and blockade may respond poorly to neostigmine during reversal
- use with caution in those with hypertension, phaeochromocytoma, kidney or liver impairment
- not recommended in those with GFR < 10 mL/minute
- not recommended in patients with pre-existing tachycardia or if increase in heart rate is undesirable
- contraindicated in those with hypersensitivity to bromide
- see General Uses/Nursing points/Cautions/Patient teaching and advice for non-depolarising blocking agents (pp. 1354–56)

ROCURONIUM BROMIDE (Esmeron, DBL Rocuronium Bromide Injection, Rocon)

Available forms
Vial: 50 mg/5 mL, 100 mg/10 mL

Action
- analogue of vecuronium with faster onset of action
- onset of action within 1–3 minutes IV, duration 30–40 minutes, half-life 66–80 minutes
- see also General Actions of non-depolarising blocking agents (p. 1353)

Dose
- 0.6 mg/kg (loading dose) IV, then 0.15 mg/kg (maintenance) **OR**
- 0.6 mg/kg IV, then 0.3–0.6 mg/kg/hr by IV infusion

Use/Adverse effects
- see General Uses and Adverse effects of non-depolarising blocking agents (p. 1354)

Interactions
- increases the onset of action of lidocaine (lignocaine)
- see General Interactions of non-depolarising blocking agents (p. 1354)

Nursing points/Cautions/Patient teaching and advice
- incompatible with amoxicillin, amphotericin B (amphotericin), azathioprine, cefazolin, dexamethasone, diazepam, erythromycin, famotidine, furosemide (frusemide), hydrocortisone, insulin, intralipid, methylprednisolone, prednisolone, propofol, thiopentone, trimethoprim or vancomycin
- ensure IV line is adequately flushed with sodium chloride 0.9% before and after administration
- solution is clear to pale yellow in colour
- should not be returned to refrigerator after being used at room temperature
- contraindicated in those with hypersensitivity to bromide
- see General Nursing points/Cautions/Patient teaching and advice for non-depolarising blocking agents (pp. 1355–56)

VECURONIUM BROMIDE (Vercure)

Available form
Vial: 10 mg

Action
- effective within 2–4 minutes IV, duration 20–40 minutes, half-life 36–117 minutes
- see also General Actions of non-depolarising blocking agents (p. 1353)

Dose
- initially 0.10 mg/kg IV, then 0.02–0.04 mg/kg at 20–40-minute intervals **OR**
- 0.8–1.4 microgram/kg/minute by IV infusion

Interactions
- may increase onset of action of lidocaine (lignocaine)
- blockade increased and duration increased if used during surgery under hypothermia
- see also General Interactions for non-depolarising blocking agents (p. 1354)

Use/Adverse effects/Nursing points/Cautions/Patient teaching and advice
- reconstitute using 5 mL water for injections
- incompatible with thiopentone
- contraindicated in those with hypersensitivity to bromide or pancuronium (as cross-sensitivity exists)
- see also General Uses/Adverse effects/Nursing points/Cautions/Patient teaching and advice for non-depolarising blocking agents (pp. 1354–56)

DEPOLARISING BLOCKING AGENTS

Suxamethonium is the only current depolarising blocking agent in clinical use.

SUXAMETHONIUM CHLORIDE (Suxamethonium Chloride Injection)

Available form
Ampoules: 100 mg/2 mL

Action
- also known as succinylcholine
- consists of two acetylcholine molecules that are joined
- binds to cholinergic receptors, resulting in persistent stimulation while maintaining depolarisation at motor end-plate, therefore receptor site is unable to respond to any other stimuli

- rapidly hydrolysed by cholinesterase (pseudocholinesterase) in liver and plasma
- onset of action within 30–60 seconds (IV) or 2–3 minutes (IM), duration 4–6 minutes (IV) or 10–30 minutes (IM), rapid half-life 2–4 minutes
- duration of action prolonged in those with low plasma cholinesterase levels
- muscle relaxation may be preceded by painful muscular fasciculations
- has no effect on consciousness, pain threshold or cerebration
- action not reversed by anticholinesterase

Use
- procedures requiring brief but profound relaxation, such as endotracheal intubation, electroconvulsive therapy (ECT), endoscopic examination or orthopaedic manipulations

Dose
- (short procedures) 0.6 mg/kg IV over 10–30 seconds **OR**
- (prolonged surgical procedures) 1–2 mg/mL solution given by IV infusion at a rate of 2.5–4.3 mg/minute **OR**
- up to 2.5 mg/kg IM (maximum 150 mg) (if IV not possible)

Adverse effects
- postoperative muscle pain (particularly chest, abdominal and shoulder girdle muscles), muscle fasciculations, hypertonia
- myoglobinuria, myoglobinaemia, rhabdomyolysis, increased creatine phosphokinase (CPK)
- trismus
- apnoea, prolongs respiratory depression, bronchospasm
- transient rise in intraocular pressure
- increase in intracranial pressure
- excessive salivation, increased gastric secretions and bowel movements, increased bronchial secretions
- hyperkalaemia, arrhythmias, hypotension, hypertension, bradycardia, tachycardia, cardiac arrest
- (rare) malignant hyperthermia (signs include muscle rigidity, tachycardia, tachypnoea, increased oxygen requirements, increased carbon dioxide production, increased temperature and metabolic acidosis), porphyria, hypersensitivity

Interactions
- may increase risk of apnoea, malignant hyperthermia and arrhythmias when given with inhalation anaesthetics, including nitrous oxide
- increased risk of bradycardia and asystole if given with fentanyl or propofol
- decreased dose required in those with hypocalcaemia or hypokalaemia
- effects may increase when given with amphotericin B (amphotericin) and thiazide diuretics because of risk of electrolyte imbalance
- causes immediate increase in serum potassium, which may be prolonged and is increased by beta-adrenoceptor blocking agents, leading to an increased risk of cardiac arrest
- intensity and duration may be altered when given before or with non-depolarising muscle relaxants
- effect may be prolonged or enhanced when given with some non-penicillin antibiotics, aprotinin, azathioprine, beta-adrenoceptor blocking agents, carbamazepine, chloroquine, cimetidine, high-dose corticosteroids, cyclophosphamide, lidocaine (lignocaine), lithium, magnesium salts, oral contraceptives, oxytocin, phenytoin, procaine, quinine, SSRIs, thiotepa or terbutaline
- increased risk of arrhythmias when given with digoxin, verapamil or in those with digoxin toxicity
- prolonged depolarisation may occur if given with cholinesterase inhibitors (e.g. donepezil, metoclopramide,

neostigmine, pyridostigmine, rivastigmine)
- duration may be decreased by atracurium or diazepam
- caution if exposed to neurotoxic insecticides and weed killers, antimalarial agents, antineoplastic agents, MAOIs, oral contraceptives, pancuronium, chlorpromazine or neostigmine as these may decrease levels of pseudocholinesterase

Nursing points/Cautions

- should only be given by experienced medical staff with immediate access to resuscitation equipment
- any known hyperkalaemia or electrolyte imbalance should be corrected before administration of suxamethonium if possible
- should not be given to conscious patient as respiratory muscles become paralysed
- administer alone
- initial test dose of 0.1 mg/kg IV may be given to test response
- for IV infusion, should be diluted using glucose 5% or sodium chloride 0.9% to a concentration of 1–2 mg/mL
- may be given IM if vein is not accessible
- if prolonged apnoea occurs after administration, neostigmine should not be used as a reversal agent as it may intensify blockade
- repeated administration is not recommended as prolonged respiratory depression and apnoea may occur
- treatment for malignant hyperthermia includes stopping the anaesthetic agent and neuromuscular agent, administration of oxygen, lowering temperature, restoring fluid and electrolyte balance, maintaining urine output, reversing any acidosis and administration of IV dantrolene
- caution if used in those with bone fractures as muscle contractions will occur before relaxation phase, causing increased pain
- caution if used in those with burns or trauma as abnormal response to suxamethonium may persist for up to 2 years post-injury with the greatest risk being between 10 and 90 days post-injury, but may also be prolonged if there is infection or prolonged healing (see contraindication below)
- caution if used in those with hypoxia, cardiovascular, liver, kidney, metabolic or lung disease or myasthenia gravis
- caution if used in those with pre-existing hyperkalaemia or electrolyte imbalance, uraemia, hemiplegia, paraplegia, head injury, encephalitis, ruptured cerebral aneurysm, tetanus, acute anterior horn disease, extensive denervation of skeletal muscle or degenerative neuromuscular disease (especially between 3 weeks and 6 months of onset) as hyperkalaemia increases risk of cardiac arrest
- caution if used in those with decreased serum levels of pseudocholinesterase (cancer, severe dehydration, malnutrition, severe hepatic disease, severe anaemia, myxoedema, burns, pregnancy, abnormal body temperature, collagen diseases, severe infection, myocardial infarction or kidney impairment)
- not recommended in those with phaeochromocytoma or during intraocular surgery in those with glaucoma
- not recommended in those with severe sepsis of greater than 7-day duration. Infection must be cleared before administering suxamethonium due to risk of hyperkalaemia
- not recommended in patients with myotonias due to unpredictable effects

- contraindicated in those who have had malignant hyperthermia or have a family history of malignant hyperthermia, a penetrating eye injury or acute narrow-angle glaucoma, myopathies associated with increased CPK, Duchenne's muscular dystrophy, genetic disorders of pseudocholinesterases
- contraindicated after multiple trauma, severe burns (acute phase), extensive muscle degeneration (e.g. recent paraplegia), severe hyperkalaemia, kidney impairment or severe long-lasting sepsis because there is an increased risk of cardiac arrhythmias and arrest because of severe hyperkalaemia resulting from administration of suxamethonium

Patient teaching and advice

- patient should be advised not to drive or operate machinery if there are any residual adverse effects
- advise patient to seek medical advice immediately if any of the following occur:
  - change in heart rate or palpitations
  - eye pain
  - muscle stiffness
- see also General Patient teaching and advice (p. xxvii)

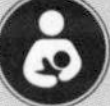

only used during pregnancy if benefits outweigh risks. Plasma pseudocholinesterase levels are decreased during pregnancy and remain low for several days after delivery

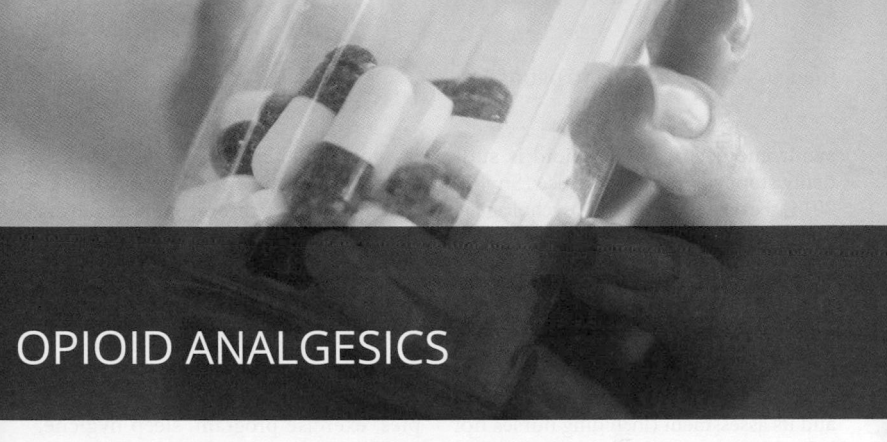

OPIOID ANALGESICS

Pain can be described as 'an unpleasant sensory and emotional experience associated with actual or potential tissue damage, or described in terms of such damage' (International Association for the Study of Pain (IASP) 2017). Pain is a subjective experience affected by a person's individual biological, psychological (including previous experience with pain) and cultural make-up, which means that ideally a person's pain management is individually tailored to their needs.

Pain may be *acute* (usually related to tissue damage and sharp in nature, also termed nociceptive), *chronic* (lasting longer than the original injury and for more than 6 months and variable in nature) or *neuropathic* (resulting from damage to nerves and presenting as burning, tingling or electric-shock type quality) (Rathmell & Fields 2018). Each of these pain types requires different management strategies. For example, neuropathic pain may not respond to traditional NSAIDs or opioid analgesics and requires adjunct medications, such as tricyclic antidepressants (TCAs) or anticonvulsant medications (Bryant et al 2019).

The opioid analgesics, as they are known today (also termed narcotic analgesics because of their sedation-producing properties), is a group of both natural and synthetic agonist drugs that have morphine-like properties and interact with specific opioid receptors (mu, delta and kappa, but predominantly the mu receptors) in the brain to lessen or remove the sensation of pain. Mu receptor activation is also responsive for other effects, including euphoria, sedation, respiratory depression, constipation and pupillary constriction. Opioid receptors are also located in other tissues, including the gastrointestinal tract, cardiovascular and immune systems (Rathmell & Fields 2018; Snyder 2014).

Drug tolerance is defined as 'a gradual decrease in effectiveness of a drug given repeatedly over a period of time; if tolerance develops, higher doses are required to achieve the same effect', and this occurs with opioids (Bryant et al 2019, p. 275). Tolerance may develop not only to the analgesic effects but also to sedation, nausea and vomiting. However, patients do not become tolerant to other adverse effects, such as constipation, confusion and hallucinations, which only worsen with increasing doses to overcome the tolerance (Bryant et al 2019). Withdrawal syndrome occurs if the opioid is suddenly stopped after chronic use (Snyder 2014). Fear of physical and psychological dependence on analgesics often leads to poor pain management (especially in the elderly), and is of little consequence in palliative or terminal care. Other reasons for poor pain management and unrelieved pain include nurses' inadequate knowledge and misconceptions about pain and its assessment (including nurses not believing it is a patient's right to expect total pain relief); poor, infrequent or unsystematic pain assessment; inadequate time to assess and manage a patient's pain (i.e. workload), irregular reassessment for pain relief (i.e. assessing the effectiveness of the analgesia); and nurses not accepting patients' report of pain (Bryant et al 2019; Pretorius et al 2015).

A 'good' pain management plan is one that incorporates treatment of the cause of the pain (if possible) rather than treating the symptoms. Accurate and ongoing pain assessment using a validated tool is essential in establishing pain levels and the efficacy of the management plan (including analgesics) (e.g. has the analgesic reduced pain levels so the patient is comfortable and able to function?). Analgesics should be administered at regular intervals (rather than prn) in order to prevent pain from occurring. Opioids such as the ones discussed in this section are prescribed for moderate-to-severe pain, where NSAIDs (see p. 11) are used for mild pain. Known adverse effects (such as constipation, nausea and vomiting) should be prevented by use of appropriate agents administered concurrently with the opioid (Bryant et al 2019).

Consideration should also be given to complementary medicine as an adjunct to traditional pain management strategies. There is strong evidence that acupuncture is effective in the management of chronic pain, resulting in a decreased usage of opioids. The evidence for other therapies, such as yoga, relaxation, tai chi and massage, is positive but weak (Lin et al 2017). The pain management plan should also consider non-pharmacological therapies, such as patient education, psychological therapies, exercise program, sleep hygiene, and looking at activities that precipitate pain and pacing or management of these activities in order to reduce the pain (e.g. timing, postural components, aides). Multidisciplinary input will often be required to facilitate these plans and include clinicians such as psychologists, physiotherapists, occupational therapists and exercise physiologists (FPM, ANZCA 2015).

General Actions of opioids

- main actions are on CNS and smooth muscle
- analgesic action is caused by binding with specific opioid receptors (mu, delta and kappa) both pre- and postsynaptically decreasing pain transmission in the spinal cord and modulating descending inhibitory pathways from the brain
- depresses respiratory centre (brainstem), decreasing the response to carbon dioxide
- suppresses cough centre (medulla)
- stimulates vomiting centre (chemoreceptor trigger zone (CTZ))
- stimulates the vagus nerve
- produces miosis
- increases smooth muscle tone in GI tract (especially the sphincters)
- reduces peristalsis and secretions
- relieves anxiety

- may produce euphoria or dysphoria, sedation and raised intracranial pressure
- causes histamine release, resulting in bronchospasm and itching
- tolerance and dependence may occur
- generally not well absorbed after oral administration due to extensive first pass metabolism in the liver

General Adverse effects of opioids

- nausea, anorexia, constipation, vomiting, dry mouth, dyspepsia
- respiratory depression, apnoea, dyspnoea, cyanosis
- urinary retention
- increased intracranial pressure
- ureteric or biliary spasm, increased intracholedochal pressure
- blurred vision, diplopia, miosis, visual disturbances
- cough suppression
- drowsiness, euphoria or dysphoria, headache, dizziness, confusion, vertigo, sedation, somnolence, mood change, slurred speech, hallucinations, delirium, tremor
- bradycardia, orthostatic hypotension (in ambulant patients), hypotension, tachycardia
- facial flushing, pruritus, urticaria
- sweating, hypothermia, chills
- muscle rigidity (including thoracic muscles), myoclonic movements
- prolongation of labour (reduction of strength, duration and frequency of contractions) or shortening of labour (increased rate of cervical dilation)
- seizures (high doses)
- tolerance and dependence (physical and/or psychological) may develop
- withdrawal symptoms (usually on rapid discontinuation)
- allergy, hypersensitivity, including rash, hives, pruritus, bronchospasm

General Interactions of opioids

- not recommended or contraindicated with alcohol, antihistamines, barbiturates, benzodiazepines, general anaesthetics, phenothiazines, sedative/hypnotics, other opioids or TCAs because CNS and respiratory depressant effects may be enhanced
- contraindicated with or within 2 weeks of MAOIs because significant respiratory depression, hypotension and hyperpyrexia may occur
- actions may be antagonised by naloxone and naltrexone
- increased risk of respiratory depression if given with neuromuscular blocking agent or benzodiazepines
- miosis may be counteracted by atropine and atropine-like agents
- use with anticholinergic agents, tricyclic antidepressants (with anticholinergic effects), anti-Parkinson's agents and antihistamines (with anticholinergic effects) may increase the risk of severe constipation, urinary retention and/or paralytic ileus
- caution if used with other agents that depress respiratory function
- increased risk of severe constipation if given with antidiarrhoeal or antiperistaltic agents (e.g. loperamide, kaolin)
- may increase hypotensive effects if given with antihypertensive agents, diuretics or other agents with hypotensive effects
- if buprenorphine is given before other opioids, therapeutic effects of opioids may be reduced
- respiratory and cardiovascular depressant effects may be potentiated

by halogenated inhalation anaesthetic agents
- metabolism may be inhibited by amiodarone, cimetidine, clarithromycin, diltiazem, erythromycin, fluconazole, itraconazole, ritonavir, verapamil and voriconazole, increasing risk of prolonged respiratory depression due to increased serum levels of opioid
- caution if an oral opioid is used with metoclopramide, because gastric emptying and absorption may be increased, potentiating the CNS effects of the opioid
- delays gastric emptying and absorption, therefore all concurrent oral medication may be affected
- caution if given with rifampicin as opioid serum levels and effects may be decreased
- may interfere with gastric emptying studies and hepatobiliary imaging

General Nursing points/Cautions for opioids

- administration and storage precautions are as per state and territory Acts and Regulations for controlled drugs
- an opioid-tolerant patient is considered to be one who takes at least 60 mg morphine daily
- patient should be assessed for any known allergy to opioids (it is important to have patient describe the allergy because some will describe the adverse effects (especially nausea and vomiting) as 'allergy')
- adverse effects are more common and severe in ambulant patients
- analgesia is more effective if given before onset of intense pain. Plan to give patient analgesia 15–30 minutes before undertaking any procedure that will cause pain or discomfort
- patient should be closely monitored for any signs of respiratory depression and drug withheld and doctor informed if the respiratory rate shows marked decline (especially if 8 breaths/minute or less). Respiratory depression can occur at any time during therapy (not just initially) and special care should be taken with opioids with long half-life (e.g. fentanyl) as respiratory depression can occur after agent has been discontinued
- any hypovolaemia should be corrected before starting therapy to reduce risk of hypotension
- even if initial dose causes vomiting, subsequent doses depress the vomiting centre
- antiemetic should be given at the same time if vomiting is likely to be a problem; laxatives should also be commenced concurrently to prevent severe constipation from developing
- urinary output, presence of bowel sounds and bowel pattern should be monitored
- if opioid is used intraoperatively, patients should be closely observed postoperatively for any signs of delayed respiratory depression
- opioid-induced hyperalgesia should be considered if there is insufficient pain control in response to increased dose
- tolerance may develop in 24–48 hours, with larger doses being required to produce the same effect
- both physical and psychological dependence may occur. If opioid is withheld, withdrawal syndrome (aggression, irritability, runny nose, body aches, yawning, fever, sweating,

pupil dilation, nausea, vomiting, diarrhoea, stomach cramps, insomnia, nervousness, restlessness, tachycardia, tremor and goosebumps) may be seen

- naloxone and resuscitation equipment should be readily available to reverse respiratory depression
- ensure that the correct strength of syrup, ampoules/vials or correct tablet type (immediate release versus sustained release) is selected as some opioids have multiple formulations
- caution if used in those with myasthenia gravis or phaeochromocytoma
- caution if used in those with hypothyroidism, adrenocortical insufficiency (e.g. Addison's disease), shock, myxoedema, as symptoms may be exacerbated and/or there may be increased risk of respiratory and/or CNS depression
- caution if used in those with pulmonary disease, decreased respiratory reserve, alcoholism or impaired liver or kidney function
- caution if used in those with hypovolaemia or shock as hypotension may occur
- caution if used in those with acute abdominal conditions (including GI obstruction or obstructive bowel disorder) or postoperatively after abdominal surgery as intestinal mobility is decreased by opioids
- caution if using opioids in the elderly as they may have reduced liver or kidney function, reduced protein binding and reduced cardiac output, which may lead to accumulation of opioid and possible toxicity
- caution if used in those with diabetes as hyperglycaemia may occur
- caution if used in those with epilepsy or at risk of seizures (e.g. head injury, metabolic disorders, alcohol or drug withdrawal) due to increased risk of seizures
- caution if used in those with prostatic obstruction/hypertrophy, urethral stricture, recent urinary tract surgery because of risk of urinary retention
- caution if prescribed to those with a known history of drug/alcohol abuse/dependence, emotional instability or suicidal ideation/attempts
- not recommended/contraindicated in those with head injury, increased intracranial pressure, impaired consciousness, brain tumour or coma as carbon dioxide retention may further increase intracranial pressure (which may obscure clinical course in those with head injury)
- contraindicated in those with biliary or renal tract spasm or after biliary tract surgery
- contraindicated in those with diarrhoea caused by pseudomembranous colitis, poisoning or other toxic organisms because the slowing of the GI tract by opioids will prolong the diarrhoea
- contraindicated in those with respiratory depression, a low respiratory reserve, acute bronchial asthma, cardiac arrhythmias, CNS depression, heart failure (secondary to chronic pulmonary disease), acute alcoholism, delirium tremens, severe liver/kidney disease, hepatic encephalopathy, diabetic acidosis with danger of coma, or convulsive disorders (including status epilepticus, pre-eclampsia or eclampsia)

General Patient teaching and advice for opioids

- advise patient not to drive or operate machinery if dizziness, drowsiness, sedation and confusion occur

- warn patient to take care when going from lying to standing position as dizziness may occur due to hypotension
- patient should be warned to avoid alcohol during therapy with opioid analgesics
- instruct patient to deep breathe, cough and move frequently (if permitted) postoperatively
- encourage patient to practise good dental hygiene as opioids can cause dry mouth increasing risk of dental caries
- advise patients with diabetes to monitor blood glucose levels closely during therapy
- see also General Patient teaching and advice (p. xxvii)

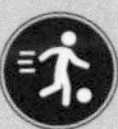

opioids are banned in sport

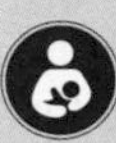

contraindicated during pregnancy as may cause respiratory depression in newborn infants, therefore naloxone should be readily available. May cause withdrawal symptoms in newborn if there has been prolonged maternal use during pregnancy

not recommended during or within 24 hours of breastfeeding. If used, baby should be observed for signs of sedation and other adverse effects

ALFENTANIL HYDROCHLORIDE (Alfentanil GH, Rapifen)

Available forms
Ampoule: 1 mg/2 mL, 5 mg/10 mL

Action
- potent short-acting synthetic opioid analgesic with mu receptor activity that is related to fentanyl (with more rapid onset)
- onset of analgesia and respiratory depression is 1–2 minutes, short duration of action (dose-related), elimination half-life is 90–110 minutes
- see General Actions of opioids (p. 1364)

Use
- anaesthetic induction
- analgesic supplement

Dose
- generally given by specialist anaesthetist

Adverse effects
- see General Adverse effects of opioids (p. 1365)
- laryngospasm
- muscle rigidity

Interactions
- may increase serum levels of propofol
- increased serum levels may occur if given with propofol
- metabolism may be decreased leading to increased serum levels by diltiazem, erythromycin, cimetidine, voriconazole and fluconazole
- increased risk of serotonin syndrome if given with SSRIs or MAOIs
- see General Interactions of opioids (p. 1365)

Nursing points/Cautions
- see General Nursing points/Cautions for opioids (p. 1366)
- oxygen, resuscitation and intubation equipment should be readily available
- if analgesia > 60 minutes is required, IV infusion is recommended
- patient should be monitored for at least 2 hours postoperatively for any signs of respiratory depression
- muscle rigidity can be avoided by slow IV administration (especially at high doses), premedication with benzodiazepines or use of muscle relaxants
- staff should be advised to wear gloves during administration. If contact with skin occurs, area should

- be thoroughly washed with water only
- not recommended in the last 10 minutes before the completion of surgery
- caution if used in those who are obese or have uncontrolled hypothyroidism as clearance may be reduced (requiring a lower dose)
- contraindicated as postoperative pain management

Patient teaching and advice

- patient should be advised to wait 3–6 hours (for 0.5–1.5 mg) or 12–24 hours (higher doses) before driving or operating machinery because of possible delayed respiratory depression
- see General Patient teaching and advice for opioids (p. 1367)

BUPRENORPHINE (Bupredermal Transdermal, Buvidal Monthly, Buvidal Weekly, Norspan Transdermal Patch, Sublocade, Subutex, Temgesic)

Available forms

Sublingual tablets: 200 microgram, 400 microgram, 2 mg, 8 mg; Transdermal patches: 5 mg, 10 mg, 15 mg, 20 mg, 25 mg, 30 mg, 40 mg; Ampoules: 300 microgram/mL; Modified-release solution (prefilled syringe): 8 mg/0.16 mL, 16 mg/0.32 mL, 24 mg/0.48 mL, 32 mg/0.64 mL, 64 mg/0.18 mL, 96 mg/0.27 mL, 100 mg/0.5 mL, 128 mg/0.36 mL, 300 mg/1.5 mL

Action

- synthetic opioid that has both opioid agonist (mu receptors) and antagonist (delta and kappa receptors) properties
- more potent than morphine and longer acting
- active metabolite (norbuprenorphine)
- see General Actions of opioids (p. 1364)

Use

- moderate-to-severe pain (short-term management) (transdermal patches, IV or IM)
- opioid dependence (detoxification or maintenance) (sublingual tablets, modified-release solution)

Dose

- (pain) 0.3–0.6 mg IM or slow IV injection (over at least 2 minutes) 6–8-hourly **OR**
- (pain) 0.2–0.4 mg sublingually 6–8-hourly **OR**
- (pain) initially 5 mg patch (releasing 5 microgram/hour), applied to skin weekly, increasing at 3–7-day interval until satisfactory analgesia is achieved (maximum 40 mg) **OR**
- (opioid dependence) initially 4–8 mg sublingually with additional 4 mg if needed (day 1, target 8–12 mg), then gradually increasing in increments of 2–8 mg according to response (daily maximum 32 mg). Dose frequency may be reduced once patient is stable **OR**
- (opioid dependence, modified-release solution) 8–32 mg slow SC weekly **OR**
- (opioid dependence, modified-release solution) 64–128 mg slow SC monthly **OR**
- (opioid dependence, modified-release solution, adults stabilised on transmucosal buprenorphine for ≥ 7 days) 300 mg SC monthly for 2 months, then 100 mg SC monthly (maintenance); however, maintenance dose can be increased to 300 mg monthly if no satisfactory response after second maintenance dose (Sublocade)

Adverse effects

- miosis more marked than for morphine and lasting > 24 hours

- (IM, IV) injection site reaction
- (SC, injection site) pain, pruritus, erythema, induration, swelling, bruising, ulceration
- (transdermal patch) erythema, oedema, rash, pruritus
- (transdermal patch, high dose) prolongation of QT interval
- liver injury (including elevated liver enzymes, hepatitis, liver failure, liver necrosis, encephalopathy) (especially in those with previous liver damage, such as hepatitis B or C, alcoholism)
- see General Adverse effects of opioids (p. 1365)

Interactions

- caution if given with rifampicin, phenytoin or carbamazepine as metabolism may be increased, decreasing serum levels
- caution if given with protease inhibitors, azole antifungals or macrolide antibiotics as serum levels may be increased
- caution if given with other hepatotoxic agents
- if given with warfarin, may increase INR, therefore this should be carefully monitored
- if buprenorphine is given before other opioids, therapeutic effects of opioids may be reduced
- elimination may be reduced if given with general anaesthetics or other agents that reduce liver blood flow
- (IV) not recommended with IV benzodiazepines
- (transdermal patch) not recommended with other agents known to prolong QT interval or cause electrolyte imbalances especially hypokalaemia or hypomagnesaemia
- see General Interactions of opioids (p. 1365)

Nursing points/Cautions

- liver function test monitoring is recommended before starting and regularly throughout therapy
- may cause withdrawal symptoms if used in patients who are dependent on other opioid analgesics, because of its antagonistic properties
- not fully reversed by naloxone, therefore if respiratory depression occurs, ensure patient is adequately ventilated
- (opioid dependence) should be part of a coordinated treatment program (medical and psychosocial), not a standalone therapy
- (opioid dependence) part of Opiate Dependence Program requiring special authority
- (opioid dependence) first dose may produce mild withdrawal symptoms in those being detoxified (i.e. with a dependence on opioids) if given too soon after opioid
- (opioid dependence) methadone dose should be reduced to 30 mg daily before starting therapy
- (opioid dependence) if transferring from methadone, a 24-hour gap should be left before starting therapy because of the long half-life of methadone. If transferring from short-acting opiates (including street heroin), there should be at least a 6-hour gap and signs of withdrawal before starting therapy
- (opioid dependence) drug should not be stopped abruptly, but gradually over 3 weeks
- (opioid dependence, SC) patient should be stabilised on sublingual therapy for at least 7 days before starting SC therapy, which can be commenced the day after last sublingual dose was administered
- (opioid dependence, SC) patient may receive an additional 8 mg SC during dosing period if required (maximum dose 128 mg)
- (opioid dependence, SC) if transitioning from sublingual tablets to weekly or monthly SC injections, the following is recommended:
  - 2–6 mg sublingual = 8 mg SC weekly

  - 8–10 mg sublingual = 16 mg SC weekly = 64 mg SC monthly
  - 12–16 mg sublingual = 24 mg SC weekly = 96 mg SC monthly
  - 18–24 mg sublingual = 32 mg SC weekly = 128 mg SC monthly
- (opioid dependence) if transitioning from SC monthly to daily sublingual, dose should be administered on month after last monthly SC injection was given
- (opioid dependence) SC injections must only be administered by health professionals
- (opioid dependence, SC) SC sites include buttock, thigh and upper arm and should be rotated
- (transdermal patch) not suitable as an 'as needed (PRN)' analgesic because of delayed onset of action, including as pain relief immediately postsurgery
- (transdermal patch) if adequate analgesia cannot be achieved using 40 mg patch, therapy should be discontinued and stronger opioid used
- (transdermal patch) patient with severe febrile illness should be closely monitored as increased skin blood flow may increase drug absorption
- (transdermal patch) during titration of dose, dose should not be increased at less than 3-day intervals. Patch can be removed and stronger strength patch applied, or a second patch can be added. However, no more than 2 patches should be applied to any one site and dose should not be greater than 40 mg
- (transdermal patch) when discontinuing therapy, dose should be tapered downwards at 7-day intervals
- (transdermal patch) when therapy is stopped, another opioid should not be given within 24 hours
- IV/IM route should only be used when sublingual route is not available
- (prefilled syringes) needle cap may contain rubber latex which may cause hypersensitivity reaction in sensitive individuals
- risk of abuse/misuse is present
- (transdermal patches or IV/IM administration) not recommended for opioid dependence/withdrawal management
- (SC, modified-release solution) must not be administered IV or intradermally. Gel depot will form on contact with body fluids causing occlusion, local tissue necrosis and/or thromboembolic events
- (modified-release solution) contraindicated in those with history of hypersensitivity reactions
- see General Nursing points/Cautions for opioids (p. 1366)

Patient teaching and advice

Sublingual tablets

- advise patient that tablets should be kept under the tongue for at least 10 minutes before swallowing and nothing else to eat or drink until tablet is completely dissolved. Warn patient that tablets are less effective if chewed or swallowed

Transdermal patch

- patient should be instructed to stop any other opioid analgesics when starting therapy with transdermal patches. However, the patient should be encouraged to take analgesics until transdermal patch takes effect
- if patient develops a fever, he/she should be advised to monitor for any opioid adverse effects, because heat increases the release of the drug from the buprenorphine transdermal patch (increasing the risk of overdose and respiratory depression)
- advise patient to continue swimming, bathing or showering as normal as these have no effect on transdermal patches
- patient should be advised that transdermal patches should:
  - not be cut or damaged

 - be applied to skin on upper outer arms, upper chest or back or side of chest. Application area should not be red, irritated, burnt, scarred or damaged in any way. Application sites should be rotated and not reused within 3 weeks
 - be applied to cleaned (using water only) skin, with area completely dried before application. Hair can be clipped (not shaved) for application if necessary
 - be removed from pouch, then silver backing foil removed and patch applied to skin with pressure from the palm for 30 seconds, taking care not to touch sticky section. If the edges of the patch start to peel, they can be taped to the skin
 - be changed weekly
 - be replaced by new patch if old one falls off accidentally
 - not be exposed to external heat source(s) (e.g. electric blanket, hot water bottle, saunas, spas, sunbathing), because heat increases release of buprenorphine, increasing risk of overdose and respiratory depression
 - be carefully/safely disposed of (used patches should be folded (with adhesive sides sticking together), wrapped and disposed of carefully to prevent any misuse of product by non-patients)
- wash hands after applying patch
- ensure that patient understands which patch or combination of patches should be applied to skin, including no more than 2 patches being applied to same site
- patient should be instructed to rotate application sites to prevent irritation to area and patch not reapplied to same area within 3–4 weeks
- instruct patient to seek medical advice immediately if any of the following occur:
 - severe skin reaction after applying transdermal patch, including severe reddening, blistering or burning sensation
 - sudden fainting for no reason or after exercise/emotional excitement, rapid or erratic heartbeat
- warn patient against stopping therapy suddenly
- see General Patient teaching and advice for opioids (p. 1367)

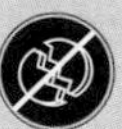

sublingual tablet can be dissolved under tongue or in cheek, but must not be chewed or swallowed

Note
- contained in Suboxone with naloxone

CODEINE PHOSPHATE HEMIHYDRATE (CODEINE PHOSPHATE) (Actacode Linctus, Codeine Linctus, Codeine Phosphate Tablets)

Available forms
Linctus: 5 mg/mL; Tablets: 30 mg

Action
- structurally similar to morphine and oxycodone
- 1/6 analgesic action of morphine
- metabolised in the liver to morphine and norcodeine
- antitussive action occurs as a result of suppression directly on cough centre in medulla, dries respiratory tract mucus and increases viscosity of bronchial secretions
- onset of analgesic action 15–30 minutes, duration 4–6 hours
- onset of antitussive action 1–2 hours, duration up to 4 hours
- half-life 2–4 hours
- withdrawal symptoms occur more slowly than morphine
- less euphoria or sedation than morphine

Use

- antitussive for unproductive dry and intractable cough
- relieves mild-to-moderate pain

Dose

- (pain relief) 30–60 mg orally 4–6-hourly **OR**
- (antitussive) 5 mL (25 mg) linctus orally 4–6-hourly

Adverse effects

- may increase plasma levels of amylase and/or lipase
- see also General Adverse effects of opioids (p. 1365)

Interactions

- metabolism may be decreased by cimetidine increasing risk of toxicity
- see also General Interactions of opioids (p. 1365)

Nursing points/Cautions/Patient teaching and advice

In 2018, the Department of Therapeutic Goods Administration (TGA) (Australia), amended previously Schedule 2 (Pharmacy Only) and Schedule 3 (Pharmacist Only) preparations containing codeine (e.g. Panadeine = paracetamol plus codeine) to become prescription-only (Schedule 4) (TGA 2018). This has resulted in a number of codeine-containing products no longer being produced by manufacturers.

- analgesic effect is variable between patients
- no benefit is gained by exceeding 60 mg per dose
- naloxone blocks the effects of codeine phosphate hemihydrate
- not recommended for chronic pain
- contraindicated in those under 12 years, or 12–18 years if respiratory function is compromised (e.g. post-tonsillectomy and/or adenoidectomy)
- contraindicated in those with hypersensitivity to morphine or oxycodone
- contraindicated in patients with acute respiratory depression with cyanosis and excessive bronchial secretions as these may be exacerbated
- see General Nursing points/Cautions for opioids (p. 1366) and General Patient teaching and advice for opioids (p. 1367)

linctus is available. Tablet can be crushed and mixed with water or spoonful of yoghurt or apple puree

Note

- contained in Aspalgin, Brufen Plus, Codalgin Forte, Codapane, Codapane Forte, Codapane Xtra, Codral Original Cold and Flu Tablets, Codral Original Day & Night Cold & Flu, Comfarol Forte, Dolased Forte, Ibudeine, Mersyndol, Mersyndol Day Strength, Mersyndol Forte, Mydol 15, Nurofen Plus, Painstop Day-Time Pain Reliever, Painstop Night-Time Pain Reliever, Panadeine Forte, Panamax Co., Prodeine, Prodeinextra, Prodeine Forte

FENTANYL (Denpax, Dutran, Durogesic, Fenpatch, Fentora)

FENTANYL CITRATE (Abstral, Actiq, DBL Fentanyl Injection, Sublimaze)

Available forms

Transdermal patches: 12 microgram/hour, 25 microgram/hour, 50 microgram/hour, 75 microgram/hour, 100 microgram/hour; Ampoules: 100 microgram/2 mL, 500 microgram/10 mL; Lozenges: 200 microgram, 400 microgram, 600 microgram, 800 microgram, 1.2 g, 1.6 g; Sublingual tablets: 100 microgram, 200 microgram, 300 microgram, 400 microgram, 600 microgram, 800 microgram; Orally disintegrating tablets: 100 microgram, 200 microgram

Action

- potent opioid analgesic that acts on mu receptors (brain, spinal cord, smooth muscle)
- more potent analgesic effect than morphine
- peak respiratory depression seen in 15–30 minutes after administration and lasts for several hours (longer than analgesic effects)
- duration of action 0.5–2 hours (SC, IM, IV, IT), 6–8 hours (oral) or 3 days (transdermal patch)
- half-life 3–12 hours (IV), 22–25 hours (transdermal patch, after 72-hour application) and 7 hours (oral)
- clearance is reduced and half-life increased in the elderly
- rarely produces histamine release and related adverse effects
- 157 microgram fentanyl citrate = 100 microgram fentanyl

Use

- premedication
- induction and maintenance of anaesthesia
- adjunct to general/regional anaesthesia
- postoperatively (in recovery room)
- chronic pain, including breakthrough pain

Dose

- (premedication) 50–100 microgram IM 30–60 minutes before surgery **OR**
- (adjunct to general anaesthesia) 50–100 microgram IV, repeated at 2–3-minute intervals until desired effect is achieved, then 25–50 microgram IV or IM (maintenance) **OR**
- (adjunct to regional anaesthesia) 50–100 microgram IM or slow IV if additional anaesthesia is required during procedure **OR**
- (postoperatively) 50–100 microgram IM repeated 1–2-hourly as necessary **OR**
- (transdermal patches) initially 25 microgram/hour patch replaced 72-hourly, then titrate up or down by 12–25 microgram/hour patch every 3 days **OR**
- (breakthrough pain (sublingual tablets)) initially 100 microgram orally sublingually, if adequate pain relief is achieved after 30 minutes; this dose should be used for further episodes of breakthrough pain. If adequate pain relief is not achieved after 30 minutes, a second 100 microgram dose may be given (no more than 2 tablets/episode of breakthrough) pain. If this does not relieve pain, next dose should be higher (daily maximum 800 microgram) **OR**
- (breakthrough pain (lozenge)) initially 200 microgram lozenge orally over 15 minutes; after waiting 15 minutes, if analgesia is inadequate, a second 200 microgram lozenge may be consumed. This dose (200 or 400 microgram) may then be used for several episodes of breakthrough pain, but if still inadequate, the dose may be increased (maximum daily dose 4 lozenges (4 episodes of breakthrough pain))

Adverse effects

- (IV) bradycardia, myoclonic movements, muscle rigidity
- (patches) skin irritation, rash, pustules, redness, oedema, itching
- (lozenge) gum bleeding, irritation, pain, ulcer, dental caries, gingivitis
- see General Adverse effects of opioids (p. 1365)

Interactions

- increased risk of respiratory depression and hypotension (and sometimes hypertension) if given with droperidol, therefore blood pressure should be closely monitored during concurrent therapy
- (IV) increased risk of severe bradycardia, hypotension and sinus arrest if given with amiodarone

- increased risk of serotonin syndrome if given with SSRIs, SNRIs and other serotoninergic agents
- cardiovascular depression may occur if given in high doses with nitrous oxide
- (IV) increased risk of severe hypotension if given with calcium-channel blockers or beta-adrenoceptor blocking agents
- see General Interactions of opioids (p. 1365)

Nursing points/Cautions

- see General Nursing points/Cautions for opioids (p. 1366)
- (transdermal patch) opioid-naive patient should be initially managed using immediate-release opioid to establish dose before commencing transdermal patch
- background persistent pain should be controlled with other opioid analgesics before starting therapy with lozenges for breakthrough pain. If patient experiences more than 4 episodes of breakthrough pain per day, a dose of background (long-acting) opioid analgesic will need adjusting. If this occurs, fentanyl lozenge dose may also require adjusting
- patients experiencing adverse effects should be monitored for at least 24 hours post-discontinuation due to long half-life
- lozenges and sublingual tablets are only recommended in those who have been previously treated with opioid analgesics (not opioid-naive patients)
- (sublingual tablets) no more than 2 sublingual tablets and an interval of at least 2 hours is recommended per episode of breakthrough pain
- to convert from oral formulations to transdermal patches, calculate the previous 24-hour analgesic amount, then convert to equi-analgesic oral morphine dose using the manufacturer's instructions (e.g. 45 mg morphine orally daily is roughly equivalent to 12 microgram/hour patch) (equi-analgesic dose refers to dose of one analgesic that is equivalent in pain-relieving effect to that of another analgesic)
- switching from one brand of transdermal patch to another should be done cautiously because of different properties and should be carried out under medical supervision
- respiratory depression may occur within 15–30 minutes of administration and persist for several hours in non-tolerant (opioid naive – no previous exposure to opioids) patients. Risk of respiratory depression is less in those who have developed tolerance to opioids
- (lozenge) if respiratory depression occurs, lozenge should be removed immediately
- (lozenge) contains almost 2 g glucose per lozenge which may be important in blood glucose level management in those with diabetes
- (sublingual tablets) caution if used in those with mouth ulcers or mucositis
- (IV) patient should be closely monitored during therapy for any signs of respiratory depression. Resuscitation equipment should be readily available
- (IV) when fentanyl and a neuroleptic agent (e.g. droperidol) are given in combination, adverse effects that may be observed include chills, shivering, restlessness, postoperative hallucinations (sometimes with transient mental depression) and extrapyramidal symptoms (up to 24 hours postoperatively)
- (IV) incompatible with thiopentone
- (transdermal patches, lozenges) not recommended for use in those who are non-tolerant (opioid naive) with non-cancer pain
- caution if used in those with liver or kidney impairment or the elderly

(because of reduced clearance and prolonged half-life)

- (transdermal patch) contraindicated for acute or postoperative pain where dose cannot be titrated, where pain can be managed by non-opioid agent, where prn analgesia/starting dose > 25 microgram/hour, or in those with acute respiratory disease and respiratory depression
- (IV) contraindicated in those with myasthenia gravis

Patient teaching and advice

- see General Patient teaching and advice for opioids (p. 1367)
- advise patient to take extra care in storage and disposal of lozenges/patches if children are in the household as dose can be fatal in children

Lozenge

- advise patient that lozenges should be sucked, not chewed, moved around inside cheek (using applicator provided) to maximise surface area exposure and held for 15 minutes
- instruct patient that lozenge should be used before or after food, but not with food or drink
- advise patient to moisten mouth with water before using lozenge if dry mouth is a problem
- lozenges contain glucose (1.89 g/dose) and it is therefore important to instruct patient to brush teeth regularly during therapy to prevent dental caries
- patients with diabetes should be warned about glucose content (1.89 g/dose) of lozenge
- instruct patient to tell doctor if lozenge is required more than 4 times per day

Sublingual tablets

- instruct patient that sublingual tablets should be:
  - removed carefully from foil container so as not to damage tablet
  - placed under the tongue as far back as possible and allowed to dissolve, not sucked, chewed or swallowed
  - not taken with food or drink
- advise patient to moisten mouth with water before using sublingual tablet if dry mouth is a problem
- patient should be instructed not to take more than 2 tablets per episode of breakthrough pain and to wait at least 2 hours before taking more tablets
- instruct patient to tell doctor if sublingual tablets are required more than 4 times per day for 4 consecutive days

Transdermal patches

- patient should be advised that patches should:
  - not be cut or damaged
  - be applied to non-irritated, non-scarred and non-irradiated skin (torso or upper arms)
  - be changed every 72 hours
  - only be worn one at a time
  - be dated to remind patient when next patch is due
  - not be exposed to external heat source(s) (e.g. electric blanket, hot water bottle, saunas, spas, sunbathing), because heat increases release of fentanyl, increasing risk of overdose and respiratory depression
  - be carefully/safely disposed of (used patches should be folded (with adhesive sides sticking together), wrapped and disposed of carefully to prevent any misuse of product by non-patients)
- patient should be instructed to rotate application sites to prevent irritation to area
- advise patient that hair can be clipped (not shaved) for application if necessary. Skin should be cleaned (using water only) and area completely dried before application
- instruct patient to remove patch from pouch, apply to skin with pressure

from the palm for 30 seconds, avoiding contact with the adhesive
- if gel contacts the skin of the carer or healthcare worker, it should be washed with copious amounts of water only
- instruct patient to wash hands after applying patch
- advise patient to wait until patch has been in situ (in place) for at least 24 hours and other analgesic doses have been titrated accordingly before making initial evaluation of effectiveness of patch
- if removed because of adverse effects, continue to monitor patient for at least 24 hours
- if patient develops a fever, he/she should be advised to monitor for any opioid adverse effects, because heat increases the release of fentanyl from transdermal patch (increasing risk of overdose and respiratory depression)

sublingual tablets can be placed under the tongue and allowed to dissolve. Lozenge should be allowed to dissolve over 15 minutes

Note
- contained in Marcain with Fentanyl (with bupivacaine) and in Naropin with Fentanyl (with ropivacaine)

HYDROMORPHONE HYDROCHLORIDE (Dilaudid, Jurnista)

Available forms
Tablets: 2 mg, 4 mg, 8 mg; Tablets (modified release): 4 mg, 8 mg, 16 mg, 32 mg, 64 mg; Oral liquid: 1 mg/mL; Ampoules: 2 mg/mL, 10 mg/mL, 50 mg/5 mL, 50 mg/mL

Action
- opioid mu receptor agonist that is related to morphine, but 5–8 times more potent
- duration of action 2–4 hours (orally) or 4–5 hours (IM, SC or IV)
- half-life is approximately 2.6 hours

Use
- moderate-to-severe pain

Dose
Non-tolerant (opioid-naive) patients
- 4–8 mg orally daily, titrating dose upwards/downwards by 4–8 mg increments every 4 days if needed (modified-release tablets) **OR**
- 2–4 mg orally 4-hourly **OR**
- 1–2 mg IM or SC 4–6-hourly **OR**
- 0.5–1 mg by slow IV over 2–3 minutes **OR**
- 0.3 mg/hr by IV infusion **OR**
- (patient-controlled analgesia) 0.1 mg/hr IV (background infusion) plus patient-administered bolus 0.2 mg at 5-minute intervals (1.2 mg/hour maximum)

Patients currently receiving opioids
- starting dose is based on previous day's opioid dose (converted using manufacturer's instructions)

Adverse effects
- (IV) injection site irritation
- see General Adverse effects of opioids (p. 1365)

Interactions
- see General Interactions of opioids (p. 1365)

Nursing points/Cautions
- in opioid-naive patient, dose should be established using immediate-release preparation before commencing on modified-release tablets
- (modified-release tablets) patient may require immediate-release opioid for breakthrough pain in addition to regular modified-release preparation
- (IV) Dilaudid-HP is a high-potency preparation and is only recommended for use in opioid-tolerant patients, therefore use caution when selecting correct formulation

- (IV) incompatible with soluble barbiturates
- oral solution contains hydrobenzoate which may cause allergic reaction in sensitive patients
- caution if used pre- or intra-operatively or within 24 hours postoperatively
- not recommended within 24 hours of chordotomy or other pain-relieving procedures
- see General Nursing points/Cautions for opioids (p. 1366)

Patient teaching and advice

- patient to be advised to swallow modified-release tablets whole, not crushed, chewed or divided
- see General Patient teaching and advice for opioids (p. 1367)

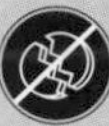

oral liquid available. Plain tablet can be crushed and mixed with water, but modified-release tablet should not be crushed, broken or chewed

METHADONE HYDROCHLORIDE (Aspen Methadone Syrup, Biodone Forte, Physeptone)

Available forms

Oral liquid: 5 mg/mL; Tablets: 10 mg; Ampoules: 10 mg/mL

Action

- synthetic opioid with properties similar to morphine, but less hypnotic
- duration of action 4–24 hours (oral, IM or IV)
- long half-life of 15 hours in non-tolerant (opioid naive) people, increasing to 22 hours with chronic use (with variation of 15–60 hours being reported)

Use

- severe pain (especially visceral)
- substitution therapy in the treatment of opioid dependence (Biodone Forte)

Dose

- (analgesia) initially 5–10 mg orally, SC or IM 6–8 hourly **OR**
- (opioid dependence) initially 10–20 mg orally, increasing by 5–10 mg daily, then 30–50 mg as maintenance (daily maximum 80 mg)

Adverse effects

- see General Adverse effects of opioids (p. 1365)
- (injection site) pain, induration, local irritation
- (rare, high dose) prolongation of QT interval
- (prolonged use) gynaecomastia

Interactions

- contraindicated with other agents that prolong QT interval or cause electrolyte disturbance especially hypokalaemia or hypomagnesaemia
- phenytoin, rifampicin, St John's wort, protease inhibitors, efavirenz, nevirapine and carbamazepine may increase metabolism of methadone, lowering the serum level and increasing the risk of withdrawal symptoms
- metabolism may be decreased by fluconazole and some SSRIs (particularly fluvoxamine)
- may increase serum levels of fluconazole, nelfinavir, desipramine and zidovudine
- may decrease serum levels of abacavir and amprenavir
- may cause false positive urine test (using Gravindex test)
- see General Interactions of opioids (p. 1365)

Nursing points/Cautions

- (opioid dependence) dose increases should not be greater than 5–10 mg daily or 30 mg in a 7-day period
- (opioid dependence) part of the Opiate Dependence Program requiring special authority
- addition of non-opioid analgesic to methadone improves analgesia

- because of long half-life, repeated doses should be given with caution
- IV infusion of naloxone is recommended if overdose occurs because of ongoing risk of respiratory depression associated with methadone's long half-life. Patient should be observed for at least 48 hours after recovery in case of relapse
- caution if used in those with phaeochromocytoma
- (syrup) contraindicated in those with hypersensitivity to permicol red
- contraindicated in those with congenital long QT syndrome or at risk of long QT syndrome (e.g. cardiac hypertrophy), hypokalaemia or hypomagnesaemia
- see General Nursing points/Cautions for opioids (p. 1366)

Patient teaching and advice

- advise patient to immediately seek medical advice if sudden fainting for no reason or after exercise/ emotional excitement, rapid or erratic heartbeat occurs
- see General Patient teaching and advice for opioids (p. 1367)

oral liquid available. Tablet can be dispersed in water or crushed and mixed with spoonful of yoghurt or apple puree

MORPHINE HYDROCHLORIDE TRIHYDRATE (MORPHINE HYDROCHLORIDE) (Morphine Juno, Ordine)

MORPHINE SULFATE PENTAHYDRATE (MORPHINE SULFATE) (Anamorph, DBL Morphine Sulfate Injection BP, Kapanol, Momex SR, Morphine MR, MS Contin, MS Mono, Sevredol)

Available forms

Oral solution: 1 mg/mL, 2 mg/mL, 5 mg/mL, 10 mg/mL; Oral solution (controlled-release granules): 20 mg, 30 mg, 60 mg, 100 mg, 200 mg; Tablets: 10 mg, 20 mg, 30 mg; Capsules: 10 mg, 20 mg, 50 mg, 90 mg, 100 mg, 120 mg; Capsules (controlled-release): 10 mg, 20 mg, 30 mg, 50 mg, 60 mg, 90 mg, 100 mg, 120 mg; Tablets (controlled-release): 5 mg, 10 mg, 15 mg, 30 mg, 60 mg, 100 mg; Ampoules: 5 mg/mL, 10 mg/mL, 15 mg/mL, 20 mg/mL, 30 mg/mL, 50 mg/mL, 100 mg/mL, 120 mg/1.5 mL, 400 mg/5 mL

Action

- opioid analgesic derived from opium with high affinity for mu receptors
- poor oral availability, undergoes extensive first-pass metabolism and has multiple active metabolites
- morphine-induced analgesia increases both pain threshold and pain tolerance
- alters response where patient is still aware of pain but not distressed by it
- peak effect 30–60 minutes (IM), 50–90 minutes (SC), 20 minutes (IV)
- duration of action varies with formulation (2–4 hours (oral solution, tablets), 12–24 hours (sustained-release preparations), 4–6 hours (IV, IM or SC))
- half-life is 1.5–2 hours

Use

- moderate-to-severe pain
- premedication (with atropine or hyoscine)
- supplementary analgesia during general anaesthesia
- chronic breathlessness

Dose

- 10–30 mg orally 4–6-hourly (immediate-release tablets) **OR**

- 5–20 mg orally 4-hourly (oral solution) **OR**
- initially 30 mg orally 12-hourly, then adjusted at 48-hour intervals according to breakthrough pain (sustained-release tablets) **OR**
- initially 20 mg orally 12-hourly or 40 mg orally daily, increasing the dose at 24-hour intervals minimum as needed (sustained-release capsules) **OR**
- initially 60 mg orally daily, increasing dose at 3-day intervals if needed (controlled-release capsules) **OR**
- (chronic breathlessness) 10 mg orally daily, increasing dose after 7 days if needed (maximum daily dose 30 mg) (sustained-release capsules) **OR**
- 5–20 mg SC or IM 4–6-hourly **OR**
- 2.5–15 mg by slow IV injection (over 4–5 minutes) diluted to at least 5 mL with water for injections **OR**
- 0.5–2 mg/hour by continuous IV infusion **OR**
- (patient-controlled analgesia (PCA)) 1 mg/hr background infusion, with 0.5–1.5 mg bolus doses via PCA pump, with lock-out interval of 6–10 minutes

Adverse effects
- (injection site) pain, induration, irritation
- (rare) supraventricular tachycardia
- see also General Adverse effects of opioids (p. 1365)

Interactions
- increased risk of severe hypotension and CNS depression if given with diazepam
- may decrease efficacy of diuretics by increasing release of antidiuretic hormone
- may potentiate effects of warfarin, therefore INR should be closely monitored, especially when starting or stopping therapy
- not recommended with zidovudine
- decreased serum levels may occur if given with ritonavir or rifampicin
- caution if given with cimetidine due to risk of apnoea, decreased respiratory rate and seizures
- if given with dexamphetamine, analgesic effect may be enhanced with reduced sedation
- may interfere with hepatobiliary imaging
- see also General Interactions of opioids (p. 1365)

Nursing points/Cautions
- shorter acting opioid should be tried before starting therapy with sustained-release preparation
- first dose of sustained-release preparation can be taken with last dose of immediate-release preparation
- (cancer pain) should be given around the clock (including waking patient at night to prevent morning pain)
- (sustained-release preparations) if breakthrough pain occurs at the end of the time interval the dose should be increased, NOT the frequency of administration
- (chronic breathlessness) breathlessness should be reviewed weekly using a validated tool to determine clinical effectiveness
- ensure that correct strength of tablets, syrup and controlled-release capsules and granules is selected, as they are available in varying strengths
- formulations are not bioequivalent
- 200 mg sustained-release preparation is only suitable for opioid-tolerant patients
- for patients using PCA, adequate assessment and education should be conducted before surgery to ascertain the patient's suitability. Only staff who have completed the required in-service sessions and associated assessment should care for patients with PCA, according to individual institution policy
- conversion from/to other opioid analgesics or other formulations of morphine should be done according to manufacturer's recommendations

(e.g. 10 mg morphine IM = 30 mg oral morphine). There may not be bioequivalence between different brands of same formulation (e.g. sustained-release capsules/tablets)

- (IM, SC) rotate injection sites to decrease pain and induration
- (IM, SC, IV) once analgesia is achieved, parenteral route should be changed to oral
- (IM, SC, IV) increases in dose should be made at no less than 24-hour intervals
- (IM, SC, IV) not normally mixed in the same syringe with other drugs, but is compatible with chlorpromazine, metoclopramide or prochlorperazine, as long as the resultant solution is used within 15 minutes and there is no precipitation
- (IV) incompatible with thiopentone, promethazine, barbiturates, pethidine and phenytoin
- have naloxone and resuscitation equipment readily available to reverse respiratory depression
- those over 50 years usually require lower doses
- (MS Contin, Momex SR) tablets contain lactose and are therefore not recommended in those with galactose intolerance, Lapp lactase deficiency or glucose–galactose malabsorption
- (chronic breathlessness, sustained-release preparations) not recommended for acute or acute-on-chronic breathlessness
- (sustained-release preparations) not recommended within 24 hours of cordotomy or other procedures that interrupt pain transmission pathway
- (SC, IM) caution if used in those with shock, especially if repeated doses are given, as overdose may occur when circulation is restored
- caution if used in those with kidney impairment due to risk of accumulation of active metabolite which may cause respiratory and CNS depression
- caution if used in those with atrial flutter or other supraventricular tachycardias
- (IV) continuous IV infusion is contraindicated in those with liver or kidney disease
- contraindicated in those with cardiac arrhythmias
- see General Nursing points/Cautions for opioids (p. 1366)

Patient teaching and advice

- advise patient to swallow sustained-release tablets whole, not chewed, crushed or broken/divided
- patient should be advised that sustained-release capsules should be swallowed whole, not chewed, crushed or broken. If swallowing is difficult, capsules may be opened and pellets sprinkled into 30 mL liquid (water, orange juice or milk) or soft food (yoghurt, custard, ice-cream, jam, apple sauce) and consumed within 30 minutes, taking care not to chew pellets. Another 30 mL of water should be used to rinse container to ensure entire dose has been taken. Pellets may also be sprinkled into water and administered via gastrostomy tube (not nasogastric tube), ensuring tube is flushed well before and after administration
- instruct patient to mix controlled-release granules with water (20, 30 and 60 mg in 10 mL; 100 mg in 20 mL and 200 mg in 30 mL) and take immediately with food. The resultant mixture should smell like raspberries and be an even red colour
- advise patient to use measuring cup or oral syringe to measure correct oral solution/syrup dose
- instruct patient to date bottle and discard oral solution/syrup 6 months after opening
- see General Patient teaching and advice for opioids (p. 1367)

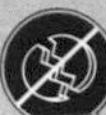

oral liquid is available. Sustained/modified-release tablets/capsules should not be crushed, broken or chewed. Plain (immediate-release) tablet can be crushed and mixed with water or spoonful of yoghurt or apple puree. Capsules can be opened and pellets dispersed in 30 mL of water, milk or apple juice or sprinkled on spoonful of yoghurt, apple puree, custard, ice cream or jam. Pellets should not be chewed

OXYCODONE (Proladone)

OXYCODONE HYDROCHLORIDE (Endone, OxyContin, OxyNorm)

Available forms

Tablets: 5 mg; Tablets (controlled-release): 5 mg, 10 mg, 15 mg, 20 mg, 30 mg, 40 mg, 80 mg; Capsules: 5 mg, 10 mg, 20 mg; Ampoules: 10 mg/mL, 20 mg/2 mL, 50 mg/mL; Suppositories: 30 mg

Action

- semi-synthetic opioid analgesic with actions similar to morphine
- (oral) onset of action 10–15 minutes, peak effect 30–60 minutes, duration of action 3–6 hours
- duration of action 4–6 hours (SC, IV) or 6–8 hours (rectal)
- half-life is about 2–4 hours
- see General Actions of opioids (p. 1364)

Use

- moderate-to-severe pain

Dose

- initially 5 mg orally after food 4–6-hourly, increasing dose as required (daily maximum 400 mg) (immediate-release tablet, oral solution) **OR**
- initially 5–10 mg orally 12-hourly, increasing dose as required (controlled-release tablets) **OR**
- 1 rectal suppository (30 mg) 6–8-hourly **OR**
- (10 mg/mL, 20 mg/mL) 1–5 mg IV bolus over 1–2 minutes, further doses may be given at 5–10-minute intervals if needed while monitoring patient, then 4-hourly (maintenance) **OR**
- 2 mg/hr by IV infusion **OR**
- (10 mg/mL) initially 5–10 mg SC, repeated 4-hourly as needed **OR**
- (patient-controlled analgesia (PCA)) 0.03 mg/kg IV bolus (patient lock-out 5 minutes) **OR**
- (50 mg/mL, opioid-tolerant patient in palliative care setting) initially 2 mg/hr IV infusion, then increasing dose as needed

Adverse effects

- injection site pain and hypersensitivity
- see also General Adverse effects of opioids (p. 1365)

Interactions

- may increase effects of warfarin, therefore INR should be carefully monitored especially when starting or stopping therapy
- see also General Interactions of opioids (p. 1365)

Nursing points/Cautions

- not recommended as first-line management for non-malignant pain; however, it can be used if patient assessment shows other analgesics to be ineffective, pain continues impacting on quality of life, there is no history of drug abuse or drug-seeking behaviour
- shorter acting opioid should be trialled before using controlled-release preparation
- if patient was previously on morphine, 1 mg IV oxycodone = 1 mg IV morphine; 2 mg oral oxycodone = 1 mg parenteral oxycodone
- if patient was previously on transdermal fentanyl, 10 mg oxycodone

oral (controlled-release) = 25 microgram fentanyl/hour (transdermal patch)
- IV bolus doses 5–15 mg are not recommended due to risk of sedation and respiratory depression
- IV solution should be diluted to 1 mg/mL with sodium chloride 0.9%, glucose 5% or water for injections before administering as IV bolus, infusion or as patient-controlled analgesia
- antagonised by acidifying agents and potentiated by alkalising agents
- incompatible with prochlorperazine and fluorouracil (5FU)
- 10 mg/mL and 20 mg/mL formulations are recommended via IV/SC injection or IV/SC infusion; 50 mg/mL formulation is recommended as IV/SC infusion, in palliative care setting
- (50 mg/mL) not recommended for more than 28 days consecutively
- 80 mg, 120 mg and 160 mg controlled-release tablets are recommended for opioid-tolerant patients only
- (controlled-release tablets) not recommended preoperatively or 24 hours postoperatively
- see General Nursing points/Cautions for opioids (p. 1366)

Patient teaching and advice

- patient should be advised to take controlled-release tablet whole, not crushed, broken or divided, as this may result in rapid release, overdose and respiratory depression
- advise patient to take tablets (immediate-release) whole with milk or food to reduce gastric upset
- instruct adult patient in correct technique for suppository insertion, including:
  - the need to empty bowel if possible before suppository insertion
  - wash hands with soap and water
  - if suppository feels soft, place it (unwrapped) in the fridge or hold it under cold water to firm it up
  - put on disposable glove if wanted
  - remove wrapper from suppository and moisten slightly by dipping in cool water
  - lie on side with knees raised to chest
  - push suppository (blunt end first) gently into rectum taking care not to break suppository
  - remain lying down for a few minutes to allow suppository to dissolve
  - wash hands thoroughly after insertion
- advise patient not to use bowels for at least 1 hour (if possible) after suppository insertion
- see also General Patient teaching and advice for opioids (p. 1367)

plain (immediate-release) tablet can be dispersed in water or crushed and mixed with spoonful of yoghurt or apple puree. Capsules can be opened and contents dispersed in water or mixed with spoonful of yoghurt or apple puree

Note

- contained in Targin with naloxone

PETHIDINE HYDROCHLORIDE (known as meperidine in the USA) (DBL Pethidine Injection BP, Pethidine Injection BP)

Available forms

Ampoules: 50 mg/mL, 100 mg/2 mL

Action

- synthetic opioid analgesic that acts on mu receptors with similar properties to morphine (not as effective in management of cough or diarrhoea)
- pethidine 75–100 mg = 10 mg morphine = 120 mg codeine = 200

microgram fentanyl = 8–10 mg methadone
- analgesia onset 10–15 minutes (IM, SC), 1 minute (IV), duration 3–5 hours (IM, IV, SC) (non-tolerant (opioid-naive) patients)
- active metabolite, norpethidine (half analgesic properties, but twice convulsant properties of pethidine)
- half-life 3.5 hours (pethidine) and 8–21 hours (norpethidine), therefore risk of accumulation and associated adverse effects is high (especially in those with liver impairment)

Use
- moderate-to-severe pain (short-term (24–36 hours) management)
- obstetric analgesia
- premedication
- adjunct to general anaesthesia

Dose
- (analgesia) 25–100 mg SC or IM 3–4-hourly, up to 150 mg for severe pain **OR**
- 25–50 mg 3–4-hourly by slow IV injection or infusion (diluted to at least 5 mL with sodium chloride 0.9%) (up to 200 mg daily) **OR**
- 0.3 mg/kg/hr as IV infusion **OR**
- (premedication) 50–100 mg IM or SC 30–90 minutes before start of anaesthesia **OR**
- (obstetric analgesia) 50–100 mg IM or SC when labour becomes regular; may be repeated 1–3-hourly (maximum daily dose 400 mg) **OR**
- (adjunct to analgesia) repeated slow IV injection of 10 mg/mL solution, not exceeding 25–50 mg **OR**
- (patient-controlled analgesia (PCA)) 5–20 mg bolus dose with 6–20-minute lock-out period (with or without background infusion) (not exceeding 800 mg/day)

Adverse effects
- see General Adverse effects of opioids (p. 1365), but has less constipation and urinary retention effects than morphine
- transient increase in BP and systemic vascular resistance
- (large dose, rapid administration) rapid respiratory depression, apnoea, hypotension, peripheral circulatory collapse, bradycardia, cardiac arrest
- pethidine-associated neurotoxicity (related to the long-acting metabolite norpethidine with symptoms including irritability, agitation, hypomania, tremor, paranoia, delirium, vertigo, headache, sweating, cold/clammy skin, pallor, hallucinations, seizures, respiratory depression)
- (IM) irritation, induration, fibrosis (with repeated injections)

Interactions
- contraindicated with anticoagulants
- phenobarbital (phenobarbitone) and phenytoin may increase metabolism and generation of norpethidine and increase risk of pethidine-associated neurotoxicity
- may cause recurrence of seizures if given with phenothiazines if the two are used in eclampsia
- metabolism inhibited by cimetidine
- see General Interactions of opioids (p. 1365)

Nursing points/Cautions

- IM is the preferred route of administration
- avoid intra-arterial route as this may result in necrosis and gangrene
- should be given slowly IV to prevent respiratory depression, hypotension, apnoea and bradycardia
- (IV) opioid antagonist and resuscitation equipment should be readily available
- (PCA) adequate assessment and education should be conducted before surgery to ascertain the patient's suitability. Only staff who

have completed the required in-service sessions and associated assessment should care for patients with PCA, according to individual institution policy
- compatible with chlorpromazine, metoclopramide, prochlorperazine or promethazine when mixed in the same syringe, as long as the resultant solution is used within 15 minutes and there is no precipitation
- physically or chemically incompatible with aciclovir, aminophylline, doxorubicin, furosemide (frusemide), heparin, idarubicin, imipenem, iodine, morphine, phenobarbital (phenobarbitone), phenytoin, sodium bicarbonate, sodium iodide, thiopentone, alkali, iodine and iodide solutions
- therapy should be limited to 24–36 hours to prevent pethidine-associated neurotoxicity due to accumulation of metabolite (norpethidine)
- (PCA) if dose is > 800 mg/day, the patient should be closely monitored for signs of pethidine-associated neurotoxicity (initial signs include anxiety and twitching)
- it is recommended that intraocular pressure is monitored if used in patients with glaucoma
- not recommended for pain associated with myocardial infarction
- contraindicated as IV infusion or patient-controlled analgesia in those with kidney impairment
- (PCA) contraindicated in patients with poor cognitive function
- contraindicated in patients with supraventricular tachycardia or cor pulmonale due to vagolytic action
- contraindicated during eclampsia or pre-eclampsia, during convulsive conditions (e.g. tetanus, strychnine poisoning, status epilepticus), during diabetic acidosis (with coma) or if patient has low platelet count or coagulation disorder
- see General Nursing points/Cautions for opioids (p. 1366)

Patient teaching and advice

- see General Patient teaching and advice for opioids (p. 1367)

REMIFENTANIL (DBL Remifentanil, Ultiva for Injection)

Available forms
Vial: 1 mg, 2 mg, 5 mg

Actions
- potent opioid analgesic
- selective mu opioid receptor agonist with rapid onset and very short duration of action with similar properties to fentanyl
- does not produce histamine release
- opioid and analgesic effect disappear within 5–10 minutes of stopping or reversal
- elimination half-life 3–10 minutes
- clearance is decreased during hypothermic cardiopulmonary bypass (decrease is about 3% per degree Celsius)
- see General Actions of opioids (p. 1364)

Use
- opioid adjunct during induction and/or maintenance of general anaesthesia
- analgesia and sedation in mechanically ventilated patients or in immediate postoperative period

Dose
- generally given by specialist anaesthetist

Adverse effects
- skeletal muscle rigidity, shivering
- hypotension, bradycardia, hypertension, tachycardia
- postoperative nausea, vomiting
- respiratory depression, apnoea, hypoxia

- pruritus
- (infusion site) erythema, pruritus, rash
- (post-procedure) fever, dizziness, headache, visual disturbances

Interactions

- increased sedation may occur if given with other CNS depressants
- may decrease dose requirements of inhaled or IV anaesthetics, hypnotics and/or benzodiazepines
- increased hypotension and bradycardia may occur if given with beta-adrenoceptor blocking agents or calcium-channel blocking agents

Nursing points/Cautions

- respiratory depression can occur for up to 30 minutes after administration, therefore it is important that the patient is fully conscious and spontaneously breathing before discharge from recovery area
- bolus dose should be given slowly (over at least 60 seconds) to prevent muscle rigidity (especially chest wall)
- depending on severity, muscle rigidity can be treated by decreasing rate or stopping remifentanil, using antagonist (naloxone), neuromuscular blocking agent and/or additional hypnotic. Patient may require intubation and ventilation
- reconstitute using water for injections, glucose 5% or sodium chloride 0.9% and then further dilute before administration
- if possible, should be administered via dedicated line which is removed after administration. If this is not possible, should be administered into fast-flowing IV close to venous cannula to prevent bolus dose being given if IV line is flushed
- incompatible with lactated Ringer's solution or propofol (in same infusion bag) or blood or blood products
- abrupt stopping is not recommended after prolonged administration
- caution if used in those with known sensitivity to opioids
- not recommended during labour or Caesarean section
- not recommended as sole agent during general anaesthesia, spontaneous ventilation anaesthesia or as analgesic in postoperative period
- contraindicated in those with hypersensitivity to fentanyl analogues or for epidural or intrathecal use
- see General Nursing points/Cautions for opioids (p. 1366)

Patient teaching and advice

- see General Patient teaching and advice for opioids (p. 1367)

TAPENTADOL HYDROCHLORIDE (Palexia IR, Palexia SR)

Available form

Tablets (sustained release): 50 mg, 100 mg, 150 mg, 200 mg, 250 mg; Tablets (immediate release): 50 mg

Action

- centrally acting synthetic analgesic with opioid and non-opioid activity
- binding affinity to mu receptors much less than morphine; however, only slightly less analgesic action
- noradrenaline (norepinephrine) reuptake inhibiting activity
- antagonised by naloxone
- no active metabolite
- elimination half-life 5–6 hours
- see also General Actions of opioids (p. 1364)

Use

- moderate-to-severe pain (unresponsive to non-opioid analgesia)

Dose

- initially 50 mg orally twice daily, increasing by 50 mg at 3-day intervals if needed (daily maximum 500 mg) (sustained-release tablets) **OR**
- initially 50 mg orally every 4–6 hours (daily maximum 700 mg), increasing

to 50–100 mg every 4–6 hours (to maintain adequate analgesia) (daily maximum 600 mg) (immediate-release tablets)

Adverse effects

- see General Adverse effects of opioids (p. 1365)
- (rare) suicidal ideation

Interactions

- see General Interactions of opioids (p. 1365)
- increased risk of serotonin syndrome if given with serotoninergic agents such as SSNIs, SNRIs, TCAs, MAOIs or triptans

Nursing points/Cautions

- in those already taking opioids, the dose should be initiated taking into account type, dose and frequency of previous opioid
- (immediate-release tablet) on first day, if pain control is not achieved within 1 hour, a second dose may be given
- withdrawal should be gradual to avoid withdrawal symptom
- not recommended in those under 18 years
- contraindicated in those with or suspected of having paralytic ileus or intoxication with alcohol, hypnotics, centrally acting analgesics or psychotropic agents
- see General Nursing points/Cautions for opioids (p. 1366)

Patient teaching and advice

- see General Patient teaching and advice for opioids (p. 1367)
- advise patient that sustained-release tablets should be swallowed whole, not chewed, broken or divided
- warn patient that shell of sustained-release tablet may not be totally digested and appear in bowel motion

plain (immediate-release) tablet can be crushed and mixed with water or spoonful of yoghurt or apple puree

TRAMADOL HYDROCHLORIDE (GA Tramadol Tramal, Tramal SR, Tramedo, Tramedo SR, Zaldiar, Zydol, Zydol SR)

Available forms

Capsules: 50 mg; Tablets (sustained release – once daily): 100 mg, 200 mg, 300 mg; Tablets (sustained release – twice daily): 50 mg, 100 mg, 150 mg, 200 mg; Ampoules: 100 mg/2 mL; Oral drops: 100 mg/mL

Action

- centrally acting synthetic analgesic with opioid-like properties without being chemically related to the opioids
- binds to mu opioid receptors
- blocks reuptake of noradrenaline (norepinephrine) and serotonin
- does not cause histamine release
- produces less respiratory depression than morphine
- little evidence to suggest drug abuse and dependence occurs
- active metabolite (desmethyltramadol) has a greater affinity for mu receptors and is more potent than tramadol. Elimination half-life of metabolite is 6–8 hours
- duration of action is 3–6 hours (oral) or 5–6 hours (IM)
- half-life is 5–7 hours
- half-life of both tramadol and its active metabolite are both increased in those with liver or kidney impairment

Use

- moderate-to-severe pain

Dose

- (postoperative) initially 100 mg IM or IV over 2–3 minutes, then 50–100 mg 4–6-hourly (maximum daily dose 600 mg) **OR**

- (less severe pain) 50–100 mg IM or IV over 2–3 minutes 4–6-hourly (maximum daily dose 400 mg) **OR**
- (moderate pain) 50–100 mg orally 2–3 times daily **OR**
- (moderate-to-severe pain) initially 100 mg orally, then 50–100 mg 4–6-hourly (maximum daily dose 400 mg) **OR**
- (SR preparations) 100–200 mg orally 1–2 times daily (depending on daily or twice daily preparations), increasing in 100 mg increments if needed (maximum daily dose 400 mg)

Adverse effects

- see General Adverse effects of opioids (p. 1365), but with less respiratory depression
- (rare) anaphylactoid reaction (sometimes after first dose), seizures

Interactions

- contraindicated with linezolid
- contraindicated with or within 14 days of MAOIs
- metabolism may be increased, lowering the serum level, if given with carbamazepine
- increased risk of convulsions if given with SSRIs, SNRIs, TCAs, antipsychotics or other agents that lower the seizure threshold
- caution if used with CNS depressants (alcohol, opioids, anaesthetics, phenothiazines, tranquillisers, sedatives/hypnotics)
- analgesic effect may be reduced by ondansetron
- increased risk of serotonin syndrome if given with SSRIs, SNRIs, TCAs, mirtazapine, and other serotonineric agents
- caution if used with warfarin, INR should be closely monitored, especially when starting or stopping therapy
- increased serum levels may occur if given with phenothiazine or antipsychotic agents, increasing risk of adverse effects
- not recommended with buprenorphine as analgesic action will be reduced
- not recommended with very light anaesthetics

Nursing points/Cautions

- IV injection should be given over at least 2–3 minutes
- (IV) incompatible with diclofenac, indometacin (indomethacin), diazepam, flunitrazepam, midazolam and glyceryl trinitrate
- naloxone reverses respiratory depression but not other symptoms of overdose
- caution if used for pain relief after throat surgery, tonsillectomy and/or adenoidectomy as patients are more susceptible to toxicity or overdose and should be carefully monitored
- (Tramal) SR tablets contain galactose and therefore should be used with caution in those with galactose intolerance, Lapp lactase deficiency or glucose–galactose intolerance
- not recommended for opioid withdrawal treatment
- contraindicated in those with acute alcohol intoxication
- see General Nursing points/Cautions for opioids (p. 1366)

Patient teaching and advice

- advise patient to take sustained-release preparations whole, not chew, crush, divide or break tablets
- see also General Patient teaching and advice for opioids (p. 1367)

oral drops are available. Capsules can be opened and contents dispersed in water or mixed with yoghurt or apple puree

Note

- contained with paracetamol in APO-Tramadol/Paracetamol

PREGNANCY, CHILDBIRTH AND BREASTFEEDING

The agents discussed in this section are those commonly used to treat infertility, to prevent premature labour or pre-eclampsia, are used during labour, or to suppress lactation.

AGENTS USED TO TREAT INFERTILITY

During the follicular stage, luteinising hormone (LH) stimulates ovarian theca cells to produce androgens, which are then used by ovarian granulosa cells to make estradiol (oestradiol), which supports the induction of follicle development by follicle-stimulating hormone (FSH). At mid-cycle, when LH levels are high, ovulation and subsequent corpus luteum formation are triggered, after which LH stimulates the production of progesterone by the corpus luteum. If fertilisation occurs, the progesterone level remains high, sustaining the endometrium and maintaining the pregnancy. However, if fertilisation does not occur, the production of progesterone by the corpus luteum decreases.

Infertility is defined as 'the inability to conceive after 12 months of unprotected sexual intercourse or after 6 months in women aged 35 years and over' (Hall 2018). Infertility may be due to male factors (e.g. sperm transport problems, hypogonadism, testicular disease, genetic disorders), female factors (e.g. insufficient LH, FSH or progesterone; tubal defects; endometriosis, polycystic ovary syndrome), both male and female factors and, in some cases, it may be unexplained.

Before starting any infertility treatment:

- discussion should take place about timing of intercourse and any modifiable factors, such as smoking, alcohol, caffeine and obesity (however, both high and low BMI can be associated with female infertility, as well as increased morbidity during pregnancy)
- the couple should have their infertility thoroughly investigated, and this may include:
  - confirmation of ovulation and tubal patency

  - identification of any menstrual cycle disorder or abnormal vaginal bleeding
  - evaluation of sperm quality and quantity via semen analysis
  - identification of any issues, such as ovarian failure, malformation of sexual organs or uterine fibroid tumours, that would be incompatible with pregnancy, otherwise LH preparations will be ineffective
  - identification and treatment of hypothyroidism, adrenocortical deficiency, hyperprolactinaemia, pituitary or hypothalamic tumours.
- any systemic disease which may worsen with pregnancy should be identified, and
- any contraindications to pregnancy identified (Hall 2018).

Infertility treatment may involve stimulation of ovulation with agents such as clomifene (clomiphene), intrauterine insemination, use of gonadotropins, in vitro fertilisation (IVF), or other assisted reproductive technologies. Success of infertility treatment is dependent on the age of the woman and the cause of the infertility. Because infertility, infertility treatment and its consequences can be extremely stressful, counselling and stress management should also be instigated early on as part of a holistic management plan (Hall 2018).

During infertility treatment:

- ultrasound monitoring (fluid in cul-de-sac, ovarian stigmata, collapsed follicle and secretory endometrium) and estradiol (oestradiol) measurement are recommended to minimise the risk of ovarian hyperstimulation syndrome and multiple pregnancy, and
- treatment should be individualised according to follicle size (determined by ultrasound) and oestrogen response.

General Adverse effects of infertility agents

- ovarian hyperstimulation syndrome (OHSS), resulting in large ovarian cysts that are prone to rupturing. OHSS commonly occurs 7–10 days after treatment with hCG and therefore the patient should be monitored (by ultrasound and estradiol (oestradiol) levels) for 14 days post-treatment for any signs and symptoms. Early symptoms begin with variable ovarian enlargement which progresses to abdominal pain and distension, nausea, vomiting, diarrhoea and weight gain. In its severest form, OHSS symptoms can include pericardial effusion, generalised massive oedema, hydrothorax, acute abdomen, pulmonary oedema, ovarian haemorrhage, DVT, ovarian torsion and acute respiratory distress. Progression to the most severe form of OHSS occurs if conception takes place, therefore it is imperative that any hyperstimulation is detected early and conception prevented. Treatment for OHSS includes rest, IV infusion with electrolytes or colloids and heparin. OHSS resolves spontaneously with the onset of menses, therefore the patient should refrain from intercourse or use barrier contraceptive methods for at least 4 days. Risk factors for OHSS include polycystic ovaries, previous episodes of OHSS, many follicles and a high level of estradiol (oestradiol).

If the woman has polycystic ovaries, it is recommended that the ovaries are monitored by ultrasound before and during stimulation to prevent OHSS
- increased risk of multiple pregnancies and births (related to number of embryos transferred)
- higher rate of miscarriage and congenital malformations (compared to the normal population)
- ectopic pregnancy
- thromboembolism
- headache, dizziness, fatigue
- (uncommon) mood swings, depression
- rash
- nausea, vomiting, abdominal pain
- ovarian disorder (including ovarian torsion), ovarian cysts, ovarian enlargement (with/without abdominal pain/distension), intermenstrual bleeding
- (injection site reaction) pain, redness, swelling, irritation, bruising, itching
- (rare) hypersensitivity, benign or malignant reproductive system neoplasms
- caution if used in those with porphyria as gonadotropins can increase risk of acute attack
- caution in those who have shown previous sensitivity to gonadotropin preparations (without FSH) because cross-sensitivity may occur. If given, patient should be closely observed after first injection
- contraindicated in those who have had prior hypersensitivity reaction to hCG or FSH preparations, primary ovarian failure, uncontrolled thyroid or adrenal dysfunction, uncontrolled hypothalamic or pituitary tumours, ovarian enlargement or cyst (not caused by polycystic ovarian disease), hormone-dependent tumours of the reproductive tract and accessory organs (including ovarian, breast and uterine cancer), uterine fibroid tumours (incompatible with pregnancy), post-menopausal, ectopic pregnancy (previous 3 months), active thromboembolic disorders or gynaecological haemorrhage (of unknown cause)

General Nursing points/Cautions for infertility agents

- pregnancy should be excluded before the start of therapy
- (ovulation induction) treatment regimen is highly individualised and requires clinical, biochemical (e.g. oestrogen levels) and ultrasonic monitoring
- first dose should be administered under supervision
- rotate SC injection sites
- caution if used in those with risk of thromboembolism or polycystic ovarian syndrome

General Patient teaching and advice for infertility agents

- before starting therapy, the patient and partner should receive counselling regarding the potential risk of multiple birth occurring
- patient should be advised to immediately seek medical advice if any of the following occur:
  - nausea, vomiting, diarrhoea, pelvic or abdominal pain, discomfort or distension (which may be early symptoms of OHSS)
  - swelling, redness, warmth or tingling in legs/arms, severe headache

or shortness of breath (possible sign of blood clot)
- patient should receive adequate education in the correct use of equipment, correct injection technique, importance of rotating sites, storage information and safe disposal of used equipment before self-administration can begin; the first injection should be under medical supervision
- warn patient against driving or operating machinery if dizziness occurs

CETRORELIX ACETATE (Cetrotide)

Available form
Vial: 250 microgram

Action
- luteinising hormone-releasing hormone (LHRH) antagonist, which controls the secretion of LH and FSH by the pituitary gland (also referred to as gonadotropin-releasing hormone (GnRH) antagonist)

Use
- prevention of premature luteinisation and ovulation in women undergoing controlled ovarian stimulation (followed by oocyte pick-up and assisted reproductive techniques)

Dose
- 250 microgram SC daily at 24-hour intervals (if given in the morning, should be started on day 5 or 6 of ovarian stimulation with FSH preparation, including day of ovulation induction with hCG or if given in the evening, should be started on day 5 of ovarian stimulation with FSH preparation and continued until evening before ovulation induction)

Adverse effects
- see General Adverse effects of infertility agents (p. 1390)

Nursing points/Cautions
- patient should be closely monitored for 30 minutes after first injection for any signs of allergic reaction
- cycle should only be repeated after risk benefit has been evaluated
- reconstitute with water for injections, and avoid vigorous shaking because it will denature product
- caution if used in those with any hypersensitivity to other GnRH products or any allergic predisposition
- contraindicated in those who have a hypersensitivity to extrinsic peptide hormone or mannitol or those with moderate or severe kidney/liver impairment
- see also General Nursing points/Cautions for infertility agents (p. 1391)

Patient teaching and advice
- see General Patient teaching and advice for infertility agents (p. 1391)

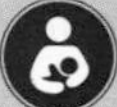
contraindicated during pregnancy and breastfeeding

CHORIOGONADOTROPIN ALFA (Ovidrel Pen)

Available form
Prefilled syringe: 250 microgram

Action
- recombinant hCG that stimulates late follicular maturation, resumption of oocyte meiosis and initiates rupture of pre-ovulatory ovarian follicle
- 250 microgram choriogonadotropin alfa is equivalent to urinary derived hCG 5000–10,000 IU in terms of number of oocytes retrieved

Use
- women undergoing superovulation prior to assisted reproductive

techniques, such as in vitro fertilisation (IVF)
- anovulatory or oligo-ovulatory women

Dose
- (women undergoing superovulation) 250 microgram SC 24–48 hours after last dose of FSH preparation **OR**
- (anovulatory or oligo-ovulatory women) 250 microgram SC 24–48 hours after optimal follicular growth stimulation has been achieved

Adverse effects
- see General Adverse effects of infertility agents (p. 1390)

Interactions
- may interfere with immunological determination of serum/urinary hCG for up to 10 days resulting in a false positive pregnancy test

Nursing points/Cautions
- if ovaries are abnormally large after FSH therapy, chorigonatropin alfa should be withheld because of increased risk of OHSS
- see General Nursing points/Cautions for infertility agents (p. 1391)

Patient teaching and advice
- (anovulatory or oligo-ovulatory women) the patient is advised to have intercourse on day of and day following administration
- see also General Patient teaching and advice for infertility agents (p. 1391)

permitted in sport for females only

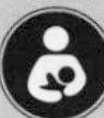
not recommended during pregnancy or breastfeeding

CHORIONIC GONADOTROPIN (HUMAN) (Pregnyl)

Available forms

Ampoules: 1500 IU, 5000 IU

Action
- action is identical to that of pituitary LH, although it also has some action on FSH
- hormone produced by placenta and is obtained from urine of pregnant women
- stimulates interstitial testicular cells to produce testosterone (males) and progesterone and oestrogens (females)

Use
- (males) hypogonadotropic hypogonadism, cryptorchism (not caused by obstruction), delayed puberty (because of insufficient gonadotropic pituitary function), sterility
- (females) improves function of the corpus luteum; sterility, inducing ovulation

Dose
- (anovulatory sterility) 5000–10,000 IU IM given in sequence with FSH to induce maturation of ovary, with a further 5000 IU given 7 days later if necessary to prevent insufficiency of corpus luteum **OR**
- (cryptorchism > 6 years) 1000 IU IM twice weekly for 6 weeks, course may be repeated if necessary **OR**
- (hypogonadotropic hypogonadism) 500–1000 IU IM 2–3 times weekly **OR**
- (delayed puberty) 1500 IU IM twice weekly for 6 months or more **OR**
- (sterility because of deficient spermatogenesis) 3000 IU IM weekly (with FSH-containing preparation)

Adverse effects
- (males, high dose) salt and water retention
- (male) antibody production resulting in ineffective results

- (males, rare) gynaecomastia
- see also General Adverse effects of infertility agents (p. 1390)

Interactions

- may interfere with immunological determination of serum/urinary hCG for up to 10 days resulting in a false positive pregnancy test

Nursing points/Cautions

- skeleton development should be monitored in pre-pubertal boys
- because active ingredient has been extracted from human urine, possibility of transmission of known or unknown pathogen exists
- caution if used in pre-pubertal boys because of increased risk of premature closure of epiphyses or precocious sexual development
- caution if used in those with cardiac failure, hypertension, kidney dysfunction, epilepsy or migraine as salt/water retention may aggravate these conditions
- contraindicated in males with known/suspected androgen-dependent tumours (e.g. prostate cancer, mammary)
- see also General Nursing points/Cautions for infertility agents (p. 1391)

Patient teaching and advice

- advise male patient to seek medical advice if any breast swelling or tenderness occurs
- see General Patient teaching and advice for infertility agents (p. 1391)

permitted in sport for females only

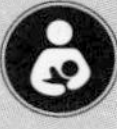

not recommended during breastfeeding

CLOMIFENE (CLOMIPHENE) CITRATE (Clomid)

Available form

Tablets: 50 mg

Action

- acts by stimulating output of pituitary gonadotropins, stimulating maturation of ovarian follicle and then development and function of corpus luteum

Use

- stimulate ovulation in infertile women with ovarian dysfunction

Dose

- initially 50 mg orally daily for 5 days starting on the 5th day of the menstrual cycle (any time if there is amenorrhoea), increasing to 100 mg for subsequent cycles if ovulation does not occur, repeated for a total of 3 cycles

Adverse effects

- hot flushes
- insomnia, increased nervous tension
- visual blurring, visual spots/flashes, 'after' images
- breast discomfort
- enlargement of existing uterine fibroids
- increased risk of ovarian cancer
- hypertriglyceridaemia, pancreatitis
- see also General Adverse effects of infertility agents (p. 1390)

Nursing points/Cautions

- pelvic examination is recommended before each cycle of treatment (to assess for ovarian cyst, ovarian cancer or pregnancy)
- therapy should be stopped if no ovulation occurs after 3 consecutive courses of therapy. Diagnosis should be re-evaluated
- record weight and record basal temperature to determine day of ovulation
- liver function and serum triglycerides should be assessed before starting therapy
- ophthalmic examination is recommended if visual disturbances occur

- caution if used in women with known uterine fibroids as they may enlarge during therapy
- caution if used in those with family history or pre-existing hyperlipidaemia (especially in those undergoing prolonged therapy)
- contraindicated in those women with liver dysfunction or disease
- see also General Nursing points/Cautions for infertility agents (p. 1391)

Patient teaching and advice

- patient should be advised to report any blurred vision or other visual symptoms immediately and stop therapy if they occur. Visual disturbances may be worse in brightly lit environments
- warn patient not to drive or operate machinery if visual blurring or headache occurs
- see General Patient teaching and advice for infertility agents (p. 1391)

banned in sport

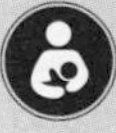
contraindicated during pregnancy and breastfeeding

tablet can be crushed and mixed with spoonful of yoghurt or apple puree

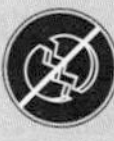
pregnant staff should not crush tablets

CORIFOLLITROPIN ALFA (Elonva)

Available forms

Prefilled syringe: 100 microgram/0.5 mL, 150 microgram/0.5 mL

Action

- gonadotrophin with sustained follicle-stimulating properties allowing once-weekly administration

Use

- controlled ovarian stimulation for follicle development and pregnancy in women undergoing assisted reproductive techniques

Dose

- (body weight ≤ 60 kg and ≤ 36 years) 100 microgram SC on day 1, followed by GnRH antagonist on day 5 or 6 depending on ovarian response (e.g. number/size of follicles and/or serum estradiol (oestradiol)), then on day 8, daily 150 IU FSH until there are 3 follicles ≥ 17 mm, followed by 5000–10,000 IU hCG (to induce final maturation) **OR**
- (body weight > 60 kg (regardless of age) or body weight > 50 kg and > 36 years) 150 microgram SC on day 1, then as above

Adverse effects

- see General Adverse effects of infertility agents (p. 1390)

Interactions

- not recommended with GnRH agonist

Nursing points/Cautions

- only one SC injection is recommended per cycle
- no FSH is recommended in first 7 days after SC administration
- not recommended in those with kidney impairment
- contraindicated in those with previous controlled ovarian stimulation resulting in > 30 follicles ≥ 11 mm (on ultrasound) or basal antral follicle count > 20
- see also General Nursing points/Cautions for infertility agents (p. 1391)

Patient teaching and advice

- see General Patient teaching and advice for infertility agents (p. 1391)

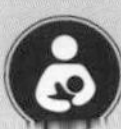

contraindicated during pregnancy and breastfeeding

FOLLITROPIN ALPHA (Bemfola, Gonal-f Pen)

Available forms

Prefilled syringes: 75 IU/0.125 mL, 150 IU/ 0.125 mL, 225 IU/0.375 mL, 300 IU/ 0.5 mL, 450 IU/0.75 mL, 900 IU/1.5 mL

Action

- recombinant human FSH that stimulates development of mature follicles (in females) and spermatogenesis (in males)

Use

- infertility in women (where clomifene (clomiphene) has failed or is contraindicated)
- controlled ovarian hyperstimulation (assisted reproductive technology)
- hypogonadotropic hypogonadism (where hCG alone is ineffective)

Dose

- (anovulatory infertility) starting in first 7 days of menstrual cycle, initially 75–150 IU SC daily, increasing if necessary by 37.5–75 IU at 7- or 14-day intervals until adequate response is achieved, followed by hCG preparation 24–48 hours after last injection (to induce follicular maturation) **OR**
- (controlled ovarian hyperstimulation) initially 150–225 IU SC daily, starting on day 2 or 3 of cycle and continued until adequate follicle development has occurred followed by hCG preparation 24–48 hours after last injection (to induce follicular maturation). Dose should be adjusted according to response (daily maximum 450 IU) **OR**
- (hypogonadotropic hypogonadism) 150 IU SC 3 times weekly with hCG preparation for at least 4 months

Adverse effects

- (males) gynaecomastia, acne, weight gain
- see also General Adverse effects of infertility agents (p. 1390)

Nursing points/Cautions

- (males) pre-treatment with hCG alone should be started to achieve testosterone level > 9–10 nanomol/L for up to 6 months, increasing dose if this is not achieved
- (males) serum should be analysed to determine clinical response
- (males) therapy can be continued for up to 24 months to achieve spermatogenesis
- (anovulatory infertility) if response is inadequate in 5 weeks, treatment should be stopped
- reconstitute with water for injections, and avoid vigorous shaking because it will denature product
- caution if used in those with porphyria as acute crisis may be triggered
- (males) contraindicated in men with primary testicular failure (elevated gonadotrophin levels) or infertility (from causes other than hypogonadotropic hypogonadism) or tumours of the hypothalamus or pituitary gland
- see also General Nursing points/Cautions for infertility agents (p. 1391)

Patient teaching and advice

- (anovulatory infertility) patient should be advised to have intercourse on day of and day following administration of hCG preparation
- advise male patient to seek medical advice if any breast swelling or tenderness occurs
- see General Patient teaching and advice for infertility agents (p. 1391)

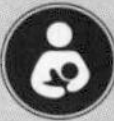

contraindicated during pregnancy and breastfeeding

Note

- contained in Pergoveris with lutropin alfa

FOLLITROPIN BETA (Puregon)

Available forms

Multidose cartridges: 300 IU/0.36 mL, 600 IU/0.72 mL, 900 IU/1.08 mL

Action

- recombinant human FSH

Use

- (females) anovulatory infertility; controlled ovarian hyperstimulation
- (males) hypogonadotropic hypogonadism

Dose

- (anovulatory infertility) initially 75–150 IU SC daily for 5–7 days, increasing dose if needed to achieve a rise in oestrogen level (40–100% increase is considered optimal), daily dose is maintained to achieve pre-ovulatory conditions estradiol (oestradiol) level 300–900 picogram/mL or total urinary estradiol (oestradiol) excretion 75–200 microgram/day and/or follicle ≥ 18 mm is present), followed by 5000–10,000 IU hCG. hCG (1000–3000 IU) may be repeated up to 3 times in the following 9 days to support the luteal phase **OR**
- (controlled ovarian hyperstimulation) 75–300 IU SC daily (alone, with clomifene (clomiphene) citrate or GnRH agonist), continued until adequate follicle development has occurred (≥ 3 follicles 16–20 mm), followed by hCG 5000–10,000 IU preparation 30–40 hours after last injection and oocytes retrieved 34–35 hours later. hCG (1000–3000 IU) may be repeated up to 3 times in the following 9 days to support the luteal phase after embryo transfer **OR**
- (hypogonadotropic hypogonadism) 75 IU SC daily or 2–3 times weekly (with 1000–2000 IU hCG preparation 2–3 times weekly) and continued for at least 12 weeks

Adverse effects

- (male) gynaecomastia, acne
- see General Adverse effects of infertility agents (p. 1390)

Interactions

- enhanced follicular response may be seen if given with clomifene (clomiphene)
- higher dose may be required following treatment with GnRH agonists

Nursing points/Cautions

- if oestrogen levels rise too fast (i.e. doubling daily for 2–3 days), dose should be decreased
- (male) testosterone should be stopped before starting therapy
- (male) semen analysis should be conducted 4–6 months after starting therapy
- caution if used in those with hypersensitivity to streptomycin or neomycin
- (male) contraindicated in those with primary testicular failure
- see also General Nursing points/Cautions for infertility agents (p. 1391)

Patient teaching and advice

- advise male patient to seek medical advice if any breast swelling or tenderness occurs
- see General Patient teaching and advice for infertility agents (p. 1391)

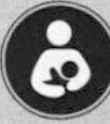

contraindicated during pregnancy and breastfeeding

GANIRELIX ACETATE (Orgalutran)

Available form

Prefilled syringes: 250 microgram/0.5 mL

Action
- GnRH antagonist that binds to GnRH receptors in the pituitary gland
- inhibitory effect is greater for LH release than for FSH
- pituitary recovers within 2 days of stopping therapy

Use
- prevention of premature luteinisation and ovulation in women undergoing controlled ovarian stimulation (followed by oocyte pick-up and assisted reproductive techniques)

Dose
- 250 microgram SC daily starting on day 5 or 6 of FSH therapy (depending on level of ovarian response) and continued until there are sufficient follicles of adequate size, followed by hCG to induce maturation and ovulation

Adverse effects
- headache, malaise
- nausea
- (injection site) redness (with or without swelling)
- (rare) OHSS, ectopic pregnancy, pelvic pain, abdominal distention

Nursing points/Cautions
- should not be mixed in same syringe with FSH, but should be administered at same time
- time between last ganirelix and hCG administration should not exceed 30 hours
- not recommended in those with allergy to latex rubber
- contraindicated in those with hypersensitivity to GnRH or GnRH analogues or with moderate-to-severe kidney or liver impairment
- see General Nursing points/Cautions for infertility agents (p. 1391)

Patient teaching and advice
- see General Patient teaching and advice for infertility agents (p. 1391)

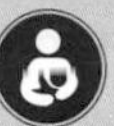
contraindicated during pregnancy and breastfeeding

LUTROPIN ALFA (Luveris 75 IU)

Available form
Vial: 75 IU

Action
- recombinant human LH
- binds to receptor shared with hCG

Use
- stimulation of follicular development in women with severe LH and FSH deficiency (usually with FSH preparation)

Dose
- 75 IU SC daily (with FSH preparation 75–150 IU) followed by hCG (5000–10,000 IU) when adequate response is obtained

Adverse effects
- see General Adverse effects of infertility agents (p. 1390)

Nursing points/Cautions
- if there is no response in 3 weeks, therapy should be stopped and restarted at a higher dose
- should not be mixed in same syringe with any other products except follitropin alfa
- treatment should be stopped if excessive response occurs and FSH levels may be decreased for next cycle
- contraindicated in those with hypersensitivity to gonadotrophins
- see General Nursing points/Cautions for infertility agents (p. 1391)

Patient teaching and advice
- patient should be advised to have intercourse on the day of and day following hCG administration. Alternatively, intrauterine (artificial)

insemination may be performed at this time
- see also General Patient teaching and advice for infertility agents (p. 1391)

permitted in sport for females only

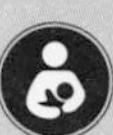
contraindicated during pregnancy or breastfeeding

Note
- contained in Pergoveris with follitropin alfa

MENOPAUSAL GONADOTROPHIN (HUMAN) (Menopur)

Available forms
Vial: 600 IU, 1200 IU

Action
- gonadotrophin that induces ovarian follicular growth and development and gonadal steroid production in women without primary ovarian failure

Use
- anovulatory infertility (including polycystic ovarian disease) in women unresponsive to clomifene (clomiphene) citrate
- controlled ovarian hyperstimulation to induce multiple follicle stimulation for assisted reproductive technologies

Dose
- (anovulatory infertility) initially 75–150 IU SC daily for at least 7 days, with subsequent doses depending on clinical monitoring and patient response. Dose may be increased by 37.5 IU at intervals not less than 7 days (daily maximum 225 IU). When optimal response is achieved, 5000–10,000 IU hCG should be given 1 day after last SC injection **OR**
- (controlled ovarian hyperstimulation) initially 150–225 IU SC daily for at least 5 days of therapy, with subsequent dose depending on clinical monitoring and patient response. Dose may be increased by not more than 150 IU per adjustment (daily maximum 450 IU)

Adverse effects
- see General Adverse effects of infertility agents (p. 1390)

Nursing points/Cautions
- may be used alone or with gonadotrophin-releasing hormone (GnRH) agonist or antagonist
- (anovulatory infertility) therapy should be started within 7 days of menstrual cycle
- (anovulatory infertility) if no response after 4 weeks of therapy, cycle should be stopped and restarted at higher starting dose than abandoned cycle
- (controlled ovarian hyperstimulation) should be started 2 weeks after the start of agonist treatment (protocol using downregulation with GnRH agonist) or on day 2 or 3 of menstrual cycle (protocol using downregulation with GnRH antagonist)
- (controlled ovarian hyperstimulation) therapy $>$ 20 days is not recommended
- to reconstitute, use one prefilled syringe of solvent (provided) for 600 IU vial and two prefilled syringes for 1200 IU vials
- roll vial between hands to dissolve any remaining powder after solvent has been added but avoid shaking
- see also General Nursing points/Cautions for infertility agents (p. 1391)

Patient teaching and advice
- (anovulatory infertility) patient should be advised to have sexual intercourse on the day of and day following hCG administration (or artificial insemination may be performed)

- see General Patient teaching and advice for infertility agents (p. 1391)

permitted in sport for females only

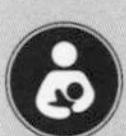
contraindicated during pregnancy

not recommended during breastfeeding

NAFARELIN ACETATE (Synarel)

Available form

Metered-dose nasal spray: 200 microgram/dose

Action

- GnRH analogue
- suppression of pituitary-gonadal system is restored 4–8 weeks after stopping treatment

Use

- endometriosis (visually proven) management (e.g. pain relief, reduce lesions)
- controlled ovarian stimulation program

Dose

- (endometriosis) initially 200 microgram to one nostril in the morning, then 200 microgram to the other nostril at night (total daily dose 400 microgram), starting on days 2–4 of the menstrual cycle, increasing to 400 microgram (given as 200 microgram to each nostril morning and night) (total daily dose 800 microgram) if symptoms of endometriosis are not controlled, for up to 6 months **OR**
- (controlled ovarian stimulation) 400 microgram twice daily given as 1 spray (200 microgram) to each nostril, morning and night, starting either day 2 or day 21 of the menstrual cycle. Once downregulation is achieved, gonadotrophin is commenced and nafarelin continued until hCG is given for follicular maturation (8–12 days)

Adverse effects

- hot flushes, headache, mood swings, insomnia
- changes in libido, vaginal dryness, decreased breast size
- acne, hirsutism, oily skin
- change in weight
- oedema
- myalgia
- irritation to nasal mucosa
- decreased bone density
- transient ovarian cysts
- increased cholesterol levels
- (rare) hypersensitivity, OHSS, multiple pregnancy

Nursing points/Cautions

- (endometriosis) bone density should be measured if symptoms recur and retreatment is necessary. Two-year interval between treatment cycles is recommended
- (controlled ovarian stimulation) should be stopped for 3 days before embryo transfer
- (controlled ovarian stimulation) if downregulation does not occur in 12 weeks, therapy should be stopped
- (controlled ovarian stimulation) caution if used in those with polycystic ovarian syndrome due to increased risk of excessive follicle development
- caution if used in women who are at risk of reduced bone mass (e.g. menstrual disturbances due to low weight or weight loss, athletic or other forms of hypothalamic amenorrhoea, immobilisation, glucocorticoid use or strong family history of osteoporosis). Baseline bone density should be measured before starting therapy in these at-risk women
- not recommended in women < 18 years

- contraindicated in women with undiagnosed abnormal vaginal bleeding or with hypersensitivity to GnRH or GnRH analogues

Patient teaching and advice

- if patient has rhinitis (runny nose), absorption of nafarelin may be decreased and may require use of nasal decongestant
- patient should be advised to allow at least 30 minutes between using nasal decongestant and nafarelin
- patient should be instructed regarding correct use of the nasal pump, including:
  - priming pump with 5–10 sprays to obtain even spray before first use
  - blowing nose before administration of nasal spray
  - correct technique
  - cleaning and storage requirements
- warn patient that symptoms of endometriosis may be exacerbated during the first few weeks of treatment
- patient should be advised to immediately contact doctor if one or more doses are missed as there is a potential for breakthrough ovulation to occur. A pregnancy test may be recommended in this situation
- patient should be counselled to use barrier methods of contraception during therapy and pregnancy should be excluded before starting therapy

permitted in sport for females only

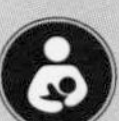

contraindicated during pregnancy due to risk of abortion or fetal abnormality

contraindicated during breastfeeding

PROGESTERONE (Crinone 8%, Endometrin, Oripro, ProFeme Cream, Prometrium, Utrogestan)

Available forms

Vaginal gel (prolonged release): 90 mg/applicator; Vaginal pessaries: 100 mg, 200 mg; Cream: 32 mg/g, 100 mg/g; Capsules: 100 mg

Action

- naturally occurring female sex hormone secreted from the ovary, placenta and adrenal gland
- if fertilisation occurs, progesterone levels remain high and this sustains the endometrium and maintains pregnancy
- rapidly absorbed from vagina

Use

- assisted reproductive technology in infertile women with progesterone deficiency (requiring supplementation to support embryo implantation and maintenance of pregnancy)
- preterm birth prevention with singleton pregnancy (in women with short cervix ≤ 25 mm)
- progesterone-deficient conditions (e.g. natural or surgical menopause)
- menstrual irregularities
- hormone replacement therapy (HRT) (with oestrogen product)

Dose

- (pessary) 100 mg intravaginally 1–2 times daily, starting within several days of ovulation and continued until approximately 11 weeks gestation (daily maximum 400 mg twice daily) (Oripro) **OR**
- (pessary) 100 mg intravaginally 3 times daily, starting at oocyte retrieval and continuing for 10 weeks (Endometrin) **OR**
- (pessary) 200 mg intravaginally 3 times daily from embryo transfer until at least 7th week of pregnancy

(and no later than 12th week) (Utrogestan) **OR**
- (prevention of preterm labour) 200 mg intravaginally nightly, from 16–24 weeks gestation and continued to 36 weeks or until delivery (Oripro, Utrogestan) **OR**
- (threatened miscarriage) 200–400 mg intravaginally daily as 2 divided doses until week 12 (Utrogestan) **OR**
- (gel) 90 mg (one application) intravaginally 1–2 times daily, starting 2 days after hCG administration, and continuing for 10–12 weeks if pregnancy occurs **OR**
- (HRT, intact uterus) 200 mg orally at night, from day 15–26, withdrawal bleeding following next week (with oestrogen) **OR**
- (HRT, intact uterus) 100 mg orally at night, from day 1–25, withdrawal bleeding following next week (with oestrogen) **OR**
- (secondary amenorrhoea) 400 mg orally nightly for 10 days **OR**
- (menstrual irregularities due to ovulation disorder, anovulation) 200–300 mg orally daily as single or divided dose (200 mg orally nightly, 100 mg morning (if needed)) for days 17–26 of menstrual cycle **OR**
- (menopause) 0.3 mL (30 mg) (10% cream) or 1 mL (32 mg) (3.2% cream) daily or in divided doses for either 25 days per calendar month or 3 weeks on and 1 week off (Profeme) **OR**
- (peri-menopause) 0.3 mL (30 mg) (10% cream) or 1 mL (32 mg) (3.2% cream) daily or in divided doses from day 12–26 of menstrual cycle (if menstrual cycle begins before day 26) (Profeme) **OR**
- (premenstrual syndrome) 0.3 mL (30 mg) (10% cream) or 1 mL (32 mg) (3.2% cream) daily or in divided doses from day 12–26 of menstrual cycle (Profeme) **OR**
- (premenstrual dysphoric disorder) 0.5–1 mL (50–100 mg) daily or in divided doses from day 12 to 26 (Profeme 10% only) **OR**
- (endometriosis, menorrhagia, postpartum depression) 1–2 mL (100–200 mg) daily or in divided doses (depending on condition severity), can be started day 12–26, but frequency can be increased to 3 weeks in 4 if symptoms recur after stopping therapy (Profeme 10% only) **OR**
- (infertility) 1 mL (100 mg) daily or in divided doses from day 12–26 until pregnancy is confirmed and then continued at 1–2 mL until at least week 13 or full term (Profeme 10%) **OR**
- (repeated first term miscarriage) 0.3 mL (30 mg) daily or in divided doses from day 12–26 until pregnancy is confirmed. If spotting occurs at week 6 or 7, 1–2 mL (100–200 mg) 2–3 times daily can be used until full term (Profeme 10%)

Adverse effects

- amenorrhoea, abnormal breakthrough bleeding, metromenorrhagia, spotting, genital itchiness, dyspareunia, perineal pain, uterine spasm, vaginal discomfort/burning/dryness, vaginal discharge
- abdominal cramping/distention/pain, bloating, weight gain
- breast pain/tenderness, breast swelling/enlargement, galactorrhoea
- fluid retention
- papillary oedema, retinal haemorrhage
- rash, pruritus
- arthralgia
- nocturia
- headache, dizziness, drowsiness
- depression, decreased libido, nervousness, somnolence, insomnia
- nausea, vomiting, diarrhoea
- hyperglycaemia, hyperlipidaemia
- ovarian enlargement, ovarian cyst formation
- (rare) thromboembolism

- (abrupt discontinuation) anxiety, moodiness, seizures

Interactions

- effects may be decreased if given with carbamazepine, phenobarbital (phenobarbitone), phenytoin, rifabutin, rifampicin or St John's wort
- may decrease serum levels of ciclosporin
- effects may be increased by itraconazole
- may potentiate levothyroxine levels potentially leading to hyperthyroidism
- glucose tolerance test and coagulation test results may be affected
- liver, thyroid and endocrine function tests may be affected
- serum levels may be decreased by aminoglutethimide
- metyrapone test may show lower response than usual
- not recommended with other vaginal products

Nursing points/Cautions

- before starting therapy, breast, abdominal and pelvic organ examination is recommended, as well as a Papanicolaou (Pap) smear
- (cream) symptoms generally diminish 8–12 weeks after starting therapy
- (secondary amenorrhoea) causes of secondary amenorrhoea, such as outflow obstruction, prolactinoma, thyroid disorders, pituitary and hypothalamic disorders, should be excluded before starting therapy
- (Endometrin) women under 35 years with adequate ovarian reserve, twice daily application is appropriate; women over 35 years with decreased ovarian reserve, 3 times daily application is necessary
- caution if used in women with history of depression
- caution if used in women with diabetes mellitus as glucose tolerance may be altered during therapy
- caution if used in those women whose conditions would be aggravated by fluid retention (e.g. asthma, cardiac, migraine, renal dysfunction), or with a history of depression, diabetes mellitus or hyperlipidaemia
- caution if used in those with myocardial infarction, cardiovascular disorders or retinal thrombosis, mild-to-moderate liver dysfunction
- caution if used in those > 35 years, smokers or with risk factors for atherosclerosis due to risk of retinal vascular lesions
- contraindicated in women with a hypersensitivity to hard fat or with porphyria, vaginal or urinary tract bleeding (of unknown origin), liver impairment, deep vein thrombosis, pulmonary embolism, previous hormone-associated thrombophlebitis or thromboembolism, seizure disorder, missed abortion or ectopic pregnancy, or cancer (ovary, breast or uterine)
- contraindicated in pregnancy during assisted reproductive technology when normal progesterone levels are present

Patient teaching and advice

- instruct patient that pessary should be inserted deep into vagina while squatting or lying on back or side and that no other intravaginal preparations should be used at the same time
- advise patient that if pessary is used once daily, preferably administer in the evening
- patient should be instructed to seek medical advice immediately if any sudden severe headache and/or visual disturbances occur
- (vaginal gel) instruct patient to shake down gel applicator, holding on to the thick end without removing cap. When gel is in the thin end, twist off

tab and insert applicator deep into vagina and press thick end to deposit prolonged-release gel. Remove applicator and discard appropriately

- warn patient not to drive or operate machinery if dizziness or drowsiness occurs
- instruct patient that capsules should be taken at bedtime without food
- ensure patient has the following information regarding application of cream:
  - maximum absorption occurs when applied over large skin area (e.g. inner aspects of arms, upper thighs, abdomen, upper chest and neck)
  - cream should be massaged until completely absorbed
  - peri-menopausal women with irregular menstrual cycle should be warned that menses may return
  - for peri-menopausal women, therapy should be synchronised with normal progesterone production (days 12–26 menstrual cycle). If menstruation occurs after 5–10 days, cream should be stopped and restarted 12 days later

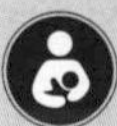

contraindicated during pregnancy in which progesterone levels are normal

not recommended during breastfeeding

AGENTS USED TO TREAT PRE-ECLAMPSIA AND ECLAMPSIA

Pre-eclampsia is defined as the 'presence of elevated blood pressure and proteinuria during pregnancy' (Rogers & Worley 2021) with eclampsia being the progression of pre-eclampsia with the addition of seizures. Australian prevalence estimates of early onset (< 34 weeks) pre-eclampsia as about 0.4%, increasing to 2.4% with late onset (≥ 34 weeks) with prevalence influenced by mental health (higher in those with schizophrenia or bipolar disorder), body mass index and country of birth (e.g. less in women from Western or Eastern Europe compared to Australia) (Australian Government Department of Health 2019).

The exact cause of pre-eclampsia is still unknown, although it is thought that placental dysfunction may start the systemic vasospasm, ischaemia and thrombosis that ultimately results in damage to maternal organs. Risk factors for developing pre-eclampsia include previous history of pre-eclampsia, chronic hypertension, pre-existing diabetes, autoimmune disease such as SLE or antiphospholipid syndrome. Other possible risk factors include nulliparity, BMI > 30, pre-existing kidney disease, maternal family history of pre-eclampsia and increasing maternal glucose levels (Australian Government Department of Health 2019). However, any pregnant woman is at risk.

MAGNESIUM SULFATE HEPTAHYDRATE (MAGNESIUM SULFATE) (DBL Magnesium Sulfate Concentrated Injection, Magnesium Sulfate Heptahydrate 50% Injection)

Available forms

Ampoules: 2.465 g/5 mL, 2.5 g/5 mL, 5 g/10 mL

Action

- second most abundant intracellular cation that is essential in more than

300 enzymatic processes, glycolysis, Krebs' cycle, protein and nucleic acid synthesis
- neuroprotective mechanism of action is unclear, but thought to be related to blockade of glutamate receptors preventing post-hypoxic brain injury
- anticonvulsant effects
- (IV) onset of action 30 minutes

Use

- prevent and treat hypomagnesaemia (see Vitamins, minerals and electrolytes, p. 1575)
- prevent and treat seizures associated with toxemias of pregnancy (pre-eclampsia and eclampsia)

Dose

- initially 4 g IV over 10–15 minutes (loading dose), followed by IV infusion of 1–2 g/hour **OR**
- initially 4 g IV over 5–10 minutes (loading dose), followed by 4–5 g IM into each buttock, then 4–5 g IM into alternate buttocks 4-hourly if needed
- (neuroprotection of fetus) initially 4 g IV over 20–30 minutes, followed by 1 g per hour by IV infusion for 24 hours or birth (whichever comes first)

Adverse effects

- flushing (hands, face, neck), sensation of warmth
- nausea, vomiting
- (uncommon) headache, dizziness
- (IM) pain, irritation at injection site
- (excess, hypermagnesaemia) thirst, nausea, vomiting, flushing, hypotension, bradycardia, slurred speech, muscle weakness and paralysis, blurred/double vision, loss of deep tendon reflexes, respiratory and CNS depression, cardiac arrest, coma

Interactions

- caution if given with cardiac glycosides
- increased CNS depression may result if given with CNS depressants
- increased neuromuscular blockade may occur if given with neuromuscular-blocking agents
- increased hypotension and neuromuscular blockade may occur if given with nifedipine

Nursing points/Cautions

- pulse, BP, respiratory rate, patellar reflexes and urine output should be checked before loading dose is given (as baseline), 10 minutes after loading dose has started and at the end of the loading dose (or according to hospital/facility protocol). Respiratory rate should be at least 16 breaths/minutes before start of infusion. During maintenance infusion, pulse, BP, respiratory rate, patellar reflexes and urinary output should be checked at least 4-hourly and infusion stopped if respiratory rate is less than 12 breaths/minute, patellar reflexes are absent, if hypotension occurs or urine output is less than 100 mL/4 hours
- serum magnesium should be measured regularly to ensure normal serum levels are not exceeded
- calcium salt (e.g. calcium gluconate monohydrate) should be available when IV magnesium sulfate heptahydrate is given (to treat hypermagnesaemia)
- IV doses should be diluted to concentration of 20% or less
- total daily dose should not exceed 30–40 g
- incompatible with calcium salts and will precipitate if mixed in the same IV infusion. Also incompatible with alkali carbonates, bicarbonates and soluble phosphates
- caution if given to those with myasthenia gravis because it may precipitate an acute crisis
- caution if used in those with impaired kidney function

- contraindicated in those with heart block, kidney failure (creatinine clearance < 20 mL/minute) or within 2 hours of delivery (unless it is the only therapy available)

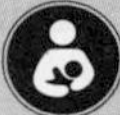

may cause hypermagnesaemia and depressed breathing in the newborn as it readily crosses the placenta and fetal serum levels are similar to the maternal levels. If given parenterally for a prolonged time (5–7 days), neonate may have bony abnormalities and congenital rickets

caution if given during breastfeeding because the concentration in breastmilk may reach twice the maternal serum concentration. Cleared from breastmilk within 24 hours of stopping therapy

AGENTS USED TO MANAGE PREMATURE LABOUR

Tocolytic agents are used to inhibit preterm labour in order to allow time for co-interventions (such as transferring to a facility with neonatal intensive care services and the administration of corticosteroids) in order to improve neonatal outcomes; however, are not recommended if pregnancy prolongation is dangerous for either mother or fetus (Bryant et al 2019).

Corticosteroids (e.g. betamethasone or dexamethasone) may be given to women at 24–34 weeks gestation who are at risk of preterm delivery within 7 days. The aim is to accelerate fetal lung maturity, reducing the risk of neonatal death, respiratory distress syndrome and cerebroventricular haemorrhage (Bryant et al 2019).

NIFEDIPINE (Adalat, Addos XR, Adefin, Adefin XL)

Available forms

Tablets: 10 mg, 20 mg; Tablets (controlled release): 20 mg, 30 mg, 60 mg

Action

- calcium-channel blocker that relaxes smooth muscle via blockade of calcium channels
- evidence suggests that it appears to be more effective than salbutamol (with fewer births within 7 days of treatment), fewer maternal adverse effects and decreased neonatal morbidity (Flenardy et al 2014)
- half-life 6–12 hours

Use

- threatened or established preterm labour (< 34 weeks gestation)

Dose

- initially 20 mg orally, then dose repeated after 30 minutes if contractions continue (maximum dose in first hour 40 mg). If contractions continue after 3 hours, 20 mg orally every 3–6 hours for 48 hours, unless contractions cease or labour is established (daily maximum dose 160 mg)

Adverse effects

- hypotension and possible fetal hypoxia
- headache, fatigue, dizziness
- flushing
- tachycardia, palpitations
- nausea, heartburn, constipation
- peripheral oedema (secondary to arteriolar vasodilation)
- transient risk in liver function tests

Interactions

- caution if given with magnesium sulfate heptahydrate as significant hypotension and neuromuscular weakness may occur
- caution if used with IV salbutamol or glyceryl trinitrate (GTN)

Nursing points/Cautions

- maternal BP, temperature, pulse and respiratory rate and fetal heart rate should be measured before starting therapy, then maternal BP, temperature and heart rate should be measured hourly for 4 hours. BP should be measured before administration of nifedipine (regularity of observations can be tapered according to clinical situation and/or hospital protocol)
- cardiotocograph (CTG) monitoring should be continuous during contractions and if there is regular abdominal pain/tenderness, change in the amount/colour of liquor or antepartum haemorrhage occurs
- tablets may be crushed or chewed to increase absorption
- if given with magnesium sulfate heptahydrate, BP, deep tendon reflexes and respiratory function should be closely monitored
- therapy should be stopped if there is marked hypotension (< 90 mm Hg) or significant dyspnoea
- caution if there is suspected intrauterine infection, fetal growth restriction, multiple pregnancy, preterm labour with placenta praevia or undiagnosed significant vaginal bleeding
- (fetal) contraindicated if there is proven intrauterine infection, fetal compromise during delivery, placental abruption, severe growth restriction, lethal fetal anomalies or intrauterine fetal death
- (maternal) contraindicated if woman has hypotension (BP < 90 mmHg) or cardiac disease, if any condition exists that would make prolongation of pregnancy dangerous, advanced cervical dilation or liver dysfunction

plain tablets can be crushed or chewed for rapid absorption

SALBUTAMOL SULFATE (known as albuterol in the USA) (Ventolin Obstetric Injection)

Available form

Ampoules: 1 mg/mL

Action

- direct-acting sympathomimetic agent related to adrenaline (epinephrine), noradrenaline (norepinephrine) and isoprenaline, with a longer duration of action
- causes bronchodilation
- relaxes uterine smooth muscle via effect on uterine beta-2 adrenoreceptors
- (IV) half-life 4–6 hours
- crosses placenta, increasing fetal heart rate

Use

- relief of reversible bronchospasm in asthma, chronic bronchitis and emphysema (see Antiasthma agents, bronchodilators and respiratory agents, p. 97)
- management of threatened or established uncomplicated premature labour (24–33 weeks gestation)

Dose

- initially 10 microgram/minute by IV infusion, increasing at 10-minute intervals until there is a decrease in strength, frequency or duration of contraction, then increasing infusion slowly until contractions have ceased. Infusion is then maintained for 1 hour at the same rate as when contractions ceased, then reducing rate by 50% 6-hourly

Adverse effects (for obstetric use)

- fine skeletal muscle tremor, especially in the hands
- nervousness, restlessness, anxiety
- dyspnoea
- oliguria
- maternal sinus tachycardia, palpitations, peripheral vasodilation, increased maternal pulse pressure and cardiac output, conduction disturbance (at high doses), hypotension
- nausea, vomiting
- headache, dizziness, flushing
- hypokalaemia, ketosis, disturbed carbohydrate metabolism, hyperglycaemia, exacerbation of diabetes
- (uncommon) maternal pulmonary oedema, myocardial ischaemia
- (neonatal) tachycardia, and rarely hypoglycaemia, ileus
- (rare) hypersensitivity, muscle cramps, maternal ileus

Interactions

- caution in patients who have already received therapy with high doses of other sympathomimetic agents
- may potentiate effects of chlorpromazine
- increased risk of hypokalaemia if given with xanthines, corticosteroids and diuretics

Nursing points/Cautions

- cardiovascular status should be assessed before starting therapy
- infusion should be started as soon as possible after diagnosis of premature labour
- hydration status (including fluid balance) should be closely monitored to prevent overhydration and maternal pulmonary oedema
- patient should lie on side during infusion to prevent aortocaval compression and hypotension
- electrolytes (especially serum potassium), glucose (especially in women with diabetes mellitus) and lactate should be monitored throughout therapy. If patient has diabetes, she should be closely monitored for any signs of ketoacidosis
- monitor vital signs (HR, BP and ECG) throughout therapy (initially every 15 minutes), noting that an elevation of heart rate may be a side-effect and a reduced heart rate a sign of improvement. Maternal pulse rate should be monitored throughout therapy and adjusted to prevent an increase over 120 beats/minute. Effect on diastolic BP is usually greater than on systolic
- fetal heart rate should be monitored continuously throughout therapy. If fetal distress occurs, acid–base balance and oxygen saturation should be closely monitored to prevent fetal acidosis and hypoxia
- symptoms of overdose are eased by rest and reassurance
- note and report any cardiac arrhythmias, especially in patients receiving digoxin, because these may result from salbutamol-induced hypokalaemia
- for patients with diabetes, IV fluids containing glucose should be avoided
- infusion should be given via infusion pump and administered alone
- infusion is not recommended for more than 48 hours. If continuation is necessary, then consideration should be given to changing to oral therapy
- if membranes rupture or cervix dilates to greater than 4 cm, salbutamol effectiveness is reduced and is not recommended
- therapy is generally stopped if strong contractions occur and labour progresses
- caution if used in those women with angina, hypertension or heart disease (especially tachyarrhythmias),

coronary artery disease, congestive heart failure or thyrotoxicosis

- caution if used in those with impaired liver or kidney function; dose reduction is recommended
- contraindicated in women with sensitivity to salbutamol and related amines, if gestational age is < 24 weeks or in those with pulmonary hypertension, diabetes mellitus, asthma, pre-existing ischaemic heart disease (or with risk factors for), pulmonary hypertension, uncontrolled hypertension, ileus, is unconscious, uncompensated potassium depletion, hypercalcaemia, hyperthyroidism, glaucoma, paroxysmal tachycardia, any condition where prolonged pregnancy could be dangerous for mother or fetus (e.g. severe pre-eclampsia, active uterine bleeding, premature rupture of membranes (with chorioamnionitis), cervical dilation > 4 cm, compression of umbilical cord, intrauterine fetal oedema, fetal acidosis or hypoxia, fetal distress, fetal death, known congenital or chromosomal malformations) or kidney insufficiency

Patient teaching and advice

- warn patient that tremor and palpitation may be experienced

banned in sport

Note

- salbutamol is available as Airomir Autohaler and Inhaler, Asmol CFC-free Inhaler and Ventolin preparations for management of asthma

AGENTS USED TO INDUCE LABOUR

DINOPROSTONE (prostaglandin E_2) (Cervidil, Prostin E_2 Vaginal Gel)

Available forms

Vaginal pessaries: 10 mg; Vaginal gel: 1 mg/2.5 mL, 2 mg/2.5 mL

Action

- releases prostaglandin E_2 into cervical tissue, which promotes softening and effacement (ripening) of the cervix (relaxation of cervical smooth muscle) to allow passage of fetus through the birth canal

Use

- induction of labour (single pregnancy with vertex presentation) at or near term

Dose

- 1 mg intravaginally, with 1–2 mg after 6 hours if necessary (not exceeding 3 mg/6 hours) **OR**
- 10 mg pessary inserted high into posterior vaginal fornix (leaving sufficient withdrawal tape for easy removal)

Adverse effects

- fetal distress
- uterine hypertonus, hypercontractility, arrested labour
- headache
- fever
- (rare) postpartum haemorrhage, amniotic fluid embolism, uterine rupture, disseminated intravascular coagulation (DIC), infection

Interactions

- not recommended with or within 30 minutes of other IV oxytocic agents since effects are potentiated
- NSAIDs (including aspirin) should be stopped before using dinoprostone

Nursing points/Cautions

- patient should be assessed before administration and have a cervical score (Bishop) of 8 or more
- should only be administered in facilities where continuous fetal and uterine monitoring is available
- (pessary) only a small amount of water-based lubricant should be applied before insertion
- (pessary) remove from freezer just before use and can be used without warming
- (pessary) should not be inserted if retrieval tape is not in place
- (gel) warm to room temperature for at least 30 minutes before administration
- (gel, pessary) insert transversely high into the posterior fornix, avoiding the cervical canal. With pessary, sufficient tape should remain outside vagina for easy removal (not tucked inside). If pessary is not correctly inserted, it will not make sufficient contact to be effective
- (gel, pessary) patient should remain recumbent for at least 30 minutes after insertion
- monitor patient (uterine activity, progression of cervical dilation and effacement, fetal condition) closely after insertion
- pessary should be removed immediately (by applying gentle traction on retrieval tape) if labour (painful uterine activity) commences (regardless of cervical state) before membranes rupture, if there are any adverse effects (maternal or fetal), or if there is insufficient cervical ripening in 12 hours or prior to amniotomy
- if oxytocin is to be used, a 30-minute interval should be allowed to elapse after removal of the pessary
- pessary is effective over 12 hours
- second dose is not recommended
- caution if used in women aged 35 years or more, or with gestational diabetes, arterial hypotension, hypothyroidism, gestation greater than 40 weeks, compromised cardiovascular function, previous uterine hypertony, asthma, glaucoma or epilepsy or who have had > 3 full term deliveries
- caution if used in those with a cervical Bishop score ≥ 8 (i.e. greater chance of having a vaginal delivery)
- contraindicated in women with multiple pregnancy, who have had three or more deliveries, previous uterine or cervical surgery, cervical rupture or current pelvic inflammatory disease (untreated), unexplained vaginal bleeding during pregnancy, if labour has started, membranes are ruptured or after amniotomy, if oxytocin will be given IV within 30 minutes, if the fetus is distressed, compromised or malpresented (non-vertex), if vaginal delivery is inappropriate (e.g. placenta praevia, active genital herpes), if strong prolonged contractions are inappropriate, if there is cephalopelvic disproportion, uterine hyperstimulation or hypertonic uterine contractions

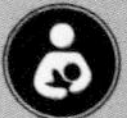

not recommended for any other stage of pregnancy or breastfeeding

OXYTOCIC AGENTS

CARBETOCIN (Duratocin)

Available form
Ampoules: 100 microgram/mL

Action
- long-acting synthetic oxytocin analogue that stimulates uterine muscle contraction
- properties similar to oxytocin with less potent but more prolonged action
- contractions established within 2 minutes of IV or IM administration, duration of action about 1 hour (IV) or 2 hours (IM)

Use
- prevention of uterine atony and excessive bleeding after elective delivery via caesarean section (under spinal or epidural anaesthesia) or vaginal delivery

Dose
- (caesarean section) 100 microgram slowly IV over 1 minute as single dose after delivery of infant (before or after delivery of placenta) **OR**
- (vaginal delivery) 100 microgram IM or slowly IV over 1 minute as single dose after delivery of infant (before or after delivery of placenta)

Adverse effects
- nausea, vomiting, abdominal pain, metallic taste
- pruritus
- flushing, feeling of warmth, sweating, fever, chills
- hypotension, tachycardia, chest pain
- headache, dizziness
- tremor, anxiety
- dyspnoea
- anaemia
- back pain

Interactions
- may cause severe hypertension if given within 3–4 hours of vasoconstricting agent with caudal block anaesthesia

Nursing points/Cautions
- if bleeding persists, patient should be closely examined for retained placental fragments, coagulopathy or genital tract trauma
- repeat administration is not recommended if uterine contraction post-delivery is not adequate. Other uterotonic agents such as oxytocin or ergometrine should be used
- (vaginal delivery) may be given IM
- caution if used in women with eclampsia or pre-eclampsia as BP should be closely monitored
- not recommended post-emergency delivery via caesarean section or after vaginal delivery
- caution if used in those with epilepsy, migraine, asthma or if rapid addition of extracellular water may be problematic
- contraindicated in those with known hypersensitivity to oxytocin, before delivery of infant or in those with cardiovascular disease (especially coronary artery disease), valvular heart disease, heart failure or cardiomyopathy

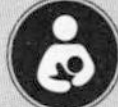

contraindicated during pregnancy

ERGOMETRINE MALEATE (DBL Ergometrine Injection)

Available form
Ampoules: 500 microgram/mL

Action

- ergot alkaloid that stimulates contraction of uterine and vascular smooth muscle
- increases amplitude and frequency of uterine contractions and tone, impeding uterine blood flow, producing haemostasis
- increases strength and frequency of cervical contractions
- produces some arterial vasoconstriction by stimulating alpha-adrenergic and serotonin receptors
- may decrease prolactin level post-delivery
- (IV) onset of action less than 1 minute, lasting for up to 45 minutes
- (IM) onset of action 2–5 minutes, lasting 3 hours

Use

- prevention and treatment of postpartum haemorrhage following delivery of placenta

Dose

- (prophylaxis of postpartum haemorrhage) 200 microgram IM after delivery is complete (after exclusion of second twin) **OR**
- (treatment of postpartum haemorrhage) 200 microgram IM **OR**
- (emergency) 200 microgram slowly IV over 1 minute

Adverse effects

- headache, dizziness, hallucination
- tinnitus, vertigo
- sweating
- nausea, vomiting, unpleasant taste, diarrhoea, abdominal pain, oesophageal spasm
- dyspnoea, nasal congestion, pulmonary oedema
- leg cramps
- bradycardia, palpitations, arrhythmias, chest pain (transient), hypotension, thrombophlebitis, peripheral vasospasm
- water intoxication
- haematuria
- (rapid or undiluted IV infusion) hypertension (sometimes sudden and/or severe)
- (prolonged therapy) gangrene, numbness/tingling of extremities
- (rare) allergy, uterine rupture, amniotic fluid embolism

Interactions

- may precipitate angina and reduce effects of antianginal agents
- may cause additive peripheral vasoconstriction if given with beta-adrenoceptor blocking agents, general anaesthetics, some local anaesthetics, sympathomimetic agents and vasoconstricting agents
- may cause hypertension, stroke, seizures or myocardial infarction if given with bromocriptine
- use caution if given with methysergide, because the combination may cause severe persistent spasm in major arteries
- vasoconstriction may increase if given with nicotine (heavy smokers)
- effectiveness is reduced in calcium deficiency states
- not recommended with sumatriptan due to increased risk of coronary vasoconstriction
- increased risk of ergotism if given with erythromycin or doxycycline
- increased risk of hypertension, peripheral ischaemia and gangrene if given with dopamine, therefore not recommended together

Nursing points/Cautions

- uterus should be inspected before administration for any retained placenta or second fetus. If administered before delivery, infant may develop hypoxia and/or intracranial haemorrhage
- response may not be seen if hypocalcaemia is present

- IV route should be restricted to emergency situations, because the risk of adverse effects is increased
- if IV route is used, should be given slowly or diluted with 5 mL sodium chloride 0.9% before administration and given slowly over 1 minute to avoid hypertension
- prolactin level may be decreased in postpartum period if multiple doses are given
- should be administered alone because of incompatibilities with many agents including adrenaline (epinephrine), ampicillin, cefalotin, chloramphenicol, heparin, metaraminol, sulfadiazine, thiopentone, vitamin B complex with C and warfarin
- should not be given for prolonged period, because ergotism and/or gangrene may result
- caution if used in those with porphyria because exacerbation may occur
- caution if used in those with Raynaud's phenomenon
- great caution if used in those with coronary artery disease, including mitral valve stenosis or venoatrial shunts
- caution if used in those with eclampsia or hypertension as hypertensive effects may be exaggerated
- contraindicated in those with hypersensitivity to ergot alkaloids, during induction of labour or in the first or second stage of labour, if there is any suspicion of retained placenta, during eclampsia, pre-eclampsia or threatened spontaneous abortion, severe or persistent sepsis, peripheral vascular disease, heart disease, hypertension, liver or kidney impairment

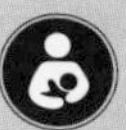

contraindicated during pregnancy (if given before delivery, may result in fetal hypoxia or intracranial haemorrhage)

contraindicated during breastfeeding (secretion in breastmilk may result in fetal ergotism although single dose to prevent haemorrhage should not prevent women from breastfeeding)

Note

- combined with oxytocin in Syntometrine

OXYTOCIN (Oxytocin Solution for Injection, Syntocinon, Viatocinon)

Available forms

Ampoules: 5 IU/mL, 10 IU/mL

Action

- synthetic oxytocin with similar actions to endogenous oxytocin, but with little vasopressin (anti-diuretic) activity
- stimulates uterine contraction and lactating breast to eject milk

Use

- induction and maintenance of labour (third stage)
- controlling postpartum bleeding

Dose

- (induction of labour) initially 1–4 milliunits/minute (0.1–0.4 mL/minute) by IV infusion, increasing at intervals of at least 20 minutes and increments of 1–2 milliunits/minute (to a maximum of 20 milliunits/minute) until contractions are similar to normal labour, then reducing infusion rate **OR**
- (management of the third stage of labour or postpartum haemorrhage) 5–10 IU IM or 5 IU slowly IV after delivery of shoulder **OR**
- (caesarean section) 5 IU by slow IV injection or IV infusion after delivery of the fetus

Adverse effects

- nausea, vomiting
- headache
- (large doses) violent uterine contractions, leading to uterine rupture, fetal distress, asphyxia and death
- (rapid infusion) severe hypotension, flushing and reflex tachycardia
- tachycardia, bradycardia and rarely ECG changes, QT prolongation
- (high dose, prolonged infusion) water intoxication, maternal hyponatraemia
- (rare) hypertension, cardiovascular collapse, amniotic fluid embolism, disseminated intravascular coagulation (DIC), rash, anaphylaxis
- (fetal) neonatal hyponatraemia, fetal distress, asphyxia, death

Interactions

- contraindicated within 6 hours of vaginal prostaglandins
- some inhalation anaesthetics (e.g. isoflurane) may reduce the action of oxytocin as well as potentiating hypotensive action and causing arrhythmias
- caution if used with other agents known to prolong QT interval
- oxytocin may potentiate pressor action of sympathomimetic vasoconstrictors if given during or after caudal block
- may enhance vasopressor effects of sympathomimetic or vasoconstricting agents (including if included in local anaesthetics)

Nursing points/Cautions

- 1000 milliunits = 1 unit (IU)
- not recommended SC, IM or by IV bolus
- multiple pregnancy should be excluded and maturity of the fetus should be established before starting infusion
- notify doctor if contractions become prolonged and unduly strong and be ready to reduce rate or stop infusion
- induction of labour should be stopped if infusion of 5 IU does not establish contractions
- during infusion, monitor maternal heart rate, blood pressure, strength, duration and frequency of uterine contractions, as well as fetal heart rate and rhythm
- infusion volume should be kept to a minimum if woman has cardiovascular problems
- (high dose or prolonged administration) oral fluid restriction and strict fluid balance chart are recommended. Serum electrolytes should be measured 8–12-hourly to prevent water intoxication. If water intoxication occurs, oxytocin should be stopped, fluids restricted, any electrolyte imbalance corrected, diuresis promoted and any seizures treated. Signs of water intoxication include headache, anorexia, nausea, vomiting, abdominal pain, lethargy, drowsiness, seizures, unconsciousness, hyponatraemia and acute pulmonary oedema (without hyponatraemia)
- burette and infusion pump should be used to deliver the solution to prevent inadvertent overdose. This also avoids rapid administration decreasing risk of cardiovascular effects
- solution should be prepared using glucose 4% with sodium chloride 0.18% and made to a solution strength of 10 IU/L. Glucose 5% is not recommended
- not compatible with solutions containing metasulfites or bisulfites
- gently rotate IV container to distribute oxytocin evenly in admixture
- administer alone
- prolonged administration is not recommended in those with oxytocin-resistant uterine inertia, cardiovascular disorders or severe pre-eclampsia
- increased risk of amniotic fluid embolism in women with fetal death in utero and/or meconium-stained amniotic fluid
- caution if used in those with borderline cephalopelvic disproportion,

secondary uterine inertia, mild–moderate pregnancy-induced hypertension, cardiovascular disease (especially if affected by changes in HR or BP), over 35 years or with known QT syndrome or history of lower segment caesarean section
- caution if patient has latex allergy or intolerance as there is an increased risk of anaphylaxis
- caution if used in women with predisposing factors for myocardial infarction (e.g. hypertrophic cardiomyopathy, valvular heart disease, ischaemic heart disease). If given, significant changes in HR and BP should be avoided
- caution if used in women with kidney impairment as there is increased risk of water retention and oxytocin accumulation
- contraindicated if there is fetal distress, abnormal presentation, cephalopelvic disproportion, elderly multiparae, excessive distension of uterus, parity greater than four, multiple pregnancy, hydramnios, previous uterine surgery (including caesarean section), severe toxaemia, placenta praevia or prolapse, hypertonic contractions or predisposition to amniotic fluid embolism (e.g. fetal death in utero, presence of meconium-stained amniotic fluid)

Note
- contained in Syntometrine with ergometrine

AGENTS USED IN TERMINATION OF PREGNANCY

GEMEPROST (prostaglandin E_1) (Cervagem)

Available form
Vaginal pessaries: 1 mg

Action
- prostaglandin E analogue which is more potent than biological prostaglandins E_1, E_2 or F_2-alpha

Use
- soften and dilate the cervix before transcervical intrauterine operative procedures during the first trimester
- therapeutic termination during the second trimester

Dose
- (cervical dilation (first trimester)) vaginal pessary (1 mg) inserted into posterior vaginal fornix 3 hours before surgery **OR**
- (therapeutic termination (second trimester)) vaginal pessary (1 mg) inserted into posterior vaginal fornix 3-hourly (to a maximum of 5 pessaries). If ineffective, may be repeated 24 hours later

Adverse effects
- vaginal bleeding, uterine pain (mild)
- nausea, vomiting, diarrhoea (mild), lower abdominal pain
- headache, flushing, mild fever
- back pain
- (uncommon) hypotension, chest pain, palpitations, tachycardia
- (rare) uterine rupture, myocardial infarction, coronary artery spasm

Interactions
- potentiated by oxytocin or other labour inducers

Nursing points/Cautions
- cervical softening and dilation usually occurs within 3 hours and lasts for 9 hours

- monitor patient carefully throughout procedure and ensure that no products of conception are retained (especially in second trimester termination)
- adverse effects such as uterine pain and bleeding, nausea and vomiting increase after 3 hours. If surgery is delayed > 3 hours after administration, patient should be closely monitored
- pessaries should be allowed to warm to room temperature for 30 minutes (away from sunlight and heat) before insertion
- should not be refrozen if not used
- should be discarded after 12 hours if not used
- not recommended for induction of labour
- caution if used in women with vaginal bleeding (of unknown origin), multiple pregnancy, multiparity or cervical stenosis, because the risk of uterine rupture is increased and necessitates close monitoring
- caution if used in women with raised intraocular pressure, cervicitis, vaginitis, cardiovascular insufficiency or obstructive airways disease
- contraindicated in women who have a known hypersensitivity to prostaglandins or uterine scarring (including caesarean section), placenta praevia or for the induction of labour at term

MIFEPRISTONE (Mifepristone Linepharma)

Available form

Tablets: 200 mg

Action

- synthetic steroid with antiprogestogen activity
- antagonises progesterone effect on endometrium and myometrium
- when used in first trimester of pregnancy, enables dilation and opening of the cervix
- when combined with a prostaglandin analogue after mifepristone, there is an increase in success rate and hastens the expulsion of fetus
- also binds to glucocorticoid receptor
- some anti-androgenic activity

Use

- medical termination of intrauterine pregnancy (in sequential combination with oral prostaglandin analogue) up to 49 days of gestation

Dose

- 200 mg orally either 2 hours before or 2 hours after food, followed 36–48 hours later with oral prostaglandin analogue (e.g. misoprostol)

Adverse effects

- nausea, vomiting, diarrhoea, gastric discomfort, abdominal pain
- dizziness, headache
- vaginal bleeding, uterine spasm, prolonged post-abortion bleeding, spotting, severe haemorrhage, endometritis, heavy bleeding
- breast tenderness
- fatigue, chills, fever
- fainting
- (uncommon) rash, pruritus, hot flush, infection, haemorrhagic shock, hypotension
- (rare) myocardial infarction, uterine rupture, toxic shock syndrome, seizures

Interactions

- may decrease efficacy of corticosteroids (including inhaled) for 3–4 days after administration, which may require dose adjustment in those receiving long-term therapy
- increased serum levels may occur if given with itraconazole, erythromycin and grapefruit juice
- decreased serum levels may occur if given with dexamethasone, St John's wort and phenytoin, phenobarbital (phenobarbitone), carbamazepine

- caution if used with agents with narrow therapeutic index

Nursing points/Cautions

- ectopic pregnancy should be excluded and gestation age confirmed before administration
- rhesus factor should be determined before procedure to prevent rhesus alloimmunisation
- women undergoing medical termination must be fully counselled regarding the need for combination therapy with oral prostaglandin, follow-up therapy within 14–21 days to confirm complete abortion, risk of procedure failure, bleeding, infection and effects on fertility
- not recommended in those with anaemia, kidney failure, liver impairment or failure or if malnourished
- not recommended if there is an intrauterine contraception device (IUD) in place. The IUD must be removed first
- caution if used in those with asthma using long-term corticosteroid therapy (including inhaled) as efficacy may be reduced for 3–4 days after administration
- caution if used in women with cardiovascular disease due to increased risk of cardiovascular events
- caution if used in women ≥ 35 years who are smokers
- contraindication if there is any uncertainty about pregnancy age or suspected ectopic pregnancy or in those with chronic adrenal failure, severe disease requiring exogenous glucocorticoid administration, known or suspected hypocoagulation diseases or treatment with anticoagulants or hypersensitivity to prostaglandin analogue which will be given sequentially with mifepristone or if there is lack of access to emergency care until complete expulsion has occurred

Patient teaching and advice

- advise patient to take mifepristone either 2 hours before or 2 hours after food
- ensure patient fully understands all of the following:
  - oral prostaglandin (misoprostol) needs to be taken 36–48 hours after mifepristone
  - in a small number of cases, the fetus is expelled before taking the prostaglandin
  - importance of attending follow-up appointment 14–21 days after taking mifepristone to ensure abortion is complete (even if fetus was expelled before taking prostaglandin). This follow-up may involve clinical examination, ultrasound or beta hCG measurement
  - risk of failure (if treatment does not work, a termination can be arranged using a different method. If treatment does not work and the patient decides to continue with the pregnancy, she should be counselled regarding possible risks to fetus and needs to be carefully monitored for the pregnancy)
  - if patient is Rh (Rhesus) negative, the doctor will need to take extra measures to prevent Rh factor sensitisation occurring
  - vaginal bleeding usually starts 1–2 days after taking mifepristone. Bleeding may be prolonged (10–16 days) and heavy. If patient is concerned, she should contact doctor or clinic
  - advise patient not to travel away from home during time that bleeding is occurring in case there is a need to visit or contact doctor/clinic immediately (patient should be provided with precise instructions with whom to contact (24-hour help line) and where

to go if prolonged heavy bleeding, pain or high temperature occurs)
- patient should be given a letter outlining information about the procedure to allow another practitioner to deal effectively with the case if the need arises
- importance of seeking medical advice immediately if patient develops any fever, abdominal pain or discomfort, pelvic tenderness, general malaise, weakness, nausea, vomiting or diarrhoea more than 24 hours after taking prostaglandin
- counsel patient regarding the need to avoid pregnancy in the next menstrual cycle and reliable contraceptive precautions should start as soon as possible after mifepristone administration

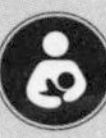

should be avoided during breastfeeding

tablet can be crushed and mixed with water or spoonful of yoghurt or apple puree

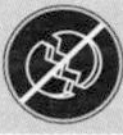

pregnant staff should not crush tablet

Note
- contained in MS-2 Step (combination pack) with misoprostol

MISOPROSTOL (Cytotec, GyMiso)

Available forms
Tablets: 200 microgram; Pessary (modified release): 200 microgram

Action
- prostaglandin E_1 analogue that induces contraction of myometrial smooth muscle and relaxation of uterine cervix
- facilitates cervical opening and evacuation of intrauterine contents
- when given sequentially with mifepristone, there is an increased success rate and hastened expulsion of fetus (GyMiso)

Use
- medical termination of developing intrauterine pregnancy (≤ 49 days gestation) (with mifepristone 200 mg) (GyMiso)
- prevention of gastric ulcers associated with NSAIDs or post-surgical stress (see Antiulcer agents, p. 818) (Cytotec)

Dose
- 800 microgram orally 2 hours before or 2 hours after food, as single or in 2 divided doses, 36–48 hours after mifepristone. May be repeated after 1–7 days if abortion has not occurred

Adverse effects
- transient and mild nausea, vomiting, diarrhoea, abdominal pain, gastric discomfort
- headache, dizziness
- vaginal bleeding, uterine spasm, prolonged post-abortion bleeding, spotting, severe haemorrhage, endometritis, heavy bleeding
- fainting
- breast tenderness
- fatigue, chills, fever
- (rare) uterine rupture,
- myocardial infarction, seizures, bronchospasm

Nursing points/Cautions
- should not be given if intrauterine contraceptive device (IUD) is in place. If present, IUD should be removed before therapy is given
- if given as a divided dose, should be given as 400 microgram, then second 400 microgram 2 hours later
- may be administered buccally (kept between cheek and gum for 30 minutes and any remainder swallowed with water)

- caution if used in those women with or with risk factors of cardiovascular disease, asthma or epilepsy
- not recommended in those women with viable pregnancy who intend to carry pregnancy to term
- contraindicated in those with known or suspected hypocoagulation diseases, treatment with anticoagulants, uncertainty about pregnancy age, suspected ectopic pregnancy or any hypersensitivity to mifepristone (which is administered first)

Patient teaching and advice

- advise patient that tablets should be taken either 2 hours before or 2 hours after food. Tablets may be placed between cheek and gum for 30 minutes and any remainder swallowed with water
- if patient prefers, tablets can be taken as 2 doses (400 microgram each) 2 hours apart
- see also Patient teaching and advice for mifepristone (p. 1417)

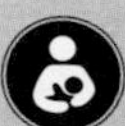

not recommended during breastfeeding as may cause diarrhoea in infant

tablet can be given buccally (between cheek and gum for 30 minutes and remaining fragments swallowed with water)

Note

- contained orally in MS-2 Step (combination pack) with mifepristone

LACTATION INHIBITORS

BROMOCRIPTINE MESILATE (MESYLATE) (Parlodel)

Available form

Tablets: 2.5 mg

Action

- ergot derivative with no uterotonic and little vasoconstrictor activity
- stimulates dopaminergic receptors
- inhibits release of prolactin
- increases release of growth hormone for several hours after administration
- decreases size and growth of prolactin-secreting pituitary tumours (prolactinomas)

Use

- preventing onset of lactation (for clearly defined medical reasons as routine use of dopaminergic agents for lactation suppression is not recommended)
- hyperprolactinaemia (where surgery/radiotherapy are ineffective or inappropriate)
- prolactinoma (conservative treatment before surgery to reduce size, and post-surgery if prolactin levels remain high)
- adjunctive therapy in acromegaly, Parkinson's disease (see Anti-Parkinson's agents, p. 740)

Dose

- (inhibition of physiological lactation) 2.5 mg orally twice daily with food for 14 days (starting more than 4 hours after delivery) **OR**
- (hyperprolactinaemia) initially 1.25 mg orally 2–3 times daily with food, increasing to 2.5 mg 2–3 times daily if needed **OR**
- (prolactinoma) initially 1.25 mg orally twice daily with food, gradually

increasing doses up to 15 mg daily in divided doses if needed to reduce prolactin levels

Adverse effects

- nausea, vomiting, constipation
- dizziness, headache (transient), somnolence
- postural hypotension, syncope
- nasal congestion
- (uncommon) confusion, hallucinations, dyskinesias
- (rare) gastrointestinal bleeding and ulceration, diabetic retinopathy, psychiatric disturbances, blurred vision, visual disturbances, impulse control disorders
- (long-term, high dose) retroperitoneal fibrosis, pleural/pericardial effusions, pleural/pulmonary fibrosis
- (very rare) sudden sleep onset, neuroleptic malignant syndrome (abrupt withdrawal), reversible pallor of toes/fingers on exposure to cold

Interactions

- tolerability may be decreased by alcohol
- hypotensive effect may be enhanced by antihypertensive agents
- increased plasma levels may result if given with erythromycin, octreotide or macrolide antibiotics
- effects may be antagonised by phenothiazines, butyrophenones, metoclopramide, methyldopa sesquihydrate, TCAs, domperidone, oestrogens and thyrotropin-releasing factor
- effects may be increased if given with levodopa or clonidine
- increased risk of headache, nausea and vomiting if given with ergometrine
- increased risk of hypertension and severe headache if given with sympathomimetic agents
- increased risk of vasospastic reaction if given with sumatriptan

Nursing points/Cautions

- hypoprolactinaemia should be thoroughly investigated before starting therapy to ensure cause is not severe hypothyroidism
- BP should be monitored during first week of therapy (hypotension is most common in first weeks of therapy) and then supine and standing BP checked regularly for postural hypotension
- gastric irritation is reduced if bromocriptine is taken with or immediately after food
- dosage increases are made gradually, usually over several days, to reduce the incidence of adverse effects
- (prolactin-secreting adenomas) visual fields should be monitored throughout therapy
- (prolactinoma) dosage is sufficient when serum prolactin level falls and tumour reduces in size
- when used for inhibiting physiological lactation, bromocriptine should not be used within 4 hours of delivery and only after vital signs have stabilised (especially BP). Therapy should be continued for 14 days to prevent rebound lactation. If secretion recurs, therapy may be restarted for another week at same dose
- when given for hyperprolactinaemia associated with galactorrhoea or amenorrhoea, treatment is continued until breast secretions have ceased or the menstrual cycle has recommenced. May be continued over several menstrual cycles to prevent relapse if needed
- when given for hyperprolactinaemia, return of ovulation postpartum may be hastened, therefore adequate contraceptive methods should be used if pregnancy is not wanted
- (long-term therapy) female patients should have regular gynaecological

examination and all patients should have a regular chest X-ray (to monitor for pulmonary fibrosis)
- caution if used in those with suspected/known peptic ulceration, impaired liver function, diabetes mellitus or Raynaud's phenomenon
- not recommended in those with galactose intolerance, severe lactase deficiency or glucose–galactose malabsorption
- contraindicated in those with sensitivity to ergot alkaloids, uncontrolled hypertension, toxaemia, hypertensive disorders associated with pregnancy (including postpartum), coronary artery disease, severe cardiovascular conditions or serious psychiatric disorders

Patient teaching and advice

- warn patient that alcohol should be avoided during therapy
- advise patient to take initial doses at bedtime, to reduce the incidence of hypotension and loss of consciousness
- warn patient against driving a vehicle or operating machinery if drowsy, dizzy or experiencing daytime somnolence
- advise patient to avoid postural hypotension by moving gradually to a sitting or standing position, especially after sleep, otherwise light-headedness and fainting may occur
- patient should be warned that milk secretion may recur 2–3 days after stopping treatment, which may necessitate restarting treatment at the same dosage for a further 7 days
- patient should be advised to seek medical advice immediately if any of the following occur:
  - any shortness of breath, persistent cough or chest pain (signs of pulmonary fibrosis)
  - loin/flank pain, lower limb swelling or abdominal tenderness (signs of retroperitoneal fibrosis)
- family/carers should be asked to observe for any:
  - sudden sleep onset as patients are often unaware that this occurs and it may be dangerous if the person drives or operates machinery, or
  - persistent/recurring gambling, increased libido, hypersexuality, binge eating, compulsive buying or spending, or repetitive behaviours with no purpose (punding)
- women of childbearing years not wishing to become pregnant should be advised to use adequate contraception during therapy

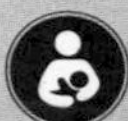

caution if used during pregnancy

not recommended during breastfeeding (if mother wishes to breastfeed)

tablet can be dispersed in water or crushed and mixed with spoonful of yoghurt or apple puree

CABERGOLINE (Cabaser, Dostinex)

Available forms

Tablets: 500 microgram, 1 mg, 2 mg

Action

- ergot derivative that stimulates D_2 dopamine receptors, inhibiting prolactin secretion
- central dopaminergic effect

Use

- Parkinson's disease (Cabaser) (see Anti-Parkinson's agents, p. 742)
- inhibiting physiological lactation (for clearly defined medical reasons as routine use of dopaminergic agents for lactation suppression is not recommended) (Dostinex)
- hyperprolactinaemia (Dostinex)

Dose

- (preventing onset of physiological lactation) 1 mg orally with food as a once-only dose first day after delivery **OR**
- (hyperprolactinaemia) initially 0.25 mg orally with food twice weekly (e.g. Monday and Thursday), increasing gradually by 0.5 mg weekly at 1-month intervals until therapeutic response is achieved

Adverse effects

- nausea, vomiting, abdominal pain, constipation, dyspepsia, epigastric pain
- headache, dizziness, vertigo
- depression, somnolence, fatigue, asthenia
- paraesthesia
- breast pain
- hot flushes
- hypotension
- (rare) pleural/pulmonary fibrosis, pleural effusions, palpitations, transient hemianopia, leg cramps, digital vasospasm, impulse control disorder, sudden sleep disorder

Interactions

- not recommended with other ergometrine
- not recommended with agents that antagonise dopamine receptors (e.g. metoclopramide, phenothiazines, butyrophenones, thioxanthines)
- not recommended with macrolide antibacterial agents (e.g. erythromycin) as bioavailability may be increased

Nursing points/Cautions

- (hyperprolactinaemia) before starting therapy, patients should have a cardiovascular assessment (including ECG/echocardiogram), ESR, lung function test, chest X-ray and renal function
- (hyperprolactinaemia) ECG/echocardiogram should be monitored within 3–6 months of starting therapy, then 6–12-monthly
- (hyperprolactinaemia) chest X-ray and ESR are recommended if patient develops any pulmonary symptoms
- evaluation of pituitary function is recommended before starting therapy for hyperprolactinaemia
- BP should be monitored regularly
- administration with food may lessen GI disturbances
- weekly doses may be given as single or divided doses, although doses over 1 mg/week should be divided to decrease GI disturbances
- caution if used in those with cardiovascular disease, Raynaud's syndrome, liver/renal disease, peptic ulcer, GI bleeding, pre-eclampsia, postpartum hypertension or psychiatric disorders
- contraindicated in those with history of pulmonary, pericardial or retroperitoneal fibrotic disease, anatomical evidence of cardiac valvulopathy or hypersensitivity to other ergot alkaloids

Patient teaching and advice

- warn patient that adverse effects usually disappear with continued therapy
- patient should be advised not to drive or operate machinery during first days of therapy, or if vertigo, dizziness or somnolence are ongoing problems
- patient should be advised to immediately report:
  - any shortness of breath, persistent cough or chest pain (signs of pulmonary fibrosis)
  - loin/flank pain, lower limb swelling or abdominal tenderness (signs of retroperitoneal fibrosis)

- family/carers should be asked to observe for any:
  - sudden sleep onset as patients are often unaware that this occurs and it may be dangerous if the person drives or operates machinery, or
  - persistent/recurring gambling, increased libido, hypersexuality, binge eating, compulsive buying or spending, or repetitive behaviours with no purpose (punding)
- women of childbearing years not wishing to become pregnant should be advised to use adequate contraception during therapy

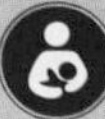

pregnancy should be excluded before starting and for 1 month after stopping therapy. Pregnancy test is recommended every 4 weeks or if menstrual period is overdue by more than 3 days

not recommended during breastfeeding (if mother wishes to breastfeed)

tablet can be crushed and mixed with water or spoonful of yoghurt or apple puree

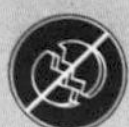

pregnant staff should not disperse or crush tablets

PULMONARY HYPERTENSION AGENTS

Pulmonary hypertension is defined as being an elevated pulmonary arterial pressure (> 22 mmHg) or an estimated systolic pulmonary arterial pressure > 36 mmHg (Waxman & Loscalzo 2019). In the past, those with pulmonary hypertension often died due to misdiagnosis and/or lack of appropriate management. The early symptoms of pulmonary hypertension can be non-specific (e.g. dyspnoea, fatigue) and easily attributed to other conditions. Symptoms of advanced disease present as oedema, chest pain, pre-syncope and syncope. Diagnosis is based on clinical symptoms and tests such as echocardiogram, lung function tests and chest imaging (e.g. chest X-Ray, CT and CT angiogram) (Waxman & Loscalzo 2019).

The development of medical treatments has improved both the quality of life and survival rates in patients with pulmonary hypertension; however, there is no known cure (Waxman & Loscalzo 2019). The agents discussed in this section are used in the management of pulmonary arterial hypertension (PAH) and include prostacyclin (epoprostenol), prostacyclin analogues, phosphodiesterase-5 (PDE5) inhibitors (see Erectile dysfunction agents, p. 1053) and endothelin receptor antagonists (Waxman & Loscalzo 2019).

AMBRISENTAN (Pulmoris, Volibris)

Available forms
Tablets: 5 mg, 10 mg

Action
- endothelin receptor (type A) antagonist that inhibits the potent vasoconstrictor endothelin-1, which is increased in those with pulmonary arterial hypertension
- half-life 13.6–16.5 hours

Use
- familial pulmonary arterial hypertension (PAH), PAH associated with connective tissue disease or in patients with functional WHO Class II, III or IV symptoms

Dose
- initially 5 mg orally daily, increasing to 10 mg if needed

Adverse effects
- hypotension, peripheral oedema, fluid retention, heart failure, palpitations, chest pain
- headache, dizziness, fatigue
- nasal congestion, sinusitis, nasopharyngitis, epistaxis
- dyspnoea, cough, bronchitis

- elevated liver enzymes, hepatitis
- flushing
- anaemia
- constipation, abdominal pain, nausea
- (rare) rash, hypersensitivity

Interactions

- caution if given with other hepatotoxic agents
- caution if given with ciclosporin. If given together, dose of ambrisentan should be limited to 5 mg daily
- increased risk of anaemia if given with tadalafil
- transient increase in serum levels may occur if given with rifampicin

Nursing points/Cautions

- liver function tests (serum liver enzymes and bilirubin) should be measured before starting and then monthly during therapy
- haemoglobin should be measured before starting therapy, after 1 month and then regularly
- BP should be monitored during therapy (especially in those with pre-existing hypotension)
- patient should be monitored for any signs of fluid retention and pulmonary oedema (especially if patient has severe systolic dysfunction in addition to PAH)
- pregnancy must be excluded before starting therapy
- caution if used in those with pre-existing hypotension or kidney impairment (especially if severe)
- caution if used in those with right heart failure, pre-existing liver disease, previous medication-induced elevation of liver enzymes or currently taking medications which may elevate liver enzymes
- not recommended in those with functional Class I symptoms
- contraindicated in those with severe liver impairment (with or without cirrhosis), elevated liver enzymes (3 times above normal) or idiopathic pulmonary fibrosis (with or without pulmonary hypertension)

Patient teaching and advice

- patient should be advised to seek medical advice immediately if any of the following occur:
  - loss of appetite, nausea, upper abdominal pain, unusual tiredness, yellowing of eyes or skin, dark urine or pale stools
  - tiredness, weakness, shortness of breath, feeling unwell
  - swollen ankles or legs
- warn patient not to drive or operate heavy machinery if dizziness or fatigue occur
- women of childbearing potential should be counselled regarding the high risk of birth defects if conception occurs while taking therapy and be willing to perform monthly pregnancy tests and use two forms of reliable contraception if sexually active (oral contraceptive may not be reliable). Pregnancy must be avoided for 3 months after stopping therapy
- see also General Patient teaching and advice (p. xxvii)

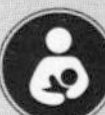

contraindicated during pregnancy. Monthly pregnancy tests are recommended. Pregnancy must be avoided for 3 months after stopping therapy

not recommended during breastfeeding

tablet can be crushed and mixed with water or spoonful of yoghurt or apple puree

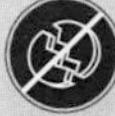

pregnant staff must not crush or disperse tablets

BOSENTAN MONOHYDRATE (Tracleer)

Available forms

Tablets: 62.5 mg, 125 mg

Action

- endothelin receptor antagonist that inhibits the potent vasoconstrictor endothelin-1 (ET-1), which is increased in those with pulmonary arterial hypertension
- slightly higher affinity for ETA receptors than ETB

Use

- idiopathic or familial pulmonary arterial hypertension (PAH), PAH associated with connective tissue disease or in patients with functional WHO Class II, III or IV symptoms, PAH associated with congenital systematic to pulmonary shunt (including Eisenmenger's physiology)

Dose

- (adults) initially 62.5 mg orally twice daily for 4 weeks, then increasing to 125 mg twice daily (maintenance) **OR**
- (children, weight 10–20 kg) initially 31.25 mg orally daily, increasing to 31.25 mg twice daily after 4 weeks **OR**
- (children > 20 kg–40 kg) initially 31.25 mg twice daily, increasing to 62.5 mg twice daily after 4 weeks **OR**
- (children > 40 kg) initially 62.5 mg twice daily, increasing to 125 mg twice daily after 4 weeks

Adverse effects

- joint swelling, arthralgia
- fever
- flushing, headache
- elevated liver enzymes and bilirubin
- anaemia
- peripheral oedema, fluid retention
- palpitations, chest pain, syncope, hypotension
- upper and lower respiratory tract infections, nasopharyngitis, sinusitis, nasal congestion, rhinitis, epistaxis
- pruritus, rash
- diarrhoea
- (uncommon) thrombocytopenia
- (rare) liver cirrhosis, liver failure

Interactions

- contraindicated with ciclosporin and glibenclamide
- not recommended with epoprostenol, fluconazole, itraconazole, voriconazole or ritonavir
- caution if given with other hepatotoxic agents including antiretroviral agents
- caution if given with tacrolimus or sirolimus
- increased serum levels may occur if given with itraconazole, voriconazole, ritonavir, sildenafil or rifampicin
- may decrease serum levels of digoxin, nimodipine, sildenafil, tacrolimus, sirolimus and simvastatin (and its active metabolite)
- may decrease efficacy of hormonal contraceptives (oral, injectable, transdermal, implantable)
- increased INR monitoring is recommended if given with warfarin
- caution if used with carbamazepine, phenobarbital (phenobarbitone), phenytoin and St John's wort

Nursing points/Cautions

- liver function tests (serum liver enzymes and bilirubin) should be measured before starting and then monthly during therapy
- haemoglobin should be measured after 1 and 3 months and then 3-monthly
- patient should be monitored for any signs of fluid retention (especially if patient has severe systolic dysfunction in addition to PAH)
- oxygen saturation monitoring is recommended in those with coronary heart disease
- discontinuation should be gradual over 3–7 days at a reduced dose
- pregnancy must be excluded before starting therapy
- caution if used in those with pre-existing anaemia or hypotension or with mild liver impairment

- contraindicated in those with moderate-to-severe liver impairment

Patient teaching and advice

- patient should be advised to seek medical advice immediately if any of the following occur:
  - nausea, vomiting, fever, lethargy, fatigue, abdominal pain, dark urine, pale stools (bowel motions) or yellowing of eyes or skin
  - swelling of ankles or legs
- advise patient not to stop therapy abruptly
- women of childbearing potential should be counselled regarding the high risk of birth defects if conception occurs while taking bosentan and be willing to perform monthly pregnancy tests and use two reliable types of contraception if sexually active (oral contraceptive may not be reliable). Pregnancy must be avoided for 3 months after stopping therapy
- see also General Patient teaching and advice (p. xxvii)

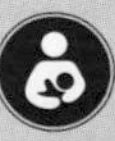

contraindicated during pregnancy. Monthly pregnancy tests are recommended. Pregnancy must be avoided for 3 months after stopping therapy

not recommended during breastfeeding

tablet can be crushed and mixed with water or spoonful of yoghurt or apple puree

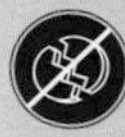

pregnant staff must not crush or disperse tablets

EPOPROSTENOL (Flolan, Veletri)

Available forms

Vial: 500 microgram, 1.5 mg (with diluent and filter)

Action

- prostacyclin
- direct vasodilation of pulmonary and systemic arterial vascular beds
- inhibits platelet aggregation
- elimination half-life less than 6 minutes

Use

- idiopathic or familial pulmonary arterial hypertension (PAH) (WHO functional Class III or IV) or PAH associated with connective tissue disease

Dose

- (short-term (acute) dose, used to determine long-term infusion rate) initially 2 nanogram/kg/minute by IV infusion, increasing by 2 nanogram/kg/minute at 15-minute intervals until dose-limiting effects or maximum haemodynamic benefit is reached **OR**
- (long term) initially 4 nanogram/kg/minute less than the maximum dose achieved with acute dose. If acute dose was less than 5 nanogram/kg/minute, then dose should be started at 1 nanogram/kg/minute

Adverse effects

- flushing, headache, dizziness, fatigue
- anorexia, nausea, vomiting, abdominal pain, diarrhoea
- hypotension, bradycardia, tachycardia, syncope
- anxiety, nervousness, agitation
- chest pain, back pain, jaw pain, neck pain
- dyspnoea
- arthralgia, myalgia
- fever
- hypoaesthesia, paraesthesia
- skin ulcer, rash, pruritus
- (injection site) pain, reaction

Interactions

- may increase vasodilatory effects if given with other vasodilators
- may decrease clearance of digoxin leading to increased serum levels and risk of toxicity (especially in the early weeks of therapy)
- may reduce efficacy of tissue plasminogen activator by increasing clearance

- increased risk of bleeding if given with NSAIDs or antiplatelet agents

Nursing points/Cautions

- short-term (acute) dose-ranging procedure should be given via peripheral or central venous access device and completed in hospital setting with equipment for haemodynamic monitoring and emergency care readily available
- (long term) infusion should be via permanent indwelling CVC and small, portable infusion pump
- risk of pulmonary thromboembolism or systemic embolism may be reduced if patient is also given anticoagulant therapy (if not contraindicated)
- cardiovascular effects disappear within 30 minutes of finishing the infusion
- if severe hypotension occurs, infusion rate should be reduced or stopped as this may be a sign of overdose
- BP (supine and erect) and heart rate should be monitored during infusion (especially if altering infusion rate), as well as observing patient for any signs of pulmonary oedema. If sudden bradycardia, nausea, sweating and hypotension occur, infusion should be stopped
- abrupt stopping of chronic infusion is not recommended as it may cause rapid clinical deterioration, which can be fatal. This also includes sudden large reductions in infusion rate
- (long-term therapy) any dose adjustment should be based on recurrence or worsening of symptoms or occurrence of adverse effects
- if no response after 12 weeks, alternative options should be considered
- infusion rate is determined by dosage, patient's weight and concentration of reconstituted solution
- IV administration set should contain 0.20–0.22 micron filter
- extravasation should be avoided as tissue damage may occur
- administer alone
- (Veletri) reconstitute using sodium chloride 0.9% or water for injections
- (Flolan) should only be reconstituted using diluent provided
- (Flolan) incompatible with sodium chloride 0.9%
- (Flolan) if reconstituted concentrated solution requires further dilution, this should be done with the provided diluent and sterile filter (supplied) should be used to dispense solution into cassette
- contraindicated in those with congestive heart failure (caused by severe left ventricular dysfunction) or long term in those who develop pulmonary oedema during therapy

Patient teaching and advice

- (Flolan) patient may self-administer after appropriate and comprehensive training in preparation of solution, catheter and pump care. This should include the use of a cold pouch with infusion pump (if available), which allows infusion to run over 24 hours as long as the cold pouch is changed regularly
- warn patient not to stop therapy suddenly as dizziness, weakness and difficulty breathing may occur
- patient should be advised not to drive or operate machinery if adverse effects occur
- instruct patient to seek medical advice immediately if any of the following occur:
  - jaw/muscle/back pain, sweating, chest pain/tightness
  - tingling or numbness in feet or hands
  - change in skin sensitivity (e.g. more sensitive, less sensitive)

- headaches, dizziness (especially on standing), fever, fatigue
- stomach upset
- shortness of breath
- facial flushing
- chills/flu-like symptoms
- redness or pain at the infusion site

- see also General Patient teaching and advice (p. xxvii)

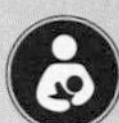

should only be given during pregnancy if benefits outweigh potential risks

caution if used during breastfeeding

ILOPROST TROMETAMOL (Ventavis)

Available form
Nebuliser solution: 20 microgram/2 mL

Action
- synthetic prostaglandin analogue
- direct vasodilation of pulmonary arterial bed, improving pulmonary artery pressure, pulmonary vascular resistance and cardiac output
- duration 1–2 hours, biphasic half-life (3–5 minutes, 15–30 minutes)

Use
- moderate-to-severe idiopathic pulmonary hypertension (PH), PH secondary to drugs or connective tissue disease
- chronic pulmonary thromboembolism (where surgery is not possible)

Dose
- initially 2.5 microgram via inhalation device over 4–10 minutes 6–9 times daily, increasing to 5.0 microgram if needed and tolerated

Adverse effects
- vasodilation, hypotension, syncope, dizziness, tachycardia, palpitations
- cough, dyspnoea
- pharyngolaryngeal pain
- epistaxis, haemoptysis, bleeding
- headache, dizziness
- trismus/jaw pain, back pain, chest pain
- peripheral oedema
- rash
- nausea, vomiting, diarrhoea, irritation of mouth/tongue/throat
- (rare) bronchospasm

Interactions
- may increase antihypertensive or vasodilatory effects of vasodilators or antihypertensive agents
- increased risk of bleeding if given with anticoagulants, antiplatelet agents, nitrates (such as glyceryl trinitrate), phosphodiesterase (PDE-5) inhibitors (e.g. sildenafil), aspirin or NSAIDs

Nursing points/Cautions
- vital signs should be monitored when starting therapy
- patient should be monitored for rebound effect if therapy is interrupted or stopped
- administered via nebuliser
- if patient has concurrent lung infection, severe asthma or chronic obstructive pulmonary disease, close monitoring for any bronchial hyperreactivity is recommended
- avoid contact with skin and eyes
- caution if used in those with liver or kidney dysfunction
- not recommended in those under 18 years
- not recommended in those with unstable pulmonary hypertension with advanced right heart failure or in those with hypotension (systolic BP < 85 mmHg)
- contraindicated in those who have an increased risk of haemorrhage (e.g. active peptic ulcer), unstable angina, myocardial infarction within the past 6 months, severe cardiac failure (not managed), severe arrhythmias,

pulmonary congestion, stroke or transient ischaemic attack (TIA) within the past 3 months, pulmonary hypertension because of venous occlusive disease, congenital/acquired valvular defects with myocardial function disorder not related to pulmonary hypertension

Patient teaching and advice

- warn patient to avoid the solution making contact with eyes and skin and it should not be taken orally
- ensure patient understands how to use the nebuliser device, including only using a mouthpiece (not a face mask that would increase contact with eyes and skin)
- instruct patient to discard any unused solution at the end of nebulisation
- those with syncope associated with pulmonary hypertension should be advised to avoid unusual strain. If syncope usually occurs when getting out of bed, first dose should be administered while still in bed
- patient should be advised to avoid driving or operating machinery if dizziness or fainting persists
- females of childbearing years should be counselled regarding the use of effective contraception during therapy to prevent pregnancy
- see also General Patient teaching and advice (p. xxvii)

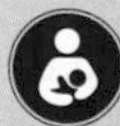

not recommended during pregnancy and breastfeeding

MACITENTAN (Opsumit)

Available form

Tablets: 10 mg

Action

- endothelin (ET)-1 and its receptors (ETA, ETB) trigger vasoconstriction, fibrosis, proliferation, hypertrophy and inflammation. In pulmonary arterial hypertension, ET is upregulated and is involved in vascular hypertrophy and organ damage
- endothelin receptor (ETA, ETB) antagonist that binds to ET receptors in human pulmonary arterial smooth muscle cells and prefers penetration into lung tissue (particularly if diseased)
- maximum plasma concentration reached in about 8 hours after administration
- active metabolite
- half-life about 18 hours (48 hours for metabolite)

Use

- idiopathic and heritable pulmonary arterial hypertension (PAH), PAH associated with connective tissue disease or in patients with PAH associated with congenital heart disease with repaired shunt) with functional WHO Class II, III or IV symptoms (monotherapy or with phosphodiesterase-5 inhibitors or inhaled prostanoids)

Dose

- 10 mg orally daily

Adverse effects

- anaemia, thrombocytopenia
- hypotension
- headache, insomnia, depression
- pruritus, urticaria, flushing, skin ulceration
- bronchitis, nasopharyngitis, pharyngitis, influenza, nasal congestion, upper respiratory tract infection, rhinitis
- arthralgia, myalgia
- peripheral oedema, fluid retention
- diarrhoea, abdominal pain, gastroenteritis
- increased liver enzymes, hypokalaemia
- fever

Interactions

- caution if given with other hepatotoxic agents

- increased serum levels may occur if given with itraconazole, voriconazole, clarithromycin, ritonavir and saquinavir
- serum levels may be decreased if given with rifampicin, St John's wort, carbamazepine and phenytoin

Nursing points/Cautions

- liver function tests and FBC are recommended before starting and monthly during therapy
- BP and haemoglobin monitoring are recommended in those with kidney impairment or pre-existing hypotension due to increased risk of anaemia and hypotension
- pregnancy must be excluded before starting therapy
- caution if used in those with pre-existing hypotension
- not recommended in those with significant anaemia, on dialysis or with severe kidney impairment
- not recommended in those under 12 years
- contraindicated in those with severe liver impairment (with or without cirrhosis) or clinically significant elevated liver aminotransferases (> than 3 times upper limit of normal)

Patient teaching and advice

- instruct patient to seek medical advice immediately if any if the following occur:
  - nausea, vomiting, fever, abdominal pain, yellowing eyes or skin, itching skin, dark urine, tiredness, exhaustion
  - flu-like syndrome, including chills, fever, joint and muscle pain
  - weight gain, swelling of feet or legs
- women of childbearing potential should be counselled regarding the high risk of birth defects if conception occurs during therapy, be willing to perform monthly pregnancy tests and use two reliable types of contraception if sexually active (oral contraceptives may not be reliable). Pregnancy must be avoided for 3 months after stopping therapy
- see also General Patient teaching and advice (p. xxvii)

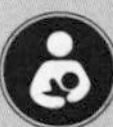

contraindicated during pregnancy. Monthly pregnancy tests are recommended. Pregnancy must be avoided for 3 months after stopping therapy

not recommended during breastfeeding

tablet can be crushed and mixed with water or spoonful of yoghurt or apple puree

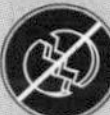

pregnant staff must not crush or disperse tablets

RIOCIGUAT (Adempas)

Available form

Tablet: 0.5 mg, 1 mg, 1.5 mg, 2 mg, 2.5 mg

Action

- stimulates soluble guanylate cyclase (sGC) (enzyme found in most tissue and receptor for nitric oxide (NO)). When sGC binds to NO, cyclic guanosine monophosphate (cGMP) is synthesised. cGMP regulates processes that influence vascular tone, proliferation, fibrosis and inflammation
- pulmonary hypertension is associated with endothelial dysfunction, impaired NO synthesis and insufficient NO-sGC-cGMP pathway stimulation
- active metabolite
- half-life 7 hours (healthy patients) and 13 hours (patients with PAH)

Use

- idiopathic or heritable pulmonary arterial hypertension (PAH), PAH associated with connective tissue diseases, PAH associated with congenital heart

disease in adults with WHO functional class II, III or IV symptoms
- chronic thromboembolic pulmonary hypertension (CTEPH) after surgical treatment, or inoperable CTEPH

Dose
- initially 1 mg orally 3 times daily (doses 6–8 hours apart) for 2 weeks, increasing at 2-week intervals by 0.5 mg increments (maximum 2.5 mg 3 times daily if patient has no signs or symptoms of hypotension and systolic BP ≥ 95mmHg)

Adverse effects
- hypotension, palpitations, chest pain or discomfort
- headache, dizziness, fatigue
- dyspepsia, nausea, diarrhoea, vomiting gastro-oesophageal reflux disease (GORD), abdominal pain, constipation, gastritis, abdominal distension
- peripheral oedema
- nasopharyngitis, dyspnoea, cough, nasal congestion, epistaxis, haemoptysis
- anaemia
- pain in extremity
- (uncommon) pulmonary oedema, pulmonary haemorrhage

Interactions
- contraindicated with nitrates or nitric oxide donor
- contraindicated with sildenafil, tadalafil, vardenafil, dipyridamole or theophylline
- increased risk of respiratory tract bleeding if patient is taking anticoagulants
- not recommended with azole antifungal agents (e.g. itraconazole) or HIV protease inhibitors (e.g. ritonavir)
- caution if used with ciclosporin, erlotinib and gefitinib
- plasma levels are reduced by smoking
- plasma levels may be reduced if given with antacids, phenytoin, carbamazepine, phenobarbital (phenobarbitone) and St John's wort

Nursing points/Cautions
- therapy should be initiated in hospital setting with equipment for haemodynamic monitoring and emergency care readily available
- blood pressure should be measured before starting therapy
- pregnancy should be ruled out before starting therapy
- if patient is thought not to be able to tolerate hypotensive action, dose should be started at 0.5 mg 3 times daily
- during titration:
    - if systolic BP ≥ 95 mmHg and patient has signs and symptoms of hypotension, dose should be reduced by 0.5 mg 3 times daily
    - if systolic BP < 95 mmHg and patient has no signs or symptoms of hypotension, dose should be maintained
    - if systolic BP < 95 mmHg and patient has signs and symptoms of hypotension, dose should be reduced by 0.5 mg 3 times daily
- if patient develops signs and symptoms of hypotension at any time during therapy, dose should be reduced by 0.5 mg 3 times daily
- if therapy is interrupted for 3 or more days, treatment should be restarted at 1 mg 3 times daily for 2 weeks, and titration continued as previously
- if patient was previously taking sildenafil, it should be stopped for at least 24 hours before starting riociguat and patient closely monitored for any signs of hypotension
- if patient was previously taking tadalafil, it should be stopped for at least 48 hours before starting riociguat and patient closely monitored for any signs of hypotension

- if patient is transitioning from riociguat to sildenafil or tadalafil, riociguat should be stopped for at least 24 hours before starting sildenafil or tadalafil, and patient closely monitored for any signs of hypotension
- caution if used in those ≥ 65 years
- caution if used in those with mild-to-moderate kidney impairment. If used, kidney function should be monitored regularly during therapy
- not recommended in patients who have had recent episodes of serious haemoptysis or bronchial arterial embolisation due to increased risk of respiratory tract bleeding
- not recommended in those with severe liver or kidney impairment, if systolic BP is < 95 mmHg, if patient has pulmonary veno-occlusive disease
- contraindicated in those with pulmonary hypertension associated with idiopathic interstitial pneumonias

Patient teaching and advice

- advise patient against driving or operating heavy machinery if dizziness, palpitations or hypotension occurs
- patient should be advised to stop smoking. However, if they do not, patient should be advised to let doctor know if there is any change to smoking habit as this will affect blood levels of riociguat
- if patient requires antacid, recommend that it is taken at least 1 hour after riociguat
- instruct patient to seek medical advice immediately if any of the following occur:
  - shortness of breath with activity or lying down, cough, pink frothy sputum, anxiety or sense of apprehension, feeling of drowning when lying down
- women of childbearing potential should be counselled regarding the high risk of birth defects if conception occurs during therapy, be willing to perform monthly pregnancy tests and use two reliable types of contraception if sexually active (oral contraceptives may not be reliable). Pregnancy must be avoided for 4 weeks after stopping therapy
- see also General Patient teaching and advice (p. xxvii)

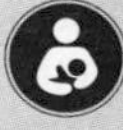

contraindicated during pregnancy and breastfeeding. Monthly pregnancy tests are recommended. Pregnancy must be avoided for 4 weeks after stopping therapy

tablet can be crushed and mixed with water or spoonful of yoghurt or apple puree

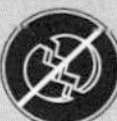

pregnant staff must not crush or disperse tablets

SEDATIVES AND HYPNOTICS

Insomnia is a very common sleep disorder that can be associated with considerable health impacts on the individual and is one of the most common psychological reasons for a person seeing a GP (Appleton et al 2018; RACGP 2015). Insomnia is 'a difficulty getting to sleep, staying asleep or having non-restorative sleep despite having adequate opportunity for sleep, together with associated impairment of daytime functioning with symptoms being present for at least 4 weeks' (RACGP 2015, p. 24). Acute insomnia generally has symptoms lasting less than 4 weeks, while chronic insomnia is a longer-term condition that can prolong, exacerbate or exist with other co-morbidities. Acute insomnia can be caused by *physiological* factors (e.g. stress, being 'on-call', caring for sick relative, being in an unknown environment such as hospital), *pharmacological* factors (including prescribed medications (e.g. new diuretic causing nocturia, ACE inhibitors, phenytoin, xanthines) and non-prescribed agents (e.g. caffeine, alcohol)), *physical* factors (e.g. coughing, noise, temperature) and *disruption to circadian rhythm* (e.g. jet lag). While the factors contributing to chronic insomnia are similar, they are longer term (e.g. depression, anxiety, dementia, substance abuse, ongoing medical conditions (e.g. pain, movement disorders, respiratory or cardiac disorders), working shift work, caffeine and alcohol use) (RACGP 2015).

Treating insomnia is not always straightforward, but it is important to treat any underlying conditions (such as pain, anxiety, medical conditions and depression), as well as receiving counselling regarding sleep hygiene and stimulus control. This education can include adequate exercise during the day (and avoiding vigorous exercise before bed), relaxation exercises, avoiding daytime napping, going to bed and getting up at the same time (routine), removal of computers, telephone, televisions and pets from the bedroom, and reducing caffeine and alcohol intake before retiring. Alcohol can cause insomnia, as well as being responsible for sleep disturbances and sedation (Bryant et al 2019).

Pharmacological agents should be used as adjuncts to the counselling described above and used in the short term (less than 4 weeks) to return a person's sleep pattern to normal and then ceased. Agents used to treat the short-term symptoms of insomnia are generally sedatives and hypnotics, with there being little distinction between them. Hypnotics produce drowsiness and help the onset of sleep, whereas sedatives are calming, decreasing activity and curbing excitement. Often the same drug can produce both effects, depending on the dosage (Bryant et al 2019).

Short-acting benzodiazepines (e.g. temazepam, alprazolam, oxazepam, zolpidem or zopliclone) are often used in the management of insomnia, because they do not have active metabolites or 'hangover' symptoms, but the risk of abuse, dependence and tolerance means they should only be used for short-term management. Withdrawal should be gradual, because an increase in sleep disturbance may occur if withdrawal is abrupt (Bryant et al 2019).

Use in the elderly should be with great caution (if at all) because of the risk of interaction with other medications, as well as the risk of delayed elimination leading to accumulation and potential side-effects, such as prolonged sedation, ataxia (and falls) and confusion. Therefore, the safest agents to use in the elderly are those with a short half-life and no active metabolites that might accumulate and cause adverse effects (Bryant et al 2019).

General Adverse effects of sedatives and hypnotics

- withdrawal reaction (prolonged use and abrupt withdrawal)
- tolerance, dependence, abuse
- memory impairment (transient)
- slurred speech, hangover, tiredness, drowsiness, dizziness, headache, unusual or unpleasant dreams, fatigue, lethargy, difficulty concentrating, decreased alertness
- anxiety, nervousness, confusion, excitation, numbed emotions
- double vision
- hypotension
- falls, ataxia, decreased physical performance, tremor
- nausea, vomiting, diarrhoea, flatulence, abdominal distension, dry mouth
- (uncommon) rash, sweating
- (rare) blood dyscrasias, elevated liver enzymes, paradoxical reactions (rage, excitement, stimulation), angioedema, complex sleep-related behaviours (e.g. sleep walking, sleep driving, preparing and eating food, making phone calls, having sex), rebound phenomenon (increase in insomnia or anxiety above pre-treatment level when therapy is stopped), angioedema, depression, suicidal ideation

General Interactions of sedatives and hypnotics

- may potentiate anticholinergic effects of atropine and related drugs, antihistamines and antidepressants
- may have additive CNS-depressant effects if given with alcohol, barbiturates, sedatives, antidepressants, MAOIs, phenothiazines, antipsychotics, antiepileptics, hypnotics, muscle relaxants, antihistamines, TCAs, opioid analgesics and anaesthetic agents
- caution if given with antiepileptic agents because levels of both antiepileptic and benzodiazepine may be altered, therefore monitoring of antiepileptic serum levels is recommended
- increased euphoria may occur if given with opioid analgesics

- abrupt withdrawal may increase frequency and severity of seizures in those with epilepsy
- serum levels may increase if given with erythromycin, clarithromycin, diltiazem, saquinavir, ritonavir, azole antifungals, fluoxetine, omeprazole, atorvastatin, verapamil, cimetidine or disulfiram
- sedative effects may be reduced if given with xanthines (e.g. aminophylline, theophylline, caffeine)
- metabolism can be increased by carbamazepine, phenytoin, rifampicin and St John's wort reducing serum levels
- benzodiazepines have an unpredictable effect on phenytoin levels and these should be closely monitored during therapy
- may cause delirium in the elderly (especially if given with anticholinergic agents)

General Nursing points/Cautions for sedatives and hypnotics

- FBC, liver and renal function should be monitored regularly during therapy with benzodiazepines
- if there is no improvement to sleep in 7–10 days, underlying causes for insomnia should be investigated
- prolonged use is not recommended
- withdrawal should be gradual; if stopped suddenly, sleep disturbance may occur
- tolerance and dependence may occur
- agent should be stopped if paradoxical reaction (acute rage, stimulation, excitation) occurs
- may increase depression in some patients or cause deterioration in severely disturbed patients with schizophrenia
- lower doses are usually required for older people
- transient amnesia may occur, especially with parenteral administration of benzodiazepines
- patients with cardiac or cerebral disease should be monitored closely if hypotension is likely to cause complications
- caution if used in the elderly or those where a fall in blood pressure may lead to cardiac or cerebral complications
- caution if used in those with depression, psychosis, schizophrenia, suicidal tendencies or drug/alcohol abuse
- caution if used in those with epilepsy as abrupt withdrawal may lead to increase in frequency or severity of seizures and there are also interactions with some antiepileptic agents (see Interactions)
- caution if used in those with blood dyscrasias, liver or kidney impairment, or respiratory insufficiency
- contraindicated in those with myasthenia gravis, severe liver insufficiency, sleep apnoea, chronic obstructive airways disease (with insipient respiratory failure) or in those with hypersensitivity to any benzodiazepine
- benzodiazepines are contraindicated in those with acute narrow-angle glaucoma (but can be used in those with open-angle glaucoma that is being treated)

General Patient teaching and advice for sedatives and hypnotics

- caution patient against increasing the dose or abruptly stopping medication without first seeking medical advice

- advise patient to seek medical advice immediately if any swelling of tongue, glottis or larynx occurs
- warn patient against driving a vehicle or operating machinery if drowsy or experiencing decreased alertness
- patient should be warned about the reduced tolerance to alcohol and other CNS depressants
- counsel patient about reliance on sleeping pills and rebound insomnia that may occur on first and second nights after stopping medication
- patient should be warned about ataxia and muscle weakness, which increases the risk of falls (especially in the elderly)
- advise patient that some sleep medication can cause short-term memory loss
- instruct patient in ways to improve sleep hygiene, including:
  - only using bed for sleep and sex
  - removing all computers, laptops, tablets, televisions, radios, videogames and smartphones from bedroom
  - if sleep doesn't occur within 20 minutes, get out of bed and read or do something relaxing (e.g. listening to relaxing music) in dim light before returning to bed
  - avoid napping in the afternoon or early evening
  - go to bed and get up at the same time every day
  - ensure environment is restful (comfortable bed, quiet, temperature not too hot or cold, dark)
  - prepare for sleep with 20–30 minutes of relaxation (e.g. warm bath, reading, listening to music, meditation, yoga)
  - avoid alcohol, caffeine, smoking, vigorous exercise or heavy eating 2–3 hours before bedtime
  - when trying to fall asleep avoid problem-solving, reviewing the day or thinking about life issues
- patient/carer/partner should be advised to immediately report any unusual activities such as sleep walking, sleep driving, preparing and eating food, making phone calls or having sex without any memory of the event (especially zolpidem and zopiclone)
- women of childbearing potential should be counselled to use adequate contraception during therapy to avoid pregnancy. If pregnancy occurs, woman should seek medical advice immediately
- see also General Patient teaching and advice (p. xxvii)

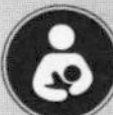

benzodiazepines cross the placental barrier and may cause hypotonia, decreased respiratory function and hypothermia in the newborn. Withdrawal symptoms in the newborn may also occur if there has been prolonged maternal use during pregnancy

not recommended during breastfeeding

CHLORAL HYDRATE (Chloral Hydrate Mixture)

Available form

Syrup: 1 g/10 mL

Action

- sedative, hypnotic
- related to chloroform and ethanol
- active metabolite (trichloroethanol) appears to be responsible for CNS depression and has a half-life of 4–12 hours. Metabolite inhibits alcohol metabolism prolonging its actions

- effective within 30 minutes, duration 4–8 hours
- has been superseded by more effective and less toxic agents

Use

- insomnia (short term)
- preoperative sedation

Dose

- (hypnotic) 0.5–1 g orally nocte 15–30 minutes before bedtime (daily maximum 2 g) **OR**
- (preoperatively) 0.5–1 g orally 30 minutes before surgery (daily maximum 2 g)

Adverse effects

- nausea, vomiting, diarrhoea, flatulence, unpleasant taste, abdominal distention
- residual sedation, hangover
- (uncommon) leucopenia, eosinophilia, disorientation, tolerance, dependence
- (prolonged therapy) gastritis, skin eruptions, kidney damage
- (rare) rash, urticaria, pruritus, angioedema, ketonuria, paradoxical reactions

Interactions

- CNS-depressant effects increased by other CNS depressants, including alcohol, benzodiazepines, barbiturates, antihistamines, TCAs, sedatives, hypnotics, opioids or antipsychotics
- caution if given with warfarin as there may be a transient increase in serum levels, therefore INR should be monitored closely, especially when starting or stopping therapy
- hypermetabolic state (sweating, flushing, labile BP, sense of unease) may result if IV furosemide (frusemide) is given after chloral hydrate
- increased risk of vasodilation reaction (tachycardia, palpitations, facial flushing, dysphoria) if given with alcohol
- increased risk of delirium if given with psychotropic or anticholinergic agents (especially in the elderly)
- may interfere with some laboratory tests (including urinary glucose using Clinitest)

Nursing points/Cautions

- contraindicated in children with obstructive sleep apnoea
- contraindicated in those with liver or kidney impairment, severe cardiac disease, gastritis, oesophagitis, gastric or duodenal ulcers or porphyria
- see General Nursing points/Cautions for sedatives and hypnotics (p. 1436)

Patient teaching and advice

- advise patient that gastric irritation may be minimised by taking mixture immediately after food or diluting with a full glass of water, fruit juice or ginger ale
- see General Patient teaching and advice for sedatives and hypnotics (p. 1436)

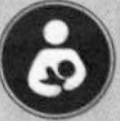

not recommended during pregnancy or breastfeeding as it may cause sedation in newborn

DEXMEDETOMIDINE (Precedex)

Available forms

Ampoules: 100 microgram/mL (concentrate), 4 microgram/mL (ready to use solution)

Action

- selective alpha-2 adrenoreceptor antagonist with sedative and analgesic actions but no amnesic properties
- half-life is approximately 2 hours

Use

- ICU sedation (intubated patients)
- procedural sedation (non-intubated patients)

Dose

- initially 1 microgram/kg IV over 10–20 minutes (loading dose), followed by 0.2–1.0 microgram/kg/hour (maintenance) (titrating maintenance dose according to response)

Adverse effects

- hypotension, transient hypertension, bradycardia, tachycardia, atrial fibrillation, sinus arrest
- fever, rigors
- agitation, confusion
- hypoxia, respiratory depression
- dry mouth, nausea, vomiting, thirst
- decreased lacrimation, corneal dryness
- oliguria
- hyper or hypoglycaemia
- anaemia

Interactions

- increased effects may occur if given with anaesthetics, sedatives, hypnotics or opioid analgesics
- bradycardia and/or hypotension may be potentiated if given with propofol or midazolam

Nursing points/Cautions

- should only be administered by anaesthetist or in ICU setting
- ECG, BP and oxygen saturation should be monitored throughout infusion. Transient hypertension (due to initial vasoconstriction) may occur with loading dose
- any hypovolaemia should be corrected before starting therapy
- lubrication of eyes is recommended to prevent corneal dryness and damage
- if amnesia is also required, an amnesic agent should also be administered
- onset of sedation is 10–15 minutes after start of infusion
- patients receiving dexmedetomidine are easily rousable and alert when stimulated. However, this does not indicate a lack of drug efficacy
- IV therapy should only continue for 24 hours
- loading dose may not be required if other sedative agents have been used previously
- use of loading dose has been associated with increased risk of adverse effects
- therapy does not need to be ceased for extubation
- not recommended as bolus or rapid IV administration due to increased risk of bradycardia and sinus arrest
- use a controlled infusion device
- 2 mL of solution is added to 48 mL of sodium chloride 0.9% and gently shaken to make up IV solution (100 microgram/mL concentrate solution)
- not recommended with blood or blood products
- caution if used in those with pre-existing bradycardia, heart block or ventricular dysfunction, > 65 years or those with diabetes
- caution if used in those with liver failure (dose reduction is required), severe cardiac disease or chronic hypertension
- see General Nursing points/Cautions for sedatives and hypnotics (p. 1436)

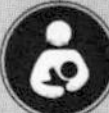

should only be used during pregnancy or breastfeeding if benefits outweigh potential risks

FLUNITRAZEPAM (Hypnodorm)

Available form

Tablets: 1 mg

Action

- long-acting benzodiazepine related to nitrazepam and clonazepam with marked hypnotic and sedative properties, as well as anxiolytic and muscle-relaxant properties
- rapid onset of action, half-life 20–30 hours

- two active metabolites, but less active than parent but have half-lives ranging from 10–33 hours

Use
- severe insomnia (short-term management)

Dose
- (adult) 1–2 mg orally nocte, immediately before going to bed **OR**
- (elderly) 0.5–1 mg orally nocte, immediately before going to bed

Adverse effects/Interactions/ Nursing points/Cautions/Patient teaching and advice
- see general points for sedatives and hypnotics (pp. 1434–37)

tablet can be dispersed in water or crushed and mixed with spoonful of yoghurt or apple puree

MELATONIN (Circadin, Melotin MR, Slenyto)

Available form

Tablets (prolonged release): 2 mg

Action
- naturally occurring hormone produced by pineal gland
- related to serotonin
- naturally secreted soon after onset of darkness, peaks between 2 am and 4 am, diminishing during second half of night
- associated with circadian rhythm control, hypnotic effect and increased sleep tendency
- acts at melatonin receptors (MT1-inhibit neuron firing, MT2-phase shifting response) in the hypothalamus
- inactive metabolite
- half-life 3.5–4 hours
- melatonin metabolism declines with age

Use
- insomnia (short-term management) in those aged 55 years and over

Dose
- 2 mg orally 1–2 hours before bedtime and after food

Adverse effects
- headache, asthenia, dizziness, migraine, drowsiness, nightmares
- anxiety
- nasopharyngitis, influenza, upper and lower respiratory tract infection, rhinitis, cough, nasopharyngeal pain
- urinary tract infection
- back ache, arthralgia, muscle cramp, neck pain, pain in extremity
- abdominal pain, constipation, diarrhoea, nausea, vomiting

Interactions
- not recommended with alcohol
- may enhance sedative properties of other sedatives and hypnotics
- increased sensation of fuzzy-headedness when given with imipramine
- serum levels may be reduced by carbamazepine, rifampicin and smoking
- increased serum levels may occur if given with fluoroquinolone antibiotics, cimetidine and oestrogen-containing agents (e.g. oral contraceptives, hormone replacement therapy)
- not recommended with fluvoxamine

Nursing points/Cautions
- caution if used in those with kidney insufficiency
- tablets contain lactose, therefore are not recommended in those with rare hereditary problems of galactose intolerance, Lapp lactase deficiency or glucose–galactose malabsorption
- not recommended in those under 18 years
- not recommended in those with autoimmune diseases or liver impairment

Patient teaching and advice

- advise patient that tablet should be swallowed whole, not chewed or split
- see General Patient teaching and advice for sedatives and hypnotics (p. 1436)

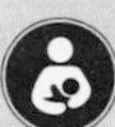

not recommended during pregnancy or breastfeeding

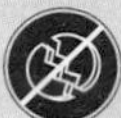

tablet should not be divided, crushed or chewed

MIDAZOLAM HYDROCHLORIDE (Hypnovel, Midazolam Solution for Injection)

Available forms

Ampoules: 5 mg/5 mL, 5 mg/mL, 15 mg/3 mL, 50 mg/10 mL

Action

- very short-acting benzodiazepine with rapid onset
- induces sedation, hypnosis, amnesia, anaesthesia, muscle relaxation
- induces sedation in 15 minutes (IM), peak effect 30–60 minutes, half-life 1.4–2.4 hours
- induces anaesthesia (IV), onset of action is 1.5–2.5 minutes (depending on dose and/or opioid premedication)
- approximately 2 hours are required for full recovery after anaesthesia (time dependent on dose and usage of other drugs)
- active metabolite (half-life 1–3 hours)
- half-life prolonged in the elderly, obese, critically ill, and those with congestive heart failure

Use

- preoperative sedation, relief of anxiety and to impair memory of perioperative events (IM)
- conscious sedation before endoscopy (lung, stomach, bladder), coronary angiography and cardiac catheterisation (IV) (alone or with opioid)
- induction of anaesthesia before anaesthetic agent (IV)
- sedation in ICU (IV)

Dose

- (preoperative sedation) 0.07–0.08 mg/kg IM 1 hour before surgery **OR**
- (endoscopic/cardiovascular procedures) initially 1 mg by slow IV injection (starting with lowest dose and titrating dose to desired sedation at 2–3-minute intervals) **OR**
- (induction of anaesthesia) 0.15–0.2 mg/kg by slow IV at a rate of 2.5 mg/10 seconds. A further dose may be given if needed (to a total of 0.35 mg/kg) **OR**
- (sedation in ICU) 0.03–0.2 mg/kg/hour by IV infusion

Adverse effects

- see General Adverse effects of sedatives and hypnotics (p. 1435)
- (IV) hiccups, acid taste, coughing, phlebitis
- (IV, IM injection site) induration, redness, pain, muscle stiffness, headache, tenderness
- (surgical procedures) respiratory depression, apnoea, variation in HR and BP

Interactions

- thiopental sodium induction dose requirement may be reduced when IM midazolam is used as premedication
- erythromycin, other macrolide antibiotics and cimetidine inhibit metabolism of midazolam prolonging duration of sedation
- increased effect if given with sodium valproate
- not recommended with St John's wort
- half-life may be increased if given with aprepitant

- see General Interactions of sedatives and hypnotics (p. 1435)

Nursing points/Cautions

- continuous cardiorespiratory function monitoring is recommended during IV administration
- any fluid or electrolyte imbalance should be corrected before administration or dose reduced
- extravasation and intra-arterial administration should be avoided
- not recommended as IV bolus or by rapid IV administration
- vital signs should be monitored carefully during administration and recovery period
- for conscious sedation, dose should be titrated until patient slurs speech, then wait for 2–3 minutes to establish effect and give further dose if needed
- patient should not be discharged until at least 3 hours post-procedure and any information given immediately post-procedure repeated on discharge as anterograde amnesia may last longer than sedation, therefore patient may not remember what was said to them in the immediate post-procedure period
- may be mixed in the same syringe with morphine, pethidine, atropine or hyoscine
- contraindicated in those in shock or coma, or with acute alcohol intoxication with depressed vital signs
- see General Nursing points/Cautions for sedatives and hypnotics (p. 1436)

Patient teaching and advice

- patient should be advised to avoid alcohol for at least 12 hours after administration, because mutual potentiation can cause unpredictable reactions
- see General Patient teaching and advice for sedatives and hypnotics (p. 1436)

NITRAZEPAM (Alodorm, Mogadon)

Available form

Tablets: 5 mg

Action

- long-acting benzodiazepine with no active metabolites
- sedative, anxiolytic, antiepileptic and muscle-relaxing properties
- facilitates action of GABA in the brain
- effective as a hypnotic within 30–60 minutes, duration 6–8 hours, long half-life (average 27 hours)

Use

- insomnia (short-term management)

Dose

- (adult) 5–10 mg orally nocte, 20–30 minutes before bedtime **OR**
- (elderly) 2.5–5 mg orally nocte, 20–30 minutes before bedtime

Adverse effects/Interactions/ Nursing points/Cautions

- dose may be increased to 20 mg in hospitalised patients if needed
- see general points for sedatives and hypnotics (pp. 1434–37)

tablet can be dispersed in water or crushed and mixed with spoonful of yoghurt or apple puree

PARALDEHYDE (Paraldehyde Injection BP)

Available form

Ampoules: 1000 microgram/mL (100% paraldehyde/5 mL = antioxidant dose of 100 micrograms/mL)

Action

- sedative and hypnotic that acts on the reticular activating system in the brain

- some antiepileptic properties
- effective within 5–15 minutes (IM), duration 8 hours, half-life about 7.5 hours
- has been largely replaced by safer, more effective agents

Use

- sedative and hypnotic in acute agitation because of alcohol or drug withdrawal (when other agents are inappropriate or ineffective)
- control convulsions of tetanus or poisons; status epilepticus (when other agents are inappropriate or ineffective)

Dose

- (hypnotic) 10 mg (10 mL) IM **OR**
- (sedative) 5 mg (5 mL) IM **OR**
- (convulsions) 5–10 mg (5–10 mL) IM **OR**
- (alcohol withdrawal) 5 mg (5 mL) IM 4–6-hourly for first 24 hours, then 6-hourly (maximum 30 mg (30 mL) first day and 20 mg (20 mL) thereafter)

Adverse effects

- dizziness, muscle cramps, trembling, unusual sweating
- rash
- (IM) sterile abscess, fat necrosis, skin sloughing, muscle irritation, pain, severe nerve damage
- (IV) pulmonary oedema and/or bleeding, hypotension, circulatory collapse, thrombophlebitis
- (prolonged use) toxic hepatitis, nephrosis, dependence, tolerance
- (overdose) short rapid breathing, cloudy urine, oligouria, slow HR, general weakness, metabolic acidosis

Interactions

- not recommended with disulfiram
- CNS-depressant effects may be increased if given with alcohol, barbiturates, TCAs, phenothiazines and morphine derivatives

Nursing points/Cautions

- solution should not be used if it has a brownish colour or smells sharply of acetic acid, which indicates decomposition of paraldehyde. Administration of partly decomposed paraldehyde may cause metabolic acidosis
- should only be given IM, not IV or SC
- give only 5 mL deeply into any one IM site
- IM injection is very painful
- rotate injection sites
- avoid contact with skin, eyes and clothing
- patient should be carefully monitored if agitated or confused
- patient's breath will have the unmistakable characteristic odour of the drug for several hours, because it is partly eliminated by the lungs
- warm gently if crystallised
- contact with rubber and plastic should be avoided because paraldehyde has a solvent action on most plastics and should be drawn up using a glass syringe only
- caution if used in those with cardiovascular disease, asthma
- contraindicated in those with liver insufficiency, bronchopulmonary disease or during obstetric anaesthesia
- see also General Nursing points/Cautions for sedatives and hypnotics (p. 1436)

Patient teaching and advice

- pregnancy should be excluded before use. Women of childbearing potential should be advised to use adequate and effective contraception to avoid pregnancy during therapy
- see General Patient teaching and advice for sedatives and hypnotics (p. 1436)

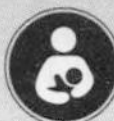

not recommended during pregnancy or breastfeeding. May result in respiratory depression of the neonate

SUVOREXANT (Belsomra)

Available forms

Tablets: 15 mg, 30 mg

Action

- highly selective orexin receptor antagonist (orexin is a neuropeptide that is a central promotor of wakefulness)
- non-active metabolite
- increases REM sleep
- does not appear to produce dependence
- half-life 12 hours

Use

- treatment of insomnia

Dose

- (adult ≥ 65 years) 15 mg orally nocte 30 minutes before bedtime **OR**
- (adult < 65 years) 20 mg orally nocte 30 minutes before bedtime

Adverse effects

- fatigue, somnolence, dizziness, headache
- abnormal dreaming, nightmares, anxiety
- nausea, dry mouth, diarrhoea
- palpitations, tachycardia
- (rare) complex behaviours, worsening of depression, suicidal ideation, sleep paralysis (inability to walk or talk for several minutes during sleep–wake transition), mild catalepsy (e.g. mild leg weakness not associated with normal triggering event such as laughter or surprise), hypnagogic/hypnopompic hallucinations (vivid and sometimes disturbing sleep hallucinations that occur at sleep–wake transition)

Interactions

- CNS depression increased if given with other CNS depressants, including alcohol, benzodiazepines, TCAs and opioid analgesics
- not recommended with other hypnotic or sedative agents
- not recommended with aprepitant, diltiazem, ciprofloxacin, erythromycin, azole antifungal agents or HIV protease inhibitors (e.g. ritonavir), imatinib, grapefruit juice or verapamil
- efficacy may be reduced if given with rifampicin, carbamazepine and phenytoin
- may increase digoxin levels slightly, therefore blood levels should be monitored especially when starting or stopping therapy

Nursing points/Cautions

- if medication is not effective in improving insomnia in 7–10 days, other causes (e.g. medical or psychiatric illness) should be investigated
- caution if used in those with compromised respiratory function (e.g. sleep apnoea, chronic obstructive pulmonary disease)
- caution in those with history of drug abuse if given for a long period
- not recommended in those with severe liver impairment
- contraindicated in those with narcolepsy

Patient teaching and advice

- patient should be instructed to take medication 30 minutes before retiring when they will get a full night's sleep (at least 7 hours) before needing to be awake
- warn patient that daytime wakefulness can be impaired, and this may persist for several days after discontinuing therapy
- patient should be instructed against driving or operating machinery if drowsy or experiencing decreased alertness

- advise patient to avoid alcohol and grapefruit juice during therapy
- patient should be warned against increasing dose
- instruct patient in ways to improve sleep hygiene (see General Patient teaching and advice for sedatives and hypnotics, p. 1436)
- patient/carer/partner should be advised to immediately report any of the following:
  - unusual activities, such as sleep walking, sleep driving, preparing and eating food and making phone calls without any memory of the activity
  - depression (new or worsening) or thoughts of self-harm
  - temporary inability to walk or talk for minutes when falling asleep or waking up
  - abnormal thoughts or behaviours, including being aggressive or more outgoing than normal, confusion, agitation or experiencing hallucinations which may be vivid and disturbing
  - sudden leg weakness or collapse

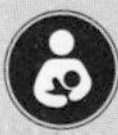

not recommended during pregnancy unless benefits outweigh risks

caution if used during breastfeeding

tablet can be crushed and mixed with water or spoonful of yoghurt or apple puree

TEMAZEPAM (Normison, Temaze, Temtabs)

Available form
Tablets: 10 mg

Action
- short-acting benzodiazepine with no long-acting active metabolite; tends not to accumulate with long-term therapy
- metabolised to oxazepam
- half-life is 8–15 hours

Use
- insomnia (short-term management)

Dose
- (adult) 10–30 mg orally nocte 20–30 minutes before retiring **OR**
- (elderly) 10 mg orally nocte 20–30 minutes before retiring

Adverse effects/Interactions/Nursing points/Cautions/Patient teaching and advice
- see general points for sedatives and hypnotics (pp. 1434–37)

tablet can be dispersed in water or crushed and mixed with spoonful of yoghurt or apple puree

ZOLPIDEM TARTRATE (Dormizol, Somidem, Stildem, Stilnox, Stilnox CR, Zolpibell)

Available forms
Tablets: 10 mg; Tablets (controlled/modified release): 6.25 mg, 12.5 mg

Action
- imidazopyridine unrelated to other hypnotic agents
- selectively bind to benzodiazepine-1 subtype receptors (omega-1 subtype), whereas benzodiazepines bind non-selectively to all three omega receptor subtypes
- no active metabolite
- rapid onset, duration 6 hours, half-life 2 hours

Use
- insomnia (short-term management)

Dose
- (adult) 10 mg orally at night 20–30 minutes immediately before bedtime (immediate-release tablets) **OR**

- (elderly) 5 mg orally at night 20–30 minutes immediately before bedtime (immediate-release tablets) **OR**
- (adult) 12.5 mg orally at night immediately before bedtime (modified-release tablets) **OR**
- (elderly) 6.25 mg orally at night immediately before bedtime (modified-release tablets)

Adverse effects

- dizziness, daytime drowsiness, headache, memory impairment, drugged feeling, abnormal dreams, fatigue, somnolence, disorientation
- nausea, vomiting, diarrhoea, abdominal pain, dry mouth
- palpitations
- myalgia, back pain
- flu-like symptoms
- visual disturbances
- (uncommon) complex sleep-related behaviours (e.g. sleep walking, sleep driving, preparing and eating food, making phone calls, having sex), rebound insomnia
- (rare) angioedema

Interactions

- additive CNS-depressant effects may occur if given with other CNS-depressant drugs including barbiturates, benzodiazepines, sedatives, hypnotics, antianxiety agents, TCAs, MAOIs, muscle relaxants, phenothiazines, antipsychotics, antihistamines, antiepileptics and anaesthetics
- caution if given with opioid analgesics due to increased CNS sedation and risk of respiratory depression and coma
- serum levels may be decreased if given with rifampicin and St John's wort
- not recommended with ciprofloxacin or fluvoxamine
- contraindicated with alcohol because of increased risk of complex sleep-related behaviours
- increased sedation may occur if given with imipramine or chlorpromazine

Nursing points/Cautions

- therapy should be limited to 4 weeks maximum under close medical supervision
- caution if used in those with long QT syndrome
- see General Nursing points/Cautions for sedatives and hypnotics (p. 1436)

Patient teaching and advice

- advise patient that modified-release tablets should be swallowed whole and not crushed or chewed
- warn patient not to take tablets with or immediately after food for maximum effect
- patient should be warned about the serious effects of drinking alcohol during therapy
- see General Patient teaching and advice for sedatives and hypnotics (p. 1436)

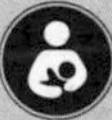

not recommended during pregnancy or breastfeeding

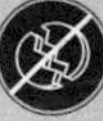

controlled-release (CR) tablets must not be crushed or chewed. Other tablets (10 mg) can be dispersed in water or crushed and mixed with spoonful of yoghurt or apple puree

ZOPICLONE (Imoclone, Imovane, Imrest)

Available form

Tablets: 7.5 mg

Action

- cyclopyrrolone with sedative, anxiolytic, muscle relaxant, antiepileptic and amnesic properties
- one metabolite has weak activity

- half-life about 5.3 hours (extended in the elderly and those with liver impairment)

Use

- insomnia (short-term treatment)

Dose

- 3.75–7.5 mg orally nocte 20–30 minutes before bedtime

Adverse effects

- bitter taste, dry mouth, anorexia, nausea, vomiting, diarrhoea/constipation, bad breath, coated tongue, heartburn, dyspepsia, epigastric pain
- drowsiness, headache, fatigue
- blurred vision
- urticaria, tingling, pruritus, rash
- impotence, ejaculation problems, libido disorder
- palpitations (elderly)
- withdrawal syndrome
- (less commonly) impaired memory, confusion, dizziness, somnolence, euphoria, hypotonia, depression, asthenia, weakness, anxiety, agitation, euphoria, rebound insomnia, lack of coordination, complex sleep-related behaviours (e.g. sleep walking, sleep driving, preparing and eating food, making phone calls, having sex), rebound insomnia
- (rare) altered micturition, altered liver enzymes, angioedema, muscle weakness

Interactions

- additive CNS-depressant effects may occur if given with other CNS-depressant drugs including barbiturates, benzodiazepines, sedatives, hypnotics, antianxiety agents, TCAs, MAOIs, muscle relaxants, phenothiazines, antipsychotics, antihistamines, antiepileptics, and anaesthetics
- not recommended with opioid analgesics due to increased CNS sedation and risk of respiratory depression and coma
- increased serum level may occur if given with erythromycin, clarithromycin, ritonavir or itraconazole
- decreased serum levels may occur if given with rifampicin, carbamazepine, phenobarbital (phenobarbitone), phenytoin or St John's wort
- contraindicated with alcohol because of increased risk of complex sleep-related behaviours

Nursing points/Cautions

- therapy for greater than 4 weeks is not recommended
- not recommended in those with thyroid dysfunction or hormonal imbalance
- contraindicated in those with acute CVA
- see General Nursing points/Cautions for sedatives and hypnotics (p. 1436)

Patient teaching and advice

- patient should be warned about the serious effects of drinking alcohol during therapy
- advise patient that tablet has a bitter taste
- see General Patient teaching and advice for sedatives and hypnotics (p. 1436)

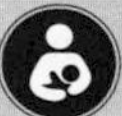

not recommended during pregnancy or breastfeeding

tablet can be dispersed in water or crushed and mixed with spoonful of yoghurt or apple puree

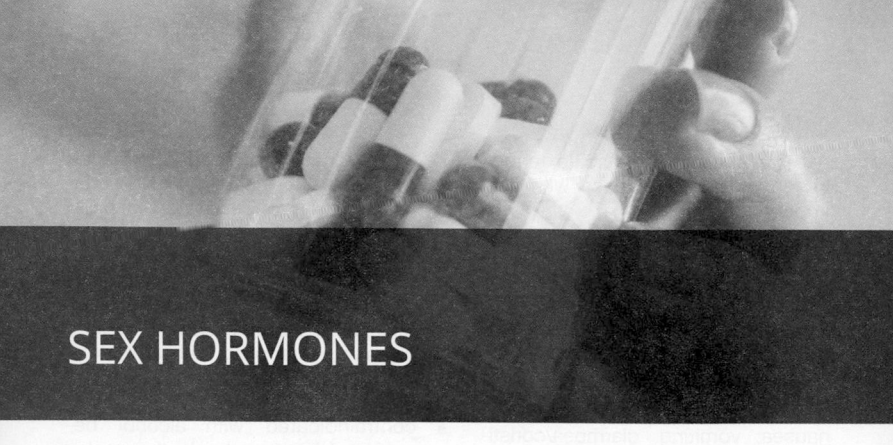

SEX HORMONES

Steroid (sex) hormones (oestrogens and androgens) are produced mainly in the ovaries and testes, but also in the adrenal cortex and the placenta. Production is controlled by gonadotrophic hormones (FSH, LH), released by the anterior pituitary gland (which is in turn controlled by the hypothalamus and circulating levels). They are generally synthesised and secreted (rather than being stored) and are lipid soluble and derived from cholesterol. The sex hormones have a role in the development and maintenance of the sex organs, as well as regulation of reproduction (Bryant et al 2019).

Other agents described in this section are the sex hormone antagonists, oral contraceptive agents and agents that do not fit into any of these categories but still have an effect on the sex hormones.

ANDROGENS AND ANABOLIC STEROIDS

General Actions of androgens and anabolic steroids

- testosterone is the main androgen produced from within the Leydig (interstitial) cells in the testes, from precursors (dehydroepiandrosterone (DHEA) and androstenedione) produced in the adrenal glands
- some testosterone acts on seminiferous tubules to produce sperm; the remainder is secreted into the bloodstream and travels to target tissue
- (before birth) androgens are responsible for masculinisation of reproductive tract and external genitalia and descent of testes into scrotum
- (reproduction-related effects) growth and sexual maturation at puberty, as well as spermatogenesis, maintenance of reproductive tract and feedback control of gonadotrophin secretion
- development of male secondary sex characteristics (e.g. deepening of voice, male pattern hair growth, muscle growth, male body shape) and behaviours. Androgens are also responsible for male accessory sex organs (e.g. prostate gland, seminal

vesicles, penis and bulbo-urethral glands)
- non-reproductive functions of androgens include anabolic effects on bone and skeletal muscle (i.e. resulting in increased skeletal weight, increased bone mass and growth), neuroprotective effect in central and peripheral nervous system, bone protection (due to decreased calcium excretion) and stimulation of vascular cell adhesion molecules in endothelial cells

General Uses of androgens and anabolic steroids
- replacement therapy in men with hypogonadism or eunuchoidism, and for the male climacteric (andropause)
- diseases in which there is protein and bone wasting (e.g. osteoporosis), and for which oestrogen therapy is contraindicated
- acute and chronic renal failure (including anaemia of chronic renal failure)
- inoperable breast carcinoma
- aplastic anaemia
- long-term corticosteroid therapy

General Adverse effects of androgens and anabolic steroids
- acne, rash, skin flushing, oily skin, greasy hair
- weight gain
- (females) virilisation (e.g. acne, hirsutism, clitoral enlargement, menstrual irregularities (e.g. oligomenorrhoea, amenorrhoea), libido changes, voice changes, increased growth of pubic hair)
- (males) increased frequency or persistence of erections, priapism
- (prepubertal male) precocious sexual development, increased frequency of penile erection, phallic enlargement, premature epiphyseal closure
- excessive sexual stimulation, increase in libido
- gynaecomastia
- abdominal pain, nausea, gastrointestinal bleeding
- altered glucose tolerance
- hyperlipidaemia, decreased serum HDL cholesterol
- headache (common), insomnia, anxiety, depression, excitation, aggression, emotional lability, mania, hypomania
- (metastatic cancer) exacerbation of hypercalcaemia/hypercalciuria
- (prolonged therapy) oligospermia, decreased ejaculatory volume, decreased sperm count, inhibition of spermatogenesis
- salt and water retention, hypertension, oedema
- (rare) bladder irritability, decreased urine flow, impotence, testicular atrophy, prostate hyperplasia
- (rare) leucocytosis, polycythaemia, hyperlipidaemia
- (rare, long term) benign or malignant liver or prostate tumours, peliosis hepatis
- (rare) liver function test abnormalities, cholestatic hepatitis, jaundice

General Interactions of androgens and anabolic steroids
- may increase effects of warfarin, therefore INR should be closely monitored, especially when starting, stopping or altering dose
- androgens may improve glucose tolerance, thereby altering requirements for insulin and/or oral hypoglycaemic agents

- may potentiate effects and also the risk of nephrotoxicity if given with ciclosporin
- caution if given with thyroxine
- increased risk of oedema if given with ACTH or corticosteroids
- may alter results of some laboratory tests including glucose tolerance test, metyrapone test (pituitary test), thyroxine and iodine studies, suppression of clotting factors

General Nursing points/Cautions for androgens and anabolic steroids

- digital rectal (prostate) examinations and measuring PSA level should be carried out before starting therapy (to rule out presence of prostate cancer) and then regularly throughout
- (hypogonadism) diagnosis (e.g. clinical and physical assessment, serum testosterone, LH and FSH levels) should be confirmed before starting therapy
- liver function, serum cholesterol and BP should be monitored regularly throughout therapy
- haemoglobin and haematocrit should be checked before starting therapy to rule out polycythaemia
- dose should be decreased if frequent or persistent erections occur
- females should be closely monitored for any signs of virilisation and therapy stopped to reverse changes
- should not be used to enhance muscle development or increase physical ability in healthy individuals due to serious health risks. Furthermore, most androgens and anabolic steroids are banned in sport
- caution if used in those with bony (skeletal) metastases as hypercalcaemia/hypercalciuria may develop or be aggravated
- caution if used in those with benign prostatic hypertrophy as urinary obstruction may occur
- caution if used in those with psychological disturbances as depression may be aggravated
- caution if used in those whose growth is incomplete, because high doses may cause premature closure of epiphyseal plates
- caution if given to those with cardiac or renal failure/impairment, hypertension, epilepsy or migraine where fluid retention/overload may aggravate conditions
- caution if given to those with a history of myocardial infarction or chronic artery disease, thrombophilia or liver dysfunction
- caution if given to those with diabetes mellitus, androgen-sensitive polycythaemia, sleep apnoea or porphyria
- contraindicated in those with hypercalcaemia, liver tumours (current or history), prostate cancer or breast cancer (males), cardiac failure, liver disease (with impaired bilirubin excretion), nephrosis or nephrotic phase of nephritis

General Patient teaching and advice for androgens and anabolic steroids

- females should be advised to report any changes, such as hoarseness or voice changes, that might be suggestive of virilisation
- instruct male patient to seek medical advice immediately if any of the following occur:
  - frequent or prolonged erection (this can become a medical emergency)
  - breast enlargement or tenderness
- patient with diabetes mellitus should be instructed to closely monitor

blood glucose levels during therapy as androgens may improve glucose tolerance decreasing requirement for insulin and/or oral hypoglycaemics
- patient (or carer) should be advised to seek medical advice immediately if any of the following occur:
  - thoughts/talk about self-harm, harm to others, suicide or death or recent attempts at self-harm or increase in aggression or hostility
  - change in mood
  - worsening of depression
- see also General Patient teaching and advice (p. xxvii)

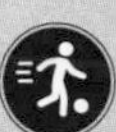
banned in sport

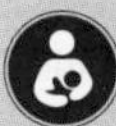
contraindicated during breastfeeding

MESTEROLONE (Proviron)

Available form
Tablets: 25 mg

Action/Use
- see General Actions of androgens and anabolic steroids (p. 1448) and General Uses of androgens and anabolic steroids (p. 1449)

Dose
- (hypogonadism) initially 25–50 mg orally 3 times daily for several months, then reduced to 25 mg 2–3 times daily (maintenance)

Adverse effects/Interactions/Nursing points/Cautions/Patient teaching and advice
- see general points for androgens and anabolic steroids (pp. 1448–51)

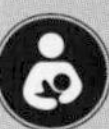
contraindicated during pregnancy. Should only be used by males

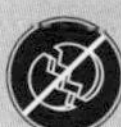
tablets should be swallowed whole

NANDROLONE DECONOATE (Deca-Durabolin)

Available form
Prefilled syringes: 50 mg/mL

Action/Use
- anabolic agent with greater anabolic but less androgenic activity than testosterone
- duration of action about 3 weeks
- see General Actions of androgens and anabolic steroids (p. 1448) and General Uses of androgens and anabolic steroids (p. 1449)

Dose
- (renal conditions) 25–50 mg deep IM every 2–3 weeks (initially 50 mg weekly may be required) **OR**
- (inoperable breast carcinoma, osteoporosis, long-term corticosteroid therapy) 50 mg deep IM every 2–3 weeks **OR**
- (aplastic anaemia) 50–150 mg deep IM weekly **OR**
- (anaemia of chronic renal failure) 200 mg IM weekly (males) or 100 mg IM weekly (females) until haemoglobin returns to normal and then therapy gradually withdrawn

Adverse effects
- urticaria at injection site
- see General Adverse effects of androgens and anabolic steroids (p. 1449)

Interactions
- not recommended with heparin
- if given with recombinant erythropoietin (especially in females) may enhance

effects requiring a decrease in dosage of erythropoietin
- see General Interactions of androgens and anabolic steroids (p. 1449)

Nursing points/Cautions/Patient teaching and advice

- for optimal effects, patient should be advised to ensure diet is rich in protein, vitamins and minerals
- contains benzyl alcohol and is not recommended in children < 3 years due to increased risk of toxicity and anaphylaxis
- contraindicated in those with peanut or soya allergy
- see General Nursing points/Cautions and Patient teaching and advice for androgens and anabolic steroids (p. 1450)

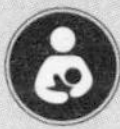

contraindicated during pregnancy

TESTOSTERONE (Androderm, AndroFeme 1, AndroForte 2, AndroForte 5, Testavan, Testogel)

TESTOSTERONE DECONAOTE (Sustanon 250)

TESTOSTERONE ENANTATE (ENANTHATE) (Primoteston Depot)

TESTOSTERONE UNDECONATE (Andriol Testocaps, Reandron 1000)

Available forms

Capsules: 40 mg; Ampoules (depot solution): 250 mg/mL, 1000 mg/4 mL; Prefilled syringes (depot): 250 mg/mL; Transdermal patches: 2.5 mg/24 hour, 5 mg/24 hour; Cream: 10 mg/g, 20 mg/g, 50 mg/g; Transdermal gel: 10 mg/g, 12.5 mg/actuation, 23 mg/1.25 mL (actuation)

Action

- androgen and anabolic
- female requirement is 10–20 times less than male
- (undeconate) maximum levels achieved after 7–14 days, then declines; half-life about 53 days
- see General Actions of androgens and anabolic steroids (p. 1448)

Use

- see General Uses of androgens and anabolic steroids (p. 1449)
- testosterone deficiency in females (AndroFem 1)

Dose

- initially 120–160 mg orally daily in divided doses after the morning and evening meals for 2–3 weeks, then 40–120 mg daily based on clinical effects **OR**
- 250 mg IM every 3 weeks (Sustanon 250) **OR**
- 250 mg IM every 2–3 weeks then 250 mg IM every 3–6 weeks as maintenance (Primoteston Depot) **OR**
- 1000 mg IM every 10–14 weeks (Reandron 1000) **OR**
- (transdermal patch) apply 5 mg/24-hour patch nightly, then dose adjusted according to serum testosterone levels **OR**
- (transdermal gel) 50 mg testosterone (5 g gel (4 actuations)) applied in the morning, then dose adjusted by 2.5 g increments if needed after 3 days, according to serum testosterone levels (Testogel) **OR**
- (transdermal gel) 23 mg (1 actuation) applied in the morning, adjusting dose by 23 mg increments according to serum testosterone levels (daily maximum 69 mg (3 actuations) (Testavan) **OR**

- (females, cream) initially 5 mg (0.5 mL) via applicator applied daily to upper outer thigh or lower torso (AndroFem 1) **OR**
- (male, cream) 100 mg (2 mL) applied daily to torso, then adjusted by 50 mg (1 mL) to achieve response (daily maximum 200 mg (4 mL) (AndroForte 5) **OR**
- (male, cream) 30 mg (1.5 mL) applied daily to scrotum with dose adjusted according to clinical response (AndroForte 2)

Adverse effects

- see General Adverse effects of androgens and anabolic steroids (p. 1449)
- (transdermal patch) erythema, pruritus, allergic contact dermatitis, rash, burning sensation, induration, vesicles
- (injection site) pain, redness, irritation, itching, haematoma
- (depot) urge to cough, coughing, respiratory distress, chest pain
- (cream) mild skin irritation, rash, redness, itching, dermatitis, dryness
- (capsules) oily stools, diarrhoea, abdominal pain
- (depot, rare) pulmonary microembolism

Interactions

- see general points for androgens and anabolic steroids (pp. 1448–51)

Nursing points/Cautions

- (depot) should be injected IM slowly to prevent coughing and respiratory distress. Oxygen may be administered to relieve any respiratory symptoms
- (depot) injection intervals may be varied for maintenance
- (capsules) if uneven number of capsules is required, higher number should be taken in the morning
- (transdermal patch/gel) serum testosterone should be measured (morning after application) before adjusting dose
- (cream) may take 3–4 weeks before clinical response is apparent
- (male, cream) if dose required is above 30 g, AndroForte 5 should be used
- (females, cream) serum testosterone levels should be measured 3 weeks after starting therapy and dose maintained at upper normal therapeutic range for females and then titrated. Follow-up is recommended at 4 and 12 weeks
- (Testavan) contains propylene glycol which may cause skin irritation
- (capsules) contain Sunset Yellow FCF (E110, FD&C Yellow No. 6) which may cause allergic reactions
- (cream) contains almond oil and is therefore contraindicated if any allergy exists
- (cream) contraindicated in females with normal reproductive function
- (depot) some preparations contain arachis (peanut) oil, which is contraindicated in those with a peanut allergy. Should also be avoided in those with soya allergy because of the relationship between peanut and soya allergies
- see General Nursing points/Cautions for androgens and anabolic steroids (p. 1450)

Patient teaching and advice

- patient should be advised to swallow capsules whole without chewing and if an uneven number of tablets is taken, the greater number should be taken in the morning
- see General Patient teaching and advice for androgens and anabolic steroids (p. 1450)

Transdermal patches

- for patients who weigh > 130 kg, 3 patches may be required
- instruct patient on correct application technique, including:
    - rotation of application sites (e.g. back, abdomen, upper arms or

legs), allowing a 7-day interval before reusing the same site
  - avoid using areas that are damaged, irritated or oily, or bony prominences such as hips or shoulders
  - if application area is hairy, hair may be clipped (but not shaved)
  - patches should not be applied to the scrotal area or over bony prominences such as hips
  - patch should be applied at night (about 10 pm)
  - press firmly in place to ensure there is good contact with skin
  - if patch falls off before midday, it should be replaced. If patch falls off after midday, it should not be replaced
  - multiple patches may be used to achieve correct dose. If using more than one patch, they should not overlap
  - patches should not be cut, torn or heated
  - showering or bathing does not affect patch
- transdermal patches should be kept out of reach of children before and after use because used patches still contain active hormone
- advise patient to remove transdermal patch before magnetic resonance imaging (MRI) procedure as aluminium backing may cause burn at site

Transdermal gel

- gel is available in sachets or metered dose pump
- advise patient to shower if skin-to-skin contact is anticipated to avoid transfer
- patient should be advised to:
  - spread gel on skin (clean, dry, healthy) and allow to dry for 3–5 minutes
  - cover area with clothing after gel has dried. This is especially important before contact with children or during sexual intercourse (patient can shower and remove gel before sexual intercourse)
  - apply gel to shoulders, arms or abdomen, but not genital area
  - avoid bathing, swimming or showering for 6 hours after application
  - thoroughly wash hands with water and soap after application
  - if using gel from metered dose pump:
    - pump should be primed before first use by depressing actuator 3–4 times and discarding any gel in these actuations
    - if using application device, applicator head should be placed under pump and then applicator used to spread gel evenly on required sites. Applicator should be cleaned with tissue and protective cap replaced
    - (Testogel pump) 50 mg = 4 actuations, 75 mg = 6 actuations, 100 mg = 8 actuations

Transdermal cream

- instruct patient to:
  - use measuring applicator to ensure correct dosage
  - apply cream to clean, dry, unbroken skin on upper outer thigh or lower torso in areas of minimal hair and body fat
  - not apply cream to genitalia or perineum (unless otherwise directed)
  - (AndroForte 2) apply cream to clean, dry scrotal skin (unshaved)
  - massage cream into skin until absorbed
  - cover area with clothing once cream is absorbed
  - wash hands well with soap and water after application
  - avoid swimming or bathing for 1 hour after application
  - avoid contact with children or partner for 1 hour after application
  - rinse applicator after use

- (AndroFeme 1) not apply perfume, deodorant or moisturiser to same area

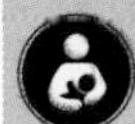

contraindicated during pregnancy. Pregnant women should avoid contact with application area (gel, cream, solution)

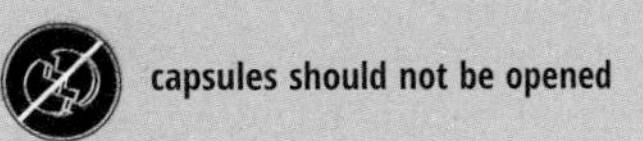

capsules should not be opened

OESTROGENS

General Actions of oestrogens

- secreted primarily by the ovarian follicles (from menarche to menopause) at a daily rate of about 70–500 microgram of estradiol (oestradiol) (depending on the phase of the menstrual cycle). Estradiol (oestradiol) is converted to oestrone and small amounts of estriol (oestriol). After menopause, oestrogen is produced from the adrenal cortex (androstenedione) and converted to oestrone in peripheral tissues
- estradiol (oestradiol) is more potent than oestrone or estriol (oestriol) at receptor sites. Oestrogen receptors are found in the uterus, hypothalamus, pituitary, vagina, urethra, breast, liver and osteoblasts
- controls ovulation and menstrual cycle and maintains pregnancy
- important for development and maintenance of accessory sex organs (e.g. breasts, uterus, vagina) and secondary sex characteristics (e.g. differences in skeletal and muscle size, body fat and hair distribution)
- oestrogen production in ovaries decreases during menopause, resulting in vasomotor symptoms (sweating, hot flushes and atrophic vaginitis)
- decreased rate of bone absorption

General Adverse effects of oestrogens

- menstrual disorders (bleeding or spotting, dysmenorrhoea), reactivation of endometriosis, endometrial hyperplasia, pelvic pain, changes to cervical secretions, increase in size of uterine fibroids, uterine spasm/disorder
- breast tenderness/discomfort/tension, enlargement, pain and discharge
- change to corneal curvature, intolerance to contact lenses, visual disturbances, double vision and, rarely, retinal vascular thrombosis
- muscle cramps, back pain, arthralgia
- nausea, vomiting, abdominal pain/cramps, bloating, diarrhoea
- changes in libido
- hypertension
- headache, migraine, mood swings, nervousness, anxiety, depression, fatigue, dizziness
- acne, pruritus, rash, hirsutism, alopecia
- fluid retention/oedema

- body weight changes
- glucose intolerance
- increased serum triglycerides and, rarely, pancreatitis, gall bladder disease, cholestatic jaundice
- venous and arterial thromboembolic events (pulmonary embolism, DVT, stroke, myocardial infarction)
- (rare/very rare) breast, ovarian or endometrial cancer, fibrocystic breast changes, dementia

General Interactions of oestrogens

- serum levels may be decreased by carbamazepine, phenobarbital (phenobarbitone), primidone, some antiviral agents, phenytoin, rifampicin, rifabutin, topiramate and St John's wort
- serum levels may be increased if given with cimetidine, erythromycin, clarithromycin, ciclosporin, itraconazole, ritonavir, paracetamol and grapefruit juice
- hot flushes and vaginal bleeding may occur if taken with St John's wort
- may affect serum levels and therefore actions of antihypertensive agents theophylline, phenothiazines, diazepam, caffeine and TCAs. For this reason serum levels should be closely monitored and the dose adjusted accordingly
- may require an increased dose of thyroid hormones if given with oestrogens
- may affect a number of laboratory tests, including serum folate level, serum triglycerides and phospholipid, response to metyrapone test, glucose tolerance, gonadotrophin, plasma cortisol, thyroid function test, prothrombin and coagulation time. It is therefore recommended that the test(s) be repeated when the person has been oestrogen-free for 1–2 months

General Nursing points/Cautions for oestrogens

- patient should have a thorough examination (including personal and family history, breast, pelvic and abdominal examination and cervical cytology) before starting therapy and at 6- to 12-monthly intervals
- BP should be monitored regularly during therapy
- prolactinoma should be ruled out before starting therapy
- any persistent or recurring abnormal bleeding should be investigated to rule out malignancy before starting therapy
- if prolonged immobilisation is foreseen (e.g. elective surgery, especially of the lower limbs), therapy should be stopped for 4–6 weeks before surgery because of the risk of thromboembolic events
- if patient is being treated for secondary amenorrhoea, presence of pituitary tumour should be excluded before starting therapy
- breast discomfort, breakthrough bleeding, water retention or bloating lasting for more than 6 weeks may indicate that the dose should be reduced
- continual therapy with oestrogen preparations (e.g. hormone replacement therapy) is thought to increase the risk of endometrial cancer and may also mask a predisposition to oestrogen-dependent breast cancer. Women with an intact uterus should also have progestogen daily for 10–14 days of each month added to oestrogen therapy. However, therapy

should be at the lowest dose and for the shortest duration to produce effective results
- if possible, oestrogens should be stopped for 4–6 weeks before surgery or other lengthy periods of immobility
- thyroid function should be monitored regularly in those treated with thyroid hormone replacement therapy
- oestrogen treatment may increase the risk of gall bladder disease
- may lead to hypercalcaemia in patients with breast cancer and bone metastases
- not recommended for prevention of cardiovascular disease and dementia
- caution if used in those with cardiac or renal dysfunction as fluid retention may exacerbate conditions
- caution if used in those with asthma, endometriosis, uterine fibroids, otosclerosis, migraine or severe headache, epilepsy, hereditary angioedema or hepatic haemangiomas as conditions may be exacerbated
- caution if used in women with risk factors for arterial vascular disease (e.g. hypertension, diabetes mellitus, tobacco use, hypercholesterolaemia, obesity) and/or venous thromboembolism (e.g. personal or family history of venous thromboembolism, obesity, SLE)
- caution if used in those with hypertriglyceridaemia, hypocalcaemia, hypothyroidism, impaired liver function, hepatic cholestasis, cholelithiasis, severe pruritus, cholestatic jaundice or history of pregnancy-induced jaundice
- caution if used in those with a history of oestrogen-dependent tumours, endometriosis (or any endometrial hyperplasia) or fibrocystic disease of the breast
- contraindicated in those with undiagnosed genital bleeding; confirmed venous thromboembolic event; recurrent venous or arterial thromboembolism; known thrombophilic disease (not receiving anticoagulants), thrombophlebitis; known, suspected or history of breast cancer; undiagnosed breast pathology; suspected or known oestrogen-dependent tumour; endometrial hyperplasia (untreated); porphyria; hyperlipoproteinaemia; pregnancy-related problems (jaundice, severe pruritus, otosclerosis, herpes gestationis); severe uncontrolled hypertension; sickle cell anaemia; severe diabetes with vascular changes; endometriosis; acute liver disease or history of liver disease (with abnormal liver function)
- contraindicated in non-hysterectomised women (unless progestogen therapy is given concurrently)

General Patient teaching and advice for oestrogens

- patient should be warned of possible weight gain
- advise patient not to smoke while having oestrogen therapy, because it increases the risk of cardiovascular effects
- instruct patient to avoid grapefruit juice during therapy
- patient should be advised to seek medical advice if any of the following occur:
  - any shortness of breath or sudden chest pain, cough, light-headedness, dizziness, rapid heart rate

  - sudden painful or tender leg swelling, increased limb warmth, skin discolouration
  - any loss of vision, double vision, bulging eyes
  - new or worsening migraine or headache
  - any yellowing of skin or eyes, loss of appetite, nausea, itching, upper abdominal pain, dark urine or pale stools
  - vaginal bleeding
- instruct patient with diabetes to closely monitor blood glucose levels, because glucose tolerance may be affected
- patient should be advised that hormone replacement therapy (HRT) is only recommended with menopausal symptoms and is not meant for long-term therapy so should be reviewed after 6 months
- warn patient that slight spotting is normal but heavier or persistent bleeding should be reported
- advise patient to avoid driving or operating machinery if dizziness occurs
- women should be aware of increased risk of heart disease and stroke associated with taking oestrogen/progestogen combination
- if patient wears contact lenses, she should be warned that intolerance to lenses may occur
- woman should be counselled to perform monthly breast self-examinations

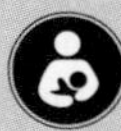
not recommended during breastfeeding

ESTRADIOL (OESTRADIOL) (Climara, Estraderm MX, Estradot, Estrofem, Estrogel, Progynova, Sandrena, Vagifem, Zumenon)

Available forms

Tablets: 1 mg, 2 mg; Transdermal patches: 25 microgram/24 hours, 37.5 microgram/24 hours, 50 microgram/24 hours, 75 microgram/24 hours, 100 microgram/24 hours; Gel: 1 mg/g 1.25 g (actuation), 0.75 mg/; Vaginal tablet (modified-release): 10 microgram

Action

- see General Actions of oestrogens (p. 1455)
- (transdermal patches) constant serum oestrogen levels produced while avoiding gastrointestinal adverse effects

Use

- oestrogen deficiency due to natural or surgically induced menopause
- prevention of post-menopausal bone mineral density loss in women at high risk of osteoporosis and fractures

Dose

- (menopausal symptoms) 1–2 mg orally daily with a drug-free interval every 6 months to establish if symptoms are still present **OR**
- (menopausal symptoms) 0.75–1.5 mg (1–2 actuations) once daily, increasing dose after 4 weeks if needed (gel) (Estrogel) **OR**
- (menopausal symptoms) initially 0.5 mg daily, applied to the lower trunk or thigh, increasing dose to 1.5 mg if needed (gel) (Sandrena) **OR**
- (atrophic vaginitis) initially 10 microgram PV daily for 14 days, then 10 microgram twice weekly (vaginal tablet) **OR**

- (oestrogen deficiency due to menopause) initially 50 microgram/24-hour patch applied every 3–7 days, then dose adjusted according to symptoms (transdermal patch) **OR**
- (prevention of bone mineral density loss) initially 50–100 microgram/24-hour patch applied every 3–7 days, then dose adjusted according to symptoms (transdermal patch) **OR**
- (prevention of bone mineral density loss) 1.5 mg (2 actuations) once daily (gel) (Estrogel)

Adverse effects

- see General Adverse effects of oestrogens (p. 1455)
- (transdermal patches) skin redness, itching, stinging, vesicle formation
- (gel) skin irritation, itching, erythema

Interactions

- see General Interactions of oestrogens (p. 1456)
- (gel) not recommended with other medications that alter skin production

Nursing points/Cautions

- see General Nursing points/Cautions for oestrogens (p. 1456)
- (oral therapy, no uterus) therapy can be started on any day
- (oral therapy, oligomenorrhoea) therapy should start on day 5 of bleeding
- Estraderm MX 25 transdermal patch is not recommended for prevention of bone mineral density loss in post-menopausal women
- in women not taking oral oestrogen currently, therapy with transdermal patch can be started immediately. If taking oral oestrogens, therapy can be started 5–7 days after stopping therapy
- (post-menopausal bone mineral density loss) if patient has established bone mineral loss, therapy should be started using 100 microgram/24 hour-transdermal patch
- (woman with intact uterus) progestogen should be taken for 10 days to avoid overstimulation of endometrial tissue
- if hot flushes have ceased, consideration should be given to changing to local vaginal therapy

Patient teaching and advice

- see General Patient teaching and advice for oestrogens (p. 1457)

Transdermal patch

- patches are available in different strengths that have different application intervals (e.g. Climara is applied weekly, whereas Estraderm is applied twice weekly)
- instruct patient on correct application technique, including:
  - rotation of application sites (e.g. upper buttock, lower part of the back or abdomen), allowing a 7-day interval before reusing the same site
  - applying patch to a clean, dry area of the lower trunk or buttocks that will be covered by clothing (not waistline or skin folds where patch may be easily rubbed loose)
  - pressing patch firmly and holding it in place for 10 seconds
  - if the patch falls off, it should be replaced for the remaining time
  - patch should not be applied to breasts or broken skin
  - patch should not be cut or torn
  - patch should not be exposed to sunlight or solariums
  - patient can bathe or shower as normal if the patch is correctly applied; however, it may fall off if exposed to hot bath or sauna
- transdermal patches should be kept out of reach of children before and after use, because used patches still contain active hormone

Gel

- (Sandrena) gel should be applied and spread over an area 2–3 times the size of the hand
- advise patient to wash hands well after application of gel and avoid applying to breasts, face, vulval area or any broken or irritated skin
- patient should be instructed to vary application sites to avoid skin irritation
- instruct patient that other skin products should not be applied within 1 hour of gel application
- gel should be allowed to dry for at least 5 minutes
- skin contact with others (e.g. partner, children) should be avoided for at least 1 hour after gel application. If contact is made, person should wash area well with soap and water
- instruct patient to avoid use of strong skin cleansers or detergents, products with high alcohol content or keratolytics
- advise patient if dose is forgotten (≤ 12 hours) it may be applied as soon as possible; if > 12 hours, apply gel next day as per routine. Warn patient not to apply double dose
- if using pump, patient should be instructed to:
  - prime pump before first use and discard gel from this actuation
  - apply to intact skin (e.g. arms, shoulder, inner thighs)

Intravaginal tablets

- patient should be instructed in the correct technique for application and insertion of intravaginal tablets, including correct care of the applicator

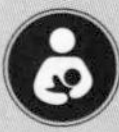

contraindicated during pregnancy

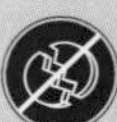

tablet can be crushed and mixed with water or spoonful of yoghurt or apple puree. Mask and gloves must be worn and closed tablet crusher used. Pregnant staff must not disperse or crush tablets

Note

- contained in Angeliq 1/2, Estalis preparation, Estrogel Pro Combination, Femoston preparations, Kliogest, Kliovance, Trisequens preparations, Qlaira and Zoely

ESTRIOL (OESTRIOL) (Ovestin Cream, Ovestin Ovula Pessaries, Ovestin Tablets)

Available forms

Tablets: 1 mg; Pessaries: 0.5 mg; Vaginal cream: 1 mg/mL

Action

- see General Actions of oestrogens (p. 1455)
- short-acting
- particularly effective in managing urogenital symptoms
- increases urogenital epithelial cell resistance to infection and inflammation reducing vaginal complaints
- half-life 5–7 hours

Use

- vulvo-vaginal complaints due to oestrogen deficiency (e.g. atrophic vaginitis, pruritus vulvae, dyspareunia due to vulvovaginal atrophy)
- adjunct to vaginal infection treatment
- pre-vulvovaginal surgery
- suspect cytological smear

Dose

- initially up to 4 mg orally daily for the first 5–7 days, then reduced to 1–2 mg daily during the next 1–3 weeks as required **OR**
- (vulvovaginal symptoms associated with menopause) initially 0.5 mg vaginal cream or pessary daily PV for 2–3 weeks then 1–2 weekly for 2–3 months. Discontinued for 4 weeks every 2–3 months to assess necessity for further treatment **OR**
- (before vulvovaginal surgery) 0.5 mg vaginal cream or pessary daily PV, starting 2 weeks preoperatively **OR**

- (suspect cytological smear) 0.5 mg vaginal cream or pessary daily PV for 7 days before re-evaluation of smear

Adverse effects

- flu like symptoms
- (cream, pessary) local irritation, pruritus
- see General Adverse effects of oestrogens (p. 1455)

Interactions

- see General Interactions of oestrogens (p. 1456)
- may increase effects of corticosteroids, theophylline and succinylcholine

Nursing points/Cautions

- 1 applicatorful = 0.5 mg cream
- if switching from cyclic hormone replacement therapy (HRT), therapy should be started 7 days after completion of HRT cycle
- (oral) may be given continuously or intermittently (tablet-free 5–7 days may be started after 3 weeks of treatment)
- tablets are contraindicated in those with hereditary galactose intolerance, Lapp lactase deficiency or glucose–galactose malabsorption
- see General Nursing points/Cautions for oestrogens (p. 1456)

Patient teaching and advice

- advise patient that cream and pessaries should be used at night for optimal effect
- patient should be instructed in correct insertion technique for vaginal cream or pessaries
- after use, applicator should be taken apart and washed in warm (not hot) soapy water
- (oral) patient should be advised that if a dose is missed (> 12 hours) dose should be taken when next scheduled. Warn patient not to double dose
- see also General Patient teaching and advice for oestrogens (p. 1457)

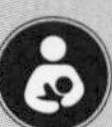
contraindicated during pregnancy

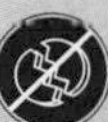
tablet can be crushed and mixed with water or yoghurt or apple puree. Mask and gloves must be worn and closed tablet crusher used. Pregnant staff must not disperse or crush tablets

OESTROGENS (CONJUGATED) (Premarin)

Available forms

Tablets: 0.3 mg, 0.625 mg

Action

- see General Actions of oestrogens (p. 1455)
- similar effects to endogenous oestrogens
- conjugated oestrogens are a mixture of natural oestrogens (of equine origin)

Use

- natural or surgically induced menopause symptoms (moderate-to-severe vasomotor symptoms and atrophic vaginitis)
- hypoestrogenic states (e.g. female hypogonadism, primary ovarian failure, female castration)
- prevention of post-menopausal osteoporosis

Dose

- (menopausal symptoms) 0.3–1.25 mg orally daily **OR**
- (female hypogonadism) 2.5–7.5 mg orally daily in divided doses for 20 days, rest for 10 days. If no bleeding has occurred, dose is repeated **OR**
- (prevention of post-menopausal osteoporosis) 0.3–0.625 mg orally daily **OR**
- (female castration, primary ovarian failure) initially 0.3–1.25 mg orally

daily, then dose adjusted according to response

Adverse effects/Interactions

- see General Adverse effects and Interactions of oestrogens (pp. 1455–56)

Nursing points/Cautions

- if used for atrophic vaginitis only, topical vaginal products should be considered first
- (female hypogonadism) number of courses needed to produce bleeding varies between women. If bleeding occurs before end of 10-day period, a 20-day combined oestrogen-progestogen regimen is suggested (with 2.5–7.5 mg daily in divided doses with progestogen added in last 5 days)
- should only be used for post-menopausal osteoporosis in women who are at high risk of osteoporosis and fractures where non-oestrogen therapies were contraindicated or the patient was intolerant of them
- see also General Nursing points/Cautions for oestrogens (p. 1456)

Patient teaching and advice

- advise patient to swallow tablets whole, not chewed, crushed, divided or dissolved
- (post-menopausal osteoporosis) women should be encouraged to maintain weight-bearing exercise and adequate intake of calcium and vitamin D (with supplements if required)
- see also General Patient teaching and advice for oestrogens (p. 1457)

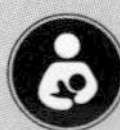

contraindicated during pregnancy

not recommended during breastfeeding

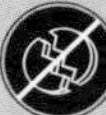

tablets should not be divided, chewed, crushed or dispersed

Note

- contained in Duavive with bazedoxifene (selective oestrogen receptor modulator (SERM))

PROGESTOGENS

General Actions of progestogens

- convert the endometrial proliferative phase to the secretory phase in preparation for the fertilised ovum
- progestogens are synthetic derivatives of progesterone
- suppress uterine motility
- alters cervical mucus hindering passage of sperm and/or ova
- promotes breast development
- raises core body temperature (thermogenic)
- affects glucose tolerance and insulin resistance
- prevents further ovulation

General Uses of progestogens

- alone or with oestrogen in menstrual disorders (e.g. primary or secondary amenorrhoea, uterine bleeding caused by hormonal imbalance, primary dysmenorrhoea)
- endometriosis

- oral contraception (either alone or combined with an orally active oestrogen)
- post-coital emergency contraception
- adjunct to oestrogen replacement therapy (to prevent endometrial hyperplasia)
- recurrent and/or metastatic breast or renal cell cancer, inoperable recurrent or metastatic endometrial carcinoma

General Adverse effects of progestogens

- dizziness, depression, fatigue, malaise, emotional lability, headache, migraine, insomnia, somnolence, nervousness, tremor
- breast pain, tension, tenderness, enlargement, galactorrhoea
- hirsutism, acne, sweating, alopecia, oily hair, hot flushes, urticaria, rash, pruritus, eczema, melasma (chloasma) (blotchy brown pigmentation)
- menstrual changes (frequent, longer and/or irregular bleeding), spotting, breakthrough bleeding, amenorrhoea, dysmenorrhoea, changes in cervical secretions, vulvovaginitis, (low dose) benign ovarian cysts
- muscle cramps
- dyspnoea
- increased triglyceride levels
- hypertension
- visual disorders (including loss of vision (partial or complete), diplopia, retinal vascular lesions, optic neuritis) and, rarely, retinal vascular thrombosis
- weight gain, fluid retention, oedema
- nausea, constipation, diarrhoea, dry mouth, abdominal pain/cramp, bloating, flatulence, weight changes
- decreased glucose tolerance, exacerbation of diabetes mellitus, glycosuria
- arterial or venous thromboembolic disease, thrombophlebitis
- (cancer treatment) Cushingoid symptoms
- (rare) cholestatic jaundice, changes in liver function, liver tumours (benign or malignant), gall bladder disease, hypercalcaemia, ectopic pregnancy, exacerbation of porphyria
- (rare) anaphylactoid-like reaction, anaphylaxis, angioedema

General Interactions of progestogens

- contraindicated with ombitasvir, paritaprevir or dasabuvir
- decreased serum levels may occur if given with phenytoin, barbiturates, primidone, carbamazepine, rifampicin, oxcarbazepine, rifabutin, griseofulvin, topiramate, bosentan and St John's wort
- increased serum levels may occur if given with itraconazole, fluconazole, voriconazole, erythromycin, clarithromycin, diltiazem, verapamil or grapefruit juice
- caution if given with HIV protease (e.g. ritonavir) and non-nucleoside transcript inhibitors (e.g. efavirenz) because of variable effects
- may increase serum levels of ciclosporin increasing risk of toxicity
- may interfere with a number of laboratory tests, including plasma testosterone level (males), plasma progestogen and oestrogen levels (females), gonadotrophin level, cortisol level, glucose tolerance, metyrapone test, sex hormone binding globulin level and coagulation test values for prothrombin and factors VII, VIII, IX and X

General Nursing points/Cautions for progestogens

- patient should have a thorough examination (including personal and family history, BP, breast, pelvic and abdominal examination and cervical cytology) before starting therapy and at 6- to 12-monthly intervals
- pregnancy should be excluded before starting therapy
- therapy should be stopped if there is a constantly elevated BP or if raised BP does not respond to antihypertensive therapy
- fluid retention occurs frequently, therefore some patients, including those with cardiac and renal disorders, asthma, epilepsy or migraine, may require closer than usual monitoring, especially in the initial phases of the therapy
- patients with an intact uterus should be given a progestogen daily for 10–14 days of each month of oestrogen therapy
- therapy should be stopped 4 weeks before planned surgery and restarted 2 weeks after complete mobilisation
- prolactin-producing tumour should be excluded before starting therapy for amenorrhoea
- caution if used in those with liver impairment as progestogens may be poorly metabolised
- caution if used in women with previous history of extrauterine pregnancy or impaired tube function due to increased risk of ectopic pregnancy
- caution if used in women with hyperlipidaemia as some progestogens may increase LDL levels and increase risk of pancreatitis
- caution if used in patients with pre-existing depression
- caution if used in patients with pre-existing diabetes mellitus, because glucose tolerance may be affected by progestogens
- caution if used in women with history of chloasma gravidarum
- caution if used in women with endometriosis because of increased risk of breakthrough bleeding
- risk of thromboembolic events increases with age, obesity, positive family history, prolonged immobilisation, major surgery or trauma, leg surgery, smoking (especially if women $>$ 35 years), valvular heart disease, migraine, atrial fibrillation and dyslipoproteinaemia
- contraindicated in those with history of or active severe liver disease or dysfunction (where liver function tests have not returned to normal), Dubin–Johnson syndrome, Rotor syndrome, active venous or arterial thromboembolic disorders, thrombophlebitis, severe hypertension, sickle cell anaemia, migraine (with focal neurological symptoms), diabetes mellitus (with nephropathy, retinopathy, neuropathy or vascular disease), undiagnosed abnormal vaginal or urinary tract bleeding, cervical dysplasia, cerebrovascular or coronary artery disease, carcinoma of breast or genital organ, benign or malignant liver tumours or hormone-dependent tumour

General Patient teaching and advice for progestogens

- women treated for endometriosis should be warned that breakthrough bleeding may occur

- patient should be advised to seek medical advice immediately if any of the following occur:
  - migraine headache for the first time or an increase in frequency or severity of headache
  - dizziness, weakness, numbness (especially if marked and one-sided), slurred speech or difficulty speaking
  - disturbed vision, including asymmetrical vision loss or double vision
  - pain/tenderness or swelling in leg, increased limb warmth, discolouration
  - pain/tightness in chest (especially if radiating down left arm), unexplained cough, breathlessness or difficulty breathing
  - depression, sadness, change in appetite, loss of interest in previously pleasurable activities, social withdrawal
  - yellowing of skin or eyes or itching of skin
- patient should be warned about increase in weight and changes to menstrual bleeding pattern (frequency, duration and/or heaviness)
- advise patient to avoid driving or operating machinery if dizziness occurs
- instruct patient to avoid grapefruit juice during therapy
- instruct patient with diabetes mellitus to monitor blood glucose levels more frequently
- if patient has a tendency to melasma (chloasma) (blotchy brown pigmentation), she should be advised to avoid excessive sunlight or UV exposure during therapy
- patient should be warned that withdrawal bleeding usually occurs on discontinuation of treatment
- women should be advised that oral contraceptives do not protect against HIV infection, AIDS and other sexually transmitted diseases
- barrier method contraception is recommended during combined therapy and for 28 days after stopping some medication such as rifampicin

ETONOGESTREL (Implanon NXT)

Available form

Implants: 68 mg

Action

- see General Actions of progestogens (p. 1462)
- biologically active metabolite of desogestrel that inhibits ovulation
- effects reversible on removal of implant

Use

- long-term contraception

Dose

- implants (68 mg) are inserted under the skin (inner side of upper arm) after area is locally anaesthetised, replaced every 3 years

Adverse effects

- (insertion site) pain, redness, swelling, bruising, irritation, itching, fibrosis, abscess, scar
- expulsion (if insert not correctly inserted) or migration (if inserted too deeply)
- see General Adverse effects of progestogens (p. 1463)

Interactions

- see General Interactions of progestogens (p. 1463)

Nursing points/Cautions

- inserted sub-dermally into non-dominant arm
- medical review is recommended 3 months after insertion to monitor BP and any side-effects

- plasma levels are inversely related to woman's weight, therefore some consideration should be given to replacing insert earlier in women with heavier body weight as implant may be less effective by third year
- if no hormonal contraceptive was taken during preceding month, implant should be inserted on day 1 to 5 of menstrual cycle (day 1 = first day of bleeding)
- if changing from combination oral contraceptive, vaginal ring or transdermal patch, implant should be inserted on next day after last day of active tablet of combination contraceptive, day of removal or when application was due
- if changing from progestogen-only contraceptive, implant should be inserted immediately with no break from progestogen-only tablets
- if changing from non-oral progestogen-only contraception (i.e. injection or implant), implant should be inserted on removal of different implant or when next injection was due
- if following first-trimester abortion/ miscarriage, implant should be inserted immediately
- if following second trimester abortion/miscarriage, implant should be inserted on day 21 to 28 after abortion/miscarriage
- if postpartum and not breastfeeding, implant should be inserted on day 21 to 28 after delivery
- if postpartum and breastfeeding, implant should be inserted after 4th postpartum week
- see also General Nursing points/ Cautions for progestogens (p. 1464)

Patient teaching and advice

- women should be given User Card which records batch number and date of insertions
- until presence and effect of the implant has been confirmed, it is recommended that barrier contraception is used
- barrier method contraception is recommended for first 7 days if avoiding pregnancy when changing from another method to etonogestrel implant
- warn patient that bleeding pattern during first 3 months after implant insertion is likely to be future pattern of bleeding
- advise patient that she should be able to feel implant under skin
- warn patient that effects wear off quickly after implant is removed
- see also General Patient teaching and advice for progestogens (p. 1464)

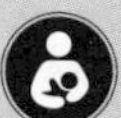

contraindicated during pregnancy; implant should be removed if pregnancy occurs

Note

- contained in NuvaRing (controlled-release vaginal contraceptive ring with ethinylestradiol)

LEVONORGESTREL (Kyleena, Levonelle-1, Microlut, Mirena, NorLevo-1, Postella-1, Postinor-1, Postrelle-1)

Available forms

Tablets: 30 microgram, 1.5 mg; Intrauterine device (IUD): 19.5 mg, 52 mg

Action

- inhibits ovulation
- may also cause endometrial changes that prevent implantation
- (post-coital emergency contraception) efficacy decreases with time after intercourse (95% efficacy if used within 24 hours, reduces to 58% between 48–72 hours)
- (intrauterine device) low-dose release directly into uterine cavity

- no antiandrogenic or glucocorticoid properties but some partial androgenic activity
- see General Actions of progestogens (p. 1462)

Use

- post-coital emergency contraception (within 72 hours) (Levonelle-1, NorLevo-1, Postella-1, Postinor-1, Postrelle-1)
- see General Uses of progestogens (p. 1462)

Dose

- (long-term contraception) 52 mg device inserted into uterine cavity (intrauterine device (IUD)) (Mirena) **OR**
- (long-term contraception) 19.5 mg device inserted into uterine cavity (intrauterine device (IUD)) (Kyleena) **OR**
- (oral contraception) 30 microgram orally daily **OR**
- (post-coital emergency contraception within 72 hours) 1.5 mg orally as soon as possible after unprotected sexual intercourse and within 72 hours

Adverse effects

- see General Adverse effects (p. 1463)
- (IUD) expulsion, bleeding, pain, and rarely, infection, perforation or penetration of uterus or cervix, ectopic pregnancy
- (high dose) nausea, vomiting, vaginal bleeding, headache, breast pain

Interactions

- see General Interactions of progestogens (p. 1463)

Nursing points/Cautions

- see General Nursing points/Cautions for progestogens (p. 1464)
- (contraception) pregnancy should be excluded before starting therapy
- (IUD) any genital infection should be treated before insertion of IUD
- (IUD) patient should be assessed for any pelvic infection risk factors (e.g. previous history of pelvic infection, sexually transmitted disease, multiple sexual partners)
- (post-coital contraception) BP should be measured before therapy is given
- (post-coital contraception) efficacy may be impaired if patient has severe diarrhoea, vomiting or malabsorption such as Crohn's disease
- (post-coital emergency contraception only) can be taken at any time during menstrual cycle
- for oral contraception:
    - if no hormonal contraceptive was taken during preceding month, oral therapy should be started on first day of menstrual cycle
    - if changing from combination oral contraceptive, oral therapy should be started on next day after last day of active tablet of combination contraceptive and omit pill-free interval
    - if changing from progestogen-only contraceptive, oral therapy can be started immediately with no break from progestogen-only tablets
    - if changing from non-oral progestogen-only contraception, oral therapy can be started on day of implant removal or when next injection was due. Barrier method contraception is recommended for first 7 days if avoiding pregnancy
    - if following abortion, oral therapy can be started immediately
    - if following delivery, oral therapy can be started 4 weeks after delivery if not breastfeeding. Barrier method contraception is recommended for first 7 days if avoiding pregnancy
- (IUD) levonorgestrel is slowly released and contains sufficient quantities to be effective for up to 5 years

- IUD should be inserted within 7 days of onset of menstruation or immediately after first-trimester abortion
- postpartum IUD insertion should be postponed for at least 6 weeks after delivery or longer until uterus is fully involuted
- for those with amenorrhoea, IUD insertion can be at any time or last day of menstruation or withdrawal bleeding
- insertion/removal of IUD is associated with pain and bleeding and this may precipitate vasovagal reaction (or seizure if patient has epilepsy)
- (IUD) patient should be examined after 4–12 weeks post insertion and then yearly (or more frequently if needed)
- (IUD) infection may occur within 4 weeks of insertion. If infection recurs, is severe or does not respond to antibiotics, IUD should be removed
- (IUD) should be removed after 5 years and new system re-inserted if patient wants to continue with IUD therapy
- (IUD) should not be first-line treatment for nulligravid women or postmenopausal women with advanced uterine atrophy (making insertion difficult)
- (IUD) caution if used in those with history of ectopic pregnancy, congenital heart disease or valvular heart disease at risk of infectious endocarditis. Antibiotic prophylaxis is required when inserting or removing IUD
- (IUD) caution if used in women with migraine, focal migraine with asymmetrical visual loss (or other symptoms of transient cerebral ischaemia), severe headache, jaundice, increased blood pressure, stroke or myocardial infarction. If any of these occur for the first time, consideration should be given to removing IUD
- (IUD) contraindicated in those women with pelvic inflammatory disease (current or recurrent history), lower genital tract infection, postpartum endometriosis, infected abortion in last 3 months, cervicitis, cervical dysplasia, uterine or cervical neoplasm, confirmed or suspected hormone-dependent tumour, undiagnosed abnormal uterine bleeding, congenital or acquired uterine anomaly, predisposition to infection or active liver disease or tumour

Patient teaching and advice

- see General Patient teaching and advice for progestogens (p. 1464)

Post-coital emergency contraception

- if patient presents multiple times for post-coital contraception she should be counselled to consider long-term contraception
- if patient vomits within 2 hours, she should be advised to return to doctor, pharmacy or clinic

Oral contraception

- patient should be advised to take oral medication at same time every day
- barrier method contraception is recommended until onset of next period
- if vomiting or diarrhoea occurs within 4 hours of oral administration, advise patient to replace it using last tablet from pack
- if tablet is forgotten (more than 27-hour interval between doses), it should be taken when remembered regardless of timing and barrier method contraception used during sexual intercourse for next 7 days if avoiding pregnancy
- warn women that ectopic pregnancy may occur if pregnancy occurs during treatment

IUD

- patient should be instructed to feel for two threads at the end of the device after each menstrual period

- patient should be warned that irregular bleeding or spotting (in addition to normal menstrual bleeding) is common with IUD for first 3–6 months after insertion
- patient should be advised that re-examination should occur 4–12 weeks after insertion and then yearly until removed after 5 years
- advise patient that if IUD is removed mid-cycle and patient has sexual intercourse, there is an increased risk of pregnancy occurring
- patient should be advised to seek medical advice immediately if any of the following occur:
  - length of removal threads increases or stem of IUD becomes visible in the cervix (expulsion may be imminent)
  - there is a noticeable increase in menstrual flow
  - removal threads cannot be felt
  - there is persistent lower abdominal pain, fever, abnormal bleeding or discharge and/or pain during sexual intercourse (especially in first 4 weeks after IUD insertion, may indicate infection)

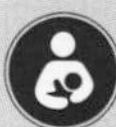

(IUD) not recommended during pregnancy. If pregnancy occurs, IUD should be removed

(oral contraception) contraindicated during pregnancy

(post-coital emergency contraception) not recommended during pregnancy

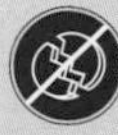

crushing tablet is not recommended as dose may be altered

Note

- contained in Eleanor 150/30 ED, Evelyn 150/30 ED, Femme-Tab ED 20/100, Femme-Tab 30/150, Lenest 20 ED, Levlen ED, Loette, Logynon ED, Microgynon Preparations, Microlevlen, Micronelle 30 ED, Monofeme 28, Nordette 28, Seasonique, Trifeme, Triphasil and Triquilar ED

MEDROXYPROGESTERONE ACETATE (Depo-Provera, Depo-Ralovera, Provera, Ralovera)

Available forms

Vial: 150 mg/mL; Tablets: 2.5 mg, 5 mg, 10 mg, 100 mg, 200 mg, 250 mg, 500 mg

Action

- see General Actions of progestogens (p. 1462)
- more potent than progesterone
- has anabolic effects with little to no androgenic or oestrogenic activity

Use

- see General Uses of progestogens (p. 1462)

Dose

- (inoperable, recurrent metastatic endometrial and renal carcinoma) 600–1200 mg IM weekly, then 450–600 mg every 1–4 weeks (maintenance) **OR**
- (breast cancer) 500 mg IM daily for 4 weeks then 500–1000 mg at weekly intervals (maintenance) **OR**
- (endometriosis) 50 mg IM weekly or 100 mg IM 2-weekly for at least 6 months **OR**
- (endometrial or renal cell carcinoma) 200–400 mg orally daily **OR**
- (breast cancer) 500 mg orally daily until progression of disease **OR**
- (endometriosis) 10 mg orally 3 times daily for 90 consecutive days starting day 1 of the menstrual cycle **OR**
- (secondary amenorrhoea) 2.5–10 mg orally daily for 5–10 days beginning with day 16–21 of cycle and repeated for 3 consecutive cycles **OR**

- (abnormal uterine bleeding) 2.5–10 mg orally daily for 5–10 days, beginning day 16–21 of the cycle and repeated for 3 consecutive cycles **OR**
- (adjunct to oestrogen therapy) 10–20 mg orally daily for at least 10 days of the cycle **OR**
- (adjunct to oestrogen therapy) 5 mg orally daily for 28 days of the cycle **OR**
- (contraception) 150 mg IM every 3 months

Adverse effects

- (IM) gluteal infiltration, abscess formation
- decreased bone mineral density
- see General Adverse effects of progestogens (p. 1463)

Interactions

- see General Interactions of progestogens (p. 1463)

Nursing points/Cautions

- (IM, contraception) if interval between IM injections is > 14 weeks, pregnancy should be excluded
- (IM, contraception) first injection should be given during first 5 days of onset of normal menstrual period, within 5 days post-partum (if not breastfeeding) or if breastfeeding, at sixth week post-partum (after pregnancy has been excluded)
- volumes of 2.5 mL or greater should be given IM in divided doses to prevent gluteal infiltration and abscess formation
- vial should be well shaken before use
- administration should be by deep IM injection into the gluteal muscle
- bone mineral density should be measured regularly if prolonged therapy is indicated
- (endometriosis, contraception) should only be used long term (> 2 years) if other methods are inadequate
- (Depo-Provera/Depo-Ralovera) not recommended for secondary amenorrhoea or dysfunctional uterine bleeding
- (endometriosis, contraception) caution if used in those with chronic alcohol and/or tobacco use, strong family history of osteoporosis or chronic use of agents that decrease bone mass (e.g. antiepileptic agents, corticosteroids) due to increased risk of osteoporosis
- see General Nursing points/Cautions for progestogens (p. 1464)

Patient teaching and advice

- women with endometriosis should be advised that breakthrough bleeding is likely to occur
- women should be warned that therapy may result in prolonged contraception. Median time to conceive was 10 months (range 4–31 months) after last injection and was not related to duration of use
- (oral) advise patient to swallow tablets whole and not crush or chew
- (prolonged therapy) all patients should be advised to have sufficient calcium and vitamin D in diets
- see General Patient teaching and advice for progestogens (p. 1464)

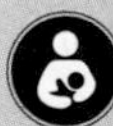

contraindicated during pregnancy

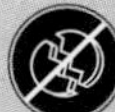

tablets can be dispersed in water or crushed and mixed with spoonful of yoghurt or apple puree. Mask and gloves must be worn and closed tablet crusher used. Pregnant staff must not disperse or crush tablets

NORETHISTERONE (Noriday 28, Primolut N)

Available forms
Tablets: 350 microgram, 5 mg

Action
- little androgenic effect
- thermogenic, altering basal body temperature
- partly metabolised to ethinylestradiol
- see General Actions of progestogens (p. 1462)

Use
- see General Uses of progestogens (p. 1462)

Dose
- (dysfunctional bleeding) 5 mg orally 3 times daily for 10 days (Primolut N) **OR**
- (prevention of recurrence of dysfunctional bleeding) 5 mg orally 1–2 times daily from day 16 to day 25 of menstrual cycle (Primolut N)
- (primary or secondary amenorrhoea) endometrial priming with oestrogen product for 14 days, then 5 mg norethisterone orally 1–2 times daily for 10 days and continued for 2–3 cycles (Primolut N) **OR**
- (premenstrual syndrome) 5 mg orally 1–3 times daily from day 19 to day 26 of the menstrual cycle (Primolut N) **OR**
- (endometriosis) 5 mg orally twice daily starting between day 1 and day 5 of menstrual cycle for 4–6 months. If spotting occurs, dose can be increased to 10 mg twice daily, then decrease dose when bleeding has decreased (Primolut N) **OR**
- (timing of menstruation) 5 mg orally 2–3 times daily for 10–14 days, starting 3 days before expected menstruation. Bleeding should occur in 2–3 days after stopping medication (Primolut N) **OR**
- (contraception) 350 microgram orally daily, starting on first day of menstrual cycle (Noriday 28)

Adverse effects
- see General Adverse effects of progestogens (p. 1463)

Interactions
- see General Interactions of progestogens (p. 1463)

Nursing points/Cautions
- (dysfunctional bleeding) bleeding usually stops in 1–3 days; however, if it does not stop, organic or extragenital cause should be investigated
- see also General Nursing points/Cautions for progestogens (p. 1464)

Patient teaching and advice
- (contraception) if tablet is forgotten (more than 27-hour interval between doses), patient should be instructed to take it when remembered, regardless of timing, and barrier method contraception used for next 7 days if avoiding pregnancy
- see General Patient teaching and advice for progestogens (p. 1464)

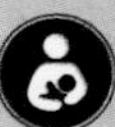
contraindicated during pregnancy as progestogens can cause masculinisation of female fetus

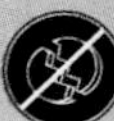
tablets can be dispersed in water or crushed and mixed with spoonful of yoghurt or apple puree. Mask and gloves must be worn and closed tablet crusher used. Pregnant staff must not disperse or crush tablets

Note
- contained in Brevinor preparations, Estalis Continuous, Estalis Sequi, Kliogest, Kliovance, Norimin, Norimin-1, Norinyl-1, Trisequens

OTHER AGENTS

CYPROTERONE ACETATE (Androcur, Anterone, Cyprone, Cyprostat, Cyrotone)

Available forms

Tablets: 50 mg, 100 mg

Action

- antiandrogenic agent with progestogenic and antigonadotrophic properties

Use

- (women) moderate-to-severe signs of androgenisation (hirsutism, androgenic alopecia, acne and/or seborrhoea)
- (men) reduce drive for men with sexual deviations, inoperable prostatic carcinoma (with a luteinising hormone-releasing hormone (LHRH) agonist)

Dose

Women

- (hirsutism, secondary to androgenisation in pre-menopausal women) 50 mg orally daily for 10 days from days 1–10 of the menstrual cycle until there is satisfactory response, then reduce dose **OR**
- (signs of androgenisation in pre-menopausal women) 100 mg orally at the same time each day with some liquid after a meal from days 1–10 of the menstrual cycle, reducing to 10–50 mg with clinical improvement (with progestogen/oestrogen contraceptive starting on day 1 of cycle) **OR**
- (androgenisation in post-menopausal/hysterectomised women) 25–50 mg orally daily for 21 days followed by 7 days drug-free, continuing for several months

Men

- (reduction of sexual drive) initially 50 mg orally twice daily, then increasing dose to 100 mg 2–3 times daily to achieve satisfactory response; dose may then be gradually reduced to 25–50 mg (maintenance) **OR**
- (prostate cancer: to decrease 'flare' associated with LHRH agonists) initially 100 mg orally twice daily for 5–7 days, then 100 mg twice daily for 3–4 weeks with LHRH agonists **OR**
- (prostate cancer, advanced without orchiectomy) 100 mg orally 2–3 times daily **OR**
- (prostate cancer, treatment for hot flushes associated with LHRH agonists or in those who have had orchiectomy) 50 mg orally 1–3 times daily, increasing gradually to 100 mg 3 times daily if needed

Adverse effects

- tiredness, headache, depression, fatigue, restlessness
- GI disturbances, nausea
- increased or decreased weight
- reduced libido
- hot flushes, sweating
- anaemia
- (high dose) shortness of breath
- (women) inhibited ovulation, menstrual cycle irregularity, spotting, breast pain, breast tension
- (men) impaired spermatogenesis, gynaecomastia, breast tenderness, osteoporosis, erectile dysfunction
- arterial or venous thromboembolic events
- (rare) benign or malignant liver tumours, liver toxicity, rash, meningioma

Interactions

- may alter requirements for insulin or oral hypoglycaemic agents
- increased risk of myopathy and/or rhabdomyolysis if given with HMG-CoA inhibitors (statins)

- metabolism may be inhibited by itraconazole, ritonavir and clotrimazole increasing serum levels
- increased metabolism may occur if given with rifampicin, phenytoin and St John's wort decreasing serum levels

Nursing points/Cautions

- (female) complete medical examination, including cervical cytological smear and breast examination, should be completed before start and regularly throughout therapy. Other causes of androgenisation (e.g. adrenal or ovarian cancer) should be ruled out before starting therapy
- pregnancy should be excluded before starting therapy
- baseline liver function tests, blood counts, blood clotting, thyroid function, adrenal function, blood glucose and agglutination should be measured before starting therapy and regularly throughout
- in pre-menopausal women (of child-bearing potential) an oestrogen/progestogen combination should be added to ensure contraception and stabilise the cycle
- (women) treatment should start on first day of menstrual cycle (first day of bleeding). Women with amenorrhoea or irregular menstrual cycle can start therapy immediately
- (men) one control spermatogram is made before start of treatment; spermatogenesis may take 3–20 months to return to normal after discontinuing treatment
- tablets contain lactose and are not recommended in those with rare hereditary problems of galactose intolerance, Lapp lactase deficiency or glucose–galactose malabsorption
- caution when used to treat prostate cancer, because there is an increased risk of liver toxicity
- caution if used in those with diabetes mellitus
- not recommended before conclusion of puberty
- contraindicated in those with liver disease (including jaundice and pruritus associated with pregnancy), previous or current liver tumours, history of herpes in pregnancy, wasting diseases (not prostate cancer), severe chronic depression, predisposition to thromboembolic events, severe diabetes mellitus (with vascular changes), sickle cell anaemia, present or history of meningioma, Dubin–Johnson syndrome or Rotor syndrome

Patient teaching and advice

- patient should be advised to avoid driving or operating machinery if tiredness or inability to concentrate occurs
- instruct women to seek medical attention if any persistent or recurrent bleeding occurs at irregular intervals
- women should be warned that hirsutism and alopecia may recur when therapy is stopped
- patient should be advised to report any unusual tiredness, dark urine, persistent loss of appetite, yellowing of skin or eyes, upper abdominal pain or unexplained flu-like symptoms
- women should be instructed to take medication at the same time every day
- if tablets are missed, contraceptive effectiveness may be reduced and patient should be advised to use barrier contraceptive methods, and continue to take tablets according to the normal regimen
- instruct female patient that if unscheduled bleeding occurs during the 3-week cycle in which the tablets are being taken, tablet taking should not be interrupted

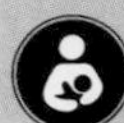

pregnancy must be excluded at the start of treatment and ethinylestradiol taken as well to ensure contraception. If taken during pregnancy, may lead to feminisation of male fetus, therefore is contraindicated

contraindicated during breastfeeding

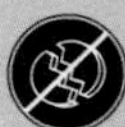

tablet can be dispersed in water or crushed and mixed with yoghurt or apple puree. Mask and gloves must be worn and closed tablet crusher used. Pregnant staff must not disperse or crush tablets

Note
- contained in Brenda-35 ED, Diane-35 ED, Estelle-35 ED, Jene-35 ED, Juliet-35 ED

FLUTAMIDE (Flutamin)

Available form
Tablets: 250 mg

Action
- non-steroidal antiandrogen with specific effects on the prostate

Use
- advanced prostatic carcinoma (with LHRH agonist) in previously untreated patients
- prophylaxis of disease 'flare' associated with LHRH agonist

Dose
- 250 mg orally 3 times daily, starting 24 hours before taking LHRH agonist

Adverse effects
- anorexia, constipation, diarrhoea
- insomnia, tiredness, headache, dizziness, malaise, drowsiness, depression, confusion
- peripheral oedema
- urine colour change (amber to yellow-green)
- blood dyscrasias, anaemia
- gynaecomastia, breast tenderness, galactorrhoea
- elevated liver enzymes and blood urea nitrogen (BUN)
- decreased glucose tolerance
- cholestatic jaundice, hepatic encephalopathy, hepatic necrosis
- (with LHRH agonist) hot flushes, decreased libido, impotence, nausea, vomiting, diarrhoea, decreased bone density
- (rare) prolongation of QT interval, increased risk of cardiovascular disease

Interactions
- may increase prothrombin time if given with warfarin, therefore should be monitored carefully, especially when starting or stopping therapy
- caution if given with paracetamol, NSAIDs or opioids
- caution if used with agents known to prolong QT interval
- may increase serum levels of theophylline

Nursing points/Cautions
- only for use in males
- before starting therapy, cardiovascular and osteoporosis risk factors should be evaluated
- haemoglobin should be monitored regularly during therapy
- liver function tests are recommended before starting, monthly for 4 months and throughout therapy. If serum transaminases are 2–3 times normal, therapy should not be started
- blood glucose levels and/or glycated haemoglobin (HbA1c) should be monitored if combined with LHRH analogues
- caution if used in men at risk of cardiovascular disease or with congenital QT interval, electrolyte imbalance or congestive cardiac failure
- caution if used in those with chronic alcohol and/or tobacco use, strong family history of osteoporosis or

- chronic use of agents that decrease bone mass (e.g. antiepileptic agents, corticosteroids)
- contraindicated in those with severe liver impairment

Patient teaching and advice

- patient should be advised to seek medical advice if any unusual tiredness, itching, dark urine, persistent loss of appetite, yellowing of eyes or skin, upper abdominal pain or unexplained flu-like symptoms occur
- warn patient that urine colour change (amber to yellow-green) is harmless
- advise patient to avoid driving or operating machinery if dizziness, drowsiness or confusion occurs
- patient should be warned that he may experience an increase in breast size, breasts may become tender and sometimes secrete fluid

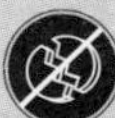

tablets can be dispersed in water or crushed and mixed with spoonful of yoghurt or apple puree. Mask and gloves must be worn and closed tablet crusher used. Pregnant staff must not open capsules

NILUTAMIDE (Anandron)

Available form

Tablets: 150 mg

Action

- non-steroidal antiandrogen which acts by competing at prostate androgen receptor site thereby blocking androgenic stimulation of prostate cancer cell differentiation
- also acts on other androgen receptor sites in pituitary and hypothalamus interrupting negative feedback
- long half-life (56 hours)

Use

- previously untreated metastatic prostate cancer (with surgical or medical castration)
- prevention of disease flare associated with LHRH agonist

Dose

- initially 300 mg orally daily as single or divided dose for 4 weeks, then 150 mg daily (starting same day as LHRH agonist or surgical castration)

Adverse effects

- nausea, vomiting
- impairment of dark or light adaptation
- dizziness
- altered liver enzymes
- impotence, decreased libido, hot flushes, loss of body hair, sweating, gynaecomastia
- interstitial pneumonia (with dyspnoea, coughing, fever and chest pain), pulmonary fibrosis
- (uncommon) hepatitis
- (rare) aplastic anaemia, QT prolongation

Interactions

- may cause alcohol intolerance (malaise with vasomotor flushes) if given together
- may increase serum levels of phenytoin, propranolol, diazepam and theophylline, increasing the risk of toxicity
- caution if given with warfarin. Monitoring of INR is recommended especially when starting or stopping therapy
- caution if given with agents known to prolong QT interval including Class IA or Class III antiarrhythmic agents, methadone, moxifloxacin and some antipsychotic agents

Nursing points/Cautions

- for use in male patients only
- patient should be examined for any signs of or predisposition to liver or respiratory impairment before starting therapy

- liver enzymes should be monitored before starting and then regularly during therapy
- caution if used in those at risk of QT prolongation, including those taking medications that may prolong QT interval or cause electrolyte imbalance (especially hypokalaemia)
- caution if used in Japanese men as there is an increased risk of interstitial pneumonia
- contraindicated in those with severe liver impairment, severe respiratory insufficiency or those who have failed to respond previously to hormone treatment

Patient teaching and advice

- warn patient to avoid alcohol during therapy
- advise patient to avoid driving (especially at night or through tunnels) or operating machinery if dizziness and visual disturbances occur
- patient should be advised to wear sunglasses
- advise patient to seek medical advice immediately if any of the following occur:
  - shortness of breath, difficulty breathing, coughing, fever or chest pain, especially in the first 12 weeks of therapy (signs of interstitial pneumonia)
  - loss of appetite, nausea, vomiting, abdominal pain, unusual tiredness, dark urine or yellowing of skin or eyes (signs of hepatitis)
  - fast or irregular heartbeat

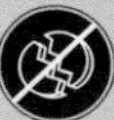

tablets can be crushed and mixed with water or spoonful of yoghurt or apple puree. Mask and gloves must be worn and closed tablet crusher used. Pregnant staff must not crush tablets

TIBOLONE (Livial, Livilan, Xyvion)

Available form

Tablets: 2.5 mg

Action

- related to naturally occurring steroids with progestogenic and androgenic properties
- three active metabolites (two with oestrogenic properties and one with progestogenic/androgenic properties)
- oestrogenic effects on vagina, bone and thermoregulatory centre
- androgenic effect on some metabolic and haematological factors
- improves vaginal dryness and atrophy, as well as mood and libido

Use

- relief of symptoms of natural or surgical menopause (short term)
- second-line treatment in prevention of post-menopausal bone mineral density loss (in those at high risk of fractures where other treatment is contraindicated or not appropriate)

Dose

- (natural or surgical menopause, prevention of post-menopausal bone mineral density loss) 2.5 mg orally daily

Adverse effects

- fluid retention, oedema, weight gain
- headache, dizziness, depression
- lower abdominal pain
- breast tenderness
- cervical dysplasia, vulvo-vaginitis, vaginal bleeding/discharge, genital pruritus/discharge, pelvic pain, endometrial wall thickening
- hypertension
- abnormal hair growth
- altered HDL cholesterol, total triglycerides and lipoprotein (a)
- rash, pruritus, acne
- blurred vision
- arthralgia, myalgia
- (long-term use > 3 years, uncommon) endometrial, ovarian or breast

cancer, venous or arterial thromboembolism, stroke
- (rare) jaundice, impaired liver function

Interactions
- anticoagulant effect of warfarin may be increased, therefore INR should be carefully monitored especially when starting or stopping therapy
- decreased serum levels may occur if given with phenobarbital (phenobarbitone), carbamazepine, phenytoin, rifampicin or St John's wort

Nursing points/Cautions

- patients should have a thorough medical examination, including breast, abdominal and pelvic examination to rule out presence of carcinoma before starting therapy. Assessment should also include personal and family history. Yearly breast and pelvic examinations are recommended while on therapy
- BP should be monitored regularly during therapy
- serum cholesterol and triglycerides should be monitored regularly if patient has pre-existing hypertriglyceridaemia
- therapy should be stopped immediately if there is any decrease in liver function, jaundice, increase in blood pressure or new onset of migraine-type headache
- treatment duration should be as short as possible and reviewed after 6 months. Symptoms usually improve after first few weeks of therapy but may take up to 12 weeks to be optimal
- (menopause) started within 12 months after last natural bleed, or immediately after surgically induced menopause
- if switching from oestrogen-only therapy, a withdrawal bleed should be induced before starting therapy
- if switching from continuous HRT, therapy can be started at any time
- if switching from sequential HRT preparations, therapy should be started after progestogen phase
- tablets contain lactose and are therefore not recommended in those with galactose intolerance, Lapp lactase deficiency or glucose–galactose malabsorption
- caution and increased monitoring in those with uterine fibroids or endometriosis, risk factors for thromboembolic disorders or oestrogen-dependent tumours (e.g. first degree relative with breast cancer), hypertension, liver disorders, diabetes mellitus (with or without vascular involvement), cholelithiasis, migraine or severe headache, SLE, epilepsy, asthma, otosclerosis or history of endometrial hyperplasia
- caution if used in those with cardiac or renal failure that may be aggravated by fluid retention
- caution if used in those with pre-existing hypertriglyceridaemia
- contraindicated in those with a history of (or suspicion of) breast cancer, oestrogen-dependent malignant tumours, undiagnosed genital bleeding, endometrial hyperplasia (untreated), idiopathic/current venous thromboembolism, arterial thromboembolic disease, known thrombophilic disorders, acute liver disease or history of liver disease (with abnormal liver function) or porphyria

Patient teaching and advice

- advise patient to avoid driving or operating machinery if blurred vision or dizziness occur
- patient should be advised to seek medical advice immediately if any of the following occur:
  - loss of appetite, nausea, vomiting, abdominal pain, unusual tiredness, dark urine or yellowing of skin or eyes

- new or worsening headache/migraine
- painful leg swelling
- sudden onset of chest pain or difficulty breathing
- any vaginal bleeding is present 6 months after starting therapy, starts after 6 months of therapy or continues after therapy has been stopped

- warn patient that vaginal bleeding or spotting may occur when starting therapy
- patient should be instructed that if missed dose is noticed within 12 hours, it should be taken; if > 12 hours has elapsed, patient should wait until next dose. Patient should be aware that there will be an increased risk of breakthrough bleeding and spotting

banned in sport

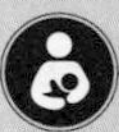
contraindicated during pregnancy or breastfeeding

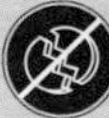
tablets can be crushed and mixed with water or spoonful of yoghurt or apple puree. Mask and gloves must be worn and closed tablet crusher used. Pregnant staff must not crush tablets

COMBINED ORAL CONTRACEPTIVES (COC)

Available forms
Tablets (see table 1483–84)

General Actions of oral contraceptives
- oral contraceptives are a combination of oestrogens (e.g. ethinylestradiol, mestranol) and progestogens (e.g. norethisterone, levonorgestrel, cyproterone, drospirenone, desogestrel)
- oestrogens inhibit the secretion of FSH, preventing follicular development and release of LH
- progestogens, in combination, appear to inhibit the pre-ovulatory rise of LH
- combination preparations decrease the likelihood of conception and implantation by causing changes in both the cervical mucus and the endometrium
- most widely used form of hormonal contraception
- progestogen-only preparations alter the cervical mucus and endometrium without influencing ovulation and are used when oestrogen is not wanted (e.g. during breastfeeding). Levonorgestrel is the most androgenic, with third generation progestogens (desogestrel, gestodene, drospirenone) less androgenic
- available in three formulations – fixed-dose oestrogen–progestogen combination, phasic oestrogen–progestogen combination and progestogen only
- menstrual cycle becomes regular, less painful and bleeding lighter

General Uses of oral contraceptives
- oral contraception (regular or emergency)

- androgenisation in women (e.g. treatment of severe acne (with inflammation, nodularity and/or at risk of scarring) where prolonged oral antibiotics or local treatment have been unsuccessful; mild-to-moderate hirsutism)
- menstrual disorders, endometriosis

General Adverse effects of oral contraceptives

- nausea, abdominal pain or bloating, weight gain and, uncommonly, vomiting, diarrhoea
- mental depression, altered mood, nervousness, dizziness
- headache and, uncommonly, migraine
- oedema and, uncommonly, fluid retention
- acne, rash, pruritus, urticaria
- spotting, breakthrough bleeding, abnormal withdrawal bleeding, pelvic pain
- leucorrhoea, vaginal candidiasis, vaginitis
- breast tenderness, pain or engorgement
- changes to libido
- (uncommon) hypertension
- (rare) increased risk of cervical, endometrial, ovarian, liver or breast cancer
- (rare) venous or arterial thromboembolic or thrombotic disorders, ocular lesions, dry eyes, intolerance to contact lenses (changed corneal curvature), chloasma (blotchy dark pigmentation), cholestatic jaundice, benign hepatic adenomas, gall bladder disease

General Interactions of oral contraceptives

- contraindicated with ombitasvir, paritaprevir or dasabuvir
- efficacy may be reduced by some broad-spectrum antibiotics, therefore additional contraception is recommended
- may increase serum levels of benzodiazepines, tacrolimus or ciclosporin increasing risk of toxicity
- may decrease serum levels of lamotrigine
- decreased serum levels, pregnancy and menstrual irregularities may occur if given with barbiturates, carbamazepine, griseofulvin, phenobarbital (phenobarbitone), phenytoin, primidone, rifabutin, rifampicin, St John's wort or topiramate. A different or additional form of contraception is recommended during therapy with these agents
- if used with rifampicin, a barrier method should be used during therapy and for 28 days after stopping
- increased serum levels may occur if given with azole antifungals, verapamil, diltiazem, macrolide antibiotics, atorvastatin and grapefruit juice
- HIV protease and non-nucleoside transcriptase inhibitors may have a variable (increase or decrease) effect on serum levels of oral contraceptives and should therefore be given with caution
- may affect a number of laboratory tests, including serum folate, triglycerides and phospholipid, response to metyrapone test, glucose tolerance, thyroid, renal, adrenal and liver function tests, prothrombin and coagulation time. It is therefore recommended that the test(s) be repeated when the person has been oestrogen-free for 1–2 months

General Nursing points/Cautions for oral contraceptives

- complete medical examination (including family history, BP and examination of breasts, pelvis and abdomen, cervical cytology and urinalysis) should occur before starting oral contraceptives. Clotting tests should be performed on any women with a family history of thromboembolic disease
- pregnancy should be excluded before starting therapy
- (androgenisation of women) androgen-producing tumour or adrenal enzyme defect should be excluded before starting therapy (especially if hirsutism has only recently appeared or intensified)
- increase in frequency or severity of migraine, loss of vision, double vision, slurred speech, aphasia, weakness or marked numbness on one side, or collapse (with or without focal seizures) could also be a sign of imminent stroke
- patient should be monitored for signs of depression, especially if pre-existing depression
- therapy should be discontinued for at least 4 weeks before elective surgery and restarted 2 weeks after complete mobilisation. Other causes of immobilisation that require stopping therapy include long-haul flights, major trauma or emergency surgery
- many oral contraceptives contain lactose and are therefore not recommended in those with rare hereditary problems of galactose intolerance, Lapp lactase deficiency or glucose–galactose malabsorption
- caution if used in women with porphyria, SLE, haemolytic uraemic syndrome, Crohn's disease, ulcerative colitis, cholestasis, gall stones or otosclerotic related hearing loss
- caution if used in women with hypertension
- caution if used in women with diabetes mellitus because of decreased glucose tolerance
- caution if used in women with hereditary angioedema as condition may be exacerbated
- caution if used in women post-bariatric surgery due to possibility of malabsorption
- caution if used in women with hypertriglyceridaemia due to increased risk of pancreatitis
- caution if used in women who may be affected by fluid retention (e.g. cardiac or renal disease, asthma, migraine)
- risk of venous or arterial thrombotic, thromboembolic or cerebrovascular accidents increases with age, smoking (further risk increase if over 35 and heavy smoker), family history of venous/arterial thromboembolism (especially at early age), obesity or overweight, hypertension, migraine, dyslipoproteinaemia, valvular heart disease, atrial fibrillation, prolonged immobilisation (including post-surgery or after any leg surgery), recent delivery or second trimester abortion, or temporary immobilisation (e.g. air travel > 4 hours)
- contraindicated in those with or who have a history of thrombophlebitis or thromboembolic disorder, predisposition to thromboembolism (including acquired or hereditary disorders such as antithrombin III deficiency or protein C deficiency), past history of DVT, cerebrovascular

or coronary artery disease, history of migraine with focal neurological symptoms, known/suspected breast/uterine/vaginal or cervical cancer, known/suspected/previous oestrogen-dependent tumour, undiagnosed abnormal vaginal bleeding, liver disease (if liver function has not returned to normal), cholestatic jaundice, pruritus in pregnancy or with contraceptive use, Dubin–Johnson or Rotor syndrome, benign or malignant liver tumour, otosclerosis (which deteriorated during pregnancy), herpes in pregnancy, abnormal lipid metabolism or hypertriglyceridaemia, pancreatitis or history of pancreatitis with severe hypertriglycidaemia, severe hypertension or severe diabetes mellitus (with or without vascular changes)

General Patient teaching and advice for oral contraceptives

- instruct patient in the importance of telling health professionals that oral contraceptive is being used when being questioned during routine medical examination
- recommend a routine of taking oral contraceptive pill at the same time each day so that it is taken regularly, including when to start (i.e. day 1 is first day of menstrual bleeding), following arrows on packet. Patient should also be advised on what to do if a dose is missed or if vomiting or diarrhoea occurs
- advise patient to keep follow-up appointments so that blood pressure can be checked and breasts may be examined (and cytology smear taken if needed)
- teach the patient how to examine her own breasts immediately after each menstrual period
- advise patient to seek medical advice immediately if any of the following occur:
  - any sudden leg/foot pain, tenderness or swelling, increased warmth and/or discolouration of leg/foot (these may be signs of deep vein thrombosis)
  - sudden chest pain, sudden breathlessness or unexplained sudden cough, light-headedness, dizziness, rapid heart rate (these may be signs of pulmonary embolism)
  - loss of appetite, nausea, unusual tiredness, upper abdominal pain, yellowing of skin or eyes, dark urine or whole body itching (signs of jaundice)
  - blurred or double vision, loss of vision
  - any changes in migraine/headache frequency and/or severity
  - change in mood, or worsening of depression
  - sudden numbness/weakness of face/arm/leg (especially if one-sided), dizziness, loss of balance or coordination, trouble walking, prolonged or severe headache, loss of consciousness
- patient who is a heavy smoker (>15 cigarettes/day) and taking oral contraceptives should be advised that she runs a higher risk of developing DVT than those who do not smoke
- women who wear contact lenses should be warned that intolerance to lenses sometimes occurs

- women should be advised that oral contraceptive efficacy may be reduced if dose is missed, during severe vomiting or diarrhoea or with some concurrent medications (including some OTC, antibiotics or herbal preparations)
- advise woman that not all women experience withdrawal bleeding during placebo/no tablet period
- women should be warned that slight spotting is common; however, persistent or heavy bleeding should be reported to doctor
- advise patient to contact her doctor if she has missed a dose or if, despite following the prescribed dose pattern, she has missed two consecutive 'periods'
- women should be advised that oral contraceptives do not protect against HIV infection, AIDS and other sexually transmitted diseases
- see also General Patient teaching and advice (p. xxvii)

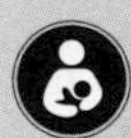
contraindicated during pregnancy or breastfeeding

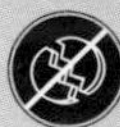
tablets should not be crushed

ORAL CONTRACEPTIVES

	Oestrogen	Progestogen
Fixed-dose combinations		
Brenda-35 ED	ethinylestradiol 35 microgram	cyproterone acetate 2 mg
Brevinor	ethinylestradiol 35 microgram	norethisterone 500 microgram
Brevinor-1	ethinylestradiol 35 microgram	norethisterone 1 mg
Diane- 35ED	ethinylestradiol 35 microgram	cyproterone acetate 2 mg
Eleanor 150/35 ED	ethinylestradiol 30 microgram	levonorgestrel 150 microgram
Estelle 35 ED	ethinylestradiol 35 microgram	cyproterone acetate 2 mg
Evelyn 35 ED	ethinylestradiol 30 microgram	levonorgestrel 150 microgram
Femme-Tab ED 20/100	ethinylestradiol 20 microgram	levonorgestrel 100 microgram
Femme-Tab ED 30/150	ethinylestradiol 30 microgram	levonorgestrel 150 microgram
Jene-35 ED	ethinylestradiol 35 microgram	cyproterone acetate 2 mg
Juliet-35 ED	ethinylestradiol 35 microgram	cyproterone acetate 2 mg
Lenest 20 ED	ethinylestradiol 20 microgram	levonorgestrel 100 microgram
Levlen ED	ethinylestradiol 30 microgram	levonorgestrel 150 microgram
Loette	ethinylestradiol 20 microgram	levonorgestrel 100 microgram
Madeline	ethinylestradiol 30 microgram	desogestrel 150 microgram
Marvelon 28	ethinylestradiol 30 microgram	desogestrel 150 microgram
Microgynon 20 ED	ethinylestradiol 20 microgram	levonorgestrel 100 microgram
Microgynon 30 ED	ethinylestradiol 30 microgram	levonorgestrel 150 microgram
Microgynon 50 ED	ethinylestradiol 50 microgram	levonorgestrel 125 microgram
Microlevlen ED	ethinylestradiol 20 microgram	levonorgestrel 100 microgram
Micronelle 20 ED	ethinylestradiol 20 microgram	levonorgestrel 100 microgram
Micronelle 30 ED	ethinylestradiol 30 microgram	levonorgestrel 150 microgram
Minulet	ethinylestradiol 30 microgram	gestodene 75 microgram
Monofeme 30 ED	ethinylestradiol 30 microgram	levonorgestrel 150 microgram
Nordette	ethinylestradiol 30 microgram	levonorgestrel 150 microgram
Norimin	ethinylestradiol 35 microgram	norethisterone 500 microgram
Norimin-1	ethinylestradiol 35 microgram	norethisterone 1 mg
Norinyl-1	mestranol 50 microgram	norethisterone 1 mg
Petibelle	ethinylestradiol 30 microgram	drospirenone 3 mg
Valette	ethinylestradiol 30 microgram	dienogest 2 mg

ORAL CONTRACEPTIVES—cont'd

	Oestrogen	Progestogen
Yasmin	ethinylestradiol 30 microgram	drospirenone 3 mg
Yaz	ethinylestradiol 20 microgram	drospirenone 3 mg
Yaz Flex	ethinylestradiol 20 microgram	drospirenone 3 mg
Zoely	estradiol valerate 1.5 mg	nomegestrol 2.5 mg
Phasic oestrogen–progestogen combination		
Logynon ED	ethinylestradiol 30 microgram	levonorgestrel 50 microgram
	ethinylestradiol 40 microgram	levonorgestrel 75 microgram
	ethinylestradiol 30 microgram	levonorgestrel 125 microgram
Trifeme	ethinylestradiol 30 microgram	levonorgestrel 50 microgram
	ethinylestradiol 40 microgram	levonorgestrel 75 microgram
	ethinylestradiol 30 microgram	levonorgestrel 125 microgram
Triphasil	ethinylestradiol 30 microgram	levonorgestrel 50 microgram
	ethinylestradiol 40 microgram	levonorgestrel 75 microgram
	ethinylestradiol 30 microgram	levonorgestrel 125 microgram
Triquilar ED	estradiol valerate 3 mg	dienogest nil
Qlaira	estradiol valerate 2 mg	dienogest 2 mg
	estradiol valerate 2 mg	dienogest 3 mg
	estradiol valerate 1 mg	dienogest nil
	estradiol valerate 1 mg	dienogest nil
Progestogen only		
Microlut		levonorgestrel 30 microgram
Noriday 28		norethisterone 350 microgram

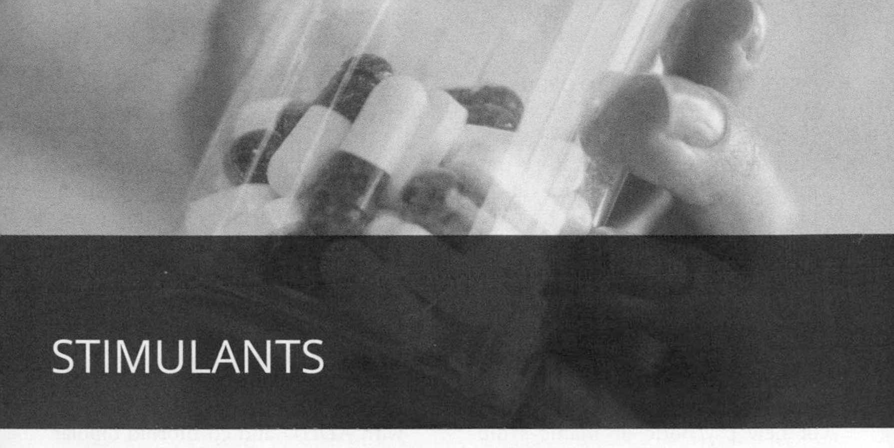

STIMULANTS

The main group of drugs used as central nervous stimulants are the amphetamines and methylxanthines (e.g. caffeine). The amphetamines are mainly used in the management of narcolepsy and some hyperkinetic states in children (e.g. attention deficit hyperactivity disorder (ADHD), previously known as attention deficit disorder (Bryant et al 2019). Amphetamines such as phentermine are utilised as appetite suppressants and discussed in Anorectics and Weight-Loss agents (p. 42).

ADHD is characterised by a persistent short attention span, impulsive behaviour and hyperactivity, resulting in a child who may be irritable, moody, have low self-esteem and experience learning difficulties. Management of ADHD involves family therapy and support, educational programs and directed activities, speech and occupational therapy, with pharmacological therapy being an adjunct if needed. It should be noted that a number of patients with ADHD will either not respond or be intolerant to a stimulant and another therapy may need to be trialled (Bryant et al 2019).

Narcolepsy is an incurable neurological condition in which the person experiences excessive drowsiness and uncontrollable 'sleep attacks' that can occur at any time, including during everyday activities such as eating, working and driving. Patients may also experience sleep paralysis (inability to move that occurs when just falling asleep or waking up), cataplexy (stress-induced, generalised muscle weakness) and vivid auditory or visual dreams when falling asleep (Bryant et al 2019).

General Adverse effects of stimulants

- palpitations, increase in BP, tachycardia
- depression, agitation, irritability, nervousness, restlessness, hostility, aggression (or worsening of aggression or hostility)
- headache, migraine, dizziness, somnolence, insomnia, sedation
- fatigue, asthenia
- loss of appetite, anorexia, nausea,
- vomiting, abdominal pain, dry mouth or unpleasant taste, thirst, weight loss, dyspepsia, constipation, diarrhoea
- (children) retarded growth (height and weight)
- fever
- sweating, flushing

- pharyngitis, upper respiratory tract infection, cough, dyspnoea, flu-like illness
- erectile dysfunction, decreased libido, impotence, menstrual irregularities
- pruritus, dermatitis, rash, urticaria
- (rare) angioedema, anaphylactic reactions
- (rare) seizures
- (rare) suicidal ideation, emergence of new psychotic or manic symptoms (e.g. hallucinations, delusional thinking, mania), onset/exacerbation of motor or vocal tics
- (rare) peripheral vasculopathy, including Raynaud's phenomenon

General Nursing points/Cautions for stimulants

- before starting therapy, patient should have a thorough assessment to identify any pre-existing or underlying cardiovascular (e.g. hypertension, cardiac abnormalities, sudden death) or psychiatric history (e.g. history of depression, bipolar disorder, suicide attempts)
- blood pressure, heart rate and psychiatric status should be regularly reviewed throughout therapy
- children should have height and weight monitored regularly throughout therapy. Growth and weight will return to normal when medication is stopped, and some specialists recommend drug-free periods to minimise these complications
- if therapy is stopped for more than 1 week, it should be restarted at the initial dose
- (narcolepsy) evaluation of excessive sleepiness and diagnosis of narcolepsy, obstructive sleep apnoea/hypopnea syndrome (OSAHS) and chronic shiftwork sleep disorder (SWSD) should be made according to diagnostic criteria, including history, physical examination and may also be supplemented by laboratory testing (e.g. sleep studies)
- patients should be closely monitored for any suicidal thoughts or behaviours during therapy
- (ADHD) caution if used in those with ADHD and co-morbid bipolar disorder as mixed/mania episodes may be induced
- caution if used in those who partake in strenuous exercise, use stimulants and/or have family history of sudden/cardiac death, due to increased risk of sudden/cardiac death
- caution if used in those with pre-existing depression, mania, psychosis, hyperthyroidism, epilepsy, mild hypertension, tachycardia, ventricular arrhythmias, recent myocardial infarction, cardiovascular disease (including unstable angina and significant cardiac abnormalities), liver or kidney dysfunction or family history of cardiac arrest or sudden death (including congenital or acquired QT syndrome), or conditions that could be worsened by increasing blood pressure and/or heart rate
- contraindicated in those with moderate-to-severe hypertension, severe cardiovascular disease, atrial fibrillation/ flutter, ventricular tachycardia, ventricular fibrillation/flutter, advanced atherosclerosis, pheochromocytoma or uncontrolled hyperthyroidism, arteriosclerosis, glaucoma, severe anxiety, tension or agitation, motor tics, Tourette's syndrome, severe depression, anorexia nervosa, psychotic or suicidal tendencies,

hypersensitivity to sympathomimetic amines or a history of drug or alcohol abuse

General Patient teaching and advice for stimulants

- patient (or carer) should be advised to report any:
  - dark urine, itching, yellowing of eyes or skin, right upper abdominal pain or tenderness, nausea, loss of appetite or flu-like illness
  - thoughts/talk about self-harm, harm to others, suicide or death or recent attempts at self-harm
  - increase in aggression, agitation, irritability, panic attacks or hostility
  - occurrence of fitting, confusion or hallucinations
  - exertional chest pain, unexplained fainting
  - discolouration of toes and/or fingers on exposure to temperature change (cold or heat) or emotional events accompanied by numbness in same area
- adult patients should be advised not to drive or operate machinery if dizziness, drowsiness, tiredness or visual disturbances occur
- warn patient to take care getting out of bed or suddenly standing up as dizziness, light-headedness and/or fainting may occur
- adult patients should be advised to avoid (or reduce) alcohol intake during therapy
- (ADHD) parent/carer should regularly monitor child's growth (height and weight) and discuss any concerns with doctor as therapy may need to be temporarily interrupted
- warn patient/carer not to suddenly stop therapy as unwanted side-effects will occur. Any interruption or stopping of therapy should be gradual and under medical supervision
- counsel adult patient that there may be changes to sexual function during therapy
- see also General Patient teaching and advice (p. xxvii)

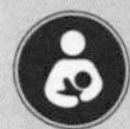
not recommended during pregnancy or breastfeeding

ARMODAFINIL (Nuvigil)

Available forms

Tablets: 50 mg, 150 mg, 250 mg

Action

- non-amphetamine that promotes wakefulness by an unknown action that is different to that of the sympathomimetic amines, but thought to involve histaminergic systems
- chemically related to modafinil (R-enantiomer) with similar properties
- indirect dopamine receptor agonist
- half-life about 15 hours

Use

- narcolepsy
- obstructive sleep apnoea/hypopnoea syndrome (OSAHS) with continuous positive airway pressure (CPAP) (adjunct)
- treatment of excessive sleepiness associated with moderate-to-severe chronic shiftwork sleep disorder (SWSD) (where non-pharmacological interventions were ineffective or inappropriate)

Dose

- (narcolepsy) 150 mg or 250 mg orally daily (in the morning) 1 hour before or 2 hours after food **OR**
- (OSAHS) 150 mg or 250 mg orally daily (in the morning) 1 hour before

or 2 hours after food (with continuous positive airway pressure (CPAP))
OR
- (SWSD) initially 150 mg orally daily 1 hour before or 2 hours after food, 1 hour before starting shiftwork

Adverse effects
- see General Adverse effects of stimulants (p. 1485)
- abuse, dependence
- (rare, high dose) serious skin reactions, angioedema, multi-organ hypersensitivity reaction

Interactions
- decreased serum levels may occur if given with carbamazepine, oxcarbazepine, phenytoin, rifabutin, phenobarbital (phenobarbitone), rifampicin and St John's wort
- increased serum levels may occur if given with ritonavir, indinavir, saquinavir, nelfinavir, chloramphenicol, clarithromycin, erythromycin, itraconazole, diltiazem and verapamil
- may increase serum level of diazepam, phenytoin, propranolol, omeprazole, esomeprazole and clomipramine
- caution if used with MAOIs
- increased monitoring of INR is recommended if given with warfarin, especially when starting or stopping therapy
- may decrease serum level of oral contraceptives, midazolam, triazolam, ciclosporin, quetiapine and carbamazepine

Nursing points/Cautions
- patients with sleep apnoea should be fully investigated by experienced doctor with access to sleep laboratory diagnostic facilities before starting therapy
- armodafinil and modafinil are not bioequivalent or interchangeable
- patient with persistent sleepiness should have their levels assessed frequently to determine the effectiveness of the medication
- therapy should not be started unless negative pregnancy test is confirmed at least 1 week before starting therapy
- not recommended in those under 18 years
- caution if used in those with a psychiatric history (including anxiety), history of drug/stimulant abuse or liver dysfunction
- caution if used in the elderly as lower dosage may be required
- not recommended in those with history of left ventricular hypertrophy or mitral valve prolapse who have history of CNS stimulant-induced valve prolapse
- contraindicated in those with hypersensitivity to modafinil
- see General Nursing points/Cautions for stimulants (p. 1486)

Patient teaching and advice
- ensure patient has an understanding of good sleep hygiene principles, such as limiting alcohol and caffeine intake before bedtime, regular bed and waking time and comfortable sleeping environment (no TV or electronics, cool room temperature)
- patient should be advised to seek medical attention immediately if any of the following occur:
  - rash or mouth blistering, fever or hives, abnormal physical weakness or lack of energy
  - swelling of face, eyes, lips, tongue or throat, hoarseness, difficulty swallowing
  - chest pain or unusual heartbeat
- if patient has abnormal levels of sleepiness, advise that medication may not return wakefulness to normal levels
- women of childbearing potential who use oral contraceptives should be warned that their effectiveness may be impaired, and therefore an

additional form of contraception is recommended to prevent pregnancy occurring. Contraception should be continued for 4 weeks after discontinuing therapy
- see General Patient teaching and advice for stimulants (p. 1487)

banned in sport

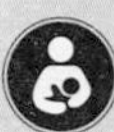

contraindicated during pregnancy

not recommended during breastfeeding

tablets can be crushed and mixed with water or spoonful of yoghurt or apple puree. Crushed tablets have very bitter taste

ATOMOXETINE (Strattera)

Available forms
Capsules: 10 mg, 18 mg, 25 mg, 40 mg, 60 mg, 80 mg, 100 mg

Action
- sympathomimetic agent that inhibits noradrenaline (norepinephrine) uptake, serotonin (5-HT) uptake and (weakly) dopamine
- non-stimulant
- has an active equipotent metabolite
- half-life 5–22 hours
- considered second-line treatment
- does not cause dependence

Use
- ADHD (in those aged 6 years and over) as part of total treatment program

Dose
- (≤ 70 kg) initially 0.5 mg/kg orally daily for at least 3 days, then increasing to 1.2 mg/kg as a single or divided dose (morning and late afternoon or early evening), increasing to a maximum 1.4 mg/kg or 100 mg after a further 2–4 weeks if optimal results have not been achieved **OR**
- (> 70 kg) initially 40 mg orally daily for at least 3 days, then increasing to 80 mg as a single or divided dose, increasing to a maximum 100 mg after a further 2–4 weeks if optimal results have not been achieved

Adverse effects
- urinary retention, urinary hesitancy
- sexual dysfunction
- chest pain
- (rare) liver injury, seizures, stroke, myocardial infarction
- see also General Adverse effects of stimulants (p. 1485)

Interactions
- contraindicated with or within 2 weeks of stopping/starting MAOIs
- may increase serum levels of diazepam, paroxetine and phenytoin
- caution if used with salbutamol or other beta-adrenoceptor agonists, because cardiovascular effects (e.g. palpitations) may be potentiated
- additive effect may occur if given with alpha-1-agonist or noradrenaline (norepinephrine) uptake inhibitors
- increased serum level may occur if given with fluoxetine or paroxetine
- not recommended with TCAs because of increased risk of cardiovascular adverse effects
- not recommended with other agents that prolong QT interval or cause electrolyte imbalance
- caution if given with antihypertensive or pressor agents

Nursing points/Cautions
- may be discontinued without tapering dose
- caution if used in males with enlarged prostate or have a history of urinary retention
- caution if used in those with history of seizures

- see General Nursing points/Cautions for stimulants (p. 1486)

Patient teaching and advice

- advise patient (or carer) to take divided dose in the morning and late afternoon/early evening for best effect
- patient (or carer) should be advised not to open capsules as powder is irritating to the eyes. Eyes should be immediately flushed with water if contact occurs
- see General Patient teaching and advice for stimulants (p. 1487)

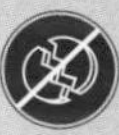

capsules can be opened and contents dispersed in water or mixed with spoonful of yoghurt or apple puree. Gloves and safety glasses must be worn when opening capsules or dispersing in water

CAFFEINE (No Doz)

Available form

Tablets: 100 mg

Action

- methylxanthine, related to theophylline
- stimulant effect on CNS, producing wakefulness and increased mental activity
- antagonises adenosine receptors leading to contraction of cardiac muscle and relaxation of airway smooth muscle
- may indirectly stimulate dopamine activity
- weak vasodilator and weak diuretic effect

Use

- relieve mental fatigue and drowsiness and increase alertness
- adjunct to enhance analgesic actions
- respiratory stimulant in premature infants (see Antiasthma agents, bronchodilators and respiratory agents p. 117)

Dose

- 100 mg orally, may be repeated after 3–4 hours (daily maximum 600 mg)

Adverse effects

- insomnia, anxiety, tremor, palpitations, increased BP, nervousness, withdrawal syndrome (including headache, irritability, weakness)
- gastric irritation, nausea, dyspepsia

Interactions

- may antagonise effects of dipyridamole when used during cardiac stress testing
- antagonises adenosine
- may increase CNS stimulation if given with other CNS-stimulating agents or other caffeine-containing products

Nursing points/Cautions

- standard cup of coffee contains 50–150 mg caffeine, with espresso coffee containing 145 mg/50 mL
- intake of chocolate or beverages that contain caffeine, including coffee, tea, energy drinks, cola and cocoa, or any products containing guarana may require a reduction in dose
- caution if used in those with insomnia, nervousness and tachycardia
- not recommended in those with severe anxiety, severe cardiac disease, liver impairment or hypertension
- contraindicated in children under 12 years or those with caffeine/xanthine sensitivity

Patient teaching and advice

- instruct patient that dose should not be repeated within 3 hours

Note

- contained in Endura Sports Energy Gels, No Doz Plus, Panadol Extra, Travacalm Original (as well as commercial products such as energy drinks)

DEXAMFETAMINE (DEXAMPHETAMINE) SULFATE (Dexamfetamine Tablets)

Available form

Tablets: 5 mg

Action

- centrally acting sympathomimetic agent with alpha and beta-adrenergic activity
- CNS stimulation, especially of the cerebral cortex, respiratory and vasomotor centres, causing increased motor activity, mental alertness and wakefulness and producing euphoria. Peripheral actions include elevation of systolic and diastolic BP and some weak bronchodilator and respiratory activity
- excretion half-life is about 16–31 hours (with excretion increased in acidic urine and decreased in alkaline urine)

Use

- ADHD (in children 3 years or over) as part of total treatment program
- narcolepsy

Dose

Narcolepsy

- (adult) 5–60 mg orally daily in divided doses **OR**
- (6–12 years) initially 5 mg orally daily, increasing by 5 mg at weekly intervals if needed **OR**
- (12 years and over) initially 10 mg orally daily, increasing by 10 mg at weekly intervals if needed

ADHD (over 3 years)

- initially 2.5 mg orally daily, increasing at weekly intervals by 2.5 mg until satisfactory response is achieved (maximum daily dose 40 mg in 2 divided doses)

Adverse effects

- tolerance, dependence, abuse potential
- (high dose, abrupt withdrawal) extreme fatigue, depression, changes on sleep EEG
- see General Adverse effects of stimulants (p. 1485)

Interactions

- contraindicated with or within 2 weeks of stopping MAOIs
- urinary excretion may be increased by urinary acidifiers
- urinary excretion may be decreased by acetazolamide, sodium bicarbonate and some thiazide diuretics
- absorption may be lowered by GI acidifying agents, including fruit juices, decreasing serum levels
- may enhance activity of TCAs (including cardiovascular effects), sympathomimetic agents and other CNS-stimulating agents and therefore combined use is not recommended
- may decrease the sedative effect of antihistamines
- may antagonise the hypotensive action of antihypertensive agents
- CNS-stimulant effects may be antagonised by haloperidol, chlorpromazine and lithium
- may slow absorption of ethosuximide
- may potentiate the analgesic effect of pethidine
- may enhance the effects of adrenaline (epinephrine) and noradrenaline (norepinephrine)
- may delay the absorption of phenobarbital (phenobarbitone) and phenytoin and may also produce a synergistic antiepileptic effect
- may cause elevation in serum corticosteroid levels (especially in the evenings) and therefore interfere with urinary steroid test

Nursing points/Cautions

- under same control as drugs of addiction (S8) (Drugs, Poisons and Controlled Substances Regulations)

- limited, by law, to the above uses in most Australian states and territories. Requires special authority
- (ADHD) a drug-free interval is suggested to determine if there are changes in behavioural patterns. If therapy is stopped for more than a week, it should be restarted at the initial dose
- any withdrawal should be gradual
- caution if used in those with mild hypertension. If used, BP should be closely monitored throughout therapy
- not recommended in those with lactose allergy
- possibility for abuse and dependence exists, especially in those with a history of drug or alcohol abuse, therefore contraindicated
- see General Nursing points/Cautions for stimulants (p. 1486)

Patient teaching and advice

- to avoid sleep disturbances, doses should not be given in the evening
- (ADHD) first dose should be given on awakening, second dose should then be given 4–6 hours later
- female patients of childbearing potential should be counselled to use adequate and reliable contraception during therapy to avoid pregnancy occurring
- see General Patient teaching and advice for stimulants (p. 1487)

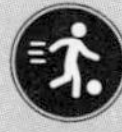

banned in sport

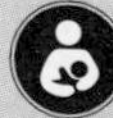

not recommended during pregnancy or breastfeeding. If used during pregnancy, increased risk of premature delivery, low birth weight and infants may experience withdrawal symptoms after birth including agitation and lassitude

tablet can be crushed and mixed with water or spoonful of yoghurt or apple puree

GUANFACINE (Intuniv)

Available forms

Tablets (modified-release): 1 mg, 2 mg, 3 mg, 4 mg

Action

- selective alpha-2A-adrenergic receptor agonist
- not a CNS stimulant
- modulates signalling in prefrontal cortex and basal ganglia through direct modification of synaptic noradrenaline (norepinephrine) transmission at the alpha-2-adrenergic receptors
- elimination about 18 hours

Use

- ADHD as monotherapy (when stimulants or atomoxetine are not suitable, not tolerated or have been ineffective) or as adjunctive therapy (with psychostimulants where the response has been suboptimal) (as part of total treatment program)

Dose

- initially 1 mg orally daily, increasing by increments of 1 mg at weekly intervals (daily maximum 4 mg if given with psychostimulants or 4–7 mg as monotherapy)

Adverse effects

- syncope, hypotension, orthostatic hypotension, bradycardia
- somnolence, sedation, nightmares
- enuresis
- (abrupt discontinuation) rebound effects (increased blood pressure and heart rate)
- see also General Adverse effects of stimulants (p. 1485)

Interactions

- caution if used with antihypertensive agents or other agents that lower blood pressure or heart rate
- caution if used with alcohol, sedatives, hypnotics, antipsychotics, phenothiazines, barbiturates or benzodiazepines as additive sedation may occur
- decreased serum levels may occur if given with rifampicin
- may increase serum levels of sodium valproate
- not recommended with grapefruit juice

Nursing points/Cautions

- before starting therapy, heart rate and blood pressure should be measured and repeated during dose increases and then regularly throughout therapy
- height, weight and BMI should be measured before starting, every 3 months for first 12 months, then 6-monthly (or more frequently during dose adjustment)
- therapy should be re-evaluated regularly to determine long-term usefulness
- if two or more consecutive doses are missed, re-titration starting at initial dose is recommended
- abrupt discontinuation is not recommended due to rebound effects including increased blood pressure and heart rate
- if discontinuation is required, daily dose should be tapered downwards in increments of 1 mg every 3–7 days to minimise risk of blood pressure increasing when therapy is stopped altogether. Blood pressure and pulse should be monitored when reducing or stopping therapy
- dose reduction may be required in those with liver or kidney impairment
- caution if used in those with history of hypotension, heart block, bradycardia and other cardiac conditions including arrhythmia, sick sinus syndrome, ischaemic heart disease, congestive heart failure or congenital long QT syndrome
- caution if used in those with history of syncope or condition which might predispose to syncope (e.g. hypotension, orthostatic hypotension, dehydration)
- caution if used in those with gastrointestinal illnesses that lead to vomiting because inability to take medication may result in rebound effects
- not recommended in those under 6 years
- see also General Nursing points/Cautions for stimulants (p. 1486)

Patient teaching and advice

- advise patient/parent/carer that medication should not be given with high-fat meal, nor tablets chewed, crushed or broken
- patient/parent/carer should be advised to avoid becoming dehydrated or overheated
- warn patient/parent/carer against abrupt discontinuation of medication to avoid rebound effect
- advise patient/parent/carer to avoid grapefruit juice during therapy

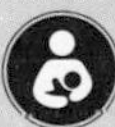
should only be used during pregnancy and breastfeeding if benefits outweigh risks

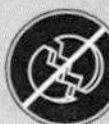
tablets should not be chewed, crushed or broken

LISDEXAMFETAMINE DIMESILATE (Vyvanse)

Available forms

Capsules: 20 mg, 30 mg, 40 mg, 50 mg, 60 mg, 70 mg

Action

- inactive prodrug
- rapidly absorbed and hydrolysed in the blood to dexamfetamine (dexamphetamine)
- non-catecholamine sympathomimetic amine with CNS-stimulant activity thought to be due to blocking noradrenaline (norepinephrine) and dopamine reuptake
- short half-life (less than 1 hour)

Use

- treatment of ADHD as part of total treatment program
- binge eating disorder (BED) where non-pharmacological therapy is unavailable or unsuccessful

Dose

- (ADHD) initially 30 mg orally in the morning, increasing by 20 mg at weekly intervals if needed (daily maximum 70 mg) **OR**
- (BED) initially 30 mg orally in the morning, increasing to 50–70 mg

Adverse effects

- see General Adverse effects of stimulants (p. 1485)
- blurred vision, accommodation difficulty
- teeth grinding at night (bruxism)
- fever
- abuse, dependence

Interactions

- contraindicated with or within 14 days of MAOIs
- stimulant effects may be blocked by haloperidol, lithium and chlorpromazine
- may potentiate analgesic actions of opioid analgesics
- urinary acidifiers (e.g. ascorbic acid) increase excretion, decreasing serum levels
- urinary alkalinisers (e.g. sodium bicarbonate) decrease excretion, increasing serum levels
- may increase serum levels of guanfacine
- may decrease effect of antihypertensive agents
- caution if used with SSRIs, SNRIs or other serotonergic agents due to risk of serotonin syndrome
- may interfere with estimation of urinary steroid test

Nursing points/Cautions

- (ADHD) therapy should be reviewed on a yearly basis
- (BED) should be prescribed for shortest amount of time and reassessed for effectiveness after 12 weeks
- under same control as drugs of addiction (S8) (Drugs, Poisons and Controlled Substances Regulations)
- limited, by law, to the above uses in most Australian states and territories. Requires special authority
- caution if used in those with kidney insufficiency. Maximum daily dose should not exceed 50 mg if glomerular filtration rate is between 15 and 30 mL/min
- not recommended in children under 6 years or adults over 55 years
- contraindicated in those with severe depression, anorexia nervosa, psychotic symptoms or suicidal tendencies
- see General Nursing points/Cautions for stimulants (p. 1486)

Patient teaching and advice

- see General Patient teaching and advice for stimulants (p. 1487)
- advise patient/carer that capsule should be swallowed whole or can be opened and contents mixed in a glass of water. The mixture should be stirred to ensure mixing and drunk immediately (not stored)
- female patients of childbearing potential should be counselled to use effective and reliable contraception during therapy

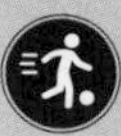

banned in sport

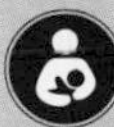

not recommended during pregnancy or breastfeeding. If used during pregnancy, increased risk of premature delivery, low birth weight and infants may experience withdrawal symptoms after birth including agitation and lassitude

capsule can be opened and given with spoonful of yoghurt or apple puree

METHYLPHENIDATE HYDROCHLORIDE (Artige, Concerta Extended-Release Tablets, Ritalin 10, Ritalin LA)

Available forms

Tablets: 10 mg; Tablets (extended release): 18 mg, 27 mg, 36 mg, 54 mg; Capsules (modified release): 10 mg, 20 mg, 30 mg, 40 mg

Action

- sympathomimetic agent that stimulates the CNS by inhibiting dopamine and noradrenaline (norepinephrine) uptake, elevating mood and improving the powers of judgement and concentration
- half-life 3.5 hours

Use

- ADHD as part of total treatment program
- narcolepsy

Dose

- (ADHD, children > 6 years, adolescents) initially 5 mg orally daily 1–2 times daily (breakfast and lunch) increasing at 5–10 mg increments at weekly intervals if needed (daily maximum 60 mg) (immediate-release tablets) **OR**
- (ADHD, children > 6 years, adolescents) initially 18 mg orally daily, then increasing at 9 mg increments at weekly intervals to 36 mg, then increasing at 18 mg increments at weekly intervals if needed (daily maximum 54 mg) (extended-release tablets) **OR**
- (ADHD, children > 6 years, adolescents) initially 10 mg orally daily, increasing at 10 mg increments at weekly intervals if needed (daily maximum 60 mg) (modified-release capsules) **OR**
- (ADHD, adults) 10–60 mg orally daily in 2–3 divided doses (immediate-release tablets) **OR**
- (ADHD, adults) initially 18–36 mg orally daily, increasing at 18 mg increments at weekly intervals if needed (daily maximum 72 mg) (extended-release tablets) **OR**
- (ADHD, adults) initially 20 mg orally daily, increasing at 20 mg increments at weekly intervals if needed (daily maximum 80 mg) (modified-release capsules) **OR**
- (narcolepsy, adults) 20–60 mg orally daily in 2–3 divided doses (daily maximum 60 mg) (immediate-release tablets)

Adverse effects

- fever
- vertigo
- arthralgia, muscle twitching, myalgia
- tachycardia, palpitations
- teeth grinding at night (bruxism)
- dyskinesia, paraesthesia, tremor
- (rare) priapism
- tolerance, dependence, potential for abuse
- (rare) leucopenia, thrombocytopenia, anaemia
- see General Adverse effects of stimulants (p. 1485)

Interactions

- contraindicated with or within 2 weeks of MAOIs

- not recommended on same day as halogenated anaesthetics due to sudden increase in blood pressure
- may decrease effects of antihypertensive agents
- may enhance effects of phenytoin, primidone, phenobarbital (phenobarbitone) and TCAs
- may enhance effects of warfarin, therefore INR should be closely monitored, especially when starting and stopping therapy
- not recommended with SSRIs, SNRIs or other serotonergic agents due to risk of serotonin syndrome
- not recommended with antipsychotic agents
- alcohol may increase CNS effects and is therefore not recommended
- not recommended with clonidine or other alpha agonists
- may cause false positive on laboratory test for amphetamine, particularly immunoassay screening tests

Nursing points/Cautions

- see General Nursing points/Cautions for stimulants (p. 1486)
- FBC, differential and platelet counts should be monitored regularly during prolonged therapy
- has possibility for abuse, tolerance and habit formation
- under same control as drugs of addiction (S8) (Drugs, Poisons and Controlled Substances Regulations)
- limited, by law, to the listed uses in most Australian states and territories. Requires special authority
- drug should be discontinued if there is no improvement after 1 month of stable dosage
- single doses > 20 mg should be avoided because of adverse effects
- should be stopped on day of surgery
- when patient is converting from immediate-release formulation to extended- or modified-release formulation, follow manufacturer's conversion table
- (modified-release capsules) contain both immediate-release and extended/delayed release beads
- (extended release tablets) not recommended in those with pre-existing GI narrowing, dysphagia or significant swallowing difficulties
- not recommended in children under 6 years of age
- not recommended for prevention or treatment of normal fatigue states
- contraindicated in those with severe depression, anorexia nervosa, psychotic symptoms or suicidal tendencies

Patient teaching and advice

- see General Patient teaching and advice for stimulants (p. 1487)
- if using 10 mg tablets and sleeplessness is a problem, patient should be advised to take last dose before 6 pm
- advise patient that extended-release tablets should be swallowed whole, not chewed, crushed or divided. Patient should also be warned that tablet shell may appear in their stools
- patient should be advised that modified-release capsules should be swallowed whole. However, contents may be sprinkled on cold soft food (e.g. apple sauce) and eaten unchewed. Uneaten food containing capsule contents should not be stored
- instruct male patient/carer to immediately seek medical attention if prolonged and painful erection occurs as this is a medical emergency

banned in sport

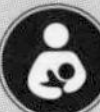

not recommended during pregnancy or breastfeeding unless benefits outweigh risks

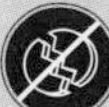

plain tablet (10 mg) can be dispersed in water or crushed and mixed with spoonful of yoghurt or apple puree. Ritalin LA capsules can be opened and beads mixed with cold apple puree. Beads must not be chewed or mixed with warm food

MODAFINIL (Modafin, Modavigil)

Available form

Tablets: 100 mg

Action

- non-amphetamine that promotes wakefulness by an unknown action that is different to that of the sympathomimetic amines but thought to involve histaminergic systems
- no effect on appetite, behaviour, nocturnal sleep or autonomic nervous system
- half-life 10–12 hours
- clearance delayed in the elderly

Use

- narcolepsy
- obstructive sleep apnoea/hypopnoea syndrome (OSAHS) with continuous positive airway pressure (CPAP) (adjunct)
- treatment of excessive sleepiness associated with moderate-to-severe chronic shiftwork sleep disorder (SWSD)

Dose

- (narcolepsy) 200–400 mg orally daily as single dose (morning) or divided doses (morning and noon) **OR**
- (OSAHS) 200–400 mg orally daily as single dose (morning) or divided doses (morning and noon) (with CPAP) **OR**
- (SWSD) initially 200 mg daily, 1 hour before starting shiftwork

Adverse effects

- see General Adverse effects of stimulants (p. 1485)
- neck rigidity
- dependence, euphoria, abuse potential
- (rare) paraesthesia
- (rare, high dose) serious skin reactions, multi-organ hypersensitivity reaction, serious rash

Interactions

- absorption may be delayed if given with methylphenidate
- caution if used with MAOIs
- caution if used with carbamazepine, phenobarbital (phenobarbitone), rifampicin and itraconazole as decreased serum modafinil levels may occur
- may increase serum level of diazepam, phenytoin, propranolol, TCAs and SSRIs
- may decrease serum level of oral contraceptives, triazolam, ciclosporin and theophylline
- INR should be closely monitored if given with warfarin, especially when starting or stopping therapy or if adjusting dose
- if given with phenytoin, serum level of phenytoin should be closely monitored to prevent toxicity

Nursing points/Cautions

- patients with obstructive sleep apnoea should be fully investigated by experienced doctor with access to sleep laboratory diagnostic facilities before starting therapy
- ECG monitoring is recommended before starting therapy
- not recommended in those under 18 years
- caution if used in those with a psychiatric history (including anxiety), history of drug/stimulant abuse or liver dysfunction
- see General Nursing points/Cautions for stimulants (p. 1486)

Patient teaching and advice

- ensure patient has an understanding of good sleep hygiene principles, such as limiting alcohol and caffeine intake before bedtime, regular bed and waking time and comfortable sleeping environment (no TV or electronics, cool room temperature)

- patient should be advised to report any rash, skin blistering, fever or hives immediately
- instruct patient to swallow tablets whole with glass of water
- women of childbearing potential who use oral contraceptives should be warned that their effectiveness may be impaired, and therefore an additional form of contraception is recommended to prevent pregnancy from occurring. Contraception should be continued for 4 weeks after discontinuing therapy
- see General Patient teaching and advice for stimulants (p. 1487)

banned in sport

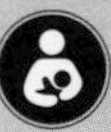

contraindicated during pregnancy

not recommended during breastfeeding

tablet can be crushed and mixed with water or spoonful of yoghurt or apple puree

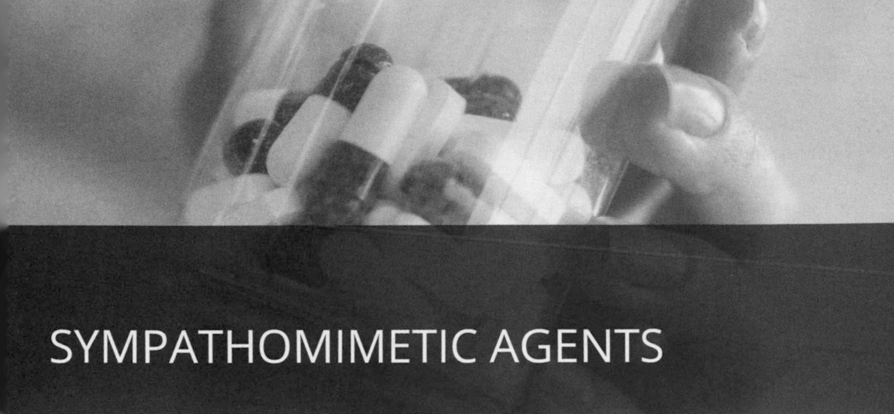

SYMPATHOMIMETIC AGENTS

The autonomic nervous system is divided into the sympathetic and parasympathetic nervous systems. The sympathetic nervous system is responsible for the basic human 'fight or flight' mechanism (e.g. increased HR and respiration, dilated pupils, increased blood glucose levels), which enables a person to be ready to deal with any oncoming stressor.

The main transmitter substance of the sympathetic nervous system is noradrenaline (norepinephrine); however, adrenaline (epinephrine) is also released from the adrenal cortex in times of stress and produces the same effects. Noradrenaline (norepinephrine) acts on postsynaptic receptors (adrenoceptors), which can be divided into alpha (α) and beta (β). Alpha adrenoceptors can be further subdivided into α_{1A}, α_{1B}, α_{1D}, α_{2A}, α_{2B} and α_{2C}, while beta adrenoceptors are subdivided into β1 (found in the heart), β2 (found in smooth muscle of bronchioles, arteries and skeletal muscle blood vessels) and β3 (found in plasma membrane of adipocytes and mediate lipolysis; also found in brain, heart, prostate, urinary bladder detrusor and GI tract) (Bryant et al 2019).

Sympathomimetic (adrenergic) agents include naturally occurring catecholamines (adrenaline (epinephrine), noradrenaline (norepinephrine) and dopamine) and drugs that mimic the effects of sympathetic nerve stimulation. Direct-acting agents stimulate the adrenergic receptors, whereas indirect-acting agents release stored noradrenaline (norepinephrine) from nerve endings, block its uptake from nerve terminals or block monoamine oxidase (MAO) or catechol-O-methyltransferase (COMT) enzymes which metabolise the catecholamines (Bryant et al 2019).

General Interactions of sympathomimetic agents

- contraindicated with halogenated general anaesthetics because they may provoke ventricular arrhythmias
- not recommended with agents that sensitise the heart to arrhythmias, such as digoxin. If given together, ECG monitoring is recommended
- not recommended with MAOIs, TCAs, some antihistamines, thyroid hormones or cocaine as sudden hypertension, tachycardia, arrhythmias and/or hyperpyrexia may occur because of potentiated effect
- additive effect may occur if given with other sympathomimetic agents

and therefore are not recommended together
- actions may be antagonised if given with rapidly acting vasodilating agents
- increased serum levels may occur if given with entacapone, increasing risk of arrhythmias
- severe hypertension may occur if given with oxytocin
- hypotension and cardiac acceleration may occur if given with alpha-adrenoceptor blocking agents (e.g. prazosin)
- severe hypertension and reflex bradycardia (and possibly heart block) may occur if given with non-specific beta-adrenoceptor blocking agents (e.g. propranolol)
- increased hypokalaemia may occur if given with other agents known to deplete potassium (e.g. diuretics, corticosteroids, aminophylline, theophylline)
- may affect control of blood glucose levels in those with diabetes managed with hypoglycaemic agents, so careful monitoring is required
- caution if used with antihypertensive agents as severe hypertension may occur

General Nursing points/Cautions for sympathomimetic agents

- any hypovolaemia, hypercapnia, hypoxia or acidosis should be corrected before starting therapy or at the same time
- frequently monitor BP, arterial blood gases, heart rate and rhythm (ECG), arterial pressure, cardiac output, CVP (central venous pressure) or pulmonary wedge pressure, mental status, skin temperature and urinary output
- serum potassium should be monitored frequently throughout therapy
- if there is a disproportionate increase in diastolic BP, the infusion rate should be slowed or infusion stopped and the patient carefully observed (unless this is the desired effect)
- shock state may continue if vasopressor amines are given for a prolonged period, because resultant vasoconstriction may prevent adequate expansion of circulating volume
- burette, infusion pump or drip regulator should be used to deliver the solution
- monitor infusion for rate and free flow to avoid extravasation
- should be given into large blood vessels and if infiltration or thrombosis occurs at IV site, infusion should be stopped immediately
- administer alone
- reduce rate gradually before discontinuing infusion to avoid rebound hypotension
- contraindicated in those with sulfite/metasulfite allergy, which may evoke allergic reaction in susceptible individuals, including those with asthma (adrenaline (epinephrine), dobutamine, dopamine, isoprenaline, metaraminol, phenylephrine)

ADRENALINE (EPINEPHRINE) (Adrenaline Aguettant, Adrenaline Jr Mylan, Adrenaline-Link Injection BP, Adrenaline Mylan, Emerade, Epipen, Epipen Jr, Min-I-Jet Adrenaline)

Available forms

Autoinjector: 150 microgram/0.3 mL, 300 microgram/0.3 mL; Ampoules: 0.1 mg/mL, 1 mg/mL, 1 mg/10 mL; Prefilled syringe: 0.1 mg/mL, 1 mg/10 mL

Action

- direct-acting sympathomimetic agent that stimulates both alpha- and beta-adrenoceptors
- cardiac stimulant causing increased heart rate, output, myocardial contractility and BP
- relaxes bronchial smooth muscle, causing bronchodilation
- constricts blood vessels in skin and mucous membranes
- relaxes gastrointestinal smooth muscle
- increases secretion of renin
- stimulates lipolysis, increasing free fatty acids in blood
- inhibits insulin secretion, increases glycogenolysis, resulting in hyperglycaemia
- inhibits uterine contraction
- decreases desire to void, which can lead to urinary retention
- crosses placenta but not blood–brain barrier
- rapid onset (IV)
- half-life about 2 minutes

Use

- adjunct in treatment of cardiac arrest
- emergency management of severe anaphylactic reactions and severe acute reactions to allergens (first-line management)
- relief of respiratory distress due to bronchospasm, angioedema, croup, mucosa and upper airway obstruction (e.g. laryngeal oedema)
- provide inotropic support in acute chronic heart failure and septic shock
- adjunct to local anaesthetic, prolonging action by delaying absorption
- as a haemostatic agent, applied topically to control superficial bleeding from arterioles and capillaries in skin, mucous membranes and other tissue
- in ocular surgery to control bleeding, relieve mucosal and conjunctival congestion, decrease intraocular pressure and produce mydriasis

Dose

Anaphylaxis

- 100–500 microgram (0.1–0.5 mL of 1 : 1000 solution) SC or IM (SC dose may be repeated at 20-minute to 4-hour intervals if required) **OR**
- (severe anaphylaxis) 100–250 microgram (1–2.5 mL of 1 : 10,000 solution) IV slowly over 10 minutes **OR**
- 500 microgram SC or IM initially, then 25–50 microgram (0.25–0.5 mL of 1 : 10,000 solution) IV every 5–15 minutes until relief **OR**
- 150–300 microgram IM, which may be repeated at 5–15-minute intervals if symptoms have not subsided or recur (autoinjector)

Cardiopulmonary resuscitation (in absence of ventricular fibrillation)

- 1 mg (10 mL of 1 : 10,000 solution) IV, repeated every 3–5 minutes during cardiopulmonary resuscitation. Line should be flushed with 20 mL of sodium chloride 0.9% to ensure that patient receives the full dose

Adverse effects

- tachycardia, palpitations, ectopic beats, ventricular fibrillation, arrhythmias, severe hypertension, anginal pain, non-specific chest pain, vasodilation with hypotension, hypertension with reflex bradycardia
- anxiety, fear, restlessness, irritability, impaired memory, psychosis, hallucinations, confusion, nervousness, disorientation, exacerbation of psychiatric disorders
- pallor, sweating, flushing of face and skin
- headache, weakness, dizziness, insomnia
- nausea, vomiting, anorexia, hypersalivation
- peripheral vasoconstriction, coldness of extremities, gangrene of the

feet if there is pre-existing peripheral vascular disease
- muscle tremor
- hypokalaemia, hyperglycaemia
- difficulty with micturition, urinary retention
- increased rigidity and tremor (if given to those with Parkinson's disease)
- (children) syncope
- (high doses) ventricular arrhythmias, severe hypertension, cerebral haemorrhage, pulmonary oedema
- (repeated injections) skin necrosis
- (accidental IV injection) convulsions, metabolic acidosis, renal failure with anuria
- (prolonged use, overdose) severe metabolic acidosis

Interactions

- see General Interactions of sympathomimetic agents (p. 1499)

Nursing points/Cautions

- see General Nursing points/Cautions for sympathomimetic agents (p. 1500)
- select correct type of solution and note concentration, dose and route carefully
- 1 : 1000 solution means 1 g in 1000 mL or 1 mg in 1 mL
- 1 : 10,000 solution means 1 g in 10,000 mL or 0.1 mg in 1 mL
- discard any discoloured (brown) or precipitated solutions
- if given SC, aspirate to ensure needle is not in a vein and inject very slowly. If SC formulation is given IV, hypertension may occur
- if giving injection IM, do NOT give into the buttocks
- SC route is not recommended due to variable absorption
- intracardiac administration is no longer recommended
- rotate injection sites to avoid local ischaemic necrosis
- if given IV, monitor cardiac rate and BP, especially in the first 5 minutes
- avoid inter-arterial administration as gangrene may occur from vasoconstriction of vessel
- adrenaline (epinephrine) is incompatible with alkaline solutions (e.g. sodium bicarbonate), metals (e.g. copper, iron, zinc, silver) and with a large number of drugs, and is therefore best infused alone
- (autoinjector) junior formulation is recommended in children weighing 15–30 kg
- contains sodium metabisulfite, which may cause allergic reactions in those with hypersensitivity
- extreme caution if used in the elderly, or those with cardiovascular disease, hypertension, cerebrovascular insufficiency, circulatory collapse (induced by phenothiazines), chronic lung disease, angina, prostatic hypertrophy, urinary retention, Parkinson's disease, asthma/emphysema (with degenerative heart disease) or psychoneurosis
- contraindicated with local anaesthetics for use in infiltration injection for digits, ears, nose, penis or scrotum, owing to risk of ischaemic tissue necrosis
- contraindicated in those with hypersensitivity to other sympathomimetic agents, shock (except anaphylaxis), hypertension, ischaemic heart disease, arrhythmias, cardiac dilation, coronary insufficiency, cerebral arteriosclerosis, narrow-angle glaucoma, diabetes mellitus, organic brain damage, hyperthyroidism, pheochromocytoma, thyrotoxicosis or in obstetrics (where maternal BP > 130/80 mmHg)

Patient teaching and advice

- warn patient against driving or operating machinery due to dizziness, weakness and tremor

- ensure patient/family member has been instructed in correct use of autoinjector, including:
  - carry autoinjector at all times
  - it is important to seek medical emergency care/assistance immediately
  - check expiry date and colour of solution before use (cloudy or brown solutions should not be used)
  - injection technique into outer thigh only (through clothing if necessary) (training autoinjector is available to assist with education, demonstration and practising technique)
  - record time injection was given
  - once-only use per autoinjector (however, more than one injection may be required)
  - storage conditions (not in fridge, protect from light and heat)
  - safe disposal
  - if accidental injection of other sites (e.g. hands, feet, nose, ears, genitalia) occurs, seek medical treatment immediately because of potential loss of blood supply to the area
- those with diabetes mellitus should be advised to monitor BGLs carefully after adrenaline (epinephrine) use as hyperglycaemia may occur

banned in sport

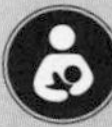

contraindicated during labour, because it may delay the second stage. Contraindicated when maternal BP is greater than 130/80 mmHg

excreted in breastmilk and therefore not recommended during breastfeeding

Note

- contained in Articadent Dental with Adrenaline, Bupivacaine with Adrenaline, Bupivadren w/v with Adrenaline, Deltazine, Lignospan Special, Marcain with Adrenaline (epinephrine), Scandonest 2% Special, Septanest, Ubistesin, Ubistesin Forte, Xylocaine (with Adrenaline (epinephrine)), 2% Xylocaine Dental with Adrenaline (epinephrine) 1 : 80,000

DOBUTAMINE HYDROCHLORIDE (DBL Dobutamine Hydrochloride Injection, Dobutamine Concentrated Solution, Dobutrex)

Available forms

Vial: 250 mg; Ampoules: 250 mg/20 mL

Action

- synthetic catecholamine that acts directly on beta1-adrenoceptors, resulting in potent inotropic effects and mild vasodilatory effects
- little increase in heart rate or peripheral resistance (and therefore BP)
- does not cause release of noradrenaline (norepinephrine)
- no effect on dopamine receptors
- does not cause renal vasodilation
- onset 1–2 minutes, peak effect within 10 minutes, duration of action up to 10 minutes, plasma half-life < 3 minutes

Use

- short-term treatment of cardiac failure secondary to acute myocardial infarction or cardiac surgery

Dose

- 2.5–10 microgram/kg/minute IV infusion (rate and duration of therapy adjusted according to patient response)

Adverse effects

- marked increased heart rate, increased systolic BP, ventricular ectopic beats, hypotension (occasionally), angina, palpitations, chest pain (non-specific)

- shortness of breath
- nausea
- headache
- mild decrease in serum potassium and rarely, hypokalaemia
- (hypersensitivity) rash, bronchospasm, fever, eosinophilia
- (IV site) phlebitis, necrosis (rare)
- (rare) cardiac rupture (during dobutamine stress testing)

Interactions

- when given with sodium nitroprusside or glyceryl trinitrate, may increase cardiac output and lower pulmonary wedge pressure
- contraindicated with halogenated general anaesthetics because they may provoke ventricular arrhythmias

Nursing points/Cautions

- see General Nursing points/Cautions for sympathomimetic agents (p. 1500)
- loading dose/bolus not recommended
- available as a powder or solution
- solution should be diluted to 50 mL with either glucose 5% or sodium chloride 0.9% before IV administration
- reconstitute powder with 10 mL water for injections (add another 10 mL if not completely dissolved) then add to at least 50 mL glucose 5%, Ringer's solution or sodium lactate. Sodium chloride 0.9% should not be used to reconstitute powder
- incompatible with sodium bicarbonate or any other strongly alkaline solution
- pink discolouration does not indicate loss of potency
- if patient has atrial fibrillation with rapid ventricular response, digitalisation is recommended before starting therapy
- solution contains sodium metabisulfite, which may cause allergic reactions in those with hypersensitivity
- caution if used in those with pre-existing hypertension, atrial flutter/fibrillation, ventricular ectopics or with any risk factors for cardiac rupture (e.g. within 4–12 days of myocardial infarction)
- contraindicated in those with idiopathic hypertrophic subaortic stenosis

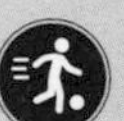

banned in sport

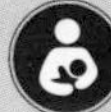

not used during pregnancy or breastfeeding unless expected benefit outweighs any potential risk

DOPAMINE HYDROCHLORIDE (DBL Sterile Dopamine Concentrate)

Available form

Ampoules: 200 mg/5 mL

Action

- both direct and indirect sympathomimetic effects
- stimulates alpha- and beta-adrenergic and dopamine receptors (depending on dose)
  - (0.5–2 microgram/kg/minute) dopaminergic (D_1) receptors are selectively activated, leading to renal and mesenteric vasodilation resulting in increased renal blood flow and urine output
  - (2–10 microgram/kg/minute) β1-receptors are activated, increasing cardiac output and systolic BP
  - (> 10 microgram/kg/minute) α receptors are activated, resulting in peripheral vasoconstriction, increases in both systolic and diastolic BP and decreased urine flow (because of decreased renal blood flow)

- inotropic effect on the heart increases cardiac output and systolic BP
- physiological precursor of noradrenaline (norepinephrine) and adrenaline (epinephrine)
- physiological neurotransmitter, mainly in the brain; however, does not cross blood–brain barrier when given systemically
- rapid onset of action (within 5 minutes), duration 5–10 minutes, half-life 2 minutes

Use
- correction of haemodynamic imbalance in acute hypotension/shock (e.g. acute myocardial infarction, endotoxic shock, trauma, renal failure)
- adjunct after open-heart surgery (when there is persistent hypotension despite correction of hypovolaemia)
- chronic cardiac decompensation in severely refractory congestive cardiac failure (short-term management)

Dose
- initially 2–5 microgram/kg/minute IV, increasing by 5–10 microgram/kg/minute increments, up to 50 microgram/kg/minute as required **OR**
- (severe refractory cardiac failure) 0.5–2 microgram/kg/minute IV, increasing to 1–3 microgram/kg/minute as urine flow increases (maintenance) as required. Rate should be decreased if diastolic BP or HR increases

Adverse effects
- tachycardia, palpitations, ectopic beats, angina, hypotension, vasoconstriction
- nausea, vomiting
- headache
- dyspnoea
- gangrene of feet (in pre-existing peripheral vascular disease or high doses)
- (rare) ventricular arrhythmias
- (IV site extravasation) skin/tissue necrosis

Interactions
- contraindicated with ergot alkaloids or methysergide because of increased vasoconstriction, resulting in ischaemia and gangrene
- bradycardia, hypotension and possible cardiac arrest may occur if given with phenytoin (IV)
- hypotension may occur if given with calcium-channel blockers, nitroprusside or glyceryl trinitrate
- if given with or within 3 weeks of MAOIs, dopamine dose should be reduced to 1/10th normal dose
- may interfere with urine tests for amino acids, catecholamines, uric acid or urobilinogen
- see General Interactions of sympathomimetic agents (p. 1499)

Nursing points/Cautions
- see General Nursing points/Cautions for sympathomimetic agents (p. 1500)
- frequently check conscious state and nail bed capillary filling
- note changes in temperature or colour of extremities if there is pre-existing peripheral vascular disease
- urine output should be carefully monitored during therapy and if it decreases without any associated hypotension, dose reduction is recommended
- must be diluted before administration; 200 mg may be added to 250 mL of the recommended infusion solution to make a concentration of 800 microgram/mL or to 500 mL for a concentration of 400 microgram/mL
- to avoid tissue necrosis, administer into a large vein high up in a limb, preferably the arm
- incompatible with amphotericin B (amphotericin) and ampicillin and alkaline solutions such as sodium bicarbonate
- hypotension may occur when weaning from dopamine and this may require an increase in blood volume

or changing to another pressor agent while slowly decreasing dose
- have phentolamine available as an antidote for peripheral ischaemia resulting from extravasation (phentolamine 5–10 mg in sodium chloride 0.9%; infiltrate area with 10–15 mL)
- contains sodium metabisulfite, which can cause allergic reactions in those with hypersensitivity
- caution if used in those with pulmonary hypertension as condition may be worsened with therapy
- caution if given to those with cardiac ischaemia or pre-existing peripheral vascular disease (including atherosclerosis, frostbite and Raynaud's disease) as these people may be at greater risk of peripheral ischaemia and gangrene
- contraindicated in those with pheochromocytoma, atrial/ventricular arrhythmias or hyperthyroidism

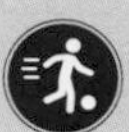
banned in sport

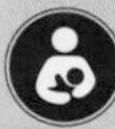
not used during pregnancy or breastfeeding unless expected benefit outweighs any potential risk

EPHEDRINE HYDROCHLORIDE (Ephedrine Hydrochloride Solution for Injection)

EPHEDRINE SULFATE (DBL Ephedrine Sulfate Injection)

Available form
Ampoules: 30 mg/mL

Action
- direct and indirect sympathomimetic effects on both alpha- and beta-adrenoceptors
- more prolonged, but less potent than adrenaline (epinephrine)
- CNS and respiratory centre stimulant
- increases cardiac output and peripheral vasoconstriction increasing systolic and diastolic BP
- causes bronchodilation
- reduces intestinal tone and motility
- relaxes bladder wall, contracts sphincter muscle and relaxes detrusor muscle
- usually reduces activity of the uterus
- onset 10–20 minutes (IM) or 3–5 minutes (IV) duration 1 hour (IM) or 10–15 minutes (IV)
- half-life 3–6 hours (increased in acidic urine)

Use
- hypotension associated with spinal anaesthesia
- shock unresponsive to fluid replacement
- treatment of bronchospasm in asthma (although more selective agents are now available)

Dose
- (hypotension secondary to spinal anaesthetic) 3–7.5 mg by slow IV, repeated if needed every 3–4 minutes (maximum 30 mg) (Ephedrine Hydrochloride) **OR**
- (pressor) 10–50 mg IM or SC, or 10–25 mg slow IV, repeated 5–10 minutes until desired response (maximum daily dose 150 mg) (Ephedrine Sulfate) **OR**
- (bronchospasm) 12.5–25 mg IM, SC or slow IV, then determined by response (maximum daily dose 150 mg) (Ephedrine Sulfate)

Adverse effects
- pallor, fever, sweating
- headache, insomnia
- angina, palpitations, bradycardia, tachycardia, hypertension, hypotension, chest pain
- nausea, vomiting, epigastric distress, increased salivation
- shortness of breath, dyspnoea
- dry mouth, nose, throat
- urinary retention, dysuria

- nervousness, anxiety, restlessness, fear, mood changes, irritability, trembling
- hyperglycaemia, hypokalaemia
- (high dose) dizziness, lightheadedness, vertigo, confusion, delirium, euphoria
- (long-term use) physical addiction
- (IV) necrosis (if extravasation occurs)

Interactions

- see General Interactions of sympathomimetic agents (p. 1499)
- contraindicated with or within 2 weeks of MAOIs
- contraindicated with linezolid
- increased risk of paroxysmal hypertension and arrhythmia if given with venlafaxine or sibutramine
- cardiac and bronchodilator effects may be reduced if given with beta-adrenergic blocking agents
- may increase serum levels of phenytoin, primidone and phenobarbital (phenobarbitone) if given together
- increased risk of headache, palpitations and hypertension if given with moclobemide
- decreased vasopressor effects may occur if given with methyldopa sesquihydrate
- increased effect may occur if pretreated with clonidine
- elimination may be reduced if given with urinary alkalinisers (e.g. acetazolamide, sodium bicarbonate and sodium citrate)
- increased risk of adverse effects of both agents if given with theophylline
- vasopressor effects may be increased by atropine sulfate monohydrate, oxytocin and ergot alkaloids
- increased risk of peripheral vascular ischaemia and gangrene if given with oxytocin or ergot alkaloids

Nursing points/Cautions

- see General Nursing points/Cautions for sympathomimetic agents (p. 1500)
- any hypoxia, hypercapnia and acidosis should be corrected before starting therapy
- IV route is recommended for those in shock to ensure adequate absorption
- avoid extravasation
- (IV, ephedrine hydrochloride) dilute 1 mL with 10 mL sodium chloride to give a concentration of 2.5 mg/mL
- (IV, ephedrine hydrochloride) if maximum dose of 30 mg does not produce required effect, another therapeutic agent should be considered
- incompatible with phenobarbital (phenobarbitone), thiopentone and hydrocortisone
- caution if used in those with prostatic hypertrophy, diabetes mellitus, cardiovascular disease (e.g. angina, arrhythmias or cardiac insufficiency) or myocardial infarction (as ischaemia may be increased)
- extreme caution (if given at all) to those with hyperthyroidism or hypertension due to increased of adverse effects
- contraindicated in those with closed-angle glaucoma, pheochromocytoma, asymmetric septal hypertrophy, tachyarrhythmias, ventricular fibrillation or psychoneurosis

Patient teaching and advice

- patient with diabetes mellitus should be warned that blood glucose levels may become unstable during therapy

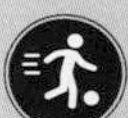

banned in some sports, while permitted in other sports subject to restrictions

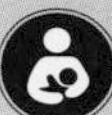

may increase fetal heart rate if used during delivery. Not recommended if maternal BP is greater than 130/80 mmHg

not recommended during breastfeeding

Note

- also available as nasal instillation (Ephedrine Nasal Instillation) for relief of nasal congestion

ISOPRENALINE HYDROCHLORIDE (known as isoproterenol in USA) (Isuprel)

Available forms

Ampoules: 200 microgram/mL; 1000 microgram/5 mL

Action

- non-selective synthetic catecholamine structurally related to adrenaline (epinephrine), but acts almost exclusively on beta-adrenergic receptors
- increased cardiac output because of positive inotropic and chronotropic actions, increases venous return
- increased peripheral vasodilation resulting in lower diastolic BP in normal individuals
- relaxes bronchial smooth muscle causing bronchodilation, as well as relaxation of skeletal muscle, GI tract and splanchnic bed
- stimulates insulin release
- metabolite has weak beta-adrenergic blocking activity
- half-life 2–3 minutes (IV) or up to 2 hours (SC)

Use

- mild or transient heart block (not requiring electric shock or pacemaker)
- cardiac arrest (until electric shock or pacemaker is available)
- serious heart block or Stokes–Adams attack (unless caused by ventricular tachycardia or fibrillation)
- bronchospasm during anaesthesia
- adjunct in management of cardiogenic, hypovolaemic and septic shock or congestive heart failure

Dose

- (bronchospasm during anaesthesia) 0.01–0.02 mg by IV bolus (diluted solution 0.2 mg in 10 mL of sodium chloride 0.9% or glucose 5%), repeated as necessary **OR**
- (shock, hypoperfusion) 1 mg (5 mL) in 500 mL glucose 5% by IV infusion at a rate of 0.5–5 microgram/minute **OR**
- (heart block, cardiac arrest, Stokes–Adams attack) initially 0.2 mg IM or SC, then 0.02–1 mg IM or 0.15–0.2 mg SC (undiluted solution) **OR**
- (heart block, cardiac arrest, Stokes–Adams attack) initially 0.02–0.06 mg by IV bolus, then 0.01–0.2 mg (diluted solution 0.2 mg in 10 mL of sodium chloride 0.9% or glucose 5%) **OR**
- (heart block, cardiac arrest, Stokes–Adams attack) 5 microgram/minute by IV infusion (diluted solution 2 mg in 500 mL glucose 5%) **OR**
- (heart block, cardiac arrest, Stokes–Adams attack) 0.02 mg by intracardiac injection (undiluted solution)

Adverse effects

- tachycardia, palpitations, angina, hypertension, hypotension, ventricular arrhythmias, Stokes–Adams attack, pulmonary oedema
- hot flashes, skin flushing, sweating
- mild tremor, weakness
- nervousness, restlessness, fear, tension
- headache, dizziness
- (rare) tinnitus, asthenia, light-headedness, nausea, vomiting

Interactions

- increased risk of cardiotoxicity if given with IV corticosteroids or IV aminophylline
- not recommended with chlorpromazine or MAOIs
- not recommended with adrenaline (epinephrine) or digoxin due to increased risk of cardiac arrhythmias (although may be given separately with adequate time interval separating agents)

Nursing points/Cautions

- see General Nursing points/Cautions for sympathomimetic agents (p. 1500)

- if time is not an essential factor, IM or SC administration is preferred
- if patient has pre-existing asthma, oxygen should be administered at the same time as IV infusion
- infusion rate is adjusted according to the heart rate, ECG, CVP, systemic BP, arterial blood gases and urine output (reduce infusion rate if adult heart rate exceeds 110 beats/minute or ventricular hyperexcitability is apparent on ECG). Cardiac enzyme (CPK MB) should be measured if ECG shows any signs of myocardial ischaemia
- caution if given to the elderly or those with coronary insufficiency, ischaemic heart disease, cardiogenic shock (due to coronary arterial occlusion or myocardial infarction), hypertension, diabetes mellitus or hyperthyroidism or if sensitive to other sympathomimetic agents
- contraindicated in those with digitalis-induced tachycardia/heart block, tachyarrhythmias, ventricular arrhythmias (requiring inotropes), recent myocardial infarction or angina

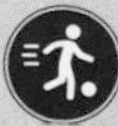
banned in sport

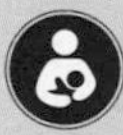
not used during pregnancy unless expected benefit outweighs any potential risk

caution if used during breastfeeding

METARAMINOL TARTRATE (Aramine, Metaraminol Solution for Injection)

Available forms
Ampoules: 3 mg/6 mL, 5 mg/mL, 10 mg/mL

Action
- direct and indirect sympathomimetic effects on both alpha- and beta-adrenoreceptors
- mainly alpha-adrenergic stimulant effects, with some beta effects, resulting in potent effects that increase systolic and diastolic BP and peripheral vasoconstriction
- increases coronary blood flow, slows heart rate
- less potent than noradrenaline (norepinephrine)
- effective within 1–2 minutes (IV), lasting 20–60 minutes

Use
- prevention or treatment of acute hypotension following spinal anaesthesia
- adjunct to treatment of hypotension associated with haemorrhage, septicaemia, reaction to medications, surgical complications or cardiogenic shock

Dose
- (adjunctive treatment of hypotension) 15–100 mg diluted in 500 mL of sodium chloride 0.9% or glucose 5% regulated by burette or microdrip with IV infusion rate adjusted to maintain BP at desired level **OR**
- (emergency treatment of severe shock) 0.5–5 mg IV bolus, followed by infusion as above

Adverse effects
- tachycardia, arrhythmias
- (IV site, rare) abscess formation, tissue necrosis, sloughing

Interactions
- contraindicated with halogenated hydrocarbon anaesthetics
- caution if used with digoxin as ectopic arrhythmias may occur
- effects may be potentiated by MAOIs and TCAs and therefore not recommended together

Nursing points/Cautions
- see General Nursing points/Cautions for sympathomimetic agents (p. 1500)

- monitor heart rate and systemic BP every 5 minutes until stabilised, then every 15 minutes during and for several hours after infusion is completed
- avoid excessive BP response
- allow at least 10 minutes to elapse between altering dosage
- IV bolus should only be used as life-saving measure
- response may be poor in those with shock and acidosis
- not used regularly in routine clinical practice
- caution if used in those with cirrhosis, heart or thyroid disease, hypertension or diabetes mellitus
- contains sodium metabisulfite, therefore is contraindicated in those with sulfite hypersensitivity

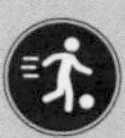

banned in sport

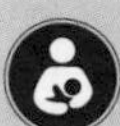

should only be used during pregnancy if benefits outweigh the potential risks to the fetus

caution if used during breastfeeding

NORADRENALINE (NOREPINEPHRINE) ACID TARTRATE (also called levarterenol in USA) (Levophed 1:1000, Noradrenaline Concentrate for Infusion, Noralin)

Available forms

Ampoules: 2 mg/2 mL, 4 mg/mL

Action

- direct-acting sympathomimetic agent with action on alpha- and beta-adrenoceptors
- dilates coronary arteries, increasing blood flow
- peripheral vasoconstriction resulting in increase in both systolic and diastolic BP
- no changes in heart rate or cardiac output
- physiological neurotransmitter released from post-ganglionic adrenergic nerve fibres when stimulated
- rapid onset of action, half-life 30 seconds to 3 minutes

Use

- treatment of acute hypotensive states when blood volume is adequate
- adjunct to cardiac arrest treatment (to restore and maintain adequate BP after effective cardiac arrest management measures)

Dose

- initially 8–12 microgram/minute IV, then adjusted to maintain the BP at the desired level, then 2–4 microgram/minute (maintenance)

Adverse effects

- arrhythmias, palpitations, reflex bradycardia, hypotension
- anxiety, transient headache
- respiratory distress
- (IV site) necrosis (if extravasation occurs)
- (rare) gangrene of extremities
- (overdose or in those who are hypersensitive) severe hypertension, violent headache, photophobia, stabbing retrosternal pain, pallor, intense sweating, vomiting

Interactions

- prolonged hypertension may result if given with MAOIs or TCAs and should be given with extreme caution if at all
- contraindicated with halogenated hydrocarbon general anaesthetics

Nursing points/Cautions

- see General Nursing points/Cautions for sympathomimetic agents (p. 1500)
- monitor conscious state, temperature and colour of extremities, urinary output and infusion site every 15 minutes (for any signs of blanching; IV should be re-sited if this occurs)

- monitor heart rate and BP every 2 minutes until stabilised at desired level, then every 5 minutes. Patient should not be left unattended
- preferably given via central venous catheter (CVC) to decrease risk of extravasation and necrosis
- must be diluted before use. Add 2 mg to 500 mL or 4 mg to 1000 mL of glucose 5% to make a concentration of 4 microgram/mL
- therapy should be continued until adequate BP and tissue perfusion can be maintained, then rate reduced gradually, avoiding abrupt withdrawal
- noradrenaline (norepinephrine) should not be added to whole blood, plasma or saline solutions
- should not be used if solution is brown
- incompatible with alkalis, barbiturates, chlorpheniramine, iron salts, nitrofurantoin, phenytoin, sodium bicarbonate or sodium iodide
- have phentolamine (5–10 mg in 10–15 mL of sodium chloride 0.9%) available if extravasation occurs
- increased risk of hypersensitivity reaction in those with hyperthyroidism
- contains sodium metabisulfite, which may cause allergic reaction in hypersensitivity individuals, therefore is not recommended
- not recommended for infusion via leg veins in those > 65 years
- contraindicated in those with hypotension (because of hypovolaemia) or mesenteric or peripheral vascular thrombosis (due to risk of increased ischaemia)

banned in sport

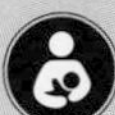

not recommended during pregnancy unless benefits outweigh risk

caution if used during breastfeeding

PHENYLEPHRINE HYDROCHLORIDE (Neo-Synephrine, Phenylephrine BNM)

Available forms

Ampoules: 10 mg/mL (1%), 0.5 mg/5 mL (0.01%)

Action

- synthetic sympathomimetic structurally related to adrenaline (epinephrine) and ephedrine
- vasoconstrictor, pressor
- slows heart rate and increases stroke output with no effect on rhythm
- main actions are on postsynaptic alpha-receptors
- little effects on coronary beta-receptors
- increases systolic and diastolic BP, marked reflex bradycardia
- constricts vascular beds, but coronary blood flow is increased
- constricts pulmonary vessels, increasing pulmonary arterial pressure
- more sustained action than adrenaline (epinephrine) (20 minutes (IV) or 50 minutes (SC))

Use

- maintain BP during spinal and inhalation anaesthesia
- vascular failure in shock, shock-like states or drug-induced hypotension
- overcome paroxysmal supraventricular tachycardia
- prolong spinal anaesthesia
- vasoconstrictor in regional anaesthesia
- mydriatic (see Eye, Ear, Nose and Throat agents, p. 1064)

Dose

- (mild/moderate hypotension) 2–5 mg SC or IM (initial dose not greater than 5 mg) **OR**
- (mild/moderate hypotension) 0.1–0.5 mg IV (initial dose not greater than 0.5 mg) increasing dose at 15-minute intervals if needed **OR**
- (severe hypotension and shock) 100–180 microgram/minute by IV

infusion (10 mg (of 1% solution) diluted in 500 mL glucose 5% or sodium chloride 0.9%) until BP is stabilised, then reduced to 40–60 microgram/minute **OR**

- (spinal anaesthesia – hypotension) 2–3 mg IM or SC given 3–4 minutes before spinal anaesthetic **OR**
- (hypotensive emergency during spinal anaesthesia) initially 0.2 mg IV, increasing dose by 0.1–0.2 mg if needed (maximum single dose 0.5 mg) **OR**
- (prolong spinal anaesthesia) 2–5 mg added to anaesthetic solution **OR**
- (vasoconstrictor for regional anaesthesia) optimal strength is 1 : 20,000 (add 1 mg (1% solution) phenylephrine to 20 mL local anaesthetic) **OR**
- (paroxysmal supraventricular tachycardia) initially up to 0.5 mg rapid IV, then increasing dose by not more than 0.1–0.2 mg of initial dose (depending on BP) (maximum dose 1 mg)

Adverse effects

- headache, excitability, restlessness
- reflex bradycardia
- (rare) arrhythmias

Interactions

- see General Interactions of sympathomimetic agents (p. 1499)

Nursing points/Cautions

- see General Nursing points/Cautions for sympathomimetic agents (p. 1500)
- can be given SC, IM, IV injection or IV infusion
- (Phenylephrine BNM) not recommended SC or IM
- (spinal anaesthesia prolongation) phenylephrine hydrochloride prolongs duration of motor block by up to 50% with no increase in adverse effects
- 5 mg IM will produce increased BP for 1–2 hours while 0.5 mg IV will produce an increase for 15 minutes
- extreme caution if used in the elderly or those with hyperthyroidism, bradycardia, partial heart block, myocardial disease or severe arteriosclerosis
- contraindicated in those with severe hypertension or ventricular tachycardia

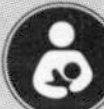

only used in pregnancy if potential benefits outweigh risks. May cause persistent hypertension if given with some oxytocic agents, which may result in cerebral vessel rupture post delivery

caution if used during breastfeeding

Note

- contained in CoPhenylcaine Forte with lidocaine (lignocaine) and in many cough and flu preparations and eye preparations (see Eye, Ear, Nose and Throat agents, p. 1067)

THYROID AND ANTITHYROID AGENTS

The thyroid gland is a highly vascular organ consisting of two connected lobes which have small parathyroid glands on the posterior surface. The thyroid gland produces two hormones, thyroxine sodium (T_4) (precursor) and liothyronine (T_3) (active hormone), which influence growth, development and metabolic processes (Jameson et al 2018c). Iodine is needed for the synthesis of both hormones and is generally acquired via the diet, with an adult requiring approximately 1 mg/week. Iodine can be found in foods such as dairy products, seafood, kelp, eggs, bread (since 2009, all breads made in Australia are made with iodised salt, except for organic bread), some vegetables (if grown in iodine-rich soil) and iodised salt (NHMRC, NZ MoH 2017). Over the past few decades, iodine intake levels have dropped and reasons are thought to include the increased consumption of processed food (manufacturers generally do not use iodised salt), less iodine in milk (treatment methods have changed), a reduction in iodine in soil, and less use of salt in cooking and eating (particularly iodised salt; sea salt and 'boutique' salts do not contain iodine) (NHMRC, NZ MoH 2017).

Control of thyroid hormone secretion is via a complex feedback system that involves both the hypothalamus and the pituitary gland. Decreased blood concentrations of thyroid hormone are detected by receptors in the hypothalamus, leading to the release of thyrotropin-releasing hormone (TRH). TRH stimulates the anterior pituitary gland to release thyroid-stimulating hormone (TSH), which in turn stimulates the thyroid gland to release T_3 and T_4. T_4 is de-iodinated in the liver to T_3, further increasing the concentration of T_3 (active) in the blood. This then feeds back to the hypothalamus and pituitary gland to stop production (negative feedback) (Jameson et al 2018c). It should be noted that goitrogenic foods, such as cruciferous vegetables (e.g. cabbage, broccoli, Brussels sprouts, cauliflower, kale, bok choy), interfere with thyroid hormone synthesis by impairing the binding of iodine to thyroglobuline (NHMRC, NZ MoH 2017).

Thyroid hormones are needed for normal growth and development and to maintain metabolic rate. Effects of thyroid hormones include activation of osteoclast and osteoblast activities in the bones; increase in cardiac output and blood volume and decrease in systemic vascular resistance; regulation of lipolysis; regulation of triglyceride and cholesterol metabolism; regulation of pituitary hormone synthesis, inhibition of TSH and stimulation of production of growth hormone; and stimulation of axonal growth and development in the brain (Jameson et al 2018c).

Thyroid gland dysfunction can manifest as hypo- or hyperthyroidism.

Hypothyroidism is a decrease in thyroid gland activity from a range of causes, including congenital, autoimmune disease (e.g. Hashimoto's disease), surgery, iodine deficiency or excess intake, some medications and radioactive iodine ingestion. Symptoms include tiredness, weakness, weight gain with poor appetite, constipation, intolerance to heat, feeling cold, cool peripheries, decreased libido, dry and coarse skin, brittle nails, hoarse/husky voice, bradycardia, difficulty concentrating and poor memory (Jameson et al 2018b). Hypothyroidism is treated using thyroid hormone replacement therapy. The term myxoedema refers to those patients with thyroid hormone deficiency of such severity that profound hypothermia, hypoventilation, hypotension and central nervous system signs are evident on physical examination and can be life threatening.

Thyroid dysfunction occurs commonly in women of childbearing years, second only to diabetes mellitus, with the incidence of hyperthyroidism in pregnancy ranging from 0.1 to 0.4%. It is important to note that overt hypothyroidism and hyperthyroidism have been associated with some adverse obstetric outcomes, including pre-eclampsia, miscarriage and low birth weight babies, and subclinical hypothyroidism associated with pre-eclampsia and perinatal mortality (Australian Government Department of Health 2019). If a woman with pre-existing thyroid disease becomes pregnant, thyroid hormone levels should be closely monitored and medications adjusted accordingly to maintain a euthyroid state (Australian Government Department of Health 2019).

Hyperthyroidism is caused by an over-functioning thyroid gland (e.g. Graves' disease), toxic adenoma, toxic multinodular goitre or excessive intake of thyroid agents or iodine. Symptoms include palpitations, tachycardia, palpably enlarged thyroid gland, ophthalmopathy, nervousness, irritability, labile emotions, heat intolerance and sweating, weight loss (in spite of increased food intake), loose stools/diarrhoea, decreased or absent menstrual flow, decreased libido, muscle weakness, warm, moist skin, fine hair, diffuse alopecia, fine tremor and excessive sweating (Jameson et al 2018a). Hyperthyroidism treatment is aimed at reducing thyroid hormone production and blocking the peripheral effects of excessive thyroxine sodium, such as tachycardia, tremor and sweating. Treatment may include surgery (subtotal resection of thyroid gland), radioactive iodine therapy or medial management using antithyroid agents (Jameson et al 2018a).

Thyrotoxicosis is defined as the state of thyroid hormone excess and is not synonymous with *hyperthyroidism*, which is the result of excessive thyroid function (Jameson et al 2018c).

Antithyroid agents inhibit the synthesis of thyroid hormones, but do not affect the thyroid hormones that are already stored or circulating in the blood. Antithyroid agents are usually given in high doses for 3–4 months until thyroid function returns to normal (euthyroid) and the dose is then reduced to the minimum dose required to maintain the euthyroid state. Treatment is sometimes a combination of antithyroid agents and thyroid hormones.

Antithyroid compounds (also termed thyrostatic compounds) can be subdivided into thioureas (also called thionamides) (e.g. carbimazole, propylthiouracil) and anion inhibitors (e.g. iodine, potassium perchlorate).

THYROID AGENTS

LEVOTHYROXINE SODIUM (Eltroxin, Eutroxsig, Oroxine)

Available forms

Tablets: 25 microgram, 50 microgram, 75 microgram, 100 microgram, 125 microgram, 200 microgram

Action

- also called L-thyroxine sodium
- converted to more active T_3 form
- slow onset of action (3–4 weeks)
- long duration of action 7–21 days (even when thyroxine sodium is stopped)
- elimination half-life 6–7 days (euthyroid patient), 9–10 days (hypothyroidism) or 3–4 days (hyperthyroidism)

Use

- thyroid hormone deficiencies
- TSH-responsive thyroid tumours

Dose

- (adult $\geq$ 70 kg) initially 50–100 microgram orally daily 30–60 minutes before food, increasing by 25–50 microgram and at least 4-weekly intervals to 100–200 microgram daily as maintenance **OR**
- (> 60 years or with ischaemic heart disease) initially 25–50 microgram orally daily 30–60 minutes before food, then increasing 75–125 microgram orally daily as maintenance

Adverse effects

- usually associated with overdosage and consists of the following:
  - nervousness, tremor, restlessness, anxiety, irritability, fatigue
  - sweating, flushing, intolerance to heat, fever
  - headache, insomnia, sleep disturbance, poor concentration, emotional lability
  - mania, psychosis, psychotic depression
  - seizures
  - tachypnoea, shortness of breath
  - tachycardia, palpitations, cardiac arrhythmias, angina pectoris, chest pain
  - myopathy, muscle cramps and weakness
  - eyelid lag
  - diarrhoea, nausea, vomiting, abdominal pain, weight loss, malabsorption
  - alopecia, hyperpigmentation
  - amenorrhoea, menstrual irregularities, decreased libido, gynaecomastia (males)
  - decreased glucose tolerance

Interactions

- may enhance clinical effects of warfarin requiring close monitoring of INR, especially when starting therapy
- may reduce the effect of digoxin

- use with ketamine may result in marked hypertension and tachycardia
- effect may be reduced by colestyramine (cholestryramine), colestipol, soya flour, soy-containing foods, high fibre diet, sucralfate, aluminium hydroxide, calcium carbonate, magnesium hydroxide, ferrous sulfate heptahydrate and proton pump inhibitors
- coronary insufficiency may occur if given with sympathomimetic agents
- increased dosage of oral hypoglycaemics and insulin may be needed. Blood glucose levels should be carefully monitored, especially when starting, stopping or changing doses of thyroxine sodium
- effect may be reduced by beta-adrenoceptor blocking agents and amiodarone, because peripheral conversion of thyroxine sodium to T_3 is decreased
- increase in therapeutic and toxic effects of thyroxine sodium and TCAs may occur if given together
- absorption may be decreased if given with ciprofloxacin
- an increase in dose of thyroxine sodium may be required if given with oestrogen (in those with a non-functioning thyroid gland)
- dose adjustment of corticosteroids may be required if given with thyroxine sodium
- decreased plasma levels may result if given with phenytoin, carbamazepine, barbiturates, rifampicin, proguanil or ritonavir
- effects may be reduced if given with sertraline or other SSRIs
- caution if given with lithium, as hypothyroidism may result
- decreased dose may be required if given with androgens
- absorption may be decreased by orlistat
- thyroid function tests can be modified by NSAIDs, salicylates, fenclofenac, diazepam and heparin

Nursing points/Cautions

- formulations are not interchangeable (Eltroxin versus Oroxine/Eutroxsig). If patient is switched between formulations, careful TSH monitoring is required
- where possible, patient should be administered whole tablets
- monitor heart rate, reporting if it is more than 100 beats/minute or if there is any marked change in rate or rhythm
- signs of overdose may take 3–6 days to be manifested
- T_4, T_3, TSH and response to TRH should be monitored regularly throughout therapy
- blood sampling times should be related to ingestion time
- if patient has hypopituitarism or adrenal insufficiency, corticosteroid replacement therapy should be started before thyroxine sodium to prevent Addisonian crisis
- therapy should be started at a low dose (25–50 microgram/day) and increased gradually. If the patient has cardiac disease or is elderly, the starting dose should be 12.5–25 microgram/day and increased in increments of not more than 25 microgram, at intervals of not less than 14 days. If not tolerated because of angina, increments should be reduced and/ or angina controlled with beta-adrenoceptor blocking agents
- caution if used in post-menopausal women as a decrease in bone mineral density may occur
- caution if used in those with diabetes insipidus or diabetes mellitus, history of hyperthyroidism or thyrotoxicosis, long-standing hypothyroidism or myxoedema or cardiac disease
- caution if given to those with malabsorption syndromes as absorption may be reduced
- not recommended for treatment of obesity or weight loss

- contraindicated in those with untreated hyperthyroidism, thyrotoxicosis, uncorrected adrenal insufficiency, acute myocarditis, acute pancreatitis or acute myocardial infarction uncomplicated by hypothyroidism

Patient teaching and advice

- patient should be warned that it may take a few weeks for therapy to be effective and changes in symptoms to occur
- instruct patient to take as a single daily dose 30–60 minutes before breakfast (on an empty stomach)
- advise patient that the replacement therapy is lifelong and that follow-up appointments need to be kept. The importance of regular blood tests should also be emphasised
- patient should be warned that therapy interacts with a number of other medications, including over-the-counter (OTC) preparations such as antacids, calcium and iron supplements and it is therefore important to discuss dosing schedule in relation to these. Patient should also be instructed to allow a 6-hour interval if prescribed ciprofloxacin or 5-hour interval if prescribed colestyramine (cholestryramine) or colestipol with thyroxine sodium
- patient should be directed to report palpitations, difficulty breathing (dyspnoea) or chest pain
- if patient has diabetes mellitus, it is important to remind him/her that insulin and/or oral hypoglycaemic agent requirements will increase with therapy and blood glucose levels should be monitored frequently, especially when starting therapy
- (Oroxine/Eutroxsig) instruct patient to store tablets in refrigerator (2–8 °C); however, a single blister strip can be stored at up 25° C for up to 2 weeks and then any remaining tablets should be discarded
- see also General Patient teaching and advice (p. xxvii)

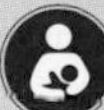

increased dose may be required if used during pregnancy. Serum thyroxine sodium and TSH levels should be monitored 3–4-weekly during pregnancy as an increase in dosage requirements is usually required. Requirements then decrease postpartum. If possible, thyroxine sodium therapy should be optimised before conception

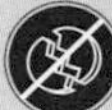

if tablet is crushed and dispersed in water, it should be taken immediately as the dispersion settles quickly and is sensitive to light

LIOTHYRONINE SODIUM (Tertroxin)

Available form
Tablets: 20 microgram

Action
- also called L-triiodothyronine
- similar to that of thyroxine sodium, but much more potent and rapid in onset (within a few hours of administration), briefer duration of action and disappears within 24–48 hours of stopping therapy
- half-life 1–2 days (in euthyroid patient), prolonged in hypothyroidism

Use
- severe and acute hypothyroid states
- myxoedema coma
- thyrotoxicosis (as an adjunct to carbimazole to prevent subclinical hypothyroidism)

Dose
- (myxoedema) 10–20 microgram orally 8-hourly, increasing gradually to a total of 60 microgram daily in 2–3 divided doses **OR**
- (myxoedema coma) 60 microgram via stomach tube, then 20 microgram 8-hourly **OR**

- (thyrotoxicosis) 20 microgram orally 8-hourly (with carbimazole)

Adverse effects

- headache, restlessness, flushing, sweating, excitability
- diarrhoea, excessive weight loss
- palpitations, anginal pain, tachycardia, cardiac arrhythmias
- skeletal muscle cramps and/or weakness

Interactions

- may enhance activity of oral anticoagulants, therefore prothrombin times should be closely monitored when therapy with liothyronine is started or dose altered
- absorption may decrease if given with colestyramine (cholestryramine)
- may increase plasma levels of phenytoin increasing risk of toxicity
- metabolism may be increased by phenytoin and carbamazepine
- increased risk of cardiac arrhythmias if given with TCAs
- may require adjustment to dose of cardiac glycoside (as liothyronine may potentiate digitalis toxicity)
- decreased serum levels may result if given with oral contraceptives
- ketamine may cause hypertension and tachycardia when given with thyroid replacement therapy
- increased oral hypoglycaemics and insulin may be needed. Blood glucose levels should be carefully monitored

Nursing points/Cautions

- regular thyroid function tests are recommended
- adverse effects are uncommon
- adrenal deficiency should be corrected with adrenocorticotrophic hormones before starting therapy
- if treating myxoedema coma, ECG monitoring, assisted ventilation and corticosteroids are also required
- caution if used in the elderly, who may be more sensitive to thyroid replacement therapy
- caution if used in those with endocrine disorders (e.g. diabetes mellitus, adrenocortical insufficiency)
- contraindicated in those with angina, cardiovascular disorders, untreated adrenal cortical insufficiency or untreated hyperthyroidism

Patient teaching and advice

- patient should be advised of the importance to continue therapy, keep follow-up appointments and have regular blood tests
- warn patient to report any chest pain or palpitations, excessive sweating or weight loss immediately
- if patient has diabetes mellitus, it is important to remind him/her that insulin and/or oral hypoglycaemic agent requirements will increase with therapy and blood glucose levels should be monitored frequently, especially when starting therapy
- if patient is taking anticoagulant medication (e.g. warfarin), blood test for prothrombin should be monitored frequently when starting therapy
- see also General Patient teaching and advice (p. xxvii)

tablet may be crushed and mixed with water (does not disperse well) or a spoonful of yoghurt or apple puree

ANTITHYROID AGENTS

CARBIMAZOLE (Neo-Mercazole)

Available form
Tablets: 5 mg

Action
- depresses thyroid hormone synthesis by inhibiting the binding of iodine to tyrosine
- clinical response does not occur until circulating and stored thyroid hormone has been used
- has no effect on iodine uptake by thyroid gland
- active metabolite (methimazole) is responsible for antithyroid activity, half-life 3–6 hours

Use
- hyperthyroidism (induction of remission in either primary or secondary thyrotoxicosis)
- preparation for thyroidectomy
- pre- and post-radioactive iodine treatment

Dose
- (hyperthyroidism, mild cases) initially 15–20 mg orally daily in divided doses; (moderate cases) 30 mg orally daily in divided doses; (severe cases) 40–45 mg orally daily in divided doses (up to 60 mg) until euthyroid, then 10–15 mg daily as maintenance for 1–2 years **OR**
- (changeover from thiouracils) 5 mg of carbimazole is equivalent to 50 mg of propylthiouracil **OR**
- (preparation for thyroidectomy) preoperatively carbimazole is prescribed in doses that will make patient euthyroid and continued until surgery, with iodide being added in the last 2 weeks

Adverse effects
- nausea, mild gastric disturbances, loss of taste
- headache, neuritis
- mild rash, pruritus, urticaria, hair loss
- arthralgia
- bone marrow depression, agranulocytosis
- jaundice, hepatitis, abnormal liver function tests
- (rare) aplastic anaemia, myopathy, vasculitis, severe hypersensitivity reaction

Interactions
- may increase serum levels of theophylline increasing risk of toxicity
- caution if given with other agranulocytosis-inducing agents
- may increase effects of anticoagulants, therefore prothrombin time should be carefully monitored especially when starting or stopping therapy
- may increase clearance of prednisolone
- may decrease clearance of erythromycin
- may increase digoxin and beta-adrenergic blocking agent levels when hyperthyroid patients become euthyroid

Nursing points/Cautions
- dosage is titrated to thyroid function until patient is euthyroid and maintenance dose continued for 12–24 months
- patient monitoring should be monthly for the first year, then 3–6-monthly
- adverse reactions usually occur within 8 weeks of starting therapy
- if patient complains of myalgia, creatine phosphokinase (CPK) levels should be monitored
- therapy is usually stopped when radioactive iodine is administered
- response to carbimazole may be delayed (weeks to months) if there are large amounts of thyroid hormones present (e.g. nodular goitre), whereas

response in thyrotoxicosis is seen in 3–4 days
- caution if given to those with memory loss or confusion as they may not be able to report symptoms of adverse effects. Regular monitoring of full blood counts is recommended
- caution if used in those with mild-to-moderate liver impairment
- caution if used in those with tracheal obstruction as high doses may lead to thyroid enlargement which in turn may exacerbate symptoms of obstruction
- not recommended in those with galactose intolerance, Lapp lactase deficiency or glucose–galactose malabsorption
- contraindicated in those with severe liver impairment or pre-existing blood disorders
- contraindicated in those with previous acute pancreatitis due to carbimazole/active metabolite
- contraindicated in those with hypersensitivity to thiamazoles or propylthiouracil as cross-allergy may exist

Patient teaching and advice

- advise patient to keep appointments throughout therapy, including the need for blood tests
- warn patient to immediately report any of the following:
    - rash, fever, mouth ulcers, malaise, sore throat, bruising or bleeding immediately (early signs of bone marrow depression)
    - muscle pain (possible myopathy)
    - yellow eyes or skin, itchiness, upper abdominal pain, nausea, vomiting or loss of appetite, loss of weight, fever or dark urine (signs of liver dysfunction)
- women of childbearing potential should be advised to use effective contraception during therapy
- also see General Patient teaching and advice (p. xxvii)

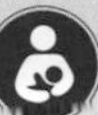

should only be given during pregnancy if benefits (mother's needs) outweigh risk to the fetus, and if propylthiouracil is unsuitable. Dose may need to be adjusted during pregnancy, because of the increase in basal metabolic rate (BMR). Dose should not exceed 15 mg twice daily during last trimester. Administration should stop 3–4 weeks before delivery date, because carbimazole may inhibit thyroid hormone synthesis in the fetus leading to congenital goitre and substituted with iodine

contraindicated during breastfeeding

tablet can be crushed and mixed with water (does not disperse easily) or mixed with spoonful of yoghurt or apple puree

PROPYLTHIOURACIL (PTU)

Available form
Tablets: 50 mg

Action
- depresses thyroid hormone synthesis by inhibiting the binding of iodine to tyrosine
- clinical response does not occur until circulating and stored thyroid hormone has been used
- has no effect on iodine uptake by thyroid gland
- half-life about 2 hours
- may become euthyroid in 4–6 weeks

Use
- hyperthyroidism (induction of remission in either primary or secondary thyrotoxicosis)
- preparation for thyroidectomy
- pre- and post-radioactive iodine treatment

Dose
- initially 200–400 mg orally daily in 3–4 divided doses until euthyroid, then 50–800 mg daily in 2–4 divided doses **OR**
- (thyrotoxic crisis) 800–1200 mg daily in divided doses (orally or via nasogastric

tube) together with other agents such as iodine, and general supportive measures

Adverse effects

- itching
- dizziness
- joint pain
- loss of taste, nausea, vomiting, stomach pain
- agranulocytosis, mild leucopenia. granulocytosis, thrombocytopenia
- (rare) cholestatic jaundice, hepatotoxicity, ototoxicity, lymphadenopathy, hypoprothrombinaemia, nephritis, vasculitis, peripheral neuropathy, severe hypersensitivity reaction
- (rare) hyperplasia of thyroid gland

Interactions

- patients receiving heparin or oral anticoagulants require close monitoring of prothrombin time, because propylthiouracil can cause hypoprothrombinaemia
- risk of agranulocytosis is increased if propylthiouracil is taken with another agranulocytosis-inducing agent

Nursing points/Cautions

- regular thyroid function tests are recommended before starting therapy, monthly during stabilisation and then 2–3-monthly. Liver function tests and full blood count monitoring are also recommended
- women under 30 should be closely monitored as they are at greater risk of hepatotoxicity (especially in first 3 months of therapy). Liver function tests monthly for first 6 months of therapy are recommended
- iodine is given with propylthiouracil in preparation for surgery to decrease friability and vascularity of thyroid gland
- caution if used in those with asthma
- contraindicated in those with hypersensitivity to thioamide derivatives

Patient teaching and advice

- advise patient to keep appointments during initial therapy
- patient should be warned not to drive or operate machinery if dizziness occurs
- patients should be instructed to seek medical advice immediately if any of the following occur:
  - rash, fever, chills, headache, malaise, mouth ulcers, sore throat, bleeding or bruising (signs of agranulocytosis)
  - upper abdominal discomfort, fever, nausea, vomiting, weight loss, yellowing of eyes or skin, dark urine (signs of hepatotoxicity)
  - diarrhoea, fever, vomiting, rapid heartbeat, irritability, weakness, listlessness (signs of excess thyroid hormone)
  - tiredness, lethargy, muscle weakness/cramping, slow heartbeat, feeling cold, dry/flaky skin, hair loss, deep/husky voice, weight gain, change in menstrual cycle, headache (signs of hypothyroidism)
- signs of hepatotoxicity should be emphasised in women under 30 because of their increased risk
- patients should be informed to keep dosing intervals equal (e.g. 6- or 8-hour intervals)
- see also General Patient teaching and advice (p. xxvii)

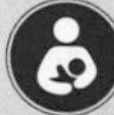

may cause damage to fetal thyroid causing fetal hypothyroidism and neonatal goitre, or congenital abnormalities, therefore should be avoided during pregnancy unless the benefits to the mother outweigh risks to the fetus. If used, dose should be as low as possible to provide therapeutic effects and discontinued if patient shows any signs of hypothyroidism

breastfeeding should be stopped before starting therapy

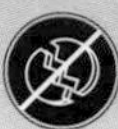

if crushing tablets, mask, gloves and closed tablet crusher should be used. May be dispersed in water or crushed tablet mixed with yoghurt or apple puree

SODIUM IODIDE (^{131}I) (Sodium Iodide (^{131}I) Capsules (Therapy), Sodium Iodide (^{131}I) Solution BP (For Therapy), Sodium Iodide (^{131}I) Injection)

Available forms

Capsule (contained in a glass vial and lead container): 50 MBq–6000 MBq; Oral solution (contained in a glass vial and lead container): 50 MBq–16 000 MBq; Injection (contained in 10 mL glass vial): 200 MBq–1600 MBq

MBq (megabecquerel) is a measure of radiation

Action

- radioactive iodide that concentrates in thyroid tissue. Therapeutic effect is due to beta radiation
- mostly excreted via kidneys but also via sweat and saliva

Use

- hyperthyroidism in patients who have a poor surgical risk or have not responded well to therapy
- detection and ablation of residual thyroid tissue (thyroid cancer)

Dose

- (thyrotoxicosis) 150–600 MBq orally (capsules, oral solution) **OR**
- (thyroid ablation) 800–2000 MBq orally (capsules, oral solution) **OR**
- (thyroid carcinoma) 2000–6000 MBq in 2 capsules orally **OR**
- (hyperthyroidism, wt ≥ 70 kg) 148–370 MBq IV **OR**
- (thyroid imaging) 0.185–3.7 MBq IV

Adverse effects

- vomiting, nausea
- tachycardia
- rash, pruritus
- (elderly patient with total thyroidectomy) hyponatraemia
- (rare) radiation-induced thyroiditis, inflamed salivary glands, transient worsening of hyperthyroidism
- (potential) radiation sickness, bone marrow depression, acute leukaemia, anaemia, pulmonary fibrosis, acute thyroid crisis

Interactions

- uptake may be affected by intake of stable iodine within last 4 weeks (e.g. seafood, radiographic contrast media, antithyroid drugs, thyroxine sodium)
- contraindicated with thyroid hormones or antithyroid agents

Nursing points/Cautions

- patient should be well hydrated before and during therapy to promote excretion
- patient should be encouraged to urinate as often as possible for 4–6 hours post administration to reduce exposure of bladder, kidney and stomach to radiation
- antithyroid drugs should be withheld for 3 days before treatment with radioactive iodide
- thyroxine sodium should be withheld for 4 weeks before treatment with radioactive iodide
- patient should be screened for any recent intake of stable iodine (e.g. seafood, radiographic contrast media, antithyroid drugs, thyroxine sodium). Patient should also be screened for any risk of hyponatraemia, including age, being female, use of thiazide diuretics and previous thyroidectomy
- women of childbearing age should have pregnancy test before administration
- patient should be managed in a single room (according to hospital protocol) to prevent unwanted radiation

exposure to others. Isolation precautions are recommended for those receiving greater than 600 MBq
- only doctor qualified and licensed to handle radioisotopes should administer dosage
- staff exposure should be minimised
- disposable gloves (for staff and patient), disposal cup with water and tissues should be prepared before removal of vial from lead container
- handling and disposal of radioactive waste (including disposable gloves, paper cup, empty vial, stopper and cap) is according to hospital policy and NHMRC 'Code of Practice for the disposal of radioactive wastes by the user' (1985, 1990)
- patient will require lifelong follow-up
- capsules and IV solution have a 14-day expiry from the day of calibration and should not be administered if expired
- iodine allergy IS NOT a contraindication to the use of sodium iodide as there is only a very small amount of iodine in the capsule (3 microgram in a 500 MBq capsule)
- not recommended in those with renal insufficiency or under 18 years
- caution if given to those with nephrosis, decreased kidney function or who eat goitrogenic foods (see p. 1513) as these interfere with accumulation of iodine by thyroid
- contraindicated in those currently undergoing treatment with thyroid or antithyroid agents, or if the person is vomiting or has diarrhoea

Patient teaching and advice

- patient should be advised to swallow capsule whole
- patient should be encouraged to drink copious amounts of fluid before and after treatment to reduce dose (radioactivity) to kidney, bladder and stomach
- secreted in saliva, therefore kissing is discouraged for at least 10 days after therapeutic dose (especially children)
- double flushing of toilet and careful washing of hands should be encouraged strongly
- patient should be instructed that he/she will require lifelong follow-up
- women of childbearing age should be advised to use appropriate contraceptive measures to prevent pregnancy and should have a negative pregnancy test at time of therapy
- see also General Patient teaching and advice (p. xxvii)

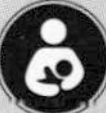

contraindicated during pregnancy or breastfeeding

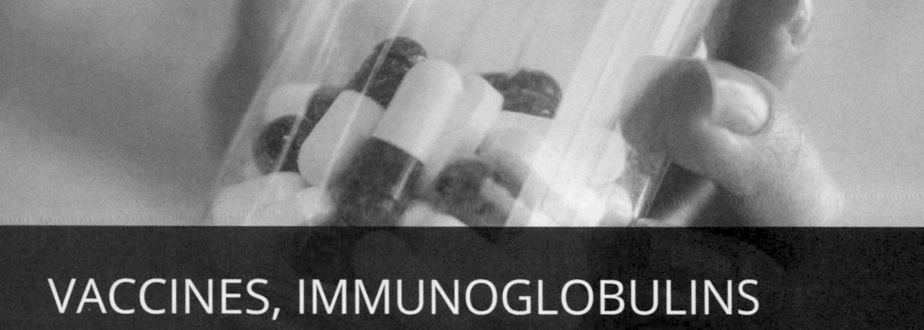

VACCINES, IMMUNOGLOBULINS AND ANTIVENOMS

Vaccination is the administration of a vaccine, and *immunisation* is the development of protective levels of antibodies (confirmed by serological testing). Immunological agents are used for both active and passive immunity. Active immunity results when the body itself responds to an antigenic agent, producing antibodies. This may happen naturally as a result of an infection or artificially after immunisation. Agents used for immunisation are vaccines, which may be live organisms, killed organisms or toxoids. Obviously, a live organism would be dangerous, so it is rendered harmless (attenuated) before use and the vaccine contains a weakened form of the pathogen. However, they can still cause problems to immunosuppressed patients, including those with HIV, and care should also be taken when administering to pregnant women. Passive immunisation is immunity given as already formed antibodies. These antibodies may be of animal origin (antivenom, also known as antisera) or human origin (immunoglobulins) and provide temporary protection.

VACCINES

General Actions of vaccines

- antigenic materials that induce a specific active artificial immunity to infection by the corresponding infecting agent
- subsequent doses of vaccine (booster doses) provide protection by increasing declining antibody levels
- live attenuated vaccines include oral typhoid, oral rotavirus, BCG, yellow fever, monovalent rubella vaccine, Japanese encephalitis vaccine, varicella vaccine, zoster vaccine and measles–mumps–rubella vaccine

General Uses of vaccines

- specific vaccine affords prophylaxis against some infectious diseases by providing complete or partial protection for months or years

- primary immunisation schedule is started early in life and is lifelong (see National Immunisation Program Schedule, p. 1529–30)

General Interactions of vaccines

- vaccination should not be given within 7 months of blood transfusion because of the risk of vaccine failure due to the presence of naturally occurring circulating antibodies
- re-vaccination may be required if an immunoglobulin is given within 2 weeks of vaccine
- vaccination with live attenuated virus vaccine should not be given within 3 months of immunoglobulin
- not recommended within 4 weeks of live vaccines or BCG (4 weeks or more should be allowed between the administration of any two live attenuated vaccines or BCG; however, if it is necessary to administer two live vaccines within 1 month, the injections should be given in different sites)
- not recommended within 14 days of high-dose corticosteroid therapy
- some live attenuated vaccines are contraindicated during corticosteroid or immunosuppressive therapy, including radiation, as they may result in an extensive vaccine-related rash or disseminated disease
- may temporarily depress tuberculin skin sensitivity for 4–6 weeks, giving a possible false negative response

General Nursing points/Cautions for vaccines

- conjugate vaccines provide improved antibody response compared to polysaccharide vaccines, induce immune memory and are more effective in young children (a conjugate vaccine is one where a bacterial capsular polysaccharide is attached to a protein to increase its immunogenicity)
- if the person to be vaccinated has an acute systemic or febrile (temperature currently ≥ 38.5°C) illness, vaccination should be postponed until the person is well and afebrile. However, children with minor illnesses (e.g. colds) should be vaccinated at the time (ATAGI 2018)
- valid consent should be obtained before each vaccination. A parent or legal guardian is able to consent for a child. However, if a child/adolescent refuses a vaccination that has been consented to by a parent or legal guardian, his or her wishes should be respected, and the parent or legal guardian informed. Consent may be written or verbal (depending on the protocols of the health facility) and should be obtained after the person has been given information (verbal and/or written) about the vaccine, its use, risks and benefits and any possible adverse effects. The person should have sufficient time to consider the information and ask questions before consent is obtained. This consent should be documented in clinical records (as per protocol of the health facility) (ATAGI 2018)
- immunisation records should contain clear documentation of the person's full name and date of birth, details of vaccine (brand name, batch number, dose number), date and time of vaccination, site of administration, name of the person providing the vaccination and the date the next vaccination is due

- some state/territory health departments have specific documentation requirements for vaccines administered to healthcare workers or healthcare students on clinical placement with state/territory health facilities
- Australian Immunisation Register is a national database that records details of vaccinations given to all Australians (ATAGI 2018)
- premature infants should be immunised as per the normal schedule (not adjusted for prematurity), although some (depending on gestation or birth weight) may require extra doses of some vaccines as preterm infants may be at increased risk of vaccine-preventable diseases (e.g. pneumococcal disease) and may not develop sufficient antibodies after some vaccinations (e.g. hepatitis B)
- because smallpox has been eradicated worldwide, only laboratory workers directly involved with smallpox are vaccinated
- vasovagal episodes (fainting) occur commonly in adolescents and adults post-vaccination, but not infants or children. If an infant or child loses consciousness, anaphylactic reaction should be presumed if strong central (carotid) pulse is not present
- vasovagal episodes tend to occur within minutes of vaccination, whereas anaphylactic reaction usually occurs with 15 minutes, although can be delayed
- ensure recipient is seated comfortably (or being held adequately by parent/carer) before administration
- use strict aseptic technique
- skin disinfectant/alcohol (if used) should be allowed to dry before any injection to reduce pain and/or irritation at the injection site
- vaccines should not be mixed in the same syringe, but can be administered in different sites (usually different limbs)
- vaccines should not be mixed with local anaesthetic
- topical anaesthetic agents not recommended routinely (unless child has excessive fear or dislike of needles) because they take 30–60 minutes to be effective
- all vaccines should be inspected before administration for any signs of discolouration or particulate matter, and only given if clear
- ensure correct siting and route of administration (anterolateral thigh is the preferred IM site in those $<$ 12 months; deltoid muscle is preferred IM site for $>$ 12 months, including adolescents and adults; anterolateral thigh can also be used in older children and adults)
- deltoid muscle is not recommended for IM administration in those $<$ 12 months
- buttocks are not recommended for IM administration due to unreliable absorption
- avoid intravascular injection by withdrawing the syringe plunger to check for blood
- site should not be rubbed after injection; however, gentle pressure can be applied for 1–2 minutes if needed
- if the person is receiving more than one vaccine, the most painful vaccine should be administered last. Different sites can be used (e.g. one injection into each of the deltoid muscles). If the same muscle (muscle mass needs to be sufficiently large) is used

for multiple injections, at least 2.5 cm should be allowed between sites

- patient should be observed for 30 minutes after any vaccination for any signs of allergic reaction; resuscitation equipment (including adrenaline (epinephrine) 1 : 1000) should also be readily available in the event of anaphylaxis occurring
- ensure products are kept at the required temperature, not exposed to direct sunlight or high humidity according to the manufacturers' instructions to retain potency, activity and antigenicity
- vaccines should never be frozen
- freeze-dried preparations should be stored in the dried state at 2–8°C. Vaccines should not be used if they have been exposed to temperatures below 2°C or above 8°C. These vaccines should not be discarded until the correct disposal has been recommended by the manufacturer/supplier or state/territory authority
- any vials with a stopper containing dry natural rubber may provoke a hypersensitivity reaction in those with latex sensitivity
- standard precautions should be strictly followed to prevent transmission of any blood-borne viruses (e.g. single-use disposable needle and syringe should be used for a single patient; needles should not be recapped after use and should be disposed of appropriately to prevent needlestick injury)
- any remains of a multidose vial should be discarded at the end of the immunisation session
- IM injections are contraindicated or given with great caution in those with bleeding disorders who are at risk of bleeding from IM administration. SC route should be considered as an alternate route of administration
- inactivated vaccines may have poor response in those who are immunocompromised
- live attenuated vaccines are not recommended in those with significantly impaired immune systems (e.g. oncology or transplant patients, those taking cytokine modulators or high-dose corticosteroids), but inactivated vaccines should be considered (e.g. measles–mumps–rubella may be given to a person with HIV (with mild immune impairment) on specialist advice)
- close contacts of immunosuppressed people should also be vaccinated against pertussis, measles, mumps, rubella, rotavirus (if indicated), chicken pox and shingles (> 50 years). Annual influenza vaccine is also recommended
- caution if given to those with compromised cardiopulmonary function as there is an increased risk of fainting (syncope)
- caution if pertussis-containing vaccines are used in infants with infantile spasm, uncontrolled epilepsy or progressive encephalopathy. Vaccination with pertussis should be deferred until condition is stable
- contraindicated in those who have had anaphylaxis following the previous dose or anaphylaxis following exposure to any component of the relevant vaccine

General Patient teaching and advice for vaccines

- patient/parent/carer should be advised that vaccination may not confer

100% protection (e.g. immunised children may still develop chicken pox after exposure, but the number of vesicles and duration of illness is reduced)
- the doctor or maternal and/or child health nurse should discuss benefits and possible adverse effects and take a careful history, with special regard to previous reactions, allergies in the patient or family (e.g. asthma, eczema, allergic or seasonal rhinitis) and current medical status (e.g. any current illness, immune system status) and make a decision about the appropriateness of vaccination on that particular date (see end of this section for cautions and contraindications to vaccination)
- parent/carer should be warned that vaccination often results in soreness, itching, swelling or burning at injection site, which lasts for 1–2 days
- adult patient should be warned not to drive or operate machinery after vaccination if drowsiness or dizziness occurs
- advise patient to avoid vigorous exercise and excessive alcohol consumption for several hours after vaccination

Notes

Overseas travel and vaccination

- the individual's doctor will decide on the type, dosage and timing of vaccination in consultation with the patient (or parents in the case of a child), and this decision is generally made according to such factors as length of stay overseas, risk of exposure, age of the patient and how endemic the disease is in the country to be visited

Healthcare workers and vaccination

- healthcare workers may be exposed to a range of vaccine-preventable diseases
- it is recommended that all healthcare workers (including students) involved in direct patient care or who come into contact with human tissue (e.g. laboratory staff, mortuary staff) are vaccinated against hepatitis B, influenza, pertussis, MMR (if non-immune) and varicella (if seronegative). In addition, those working with remote Aboriginal and Torres Strait Islander communities in the Northern Territory, Western Australia, Queensland and South Australia should also be vaccinated against hepatitis A. Staff who may be at high risk of exposure to drug-resistant tuberculosis should also receive BCG. There are also recommendations for people who work with animals
- healthcare workers should consider that vaccination may protect not only themselves from developing diseases and requiring time away from the workplace, but also protect the patients they care for from the potential spread of illness (e.g. influenza), which may be potentially life threatening in some groups of particularly vulnerable patients (e.g. the elderly, immunocompromised, after transplantation, after radiation or chemotherapy)
- some workplaces have immunisation requirements with comprehensive occupational vaccination programs in place. This may include the management of vaccine refusal by the healthcare worker (e.g. reducing the risk of the healthcare worker

transmitting a disease to vulnerable individuals)

- BCG vaccination is recommended in staff at high risk of TB (e.g. staff working in chest clinics, infectious diseases wards, physiotherapist, diagnostic laboratory staff, autopsy room staff, medical and nursing staff in public hospitals)

NATIONAL IMMUNISATION PROGRAM SCHEDULE

Age	Disease
Birth (preferably within 24 hours for the greatest benefit, but within 7 days of birth)	Hepatitis B
2 months (can be given from 6 weeks)	Hepatitis B, diphtheria, tetanus, pertussis (whooping cough), *Haemophilus influenzae* type b, poliomyelitis, pneumococcal, rotavirus
Aboriginal and Torres Strait Island children	Meningococcal B
4 months	Hepatitis B, diphtheria, tetanus, pertussis (whooping cough), *H. influenzae* type b, poliomyelitis, pneumococcal, rotavirus
Aboriginal and Torres Strait Island children	Meningococcal B
6 months	Hepatitis B, diphtheria, tetanus, pertussis (whooping cough), *H. influenzae* type b, poliomyelitis,
Additional dose for children with specified medical risk conditions and Aboriginal and Torres Strait Island children from WA, SA and Queensland	Pneumococcal
Additional dose for children with specified medical risk conditions (Aboriginal and Torres Strait Island children)	Meningococcal B
12 months	Measles, mumps and rubella, meningococcal ACWY, Pneumococcal, *H. influenzae* type b
Aboriginal and Torres Strait Island children	Meningococcal B
18 months	Diphtheria, tetanus, pertussis (whooping cough), measles, mumps, rubella and varicella (chickenpox)
Additional vaccine for Aboriginal and Torres Strait Island children in WA, NT, SA and Queensland	Hepatitis A
4 years	poliomyelitis, diphtheria, tetanus, pertussis (whooping cough)
Additional dose for children with specified medical risk conditions, and Aboriginal and Torres Strait Island children in WA, SA and Queensland	Pneumococcal

Age	Disease
Additional vaccine for Aboriginal and Torres Strait Island children in WA, NT, SA and Queensland	Hepatitis A
12–13 years	Human papillomavirus Diphtheria, tetanus, pertussis (whooping cough)
14–16 years	Meningococcal ACWY
50 years and over (Aboriginal and Torres Strait Island adults)	Pneumococcal
70 years and over	Pneumococcal
70–79 years	Shingles (herpes zoster)
Pregnant women (ideally between 20–32 weeks, but may be given up to delivery)	Pertussis (whooping cough)

National Immunisation Program Schedule © 2020 Commonwealth of Australia as represented by the Department of Health.

BACILLUS CALMETTE-GUERIN (BCG) VACCINE (BCG Vaccine)

Action

- prepared from attenuated strain of *Mycobacterium bovis*

Use

- recommended for Aboriginal and Torres Strait Islander neonates in high-risk areas, neonates born to parents with leprosy or with household contacts with leprosy; children travelling to settings with high tuberculosis (TB) prevalence or infants born to parents with high TB incidence (based on risk assessment)
- recommended for staff at high risk of TB (e.g. staff working in chest clinics, infectious diseases wards, physiotherapist, diagnostic laboratory staff, autopsy room staff, medical and nursing staff in public hospitals)
- treatment of in situ bladder cancer BCG (non-vaccine) (OncoTICE)

Dose

- 0.1 mL intradermally

Adverse effects

- local reaction of a small indurated red papule occurs in 1–3 weeks, which softens then ulcerates and heals over several weeks leaving superficial scar, lymphadenopathy
- (rare) keloid scarring, local or generalised infection, anaphylactoid reaction

Interactions

- response may be inhibited if given within 4–6 weeks of measles-containing vaccine or measles infection

Nursing points/Cautions

- tuberculin test (Mantoux test) is recommended before vaccination (unless under 6 months old) and vaccine given if induration is less than 5 mm with test dose of 10 units
- given intradermally using specialised tuberculin syringe

- those with latent or previous TB infection will have accelerated response to BCG
- does not prevent TB if patient is already infected, but reduces mortality
- not used in TB treatment
- re-vaccination is not recommended
- contains polysorbate 80 and is not recommended in those with known hypersensitivity to these
- contraindicated in people who have an immunodeficiency disorder or have had TB or a positive tuberculin reaction > 5 mm
- see general points for vaccines (pp. 1524–29)

Patient teaching and advice

- patient should be advised that small red lump will form and ulcerate in about 2–3 weeks after vaccination and will heal with a small scar. Swelling and tenderness under the arm also commonly occurs
- see General Patient teaching and advice for vaccines (p. 1527)

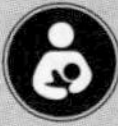

live vaccine, therefore not recommended in pregnancy

CHOLERA VACCINE (Dukoral)

Action

- protection against cholera (serogroup O1 *Vibrio cholerae*), which is one of the virulent strains of the disease
- not active against other species of cholera
- cholera is an acute diarrhoeal disease that can kill a person within hours if untreated with oral rehydration salts
- confers 85% protection for 4–6 months in all age groups

Use

- travellers to high-risk areas where cholera is endemic or the person is at high risk (e.g. immunocompromised)

Dose

- (adults, children > 6 years) 2 doses orally, at least 1 week apart **OR**
- (children 2–6 years) 3 doses orally, at least 1 week apart

Adverse effects

- (uncommon) diarrhoea, abdominal pain/cramps/discomfort, gas/gurgling
- (rare) nausea, vomiting

Interactions

- see General Interactions of vaccines (p. 1525)
- should be separated by at least 8 hours from oral typhoid vaccine

Nursing points/Cautions

- should be started at least 2 weeks before arrival at destination
- if more than 6 weeks elapse between doses, immunisation should be restarted
- offers protection for about 6 months after vaccination. Booster dose is recommended after 2 years for repeated travel or ongoing risk
- contains 1.1 g sodium/dose, which may need to be considered if patient requires sodium-/salt-restricted diet
- administration should be delayed if person has acute gastrointestinal illness
- not recommended for children under 2 years
- contraindicated in those with hypersensitivity to formaldehyde
- see General Nursing points/Cautions for vaccines (p. 1525)

Patient teaching and advice

- instruct patient to mix effervescent granules with 150 mL of cool water (buffer solution). Mix vaccine vial well and then add to buffer solution and drink. If patient is a child, half amount of cool water can be used
- advise patient to avoid food and drink for 1 hour before and after taking vaccine (because it is acid labile)

- patient should be warned to take care with selection of food and water while travelling in endemic areas
- see also General Patient teaching and advice for vaccines (p. 1527)

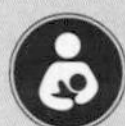

should only be given during pregnancy if benefits outweigh risks

COVID-19 VACCINE (Comirnaty, COVID-19 Vaccine AstraZeneca)

Action

- single stranded messenger RNA (mRNA) encoding the viral spike (S) protein of severe acute respiratory syndrome coronavirus 2 (SARS-CoV-2) (Comirnaty)
- monovalent vaccine recombinant adenovirus encoding the viral spike (S) protein of severe acute respiratory syndrome coronavirus 2 (SARS-CoV-2) (COVID-19 Vaccine AstraZeneca)

Use

- active immunisation to prevent coronavirus disease 2019 (COVID-19) caused by SARS-CoV-2

Dose

- 2 doses IM at least 21 days apart (Comirnaty) **OR**
- 2 doses IM given between 4 and 12 weeks apart (COVID-19 Vaccine AstraZeneca)

Adverse effects

- headache, fatigue, malaise
- pyrexia, chills
- nausea
- myalgia, arthralgia
- injection site tenderness, warmth, pain, swelling, redness
- (rare) hypersensitivity, anaphylaxis
- (COVID-19 Vaccine AstraZeneca) (very rare) thrombosis and thrombocytopenia with bleeding, including venous thrombosis

Nursing points/Cautions

- name and batch number should be recorded to assist traceability of vaccine
- antibody production does not interfere with SARS-CoV-2 PCR testing results
- preferred vaccination site is deltoid muscle of upper arm
- medical recommendations regarding preferred vaccine according to patient's age should be considered before vaccination
- (Comirnaty) stored frozen at –90°C to –60°C and thawed at 2–8°C prior to dilution
- (Comirnaty) thawed vial should be gently inverted (not shaken) 10 times before dilution, and again after dilution. Diluted vial should be marked with date and time of dilution and administered within 6 hours and any unused vaccine discarded after that time
- (COVID-19 Vaccine AstraZeneca) vials should be stored between 2°C and 8°C and not frozen
- (COVID-19 Vaccine AstraZeneca) contraindicated in those who have experienced major venous and/or arterial thrombosis in combination with thrombocytopenia after vaccination with any COVID-19 vaccine
- see General Nursing points/Cautions for vaccines (p. 1525)

Patient teaching

- paracetamol can be recommended to patient to provide relief from post-vaccination adverse reactions such as headache and fever
- (COVID-19 Vaccine AstraZeneca) advise patient that second dose adverse effects are milder than with first dose
- (COVID-19 Vaccine AstraZeneca) warn patient to seek medical advice immediately if any of the following occur:
  - severe or persistent headache
  - blurred vision

  - confusion, seizures
  - shortness of breath, chest pain
  - leg swelling or leg pain
  - persistent abdominal pain
  - unusual skin bruising and/or tiny purple/red/brown spots on skin
- see General Patient teaching and advice for vaccines (p. 1527)

DIPHTHERIA–TETANUS VACCINE (ADT Booster)

Action/Use

- re-vaccination of adults and children over 5 who have received at least 3 doses of vaccine for immunisation against diphtheria and tetanus
- tetanus prophylaxis after injury (see Tetanus-prone wounds p. 1566)

Adverse effects

- (injection site) redness, swelling
- headache, fever, lethargy, malaise, myalgia
- (rare) urticaria, peripheral neuropathy, anaphylaxis

Interactions/Nursing points/ Cautions/Patient teaching and advice

- given IM
- not recommended as primary immunisation
- laboratory workers should have serology tests for diphtheria antibody levels every 10 years and booster given if diphtheria antitoxin < 0.1 IU/mL
- caution if used in those with formaldehyde sensitivity
- see also general points for vaccines (pp. 1524–29)

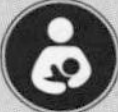

only used in pregnancy if benefits outweigh risks

DIPHTHERIA–TETANUS–PERTUSSIS (DTP) VACCINE (Adacel, Boostrix, Infanrix, Tripacel)

Action

- active immunisation against diphtheria, tetanus and pertussis (whooping cough)
- effect of diphtheria and tetanus vaccines is enhanced when administered with pertussis vaccine
- adult formulations provide lower diphtheria and pertussis antigens than formulations for children, which reduces risk of adverse effects

Use

- as primary immunisation in infants aged 2–12 months
- recommended in those over 10 years as a booster after primary immunisation

Adverse effects

- (injection site) pain, swelling, redness
- (children) crying, irritability, somnolence, extensive limb swelling, loss of appetite, diarrhoea, vomiting, headache
- fever, chills, body aches
- headache, lethargy, malaise
- nausea, diarrhoea
- myalgia
- (children, rare) febrile convulsion, hypotonic–hyporesponsive episodes (child becomes pale, limp and unresponsive)
- (rare) limb/joint swelling

Interactions

- see General Interactions of vaccines (p. 1525)

Nursing points/Cautions

- given by deep IM injection
- any reaction is likely to be caused by pertussis component and any further diphtheria–tetanus–pertussis or pertussis-only vaccines should be avoided

- diphtheria and tetanus toxoid-containing vaccines should be avoided within 5 years of previous booster dose to avoid risk of local adverse reactions
- paracetamol (15 mg/kg 3–4-hourly up to 4 times daily) can be given (at time of vaccination and for following 24 hours) to reduce febrile reaction if child has previously experienced febrile seizure post-vaccination, but is not routinely recommended
- (Boostrix, Adacel) not to be used as primary immunisation for those with no or incomplete primary immunisation
- not recommended if encephalopathy occurred after prior immunisation with pertussis-containing vaccine or neurological complications after diphtheria–tetanus–pertussis combination or in those with progressive or unstable neurological disorders, uncontrolled epilepsy or progressive encephalopathy until condition has stabilised
- contraindicated in those with allergy to formaldehyde or glutaral (glutaraldehyde)
- see also general points for vaccines (pp. 1524–29)

Patient teaching and advice

- parent should be advised that limb swelling occurs commonly in children, especially after fourth dose. Swelling can be extensive, as well as redness and pain, and usually occurs within 48 hours of vaccination and may last for 1–7 days
- see General Patient teaching and advice for vaccines (p. 1527)

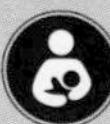

vaccination is not recommended during pregnancy unless there is a definite risk of acquiring pertussis. Risk of administration should be weighed up against risk of disease

Note

- contained in Infanrix Hexa with hepatitis B vaccine and Haemophilus influenza type B vaccine
- contained in Adacel Polio, Boostrix-IPV, Infanrix-IPV and Quadacel with poliomyelitis vaccine

HAEMOPHILUS INFLUENZAE TYPE B VACCINE (Act-HIB, Hiberix)

Action/Use

- immunisation against *Haemophilus influenzae* type B (Hib) in infants and children between 2 months and 5 years

Dose

- (Hiberix) 3 doses given IM at 2, 4 and 6 months, with booster recommended at 12 months **OR**
- (Act-HIB) (2–6 months) 3 doses IM at 1–2 month intervals, (7–11 months) 2 doses IM at 1–2 month intervals, followed by booster at 18 months, (> 12 months) 1 dose IM

Adverse effects

- (injection site reaction) pain, swelling
- vomiting, prolonged crying, irritability, unusual tiredness, runny nose, cough, otitis media, conjunctivitis, fever, rash, loss of appetite, diarrhoea

Interactions/Nursing points/ Cautions/Patient teaching and advice

- does not protect against all strains of *Haemophilus*
- see general points for vaccines (pp. 1520–29)

Note

- combined with hepatitis B and poliomyelitis in Infanrix Hexa and with hepatitis B, poliomyelitis and Haemophilus B in Hexaxim

HEPATITIS A VACCINE (Avaxim, Havrix 1440, Havrix Junior, VAQTA Adult Formula)

Action

- inactivated hepatitis A virus
- hepatitis A is a highly contagious disease that is generally spread via faecal-oral route through contact with contaminated food and/or water or direct contact with an infectious person

Use

- for use in susceptible people over the age of 2 years at risk of exposure to hepatitis A virus (e.g. travellers to endemic areas, occupational risk, lifestyle risk factors, medical risk factors, Aboriginal and Torres Strait Island children)

Dose

- usually given as a single dose IM

Adverse effects

- (local reaction) pain, redness, swelling, induration, haematoma
- headache, malaise, fatigue, fever, asthenia
- diarrhoea, loss of appetite, nausea, vomiting
- (uncommon) rash, myalgia, arthralgia

Interactions/Nursing points/ Cautions/Patient teaching and advice

- if person has had previous hepatitis or unexplained jaundice, was born before 1950 or lived childhood in endemic area, vaccination may not be required. Screening is recommended
- should be given 2 weeks before expected exposure
- immunity occurs after about 4 weeks and persists for up to 12 months and may be reinforced by booster dose given 6–36 months after initial vaccination
- does not protect against other strains of hepatitis
- not given IV or intradermally
- (Avaxim) caution if used in those with hypersensitivity to neomycin or formaldehyde
- (Havrix) caution if used in those with hypersensitivity to neomycin
- (Havrix, VAQTA) available in both an adult (≥ 16 years) and a paediatric (2–15 years) formulation
- see general points for vaccines (pp. 1524–29)

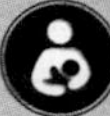
should only be used during pregnancy if clearly needed

Note

- combined with hepatitis B in Twinrix vaccine and with typhoid fever in Vivaxim vaccine (recommended for patients > 16 years)

HEPATITIS B VACCINE (Engerix-B, H-B-Vax II)

Action

- recombinant DNA hepatitis B vaccine that causes seroconversion in 97–99% of normal adults
- will not protect against other hepatitis viruses such as A, C or E

Use

- recommended in those with chronic liver impairment or transplantation, hepatitis C, post-exposure prophylaxis or other susceptible groups (including high-risk occupational groups, infants born to hepatitis B-positive mothers, susceptible sexual contacts, injecting drug users)

Dose

- (adult) 3 doses IM at 0, 1- and 6-month intervals **OR**

- (infants) 4 doses IM at birth, and 2, 4 and 6 months

Adverse effects

- (injection site) redness, swelling, pain
- fever, headache, drowsiness, irritability, fatigue
- loss of appetite, nausea, vomiting, diarrhoea, abdominal pain
- (uncommon) myalgia
- (rare) lymphadenopathy

Interactions/Nursing points/Cautions/Patient teaching and advice

- will not prevent disease if infection was already present when vaccination occurred (long incubation period) or if protective antibody titres are not achieved
- available in both adult and paediatric formulations. Paediatric formulation can be used in young adults ≤ 20 years (Energix-B)
- antibody titres should be measured after primary course in those at high occupational risk, at high risk of serious disease, household contacts or where response is expected to be poor
- reduced response may occur in those > 40 years, male, smokers or those who are obese
- if more rapid protection is required (e.g. travel to endemic area within 4 weeks), vaccination may be given at 0, 7 and 21 days (adult)
- (low birthweight (< 2000 g) and preterm infants (< 32 weeks regardless of weight) doses as per infants (above) plus booster at 12 months **OR** surface antigen measured at 7 months and booster given if level is < 10 IU/mL
- neonates should be vaccinated within 24 hours of birth (and no later than 7 days).
- if neonate is born of hepatitis B-positive mother, hepatitis B immunoglobulin should also be given within 12 hours of birth as efficacy decreases if given after 48 hours
- booster doses are recommended in immunocompromised people (especially if HIV positive) or dialysis-dependent. Antibody levels should be measured every 6–12 months
- for post-exposure prophylaxis, vaccine should be given within 7 days of exposure and then course completed as usual. Hepatitis B immunoglobulin should be given within 72 hours of exposure (and in different limb if administered at the same time)
- larger doses may be required in those with renal failure due to impaired immune response
- HIV infection is not a contraindication to vaccine
- see also general points for vaccines (pp. 1524–29)

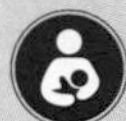
not recommended during pregnancy unless benefits outweigh risks

Note

- combined with hepatitis A in Twinrix and Haemophilus influenzae, DTP and poliomyelitis vaccines in Infanrix Hexa and Hexaxim

HUMAN PAPILLOMAVIRUS (HPV) VACCINE (Cervarix, Gardasil-9)

Action

- persistent infection with HPV appears to be primary cause of cervical cancer and most precursor lesions with HPV types 16 and 18 being responsible for about 70% of cervical cancers worldwide
- contains recombinant virus-like particles which are not capable of causing

infection as they are not viruses and not able to reproduce

Use

- prophylactic vaccine against several strains (HPV types 6, 11, 16, 18, 31, 33, 45, 52, 58 (Gardasil-9) or HPV types 16 and 18 (Cervarix)) of human papillomavirus thought to be responsible for persistent infection, pre-malignant lesions, genital warts, cervical, vaginal, vulval and anal cancers
- (males, 9–26 years) prevention of anal cancer, pre-malignant or dysplastic lesions, external genital lesions caused by HPV types 6, 11, 16, 18, 31, 33, 45, 52, 58 (Gardasil-9)

Dose

- 3 doses given IM at 0, 2- and 6-month intervals (Gardisil-9) **OR**
- (10–14 years) 2 doses given IM at 0 then 5–13 months after (Gardisil-9, Cervarix) **OR**
- (15–45 years) 3 doses given IM at 0, 1- and 6-month intervals (Cervarix)

Adverse effects

- (injection site reaction) pain, redness, swelling, bruising
- arthralgia, myalgia,
- fatigue, headache, dizziness
- nausea, vomiting, abdominal pain, diarrhoea
- rash, urticaria, pruritus
- fever

Interactions/Nursing points/ Cautions/Patient teaching and advice

- most effective if given before sexually active
- regular cytological screening (every 5 years for women aged 25–70 years) is still recommended as vaccine does not protect against cancer
- will not protect against diseases not caused by HPV or if established lesions are present
- (Gardasil) vaccine is not recommended for treatment of active genital lesions, cervical, vulval, vaginal or anal cancers
- see also general points for vaccines (pp. 1524–29)

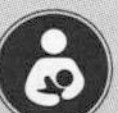

women who are pregnant or trying to become pregnant should postpone vaccination

INFLUENZA VACCINE (Afluria Quad, Fluad, Fluad Quad, Fluarix Tetra, FluQuadri, Influvac Tetra, Vaxigrip Tetra)

Action

- prevents influenza caused by influenza virus types A and B
- vaccine is composed of two current influenza A subtypes and influenza B, representing recently circulating viruses (in Australia, these tend to be those circulating in the European winter season) with composition being revised annually
- protection occurs within 2–3 weeks and lasts for 6–12 months

Use

- prevention of influenza type A and B
- recommended for everyone aged over 6 years, but particularly those aged ≥ 65 years, all Aboriginal and Torres Strait Islander people, children aged 6 months to 5 years, pregnant or breastfeeding women, people with medical conditions increasing their risk of influenza (e.g. being immunocompromised, chronic medical conditions, chronic liver or kidney failure, chronic alcohol misuse, obesity), occupational groups (e.g. healthcare workers, carers, staff, volunteers and visitors to long-term or aged care facilities, essential

services providers), residents of long-term or aged care facilities, those travelling during influenza season and homeless people

Dose

- 1 dose annually **OR**
- (children under 9 years and over 6 months receiving first influenza vaccine, first influenza vaccine after solid organ or stem cell transplant) 2 doses annually 4 weeks apart

Adverse effects

- (injection site reaction) pain, redness, swelling, induration
- fever, malaise, fatigue, headache, sweating, shivering
- myalgia, arthralgia
- (rare) allergic reaction

Interactions

- may cause false positive serological test for hepatitis C
- see General Interactions of vaccines (p. 1525)

Nursing points/Cautions

- vaccination usually recommended from autumn before the start of the influenza season
- (Afluria Quad, Fluarix Tetra, Fluad Quad, FluQuadri, Influvac Tetra, Vaxigrip Tetra) provide protection against 4 strains (two A subtypes and two B subtypes)
- (Influvac Tetra) recommended in children aged 3 years and over
- (Vaxigrip Tetra) caution if used in those with hypersensitivity to neomycin or formaldehyde
- (Fluad, Fluad Quad) recommended for patients aged 65 years and over
- not recommended in those who developed Guillain-Barre syndrome within 6 weeks of previous influenza vaccination
- (Afluria Quad) contraindicated in children under 5 years
- (Influvac Tetra) contraindicated in those with hypersensitivity to formaldehyde, gentamicin, cetrimonium or polysorbate 80
- (all influenza preparations) contraindicated in those with hypersensitivity to eggs or chicken feathers
- see also General Nursing points/Cautions for vaccines (p. 1525)

Patient/staff teaching and advice

- all healthcare workers who have direct patient contact should be vaccinated against influenza on a yearly basis. This is not just to protect the healthcare worker against influenza but to prevent transmission of influenza to patients, particularly those who are elderly or immunosuppressed, for whom influenza can be fatal, as was seen in the influenza pandemic of 1918 when almost 23 million people died worldwide (more than died as a result of the First World War, which had just finished)
- unfortunately, many myths surround the influenza vaccine and influenza itself and people (healthcare workers among them) often confuse the 'common cold' with true influenza
- influenza vaccine cannot give anyone the 'flu'. It may give the person a sore arm, mild fever or muscle ache, but it does not give anyone the flu or a cold
- influenza vaccine does not protect against coughs, colds or any other viral diseases, nor from influenza caused by strains not contained in the vaccine. The person is also not protected if they are incubating influenza at the time of immunisation
- influenza vaccine is only effective for that year, because each year a new vaccine is developed from the most common influenza strains from the previous winter (e.g. in Australia the vaccine contains the most common

influenza strains from the previous northern hemisphere winter)

- influenza is not just the common cold, is highly contagious and is spread by direct contact with respiratory secretions or respiratory aerosol droplets (i.e. coughing and sneezing)
- influenza incubation period is usually 1–3 days
- influenza symptoms vary from mild-to-severe illness lasting for 7–10 days, high fever, loss of appetite, malaise, chills and shivering, muscle pains, need for bed rest, dry sensation in the nose and throat initially, severe headache and dry cough that may become moist; pneumonia may be a secondary bacterial complication
- common cold symptoms include symptoms that last for 1–2 days generally, mild fever (if at all), no muscle pain, runny nose and sneezing, mild headache, which is generally because of congested sinuses, cough with mild or no complications
- management of influenza includes bed rest until temperature has returned to normal, drinking plenty of fluids and using paracetamol to control fever, aches and pains. If cough worsens or phlegm becomes green/yellow or breathing becomes difficult, a doctor should be consulted

JAPANESE ENCEPHALITIS VIRUS VACCINE (Imojev, Jespect)

Action

- live attenuated virus vaccine (Imojev) or adsorbed inactivated virus vaccine (Jespect)
- does not protect against other forms of encephalitis

Use

- usually given to people who plan to live in or travel to areas where Japanese encephalitis is endemic or epidemic during the transmission season (e.g. workers who work in the outer Torres Strait Islands for a total of 30 days or more during the wet season)
- laboratory workers with potential exposure to infected material

Dose

- 2 doses given IM 28 days apart (Jespect) **OR**
- single SC dose (Imojev)

Adverse effects

- (injection site) redness, swelling, bruising, pruritus, pain
- diarrhoea, nausea, vomiting, abdominal pain
- dyspnoea, runny nose, cough, wheezing, nasal congestion, pharyngeal pain
- fatigue, malaise, headache, dizziness, feeling hot, chills
- myalgia, arthralgia

Interactions/Nursing points/ Cautions

- should be given at least 14 days before exposure (adults) or 28 days (children) (Imojev) or 7 days (Jespect)
- (Imojev) booster given at 12–24 months (if under 18 years) or 5 years (if > 18 years) if risk is ongoing
- immunity last for at least 5 years (adults) or 3 years (children) (Imojev) or 12 months (Jespect)
- Japanese encephalitis virus during second or third trimester has been associated with miscarriage
- contraindicated in those with immunodeficiency disorders, including HIV
- see general points for vaccines (pp. 1524–29)

Patient teaching and advice

- patient should be advised to avoid mosquito bites while travelling in endemic areas by using insect repellent, protective clothing and mosquito netting and also avoiding

outdoor activities during twilight or in the evening
- female patients of childbearing age should be advised to avoid pregnancy for 28 days after vaccination (Imojev)
- see also General Patient teaching and advice for vaccines (p. 1527)

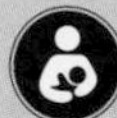

contraindicated during pregnancy and breastfeeding (Imojev)

not recommended during pregnancy unless benefits outweigh risks (Jespect)

MEASLES-MUMPS-RUBELLA (MMR) VACCINE (MMRII, Priorix)

Action
- live attenuated virus

Use
- active immunisation against measles, mumps and rubella

Dose
- (child) dose SC or IM at 12 months with booster at 4–6 years **OR**
- (adult with no immunity) 1 dose IM or SC

Adverse effects
- (injection site) redness, pain, swelling
- headache, fever, rash
- pharyngitis, bronchitis, rhinitis, cough, otitis media, upper respiratory tract infection
- vomiting, diarrhoea
- (uncommon) parotid swelling
- (rare) febrile seizures, arthralgia, lymphadenopathy

Interactions
- measles virus inhibits tuberculin skin response. Mantoux test may be unreliable for 4–6 weeks after vaccination
- see General Interactions of vaccines (p. 1525)

Nursing points/Cautions
- limited protection if vaccination is given within 72 hours of contact with measles (and no protection against contact with mumps or rubella in this timeframe)
- non-immune pregnant women should be vaccinated post-partum
- may be given to asymptomatic HIV infected people (however, it should be noted that immunisation is less effective in this group)
- caution if used in those with history of convulsions or cerebral injury where fever should be avoided
- contraindicated if used in those with untreated TB as condition may be exacerbated
- contraindicated in those with hypersensitivity to eggs and chicken feathers, history of allergic diseases or neomycin (but not contact dermatitis due to neomycin)
- see also general points for vaccines (pp. 1524–29)

Patient teaching and advice
- parents should be warned that children may experience fever 7–10 days after vaccination, which may be accompanied by non-infectious rash and/or a general feeling of being unwell. Paracetamol may be given to manage fever
- female patient of childbearing age should be advised to avoid pregnancy for a month after vaccination

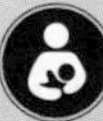

women of childbearing potential should be tested for rubella antibodies before pregnancy and if negative and not pregnant, should be offered rubella vaccine and instructed to avoid pregnancy for 3 months

contraindicated during pregnancy, and pregnancy should be avoided for at least 1 month after vaccination

Note
- contained in Priorix-Tetra and Pro-Quad with varicella zoster virus vaccine

MENINGOCOCCAL VACCINE (Bexsero, Menactra, Menveo, NeisVac-C, Nimenrix, Trumenba)

Action
- meningococcal disease is caused by *Neisseria meningitidis* (meningococcus) with serogroups A, B, C, W 135 and Y the most likely cause of disease (Serogroup B causes the most cases in Australia)
- vaccine against groups A, C, W135 and Y *N. meningitidis* (meningococcus) (Menactra, Menveo, Trumenba)
- vaccine against group C *N. meningitidis* (meningococcus) (NeisVac-C)
- vaccine against group B *N. meningitidis* (meningococcus) (Bexsero, Trumenba)

Use
- infants, children, adolescents and young adults (especially smokers and those who live in close contact with each other (e.g. student accommodation, new military recruits)), travellers where disease is endemic, laboratory workers frequently handling specimens, those with medical risk factors increasing risk of invasive meningococcal disease
- inherited disease of properdin or factor H or D deficiency, HIV, stem cell transplantation, asplenia (functional or anatomical), treatment with eculizumab), Aboriginal and Torres Strait Islander people
- controlling epidemic caused by *N. meningitides* in confined communities

Adverse effects
- (injection site) tenderness, redness, pain, swelling
- fever, chills, sleepiness, irritability, malaise, fatigue, headache, unusual crying
- nausea, vomiting, changes in appetite
- rash
- myalgia, arthralgia
- (Bexsero) fever (highest 6 hours after vaccination, decreasing by day 2)

Interactions/Nursing points/ Cautions
- not recommended for treatment of meningococcal infection or meningitis caused by other organisms
- given IM
- (Menactra, Menveo) caution in those with Guillain-Barre syndrome
- (Menveo) contraindicated in those with latex hypersensitivity or diphtheria-containing vaccines
- (NeisVac-C) contraindicated in those with known hypersensitivity to tetanus toxoid
- see also general points for vaccines (pp. 1524–29)

Patient teaching and advice
- (Bexsero) parents should be advised that children under 2 can be given paracetamol (15 mg/kg) prophylactically with each dose of vaccine, either 30 minutes before or as soon as practicable after injection. Two more doses of paracetamol can be given 6 hours apart (ATAGI 2018)

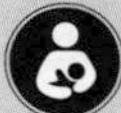
not recommended during pregnancy unless benefits outweigh risks

PNEUMOCOCCAL VACCINE (Pneumovax 23, Prevenar 13)

Action

- polysaccharide (Pneumovax 23) or conjugate (Prevenar 13)
- polyvalent vaccine covering most prevalent or invasive pneumococcal species (*Streptococcus pneumoniae*)
- number of species is dependent on formulation (e.g. Pneumovax 23 covers 23 species)

Use

- active immunisation in adults and children over 6 weeks for prevention of pneumococcal disease (Prevenar 13)
- prevention of pneumococcal disease in those aged over 65 years, immunocompromised, Aboriginal and Torres Islander people over 50 years, with asplenia or CSF leak, or at risk from pneumococcal disease complications (e.g. diabetes, alcohol dependence, heart, kidney and lung disease, smokers) (Pneumovax 23)

Adverse effects

- (injection site) redness, swelling, pain/tenderness, induration
- fever, chills, drowsiness, irritability, headache, fatigue
- rash
- diarrhoea, vomiting, loss of appetite
- (premature infants ≤ 30 weeks gestation) sleep apnoea

Interactions

- not recommended with zoster vaccine (Zostavax) as it may decrease responsiveness of zoster vaccine (Pneumovax 23)
- see General Interactions of vaccines (p. 1525)

Nursing points/Cautions/Patient teaching and advice

- does not prevent diseases caused by other capsular types of pneumococcus
- should be given 2 weeks before splenectomy or immunosuppressant therapy (including bone marrow transplantation) or as soon as possible after diagnosis of HIV
- (premature infants ≤ 30 weeks gestation) infants should be closely monitored for 48–72 hours after vaccination
- protection lasts for 5–10 years
- (Pneumovax 23) caution if used in those with severely compromised cardiac and/or respiratory function
- see general points for vaccines (pp. 1524–29)

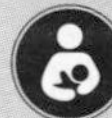

not recommended during pregnancy unless clearly needed

POLIOMYELITIS VACCINE (Ipol)

Action

- inactivated polio virus (IPV)
- vaccine against the three types of polio virus
- oral polio vaccine is no longer used in Australia
- Australia was declared polio-free in 2000; however, wild polio virus can be imported from countries where it is still endemic

Use

- all infants, unimmunised children and adolescents not previously vaccinated or those where oral polio vaccine was refused or contraindicated
- travellers to countries where poliomyelitis is epidemic or endemic
- healthcare workers (who may come into contact with those who might be excreting poliovirus) or laboratory workers (who may handle specimens)

Dose

- (child > 6 years) 3 doses SC with a 2-month interval between each

dose and the fourth dose at 4 years
OR

- (adult) 3 doses SC at 1–2 month intervals (if unvaccinated) or remaining doses (if partially vaccinated)

Adverse effects

- (injection site) redness, pain, induration
- fever, irritability, drowsiness
- diarrhoea, vomiting

Interactions/Nursing points/ Cautions/Patient teaching and advice

- booster dose not required in adults unless at high risk (e.g. travelling to endemic area, laboratory workers, healthcare workers)
- contraindicated in those with hypersensitivity to formaldehyde, neomycin, streptomycin or polymyxin B
- see also general points for vaccines (pp. 1524–29)

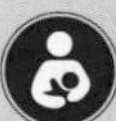

not recommended during pregnancy unless clearly needed

Note

- contained in Adacel Polio, Boostrix-IPV, Infanrix Hexa, Hexaxim, Infanrix-IPV and Quadracel

Q FEVER (COXIELLA BURNETI) VACCINE (Q-Vax)

Available forms

Prefilled syringe: 25 microgram/0.5 mL (vaccine); Prefilled vial: 2.5 microgram/mL (skin test)

Action

- protects against infection by *Coxiella burnetii* which causes Q fever
- transmitted from both wild and domesticated animals, including sheep, cattle, goats, kangaroos, feral camels and cats
- infection is via inhalation of infected aerosol or dust
- vaccination during incubation period does not prevent onset of disease

Use

- recommended for those susceptible to Q fever (e.g. abattoir workers, veterinarians, veterinary nurses, veterinary students, laboratory workers, goat, cattle, sheep and dairy farmers, shearers, livestock transporters or sale yard workers, professional cat and dog breeders, agricultural college staff and students, wildlife and zoo workers working with high-risk animals, animal refuge workers)
- skin test for pre-testing for previous sensitisation to Q fever antigens

Adverse effects

- (local reaction) redness, tenderness, induration
- headache, fever, chills, minor sweating
- delayed skin reaction (up to 6 months after vaccination at either test or injection site)
- (uncommon) nausea, vomiting, diarrhoea

Interactions/Nursing points/ Cautions/Patient teaching and advice

- before vaccination, patient should be questioned regarding any prior possible exposure to Q fever and duration of any such illness
- risk of Q fever is greatest in first year of exposure, therefore vaccination should be given as soon as possible after starting employment
- serum antibody levels and a skin test are recommended before vaccination to prevent serious hypersensitivity reactions from occurring
- (skin test) skin testing and interpretation should only be done by immunisation providers who are trained to administer Q fever skin testing. The

site is read after 7 days and any induration is considered positive and the vaccine should therefore not be given
- re-vaccination is not recommended because of risk of severe hypersensitivity reaction
- contraindicated in those with history of or previous vaccination to Q fever, history of likely exposure to or symptoms of Q fever, positive serology or skin test for Q fever or hypersensitivity to egg proteins
- see also general points for vaccines (pp. 1524–29)

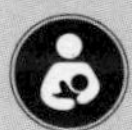

effects in pregnancy not established, therefore vaccination should be deferred

RABIES VACCINE (Merieux Inactivated Rabies Vaccine, Rabipur)

Action
- rabies is almost always fatal
- inactivated rabies vaccine against zoonotic disease caused by exposure of saliva or nerve tissue of infected animal (e.g. animal scratch, direct contact to mucosal surface (e.g. lick))

Use
- post-exposure to the rabies virus
- prophylaxis for those who work with animals (e.g. veterinarians, veterinary students or veterinary nurses – depending on animals they come in contact with) or those who come into regular contact with bats (both 'flying foxes' and microbats), bat handlers, bat scientists, wildlife officers and zoo curators, as well as laboratory personnel who handle bat tissues or lyssaviruses
- prophylaxis for travellers to rabies-enzootic regions based on risk assessment

Dose
- (primary immunisation) 3 deep SC or IM injections at days 0, 7 and 21 or 28 **OR**
- (post-exposure with no previous vaccination) 4 deep SC or IM injection at days 0, 3, 7 and 14 and a booster at days 30 and 90 (to maintain antibody levels). If infection is severe, 20 IU/kg human rabies immunoglobulin should also be given on day 0 (Merieux) **OR**
- (post-exposure, previously immunised with demonstrated antibodies) 2 deep SC or IM injection at day 0 and 3 (Merieux) **OR**
- (post-exposure, previously immunised) IM injection at day 0 and 3 (Rabipur) **OR**
- (post-exposure with no previous vaccination or at high risk of rabies, e.g. multiple bites/scratches) IM injection at days 0, 3, 7, 14 and 28, or 2 IM injections on day 0 (one in each deltoid muscle) followed by single injections on days 7 and 21. Human rabies immunoglobulin (20 IU/kg) should be given with first dose if infection is severe (Rabipur)

Adverse effects
- (local reaction) redness, swelling, tenderness, induration, pruritus, bruising
- fever, headache, dizziness, fatigue, malaise
- arthralgia, myalgia
- rash
- nausea, abdominal pain, decreased appetite

Interactions
- anti-rabies immunoglobulin may decrease response to vaccine
- see also General Interactions of vaccines (p. 1525)

Nursing points/Cautions
- immediate first aid treatment should include cleaning area with soap and copious amounts of water and then

applying 70% alcohol or iodine-containing antiseptic/disinfectant
- suturing bite(s) is not recommended
- deltoid should be used rather than buttock (as vaccine failure has been reported using this site)
- tetanus prophylaxis is also recommended post-exposure
- vaccination should be stopped if animal remains healthy for 10 days or the animal is euthanised humanely and found to be negative for rabies
- booster is recommended in those with ongoing risk (e.g. veterinarians, wildlife workers) if antibody level falls below 0.5 IU/mL
- antibody levels should be tested 6-monthly for those where risk remains high (e.g. laboratory workers) or every 2 years in those who are at continuing risk of exposure (e.g. veterinarians, wildlife workers)
- (Merieux) contains albumin
- (Merieux) contraindicated in those with hypersensitivity to neomycin
- (Rabipur) (as pre-exposure prophylaxis) contraindicated in those with hypersensitivity to neomycin or bovine gelatin, egg or chicken proteins, chlortetracycline and amphotericin B (amphotericin)
- see also general points for vaccines (pp. 1524–29)

Patient teaching and advice

- travellers should be given advice about avoiding contact with bats, wild and domestic animals (including feeding and patting monkeys at tourist spots such as temples). Travellers should also be discouraged from carrying food and they should be aware of immediate first aid measures if contact or injury occurs. Parents travelling with children should be given advice about the increased risk in children of facial injuries because of their height and the importance of discouraging children to pat or touch animals
- (Merieux) inform patient that any product prepared from human blood or plasma (such as albumin) has the potential for transmission of blood-borne viral or prion diseases (e.g. Creutzfeldt-Jakob disease), although stringent procedures now exist for careful selection of blood donors and removal and inactivation of known enveloped viruses from blood products (e.g. HIV, hepatitis B and C) and non-enveloped viruses (e.g. hepatitis A)

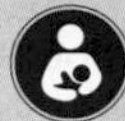

benefits of use in pregnancy clearly outweigh risks for post-exposure situation

ROTAVIRUS VACCINE (Rotarix Oral Liquid)

Action
- live attenuated virus vaccine
- rotavirus infection commonly occurs in children under 5 years, especially between 6 and 24 months causing sudden vomiting and diarrhoea

Use
- prevention of rotavirus gastroenteritis which can lead to dehydration and hospitalisation in infants < 6 months

Dose
- 2 oral doses at 2 and 4 months of age

Adverse effects
- vomiting, loss of appetite, diarrhoea
- fever, irritability
- cough, runny nose
- (rare) intussusception

Interactions
- see General Interactions of vaccines (p. 1525)

Nursing points/Cautions

- administered orally inside infant's cheek directly from tube with no dilution needed
- dose should **not** be readministered if infant spits or regurgitates the dose
- vaccination should be postponed if infant has moderate-to-severe vomiting or diarrhoea
- does not protect against gastroenteritis due to other pathogens
- not recommended in infants > 24 weeks
- contraindicated in those with chronic gastrointestinal history, including uncorrected gastrointestinal congenital malformation that might lead to intussusception, intussusception or combined immunodeficiency disorder
- see also General Nursing points/Cautions for vaccines (p. 1525)

Parent teaching and advice

- parent/carer should be advised to immediately report if child experiences any abdominal pain or distress, persistent vomiting, blood in stools (bowel motions), high fever and/or bloated stomach
- see General Patient teaching and advice for vaccines (p. 1527)

TYPHOID (SALMONELLA TYPHI) VACCINE (Typhim Vi, Vivotif (Oral))

Action

- live attenuated typhoid vaccine
- typhoid fever is spread via faecally contaminated food and water

Use

- active immunisation against typhoid fever caused by *Salmonella typhi* and recommended for military personnel, travellers (≥ 2 years) going to typhoid-endemic areas and laboratory workers routinely working with *S. typhi*

Dose

- 1 capsule on days 1, 3 and 5 **OR**
- 25 microgram IM

Adverse effects

- (IM) (common) local site reaction (tenderness/pain, redness, induration) headache, nausea, malaise, fever
- (oral) (uncommon) diarrhoea, constipation, nausea, vomiting, loss of appetite, abdominal cramps, fever, headache, rash
- (rare) allergic reaction

Interactions

- (oral) not recommended with antimalarials or sulfonamides that may be active against *Salmonella* spp. A 3-day gap should be allowed between vaccination and the administration of these agents
- (oral) should be given at least 8 hours apart from oral cholera vaccine
- see General Interactions of vaccines (p. 1525)

Nursing points/Cautions

- IM dose should be given 2 weeks before expected exposure
- repeat vaccination is recommended 2–3-yearly in those who have continued or repeated exposure
- (Typhim Vi) contains traces of formaldehyde, therefore should be given with caution in anyone with a formaldehyde sensitivity
- see also general points for vaccines (pp. 1524–29)

Patient teaching and advice

- advise patient to swallow capsules whole, not chewed or crushed, and take 1 hour before meals with cold or lukewarm (not hot) drink or food
- female patients of childbearing age should be counselled to avoid pregnancy for 12 weeks after vaccination

- see General Patient teaching and advice for vaccines (p. 1527)

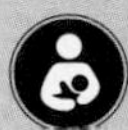

not recommended during pregnancy and pregnancy should be avoided for 12 weeks after vaccination

Note

- combined with hepatitis A in Vivaxim vaccine

VARICELLA ZOSTER VACCINES (Varilrix, Varivax Refrigerated, Zostavax)

Action

- live attenuated vaccine given as active immunisation against varicella zoster
- herpes zoster (shingles) is a reactivation of varicella zoster virus with primary infection producing chicken pox
- post-herpetic neuralgia (PHN) is a serious complication of herpes zoster viral infection and can persist long after rash appearance
- (Varilrix, Varivax Refrigerated) varicella vaccine
- (Zostavax) zoster vaccine

Use

- (varicella vaccine) non-immune adults in at-risk occupations, non-immune parents of young children and non-immune household contacts of immunocompromised patient with no history of disease
- (zoster vaccine) prevention of herpes zoster in those > 50 years
- (zoster vaccine) prevention of postherpetic neuralgia and reduction of pain associated with varicella zoster (shingles) (> 60 years)

Dose

- 2 doses SC 4 weeks apart (Varilrix, Varivax Refrigerated) **OR**
- single dose SC (Zostavax)

Adverse effects

- (injection site) pain, swelling, redness, swelling, pruritus, induration, haematoma
- (varicella vaccine) mild vesicular rash (within 5–26 days of vaccination), fever, rash, pruritus
- (zoster vaccine) headache, fatigue, pain in extremity

Interactions

- salicylates (e.g. aspirin) should not be given for 6 weeks after vaccination due to increased risk of Reye's syndrome (Varilrix)
- zoster vaccine is not recommended concurrently with inactivated influenza vaccine
- antiviral medication may interfere with vaccine, therefore should be stopped for at least 24 hours before vaccination and withheld for at least 14 days after
- see General Interactions of vaccines (p. 1525)

Nursing points/Cautions

- varicella vaccine and zoster vaccine are not interchangeable
- (varicella vaccine) can prevent infection if given with 5 days of exposure (preferably within 3 days). Some contacts may require immunoglobulin
- (zoster vaccine) protection for about 4–5 years
- (zoster vaccine) efficacy of vaccine decreases with age with prevention of shingles (64% in 60–69 year group, compared to 38% in those over 70 years)
- (zoster vaccine) reduces post-herpetic neuralgia in over 66% of those aged 60 years and over
- zoster vaccination is not currently recommended for those who have received varicella vaccine
- after vaccination, avoid contact with susceptible individuals for up to

6 weeks (i.e. those who are immunocompromised)
- (Zostavax) not recommended in children or as treatment for post-herpetic neuralgia or zoster varicella (shingles)
- contraindicated in those with active untreated TB
- contraindicated in those with hypersensitivity to neomycin (not contact dermatitis)
- see also general points for vaccines (pp. 1524–29)

Patient teaching and advice

- female patients of childbearing age should be counselled to avoid pregnancy for 12 weeks after vaccination
- see General Patient teaching and advice for vaccines (p. 1527)

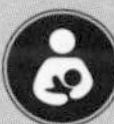

contraindicated during pregnancy and pregnancy should be avoided for 12 weeks after vaccination

Notes

- contained in Priorix-Tetra and ProQuad with measles, mumps and rubella

YELLOW FEVER VACCINE (Stamaril)

Action

- live attenuated virus vaccine for active immunisation against yellow fever
- immunity appears 7–10 days after vaccination and lasts for at least 10 years

Use

- prevention of yellow fever in those living or travelling through endemic areas or laboratory workers handling infected material

Adverse effects

- (injection site reaction) pain, tenderness, redness, induration, swelling, haematoma
- fever, headache, asthenia
- myalgia
- nausea, vomiting
- rash
- (very rare) yellow fever vaccine-associated viscerotropic disease (fever, fatigue, myalgia, headache, hypotension, metabolic acidosis, muscle and liver cytolysis, lymphocytopenia, thrombocytopenia, renal failure, respiratory failure), yellow fever vaccine-associated neurotropic disease (high fever, headache, confusion, encephalopathy, meningitis and seizures)

Interactions

- not recommended within 4 weeks of cholera or typhoid vaccines (unless given at the same time into different sites)
- can cause false positive results for other flaviviruses (e.g. dengue, Japanese encephalitis)
- may be given at same time as Japanese encephalitis vaccine (in separate sites)
- see General Interactions of vaccines (p. 1525)

Nursing points/Cautions

- given SC or IM
- immunity appears in 14–28 days after vaccination and lasts for at least 10 years (may be lifelong)
- must be given by approved vaccination centre and registered on international certificate, which is valid for 10 years
- reconstituted using sodium chloride 0.4%
- caution if used in those > 60 years or with thymus disease as there is an increased risk of yellow fever-associated viscerotropic disease

- contains lactose and sorbitol and therefore contraindicated in those with fructose intolerance
- contraindicated in infants under 6 months due to risk of encephalitis
- contraindicated in those who have an allergy to egg or egg proteins or with thymus disorders (e.g. myasthenia gravis)
- see also general points for vaccines (pp. 1524–29)

Patient teaching and advice

- instruct patient to seek medical advice immediately if any of the following occur:
  - fever, fatigue, myalgia or headache occur within 10 days of vaccination
  - high fever, headache, confusion, stiff neck, fitting (seizures) within 30 days of vaccination
- yellow fever is transmitted by mosquitoes, therefore patient should be encouraged to use insect spray, protective clothing and mosquito nets while sleeping to avoid mosquito bites while in endemic areas
- see General Patient teaching and advice for vaccines (p. 1527)

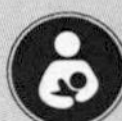

contraindicated during pregnancy and breastfeeding unless benefits outweigh risks

ANTIVENOMS

General Actions of antivenoms

- snake antivenom is produced by 'milking' venom from the snake and then injecting small quantities repeatedly into horses over 10–12 months. Blood is then removed and the plasma containing antibodies extracted and purified
- monovalent snake antivenom is produced against a single snake (or related) species and a smaller dose is usually required to neutralise the venom. It is, however, important to identify the snake species. It is important to note that many Australian snakes are protected species and should not be killed
- polyvalent snake antivenom is useful for a broad range of snake species; however, larger doses are required to neutralise the venom
- spider bites generally cause less mortality than snake bites
- spider antivenom is produced in a similar way to snake antivenom, but in different animal species (rabbit, sheep)
- administration of repeated or large dose (> 1 vial) has not been shown to shorten the recovery period

General Uses of antivenoms

- to neutralise specific toxins when envenomation has clearly occurred

General Adverse effects of antivenoms

- anaphylaxis (including hypotension, pallor, angioedema, rash, dyspnoea and cough (because of bronchospasm and laryngeal oedema), urticaria, shock and, less commonly, nausea, vomiting and abdominal pain

- serum sickness (delayed) occurring 8–13 days later (but can occur 12 hours after second injection of animal protein) (consisting of urticaria, fever, joint pains, enlarged lymph nodes and albuminuria and, less commonly, arthritis, nephritis, neuropathy and vasculitis)
- (common) fever, chills, headache, hypotension, urticaria, rash
- (uncommon) arthralgia, myalgia, abdominal pain, nausea, vomiting, diarrhoea, chest pain, cyanosis, angioedema, pain or tenderness at injection sites

General Nursing points/Cautions for antivenoms

- antivenom should only be used if there are clear signs of systemic envenomation (usually occur within 2 hours of bite or sting)
- enquire about any previous injections of antivenom (including equine tetanus antitoxin before 1974 in Australia) or any allergies in the patient or family, especially asthma, hay fever and infantile eczema, because the risk of anaphylactoid reaction is increased
- suspected snake-bite cases should be observed for at least 6 hours after the bite or removal of the splint and bandage and, in known snake-bite cases, observation should be for 12 hours, preferably in an ICU setting
- dose for children is the same as the adult dose (as the dose is snake dependent, not weight of victim dependent); however, it should be noted that children can become critically ill faster than adults
- patient should be carefully monitored for any signs or symptoms of neurotoxicity (flaccid paralysis (within 1–3 hours), ptosis and/or diplopia, dysphagia, and if severe, paralysis of respiratory muscles (3–18 hours)), coagulopathy (regular monitoring of INR, APTT, fibrinogen, platelets), neuromuscular impairment, myolysis (myotoxin destroys muscle cells (rhabdomyolysis) causing pain, weakness, red discolouration of urine, and increase in creatine kinase) and nephrotoxicity (resulting from rhabdomyolysis, hypotension and coagulopathy)
- pressure bandage and splint should not be removed until antivenom is ready to be administered
- antivenom is diluted in sodium chloride 0.9%, or preferably Hartmann's solution 1 in 10, and given by slow IV infusion without testing for sensitivity to horse serum. Dilution of the antivenom reduces risk of anaphylactoid reaction
- if the person has a fluid restriction, dilution may be 1 in 5 (with medical advice)
- antivenom is usually not required if envenomation is mild
- IV administration is more likely to cause anaphylaxis than SC or IM
- skin testing is NOT recommended
- IV antihistamine (non-sedating) and 0.25 mL of 1 : 1000 adrenaline (epinephrine) SC may be used before antivenom administration, but this practice is contentious and is no longer recommended
- have available adrenaline (epinephrine) 1 in 1000 (drawn up), antihistamines, IV corticosteroid, oxygen, suction and resuscitation equipment whenever antivenom is administered. If anaphylaxis occurs, antivenom

should be stopped immediately and oxygen and IM adrenaline (epinephrine) administered. If no response to IM administration, adrenaline (epinephrine) should be readministered IV and repeated at 5-minute intervals if needed
- expired antivenom should not be used
- avoid intravascular injection (when not intended) by withdrawing the syringe plunger
- repeated or larger doses are not generally recommended as these do not shorten recovery period
- serial coagulation tests are recommended as indicators of recovery (where venom contains procoagulants or anticoagulants)
- in those with known hypersensitivity (e.g. to horse protein, rabbit or rabbit products, sheep or sheep products), antivenom should be given with caution and patient monitored closely (e.g. airway and vital signs). Antivenom should not be withheld
- because antivenom has been produced from animal plasma, there is always a risk of transmitting infectious agents (possibly unknown) and the patient should be informed of this potential risk before administration
- any deterioration in the patient's condition may indicate the necessity for further administration of antivenom
- envenomation may have significant effects on both mother and fetus and therefore benefits of antivenom should be weighed against risks of envenomation

Patient teaching and advice for antivenoms

- patient should be advised to seek medical attention immediately if any signs of delayed serum sickness occur (e.g. rash, fever, joint pain, swollen lymph glands, flu-like illness) as this can be days or weeks after the antivenom was given

Pressure immobilisation first aid technique (Guideline 9.4.8, Australian Resuscitation Council, 2011)

- this technique was first developed to manage snake bite as a way to delay the movement of venom from the bite site to the circulation; however, it is suitable for all species of Australian snakes (including sea snakes), funnel-web spiders, blue ringed octopus and cone shell stings
- this technique is **not** suitable for spider bites (other than funnel-web spider), jelly fish stings, stonefish or other fish stings, scorpion, centipede or beetle bites
- bitten or stung area should not be washed, cut or excised
- in the event of envenomation, the person should be as immobilised as soon as possible (e.g. person not allowed to walk or move limb; if possible, transport such as a stretcher should be brought to the person, rather than the person walking to the stretcher)
- call Triple Zero (000)
- bite area should not be washed as any venom can be used to identify the snake species using snake venom detection kit
- wide bandage (e.g. elasticised bandage is preferred over crepe bandage; however, clothing and other material can be torn into wide strips) should be applied to area as soon as possible to reduce venom from spreading through lymphatics. Bandage should be firm, but not tight enough to impair circulation (you should not be

able to slide finger between bandage and skin). Clothing should not be removed as movement may promote movement of venom into bloodstream, therefore limb and patient should be kept as still as possible

- bandage should be applied upwards from lower portion of bitten/stung limb (as this is more comfortable and can be tolerated for longer, even though a small amount of venom may be squeezed upwards). Bandage should be extended as high as possible on the limb (if leg). If arm or hand is affected, bandage should start at fingers and extend upwards, with splint applied to elbow. A sling may also be used to immobilise the arm
- if the bite is not on a limb, firm pressure can be applied as long as breathing or chest movement is not restricted. Firm pressure should not be applied to neck or head area
- apply splint to leg (if bitten/stung), and this should then be bound to limb. Splint can be anything that is firm and at hand (e.g. rolled up newspaper, tree branch, piece of wood)
- if possible, area of bite should be marked on the bandage so that venom sample can be accessed for testing without having to remove compression bandage
- person should be transported to hospital and bandage not removed until antivenom is ready for administration (removal may bring on the systemic effects of the venom). Treating doctor should make the decision to remove the bandage
- snake venom detection kit may be useful in identifying specific venom from snake-bite site as puncture marks can be difficult to see. The detection kit uses a swab to identify the presence of venom; however, urine can also be used if no venom sample is available (as blood can be unreliable). Snake venom detection kit can detect venom from brown snakes, black snakes, tiger snakes, death adders and taipans

BLACK SNAKE ANTIVENOM

Available form
Vial: 18,000 units

Action
- see General Actions of antivenoms (p. 1549)
- venom contains neurotoxins, myotoxins, procoagulants and anticoagulants
- local reaction (pain, swelling, redness) is a major feature
- produced from horse plasma

Use
- may be used for mulga (King brown) snake, Butler's mulga snake, Papuan black snake
- can also be used for Collett's snake but tiger snake antivenom is the preferred treatment option

Dose
- 18,000 units diluted 1 in 10 with Hartmann's solution and given IV

Adverse effects/Nursing points/Cautions
- not given IM
- see General Adverse effects/Nursing points/Cautions for antivenoms (including pressure immobilisation first aid technique, pp. 1549–50)

BOX JELLYFISH ANTIVENOM

Available form
Vial: 20,000 units

Action

- box jellyfish are found in tropical coastal waters from Gladstone (Queensland) to Broome (Western Australia), but not the Great Barrier Reef from December to March generally, or October to end of May in the Northern Territory
- box jellyfish are transparent and difficult to see in water. They are large (20–30 cm), and weigh up to 6 kg with tentacles ≥ 3 metres (containing nematocysts (stinging cells)). Upon contact the nematocysts discharge tubules loaded with venom (which act as mini-harpoons)
- severity of envenomation is related to the surface area that the tentacles containing nematocysts make contact with and the age of the victim
- in severe cases, death can occur in 20 minutes; however, most cases, while painful, are not life threatening
- venom contains toxin, which can affect myocardium and respiratory system as well as causing severe and intense pain
- prepared from sheep plasma

Use

- treat envenomation by box jellyfish (*Chironex fleckeri*)

Dose

- 20,000 units diluted 1 in 10 with Hartmann's solution and given IV or 60,000 units IM into 3 separate sites (if IV is not practical)

Adverse effects/Nursing points/ Cautions

- vinegar (NOT ALCOHOL) should be applied to any tentacles sticking to the skin and first aid measures taken immediately to ensure an adequate airway is maintained. Vinegar will not ease pain, but will inactivate any stinging cells still present. Any remaining tentacles should be picked off. Cold pack or ice in a dry plastic bag can be applied for pain relief. Fresh water should not be applied to area as it may cause further discharge of venom from undischarged nematocysts
- IM administration may be used as emergency treatment pre-hospitalisation
- see General Adverse effects/Nursing points/Cautions for antivenoms (pp. 1549–50)

BROWN SNAKE ANTIVENOM

Available form

Vial: 1000 units

Action

- see General Actions of antivenoms (p. 1549)
- brown snakes are the most common cause of bites and account for the majority of deaths in Australia
- venom contains neurotoxins and procoagulants, but local reactions (pain, swelling, redness) rarely occur
- prepared from horse plasma

Use

- may be used for all brown snake species (except King brown, which is a black snake), dugite or Western brown (Gwardar) snake bite

Dose

- initial dose is 1000 units slowly IV after dilution of 1 : 10 with Hartmann's solution

Adverse effects/Nursing points/ Cautions

- see General Adverse effects/Nursing points/Cautions for antivenoms (including pressure immobilisation first aid technique, pp. 1549–50)

DEATH ADDER ANTIVENOM

Available form

Vial: 6000 units

Action

- see General Actions of antivenoms (p. 1549)

- venom contains neurotoxin with local reactions (pain, redness, swelling) rarely reported

Use
- used for death adder species envenomation

Dose
- initial dose is 6000 units by slow IV after dilution 1 : 10 with Hartmann's solution

Adverse effects/Nursing points/Cautions
- see General Adverse effects/Nursing points/Cautions for antivenoms (including pressure immobilisation first aid technique, pp. 1549–50)

FUNNEL-WEB SPIDER ANTIVENOM

Available form
Vial: 125 units

Action
- funnel-web spiders consist of 30 species in two genera, *Atrax* and *Hadronyche*. The male spider (*Atrax robustus*) is responsible for most, if not all, of the known funnel-web deaths, which can result within 30 minutes of bite. There have been no recorded deaths since 1980 due to the availability of the antivenom
- venom contains neurotoxins
- prepared from rabbit plasma

Use
- treatment of funnel-web spider envenomation

Dose
- 250 units (2 vials) given slowly IV after reconstitution with water for injections

Adverse effects/Nursing points/Cautions
- hypersensitivity reactions are not common
- should not be used without clear evidence of systemic envenomation with potential for serious toxic effects
- see General Adverse effects/Nursing points/Cautions for antivenoms (including pressure immobilisation first aid technique, pp. 1549–50)

POLYVALENT SNAKE ANTIVENOM

Available form
Vial: 40,000 units

Action
- contains antivenom against black snakes (18,000 units), tiger (3000 units) and brown snakes (1000 units), taipan (12,000 units) and death adder (6000 units)
- prepared from horse plasma

Use
- for use in Papua New Guinea and Australia (except for Victoria and Tasmania) when the snake has not been definitely identified. In Victoria, a combination of tiger snake and brown snake antivenom is the preferred treatment, whereas in Tasmania, tiger snake antivenom is used in preference to polyvalent antivenom

Dose
- 40,000 units by slow IV after dilution 1 : 10 with Hartmann's solution

Adverse effects/Nursing points/Cautions
- see General Adverse effects/Nursing points/Cautions for antivenoms (including pressure immobilisation first aid technique, pp. 1549–50)

RED BACK SPIDER ANTIVENOM

Available form
Vial: 500 units

Action/Use
- used for red back spider (*Latrodectus hasselti*) bite
- venom causes intense pain that can last for days to weeks, redness or red marks and itchiness
- venom contains alpha-latrotoxin causing latrodectism (local pain, local and general sweating, nausea, vomiting, headache, dizziness and malaise, and less commonly, hypertension, hyperthermia, abdominal rigidity and agitation/irritability)
- prepared from horse plasma

Dose
- 500 units IM or 500 units by slow IV after dilution 1 : 10 with Hartmann's solution (if envenomation is life threatening)

Adverse effects/Nursing points/ Cautions
- adverse effects are more common if given IV
- ice or cold compress can be applied for up to 20 minutes to decrease pain of spider bite
- (first aid) pressure immobilisation technique should not be used as venom acts slowly
- see General Adverse effects/Nursing points/Cautions for antivenoms (pp. 1549–50)

SEA SNAKE ANTIVENOM

Available form
Vial: 1000 units

Action
- sea snakes are commonly found in tropical water ≥ 20°C
- bite can be painless with no local swelling, although small teeth marks can be obvious
- venom contains neurotoxins and myotoxins with minor reaction (pain, redness, swelling) reported
- prepared from horse plasma

Use
- used for envenomation due to a variety of sea snakes found in the northern Australian waters

Dose
- 1000 units by slow IV after dilution 1 : 10 with Hartmann's solution or sodium chloride 0.9%
- (severe envenomation with myalgia, weakness, trismus, ptosis) 3000–4000 units by slow IV after dilution 1 : 10 with Hartmann's solution or sodium chloride 0.9%

Adverse effects/Nursing points/ Cautions
- tiger snake antivenom may also be used if sea snake antivenom is not available
- see General Adverse effects/Nursing points/Cautions for antivenoms (including pressure immobilisation first aid technique) (pp. 1549–50)

STONE FISH ANTIVENOM

Available form
Vial: 2000 units

Action
- stonefish are found in tropical Australian waters and prefer calm shallow water where they bury themselves in the sand
- envenomation usually occurs by standing on stone fish buried in sand
- venom contains cardiotoxins, neurotoxins and myotoxins

Use
- envenomation by stone fish (*Synanceia horrida* and *Synanceia verrucosa*) not responding to first aid measures

Dose
- dose given is dependent on the number of puncture wounds and given IM or slowly IV after dilution

1 : 10 with Hartmann's solution in severe cases
  - (1–2 punctures) 2000 units
  - (3–4 punctures) 4000 units
  - (> 5 punctures) 6000 units

Adverse effects/Nursing points/ Cautions

- initially, severe pain, redness and swelling occurs at site of puncture, then spreads to limb and local lymph nodes
- first aid includes immersing puncture wounds in hot water (50°C) to relieve pain as the toxin is heat labile
- tourniquet and/or compression bandage are not recommended
- local anaesthetic injected around puncture site or region may also relieve pain
- see General Adverse effects/Nursing points/Cautions for antivenoms (pp. 1549–50)

TAIPAN ANTIVENOM

Available form
Vial: 12,000 units

Action
- taipan venom is thought to be the most potent snake venom worldwide
- venom contains neurotoxin, myotoxins and procoagulants with minor local reaction (pain, swelling, redness) reported
- prepared from horse plasma

Use
- used for envenomation by coastal taipan (*Oxyuranus scutellatus*) and inland taipan (*Oxyuranus microlepidotus*) (Fierce snake)

Dose
- initial dose is 12,000 units slowly IV after dilution 1 : 10 with Hartmann's solution
- (severe defibrination) 36,000 units slowly IV after dilution 1 : 10 with Hartmann's solution

Adverse effects/Nursing points/ Cautions

- see General Adverse effects/Nursing points/Cautions for antivenoms (including pressure immobilisation first aid technique) (pp. 1549–50)

TIGER SNAKE ANTIVENOM

Available form
Vial: 3000 units

Action
- venom contains neurotoxin, myotoxin and procoagulants with minor local reactions (pain, swelling, redness) also reported
- prepared from horse plasma

Use
- envenomation due to tiger snakes, as well as copperhead snakes, black snakes, rough-scaled snakes and Collett's snake (red and blue-bellied black snakes)

Dose
- initial dose is 3000 units slowly IV after dilution 1 : 10 with Hartmann's solution

Adverse effects/Nursing points/ Cautions

- see General Adverse effects/Nursing points/Cautions for antivenoms (including pressure immobilisation first aid technique) (pp. 1549–50)

IMMUNOGLOBULINS

General Actions of immunoglobulins

- immunoglobulins provide acquired passive immunity as they contain high titres of antibodies which can be against a specific antigen or pooled (containing a number of antibodies)
- protection using immunoglobulins is immediate but only lasts for 3 to 4 weeks

General Uses of immunoglobulins

- individuals who are unable to produce antibodies
- prevention of disease when time does not permit active immunity (post-exposure)
- treatment of some diseases that are normally prevented by immunisation
- treatment of conditions where active immunisation is not available or is impractical

General Adverse effects of immunoglobulins

- (IM site) redness, stiffness, tenderness, induration, pain, irritation, bruising
- (IV site, high dose, prolonged administration) thrombophlebitis
- headache, malaise, drowsiness
- chest tightness
- fever
- facial flushing or pallor, feeling hot, chills, sweating
- abdominal pain, nausea, vomiting
- dyspnoea
- rash, pruritus
- hypotension (transient)
- (delayed reaction, within 24 hours) nausea, vomiting, chest pain, chills or shivering, dizziness, aching legs
- (infrequently, high dose) aseptic meningitis syndrome occurring from several hours up to 2 days after administration and consisting of headache, nuchal rigidity, drowsiness, fever, photophobia, painful eye movement, nausea and vomiting
- (rare) renal dysfunction, acute renal failure, haemolysis, haemolytic anaemia, thrombotic events, abscess
- (very rare) anaphylactic reaction, transfusion-related acute lung injury
- any human serum carries the risk of transmitting blood-borne viral or prion diseases

General Interactions of immunoglobulins

- caution if immunoglobulins are given with nephrotoxic agents due to increased risk of renal dysfunction and acute renal failure
- immunoglobulins should not be given within 14 days of vaccines (if possible) as effectiveness may be reduced requiring re-vaccination
- vaccination with live attenuated vaccines (e.g. measles, poliomyelitis) should not be given within 3 months of immunoglobulin
- may produce misleading positive (false positive) results on serological testing
- some immunoglobulins contain maltose or glucose, which may interfere with measurements of blood glucose levels

General Nursing points/Cautions for immunoglobulins

- patient should be adequately hydrated before starting therapy

- vital signs should be closely monitored and patient observed during and for at least 20 minutes after administration
- transfusion-related acute lung injury occurs 1–6 hours after administration and patient should be monitored for any signs of respiratory distress or fever
- infusion rate should commence slowly and rate gradually increased after 15–30 minutes if tolerated by patient
- if patient is at risk of thromboembolic events, therapy should be administered at minimal dose infused at a slow rate while observing patient closely. Consideration should be given to evaluation of blood viscosity
- if adverse reactions occur, infusion should be stopped for 5–10 minutes and restarted at slower rate, monitoring patient carefully
- batch number of product should be recorded each time it is administered to enable linking between patient and product if untoward event occurs
- if given IM, no more than 5 mL should be given per site
- reconstituted solutions should not be shaken as this denatures the protein
- have readily available adrenaline (epinephrine) 1 in 1000 (drawn up), antihistamines, IV corticosteroid, oxygen, suction and resuscitation equipment in the event of anaphylaxis occurring
- allow preparation to reach room temperature before injection/infusion
- turbid-looking preparation should not be administered and should be returned to manufacturer (Australian Red Cross)
- immunoglobulin should not be used if it has been frozen
- administer alone
- if container breaks and/or spillage occurs, it should be cleaned with sodium hypochlorite 1% for 15 minutes, avoiding inhalation or any contact with spill. Standard precautions should be strictly applied
- produced from human plasma, therefore there is a potential risk of disease transmission (e.g. viruses, Creutzfeldt-Jacob disease)
- caution if immunoglobulins are used in those with pre-existing renal impairment, diabetes mellitus, volume depletion, sepsis or paraproteinaemia or who are older than 65 years due to increased risk of renal dysfunction and possible acute renal failure
- caution if used in those with increased risk of thrombotic events (e.g. immobile, elderly, cardiovascular risk factors (e.g. impaired cardiac output, atherosclerosis), hypertriglyceridaemia, monoclonal gammopathies, previous history of thrombotic event, severe hypovolaemia, hyperviscosity, oestrogen use, acquired/inherited hypercoagulation states) or if the person has an in-dwelling vascular catheter
- caution if used in those with non-O blood group, with underlying associated inflammatory conditions or receiving high cumulative doses of immunoglobulins over several days due to increased risk of haemolysis
- IM administration is contraindicated in those with severe thrombocytopenia or coagulation disorders
- immunoglobulins are contraindicated in those who have had a previous anaphylactic reaction following

administration of immunoglobulins or in those with IgA deficiency (unless tested and found to be negative for anti-IgA antibodies)

General Patient teaching and advice for immunoglobulins

- warn patient that nausea, vomiting, chills or shivering, chest pain, dizziness and/or aching legs may occur with 24 hours of immunoglobulin administration
- patient should be advised to immediately seek medical advice if any of the following occur:
  - headache, nausea, vomiting, drowsiness, fever, stiff neck, painful eye movement or inability to tolerate bright light (especially within 2 days of immunoglobulin administration) (may be signs of aseptic meningitis syndrome)
  - fatigue, fever, pallor, confusion, dizziness, light-headedness and weakness/inability to complete any physical activity (signs of haemolysis)
  - fever or any signs of respiratory difficulty (signs of transfusion-related acute lung injury)
- inform patient that any product prepared from human blood or plasma has the potential for transmission of blood-borne viral or prion diseases (e.g. Creutzfeldt-Jakob disease), although stringent procedures now exist for careful selection of blood donors and removal and inactivation of known enveloped viruses from blood products (e.g. HIV, hepatitis B and C) and non-enveloped viruses (e.g. hepatitis A)
- if patient has diabetes mellitus, it is important to instruct him/her to seek advice from doctor regarding the possibility that maltose/glucose contained in some immunoglobulins may interfere with estimation of blood glucose levels

CYTOMEGALOVIRUS (CMV) IMMUNOGLOBULIN (CMV Immunoglobulin-VF)

Available form
Vial: 1.5×10^6 U

Action
- see General Actions of immunoglobulins (p. 1557)
- trace of IgA present
- half-life about 3 weeks (but less if patient is immunocompromised)

Use
- prevention of CMV infection in those with bone marrow or kidney transplantation when the donor is CMV positive and the recipient is CMV negative
- (adjunct) treatment of established CMV infection (e.g. CMV pneumonitis)

Dose
- (prophylaxis) 25,000 U/kg IV given on days –4, –2, day of transplant (intraoperatively) and then weekly for 8 weeks **OR**
- (therapy) 50,000 U/kg IV, repeated after 4–5 days and then every 10–14 days until clinical improvement is seen

Adverse effects/Interactions/Nursing points/Cautions/Patient teaching and advice
- may be given undiluted or diluted with glucose 5% or sodium chloride 0.9%. Infusion rate should start at 1 mL/minute for 15 minutes, then increased gradually to 3–4 mL/minute if patient's vital signs remain stable
- administer alone
- only given IV

- contains maltose
- see General Adverse effects/Interactions/Nursing points/Cautions/Patient teaching and advice for Immunoglobulins (pp. 1557–59)

HEPATITIS B IMMUNOGLOBULIN (Hepatitis B Immunoglobulin-VF)

Available forms
Vial: 100 IU, 400 IU

Action
- see General Actions of immunoglobulins (p. 1557)
- contains specific neutralising antibodies against hepatitis B surface antigen (HBsAg)

Use
- post-exposure prophylaxis in those never previously vaccinated, incomplete vaccination or HBsAg antibody level is inadequate (< 10 IU/L)
- prophylaxis in infants born to HBsAg-positive mothers

Dose
- (prophylaxis in infants born to HBsAg-positive mother) 100 IU IM at birth and hepatitis B vaccination started at same time (in different limbs) **OR**
- (confirmed exposure to HBsAg, person has no/incomplete immunisation) 400 IU IM stat within 72 hours of exposure, start hepatitis B vaccination at same time (in different limbs) **OR**
- (confirmed exposure to HBsAg, person has complete immunisation) antibody level should be measured and if inadequate (< 10 IU/L), 400 IU IM stat and hepatitis B vaccine booster dose (in different limbs) **OR**
- (high risk for HBsAg but not confirmed, person has no/incomplete immunisation) start hepatitis B vaccination regimen, test potential source of infection; if positive, give 400 IU IM stat **OR**
- (high risk for HBsAg but not confirmed, person has complete immunisation) antibody level should be measured and if inadequate (< 10 IU/L), source tested and, if positive, 400 IU IM stat and hepatitis B vaccine booster dose (in different limbs) **OR**
- (uncertain or low risk of exposure, person has no/incomplete immunisation) start hepatitis B vaccination regimen **OR**
- (uncertain or low risk of exposure, person has complete immunisation) no treatment required

Adverse effects/Interactions
- see General Adverse effects/Interactions of immunoglobulins (p. 1557)

Nursing points/Cautions
- post-exposure prophylaxis should be considered after percutaneous or permucosal exposure to HBsAg positive or suspected positive material (e.g. needlestick, sexual exposure, oral ingestion)
- only given IM as IV administration has high risk of anaphylaxis
- if given with hepatitis B vaccine, different limbs should be used
- immunoglobulin is not necessary if hepatitis B antibodies are present in adequate levels
- contraindicated in those who are HBsAg positive or have adequate hepatitis B antibodies (≥ 10 IU/L)
- see also General Nursing points/Cautions for immunoglobulins (p. 1557)

Patient teaching and advice
- warn patient that local reaction (pain, redness, tenderness, induration) is normal and may persist for some hours after IM administration
- see also General Patient teaching and advice for immunoglobulins (p. 1559)

NORMAL (HUMAN) IMMUNOGLOBULIN (Cuvitru, Evogam, Flebogamma 5% DIF, Flebogamma 10% DIF, Gammanorm, Gamunex, Hizentra, Hyqvia, Intragam 10, Kiovig, Normal Immunoglobulin-VF, Octagam, Privigen)

Available forms

Solution for Infusion: 320 mg/2 mL, 1 g/5 mL, 0.8 g/10 mL, 1 g/10 mL, 1.6 g/2 mL, 2 g/10 mL, 1 g/20 mL, 2 g/20 mL, 3.3 g/20 mL, 4 g/20 mL, 2.5 g/25 mL, 2.5 g/50 mL, 5 g/50 mL, 10 g/50 mL, 5 g/100 mL, 10 g/100 mL, 10 g/200 mL, 20 g/200 mL, 40 g/400 mL, 0.16 g/mL, 165 mg/mL; Prefilled syringe: 1 g/5 mL, 2 g/10 mL

Action

- contains a range of IgG antibodies collected from pooled plasma from at least 1000 donors

Use

- replacement therapy in primary immunodeficiency (e.g. severe combined immunodeficiency, congenital agammaglobinaemia and hypogammaglobinaemia, common variable immunodeficiency)
- replacement therapy in secondary immunodeficiency (e.g. myeloma, children with AIDS, allogenic bone marrow transplantation)
- immunomodulation (e.g. Guillain-Barre syndrome, Kawasaki disease, idiopathic thrombocytopenic purpura at high risk of bleeding or before surgery, susceptible contacts of hepatitis A, measles and poliomyelitis)

Dose

- (primary immunodeficiency replacement) 0.2–0.8 g/kg IV every 3–4 weeks to achieve IgG trough of ≥ 5 g/L (Intragam 10) **OR**
- (primary immunodeficiency replacement) initially 0.4–0.8 g/kg IV every 2–4 weeks, then 0.2–0.8 g/kg IV every 2–4 weeks, to achieve IgG trough level of ≥ 4–6 g/L (Flebogamma, Kiovig, Octagam 5% or 10%, Privigen) **OR**
- (primary immunodeficiency replacement) 300–600 mg/kg by SC infusion weekly (first week), second dose after 2 weeks, third dose after 3 weeks, fourth dose after 4 weeks, then every 3–4 weeks. Therapy should start 1 week after treatment with previous immunoglobulin (with infusion of vorhyaluronidase alfa) (Hyqvia) **OR**
- (primary immunodeficiency replacement) ≥ 0.2–0.5 g/kg by SC infusion, divided over several days (loading dose), then repeated to achieve 0.3–1 g/kg cumulative monthly dose (Cuvitru) **OR**
- (primary immunodeficiency replacement in children) initially 0.2–0.5 g/kg SC to achieve steady-state IgG levels, then repeated to achieve 0.4–0.8 g/kg cumulative monthly dose (Gammanorm) **OR**
- (primary immunodeficiency replacement) 0.3–0.6 mg/kg IV or SC every 3–4 weeks to reach IgG trough level of ≥ 5 g/L (Gamunex) **OR**
- (primary immunodeficiency replacement) 0.05–0.15 g/kg SC weekly (total maintenance dose 0.2–0.6 g/kg) (Evogam) **OR**
- (primary immunodeficiency replacement or hypogammaglobinaemia in children) 0.2–0.5 g/kg SC over several days until steady-state IgG trough level is achieved, maintenance doses administered to achieve 0.4–0.8 g/kg cumulative monthly dose (Hizentra) **OR**
- (primary immunodeficiency replacement in children) 100 mg (0.6 mL)/kg weekly via syringe driver at 10 mL/hour. Rate may be increased by 1 mL/hour/pump every 3–4 weeks (maximum

dose 40 mL/hour using 2 pumps) (Gammanorm) **OR**

- (secondary immunodeficiency replacement, symptomatic hypogammaglobinaemia) 0.2–0.4 g/kg IV every 3–4 weeks to achieve IgG trough level of ≥ 4–6 g/L (Flebogamma, Gamunex, Kiovig, Octagam 5% or 10%, Privigen) **OR**
- (allogenic bone marrow transplantation (infection, graft vs host disease)) 0.5 g/kg/week IV, starting 7 days pretransplant up to 12 weeks post-transplant (Flebogamma, Octagam 5% or 10%) **OR**
- (allogenic bone marrow transplantation (persistent lack of antibody production)) 0.5 g/kg IV monthly until antibody levels return to normal (Flebogamma, Intragam 10, Octagam 5% or 10%) **OR**
- (Kawasaki disease) 1.6–2.0 g/kg IV as a single dose or in divided doses over 2–5 days with aspirin (Gamunex, Octagam 5% or 10%, Intragam 10, Privigen, Flebogamma) **OR**
- (Kawasaki disease) 2 g/kg IV as a single dose with aspirin (Kiovig, Intragam 10, Octagam 10%, Privigen) **OR**
- (idiopathic thrombocytopenic purpura) 0.8–1 g/kg IV, repeated once in next 3 days if needed (Flebogamma, Kiovig, Octagam 5% or 10%, Privigen) **OR**
- (idiopathic thrombocytopenic purpura) 2 g/kg IV as single dose, 1 g/kg over 2 consecutive days or 0.4 g/kg over 5 consecutive days (Intragam 10, Gamunex) **OR**
- (idiopathic thrombocytopenic purpura) 0.4 g/kg/day IV for 2–5 days (Flebogamma, Kiovig, Octagam 5% or 10%, Privigen) **OR**
- (Guillain-Barre syndrome) 0.4 g/kg/day IV for 3–7 days starting within 14 days of symptom onset (Gamunex, Flebogamma, Kiovig, Octagam 5% or 10%, Intragam 10, Privigen) **OR**
- (children with AIDS and recurrent infection) 0.2–0.4 g/kg IV every 3–4 weeks (Flebogamma, Octagam 5% or 10%) **OR**
- (hepatitis A household contact/institutional contact/staff in institution where hepatitis A is endemic) 0.06 mL/kg deep IM 5–6-monthly (or until active immunity develops or risk no longer exists (long-term protection) (Normal Immunoglobulin-VF) **OR**
- (hepatitis A household contact) 0.03 mL/kg deep IM (short-term protection) (Normal Immunoglobulin-VF) **OR**
- (measles) 0.2 mL/kg deep IM (Normal Immunoglobulin-VF) **OR**
- (poliomyelitis) 0.3 mL/kg deep IM (Normal Immunoglobulin-VF) **OR**
- (hypogammaglobinaemia) 0.6 mL/kg at monthly intervals (with an extra dose during first month) (Normal Immunoglobulin-VF) **OR**
- (chronic inflammatory demyelinating polyneuropathy) initially 2 g/kg in divided doses over 2–4 consecutive days (loading dose), then 1 g/kg over 1 day or 500 mg/kg over 2 consecutive days, every 3 weeks (Gamunex, Privigen) **OR**
- (chronic inflammatory demyelinating polyneuropathy) initially 2 g/kg IV in divided doses over 2–5 weeks (induction), then 0.4–1 g/kg every 2–6 weeks (Intragam 10) **OR**
- (multifocal motor neuropathy (MMN)) initially 2 g/kg in divided doses over 2–5 days, then 0.4–2 g/kg every 2–6 weeks for 3–6 months (Kiovig, Privigen, Intragam 10) **OR**
- (myasthenic gravis exacerbation (e.g. before surgery, during myasthenic crisis) initially 1–2 g/kg IV in divided doses over 2–5 days, then 0.4–1 g/kg every 4–6 weeks (maintenance) (Privigen, Intragam 10) **OR**
- (Lambert-Eaton myasthenic syndrome) initially 2 g/kg IV in divided doses over 2–5 days, then 0.4–1 g/kg

every 2–6 weeks (maintenance) (Privigen, Intragam 10) **OR**

- (Stiff person syndrome) initially 2 g/kg IV in divided doses over 2–5 days, then 1–2 g/kg every 4–6 weeks (maintenance) (Privigen)

Adverse effects/Interactions

- see General Adverse effects/ Interactions of immunoglobulins (p. 1557)

Nursing points/Cautions

- higher doses may be required at the start of therapy to provide rapid protection
- IgG trough levels should be measured before next infusion. It may take 3–6 months for IgG trough levels to equilibrate
- patient should be closely monitored if new to immunoglobulin therapy, if there has been a large time interval between administrations or if changing from one formulation to another
- (SC) patient and/or carer/family member may be taught SC administration technique
- (Hyqvia) only given SC
- (Hyqvia) infusion of vorhyaluronidase alfa (160 U/mL) is administered first at 1–2 mL/minute, followed within 10 minutes by infusion of immunoglobulin through same needle. Vorhyaluronidase alfa acts increases permeability of subcutaneous tissue allowing better absorption of immunoglobulin
- (Hyqvia) if using two sites, doses of both should be divided and contralateral sites used
- (Evogam) administered SC (not IV) starting at rate of 10 mL/hour and increasing up to 20 mL/hour (as tolerated by patient)
- (Evogam) doses over 20 mL should be administered into two different sites
- (Flebogamma) initial infusion rate should be 0.01–0.02 mL/kg/minute for first 30 minutes, then increasing gradually to maximum of 0.08–0.1 mL/kg/minute if tolerated
- (Flebogamma) contains sorbitol and is not recommended in those with fructose intolerance
- (Flebogamma) SC infusion site should be changed after 5–15 mL has been administered. Multiple sites can be used simultaneously (as long as they are at least 5 cm apart)
- (Gammanorm) SC is preferred route, but IM may be used for small doses or if SC route is not applicable
- (Cuvitru) administered by SC infusion at 10 mL/hour/site initially, increasing by ≥ 10 minute intervals if well tolerated, to 20 mL/hour/site. More than one pump can be used at same time
- (Kiovig) SC route is only recommended for primary immunodeficiency replacement therapy. Initial recommended infusion rate is 0.5 mL/kg/hour increasing to < 6 mL/kg/hour if tolerated
- (Kiovig, MMN) therapy should continue for 3–6 months to establish patient response. Six months may be required if significant axonal degeneration has occurred. Regular review by neurologist is also recommended
- (Intragam 10) may be given undiluted or diluted with glucose 5% or sodium chloride 0.9% (up to 2 parts) and infused at 1 mL/minute for first 15 minutes, increasing to maximum of 3–4 mL/minutes if tolerated
- (Gamunex) may be diluted with glucose 5% (not sodium chloride 0.9%) and infused IV at an initial rate of 1 mg/kg/minute for 30 minutes, then increasing gradually to 8 mg/kg/minute if tolerated
- (Gamunex) high-dose regimen (1 g/kg over 1–2 days) for idiopathic thrombocytopenic purpura is not recommended if there is any concern about patient's fluid volume
- (Gamunex – idiopathic thrombocytopenic purpura) after first dose (of

2 consecutive day regimen), platelet count should be measured and if adequate, second dose not given. This also applies to 0.4 g/kg regimen
- (Hizentra) only given SC
- (Hizentra) doses greater than 25 mL should be administered over multiple sites, at least 5 cm apart
- (Hizentra) infusion rate ≤ 20 mL/hour/site, gradually increasing to 35 mL/hour/site if tolerated
- (Octagam 10%) infusion rate 0.6–1.2 mL/kg/hour for first 30 minutes, increasing gradually to 7.2 mL/kg/hour if tolerated
- (Octagam 5%) infusion rate 1 mL/kg/hour for first 30 minutes, increasing gradually to 5 mL/kg/hour if tolerated
- (Octagam 5% or 10%) contain maltose
- (Privigen) not given with sodium chloride 0.9%
- (Privigen – primary immunodeficiency replacement) infusion rate 0.3 mL/kg/hour, increasing gradually to 4.8 mL/kg/hour, and finally to 7.2 mL/kg/hour if very well tolerated
- (Privigen, Hizentra) contraindicated in those with hypoprolinaemia type I or II
- (Evogam, Kiovig, Normal Immunoglobin-VF) contain glycine and are therefore contraindicated if glycine hypersensitivity exists
- (Hyqvia) contraindicated in those with hypersensitivity to vorhyaluronidase or hyaluronidase (as this is given as infusion before immunoglobulin)
- see also General Nursing points/Cautions for immunoglobulins (p. 1557)

Patient teaching and advice

- instruct patient in SC administration technique, including importance of:
    - allowing solution to come to room temperature before use (usually 20–60 minutes)
    - not shaking vial
    - collecting all equipment before starting procedure (e.g. infusion pump, administration tubing, SC needle or catheter set, Y-connector, alcohol swab, syringe, vial adapter, gauze or transparent dressing, tape, sharps disposal container, treatment diary (if used))
    - checking expiry date and solution for any turbidity or sediment (not used if out of date, turbid or contains sediment)
    - washing hands with soap and water before starting
    - drawing up of solution technique and preparation of infusion tubing
    - insertion of SC needle (including choice of sites and technique and use of multiple sites e.g. at least 5 cm apart if multiple sites are administered at same time)
    - starting infusion at correct infusion rate
    - use of syringe driver or other infusion pumps (if used)
    - correct disposal of used equipment
    - recording treatment (including recording label information or removing label and putting this in diary/log book)
- see also General Patient teaching and advice for immunoglobulins (p. 1559)

RABIES IMMUNOGLOBULIN (Imogam Rabies (Pasteurized))

Available form

Vial: 150 IU/mL

Action

- see General Actions of immunoglobulins (p. 1557)
- rabies virus is transmitted via saliva of infected mammals

Use

- given immediately after exposure to virus (single or multiple bites or scratches or if contamination with mucous membrane (e.g. licks)) occurs (unless person already has adequate antibody levels from previous vaccination)

Dose

- 20 IU/kg with largest portion infiltrated around wound(s) (if possible) and remainder IM at a site distant to vaccination site (at time of first vaccine dose)

Adverse effects/Nursing points/Cautions/Patient teaching and advice

- bites/scratches should be washed with copious amount of water and detergent, and then treated with disinfectant. Tetanus prophylaxis is also recommended
- may be given up to 8 days after initial dose of rabies vaccine
  - should not be given in same syringe or same anatomical site as rabies vaccine
- repeated doses of immunoglobulin should not be given once vaccination schedule has started
- may be diluted with sodium chloride 0.9% before administration
- given IM
- not given IV due to risk of shock
- should be given with rabies vaccine (see Vaccines, p. 1544) (different limb)
- see General Adverse effects/Nursing points/Cautions/Patient teaching and advice for immunoglobulins (pp. 1557–59)

RHESUS (RH(D)) IMMUNOGLOBULIN (Rh(D) Immunoglobulin-VF, Rhophylac)

Available forms

Vial (solution): 250 IU; Vial (powder): 625 IU; Prefilled syringe: 1500 IU/2 mL

Action

- when mother is Rh(D)-negative and fetus is Rh(D)-positive, mother can become immunised to Rh(D) antigen producing anti-Rh(D) antibodies which may cross the placenta and cause haemolytic anaemia in the newborn

Use

- prevention of Rh sensitisation in Rh(D)-negative female (at or below childbearing age). Sensitising events include antepartum haemorrhage, maternal abdominal trauma (likely to cause bleeding to both mother and fetus (feto–maternal haemorrhage)), external cephalic version, cordocentesis, amniocentesis or chorionic villi sampling, normal delivery, miscarriage, pregnancy termination and ectopic pregnancy
- treatment of Rh(D)-negative person after incompatible transfusion of Rh(D)-positive blood or other products containing red blood cells (RBC)

Dose

- (sensitising event in pregnancy unless fetus is confirmed Rh(D)-negative) 250 IM (in first trimester) or 625 IU IM (in second or third trimester or if multiple pregnancy) (Rh(D) Immunoglobulin-VF) **OR**
- (gestational age is unknown but possibly ≥ 13 weeks) 625 IU IM (Rh(D) Immunoglobulin-VF) **OR**
- (abdominal trauma causing haemorrhage > 6 mL) 100 IU/mL of Rh(D)-positive RBC (Rh(D) Immunoglobulin-VF) **OR**
- (abdominal trauma causing haemorrhage ≤ 6 mL) 625 IU IM (Rh(D) Immunoglobulin-VF) **OR**
- (transfusion of Rh(D)-positive blood) 100 IU/mL IM of Rh(D)-positive RBC (Rh(D) Immunoglobulin-VF) **OR**
- (antepartum prophylaxis, 28–30-week gestation) 1500 IU IM or IV (Rhophylac) **OR**

- (post-partum prophylaxis if newborn is Rh(D)-positive) 1500 IM or IV within 72 hours of delivery (Rhophylac) **OR**
- (prophylaxis after pregnancy complication or invasive procedure) 1500 IU IM or IV within 72 hours of event (Rhophylac) **OR**
- (large haemorrhage $>$ 15 mL) 1500 IU IM or IV within 72 hours of haemorrhage plus 100 IU/mL fetal RBC $>$ 15 mL (Rhophylac) **OR**
- (incompatible blood transfusion) 100 IU per 2 mL of transfused Rh(D)-positive blood or 1 mL erythrocyte concentrate IV (maximum dose 15,000 IU) (Rhophylac)

Adverse effects/Interactions/Nursing points/Cautions/Patient teaching and advice

- dose should be given within 72 hours of sensitising event
- (IM administration) local anaesthetic may be added to lessen pain
- if $>$ 5 mL is required IM, dose should be divided and given into different sites
- if patient body mass index (BMI) $\geq$ 30, IV route is recommended as IM administration may be ineffective
- contraindicated in those who are Rh(D)-positive or Rh(D)-negative and have been immunised or in Rh(D)-positive post-partum babies
- see General Adverse effects/Interactions/Nursing points/Cautions/Patient teaching and advice for immunoglobulins (pp. 1557–59)

TETANUS IMMUNOGLOBULIN (Tetanus Immunoglobulin-VF (For Intramuscular Use), Tetanus Immunoglobulin-VF (For Intravenous Use))

Available forms

Vial: (for IM use) 250 IU, (for IV use) 4000 IU

Action

- see General Actions of immunoglobulins (p. 1557)

Use

- passive protection in those with a tetanus-prone wound (see Tetanus prone wounds below) with no or doubtful tetanus immunity or greater than 10 years since last booster dose
- treatment of clinical tetanus

Dose

- 250 IU IM or 500 IU IM if wound is grossly contaminated or 24 hours has elapsed before seeking medical advice (Tetanus Immunoglobulin-VF (For Intramuscular Use)) **OR**
- (clinical tetanus) 4000 IU by IV infusion starting at 1 mL/minute for 15 minutes, then increasing rate to 3–4 mL/minute if tolerated (Tetanus Immunoglobulin-VF (For Intravenous Use))

Adverse effects/Nursing points/Cautions/Patient teaching and advice

- may be diluted using sodium chloride 0.9% or glucose 5% or may be given undiluted IV (IV preparation) or by IM injection (IM preparation)
- local anaesthetic can be added to IM to lessen pain
- IV formulation contains maltose
- administer IV alone
- IV preparation should not be given IM
- IM preparation should not be given IV
- see General Adverse effects/Nursing points/Cautions/Patient teaching and advice for immunoglobulins (pp. 1557–59)

Tetanus-prone wounds

- *Clostridium tetani* is a gram-positive organism responsible for tetanus. It forms spores which can easily enter a wound where they can then grow anaerobically and produce a toxin that contains both a neurotoxin and haemolysin. The neurotoxin acts on the CNS, producing muscle rigidity and painful spasms. Incubation period is 3–21 days, the median being 10 days after injury (or less with heavily contaminated wounds). Early signs of tetanus include trismus (lockjaw), dysphagia and pain or stiffness in the neck, back or shoulder muscles. Violent, painful generalised muscle spasms may also occur. The person may or may not be febrile and mental status is generally not impaired. Death usually results from respiratory failure, hyper/hypotension or cardiac arrhythmias

- most deaths occur in those $>$ 70 years and is often associated with apparently minor injuries (e.g. prick with a rose thorn while gardening) in those who may never have been vaccinated or vaccinated $>$ 10 years ago
- all wounds (except clean minor cuts) should be considered tetanus-prone
- growth of *C. tetani* is favoured in compound fractures, bite wounds, deep penetrating wounds, wounds complicated by extensive tissue damage (such as burns), pyogenic infection or with foreign bodies (particularly wood splinters) or superficial wounds contaminated with soil, dust or horse manure that have remained untreated for 4 hours. Re-implantation of an avulsed tooth is considered a tetanus-prone event as washing and cleaning is often minimised to improve implantation of the tooth. Depot injections (SC or intradermal) in those who inject drugs may also cause tetanus-prone wounds
- wound should be thoroughly cleaned and any foreign or necrotic material removed
- regardless of the patient's immune status, local disinfection and, if needed, surgical treatment should be included as part of the overall management plan. Antibiotic prophylaxis is usually not required; however, may be needed if bacterial infection is present
- booster doses are recommended for adults $>$ 50 years who have not received a booster dose in previous 10 years (with pertussis), in those $\geq$ 65 years (if not received in previous 10 years) or in travellers to countries where health services may be difficult to access (if more than 10 years has elapsed since last dose of tetanus-containing vaccine)
- when tetanus vaccine and immunoglobulin are administered at the same time, each is given into a different limb and a separate syringe is used
- tetanus prophylaxis is dependent on the person's history of active immunisation, time since last dose of tetanus-containing vaccine and the type of wound. The following table shows the current recommendations.

RECOMMENDATIONS FOR TETANUS PROPHYLAXIS IN WOUND MANAGEMENT

History of tetanus vaccination	Time since last dose	Type of wound	Tetanus vaccine	Tetanus immunoglobulin
$\geq$ 3 doses	$<$ 5 years	Clean minor wound	NO	NO
$\geq$ 3 doses	$<$ 5 years	All other wounds	NO	NO (unless person is immunodeficient)

History of tetanus vaccination	Time since last dose	Type of wound	Tetanus vaccine	Tetanus immunoglobulin
≥ 3 doses	5–10 years	Clean minor wound	NO	NO
≥ 3 doses	5–10 years	All other wounds	YES	NO (unless person is immunodeficient)
≥ 3 doses	> 10 years	Clean minor wound	YES	NO
≥ 3 doses	> 10 years	All other wounds	YES	NO (unless person is immunodeficient)
< 3 doses	Uncertain	Clean minor wound	YES	NO
< 3 doses	Uncertain	All other wounds	YES	YES

Immunodeficient: those who have humoral immune deficiency or with HIV (regardless of CD4+ count) if tetanus-prone wound has occurred regardless of when last dose of tetanus-containing vaccine was administered

Australian Technical Advisory Group on Immunisation (ATAGI). The Australian Immunisation Handbook (2018). Available from: https://immunisationhandbook.health.gov.au/resources/handbook-tables/table-guide-to-tetanus-prophylaxis-in-wound-management © Commonwealth of Australia as represented by the Department of Health.

ZOSTER IMMUNOGLOBULIN (Zoster Immunoglobulin-VF)

Available form
Vial: 200 U

Action
- see General Actions of immunoglobulins (p. 1557)
- most effective if given within 96 hours of exposure

Use
- prevention of varicella in susceptible high-risk patients (e.g. leukaemia, lymphoma, congenital or acquired immunodeficiency (e.g. AIDS), corticosteroid or antineoplastic therapy), after exposure to chicken pox or shingles, with no/unknown history of prior exposure to chicken pox

Dose
- (patient weight > 40 kg) 600 IU IM **OR**
- (patient weight 30.1–40 kg) 500 IU IM **OR**
- (patient weight 20.1–30 kg) 375 IU IM **OR**
- (patient weight 10.1–20 kg) 250 IU IM **OR**
- (patient weight 0–10 kg) 125 IU IM

Adverse effects/Interactions/Nursing points/Cautions/Patient teaching and advice
- should be administered within 96 hours of exposure
- not given IV
- not recommended prophylactically in those who are immunodeficient
- if greater than 5 mL is required, dose should be administered over several sites
- local anaesthetic can be added to lessen pain
- see General Adverse effects/Interactions/Nursing points/Cautions/Patient teaching and advice for immunoglobulins (pp. 1557–59)

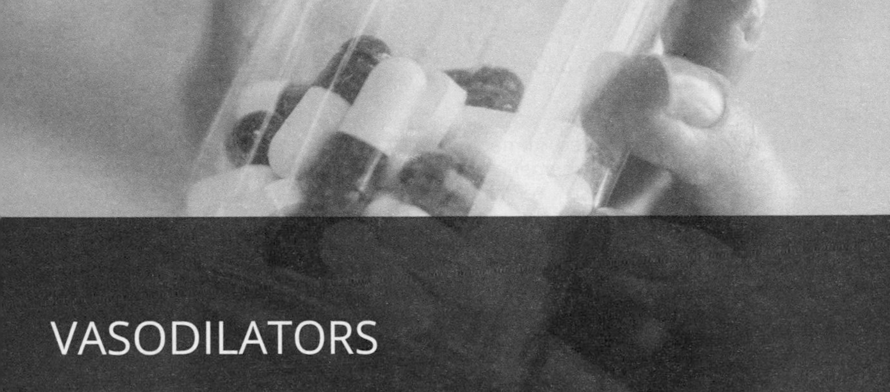

VASODILATORS

The vasodilators are a heterogeneous (diverse) group of agents that act either directly or indirectly, resulting in vasodilation and improved circulation. Directly acting vasodilators include those that affect the smooth muscle within blood vessels, such as the nitrates (e.g. glyceryl trinitrate; see Antianginal agents, p. 61); calcium-channel blockers, which act by inhibiting the cellular influx of calcium ions into vascular smooth muscle, thereby reducing contractile ability (e.g. diltiazem; see Antihypertensive agents, p. 523); and potassium-channel activators (e.g. nicorandil; see Antianginal agents, p. 70). Indirectly acting vasodilators include centrally acting agents (e.g. clonidine; see Antihypertensive agents, p. 530), ACE inhibitors (e.g. captopril; see Antihypertensive agents, p. 496) or angiotensin II receptor antagonists (e.g. losartan; see Antihypertensive agents, p. 505).

Other vasodilators that do not fall into these categories are included in this chapter.

ALPROSTADIL (prostaglandin E1) (Caverject Impulse, Prostin VR)

Available forms

Ampoules: 500 microgram/mL; Vial: 10 microgram, 20 microgram

Action

- prostaglandin
- vasodilator, prevents platelet aggregation
- relaxes ductus arteriosus, supporting patency
- elevates body temperature
- most effective if used within 96 hours of birth
- (IV) half-life 5–10 minutes

Use

- maintain patency of the ductus arteriosus in neonates with congenital heart failure until surgery is possible (Prostin VR)
- erectile dysfunction in adult men (see Erectile dysfunction agents, p. 1057) (Caverject Impulse)

Dose

- (ductus arteriosus) 0.1 microgram/kg/minute IV until effective, then dose is decreased

Adverse effects

- (IV) apnoea, fever, flushing, hypotension, bradycardia, tachycardia, seizures, diarrhoea, oedema, cardiac arrest, hypokalaemia, disseminated intravascular coagulation (DIC), sepsis
- (long term) reversible cortical proliferation of long bones

Nursing points/Cautions

- use is only recommended in facilities where intubation and ventilatory

support can be accessed immediately in the event of an emergency
- babies (especially those weighing < 2 kg) should be closely monitored for apnoea (especially during first 60 minutes of infusion)
- arterial pressure should be monitored during therapy and infusion rate decreased if there is a significant fall
- if therapy > 120 hours, babies should be monitored for antral hyperplasia and gastric outlet obstruction
- solution should be replaced every 24 hours
- should be given into a large blood vessel or via umbilical artery catheter
- dilute with sodium chloride 0.9%
- infusion rate is calculated using dosage, neonate's weight and final concentration to be used
- administer using infusion pump
- avoid Prostin VR (undiluted) coming into contact with a plastic container, because a hazy solution will result which should be discarded
- caution if used in neonates with a history of bleeding because of the risk of DIC
- not recommended in neonates with respiratory distress syndrome or for more than 2–3 days continuously
- contraindicated in neonates with persistent fetal circulation (with cyanosis) or with total anomalous pulmonary venous return (below diaphragm), or with asplenia or polysplenia in whom pulmonary atresia is combined with anomalous pulmonary venous return that may be obstructed

BETAHISTINE DIHYDROCHLORIDE (Betaserc, Serc, Setear)

Available forms
Tablets: 16 mg, 24 mg

Action
- histamine-like drug that increases blood flow in the microcirculation in the inner ear
- half-life about 3.5 hours

Use
- Ménière's syndrome (symptoms include vertigo with nausea and/or vomiting, tinnitus and hearing loss)

Dose
- initially 8–16 mg orally 3 times daily (maximum daily dose 48 mg) **OR**
- 24 mg twice daily (maximum daily dose 48 mg)

Adverse effects
- headache
- nausea, dyspepsia
- (rare) dizziness, malaise, tiredness, mild skin or GI disturbances, hypersensitivity

Interactions
- may antagonise antihistamines
- caution if used with MAO inhibitors (including MAO B selective)

Nursing points/Cautions
- monitoring is required if patient has asthma
- caution if used in those receiving antihistamines or who have asthma
- contraindicated in those with a history of or current active peptic ulcer or pheochromocytoma or under 18 years

Patient teaching and advice
- advise patient that improvement in condition should be seen within a few days of starting therapy
- warn patient not to drive or operate machinery if dizziness or tiredness occur
- patient should be advised to take with meals if GI disturbances occur
- female patients should be counselled to use adequate contraception to prevent pregnancy occurring

- see also General Patient teaching and advice (p. xxvii)

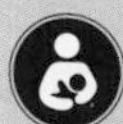

contraindicated during pregnancy and breastfeeding

tablet can be crushed and mixed with water or spoonful of yoghurt or apple puree

PENTOXIFYLLINE (OXPENTIFYLLINE) (Trental 400)

Available form

Tablets (controlled release): 400 mg

Action

- xanthine derivative thought to improve blood flow in the affected microcirculation by reducing blood viscosity, platelet adhesion and aggregation and increasing tissue oxygenation
- half-life 0.4–0.8 hours
- active metabolites (elimination half-lives 1–1.6 hours)

Use

- intermittent claudication in peripheral arterial disease of limbs

Dose

- 400 mg orally 3 times daily with or after food

Adverse effects

- nausea, dyspepsia, vomiting, bloating, flatulence, belching, abdominal pain, diarrhoea
- dizziness, headache, tremor
- pruritus, rash, urticaria
- (uncommon) angina/chest pain
- (rare) jaundice, cholestasis

Interactions

- combined use with other xanthine derivatives or with sympathomimetics may cause excessive CNS stimulation
- may increase serum levels of theophylline and risk of adverse effects
- may increase effects of hypoglycaemic agents, requiring a dose adjustment to prevent hypoglycaemia occurring in patients with diabetes
- may cause bleeding if given with oral anticoagulants or antiplatelet agents. Those on warfarin should have INR time monitored more frequently than normal
- effects of antihypertensive agents may be enhanced
- serum levels may increase if given with ciprofloxacin or cimetidine
- may cause false positive result on urinary assay for pregnanediol

Nursing points/Cautions

- blood pressure (BP) should be measured regularly during therapy, especially in those with pre-existing low or labile BP
- observe for improvement of skin colour, temperature and peripheral pulses
- note if patient can walk further without pain after treatment
- treatment is recommended for at least 8 weeks to assess effectiveness
- caution if used in the elderly, those with low/labile blood pressure, at risk of bleeding, severe coronary heart disease, stenosis of cerebral blood vessels or impaired kidney function (creatinine clearance < 30 mL/min)
- not recommended in those with severe liver or kidney impairment
- contraindicated in those with or history of peptic ulceration or myocardial infarction or who have recently experienced a severe haemorrhage or have an intolerance to other methylxanthines (e.g. caffeine, theophylline)

Patient teaching and advice

- advise patient to avoid smoking and alcohol

- instruct patient that controlled-release tablet is swallowed whole (not broken, chewed or crushed) with a glass of water
- suggest taking with food to reduce stomach disturbances if they occur
- advise patient against driving or operating heavy machinery if dizziness or tremor occurs
- those with diabetes should be instructed to monitor blood glucose levels regularly during therapy as adjustment to hypoglycaemic agent (insulin or oral medication) may be required
- prevent ulceration of affected lower extremities by advising good skin care, close attention to toenails, properly fitting shoes and hosiery and by avoiding garters, hot water bottles and any trauma
- see also General Patient teaching and advice (p. xxvii)

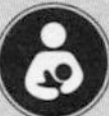

not used in pregnancy or breastfeeding unless expected benefit outweighs potential risk

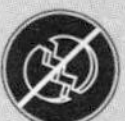

tablet should not be crushed, broken or chewed

VITAMINS, MINERALS AND ELECTROLYTES

Vitamins are organic substances required by the body in small amounts for various metabolic processes. Minerals are inorganic nutrients or trace elements, also required in small quantities, which act as essential co-factors in various enzyme systems. Deficiency states are rare in people who have an adequate diet. However, oral vitamin and mineral supplements may be necessary in cases of restricted diet, malabsorption syndrome and where there are increased requirements, such as in pregnancy, lactation, fever, hyperthyroidism, burn injuries, large wounds and wasting diseases. They may also be added to parenteral and enteral nutrition solutions.

The vitamin B group and vitamin C are water soluble, whereas vitamins A, D, E and K are fat soluble. Many mixed vitamin (multivitamin) preparations containing vitamins A, B group, C, D and E are available, and some also containing minerals. Prolonged courses of high-dose multivitamins are of little value if the diet is well balanced, and can have serious consequences in the case of excessive intake of the fat-soluble vitamins A and D.

VITAMINS

VITAMIN A

VITAMIN A (also known as Retinol) (Bio-Logical Vitamin A, Blackmores Vitamin A 5000)

Available forms

Capsules: 5000 IU; Oral solution: 2.75 mg/0.2 mL (5000 IU)

Action

- fat-soluble vitamin necessary for normal formation and function of epithelial and mucosal cells, normal bone growth, embryonic development (particularly spinal cord, vertebrae, limbs, eyes, ears and heart) and immune function
- necessary for formation and regeneration of rhodopsin (visual purple), which is needed for vision, particularly in dim light

- available in a number of forms (retinol, retinal, retinoic acid, retinyl ester)
- preformed vitamin A is only available in animal-derived foods, oils, fruits and vegetables contain provitamin A carotenoid (precursor of retinol)

Deficiency
- night blindness; later, xerophthalmia
- dry rough skin (follicular hyperkeratosis)
- infection due to immune dysfunction

Use
- deficiency states, night blindness
- some skin diseases (e.g. dermatitis, skin ulcers), chronic infection (e.g. acne)
- premenstrual tension
- prophylaxis against respiratory infection
- replacement in decreased intestinal absorption conditions (e.g. steatorrhoea, biliary obstruction, coeliac disease)
- xerophthalmia

Optimal daily requirements
- 700 microgram (women), 900 microgram (men)

Dose
- 5000 IU orally daily with food **OR**
- (severe deficiency) 50,000 IU orally twice daily for 3 days, then daily for 14 days

Adverse effects

Acute toxicity (very high doses)
- drowsiness, sedation, dizziness, irritability, severe headache (because of increased intracranial pressure), papilloedema
- nausea, vomiting, hepatomegaly
- erythema, pruritus, desquamation
- (infants) vomiting, bulging fontanelles

Chronic toxicity (excessive amounts over prolonged period)
- anorexia, weight loss
- irritability, headache, fatigue
- cracking and bleeding lips
- dry itching peeling skin, dermatitis, disturbed hair growth
- bone pain, hyperostosis
- papilloedema
- haemorrhage

Nursing points/Cautions
- contraindicated in those with hypervitaminosis A

Patient teaching and advice
- (oral solution) advise patient that oral solution can be mixed in water or juice

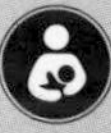

not recommended during pregnancy. High doses can cause birth defects

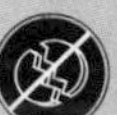

vitamin A capsules should not be opened. Available as oral solution

Note
- contained in multivitamin preparations

VITAMIN B

THIAMINE HYDROCHLORIDE (Vitamin B_1) (Betamin, Betavit)

Available form

Tablets: 100 mg

Action
- member of the water-soluble vitamin B group necessary for carbohydrate metabolism, including detoxification of oestrogen in the liver
- not stored in any significant amounts (about 30 g), therefore any excess is excreted in the liver
- found predominantly in cereal foods; thiamine-enrichment of baking flour exists in Australia (not New Zealand)

Deficiency

- dietary deficiency (e.g. beriberi, chronic alcoholism (as alcohol metabolism requires thiamine), anorexia)
- (chronic) peripheral neuropathy, Wernicke's encephalopathy, Korsakoff's syndrome, psychosis, cardiac failure
- (acute) weakness, fatigue, nausea, anorexia, hypotension, decreased reflexes and sensation, paralysis

Use

- thiamine deficiency due to restricted diet (including those receiving total parenteral nutrition), extensive burns, diabetes, impaired kidney or liver function, hyperthyroidism, alcoholism, benign breast dysplasia

Optimal daily requirements

- 1.2 mg (male), 1.1 mg (female), 1.4 mg (during pregnancy)

Dose

- 50–100 mg orally daily as a single dose or 2 divided doses

tablets can be crushed and mixed with water or spoonful of yoghurt or apple puree

Note

- contained in B-Dose 2 mL injection and B-Dose Forte 2 mL injection with other B vitamins cyanocobalamin (B_{12}), (nicotinamide (B_3), pyridoxine (B_6), riboflavine (B_2) and dexpanthenol (B_5)) for treatment of beriberi, Wernicke's encephalopathy (Forte formulation), pellagra (as patients often have other vitamin B deficiencies), peripheral neuritis, pernicious anaemia and chronic alcoholism
- contained in multivitamin preparations

NICOTINAMIDE (also known as Vitamin B_3, Nicotinic acid and Niacin) (Blackmores InSolar)

Available form

Tablets: 500 mg

Action

- member of the water-soluble vitamin B group
- peripheral vasodilator
- hypolipidaemic, hypotriglyceridaemic and hypocholesterolaemic
- forms co-enzymes important in tissue respiration
- available in a wide range of foods, including beef, pork, wholegrain cereals, eggs and cow's milk

Deficiency

- pellagra (glossitis, dermatitis, diarrhoea, and, in severe cases, dementia or delirium)

Use

- pellagra
- skin health
- hypercholesterolaemia, hypertriglyceridaemia, hyperlipoproteinaemia (most types) (see Lipid regulating agents, p. 1261)

Optimal daily requirements

- 16 mg (males), 14 mg (females), 18 mg (pregnancy), 17 mg (breastfeeding)

Dose

- (pellagra) 250 mg orally twice daily after meals **OR**
- 500 mg orally daily **OR**
- (solar damaged skin, prevention recurrence of skin cancers) 500 mg orally twice daily

Adverse effects/Interactions/ Nursing points/Cautions/Patient teaching and advice

- it is important to differentiate between nicotinic acid (niacin) and nicotinamide (niacinamide e.g. Insolar).

Nicotinic acid is used for treating hyperlipidaemia; nicotinamide is used for treating solar damaged skin. These uses are not interchangeable; however, either can be used for treating B_3 deficiency

- not recommended in those < 18 years
- see nicotinic acid in Lipid-regulating agents (p. 1261)
- see also general points for thiamine (pp. 1574–75)

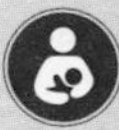

not recommended during pregnancy or breastfeeding

PYRIDOXINE (VITAMIN B_6) (Blackmores Vitamin B6, Pyridox)

Available forms

Tablets: 25 mg, 100 mg; Tablets (sustained-release): 240 mg

Action

- member of the water-soluble vitamin B group, important in carbohydrate, lipid and protein metabolism
- assists in formation of haemoglobin
- made up of 6 compounds (pyridoxal, pyridoxine, pyridoxamine and their phosphates)
- found in a wide range of foods (e.g. organ meats, muscle meats, breakfast cereals, vegetables, fruits)

Deficiency

- irritability, convulsions, depression, confusion
- hypochromic (microcytic) anaemia
- seborrhoeic dermatitis

Use

- some types of anaemia
- nausea and vomiting in pregnancy
- radiation sickness
- symptoms associated with premenstrual tension
- acute alcoholism
- homocystinuria

Optimal daily requirements

- 1.3–1.7 mg (males), 1.3–1.5 mg (females), 1.9 mg (pregnancy), 2.0 mg (breastfeeding)

Dose

- 25–100 mg orally daily or as prescribed

OR

- 240 mg orally daily (sustained-release)

Adverse effects

- gastrointestinal upset, headache
- (high dose, prolonged therapy) peripheral neuropathy, nervousness, tremors, abnormal ECG

Interactions

- may reduce effects of levodopa (not if a dopa decarboxylase inhibitor is also given)

Nursing points/Cautions

- contraindicated if there is inadequate dietary protein intake to avoid undesirable increase in amino acid catabolism
- see general points for thiamine (pp. 1574–75)

Patient teaching and advice

- (premenstrual tension) patient should be advised to take pyridoxine daily for the number of days the symptoms occur before onset of menstruation
- advise patient to seek medical advice if any tingling, burning, prickling or tightening sensation of hands or feet occur

plain tablets can be dispersed in water or crushed and mixed with spoonful of yoghurt or apple puree

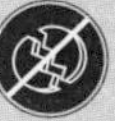

sustained-release tablets should not be chewed, broken or crushed

CYANOCOBALAMIN (VITAMIN B_{12}) (B12 Liquid, Blackmores B12, Cyanocobalamin 1 mg in 1 mL Injection, Cyanocobalamin 20 mg in 2 mL Injection, Eagle Sublingual B12, Methylcobalamin 10 mg in 2 mL injection, Methyl B12 Chewable, NanoCelle B12)

Available forms

Tablets: 100 microgram; Tablets (sublingual): 1 mg; Ampoules: 1 mg/mL, 10 mg/2 mL, 20 mg/2 mL; Sublingual spray: 500 microgram/spray

Action

- member of the water-soluble vitamin B group, essential for normal cell growth, production of epithelial cells, haemopoiesis and maintenance of myelin throughout the nervous system
- acts as a co-enzyme in nucleic acid synthesis
- dietary sources include red meats, milk and milk products

Deficiency

- megaloblastic anaemia (macrocytosis) (similar to folate deficiency)
- neurological damage (e.g. sensory disturbance of feet and hands, motor disturbance, cognitive changes, visual disturbance)
- GI disturbance

Use

- pernicious anaemia
- prophylaxis and treatment of other macrocytic anaemias associated with vitamin B_{12} deficiency (unable to be corrected orally)
- peripheral neuropathy, diabetic polyneuropathy (adjunct)
- diet supplement for vegan and vegetarian diets

Optimal daily requirements

- 2.4 microgram; (pregnancy) 2.6 microgram; (breastfeeding) 2.8 microgram

Dose

- 20 mg slow IM stat **OR**
- 5 mg slow IM daily for 5 days **OR**
- 10 mg slow IM, repeated as needed **OR**
- 1 mg slow IM, repeated as needed **OR**
- 1 mg daily orally (dissolved under tongue) (sublingual tablets) **OR**
- 100 microgram orally twice daily with food or as prescribed **OR**
- 500–1000 microgram sublingually 1–2 times daily after meals (or as prescribed) (sublingual spray)

Adverse effects

- diarrhoea, prolonged nausea or vomiting, abdominal pain
- IM pain, redness, induration
- (rare) hypersensitivity reaction, anaphylaxis, pulmonary oedema, congestive cardiac failure, hypokalaemia, cardiac arrest

Interactions

- malabsorption may occur if given with colchicine or heavy alcohol use (> 2 weeks)
- serum levels by decreased by combined oral contraceptives or folic acid (high dose, prolonged use)
- response may be decreased if given with methotrexate

Nursing points/Cautions

- diagnosis of pernicious anaemia should be made before starting therapy
- before starting therapy, haematocrit, reticulocyte count, vitamin B_{12}, folate and iron levels should be checked. Haematocrit and reticulocyte count should also be checked daily from day 5 to 7 of therapy, then regularly depending on haematocrit. If reticulocyte

count does not increase or reticulocyte count remains elevated with haematocrit < 35%, therapy should be re-evaluated
- serum potassium levels should be monitored during therapy, especially initially, and any hypokalaemia corrected immediately
- FBC and serum vitamin B_{12} should be monitored 6–12-monthly (if the patient is well), or more frequently if the patient has some condition that may increase the need for vitamin B_{12}. Monitoring of levels should continue for life
- oral administration may be insufficient to treat pernicious anaemia, malabsorption disorders, gastrectomy and gastrointestinal pathologies
- if patient has an allergic disposition to B vitamins, this can be checked giving a dermal dose
- antihistamines, corticosteroids and adrenaline (epinephrine) (1:1000) should be readily available in the event of anaphylaxis
- not given IV
- solution should be warmed before use to reduce pain
- solution is a crimson–red colour
- not recommended in children < 12 years
- caution if used in those with liver disease or myeloproliferative disorders or Leber's disease
- contraindicated in those with hypersensitivity to cobalt, hypervitaminosis, megaloblastic anaemia of pregnancy

Patient teaching and advice

- patient should be advised to allow sublingual tablets to dissolve under the tongue
- advise patient with pernicious anaemia that therapy is for life to prevent nerve damage to spinal cord

available as chewable or sublingual tablets

HYDROXOCOBALAMIN (VITAMIN B_{12}) (Cobal-B12, Hydroxo-B12, Neo-B12 Injection, Vita B12)

Available form

Ampoules: 1000 microgram/mL

Action

- as for cyanocobalamin (p. 1577), but produces a higher and more prolonged vitamin B_{12} level when given IM at the same dose
- excreted slowly via bile and urine

Use

- prevention and treatment of pernicious anaemia and other macrocytic anaemias associated with vitamin B_{12} deficiency
- treat optic neuropathies (e.g. tobacco amblyopia, Leber's disease, optic atrophy)

Dose

- (pernicious anaemia, macrocytic anaemias without neurological involvement) initially 250–1000 microgram IM alternate days for 1–2 weeks, then 250 microgram IM weekly until RBC count is normal, then 1000 microgram every 2–3 months for life (maintenance) **OR**
- (pernicious anaemia, macrocytic anaemia with neurological involvement) initially 1000 microgram IM alternate days for 1–2 weeks, then 1000 microgram every 2 months for life (maintenance) **OR**
- (optic neuropathies) initially 1000 microgram IM daily for 2 weeks, then twice weekly for 4 weeks, then monthly for life (maintenance) **OR**

- (prevention of macrocytic anaemia and associated B_{12} deficiency) 1000 microgram IM every 2–3 months

Adverse effects

- itching, sensation of hot and cold, urticaria, eczema, acne, folliculitis
- nausea, vomiting, diarrhoea
- headache, dizziness, malaise
- chest pain/discomfort, hypokalaemia, arrhythmias (secondary to hypokalaemia), cardiac arrest
- feeling of body swelling
- development of antibodies
- peripheral vascular thrombosis
- IM site reaction
- (rare) anaphylaxis, pulmonary oedema, congestive cardiac failure

Interactions

- poor response if given with chloramphenicol or other agents with bone marrow depressing properties
- serum levels may be decreased by oral contraceptives
- vitamin B_{12} levels may be lowered by large, continuous doses of folic acid, as well as potentiating neurological complications
- vitamin B_{12} blood assay may be invalidated by antibacterial agents

Nursing points/Cautions

- diagnosis of pernicious anaemia should be made before starting therapy
- intradermal test is recommended in those with sensitivity to cobalamins
- not given IV
- serum potassium should be monitored during therapy, especially initially, and any hypokalaemia corrected immediately
- serum vitamin B_{12} should be monitored regularly during therapy
- therapy may unmask polycythaemia vera
- solution is dark red in colour
- iron and folic acid supplements may also be necessary if there is severe anaemia
- caution if used in those with iron or folate deficiency, uraemia or a concurrent infection because therapeutic effect may be decreased
- contraindicated in those with hypersensitivity to cobalt or with megaloblastic anaemia of pregnancy

Patient teaching and advice

- patient should be advised to seek medical advice if any of the following occur:
  - breathlessness that worsens on lying down
  - changes in heart rate
  - chest tightness or pain

FOLIC ACID (FOLATE) (Blackmores Folate, Foltabs, Megafol)

Available forms

Vial: 5 mg/mL; Tablets: 500 microgram

Action

- member of the water-soluble vitamin B group, required for the maturation of RBC and necessary for DNA synthesis and mitosis and hence growth
- available in different forms in foods; dietary sources include cereals, cereal products, vegetables, fruits and legumes
- stored in the liver and excreted in the urine (4–5 microgram/day)
- folate utilisation increased in pregnancy and lactation, haemolytic anaemia, hyperthyroidism, exfoliative dermatitis and chronic infection

Deficiency

- megaloblastic anaemia

Use

- to prevent or treat megaloblastic anaemia caused by folic acid deficiency
- prevention of deficiency during pregnancy and breastfeeding
- decreases risk of spina bifida (neural tube defect in fetus) if taken 4 weeks before conception and during pregnancy

Optimal daily requirements

- 400 microgram (males and females), 600 microgram (pregnancy), 500 microgram (breastfeeding)

Dose

- (prevention during pregnancy and breastfeeding) 0.5 mg orally daily **OR**
- (treatment of megaloblastic anaemia) 1–5 mg orally or IM adjusted according to severity of anaemia **OR**
- (prevention of spina bifida) 0.5 mg orally daily starting 4 weeks before conception

Adverse effects

- (uncommon) nausea, flatulence, diarrhoea
- (uncommon) sleep disturbance, irritability
- (uncommon) rash, bronchospasm
- (IV) seizures, EEG changes
- (rare) anaphylaxis

Interactions

- absorption decreased by chronic alcohol intake and sulfasalazine
- metabolism may be inhibited by methotrexate, trimethoprim and pyrimethamine
- may decrease serum levels of phenytoin and phenobarbital (phenobarbitone) leading to possible loss of seizure control

Nursing points/Cautions

- vitamin B_{12} deficiency should be excluded before starting therapy
- folic acid does not correct folate deficiency due to methotrexate; folinic acid should be used
- (parenteral) usually given IM, but may be given IV or SC
- (parenteral) may be diluted with 49 mL of water for injections for IV administration
- contains 34.5 mg of sodium/mL
- caution if used in those with folate dependent tumours
- contraindicated for treatment of megaloblastic anaemia caused by vitamin B_{12} deficiency

Patient teaching and advice

- advise patient to avoid alcohol during therapy

tablets can be dispersed in water or crushed and mixed with spoonful of yoghurt or apple puree

Note

- contained with iron in Blackmores I-Folic, Fefol and Ferro-F tab
- contained in multivitamin preparations

VITAMIN C

ASCORBIC ACID (VITAMIN C) (Biological Therapies Sodium Ascorbate Solution, Blackmores Vitamin C, Cenovis MegaC 1000 mg Chewable Tablets, Cenovis Sugarless C 500 mg Chewable Tablets)

Available forms

Tablets: 250 mg, 500 mg, 1 g; Tablets (chewable): 250 mg, 500 mg; 1 g; Vial: 90 mg/mL, 150 mg/mL, 300 mg/mL (as calcium ascorbate)

Action

- water-soluble agent essential for synthesis of collagen and intercellular material

- necessary for wound healing and resistance to infection
- necessary for the conversion of folic acid to folinic acid, carbohydrate and iron metabolism, lipid and protein synthesis
- necessary for maintenance of teeth, bone matrix and capillary walls
- antioxidant properties
- facilitates absorption of iron and copper
- necessary for RBC production
- dietary sources include fruit (e.g. blackcurrants, guava, citrus, kiwi fruit) and vegetables (e.g. broccoli and sprouts)

Deficiency
- scurvy (petechiae, coiled hairs, inflamed and bleeding gums, joint effusion, fatigue, poor wound healing, lesions, pain in extremities, haemorrhage, oedema)

Use
- prevention of ascorbic acid (vitamin C) deficiency
- as a supplement when on a restricted diet
- treatment of scurvy
- promotion of healing of wounds and fractures at times of increased requirement that cannot be met by normal dietary intake (e.g. burns, trauma, postoperatively, thyrotoxicosis)
- adjunct in treatment of idiopathic methaemoglobinaemia

Optimal daily requirements
- 45 mg (males, females), 60 mg (pregnancy), 85 mg (breastfeeding)

Dose
- (dietary supplement) 1–3 tablets orally daily or as prescribed **OR**
- (IV when oral treatment is not feasible) 100–500 mg IV as bolus or IV infusion **OR**
- (antioxidant) 500 mg orally 1–2 times daily or as prescribed

Adverse effects
- headache, dizziness
- (large doses) diarrhoea, renal calculi
- (doses > 600 mg) diuretic action
- stomach cramps, nausea, vomiting
- (high dose) may precipitate gout or sickle cell crisis
- (IV) pain, thrombophlebitis, dehydration
- (IV, rapid infusion) temporary dizziness or faintness

Interactions
- may increase absorption of aluminium hydroxide from gut and therefore not recommended together in those with renal failure
- increased urinary excretion may occur if given with aspirin, primidone or barbiturates
- may decrease excretion of aspirin increasing serum levels
- caution if given with warfarin
- (oral) may increase bioavailability of ethinyloesterol
- (oral) may increase absorption of iron
- increases excretion of desferrioxamine when given together. Vitamin C should be given 1–2 hours after desferrioxamine infusion has started
- decreases chronotropic effect of isoprenaline
- decreased serum levels may occur if given with alcohol
- (chronic/high dose) may interfere with disulfiram
- may decrease effects of phenothiazines
- may interfere with some laboratory tests including theophylline serum levels and occult blood

Nursing points/Cautions/Patient teaching and advice

- (IV) ensure patient is adequately hydrated during therapy
- (IV) large vein should be used
- (IV) pain at infusion site can be minimised by decreasing infusion rate or

diluting infusion (50:50) with water for injections or warming solution to body temperature before administration
- (IV) avoid extravasation
- caution if used in those with iron overload (e.g. haemochromotosis, thalassaemia, polycythaemia, sideroblastic anaemia), G6PD deficiency, sickle cell anaemia (high dose), diabetes mellitus, gout, active peptic ulcer, advanced cancer, congestive cardiac failure, severely impaired kidney function, hypernatraemia, hyperoxaluria or prone to kidney stones

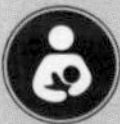

high doses should not be used during pregnancy or breastfeeding

chewable, dispersible and effervescent formulations are available

Note
- contained in multivitamin preparations

VITAMIN D

General Actions of vitamin D
- endogenous vitamin D is obtained from sunlight's action on the skin, and is then activated in the liver and kidneys (D_3 or colecalciferol (cholecalciferol)); also found in some foods (D_2 or ergocalciferol)
- group of closely related fat-soluble sterol compounds involved in the regulation of calcium and phosphate homeostasis and bone mineralisation
- enhances calcium absorption from the small intestine
- immune function

Optimal daily requirements
- 5 microgram (males, females, pregnancy, breastfeeding)
- 10 microgram (males, females 51–70 years)
- 15 microgram (males, females over 70 years of age)

Deficiency
- osteomalacia (adults)
- rickets (children)
- studies have found deficiencies in elderly people with restricted access to sunlight, many of whom live in residential care (Australian NHMRC & New Zealand MoH 2006)

COLECALCIFEROL (CHOLECALCIFEROL) (VITAMIN D_3) (Bio-Logical Vitamin D3 Solution, Blackmores Vitamin D3, Caltrate Vitamin D 1000 IU, D3 Capsules and Drops Forte, Ostelin Vitamin D, OsteVit-D, OsteVit-D Vitamin D3 Oral Drops for Children, OsteVit-D One-A-Week, Phyta D)

Available forms
Tablets: 25 microgram (1000 IU), 175 microgram (7000 IU); Capsules: 25 microgram (1000 IU); Drops: 5 microgram (200 IU), 25 microgram (1000 IU); Oral spray: 25 microgram/spray (1000 IU); Oral solution: 25 microgram/0.5 mL

Use
- treatment and prevention of vitamin D deficiency states, including those associated with malabsorption, hypocalcaemia, hypophosphataemic rickets, hypoparathyroidism and metabolic disorders
- osteoporosis
- prevention of osteoporosis associated with corticosteroids

Dose

- 25 microgram (1000 IU) orally daily with food or as prescribed **OR**
- 175 microgram (7000 IU) orally with food once per week **OR**
- 1 spray (25 microgram (1000 IU)) once daily **OR**
- (adult) 1 drop (25 microgram (1000 IU)) once daily (Forte drops)

Adverse effects

- nausea, abdominal pain
- headache, drowsiness, weakness
- hypercalcaemia, hypercalciuria
- (high dose, prolonged therapy) vitamin D intoxication
- severe dehydration
- (uncommon) ectopic calcification, nephrocalcinosis, proteinuria, casts in urine
- (uncommon) diarrhoea, constipation, rash, pruritus, urticaria
- (children, high dose, rare) retarded growth

Interactions

- not recommended with other vitamin D-containing preparation due to risk of vitamin D intoxication
- phenobarbital (phenobarbitone), phenytoin, primidone and cimetidine may increase metabolism and decrease effects
- caution if used with calcitonin, gallium nitrate, pamidronate, calcium-containing preparations, thiazide diuretics due to risk of hypercalcaemia
- mineral oil, orlistat or lipid-lowering agents (e.g. colestipol or colestyramine (cholestryramine)) may decrease absorption of fat-soluble vitamins including vitamin D
- hypermagnesaemia may develop if calcitriol is used concurrently with magnesium-containing antacids
- may increase aluminium levels and risk of toxicity if given with aluminium-containing antacids (if used as phosphate binders in hyperphosphataemia)
- caution if vitamin D and digoxin are given together as this may precipitate cardiac arrhythmias
- may decrease effectiveness of calcium-channel blockers

Nursing points/Cautions

- monitor serum calcium and phosphate levels regularly (twice weekly when starting therapy) then 2–3-monthly. Magnesium, alkaline phosphatase and urinary calcium and phosphorus (24-hour) should also be monitored
- if possible, bloods should be drawn without using a tourniquet to minimise local calcium effects
- parathyroid hormone (PTH) levels should be monitored regularly during therapy
- patients who are immobile (e.g. post-surgery) are at increased risk of hypercalcaemia
- vitamin D-resistant state may exist in uraemic patient due to failure of kidneys to convert precursor to active component
- caution if used in those with hyperphosphataemia due to risk of ectopic calcifications occurring
- caution if used in those with impaired renal function or renal calculi, history of raised urinary oxalates, sarcoidosis and granulomas
- caution if used in those with arteriosclerosis or cardiac function impairment
- contraindicated in those with vitamin D toxicity, hypercalcaemia or renal osteodystrophy with hyperphosphatemia

Patient teaching and advice

- advise patient to take 1 hour before or 4–6 hours after colestyramine (cholestryramine) or orlistat
- patient should be instructed to seek medical advice immediately if any of the following occur:

  - loss of appetite, nausea, vomiting, diarrhoea
  - profuse sweating, excessive thirst or urination
  - headache, muscle weakness or bone pain
- instruct patient/parent/carer that drops should be dispensed using graduated dropper; can be taken directly or added to water or juice
- patient should be advised to avoid magnesium or aluminium-containing antacids during therapy
- inform patient that daily dietary calcium intake should not exceed 1000 mg (calcitriol therapy) and that calcium supplements are not required unless diet is clearly inadequate
- advise patient that vitamin D supplements are not required if he/she receives sufficient daily sunlight exposure (20 minutes daily)
- instruct patient to shake spray or oral solution well before use

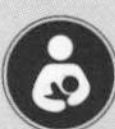

not recommended during breastfeeding

oral solution is available. Tablets can be crushed and mixed with spoonful of yoghurt or apple puree

Note

- Calcitriol (1, 25-dihydroxycholecalciferol) is discussed in Bone and calcium regulating agents (p. 895)
- contained in multivitamin preparations

VITAMIN E

VITAMIN E (ALPHA TOCOPHERYL) (Blackmores Natural E, Cenovis MegaE, Cenovis Vitamin E 250 IU, E-Prime)

Available forms

Capsules: 100 IU, 200 IU, 250 IU, 500 IU, 1000 IU

Action

- water-soluble vitamin consisting of several tocopherols that function as antioxidants
- doses of vitamin E, no matter which tocopherol, should be expressed as d-alpha tocopherol equivalents
- 10 mg of d-alpha-tocopherol is ~15 IU (= 14.9)
- main dietary sources are fats and oils

Deficiency (very uncommon)

- peripheral neuropathy, ataxia, skeletal muscle atrophy, retinopathy (symptoms include hyporeflexia, gait disturbances, reduced sensitivity to vibration and proprioception, ophthalmoplegia) (this is due to genetic abnormalities rather than dietary deficiency)

Use

- impairment of fat-soluble vitamin absorption (cystic fibrosis, chronic cholestasis, A-beta-lipoproteinaemia)
- antioxidant

Optimal daily requirements

- 10 mg (males), 7 mg (females), 7 mg (pregnancy), 11 mg (breastfeeding)

Dose

- 100 IU orally with food 1–3 times daily or as prescribed **OR**
- 200 IU orally with food twice daily or as prescribed **OR**
- 250 IU orally with food 1–3 times daily or as prescribed **OR**
- 500 IU orally with food 1–2 times daily or as prescribed **OR**
- 1000 IU orally daily with food or as prescribed

Adverse effects

- (high dose) nausea, diarrhoea, abdominal pain, fatigue and weakness

Interactions

- may antagonise effects of vitamin K, leading to increased blood clotting time

- caution if used with warfarin, INR should be monitored
- caution if given with ciclosporin as ciclosporin levels may decrease or increase. Serum levels should be monitored if given together

Nursing points/Cautions/Patient teaching and advice

- should be taken with food

VITAMIN K

General Actions of vitamin K

- a group of fat-soluble compounds that promote the hepatic biosynthesis of prothrombin (factor II) and coagulation factors VII, IX and X and anticoagulant proteins C and S
- antagonises the effects of indirect-acting oral anticoagulants
- dietary sources include leafy green vegetables (e.g. spinach, salad greens, broccoli, cabbage, brussels sprouts) and some plant oils (e.g. soybean and canola oils and products derived from them)

General Uses of vitamin K

- prothrombin deficiency
- prevention and therapy of vitamin D deficiency bleeding of the newborn
- haemorrhage (or threatened haemorrhage) resulting from hypoprothrombinaemia
- hypovitaminosis K
- to reverse the effects of oral anticoagulants (as an adjunct to blood transfusion)

Deficiency

- hypoprothrombinaemia, bleeding
- haemorrhagic disease of the newborn (neonates)

Optimal daily requirements

- 70 microgram (males), 60 microgram (females, pregnancy, breastfeeding)

PHYTOMENADIONE (VITAMIN K1) (Konakion MM Adult, Konakion MM Paediatric)

Available forms

Ampoules (adult): 10 mg/mL; Ampoules (newborn): 2 mg/0.2 mL

Dose

- (adult, asymptomatic high INR with/without mild haemorrhage) (INR 5–9) 0.5–1.0 mg IV **OR**
- (adult, asymptomatic high INR with/without mild haemorrhage) (INR > 9) 1.0 mg IV **OR**
- (adult, major haemorrhage) 5–10 mg slowly IV with fresh frozen plasma (FFP) and prothrombin complex concentrate (PCC) **OR**
- (adult, life-threatening haemorrhage) 10 mg slowly IV with fresh frozen plasma (FFP) and prothrombin complex concentrate (PCC) **OR**
- (prophylaxis, neonate) 1 mg IM at birth (Konakion MM Paediatric) **OR**
- (prophylaxis, neonate) 2 mg orally at birth, then at 3–5 days old and at 4 weeks (Konakion MM Paediatric) **OR**
- (prophylaxis, neonate weight < 1.5 kg) 0.5 mg IM at birth (Konakion MM Paediatric) **OR**
- (bleeding, neonate) 1 mg IV, repeated if needed (Konakion MM Paediatric)

Adverse effects

- unusual taste, facial flushing, sweating
- (adult, IV injection site) phlebitis
- (neonate, IM) (rare) injection site reaction
- (rare) anaphylactoid reaction

Interactions

- antagonises warfarin
- action may be impaired by phenobarbital (phenobarbitone), phenytoin, rifampicin and isoniazid

- effects may be decreased by cephalosporins, aspirin and salicylates

Nursing points/Cautions/Patient teaching and advice

- ineffective in heparin overdose
- IV rate not more than 1 mg/minute
- (IV) administer alone and should not be diluted
- (adult, major or life-threatening haemorrhage) prothrombin time should be measured after 3 hours and dose repeated if needed
- (adult) if patient has severe liver impairment, INR should be closely monitored after administration
- (adult) should be discontinued if ineffective after 1–2 days in those with severe liver disease
- (neonate, oral) dispenser is supplied with ampoule. Open ampoule and place dispenser in it vertically. Withdraw solution to 2 mL mark on dispenser. Contents can be given directly into infant's mouth. If infant spits it out or vomits, dose can be readministered
- important to check expiry date as impurities may develop over time
- (adult) caution as risk of thromboembolism will return if given to reverse anticoagulant action in those being treated for thromboembolism
- (neonate) increased risk of kernicterus if given to premature infants weighing < 2.5 kg
- (adult) contraindicated IM because of variable absorption (may act as a depot) and also increased risk of haematoma if given to those receiving anticoagulant therapy
- (adult) contraindicated in those with severe allergic predisposition
- see general points for vitamin K (p. 1585)

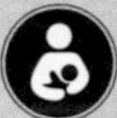

contraindicated during pregnancy

not recommended during breastfeeding as prophylaxis of haemorrhagic disease of the newborn

MINERAL SUPPLEMENTS

CALCIUM

General Actions of calcium

- essential for functioning of muscular, skeletal and nervous systems, and cardiac function
- involved as a co-factor in blood coagulation and transmission of nerve impulses, contraction of cardiac, smooth and skeletal muscle, renal function and respiration
- storage and release of hormones and neurotransmitters
- absorbed from small intestine
- absorption of vitamin B_{12}
- bone has 99% of body's calcium stores
- main dietary sources are milk and milk products, with smaller amounts in bony fish, legumes, some nuts, fortified soy products and breakfast cereals

Optimal daily requirements

- 1000–1300 mg (males, females, pregnancy, breastfeeding)

CALCIUM CARBONATE (CAL-500 Tablets, CAL-600 Tablets, Cal-Care, Calci-Tab 600, Cal-Sup Chewable, Caltrate 600 mg)

Available forms
Tablets: 500, 600 mg (of elemental calcium)

Action
- See General Actions of calcium (p. 1586)

Use
- antacid (see Antacids in Antiulcer agents, p. 820)
- calcium supplement in prevention and treatment of calcium deficiency (e.g. osteoporosis)
- supplement in pregnancy
- phosphate binder in chronic renal failure

Dose
- 1–2 tablets orally daily after food or as prescribed

Adverse effects
- GI irritation, nausea, vomiting, diarrhoea, abdominal pain and distension, flatulence, constipation

Interactions
- may interfere with absorption of oral iron
- forms a complex when given with tetracyclines, therefore should not be given together

Nursing points/Cautions
- contraindicated in those with hypercalcaemia, hypercalciuria, severe renal failure

Patient teaching and advice
- advise patient that chewable tablets can be chewed, sucked or swallowed whole (Cal-Sup Chewable)
- advise patient to take oral calcium at least 2 hours apart from oral iron compounds and oral tetracyclines
- chewable tablets are available. Tablets are difficult to crush

Note
- combined with risedronate in Acris Combi, Actonel EC, Actonel EC Combi and Actonel EC Combi D, as well as in multivitamin supplements (including sports liquids) and antacids

CALCIUM GLUCONATE MONOHYDRATE (CALCIUM GLUCONATE) (Calcium Gluconate 953 mg/10 mL Injection)

Available form
Ampoules: 100 mg/mL (contains 8.9 mg (or 0.44 mEq) elemental calcium/mL)

Actions
- See General Actions of calcium (p. 1586)

Use
- prevention and treatment of hypocalcaemia
- acute hypocalcaemia
- hypocalcaemic tetany
- severe hyperkalaemia
- cardiac resuscitation
- magnesium sulphate toxicity
- acute renal, biliary or intestinal colic

Dose
- (hypocalcaemia) 7–14 mEq IV repeated every 1–3 days if needed **OR**
- (hypocalcaemic tetany) 4.5–16 mEq IV until response occurs (daily maximum 15 g calcium gluconate (calcium ion 67.5 mEq)) **OR**
- (hypermagnesaemia) initially 7 mEq IV, may be repeated if necessary **OR**
- (severe hyperkalaemia) 4.5–9.0 mEq IV, as an adjunct (with ECG monitoring)

Adverse effects
- (high dose) hypercalcaemia (anorexia, nausea, vomiting, constipation, abdominal pain, muscle weakness, polydipsia, polyuria, mental

disturbances, bone pain, renal calculi, cardiac arrhythmias, coma, cardiac arrest), nephrolithiasis
- (IV) sweating, hypotension, irregular heart rate, hot flushed sensation, tingling, 'chalky' taste, feeling of oppression, dizziness, nausea, vomiting, sweating
- (rapid IV) peripheral vasodilation, hot flushes, bradycardia, arrhythmias, hypotension, syncope, cardiac arrest, skin necrosis
- transient increase in BP (elderly or hypertensive patient)
- (IV) burning, redness, rash, pain
- (IM/SC) sloughing, necrosis, burning, cellulitis
- (extravasation) skin redness, rash, pain, burning, soft tissue calcification

Interactions

- (parenteral) contraindicated with digoxin due to calcium's effects on the heart and increased risk of digoxin toxicity
- may interfere with absorption of oral iron
- may reduce response to verapamil and other calcium-channel blockers
- increased risk of calcium deposition in soft tissue if given with potassium and/or sodium phosphate
- forms a complex when given with tetracyclines, therefore should not be given together
- increased risk of hypercalcaemia and hypermagnesaemia if given with other calcium-containing agents or magnesium-containing agents (especially in those with impaired renal function)
- increased risk of hypercalcaemia if given with high doses of vitamin A (as vitamin A stimulates bone loss of calcium)
- vitamin D increases absorption of calcium from the diet, therefore high doses of vitamin D should be avoided during therapy
- may reverse actions of non-depolarising neuromuscular-blocking agents
- may antagonise effects of calcitonin (if used to treat hypercalcaemia)
- increased risk of hypercalcaemia if given with thiazide diuretics
- increased calcium serum levels (but not risk of toxicity) if calcium is given to patients who have recently received citrated blood transfusions

Nursing points/Cautions

- any hyperphosphataemia should be corrected before treating hypocalcaemia in patients who have both conditions
- any fluid or electrolyte imbalance corrected before starting IV therapy, including adequate hydration to prevent formation of renal calculi
- ECG monitoring is recommended during IV injection to detect bradycardia (especially if given to treat hyperkalaemia), and therapy discontinued if significant bradycardia occurs
- patient should remain recumbent during IV therapy to prevent dizziness and should be cautioned to move slowly when first standing
- serum levels of calcium and kidney function should be measured regularly throughout therapy, especially if large doses are given
- solution should be warmed to body temperature (if possible) before IV administration
- do not dilute using any phosphate-containing solutions as precipitate may form
- do not use if a precipitate is present
- vitamin D analogues may be given concurrently with calcium, especially when hypocalcaemia is caused by vitamin D deficiency; however, high vitamin D intake should be avoided

- injected very slowly into a large vein. IV infusion rate should not exceed 2 mL/minute (or calcium ion 0.9 mEq/minute). May also be given by direct IV injection at a rate of 1.5–3 mL/minute
- avoid extravasation, IM or SC injection, because they may cause necrosis
- incompatible with 10% IV fat emulsions, cephalosporins, dobutamine, methylprednisolone, prochlorperazine, metoclopramide, indometacin (indomethacin), soluble carbonates, sulphates and phosphates
- caution if used in those with sarcoidosis or other diseases associated with elevated vitamin D levels, mild hypercalcaemia, impaired renal function, cardiac disease or history of calcium-containing renal calculi
- contraindicated in galactosaemic patients
- contraindicated in those with hypercalcaemia, hypercalciuria, severe renal failure, severe cardiac disease, severe calcium loss due to immobilisation or calcium level above normal (4.2–5.2 mEq/L)

Patient teaching and advice

- patient should be advised to immediately report any loss of appetite, nausea, vomiting, increased thirst and urination, constipation, confusion, muscle or joint pain or general weakness (early signs of hypercalcaemia)

IRON AND IRON COMPOUNDS

General Actions of iron and iron compounds

- approximately 15–20 g of iron is absorbed from the diet, with the main site of absorption being the duodenum and jejunum, and this iron more than adequately replaces the small amount that is lost in the faeces, urine, skin and sweat
- rate of absorption is dependent on acid secretion from the stomach, as well as the amount of iron already stored within the body. The actual amount needed depends on such factors as loss through menstruation, whether a child/adolescent is growing or whether a woman is pregnant or breastfeeding
- approximately 4 g of the iron is present in the body in the form of haemoglobin or stored as ferritin, haemosiderin or myoglobin, as well as small amounts in the plasma (bound to transferrin) and in haem-containing enzymes
- only very small amounts of iron are excreted, hence the risk of iron overload
- main dietary sources of iron include meat, fish and poultry and some leafy vegetables, wholegrain cereals and legumes; however, iron from plant sources is less bioavailable. Phytates (found in legumes, rice and other grains), calcium and zinc can inhibit absorption of iron
- iron (as oxide or hydroxide) is used as a colouring agent

General Uses of iron and iron compounds

- iron deficiency anaemia
- iron deficiency
- (IV) when oral therapy is contraindicated or impractical or if patient is non-adherent with oral therapy

Optimal daily requirements

- 8 mg (males), 8–18 mg (females), 27 mg (pregnancy), 9 mg (breastfeeding)

- requirements increase during periods of rapid growth such as early childhood and adolescence

General Adverse effects of iron and iron compounds

- metallic taste, GI irritation, nausea, vomiting, constipation, dark/discoloured stools, diarrhoea, abdominal pain
- (oral) teeth or skin staining
- generalised lymph node enlargement
- rash, urticaria, pruritus, angioedema
- bronchospasm, dyspnoea
- transient hypophosphataemia
- sensation of stiffness in arms, legs and/or face, joint and muscle pain, muscle spasm, arthralgia
- headache, dizziness, faintness
- tachycardia, faintness, syncope, hypotension, hypertension
- elevated liver enzymes
- (parenteral) flushing, sweating, chills, fever, chest and back pain, fatigue
- (IV) hypersensitivity, anaphylactoid reaction, anaphylaxis, phlebitis, thrombophlebitis
- (IM) pain, bruising, burning, irritation, lower quadrant abdominal pain, local inflammation, sterile abscess formation, enlarged inguinal lymph nodes, permanent skin discolouration, pain (if incorrectly administered)

General Interactions of iron and iron compounds

- (oral) absorption may be reduced by antacids, colestipol, colestyramine (cholestryramine) and tetracyclines
- (oral) absorption of oral tetracyclines, quinolones, penicillamine, levodopa and methyldopa sesquihydrate may be reduced by oral iron compounds
- parenteral iron is not recommended with oral iron, because the absorption of oral iron is decreased
- oral iron should not be given within 7 days of parenteral iron
- increased risk of erythema, abdominal cramps, nausea, vomiting and hypotension if given with ACE inhibitors
- parenteral iron interferes with a number of laboratory tests (and continues for up to 3 weeks post-administration), including serum bilirubin (falsely elevated) and serum calcium (falsely decreased). Scanning using gallium or technetium (Tc-99m) may be affected. Blood samples appear brown colour within hours of administration. Darkened stools may mask GI bleeding; however, this darkening does not affect haemoccult test

General Nursing points/Cautions for iron and iron compounds

- the type of anaemia should be investigated to determine the cause before starting treatment with iron
- regular monitoring of haemoglobin, haematocrit, serum ferritin and transferrin saturation is recommended to prevent iron overload as excretion is limited
- observe the patient carefully for any breathing difficulties, tachycardia or hypotension (frequently reported in haemodialysis patients) during the initial stages of IV injection or infusion in case of anaphylactoid reaction. Patient should be observed for at least 30 minutes post infusion for any reaction
- IM injection should not be given into arm or exposed area

- give IM injection by drawing subcutaneous tissue to one side before inserting needle (5–6 cm long) (Z track technique) to promote absorption and prevent skin staining and pain. Pressure should be applied to injection site for 1 minute. Consult manufacturer's instructions for recommended injection sites
- extravasation should be avoided as it may result in brown discolouration of the skin
- administer alone
- have available adrenaline (epinephrine), IV corticosteroids, oxygen and resuscitation equipment; antihistamines may be used for minor allergic reactions
- overdose is very serious in young children, because the gut lining may be destroyed and should be treated urgently by emptying the stomach and giving milk to form an iron-protein complex (first aid) and then the iron-chelating agent, desferrioxamine (see Antidotes, antagonists and chelating agents, p. 332)
- caution if used in those with rheumatoid arthritis and other inflammatory disease because there is increased risk of delayed reaction, including fever and exacerbation or reactivation of joint pain
- caution if used in those with asthma or history of allergic disorders (e.g. eczema, atopic allergies), low iron binding capacity or folic acid deficiency, because they are at increased risk of allergy or anaphylactoid reaction
- (IM/IV) caution if used in those with acute or chronic infection and should be discontinued if any bacteraemia occurs
- caution if used in those with severe liver or kidney inflammation as iron accumulates in inflamed tissue
- caution if used in those with GI disease resulting from the gastrointestinal irritation because oral iron may exacerbate mucosal irritation
- not recommended in those with liver dysfunction related to iron overload such as porphyria cutanea tarda
- not recommended in those who have had previous reactions to parenteral iron
- contraindicated in those with anaemia not caused by simple iron deficiency, iron overload, chronic polyarthritis, asthma, uncontrolled hyperparathyroidism, acute kidney infection, infectious hepatitis, haemosiderosis, haemochromatosis or thalassaemia

General Patient teaching and advice for iron and iron compounds

- warn patient not to drive or operate machinery until any dizziness or faintness subsides
- advise patient to keep iron preparations out of the reach of children as they are particularly sensitive to high doses
- inform the patient that gastrointestinal irritation can be reduced if oral iron preparations are taken with or immediately after food (although iron is absorbed better if taken between meals)
- instruct the patient that oral iron, tetracyclines, zinc salts and aluminium salts are each given at least 2 hours apart to allow adequate absorption
- instruct the patient that iron mixtures should be taken in milk or

through a straw to avoid temporary staining of teeth and teeth staining may be minimised by brushing teeth with baking soda
- warn patient that faeces become darker/discoloured during treatment
- if patient was receiving oral iron before receiving parenteral iron, advise patient not to restart oral therapy until at least 5 days post-infusion/injection

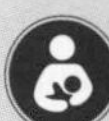

(parenteral) contraindicated in first trimester of pregnancy. Use during second or third trimester only if benefits outweigh potential risks. May cause transient fetal bradycardia. Unborn child should be monitored if pregnant mother is given IV iron during second or third trimester

caution if used during breastfeeding

FERRIC CARBOXYMALTOSE (Ferinject)

Available forms
Ampoule: 100 mg/2 mL, 500 mg/10 mL, 1 g/20 mL (as elemental iron)

Use
- parenteral administration is recommended when oral route is not available or is impractical

Dose
- cumulative dose calculated according to following formula (Ganzoni):

Cumulative iron deficit (mg) = body weight (kg) × (target Hb − actual Hb (in mg/L) × 0.24 + iron storage (mg)

Adverse effects/Interactions
- see General Adverse effects/Interactions for iron (p. 1590)

Nursing points/Cautions/Patient teaching and advice
- maximum weekly dose 1 g
- if patient is overweight, normal body weight and blood volume relation should be assumed when calculating iron requirements
- target Hb = 130 g/L if < 35 kg or 150 g/L if ≥ 35 kg
- iron stores (depot) = 15 mg/kg if < 35 kg or 500 mg if ≥ 35 kg
- for patient ≤ 66 kg, calculated cumulative dose should be rounded down to nearest 100 mg
- for patient > 66 kg, calculated cumulative dose should be rounded up to nearest 100 mg
- 1 mL (undiluted) contains up to 5.5 mg (0.24 mmol) sodium, which may need to be considered if patient has sodium restriction
- not for IM or SC use
- administer alone
- IV dilution with sodium chloride 0.9% only as follows: 100–200 mg iron diluted in 50 mL and given over 3 minutes; > 200–500 mg iron diluted in 100 mL and given over 6 minutes; > 500 mg–1 g iron diluted in 250 mL and given over 15 minutes
- may be given as IV bolus injection to a daily maximum of 200 mg (4 mL) and not repeated more than 3 times per week
- may be given at IV infusion (not greater than 20 mg/kg or maximum 1 g (20 mL)), should only be given weekly
- may be given during haemodialysis undiluted via venous limb of dialyser
- contains 5.5 mg (0.24 mmol) sodium/mL which should be considered if person has sodium restriction
- see also General Nursing points/Cautions and Patient teaching and advice for iron (pp. 1590–91)

FERROUS FUMARATE (Ferro-tab)

Available form

Tablets: 200 mg (= elemental iron 65.7 mg)

Dose

- (prophylaxis) 1 tablet orally daily **OR**
- (treatment) 1 tablet orally 2–3 times daily

Patient teaching and advice

- advise patient that tablets may be taken with or without water. However, if taken between meals, the patient should take them with at least 240 mL water and avoid lying down for ≥ 30 minutes
- see General Patient teaching and advice for iron (p. 1591)

Use/Adverse effects/Interactions/ Nursing points/Cautions

- see general points for iron (pp. 1589–92)

tablets can be crushed and mixed with water or spoonful of yoghurt or apple puree

Note

- contained in Ferro-F Tab with folic acid, as well as part of multivitamin preparations

FERROUS SULFATE HEPTAHYDRATE (FERROUS SULFATE) (Ferro-Grad, Ferro-Liquid)

Available forms

Oral solution: 150 mg (= 30 mg elemental iron)/5 mL; Tablets (slow-release): 325 mg (= 105 mg elemental iron)

Dose

- 325 mg orally daily before food or as prescribed **OR**
- 450–900 mg (15–30 mL) orally daily or as prescribed (oral liquid)

Use/Adverse effects/Interactions

- see general points for iron (pp. 1589–92)

Nursing points/Cautions/Patient teaching and advice

- advise patient that tablets should be swallowed whole (not crushed or chewed) and if gastric irritation occurs, may be taken with food
- (oral solution) contains sorbitol and bisulfite and may cause diarrhoea and allergic reaction in susceptible individuals
- tablets contain lactose
- prolonged administration > 12 months is not recommended
- see general points for iron (pp. 1589–92)

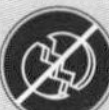

oral solution available. Slow-release tablets should not be chewed, broken or crushed

Note

- contained in Fefol, Ferrograd F, Ferrograd C, Ferro-Max C and other multivitamin preparations

IRON POLYMALTOSE COMPLEX (Ferrosig Injection, Ferrum H Injection, Maltofer)

Available forms

Ampoules: 100 mg/2 mL (as elemental iron); Tablets: 370 mg (= 100 mg elemental iron); Syrup: 185 mg/5 mL (= 50 mg elemental iron/5 mL)

Action

- (IM) evokes local inflammatory response and is transported to regional lymph nodes without being broken down. Then enters blood reaching maximum concentration in 24 hours

- half-life 22.4 hours
- see General Actions of iron (p. 1589)

Dose

- (treatment) 100–200 mg orally daily with food or as prescribed **OR**
- (prophylaxis) 100 mg orally daily with food or as prescribed **OR**
- 100 mg of iron IM every second day until total dose is achieved **OR**
- 200 mg IM at intervals longer than 2 days until total dose is achieved **AND**
- (IM) total dose is calculated using the formula:

Iron dose (mg) = body weight (kg) × target Hb − actual Hb (in g/L) × 0.24 + iron depot

Adverse effects/Interactions

- see General Adverse effects and Interactions for iron (p. 1590)

Nursing points/Cautions

- 100 mg = 1 tablet = 10 mL syrup. If dose is less than 100 mg, syrup should be used
- (IV) administer alone
- (Ferrosig) for IV use, dilute in 500 mL of sodium chloride 0.9% and infuse first 50 mL at a rate of 5–10 drops/minute, then carefully observe the patient. If tolerated, continue infusion at 30 drops/minute
- for body weight > 34 kg, target Hb = 150 g/L and iron depot = 500 mg; for body weight < 34 kg, target Hb = 130 g/L and iron depot 15 mg/kg
- for adult > 45 kg, daily maximum is 200 mg
- test dose of 25 mg may be given before first therapeutic dose
- dose given by IM injection is 2 mL (100 mg) on alternate days until total dose is attained, or 4 mL (200 mg) at longer intervals
- monitor treatment by regular determination of haemoglobin
- adverse effects may occur up to 1–2 days after administration
- IV route can be used if IM is impractical or unacceptable and when bone marrow stores show no iron
- (oral solution) contains hydroxybenzoates which may cause allergic reactions in sensitive individuals
- (oral solution) contains small amount of alcohol (3.25 mg/mL)
- (oral solution) contains sorbitol and sucrose and is therefore not recommended in those with rare hereditary problems of fructose intolerance, glucose–galactose malabsorption or sucrase–isomaltase insufficiency
- contraindicated in those with any hypersensitivity to iron (III) hydroxide polymaltose complex
- see also General Nursing points/Cautions for iron (p. 1590)

Patient teaching and advice

- advise patient to swallow tablets whole, not chewed or crushed
- instruct the patient that oral solution can be mixed with fruit or vegetable juice. This may show a slight discolouration, but is fine to ingest
- see General Patient teaching and advice for iron (p. 1591)

oral solution available

IRON SUCROSE (Venofer)

Available form

Ampoules: 100 mg/5 mL (as elemental iron)

Use

- treatment of iron deficiency anaemia in patients receiving chronic haemodialysis and supplemental erythropoietin therapy

Dose

- 100 mg by IV infusion or slow IV injection into venous limb of dialysis line during dialysis session, no more than 3 times weekly until haemoglobin, haematocrit and laboratory parameters of iron storage are within acceptable limits

Action/Adverse effects/Interactions/Patient teaching and advice

- see general points for iron (pp. 1589–91)

Nursing points/Cautions

- most patients require a cumulative dose of 1 g over 10 sequential dialysis sessions
- dilute with 100 mL sodium chloride 0.9% just before IV infusion and administer over at least 15 minutes
- slow IV injection should be at least 5 minutes into venous line of dialysis machine
- not given IM or SC because of strong alkaline nature
- administer alone
- if not effective in 1–2 weeks, original diagnosis should be reconsidered
- see General Nursing points/Cautions for iron (p. 1590)

MAGNESIUM

General Actions of magnesium

- second most abundant cation
- essential for more than 300 enzyme processes
- necessary for glycolysis, the Krebs cycle, protein and nucleic acid synthesis
- neurochemical transmission
- anticonvulsant effect
- role in calcium homeostasis and bone mineralisation
- 90% stored in bone, muscle and soft tissue
- dietary sources include most green vegetables, legumes, peas, beans and nuts, some shellfish and spices, unrefined cereals

Optimal daily requirements

- 400–420 mg (males), 310–320 mg (females), 350–360 mg (pregnancy), 310–320 mg (breastfeeding)

General Adverse effects of magnesium

- hypermagnesaemia (nausea, vomiting, flushing, hypotension, muscle weakness and paralysis, blurred or double vision, loss of reflexes and CNS depression; more severe, respiratory depression/paralysis, renal failure, coma, arrhythmias, cardiac arrest)
- hypocalcaemia with tetany (secondary to hypermagnesaemia)
- (IM injection site) irritation and pain

General Interactions of magnesium

- increased CNS depression may occur if given with CNS depressant drugs
- not recommended with other agents containing magnesium, including antacids due to increased risk of magnesium toxicity
- excessive neuromuscular blockade may occur if given with neuromuscular-blocking agents or aminoglycosides
- caution if used with digoxin as heart block may occur
- increased hypotension can occur if given with nifedipine and other antihypertensive agents

General Nursing points/Cautions for magnesium

- patient should be adequately hydrated before starting therapy and

urine output should be at least 100 mL for the preceding 4 hours before the infusion is started
- serum magnesium levels and renal function should be monitored frequently during therapy
- patellar reflexes should be assessed before repeating doses, because decreased reflexes are indicative of toxicity
- respiratory rate should be monitored throughout infusion (maintained at a rate of at least 16 breaths/minute)
- have IV calcium salts (e.g. calcium gluconate) readily available to treat any toxicity when parenteral magnesium chloride is administered
- incompatible with carbonates, bicarbonates, phosphates and calcium salts
- may precipitate myasthenic crisis
- caution if used in those with renal or liver impairment due to risk of hypermagnesaemia
- contraindicated in those with heart block or renal failure (creatinine clearance < 20 mL/min)
- contraindicated in those with hypermagnesaemia

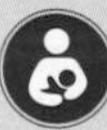

(parenteral) should not be given within 2 hours of delivery, because respiratory depression may occur in the newborn (unless there are no other options in treatment of eclamptic seizures). Readily crosses the placenta and fetal serum levels are similar to maternal; bony abnormalities and congenital rickets may occur in neonates if given for prolonged periods (4–13 weeks) during pregnancy

not recommended during breastfeeding as concentration in breastmilk is twice maternal serum levels. Cleared from breastmilk within 24 hours of stopping IV therapy

Note
- contained in many multi vitamin preparations

MAGNESIUM ASPARTATE (Mag-A, Magmin, Mag-Sup)

Available form
Tablets: 500 mg (= elemental magnesium 37.4 mg)

Use
- magnesium deficiency
- symptom relief of muscle cramps and spasm

Dose
- 1–3 g daily orally with meals or as prescribed

Action/Adverse effects/Nursing points/Cautions/Patient teaching and advice
- see general points for magnesium (p. 1595–96)

tablets can be crushed and mixed with water or spoonful of yoghurt or apple puree

MAGNESIUM CHLORIDE (DBL Magnesium Chloride Concentrated Injection)

Available form
Ampoules: 480 mg/5 mL

Use
- acute hypomagnesaemia
- prevention of hypomagnesaemia in those receiving total parenteral nutrition (TPN)

Dose
- (acute hypomagnesaemia) initially 3.3–7.2 g (70–150 mEq) by slow IV infusion (day 1), then reduced to 2.4 g (50 mEq) daily until hypomagnesaemia

has been corrected (maximum daily dose 18.7 g) **OR**

- (prevention of hypomagnesaemia in those receiving TPN) 0.2–1.2 g (4–24 mEq) by slow IV infusion daily

Action/Adverse effects/Interactions/Nursing points/Cautions/Patient teaching and advice

- administer alone
- IV dose should be diluted with glucose 5%
- 1 mL = 1 mmol = 2 mEq magnesium ions
- see general points for magnesium (p. 1595–96)

Note

- contained in Cardioplegia A solution and DBL Sterile Cardioplegia Concentrate used in cardiac surgery to induce cardiac arrest

MAGNESIUM SULFATE HEPTAHYDRATE (DBL Magnesium Sulfate Concentrated Injection, Magnesium Sulfate Heptahydrate Concentrated 50% Injection)

Available forms

Ampoules: 2.465 g/5 mL; Vial: 2.5 g/5 mL, 5 g/10 mL

Use

- acute hypomagnesaemia
- prevention of hypomagnesaemia in those receiving total parenteral nutrition (TPN)
- seizures associated with pre-eclampsia and eclampsia (see Pregnancy, childbirth and breastfeeding, p. 1404)
- cardiac arrhythmias

Dose

- (severe hypomagnesaemia) 0.25 mg/kg IM over 4 hours **OR**
- (severe hypomagnesaemia) 5 g by slow IV infusion over 3 hours **OR**
- (mild hypomagnesaemia) 1 g (8 mEq) IM 6-hourly for 4 doses **OR**
- (arrhythmias) 2 g (8.2 mmol) by slow IV infusion over 20 minutes **OR**
- (prevention of hypomagnesaemia in those receiving TPN) 0.5–3.0 g daily IV or IM

Action/Adverse effects/ Interactions/Nursing points/Cautions/Patient teaching and advice

- total daily dose should not exceed 30–40 g
- given IV or IM only
- IV dose should be diluted to 20% before administration
- IM administration may be given diluted or undiluted
- 2 mL = 1 g = 4 mmol = 8 mEq magnesium ions
- see general points for magnesium (p. 1595–96)

OTHER MINERALS

PHOSPHORUS/PHOSPHATE (DBL Potassium Dihydrogen Phosphate Concentrated Injection, DBL Potassium Phosphate – Monobasic and Potassium Phosphate – Dibasic Concentrated Injection, Phosphate Phebra Tablets, Potassium Dihydrogen Phosphate 13.6% Concentrated Injection, Sodium Phosphate and Potassium Phosphate Concentrated Injection)

Available forms

Tablets (effervescent): 500 mg; IV solution contains phosphate, potassium and sodium ions

Action

- most of the body's phosphate is found in bones, giving rigidity, and some is also in soft tissue
- main anion of intracellular fluid
- involved in metabolic and enzymatic pathways
- involved in energy storage and transfer, utilisation of vitamin B, buffering and renal excretion of hydrogen ions
- excretion controlled by parathyroid gland
- mainly (85%) stored in bone, rest in soft tissue
- inverse relationship with serum calcium (i.e. increased phosphate level leads to decreased calcium level)
- normal serum concentration 0.8–1.5 mmol/L
- widely distributed in foods; plant seeds (e.g. beans, peas, cereals, nuts) have phosphate stored in a form (phytic acid) that is not bioavailable to mammals

Use

- hypercalcaemia (associated with hyperparathyroidism, metastatic bone disease)
- hypophosphataemia associated with vitamin D-resistant rickets
- hypophosphataemia (serum level < 0.3 mmol/L)

Optimal daily requirement

- 1000 mg

Dose

- (hypercalcaemia) up to 3 g orally daily **OR**
- (vitamin D-resistant rickets) 2–3 g orally daily **OR**
- (hypophosphataemia) up to 10 mmol by slow IV infusion over 12 hours, may be repeated until serum level > 0.3 mmol/L

Adverse effects

- (oral) diarrhoea, nausea, vomiting, abdominal pain
- (IV) hypotension, fluid retention, weight gain
- (IV) hyperkalaemia (confusion, weakness, irregular or slow heartbeat, numbness/tingling of lips, hands or feet, anxiety, difficulty breathing or shortness of breath, heaviness of legs)
- (IV) hypernatraemia (confusion, tiredness, weakness, convulsions, oliguria, tachycardia, headache, dizziness, increased thirst)
- (IV) hyperphosphataemia, hypocalcaemia or hypomagnesaemia (convulsions, muscle cramps, numbness, tingling, pain or weakness of feet or hands, shortness of breath, tremor)
- (IV) soft tissue calcification, nephrocalcinosis
- (rare) myocardial infarction, acute renal failure

Interactions

- hyperkalaemia may occur if given with ACE inhibitors, potassium-sparing diuretics, NSAIDs, potassium-containing agents or in patients with heart block who are taking cardiac glycosides (digoxin) or renal impairment
- increased risk of calcium deposition in soft tissue if given with calcium or phosphate-containing agents (including supplements)
- oedema may occur if given with corticosteroids that have mineralocorticoid actions
- may increase serum salicylate levels leading to toxicity
- hypernatraemia may occur if given with sodium-containing agents
- hyperphosphataemia may occur if given with phosphate-containing products or vitamin D
- (oral) efficacy decreased if given with aluminium, calcium or magnesium-containing antacids
- increased urinary excretion may occur if given with parathyroid hormone
- may interfere with some bone imaging studies

Nursing points/Cautions

- cause of hypophosphataemia should be investigated and treated
- serum sodium, potassium, phosphate and calcium levels and renal function should be monitored 12–24-hourly during therapy
- parenteral therapy should be replaced with oral therapy as soon as possible
- tablets contain sodium (469 mg or 20.4 mEq) and potassium (123 mg or 3.1 mEq) in addition to phosphate
- IV solution should be diluted with sodium chloride 0.9% or glucose 5% and given by slow IV infusion to prevent toxicity
- incompatible with iron, aluminium, calcium or magnesium-containing solutions as precipitates may occur
- caution if given to those with myotonia congenita or heart disease
- caution in those with potentially high phosphate levels (e.g. rhabdomyolysis, hypoparathyroidism, chronic renal disease), low calcium levels (e.g. osteomalacia, hypoparathyroidism, rickets, acute pancreatitis), high potassium level (e.g. acute dehydration, pancreatitis, rhabdomyolysis, severe burns or other extensive tissue damage) or high sodium levels (e.g. toxaemia of pregnancy, hypertension, congestive cardiac failure, electrolyte imbalance, peripheral oedema, liver cirrhosis, pulmonary oedema, severe liver disease)
- contraindicated in those with severe renal impairment (< 30% of normal), hyperphosphataemia, hypocalcaemia, hyperkalaemia, hypernatraemia, Addison's disease or urolithiasis

Patient teaching and advice

- patient should be advised to dissolve effervescent tablets in half a glass of water
- advise patients to avoid aluminium, calcium or magnesium-containing antacids within 2 hours of phosphate
- instruct patient to seek medical advice immediately if any of the following occur:
  - swelling of feet or lower legs, weight gain
  - increased thirst
  - muscle weakness, weakness or heaviness in hands or feet, muscle cramps
  - irregular heart rate
  - unexpected anxiety
  - tiredness
  - confusion
  - seizures
  - pain or numbness

- breathing difficulties
- tingling, prickling or burning sensation

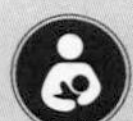

not recommended during pregnancy or breastfeeding

effervescent tablets are available

POTASSIUM

General Actions of potassium

- main intracellular ion
- involved in maintaining intracellular tonicity, nerve–muscle transmission, muscle contraction and normal renal function
- best dietary sources of potassium include leafy green vegetables, vine fruit (e.g. tomatoes, zucchini, cucumbers, pumpkin, eggplant) and root vegetables. Other sources include beans, peas, tree fruit (e.g. apples, bananas, oranges), milk, yoghurt and meats
- normal serum concentration 3.5–5 mmol/L

General Uses of potassium

- hypokalaemia
- potassium replacement therapy after long-term use or high doses of potassium-depleting diuretics, especially if the patient is also receiving digoxin
- long-term or high-dose corticosteroid therapy, ACTH or benzylpenicillin
- low-salt, low-potassium diet
- poor absorption or loss from GI tract after excessive vomiting or diarrhoea, fistula or enterostomy drainage, or use of laxatives
- metabolic alkalosis (including hypochloraemic alkalosis)
- hyperaldosteronism
- renal disease associated with increased potassium excretion
- liver cirrhosis with diuretic therapy
- electrolyte supplement with TPN

Optimal daily requirements

- 3800 mg (males), 2800 mg (females, pregnancy), 3200 mg (breastfeeding)

General Adverse effects of potassium

- (IV) nausea, vomiting, diarrhoea, abdominal discomfort, fall in BP, arrhythmias, heart block, cardiac depression, ECG abnormalities
- (IV site) pain, phlebitis
- hyperkalaemia (lethargy, listlessness, confusion, weakness and heaviness of legs, flaccid paralysis, cold skin, grey pallor, paraesthesia of extremities, hypotension, heart block, cardiac arrhythmias, ECG abnormalities, cardiac arrest) (potentially fatal hyperkalaemia can develop rapidly and be asymptomatic)

General Interactions of potassium

- contraindicated with potassium-sparing diuretics (amiloride, spironolactone or triamterene) due to risk of hyperkalaemia
- caution if given with ACE inhibitors (such as captopril and enalapril) and angiotensin II receptor antagonists due to risk of hyperkalaemia
- hyperkalaemia may result if given with NSAIDs or heparin
- caution if used with other potassium-sparing agents such as renin inhibitors or proton pump inhibitors due to risk of hyperkalaemia

- not recommended in those taking digoxin for heart block (severe or complete)
- caution if given with beta-adrenoceptor blocking agents as serum potassium levels may increase, as well as increasing time to return to basal levels
- serum potassium levels may decrease if used with insulin, sodium bicarbonate, ciclosporin or tacrolimus

General Nursing points/Cautions for potassium

- potassium replacement should be undertaken cautiously and include monitoring acid–base balance, serum electrolytes, ECG and urine output
- serum potassium level should be closely monitored during therapy
- any dehydration should be corrected before treating potassium imbalance
- any hypomagnesaemia should be treated at same time as potassium deficiency as magnesium deficiency prevents restoration of intracellular potassium deficit
- IV administration is usually given via a large vein to minimise vein irritation
- prevent extravasation
- must be diluted before using and should be diluted with sodium chloride 0.9% rather than glucose 5%, because the glucose may decrease the serum potassium concentration
- IV potassium must be given as a thoroughly mixed dilute solution of uniform concentration. This avoids a sudden increase in plasma potassium concentration, which may lead to cardiac arrest and death. If potassium chloride is to be added to a hanging IV solution, ensure that there is sufficient solution to make the correct dilution, then, after adding the potassium, invert the container several times to guarantee complete and even mixing
- ensure container is labelled carefully
- monitor IV infusion rate by using a burette or infusion pump or syringe pump
- potassium should not be added to a burette or injection port
- IV rate should be not greater than 20 mmol/hour
- (metabolic acidosis) hypokalaemia should be treated with potassium salt (with alkalinising anion e.g. potassium bicarbonate), not potassium chloride
- administer alone
- (IV) incompatible with mannitol and fat emulsions containing soya oil or lecithin
- (oral) caution if used in those with oesophageal stasis, a history of peptic ulcer, delayed intestinal transit, intestinal ischaemia or GI tract obstruction
- caution if used in those with chronic renal disease or liver impairment because of increased risk of hyperkalaemia
- caution if used in those with heart block as degree of block may be increased
- caution if used in those on low salt diet due to risk of hypokalaemic hypochloraemic alkalosis occurring
- contraindicated in those with hypersensitivity to potassium or potassium administration (e.g. congenital paramyotonia), renal impairment with oliguria or azotemia, severe tissue damage (including severe

burns), severe renal failure, untreated Addison's disease, acute dehydration, hyperkalaemia, hyperchoraemia, uncontrolled diabetes mellitus, severe or prolonged diarrhoea, slowed or obstructed GI disease, heat cramps, hyperadrenalism associated with adrenogenital syndrome, metabolic or respiratory acidosis, ventricular fibrillation or atrioventricular/intraventricular heart block

General Patient teaching and advice for potassium

- advise patient to seek medical advice immediately if any confusion, weakness, irregular or slow heartbeat, numbness/tingling of lips, hands or feet, anxiety, shortness of breath or heaviness of legs occurs

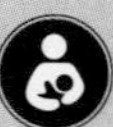

serum potassium levels should be closely monitored if used during pregnancy

caution if used during breastfeeding

POTASSIUM ACETATE (DBL Potassium Acetate Concentrated Injection)

Available form
Ampoules: 5 mEq/mL

Dose
- (IV) dose and rate are dependent on individual patient's condition with maximum concentration of 40 mmol/L

Action/Use/Adverse effects/Interactions/Patient teaching and advice
- see general points for potassium (pp. 1600–02)

Nursing points/Cautions
- must be diluted before IV use
- total dose should not exceed > 150 mEq/24 hours
- if potassium level > 2.5 mEq/L (2.5 mmol/L), infusion rate < 10 mEq/hour (10 mmol/hour)
- see General Nursing points/Cautions for potassium (p. 1601)

POTASSIUM CHLORIDE (Chlorvescent, Potassium Chloride (2.23 g/10 mL) Injection, Span-K)

Available forms
Tablets (slow-release): 600 mg; Effervescent tablets: 548 mg (14 mmol); Vials: 2.23 g/10 mL; Ampoules: 75 mg/mL, 150 mg/mL; 10 mmol (0.75 g)/10 mL, 13.4 mmol (1 g)/10 mL, 20 mmol (1.5 g)/10 mL, 13.4 mmol (1 g)/4 mL, 26.8 mmol (2 g)/8 mL

Action/Use
- see General Actions and Uses for potassium (p. 1600)

Dose
- (with potassium-losing diuretic) 600 mg–1.2 g orally daily with or after food (slow-release tablets) **OR**
- (potassium deficiency) 600 mg–1.2 g orally daily 2–3 times daily with or after food (slow-release tablets) **OR**
- (potassium deficiency) 1–2 tablets orally daily 2–3 times daily with or after food (effervescent tablets) **OR**
- (IV) dose and rate are dependent on individual patient's condition with maximum concentration of 40 mmol/L

Adverse effects
- (SR tablets) nausea, vomiting, diarrhoea, abdominal pain, flatulence, gastrointestinal bleeding and, rarely, stricture, ulceration or perforation of bowel

- (effervescent tablets) nausea, vomiting, diarrhoea, abdominal pain
- see also General Adverse effects for potassium (p. 1600)

Interactions

- (oral, slow-release) caution if given with anticholinergic agents that reduce intestinal motility due to increased risk of gastrointestinal ulceration and haemorrhage
- see also General Interactions for potassium (p. 1600)

Nursing points/Cautions

- dilute well before IV use
- if serum potassium > 2.5 mmol/L, rate should not exceed 10 mmol/hour and daily dose maximum 150–200 mmol
- if serum potassium < 2 mmol/L with ECG changes or paralysis, rate can be increased to 40 mmol/hour and daily dose maximum 400 mmol
- (IV) incompatible with amikacin, amphotericin B, amoxycillin, benzylpenicillin, diazepam, dobutamine, etoposide with mannitol and cisplatin, methylprednisolone, phenytoin, promethazine or sodium nitroprusside
- see General Nursing points/Cautions for potassium (p. 1601)

Patient teaching and advice

- advise patient to stop medication and seek medical advice immediately if there are any GI symptoms, including marked nausea, vomiting, flatulence, abdominal pain, diarrhoea with black or blood-stained stools
- advise patient to swallow SR tablets whole (not chewed, crushed or broken) with water and not to allow to dissolve in the mouth
- warn patient that if taking SR preparations, potassium is released gradually from an insoluble wax core or matrix, which is excreted (and may be seen) in the faeces
- (oral) warn patient against using potassium salt substitutes during therapy
- (effervescent tablets) instruct patient to dissolve tablets in 120–240 mL cold water and take with or after food
- see General Patient teaching and advice for potassium (p. 1602)

(IV) this product is permitted in some sports and prohibited in others

effervescent tablets can be dissolved in 5 mL water and then added to 120 mL thickened fluids

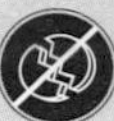

slow-release tablet should not be chewed, crushed or broken

BICARBONATE

SODIUM BICARBONATE (Sodibic, Sodium Bicarbonate Injection, Sodium Bicarbonate Injection 8.4%)

Available forms

Capsules: 840 mg; Prefilled syringe (Min-I-Jet): 1 mmol/mL; Vials: 84 mg/mL (1 mmol/mL)

Actions

- bicarbonate is a normal constituent of body fluids
- part of the buffering system that maintains the acid–base balance in the body
- can cause redistribution of potassium ions into cells
- increases urinary pH
- normal plasma concentration 24–31 mmol/L

Uses

- renal tubular acidosis
- alkaliniser used in treatment of metabolic acidosis (e.g. cardiac arrest, shock, severe dehydration, diabetes mellitus)

- urinary alkaliniser to increase solubility of some weak acids (e.g. cysteine, uric acid, sulphonamides)
- forced alkaline diuresis in acute poisoning from weakly acidic drugs (e.g. salicylates, methanol, phenobarbital (phenobarbitone)) resulting in decreased renal absorption of the drug

Dose

- (renal tubular acidosis) 840 mg orally daily **OR**
- (cardiac arrest) initially 1 mmol/kg IV, followed by 0.5 mmol/kg at 10-minute intervals during arrest (depending on arterial blood gases) **OR**
- (non-urgent metabolic acidosis) 2–5 mmol/kg by IV infusion over 4–8 hours

Adverse effects

- (oral) anorexia, nausea
- (IV) alkalosis, hypokalaemia, sodium and water retention, oedema, congestive heart failure, hypernatraemia, hyperosmolality, hyperirritability, tetany, cerebral oedema and rarely, intracranial haemorrhage
- hypercapnia (if patient is on fixed ventilation)
- (IV, extravasation) vascular irritation, chemical cellulitis, tissue necrosis, ulceration

Interactions

- caution if used in those taking corticosteroids or corticotrophin
- urinary alkalinisation will increase clearance of tetracyclines (especially doxycycline)
- urinary alkalinisation will increase half-life and action of amphetamines, ephedrine and pseudoephedrine
- if used with thiazide diuretics, frusemide or etacrynic acid, hypochloraemic alkalosis may occur
- may enhance or prolong action of flecainide because of decreased excretion due to alkalinisation of urine
- may decrease effects of aspirin and other salicylates, barbiturates or lithium because of increased excretion due to alkalinisation of urine
- may produce false positive on urine protein test

Nursing points/Cautions

- any hypokalaemia or hypocalcaemia should be corrected before starting therapy
- arterial blood gases (especially carbon dioxide and arterial/venous blood pH) and serum electrolytes should be monitored before starting and during therapy to prevent alkalosis
- levels should be monitored frequently to avoid excessively elevated plasma sodium levels occurring, which can lead to brain dehydration, confusion, somnolence, convulsions and coma
- therapy should be carried out in a slow step-wise manner to prevent alkalosis
- if patient has respiratory acidosis and metabolic acidosis, pulmonary ventilation and perfusion should be supported to ensure carbon dioxide is removed
- avoid extravasation. However, if it occurs, treat extravasation by elevating and warming the limb and giving a local injection of lidocaine (lignocaine) or hyaluronidase
- excessive sodium-containing solution may cause fluid overload, electrolyte dilution and pulmonary oedema
- see manufacturer's instructions for dilution and compatibility with solutions and other drugs as there are a large number of incompatibilities
- ensure IV is flushed with sodium chloride 0.9% before and after administration
- may be diluted with sodium chloride 0.9% or glucose 5%

- not recommended with IV calcium-containing solutions as precipitation will occur
- caution if used in those with cirrhosis
- caution if used in those with tissue hypoxia (type A lactic acidosis) as increased lactate production will occur worsening acidosis
- extreme caution if used in those predisposed to sodium retention and oedema or those with congestive heart failure or renal insufficiency because of the sodium content (12 mEq/g)
- not recommended for diabetic ketoacidosis with pH between 6.9 and 7.1
- contraindicated in those with renal failure, metabolic/respiratory alkalosis, hypertension, oedema, congestive heart failure, hypoventilation, chloride depletion, hypernatraemia, hypocalcaemia, coexisting potassium depletion, history of urinary calculi, eclampsia or aldosteronism

permitted in some sports but prohibited in others

capsules can be opened and mixed with water or spoonful of yoghurt or jam

Note

- contained in Citravescent and Ural for the treatment of cystitis
- contained in antacids and laxatives and multi-electrolyte preparations

SODIUM

General Actions of sodium

- sodium is a principal electrolyte
- major cation involved in maintenance of extracellular volume and serum osmolality
- 95% found in extracellular fluid, maintained with sodium/potassium-ATPase pump
- maintains membrane potential
- absorption (with chloride) is in small intestine
- found in most foods in a variety of forms
- mainly excreted in the urine and sweat

Recommended daily intake

- 460–920 mg (20–40 mmol) (males, females, pregnancy, breastfeeding)
- daily intake should not exceed 2300 mg (100 mmol)

SODIUM CHLORIDE (Sodium Chloride 0.9% (Normal Saline) Sterile Injection, Sodium Chloride (0.9%) for Irrigation Solution BP, Saltabs, Toppin Salt Tablets)

Available forms

Tablets: 600 mg; IV solution: 0.45%, 0.9%, 3%; Ampoules: 0.9%; Vial: 0.9%

Action

- source of sodium and chloride ions
- sodium is a principal electrolyte

Use

- prevention and/or correction of fluid and electrolyte deficits or imbalance
- diluent for drugs and vehicle for drug admixtures
- prevention or treatment of sodium chloride loss in sweat when heavy work is being done in a hot environment
- replacement of urinary sodium chloride loss in Addison's disease (adrenocortical atrophy)
- dialysis fluid
- priming fluid for haemodialysis procedures
- eye lotion, mouth wash and irrigating solution

Dose
- mainly given by IV infusion as sodium chloride 0.9% (isotonic saline) **OR**
- (prophylaxis during light work) 2.4–3.6 g (4–6 tablets) orally daily or as prescribed **OR**
- (prophylaxis during heavy work) 7.2–9 g (12–15 tablets) orally daily

Adverse effects
- electrolyte imbalance, fluid overload, acid–base imbalance
- (IV site) phlebitis, burning sensation, itching

Interactions
- caution if given with lithium as clearance may be increased reducing serum levels
- caution if given with corticosteroids or corticotropin because of potential sodium and fluid retention
- increased risk of hyponatraemia if given with antiepileptic agents, antipsychotics, SSRIs, NSAIDs, opioids, cyclophosphamide, vincristine, clofibrate

Nursing points/Cautions
- select the correct concentration of sodium chloride: isotonic (0.9%), hypotonic (less concentrated) or hypertonic (more concentrated), noting also that sodium chloride is often combined with glucose
- monitor heart rate, BP, fluid intake and output and serum electrolytes, especially throughout prolonged IV therapy
- rapid correction of hyponatraemia or hypernatraemia is potentially dangerous
- (IV) not recommended with blood products
- caution if used in the elderly or those with cardiac failure, hypertension, kidney impairment, oedema (peripheral, pulmonary, cerebral), cirrhosis or pre-eclampsia
- caution if used in children or the elderly, women or postoperatively due to risk of hyponatraemia
- caution if used in those at risk of hypernatraemia, hyperchloraemia or hypervolaemia
- contraindicated in those for whom salt retention may be undesirable (e.g. heart disease, oedema, renal impairment, primary/secondary aldosteronism)

Patient teaching and advice
- patient should be advised to maintain an adequate water intake with oral preparations to prevent high salt levels, especially during hot weather, fever, diarrhoea, exercise or heavy manual labour
- advise patient to seek medical advice immediately if any of the following occur:
  - swelling in arms or legs, difficulty breathing or frothy pink sputum, or
  - thirst, swollen tongue, decreased saliva, dry eyes, flushing, fever, rapid breathing, rapid heart rate, weakness, dizziness, decreased urination and/or headache

tablets can be dispersed in water or crushed and mixed with spoonful of yoghurt or apple puree

Note
- available nasal spray or drops, eye drops

ZINC

General Actions of zinc
- co-factor in multiple biochemical pathways
- involved in wound healing, and protein, DNA and collagen synthesis
- enzyme reactions necessary for normal skin gland function

- mobilisation of vitamin A
- essential for immune function
- involved in normal prostate function
- aids in maintenance of taste and smell
- present with insulin in the pancreas
- normal serum levels 0.7–1.5 mg/L

General Uses of zinc

- zinc deficiency (growth deterioration, skin lesions, alopecia, delayed wound healing, impaired prostate gland development and function)

Optimal daily requirements

- 14 mg (males), 8 mg (females), 11 mg (pregnancy), 12 mg (breastfeeding)

ZINC CHLORIDE (DBL Zinc Chloride Injection, Zinc Chloride Concentrated Injection)

Available forms

Ampoules: 5.1 mg/2 mL, 10.6 mg/2 mL

Action/Use

- see General Actions and Uses for zinc (p. 1606–07)

Dose

- 2.5–4 mg daily by IV infusion over 8–24 hours, with additional 2 mg daily for acute catabolic states

Adverse effects

- (prolonged therapy) copper deficiency, anaemia
- increased serum amylase, lipase and alkaline phosphatase

Interactions

- if given without copper, may cause decrease in serum copper levels

Nursing points/Cautions

- serum copper and zinc levels should be regularly monitored
- increased amount is required in those on a vegetarian diet as there is lower zinc absorption
- further zinc supplementation may also be required in situations of acute catabolism (2 mg per day) or for fluid loss from small intestine (12.2 mg/L of fluid lost or 17.1 mg/kg of stool/ileostomy output)
- (IV solution) avoid contact with eyes and skin. If contact occurs, wash area immediately with copious amounts of water
- not recommended undiluted
- for IV use, dilute in 1000 mL of glucose 5% or sodium chloride 0.9% and infuse over 8–24 hours
- caution if given to those with renal impairment as zinc may accumulate
- contraindicated by IM or IV bolus injection

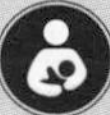

only used during pregnancy or breastfeeding if benefits outweigh potential risks. May induce copper deficiency in newborn if breastfed

ZINC SULFATE (ZinCaps)

Available form

Capsules: 50 mg

Action/Use

- see General Actions and Uses for zinc (p. 1606–07)

Dose

- 50 mg orally daily with food

Adverse effects

- nausea, mild epigastric discomfort

Interactions/Nursing points/Cautions

- see Interactions/Nursing points/Cautions/Patient teaching and advice for zinc chloride above

Patient teaching and advice

- advise patient that capsules may be taken with food to overcome gastric irritation capsules can be opened and contents dispersed in water or mixed with spoonful of yoghurt or apple puree

AMINO ACIDS

ARGININE (Arginine Hydrochloride 60% Concentrated Injection)

Available form
Vial: 15 g/25 mL

Action
- essential amino acid
- absorbed from GI tract and processed by liver
- important part of urea cycle enabling body to safely store and excrete ammonia

Use
- stimulates release of growth hormone and may be used instead of, or in addition to, other tests to evaluate growth disorders
- acidifying agent in severe metabolic alkalosis
- severe deficiency of ornithine carbamoyl transferase or carbamoyl phosphate synthetase where respiratory alkalosis is present

Dose
- 30 g by IV infusion over 30 minutes

Adverse effects
- nausea, vomiting
- flushing
- headache, numbness
- (rare) hypotension, anaphylaxis, allergic reactions, severe hyperkalaemia
- (IV site) irritation (if infused too rapidly)

Interactions
- caution if given with spironolactone

Nursing points/Cautions
- BP should be monitored during and for 24 hours after IV infusion due to risk of hypotension
- antihistamines should be readily available in the event of allergic reaction
- single test should not be used as evaluation for growth disorders as false positive and false negative results are common
- should be diluted with sodium chloride 0.9% or glucose 5% before IV administration
- caution if used in those with electrolyte disturbance due to risk of hyperchloraemic acidosis
- caution if used in those with severe liver disease or moderate kidney insufficiency
- caution if used in those with uraemia, anuria or kidney disease due to risk of elevated potassium levels
- contraindicated in those who are highly allergic or with hypersensitivity to arginine, severe acidosis, hypotension or any disease/defect related to nitric oxide production

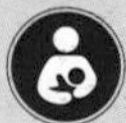
caution if used during pregnancy or breastfeeding

Note
- contained in Arginaid and Arginine Amino Acid supplements

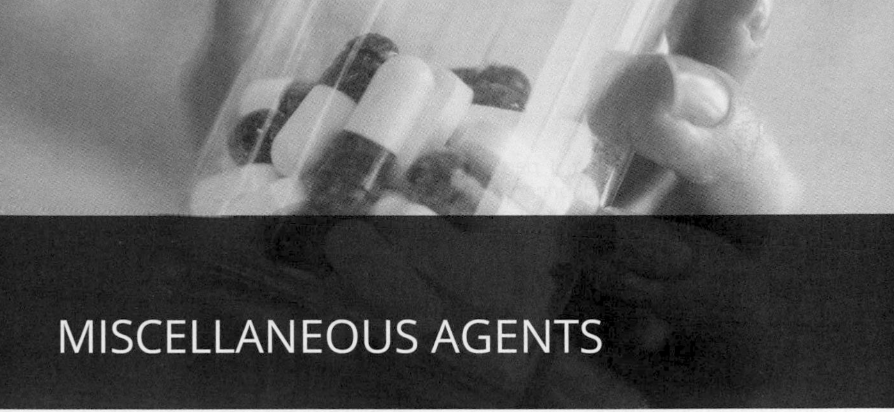

MISCELLANEOUS AGENTS

The agents included in this section are a heterogeneous group of drugs which do not fit into any of the other more clearly defined chapters.

BEZLOTOXUMAB (Zinplava)

Available form
Vial: 1 g/40 mL

Action
- antitoxin that binds with high affinity to *Clostridium difficile* toxin B preventing binding to host cell and therefore neutralising its activity. (*C. difficile* produces two endotoxins (toxin A and toxin B) that cause the release of inflammatory mediators and recruitment of immune cells to the infection site leading to tissue damage in the gut)

Use
- prevention of recurrence of *C. difficile* infection in adults who are receiving antibacterial therapy and are at risk of recurrence

Dose
- 10 mg/kg IV over 60 minutes (with antibacterial therapy)

Adverse effects
- nausea, diarrhoea
- fever
- headache, fatigue, dizziness
- dyspnoea
- hypertension
- heart failure

Nursing points/Cautions
- do not shake vial
- dilute required amount (based on patient weight) with sodium chloride 0.9% or glucose 5% to give a final concentration of 1–10 mg/mL and administer IV over 60 minutes
- not recommended as an IV push or bolus
- should be administered using a low-protein binding 0.2–5 micron inline or add-on filter
- administer alone
- caution if used in those with heart failure and should only be used if benefits are thought to outweigh risks
- not an antibacterial agent, therefore is not recommended for management of acute *C. difficile* infection

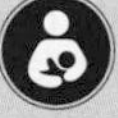
only used during pregnancy or breastfeeding if benefits outweigh risks

HYALURONIC ACID (Durolane)

Available form
Glass syringe: 20 mg/mL

Action

- hyaluronic acid is a normal part of synovial fluid, acting as lubricant for cartilage and ligaments, as well as a shock absorber
- in joints affected by osteoarthritis (OA), synovial fluid has a lower viscosity and elasticity, therefore hyaluronic acid is used to restore viscosity and elasticity, reducing pain and improving mobility
- half-life is about 4 weeks

Use

- symptomatic treatment of mild-to-moderate OA

Dose

- 60 mg (3 mL) intra-articular injection into knee

Adverse effects

- transient knee pain, swelling or stiffness

Interactions

- not recommended with other intra-articular injections

Nursing points/Cautions

- any joint effusion should be removed before intra-articular injection
- same needle can be used for both removal of effusion and intra-articular injection
- if both limbs are being treated, a separate syringe should be used for each limb
- re-injection in less than 6 months is not recommended
- caution if used in those with venous or lymphatic stasis of the limb
- caution if used in those with pre-existing chondrocalcinosis as administration may lead to acute attack
- not recommended if there is any infection or severe inflammation of the knee joint or skin infection/disease at or near injection site
- not recommended IV, extra-articularly or in synovial tissue or capsule
- not recommended in those with known hypersensitivity to hyaluronic acid

Patient teaching and advice

- patient should be instructed to avoid strenuous exercise (e.g. tennis, jogging, long walks) for 48 hours after injection
- warn patient that there may be some transient mild-to-moderate pain, swelling or stiffness during first week after injection. If these symptoms persist for more than 1 week, patient should be advised to seek medical advice

HYDROXYETHYLRUTOSIDES (Paroven, Paroven Forte)

Available forms

Capsules: 250 mg; Tablets: 500 mg

Action

- semi-synthetic flavonoids thought to decrease microvascular fragility and permeability, resulting in reduced fluid leakage from capillaries, reducing oedema and tissue congestion and improving capillary circulation

Use

- relieves symptoms of venous insufficiency, such as tired, aching, heavy, painful or swollen legs

Dose

- initially 250 mg orally 3–4 times daily with food for 3–4 weeks, reducing to 250 mg 1–2 times daily and discontinuing after 12 weeks. If symptoms recur, restart therapy with 250 mg 3–4 times daily with food until remission is achieved (Paroven) **OR**
- initially 500 mg orally twice daily with food for 3–4 weeks, then reducing to 500 mg daily. If symptoms recur after ceasing therapy, restart with 500 mg twice daily for 3–4 weeks (Paroven Forte)

Adverse effects
- nausea, indigestion, diarrhoea
- rash, pruritus, flushing
- headache, dizziness, fatigue
- (rare) hypersensitivity

Interactions
- caution if given with calcium-channel blockers (dihydropyridine)

Nursing points/Cautions
- clinical response is usually seen in 7–10 days, with maximum response occurring in 3–4 weeks
- caution if used in those with severe circulatory problems or heart, kidney or liver conditions associated with lower leg oedema

Patient teaching and advice
- advise patient to swallow tablets/capsules whole with food (not break, chew or crush)
- instruct patient not to drive or operate machinery if dizziness occurs
- patient should be advised to seek medical advice if symptoms persist or worsen after 2 weeks

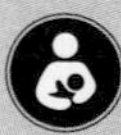
not recommended during pregnancy or breastfeeding

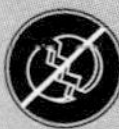
tablets/capsules should be swallowed whole, not crushed, chewed or broken

LAURETH-9 (LAUROMACROGOL 400) (Aethoxysklerol)

Available forms
Ampoules: 10 mg/2 mL, 20 mg/2 mL, 60 mg/2 mL

Action
- irritates vein wall intima, causing thrombus, which permanently occludes vessel by causing fibrosis when compression is applied

Use
- treatment of varicose veins (up to 6 mm) in lower limbs (with compression therapy)

Dose
- injected slowly into lumen of affected vein (daily maximum 2 mg/kg)

Adverse effects
- (immediate) pain, inflammation, swelling, haematoma, local allergic reaction
- (delayed) hyperpigmentation, vein thrombosis, ecchymosis, neovascularisation
- (rare) allergic reaction, angioedema, anaphylactoid reaction

Interaction
- may intensify effects of anaesthetics especially cardiac effects

Nursing points/Cautions
- before therapy, valvular competence and deep vein patency should be assessed
- before injection, leg should be elevated 30–45 degrees above horizontal
- if patient has a history of hypersensitivities or allergies, only 1 injection should be given initially under careful observation
- amount injected is dependent on size of vessel (e.g. spider veins 0.1–0.2 mL of 0.5% solution, whereas medium-sized varices require 0.5–1 mL of 2–3% solution)
- once injections are complete and sites covered, firm compression bandage is applied and patient should walk under observation for at least 30 minutes
- bandage should remain in situ for 2–3 days (spider veins), 3–7 days (small varices) and 4–6 weeks (medium-to-large sized varices)
- repeat treatments at 1–2-week intervals may be necessary depending on size and extent of varices

- contains alcohol which may need to be considered in patients with alcoholism
- oxygen, adrenaline (epinephrine), IV corticosteroids and resuscitation equipment should be available in the event of anaphylaxis
- caution if injecting into malleolus area. Small quantities of low concentration solution should be used
- contraindicated intra-arterially
- caution or contraindicated (depending on severity) in those with leg oedema (that can't be compressed), symptoms of microangiopathy or neuropathy, hypercoagulability, spider veins, inflammatory skin reaction at injection site, acute severe cardiac disease, febrile states or advanced age (with impaired mobility or very poor general condition) or right-to-left shunt (asymptomatic)
- contraindicated in those who are bedridden or unable to walk or those with arterial occlusive disease, acute superficial thrombophlebitis, thromboembolic disorders or high risk of thromboembolic disorders, significant valvular or deep vein incompetence, huge superficial veins that communicate to deeper veins, acute cellulitis or infections, phlebitis migrans, varicosities caused by abdominal/pelvic tumours (unless tumour has been removed), uncontrolled systemic disease (e.g. diabetes mellitus, hypertension), tuberculosis, toxic hyperthyroidism, asthma, blood dyscrasias, acute respiratory or skin disease or strong predisposition to allergies

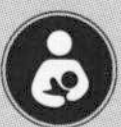

not recommended during pregnancy

caution if used during breastfeeding

METYRAPONE (Metopirone)

Available form
Capsules: 250 mg

Action
- reversibly inhibits production of cortisol, corticosterone and aldosterone by the adrenal cortex
- if pituitary feedback control system is intact, causes a compensatory increase in ACTH, resulting in increased cortisol precursor production
- rapidly absorbed orally
- elimination half-life is 20–26 minutes
- active metabolite

Use
- diagnostic agent for assessing anterior pituitary and adrenocortical function
- differential diagnosis of adrenal hyperfunction in Cushing's syndrome

Dose
Short single-dose test (ambulant patient)
- 1–2 g (based on 30 mg/kg) orally at approximately midnight with yoghurt or milk; 8 hours later, take blood for estimation of ACTH and/or 11-deoxycortisol, then give cortisone acetate 50 mg prophylactically

Multiple-dose test (in hospital setting)
- obtain urine samples in the 24 hours preceding the test (for control values of urinary steroid excretion)
- 500–750 mg orally 4-hourly for 6 doses after food or with milk (total 3.0–4.5 g/24 hours)
- collect all urine for the next 24 hours and store at −10°C until analysis

Adverse effects
- nausea, vomiting
- headache, dizziness, sedation
- hypotension
- (rare) skin reactions

Interactions
- may potentiate paracetamol increasing risk of toxicity
- test results may be influenced by phenytoin, barbiturates, amitriptyline, chlorpromazine, alprazolam, hormone preparations, corticosteroids,

cyproheptadine and antithyroid agents

Nursing points/Cautions

- requires some functioning of the adrenal cortex for satisfactory results, otherwise acute adrenal insufficiency may be induced
- drugs affecting pituitary or adrenocortical function (e.g. antiepileptics, psychoactive drugs, hormone preparations, corticosteroids, antithyroid drugs) must be withdrawn before the test
- if adrenocortical insufficiency is suspected, patient should be observed overnight in hospital if carer/supervision is not available
- caution if used in those with ectopic Cushing's syndrome due to risk of opportunistic infection
- caution if used in those with liver damage (response may be delayed) or thyroid hypofunction (urinary steroid excretion may not increase at all or very slowly)
- contraindicated in those with adrenocortical insufficiency

Patient teaching and advice

- patient should be advised against driving or operating machinery if dizziness or sedation occurs
- see also General Patient teaching and advice (p. xxvii)

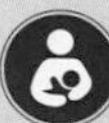

not used during pregnancy unless benefit outweighs any potential risk

contraindicated with breastfeeding during this test

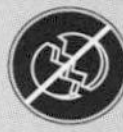

contents of capsule can be squeezed into water or spoonful of yoghurt; however, content is very thick and dose may not be correct. Mask, gloves and safety glasses should be worn if opening capsule

PHENOL (Haemorol)

Available form

Ampoules: 250 mg/5 mL

Action

- sclerosing agent

Use

- first- to second-degree symptomatic haemorrhoids (unresponsive to conservative treatment such as dietary manipulation)

Dose

- 100–250 mg (2–5 mL) into submucosal space above each of the 3 main haemorrhoids (maximum per treatment 500 mg (10 mL))

Adverse effects

- pain, discomfort
- dizziness
- local ulceration, sterile abscess
- (rare) necrotising fasciitis

Interactions

- incompatible with alkaline salts and non-ionic surfactants
- interferes with a number of laboratory tests, including plasma estimation for adrenaline (epinephrine) and noradrenaline (norepinephrine), ferric chloride test for urinary ketones or salicylates, serum calcium, serum sulfonamides and Benedict's test for glycosuria

Nursing points/Cautions

- not for intrathecal use, or injection into blood vessels or deep tissue
- not recommended over large areas of skin due to absorption and toxicity
- glass syringes are recommended; however, plastic syringes with plastic hubs can be used if administered immediately
- contraindicated in those with hypersensitivity to phenol or almond oil or over large areas

Patient teaching and advice

- warn patient to avoid driving or operating machinery if dizziness occurs

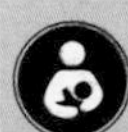

not recommended during pregnancy or breastfeeding

POVIDONE–IODINE (Betadine Preparations, Difflam Sore Throat Gargle with Iodine Concentrate, Herron Riodine Concentrated Gargle, Inadine, Microshield PVP)

Available forms

Surgical body wash solution: 7.5%; Cream: 5%; Ointment: 10%; Cold sore ointment: 10%; Spray: 5%; Liquid throat gargle: 1%, 7.5%; Solution: 7.5%, 10%; Dressing

Action

- rapidly effective against bacteria, viruses and fungal spores
- low concentration solutions provide kill-rate equal to or greater than concentrated solutions

Use

- broad spectrum antiseptic and disinfectant

Dose

- (sore throat) dilute 7.5% solution according to instructions (1 in 20) and gargle for greater than 30 seconds, then expel. Repeat 3–4-hourly (some solutions (1%) do not need to be diluted) **OR**
- (pre-surgical body wash) wet body and hair, apply solution and work into a lather (paying particular attention to hair, groin and axilla) for at least 2 minutes, rinse thoroughly with running water and dry. Should be repeated at least twice before surgery **OR**
- (minor burns, wounds, cuts, abrasions) apply to affected area according to the manufacturer's instructions and cover with dressing, if required **OR**
- (surgical hand scrub) apply 3.5 mL (1 pump) to 5 mL to wet hands and arms and wash for at least 2 minutes, scrub nails with nail brush, rinse, then repeat, and dry with sterile towel **OR**
- (surgical skin preparation) operative field is painted with skin preparation (10%) and allowed to dry before starting procedure **OR**
- (cold sore ointment) ointment applied to cold sore at least 4 times per day **OR**
- (dressing) apply dressing to cleansed wound

Adverse effects

- irritation, redness, swelling

Nursing points/Cautions

- (skin preparation) 10% solution contains alcohol and may be hazardous if allowed to pool on surgical drapes or under patient before diathermy
- (dressing) dressing should be changed when colour fades. For highly exuding or infected wounds, dressing may require changing twice daily with frequency reducing as healing occurs
- multiple preparations and strengths are available, therefore care should be taken to select the correct preparation and strength
- (solution) avoid contact with mucous membranes, eyes or ears
- (dressing) caution if used in deep ulcers, burns or over large areas
- prolonged (> 14 days) or extensive use (> 10% total body surface) should be avoided
- not recommended or used on premature newborns and caution if used on full-term infants due to risk of transient hypothyroidism if used

for extended time or over large area of body
- contraindicated if used in those with thyroid disorders or within 4 weeks of thyroid cancer treatment
- contraindicated in those with known iodine sensitivity

Patient teaching and advice

- (cold sore ointment) warn patient not to apply close to eyes, ears or mucous membranes
- (gargle solution) advise patient not to swallow solution
- (sore throat) instruct patient that if symptoms persist for > 2 days, medical advice should be sought

Note

- contained with ethanol in Betadine Cold Sore Paint Pain Relief Formula

SODIUM TETRADECYL SULFATE (Fibro-Vein)

Available forms

Solution: 0.2%, 0.5%, 1%, 3%

Action

- sclerosing agent that irritates the intima of the vein wall so that when compressed the vein is permanently occluded because of vein fibrosis

Use

- compression sclerotherapy of varicose veins

Dose

- 0.5–1.0 mL IV into lumen of emptied, isolated segment of superficial vein, followed by immediate compression (maximum 4 sites (4 mL) per treatment) (3% solution) **OR**
- 0.25–1.0 mL IV into lumen of emptied, isolated segment of superficial vein, followed by immediate compression (maximum 10 sites (10 mL) per treatment) (1% solution) **OR**
- 0.25–1.0 mL IV into lumen of emptied, isolated segment of superficial vein (medium venules), followed by immediate compression (maximum 10 sites (10 mL) per treatment) (0.5% solution) **OR**
- 0.1–1.0 mL IV into lumen of emptied, isolated segment of superficial vein (minor venules, spider veins), followed by immediate compression (maximum 10 sites (10 mL) per treatment) (0.2% solution)

Adverse effects

- superficial thrombophlebitis
- (local) pain, burning sensation, skin pigmentation, necrosis, ulceration (superficial extravasation)
- (rare) anaphylaxis, allergy, deep vein thrombosis, pulmonary embolism

Interactions

- contraindicated in those taking oral contraceptives or hormone replacement therapy

Nursing points/Cautions

- pre-injection assessment for valvular competence and deep vein patency must be carried out. Allergy history should also be taken from patient before administration, including any previous treatment with sodium tetradecyl sulfate, because there is an increased risk of allergic reaction with repeated treatments
- strength of solution used is dependent on size of vein to be sclerosed
- not given intra-arterially due to risk of tissue necrosis and ischaemia
- caution if used in those with history of allergy/anaphylaxis. If deemed necessary, test dose (0.25–0.5 mL) can be given 24 hours before treatment
- because the possibility of anaphylaxis exists (although rare), it is necessary to have ready availability of adrenaline (epinephrine), aminophylline, hydrocortisone, an antihistamine

and equipment for mucous extraction and endotracheal intubation in the event of a reaction occurring
- class 1 compression stocking can be applied over bandages for retention and compression
- (fibrovein 1%) bandages can be replaced by class 2 or 3 compression stockings at an early stage but must be worn for at least 6 weeks
- available in four strengths, therefore ensure that correct solution is selected
- patient should walk for 30–60 minutes immediately post-procedure
- extreme caution if used in those with arterial disease including peripheral atherosclerosis and thromboangiitis obliterans
- contraindicated in those who are bedridden or unable to walk 5 km/day, or those with arterial occlusive disease, acute superficial thrombophlebitis, thromboembolic disorders or high risk of thromboembolic disorders, significant valvular or deep vein incompetence, high superficial veins that communicate to deeper veins, acute cellulitis or infections, phlebitis migrans, varicosities caused by abdominal/pelvic tumours (unless tumour has been removed), uncontrolled systemic disease (e.g. diabetes mellitus, hypertension), tuberculosis, toxic hyperthyroidism, asthma, blood dyscrasias, recent surgery, acute respiratory or skin disease or strong predisposition to allergies

Patient teaching and advice

- patient should be advised to seek medical attention immediately if any of the following occur:
  - sudden shortness of breath, sudden chest pain which worsens on deep breathing or coughing, coughing up pinky frothy sputum, rapid heart rate and/or breathing, anxiety, fainting, sweating
  - pain in calf, foot or leg, swelling of extremity (usually one side), tenderness, warmth
- after procedure, patient should be given the following instructions:
  - bandages/stockings must not be removed for at least 6 weeks after injection, and then only removed once doctor has specified this can occur
  - bandages/stockings should be kept dry during bathing or showering
  - daily exercise (walking) for at least 1 hour or 5 km is recommended from day of injection and should be continued after removal of bandages/stockings
  - standing still for any period of time is not recommended

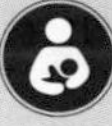

caution if used during pregnancy or breastfeeding as use should be limited to single application or over small area for short time

THYROTROPHIN ALFA (RCH) (Thyrogen)

Available form
Vial: 0.9 mg/mL

Action
- human thyroid-stimulating hormone (TSH) produced by recombinant DNA technology
- similar to human pituitary TSH
- binds to TSH receptors on normal thyroid epithelial cell or well-differentiated thyroid cancer cells stimulating iodine uptake, organification, synthesis of thyroglobulin (Tg), triiodothyronine (T3) and thyroxine (T4)

Use
- use with serum thyroglobulin (Tg) testing (with or without radioactive iodine imaging) to detect thyroid remnants or

well-differentiated thyroid cancer in post-thyroidectomy patients on hormone suppression therapy
- combined with radioactive iodine in the ablation of thyroid remnant tissue post-thyroidectomy on hormone suppression therapy

Dose
- 0.9 mg IM, followed by 0.9 mg after 24 hours

Adverse effects
- nausea, vomiting, diarrhoea
- headache, fatigue, dizziness, asthenia, paraesthesia
- transient flu-like symptoms (including fever (> 38°C), chills, shivering, myalgia, arthralgia, fatigue, malaise, headache)
- elevated (short term) TSH levels which may stimulate tumour or metastatic growth (where thyroid hormones have been withdrawn for diagnostic purpose)
- (rare) hypersensitivity

Nursing points/Cautions

- use should be restricted to patients who are at low risk of disease recurrence
- Tg levels are generally lower and do not correlate with Tg levels after thyroid hormone withdrawal. If detectable Tg level appears or rises after administration, or there is a high index of suspicion of metastatic disease, further evaluation is recommended immediately
- in clinical trials, undetectable thyrotrophin alfa-stimulated Tg levels (< 2.5 nanogram/mL) suggested the absence of clinically significant disease
- whole body scanning with thyroglobulin testing after administration increased detection rate of remnant cancer when compared to either method alone
- reconstitute with 1.2 mL water for injections
- administer by deep IM into buttocks
- radioactive imaging or treatment, radioactive administration is recommended 24 hours after second IM injection
- diagnostic scanning should be performed 48 hours after radioactive administration (72 hours after last IM injection)
- for serum Tg testing, serum sample should be collected 72 hours after final IM injection
- thyroglobulin antibodies will interfere with Tg assay leading to uninterpretable results. If this occurs, a thyroid hormone withdrawal scan is recommended to determine the site and extent of thyroid cancer
- administer alone
- caution if used in those who have previously experienced hypersensitivity reaction to bovine TSH
- caution if used in those with history of heart disease with residual thyroid tissue as a rise in thyroid hormone levels may lead to thyrotrophin alfa-induced hyperthyroidism
- caution if used in those with thyroid cancer with metastases in confined spaces (e.g. brain, spinal cord, orbit, neck infiltration) as elevated TSH levels after administration may result in symptoms such as acute hemiplegia, hemiparesis, pain or swallowing difficulties. Pre-treatment with corticosteroids may prevent this from occurring

Patient teaching and advice

- warn patient to avoid driving or operating machinery if dizziness or fatigue are ongoing
- patient should be warned that flu-like symptoms may occur for up to 48 hours after procedure

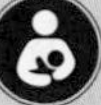

not recommended during pregnancy or breastfeeding

APPENDIX 1: POISONING AND ITS TREATMENT

A poison can be defined as 'a substance (other than an infectious substance) that is harmful if ingested, inhaled, injected or absorbed through the skin' (Australian Resuscitation Guidelines (ARC) 2021, p. 3). It should be noted, however, that any substance can be poisonous if the dose is large enough.

Poisons can include:

- prescription, over-the-counter (OTC) medications or other readily available substances taken in doses that are higher than recommended (e.g. alcohol, paracetamol, aspirin)
- illegal drug overdoses (e.g. heroin, morphine, ecstasy)
- gases (e.g. carbon monoxide from gas appliances or car emissions, bromine or chlorine gas)
- household products (e.g. cleaning products, furniture polish)
- pesticides
- plants (including mushrooms)
- metals (e.g. lead, mercury).

It is essential to prevent poisoning by:

- surveying home or workplace to identify any poisonous substances present
- minimising the amount of poisonous substances stored in the house
- correctly disposing of unwanted and out-of-date medicines by returning them to the local pharmacy (and not disposing in domestic waste or flushing down the toilet)
- leaving medicines and chemicals in the original containers (and not decanted into other containers such as soft drink bottles)
- ensuring medicines and chemicals are stored safely out of reach of children in locked or child-proof cupboards
- never leaving medicines unattended or within reach of children
- storing medicines separately from household products
- not referring to medicines as 'lollies'
- not taking other people's medicine
- checking with a pharmacist or doctor if uncertain about when or how to take medicines
- using appropriate protection (personal protective equipment) and ensuring adequate ventilation when using toxic or caustic chemicals (e.g. over-cleaning, spraying pesticides, painting) (ARC 2021).

Diagnosis of poisoning is usually made from the history and circumstantial evidence. Signs and symptoms of poisoning may include:

- burns or redness around the mouth and/or lips
- breath that smells like chemicals
- burns, stains and/or odour on the person or his/her clothing, furniture, floor or other surrounding area
- empty container(s), medication bottles or scattered pills
- person unexpectedly vomiting, becoming sleepy, restless or agitated, confused or having breathing difficulty, having either pinpoint or dilated

pupils, unusual heart rate (slow or fast depending on the poisoning agent), having a seizure or becoming unconscious.
- some poisons have delayed symptoms (hours, days or even months), which may make it difficult to connect the signs and symptoms with the offending agent(s) (e.g. paracetamol, lead, sustained/modified-release preparations).

Aims

The aims in treating poisoning are to:
- assess the severity of the poisoning
- identify the poison or poisons, if possible
- prevent poisoning of the rescuer
- remove or neutralise the poison before absorption or corrosion occurs
- apply first aid treatment.

Action

When treating poisoning, the Australian Resuscitation Council (2021) makes the following recommendations:
- If the person has collapsed, ring for an ambulance NOT the Poisons Information Centre.
- Do not put yourself in any danger (e.g. poorly ventilated room, contact with chemicals on the person's skin).
- Ensure that the person's airway, breathing and circulation are maintained. Commence cardiopulmonary resuscitation (CPR) if necessary and if the environment is safe to do so.
- Protect the spine, especially in an unconscious patient.
- If possible, obtain a history to ascertain the name of the product (and manufacturer), the type of contact with the poison (ingestion, inhalation, skin contamination), the amount ingested, the length of time elapsed since contact, any existing illnesses or allergies, current medications, any symptoms since contact and the weight of the person (especially if a child is involved). However, if the person is unconscious and the event was unwitnessed, this information may be difficult, if not impossible, to obtain. At times, some of this information may be obtained by counting missing tablets or questioning partners, carers or family members regarding what was available and/or quantities.
- Observe level of consciousness (e.g. conscious, unconscious, drowsy, responding to questions and commands), any seizure activity, colour (flushed, pallor, cyanotic), heart rate (is pulse present? rapid, slow, strong and bounding, weak and thready), peripheral perfusion, breathing (including any increased or decreased respiratory rate, breathing is laboured, wheezing or stridor present), difficulty swallowing, voice alteration, temperature (increased or decreased), hydration status and urine output.
- Collect evidence (e.g. medication containers, spilled pills) and samples of gastric contents, urine and blood, if required, possible and appropriate.

Swallowed poison

- Do not try and make the person vomit. Adsorbing with activated charcoal lowers blood concentrations more effectively than inducing vomiting. Vomiting is not recommended in all cases as severe damage to the oesophagus may occur if the substance taken is corrosive. Activated charcoal is not recommended in ALL cases of poisoning, so it is important to seek advice before taking any action.

- A sip of water may be used to wash out mouth.
- If the ingested poison is a button battery, it is time critical that an X-ray of neck, chest and abdomen is conducted. Endoscopic removal of the battery may be needed urgently.
- Seek advice from the Poisons Information Centre (see Appendix 2, p. 1637).

Inhaled poison

- Move patient into fresh air or admit fresh air to the area, if safe to do so. Avoid breathing in fumes.
- Check for any stridor or hoarse voice.
- Call for ambulance.

Poison in contact with skin

- Remove contaminated clothing and shoes and socks, avoiding contact with the poison/chemical.
- Drench contaminated area with tepid running water for at least 15–20 minutes, then wash area gently with soap and water and rinse well, taking care to wash behind ears, under nails and in skin folds.
- Use soap or shampoo if the poison was oily.
- Call for ambulance.

Poison in contact with eyes

- Timing is important as the corneal surface can be damaged rapidly and permanently scarred.
- Contact lenses should be removed if present.
- Holding eyelids apart, wash eyes thoroughly with copious amounts of water or saline for 15–20 minutes.
- Evert the lids to ensure adequate removal of the agent.
- Cover the eye(s) and transport patient for medical assessment.

Hospital management

- After the person has been transferred to hospital, Murray and collegues (2015) outline the following as being priorities of care:
  - airway, breathing and circulation
- assessment and correction of any:
  - seizure activity (generally managed with IV benzodiazepines; phenytoin is contraindicated in seizure management due to acute poisoning)
  - hypoglycaemia (may be associated with poisoning/overdose due to insulin, oral hypoglycaemic agents, chloroquine, salicylates, beta-adrenoceptor blocking agents and sodium valproate)
  - hypo- or hyperthermia (temperature $> 39.5°C$ is life threatening and requires immediate management to prevent organ damage or failure; severe hypothermia $< 29°C$ can imitate or cause cardiac arrest)
- administration of antidote – this is not always part of the resuscitation phase of poisoning management; however, it is dependent on the agent used (e.g. naloxone for opioid overdose; atropine for organophosphate poisoning)
- risk assessment is the next element of hospital management and involves identifying potential problems and making decisions about subsequent care (Murray et al 2015), involving steps identified earlier

(identifying agent(s), amount ingested, time since ingestion, clinical features and progress, as well as patient-specific factors such as weight and co-morbidities)
- initial hospital investigations should include:
  - 12-lead ECG (assessing rate, rhythm, PR interval, QRS interval, QT interval)
  - serum paracetamol level (normally done if 4 hours has elapsed and is implicated in overdose; however, non-detectable paracetamol levels more than 1 hour after ingestion excludes significant ingestion). Alanine amino-transferase (ALT) should also be measured in all patients along with serum paracetamol levels (Toxicology and Toxinology Expert Group 2020)
  - other investigations may include arterial blood gases, urine blood screen, baseline blood count, electrolytes, renal function, blood sugar, creatine kinase, troponins (especially if cocaine was used), and, if indicated, coagulation studies, liver function tests, and/or specific drug tests
- the patient should be closely and continuously monitored, including the circulation (pulse, blood pressure, peripheral perfusion), urine output, temperature, hydration, respiration (airway protective reflexes, respiratory rate, air entry, breath sounds, pulse oximetry) and neurological status (including conscious state) (Glasgow Coma Scale, seizure activity)
- duration of observation is dependent on agent(s) ingested, formulation (e.g. immediate-release tablets or sustained release) and potential complications
- determine the time of poison ingestion (if possible), because there is little benefit in emptying the stomach if more than 3 hours has elapsed since ingestion
- stomach should not be emptied if the airway cannot be protected or if a petroleum distillate or corrosive substance has been ingested
- specific antidotes may be given for a limited number of drugs (e.g. naloxone for opiates, acetylcysteine for paracetamol, fresh frozen plasma and vitamin K for warfarin, chelating agents for heavy metals, flumazenil for benzodiazepines, hyperbaric oxygen for carbon monoxide, glucagon, isoprenaline and pacing for beta-adrenergic blocking agents) (see Antidotes, antagonists and chelating agents, p. 332)
- the patient may also need fluid therapy and oxygen
- enhanced removal techniques may be used to remove some agents. These include repeat doses of activated charcoal, forced diuresis, alkalinisation of the urine, peritoneal or haemodialyis or haemoperfusion
- admission to ICU may be required if haemodialysis, prolonged or invasive haemodynamic monitoring is required and/or the patient is ventilated
- formal psychiatric and social work assessments may be necessary before discharge, with the patient given access to social work, counselling and other resources (e.g. drug and alcohol counselling) if the poisoning was a deliberate attempt at self-harm.

TREATMENT WITH ACTIVATED CHARCOAL (CARBOSORB X)

Action and use

- absorbs most inorganic and organic compounds in the alimentary tract, so reducing or preventing systemic absorption. Drugs that are well absorbed include aspirin, amphetamines, barbiturates, cocaine, digoxin, morphine and phenothiazines. Drugs that are poorly bound to activated charcoal include corrosive acids or alkalis, metals (e.g. lithium, iron, potassium, lead, arsenic and mercury), alcohols and hydrocarbons
- may be given after emptying stomach contents by emesis or washout (gastric lavage), although activated charcoal is increasingly being used in emergency departments as first-line management of ingested poisoning. The earlier the charcoal is given, the more effective it is likely to be. Emesis should not be used if the person is drowsy, unconscious, fitting or likely to become drowsy within 30 minutes of taking an emetic.

Adult dose

- 1 g/kg orally or via nasogastric/orogastric tube as soon as possible after ingestion or suspected ingestion of the potential poison or after induced emesis or stomach washout (may be repeated 2–6-hourly until first black stool has been passed (maximum dose 50 g)).

Paediatric dose

- 1 g/kg orally or via nasogastric tube.

Nursing points/Cautions

- if antidote to a specific drug is available, it should be used as first-line treatment. Specific antidotes should not be given with activated charcoal as they may be adsorbed
- risk versus harm should be assessed before administration
- activated charcoal should be administered as soon as possible after poison ingestion or up to 2 hours after immediate-release or 4 hours after sustained-release preparations
- any concurrent medication should preferably be given parenterally
- bowel sounds should be assessed before any dose (or repeat dose) of activated charcoal
- colours faeces black
- caution if given to patients with diabetes as Carbosorb X contains 0.46 g sucrose/mL
- contraindicated in poisoning due to strong acids and alkalis and where adsorptive capacity is too low to treat poisoning (e.g. iron salts, ferrous sulfate, cyanides, other sulfonylureas, malathion, lithium, ethanol, methanol, ethylene glycol and hydrocarbons)
- contraindicated if airway is not protected, corrosive agent was ingested or the gastrointestinal tract is not intact
- see also Antidotes, antagonists and chelating agents (p. 332)

Note

- contained in Carbosorb XS with sorbitol.

APPENDIX 2: POISONS INFORMATION CENTRES

When contacting the Poisons Information Centre, it is useful to provide the following information if possible or available:

- name of toxin or drug (with exact name and spelling, if possible)
- patient details (age, weight, sex, medical history, medication history)
- whether the poisoning was deliberate, intentional or accidental
- exposure details (e.g. time since exposure, route, dose)
- any immediate first aid action taken,
- basic observations if possible (including heart rate, respiratory rate, temperature, consciousness level) and
- any clinical symptoms (Toxicology and Toxinology Expert Group 2020).

Australia

Please call: 13 11 26

(24-hour line, Australia-wide) (cost of a local call excluding mobile phones) for information and advice on emergency treatment of poisoning, bites and stings in all Australian states and territories.

New Zealand

In New Zealand call: 0800 764 766 (0800 POISON)

APPENDIX 3: CHANGES TO DRUG NAMES

From April 2016, drug ingredient names are being updated to bring Australia in line with the rest of the world. The goal of this is to ensure international conformity in order to promote patient safety by eliminating major name differences between Australia and other countries. It is expected that these changes will be completed by 2023, with products displaying dual labelling until that time. The table below outlines these changes.

Previous term	Current term
Adrenaline and noradrenaline	
adrenaline	adrenaline (epinephrine)
noradrenaline	noradrenaline (norepinephrine)
Other significant changes	
diclofenac diethylammonium	diclofenac diethylamine
hexamine hippurate	methenamine hippurate
insulin – human	insulin
tetrahydrozoline hydrochloride	tetryzoline hydrochloride
thyroxine sodium	levothyroxine sodium
Minor spelling changes	
amoxycillin	amoxicillin
amoxycillin sodium	amoxicillin sodium
amoxycillin trihydrate	amoxicillin trihydrate
atracurium besylate	atracurium besilate
beclomethasone	beclometasone (beclomethasone)
beclomethasone dipropionate	beclometasone dipropionate
benztropine mesylate	benztropine mesilate

Previous term	Current term
bromocriptine mesylate	bromocriptine mesilate
cephalexin	cefalexin monohydrate
cephalothin sodium	cefalotin sodium
cephazolin	cefazolin
cephazolin sodium	cefazolin sodium
chlorthalidone	chlortalidone
cholecalciferol	colecalciferol
cholestyramine	colestyramine
clomiphene citrate	clomifene citrate
cyclosporin	ciclosporin
dexamphetamine sulfate	dexamfetamine sulfate
dextropropoxyphene napsylate	dextropropoxyphene napsilate
dolasetron mesylate	dolasetron mesilate monohydrate
ethacrynic acid	etacrynic acid
ethinyloestradiol	ethinylestradiol
flumethasone	flumetasone
flupenthixol decanoate	flupentixol decanoate
glutaraldehyde	glutaral

Previous term	Current term
heparinoid	heparinoids
indomethacin	indometacin
lapatinib ditosylate monohydrate	lapatinib ditosilate monohydrate
oestradiol	estradiol
oestradiol valerate	estradiol valerate
oestriol	estriol
oestrogens – conjugated	conjugated estrogens
pentamidine isethionate	pentamidine isetionate
pericyazine	periciazaine
sorafenib tosylate	sorafenib tosilate
testosterone enanthate	testosterone enantate
thioguanine	tioguanine
Additional minor changes	
disodium pamidronate	pamidronate disodium
pramipexole hydrochloride	pramipexole dihydrochloride
samarium	samarium (153Sm)

Previous term	Current term
Dual labelling required till 2023	
actinomycin D	dactinomycin (actinomycin D)
amethocaine hydrochloride	tetracaine (amethocaine) hydrochloride
amphotericin	amphotericin B (amphotericin)
Bacillus Calmette and Guerin	Mycobacterium bovis (Bacillus Calmette and Guerin (BCG) strain)
benzhexol hydrochloride	trihexyphenidyl (benzhexol) hydrochloride

Previous term	Current term
colaspase	asparaginase (colaspase)
cysteamine bitartrate	mercaptamine (cysteamine) bitartrate
dothiepin hydrochloride	dosulepin (dothiepin) hydrochloride
doxycycline hydrochloride	doxycycline hyclate (hydrochloride)
eformoterol fumerate	formoterol (eformoterol) fumerate
eformoterol fumerate dihydrate	formoterol (eformoterol) fumerate dihydrate
frusemide	furosemide (frusemide)
glycopyrrolate	glycopyrronium bromide (glycopyrrolate)
hydroxyurea	hydroxycarbamide (hydroxyurea)
lignocaine	lidocaine (lignocaine)
lignocaine hydrochloride	lidocaine (lignocaine) hydrochloride monohydrate
oxpentifylline	pentoxifylline (oxpentifylline)
phenobarbitone	phenobarbital (phenobarbitone)
procaine penicillin	procaine benzylpenicillin (procaine penicillin)
salcatonin	calcitonin salmon (salcatonin)
tetracosactrin	tetracosactide (tetracosactrin)
trimeprazine tartrate	alimemazine (trimeprazine) tartrate

Source: Therapeutic Goods Administration (TGA) (2020). Updating medicine ingredient names – list of affected ingredients. Therapeutic Goods Administration, Department of Health, Australian Government, www.tga.gov.au/updating-medicine-ingredient-names-list-affected-ingredients

BIBLIOGRAPHY

Anderson, I. (2013). How to ... Ten top tips on compliance, concordance and adherence. Wounds International 4(2), 9–12.

Andrews, G., Bell, C., Boyce, P. et al (2018). Royal Australian and New Zealand College of Psychiatrists clinical practice guidelines for the treatment of panic disorder, social anxiety disorder and generalised anxiety disorder. Australian and New Zealand Journal of Psychiatry 52(12), 1109–1172.

Antman, E. & Loscalzo, J. (2019). Ch. 267. Ischaemic heart disease. In: J.L. Jameson, A.S. Fauci, D.L. Kasper et al (eds). Harrison's principles of internal medicine, 20th edn. McGraw-Hill (Online edition).

Appleton, L., Gill, T., Lang, C. et al (2018). Prevalence and comorbidity of sleep conditions in Australian adults: 2016 Sleep Health Foundation national survey. Sleep Health 4, 13–19.

Arruda, V. & High, K. (2018). Ch. 112. Coagulation disorders. In: J.L. Jameson, A.S. Fauci, D.L. Kasper et al (eds). Harrison's principles of internal medicine, 20th edn. McGraw-Hill. (Online edition).

Atik, A. (2013). Adherence to the Australian National Inpatient Medication Chart: the efficacy of a uniform national drug chart on improving prescription error. Journal of Evaluation in Clinical Practice 19(5), 769–772.

Australian Bureau of Statistics (ABS) (2019). Australian Health Survey: first results, 2017–2018. Cat. no. 4364.0.55.001. Online. Available: www.abs.gov.au/ausstats/abs.

Australian Commission on Safety and Quality in Health Care (ACSQHC) (2019a). National inpatient medication chart – development and background. Online. Available: www.safetyandquality.gov.au/our-work/medication-safety/medication-charts/background-and-development-medication-charts/national-inpatient-medication-chart-development-and-background.

Australian Commission on Safety and Quality in Health Care (ACSQHC) (2019b). National standard medication charts. Online. Available: www.safetyandquality.gov.au/our-work/medication-safety/medication-charts/national-standard-medication-charts.

Australian Commission on Safety and Quality in Health Care (ACSQHC) (2016a). National recommendations for user-applied labelling of injectable medicines, fluids and lines. Online. Available: www.safetyandquality.gov.au/our-work/medication-safety/safer-naming-labelling-and-packaging-medicines/recommendations-terminology-abbreviations-and-symbols-used-medicines-documentation.

Australian Commission on Safety and Quality in Health Care (ACSQHC) (2016b). Recommendations for terminology, abbreviations and symbols used in the prescribing and administration of medicines. Online. Available: www.safetyandquality.gov.au/sites/default/files/migrated/Recommendations-for-terminology-abbreviations-and-symbols-used-in-medicines-documentation-Summary-sheet-December-2016.pdf.

Australian Commission on Safety and Quality in Health Care (ACSQHC) (2002). Second national report on patient safety: improving medication safety. Australian Department of Health and Ageing, Canberra.

Australian Government, Department of Health (2020). National Immunisation Program. Online. Available: www.health.gov.au/health-topics/immunisation/immunisation-throughout-life/national-immunisation-program-schedule.

Australian Government, Department of Health (2019). Clinical practice guidelines: pregnancy care. Online. Available: www.health.gov.au/resources/pregnancy-care-guidelines.

Australian Institute of Health and Welfare (AIHW) (2020). Australia's health – causes of death. Online. Available: www.aihw.gov.au/reports/australias-health/causes-of-death.

Australian Institute of Health and Welfare (AIHW) (2019a). Arthritis. Cat. no. PHE 234. AIHW, Canberra. Online. Available: www.aihw.gov.au/reports/chronic-musculoskeletal-conditions/arthritis.

Australian Institute of Health and Welfare (AIHW) (2019b). Asthma. AIHW, Canberra. Online. Available: www.aihw.gov.au/reports/chronic-respiratory-conditions/asthma/contents/asthma.

Australian Institute of Health and Welfare (AIHW) (2019c). Dementia. Online. Available: www.aihw.gov.au/reports-data/health-conditions-disability-deaths/dementia/overview.

Australian Institute of Health and Welfare (AIHW) (2019d). Diabetes. AIHW, Canberra. Online. Available: www.aihw.gov.au/reports/diabetes/diabetes/contents/what-is-diabetes.

Australian Institute of Health and Welfare (AIHW) (2019e). Incidence of gestational diabetes in Australia. AIHW, Canberra. Online. Available: www.aihw.gov.au/reports/diabetes/incidence-of-gestational-diabetes-in-australia/contents/what-is-gestational-diabetes.

Australian Institute of Health and Welfare (AIHW) (2019f). Osteoporosis. Cat. no. PHE 178. AIHW, Canberra. Online. Available: www.aihw.gov.au/reports/chronic-musculoskeletal-conditions/osteoporosis/contents/what-is-osteoporosis.

Australian Institute of Health and Welfare (AIHW) (2019g). Rheumatoid arthritis. Cat. no. PHE 252. AIHW, Canberra. Online. Available: www.aihw.gov.au/reports/chronic-musculoskeletal-conditions/rheumatoid-arthritis.

Australian Institute of Health and Welfare (AIHW) (2017). Gout. AIHW, Canberra. Online. Available: www.aihw.gov.au/.

Australian Resuscitation Council (ARC) (2011). Guideline 9.4.8. Envenomation – pressure immobilization technique. Online. Available: resus.org.au/?wpfb_dl=44.

Australian Resuscitation Council (ARC) (2011, amended 2019). Guideline 9.5.1. Emergency management of a patient who has been poisoned. Online. Available: resus.org.au/guidelines/.

Australian Technical Advisory Group on Immunisation (ATAGI) (2018). Australian immunisation handbook. Australian Government Department of Health, Canberra. Online. Available: immunisationhandbook.health.gov.au.

Austroads (2017). Assessing fitness to drive. Online. Available: austroads.com.au/publications/assessing-fitness-to-drive/ap-g56/neurological-conditions/seizures-and-epilepsy/medical-standards-for-licensing-6.

Banga, S. & Chalfoun, N.T. (2018). Ch. 9. Arrhythmias and antiarrhythmic drugs. In: A. Elmoselhi (ed). Cardiology: an integrated approach. McGraw-Hill. (Online edition).

Barbieri, R. & Repke, J. (2018). Ch. 466. Medical disorders during pregnancy. In: J.L. Jameson, A.S. Fauci, D.L. Kasper et al (eds). Harrison's principles of internal medicine, 20th edn. McGraw-Hill. (Online edition).

Brenner, G. & Stevens, C. (2017). Brenner & Stevens' pharmacology, 5th edn. Elsevier, Philadelphia.

Bringhurst, F.R., Demay, M. & Kronenberg, H. (2019). Ch. 402. Bone and mineral metabolism in health and disease. In: J.L. Jameson, A.S. Fauci, D.L. Kasper et al (eds). Harrison's principles of internal medicine, 20th edn. McGraw-Hill. (Online edition).

Brown, R.H. (2019). Ch. 429. Amyotrophic lateral sclerosis and other motor neuron diseases. In: J.L. Jameson, A.S. Fauci, D.L. Kasper et al (eds). Harrison's principles of internal medicine, 20th edn. McGraw-Hill. (Online edition).

Bryant, B., Knights, K., Darrouch, S. et al (2019). Pharmacology for health professionals, 5th edn. Elsevier, Chatswood.

Butterworth, J., Mackey, D. & Wasnick, J. (2018). Morgan & Mikhail's clinical anesthesiology, 6th edn. McGraw-Hill. (Online edition).

Camilleri, M. & Murray, J. (2018). Ch. 42. Diarrhea and constipation. In: J.L. Jameson, A.S. Fauci, D.L. Kasper et al (eds). Harrison's principles of internal medicine, 20th edn. McGraw-Hill. (Online edition).

Carruthers, A., Naughton, K. & Mallarkey, G. (2008). Accuracy of packaging of dose administration aids in regional aged care facilities in the Hunter area of New South Wales. Medical Journal of Australia 188(5), 280–282.

Centers for Disease Control & Prevention (CDC) (2016). About parasites. Online. Available: www.cdc.gov/parasites/about.html.

Cree, B. & Hauser, S. (2019). Multiple sclerosis. In: J.L. Jameson, A.S. Fauci, D.L. Kasper et al (eds). Harrison's principles of internal medicine, 20th edn. McGraw-Hill. (Online edition).

Del Valle, J. (2018). Ch. 317. Peptic ulcer disease and related disorders. In: J.L. Jameson, A.S. Fauci, D.L. Kasper et al (eds). Harrison's principles of internal medicine, 20th edn. McGraw-Hill. (Online edition).

Deloitte Access Economics (2019). The cost of pain in Australia. Online. Available: www2.deloitte.com/au/en/pages/economics/articles/cost-pain-australia.html.

Deloitte Access Economics (2018). Migraine in Australia Whitepaper. Online. Available: www.painaustralia.org.au/static/uploads/files/deloitte-au-economics-migraine-australia-whitepaper-101018-wfsydysdysky.pdf.

Derry, S., Wiffen, P., Kalso, E. et al (2019). Topical analgesics for acute and chronic pain in adults – an overview of Cochrane reviews. Cochrane Database of Systematic Reviews 2017, 5, CD008609; CD008609.pub2 (updated).

Edwards, J.E. (2018). Ch. 206. Diagnois and treatment of fungal infections. In: J.L. Jameson, A.S. Fauci, D.L. Kasper et al (eds). Harrison's principles of internal medicine, 20th edn. McGraw-Hill. (Online edition).

Elliott, R. (2014). Appropriate use of dose administration aids. Australian Prescriber, 37, 46–50.

Faculty of Pain Medicine (FPM), Australian and New Zealand College of Anaesthetists (ANZCA) (2015). Recommendations regarding the use of opioid analgesics in patients with chronic non-cancer pain. Online. Available: http://fpm.anzca.edu.au/documents/pm1-2010.

Favus, M. & Vokes, T. (2019). Ch. 405. Paget's disease and other dysplagias of bone. In: J.L. Jameson, A.S. Fauci, D.L. Kasper et al (eds). Harrison's principles of internal medicine, 20th edn. McGraw-Hill. (Online edition).

Flenady, V., Wojcieszek, A.M., Papatsonis, D.N.M. et al (2014). Calcium channel blockers for inhibiting preterm labour and birth. Cochrane Database of Systematic Reviews 6, CD002255.

Gelber, R.H. (2018). Ch. 203. Leprosy. In: J.L. Jameson, A.S. Fauci, D.L. Kasper et al (eds). Harrison's principles of internal medicine, 20th edn. McGraw-Hill. (Online edition).

Gilmartin, J.F-M., Marriott, J.L., Hussainy, S.Y. (2016). Improving Australian care home medicine supply services: evaluation of quality improvement intervention. Australian Journal of Ageing 35(2), E1–6.

Gowan, J. & Roller, L. (2010). Crushing medications: dose delivery challenges for people with impaired swallowing. Australian Journal of Pharmacy 91, 50–4.

Grosser, T., Smyth, E. & FitzGerald, G. (2018). Ch. 38. Pharmacotherapy of inflammation, fever, pain and gout. In: L. Brunton, R. Hilal-Dandan & B.C. Knollman (eds). Goodman and Gilman's: the pharmacological basis of therapeutics, 13th edn. (Online edition).

Gunning, K., Pippitt, K., Kiraly, B. et al (2012). Pediculosis and scabies: a treatment update. American Family Physician 86(6), 535–541.

Hall, J. (2018). Ch. 389. Infertility and contraception. In: J.L. Jameson, A.S. Fauci, D.L. Kasper et al (eds). Harrison's principles of internal medicine, 20th edn. McGraw-Hill. (Online edition).

Harris, B.R. & Cooper, A.J. (2017). Modern management of acne. Medical Journal of Australia 206(1), 41–45.

Hasler, W. (2018). Ch. 41. Nausea, vomiting and indigestion. In: J.L. Jameson, A.S. Fauci, D.L. Kasper et al (eds). Harrison's principles of internal medicine, 20th edn. McGraw-Hill. (Online edition).

Hempenstall, A., Smith, S. & Hanson, J. (2019). Leprosy in Far North Queensland: almost gone, but not to be forgotten. Medical Journal of Australia 211(4), 182–183.

Hendrick, L. (2017). Ch. 16. The structure and function of the haematological system. In: J. Craft & C. Gordon (eds). Understanding pathophysiology, 3rd edn. Elsevier, Chatswood.

Hogg, K. & Weitz, J. (2018). Ch. 32. Blood coagulation, anticoagulant, fibrinolytic and antiplatelet drugs. In: L. Brunton, R. Hilal-Dandan & B.C. Knollman (eds). Goodman and Gilman's: the pharmacological basis of therapeutics, 13th edn. (Online edition).

Holland, S. (2018). Ch. 175. Nontuberculous mycobacterial infections. In: J.L. Jameson, A.S. Fauci, D.L. Kasper et al (eds). Harrison's principles of internal medicine, 20th edn. McGraw-Hill. (Online edition).

Hopkins, R. & Grabowski, G. (2019). Ch. 411. Lysosomal storage diseases. In: J.L. Jameson, A.S. Fauci, D.L. Kasper et al (eds). Harrison's principles of internal medicine, 20th edn. McGraw-Hill. (Online edition).

Hotham, N. & Hotham, E. (2015). Drugs in breastfeeding. Australian Prescriber 38(5), 156–160.

International Association for the Study of Pain (IASP) (2017). IASP terminology. Online. Available: www.iasp-pain.org/Education/Content.aspx?ItemNumber=1698#Pain.

International Headache Society (2019). The international classification of headache disorders, 3rd edn. Online. Available: https://ichd-3.org/.

Jameson, J.L., Fauci, A.S., Kasper D.L. et al (eds). (2020). Ch. 123. Chronic stable angina. In: J.L. Jameson, A.S. Fauci, D.L. Kasper (eds). Harrison's manual of medicine, 20th edn. McGraw-Hill. (Online edition).

Jameson, J.L., Mandel, S. & Weetman, A. (2018a). Ch. 377. Hyperthyroidism. In: J.L. Jameson, A.S. Fauci, D.L. Kasper et al (eds). Harrison's principles of internal medicine, 20th edn. McGraw-Hill. (Online edition).

Jameson, J.L., Mandel, S. & Weetman, A. (2018b). Ch. 376. Hypothyroidism. In: J.L. Jameson, A.S. Fauci, D.L. Kasper et al (eds). Harrison's principles of internal medicine, 20th edn. McGraw-Hill. (Online edition).

Jameson, J.L., Mandel, S. & Weetman, A. (2018c). Ch. 375. Thyroid gland physiology and testing. In: J.L. Jameson, A.S. Fauci, D.L. Kasper et al (eds). Harrison's principles of internal medicine, 20th edn. McGraw-Hill. (Online edition).

Jokanovic, N., Ferrah, N., Lovell, J. et al (2019). A review of coronial investigations into medication-related deaths in residential care. Research in Social and Administrative Pharmacy 15, 410–416.

Karsan, N., Bose, P. & Goadsby, P. (2018). The migraine premonitory phase. Continuum: Lifelong Learning in Neurology 24(4), 996–1008.

Katzung, B. (2018). Ch. 12. Vasodilators and the treatment of angina pectoris. In: B. Katzung (ed). Basic and clinical pharmacology, 14th edn. (Online edition).

Keiser, J., McCarthy, J. & Hotez P.J. (2018). Chemotherapy of helminth infections. In: L. Brunton, R. Hilal-Dandan & B.C. Knollman (eds). Goodman and Gilman's: the pharmacological basis of therapeutics, 13th edn. (Online edition).

Khosla, S. (2019). Ch. 50. Hypercalcemia and hypocalcemia. In: J.L. Jameson, A.S. Fauci, D.L. Kasper et al (eds). Harrison's principles of internal medicine, 20th edn. McGraw-Hill. (Online edition).

Konkie, B. (2018). Ch. 111. Disorders of platelets and vessel wall. In: J.L. Jameson, A.S. Fauci, D.L. Kasper et al (eds). Harrison's principles of internal medicine, 20th edn. McGraw-Hill. (Online edition).

Kruidering-Hall, M. & Campbell, L. (2018). Ch. 27. Skeletal muscle relaxants. In: B. Katzung & A. Trevor (eds). Basic and clinical pharmacology, 14th edn. McGraw-Hill, New York.

Kushner, R. (2018). Ch. 395. Evaluation and management of obesity. In: J.L. Jameson, A.S. Fauci, D.L. Kasper et al (eds). Harrison's principles of internal medicine, 20th edn. McGraw-Hill. (Online edition).

Lander, C. (2008). Antepileptic drugs in pregnancy and lactation. Australian Prescriber 31(3), 70–72.

Lawley, L., McCall, C. & Lawley, T. (2018). Ch. 53. Eczema, psoriasis, cutaneous infections, acne and other common skin infections. In: J.L. Jameson, A.S. Fauci, D.L. Kasper et al (eds). Harrison's principles of internal medicine, 20th edn. McGraw-Hill. (Online edition).

Levison, W. (2014). Review of medical microbiology and immunology, 13th edn. McGraw-Hill. (Online edition).

Lin, Y.C., Wan, L. & Jamison, R. (2017). Using integrative medicine in pain management: an evaluation of current practice. Anesthesia and Analgesia 125(6), 2081–2093.

Lindsay, R. & Cosman, F. (2019). Ch. 404. Osteoporosis. In: J.L. Jameson, A.S. Fauci, D.L. Kasper et al (eds). Harrison's principles of internal medicine, 20th edn. McGraw-Hill. (Online edition).

Loosen, P. & Shelton, R. (2019). Ch. 17. Mood disorders. In: M. Ebert, J. Leckman & I. Petrakis (eds). Current diagnosis and treatment: psychiatry, 3rd edn. McGraw-Hill. (Online edition).

Lowenstein, D. (2019). Ch. 418. Seizures and epilepsy. In: J.L. Jameson, A.S. Fauci, D.L. Kasper et al (eds). Harrison's principles of internal medicine, 20th edn. McGraw-Hill. (Online edition).

Mahli, G., Outhred, T., Hamilton, A. et al (2018). Royal Australian and New Zealand College of Psychiatrists clinical practice guidelines for mood disorders: major depression summary. Medical Journal of Australia 208(4), 175–180.

McQuaid, K. (2018). Ch. 62. Drugs used in the treatment of gastrointestinal diseases. In: B.G. Katzung (ed.). Basic and clinical pharmacology, 14th edn. (Online edition).

MIMS Australia. MIMS Online. Available: www.mims.com.au.

Mitchell, H. & Katelaris, P. (2016). Epidemiology, clinical impacts and current clinical management of Helicobacter pylori infection. Medical Journal of Australia 204(10), 376–380.

MND Australia (n.d.). What is MND? Facts and figures. Online. Available: www.mndaust.asn.au/Get-informed/What-is-MND/Facts-and-figures.aspx.

MS Australia (2019). Key facts and figures about multiple sclerosis. Online. Available: www.msaustralia.org.au.

Murray, L., Little, M., Pascu, O. et al (2015). Toxicology handbook, 3rd edn. Elsevier, Chatswood.

National Asthma Council Australia (2019). Australian asthma handbook (Version 2). Online. Available: www.nationalasthma.org.au/health-professionals/australian-asthma-handbook.

National Heart Foundation of Australia (2016). Guidelines for the diagnosis and management of hypertension in adults. Online. Available: www.heartfoundation.org.au.

National Health & Medical Research Council (NHMRC), New Zealand Ministry of Health (NZ MoH) (2017). Sodium. Online. Available: www.nrv.gov.au/nutrients/sodium.

National Vascular Disease Prevention Alliance (2012). Guidelines for the management of absolute cardiovascular disease risk. Online. Available: www.cvdcheck.org.au/pdf/Absolute_CVD_Risk_Full_Guidelines.pdf.

Newman-Casey, P. & Myers, J. (2019). Preliminary steps to address glaucoma medication adherence beginning to tackle the elephant in the room. JAMA Ophthalmology 137(3), 246–247.

Nursing and Midwifery Board of Australia (NMBA), Australian Health Practitioner Regulation Agency (AHPRA) (2020a). Fact sheet: endorsement for scheduled medicines for midwives. Online. Available: www.nursingmidwiferyboard.gov.au/codes-guidelines-statements/faq/fact-sheet-endorsement-for-scheduled-medicines-for-midwives.aspx.

Nursing and Midwifery Board of Australia (NMBA), Australian Health Practitioner Regulation Agency (AHPRA) (2020b). Fact sheet: enrolled nurses and medication administration. Online. Available: www.nursingmidwiferyboard.gov.au/Codes-Guidelines-Statements/FAQ/Enrolled-nurses-and-medicine-administration.aspx.

Olanow, C.W., Klein, C. & Schapira, A. (2019). Ch. 427. Parkinson's disease and other movement disorders. In: J.L. Jameson, A.S. Fauci, D.L. Kasper et al (eds). Harrison's principles of internal medicine, 20th edn. McGraw-Hill. (Online edition).

Powers, A. (2019). Ch. 417. Diabetes mellitus. In: J.L. Jameson, A.S. Fauci, D.L. Kasper et al (eds). Harrison's principles of internal medicine, 20th edn. McGraw-Hill. (Online edition).

Pretorius, A., Searle, J. & Marshall, B. (2015). Barriers and enablers to emergency department nurses' management of patients' pain. Pain Management Nursing 16(3), 372–379.

Psychotropic Expert Group (2021). Therapeutic guidelines: Psychotropic. eTG.

Ramasamy, S., Baysari, M., Lehnbom, E. et al (2013) Evidence briefings on intervention to improve medication safety: double checking medication administration. Online. Available: www.safetyandquality.gov.au/wp-content/uploads/2013/12/Evidence-briefings-on-interventions-to-improve-medication-safety-Double-checking-medication-administration-PDF-888KB.pdf.

Rathmell, J. & Fields, A. (2018). Ch. 10. Pain: pathophysiology and management. In: J.L. Jameson, A.S. Fauci, D.L. Kasper et al (eds). Harrison's principles of internal medicine, 20th edn. McGraw-Hill. (Online edition).

Raviglione, M. (2018). Ch. 173. Tuberculosis. In: J.L. Jameson, A.S. Fauci, D.L. Kasper et al (eds). Harrison's principles of internal medicine, 20th edn. McGraw-Hill. (Online edition).

Reddy, D. & O'Donnell, M. (2018). Ch 176. Antimycobacterial agents. In: J.L. Jameson, A.S. Fauci, D.L. Kasper et al (eds). Harrison's principles of internal medicine, 20th edn. McGraw-Hill. (Online edition).

Roach, S. (2005). Pharmacology for health professionals. Lippincott Williams & Wilkins, Philadelphia.

Roberson, E. (2018). Ch. 18. Treatment of central nervous system degenerative disorders. In: L. Brunton, R. Hilal-Dandan & B.C. Knollman (eds). Goodman & Gilman's: the pharmacological basis of therapeutics, 13th edn. (Online edition).

Robinson, P. & Stamp, L. (2016). The management of gout: much has changed. Australian Family Physician 45(5), 299–302.

Rogers, V. & Worley, K. Ch. 19.12. Preeclampsia-eclampsia. In: M. Papadakis, S. McPhee, & M. Rabow (eds) (2021). Current medical diagnosis and treatment. McGraw-Hill. (Online edition).

Roman-Rodriguez, M., Metting, E., Gacia-Pardo, M. et al (2019). Wrong inhalation technique is associated to poor asthma clinical outcomes. Is there room for improvement? Current Opinion in Pulmonary Medicine 25(1), 18–26.

Ropper, A., Samuels, M., Klein, J. et al (2019). Adams and Victor's principles of neurology, 11th edn. McGraw-Hill (Online edition).

Royal Australian College of General Practitioners (RACGP) (2015). Prescribing drugs of dependence in general practice, Part B: Benzodiazepines. RACGP, Melbourne. Online. Available: www.racgp.org.au/clinical-resources/clinical-guidelines/key-racgp-guidelines/view-all-racgp-guidelines/prescribing-drugs-of-dependence/prescribing-drugs-of-dependence-part-b/evidence-based-guidance-for-benzodiazepines/insomnia.

Salmon, J. (2018). Ch. 11. Glaucoma. In: P. Riordan-Eva & J. Augsburger (eds). Vaughan & Asbury's general ophthalmology, 19th edn. McGraw-Hill. (Online edition).

Schumacher, H.R. & Chen, L.X. (2018). Ch. 365. Gout and other crystal-associated arthropathies. In: J.L. Jameson, A.S. Fauci, D.L. Kasper et al (eds). Harrison's principles of internal medicine, 20th edn. McGraw-Hill. (Online edition).

Schwedt, T. (2018). Preventive therapy of migraine. Continuum: Lifelong Learning in Neurology 24(4), 1052–1065.

Seeley, W. & Miller, B. (2018). Ch. 423. Alzheimer's disease. In: J.L. Jameson, A.S. Fauci, D.L. Kasper et al (eds). Harrison's principles of internal medicine, 20th edn. McGraw-Hill. (Online edition).

Sharkey, K.A. & Wallace, J.L. (2018). Ch. 50. Gastrointestinal motility and water flux, emesis, and biliary and pancreatic disease. In: L. Brunton, R. Hilal-Dandan &

B.C. Knollman (eds). Goodman and Gilman's: the Pharmacological basis of therapeutics, 13th edn. (Online edition).

Skidgel, R. (2018). Ch. 39. Histamine, bradykinin and their antagonists. In: L. Brunton, R. Hilal-Dandan & B.C. Knollman (eds). Goodman and Gilman's: the pharmacological basis of therapeutics, 13th edn. McGraw-Hill. (Online edition).

Snyder, B. (2014). Revisiting old friends: update on opioid pharmacology. Australian Prescriber 17(2), 56–60.

Society of Hospital Pharmacists of Australia (SHPA) (2018). Don't rush to crush. SHPA.

The National Return & Disposal of Unwanted Medicines Ltd. (2020). Return Unwanted Medicines. Online. Available: https://returnmed.com.au/about-us/.

Therapeutic Goods Administration (TGA) (2020). No. 31 Poisons Standard October 2020. Australian Government, Department of Health. Online. Available: www.legislation.gov.au/Details/F2020L01255.

Therapeutic Goods Administration (TGA) (2018). Current list of up-scheduled codeine containing products. Australian Government, Department of Health. Online. Available: www.tga.gov.au/node/770507.

Thomas, J., Van Hove, J., Larson, A. et al (2020). Ch. 36. Inborn errors of metabolism. In: W. Hay, M. Levin, M. Abzug & M. Bunik (eds). Current diagnosis and treatment: pediatrics, 25th edn. McGraw-Hill. (Online edition).

Tortora, G. & Derrickson, B. (2018). Principles of anatomy and physiology, 15th edn. Wiley.

Traver, J. & Cheng, A. (2016). Multidrug-resistant tuberculosis in Australia and our region. Medical Journal of Australia 204(7), 251–252.

Vargas, B. (2018). Acute treatment of migraine. Continuum: Lifelong Learning in Neurology 24(4), 1032–1051.

Victorian Government (2017). Drugs, Poisons and Controlled Substances Regulations. Statutory Rule No. 29/2017 version 7. Online. Available: www.legislation.vic.gov.au/in-force/statutory-rules/drugs-poisons-and-controlled-substances-regulations-2017/007.

Waxman, A. & Loscalzo, J. (2019). Ch. 277. Pulmonary hypertension. In: J.L. Jameson, A.S. Fauci, D.L. Kasper et al (eds). Harrison's principles of internal medicine, 20th edn. McGraw-Hill. (Online edition).

Westbrook, J., Li, L., Lehnbom, E. et al (2015). What are incident reports telling us? A comparative study at two Australian hospitals of medication errors identified at audit, detected by staff and reported to an incident system. International Journal for Quality in Health Care 27(11), 1–9.

White, N.J. & Ashley, E.A. (2018). Ch. 219. Malaria. In: J.L. Jameson, A.S. Fauci, D.L. Kasper et al (eds). Harrison's principles of internal medicine, 20th edn. McGraw-Hill. (Online edition).

World Anti-Doping Agency (WADA) (2021). World Anti-Doping Code 2021. Online. Available: www.wada-ama.org/sites/default/files/resources/files/2021_wada_code.pdf.

World Anti-Doping Agency (WADA) (2020). Prohibited list. Online. Available: www.wada-ama.org/en/what-we-do/the-prohibited-list.

World Health Organization (WHO) (2019a). Leishmaniasis. Online. Available: www.who.int/mediacentre/factsheets/fs375/en/.

World Health Organization (WHO) (2019b). Leprosy. Online. Available: www.who.int/en/news-room/fact-sheets/detail/leprosy.

World Health Organization (WHO) (2019c). Malaria. Online. Available: www.who.int/news-room/fact-sheets/detail/malaria.

World Health Organization (WHO) (2019d). Soil transmitted helminth infection. Online. Available: www.who.int/news-room/fact-sheets/detail/soil-transmitted-helminth-infections.

World Health Organization (WHO) (2018). Tuberculosis. Online. Available: www.who.int/en/news-room/fact-sheets/detail/tuberculosis.

Wright, E.K., Ding, N.S. & Niewiadomski, O. (2018). Management of inflammatory bowel disease. Medical Journal of Australia 209(7), 318–323.

Zaenglein, A.L., Pathy, A.L., Schlosser, B.J. et al (2016). Guidelines of care for the management of acne vulgaris. Journal of the American Academy of Dermatology 74(5), 945–973.

GLOSSARY

Anaphylactoid reactions (pseudoallergic reactions): thought to be caused by direct release of histamine provoked by unclear non-immune mechanisms. Unlike anaphylactic reactions, there may be no prior exposure or triggering factors with anaphylactoid reactions, which may be seen with the first dose of a drug

Anaphylaxis: manifestation of immediate hypersensitivity (also called type 1 hypersensitivity). The sensitised individual (i.e. the person who has had prior exposure or contact with the drug or substance) is exposed to a specific antigen or hapten, resulting in urticaria, pruritus and angioedema, which may progress to vascular collapse, shock and respiratory distress and require immediate treatment

Angioedema: a vascular reaction involving the deep dermis or subcutaneous or submucosal tissue, leading to localised oedema and wheals. Hereditary angioedema (dominant trait) may be mediated by minor trauma, sudden increases or decreases in environmental temperature or sudden emotional stress, and the result is visceral lesions

Anhidrosis: absence of sweating

Arachnoiditis: signs and symptoms include tingling, numbness or weakness of legs, leg sensation (e.g. insects crawling, water running over limb), severe shooting pain, muscle cramps and spasms, uncontrollable twitches, bladder, bowel and sexual problems

Aseptic meningitis syndrome: occurs from several hours up to 2 days after administration of IV human immunoglobulin (high dose: 2 g/kg) and consists of headache, nuchal rigidity, drowsiness, fever, photophobia, painful eye movement, nausea and vomiting

Asthenia: loss of strength and energy, weakness

Bier's block: anaesthetic technique for surgical procedures on the extremities where a local anaesthetic is injected intravenously

Blepharitis: inflammation of eyelid glands and lash follicles

Charcot-type arthropathy: progressive degeneration of weight-bearing joint characterised by bony destruction, bone resorption and eventual deformity

'Cheese reaction': a combination of tyramine-containing food and MAOIs which can result in headache, severe hypertension and subarachnoid haemorrhage, even up to 2 weeks after discontinuation of the MAOI. Tyramine-containing foods include: products that have been aged, pickled, fermented or smoked; some types of red wines (especially those of the Chianti and Alicante types) and beer (or large quantities of beer or wine); caviar; pickled herrings; chicken liver; vegetable, yeast and meat extracts (e.g. Vegemite, Promite, Bovril, Bonox, Marmite); mature cheeses; sour cream; yoghurt; liver; dry sausage (e.g. salami); aged meats; sauerkraut; excessive amounts of coffee or chocolate; coffee substitutes; avocados; broad-bean pods; stock cubes; packet or canned soup; and dehydrated foods

Cheilitis: lip inflammation

Cryptorchism (cryptorchidism): failure of one or both testes to descend into the scrotum; may be treated with surgery (usually when the child is 5–7 years old) or with gonadotrophic hormones
Disulfiram–alcohol reaction: characterised by intense flushing of the face and neck accompanied by heat and sweating, feeling of constriction and irritation of throat and trachea, chest pains, restlessness, headache, tachycardia, palpitation, dyspnoea, hypertension initially, then hypotension; later, pallor, weakness, vertigo, nausea, vomiting, abdominal cramps, thirst, dizziness, blurred vision, numbness of hands and feet, insomnia, and, finally, in severe reactions, cardiopulmonary arrest. Disulfiram reaction is managed by giving the patient 1 g ascorbic acid IV, chlorpromazine 5–100 mg IM, and resuscitation measures as necessary
Dubin–Johnson syndrome: hereditary, chronic non-haemolytic jaundice
Eaton–Lambert syndrome: limb muscle weakness similar to myasthenia gravis, but not involving ocular or bulbar muscles
Embryotoxic: causing injury to the embryo, resulting in death, growth retardation or abnormal development in a part that may affect either its structure or function
Erythema nodosum leprosum (ENL) (lepromatous reaction) (type 2 reaction): which occurs within the first 2 years of treatment. Symptoms include high fever and raised, tender erythematous skin nodules (which may become pustular and/or ulcerate), and may also include malaise, neuritis, orchitis, albuminuria, joint swelling, iritis, epistaxis, acute vasculitis and depression. Usual treatment consists of corticosteroids, analgesics and/or other agents that suppress the reaction
Erythrasma: superficial skin infection caused by *Corynebacterium minutissimum*, resulting in brown, scaly skin patches, affecting the skin in the armpits, groin and between the toes. It may co-exist or be mistaken for tinea or Candida fungal infection. It may also be more generalised and found on the trunk of the body, under the breasts or umbilicus
Extrapyramidal reactions or syndromes: may include some or all of the following symptoms and may occur after a single dose, especially in children and young adults:

- Parkinsonian symptoms: akinesia, rigidity, tremor at rest
- akathisia: motor and mental restlessness
- acute dystonic reaction: facial grimacing, torticollis, oculogyric crisis
- tardive dyskinesia: exaggerated and persistent chewing movements, tongue protrusion. Drugs that may be used to reverse the extrapyramidal reaction include benztropine and diphenhydramine

Fanconi syndrome: syndrome of inadequate reabsorption in the proximal renal tubules which can be caused by congenital or acquired diseases, toxicity or adverse drug reactions
Glossodynia (also known as burning mouth syndrome): burning sensation, discomfort, pain, irritation or rawness of tongue, lips or oral cavity
Goodpasture's syndrome: syndrome characterised by cough, production of frothy mucus containing bright red blood, nausea, pruritus, constipation and decreased urination
Hyperostosis: excessive growth of bony tissue
Hypersensitivity: altered reactivity in which the body reacts with an exaggerated immune response to a foreign substance. It may be subdivided into immediate (type 1),

cytotoxic (type II), immune complex (type III) or delayed (type IV) reactions. Immediate (type 1) reactions are antibody mediated and occur within minutes of the sensitised person being exposed to an antigen; they may result in anaphylaxis or atopic allergy (allergic rhinitis, asthma, dermatitis, urticaria and/or angioedema). Cytotoxic (type II) reactions occur when an antigen combines with an antibody resulting in a complement-mediated lysis (e.g. transfusion reaction). Immune complex (type III) reactions result in a complement being activated when antigen–antibody immune complexes are deposited into tissues. Polymorphonuclear cells are then attracted to the site, resulting in the release of lysosomal enzymes and tissue damage. Delayed (type IV) reactions take 12–48 hours to develop and are produced by natural infection, vaccination with live attenuated virus vaccines or by injection of antigens and are mediated through T lymphocytes

Lepra reaction, reversal reaction (type 1): usually seen early in therapy and thought to be due to a decrease in antigens where the immune system mounts a response to the remaining infection. It consists of swelling of any skin and nerve lesions and is generally treated using corticosteroids (especially if neuritis is present), analgesics or surgical decompression, if necessary. Non-treatment may result in irreversible nerve damage

Livedo reticularis: mottled discolouration of skin appearing net-like, reddish-blue in colour with surrounding pale areas, occurring mainly on arms, legs and trunk, worse in cold weather

Lymphopenia: low level of lymphocytes in the blood

Lypodystrophy syndrome: redistribution/accumulation of body fat, peripheral and facial wasting, breast enlargement, central obesity, dorsocervical fat enlargement ('buffalo hump'), elevated serum lipids and blood glucose concentration

Malignant hyperthermia (also called malignant hyperpyrexia): rare but potentially fatal condition associated mainly with halogenated general anaesthetic agents. It occurs more commonly in males and is genetically determined. There appears to be a skeletal hypermetabolic state caused by a sudden increase in calcium concentration in the muscle cytoplasm, leading to high oxygen demand. Symptoms include muscle rigidity, acidosis, hyperkalaemia, tachycardia, arrhythmias, tachypnoea, cyanosis, sweating and unstable blood pressure. The body temperature rises at a rate of at least 2°C per hour, but sometimes this is a late sign. Late complications may include renal failure, intravascular coagulopathy and pulmonary oedema. The reaction is thought to be induced by preoperative exercise, muscle trauma, fever or anxiety, or induction by inhalation anaesthetics, suxamethonium or prolonged anaesthesia

Melasma (also called chloasma): facial hyperpigmentation consisting of sharply demarcated blotchy brown macules that are symmetrically spread over cheeks and forehead and, sometimes, upper lip and neck.

Metorrhagia: abnormal uterine bleeding

Neuroleptic malignant syndrome: a potentially fatal reaction to antipsychotic drugs. Symptoms include hyperthermia and severe extrapyramidal symptoms (muscle rigidity, altered consciousness, tachycardia, labile blood pressure, profuse sweating and dyspnoea). Skeletal muscle damage may occur as a consequence. Predisposing factors include dehydration, pre-existing organic brain disease and

AIDS. Infants and the elderly are particularly susceptible. It is usually managed by discontinuing antipsychotic drugs and monitoring and treating symptoms

Oligohidrosis: decreased sweating

Paracervical block: anaesthetic procedure used in obstetrics and gynaecology where the anaesthetic is injected into between two and six sites at a depth of 3–7 mm alongside the vaginal portion of the cervix in the vaginal fornices

Peliosis hepatitis: liver, and sometimes splenic, tissue replaced by blood-filled cysts; may be associated with liver failure and life-threatening intra-abdominal haemorrhage

Phaeochromocytoma: catecholamine-producing tumour of the adrenal medulla, resulting in the excessive production of adrenaline and noradrenaline (norepinephrine) and associated symptoms, including palpitations, weight loss, sweating and high blood pressure

Porphyria: porphyrins usually combine with haem to produce haemoproteins, including haemoglobin, and the process involves multiple enzymes. Abnormal enzymes result in a build-up and excretion of porphyrin. Porphyria are inherited disorders affecting either the skin (e.g. on exposure to sun, the skin develops blisters, itching and swelling) or the nervous system (resulting in pain in the chest, abdomen, limbs or back, muscle numbness, tingling, paralysis or cramping; vomiting, constipation and personality disorders). Attacks of porphyria may be triggered by a number of agents, including some medications (e.g. sedatives, oral contraceptives, barbiturates and tranquillisers), chemicals, smoking, alcohol, infection, sun exposure, menstrual hormones, and emotional or physical stress

Pulmonary wedge pressure: indirect measure of left atrial pressure, measured by placing a catheter (Swanz Ganz) into the pulmonary artery and attaching it to a pressure transducer

Prader–Willi syndrome: genetic disorder of chromosome 15, resulting in hypotonia (e.g. floppiness and weakened/absent suck reflex in babies); poor large muscle strength, sometimes with poor coordination and balance; hypogonadism (immature development of sexual organs and sexual characteristics); hyperphagia (excessive appetite and overeating, resulting in obesity if food intake is not controlled); CNS and endocrine gland dysfunction (resulting in learning disabilities, short stature, hyperphagia, somnolence and poor emotional and social development)

Priapism: abnormal erection of penis, accompanied by pain and tenderness

Proptosis: bulging eyes

Pseudomembranous colitis: severe acute inflammation of the bowel mucosa, commonly associated with antibiotic therapy. Pseudomembranous plaques (yellow–green) in the bowel are common, and symptoms include watery diarrhoea, fever and abdominal cramps

Pyrosis: burning sensation in the stomach and oesophagus with belching (sour taste)

'Purple toe' syndrome: characterised by toes becoming dark, purple or mottled in appearance, usually within 3–10 weeks of starting therapy with warfarin or related drugs. Other symptoms include purple colour of the plantar surfaces and sides of toes. The colour blanches when moderate pressure is applied and fades when legs are elevated. Toes may also become painful and tender. In some cases, purple toes may progress to gangrene or necrosis requiring debridement or amputation

Radical cure: aims to eliminate dormant schizonts from the liver during malaria

Raynaud's disease/syndrome: a disease characterised by spasm of the arteries in the extremities (especially fingers) and brought on by cold or vibration, resulting in pallor, pain, numbness and in severe cases, gangrene
'Red man' syndrome: flushing of upper body, hypotension, angioedema, pruritus
Reye's syndrome: rare but fatal disease that may occur as a sequel of varicella or viral upper respiratory infection, and which has been associated with the taking of aspirin by children under 12 years for febrile, viral illnesses. Symptoms include recurrent vomiting, liver and visceral changes, deteriorating to encephalopathy with acute brain swelling, disturbance in consciousness and seizures
Rotor syndrome: rare, idiopathic form of hyperbilirubinaemia
Serotonin syndrome: a triad of altered mental status, autonomic dysfunction and neuromuscular abnormalities associated with the use of serotogenic antidepressants or antidepressant combination. Symptoms include agitation, coma, confusion, delirium, hallucinations, mania, mutism, fluctuating blood pressure, sweating, diarrhoea, hyperthermia, lacrimation, mydriasis, shivering, tachycardia, restlessness, hyperreflexia, clonus, myoclonus, nystagmus, oculogyric crisis, tetanic body arching, tremor, rigidity and rhabdomyolysis
Stevens–Johnson syndrome: a form of erythema multiforme that is sometimes fatal. It may be preceded by influenza-like symptoms and is characterised by systemic and more severe mucocutaneous lesions. It usually involves oronasal and anogenital mucous membranes, with characteristic grey–white pseudomembranes, and haemorrhagic crusts on the lips. Ocular lesions (iritis, uveitis, corneal vesicles, erosions and perforations) may lead to corneal opacities and blindness. There may also be pulmonary, gastrointestinal, cardiac and renal involvement
Stokes–Adams syndrome: condition caused by heart block and characterised by sudden attacks of unconsciousness with or without convulsions
Superinfection: overgrowth of non-susceptible organisms with prolonged or repeated treatment
Suppressive cure: if a suppressive drug is continued for long enough after a patient has left a malarial area, the liver cycle of the plasmodium is no longer maintained by re-infection, resulting in a cure
Suppressive prophylaxis: suppression of the erythrocyte cycle of malaria, preventing acute attacks
Teratogen: any substance that can cause a disturbance in growth and development of embryo or fetus or may cause a stop to the pregnancy altogether. Teratogens can include drugs, chemicals, radiation and maternal infection
Teratogenic: able to disturb the growth and development of the embryo or fetus
Torsades de pointes: atypical, rapid ventricular tachycardia with periodic waxing and waning of the amplitude of the QRS complex on ECG. It may be self-limiting or progress to ventricular fibrillation
Vasomotor reaction (nitritoid reaction): vasodilation, facial flushing, loss of consciousness, hypotension, syncope, nausea, vomiting and cerebrovascular accident. May occur immediately after taking ACE inhibitor or months later. Is most common when ACE inhibitor is given with systemic gold preparation, but can also occur with oral gold
Vitiligo: skin condition in which melanocytes are destroyed, resulting in patches of de-pigmented areas, often surrounded by hyperpigmentation

Water intoxication: increased water intake causes decreased sodium concentration (hyponatraemia) and the excess water is absorbed into the blood, accumulating in the brain and lungs, leading to symptoms of breathlessness and nausea
Wernicke's encephalopathy: associated with thiamine deficiency and generally related to chronic alcohol abuse, although other conditions can cause it. Symptoms include paralysis of eye muscles, diplopia, nystagmus, ataxia and mental changes
Wolff–Parkinson–White syndrome: an extra electrical pathway exists in the heart leading to the electrical signal reaching the ventricles prematurely. Symptoms include tachycardia, dizziness, chest palpitations, fainting and, rarely, cardiac arrest
Xerostomia: dry mouth associated with dysfunction of the salivary glands
Xerophthalmia: abnormal dryness and thickening of conjunctiva and cornea
Zollinger–Ellison syndrome: rare disorder causing pancreatic and duodenal tumours, as well as gastric and duodenal ulcers. The tumour secretes gastrin, which causes the stomach to produce acid and in turn causes gastric and duodenal ulcers that are less responsive than ordinary ulcers to treatment

Drug administration

Oral preparations

Capsule: gelatin container, swallowed whole, containing a drug that is to be released or has an unpleasant taste; the drug is released when the capsule is dissolved in the stomach or intestine
Elixir: flavoured, sweetened alcoholic solution of a potent or unpleasant-tasting drug in a small dose volume
Emulsion: mixture of oil and water, the oil remaining dispersed by an emulsifying agent; the container needs to be shaken before use
Extract: concentrated preparation of a drug that may remain in fluid form or be evaporated and the solid sediment incorporated into a tablet or capsule
Granule: small pellet of the active substance
Linctus: drug prepared as a sweet syrup, given in doses of small volume to be swallowed slowly without the addition of water, usually for the relief of cough
Lozenge: solid drug form that acts by slow disintegration in the mouth and is used when a local drug action in the mouth or throat is required
Mixture: contains several drugs dissolved or suspended in an aqueous vehicle
Powder: usually a mixture of two or more powdered drugs intended for internal use
Suspension: solid insoluble particles of a drug dispersed in a liquid; must be shaken well before use
Syrup: drug contained in a concentrated sugar solution
Tablet: dried, powdered drug mixed with a binding base and compressed into a variety of shapes; may be swallowed whole or crushed if required
Tablet – enteric-coated: coated tablet containing a drug that is a gastric irritant or is broken down by gastric acid; the tablet is swallowed whole
Tablet – slow-release: the tablet, swallowed whole, contains a drug that is released over a prolonged period
Tincture: drug contained in an alcoholic solution

Injections

Intra-arterial: mainly cytotoxic (antineoplastic) agents delivered directly to an organ or tissue via the feeding artery
Intra-articular: injected into a joint cavity
Intracardiac: drug is delivered directly into the ventricle or myocardium for an immediate cardiac response
Intradermal: drug is given into the superficial skin layers, mainly in skin testing
Intramuscular: delivered into muscle (e.g. oily solutions, suspensions or potentially irritant substances) or if rapid absorption is required; the site is not massaged if the Z-track technique is used
Intraperitoneal: drugs have direct contact with intraperitoneal organs during peritoneal dialysis
Intrathecal: for drugs that do not penetrate the blood–brain barrier; they may be delivered to the cerebrospinal fluid in the subarachnoid space, usually after lumbar puncture
Intravenous: if a very rapid effect is required or if the preparation is too irritating to the tissues
Subcutaneous: used if relatively slower absorption is required

Topical applications

Cream: semi-solid emulsion that may be aqueous or oily
Drops: for the eye, ear and nose; avoid touching eye, ear or nose with the dropper and return the dropper to the bottle without washing (eye drops are sterile and may be supplied with a dropper or administered directly from the container)
Dusting powder: usually a mixture of two or more substances in fine powder; should not be applied to open wounds or large areas of raw surface
Gel: aqueous preparation used to apply water soluble medicament to body surfaces for longer retention than with an aqueous solution
Inhalation: liquid preparation containing volatile substances, which, on vaporisation, are inhaled to produce a local or systemic effect via the respiratory tract (e.g. steam inhalation, nebuliser, atomiser or aerosol spray)
Insufflation: powder intended for introduction into the ear, nose, throat, body cavities or wounds
Irrigation: washing of a body cavity or wound by a stream of water or other solution
Liniment: thin cream or oily preparation applied to the intact skin by rubbing; may contain substances possessing analgesic, rubefacient, soothing or stimulating properties
Lotion: agent contained in an aqueous, alcoholic or emulsified vehicle, applied to the skin without friction, having an astringent, emollient or other therapeutic action
Ointment: semi-solid preparation in a greasy base
Paint: liquid preparation for application in limited amounts to the skin or mucous membranes
Paste: semi-solid preparation containing a high proportion of drug that is not intended to be absorbed
Pessary: solid preparation shaped suitably for vaginal administration and containing an agent intended to act locally
Suppository: solid preparation shaped suitably for rectal administration and containing an agent intended for local or systemic medication

INDEX

F

J